PRINCIPLES OF MOLECULAR MEDICINE

SECOND EDITION

Section Editors

PRINCIPLES OF
MOLECULAR
MEDICINE

SECOND EDITION

EDITED BY

MARSCHALL S. RUNGE, MD, PhD

DEPARTMENT OF MEDICINE, DIVISION OF CARDIOLOGY
CAROLINA CARDIOVASCULAR BIOLOGY CENTER
UNIVERSITY OF NORTH CAROLINA SCHOOL OF MEDICINE
CHAPEL HILL, NC

CAM PATTERSON, MD

DEPARTMENT OF MEDICINE, DIVISION OF CARDIOLOGY
CAROLINA CARDIOVASCULAR BIOLOGY CENTER
UNIVERSITY OF NORTH CAROLINA SCHOOL OF MEDICINE
CHAPEL HILL, NC

FOREWORD BY

VICTOR A. McKUSICK, MD

JOHNS HOPKINS UNIVERSITY
BALTIMORE, MD

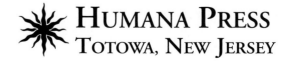

HUMANA PRESS
TOTOWA, NEW JERSEY

Library of Congress Cataloging in Publication Data

Principles of molecular medicine / edited by Marschall S. Runge ; fore-
    word by Victor A. Mckusick. -- 2nd ed.
      p. ; cm.
    Includes bibliographical references and index.
    ISBN 1-58829-202-9 (alk. paper)
    1. Medical genetics. 2. Pathology, Molecular. 3. Molecular biology.
  I. Runge, Marschall Stevens, 1954-   .
    [DNLM: 1. Genetics, Medical. 2. Gene Therapy. 3. Molecular
  Biology.   QZ 50 P9573 2006]
  RB155.P695 2006
  616'.042--dc22

                                                                        2005034346

Foreword

The concept of molecular medicine dates back to Linus Pauling, who in the late 1940s and early 1950s generalized from the ideas that came from the study of the sickle cell hemoglobin molecule. With the first cloning of human genes about 1976, molecular genetics took the molecular perspective on disease to the level of DNA. The term molecular medicine achieved wide currency in the 1980s with the assignment of this designation to journals, at least one society, institutes, and academic divisions of departments of internal medicine. Undoubtedly, molecular medicine has been abetted by the Human Genome Project, which has aided greatly in the molecular characterization of disease. Map-based gene discovery, as in positional cloning of previously unknown genes responsible for "mystery diseases," could be now replaced by sequence-based gene discovery.

What is molecular medicine? In the first edition of *Principles of Molecular Medicine*, Francis Collins seems to define it as "molecular genetics and medicine"—the last four words of his Foreword. He was referring to the pervasive relevance of genetics and genomics to all of medicine. In essence, molecular medicine is genetic medicine.

Since the publication of the first edition *Principles of Molecular Medicine* in 1998, the Human Genome Project has provided a "complete" sequence of the human genome with several surprising revelations relevant to molecular medicine.

As indicated in the Preface of the first edition, the total count of genes was thought to be 50,000 to 80,000. Scrutiny of the complete human sequence leads to a count only half that, perhaps fewer than 30,000. It has come to be realized that each gene can give rise to multiple protein gene products through alternative splicing of pre-messenger RNA, as well as through different posttranscriptional modification of the gene products. Each gene may on the average have as many as 10 different protein products. Mutations in different ones of these can cause quite different clinical disorders. Thus the focus has shifted to the transcriptome and to the proteins that constitute the proteome—a shift from genomics to proteomics.

Compilation of the rapidly expanded topic of molecular medicine since the edition of some 8 years ago is a daunting task. The rate at which new discoveries have been made

means that there are many new opportunities and challenges for clinical medicine. One of the effects of the completion of the Human Genome Project is the increasing application of the fields of molecular biology and genetics to the understanding and management of common diseases. Assimilation of the new developments since the first edition has been ably accomplished by Drs. Runge and Patterson with the help of their many knowledgeable authors.

As was evident in the first edition, molecular genetics is involved in every specialty of medicine. A recurrent theme in that edition, perhaps even more striking in the present one, is that information gleaned and research methods designed in one specialty have been highly influential on researchers and physicians in other fields—often in ways that could not have been foreseen. The editors have succeeded in considering all the disciplines while searching for connections and correlations that might otherwise be missed.

The organization selected by the editors allows for the molecular bases of disease, as well as the constantly evolving areas of ethical issues and counseling that affect all disciplines, to be covered in the opening section. Specifics in the several medical disciplines are then handled splendidly in the sections that follow. Each chapter resounds with the amazing detail of what is known and simultaneously probes the many unanswered questions that provide new avenues for research in the 21st century. The state-of-the-art focus in each specialty will be much appreciated by the reader, whether practitioner, researcher or student.

The authors and section editors that participated in this text are recognized leaders in their fields from around the globe. They and Drs. Runge and Patterson, who have led and coordinated this extraordinary effort, deserve commendation. The product is a text that will be useful for all interested in the molecular pathogenesis of disease.

Victor A. McKusick, MD

Foreword to the First Edition

Until recently, medical genetics and molecular medicine were considered the exclusive province of academic specialists in tertiary-care medical centers. Queried about their familiarity with molecular genetic aspects of clinical medicine, most primary-care providers only a few years ago would have responded that such matters were irrelevant to their daily practice.

Yet few could say that today. Few internists or general practitioners have not prescribed recombinant insulin, tPA, or erythropoietin; few pediatricians have not gone through the molecular evaluation of a child with dysmorphology or learning disability; few obstetricians have not performed amniocentesis or CVS for couples at increased genetic risk; and few general surgeons have not faced penetrating questions about the role of genetic testing or prophylactic surgery from women with a strong family history of breast or ovarian cancer.

This level of emergence of molecular genetics into clinical medicine is still quite modest, however, compared to what is coming. As the human genome project hurtles toward completion of the sequence of a reference human genome, and the identification of all human genes, by 2005, the pace of revelations about human illness will continue to accelerate. Until recently, most disease-gene discoveries have related to single-gene disorders (cystic fibrosis, fragile X syndrome, and so on) or to Mendelian subsets of more common illnesses (BRCA1 and BRCA2, the hereditary nonpolyposis colon cancer syndromes, and so on). But with the initiation in 1998 of an aggressive new genome project goal, cataloging all common human sequence variations, it is expected that the weaker polygenic contributors to virtually all diseases will begin to be discerned. Many consequences will result. Individualized preventive medicine strategies, rooted in the gene-based determination of future risk of illness, will become part of the regular practice of medicine. New designer drugs, based not on empiricism but on a detailed understanding of the molecular pathogenesis of disease, will appear. Pharmacogenomics, wherein the efficacy and toxicity of a particular drug regimen can be predicted based on patient genotype, will become a standard component of designing optimum therapy for the individual. And gene therapy, fed by a wealth of disease-gene discoveries, will mature into a significant part of the physician's armamentarium against disease.

As we watch this train coming down the track, this is an ideal time to collect information about molecular medicine into one authoritative text. *Principles of Molecular Medicine* aims to do just that, bridging the current gap between basic science and the bedside. It will thus be useful to researchers and clinicians alike. With more than 100 chapters covering a wide variety of topics, its distinguished cohort of section editors, and its abundant tables and illustrations, it provides an accessible and much needed manual to the present and the future of molecular genetics and medicine.

Francis S. Collins

Preface

Since publication of the first edition of *Principles of Molecular Medicine*, dramatic discoveries in molecular medicine along with concomitant rapid technological advances have revolutionized the diagnosis and treatment of a broad range of human diseases. Given the pace of new discovery, genetic- and cell-based therapies may well become a common part of the physicians' armamentarium in the near future. Direct links between genetic mutations and diseases are being mapped almost routinely. Genomic approaches to diseases such as breast cancer have led to identification of previously unrecognized malignancies and the ability to prognosticate outcomes to therapy. The delicate interplay between adipocytes and regulation of insulin sensitivity, the roles of bone morphogenetic proteins in pulmonary hypertension, and the discovery of mutations involved in an array of cardiomyopathies are but a few of the important recent advances that have direct implications for patient care.

It is virtually impossible to keep track of the breadth of discovery that has led to these biomedical advances. The goal of the many authors and editors of this second edition of the *Principles of Molecular Medicine* has been to present the voluminous discoveries of the past decade in a format that captures the essence of scientific discovery but allows rapid assimilation in each particular area.

This second edition again includes chapters describing advances in fields paralleling traditional medical texts, and will be especially useful to specialists who are updating their education, practicing physicians interested in keeping abreast of new developments, and students appropriately curious about what is known and what lies ahead. Although only 8 years have passed since the first edition was published, we have made every effort to comprehensively update chapters with recent advances and have added chapters for disease entities and areas in which discovery has accelerated during the past five years.

As we have participated in the assembly of this volume, we have had the good fortune to review in depth the molecular discoveries that are transforming medical practice. For example, in the interval since the first edition of this text, stem cell populations have been discovered that regenerate muscle, heart, and neural cell populations, and that have the potential to serve as cell-based therapies in chronic and degenerative diseases. New cell growth and cell death mechanisms that are dysregulated in neoplasia and that may serve as new anticancer targets have been elucidated. Advances have been made in understanding the biology of previously untreatable neurodegenerative diseases such as Huntington's disease. These and many other important advances in our understanding of human diseases are elucidated in this edition.

In addition, we have been able to note the new epistemologies in the genetic basis of human disease that are rapidly emerging. For instance, characterization of candidate genes for human diseases has expanded well beyond monogenic diseases, the study of late-onset diabetes being a notable example. Molecular alterations can have far-reaching effects on many systems. The identification of genes for epithelial sodium channels has led to a deeper understanding of their role in disorders of total body Na+ homeostasis, blood volume, and blood pressure. As a result of advances like these, views that had been held for much of the 20th century are being reconsidered. For example, hereditary hemochromatosis, a familial disease characterized by excess tissue deposits of iron leading to end-organ damage, has traditionally been thought to result from mutations in a single gene. Very recently, the identification of similar phenotypes associated with mutations of at least four different iron-metabolism genes has expanded our understanding of the pathophysiology of this relatively common genetic disease.

One common theme repeated in the chapters in this text is that the pathophysiology of disease is often a succession of genetic alterations, not just a single mutation. Although understanding these genetic relationships is never simple, their role in human diseases is all the more fascinating to consider. Human health often appears tenuous, but the discovery that a series of genetic missteps is often required to produce many disease states can be reassuring. The presence of several genetic steps in a disease process also suggests that multiple therapeutic targets may exist to modulate the course of these diseases. Less exhilarating is the knowledge that numerous diseases result not just from a complex succession of genetic missteps, but also from an individual's interaction with the environment. Abundant examples of this principle are present throughout clinical medicine, and are described in detail in this edition of *Principles of Molecular Medicine*.

Paradoxically, as new discoveries are made, new mysteries appear. The many advances described in this volume often raise as many new questions as they answer. On the one hand, this indicates that biomedical discovery and medical practice will continue to evolve. On the other hand, the changes in medical care described in the chapters of this text are an indication that the unresolved questions of today may be harbingers of new therapeutic approaches in years to come.

It has been our pleasure to bring together in-depth expositions of the most recent advances in molecular medicine. We invite you to enjoy this magnificent point in biomedical history, as genetics and molecular medicine continue to merge with clinical practice. The compendium of information in *Principles of Molecular Medicine: Second Edition,* has been made possible by the tireless efforts of our section editors. Without their expertise and commitment to this project, this textbook would not be possible. In addition, we thank the individual authors for sharing their expertise with all of us.

In addition to the phenomenal work of the editors and contributors, we would like to extend special thanks to Ms. Katie O'Brien for her commitment to this project; to Ms. Angela Clotfelter-Rego, whose tireless efforts despite numerous obstacles made this project possible; and to Ms. Carolyn Kruse, who synthesized the work of numerous authors to create a blazingly readable text. The editors thank our families, who have tolerated yet another joint effort. Finally, we would like to dedicate this volume to the first chairmen of medicine we had the privilege to serve under, Juha P. Kokko, MD, PhD, and Victor McKusick, MD. As physicians and scientists, these gentlemen nurtured many of the contributors to this edition, and their own work as scientists is frequently cited directly and indirectly in these chapters. It is on the shoulders of men like these that the principles of molecular medicine have been determined.

Marschall S. Runge, MD, PhD
Cam Patterson, MD

Contents

XIV. PSYCHIATRY

KERRY J. RESSLER AND CHARLES B. NEMEROFF

Contributors

ADRIANO AGUZZI, MD, PhD, FRCP, FRCPath, *Institute of Neuropathology, University Hospital, Zurich, Switzerland*

ERIC WFW ALTON, MD, FRCP, *Department of Gene Therapy, Imperial College London, National Heart and Lung Institute, London, UK*

CHRISTOPHER I. AMOS, PhD, *Section Head of Computational and Genetic Epidemiology, Departments of Epidemiology, and Biostatistics and Applied Mathematics, University of Texas M.D. Anderson Cancer Center, Houston, TX*

AYAD M. AL-KATIB, MD, *Lymphoma Research Laboratory, Wayne State University School of Medicine, Detroit, Michigan and Van Elslander Cancer Center, Grosse Pointe Woods, MI*

JEAN-PIERRE ALLAIN, MD, PhD, *Department of Haematology, University of Cambridge, Cambridge, UK*

NANCY C. ANDREWS, MD, PhD, *Howard Hughes Medical Institute, Children's Hospital Boston, Harvard Medical School, Boston, MA*

ANDREW ARNOLD, MD, *Center for Molecular Medicine and Division of Endocrinology and Metabolism, University of Connecticut School of Medicine, Farmington, CT*

RICHARD J. AUCHUS, MD, PhD, *Department of Internal Medicine, University of Texas Southwestern Medical Center, Dallas, TX*

YUSHI BAI, MD, PhD, *Endocrine Biology Program, Division of Biological Sciences, CIIT Centers for Health Research, Research Triangle Park, NC*

HENRY V. BAKER, PhD, *Department of Molecular Genetics and Microbiology, College of Medicine, University of Florida, Gainesville, FL*

ALEXEI G. BASNAKIAN, MD, PhD, *Department of Internal Medicine, Division of Nephrology, University of Arkansas for Medical Sciences, Central Arkansas Veterans Healthcare System, Little Rock, AR*

ROBIN L. BENNETT, MS, CGC, *Department of Medicine, Division of Medical Genetics, University of Washington Medical Center, Seattle, WA*

DANIEL G. BICHET, MD, *Department of Medicine, University of Montreal, Hôpital du Sacré-Coeur de Montreal, Quebec, Canada*

GUENTHER BODEN, MD, *Department of Medicine, Section of Metabolism, Diabetes and Endocrinology, Temple University Hospital, Philadelphia, PA*

JEAN L. BOLOGNIA, MD, *Department of Dermatology, Yale University, New Haven, CT*

ANIRBAN BOSE, MD, *Section of Nephrology, University of Rochester, Rochester, NY*

RICHARD C. BOUCHER, MD, *Division of Pulmonary Diseases, Department of Medicine, Cystic Fibrosis Research and Treatment Center, University of North Carolina, Chapel Hill, NC*

SCOTT BOWDEN, PhD, *Victorian Infectious Diseases Reference Laboratory (VIDRL), North Melbourne and Department of Microbiology, Monash University, Clayton, Victoria, Australia*

J. DOUGLAS BREMNER, MD, *Department of Psychiatry and Behavioral Sciences, Emory University School of Medicine, Atlanta, GA*

DAVID A. BRENNER, MD, *Department of Medicine, College of Physicians and Surgeons, Columbia University Medical Center, New York, NY*

ROBERT H. BROWN, JR., MD, PhD, *Day Neuromuscular Research Laboratory, Department of Neurology, Harvard Medical School, Massachusetts General Hospital, Boston, MA*

MARK G. BUCKLEY, PhD, *Respiratory Cell and Molecular Biology, University of Southampton School of Medicine, Southampton, UK*

W. TODD CADE, PT, PhD, *Department of Internal Medicine, Washington University School of Medicine, St. Louis, MO*

STEPHEN C. CANNON, MD, PhD, *Department of Neurology, University of Texas Southwestern Medical Center, Dallas, TX*

SUZANNE B. CASSIDY, MD, *Department of Pediatrics, Division of Human Genetics, University of California, Irvine, Irvine, CA*

MARINA CAVAZZANA-CALVO, *INSERM, Department of Biotherapy AP-HP, Hôpital Necker, Paris, France*

IRIS T. CHAN, MD, PhD, *Dana-Farber Cancer Institute, Brigham and Women's Hospital, Howard Hughes Medical Institute, Harvard Medical School, Boston, MA*

BERNARD S. CHANG, MD, *Division of Neurogenetics, Howard Hughes Medical Institute, Beth Israel Deaconess Medical Center, Department of Neurology, Harvard Medical School, Boston, MA*

JENNIFER CHAO, MD, PhD, *Department of Ophthalmology, University of Southern California, Los Angeles, CA*

KELLY D. CHASON, BS, *Division of Pulmonary and Critical Care Medicine, University of North Carolina, Chapel Hill, NC*

DENNIS J. CHEEK, PhD, RN, FAHA, *Texas Christian University, Harris College of Nursing and Health Sciences and School of Nurse Anesthesia, Fort Worth, TX*

ALVIN J. CHIN, MD, *Department of Pediatrics, Division of Cardiology, University of Pennsylvania School of Medicine and Joseph Stokes Research Institute, The Children's Hospital of Philadelphia, Philadelphia, PA*

DAVID C. CHRISTIANI, MD, MPH, MS, *Pulmonary and Critical Care Unit, Department of Medicine, Massachusetts General Hospital, Harvard Medical School, Environmental Health Department, Harvard School of Public Health, Boston, MA*

ANGELA M. CHRISTIANO, PhD, *Departments of Dermatology, and Genetics and Development, College of Physicians and Surgeons, Columbia University, New York, NY*

JONATHAN A. COHN, MD, *Division of Gastroenterology, Duke University, Durham, NC*

SHEILA COLLINS, PhD, *Departments of Psychiatry and Behavioral Sciences, Duke University Medical Center, Durham, NC, and Endocrine Biology Program, Division of Biological Sciences, CIIT Centers for Health Research, Research Triangle Park, NC*

KEVIN D. COOPER, MD, *Department of Dermatology, University Hospitals of Cleveland, Cleveland, OH*

ELENA CORRADINI, MD, *Center for Hemochromatosis and Hereditary Liver Diseases, Department of Internal Medicine, University of Modena and Reggio Emilia, Modena, Italy*

GILBERT COTE, PhD, *Department of Endocrine Neoplasia and Hormonal Disorders, University of Texas M.D. Anderson Cancer Center, Houston, TX*

GLENN R. CUNNINGHAM, MD, *Departments of Medicine and Molecular and Cellular Biology, Baylor College of Medicine, Houston, TX*

WILLIAM S. DALTON, MD, PhD, *Experimental Therapeutics, H. Lee Moffitt Cancer Center and Research Institute, Tampa, FL*

SAUMYA DAS, MD, *Thoracic Aortic Center and Cardiology Division, Massachusetts General Hospital, Boston, MA*

NANCY E. DAVIDSON, MD, *The Breast Cancer Program, The Sidney Kimmel Comprehensive Cancer Center, Johns Hopkins University School of Medicine, Baltimore, MD*

JANE C. DAVIES MRCP, MD, *Department of Gene Therapy, Imperial College London, National Heart and Lung Institute, London, UK*

JEAN DELAUNAY, MD, PhD, *Service d'Hématologie, d'Immunologie et de Cytogénétique, INSERM, Hôpital de Bicêtre, Le Kremlin-Bicêtre, France*

FEDERICA DEL MONTE MD, PhD, *Cardiovascular Research Center, Massachusetts General Hospital, Boston, MA*

XINGMING DENG, MD, PhD, *University of Florida Shands Cancer Center, University of Florida, Gainesville, FL*

GORDON DENT, PhD, *Institute of Science and Technology in Medicine, Keele University, Keele, UK*

CHRIS T. DERK, MD, *Division of Rheumatology, Department of Medicine, Thomas Jefferson University, Philadelphia, PA*

LUIS A. DIAZ, MD, *Department of Dermatology, School of Medicine, University of North Carolina, Chapel Hill, NC*

DAVID A. DICHEK, MD, *Department of Medicine, Division of Cardiology, University of Washington, Seattle, WA*

DONALD J. DIPETTE, MD, *Department of Medicine, Scott and White, The Texas A&M University System Health Science Center College of Medicine, Temple, TX*

SCOTT H. DONALDSON, MD, *Cystic Fibrosis Research and Treatment Center, University of North Carolina, Chapel Hill, NC*

BRIAN J. DRUKER, MD, *Oregon Health and Science University Cancer Institute is usually noted as Oregon Health and Science University Cancer Institute, Portland, OR*

DOUGLAS C. EATON, PhD, *Department of Physiology, The Center for Cell and Molecular Signaling, Emory University School of Medicine, Atlanta, GA*

RENEE E. EDKINS, MA, RN, CCRN, *Critical Care: Nursing Practice, Education and Research, University of North Carolina, Chapel Hill, NC*

JAMES T. ELDER, MD, PhD, *Departments of Dermatology and Radiation Oncology, University of Michigan, Ann Arbor, MI*

PETER B. ERNST, DVM, PhD, *Internal Medicine and Microbiology, Division of Gastroenterology and Hepatology, Digestive Health Center of Excellence, University of Virginia, Charlottesville, VA*

GREGORY J. ESPER, MD, *Department of Neurology, Washington University School of Medicine, St. Louis, MO*

JAMES P. EVANS, MD, PhD, *Department of Genetics, University of North Carolina, Chapel Hill, NC*

JANE WING-SANG FANG, MBBS, MRCP, FAAP, *Kinex Pharmaceuticals, Buffalo, NY*

STEPHEN V. FARAONE, PhD, *Medical Genetics Research Program and Department of Psychiatry and Behavioral Sciences; SUNY Upstate Medical University, Syracuse, NY*

FRANCESCA FERRARA, MD, *Center for Hemochromatosis and Hereditary Liver Diseases, Department of Internal Medicine, University of Modena and Reggio Emilia, Modena, Italy*

ALAIN FISCHER, *INSERM, Unité d'Immunologie et d'Hématologie Pédiatriques, Hôpital Necker, Paris, France*

THOMAS FORCE, MD, *Center of Translational Medicine, Jefferson Medical College, Philadelphia, PA*

BRIAN FOUTY, MD, *Division of Pulmonary Medicine, Center for Lung Biology, University of South Alabama School of Medicine, Mobile, AL*

MASON W. FREEMAN, MD, *Lipid Metabolism Unit, Massachusetts General Hospital, Harvard Medical School, Boston, MA*

ROBERT F. GAGEL, MD, *Division of Internal Medicine, University of Texas M.D. Anderson Cancer Center, Houston, TX*

JOSÉ M. GARCIA, MD, *Department of Medicine, Baylor College of Medicine, Houston, TX*

DANIEL J. GARRY, MD, PhD, *Departments of Internal Medicine and Molecular Biology, Univesity of Texas Southwestern Medical Center, Dallas, TX*

JUAN C. GEA-BANACLOCHE, MD, *Infectious Diseases Section, Experimental Transplantation and Immunology Branch, National Cancer Institute, Bethesda, MD*

DUNCAN M. GEDDES, MD, FRCP, *Department Thoracic Medicine, Royal Brompton Hospital, London, UK*

ROBERT E. GERSZTEN, MD, *Program in Cardiovascular Gene Therapy, Cardiovascular Research Center, Center for Immunology and Inflammatory Diseases, Massachusetts General Hospital, Boston, MA*

D. Gary Gilliland, MD, PhD, *Brigham and Women's Hospital, Dana-Farber Cancer Institute, Harvard Medical School, Howard Hughes Medical Institute, Boston, MA*

Robert G. Gish, MD, *Department of Hepatology and Liver Transplantation, California Pacific Medical Center, San Francisco, CA*

Stephen J. Glatt, PhD, *Center for Behavioral Genomics, Department of Psychiatry, University of California, San Diego, La Jolla, CA; and Veterans Medical Research Foundation, San Diego, CA*

Lowell A. Goldsmith, MD, MPH, *Dermatology, School of Medicine, University of North Carolina, Chapel Hill, NC*

Daniel R. Goldstein, MD, *Section of Cardiovascular Medicine, Department of Internal Medicine, Yale University, New Haven, CT*

Michelle Ng Gong, MD, MS, *Pulmonary, Critical Care and Sleep Medicine, Department of Medicine, Mount Sinai School of Medicine, New York, NY*

Maureen M. Goodenow, PhD, *Department of Pathology, Immunology, and Laboratory Medicine, Department of Pediatrics, Division of Immunology and Infectious Diseases, College of Medicine, University of Florida, Gainesville, FL*

Erynn S. Gordon, MS, CGC, *Research Center for Genetic Medicine, Children's National Medical Center, Washington, DC*

Jack M. Gorman, MD, *Partners Psychiatry and Mental Health, Harvard Medical School, McLean Hospital, Belmont, MA*

Allan Green, D.Phil., *The Mary Imogene Bassett Hospital, Bassett Research Institute, Bassett Healthcare, Cooperstown, NY*

David H. Gutmann, MD, PhD, *Department of Neurology, Washington University School of Medicine, St. Louis, MO*

Salima Hacein-Bey-Abina, INSERM, *Department of Biotherapy AP-HP, Hôpital Necker, Paris, France*

Roger J. Hajjar, MD, *Cardiovascular Research Center, Massachusetts General Hospital, Boston, MA*

Stephen R. Hammes, MD, PhD, *Department of Internal Medicine, University of Texas Medical Center, Dallas, TX*

Sian E. Harding, PhD, *Imperial College, National Heart and Lung Institute, London, UK*

John B. Harley MD, PhD, *Department of Medicine, University of Oklahoma Health Sciences Center, US Department of Veterans Affairs Medical Center, Arthritis and Immunology Program, Oklahoma Medical Research Foundation, Oklahoma City, OK*

Tomonobu Hasegawa, MD, PhD, *Department of Pediatrics, Keio University School of Medicine, Tokyo, Japan*

Thomas J. Hawke, PhD, *Department of Pure and Applied Science, York University, Toronto, Ontario, Canada*

Hironori Hayashi, MD, *University of Texas M.D. Anderson Cancer Center, Houston, TX*

Christine Heim, PhD, *Department of Psychiatry and Behavioral Sciences, Emory University School of Medicine, Atlanta, GA*

Carolyn Y. Ho, MD, *Cardiovascular Division, Brigham and Women's Hospital, Boston, MA*

Eric P. Hoffman, PhD, *Children's National Medical Center, Washington, DC*

Stephen T. Holgate, MD, FRCP, DSc, *Respiratory Cell and Molecular Biology, University of Southampton School of Medicine, Southampton, UK*

Steven M. Holland, MD, *Laboratory of Clinical Infectious Diseases, National Institute of Allergy and Infectious Disease, National Institutes of Health, Bethesda, MD*

Florian Holsboer, MD, PhD, *Max Planck Institute of Psychiatry, Munich, Germany*

Yi Huang, MD, PhD, *The Sidney Kimmel Comprehensive Cancer Center, Johns Hopkins University School of Medicine, Baltimore, MD*

Eric M. Isselbacher, MD, *Thoracic Aortic Center and Cardiology Division, Massachusetts General Hospital, Boston, MA*

Moira R. Jackson, PhD, *Department of Anatomy and Cell Biology, University of Florida College of Medicine, Gainesville, FL*

James L. Januzzi, Jr., MD, *Thoracic Aortic Center and Cardiology Division, Massachusetts General Hospital, Boston, MA*

Sergio A. Jimenez, MD, *Division of Rheumatology, Department of Medicine, Thomas Jefferson University, Philadelphia, PA*

Richard J. Johnson, MD, *Department of Medicine, Baylor College of Medicine, Houston, TX*

Kefei Kang, MD, *Department of Dermatology, Case Western Reserve University, Cleveland, OH*

Peter B. Kang, MD, *Program in Genomics, Department of Neurology, Children's Hospital, Harvard Medical School, Boston, MA*

Khurshed A. Katki, PhD, *Department of Medicine, Scott and White, The Texas A&M University System Health Science Center College of Medicine, Temple, TX*

Gur P. Kaushal, PhD, *Departments of Internal Medicine and Biochemistry and Molecular Biology, Division of Nephrology, University of Arkansas for Medical Sciences, Central Arkansas Veterans Healthcare System, Little Rock, AR*

Talmadge E. King Jr., MD, *Medical Services, San Francisco General Hospital, Department of Medicine, University of California, San Francisco, CA*

Samuel Klein, MD, *Center for Human Nutrition, Division of Geriatrics and Nutritional Sciences, Washington University School of Medicine, St. Louis, MO*

Michael R. Knowles, MD, *Division of Pulmonary Diseases, Department of Medicine, University of North Carolina, Chapel Hill, NC*

Lazaros K. Kochilas, MD, *Department of Pediatrics, Division of Pediatric Cardiology, Hasbro Children's Hospital/RIH, Brown University Medical School, Providence, RI*

James J. Kohler, PhD, *Department of Pathology, College of Medicine, Emory University, Atlanta, GA*

Peter Kopp, MD, *Division of Endocrinology, Metabolism and Molecular Medicine, Feinberg School of Medicine, Northwestern University, Chicago, IL*

Bruce R. Korf, MD, PhD, *Department of Genetics, University of Alabama, Birmingham, AL*

LOUIS M. KUNKEL, PhD, *Program in Genomics, Howard Hughes Medical Institute, Children's Hospital, Harvard Medical School, Boston, MA*

FADI G. LAKKIS, MD, *Thomas E. Starzl Transplantation Institute, University of Pittsburgh, Pittsburgh, PA*

DOLORES J. LAMB, PhD, *Scott Department of Urology and Department of Molecular and Cellular Biology, Baylor College of Medicine, Houston, TX*

HUI Y. LAN, MD, PhD, *Department of Medicine, Baylor College of Medicine, Houston, TX*

CAROL A. LANGE, PhD, *University of Minnesota Cancer Center, Minneapolis, MN*

KAREN A. LAPIDOS, PhD, *Department of Molecular Genetics and Cell Biology, The University of Chicago, Chicago, IL*

JOHNSON YIU-NAM LAU, MBBS, MD, FRCP, *Managing Director, Roth Capital Partners, Newport Beach, CA*

PHILIPPE LEBOULCH, *Harvard Medical School and Genetics Division, Brigham and Women's Hospital, Boston, MA*

VIRGINIA M.-Y. LEE, PhD, *Center for Neurodegenerative Disease Research, Department of Pathology and Laboratory Medicine, University of Pennsylvania School of Medicine, Philadelphia, PA*

DONALD Y.M. LEUNG, MD, PhD, *Department of Pediatrics, University of Colorado Health Sciences Center, Pediatric Allergy/Immunology Division, National Jewish and Medical Research Center, Denver, CO*

MICHAEL A. LEVINE, MD, *The Children's Hospital at The Cleveland Clinic, Department of Pediatrics, The Cleveland Clinic Lerner College of Medicine, Case Western Reserve University, Cleveland, OH*

CLIVE J. LEWIS, MD, *Imperial College, National Heart and Lung Institute, London, UK*

NING LI, PhD, *Department of Dermatology, School of Medicine, University of North Carolina, Chapel Hill, NC*

MIN LIU, MD, PhD, *Department of Pathology, University of Cincinnati Medical Center, Cincinnati, OH*

ZHI LIU, PhD, *Department of Dermatology, Department of Microbiology and Immunology, School of Medicine, University of North Carolina, Chapel Hill, NC*

KIRK C. LO, MD, CM, *Male Reproductive Medicine and Surgery, Scott Department of Urology, Baylor College of Medicine, Houston, TX*

STEPHEN LOCARNINI, MD, PhD, *Victorian Infectious Diseases Reference Laboratory (VIDRL), North Melbourne and Department of Microbiology, Monash University, Clayton, Victoria, Australia*

BARRY LONDON, MD, PhD, *Cardiovascular Institute, University of Pittsburgh, Pittsburgh, PA*

TAMMY L. LOUCKS, MPH, *Magee-Women's Research Institute, Pittsburgh, PA*

WILLIAM L. LOWE, JR., MD, *Division of Endocrinology, Metabolism, and Molecular Medicine, Feinberg School of Medicine, Northwestern University, Chicago, IL*

JAY LOZIER, MD, PhD, *Center for Biologics Evaluation and Research, Food and Drug Administration, Rockville, MD*

JAMES R. LUPSKI, MD, PhD, *Department of Molecular and Human Genetics, Department of Pediatrics, Baylor College of Medicine, Texas Children's Hospital, Houston, TX*

HE-PING MA, MD, *Department of Medicine, University of Alabama at Birmingham School of Medicine, Birmingham, AL*

CALUM A. MACRAE, MD, *Cardiology Division and Cardiovascular Research Center, Massachusetts General Hospital, Harvard Medical School, National Heart, Lung and Blood Institute's Framingham Heart Study, Boston, MA*

TERRY MAGNUSON, PhD, *Department of Genetics, University of North Carolina, Chapel Hill, NC*

FRANK MALDARELLI, MD, PhD, *HIV Drug Resistance Program, National Cancer Institute, National Institutes of Health, Bethesda, MD*

BELA MALIK, PhD, *Department of Physiology, The Center for Cell and Molecular Signaling, Emory University School of Medicine, Atlanta, GA*

MARCO MARCELLI, MD, *Departments of Medicine and Molecular and Cellular Biology, Baylor College of Medicine, Division of Endocrinology, Michael E. DeBakey VA Medical Center, Houston, TX*

CINDY M. MARTIN, MD, *Department of Internal Medicine, University of Texas Southwestern Medical Center, Dallas, TX*

W. STRATFORD MAY, JR., MD, PhD, *University of Florida, Shands Cancer Center, University of Florida, Gainesville, FL*

SHAWN E. MCCANDLESS, MD, *Department of Genetics, Case Western Reserve University, Center for Human Genetics, University Hospitals of Cleveland, Cleveland, OH*

ELIZABETH A. MCGEE, MD, *Magee-Women's Research Institute, Pittsburgh, PA*

ELIZABETH M. MCNALLY, MD, PhD, *Department of Medicine, Section of Cardiology, Department of Human Genetics, The University of Chicago, Chicago, IL*

MICHAEL J. MCPHAUL, MD, *Department of Internal Medicine, University of Texas Southwestern Medical Center, Dallas, TX*

DEBORAH C. MEDOFF, PhD, *Maryland Psychiatric Research Center, Department of Psychiatry, University of Maryland School of Medicine, Baltimore, MD*

SHLOMO MELMED, MD, *Academic Affairs, Cedars-Sinai Medical Center, David Geffen School of Medicine at UCLA, Los Angeles, CA*

WILLIAM E. MITCH, MD, *Division of Nephrology, Baylor College of Medicine, Houston, TX*

CHRISTOPHER B. MIZELLE, MD, *School of Medicine, University of North Carolina, Chapel Hill, NC*

MASASHI MIZOKAMI, MD, PhD, *Department of Clinical Molecular Informative Medicine, Nagoya City University Graduate School of Medical Sciences, Nagoya, Japan*

ANWAR N. MOHAMED, MD, *Cancer Cytogenetic Laboratory, Department of Pathology, Wayne State University School of Medicine, Detroit, MI*

JEFFERY D. MOLKENTIN, PhD, *Department of Pediatrics, Division of Molecular Cardiovascular Biology, Children's Hospital Medical Center, Cincinnati, OH*

STEPHAN MOLL, MD, *Department of Medicine, Division of Hematology-Oncology, University of North Carolina, Chapel Hill, NC*

KHEDOUDJA NAFA, PhD, *Memorial Sloan Kettering Cancer Center, New York, NY*

SATYA NARAYAN, PhD, *Department of Anatomy and Cell Biology, UF Shands Cancer Center, College of Medicine, University of Florida, Gainesville, FL*

CHARLES B. NEMEROFF, MD, PhD, *Department of Psychiatry and Behavioral Sciences, Emory University School of Medicine, Atlanta, GA*

ERIC J. NESTLER, MD, PhD, *Department of Psychiatry and Center for Basic Neuroscience, The University of Texas Southwestern Medical Center, Dallas, TX*

MARIA I. NEW, MD, *Adrenal Steroid Disorders Program, Department of Pediatrics, Mount Sinai School of Medicine, The Mount Sinai Hospital, New York, NY*

WILLIAM G. NEWMAN, MD, PhD, *University of Manchester, UK, St. Mary's Hospital, Manchester, UK*

PEADAR G. NOONE, MD, *Cystic Fibrosis Research and Treatment Center, Department of Medicine, Division of Pulmonary Diseases, University of North Carolina, Chapel Hill, NC*

CHRISTOPHER J. O'DONNELL, MD, MPH, *Cardiology Division, Massachusetts General Hospital, Harvard Medical School and the National Heart, Lung and Blood Institute's Framingham Heart Study, Boston, MA*

ERIC N. OLSON, PhD, *Department of Molecular Biology, University of Texas Southwestern Medical Center, Dallas, TX*

MARCELO PÁEZ-PEREDA, PhD, *Affectis Pharmaceuticals and Max Planck Institute of Psychiatry, Munich, Germany*

KEITH L. PARKER, MD, PhD, *Department of Internal Medicine, Division of Endocrinology and Metabolism, University of Texas Southwestern Medical Center, Dallas, TX*

KEVIN A. PELPHREY, PhD, *Department of Psychological and Brain Sciences, Duke University, Durham, NC*

ALEXANDER E. PERL, MD, *Division of Hematology-Oncology, Department of Medicine, University of Pennsylvania, Philadelphia, PA*

JOHN A. PHILLIPS III, MD, *Division of Medical Genetics, Department of Pediatrics, Vanderbilt University School of Medicine, Nashville, TN*

ANTONELLO PIETRANGELO, MD, PhD, *Center for Hemochromatosis and Hereditary Liver Diseases, Department of Internal Medicine, University of Modena and Reggio Emilia, Modena, Italy*

JOSEPH PIVEN, MD, *Departments of Psychiatry and Pediatrics, Neurodevelopmental Disorders Research Center, University of North Carolina, Chapel Hill, NC*

SHARON E. PLON, MD, PhD, *Departments of Pediatrics, and Molecular and Human Genetics, Baylor College of Medicine, Houston, TX*

DIDIER PORTILLA, MD, *Department of Internal Medicine, Division of Nephrology, University of Arkansas for Medical Sciences, Central Arkansas Veterans Healthcare System, Little Rock, AR*

AMY POTTER, MD, *Adult and Pediatric Endocrinology, Division of Endocrinology, Department of Pediatrics, Division of Endocrinology and Metabolism, Department of Medicine, Vanderbilt University School of Medicine, Nashville, TN*

S. RUSS PRICE, PhD, *Renal Division, Department of Medicine, Emory University, Atlanta, GA*

CHARMIAN A. QUIGLEY, MBBS, *Department of Pediatrics, Indiana University School of Medicine, Lilly Research Laboratories, Indianapolis, IN*

WILLIAM E. RAINEY, PhD, *Department of Physiology, Medical College of Georgia, Augusta, GA*

GIUSEPPE REMUZZI, MD, *Mario Negri Institute for Pharmacological Research, and Division of Nephrology and Dialysis, Azienda Ospedaliera, Ospedali Riuniti di Bergamo, Bergamo, Italy*

KERRY J. RESSLER, MD, PhD, *Department of Psychiatry and Behavioral Sciences, Emory University School of Medicine, Atlanta, GA*

GABRIELE RICHARD, MD, *Department of Dermatology and Cutaneous Biology, Jefferson Medical College, Thomas Jefferson University, Philadelphia, PA*

FRANZISKA RINGPFEIL, MD, *Department of Dermatology and Cutaneous Biology, Jefferson Medical College, Thomas Jefferson University, Philadelphia, PA*

ANTONIO M. RISITANO, PhD, *Dipartimento di Biochimica e Biotecnologie Mediche, Federico II University of Naples, Naples, Italy*

JACQUES ROBIDOUX, PhD, *CIIT Centers for Health Research, Endocrine Biology Program, Division of Biological Sciences, Research Triangle Park, NC*

DAVID M. RODMAN, MD, *Division of Pulmonary Sciences and Critical Care Medicine, University of Colorado Health Sciences Center, Denver, CO*

ANTHONY ROSENZWEIG, MD, *Program in Cardiovascular Gene Therapy, Cardiovascular Research Center, Center for Immunology and Inflammatory Diseases, Massachusetts General Hospital, Boston, MA*

BRUNO ROTOLI, MD, *Dipartimento di Biochimica e Biotecnologie Mediche, Federico II University of Naples, Naples, Italy*

DAVID S. RUBENSTEIN, MD, PhD, *Department of Dermatology, School of Medicine, University of North Carolina, Chapel Hill, NC*

DEBORAH C. RUBIN, MD, *Division of Gastroenterology, Departments of Medicine and Molecular Biology and Pharmacology, Washington University School of Medicine, St. Louis, MO*

DEEPAK M. SAMPATHU, PhD, *Center for Neurodegenerative Disease Research, Department of Pathology and Laboratory Medicine, University of Pennsylvania School of Medicine, Philadelphia, PA*

JEFF M. SANDS, MD, *Renal Division, Department of Medicine, Department of Physiology, Emory University School of Medicine, Atlanta, GA*

AMR H. SAWALHA, MD, *Department of Medicine, University of Oklahoma Health Sciences Center, US Department of Veterans Affairs Medical Center, Arthritis and Immunology Program, Oklahoma Medical Research Foundation, Oklahoma City, OK*

THOMAS E. SCAMMELL, MD, *Department of Neurology, Beth Israel Deaconess Medical Center, Boston, MA*

JULIE V. SCHAFFER, MD, *Department of Dermatology, New York Univesity School of Medicine, New York, NY*

MARCUS J. SCHULTZ, MD, PhD, *Department of Intensive Care Medicine, Laboratory of Experimental Intensive Care and Anesthesiology, Academic Medical Center, University of Amsterdam, Amsterdam, The Netherlands*

BRAHM H. SEGAL, MD, *Department of Medicine, Division of Infectious Diseases, The University at Buffalo, The State University of New York (SUNY), Roswell Park Cancer Institute, Buffalo, NY*

CHRISTINE E. SEIDMAN, MD, *Cardiovascular Division, Brigham and Women's Hospital, Howard Hughes Medical Institute and Department of Genetics, Harvard Medical School, Boston, MA*

SUDHIR V. SHAH, MD, *Department of Internal Medicine, Division of Nephrology, University of Arkansas for Medical Sciences, Central Arkansas Veterans Healthcare System, Little Rock, AR*

KENNETH H. SHAIN, MD, PhD, *Experimental Therapeutics, H. Lee Moffitt Cancer Center and Research Institute, Tampa, FL*

STEVEN D. SHAPIRO, MD, *Pulmonary and Critical Care, Department of Medicine, Brigham and Women's Hospital, Harvard Medical School, Boston, MA*

THOMAS C. SHEA, MD, *Division of Hematology and Oncology, Bone Marrow and Stem Cell Transplant Program, Lineberger Comprehensive Cancer Center, University of North Carolina, Chapel Hill, NC*

SARAH SHEFELBINE, MD, *Department of Otolaryngology, University of Florida, Gainesville, FL*

LINMARIE SIKICH, MD, *Department of Psychiatry, University of North Carolina, Chapel Hill, NC*

JONATHAN W. SIMONS, MD, *Winship Cancer Institute, Emory University, Atlanta, GA*

DONALD SMALL, MD, PhD, *Departments of Pediatrics, Oncology, Cellular and Molecular Medicine, Sidney Kimmel Comprehensive Cancer Center at Johns Hopkins, Baltimore, MD*

PETER H. ST GEORGE-HYSLOP, MD, FRCPC, FRS, *Centre for Research in Neurodegenerative Diseases, University of Toronto, Department of Medicine, Division of Neurology, University Health Network, Toronto, Ontario, Canada*

AMY STEIN, MD, *Department of Dermatology, School of Medicine, University of North Carolina, Chapel Hill, NC*

GORDON W. STEWART, MD, FRCP, *Department of Medicine, The Rayne Institute, London, UK*

STEPHEN M. STRITTMATTER, MD, PhD, *Department of Neurology, Yale University School of Medicine, New Haven, CT*

STEPHEN P. SUGRUE, PhD, *Department of Anatomy and Cell Biology, University of Florida College of Medicine, Gainesville, FL*

GREGORY M. SULLIVAN, MD, *Department of Psychiatry, Columbia University College of Physicians and Surgeons, New York, NY*

MARIJA TADIN-STRAPPS, PhD, *Department of Dermatology, College of Physicians and Surgeons, Columbia University, New York, NY*

CAROL A. TAMMINGA, MD, *Department of Psychiatry, Univesity of Texas Southwestern Medical Center, Dallas, TX*

STEPHEN J. TAPSCOTT, MD, PhD, *Fred Hutchinson Cancer Research Center, Department of Neurology, University of Washington, Seattle, WA*

GUNVANT THAKER, MD, *Maryland Psychiatric Research Center, Department of Psychiatry, University of Maryland School of Medicine, Baltimore, MD*

RAJESH V. THAKKER, MD, FRCP, FRCPath, FMedSci, *Nuffield Department of Clinical Medicine, University of Oxford, Academic Endocrine Unit, Oxford Centre for Diabetes, Endocrinology and Metabolism (OCDEM), Churchill Hospital, Headington, Oxford, UK*

SWEE LAY THEIN, DSc, FRCP, FRCPath, FMedSci, *Department of Haematological Medicine, Guy's, King's and St. Thomas' School of Medicine, London, UK*

NANCY E. THOMAS, MD, PhD, *Department of Dermatology, University of North Carolina, Chapel Hill, NC*

ADRIAN J. THRASHER, *Molecular Immunology Unit, Institute of Child Health, London, UK*

STEPHEN L. TILLEY, MD, *Department of Medicine, Division of Pulmonary and Critical Care Medicine, University of North Carolina, Chapel Hill, NC*

BRUCE C. TRAPNELL, MD, MS, *Department of Pediatrics, Division of Pulmonary Biology, Cincinnati Children's Hospital Medical Center, University of Cincinnati, Cincinnati, OH*

PATRICK TSO, PhD, *Department of Pathology, University of Cincinnati Medical Center, Cincinnati, OH*

MING T. TSUANG, MD, PhD, *Center for Behavioral Genomics, Department of Psychiatry, University of California, San Diego, La Jolla, CA; Veterans Affairs San Diego Healthcare System, San Diego, CA; and Harvard Institute of Psychiatric Epidemiology and Genetics, Harvard Departments of Epidemiology and Psychiatry, Boston, MA*

J. ERIC TURNER, MD, *Division of Hematology and Oncology, University of North Carolina, Chapel Hill, NC*

JOUNI UITTO, MD, PhD, *Department of Dermatology and Cutaneous Biology, Jefferson Medical College, Thomas Jefferson University, Philadelphia, PA*

TOM VAN DER POLL, MD, PhD, *Laboratory of Experimental Internal Medicine, Department of Infectious Diseases, Tropical Medicine and AIDS, Academic Medical Center, University of Amsterdam, Amsterdam, The Netherlands*

MARCIA VAN RIPER, PhD, RN, *School of Nursing, University of North Carolina, Carolina Center for Genome Sciences, Chapel Hill, NC*

CHRISTOPHER A. WALSH, MD, PhD, *Division of Neurogenetics, Howard Hughes Medical Institute, Beth Israel Deaconess Medical Center, Department of Neurology, Harvard Medical School, Boston, MA*

THOMAS H. WASSINK, MD, *Department of Psychiatry, Carver College of Medicine, University of Iowa, Iowa City, IA*

SUSAN E. WERT, PhD, *Department of Pediatrics, Division of Pulmonary Biology, Cincinnati Children's Hospital Medical Center, University of Cincinnati, Cincinnati, OH*

MATTHEW T. WHEELER, MD, PhD, *Department of Molecular Genetics and Cell Biology, The University of Chicago, Chicago, IL*

DAVID C. WHITCOMB, MD, PhD, *Division of Gastroenterology, Hepatology and Nutrition, University of Pittsburgh, Pittsburgh, PA*

GILBERT C. WHITE, II, MD, *Richard H. and Sarah E. Aster Chair for Medical Research, Blood Center of Wisconsin, Blood Research Institute, and Biochemistry, and Pharmacology and Toxicology, Medical College of Wisconsin*

JEFFREY A. WHITSETT, MD, *Department of Pediatrics, Division of Pulmonary Biology, Cincinnati Children's Hospital Medical Center, University of Cincinnati, Cincinnati, OH*

CHRISTOPHER S. WILCOX, MD, PhD, *Division of Nephrology and Hypertension, Cardiovascular Kidney Institute, Georgetown University, Washington, DC*

R. SANDERS WILLIAMS, MD, *Department of Medicine, Division of Cardiology, Duke University Medical Center, Durham, NC*

ROBERT W. WILLIAMS, PhD, *Department of Anatomy and Neurobiology, Department of Pediatrics, Center for Genomics and Bioinformatics, University of Tennessee, Memphis, TN*

LORNA M. WILLIAMSON, BSc, MD, FRCP, FRCPath, *Department of Haematology, University of Cambridge/ National Blood Service, Cambridge, UK*

JOHN S. WITTE, PhD, *Departments of Epidemiology and Biostatistics, and Urology, University of California, San Francisco, San Francisco, CA*

ROBERT C. WILSON, PhD, *Department of Pediatrics, Mount Sinai School of Medicine, New York, NY*

J. TIM WRIGHT, DDS, MS, *Department of Pediatric Dentistry, School of Dentistry, University of North Carolina, Chapel Hill, NC*

TERESA L. WRIGHT, MD, *Department of Medicine, University of California, San Francisco, Gastroenterology Division, Veterans Affairs Medical Center, San Francisco, CA*

LEI XIAO, PhD, *Department of Anatomy and Cell Biology, University of Florida, Gainesville, FL*

ANTHONY T. YACHNIS, MD, MS, *Department of Pathology and Laboratory Medicine, College of Medicine, University of Florida, Gainesville, FL*

ZHEN YAN, PhD, *Department of Medicine, Division of Cardiology, Duke University Medical Center, Durham, NC*

KEVIN E. YARASHESKI, PhD, *Department of Internal Medicine, Washington University School of Medicine, St. Louis, MO*

MAIMOONA ZARIWALA, PhD, *Division of Pulmonary Diseases, Department of Medicine, University of North Carolina, Chapel Hill, NC*

ANDREW R. ZINN, MD, PhD, *McDermott Center for Human Growth and Development, Department of Internal Medicine, University of Texas Southwestern Medical School, Dallas, TX*

HUDA Y. ZOGHBI, MD, *Departments of Pediatrics, Neurology, Molecular and Human Genetics, Neuroscience, Baylor College of Medicine, Howard Hughes Medical Institute, Houston, TX*

CARLA ZOJA, PhD, *Mario Negri Institute for Pharmacological Research, Bergamo, Italy*

Color Plates

Plate 1 (Fig. 2, Chapter 4). Fluorescent *in situ* hybridization of a pediatric leukemia sample demonstrating that one chromosome 5 contains a deleted segment that includes the EGR1 gene.

Plate 2 (Fig. 1, Chapter 10). The left side of the figure depicts fetal circulation in the human. The right side of the figure depicts neonatal circulation in the human.

Plate 3 (Fig. 2, Chapter 10). Dosage sensitive role of *Tbx1* in the etiology of cardiovascular defects in mice.

Plate 4 (Fig. 1A–C, Chapter 11). Gross pathological specimens of a heart with (**A**) hypertrophic cardiomyopathy (HCM) and (**C**) dilated cardiomyopathy (DCM). Note the marked increased in left ventricular hypertrophy (HCM) and chamber dimensions (DCM) as compared with (**B**) the normal heart.

Plate 5 (Fig. 2, Chapter 11). Histopathology of distinct human cardiomyopathies revealed by hematoxylin and eosin staining.

Plate 6 (Fig. 3, Chapter 15). The palmar and tuberoeruptive xanthomas are classically seen in patients with increased concentrations of intermediate density lipoproteins whereas the eruptive xanthomas are typically found in patients with massive serum triglyceride elevations resulting from excess chylomicrons and/or very low-density lipoproteins.

Plate 7 (Fig. 5, Chapter 22). Increased immunostaining for the caspase 3 p85 cleavage product of poly ADP-ribose polymerase in asthmatic mucosal biopsies and bronchoalveolar lavage epithelial cells.

Plate 8 (Fig. 4, Chapter 24). Plexiform lesion. The end-stage of pulmonary hypertension is associated with the formation of occlusive intimal lesions.

Plate 9 (Fig. 1, Chapter 29). Development of granulomatous inflammation. Antigen presenting cells interact with CD4+ T lymphocytes by presenting antigenic peptides, bound to major histocompatibility complex molecules, to T-cell receptors.

Plate 10 (Fig. 2A–D, Chapter 30). Histopathology of surfactant abnormalities found in the lungs of human patients with (**A**) mutations in the *SFTPB* gene, (**B**) mutations in the *SFTPC* gene, (**C**) mutations in the *ABCA3* gene, (**D**) and antibodies to granulocyte macrophage-colony-stimulating factor.

Plate 11 (Fig. 1, Chapter 66). Activation of MHC expression in fibroblasts expressing exogenous MyoD.

Plate 12 (Fig. 6, Chapter 66). Diagrammatic representation of somite maturation.

Plate 13 (Fig. 7, Chapter 66). Expression pattern of a myogenin-lacZ transgene in an 11.5-day mouse embryo. The myogenin promoter was linked to a β-galactosidase reporter gene and introduced into transgenic mice.

Plate 14 (Fig. 1, Chapter 84). Global epidemiology of HIV-1 subtypes and estimated number of infected individuals (in millions) at the end of 2002 according to the International AIDS Vaccine Initiative and the Joint United Nations Programme on HIV/AIDS.

Plate 15 (Fig. 1, Chapter 108). Features of the hairless phenotype in humans and mice.

Plate 16 (Fig. 1, Chapter 119). Characteristic neuropathological features of transmissible spongiform encephalopathies.

Plate 17 (Fig. 1, Chapter 129). Key neural circuits of addiction. Dotted lines indicate limbic afferents to the nucleus accumbens. Arrows represent efferents from the nucleus accumbens thought to be involved in drug reward.

GENETICS

SECTION EDITORS:
TERRY MAGNUSON AND JAMES P. EVANS

I

Abbreviations

I. MOLECULAR GENETICS

AAV   adeno-associated virus
ABGC   American Board of Genetics Counseling
ADR   adverse drug reaction
AMKL   acute megakaryocytic leukemia
AS   Angelman syndrome
BBS   Bardet-Biedl syndrome
BNSF   Burlington Northern Santa Fe Railroad
BWS   Beckwith-Wiedemann syndrome
CD   Crohn's disease
CEERs   Centers of Excellence in ELSI Research
CF   cystic fibrosis
cM   centimorgan
DPD   dihydropyrimidine dehydrogenase
DS   Down syndrome
ELSI   ethical, legal, and social implications
EM   extensive metabolizer
F1   filial 1
FAP   familial adenomatous polyposis
FDA   Food and Drug Administration
FISH   fluorescent *in situ* hybridization
HD   Huntington disease
HER2   human epidermal receptor 2
HGP   Human Genome Project
HH   hemihyperplasia
htSNP   haplotype tagging single-nucleotide polymorphism
IBD   inflammatory bowel disease

IGF   insulin-like growth factor
IND   investigational new drug
LGK   Lander-Green-Kruglyak
LOD   likelihood of the odds
MCMC   Monte-Carlo Markov Chain
MDR   multidrug resistance
MELAS   mitochondrial encephalomyopathy, lactic acidosis, and stroke-like episodes
MEN   multiple endocrine neoplasia
MEN1   multiple endocrine neoplasia type 1
MEN2   multiple endocrine neoplasia type 2
MTC   medullary thyroid carcinoma
mtDNA   mitochondrial DNA
NHGRI   National Human Genome Research Institute
PKU   phenylketonuria
PM   poor metabolizer
PWS   Prader–Willi syndrome
RP   retinitis pigmentosa
SNP   single-nucleotide polymorphism
TDT   transmission/disequilibrium test
UC   ulcerative colitis
UPD   uniparental disomy
URM   ultra rapid metabolizer
UV   ultraviolet
WAGR   Wilm's tumor, aniridia, genital–urinary abnormalities, and mental retardation
XP   xeroderma pigmentosum

1 Mendelian Inheritance

BRUCE R. KORF

SUMMARY

The basic patterns of genetic transmission in humans have been known for about a century, but are now coming to be understood at the molecular level. In addition to classical dominant, recessive, and sex-linked inheritance, more complex patterns have also been identified. These include maternal transmission of traits encoded in the mitochondrial genome, digenic traits determined by two distinct genes, and genomic imprinting. It is becoming clear that both rare and common genetic traits are determined by a complex interaction of multiple genetic and nongenetic factors.

Key Words: Digenic; dominant; expressivity; imprinting; Mendelian; mitochondrial inheritance; penetrance; recessive; X-linked.

INTRODUCTION

The existence of human traits that are transmitted from generation to generation in accordance with Mendel's laws was first recognized early in the 20th century. Understanding the mechanisms that underlie Mendelian inheritance has unfolded over the ensuing decades, and forms the basis for knowledge of human genetics. With increasing sophistication it has become clear that the seemingly straightforward rules of inheritance—for example, dominance and recessiveness—are in fact complex. With more nuanced understanding, however, comes recognition of genetic principles that have a critical role in diagnosis and counseling. This chapter reviews the basics of Mendelian inheritance and explores how insights in molecular genetics are both explicating and changing views of these fundamental principles.

PATTERNS OF GENETIC TRANSMISSION

The patterns of Mendelian transmission ensue from the fact that humans are diploid organisms, inheriting a complete set of genes from each parent. The two individual copies of a specific gene are referred to as *alleles*. The alleles on homologous chromosomes segregate at meiosis and new combinations are paired together on fertilization. The specific alleles at a locus comprise the genotype; the physical characteristic that results from action of the alleles is the phenotype.

DOMINANT AND RECESSIVE INHERITANCE The first instance of Mendelian transmission in humans was recognized by Archibald Garrod, working in the early years of the 20th century.

From: *Principles of Molecular Medicine, Second Edition*
Edited by: M. S. Runge and C. Patterson © Humana Press, Inc., Totowa, NJ

He originated the term "inborn errors of metabolism" to describe a set of disorders in which specific biochemical pathways were deranged, leading to accumulation of toxic substrates or deficiency of end products. He recognized that these conditions are familial and behave as Mendelian recessive traits. A recessive trait is only expressed in a homozygous individual who inherits a mutant allele from both parents (Fig. 1-1A). The parents are heterozygous carriers, who are asymptomatic because of the action of the dominant allele. A couple consisting of two carriers faces a 25% risk of transmission of homozygosity to any offspring.

The basis of recessive inheritance of inborn errors of metabolism is that the responsible genes encode enzymes required to catalyze specific biochemical reactions. Enzymes function in a catalytic manner, so the 50% level of activity that may occur in a heterozygote is sufficient to complete the reaction and thereby avoid the phenotype. Only a homozygote will lack sufficient activity to manifest the disorder. An example is the disorder phenylketonuria, which is because of mutation in the gene that encodes the enzyme phenylalanine hydroxylase, required to convert phenylalanine to tyrosine. Homozygotes accumulate phenylalanine to toxic levels, and also have a deficiency of phenylalanine metabolites such as dopamine and melanin. Children with this disorder detected by newborn screening can be spared the severe developmental impairment of this disorder by treatment with a low-phenylalanine diet. Carrier parents are asymptomatic, but have a 25% risk of additional affected children.

Dominant traits are expressed in both homozygous and heterozygous individuals (Fig. 1-1B). If the trait is rare, most affected individuals will be heterozygous. Moreover, many dominantly inherited medical conditions are lethal in the homozygous state, technically indicating that they are not "true" dominants. An individual who is heterozygous for a dominant trait has a 50% chance of passing either allele to any offspring.

A prototypical autosomal-dominant disorder is Marfan syndrome, resulting from mutation in the connective tissue protein fibrillin. Affected individuals are tall, lanky, and experience complications such as joint dislocation, lens subluxation, and aortic aneurysms because of weakness of connective tissue. The disorder is compatible with survival to reproductive age, and affected individuals have a 50% risk of transmitting the mutant allele to any offspring. The molecular basis for dominance is reviewed later.

SEX LINKAGE Sex determination occurs by inheritance of two X chromosomes in females or an X and a Y in males. The Y carries a limited repertoire of genes, including those involved

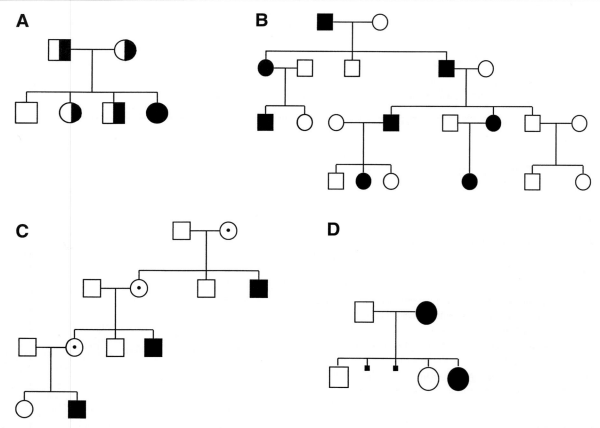

Figure 1-1   Pedigrees depicting autosomal-recessive (**A**), autosomal-dominant (**B**), X-linked-recessive (**C**), and X-linked-dominant with male lethality (**D**). By convention, squares denote males, circles females, and filled-in symbols are individuals who manifest a phenotype. Half-filled symbols in the recessive pedigree are carriers, and females with dots in the X-linked recessive pedigree are heterozygotes.

in testes determination and spermatogenesis. The X carries a larger set, most of which lack counterparts on the Y. Therefore, for these genes, females have two alleles, but males only one. There are regions at the two ends of the X chromosome where homologous loci exist on the Y. These are referred to as *pseudoautosomal*. For the other loci found only on the X males are said to be *hemizygous*.

Gene dosage is finely controlled, and, therefore, a mechanism exists to compensate for the dosage differences in males and females for X-linked genes. Most genes on the X chromosome are inactivated on one of the two X's in female cells early in development. The choice of X to be inactivated is random, but once an X is "turned off," that chromosome remains off in all descendents of a particular cell. Some genes, especially those in the pseudoautosomal regions escape inactivation. The molecular basis for X chromosome inactivation is becoming understood. It includes selection of the chromosome to be inactivated by an RNA molecule encoded by an X-linked gene called *Xist* and subsequent methylation of DNA on the inactive chromosome.

There are few Y-linked traits of medical significance. A Y-linked gene is transmitted from a male to all his sons and none of his daughters. X-linked traits are transmitted by a heterozygous female to half her offspring; a hemizygous male passes the gene to all his daughters and none of his sons (Fig. 1-1C). The concepts of dominance and recessiveness are meaningless when applied to genes on the X chromosome, which are subject to inactivation, because only one allele is expressed in any cell in either a male or a female.

Whether or not a trait is expressed in a heterozygous female depends on whether expression of the mutant gene in approx 50% of cells is sufficient to cause the phenotype, or whether expression of the wild-type allele in 50% is insufficient. Classic "X-linked-recessive" traits such as Duchenne muscular dystrophy and hemophilia A tends not to lead to a phenotype in heterozygous females, unless X chromosome inactivation has somehow been skewed toward inactivation of the wild-type allele. "X-linked-dominant" traits, such as hypophosphatemic rickets, are expressed in both sexes. X-linked traits such as Rett syndrome or incontinentia pigmenti are lethal in hemizygous males and, therefore, only are seen in heterozygous females (Fig. 1-1D).

MATERNAL TRANSMISSION   Although not a "Mendelian" pattern, maternal inheritance is another form of single gene transmission. Maternal inheritance applies to a set of genes found on the 16.5-kb circular double-stranded DNA molecules found within mitochondria. These encode 13 peptides involved in mitochondrial oxidative phosphorylation, as well as a set of transfer RNAs and ribosomal RNAs. There are thousands of DNA molecules within mitochondria in every cell. If there is a mutation in some, the cell is said to be heteroplasmic (Fig. 1-2A). Because mitochondrial DNA molecules segregate at random during cell division, the proportion of mutant and wild-type DNA molecules can vary widely between cells. Mitochondrial DNA mutations tend to interfere with cellular energy production. Because of heteroplasmy there can be a wide range of phenotypic effects, depending on the proportion of mutant mitochondria in different tissues.

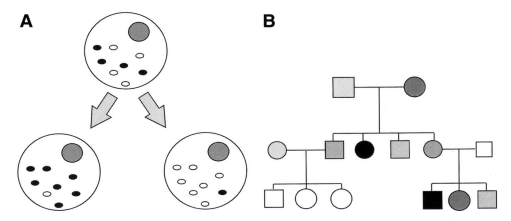

Figure 1-2 (**A**) Mutant and wild-type mitochondrial DNA may coexist in a cell, referred to as heteroplasmy. Mitochondrial DNA molecules segregate passively when a cell divides, so daughter cells may differ in their proportions of mutant and wild-type mitochondrial DNA. (**B**) Essentially, all the mitochondrial DNA is maternally transmitted. Hence, a female with a mitochondrial disorder will transmit it to all her offspring, whereas a male will not transmit the trait. Offspring may differ in their degree of expression of the phenotype because of heteroplasmy.

Most, if not all, mitochondria are transmitted through the oocyte. As a result, a female with a mitochondrial mutation will pass it to all of her offspring, whereas a male will not transmit it at all (Fig. 1-2B). Once again, however, heteroplasmy will account for variability, in this case among members of a sibship. This creates a challenge in recurrence risk counseling for mitochondrial disorders, because the likelihood that an offspring will inherit sufficient mutant DNA molecules to produce a phenotype cannot be predicted.

COMPLEXITIES OF MENDELIAN TRAITS

Although single gene traits are transmitted in accordance with Mendel's laws, a number of phenomena may lead to deviation from the expected segregation ratios. These include nonpenetrance, new mutation, mosaicism, anticipation, imprinting, and digenic inheritance.

PENETRANCE AND EXPRESSIVITY   Individuals who have the genotype associated with a particular phenotype yet do not display the phenotype are said to be nonpenetrant. For a dominant trait this may lead to a skipped generation (i.e., a trait is seen in a child and a grandparent, but the parent is not affected). Some phenotypes display age-dependent penetrance, so the probability of phenotypic expression increases with age. This is typical of disorders such as Huntington disease or adult polycystic kidney disease. Penetrance is an all-or-none phenomenon for an individual; the phenotype is either present or not at a particular time. Penetrance should not be confused with expressivity, which refers to the degree of phenotypic expression from individual to individual. The possibility of nonpenetrance or of age-dependent penetrance needs to be considered when counseling an individual at risk of a dominant trait. The lack of phenotype does not necessarily preclude one from occurring at a later age or exclude the possibility of transmission of the trait to an offspring.

MUTATION AND MOSAICISM   Sporadically affected individuals with a dominant or an X-linked trait may occur because of a new mutation in the sperm or egg cell. Neither parent will be found to carry the trait, and the affected child will be the first affected member of the family. That child, however, will be at risk of transmitting the trait to his or her offspring. Mutation rates vary among different loci, usually hovering in the range of 10^{-4} to 10^{-6}/gamete/generation. Few distinct risk factors have been

identified, although there is a slight increase in the risk of mutation with advancing paternal age.

Mutation may occur in somatic cells as well as in the germline. Somatic mutation during early development results in somatic mosaicism, in which an individual has a mixture of mutant and nonmutant cells. This may manifest as milder expression of a phenotype, or as expression of the phenotype in a limited region of the body. A dramatic example is segmental neurofibromatosis, where *café-au-lait* spots and neurofibromas may be restricted to part of the body. Germline mosaicism results in multiple sperm or egg cells carrying a new mutation. A parent with germline mosaicism can have multiple affected children despite not carrying the mutation in somatic cells.

ANTICIPATION   It has long been noted that in some families with particular dominant traits, severity increases, and age of onset decreases, from generation to generation. This phenomenon is referred to as anticipation. Although initially thought to be an artifact owing to bias of ascertainment, it is now known to be a real event that is the signature of a specific type of mutation, the triplet repeat expansion (Fig. 1-3). A number of genes include repeated triplets of bases, such as CAGCAGCAG. The exact number of repeats is a heritable polymorphism, as there is no phenotypic impact regardless of the number, up to a point. Individuals with mutations, however, have expanded numbers of repeats that lead to aberrant gene expression. Anticipation results from two characteristics of repeat expansion mutations. First, the larger the number of repeats, the more severe and earlier is the onset of the disorder. Second, the larger the repeat size, the more unstable it is, creating risk of further expansion in the next generation. The expansion, therefore, increases from generation to generation, leading to anticipation. Disorders associated with triplet repeat expansion tend to affect the nervous system, and include Huntington disease, fragile X syndrome, myotonic dystrophy, spinocerebellar ataxia, and others.

IMPRINTING   A subset of genes is expressed only from the maternal or paternal allele, but not both, and is referred to as imprinting. The "imprint" that identifies an allele as being of maternal or paternal origin is "erased" each generation. For example, if it is the maternally derived allele that is expressed, a maternally inherited allele will be turned on in a male, but will be turned off when he transmits it to the next generation. It appears that only

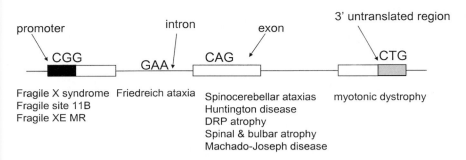

Figure 1-3 A prototypical gene, showing sites of triplet repeats that are prone to expansion, and examples of resultant disorders.

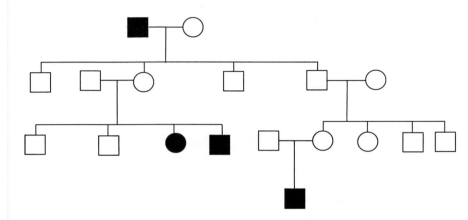

Figure 1-4 In this autosomal-dominant trait, an imprinted gene is only expressed when inherited from a female. Hence, only females can have affected offspring. Individuals who inherit the mutation from their fathers will not express the phenotype, but their daughters who carry the mutation can have affected children.

a relatively small number of genes are subject to imprinting, but these account for some distinct phenotypes and unusual patterns of transmission. A dominant trait because of an imprinted gene will only result in a phenotype when the transmitting parent is the one who transmits the expressed allele (Fig. 1-4). This gives rise to multiple examples of nonpenetrance. For example, this is the case in familial glomus tumors. Prader–Willi and Angelman syndromes result from deletions on chromosome 15 from a region that contains imprinted genes. The gene involved in Angelman syndrome is expressed from the maternal allele, so deletion of this allele results in the disorder. In contrast, paternal deletion of the same region produces Prader–Willi syndrome, reflecting the presence of one or more paternally expressed genes in the region. The same phenotypes can result from the inheritance of both copies of chromosome 15 from the same parent, referred to as uniparental disomy. In this case there will be absence of either maternally or paternally expressed genes, depending on whether there are two copies of mother's or father's chromosomes. Uniparental disomy results when a trisomic zygote produces an embryo in which disomy is restored by a second nondisjunction event. If the chromosomes that remain are from the parent in whom nondisjunction occurred, uniparental disomy will result. Aside from accounting for some cases of Prader–Willi or Angelman syndromes, uniparental disomy for several other chromosomes has been associated with a phenotype.

DIGENIC INHERITANCE In rare instances, it has been found that individuals who are doubly heterozygous for two recessive alleles may manifest a phenotype (Fig. 1-5). This has been found, for example, in some cases of the eye disorder retinitis pigmentosum. Parents who are heterozygous for two different genes can have doubly heterozygous offspring. If the genes are on different chromosomes, an affected child can transmit both mutant alleles to an offspring, producing apparent dominant transmission. Genes that are subject to digenic inheritance tend to encode proteins that interact with one another in the same pathway.

MOLECULAR BASIS OF MENDELIAN INHERITANCE

The patterns of single gene transmission have been known for a long time, but only recently the phenomena have begun to be understood at the molecular level. The bases for the Mendelian patterns as well as the complexities noted in the previous section are gradually emerging.

RECESSIVE VS DOMINANT ALLELES Recessive alleles, by definition, only exert a phenotypic effect in a homozygous state. In general, this implies that a mutation has resulted in loss of function of the gene product, and that partial loss of function is not sufficient to result in a phenotype. As noted, this is the case for most enzyme deficiencies. The mutations responsible for such disorders tend to be those that cause premature termination of translation, such as frame shifts or stop mutations, nonsense mutations, deletions, or splicing mutations, which significantly disrupt the coding sequence. Missense mutations may also cause a phenotype if they significantly disrupt the function of the gene product.

The basis for dominance can be a diverse set of genetic changes. Some mutations lead to gain of function, for example,

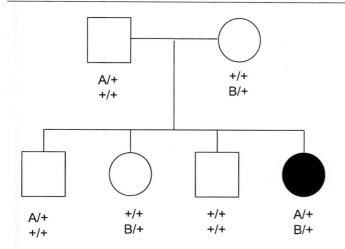

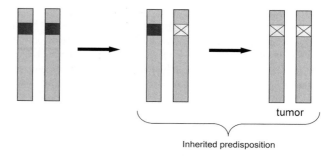

Figure 1-6 Tumor suppressor concept. A tumor suppressor gene is homozygously mutated in a tumor cell. Those who inherit a heterozygous mutation as a dominant trait are at increased risk of cancer if the remaining wild-type allele is mutated.

Figure 1-5 Pedigree illustrating digenic inheritance. Each parent is heterozygous for a different gene. The child who is heterozygous for both expresses the phenotype.

constitutive activation of a cell membrane receptor as occurs in the *FGFR3* gene in achondroplasia. Activation of just one allele is sufficient to alter the behavior of a cell. Another mechanism is referred to as dominant negative. Here, a single mutant allele produces sufficient abnormal product to disrupt cellular function. This is the hallmark of mutations in genes that encode products of multimeric proteins. Although only 50% of the protein may be abnormal, abnormal subunits may contribute to a higher proportion of proteins, resulting in a heterozygous phenotype. This is the case for some types of collagen mutations responsible for osteogenesis imperfecta. Dominant transmission may also occur with loss-of-function mutations if 50% levels of gene product are insufficient for normal function. This occurs in mild forms of Marfan syndrome because of loss-of-function fibrillin gene mutations. Interestingly, dominant negative mutations in this gene cause more severe disease, because the presence of abnormal fibrillin molecules has a more pervasive effect on connective tissue integrity than does 50% reduction of quantity.

A special case of dominant inheritance is accounted for by tumor suppressor genes. These genes account for familial susceptibility to cancers such as retinoblastoma, colon cancer, and breast or ovarian cancer. In families with an inherited susceptibility, the risk is transmitted as a dominant trait. Within a tumor cell, however, both alleles of the tumor suppressor are mutated, usually with a loss of function type mutation (Fig. 1-6). The mutation of one allele in such families is transmitted from generation to generation. An individual with heterozygous mutation faces an increased risk of cancer because somatic mutation of the remaining wild-type allele is all that is required to start a cell on the path to malignancy.

GENETIC HETEROGENEITY   There is a wide diversity of different mutation types, with a range of effects on gene function, including mutations that increase or decrease levels of gene product expression, or change the functional properties of the protein. Different mutations in the same gene may have differing impacts on phenotype. The consequence is that different individuals with a dominant trait may have distinct mutations. Furthermore, the two mutant alleles in an individual who is homozygous for a recessive mutation may differ. There are exceptions; in some cases only a very specific mutation will cause a specified phenotype. This is true for the *FGFR3* mutation in achondroplasia. In other instances,

a specific mutation may have arisen in an isolated population and remain relatively common there. This is called the founder effect, and accounts, for example, for the high prevalence of specific mutations responsible for Tay-Sachs disease in the Ashkenazi Jewish population.

Other than these instances, allelic heterogeneity is more a rule than an exception. In some cases, variable expressivity is explained by the occurrence of different mutations causing slightly different phenotypes. Study of genotype–phenotype correlations can sometimes provide information predictive of disease severity useful in genetic counseling. The difference between severe Duchenne muscular dystrophy and the milder Becker form can be predicted from whether the mutation causes complete loss of the gene product, dystrophin (Duchenne), or production of an aberrant protein (Becker). In still other cases, the different mutations result in phenotypes that would not have been regarded as the same disease. For example, different mutations in the *CFTR* gene can cause cystic fibrosis, chronic sinusitis, or male infertility resulting from congenital bilateral absence of the vas deferens.

Genetic heterogeneity extends not only to different alleles, but also to different loci. Studies to identify genes responsible for disease often reveal multiple distinct genes that are associated with the same phenotype in different individuals. In some instances, such as congenital deafness, this locus heterogeneity reflects that a large number of genes contribute to normal hearing. Many of these genes can be disrupted by mutation, all leading to deafness. In other cases, genes that encode proteins that interact with one another in the same pathway result in an indistinguishable phenotype when mutated. This is the case in tuberous sclerosis, associated with mutation in either the *TSC1* or *TSC2* genes. The protein products, hamartin and tuberin, interact with one another to form a complex that is involved in the control of cell growth. Locus heterogeneity is important in clinical genetics, because testing of the incorrect gene will fail to reveal an underlying mutation and could lead to incorrect exclusion of a diagnosis. For a recessive disorder, locus heterogeneity explains why two affected parents may have unaffected children. This is a common occurrence in hereditary deafness.

MODIFYING GENES   Although some phenotypes are reliably associated with specific genotypes, such as sickle cell anemia with the substitution of valine for glutain acid at position 6 β-globin mutation, mutations should not be thought of as totally deterministic of any specific phenotype. All mutations act within a context that is specified by factors including genetic background and the environment. Although a distinction is often made between mono-genic and multilateral phenotypes, in a sense all phenotypes are multifactorial. In some instances, a single gene exerts a major effect and in others many genes exert a more modest effect, but in virtually all cases genetic background and environment play some role.

Modifying loci may be intragenic or may occur as interactions between different gene loci. The poly T polymorphism with the *CFTR* gene exerts a modifying effect in the expression of muta-tions within this gene. Individuals may have an allele with 5, 7, or 9T's with this polymorphic site, which resides within the interval between exons 7 and 8. The 5T allele is associated with skipping of exon 9, whereas the 9T allele leads to normal splicing. Genotype at the poly T site influences phenotype associated with another *CFTR* mutation, R117H. This mutation is associated with CBAVD when in *cis* with 9T and opposite another *CFTR* mutation, but with mild cystic fibrosis if in *cis* with a 5T allele.

A dramatic example of gene–gene interaction is the phenome-non of epitasis, wherein the phenotype of one gene masks that of another. Individuals will only secrete A or B blood group antigens into saliva if they have at least one dominant Se alleles at the secretor locus. Someone with the se/se genotype will not have A or B antigen in saliva regardless of ABO genotype. Modifier loci with more subtle effects are likely to play a role in a large number of phenotypes. At least some degree of variable expression is probably the consequence of interactions between genes. Any single locus can be visualized as a node in a network. Changing the state of a single node will influence, and be influenced by, a large number of other nodes. In rare and common disorders, expression of a phenotype is a consequence of a complex web of interactions, and genetic analysis will increasingly require such complex systems.

CONCLUSIONS

The rules of Mendelian inheritance have provided the basis for the study of human genetics for a century. Studies at the molecu-lar level have provided an understanding of the basis for single gene inheritance and have uncovered some unexpected mecha-nisms. With new tools of genomics, exploration is beginning of the complexities of gene interactions as they relate to rare and common phenotypes, and knowledge of the elements of genetics is being integrated into a broader picture of biology.

SELECTED REFERENCES

Augarten A, Kerem BS, Kerem E, Gazit E, Yahav Y. Correlation between genotype and phenotype in patients with cystic fibrosis. N Engl J Med 1993;329:1308–1313.

Cassidy SB, Dykens E, Williams CA. Prader-Willi and Angelman syn-dromes: sister imprinted disorders. Am J Med Genet 2000;97(2): 136–146.

DiMauro S, Schon EA. Mitochondrial DNA mutations in human disease. Am J Med Genet 2001;106(1):18–26.

Kajiwara K, Berson EL, Dryja TP. Digenic retinitis pigmentosa due to mutations at the unlinked peripherin/RDS and ROM1 loci. Science 1994;264(5165):1604–1608.

Kiesewetter S, Macek M Jr, Davis C, et al. A mutation in CFTR produces different phenotypes depending on chromosomal background. Nat Genet 1993;5:274–278.

Levy HL, Albers S. Genetic screening of newborns. Annu Rev Genomics Hum Genet 2000;1:139–177.

Lieberman AP, Fischbeck KH. Triplet repeat expansion in neuromuscular disease. Muscle Nerve 2000;23(6):843–850.

McIntosh GC, Olshan AF, Baird PA. Paternal age and the risk of birth defects in offspring. Epidemiology 1995;6:282–288.

Monaco AP, Bertelson CJ, Liechti-Gallati S, Moser H, Kunkel LM. An explanation for the phenotypic differences between patients bearing partial deletions of the DMD locus. Genomics 1989;2:90–95.

Plath K, Mlynarczyk-Evans S, Nusinow DA, Panning B. Xist RNA and the mechanism of X chromosome inactivation. Annu Rev Genet 2002;36:233–278.

Prockop DJ, Baldwin CT, Constantinou CD. Mutations in type I procollagen genes that cause osteogenesis imperfecta. Adv Hum Genet 1990;19: 105–132.

Robinson PN, Booms P, Katzke S, et al. Mutations of FBN1 and geno-type-phenotype correlations in Marfan syndrome and related fib-rillinopathies. Hum Mutat 2002;20(3):153–161.

Ruggieri M, Huson SM. The clinical and diagnostic implications of mosaicism in the neurofibromatoses. Neurology 2001;56(11): 1433–1443.

Sampson JR. TSC1 and TSC2: genes that are mutated in the human genetic disorder tuberous sclerosis. Biochem Soc Trans 2003;31(Pt 3):592–596.

Shiang R, Thompson LM, Zhu Y-Z, et al. Mutations in the transmembrane domain of FGFR3 cause the most common genetic form of dwarfism, achondroplasia. Cell 1994;78:335–342.

Walter J, Paulsen M. Imprinting and disease. Semin Cell Dev Biol 2003;14(1):101–110.

2 Nontraditional Inheritance

Shawn E. McCandless and Suzanne B. Cassidy

SUMMARY

The "rules" of segregation of alleles originally defined by Gregor Mendel explained much of the phenomena associated with inheritance and have been dogmatically applied in the field of genetics. However, there are situations in which the rules of Mendelian inheritance cannot explain observed phenomena. A variety of molecular mechanisms have been identified that explain certain phenomena that are not easily explained by traditional Mendelian patterns of inheritance. These non-Mendelian mechanisms differ on a molecular basis, but can be described as a group by the term "nontraditional mechanisms of inheritance" or "nontraditional inheritance." Stated simply, nontraditional inheritance refers to the pattern of inheritance of a trait or phenotype that occurs predictably, recurrently, and in some cases familially, but does not follow the rules of typical Mendelian autosomal or sex chromosome inheritance. Examples discussed in this chapter are the triplet repeat expansion mutations, and genomic disorders including genetic imprinting, mitochondrial inheritance, and multi-allelic inheritance.

Key Words: Angelman syndrome (AS); fragile X; Mendelian; mitochondrial inheritance; multifactorial inheritance; non-Mendelian; Prader–Willi syndrome (PWS).

INTRODUCTION

The "rules" of segregation of alleles originally defined by Gregor Mendel explained much of the phenomena associated with inheritance and have been dogmatically applied in the field of genetics. However, there are situations in which the rules of Mendelian inheritance cannot explain observed phenomena. A variety of concepts have been suggested to explain such phenomena, including the idea that individual genes may function in cooperation with each other and with environmental factors to produce a given phenotype. This concept of multifactorial inheritance is well accepted; however, specific examples for which the various factors can be well defined have been difficult to identify. Other natural phenomena, such as anticipation, in which genetic traits or disorders become more severe or pronounced in successive generations, or genetically determined conditions that appear to depend on the sex of the parent of origin of the involved chromosome, have been difficult to explain, even using concepts of multifactorial inheritance.

From: *Principles of Molecular Medicine, Second Edition*
Edited by: M. S. Runge and C. Patterson © Humana Press, Inc., Totowa, NJ

A variety of molecular mechanisms have been identified, which explain certain phenomena that are not easily explained by traditional Mendelian patterns of inheritance. These non-Mendelian mechanisms differ on a molecular basis, but can be described as a group by the term "nontraditional mechanisms of inheritance" or "nontraditional inheritance." Stated simply, nontraditional inheritance refers to the pattern of inheritance of a trait or phenotype that occurs predictably, recurrently, and in some cases familially, but does not follow the rules of typical Mendelian autosomal or sex chromosome inheritance. Examples discussed in this chapter are the triplet repeat expansion mutations and genomic disorders including genetic imprinting, mitochondrial inheritance, and multi-allelic inheritance.

TRIPLET REPEAT EXPANSION

The first disorder identified as resulting from this form of nontraditional inheritance is fragile X syndrome (FRAXA). FRAXA is a well-recognized disorder that causes mental retardation, autistic-like behaviors, and a subtle, but characteristic, external phenotype in all males and many females possessing the mutation. Early studies confirmed that the locus of interest was on the X chromosome, and that in some cases the trait was associated with a cytogenetically visible fragile site on the X chromosome, seen only when cells were grown in a folic acid-deficient medium. The mental retardation syndrome was inherited in a classic pattern of X-linked inheritance, with carrier mothers who might have affected brothers or uncles passing the trait on to half of their male offspring. However, some unusual families caused confusion because of a pedigree pattern demonstrating what came to be known as the Sherman paradox. Specifically, there were families identified in which a male appeared to have passed the trait on to his daughters, but he himself was not affected, even though he might have affected brothers or uncles. This pattern could not be explained by typical X-linked inheritance.

The solution to the Sherman paradox became apparent when the molecular basis of the FRAXA was found to be a unique type of mutation that occurs in a region of repeated nucleotides in the genetic sequence. Specifically, in the FMR1 gene (*Xq27.3*) there is a repeated sequence of CGG nucleotides, a "triplet repeat" (Fig. 2-1). In normal individuals this sequence is repeated 5–44 times, but in an affected individual the sequence is repeated more than 200 times. Even more interesting, the mothers of the affected individuals were found to have triplet repeats with 60–200 copies. The normal allele is stably copied during the process of meiosis,

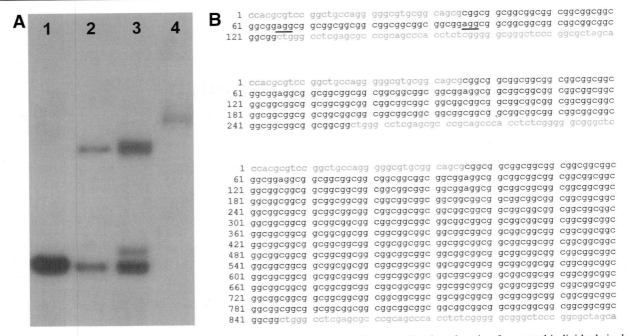

Figure 2-1 Triplet repeat expansion in fragile X syndrome. The gel (**A**) shows Southern blot-based testing for several individuals including a normal male—lane 1, a normal female—lane 2, a female premutation carrier—lane 3, and an affected male—lane 4. DNA is double digested with *Eco*RI, a restriction enzyme that cuts on either side of the triplet repeat, and *Eag*I, a methylation-sensitive enzyme that only cuts unmethylated DNA (including one site near the Fragile X triplet repeat). DNA is loaded from the top of the gel and separated by electrophoresis. A radioactively labeled probe, which binds near the triplet repeat, is used to visualize the bands of interest. Because *Eag*I only cuts unmethylated DNA, the methylated (inactive) allele is not cut and is seen as a 5.2-kb fragment (containing the triplet repeat). The unmethylated (active) allele is cut by *Eag*I and is seen as a 2.8-kb fragment (also containing the triplet repeat). Normal males have only the 2.8-kb fragment, representing the unmethylated allele from the active X chromosome, as seen in lane 1. Because they have two X chromosomes, normal females have both a 2.8-kb fragment and a 5.2-kb fragment, representing the methylated (inactive) and the unmethylated (active) alleles (lane 2). The female premutation carrier (lane 3) has two bands around 2.8 kb, one slightly larger because of the triplet repeat expansion of about 70 repeats (210 nucleotides). These additional 210 nucleotides represent approx 8% of the 2.8-kb fragment, so two lower bands are seen. The upper, methylated, fragment also has two bands, but because the 210 extra nucleotides only account for approx 4% of the whole fragment, the two bands do not separate enough to be visualized. The affected male in lane 4 has only one allele, seen as a fragment larger (above) than the 5.2-kb alleles in the female premutation carrier (lane 3) because of the increased size of the triplet repeat region of the fragment (estimated to be 330–530 repeats). Because males have only one X chromosome, this band represents a full-size expansion of the triplet repeat, which leads to methylation (inactivation) of the gene, resulting in Fragile X syndrome. Examples of the sequence (**B**) are shown for normal, a pre-expansion carrier and an affected allele, with the expansion shown in black and flanking sequence shown in gray. The normal allele in this figure has 30 CGG repeats, the premutation 74, and the full expansion 270. (Fig. 2-1A is courtesy of Stuart Schwartz and Linda Jeng.)

but alleles that are somewhat larger than normal, called "premutations," are prone to further expansion (increase in the number of repeats), leading in some cases to the full mutation. For reasons that are not well understood, the triplet repeat expansion in FRAXA appears to be much more likely to expand during female meioses than during male meioses. Occasionally, a female carrier of a premutation may pass on to her son an allele that has not undergone further expansion. He will not be affected, but can pass on the premutation to his daughters, who then will have a high risk of having an affected child by passing on a further expanded allele. It should be noted that FRAXA is caused by loss of function of the FMR1 protein and can also be caused by other inactivating mutations or deletion of the FMR1 gene.

Another interesting observation about FRAXA is that, contrary to Mendelian expectations for an X-linked recessive disorder, carrier females are often affected. In fact, as many as 50% of females who carry a full expansion will have measurable cognitive defects. This is not because of variation in the triplet repeat expansion, but is instead a result of intraindividual variation in X-chromosome inactivation. In every female cell, one or the other of the two X chromosomes is inactivated to compensate for the fact that women have double the number of X chromosomes as men. This X-inactivation is thought to occur randomly at an early stage of development when there are only 64–128 cells in the blastocyst. On average, half of the cells would be expected to maintain one of the X chromosomes as the active one, and the other half of the cells will maintain the other X. In an individual, however, merely by chance, the ratio may be skewed toward one or the other of the X chromosomes being active. This has been well documented, so that in a population of women there is a normal distribution, with a significant minority of women having one or the other X chromosome much more often inactivated. There are also likely to be different ratios of X-inactivation in a single individual when examining different tissues, with the tissue of interest for the cognitive defects (the brain) being generally unavailable for diagnostic molecular evaluation. These and other examples of the effect of X-inactivation on expression of X-linked disorders have led some to suggest that it is inaccurate to use the distinction of X-linked-recessive or X-linked-dominant. Rather, all of these disorders should be simply called "X-linked."

A number of genetic disorders caused by triplet repeat expansions have now been described. Table 2-1 shows several examples, along with the mode of apparent Mendelian inheritance, the

Table 2-1
Examples of Other Triplet Repeat Expansion Disorders

Disorder	Inheritance	Triplet sequence	Normal number of repeats	Number of repeats associated with disorder
Myotonic dystrophy	AD	CTG	5–27	>50 to >1000
Huntington disease	AD	CAG	9–37	>37
Spinocerebellar ataxia type I	AD	CAG	19–38	40 to >80
Friedreich ataxia	AR	GAA	7–20	>200
Fragile X syndrome	XLR	CGG	6–52	>200
X-linked spinobulbar atrophy	XLR	CAG	19–25	>40

AD, autosomal-dominant; AR, autosomal-recessive; XLR, X-linked-recessive.

repeated triplet of bases, and the number of repeats associated with the disease state. The molecular mechanism that causes disease is likely different, because some triplet repeat expansions are in coding regions of the gene (exons), some are in noncoding regions (introns), and others are completely outside of the gene, apparently affecting transcriptional regulation. In some cases, the triplet repeat expansion causes disease because it leads to the loss of function of the normal protein product. The triplet repeat expansion may also cause some new function or interaction, which has been shown to be the case in Huntington disease. Interestingly, the vast majority of disorders known to result from triplet repeat expansion are disorders of the neurological system, especially ataxias and other movement disorders.

This mechanistic heterogeneity extends also to the meiotic instability of the triplet repeat expansions. Some triplet repeats are more prone to expansion during female meiosis (e.g., fragile X and myotonic dystrophy) whereas others are more likely to expand when inherited from the father (e.g., Huntington disease). The FMR1 gene also has mitotic instability, so that there may be variation in the size of expansion in different cells and different tissues in the same individual. This is not a generalized trait of triplet repeat expansions, though, as it does not occur with the Huntington disease gene, Huntingtin (*4p16.3*).

Anticipation refers to an observed phenomenon where a genetic disorder appears to become more severe in successive generations, a condition not easily explained by simple Mendelian inheritance. For many years there was a controversy as to whether this observation was true, or was a result of ascertainment bias because mildly affected parents may only be identified if they have a more severely affected child. It is now known that anticipation does occur, at least in many triplet repeat expansion disorders, because of increasing size of the triplet repeat expansion in successive generations. In Huntington disease, the child of an affected father may present at a significantly earlier age than the father because of further expansion of the abnormal allele during male meiosis. A similar situation occurs with myotonic dystrophy, a disorder characterized by progressive weakness, especially in the distal extremities, associated with myotonia (difficulty relaxing a contracted muscle), cataracts, and frontal hair loss. A mildly affected mother, who may not know she has the disorder, can give birth to an infant with severe hypotonia and weakness causing respiratory compromise and often death in the neonatal period. The mother may have few symptoms, which can be as subtle as difficulty releasing a handshake. A similar pattern of a severely affected infant born to a mildly affected parent has been described with massive triplet repeat expansions occurring in genes associated with some forms of spinocerebellar ataxia.

GENOMIC DISORDERS AND IMPRINTING

Prader–Willi syndrome (PWS) and Angelman syndrome (AS) exemplify several aspects of nontraditional inheritance. In the case of PWS and AS, the parent of origin of chromosome 15 affects the expression of some genes. The discredited hypothesis of Lamarck suggested that the parental factor of inheritance is somehow "imprinted," and that acquired traits can be passed on to the offspring. Although Lamarck was incorrect, the concept of imprinting has survived, in this case meaning that expression of certain genes is determined by the sex of the parent who passed on that chromosome.

These imprinted genes, which reside on autosomes, exist in two copies, as do all autosomal genes. The inactivation of one copy of these genes resulting from imprinting makes the genes dosage dependent. Stated another way, some autosomal genes are normally expressed only from one member of the gene pair even though both genes in the pair have normal base sequence because one allele has been inactivated. This exposes at least three different, and fascinating, causes of nontraditional inheritance not because of variation in the DNA sequence of the genes involved, but instead because of changes affecting the way the genes are transcribed and expressed. "Genomic disorders" are those disorders resulting from the loss of function of a dosage-dependant gene as a result of loss, duplication, or disruption of the region of the genome in which the genes reside. Often, these events are mediated by deletions or duplications caused by aberrant recombination resulting from closely spaced low copy number repeats flanking the critical region. Points in the DNA that break are more susceptible to breakage because of intrinsic characteristics of the DNA sequence that predispose to abnormal DNA looping at the time of meiosis. The following discussion uses PWS and concerning to demonstrate these mechanisms of nontraditional inheritance.

PWS is characterized by two distinct clinical phases, both of which are seen in essentially all individuals with the disorder. The first phase, marked by profound hypotonia, can be noted prenatally with decreased fetal movement and breech position in the uterus. After birth the infant is profoundly hypotonic, sleeps excessively and has difficulty with feeding and weight gain. There is a global developmental delay, often accompanied by hypoplastic genitalia and cryptorchidism (in boys), strabismus, and evidence of growth hormone deficiency. By the end of 1 yr the feeding difficulty is generally resolved, and behavioral issues are mild.

The second phase typically begins around the age of 2–4 yr. The child is noted to have an apparently insatiable appetite leading to profound obesity if not carefully monitored. There is a typical,

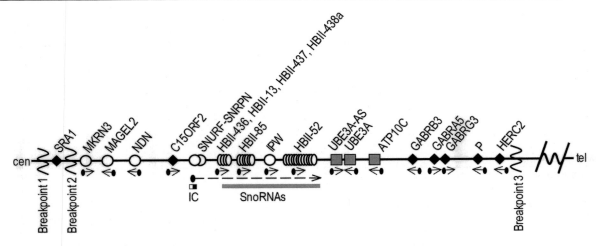

Figure 2-2   Gene map of Prader-Willi syndrome/Angelman syndrome region of chromosome 15. This represents approx 4–5 Mb of chromosome 15 just below the centromere. The common breakpoints of the recurrent deletions are shown. Open circles represent maternally imprinted (expressed only from the paternally inherited chromosome) genes. Gray squares are paternally imprinted genes, and black diamonds represent nonimprinted genes. The open ovals represent clusters of small nucleolar RNAs (SnoRNAs) that have been identified. The function of these RNAs is not known, but they are distributed in intronic regions between the 144 purported exons of SNURF/SNRPN. Arrows show the direction of transcription of genes, with the long, dashed arrow showing the direction and extent of the SNRPN exons. Any of the maternally imprinted genes potentially could contribute to the PWS phenotype, although evidence does not suggest a role for MKRN3 or IPW. The imprinting center is shown as two pieces, with the open rectangle representing the region controlling paternal imprinting (AS), and the filled portion representing the maternal imprint control (PWS) region.

but subtle, facial appearance. There is mild mental retardation or low normal intelligence and a characteristic behavioral profile with temper tantrums, obsessive behaviors, verbal perseveration, skin picking, and a variety of other traits. Management includes avoidance of obesity by careful dietary control and exercise, avoiding exposure to food except at mealtime, use of supplemental growth hormone, and an array of behavioral interventions. Without intervention, the life expectancy is significantly shortened because of complications of obesity such as obstructive sleep apnea, right-sided heart failure, and diabetes.

AS is characterized by more significant mental retardation, severe speech delay or no speech at all, marked gait disturbance with ataxia, and an unusual behavioral profile with a happy demeanor, frequent bursts of laughter for no apparent reason, and rapid escalation of behaviors. There is a characteristic facial appearance, microcephaly, commonly seizures, and there may be a typical EEG pattern.

PWS and AS were delineated clinically in the 1950s and 1960s. In the 1980s, the same recurrent chromosomal deletion was shown to cause both of these disparate clinical syndromes. Further study showed that both result from lack of expression of imprinted genes located near the centromere on the long arm of chromosome 15, but the parental origin of the deletion differed in the two disorders. These two disorders were the first abnormalities resulting from imprinted genes to be recognized in humans. Specifically, at least five different causes of these two disorders have now been delineated, all of which result because genes in the affected region of chromosome 15 are expressed differently when inherited from the mother than when inherited from the father. The known genes in the region are shown in Fig. 2-2, with the sex of the parent in whom the genes are expressed (active) indicated.

Much has been learned about the mechanism by which differential gene expression occurs in imprinted genes. Several genes in the PWS/AS region have an excess of methyl groups attached to

cytosine nucleotides. The methylation appears to block the transcriptional machinery from attaching to or acting on these genes, so that no messenger RNA is made from the highly methylated chromosome. Therefore, the only active copies of the genes in this region are those that are unmethylated. This hypermethylation is found in a parent-of-origin-specific distribution. In Fig. 2-2, genes that are hypermethylated (inactive) when inherited from the mother are shown as white circles, whereas those that appear to be inactive when inherited from the father are shown as gray squares. Any structural change that leads to loss or disruption of the active genes will lead to an absence of the gene product. Several of the genes produce a protein product, although little is known about the function of any of these proteins.

PWS is a result of the loss of genes that are only expressed from the paternally inherited chromosome 15. The most common mechanism leading to PWS is a small interstitial deletion on the chromosome 15 inherited from the father. This recurrent deletion accounts for about 70–75% of all cases of PWS, and occurs with a frequency as high as 1 in 20,000 liveborn infants (the overall incidence of PWS, resulting from all causes, is thought to be 1 in 10,000–15,000). The same deletion accounts for a similar proportion of cases of AS, when it occurs on the chromosome 15 inherited from the mother. The common deletion in both disorders has the same breakpoints, in the vast majority of cases, resulting from small duplicated sections of DNA flanking the region, spanning a distance of about 4 Mb. This type of duplication has been referred to as a "duplicon," and a number of similar situations appear throughout the genome. Several have already been identified as causing aberrant recombination leading to recurrence of other microdeletions (e.g., deletion 22q11 syndrome).

A second mechanism leading to an individual having no active copies of these imprinted genes occurs when both copies of chromosome 15 are inherited from the same parent, called "uniparental disomy" (UPD). PWS and AS were among the first disorders caused by UPD to be described. Now, several other conditions have been shown to have a similar mechanism because UPD for chromosomes containing imprinted genes results in absent expression of the imprinted genes. Other examples include some cases of Beckwith-Wiedemann syndrome resulting from UPD for chromosome 11, transient neonatal diabetes resulting from UPD of chromosome 6, some cases of Silver-Russell syndrome resulting from UPD of chromosome 7, and a mental retardation syndrome resulting from UPD for chromosome 14.

UPD most often occurs as a result of a trisomy present at fertilization. PWS occurs when there are two copies of the maternally inherited chromosome 15 present. Most often this results from malsegregation during female meiosis, leading to conception with two copies of chromosome 15 from the ovum and one copy from the sperm. This is nonviable unless there is a second postmitotic event, usually loss of one of the chromosome 15s resulting from malsegregation during mitosis (called "trisomy rescue"). This often occurs because of anaphase lag, where one chromosome fails to move along with the others as the mitotic spindles separate during cell division, and the chromosome is lost into the cytoplasm of one of the daughter cells. It is apparent that there are two possible outcomes from this event. One is the loss of one of the two chromosomes that came from the same parent, resulting in a cell that is now back to the normal and appropriate chromosomal complement, having one chromosome 15 from the father and one from the mother. Alternatively, the chromosome lost in the trisomy rescue process may be from the parent who only contributed one chromosome. This rescues the trisomy, and allows the pregnancy to continue, but if there are imprinted genes on the involved chromosome they will have abnormal expression. Specifically, as seen in PWS, although there are two copies of each gene on chromosome 15, both are from the mother so there will be no gene expression from the imprinted genes.

The point in meiosis where nondisjunction occurs is another important factor concerning UPD. Meiosis I nondisjunction is a failure of separation of the homologous chromosomes, but the sister chromatids divide normally at meiosis II (Fig. 2-3). This results in two gametes that carry one copy of each original parental chromosome (heterodisomy) and two gametes with no copies of the parental chromosome involved. The alternative is that the nondisjunction occurs in meiosis II, after the homologues have successfully separated. Meiosis II defects result in one gamete with two identical copies of the same chromosome (isodisomy), one gamete with no copy of the chromosome and two normal gametes (Fig. 2-3D). Both types of meiotic errors can lead to a trisomic fertilization that is then rescued by loss of one of the chromosomes. Isodisomy can also occur when a gamete that is missing a chromosome (nullisomic) is involved in fertilization. That fertilization results in a monosomic pregnancy, most of which are not viable, unless a mitotic segregation defect occurs that leads to a duplication of the chromosome in question. This mechanism always leads to isodisomy. In AS, the majority of UPD cases have paternal isodisomy, suggesting that the mitotic mechanism is more common. In PWS, both heterodisomy and isodisomy have been seen, making it difficult to determine the mechanism.

Heterodisomy and isodisomy cause a phenotype if there are imprinted genes in the region. Even when the two copies of the chromosome are different (heterodisomy), both carry the identical imprint (i.e., maternally derived or paternally derived) so that the imprinted genes are not expressed. Isodisomy, on the other hand, can also cause a phenotype because nonimprinted recessive disease-causing genes on the duplicated chromosome will be present

on both copies of the chromosome. The very first documented case of UPD was in a child with cystic fibrosis (CF) who was homozygous for the common ΔF508 mutation, a mutation that was only found in one of her parents. She also had short stature. Additional studies demonstrated that both copies of her chromosome 7 were inherited from the parent who carried the CF mutation. This situation has been described for other autosomal-recessive conditions. Furthermore, maternal UPD for chromosome 7 has been shown to be associated with poor growth of prenatal onset, and appears to cause some cases of the primordial dwarfing condition Silver-Russell syndrome.

Several possible evolutionary advantages of imprinting have been put forward. One hypothesis suggests a relative survival advantage to males of being physically large (the idea of the "strapping" boy) weighed against the survival advantage to the female, in this case the mother, of surviving the delivery to reproduce again by having a relatively smaller baby. Supportive evidence for this comes from the fact that pregnancies resulting from duplication of the male genome form a mass of trophoblastic tissue (placentation) with little or no recognizable embryonic tissue, the so-called "hydatidiform mole." Likewise, the parental contribution of the extra set of chromosomes in triploid pregnancies correlates with the clinical findings. Triploidy with the paternal genome duplicated is usually associated with a very small fetus and large placenta, whereas maternal genomic duplication is associated with a small placenta and an early spontaneous miscarriage. Many of the earliest imprinted genes identified were found to be associated with growth, although that generalization has not held up entirely as more imprinted genes have been found. Other hypotheses purporting an evolutionary advantage for imprinted genes suggest a role either in protection from inappropriate timing of expression of certain genes, or a role in protecting mammalian females from malignant trophoblastic disease because of parthenogenic reproduction, so that paternally contributed genes are required for normal placentation. It has been suggested that there are only 100–200 imprinted genes out of the total estimated less than 30,000 genes in the human genome.

The third mechanism for development of PWS and AS, accounting for less than 5% of cases of each, also results from an imprinting abnormality. During the normal process of gamete production, an individual must change the imprinting pattern of chromosomes inherited from their own opposite sex parent. For example, the chromosome 15 that a man inherits from his mother will be maternally imprinted, and the imprinted genes will not be expressed during that man's embryonic development. When he passes on that chromosome 15 to his children he must be able to switch the imprint and turn those genes back on. If this does not happen, his offspring will inherit a normal maternally imprinted chromosome 15 from their mother, and an abnormal maternally imprinted chromosome 15 from their father. In this case, there is biparental inheritance of chromosome 15, but both copies are maternally imprinted. When molecular testing is performed there will be no deletion of chromosome 15, nor will there be molecular evidence, usually identified by microsatellite-polymorphism analysis, of UPD. Specific analysis of the methylation pattern in the PWS/AS region of chromosome 15 will be abnormal, though. This "methylation assay" relies on the use of a methylation-sensitive method of evaluating the region, either by use of a methylation-sensitive restriction enzyme, or by use of a specialized methylation-sensitive polymerase chain reaction protocol. In either test, the result will be production of different-sized DNA fragments from

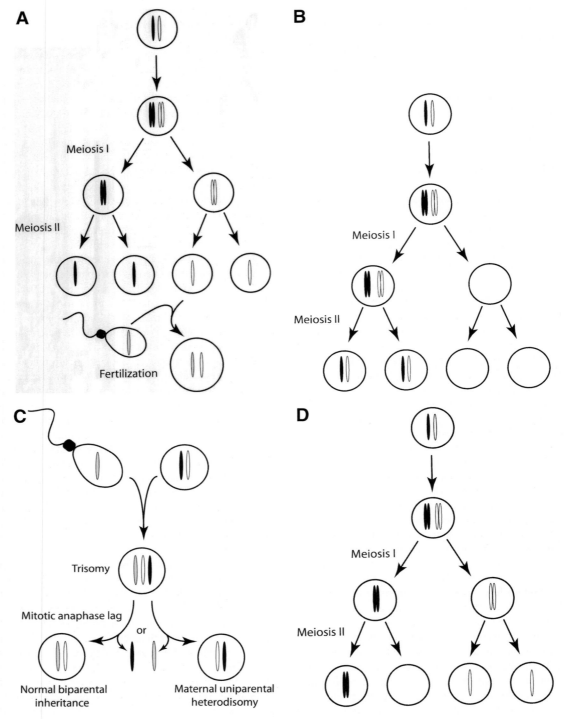

Figure 2-3 *(Continued)*

maternally and paternally imprinted DNA, demonstrating the presence (or absence) of maternally and paternally imprinted genes. This test will identify all cases of PWS and AS resulting from deletion, UPD, or imprinting defects.

The specific mechanism by which the parent of origin imprint is switched has not been elucidated. The region of chromosome 15 involved, the "imprinting center," has been defined through examination of a series of chromosome rearrangements and progressively smaller deletions. There appear to be distinct, slightly

separated, regions responsible for initiating the imprint for the maternally silenced genes and the paternally silenced genes. Unlike deletions and UPD, which occur sporadically, some imprinting defects result from imprinting mutations (mostly very small deletions of sequence around the imprinting center) that may be familial. Imprinting mutations cause a unique situation in which the first individual in a family to acquire the defect will be normal, but half of the chromosomes that they pass on will be abnormal because the imprint will not be properly switched on

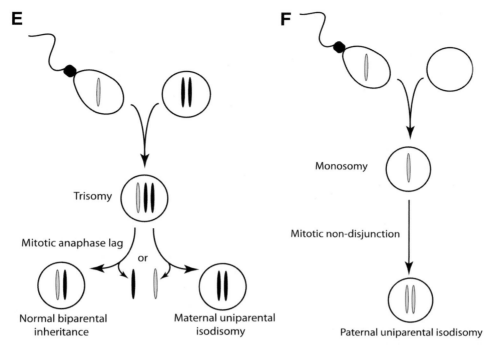

Figure 2-3 Uniparental disomy. This figure follows a single pair of chromosomes through a variety of meiotic and mitotic outcomes to demonstrate how UPD occurs. The chromosomes are shaded differently so that parent of origin for individual chromosomes can be followed easily. All of the meioses are shown in ova, but the process is similar in spermatogenesis. (**A**) Normal female meiotic gametogenesis. After duplication, the homologues separate during the first meiotic division so that each cell contains two identical chromosomes (sister chromatids). During the second meiotic division the sister chromatids separate so that each gamete contains one copy of each chromosome. (**B**) In meiosis I, errors the homologues fail to separate, but the sister chromatids do separate normally during the second meiotic division. Thus there are two potential types of gametes, those that contain one copy of each of the parental chromosomes, and those that contain no copy of the chromosome. The first produces a trisomic fertilization (**C**) that is not viable unless a second error occurs. Mitotic anaphase lag rescues the pregnancy by loss of one of the chromosomes. Depending on which chromosome is lost the result may be either normal biparental inheritance (left side) or uniparental heterodisomy (right side). (**D**) Meiosis II errors occur after the normal separation of the homologues, but with failure of separation of the sister chromatids during the second meiotic division. In this case, there are three potential chromosomal complements for the gametes, isodisomy, nullisomy, and normal. Fertilization of the disomic gamete (**E**) leads to a trisomy that can be rescued by loss of one chromosome. This results either in normal biparental inheritance (left side) or in uniparental isodisomy (right side). Note that in meiosis II errors two of the gametes are normal, whereas in meiosis I defects all of the gametes are abnormal. (**F**) Fertilization of the nullisomic gamete resulting from either type of meiotic error leads to monosomy, which can then be rescued by a mitotic nondisjunction event leading to duplication of the single chromosome. This always results in uniparental isodisomy.

one of their chromosomes. For example, if a woman acquires a new imprinting mutation she will be normal. If that mutation arose on the chromosome 15 that she inherited from her mother, there will be no problem in her offspring because the imprinting pattern does not need to switch. Likewise, each of her daughters who inherit this mutated chromosome will also be fine, as will all of their offspring. However, the son of a mother with a maternally inherited imprinting mutation will be unable to switch the imprint when he passes on that chromosome 15, so that half of his offspring will inherit a maternally imprinted chromosome 15 from their father and will have PWS. This fact makes it important that every child with PWS have the cause thoroughly investigated to rule out this 50% recurrence risk for offspring of the father who carries an imprinting mutation. When analyzing the pedigree of this family it will appear that the trait may skip generations, leading to what has been called a "grandmatrilineal" inheritance pattern for PWS. Similarly, if the original imprinting mutation arises in a male, the eventual result will be females with a 50% risk of having children with AS.

Both PWS and AS have been caused by apparently balanced translocations that either disrupt specific genes, or, more likely,

interfere with imprinting in the region. AS can also be caused by mutations in a single gene in the region, UBE3A, possibly accounting for 10% of cases. This gene is unusual in that it appears to be expressed from both alleles in most tissues, but only from the maternal allele in certain regions of the brain. This tissue-specific imprinting pattern is not typical of the genes in the region and the mechanism is poorly understood. It does not appear to be resulting from hypermethylation of CpG islands at the 5′ end of the gene, the most common silencing mechanism for imprinted genes, but may be a result of expression of an antisense transcript of UBE3A. This antisense transcript is in the area of the imprinting region, upstream of UBE3A. It is speculated that on the paternal chromosome the imprinting center allows transcription of the paternally active genes as well as allowing transcription of the paternal copies of the UBE3A antisense region. This antisense transcript, through unknown mechanisms, may interfere with expression of the UBE3A from the same chromosome. The result is that when the imprinting center is "off," the paternally expressed genes are transcribed, as is an antisense transcript that stops expression of UBE3A from that chromosome. Alternatively, when the imprinting center is "on," the maternally expressed genes are silenced, and the UBE3A antisense transcript is not expressed, thus allowing normal expression of UBE3A from that chromosome.

No mutation in a single gene has been shown to cause PWS, and the abnormal methylation pattern is almost always seen in individuals with typical PWS. This supports the idea that PWS is a true contiguous gene syndrome, meaning that the full phenotype is the result of a combination of effects from several genes that are not properly expressed. There is also support for this idea from the various mouse models of PWS as well, none of which fully recapitulate the complete PWS phenotype.

The recurrent nature of the common deletion in PWS and AS is a result of the genomic structure around the region, which is flanked by highly homologous stretches of DNA that predispose to aberrant recombination and deletion or duplication. Such areas can be found throughout the genome, and are thought to explain several recurrent deletion syndromes. It is important to note that one or more of the genes included in the deleted region must be dosage sensitive, so that the loss of a single copy can lead to disease. Developmental abnormalities resulting from this phenomenon of genomic architecture leading directly to a mechanism of disease that does not involve a traditional type of mutation, or traditional inheritance, have been called "genomic disorders." There are other examples of genomic disorders. Smith–Magenis syndrome, a recognizable mental retardation syndrome, is caused by a recurrent microdeletion on chromosome 17p11.2. Charcot-Marie-Tooth disease type 1A results from a recurrent duplication nearby on 17p11.2, involving the peripheral myelin protein 22 gene, which, when deleted instead of duplicated, causes a different disorder, a hereditary neuropathy with liability to pressure palsy. These genomic rearrangements, once they occur, segregate following Mendelian principles, as can be seen with Charcot-Marie-Tooth, long known to be inherited in an autosomal-dominant fashion. There is some evidence that this particular aspect of genomic architecture, whereas in some instances predisposing to genomic disorders, is actually part of the process of primate evolution, as some of these regions appear to be associated with new genes developing as part of gene families resulting from genomic duplication.

MITOCHONDRIAL INHERITANCE

The idea of nontraditional inheritance developed in response to contradictions between Mendel's laws and observed biological facts and was initially used to describe imprinting defects. The concept, though, can be further extended to include a variety of other interesting phenomena that lead to situations in which inheritance is not easily explained by Mendel's laws. A well-recognized example of this is the condition of mitochondrial inheritance, which appears in a matrilineal pattern. This means that the disorder can be seen in males or females, but can only be transmitted from an affected female to her children. Affected males do not transmit the disorder (although this, like most biological "rules" has not been shown to be 100% true). The cause of this inheritance pattern is now well understood, because the mitochondria contain their own small genome. Mitochondrial DNA (mtDNA) is a small, circular DNA containing only 16,569 bp, encoding 13 proteins, each of which is a part of one of the subunits of the mitochondrial electron transport chain. The mitochondrial genome also encodes a unique set of transfer RNAs (tRNAs), as well as two ribosomal RNAs. Mutations throughout the intronless genes on the mtDNA can cause disease, all of which are manifest by disturbances in energy metabolism, as would be expected by the roles of the known proteins.

During the process of gametogenesis the ovum accumulates a large number of mitochondria, each of which contains multiple copies of the mitochondrial genome. The nucleotide sequence of these mitochondrial genomes is not identical, so that in any particular ovum there may be a variety of mutations, none of which are present in every copy of the mtDNA. The sperm compartmentalizes its mitochondria to the motor unit of the tail, so that none of the mitochondria are delivered into the fertilized egg. Therefore, the mother, explaining the matrilineal inheritance pattern, supplies all of the mitochondria in the fertilized egg.

Another hallmark of mtDNA diseases is that there can be tremendous clinical variation. Different mutations may predispose to different phenotypes, but even with the same mutation the phenotype may vary. One of the reasons for this becomes clear from the fact that multiple different copies of the mtDNA exist in each egg. After fertilization, mitochondria, and their mtDNA component, replicate and segregate during cell division. In this way, different developing tissues may acquire different complements of mtDNA mutations, and, depending on the effect of the mutation and the energy requirements of the tissue in question, there may be selection for one mtDNA genome over another, leading to accumulation or loss of a particular mutation in a particular tissue type. This variation of mitochondrial complement in different tissues is referred to as heteroplasmy.

MELAS, or mitochondrial encephalomyopathy, lactic acidosis, and stroke-like episodes, is a recurrent mtDNA phenotype most often resulting from a point mutation in the mitochondrial leucine tRNA (nucleotide 3243). There is often an accumulation of mutant mtDNA in successive generations, leading to increased severity with earlier onset in the younger generations. Affected individuals may present with poor growth, lactic acidosis, seizures and ataxia, severe headaches, recurrent strokes or stroke-like episodes, cortical blindness, or muscle weakness. The symptoms tend to progress, with death resulting from respiratory complications, infections, or bowel obstruction. Affected individuals may be identified across many generations and branches of the family, always inherited through females.

Kearn-Sayre syndrome is a progressive disorder consisting of peripheral weakness, pigmentary retinopathy, progressive external ophthalmoplegia (because of weakness of the extraocular muscles), heart block or cardiomyopathy, and, occasionally, diabetes mellitus. Most cases of Kearn-Sayre are associated with large deletions of the mitochondrial genome, but some cases have been reported with point mutations in the same leucine tRNA associated with MELAS. The fact that two distinct phenotypes may result from defects in the same tRNA may be a result of tissue heteroplasmy, but it also points to the difficulty in predicting phenotype from genotype in mitochondrial diseases.

Many other phenotypes have been described with mtDNA mutations, some more predictable than others, but it is important for the clinician to remember that defects of the oxidative phosphorylation process may produce almost any symptom in almost any tissue at almost any time of life. Also, although this section discusses defects resulting from mtDNA changes, many more nuclear-encoded genes are involved in the production of electron transport protein subunits and the formation and maintenance of the mitochondrial membranes, transporters and oxidative phosphorylation complexes, defects of which are most often inherited as traditional autosomal-recessive traits.

MULTI-ALLELIC INHERITANCE

In the later 19th and early 20th century, as Mendel's ideas about the independent segregation of traits were being re-evaluated, it was understood that some traits were clearly not the result of single genes. Sir Francis Galton established that height was a trait that could not be explained by Mendelian arguments, and Ronald A. Fisher, a statistician, later showed how multiple genes, each contributing more or less to the final outcome, could explain Galton's findings on height and other quantitative traits. The concept of polygenic inheritance followed, and along with that the idea that genetic factors may interact with environmental factors to produce a trait in a multifactorial way. Multifactorial inheritance, then, can be invoked to mathematically model empirically observed incidences of a variety of traits, and the concept is now fully accepted in genetic thinking and counseling. This multifactorial model requires several assumptions, including that the genes involved all contribute something to the phenotype, without being dominant or recessive, and that they act together in an additive fashion. The number of genes and environmental factors involved in a multifactorial trait is not infinite, and may vary from just a few to a great many (as has been suggested for the development of hypertension).

Findings now point to a form of nontraditional inheritance that is neither fully Mendelian nor fully multifactorial. Three specific examples are digenic inheritance, synergistic heterozygosity, and triallelic inheritance. None of these are completely unique and independent concepts, but all serve to illustrate the complexity of genetic and biological interactions. Retinitis pigmentosa (RP) is a genetically heterogeneous condition of progressive vision loss because of degeneration of the retina associated with increased retinal pigment deposition. It can be isolated or associated with a variety of genetic syndromes, and at least 26 loci have been described in the genome that cause isolated RP, some as X-linked, others as autosomal-dominant and -recessive traits. All of them, though, result from mutations in a single gene. A unique inheritance pattern was identified when a form of RP was found in several different families because of the combination of heterozygosity for mutations in two different genes, ROM1 and RDS. Homozygosity for mutations in the RDS gene can also cause RP, but heterozygosity for a mutation in either, by itself, does not. This finding, that heterozygosity at two different unlinked loci is a requirement for the development of the phenotype, represents a newly recognized form of inheritance that is neither Mendelian nor multifactorial, but is instead digenic. Specifically, it cannot be said to be multifactorial or polygenic inheritance because it is not an additive effect of the two genes, but a synergistic effect. Similar findings have now been shown for several conditions, including one form of hereditary deafness, some cases of Hirschsprung disease, and severe insulin resistance. It is interesting to note, though, that pedigree analysis of affected families might be suggestive of autosomal-recessive inheritance, because the recurrence risk for the parents of an affected child would be 25% with each pregnancy.

In some cases digenic inheritance could result from mutations in two genes that interact in a developmental pathway, or that both contribute to the same developmental pathway although they may not physically interact with each other. An analogous situation has been described in several individuals presenting with metabolic myopathies. Investigation into the usual causes of disruption in fatty acid oxidation or electron transport pathways led to the observation that in some cases, heterozygosity for mutations in two different genes involved in cellular energy metabolism may cause myopathy. Specific genes involved include those for carnitine palmitoyl transferase II, very long chain acyl-CoA dehydrogenase gene, and some of the nuclear-encoded subunits of the electron transport chain. Each, by itself, will be considered a recessive allele, not expected to cause disease if the other partner of the gene pair were normal. It appears that in the heterozygous state the reduction in flux through a particular pathway may be tolerated, but if there is a mild (heterozygous) defect in a different part of the same pathway, the sum of the reductions in flux through the pathway may lead to insufficiency of energy production during periods of metabolic stress. This condition has been referred to as synergistic heterozygosity, but the parallel to digenic inheritance is obvious.

Although both of these forms of inheritance would lead to Mendelian (recessive) proportions of affected individuals on pedigree analysis, triallelic inheritance would not. This fascinating example of nontraditional inheritance has been described in an isolated population with a high rate of an unusual disorder called Bardet-Biedl syndrome (BBS). Individuals with BBS present with pigmentary retinal dystrophy, polydactyly, obesity, reduced cognitive function, and renal abnormalities. There is genetic heterogeneity for the disorder, with eight loci having been identified. In studying several families it was found that some affected individuals were homozygous for mutations in a previously identified BBS gene, whereas there were unaffected family members that were also homozygous for the same mutations. Further investigation revealed that the difference between the affected and the unaffected individuals was that those affected also had heterozygous mutations of another gene known to be associated with BBS. Therefore, in this population, homozygosity for mutation in the first locus was not sufficient to cause the phenotype, but required a third abnormal allele in a different gene, thus triallelic inheritance. There are different ways to interpret these findings, and debate continues whether these may really represent modifier effects; nonetheless, the complexity of inheritance is much greater than was previously imagined.

Similar arguments could be made for some complex traits. A good example is in the risk of blood clotting resulting from inherited thrombophilia. This is one area in which genetic dissection of a complex, multifactorial trait has led to the recognition of a variety of more or less common genetic factors predisposing to thrombosis. The identification of certain of these factors, including the Leiden mutation in the gene for clotting factor V and the prothrombin 20210G > A mutation, along with certain environmental factors, such as cigaret use and oral contraceptive use, allows, at least partially, for the determination of broad categories of risk of abnormal thrombosis and of the relative contribution of individual factors to that risk.

New technologies for exploring the human genome, the Human Genome Project, and the dedicated work of thousands of researchers are beginning to unravel the complexities of human inheritance in ways that could not have been imagined by Mendel, Galton, or other pioneers of genetics. This chapter has reviewed some of the complexities of non-Mendelian, nontraditional inheritance and discussed new ways of understanding old paradoxes. It is likely that more complexities will be discovered, giving new insight into genetic disorders both rare and common, and informing new therapeutic approaches. At the least, it seems likely that these new genetic findings will lead to more personalized medical information and risk assessments. The immediate impact, unfortunately, is to make the job of the physician much more complicated. Patient demands for genetic information will make it impossible to ignore these advances, so physicians need to find tools and resources to keep up to date, and to find approaches to share this information with patients in ways that will be beneficial without raising inappropriate expectations or fears.

SELECTED REFERENCES

DiMauro S, Andreu AL, Musumeci O, Bonilla E. Diseases of oxidative phosphorylation due to mtDNA mutations. Semin Neurol 2001;21: 251–260.

GeneTests: Medical Genetics Information Resource. University of Washington and Children's Health System (Seattle, OR). http://www.genetests.org 1993–2004 (updated weekly). Accessed May 21, 2004.

Goldstone AP. Prader-Willi syndrome: advances in genetics, pathophysiology and treatment. Trends Endocrinol Metab 2004;15:12–20.

Katsanis N, Ansley SJ, Badano JL, et al. Triallelic inheritance in Bardet-Biedl syndrome, a Mendelian recessive disorder. Science 2001;293: 2256–2259.

Lupski JR. Genomic disorders: structural features of the genome can lead to DNA rearrangements and human disease traits. Trends Genet 1998;14:417–422.

McCandless SE, Cassidy SB. 15q11-13 and the Prader-Willi syndrome. In: Epstein CJ, Erickson RP, Wynshaw-Boris A, eds. Inborn Errors of Development. New York: Oxford University Press, 2004; pp. 765, 766.

Ming JE, Muenke M. Multiple hits during early embryonic development: Digenic diseases and holoprosencephaly. Am J Hum Genet 2002;71: 1017–1032.

Morison IM, Reeve AE. A catalogue of imprinted genes and parent-of-origin effects in humans and animals. Hum Mol Genet 1998;7: 1599–1609.

Nicholls RD, Knepper JL. Genome organization, function, and imprinting in Prader-Willi and Angelman syndromes. Annu Rev Genomics Hum Genet 2001;2:153–175.

Online Mendelian Inheritance in Man, OMIM. McKusick-Nathans Institute for Genetic Medicine, Johns Hopkins University (Baltimore, MD) and National Center for Biotechnology Information, National Library of Medicine (Bethesda, MD). http://www.ncbi.nlm.nih.gov/omim/2000. Accessed September 23, 2004.

Preece MA, Moore GE. Genomic imprinting, uniparental disomy and foetal growth. Trends Endocrinol Metab 2000;11:270–275.

Vockley J, Rinaldo P, Bennett MJ, Matern D, Vladutiu GD. Synergistic heterozygosity: disease resulting from multiple partial defects in one or more metabolic pathways. Mol Genet Metab 2000;71:10–18.

3 Identifying Causal Genetic Factors

CHRISTOPHER I. AMOS, JOHN S. WITTE, AND WILLIAM G. NEWMAN

SUMMARY

The study of a complex disease requires careful characterization of the clinical phenotypes for study. Linkage studies, which can detect relative risks of four or greater, apply stringent diagnostic criteria and restrictive rules for family selection to assure a maximally informative collection of subjects. Clinical characterizations that are adopted for association studies must be precise and should be widely accepted to facilitate large studies. The presence of linkage disequilibrium among tightly linked loci provides a basis for genome-wide association studies. A subset of "tagging" markers that maximally characterize interindividual variability can be sought to minimize genotyping costs. Association studies can detect lower relative risks than linkage methods provided there are a limited number of causal variants at each locus and linkage disequilibrium is present (or one directly studies the causal variant). For some complex diseases there may be multiple disease variants and only moderate risks from any single locus. For these complex diseases alternative strategies using comparative genomics and animal models may be required. Admixture linkage mapping may also permit the study of larger collections of patients than is feasible using traditional linkage methods. Finally, once causal loci are identified, further genotype–phenotype studies will allow the disease to be further delineated. Such studies may also identify subsets of patients with varying responsiveness to treatments.

Key Words: Association; comparative genomics; disequilibrium; genetic linkage; genotype–phenotype correlations; linkage haplotypes.

INTRODUCTION

Identifying genetic factors that increase an individual's risk of disease is a major goal of genetic epidemiology. In this chapter, we provide an overview of the primary approaches that use information from families and individuals to discover disease-causing genes. For illustrative purposes, the chapter integrates examples from studies that are successfully deciphering the complex etiology of inflammatory bowel disease (IBD), identifying genetic factors, and providing potential new targets for therapy. The chapter concludes with a summary of clinical observations relevant to the findings from these studies of IBD. We have decided to use the success in understanding the complex etiology of IBD as an example

for which genetic studies have been particularly successful, both in identifying genetic factors as well as in providing potential new targets for therapy. We integrate examples from the study of IBD throughout the chapter and then provide a few clinical observations relevant to the findings from these studies as a summary to the chapter.

A common disease has been defined as affecting 1 or more individuals per 1000 population. A number of factors may suggest that a common disease (or related clinical traits) is inherited. Clustering of affected individuals within families often provides the initial evidence of an inherited susceptibility to disease. Such findings can be supported by studies of twins; greater disease concordance between monozygotic (identical) compared with dizygotic (nonidentical) twins suggests a genetic susceptibility as it presumes similar environmental exposures among twins. Further evidence of genetic predisposition to common disease may be indicated by studies of migrant populations who retain the level of risk for a particular disease from their area of origin rather than that of the indigenous population. Higher prevalence levels of the disease in specific ethnic populations may be accounted for by a genetic variant in an ancestor (founder effect). Occasionally, common diseases can occur as manifestations of rare single gene disorders. However, further analysis often identifies minor differences between these rare, segregating forms of common disease, and the more prevalent form. For example, segregation of mutations in BRCA1 predispose to breast cancer, but the onset is usually early and there are often distinct pathological changes that can identify cancers arising in individuals with BRCA1 mutations from those with sporadic breast cancers.

IBD is an excellent paradigm for a common disease with a significant heritable component. IBD encompasses two major inflammatory diseases of the bowel, Crohn's disease (CD, MIM 266600) and ulcerative colitis (UC, MIM 191390). The heritable nature of IBD was first described over 40 yr ago by Kirsner who noted that individuals with CD and UC were more likely to have relatives affected by these diseases compared to unaffected individuals. Such familial clustering in itself does not provide conclusive evidence for the genetic basis of a disease. However, studies of disease concordance in twins revealed that both CD and UC are present more commonly in both members of monozygotic compared with dizygotic twins. Additional evidence emerged from Asian migrants to the United Kingdom who maintained a lower level of CD risk than the indigenous population. Finally, a higher prevalence of IBD has been reported in the Ashkenazi Jewish population and IBD is a

From: *Principles of Molecular Medicine, Second Edition*
Edited by: M. S. Runge and C. Patterson © Humana Press, Inc., Totowa, NJ

Identifying Genetic Factors

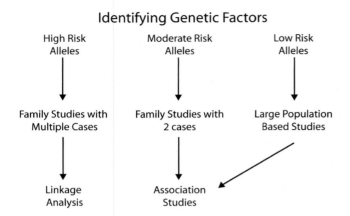

Figure 3-1 Designs for the identification of causal genetic factors influencing risk for diseases.

Table 3-1
Chromosomal Loci Containing Potential or Confirmed Susceptibility Genes for CD, UC, or Both (IBD), as Identified by Genome-Wide Scans or Subsequent Association Studies

	Chromosome locus	Gene identified	Association with CD, UC, or IBD
IBD1	16q13	CARD15	CD
IBD2	12q14	–	UC
IBD3	6p	–	CD
IBD4	14q11–q12	–	CD
IBD5	5q31–33	OCTN cluster variants	CD
IBD6	19p13	–	IBD
IBD7	1p36	–	IBD
IBD8	16p12	–	CD
IBD9	3p26	–	IBD
	3p21	–	IBD
	10q23	DLG5	IBD
	Xq21.3	–	IBD

characteristic feature of rare single gene disorders including Wiskott-Aldrich and Hermansky-Pudlak syndromes.

DEFINING THE PHENOTYPE

CLINICAL CLASSIFICATION In order to identify genetic loci predisposing for disease, studies often adopt stringent criteria for designating an individual as affected. These strict criteria are used in family studies because affected individuals provide the most information about their underlying genotype, especially when studying infrequent diseases for which the penetrance, or probability to be affected given that one has inherited a risk-increasing genotype, is decreased. Often in family studies we are interested in tracking the inheritance of disease susceptibility, and the underlying genotypes can be most effectively deduced from the affected individuals. We use strict criteria in the initial family studies to avoid misclassification of genotypes. Once genetic loci influencing disease susceptibility are identified, then interest turns to evaluating the impact that disease-increasing genotypes have on the broader spectrum of disease. Figure 3-1 displays designs for identifying genetic factors influencing risk for complex diseases. As shown, for diseases in which the risk conferred by a single factor is high (i.e., exceeding a fourfold increased risk), linkage studies are highly effective for disease localization. However, if the risk associated with a mutation is lower, then alternate strategies employing association-based approaches are more likely to be successful.

Precise diagnostic classification of phenotypes is vital to maximize one's ability to identify causal genetic variants. IBD illustrates the importance of collecting complete clinical data. Individuals with CD are 30 times more likely to have a sibling affected with CD and 16 times more likely to have a sibling with UC than a healthy individual. Patients with UC have similarly raised familial risks. This suggests that there are genes that increase the risk of CD and UC specifically and IBD generally. Genetic studies to date in IBD have supported this suggestion (Table 3-1). To dissect these different genes precise classification of CD and UC is imperative. Individuals with IBD can generally be defined as having CD or UC based on endoscopic, histological, and/or radiological criteria. However, in about 10% of patients a differentiation is not apparent and the term indeterminate colitis is applied. International diagnostic guidelines such as the Vienna Classification for the diagnosis of CD can aid consistency among studies.

Phenotypic expression of common diseases as well as susceptibility may also be inherited. These clinical characteristics may be influenced by disease susceptibility genes or by disease modifier genes, which do not alter risk of the disease itself just the expression. In IBD, epidemiological studies have demonstrated that a number of clinical characteristics may be inherited, including early age of disease onset, disease involving a specific part of the bowel, and more severe disease. Therefore, clinical and demographic data including ethnicity, gender, age of disease onset, and disease severity should all be collected. Ethnicity data are particularly important to ensure that the frequency of a particular genotype in affected individuals is matched to that in an appropriate control population. This is evidenced by variants in the CARD15 gene that have been associated with CD in North American and European but not Japanese populations. In addition, some of the extraintestinal manifestations of IBD including psoriasis and ankylosing spondylitis have a significant heritable component. Genotype–phenotype correlations for mutations in CARD15 have shown associations with the site of bowel disease and earlier age at disease onset among CD patients and with psoriatic arthropathy.

QUANTITATIVE PHENOTYPES An alternative to employing stringent criteria for identifying those families most likely to be segregating a simple cause for a genetic disease is to seek phenotypes that are correlated with the disease of interest but which show a more clear genetic component. For example, in the study of cardiovascular disease, identifying genetic causes of myocardial infarction is difficult, although identifying genetic factors influencing low- and high-density lipoprotein cholesterol levels has been more straightforward. Myocardial infarction as an end point is hard to study because it is caused by many different factors. Aberrant cholesterol levels can be strong risk factors for myocardial infarction, and the genetic causes influencing cholesterol levels are simpler to identify than the many factors influencing myocardial infarction as an endpoint. In addition, because cholesterol levels are measured and variable among subjects, each individual provides more statistical information than is provided by the dichotomous information provided by presence or absence of myocardial infarction. The simpler genetic causation influencing cholesterol levels is indicated by the higher heritability (i.e., increased similarity among closely related individuals) of these traits compared with myocardial infarction as an end point. However, heritability alone does not necessarily indicate that a trait has a genetically simple architecture because even traits that are highly heritable can be influenced by multiple genetic factors. In addition to having high heritability, traits that are known from biological studies to have biochemically or physiologically simple causes would be good candidates for genetic studies.

Although quantitative traits can provide more information than dichotomous traits, there are often sampling advantages in studying discrete traits. Individuals who have a disease may become "affected" because they are extreme for an underlying quantitative trait. Identifying individuals with a disease may provide a mechanism for identifying individuals who are extreme for an underlying quantitative phenotype. Families that include some individuals with extreme values may provide the most information in a linkage study because there are underlying genetic variants increasing the trait levels of these subjects.

GENETIC LINKAGE ANALYSIS Genetic linkage analysis has been an extremely powerful tool for identifying specific genetic factors for diseases. Linkage analysis has typically been applied for identifying novel genetic factors, by using a genome-wide analysis of the coinheritance of disease with genetic markers. Evidence in favor of linkage is typically expressed by the LOD score which is the $\log_{10}$ ratio of the likelihood of the data assuming linkage between a modeled disease susceptibility locus and a genetic marker to the likelihood of the data assuming no linkage of the disease susceptibility and genetic marker. To allow for the large number of tests that are indicated in a genome-wide analysis, several testing paradigms have been developed. If a Bayesian approach is adopted then a LOD score of about 3 leads to a 5% posterior probability of linkage assuming the existence of a single disease locus, even when many markers are genotyped over the entire genome. Morton developed an approach for sequentially combining data from multiple studies by adding LOD scores across studies that has been highly effective. From Bayesian and sequential analytical approaches, a LOD score of 3.0 was proposed as providing a meaningful critical value for declaring strong evidence for linkage. More recently, approaches to control the overall significance of genetic studies when studying multiple markers have been adopted. These criteria have been criticized for being excessively conservative particularly when candidate regions are of primary interest, for example, when prior studies indicated evidence for linkage to an area. The significance testing paradigm requires the slightly higher LOD score of 3.3 to declare that a significant result has been obtained while providing a genome-wide significance of 5%.

If a simple genetic mechanism explains inheritance of disease, then a genetic model can be specified and tested for coinheritance of disease susceptibility with genetic markers. In order for linkage studies to be informative, the families chosen for study must be able to show inheritance of a genetic factor. For uncommon diseases for which the penetrance is reduced, the affected individuals provide the majority of information about the segregation or inheritance of genetic mutations predisposing to disease. For quantitative traits, sampling through individuals with extreme phenotypes can increase the probability of sampling a genetic variant influencing the trait of interest. Sampling through extreme individuals is an effective strategy for increasing the power of a linkage study, but may only be practical if the quantitative phenotype can be assayed inexpensively. Some studies of quantitative phenotypes study many phenotypes. Sampling through extreme individuals only increases power for a single or a few correlated phenotypes.

Currently available microsatellite-based mapping platforms usually study the genome at approx 10-cM intervals, and investigators usually follow-up positive signals with denser maps. Evidence for genetic linkage in a region would often be followed by finer scale mapping to (1) improve the information for detecting linkage and to identify any recombinant individuals, and (2) using much finer maps, to search for associations between the disease or trait and particular marker alleles. Standard finer mapping panels for microsatellites provide a 5-cM interval spacing, and microsatellite sequences and technologies for approx 0.2-cM interval mapping are routinely available from DeCode genetics (www.decodegenetics.com) or by custom request for even finer mapping (e.g., by request to Invitrogen genetics). Routine genotyping platforms for the purposes of genetic linkage analysis are available from Affymetrix and Illumina and provide results from genotyping of about 11,000 and 6000 genome-wide single-nucleotide polymorphisms (SNPs), respectively. These much finer mapping panels can improve the power to detect linkages and may provide narrower intervals for positional cloning.

A wide range of genetic linkage methods is available. The diversity of methods reflects, in part, the considerable success that linkage methods have had in identifying genetic causes of disease, and the consequent value and interest in using the methods by the scientific community. Computing statistics over a large number of genetic markers in families for diseases that do not show simple inheritance patterns is computationally demanding and there are three basic approaches that are taken for the analysis of the genetic marker data. The Elston–Stewart algorithm resummarizes information about haplotypes (the set of alleles on a chromosome) sequentially in a pedigree and is, therefore, efficient for statistical analysis of large families, but limited in the number of markers that can be jointly modeled; usually fewer than five markers can be considered jointly. The Lander-Green-Kruglyak (LGK) method adopts a different approach that facilitates the analysis of multiple markers. The LGK model first identifies the possible inheritance patterns of genotypes within families and stores this information as inheritance vectors. Because the number of inheritance vectors increases rapidly according to the number of individuals in a family, this approach is only suitable for small- or medium-sized families, usually allowing at most 25 individuals in a family to be studied. In addition, because the method stores all possible inheritance vectors in memory, the approach requires considerable RAM to be efficient. The major advantage of the LGK approach is that computational speed increases only linearly in the number of markers so that it is highly efficient for genome-wide analyses.

Analyses including many markers on large pedigrees or analyses of pedigrees that include more than a few inbred individuals may not be effectively performed using the Elston–Stewart of LGK algorithms. In this case, Monte-Carlo Markov Chain (MCMC) algorithms are used to approximate the likelihood of the data. MCMC methods provide tools for sampling the haplotype configurations in data. The MCMC procedure samples possible haplotypes according to the underlying probability distribution that generated the data and provides an accurate approximation to the likelihood. A major advantage of MCMC procedures is a decreased need for memory, because they do not require summing over all possible genotypes as in the Elston–Stewart algorithm, or over all possible inheritance vectors as in the LGK. One disadvantage may include the complexity in storing output from analysis, because results from large numbers of realizations from the sampling of genotype configurations are often stored. MCMC methods infer the genotypes for all individuals that are specified as a part of the analytical file. Individuals with known genotypes have a limited number of potential haplotypes, but individuals who have not been genotyped can have a large number of potential genotypes and haplotypes. The probability distribution from which MCMC methods must sample can become quite large if many individuals who have not been genotyped are included in the analytical file. Therefore, it is often beneficial to remove the ungenotyped individuals from MCMC analyses, particularly those who are not affected, because they contribute little in most linkage analyses.

An issue in performing genetic analysis is whether to use model-dependent or model-free methods for linkage analysis. Model-dependent methods have higher power for linkage analysis if an approximately valid genetic model can be specified to describe the manner in which disease susceptibility at a given locus is expressed. One approach for estimating penetrance to be used in a linkage study is to first perform a segregation analysis of families that have been ascertained according to a specified sampling scheme. The approach estimates parameters for models describing the inheritance of genetic and environmental factors that most closely fit the dependence in family data. For uncommon conditions, random sampling of families would not result in an informative family, and a sampling scheme is usually followed in which relatives of cases with a disease are preferentially sampled. When the families are not randomly sampled, an ascertainment correction for nonrandom sampling is required in order to obtain parameter estimates that reflect the more general population of families. In order to correct for the nonrandom sampling approach that is typically used, a clearly defined sampling scheme must typically be followed. Using only a binary phenotype (e.g., affection or nonaffection) one may not be able to estimate all the parameters that are necessary to describe the penetrance of the genotypes of the loci influencing disease susceptibility, unless restrictive assumptions about the interactions among the loci are made.

Sampling families and collecting information for segregation analysis can be an arduous task and may not be fully informative about the parameters that describe the penetrance and disease allele frequencies. Therefore, investigators studying complex diseases may postulate genetic models from assumptions about the relative risks for disease that are observed from epidemiological studies. It has been shown that postulating an inaccurate genetic model for genetic linkage studies does not lead to false-positive results, in a model-based linkage study. However, if multiple models are tested, then there can be an inflation in the overall number of false-positive results from linkage studies because of the inherent multiple testing problem that is so introduced. A powerful approach for studying complex diseases is to evaluate the evidence for linkage assuming simple recessive and dominant models of disease and then to adjust the required critical value for the LOD score upward by about 0.3 for the small multiple testing problem so engendered.

If the genetic model influencing disease susceptibility cannot be inferred with any confidence, either because the genetic model appears too complex or because there is a lack of epidemiological data from which to postulate penetrance, then model-free methods are typically adopted. One approach is to set the penetrance to an artificially low level, thus restricting analysis to include only the affected subjects: with very low penetrance, unaffected individuals provide no information about their possible genotypes and so

do not contribute in the linkage analysis, but this approach still makes some modeling assumptions about disease expression. An alternative approach is to evaluate the similarity in alleles that have been inherited by common parentage (identity by descent) and test whether or not there is evidence that affected relatives share more alleles than expected identical by descent. In some cases this approach may provide a more powerful test for linkage than a model-dependent approach, particularly when multiple independent loci additively increase disease risk. Because pedigrees are usually variable in size and contain different numbers of affected relatives, a variety of different tests have been proposed and are available for testing for linkage. These tests are optimal for varying disease penetrances (which are typically unknown). As a compromise, the pairs statistic, which includes all affected relatives in a pedigree and gives only moderately higher weight to families that include multiple affected relatives is often used.

The joint analysis of covariates along with genetic markers in family studies usually has limited utility. Typically collecting covariate information in families is difficult because data cannot be directly collected from deceased or otherwise unavailable individuals. In addition, the genetic risks that are sought in linkage analyses are often large. Some nongenetic factors such as smoking and reproductive behaviors can be reliably collected through proxies (when needed) are inexpensive to collect and may have a strong effect on risk for some diseases.

One of the first major investigations to identify genes/chromosomal loci for a common disease was performed by John Todd's group at Oxford University in 1994 in families with type 1 diabetes mellitus. Siblings have a 50% chance of inheriting the same allele from a parent. A wide range of statistical methods have been developed to identify regions showing excess sharing of inherited alleles in relatives. This theory has provided the basis for numerous further investigations in a range of common diseases where panels of evenly spaced microsatellite markers are used in genome-wide linkage studies. In IBD there has been consistency between linkage study results with replication of six loci (Table 3-1).

For complex diseases, a large number of families may be needed to obtain adequate power to detect linkages. Meta-analysis combining multiple studies can assist in overcoming power limitations from a single study. However, in order for meaningful results to be obtained in meta-analysis, investigators must be studying comparable classifications of the same disease. Coordination of studies becomes necessary for the study of complex diseases.

Genetic linkage analyses of IBD have identified numerous genomic regions harboring susceptibility factors. Because of the apparent genetic complexity of these diseases, simple Mendelian models have typically not been applied. Instead, model-free methods using primarily nuclear families have been the preferred method for identifying genetic factors. Genetic linkage analysis followed by positional cloning has been effective in identifying CARD15 and OCTN1/OCTN2 causal mutations for CD. The identification of CARD15 mutations as causal resulted when genetic linkage analysis indicated the chromosome 16q region as likely to contain a genetic susceptibility factor. The CARD15 locus had previously been identified by homology to a similar locus in mice and it was an excellent candidate locus for IBD because mice homozygous for CARD15 deletions showed an IBD-like phenotype. In contrast, genetic linkage analysis identified a region of chromosome 5 encompassing the cytokine cluster on 5q. Haplotype studies, discussed below showed that a single extended haplotype was often present in CD patients. However, causal variants in OCTN1 and OCTN2 were only found after extensive sequencing of all the genes in an extended region.

ASSOCIATION STUDIES   Although parametric and nonparametric linkage analysis approaches have proved successful for mapping many disease and trait genes, in some gene mapping investigations, the limited number of meioses occurring within pedigrees limit one's ability to detect by linkage the recombination events between closely spaced (~ <1 cM) loci. One might instead map more closely spaced disease genes by using association studies. These studies generally have a case–control design, where cases are recruited from a disease registry or hospital-based populations. Controls can range from the cases' family members (e.g., parents or siblings) or unrelated individuals. Genetic variants observed in cases are contrasted with those observed among controls to determine an "association" exists between genes and disease.

Association studies may allow one to get closer to the disease-causing gene than allowed by linkage studies (i.e., more recombinant events over evolutionary time). This type of study can also be used to look directly at genetic variants in known candidate genes. That is, association studies can be used either in an "indirect" manner as a tool for mapping genes using linkage disequilibrium or in a "direct" manner for evaluating associations with postulated causal ("candidate") genes.

The growing use of association studies is driven in part by how quickly and easily they can be undertaken, and the availability of high-density SNP genotyping technology. The SNP consortium (http://snp.cshl.org) has provided sequences for 1.8 million SNPs, and at least 250,000 of these have been verified as polymorphic by Perlegen (alone), whereas polymorphisms in hundreds of thousands of additional SNPs have also been verified by the SNP consortium, Applera, and by many investigators and companies.

LINKAGE DISEQUILIBRIUM AND HAPLOTYPES   The genetic variants that cause disease arise through, for example, novel mutations or immigration of mutation carriers into a population. When a mutation initially arises, it has a particular chromosomal location and specific neighboring marker alleles. At this incipient point in time, the mutation is completely associated with the adjacent alleles: it is only observed when the marker alleles are also present. Marker alleles that were in the neighborhood of the disease gene when its mutation was introduced into the population will generally remain associated over numerous generations (i.e., in linkage disequilibrium). If specific marker allele frequencies are higher among cases vs controls, this suggests linkage disequilibrium between the corresponding loci and a disease gene. The extent of this disequilibrium depends on the number of subsequent generations because the mutation was introduced into the population, the recombination between the disease and marker alleles, mutation rates, and selective values.

Alleles in linkage disequilibrium may be parts of haplotypes, and recent work indicates that there may exist discrete chromosomal regions with low haplotype diversity, termed "haplotype blocks," which are separated by recombination hotspots. Information from some polymorphisms within each block may be redundant; in other words, having information on one SNP provides all the information about another if they are in strong linkage disequilibrium. The majority of the haplotypes within a block can thus be distinguished using a much smaller number of SNPs, known as "haplotype tagging" SNPs or htSNPs (Fig. 3-2). Using such SNPs can drastically reduce the effort required to undertake large-scale association studies. Instead of saturating an entire chromosomal region with genotypes in all study samples, an

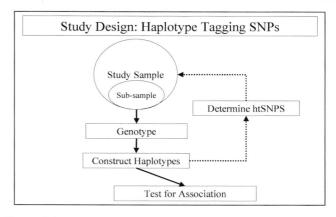

Figure 3-2 Two-phase study design based on haplotype tagging SNPs. First, one screens for SNPs within a subsample of study subjects to determine the htSNPs. Then these htSNPs, and possibly other promising SNPs, are genotyped in the entire study population.

investigator can first screen for SNPs within a subsample of study subjects to determine the htSNPs. Then only these tagging SNPs (and possibly other promising SNPs) can be genotyped in the entire study population. Several approaches have been suggested for identifying optimal htSNPs. These include simple visual inspection of haplotypes and analytic approaches.

FAMILY-BASED ASSOCIATION STUDIES   The most common familial case–control designs use parents or siblings as controls (Fig. 3-3). In the former, the parents themselves are not the controls, but the set of genotypes the parents could have transmitted to the case, given their own genotypes (the case's "pseudosibs"). For example, the Transmission/Disequilibrium Test (TDT) compares alleles transmitted from parents to diseased offspring with those alleles that are not transmitted (i.e., the "nondiseased alleles"). The TDT provides a joint test of linkage and association (i.e., linkage in the presence of association or vice versa). In doing so, when there is disequilibrium between marker and disease alleles, incorporating the additional information that the same alleles are associated across families with the TDT can provide increased power in comparison with linkage analysis. Furthermore, the use of pseudosib controls has better statistical efficiency than sibling or cousin controls (even more than population controls for a recessive gene), but the requirement that parents be available for genotyping limits its usefulness for late-onset diseases.

As with pseudosib controls, siblings are derived from the same gene pool as the cases, and, thus, provide another attractive source of controls for family-based studies. However, using siblings as controls can pose other difficulties. A major issue is that not every case will have an available sibling. If sibship size or other determinants of availability are associated with genotype, selection bias may result, possibly leading to false-negative or -positive results. Another issue is that controls should generally be selected from siblings who have already survived to the age at diagnosis of the case free of the disease. In practice, this will tend to limit control eligibility to older siblings, which can lead to confounding by factors related to year of birth, family size, or birth order. Siblings are also more likely to have the same genotype as the case than are unrelated controls, thereby leading to some loss of statistical efficiency (i.e., larger sample sizes required to attain the same statistical precision).

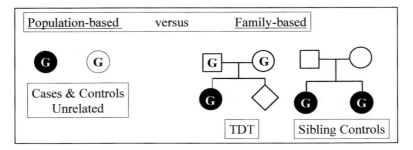

Figure 3-3   Population- and family-based association study designs.

POPULATION-BASED ASSOCIATION STUDIES   The use of unrelated controls is susceptible to a form of confounding known as "population stratification" if the gene under study shows marked variation in allele frequency across subgroups of the population and if these subgroups also differ in their baseline risk of the disease. A number of authors have proposed using genomic information to help address the problem of bias resulting from population stratification, and overdispersion owing to cryptic relatedness (Fig. 3-4). In particular, with a panel of polymorphic markers that are not linked to the candidate gene under study, one can attempt to address the issue population stratification by (1) using an overdispersion model to determine a test statistic's appropriate empirical distribution; (2) evaluating whether stratification exists; and (3) using a latent-class model to distinguish homogeneous subpopulations. Witte et al. (1999) further explore the theoretical, statistical, and practical considerations in choosing between family and unrelated population controls.

The ability to identify genetic loci through an association-based technique depends very heavily on the degree of association between the disease-causing variants and genetic markers. Many of the power calculations that have been presented suggest outstanding power to detect disease-causing loci through an association-based approach. However, the earlier, optimistic power studies make highly optimistic assumptions that one is studying the causal SNP, that there is a single disease-causing variant, and/or that the population being studied is homogeneous with respect to the association between the marker(s) being studied. Less optimistic power calculations that do not assume complete disequilibrium of the study of a causal variant lead to far more pessimistic conclusions about the power of an association study to detect genetic variants. Similarly, the presence of multiple alleles influencing trait variability or disease susceptibility leads to a dramatic loss of power. Slager et al. shows that if there are multiple disease-susceptibility alleles and one is studying a tightly linked locus but not the causal locus, then the required sample sizes for detecting association can easily become unattainable. Despite these concerns, many groups are proceeding with very large-scale association genotyping projects with the hope that at least some disease-susceptibility loci will be identified.

Although it is highly likely that this approach will identify some loci for which the underlying genetic architecture is straightforward (i.e., a single common-disease-causing variant in strong linkage disequilibrium with disease), it is also likely that some disease-causing variants will be missed because the genetic architecture is too complex (several disease-causing variants in the same locus and/or low levels of linkage disequilibrium with SNPs or extensive locus heterogeneity with multiple loci causing the same phenotype).

Alternative approaches can be used to identify genetic regions harboring some causal loci. One novel approach seeks to identify loci by evaluating ancestrally shared regions of the genome. This approach can identify evidence for genetic effects even when there are multiple distinct mutations predisposing to disease. This mapping scheme requires the study of admixed populations and the availability of genetic markers that can discriminate among ancestral founding populations. Another approach that has been effective in identifying genetic factors predisposing to mental retardation, schizophrenia, and autism searches for small regions of segmental aneusomy (i.e., duplicated or deleted segments of DNA) in affected individuals.

COMPARATIVE GENOMICS

Animal models of complex disease have provided additional information to direct the identification of gene variants relevant to human disease. Animal models and in particular, mice, have a number of advantages when trying to identify human disease genes. Breeding can be planned with the generation of large numbers of affected progeny and environmental influences can be controlled. Comparative genomics has become increasingly relevant as a number of genomes have been mapped, linkage maps created and information about SNP variation has become available. This has facilitated an explosion in linkage and association studies for both disease and quantitative trait loci.

A number of techniques and strategies have informed comparative genomics. Congenic strains allow refinement of a disease associated locus through the isolation of a chromosomal region known to predispose to a particular disease or disease parameter and through its insertion into the genome of a rodent strain that is not predisposed to the disease under study. Chromosomal synteny is the conservation of whole chromosomal segments between species. Such that the identification of a susceptibility locus in a rat model of rheumatoid arthritis on chromosome 10 led to the investigation and confirmation of an RA susceptibility locus in the syntenic region on the long arm of human chromosome 17. In addition, transgenic and knockout mice can be used to study the effects of specific gene variants on phenotype. Animal models of human disease may arise spontaneously or be induced either by mutagenesis by radiation or by chemical means using N-ethyl-N-nitrosourea or another insult, for example, injection of collagen into rodent footpads to effect arthritis.

Animal models of single gene disorders have also provided insight into pathways important in common diseases. The *ob/ob* mouse is characterized by gross obesity. Mutations in leptin have been identified to underlie this phenotype and a very rare recessive form of obesity in humans, but the study of the leptin pathway has provided significant insights in the control of body weight.

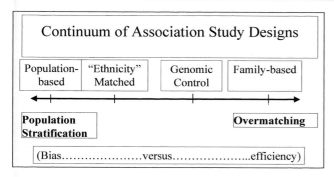

Figure 3-4 Identifying genetic regions for further positional cloning efforts. The designs range from population-based without matching to family-based, which are completely matched on ethnicity. Many forms of matching decrease efficiency, but provide increasing protection from false-positive results from population substructure.

A number of animal models of IBD have been identified including mice administered dextran sulfate and the spontaneously occurring C3H/HeJBir mouse strain. No model completely replicates the disease process in humans, but each may provide important clues to direct human gene and disease pathway identification. Multiple pathways lead to and protect against bowel inflammation. The IL-10 knockout mouse is illustrative in that one strain develops IBD, whereas another strain is resistant, demonstrating the importance of genetic background in animal models.

Linkage studies have identified loci which are syntenic to loci identified in genome-wide scans of IBD in humans, for example, the D5Mit216 locus is syntenic to the human 5q31 locus recently shown to harbor a high-risk haplotype across SLC22A4 and SLC22A5 genes for CD. Furthermore, animal models of IBD have shown the impact of nongenetic factors with disease only manifesting in animals once they are removed from a germ-free environment.

CONCLUSIONS

The search for genes that predispose to IBD has been successful. Variants in CARD15 are associated with CD in many populations and more recently variants in the OCTN gene cluster at chromosome 5q31 and DLG5 on chromosome 10 have been identified. Both positional cloning and candidate gene analysis have been successfully employed to identify these variants and the use of linkage disequilibrium mapping has been a powerful aid to refine the critical regions containing the susceptibility variants. Subsequent work has started to define the phenotypic consequences of these disease associated gene variants, for example, both CARD15 and OCTN variants increase the risk of ileal disease. In addition, the functional effects of these variants have been explored, especially in CARD15, which appears to act as a host defense mechanism to clear intracellular bacteria.

It is interesting to speculate on whether the genes identified to be associated with CD also predispose to other inflammatory diseases, for example, an intronic variant in SLC22A4 (OCTN1) has been associated with rheumatoid arthritis. This would support a proposed theory that common gene variants predispose to multiple diseases. This is compatible with the common disease: common variant hypothesis underpinning the genetic study of common diseases. This theory provides part of the justification for the HapMap project to identify SNPs and the relationships between these SNPs and is hoped that it will lead to the rapid identification of common disease associated variants. In IBD research, the discovery of variants in the OCTN gene cluster and DLG5 support this approach and provide hope for further significant advances in common disease genetics. Major challenges still lie ahead to determine the function relevance of disease associated variants and how this information may be translated into advances in clinical practice.

SELECTED REFERENCES

Ahmad T, Armuzzi A, Bunce M, et al. The molecular classification of the clinical manifestations of Crohn's disease. Gastroenterology 2002; 122:854–866.

Amos CI, Rubin LA. Major gene analysis for diseases and disorders of complex etiology. Exp Clin Immunogenet 1995;12:141–155.

Cavanaugh J. International collaboration provides convincing linkage replication in complex disease through analysis of a large pooled data set: Crohn disease and chromosome 16. Am J Hum Genet 2001;68: 1165–1171.

Cuthbert AP, Fisher SA, Mirza MM, et al. The contribution of NOD2 gene mutations to the risk and site of disease in inflammatory bowel disease. Gastroenterology 2002;122:867–874.

Daly MJ, Rioux JD, Schaffner SF, Hudson TJ, Lander ES. High-resolution haplotype structure in the human genome. Nat Genet 2001;29: 229–232.

Davies JL, Kawaguchi Y, Bennett ST, et al. A genome-wide search for human type 1 diabetes susceptibility genes. Nature 1994;371:130–136.

Devlin B, Roeder K, Bacanu SA. Unbiased methods for population-based association studies. Genet Epidemiol 2001;21:273–284.

Gu C, Province MA, Rao DC. Meta-analysis for model-free methods. Adv Genet 2001;42:255–272.

Hugot JP, Chamaillard M, Zouali H, et al. Association of NOD2 leucine-rich repeat variants with susceptibility to Crohn's disease. Nature 2001;411:599–603.

Hugot JP, Laurent-Puig P, Gower-Rousseau C, et al. Mapping of a susceptibility locus for Crohn's disease on chromosome 16. Nature 1996;379:821–823.

King RA, Rotter JI, Motulsky AG. Approach to genetic basis of common diseases. In: King RA, Rotter JI, Motulsky AG, eds. The Genetic Basis of Common Diseases. New York: Oxford University Press, 2002; pp. 3–17.

Lander ES, Schork NJ. Genetic dissection of complex traits. Science 1994;265:2037–2048.

Lesage S, Zouali H, Cezard JP, et al. CARD15/NOD2 mutational analysis and genotype-phenotype correlation in 612 patients with inflammatory bowel disease. Am J Hum Genet 2002;70:845–857.

Newman B, Silverberg MS, Gu X, et al. CARD15 and HLA DRB1 alleles influence susceptibility and disease localization in Crohn's disease. Am J Gastroenterol 2004;99:306–315.

Ogura Y, Bonen DK, Inohara N, et al. A frameshift mutation in NOD2 associated with susceptibility to Crohn's disease. Nature 2001;411: 603–606.

Orholm M, Binder V, Sorensen TI, Rasmussen LP, Kyvik KO. Concordance of inflammatory bowel disease among Danish twins. Results of a nationwide study. Scand J Gastroenterol 2000;35:1075–1081.

Ott J. Analysis of Human Genetic Linkage. Baltimore: Johns Hopkins University Press, 1999.

Rahman P, Bartlett S, Siannis F, et al. CARD15: A pleiotropic autoimmune gene that confers susceptibility to psoriatic arthritis. Am J Hum Genet 2003;73:677–681.

Rich SS, Sellers TA. Genetic epidemiologic methods. In: Richard A King, Jerome I Rotter, Arno G Motulsky, eds. The Genetic Basis of Common Diseases. Oxford University Press, 2002; pp. 39–49.

Rioux JD, Daly MJ, Silverberg MS, et al. Genetic variation in the 5q31 cytokine gene cluster confers susceptibility to Crohn disease. Nat Genet 2001;29:223–228.

Slager SL, Huang J, Vieland VJ. Effect of allelic heterogeneity on the power of the transmission disequilibrium test. Genet Epidemiol 2000;18:143–156.

Terwilliger JD and Ott J. Handbook of Human Genetic Linkage. Baltimore: Johns Hopkins University Press, 1994.

Thompson D, Goldgar D, Stram D, Witte JS. Design issues in using haplotype tagging SNPs for association studies. Hum Hered 2003;56:48–55.

Vermeire S, Satsangi J, Peeters M, et al. Evidence for inflammatory bowel disease of a susceptibility locus on the X chromosome. Gastroenterology 2001;120:834–840.

Witte JS, Gauderman WJ, Thomas DC. Asymptotic bias and efficiency in case-control studies of candidate genes and gene-environment interactions: basic family designs. Am J Epideminol 1999;149: 693–705.

Zhang K, Sun F, Waterman S, Chen T. Haplotype block partition with limited resources and applications to human chromosome 21 haplotype data. Am J Hum Genet 2003;73:63–73.

4 Cancer Genetics and Molecular Oncology

Sharon E. Plon

SUMMARY

Cancer is a genetic disease, but there are many different types of genetic changes found within a cancer cell. The study of relatively rare cancer predisposition disorders has provided crucial insights into basic mechanisms of cellular physiology and tumorigenesis. In this chapter, we review different mechanisms that result in an inherited predisposition to cancer, including chromosomal disorders, defects in imprinted genes, mutations in tumor suppressor genes, activation of oncogenes, and mutations in DNA repair genes. This research is now being accelerated through the Human Genome Project and high throughput analysis of the genetic changes found in cancer cells.

Key Words: Autosomal-dominant; autosomal-recessive; cancer susceptibility; deletions; DNA repair; imprinting; mutations; oncogenes; translocations; tumor suppressor genes.

INTRODUCTION

Overwhelming evidence demonstrates that cancer is the result of genetic changes in the DNA of the tumor cell. The mechanism of mutation and the impact of these somatic alterations on the growth of cancer cells make up the field of molecular oncology. In addition to mutational changes, a number of genes are deregulated in the cancer cell by epigenetic mechanisms including DNA methylation. Overall, the percentage of human cancers that is caused by a major inherited predisposition is low. That percentage varies with individual tumor types and is a composite of several different genetic factors. Despite their lower frequency, the ability to identify the genes mutated in these families has provided significant insight into the etiology of cancer in the general population. Our understanding of somatic mutations in cancer cells has relied heavily on identification of important genes through study of familial cases with subsequent research focused on mutations in these genes in sporadic cases (*see* Fig. 4-1). Key examples of the different forms of inherited predisposition to cancer will be reviewed.

Hereditary predisposition may include either genetic alterations that have been passed on to the individual from a parent or new mutations that occurred in the oocyte or sperm before fertilization. Therefore, hereditary predisposition to cancer is not always associated with a family history of the disease. For example, a *de novo* mutation in a cancer predisposing gene such as *RB1* can result in healthy parents having a child with the hereditary

From: *Principles of Molecular Medicine, Second Edition*
Edited by: M. S. Runge and C. Patterson © Humana Press, Inc., Totowa, NJ

form of retinoblastoma. In the case of new dominant mutations in genes that result in highly lethal tumors, there may not be a family history because the children with cancer do not live to reproduce. In these cases, the process of gene discovery can work in reverse (*see* Fig. 4-1). For example, in atypical rhabdoid tumors, it was found that the tumors frequently carry a cytogenetically visible deletion at chromosome 22q11.2. This harbors the *hSNF5/INI-1* gene. Subsequently, children who carry a point mutation in this gene in their tumor were found to actually carry the mutation in all the cells in their body. These new dominant mutations presumably occur during the production of the egg or sperm before fertilization. This results in children with a cancer predisposition syndrome without an obvious family history. The identification of the gene by tumor cytogenetics allowed the uncovering of this syndrome. Thus, there may be other apparently sporadic cancers that could be the result of *de novo* constitutional mutations.

There are a variety of mechanisms that result in inheritance of cancer susceptibility. In this chapter, we will review examples of the major types including, constitutional chromosomal abnormality, Mendelian autosomal-dominant and autosomal-recessive patterns, and non-Mendelian inheritance. Non-Mendelian patterns include multigenic disorders, mutations in mitochondrial DNA, and imprinting errors. Imprinting refers to the fact that gene expression from a given gene may differ if the gene is on a chromosome inherited from the mother or father. Conversely, for any given tumor type there may be more than one mechanism that results in an inherited predisposition to that disorder. The most commonly cited example is Wilm's tumor, a malignant cancer of the kidney frequently diagnosed in very young children. An increased risk of Wilm's tumor can be the result of a chromosomal deletion, an autosomal-dominant disorder or a disorder of imprinting.

CONSTITUTIONAL CHROMOSOMAL ABNORMALITIES

Children with constitutional chromosomal abnormalities often present with many different medical problems including abnormalities in growth, multiple congenital anomalies (birth defects), and learning abnormalities. Constitutional chromosomal abnormalities are the result of abnormal number (i.e., aneuploidy) or structural rearrangements of chromosomes. Cells normally contain 46 chromosomes (i.e., 22 pairs of autosomes and the sex chromosome pair). In addition to their other medical problems, individuals with a constitutional chromosome problem may have an increased predisposition to cancer.

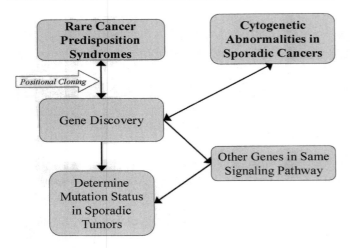

Figure 4-1   Pathway of molecular genetics research in oncology.

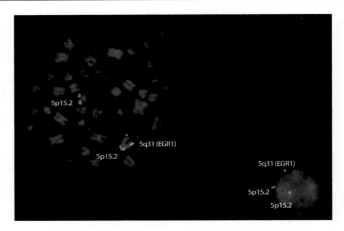

Figure 4-2   FISH of a pediatric leukemia sample demonstrating that one chromosome 5 contains a deleted segment that includes the *EGR1* gene. On the left are chromosomes from a cell in metaphase. On the right is an interphase cell. Hybridization is also performed with a probe from the short arm of chromosome 5 as a control. (Photograph courtesy of R. Naeem.) (Please *see* color insert.)

DOWN SYNDROME   Down syndrome (DS) is one of the most common chromosomal abnormalities in humans. It is the result of a child having three copies of chromosome 21 (trisomy 21). This increase in chromosome number typically results from an error in chromosome segregation during oogenesis. Thus, the child is usually the only person in the family with trisomy 21 and there is no structural abnormality in the three chromosome 21s present in the child. In addition to particular facial features and learning disabilities, it was noted quite early that children with DS have a strikingly increased predisposition to leukemia. By 5 yr of age approx 2% of children with DS will be diagnosed with leukemia. This is in contrast to approx 5/100,000 in the general population. Despite the fact that this association has been known for many years, we are still not certain which genes on chromosome 21 result in the increased leukemia risk. The completion of the sequencing of the entire chromosome 21 as part of the human genome project and large-scale expression studies of leukemia cells using microarray technology is facilitating this search. Children with DS also demonstrate another common feature of cancer predisposition syndromes, which is that they are increased risk for only certain cancer types, in spite of the fact that all cells of their body contain the extra chromosome 21. It is often the case that in inherited syndromes there are specific subtypes of cancer that show an increased predisposition. Again, scientists often do not have a molecular mechanism to explain this specificity. In the case of children with DS, they are particularly predisposed to an otherwise less common form of leukemia termed acute megakaryocytic leukemia (AMKL). AMKL is the result of malignant transformation of the megakaryocyte cell that provides platelets in the bloodstream. Outside of DS, AMKL is a very rare form of leukemia with a 400-fold increase of AMKL in children with DS. Clearly, the megakaryocyte is particularly sensitive to an extra copy of chromosome 21. Also, children with DS and AMKL show a different pattern of mutations in other genes within the cancer cell compared with other children with AMKL. In particular, the characteristic translocation between chromosomes 1 and 22 (t[1;22][p13;q13]) is absent in children with DS and AMKL.

As we will discuss for other malignancies, the leukemogenic effect of trisomy 21 is also seen in children without DS. If one looks at the pattern of chromosomes from leukemia cells in children without DS, one frequently finds that the leukemia cell has acquired a third chromosome 21. Thus, if we can understand why children with DS have an increased risk of leukemia it may help us better understand leukemogenesis in the general population.

Despite the well-documented increase in the risk of leukemia in children with DS, several large-scale population studies have not found an increased risk of other cancers in children with DS. In particular, many common cancers, including breast cancer, were less frequent in the population of adults with DS. Again we see a specific relationship between trisomy 21 and leukemia risk even though all cells in the body contain an extra chromosome 21. The reason why mutations in certain genes result in the development of cancer in only specific cell types is one of the remaining challenges in the field of cancer genetics.

STRUCTURAL CHROMOSOMAL ABNORMALITIES

Detection and Impact   The ability to detect the number and, subsequently, the overall shape of human chromosomes improved through the 1960s and 1970s. As these techniques improved it became possible to identify that deletions of certain portions of chromosomes were a frequent occurrence in human cancers. In a smaller number of patients, this deletion or chromosome loss is an inherited event and again may be associated with a specific pattern of birth defects. Over the last 20 yr, the technology has continued to improve. In particular, the development of fluorescently labeled DNA probes allowed researchers to identify chromosomes that appear normal in the microscope but are deleted for sequences that bind to the fluorescent probe. This technique is termed fluorescent *in situ* hybridization (FISH) and is in regular use in both clinical and research laboratories. Figure 4-2 demonstrates FISH analysis of leukemia cells demonstrating deletion of part of chromosome 5 that results in loss of the *EGR1* gene. Over the last several years, even newer methodologies are being developed to allow scientists to screen the entire genome of a normal or cancer cell for small areas of loss or gain. These methods combine the power of microchip arrays and fluorescent probes. Thus, we expect that our ability to detect clinically important deletions will increase exponentially in the next decade.

Deletions of a portion of a chromosome can result in the loss of several neighboring genes. The size of the deletion impacts how many of these genes are lost and how many different medical problems a patient may manifest. Chromosomal deletions may be *de novo* events or inherited from either parent.

WAGR: Wilm's Tumor, Aniridia, Genital Abnormalities, and Mental Retardation The WAGR syndrome is named after an acronym that represents the most common medical problems seen in the condition including: *W*ilm's tumor, *a*niridia, *g*enital-urinary abnormalities, and mental *r*etardation. Two early cytogeneticists noticed that children with this group of medical problems had a microscopically visible deletion of the short arm of chromosome 11 (named 11p13).

When techniques were first developed to map the location of DNA fragments onto specific chromosomes, members of the Housman laboratory laboriously defined the minimal amount of DNA that had to be deleted to result in the WAGR syndrome, termed the "critical region." They then searched for the genes contained in this region and were able to identify that a specific gene, named *WT1* for Wilm's tumor 1, was deleted in the children with WAGR and Wilm's tumor. They also found that this gene is normally expressed in the developing kidney. *WT1* was one of the first genes identified that encodes a member of the family of transcription factors called zinc finger proteins. We have subsequently learned that many different tumor types result from mutations in this class of genes. All or part of *WT1* is deleted in children with WAGR and Wilm's tumor. In contrast, mutations of a single amino acid in the *WT1* gene are the cause of another genetic condition, Denys–Drash syndrome, which also results in an increased risk of Wilm's tumor. This latter finding was the final proof that mutations in *WT1* are the cause of an increased predisposition to Wilm's tumor.

The results of identification of the genetic mechanism underlying these syndromes have lead to development of specific screening regimens for young children with these disorders. For example, all children with aniridia who are found to carry a deletion in the *WT1* gene are screened every 3–4 mo by renal ultrasound in order to detect any Wilm's tumor at an early stage, thus decreasing the intensity and potential toxicity of their cancer treatment and increasing the likelihood of a cure.

OVERGROWTH DISORDERS AND IMPRINTING ERRORS

BECKWITH–WEIDEMANN SYNDROME Not surprisingly, there has long been a recognized relation between disorders of increased growth and predisposition to cancer. Certain genetic conditions result in abnormal growth profiles and an increased risk of cancer. In particular, Beckwith–Wiedemann syndrome (BWS) and hemihyperplasia (HH) are linked to a significantly increased risk of developing abdominal tumors, including Wilm's tumor and hepatoblastoma. It is estimated that approx 3–5% of children with BWS develop one of these tumor types compared with less than 1/10,000 in the general population. BWS is characterized by excessive intrauterine and postnatal growth, organomegaly, and several specific congenital anomalies. HH (HH—also sometimes referred to as hemihypertrophy) in a child is defined as asymmetric growth owing to overgrowth of one side relative to the other. It can be limited to a limb or the face or include the whole side. Several studies have demonstrated that children with both BWS and HH had a higher risk of Wilm's tumor, than either condition alone.

The genetic basis of BWS and HH is complex but a common theme is that there are differences in development of BWS depending on the parent it is inherited from. In rare children with BWS (and no family history) part of chromosome 11p15 (distinct

from where *WT1* resides) is duplicated. This duplication always occurs on the chromosome they inherited from their father.

The dependence on whether the abnormality is inherited from the father or mother is the result of imprinting. Imprinting refers to the fact that certain genes are expressed differently, depending on whether they were inherited on the maternal or paternal chromosome. An extreme example is that some children with BWS have two normal chromosomes 11 but they inherited both copies of chromosome 11 from their father, termed uniparental disomy and none from their mother.

Extensive research efforts have identified multiple imprinted genes in this region of chromosome 11 which when deregulated result in BWS. These include a growth factor, IGF-2, a cell-cycle inhibitor, p57^{KIP1}, and RNAs, *H19* and *LIT1*. For example, *IGF-2* is expressed from the paternal chromosome and *p57^{KIP1}* is only expressed from the maternal chromosome. Thus, the study of rare disorders has shed light on a hitherto unsuspected but fundamental aspect of inheritance, that there are distinct differences in expression from the maternal and paternal chromosome. When this balance is disrupted congenital anomalies can develop as well an increased risk of cancer. Cancer biologists are now trying to understand how loss of imprinting may play a role in cancers in the general population.

MENDELIAN INHERITANCE OF A PREDISPOSITION TO CANCER

There are many families that show a Mendelian inheritance pattern of cancer predisposition consistent with inheritance of either a dominant or recessive mutation in a single gene. In the following sections, we discuss examples of both autosomal-dominant and autosomal-recessive disorders that results in family members with an increased risk of developing cancer.

AUTOSOMAL-DOMINANT DISORDERS The majority of syndromes that result in an increased susceptibility to cancer are owing to autosomal-dominant mutations. The autosomal name refers to the fact that the mutations are on an autosome as demonstrated by the mutation being equally transmitted from either the father or mother to a son or daughter. Dominant refers to the finding that cancer predisposition results from inheritance of a mutation from only one parent. Thus, one sees a multigenerational pattern of cancer risk in one lineage. However, as we also see in other autosomal-dominant conditions, the degree of cancer risk varies within the family and there may be members of the family who inherit the cancer-predisposing mutation but never develop cancer (termed incomplete penetrance). Thus, we emphasize to patients and their physicians that these are cancer predisposition or susceptibility disorders, and that simple inheritance of such a mutation does not guarantee that an individual will develop cancer. The risk of developing cancer varies with the specific syndrome from over 95% for colon cancer in familial adenomatous polyposis to 15% for ovarian cancer in women who inherit a *BRCA2* mutation.

Retinoblastoma The study of genetic predisposition to a rare pediatric eye tumor, retinoblastoma, was a turning point in our general understanding of the pathogenesis of cancer. Alfred Knudson and his colleague Louise Strong published a series of articles in the early 1970s that were based on the statistical analysis of children with retinoblastoma and other pediatric malignancies. By modeling the age of onset of retinoblastoma in children with bilateral disease in comparison with unilateral disease,

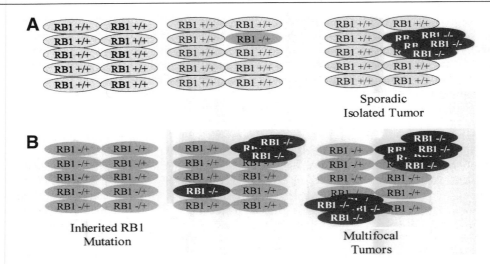

Figure 4-3 Model of the two-hit hypothesis. (**A**) illustrates the events in the retina of a child born with two normal copies of the *RB1* gene. A rare retinal cell may develop a single *RB1* mutation and eventually lose the second copy of *RB1* and become a tumor. (**B**) illustrates the events in the retina of a child born with a constitutional *RB1* mutation. All retinal cells carry this mutation and there is an increased frequency of tumors developing when the second copy of the *RB1* gene is lost.

Knudson tested the hypothesis that bilateral retinoblastoma represented the inherited form of the disorder with those patients inheriting the first event, presumably a mutation. His data were most consistent with a model that posited that the bilateral form required only one additional event or "hit" but that the unilateral form required two hits. Knudson recognized that in unilateral or sporadic forms of the disease the same two events must occur in a somatic cell, a relatively rare event (Fig. 4-3). In the inherited cases, all cells in the body contain the first hit and thus the frequency of a second hit in a somatic cell is high leading to bilateral or multifocal disease with an earlier age of onset.

The two-hit hypothesis is consistent with the finding that inherited forms of retinoblastoma present earlier and with a greatly increased percentage of bilateral and multiple primary tumors. Importantly, some patients (~15%) with unilateral disease also carry a constitutional mutation as well; presumably having only a single cell that incurred a second hit. Overall, approx 10% of people with a constitutional mutation in *RB1* do not develop retinoblastoma, yielding a "penetrance" for retinal tumors of 90%. These features of early age of onset, multifocal or bilateral disease, and incomplete penetrance are found in many different cancer predisposition syndromes that are the result of mutations in tumor suppressor genes (Table 4-1). Tumor suppressor gene is the term used to describe genes that normally function to prevent tumor development by controlling proliferation, maintaining genomic stability, or DNA repair and are inactivated in tumors.

An additional phenotype common to the autosomal-dominant conditions was also found for retinoblastoma families by long-term follow-up of childhood survivors. Individuals carrying germline mutations in the *RB1* gene are at increased risk for development of other primary tumors. In particular, there is an increased risk of osteosarcoma and malignant melanoma. This clustering of a specific subset of tumor types is found in a number of other cancer predisposition syndromes including breast and ovarian cancer in the same families.

Rare children with bilateral retinoblastoma who were found to carry a cytogenetically visible deletion of chromosome 13q14 led

Table 4-1
Clinical Features Associated With Autosomal-Dominant Cancer Susceptibility

Feature
Increased cancer risk seen in multiple generations in one lineage
Transmission of cancer risk through both men and women
Earlier onset of cancer diagnosis compared with general population
Bilateral or multifocal cancers
An individual diagnosed with more than one type of cancer
Clustering of specific cancer types within a family, for example, breast and ovarian cancer

to the cloning of the *RB1* gene. Molecular studies of this gene in both inherited and sporadic cases of retinoblastoma provided a physical confirmation of the two-hit hypothesis. Retinoblastoma requires loss or inactivation of both functional copies (i.e., two hits) of the *RB1* gene for a tumor to develop (Fig. 4-3). The *RB1* gene is a prototypical "tumor suppressor gene," whose normal function is to negatively regulate the cell division cycle. The loss of this function, called tumor suppression, is consistent with loss of cell cycle control when both copies are inactivated. In the familial form, a mutation in one *RB1* gene is inherited, and therefore all the cells in the body have only one normal allele. If during development of the eye, the remaining normal copy is mutated or lost then there is no residual *RB1* function and cell cycle control is disrupted. Many different mechanisms can lead to loss of the second copy of the *RB1* gene, such as deletion of a portion of the chromosome, loss of the whole chromosome, loss and duplication of the mutant chromosome, or smaller events within the *RB1* gene. In the sporadic form, mutation or loss of both *RB1* genes must occur in the same retinal cell for retinoblastoma to develop.

Implications   Several themes first identified in the study of retinoblastoma have been found to be true of a number of autosomal-dominant cancer predisposition syndromes. Specifically, important molecular events may be shared between the cancers that arise in those rare individuals with an inherited predisposition and the much

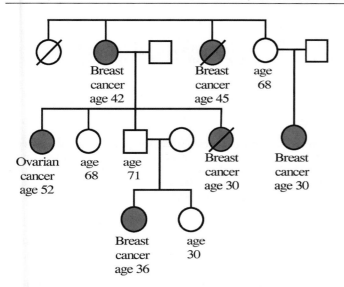

Figure 4-4 Pedigree of a family carrying a mutation in the *BRCA1* gene. Note the increased number of women diagnosed with breast cancer at young ages, the occurrence of ovarian cancer and the transmission of the risk of cancer through both men and women.

more common sporadic cancers. For example, the same genes that are mutated in inherited syndromes has also been found to be inactivated in significant percentages of kidney cancers, sarcomas, colon cancers, and skin cancers. This inactivation can be due to mutation or to epigenetic changes that silence the gene. For example, rare inherited mutations in the mismatch repair gene, *MLH1*, result in hereditary nonpolyposis colon cancer. In contrast, in about 15% of colon cancers in the general population, the *MLH1* gene is silenced by methylation. Exceptions to this relationship between inherited and sporadic cancers will be summarized in the section on breast cancer susceptibility.

A fundamental result of mutation of the *RB1* gene is inactivation or loss of function leading to cancer development. Genes that share this feature have been termed tumor suppressor genes because when present they result in decreased cancer development. The identification of tumor suppressor genes was in stark contrast to the earlier discovery of oncogenes and the genetic mechanisms that result in activation of the oncogene in human tumors including amplification, point mutation, and translocation. The majority of syndromes that result in inherited susceptibility to cancer are due to inactivating mutations in tumor suppressor genes. However, as described in the section on multiple endocrine neoplasia, there are rare syndromes that result from the inheritance of a mutation that activates a protooncogene.

BRCA1: DISCORDANCE BETWEEN INHERITED AND SPORADIC BREAST CANCER
A woman's risk of developing breast or ovarian cancer is a combination of personal risk factors (age of menarche, number of children, hormonal exposure, history of breast disease), and genetic predisposition. Statistically, one of the most significant risk factors for these cancers is family history of these cancers. *BRCA1* was the first major breast and ovarian cancer predisposition gene identified. Its chromosome location was identified as 17q21 by classic linkage analysis of a large number of families characterized by multiple cases of early onset breast cancer, ovarian cancer, and bilateral breast cancer (Fig. 4-4). Much of the impetus for identifying the *BRCA1* gene came from the expectation that mutations in this gene would also be found in

sporadic breast cancers in the general population. This idea was supported by studies of breast tumors themselves, which suggested that the 17q21 region was rearranged or lost in sporadic breast cancers.

BRCA1 is a large gene containing 24 exons and encodes a protein of 1863 amino acids. Studies of tumors from women, found to have inherited a *BRCA1* mutation, were consistent with the Knudson two-hit hypothesis. The tumors showed loss or inactivation of the remaining wild-type gene in both breast and ovarian cancers in these women. Surprisingly, studies of breast cancers from women who do not carry a constitutional mutation revealed no evidence for somatic mutations in the *BRCA1* gene. Thus, the *BRCA1* gene functions primarily as a tumor suppressor gene in women who inherit one mutation. Why mutations do not occur in sporadic breast cancer is unknown. Some studies have suggested that the BRCA1 protein may be regulated differently in sporadic cancers, although that remains unclear. Thus, one cannot predict *a priori* whether the same gene will be mutated in both inherited syndromes and sporadic cancers. As each new tumor suppressor gene is found, it is important to directly determine the frequency of mutations in both situations. In some cases, it may be that different genes in the same cellular pathway are mutated in inherited vs sporadic cancers.

Recent studies have demonstrated that the normal function of the BRCA1 protein is in recognition of DNA damage and transduction of that signal to downstream proteins that mediate cell cycle arrest (termed checkpoints) and DNA repair. Loss of *BRCA1* function results in somatic cells having an increased number of mutations and genomic instability with subsequent tumorigenesis. Other proteins encoded by tumor suppressor genes, including p53, ATM, and CHEK2 also function in the same pathway. Mutations in each of these genes have been found in women with an inherited predisposition to breast cancer and *p53* mutations are also found in sporadic breast cancers. Thus, one can generalize our understanding of breast cancer to say that women who inherit defects in the DNA damage checkpoint pathway have a significantly increased risk of breast cancer. The susceptibility of mammary tissue to DNA damage can also be demonstrated by the very high rate of breast cancer in women who were treated as adolescents with radiation therapy to the chest for Hodgkin lymphoma.

MULTIPLE ENDOCRINE NEOPLASIA: INHERITANCE OF A MUTATION IN AN ONCOGENE
Thus far we have emphasized autosomal-dominant cancer predisposition disorders that are the result of inheriting a mutation in one copy of a tumor suppressor gene with tumors resulting from the somatic loss or inactivation of the remaining copy. Like all good rules there are exceptions and multiple endocrine neoplasia (MEN) type 2 represents such an exception. The MEN disorders represent at least three different diseases, which all result in an increased risk of tumors in endocrine organs. MEN1 is characterized by parathyroid, pancreatic islet cell, and pituitary gland involvement and is due to mutations in the *MEN1* gene on chromosome 11.

MEN type 2 is divided into subtypes MEN2A and MEN2B. Both MEN2A and MEN2B syndromes present in childhood but have a different pattern of onset and tumors types. MEN2A is more common and is associated with medullary thyroid carcinoma, parathyroid adenomas, and pheochromocytomas beginning in childhood and young adults. MEN2B is a related disorder but with the onset of tumors in infancy and associated with other medical problems.

The gene for MEN2A was initially mapped using standard genetic techniques to a small region on human chromosome 10q11.2. It was assumed that mutation in a tumor suppressor gene was responsible. However, researchers noted that the *RET* protooncogene, a receptor tyrosine kinase gene, mapped in this region. *RET* had been found to be activated in papillary thyroid cancer due to a translocation. Thus, it had many features of a classic oncogene. Surprisingly, analysis of constitutional DNA from multiple MEN2A families revealed a set of highly consistent mutations in the *RET* gene. The MEN2A mutations found in these families appeared to replace one of four cysteines with another amino acid in the extracellular domain of the protein encoded by exons 10 and 11. There was also some correlation between the types of cancers seen in the families and the specific cysteine mutation. For example, a mutation in cysteine 634 results in a high risk of pheochromocytomas in the family. Patients with MEN2B did not have cysteine mutations but subsequent studies demonstrated two specific missense mutations in the highly conserved tyrosine kinase domain of the *RET* gene in over 95% of MEN2B patients.

What we see in MEN2 families is in contradiction to the two-hit hypothesis. These missense mutations do not inactivate the Ret protein and the remaining copy of the gene remains intact in the tumor cell. Laboratory tests directly demonstrated that the cysteine mutations result in constitutional activation of the Ret protein and transforming activity. Thus, the predisposition to endocrine cancers is the result of inheritance of a mutation that activates an oncogene in contrast to inactivating a tumor suppressor gene.

Clinically, the screening and treatment of MEN2A and MEN2B families have been significantly improved by these genetic discoveries. In comparison to older hormonal studies to identify which family member was at increased risk for a cancer, there is greatly improved accuracy in DNA testing, particularly for young children. The DNA test need only be performed once, and it decreases the cost and potential health risks of the older techniques. Those children found to have inherited the mutation are recommended to have removal of the thyroid gland in early childhood in order to prevent the development of medullary thyroid cancer.

AUTOSOMAL-RECESSIVE DISORDERS

Recessive disorders that predispose to cancer have distinct characteristics when compared with the autosomal-dominant disorders. Individually, these are very rare disorders. There may be specific ethnic groups with an increased risk of a specific autosomal-recessive disorder owing to a high rate of carriers for a recessive trait. Clinically, recessive disorders result when a person carries two mutant alleles, one inherited from each parent. Thus, these disorders normally occur in sibships and are not evident in multiple generations. Generally, the parents who carry a single copy of the mutation are asymptomatic without an increased cancer risk, but have a one in four chance of having a subsequent child with the same disorder.

The symptoms of autosomal-recessive disorders are often more severe than in autosomal-dominant disorders and are typically diagnosed in childhood. Many of the autosomal-recessive cancer syndromes are caused by mutations in genes that encode DNA repair enzymes or proteins that monitor the presence of DNA

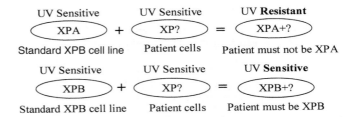

Figure 4-5 Complementation assay using UV sensitivity for cells from patients with xeroderma pigmentosum (XP). The patient sample is fused to standard cell lines from each XP subtype. If the fusion restores UV resistance then the patient must carry a mutation in another subtype. If the fusion does not restore UV resistance then the patient carries mutations in the same subtype genes.

damage. The lack of these functions results in increased mutation rates or genomic instability. The loss of a specific enzyme or surveillance function results in cells from these patients showing increased sensitivity to spontaneous and exogenous DNA damage and increased risk of specific cancer types.

XERODERMA PIGMENTOSUM   Xeroderma pigmentosum (XP) represents the classic DNA repair defect syndrome. Patients demonstrate extreme photosensitivity to even very modest sun exposure and present within the first few years of life with burns, telangiectasias, and freckling of the skin. Ocular abnormalities are common and are found in UV light-exposed areas of the cornea, lids, and conjunctivae, including corneal clouding and ocular malignancies. There is a several thousandfold increased risk of basal and squamous cell skin carcinomas and melanomas beginning in childhood in sun-exposed areas including the neck, face, and tip of the tongue.

The clinical finding of photosensitivity led investigators to test the response of cells from patients with XP to UV light. XP cells demonstrate increased UV sensitivity in vitro. More detailed analyses of the repair of UV-induced DNA damage demonstrated that in cells from different XP patients there were different defects. The determination that multiple genes caused the same clinical disorder was based on complementation assays in which fibroblasts from different patients are fused together in the laboratory (Fig. 4-5). The cell resulting from the fusion (heterokaryon) is then tested to determine if the cells remain sensitive to UV light. If the heterokaryon is sensitive that implies that both patients carry mutations in the same gene. If the heterokaryon becomes resistant to UV light (complementation) then that implies that different genes must be mutated in the two cells. It became apparent from these types of complementation assays that XP can result from mutations in at least seven different genes.

Once the different complementation groups were identified, biochemical assays revealed the specific step in repair of a UV-induced DNA lesion, which was defective in each group. One could then use this biochemical defect to identify which normal human gene could restore repair of the UV-induced lesion to the cell. Analysis of these gene products demonstrates that many of them encode proteins that are highly conserved. Similar proteins that perform similar functions can be found in prokaryotes (*Escherichia coli*) and many simpler eukaryotic organisms. It appears that developing defense mechanisms against UV-induced DNA damage is important for all organisms. This similarity between human and bacterial proteins has been found for other causes of inherited cancer. For example, mutations in mismatch repair genes cause an increased risk of colon cancer. There are similar proteins in bacteria and humans for performing this form of DNA repair. The similarity also allows scientists trying to understand the function of these cancer-suppressing proteins to carry out much of their research using simple bacterial or yeast organisms in the laboratory.

CONCLUSION

In this chapter, we have reviewed different mechanisms that result in an inherited predisposition to cancer, including chromosomal disorders, defects in imprinted genes, mutations in tumor suppressor genes, activation of oncogenes, and mutations in DNA repair genes. In each case, the analysis of a relatively rare disorder has provided crucial insights to basic mechanisms of cellular physiology and tumorigenesis. The recent development of large-scale highly automated methods including genome sequencing, microarray analysis and sophisticated hybridization techniques is aiding investigators to further apply what has been learned from these inherited disorders to cancers in the general population.

SELECTED REFERENCES

Cleaver JE, Thompson LH, Richardson AS, States JC. A summary of mutations in the UV-sensitive disorders: xeroderma pigmentosum, Cockayne syndrome, and trichothiodystrophy. Hum Mutat 1999;14(1):9–22.

DeBaun MR, Tucker MA. Risk of cancer during the first four years of life in children from The Beckwith–Wiedemann Syndrome Registry. J Pediatr 1998;132(3 Pt 1):398–400.

Eng C, Li FP, Abramson DH, Ellsworth RM, et al. Mortality from second tumors among long-term survivors of retinoblastoma. J Natl Cancer Inst 1993;85(14):1121–1128.

Gessi M, Giangaspero F, Pietsch T. Atypical teratoid/rhabdoid tumors and choroid plexus tumors: when genetics "surprise" pathology. Brain Pathol 2003;13(3):409–414.

Harbour JW. Overview of RB gene mutations in patients with retinoblastoma. Implications for clinical genetic screening. Ophthalmology 1998;105(8):1442–1447.

Hasle H, Clemmensen IH, Mikkelsen M. Risks of leukaemia and solid tumours in individuals with Down's syndrome. Lancet 2000;355(9199):165–169.

Huff V. Wilms tumor genetics. Am J Med Genet 1998;79(4):260–267.

Santoro M, Carlomagno F, Romano A, et al. Activation of RET as a dominant transforming gene by germline mutations of MEN2A and MEN2B. Science 1995;267(5196):381–383.

Wooster R, Weber BL. Breast and ovarian cancer. N Engl J Med 2003;348(23):2339–2347.

5 Pharmacogenetics

Renee E. Edkins and Dennis J. Cheek

SUMMARY

The clinical implications of pharmacogenetics are vast and many more are becoming apparent as research continues. Health-care providers will increasingly need to take pharmacogenetics into consideration when prescribing medications. Each patient's history, physical condition, gender, and ethnicity must be considered when prescribing drugs. Specific genotypic testing of patients for polymorphisms that influence drug metabolism and action will become a clinical reality. Silicone chip technology utilizing single-nucleotide polymorphisms will be able to provide a practitioner with reliable and timely information in an office setting to guide practice. Genetics and pharmacology are no longer separate sciences.

Key Words: Adverse drug event (ADE); drug development; extensive metabolizers (EM); pharmacogenetics; safety.

INTRODUCTION

Pharmacogenetics is targeted to the understanding of how genetic variation contributes to an individual's response when exposed to pharmacological agents. Pharmacogenomics takes entire populations into consideration when designing and evaluating disease and drug development. Variation or polymorphism, present in all genes, results in different forms of a protein. Such differences are especially important from the pharmacological standpoint for those proteins that are involved in the metabolism of many different medications. In addition to metabolism, receptor affinity to pharmacological agents is subject to variations. These variations can result in toxicity or loss of efficacy. As more becomes clear about the human genome, medications will be tailored to individuals, avoiding many adverse events and drug–drug interactions. Genes that code for the proteins that modulate drug targets vary. For example, genes that code for the cholesteryl ester transfer protein influence a patient's response to pravastatin (Fig. 5-1). Mutations in this protein can result in a patient's cholesterol remaining high in spite of the use of cholesterol-lowering drugs. Initial doses of pravastatin in these patients may show no effect, but this lack of response is because of genetics, not poor compliance. Increasing the dose may show no efficacy, but instead result in adverse reactions. This chapter reviews this fascinating interplay of genetics and pharmacology.

From: *Principles of Molecular Medicine, Second Edition*
Edited by: M. S. Runge and C. Patterson © Humana Press, Inc., Totowa, NJ

HISTORICAL OVERVIEW

The actual start of the field of pharmacogenetics is debatable. It is clear that a difference in the tolerance of certain people to the growing number of chemicals, both natural and pollutants, food toxins, and medications (collectively referred to as xenobiotics) in their environment had been observed long before the elucidation of the double helix in 1953. Pythagoras, as early as 510 BC, identified individuals who could not tolerate eating fava beans whereas others could. Those not tolerating fava beans developed hemolytic anemia because of a deficiency in glucose-6-phosphate dehydrogenase, a deficiency that has been well defined since 1956. In 1902, Archibald Garrod identified enzymes playing a key role in the detoxification of foreign substances. This work was expanded by Guthrie, who developed a simple blood test to identify newborns with phenylketonuria, a condition resulting from an inborn error of metabolism.

The 1950s were a defining decade for pharmacogenetics. It was becoming clear that inheritance might explain many individual differences in the efficacy of drugs and in the occurrence of adverse drug event (ADEs). In 1953, individuals were noted to experience neurological side effects from the antituberculosis drug isoniazid. Later biochemical analysis revealed that these subjects were poor metabolizers (PM) of isoniazid resulting from a deficiency in the enzyme *N*-acetyltransferase. Initial trials for the drug suxamethonium, a muscle relaxant used for surgery, evidenced no complications or adverse events. Thought to be safe, this drug was released into the larger population. Soon thereafter, prolonged and dangerous muscle relaxation was noted in an alarming number of individuals. It was found that variances in plasma cholinesterase levels left many individuals unable to clear the drug from their systems resulting in prolonged muscle relaxation.

In 1977 research on the antihypertensive agents bethanidine and debrisoquin revealed that bethanidine acted within a relatively narrow range of dosing. Debrisoquin, however, evidenced a wide effective dose range. It was discovered that bethanidine was rapidly absorbed and excreted unchanged. No metabolic transformation was required, thus the narrow range of dosage. Debrisoquin was also rapidly absorbed, but was excreted as metabolites. One subject excreted few metabolites, but mostly active parent compound. This individual evidenced a profound hypotensive response to the same dosage that caused no response in other individuals. Further work in this area led to the discovery of the first polymorphism of drug oxidation in man. The terms extensive metabolizers (EM) and PM, discussed later in this chapter, were first introduced in this research.

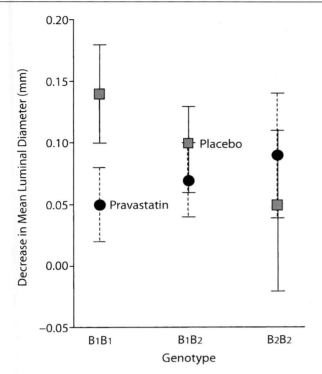

Figure 5-1 Changes in mean luminal diameter according to the CETP TaqlB genotype in patients with established coronary atherosclerosis treated with either placebo or pravastatin. (Reproduced with permission from Kuivehoven JA, Jukema JW, Zwinderman AH, et al. The role of a common variant of the cholesteryl ester transfer protein gene in the progression of coronary atherosclerosis. N Engl J Med, 1998;338[2]:1200–1205. Copyright © 1998 Massachusetts Medical Society. All rights reserved.)

Pharmacogenetics is not a new discipline. Although the term pharmacogenetics entered the lexicon in 1959 when coined by Fredreich Vogel, the effects of polymorphisms on metabolism in humans have been observed as early as the sixth century. With the mapping of the human genome, pharmacogenetics will play an increasingly important role in clinical medicine. Health-care providers will need to take variation and genetics into account when prescribing medications.

CLINICAL DEVELOPMENT AND APPROVAL

Medications are essentially prescribed through a process of trial and error. Federal law in the United States mandates that medications are approved only after going through clinical trials to prove their worth. However, clinical trial populations are of relatively small size compared to the general population. It is only after a drug has been approved for use in the general population and many more exposures have occurred that its true safety and efficacy profile becomes clear.

The development of a drug can be a long and arduous process. Basic research by chemists, pharmacologists, and molecular biologists seeks to determine if a desired chemical effect can be obtained with minimal toxicity. Hundreds of thousands of chemical compounds are screened for candidates. Likely candidate compounds that show promise move into a pipeline for development. Whether a compound has been chosen specifically to treat a disease or has simply evidenced unique properties, it must undergo a long process of research to become a new drug.

The traditional path of drug development can take 6–14 yr. At any time in this path a potential drug can be pulled from the pipeline for failing proof of concept. Thousands are rejected, but in the future the problem evidenced by these compounds may no longer present an obstacle and they will be reinvestigated. For those that succeed, the average time to market, according to the Food and Drug Administration (FDA) is 8.5 yr.

The classic clinical trial paradigm occurs in four phases following an initial preclinical stage (Table 5-1). Once a compound has cleared preclinical testing in the laboratory, it moves into Phase 1 trials. These trials consist of the initial human studies and usually involve healthy volunteers. Small populations are enrolled, averaging 20–80 subjects. At this phase study end points consist of safety, tolerability, and pharmacokinetic data. For a compound to enter this phase an investigational new drug (IND) application must be filed and approved by the FDA. The IND reference number will be linked to all future studies.

Phase 2 trials represent the start of testing in select affected populations and last 1–2 yr. These are small pilot studies, consisting of about 100–300 subjects. Safety and pharmacokinetic data continue to be evaluated, but with the addition of two new end points: dose escalation and efficacy.

Phase 3 clinical trials are the studies that attract the most public attention. These trials are large, by industry standards, and can enroll from 1000 to 10,000 affected subjects. As the exposed population grows, a profile of the investigational drug's-related adverse effects and therapeutic ranges emerges. An investigational drug remains in this phase for 2–3 yr. Even at the largest and most expensive enrollment of 10,000, this represents only a scant percentage of the total population for which a drug is usually intended.

In the last of these three phases, a new drug application is completed and submitted to the FDA for review. This review process can take up to 2 yr. If the data are positive, the investigational drug receives approval and becomes available by prescription to the general population. Approval, though, does not mean the end of evaluation. After approval, a fourth phase of evaluation is entered. Phase 4 consists of postmarketing surveillance by the pharmaceutical company. The FDA continues to monitor approved drugs for safety. Additionally, the pharmaceutical company studies pharmacoeconomic data and clinical reports to elucidate additional indications. For example, the drug minoxidil, approved for hypertension as Loniten®, was found to increase hair growth in men. After further research the drug was approved for a new indication, alopecia, and appears as Rogaine®.

SAFETY   As indicated by the paradigm discussed earlier, most drugs approved by the FDA have had only a limited exposure in humans for only a short period of time. Some drugs can cause serious ADEs at very low frequencies and thus require more exposures to detect such reactions. In 1997 bromfenac sodium (Duract®), a nonsteroidal anti-inflammatory agent developed for short-term management of acute pain was approved for short-term use. Although clinical trials had revealed some elevation of liver functions, no incidences of overt liver failure occurred and the drug was approved. Because some liver enzyme elevation had occurred, a warning was included in the packaging to only prescribe the product for short-term use. Within 1 yr of approval the FDA had received 20 reports of serious hepatotoxic events. Of these 20 reports, four patients died of liver failure and eight required liver transplant. In 1998, 1 yr after approval, Wyeth-Ayerst Laboratories withdrew Duract from the market. Duract caused serious hepatotoxicity in only 1 in 20,000 patients taking the drug for longer than

Table 5-1
Drug Development and Approval

Phase	Number of patients	Focus	Length of trials	Regulatory
Preclinical	Laboratory and animal models (no humans)	Safety, pharmacokinetics	Indeterminate	Investigational new drug application filed IND approval must be received to enter Phase 1 trials
Phase 1	Healthy human volunteers or special populations of intent (up to one hundred)	Safety, tolerability pharmacokinetics	1–2 yr	Continuing updates to IND
Phase 2	Population of intent (up to several hundreds)	Safety, dosing, efficacy, pharmacokinetics	1–2 yr	Continuing updates to IND
Phase 3	Population of intent (up to several thousands)	Safety, efficacy, pharmacoeconomic	2–3 yr	New drug application (NDA) filed
Phase 4	General population	Safety, pharmacoeconomic	Ongoing	NDA approved prior to marketing, followed by a 120 d review Continuing updates and monitoring through FDA MedWatch Program

10 d. To have reliably predicted the hepatotoxicity during clinical trials, roughly 100,000 human exposures to Duract would have had to occur. Only 2400 exposures to this drug occurred before approval. Knowing which patients were at risk for hepatic toxicity could have resulted in their exposure being limited.

The Institute of Medicine reported in January of 2000 that from 44,000 to 98,000 deaths occur annually from medical errors. Of this total, an estimated 7000 deaths occur because of ADEs. An analysis of multiple hospitalized populations has placed much higher estimates on the overall incidence of serious ADEs. This study estimates that 6.7% of hospitalized patients have a serious ADE with a fatality rate of 0.32%. These results lead to an estimate of more than 2,216,000 serious ADEs in hospitalized patients and over 106,000 deaths annually. These results do not address ADEs in the ambulatory setting, and additionally, an estimated 350,000 ADEs occur in US nursing homes each year. The exact number of ADEs is unknown, but ADEs represent a significant public health threat that can be potentially preventable.

VARIABILITY

What causes this range of response in individuals when they are exposed to the same dose of the exact same drug? Human beings are approx 99.9% identical at the genetic level, 100% in the case of monozygotic twins. Yet it is these small individual differences in the sequence of DNA that result in clinically significant variation between individuals. The issue of interindividual variability is central to pharmacogenetics. Individuals who metabolize drugs rapidly may require dosages many times larger than what is recommended in initial research performed on relatively small numbers of subjects. PM may experience toxicity at the recommended dose. If metabolism is required to transform the compound from prodrug to active metabolite, no efficacy may be seen at all. Enzymes responsible for activation and/or transformation of drugs and prodrugs show substantial individual variation.

In addition to metabolism there is also the issue of drug targets. Drugs are designed to function with specific targets such as enzymes or substrates. Because gene expression can be variable, target structures may be mutated. Polymorphisms can cause loss of function, decreased function, or in the case of multiple copies, rapid function. In such cases, drugs administered to an individual may show no benefit and actually increase the risk of ADEs. Multiple agents may be tried in this scenario with the hope that side effects may be tolerable.

Time and money are lost with this method of drug use, whereas the risk to the patient increases because of disease progression and potential ADEs.

Health-care providers must be aware of host factors that can affect how drugs react within the human system. Variability in host factors can play as important a role as metabolism and drug targets in pharmacogenetics. Each of these three areas—variability in metabolism, drug targets, and host factors—is critical in pharmacogenetics.

METABOLISM Of the two phases of metabolism (Phase I and Phase II), Phase II typically results in conjugation of a drug to a water soluble group like a sugar, peptide, or sulfur group and does not usually present the obstacles which Phase I metabolism presents. However, in ill patients Phase II metabolism can be an issue. Many drugs are bound to intracellular proteins such as albumin. In a chronically ill individual albumin levels can be low and result in dangerously high free serum levels of drugs such as phenytoin. Because there are usually an excess of peptide, sugar, and sulfur groups in a well-nourished cell, these reactions are rarely rate limiting and may be best discussed under host factors. Thus for the purposes of discussion, this chapter focuses on Phase I metabolism.

Drugs are metabolized during Phase I by oxidation or reduction reactions. Most drugs are lipophilic in composition allowing for easy movement into cellular membranes. Enzymes are responsible for the biotransformation of very lipophilic molecules in preparation for Phase II metabolism, often accomplished by adding a hydroxyl group resulting in a conjugation site. Most medications require Phase I biotransformation into water-soluble moieties. This action ultimately facilitates excretion. Biotransformation is performed primarily by the cytochrome P450 mono-oxygenase system. These heme-containing proteins are located in the smooth endoplasmic reticulum of many tissues. However, the liver is the main repository of these proteins, and so has a critical role in drug metabolism. This system has broad substrate specificity. It is induced by hundreds of different compounds including steroids and is responsible for the metabolism of up to 50% of all drugs.

In 1962, an unknown pigment was identified as a heme-containing protein. It had a unique 450-nm optical peak in its reduced carbon monoxide form. This led to the term cytochrome-P450 and a designation of "CYP." There are many cytochrome-P450 isoforms; indeed the growing number of identified isoforms led to confusion.

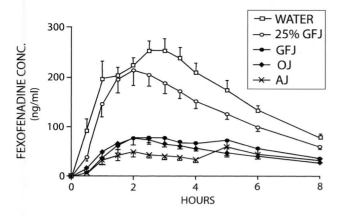

Figure 5-2 Mean plasma fexofenadine concentration–time profiles for persons ($n = 10$) orally administered fexofenadine (120 mg) with 300 mL water, grapefruit juice at 25% of regular strength (25% GFJ), grapefruit juice, orange juice, or apple juice followed by 150 mL of the same fluid every 0.5–3 h (total volume, 1.2 L). (Reprinted from Dresser GK, Bailey DG, Leake BF, et al. Fruit juices inhibit organic anion transporting polypeptide-mediated drug uptake to decrease the oral availability of fexofenadine. Clin Pharmacol Ther 2002;71:11–20, with permission from American Society for Clinical Pharmacology and Therapeutics.)

To rectify this, a classification system is in use. Twelve main cytochrome-P450 gene families have been identified in humans and are designated by a number. To increase specificity, each family is then divided further into a subfamily designated by a letter. Last, the specific location of the gene responsible for the production of that isoform is listed. Thus, CYP2D6 is a cytochrome-P450 protein located in a genetic family with at least 40% similar amino acids and is designated by the number "2." The family is further categorized to amino acids with similar sequences. This is designated by the letter "D." The gene responsible for this particular isoform can be found on chromosome 6. Nine cytochrome-P450 enzymes metabolize most medications but it is CYP3A4 that is responsible for the vast majority of this activity. Following CYP3A4 in importance is CYP2D6.

As an example of the variability in the CYP450 family, consider CYP2D6. This isoform is absent in 7% of Caucasians and 1–2% of non-Caucasians. Extra copies of the isoform are common in East Africans; up to 30% of this population evidences hyperactivity. CYP2D6 is responsible for the primary metabolism of such drugs as codeine, many β-blockers, and tricyclic antidepressants. It is inhibited by drugs such as fluoxetine, haloperidol, paroxetine, and quinidine. Keeping these factors in mind, consider a patient who presents to the emergency department after an automobile accident.

The subject is a healthy young woman, admitted for observation and prescribed codeine for pain. After receiving several doses of codeine through the night, she becomes nauseated and complains of continued unrelieved pain. In evaluating this patient would it be prudent to increase the dose of codeine and add an antiemetic? Or is it possible that she abuses narcotics and thus has developed a tolerance? In this particular case neither explanation is correct. In completing an admission history it should be noted that the patient is also taking paroxetine for depression associated with premenstrual syndrome, and this is an important clue to her lack of response to codeine.

Codeine is a prodrug which requires biotransformation by CYP2D6 to its active metabolite, morphine sulfate. Paroxetine inhibits CYP2D6. Thus, repeated doses of codeine do not relieve

this patient's pain and increase the adverse reaction of nausea. Paroxetine requires a 14 d wash-out period before it is totally eliminated from the body, so its inhibitor effects will be seen in this patient for some time. There are many such drug–drug interactions resulting from issues with the CYP450 system that should be considered. If the individual was of East African descent it would be possible that codeine would never be effective as many individuals in this population lack the required catalysts. This is a perfect example of genetic variability and the role that CYP450 plays in drug efficacy and ADEs. Even something as innocuous as fruit juices can inhibit these enzymes and leave patients to appear as if they are totally lacking the necessary proteins for drug metabolism (Fig. 5-2).

Genetic differences in individuals' ability to metabolize a drug through a given pathway are important contributors to the large interindividual differences in biotransformation within a population. There are PM, EM, and ultra rapid metabolizers, each with progressively more metabolic capacity. Genetic polymorphisms are often responsible for this variability but xenobiotics can also cause changes in the ability to metabolize a drug. For example, CYP1A2 is induced by smoking tobacco and catalyzes the primary metabolism of drugs such as theophylline. Prolonged exposure to tobacco smoke frequently results in chronic obstructive pulmonary disease, often treated with theophylline. Yet the cause of the disease may result in the treatment being ineffective.

A hypothetical example serves to illustrate the potential clinical impact of variability in drug metabolism among individuals. After drug X was tested and approved within a population and becomes commonplace, exposures increase and various patterns become evident. EMs in this population evidence normal enzyme activity. They would represent 75–85% of the hypothetical population. The EMs are homozygous (+/+) or heterozygous (+/–) for the genetic alleles most prevalent in the population and therefore would possess the enzymatic potential to safely metabolize drug X.

Ultra rapid metabolizers would constitute 1–10% of the target population. These individuals would have high-activity alleles that code for the necessary metabolic enzymes leading to very rapid metabolism of the drug. Thus, drug X will never have a chance to reach therapeutic levels. Efficacy would likely never be seen because of increased drug clearance. ADEs may occur as drug X metabolizes rapidly resulting in high metabolite concentrations.

The remaining percentage of the population would fall into the classification of PM. Genetic mutations resulting in loss of function or total absence of the alleles coding for the necessary metabolic enzymes would result in high blood level of a drug. This group would be particularly prone to ADEs as the drug reaches toxic levels.

TRANSPORTERS, TARGETS, AND RECEPTORS The journey is not finished once a drug gets past the cytochrome-P450 system. As stated, drugs must traverse other obstacles to reach their targeted sites. A key ATP-dependent drug efflux transporter (P-glycoprotein), encoded by the multidrug resistance gene (*MDR1*), can play a large role in the availability of protease inhibitors in vitro. Disrupting the function of the P-glycoprotein gene in mice caused the plasma concentration of indinavir, nelfinavir, and saquinqvir to rise dramatically. A compound that would effectively target this P-glycoprotein would result in much higher concentrations of protease inhibitors and thereby more effective HIV treatment.

The *MDR* gene results in the transport out of the cell of a variety of compounds such as cyclosporine A and fexofenadine. In addition its overexpression in a malignancy is associated with resistance to chemotherapeutic agents such as adriamycin and paclitaxel. A broad family of transporter mediators including multiple variants of the *MDR* gene is being studied for their role in drug uptake in the brain, intestine, liver, and kidneys.

Designing drugs to interact with proteins directly involved with the disease process results in more effective treatment. A prominent example of this is the drug trastuzumab (Herceptin®). Herceptin is a recombinant DNA-derived humanized monoclonal antibody that selectively binds with high affinity to the extracellular domain of the human epidermal receptor 2 (HER2). HER2, one of the members of the family of epidermal growth factor receptors, is overexpressed in about 25% of breast tumors. This overexpression portends a poor prognosis. Herceptin® has proven to be highly effective in this population. However, because the drug target is HER2, tumors that do not overexpress this receptor will not be affected by the drug. For this reason genetic testing of tumor tissue by means of fluorescent *in situ* hybridization or immunohistochemical assessment is routinely conducted to determine the value of adding Herceptin to a treatment regimen.

Another example from oncology is the chemotherapeutic agent fluorouracil. A large percentage of this agent is catabolized by the enzyme dihydropyrimidine dehydrogenase (DPD). DPD enzyme deficiency can result in the shunting of fluorouracil into an alternate pathway leading to profound cytotoxicity. This is an instance where testing for the DPD genotype would profoundly increase patient safety.

Oncology is not the only area where progress is being made in the field of pharmacogenetics. Mutations have been identified in the gene *MDR1* that can result in increased plasma concentrations of digoxin, an agent with a notoriously narrow therapeutic index. Function of the β_2 adrenergic receptor gene is a major determinant of an individual's response to albuterol, a common bronchodilator. Such clinically important genetic polymorphisms of the CYP450 system, drug targets, and transporters are being identified through continuing research.

HOST FACTORS   Last is the issue of host factors. Common single gene disorders such as Factor V Leiden need to be considered when medications are prescribed. The prescribing of oral contraceptives to individuals with this prothrombin gene variant greatly increases a woman's risk for deep vein thrombosis. Although mass screening of women for this mutation would prevent the inappropriate exposure of susceptible individuals to oral contraceptives, it would not be cost-effective and would present other problems such as an increase in unwanted pregnancies and the attendant health impacts that would follow. The best alternative is a thorough discussion between patients and practitioners to reveal any family history of thrombosis. This approach would increase patient satisfaction as well as safety.

Fetal alcohol syndrome may occur when a fetus is exposed to elevated alcohol levels although being carried by a mother with polymorphisms in alcohol dehydrogenase. Individuals with the 677C-T polymorphism in the *MTHFR* gene have reduced enzyme activity, which results in elevated plasma homocysteine levels. This inborn error of folic acid production can easily be corrected with supplemental folic acid and may also provide some explanation for the observed prevention of neural tube defects by folic acid.

SELECTED REFERENCES

Carson PE, Flanagan CL, Ickes CE, Alvong AS. Enzymatic deficiency in primaquine sensitive erythrocytes. Science 1956;124:484, 485.

Committee on Quality of Health Care in America: Institute of Medicine. To Err is Human: Building A Safer Health System. Washington, DC: National Academy Press, 2000.

Evans DA. Genetic variations in the acetylation of isoniazid and other drugs. Ann N Y Acad Sci 1968;151(2):723–733.

Flockhart DA. Drug Interactions: Defining genetic influences on pharmacologic responses. Indiana University School of Medicine, Division of Clinical Pharmacology. Indianapolis, Indiana. www.drug-interactions.com. Retrieved January 20, 2004.

Friedman MA, Woodcock J, Lumpkin MM, Shuren JE, Hass AE, Thompson LJ. The safety of newly approved medicines: Do recent market removals mean there is a problem? JAMA 1999;281(18):1728–1734.

Garrod AE, Harris H. Garrod's Inborn Errors of Metabolism. London, New York: Oxford University Press, 1963.

Gurwitz JH, Field TS, Avorn J, et al. Incidence and preventability of adverse drug events in nursing homes. Am J Med 2000;109(2):87–94.

Guthrie R. Screening for "inborn errors of metabolism" in the newborn infant—a multiple test program. Birth Defects 1968;4:92–98.

Ingelman-Sundberg M. Pharmacogenetics: an opportunity for a safer and more efficient pharmacotherapy. J Intern Med 2001;250(3):186–200.

Ingelman-Sundberg M, Oscarson M, McLellan RA. Polymorphic human cytochrome P450 enzymes: an opportunity for individualized drug treatment. Trends Pharmacol Sci 1999;20(8):342–349.

Kim RB, Fromm MF, Wandel C, et al. The drug transporter P-glycoprotein limits oral absorption and brain entry of HIV-1 protease inhibitors. J Clin Invest 1998;101(2):289–294.

Kuivenhoven JA, Jukema JW, Zwinderman AH, et al. The role of a common variant of the cholesteryl ester transfer protein gene in the progression of coronary atherosclerosis. N Engl J Med, 1998; 338(2):86–93.

Lazarou J, Pomeranz BH, Corey PN. Incidence of adverse drug reactions in hospitalized patients: A meta-analysis of prospective studies. JAMA 1998;279(15):1200–1205.

Nebert DW. Pharmacogenetics and pharmacogenomics: why is this relevant to the clinical geneticist? Clin Genet 1999;56(4):247–258.

Smith RL. The paton prize award. The discovery of the debrisoquine hydroxylation polymorphism: scientific and clinical impact and consequences. Toxicology 2001;168(1):11–19.

Trenter M. From test tube to patient: improving health through human drugs. Washington, D C: U.S. Food and Drug Administration Center for Drug Evaluation and Research, 1999 pp. 1–100.

6 Hemophilia as a Model Disease for Gene Therapy of Genetic Disorders

Jay Lozier

SUMMARY

Gene therapy offers the potential for cure of hemophilia, a sex-linked genetic bleeding disorder caused by deficiency of either coagulation factor VIII or coagulation factor IX. The features of hemophilia that make it a leading candidate for gene therapy include the fact that the factor VIII and factor IX genes have been identified and cloned, therapeutic benefit would result from achieving expression at plasma levels as low as 1% of normal, and a wide variety of gene transfer vectors and cell target types could be useful. The challenge is to obtain long-term gene expression at levels sufficient to prevent spontaneous bleeding, while avoiding unwanted toxicity or immune responses to the expressed clotting factor.

Key Words: Adenovirus; AAV; factor VIII; factor IX; gene therapy; gene transfer; hemophilia; lentivirus; retrovirus; vector.

INTRODUCTION

Hemophilia is a model disease for gene therapy of genetic disorders and has attracted tremendous attention from investigators interested in its cure as opposed to its treatment by protein replacement therapy. Hemophilia is actually two diseases, hemophilia A and hemophilia B, resulting from deficiency of factor VIII and factor IX, respectively (Fig. 6-1). The salient features of hemophilia that are attractive for gene transfer are as follows: each is a single-gene disorder, both the factor VIII and factor IX cDNAs have been cloned; active protein may be expressed from either gene in various cell types as long as the correct post-translational modifications are made. Additionally, as little as 1% of normal protein levels could moderate the bleeding phenotype significantly. Overexpression should not be a problem owing to regulation of the factor VIII/factor IX enzyme complex by other downstream enzyme reactions of the blood coagulation "cascade" such as protein C, protein S, and antithrombin III anticoagulant proteins. Although epidemiological studies suggest elevated factor VIII or factor IX levels are associated with thrombotic diseases, it is unlikely that these superphysiological levels of factor VIII or factor IX would be achieved and sustained for the long periods of time described in these studies (years). Preclinical hemophilia gene transfer testing is facilitated by various small and large animal models such as factor VIII and factor IX knockout mice and

spontaneous hemophilia A and B dog colonies. It also is possible to detect epitope-tagged human factor VIII or normal human factor IX in normal monkeys after gene transfer with various vectors, thus permitting assessment of vector safety as well as gene expression in vivo in nonhuman primates.

GENETICS OF HEMOPHILIA

Hemophilia A and B are both X-linked diseases. Thus, they are more common than bleeding disorders resulting from a deficiency of other (autosomal) coagulation factors because any male inheriting a mutation in either the factor VIII or factor IX genes will manifest disease. Inbreeding to produce two defective alleles in an affected individual is therefore not required and *de novo* disease resulting from new mutations is frequently seen. Hemophilia A is more common than hemophilia B for two reasons. First, the factor VIII gene is approx 186,000 bp long, five times the size of the factor IX gene, which is approx 34,000 bp in length. More DNA is therefore "at risk" for mutation by any mechanism in the factor VIII gene than in the factor IX gene. Second, there is a common unique inversion of the factor VIII gene that involves homologous recombination between a transcribed gene in intron 22 of the factor VIII gene and one or the other of two nontranscribed copies of this "factor VIII-associated" gene found outside the factor VIII gene. The resulting inversion puts the first 22 exons of the factor VIII gene in the opposite orientation to the last four exons, and no functional protein is produced in such affected individuals.

MOLECULAR BIOLOGY OF FACTOR VIII AND FACTOR IX

The molecular biology and physiology of factors VIII and IX are important to understand when considering gene therapy of hemophilia A or B. Factor VIII mRNA (approx 9.2 kb) is transcribed from the 186-kb gene in hepatocytes and endothelial cells of the liver and various other organs. Factor IX mRNA (approx 3 kb, half of which is untranslated) appears to be transcribed from the 34-kb gene in hepatocytes exclusively. Factor VIII circulates in trace amounts (approx 100–200 ng/mL) in plasma and has a half-life of 8–12 h in the circulation. Factor IX is found in plasma at levels of approx 5 μg/mL and has a half-life of 18–24 h. Unlike factor VIII, which remains in the circulation and does not normally enter the extravascular space, factor IX traverses blood vessels in equilibrium with the extravascular space. Both factor VIII

From: *Principles of Molecular Medicine, Second Edition*
Edited by: M. S. Runge and C. Patterson © Humana Press, Inc., Totowa, NJ

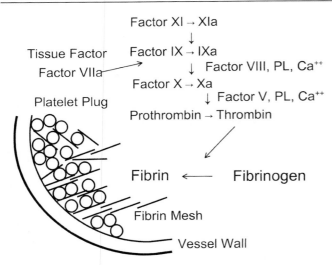

Factor XI → XIa
↓
Tissue Factor   Factor IX → IXa
Factor VIIa —————↗   ↓ Factor VIII, PL, Ca⁺⁺
                             Factor X → Xa
Platelet Plug   ↓ Factor V, PL, Ca⁺⁺
                             Prothrombin → Thrombin

Fibrin ⟵———— Fibrinogen

Fibrin Mesh

Vessel Wall

Figure 6-1 Blood coagulation and the coagulation cascade. Blood coagulation is a dynamic process in which the platelet initially forms a friable hemostatic plug at the site of damage to blood vessels; the temporary plug is reinforced by the deposition of a rigid protein mesh that consists of fibrin. Fibrin is produced by the polymerization of its precursor, fibrinogen, which is converted to fibrin through enzymatic cleavage by the enzyme thrombin. Thrombin is generated in small amounts by a series of tightly regulated enzymatic reactions (the coagulation "cascade") in which a series of serine proteases cleave one another so as to amplify an initiating signal leading to blood clotting. The physiological signal initiating blood coagulation is the subject of much debate but would seem to be mediated by the interaction of platelets with exposed vascular subendothelium followed by interactions between tissue factor (a ubiquitous, cell surface apolipoprotein) and coagulation factor VIIa, one of the coagulation enzymes that circulates in blood. A recurring theme of the coagulation cascade is the interaction of a serine protease with phospholipids in the presence of a large cofactor protein to form an enzyme complex that cleaves and thereby activates another serine protease, which in turn continues the chain of activation events until thrombin is produced. One of these complexes contains the serine protease enzyme factor IX and its cofactor protein, factor VIII. Deficiency of either factor VIII or factor IX results in the clinically indistinguishable bleeding disorders hemophilia A or hemophilia B, respectively. PL, platelets.

and factor IX undergo posttranslational modifications that include attachment of N-linked and O-linked oligosaccharide groups, phosphorylation and sulfation of certain amino acids, and, in the case of factor IX additional carboxylation of γ-carbons of certain glutamic acid residues and β-hydroxylation of a single aspartic acid residue. These properties of the factor VIII and factor IX proteins must be taken into account when designing gene therapy strategies for hemophilia A or hemophilia B.

GENERAL PRINCIPLES OF GENE TRANSFER

Gene therapy may be defined as introduction of a nucleic acid into cells or tissues of a patient with a disease in order to replace the missing function of the defective or absent gene. The process of introducing DNA or RNA into cells (gene transfer) can be accomplished using viruses that have been engineered to contain a gene (or expression cassette) in place of certain viral genes that are normally associated with virulence. This process of producing a viral vector serves the dual purpose of placing a desired gene into the vector for introduction into host cells and removing the viral genes that are required for its replication (and virulence) in the host. Two differing strategies, termed "in vivo" and "ex vivo"

have been the primary strategies employed for gene transfer therapy experiments. In the in vivo approach, a DNA vector containing the desired corrective gene is infused into the living organism in hopes that cells will take up the vector and synthesize the desired product. This strategy is simple and convenient, but suffers from low efficiency of gene transfer. The ex vivo approach consists of removing the target cells from the organism (e.g., fibroblasts from skin, hepatocytes from liver, or hematopoietic cells from the bone marrow), growing them in the laboratory, and introducing the desired vector into the cells at this stage. The altered cells are then replaced back into the organism. This approach results in far more efficient gene transfer but is obviously much more cumbersome.

Typically retroviruses, adenoviruses, and adeno-associated viruses (AAVs) have been used as vectors for gene transfer; each has intrinsic properties that confer certain advantages and disadvantages for the purposes of gene transfer (Table 6-1). For instance, retroviruses have the ability to transfer nucleic acid fragments on the order of about 7 kb in size, adenoviruses can be modified to transfer nucleic acid fragments on the order of up to 34 kb in size, but AAV can only transfer fragments of about 5 kb in length. Titers of adenovirus vectors are typically on the order of 10^{12}–10^{13} vector particles/mL and are exceptionally efficient at in vivo gene transfer into cells of epithelial origin (e.g., lung, liver, and intestinal epithelium), whereas retrovirus vectors are not typically produced in titers of more than 10^8 vector particles/mL without special concentration procedures and are much less efficient at in vivo gene transfer. Accordingly, adenoviruses have been utilized mainly for in vivo gene transfer and retroviruses have been utilized most commonly for ex vivo gene transfer, particularly into hematopoietic cells. Unfortunately, most adenovirus vectors do not have the ability to mediate integration of nucleic acids into host chromosomal DNA to effect long-term gene expression, and furthermore have been associated with significant toxicity at high doses. Therefore, adenovirus vector-mediated gene transfer for long-term correction of a genetic defect is now considered less promising than other vector systems. AAV vectors have been proposed as gene transfer agents with the theoretical ability to mediate integration of nucleic acids, but lack the efficiency of retroviruses, especially the lentiviruses under study. Production of AAV vectors requires either the use of adenovirus as a helper virus, or multiple transfections of nucleic acid constructs into producer cells, which can be problematic because of the need to remove the adenovirus or the lower efficiency of nucleic acid transfections. Potential targets for gene transfer that have been addressed in preclinical studies in vivo include cells from skin, muscle, liver, and bone marrow.

GENE TRANSFER STUDIES IN HEMOPHILIA A AND B

Skin fibroblasts or keratinocytes are easily grown and transduced by a wide variety of gene transfer vectors that may contain selectable markers (e.g., neomycin resistance). Transduced cells can then be reintroduced to the host in which the desired protein will be produced and secreted into the bloodstream. Studies of factor VIII or factor IX transduced fibroblasts or keratinocytes in rodents have shown that significant levels of factor IX or factor VIII can be achieved using retroviral vectors. However, lack of sustained factor VIII or factor IX expression has been a recurring problem and may be owing to loss of transduced cells from cell-mediated immunity or promoter shutdown in the cells that remain

Table 6-1
Properties of Gene Transfer Vectors Used for Gene Therapy

Vector/system	Category	Gene transfer capacity	Vector titer	In vivo tissue tropism/efficiency	Comments
Retrovirus (Moloney murine leukemia virus)	ssRNA virus, enveloped	approx 8.8 kb	$>10^8$ transducing particles/mL	No clear in vivo tropism	Requires cell division for integration into cellular DNA
Retrovirus (lentivirus)	ssRNA virus, enveloped	approx 9.6 kb	$>10^8$ transducing particles/mL	No clear in vivo tropism	Can integrate into cellular DNA of nondividing cells
Adenovirus	dsDNA virus, nonenveloped	up to 34 kb	$>10^{11}$ pfu/mL	Epithelial cells (liver, lung, intestine)	Adenovirus serotype 5 most commonly used as vector
Adeno-associated virus (AAV)	ssDNA virus, nonenveloped	approx 4.5–5.0 kb	10^{13} vector genomes/mL	In vivo tropism varies with serotype	AAV serotype 2 most commonly used as vector; capacity varies with serotype
Herpesvirus (HSV)-1	dsDNA virus, enveloped	approx 30 kb	Not determined	Epithelial and neural cells	HSV-1 most commonly used as vector
Molecular conjugates	"Hybrid of viral/nonviral"	Unlimited	Not applicable	Tropism may be conferred by ligands in conjugate	Adenovirus capsids linked to DNA facilitate gene transfer
Liposomes	Nonviral	Unlimited	Not applicable	No clear in vivo tropism	Low efficiency of gene transfer in vivo; direct application to mucosal surface has been performed in vivo
Naked DNA	Nonviral	Unlimited	Not applicable	No clear in vivo tropism	Typically delivered by injection (e.g., "gene gun")

viable. One clinical trial has been performed in which factor VIII-transfected skin fibroblasts were reimplanted in the omentum. The peak factor VIII levels achieved were only marginally therapeutic, however, and were not sustained. The need to make autologous transduced cells for each individual patient's treatment could be approached by the use of standardized cell lines expressing factor VIII or factor IX contained in an immunoisolation device as protected allografts; however, this has not been tried in humans.

Gene transfer to muscle can be performed using appropriate promoters to direct tissue-specific gene expression. Engineered cells can be implanted in the host, and factor IX has been expressed in mice using muscle cells transduced before reimplantation. Alternatively, muscle cells have been encapsulated in alginate compounds before implantation to protect the modified cells in vivo, permitting them to express human factor IX in immunocompetent mice. Immunodeficient (nude) hemophilia B mice have developed tumors of myoblast origin after implantation of encapsulated cells, which raises the possibility that muscle cell therapies may be tumorigenic in humans under some circumstances. It would be much more practical to transduce myocytes in vivo because there are no human myoblast/myotube cell lines suitable for use in humans.

In vivo gene transfer to muscle by intramuscular injection would be more appealing than ex vivo approaches because the methodology is simpler; one vector could be used for all patients, and there would be no need for in vitro cultivation of patient myocytes. The most extensively studied application of this approach utilizes AAV vectors. AAV vectors can only transfer DNA of total length less than 4.5 kb, which can accommodate factor IX gene transfer, but not factor VIII gene transfer. Preclinical studies with AAV vectors in hemophilia B knockout mice and hemophilia B dogs have achieved sustained, clinically relevant plasma levels of factor IX using this approach. Poor delivery of recombinant factor IX by muscle into plasma is the key problem directly related to the use of muscle as an in vivo target for gene transfer. This has been attributed to binding of factor IX by type-IV collagen, and seems to be mediated by epidermal growth factor-like domains on factor IX. It also appears that AAV gene transfer is significantly more efficient in type-X (slow-twitch) fibers as compared with type-Y (fast-twitch) fibers, perhaps as a consequence of more AAV receptors on the cell surface for the former muscle fiber type. Clinical trials of AAV-factor IX gene transfer targeting muscle have demonstrated therapeutically significant plasma factor IX levels approaching 1% of normal in patients given 2×10^{11} vector genomes/kg. Patients reported fewer joint bleeds and administered fewer doses of factor IX after treatment as compared with the period before treatment. A placebo effect cannot be ruled out because this was an open label study, however. Hopes for greater factor IX plasma levels were not realized when higher doses of AAV-factor IX vector were given to other patients, and the factor IX levels seen in the early trials gradually disappeared. It is not clear whether the loss of factor IX was because of loss of vector, adsorption of factor IX by type-IV collagen, methylation of promoter DNA, or other epigenetic events; inhibitor antibodies to human factor IX were not seen in any of these patients, however.

Nonviral gene transfer by electroporation of plasmid DNA has been studied. Using in vivo electroporation of plasmid DNA into muscle of mice and dogs it has been possible to demonstrate transient factor IX expression at levels of about 1% of normal, which was followed by an antibody response to foreign (human) factor IX. This technique requires confirmation of factor IX activity in hemophilia B animals to confirm its utility.

Factor VIII expression in muscle has not been shown to deliver active factor VIII to the circulation. The amount of factor VIII that can be expressed by muscle cells and secreted in active form into the circulation may be the chief limiting factor to this approach.

Liver hepatocytes synthesize many plasma proteins including coagulation factors VIII and IX, and make some proteins, such as albumin, in tremendous quantities. For these reasons, in vivo gene transfer to liver is one avenue being investigated for hemophilia gene therapy. Hepatocytes cannot be easily propagated in tissue culture, but in vivo gene transfer has been demonstrated in animals using adenovirus, AAV, and retrovirus vectors. Adenovirus vectors can mediate quantitative in vivo gene transfer to hepatocytes when administered intravenously. Thus, it is not surprising that adenovirus vectors have been used for in vivo gene transfer of factor VIII or factor IX to liver cells of mice, monkeys, and hemophilic dogs. Unfortunately, adenovirus-mediated gene transfer is typically characterized by a gradual decrease in gene expression. Moreover, adenovirus vector proteins in immune-competent animals induce numerous cytokines and have powerful adjuvant effects that may cause antibodies to the gene product to be formed. Efforts to create and test vectors with most of the adenovirus genes removed have been pursued, based on the observation that deletion of adenovirus vector genes may result in longer periods of gene expression and a decreased immune response. Problems with production of large quantities of these highly deleted vectors have impeded the translation to clinical trials. At least one clinical trial is testing an extensively deleted adenovirus vector for in vivo factor VIII gene transfer. Use of adenovirus vectors may be limited by neutralizing antibodies to the common serotypes, which commonly infect humans; however, the sequential use of different serotypes of adenovirus vector might be employed to circumvent this problem.

Although AAV-mediated factor VIII gene transfer to liver in vivo has been reported, gene transfer to liver hepatocytes using AAV vectors has focused largely on factor IX, because of the size constraints of vector DNA packaging. Gene transfer of factor IX DNA by intravenous, portal vein, or hepatic artery injection of AAV vectors has resulted in expression of factor IX in mice, dogs, and nonhuman primates. The results of these studies have justified clinical trials, one of which is underway in patients with hemophilia B. This trial was temporarily put on hold because of vector shedding in the semen of the first subject enrolled. After showing that the AAV vector was not incorporated in germline DNA, the trial has resumed but data on factor IX gene transfer and expression are not yet available.

In the field of AAV vector development it has sometimes been difficult to predict the effectiveness of in vivo gene transfer from the results of in vitro experiments. Accordingly, many new approaches are being evaluated. It has been shown recently that different AAV vector serotypes (e.g., AAV 1, AAV 5, AAV 7, AAV 8, and so on) may have advantages for gene transfer regarding DNA capacity or efficiency of gene transfer in particular cell types or animal species, as compared with the AAV 2 vectors that have

been more commonly utilized. Some of the "new" AAV serotypes have been identified as pathogens in nonhuman primates, and their utility in human gene therapy has yet to be proven.

Although retroviral vectors based on Moloney murine leukemia viruses are not suitable for in vivo gene transfer to hepatocytes owing to the low rate of cell division in this cell type, lentivirus vectors (which can transfer genes into nondividing cells) may be useful for hemophilia gene therapy. Pseudotyped lentiviral vectors have been used to transfer the factor VIII cDNA into liver more efficiently than nonpseudotyped vectors.

Hematopoietic cells are logical targets for gene transfer because they could be transduced ex vivo and returned to the donor by marrow transplantation, after which progeny cells would circulate in the bloodstream. In the case of platelets, an additional advantage might be realized because they would be concentrated at the site of vascular injury where factor VIII or factor IX is needed most. Such hematopoietic cell gene transfer has been attempted as an experimental approach to both hemophilia A and B. Retroviral gene transfer of the (B domain-deleted) human factor VIII gene into hemophilia A knockout mouse bone marrow did not result in detectable plasma levels of human factor VIII after transplantation with concomitant myeloablation, but immune tolerance to human factor VIII in recipients of transduced bone marrow was conferred. A nonspecific viral (long terminal repeat) promoter was used to drive expression of factor VIII, thus the vector could in theory direct expression in any progeny cell type, including many nonhematopoietic cell lineages. It is possible that expression of factor VIII in either hematopoietic or nonhematopoietic progeny cells could mediate the immune tolerance response that was seen after gene transfer in these experiments. Similar experiments using a lentiviral vector that expressed factor VIII in hematopoietic cells resulted in antibodies to human factor VIII in mice that were transplanted with transduced bone marrow; it is suggested that the immunogenic (rather than "toleragenic") effect might be owing to higher expression levels seen in lentivirus-transduced cells and/or more efficient transduction of antigen-presenting cells.

Erythroid and megakaryocytic cell lines secrete significantly higher levels of factor VIII than do B- or T-cell lines in vitro when transduced with lentivirus vectors containing factor VIII expression cassettes. Cytokine stimulators had little effect on factor VIII expression, but differentiating agents such as phorbol myristic acid, which activates protein kinase C, induce approx two- to threefold greater factor VIII expression.

Human myeloid leukemia (HL)-60, cells can express factor IX in vitro when transduced by Moloney retroviral vectors; expression from the CMV promoter is increased with phorbol myristic acid (a monocytic differentiating agent) or dimethylsulfoxide (a granulocytic differentiating agent). Human erythroleukemia cells can express factor IX in vitro when expressed under control of a megakaryocyte-specific (glycoprotein IIb) promoter, suggesting that platelets could store the expressed protein in granules that would be available for release at the site of platelet aggregation in vivo. Induction of differentiation resulted in increased levels of factor IX expression in vitro as was seen in previous work with myelomonocytic leukemia cells. However, factor IX has not been expressed at clinically significant levels in vivo by hematopoietic cells.

Stromal fibroblasts are cells from bone marrow, which can be obtained by modestly invasive methods (marrow aspiration) and can be grown easily in tissue culture and transduced by retroviral vectors in vitro. Human marrow stromal cells transduced ex vivo with a gibbon ape leukemia virus-pseudotyped Moloney retroviral vector containing a factor VIII expression cassette showed clinically significant (6% of normal) factor VIII levels after reimplantion of cells in the spleen of NOD-SCID mice. Expression of human factor VIII ceased after approx 4 mo owing to promoter inactivation, however. Reinfusion of factor IX-expressing bone marrow stromal cells in canines after irradiation of marrow (to facilitate growth of infused cells in the marrow) led to detectable levels of factor IX in plasma; it is unlikely that such a procedure would be practical in humans, however.

Under appropriate culture conditions cells that have the properties of endothelial cells can be induced to grow from nucleated peripheral blood cells. These so-called blood outgrowth endothelial cells (or BOECs) have been isolated from humans, transduced with factor VIII vectors, and infused into immunodeficient mice in which they have expressed significant amounts of factor VIII. The BOECs have been shown to persist with endothelial cell properties in the spleen and bone marrow of treated mice. Use of autologous BOECs transduced with factor VIII or factor IX vectors may be another relatively noninvasive avenue for gene therapy of hemophilia in humans.

FUTURE DIRECTIONS

Future issues to be addressed in the field of gene therapy include minimization of the risk for immune response and antibody formation, development of vectors that can sustain high levels of protein expression, and avoidance of germline transmission of vector nucleic acid sequences. It will be instructive to see whether inhibitor antibodies to factor VIII or factor IX in hemophilia gene therapy patients will be observed once the technology is applied to patients who have not had extensive exposure to clotting factor proteins. Novel viral vectors are rapidly being developed and their suitability for gene transfer is being assessed. Novel strategies for expression of relatively large genes such as factor VIII cDNA are required and so-called split vectors may someday permit hemophilia A gene therapy with AAV vectors. Another potential avenue for the introduction of large genes such as hemophilia A is the use of vectors that mediate splicing of normal mRNA in place of defective or missing 3′ mRNA in the message. This method has resulted in transient therapeutic factor VIII levels in hemophilia A knockout mice, and in principle would be an attractive approach to the problem in the common intron 22 inversion of the factor VIII gene in which the last 4 of 26 exons are missing. The hemophilia A dogs in which the same inversion mechanism occurs would be a good model in which to test this approach before clinical trials in patients.

Concerns for the safety of retroviral gene transfer to bone marrow cells have been raised by the finding of clonal T-cell proliferation in two young patients with X-linked severe combined immunodeficiency (SCID)-X1 treated with retroviral gene transfer; in both cases the vector was shown to be integrated into genomic DNA of T cells near the *LMO2* proto-oncogene promoter. It remains to be seen whether this event is specific to patients with SCID-X1, the vector construct used in the trial, or retroviral vectors in general. The lack of similar adverse events in extensive preclinical and clinical experience with retroviral vectors in other trials suggests that the problem is not generic to retroviral vectors. The problem of T-cell leukemogenesis may be related to the selective advantage that T cells gain in SCID patients after transduction with the γ-subunit of the IL-2 receptor (IL2Rγc), compared with nontransduced T cells. Further, the IL2Rγc gene sequence may preferentially integrate in the *LMO2* genomic DNA sequence.

Vector constructs that mediate integration by novel methods have also been described. Novel targets, such as intestinal epithelial cells that have been transduced in vitro by viral and/or nonviral vectors, need to be studied in vivo. These areas are being addressed by investigators throughout the world.

ACKNOWLEDGMENT

This represents the opinion of the author and does not constitute US Government policy.

SELECTED REFERENCES

Andrews JL, Shirley PS, Iverson WO, et al. Evaluation of the duration of human factor VIII expression in nonhuman primates after systemic delivery of an adenoviral vector. Hum Gene Ther 2002;13(11):1331–1336.

Antonarakis SE, Rossiter JP, Young M, et al. Factor VIII gene inversions in severe hemophilia A: Results of an international consortium study. Blood 1995;86:2206–2212.

Axelrod JH, Read MS, Brinkhous KM, Verma IM. Phenotypic correction of factor IX deficiency in skin fibroblasts of hemophilic dogs. Proc Natl Acad Sci USA 1990;87:5173–5177.

Bi L, Lawler AM, Antonarakis SE, High KA, Gearhart JD, Kazazian HH Jr. Targeted disruption of the mouse factor VIII gene produces a model of haemophilia A. Nat Genet 1995;10:119–121.

Brauker J, Frost GH, Dwarki V, et al. Sustained expression of high levels of human factor IX from human cells implanted within an immunoisolation device into athymic rodents. Hum Gene Ther 1998;9(6):879–888.

Brinkhous KM, Graham JB. Hemophilia in the female dog. Science 1950;111:723.

Bristol JA, Gallo-Penn A, Andrews J, Idamakanti N, Kaleko M, Connelly S. Adenovirus-mediated factor VIII gene expression results in attenuated anti-factor VIII-specific immunity in hemophilia A mice compared with factor VIII protein infusion. Hum Gene Ther 2001;12(13):1651–1661.

Chao H, Liu Y, Rabinowitz J, Li C, Samulski RJ, Walsh CE. Several log increase in therapeutic transgene delivery by distinct adeno-associated viral serotype vectors. Mol Ther 2000;2(6):619–623.

Chao H, Mansfield SG, Bartel RC, et al. Phenotype correction of hemophilia A mice by spliceosome-mediated RNA trans-splicing. Nat Med 2003;9(8):1015–1019.

Chao H, Mao L, Bruce AT, Walsh CE. Sustained expression of human factor VIII in mice using a parvovirus-based vector. Blood 2000;95(5):1594–1599.

Chao H, Sun L, Bruce A, Xiao X, Walsh CE. Expression of human factor VIII by splicing between dimerized AAV vectors. Mol Ther 2002;5(6):716–722.

Chao H, Walsh CE. Induction of tolerance to human factor VIII in mice. Blood 2001;97(10):3311–3312.

Choo KH, Gould KG, Rees DJ, Brownlee GG. Molecular cloning of the gene for human anti-haemophilic factor IX. Nature 1982;299(5879):178–180.

Chuah MK, Brems H, Vanslembrouck V, Collen D, Vandendriessche T. Bone marrow stromal cells as targets for gene therapy of hemophilia A. Hum Gene Ther 1998;9(3):353–365.

Chuah MK, Schiedner G, Thorrez L, et al. Therapeutic factor VIII levels and negligible toxicity in mouse and dog models of hemophilia A following gene therapy with high-capacity adenoviral vectors. Blood 2003;101(5):1734–1743.

Chuah MK, Van Damme A, Zwinnen H, et al. Long-term persistence of human bone marrow stromal cells transduced with factor VIII-retroviral vectors and transient production of therapeutic levels of human factor VIII in nonmyeloablated immunodeficient mice. Hum Gene Ther 2000;11(5):729–738.

Davé UP, Jenkins NA, Copeland NG. Gene therapy insertional mutagenesis insights. Science 2004;303:333.

Ehrhardt A, Kay MA. A new adenoviral helper-dependent vector results in long-term therapeutic levels of human coagulation factor IX at low doses in vivo. Blood 2002;99(11):3923–3930.

Evans GL, Morgan RA. Genetic induction of immune tolerance to human clotting factor VIII in a mouse model for hemophilia A. Proc Natl Acad Sci USA 1998;95(10):5734–5739.

Fang B, Eisensmith RC, Wang H, et al. Gene therapy for hemophilia B: host immunosuppression prolongs the therapeutic effect of adenovirus-mediated factor IX expression. Hum Gene Ther 1995; 6: 1039–1044.

Fewell JG, MacLaughlin F, Mehta V, et al. Gene therapy for the treatment of hemophilia B using PINC-formulated plasmid delivered to muscle with electroporation. Mol Ther 2001;3(4):574–583.

Gerrard AJ, Austen DE, Brownlee GG. Recombinant factor IX secreted by transduced human keratinocytes is biologically active. Br J Haematol 1996;95(3):561–563.

Gerrard AJ, Hudson DL, Brownlee GG, Watt FM. Towards gene therapy for haemophilia B using primary human keratinocytes. Nat Genet 1993;3:180–183.

Giannelli F, Green PM, Sommer SS, et al. Haemophilia B: database of point mutations and short additions and deletions, 7th edition. Nucleic Acids Res 1997;25:133–135.

Giles AR, Tinlin S, Greenwood R. A canine model of hemophilic (factor VIII: C deficiency) bleeding. Blood 1982;60:727–730.

Gnatenko DV, Saenko EL, Jesty J, Cao LX, Hearing P, Bahou WF. Human factor VIII can be packaged and functionally expressed in an adeno-associated virus background: applicability to haemophilia A gene therapy. Br J Haematol 1999;104(1):27–36.

Graham JB, Buckwalter JA, Hartley LJ, Brinkhous KM. Canine hemophilia: observations on the course, the clotting anomaly, and the effects of blood transfusion. J Exp Med 1949;90:97–111.

Hacein-Bey-Abina S, Von Kalle C, Schmidt M, et al. LMO2-associated clonal T cell proliferation in two patients after gene therapy for SCID-X1. Science 2003;302(5644):415–419.

Hao Q-L, Malik P, Salazar R, Tang H, Gordon EM, Kohn DB. Expression of biologically active human factor IX in human hematopoietic cells after retroviral vector-mediated gene transduction. Hum Gene Ther 1995;6:873–880.

Herzog RW, Hagstrom JN, Kung S-H, et al. Stable gene transfer and expression of human blood coagulation factor IX after intramuscular injection of recombinant adeno-associated virus. Proc Natl Acad Sci USA 1997;94:5804–5809.

Hoeben RC, van der Jagt RCM, van Tilburg NH, et al. Expression of functional factor VIII in primary human skin fibroblasts after retrovirus-mediated gene transfer. J Biol Chem 1990;265(13):7318–7323.

Hortelano G, Wang L, Xu N, Ofosu FA. Sustained and therapeutic delivery of factor IX in nude haemophilia B mice by encapsulated C2C12 myoblasts: Concurrent tumourigenesis. Haemophilia 2001;7(2):207–214.

Hortelano G, Xu N, Vandenberg A, Solera J, Chang PL, Ofosu FA. Persistent delivery of factor IX in mice: gene therapy for hemophilia using implantable microcapsules. Hum Gene Ther 1999;10(8):1281–1288.

Hough C, Kamisue S, Cameron C, et al. Aberrant splicing and premature termination of transcription of the FVIII gene as a cause of severe canine hemophilia A: similarities with the intron 22 inversion mutation in human hemophilia. Thromb Haemost 2002;87:659–665.

Hurwitz DR, Kirchgesser M, Merrill W, et al. Systemic delivery of human growth hormone or human factor IX in dogs by reintroduced genetically modified autologous bone marrow stromal cells. Hum Gene Ther 1997;8:137–156.

Kemball-Cook G, Barrowcliffe TW. Interaction of factor VIII with phospholipids: Role of composition and negative charge. Thromb Haemost 1992;67:57–71.

Koeberl DD, Alexander IE, Halbert CL, Russell DW, Miller AD. Persistent expression of human clotting factor IX from mouse liver after intravenous injection of adeno-associated virus vectors. Proc Natl Acad Sci USA 1997;94:1426–1431.

Kootstra NA, Matsumura R, Verma IM. Efficient production of human FVIII in hemophilic mice using lentiviral vectors. Mol Ther 2003;7(5):623–631.

Kundu RK, Sangiorgi F, Wu LY, et al. Targeted inactivation of the coagulation factor IX gene causes hemophilia B in mice. Blood 1998;92(1):168–174.

Lakich D, Kazazian HH, Antonarakis SE, Gitschier J. Inversions disrupting the factor VIII gene are a common cause of severe hemophilia A. Nat Genet 1993;5:236–241.

Lensen R, Bertina RM, Vandenbroucke JP, Rosendaal FR. High factor VIII levels contribute to the thrombotic risk in families with factor V Leiden. Br J Haematol 2001;114(2):380–386.

Levinson B, Kenwrick S, Lakich D, Hammonds JG, Gitschier J. A transcribed gene in an intron of the human factor VIII gene. Genomics 1990;7:1–11.

Lin Y, Chang L, Solovey A, Healey JF, Lollar P, Hebbel RP. Use of blood outgrowth endothelial cells for gene therapy for hemophilia A. Blood 2002;99:457–62.

Lin H-F, Maeda N, Smithies O, Straight DL, Stafford DW. A coagulation factor IX-deficient mouse model for human hemophilia B. Blood 1997;90:3962–3966.

Lozier JN, Csako G, Mondoro TH, et al. Toxicity of a first-generation adenoviral vector in rhesus macaques. Hum Gene Ther 2002;13(1):113–124.

Lozier JN, Dutra A, Pak E, et al. The Chapel Hill hemophilia A dog colony exhibits an inversion of the factor VIII gene. Proc Natl Acad Sci USA 2002;99(20):12,991–12,996.

Lozier JN, Metzger ME, Donahue RE, Morgan RA. The rhesus macaque as an animal model for hemophilia B gene therapy. Blood 1999;93(6):1875–1881.

Lozier JN, Metzger ME, Donahue RE, Morgan RA. Adenovirus-mediated expression of human coagulation factor IX in the rhesus macaque is associated with dose-limiting toxicity. Blood 1999;94(12):3968–3975.

Lozier JN, Yankaskas JR, Ramsey WJ, Chen L, Berschneider H, Morgan RA. Gut epithelial cells as targets for gene therapy of hemophilia. Hum Gene Ther 1997;8(12):1481–1490.

Mah C, Sarkar R, Zolotukhin I, et al. Dual vectors expressing murine factor VIII result in sustained correction of hemophilia A mice. Hum Gene Ther 2003;14(2):143–152.

Manno CS, Chew AJ, Hutchison S, et al. AAV-mediated factor IX gene transfer to skeletal muscle in patients with severe hemophilia B. Blood 2003;101(8):2963–2972.

Marshall E. Gene therapy. Panel reviews risks of germ line changes. Science 2001;294(5550):2268–2269.

McCormack MP, Rabbitts TH. Activation of the T-cell oncogene LMO2 after gene therapy for X-linked severe combined immunodeficiency. N Engl J Med 2004;350:913–922.

Nakai H, Storm TA, Kay MA. Increasing the size of rAAV-mediated expression cassettes in vivo by intermolecular joining of two complementary vectors. Nat Biotechnol 2000;18(5):527–532.

Nathwani AC, Davidoff AM, Hanawa H, et al. Sustained high-level expression of human factor IX (hFIX) after liver-targeted delivery of recombinant adeno-associated virus encoding the hFIX gene in rhesus macaques. Blood 2002;100(5):1662–1669.

Naylor JA, Brinke A, Hassock S, Green PM, Giannelli F. Characteristic mRNA abnormality found in half the patients with severe hemophilia A is due to large DNA inversions. Hum Mol Genet 1993;2:1773.

Naylor JA, Buck D, Green P, Williamson H, Bentley D, Giannelli F. Investigation of the factor VIII intron 22 repeated region (int22h) and the associated inversion junctions. Hum Mol Genet 1995;4(7):1217–1224.

Naylor JA, Nicholson P, Goodeve A, Hassock S, Peake I, Giannelli F. A novel DNA inversion causing severe hemophilia A. Blood 1996;87:3255–3261.

Nunes FA, Furth EE, Wilson JM, Raper SE. Gene transfer into the liver of nonhuman primates with E1-deleted recombinant adenoviral vectors: Safety of readministration. Hum Gene Ther 1999;10(15):2515–2526.

Palmer TD, Rosman GJ, Osborne WRA, Miller AD. Genetically modified skin fibroblasts persist long after transplantation but gradually inactivate introduced genes. Proc Natl Acad Sci USA 1991;88:1330–1334.

Palmer TD, Thompson AR, Miller AD. Production of human factor IX in animals by genetically modified skin fibroblasts: potential therapy for hemophilia B. Blood 1989;73(2):438–445.

Plantier JL, Rodriguez MH, Enjolras N, Attali O, Negrier C. A factor VIII minigene comprising the truncated intron I of factor IX highly improves the in vitro production of factor VIII. Thromb Haemost 2001;86(2):596–603.

Rodriguez MH, Enjolras N, Plantier JL, et al. Expression of coagulation factor IX in a haematopoietic cell line. Thromb Haemost 2002;87(3):366–373.

Roth DA, Tawa NE Jr, O'Brien JM, Treco DA, Selden RF. Nonviral transfer of the gene encoding coagulation factor VIII in patients with severe hemophilia A. N Engl J Med 2001;344(23):1735–1742.

Sarkar R, Tetrault R, Gao G, et al. Total correction of hemophilia A mice with canine FVIII using an AAV 8 serotype. Blood 2004;103(4):1253–1260.

Sarkar R, Xiao W, Kazazian HH Jr. A single adeno-associated virus (AAV)-murine factor VIII vector partially corrects the hemophilia A phenotype. J Thromb Haemost 2003;1(2):220–226.

Schnell MA, Zhang Y, Tazelaar J, et al. Activation of innate immunity in nonhuman primates following intraportal administration of adenoviral vectors. Mol Ther 2001;3(5 Pt 1):708–722.

Stein CS, Kang Y, Sauter SL, et al. In vivo treatment of hemophilia A and mucopolysaccharidosis type VII using nonprimate lentiviral vectors. Mol Ther 2001;3(6):850–856.

Tonn T, Herder C, Becker S, Seifried E, Grez M. Generation and characterization of human hematopoietic cell lines expressing factor VIII. J Hematother Stem Cell Res 2002;11(4):695–704.

van Hylckama Vlieg A, van der Linden IK, Bertina RM, Rosendaal FR. High levels of factor IX increase the risk of venous thrombosis. Blood 2000;95(12):3678–3682.

Van Raamsdonk JM, Ross CJ, Potter MA, et al. Treatment of hemophilia B in mice with nonautologous somatic gene therapeutics. J Lab Clin Med 2002;139(1):35–42.

Wang L, Nichols TC, Read MS, Bellinger DA, Verma IM. Sustained expression of therapeutic level of factor IX in hemophilia B dogs by AAV-mediated gene therapy in liver. Mol Ther 2000;1(2):154–158.

Wang J-M, Zheng H, Blaivas M, Kurachi K. Persistent systemic production of human factor IX in mice by skeletal myoblast-mediated gene transfer: feasibility of repeat application to obtain therapeutic levels. Blood 1997;90:1075–1082.

Wang L, Zoppe M, Hackeng TM, Griffin JH, Lee K-F, Verma IM. A factor IX-deficient mouse model for hemophilia B gene therapy. Proc Natl Acad Sci USA 1997;94:11,563–11,566.

White SJ, Page SM, Margaritis P, Brownlee GG. Long-term expression of human clotting factor IX from retrovirally transduced primary human keratinocytes in vivo. Hum Gene Ther 1998;9(8):1187–1195.

Wood WI, Capon DJ, Simonsen CC, et al. Expression of active human factor VIII from recombinant DNA clones. Nature 1984;312: 330–337.

Xiao W, Chirmule N, Berta SC, McCullough B, Gao G, Wilson JM. Gene therapy vectors based on adeno-associated virus type 1. J Virol 1999;73(5):3994–4003.

Yao SN, Farjo A, Roessler BJ, Davidson BL, Kurachi K. Adenovirus-mediated transfer of human factor IX gene in immunodeficient and normal mice: evidence for prolonged stability and activity of the transgene in liver. Viral Immunol 1996;9(3):141–153.

Yao S, Kurachi K. Expression of human factor IX in mice after injection of genetically modified myoblasts. Proc Natl Acad Sci USA 1992;89: 3357–3361.

Yao S-N, Smith KJ, Kurachi K. Primary myoblast-mediated gene transfer: persistent expression of human factor IX in mice. Gene Ther 1994;1: 99–107.

7 Genetic Counseling

ROBIN L. BENNETT

"Genetic counseling is the process of helping people understand and adapt to the medical, psychological and familial implications of genetic contributions to disease. This process integrates:

— Interpretation of family and medical histories to assess the chance of disease occurrence or recurrence.

— Education about inheritance, testing, management, prevention, resources and research.

— Counseling to promote informed choices and adaptation to the risk of condition."

—National Society of Genetic Counselors, 2006

SUMMARY

Genetic counseling is an expanding field in the age of genomic medicine. Genetic counselors provide services to clients across the lifespan, from preconception counseling to prenatal diagnosis, the diagnosis of newborns or pediatric genetic disorders, and the diagnosis of adults with inherited predisposition to diseases such as cancer, presenile dementia, psychiatric disorders, and heart disease. The approach to genetic counseling involves assessing family, medical, and environmental history to determine disease risk; assisting in genetic testing, diagnosis, and disease prevention and management; and offering psychosocial and ethical guidance to help patients make informed, autonomous health care and reproductive decisions. Genetic counseling focuses on complex issues related to the value of genetic testing, and on medical interventions and health care practices that have varying degrees of efficacy and success. The traditional dogma that genetic counseling must be nondirective is being challenged in favor of a psychosocial approach that emphasizes shared deliberation and decision making between the counselor and the client.

Key Words: Cancer genetics; genetic counseling; genetic testing; neurogenetics; prenatal genetics.

INTRODUCTION

Historically, the practice of genetic "counseling" focused on providing information about recurrence risks for particular conditions within a family. The first clinics providing information on disease inheritance were established in the early 1900s in Cold Spring Harbor, New York and the University College, London, where scientists collected data on human traits and sometimes provided information to affected families, with the primary purpose of "...accumulating and studying records of physical and mental characteristics of human families to the end that the people may be better advised as to reproduce fit and unfit marriages, and in order to establish the potentialities of an individual."

The horrendous excesses of Nazi Germany and the eugenics movement in the first half of the 20th century led to a retreat from advising families about potential hereditary conditions to a more neutral educational model. Risk information was provided to couples and families with the main options being to "take their chances" by becoming pregnant or to refrain from pregnancy. Sheldon Reed is credited with introducing the term "genetic counseling" in 1947. In the 1940s, genetics clinics were staffed by physicians and doctoral geneticists, using a medical/prevention model that primarily involved providing "facts" (risk figures, natural history, and treatment information) so that couples and families could make informed reproductive decisions.

With the advent of carrier testing and prenatal diagnosis in the 1960s and 1970s, couples and families were faced with a new range of choices. The educational model of providing genetic information did not facilitate patient decision-making. In 1969, Melissa Richter had the foresight to initiate the development of a master's degree program in genetic counseling. The provision of genetic information shifted to a more client-centered approach with information being presented within a psychological and cultural context so clients could make informed decisions regarding genetic testing and reproductive options. A tenet of nondirectiveness, particularly regarding reproductive choices, was held firmly in this genetic counseling model, to demonstrate respect for patient's autonomy and to clearly distance the genetic counselors of this era from the earlier eugenics movement.

Genetic counseling is an expanding field in the age of genomic medicine. Genetic counselors provide services to clients across the lifespan, from preconception counseling to prenatal diagnosis, the diagnosis of newborns or pediatric genetic disorders, and the diagnosis of adults with inherited predisposition to diseases such as cancer, presenile dementia, psychiatric disorders, and heart disease. The approach to genetic counseling involves assessing family and environmental history to determine disease risk; assisting in genetic testing, diagnosis, and disease prevention and management; and offering psychosocial and ethical guidance to help patients make informed, autonomous health care and reproductive

From: *Principles of Molecular Medicine, Second Edition*
Edited by: M. S. Runge and C. Patterson © Humana Press, Inc., Totowa, NJ

decisions. Genetic counseling focuses on complex issues related to the value of genetic testing, and on medical interventions and health care practices that have varying degrees of efficacy and success. The traditional dogma that genetic counseling must be nondirective is being challenged in favor of a psychosocial approach that emphasizes shared deliberation and decision-making between the counselor and the client. As genetic counselor Beth Fine noted in 1998, "Genetic counselors function within the health care system as patient advocates who aim to empower patients and families to find solutions to problems and ways of coping that are optimal for them."

WHAT IS UNIQUE ABOUT GENETIC INFORMATION?

As more tests are developed that identify a hereditary component to common chronic disorders such as cancer, heart disease and presenile dementia, genetic disorders are no longer categorized in the exclusive realm of rare, mostly pediatric diseases. Competency in genomic medicine is important for all health professionals, and an idea of "genetics exceptionalism" may no longer apply. But there are still several features of genetic information that present unique personal, family, and social consequences that distinguish genetic disorders from other nonhereditary medical conditions.

Obviously, genetic disorders are familial. A genetic diagnosis may embrace multiple generations and members of a family. Often, to provide comprehensive risk assessment to relatives, molecular testing must first be performed on an affected relative to identify the specific gene mutation. When a client seeks an opinion of a surgeon for knee surgery, no other relatives are involved; the consultation remains a private conversation between the consultant and the health provider. In contrast, a healthy woman with a strong family history of breast cancer seeking an opinion regarding her options for breast cancer risk reduction and surveillance may need to obtain medical records and death certificates on multiple affected relatives. Testing the client's affected mother or sister to identify a gene mutation may be important to provide the consultant with critical information regarding whether she has a high lifetime risk to develop breast and possibly other cancers. In medical genetics, a whole extended family often becomes the client unit, raising unique issues of confidentiality and privacy of health and personal information.

Knowledge of familial disease risks might have profound effects (both positive and negative) on interpersonal relationships among family members. Parental guilt is a common experience of the parents of affected offspring. Children might blame a parent for passing on the genetic disorder in the family, or partners may blame each other for the birth of an affected child. Survivor guilt is another common problem that is experienced by unaffected individuals in a family who have "escaped" the genetic disease in the family. The healthy individuals may wonder why they are unaffected whereas other relatives have been less fortunate. The "survivor" may feel on the outskirts of the "family team" despite knowing it is irrational to desire ill health.

The familial nature of genetic disorders may alter reproductive plans of many relatives. The parental role is often threatened by learning genetic carrier status. There may be challenges to religious and ethical belief systems between couples and their extended family as couples wrestle with core values of biological parenting and views on adoption, assistive reproductive technologies (including donor gametes and preimplantation diagnosis), prenatal diagnosis, and potential abortion.

Although remarkable advances are continuing to be made in the general understanding of the mechanism of many genetic disorders, unfortunately, durable cures such as gene therapy have been slow to become reality. The permanent nature of genetic disease may bring a sense of fatalism or hopelessness with the diagnosis or results of genetic testing.

Genetic disorders are chronic, thus there is often a continual array of new health and physical challenges over a person's lifetime. Individuals with a genetic disorder often experience increasing medical problems as they age. The individual and the family may experience "chronic sorrow" for the "healthy person who will never be."

Genetic disorders are complex, usually affecting multiple organ systems. Frequently, a multidisciplinary team approach is needed to provide comprehensive care to persons with inherited disorders. Individuals with rare genetic disorders often face continual frustration attempting to locate health professionals with experience in their condition. They may feel extremely isolated, with a sense that no one else is quite like them. Linking these individuals through disease specific support networks (such as the Genetic Alliance) can be instrumental in providing clients with the emotional and medical support they require. Genetic disorders often demonstrate enormous variability of disease expression, with some individuals having few manifestations and others have multiple disabling features of the condition. This clinical variability further confounds the understanding of appropriate management for individuals with genetic disorders and makes prognostic predictions close to impossible.

Unfortunately, genetic disorders continue to be labeling. As Francis Galton observed, "Most men and women shrink from having their hereditary worth recorded. There may be family diseases of which they hardly dare to speak, except on rare occasions, and then in whispered hints, or obscure phrases as though timidity of utterance could hush thoughts…." A genetic diagnosis still carries the potential for social stigma. A person may be considered less desirable as a mate or employee. The family may feel their heritage is "tainted." Fear of genetic discrimination (insurance, employment, and societal) may hinder the willingness of individuals and their families to participate in genetic testing and research.

The ability to test a healthy person for possible future health status provides new challenges to traditional definitions of "healthy" and "diseased." Not long ago, the usual appointment with a health professional centered on the client's specific medical symptoms. Now, a healthy person can be tested for a growing list of potential inherited diseases. Yet, the spectrum of disorders for which there is effective medical therapy remains relatively small compared with the burgeoning number of available genetic tests. None of these genetic tests predict the exact age a person will develop the genetic condition nor do they predict the specific manifestations and severity of the disease. Jonsen and colleagues coined the term the "unpatient" for this group of "genetically unwell" but outwardly healthy individuals who have inherited a gene mutation predisposing to disease. An individual with diagnostic results that are opposite of his or her preconceived affected status may be at higher risk for adverse psychological consequences. Results of genetic testing may alter the person's self-concept and self-esteem, as well as his or her perceptions of wellness and genetic or social identity.

WHO ARE GENETIC COUNSELORS?

Genetic counseling is a distinct medical specialty with the role of providing clinical health care, education and emotional support to individuals and families challenged by congenital and inherited diseases. The field of genetic counseling developed from a

Table 7-1
Resources for Locating a Genetics Professional

National Society of Genetic Counselors	www.nsgc.org
Gene Clinics	www.geneclinics.org
International Federation of Human Genetics Societies	www.ifhgs.org/genetics/ifhgs/members.htm

need to educate, manage, and counsel individuals and families diagnosed with, or at risk for genetic diseases, with respect to how these conditions affect the psychological, medical, financial, and social aspects of life.

The term "genetic counselor" is generally reserved for masters-level health professionals with extensive training in human genetics and counseling skills. The first group of ten genetic counselors graduated from Sarah Lawrence College in 1971. There are 30 programs in the United States and Canada accredited by the American Board of Genetics Counseling (ABGC) with similar programs in place in the United Kingdom, South Africa, Australia, Cuba, Norway, the Netherlands, Taiwan, Spain, Sweden, Saudi Arabia, Japan, France, Israel, and China. As of 2004, there were more than 2300 members of the professional society of genetic counselors, the National Society of Genetic Counselors.

Graduates from genetic counseling programs accredited by the ABGC demonstrate competencies in 27 areas within four critical domains: communication, critical-thinking, interpersonal counseling, and psychosocial assessment, and professional ethics and values. Didactic coursework in genetic counseling training programs involves human and medical genetics, cytogenetics, developmental biology and embryology, teratology, statistics, qualitative and quantitative research, counseling theory, communication skills, interviewing techniques, and public health. Clinical skills are obtained by a combination of role-playing and >800 h of comprehensive supervised fieldwork in a variety of practice settings. Teaching experience and completion of a thesis or other scholarly enterprise are ABGC accreditation requirements. Program lengths are approx 2 academic years.

Adopted in 1993 and revised in 2006, The Code of Ethics of the National Society of Genetic Counselors is an "ethic of care," because this approach emphasizes the interdependence of individuals and reflects the values, principles and beliefs of genetic counselors. The relationships are genetic counselors themselves; genetic counselors and their clients; genetic counselors and their colleagues; and genetic counselors and society. A primary focus is respect for client autonomy and patient advocacy.

Most genetic counselors work in university medical centers, private and public hospitals, or large medical facilities. Genetic counselors work independently or as a member of a multispecialty team. An increasing number of genetic counselors work with diagnostic laboratories and pharmaceutical companies as well as in positions related to the development of government and public policy. Genetic counselors are also uniquely trained to work as research coordinators for genetic research studies. Most genetic counselors are involved in education, including providing education to a variety of health professionals and community organizations, as well as students at all levels, from elementary schools to postgraduate programs.

Other health professionals that are specifically trained to provide genetic counseling services include physician (medical) geneticists and clinical nurse specialists in genetics. Medical geneticists attend a fellowship or residency program through a program accredited by the American Board of Medical Genetics or the Canadian College of Medical Genetics. Clinical geneticists often have particular areas of interest such as oncology, pediatrics, dysmorphology, prenatal diagnosis, neurogenetics, or metabolic disorders. Advance Practice Genetic Nurses meet genetic competencies through a portfolio process established by the International Society of Nurses in Genetics and the Genetic Nurses Credentialing Committee.

All health care professionals need to develop basic aptitude in human genetics as genomic medicine becomes incorporated into all fields of medicine. The National Coalition of Health Care Provider Education in Genetics has developed a set of core competencies that can be adapted to various health specialties. Recognizing the need for genetic counseling and referral to a genetics specialist is an important component of these competencies. Table 7-1 includes a list of resources for locating health professionals with expertise in genetic counseling and medical genetics; many of these listings include specialty areas of practice (such as cancer genetics, neurogenetics, prenatal genetics, and so on).

THE PROCESS OF GENETIC COUNSELING

Genetic counseling sessions with clients and their families may involve a one-time crisis intervention dealing with a new genetic diagnosis, or may develop into a relationship over many years if the client is treated in a specialty clinic for diseases such as hemophilia, neurofibromatosis, fragile X syndrome, or Huntington disease. The genetic counseling intervention is designed to reduce the client's anxiety, enhance the client's sense of control, and mastery over life circumstances, increase the client's understanding of the genetic disorder and options for testing and disease management, and provide the individual and family with the tools required to adjust to potential outcomes. A major paradigm of genetic counseling is that it is noncoercive. The information provided during genetic counseling helps the individual and family personalize often threatening information in order to clarify their values and strengthen their coping mechanisms.

Whether a genetic counseling session is a one-time visit or over many years, there are three broad areas that are covered in each session, assessment, education, and counseling.

ASSESSMENT   The process of genetic counseling begins with "contracting"—the merging of the counselor's and client's expectations. Why is the client here? What are their concerns? What are the mutual expectations and goals of the session? Gathering information during the phone intake or early in the visit assists in developing patient rapport and realistic expectations of the visit as well as appropriate triage to other health professionals. Explaining what will happen and who is involved in the visit can help alleviate client anxiety. What are the client's preconceived notions about patterns of inheritance, chances of testing positive or developing the family disorder? What is the perceived burden of the disease (financial, emotional, and social)? If the genetic counseling information is divergent from a client's perceptions, the client may have difficulty incorporating the information or implementing disease-management recommendations. Throughout the process of genetic counseling,

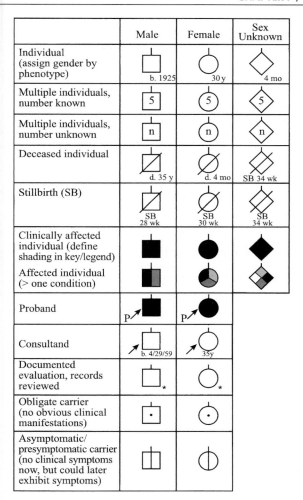

	Male	Female	Sex Unknown
Individual (assign gender by phenotype)	b. 1925	30 y	4 mo
Multiple individuals, number known	5	5	5
Multiple individuals, number unknown	n	n	n
Deceased individual	d. 35 y	d. 4 mo	SB 34 wk
Stillbirth (SB)	SB 28 wk	SB 30 wk	SB 34 wk
Clinically affected individual (define shading in key/legend)			
Affected individual (> one condition)			
Proband	P	P	
Consultand	b. 4/29/59	35 y	
Documented evaluation, records reviewed	*	*	
Obligate carrier (no obvious clinical manifestations)			
Asymptomatic/presymptomatic carrier (no clinical symptoms now, but could later exhibit symptoms)			

Figure 7-1 Pedigree symbols. Reproduced with permission from the University of Chicago, from Bennett RL, Steinhaus KA, Uhrich SB, et al. Recommendations for standardized human pedigree nomenclature. Am J Hum Genet 1995;56:745–752.

	Male	Female	Sex Unknown
Pregnancy (P)	LMP: 7/1/94	20 wk	16 wk
Spontaneous abortion (SAB), ectopic (ECT)	male	female	ECT
Affected SAB	male	female	16 wk
Termination of pregnancy (TOP)	male	female	12 wk
Affected TOP	male	female	12 wk

Figure 7-2 Additional pedigree symbols. Reproduced with permission from the University of Chicago, from Bennett RL, Steinhaus KA, Uhrich SB, et al. Recommendations for standardized human pedigree nomenclature. Am J Hum Genet 1995;56:745–752.

such as distinguishing absolute from relative risks (e.g., a 10% absolute risk but a threefold increased relative risk), and using percentages to frame the magnitude of risks from different perspectives. For example, if an autosomal-recessive pattern is the mode of inheritance, the chance of having an affected child would be framed in terms of a 25% or one in four chance of occurrence or recurrence, as well as a 75% chance or three in four chance that a son or daughter would be unaffected.

Has a diagnosis been established? Confirmation of family medical information through review of medical records and death certificates or even obtaining family photographs can be essential to ensure that the pedigree, and thus the risk assessment provided to the client, is based on accurate information. A client's recall of information about second- and third-degree relatives (e.g., aunts and uncles, grandparents, and cousins) is much less likely to be accurate than information about more closely related relatives (e.g., siblings, parents, and children).

EDUCATION AND HEALTH PROMOTION Knowledge is more than information. Genetic counselor Ann C. M. Smith noted, "Individuals and families affected by genetic diseases face a plethora of high tech information from which they seek to gain true knowledge about their genetic circumstances. What is said and how information is communicated can have a significant impact on their ability to process the information, and to their understanding and assimilation into personal life circumstances. To place more power into the hands of individuals and their families affected by genetic disease is to be sure that they have adequate knowledge—not just information—about their genetic circumstance…the genetic counselor seeks to effectively "communicate" such highly technical genetic information in a way that is compassionate, empathic, and sensitive to the ethnocultural values of the client. In this way, the genetic encounter moves from basic patient education to the multifaceted practice of genetic counseling."

Genetic education and health promotion usually involves communication about the following areas:

• Discussing options for available genetic testing or diagnostic procedures (including testing costs, sensitivity, and specificity), and arranging for testing as appropriate.

there is continual appraisal of family beliefs about causation, and of emotional, experiential, social, educational, and cultural issues that may affect the client's incorporation of information and coping patterns.

Early in the session a medical family history is recorded using standard pedigree symbols (Figs. 7-1–7-3). Usually a pedigree includes two generations of ascent from the consultant (the person seeking information) or proband (the first affected relative who brings the family to medical attention), and two generations of descent. For example, pedigree assessment for a 60-yr-old man with a family history of colorectal cancer would include information about his parents, grandparents, aunts and uncles, and possibly his cousins, as well as information regarding his siblings, children, and likely his grandchildren. A pedigree is an important method of establishing patient rapport and serves as a visual demonstration for providing patient education on variation in disease expression in the family, as well as identifying other relatives at risk for disease.

Statistical risk assessment based on pedigree analysis, epidemiology (such as Hardy-Weinberg equilibrium), various risk models (such as Bayes theorem), and the sensitivity and specificity of various genetic tests is central to genetic counseling. Genetic counseling involves explaining risks in multiple ways,

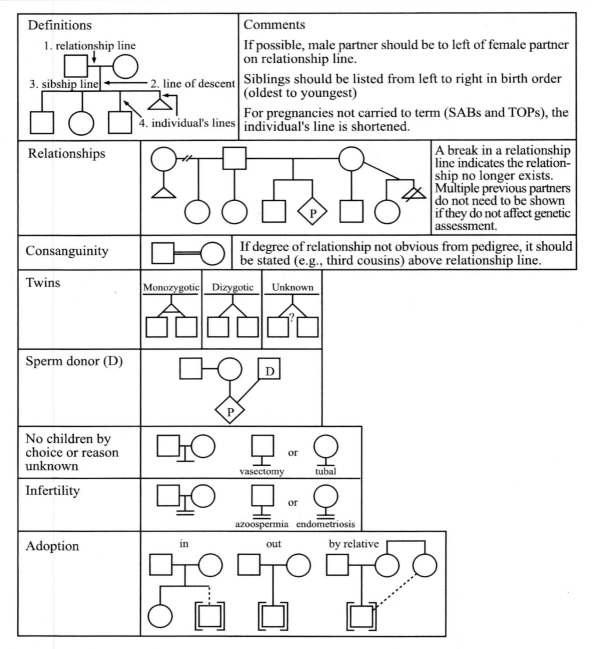

Figure 7-3   Pedigree relationships. Reproduced with permission from the University of Chicago, from Bennett RL, Steinhaus KA, Uhrich SB, et al. Recommendations for standardized human pedigree nomenclature. Am J Hum Genet 1995;56:745–752.

- Review of the inheritance pattern(s) and natural history of the condition, disease monitoring and management, available preventive measures, and reproductive options.
- Options for prenatal diagnosis and availability of assistive reproductive technologies (e.g., gamete donation, preimplantation diagnosis).
- Provision of contact information for disease specific support groups (*see* www.geneticalliance.org).
- Referral to community resources and health specialists, as needed.
- Recommendations for genetic evaluation of other relatives with information about local resources for relatives that live in other communities.

Because of the potentially profound effect that a genetic diagnosis may have on the life of the individual being evaluated, genetic test results are usually relayed in person. A support person is encouraged to attend most genetic counseling visits, especially when tests results are disclosed. A follow-up visit or phone call to discuss the client and family's reaction to the results is advisable.

Patients are likely to remember only about half of the information presented during a clinical visit. Focusing on areas of client concern that were ascertained in the initial assessment helps make the information meaningful to the client. Patients also remember best what they are told first; therefore concentrating on the most important issues in the beginning of the session aids client recall. Providing opportunity for questions and for clients to restate the

Table 7-2
Pros and Cons of Genetic Testing of an Asymptomatic Minor

Potential adverse consequences of testing (focus on positive test results)	Potential benefits of testing
Damage to the minor's self esteem	Resolution of the parent's (and possibly the child's) concerns about mutation status
Distortion of the family's perception of the child. Siblings may be treated differently depending on their genetic status	Allow child and family time to adjust to status if test is positive. No anticipation of developing disease if result is negative
Child may identify with severely affected relatives	Affected relatives can be positive role models for child
Loss of future adult autonomy and confidentiality for the tested child	Anticipatory guidance such as choosing physical activities and occupation for possibly affected child
Adverse effects on the child's capacity to form future relationships	Health status is normalized and perception of disease becomes part of the child's sense of self
Fear of rejection in forming long-term relationships. Fear/guilt if person wants biological children	Ability to make informed reproductive decisions
Fear/guilt if person wants biological children. Chronic sadness for "planned" family.	Anticipatory guidance regarding reproductive decisions (e.g., discussions of alternative forms of parenting such as adoption and donor gametes)
Discrimination (insurance, employment, education, choice of mate)	Decreased premiums for insurance because risk factor eliminated if test result is negative
Increased medical surveillance for "healthy" child. Child feels labeled	Available at earliest opportunity for medical intervention (if available)

From Bennett RL, Hart KA, O'Rourke E, et al. Fabry disease in genetic counseling practice: recommendations of the National Society of Genetic Counselors. J Genet Couns 2002;11:121–146. With kind permission of Springer Science and Business Media.

information in their own terms also allows the health professional to estimate how much of the information is understood by the patient. Providing information in several ways to accommodate different learning styles (e.g., verbal, audiovisual, written, and websites) is useful. A patient follow-up letter (that can also be sent to relevant health professionals) provides a resource after the clinic visit that may be referred to even years later, and also assists with coordination of patient care and as a resource for informing at-risk relatives.

COUNSELING Genetic counseling is multifaceted; it includes assessing personal, social, religious, and ethnocultural views on how a genetic diagnosis, genetic testing, and test results affect the client's life. Assessing possible ethical concerns such as confidentiality, disparate paternity, concerns about insurability, views on discrimination, employment issues, feeling about reproduction, and prenatal diagnosis, and testing minor individuals for adult onset conditions are some of the many areas that are explored in genetic counseling. Understanding the client's perception of risk is more important than the actual risk number. Did the client have a preconceived notion of whether the "chances" were high? What percentage risk does the client consider acceptable or too high? Is the information presented different from what the client expected? Patient decisions are supported in the context of individual values, beliefs and goals. There are several excellent books that review the many counseling issues and process of genetic counseling.

THE FUTURE OF GENETIC COUNSELING

The demands for genetic counseling will increase as new genetic tests continually become available. Pharmacogenetics and susceptibility counseling pose novel challenges to the system of genetic counseling that has traditionally concentrated on rare genetic disorders with clear patterns of Mendelian inheritance. Models of genetic counseling must continue to evolve. Can the health care system afford the time intensive previsit preparation, interviewing, assessment, and counseling intervention that the present genetic counseling model embraces? It can be argued that

the subject matter at the core of genetic counseling sessions—heart-wrenching reproductive choices or decisions centering on extreme prevention measures such as prophylactic mastectomy or oophorectomy—deserve more time than what has become the usual 10-min health encounter.

Genetic advances will challenge ethics of care. For example, it is generally thought that healthy minors should not be tested for adult-onset conditions in which there are no treatments, yet there may be benefits to testing children under certain circumstances (Table 7-2). With the advent of high-throughput genetic technologies such as tandem mass spectrometry, a growing number of disorders with limited treatments are being added to the diseases that are available for newborn screening—the potential is there for simultaneous screening for hundreds of diseases. How can parents truly be educated and counseled about the implications of so many disorders? Is there significant natural history data on these diseases to know the age that a medical intervention should be implemented? Will parents have a choice regarding which screening tests are given to their newborns?

Finally, the atrocities that were committed in the spirit of genetic research and "ethnic cleansing" in the Eugenics era must never be forgotten. By 1926, laws mandating sterilization of the "mentally defective" were implemented by 23 of the 48 United States. Federal immigration quotas limited immigration by "inferior" ethnic groups. Euthanasia was a legal program in Nazi Germany, where the lives of over 70,000 people with hereditary disorders were extinguished, in addition to the six million Jews and others who were murdered. With the clarity of hindsight modern human geneticists shudder at these early biases and abuses. Yet, genetic counselor Robert Resta notes that genetic research as all scientific research may be "influenced by the political and social beliefs of all-too-human geneticists. Those beliefs may be so ingrained that we mistake them for biological laws. It is, I suspect, beyond our ability to know which of our personal biases we are disguising as scientific truths. The whispers and hints of our biases may be heard only by future generations of geneticists." The voluntary nature of genetic testing and the availability of genetic counseling by skilled health professionals must continue.

SELECTED REFERENCES

American Board of Genetic Counseling, Bethesda, Maryland; www.abgc.net. Accessed Feb. 22, 2006.

American Board of Medical Genetics, Bethesda, Maryland; www.abmg.org. Accessed Feb. 22, 2006.

Baker DL, Schuette JL, Uhlmann WR, eds. A Guide to Genetic Counseling. New York: Wiley-Liss, 1998.

Bennett RL. The Practical Guide to the Genetic Family History. New York: John Wiley and Sons, Inc., 1999.

Bennett RL, Hampel HL, Mandell JB, Marks JH. Genetic counselors: translating genomic science into clinical practice. J Clin Invest 2003; 112:1274–1279.

Bennett RL, Hart KA, O'Rourke E, et al. Fabry disease in genetic counseling practice: recommendations of the National Society of Genetic Counselors. J Genet Couns 2002;11:121–146.

Bennett RL. Steinhaus KA, Uhrich SB, et al. Recommendations for standardized human pedigree nomenclature. Am J Hum Genet 1995;56: 745–752.

Biesecker BB. Back to the future of genetic counseling: commentary on "psychosocial genetic counseling in the post-nondirective era." J Genet Couns 2003;12:213–217.

Biesecker B, Peter K. Genetic counseling: ready for a new definition? J Genet Couns 2003;11:536, 537.

Ciarleglio LJ, Bennett RL, Williamson J, Mandell JB, Marks JH. Genetic counseling throughout the life cycle. J Clin Invest 2003;112: 1280–1286.

Claus EB, RIsch N, Thompson WD. Autosomal dominant inheritance of early-onset breast cancer: implications for risk prediction. Cancer 1994;73:643–651.

Fine BA. Genetic counseling. In: Jameson JL, ed. Principles of Molecular Medicine, Totowa, New Jersey: Humana Press, 1998, pp. 89–95.

Gail MH, Brinton LA, Byar DP, et al. Projecting individualized probabilities of developing breast cancer for white females who are being examined annually. J Natl Cancer Inst 1989;81:1879–1886.

Genetic Alliance, Washington, DC; www.geneticalliance.org Accessed Feb. 22, 2006.

Genetic Nursing Credentialing Commission, Inc., Hot Springs, Arkansas; www.geneticnurse.org. Updated April, 2005. Accessed 21-7-05.

International Society of Nurses in Genetics, Pittsburgh, PA. www.isong.org. Accessed Feb. 22, 2006.

Jonsen AR, Durfy SJ, Burke W, Motulsky AG. The advent of the "unpatients." Nat Med 1996;2:622–624.

Marymee K, Dolan CR, Pagan RA, Bennett RL, Coe S, Fisher N. Development of the critical elements of genetic evaluation and genetic counseling for genetic professionals and gerontologists in Washington state. J Genet Couns 1998;6:133–165.

Mazumdar PMH. Eugenics, Human Genetics and Human Failings. London:Routledge, 1992.

McConkie-Rosell A, DeVellis BM. Threat to parental role: a possible mechanism of altered self-concept related to carrier knowledge. J Genet Couns 2000;9:285–302.

National Coalition for Health Professional Education in Genetics, Lutherville, Maryland. www.nchpeg.org. Accessed 21-7-05.

National Society of Genetic Counselors, Chicago, IL. www.nsgc.org Accessed Feb. 22, 2006.

National Society of Genetic Counselors, Resta RG, Biesecker BB, Bennett RL, et al. A new definition of genetic counseling: National Society of Genetic Counselor's Task Force Report. J Genet Couns 15 (2), in press.

Nussbaum RL, McInnes RR, Willard HF, Thompson MW. Thompson & Thompson Genetics in Medicine, 6th ed, Philadelphia: W.B. Saunders, 2004.

Parmigiani G, Berry DA, Aguilar O. Determining carrier probabilities for breast cancer-susceptibility genes BRCA1 and BRCA2. Am J Hum Genet 1998;62:145–158.

Plumridge D, Bennett R, Dingo N, Branson C. The Student with a Genetic Disorder: Educational Implications for Special Education Teachers and for Physical Therapists, Occupational Therapists and Speech Pathologists. Springfield: Charles C Thomas, 1993.

Resta RG, ed. Psyche and Helix, Psychological Aspects of Genetic Counseling. New York: Wiley Liss, 2000.

Resta RG. Whispered hints. Am J Med Genet 1995;59:131–133.

Schild S, Black RB. Social Work and Genetics: A Guide for Practice. New York: The Hawthorth Press, 1984.

Smith ACM. Patient education. In: Baker DL, Schuette JL, Uhlmann WR, eds. A Guide to Genetic Counseling. New York: Wiley Liss, 1998; 99–121.

Walker AP. Genetic counseling. In: Emery AEH, Rimoin DL, Connor JM, Pyreitz RE, Korf BR, eds. Principles and Practice of Medical Genetics, 4th edition. New York: Churchill Livingston, 2002, pp. 842–874.

Weil J, Psychosocial Genetic Counseling. Oxford: Oxford University Press, 2000.

Weil J. Psychosocial genetic counseling in the post-nondirective era: a point of view. J Genet Couns 2003;12:199–211.

Williams JK, Schutte Dl, Evers C, Holkup PA. Redefinition: coping with normal results from predictive gene testing for neurodegenerative disorders. Res Nurs Health 2000;23:260–269.

Young ID. Introduction to risk calculation in genetic counseling, 2nd ed. Oxford: Oxford University Press, 1999.

8 Animal Models in Biomedical Research
Ethics, Challenges, and Opportunities

ROBERT W. WILLIAMS

> We are all conscious today that we are drowning in a sea of data and starving for knowledge.
>
> —Sydney Brenner (2002)

SUMMARY

Diagnostic power needs to be matched to prognostic accuracy. To accomplish this, we need robust animal models that incorporate the same level of genetic and genomic variation as highly diverse human populations. A key goal of biomedical research is to provide clinicians with sufficient knowledge to predict disease risk and choose effective treatment. We are on the cusp of having complete genome data for each patient. However, our current understanding of complex biological systems and individual differences does not allow us to predict effects of novel interventions and drugs. Animal models provide precise genetic and experimental control, and they also provide a route to more rapid discovery and validation of disease prevention and treatment. But the successful application of experimental results to diverse humans requires that models accurately represent both the underlying disease process and the impact of human genetic variation on treatment and outcome.

Key Words: Animal model; biomedical research; humanizing mice; inbred; molecular medicine.

INTRODUCTION

It has been just over 50 yr since Linus Pauling introduced the term *molecular medicine* in the context of groundbreaking work on sickle cell anemia, and since Roger Williams wrote *Biochemical Individuality*—a prescient introduction to what we now call individualized medicine. Progress in genetics and molecular biology has been relentless over these fifty years, and thanks to new technologies that range from microarrays to magnetic resonance imaging, we are acquiring information at an accelerating pace. In the next decade, patients are likely to have their individual genomes and transcriptomes stored as part of their medical records. Fine-tuning treatment on a case-by-case basis will become the norm, and we can hope that this process will involve more science than art.

Despite this upbeat assessment and the impressive size of *Principles of Molecular Medicine*, biomedical research is only now beginning to move from relatively simple qualitative analysis of single factors to well-designed studies of multiple interacting factors and a multitude of genes. In his *Foreword*, Victor McKusik points out that we still do not have an accurate inventory of the number of genes, mRNAs, or proteins that make up a human. We know even less about the interactions among these complex molecules. We have just begun to explore the intricate molecular networks that mediate between our genomes, our environment, and our health. We know comparatively little about the linkage between gene variants and the most common and pervasive diseases.

Animal models are essential for this transition to a more global and integrative approach to medical care. These models have a vital role as fast and secure routes to improving our understanding of the vocabulary and syntax of the genome and of the complex relations between gene variants and disease. Only research with animals allows us the precise experimental and genetic control required to confirm causality. Animals are also essential when cellular assays fail to provide a relevant biological context, for example, to study the regulation of blood pressure or the systemic effects of drugs or pathogens. As a result, we can expect to rely more heavily on animal models as we transition from simple approaches to more sophisticated and realistic studies that account for human genetic diversity and differences in environmental exposure. Animal models will remain a permanent part of any experimentally validated research program, and will be even more crucial to converting the sea of data alluded to by Sydney Brenner in the opening quotation into effective knowledge that will have a positive impact on human health.

USING ANIMALS IN RESEARCH: RATIONALE AND ETHICAL CONTEXT

A wide variety of unusual species have been valuable in specific areas of research. Several examples highlight serendipitous discoveries and unique animal models that are making important contributions.

- The common nine-banded armadillo has an unusually low average body temperature (approx 32°C), which makes it a unique nonhuman host for the leprosy bacillus, Mycobacterium

From: *Principles of Molecular Medicine, Second Edition*
Edited by: M. S. Runge and C. Patterson © Humana Press, Inc., Totowa, NJ

leprae. In nature, prevalence of infection reaches 30% in some coastal parts of Louisiana. For three decades, armadillos have, therefore, been the pre-eminent model used to study leprosy and to develop and test vaccines. Female armadillos also give birth to litters of monozygotic quadruplets, a unique pattern of reproduction that makes armadillos an intriguing model for the developmental biology of twinning and the limits of genetic control.

- Groundhogs have a high endogenous incidence of hepatitis B virus that leads to liver cancer virtually indistinguishable from that of humans infected with the same virus. This species is used to evaluate environmental and toxicological factors such as aflatoxin that affect susceptibility to liver pathology and cancer progression in humans.

- Two closely related species of voles provide insight into variation in neuroendocrine modulation of reproduction and social structure. Montaine voles are monogamous, whereas meadow voles are polygamous. The activity of neuroactive peptide hormone systems—vasopressin in particular—has a strong impact on pair bonding and social structure. This work continues to lead to mechanistically sound information into how neuroactive peptides modulate aspects of reproduction and behavior.

Most biomedical research, however, relies on familiar domesticated subspecies of mice, rats, hamsters, rabbits, ferrets, cats, dogs, and pigs. Although the size of these species is often confounded with their complexity and similarity to humans, mammals are not arrayed from simple to complex, from primitive to modern, or from stupid to smart. From the standpoint of evolutionary refinement or biochemical complexity, mice, rats, dogs, pigs, chimpanzees, and humans are peers—all are the latest products of roughly 200 million yr of mammalian evolution.

ANTHROPOMORPHIC LEGAL THEORY   Old-world monkeys and apes (macaques, baboons, chimpanzees, and so on) belong to a special category of genuinely wild species that share evolutionary history and biological affinity with humans. They are not more complex than mice or more deeply thoughtful than dogs or pigs, but they are incontrovertibly more similar biologically to humans. This in itself is a reason for using these species in research despite the cost and emotional qualms their use engenders.

A vocal wing of the legal community, led by Steven Wise, Laurence Tribe, and Alan Dershowitz, is exploring the idea that "humanity quotients" can be assigned to life forms as diverse as honeybees and chimpanzees, arguing that each species should be provided with scaled legal protection. For example, according to Wise's scale, the humanity quotient of parrots ranks them somewhere between elephants and dolphins. This fractional anthropomorphic legal theory clearly remains outside the scope of scientific discourse. Misapplying the results of cognitive neuroscience to scale species and perhaps even individuals will produce unintended consequences and a cascade of legal ambiguities. Being human is not an honorary degree that scientists or lawyers are poised to confer. Yet these misframed ideas have begun to exert a subtle but serious impact on scientists themselves, many of whom are willing to concede or even to formally endorse the inverted proposition that similarity to humans makes the use of an animal model inappropriate.

This is precisely wrong. The more closely an animal is related to humans, the more potential value it has as a model. Given that animal research is ethically well grounded and is not abusive,

biomedical research is a more meaningful use of animals than their alternative uses as pets, food, transport, or articles of clothing. Their contributions become a permanent part of a knowledge base. Only biological Luddites will deny the long-term positive impact animal models are having on medical care. In this context, the intrinsic barrier to using chimpanzees in research becomes clear: their use is limited by their wild origin and endangered status, their size, and their high cost.

Classification schemes based on scales of intelligence and levels of consciousness will falter because the sensory and cognitive capacity of each species is unique and of roughly equal sophistication from a neurobiological perspective. The biological quirks of human brains and the self-reported complexity of human thought are not the qualities that make humans special. Yes, humans have a slight cognitive edge, but what distinguishes humans is our highly complex cultures and unique ability to accumulate and pass knowledge from generation to generation. A sound understanding of human biology is a priceless scientific heirloom bequeathed to the next generation.

Animal rights activists exert almost continuous pressure to reduce or eliminate the use of nonhuman mammals in biomedical research. It is relatively easy and effective for this advocacy group to shift the focus away from the unequivocal benefits that have already accrued from animal research onto ethical ambiguities and the difficulties of generating effective animal models. Exploiting the emotional bonds that most humans have with domestic animals and pets, opponents of animal research paint a bleak picture of the state of biomedical research and the need for animal models.

The term "sacrifice" is used to refer to killing animals as part of research projects. This is not a euphemism; this word choice is an acknowledgment of their death and our intent to use them for common good. As individuals and as groups, humans constantly make active and passive decisions about the value of human lives compared with those of other species with which we have natural affinity and even sympathy. Animal research is an explicit and honest example of one of these decisions.

LIMITS OF USING HUMANS IN BIOMEDICAL RESEARCH Several prominent commentators, researchers, and organizations have stressed the need for more widespread and effective use of humans to study human disease. Their point is that with appropriate safeguards, new informatic methods can be harnessed to effectively mine vast clinical resources within patient records, tissue samples, and images. Massive clinical resources can in principle be merged with data on DNA sequence variants and gene expression differences to generate deep insights into disease vulnerability and environmental modulators. The systematic efforts of deCode in Iceland and the United Kingdom BioBank in Britain are beginning to provide compelling examples of the effective integration of clinical, genetic, and molecular analyses of large populations of humans. The limitation of these massive studies is that they often cannot directly test relations between cause and effect.

The critical advantage of animal models is that they can be used to directly test causal relations and mechanisms of action under well-defined experimental conditions and perturbations. The ponderous effort by the US Surgeon General to prove the causal connection between cigarette smoking and cancers in the 1950s is a compelling example of precisely why good animal models are needed. How can human association studies be expected to disprove the alternative hypotheses that a common genetic factor causes both cancer and a yearning for nicotine, or perhaps a tumor suppressor gene variant is tightly linked with a nicotinergic acetylcholine receptor gene variant? Animal models can unequivocally resolve these types of ambiguity.

The need for unequivocal mechanistically sound explanations cannot usually be circumvented by use of humans or cell lines. The effects of thalidomide, ethanol, or heavy metals on human embryonic development cannot be studied, and even unintended toxicological "experiments" of these types are unacceptable. Even voluntary participation in biomedical research by humans must be tightly constrained for ethical reasons. For example, for what period of time is it permissible to temporarily blind human volunteers to study brain reorganization and subsequent recovery—a day, a week, a month, or a year? —and what is the appropriate compensation for participation in such a project?

THE PROBLEM OF TRANSLATION Most common diseases are inherently complex and multifactorial. Elias Zerhouni stated this point clearly: "Solving the puzzle of complex diseases, from obesity to cancer, will require a holistic understanding of the interplay between factors such as genetics, infectious agents, environment, behavior, and social structures." Molecular medicine is not something usually considered holistic, but oddly enough, this direction seems likely with high throughput genomic tools that will soon provide many humans with their personal genome sequence. This advance in medicine will produce exceedingly well-informed patients who will expect customized care.

Molecular processes and organismal responses will often not extrapolate directly across individuals, strains, and species. The supposed failure to make rapid progress in research and clinical delivery—for instance, in the war on cancer initiated in 1971—often reflects a misunderstanding of the complexity of biology (a single cell can be thought of as having greater organizational complexity than the stock exchange), the current depth of ignorance of these complex systems, and the disappointment that follows from overly optimistic media reports on the latest results and potential cures. Unjustified high expectations and incautious headlines are followed by disappointment and denunciation of the models on which they are based.

Nonetheless, there are reasons to constructively critique animal models. A general problem is that the majority of models are designed to reduce genetic and environmental complexity—an unrealistic setting that fails to account for, let alone embrace, the inherent complexity of human populations. Several generations of biologists have been trained to adhere to reductionist methods in which single variables and subsystems of subsystems are studied in isolation. Although this approach is highly productive when access is limited to statistical resources and when questions and answers are focused on fundamental qualitative processes such as basic mechanisms of transcription or enzymatic pathways, it is no longer adequate.

The closer that research gets to clinical treatment—the major purpose of animal models—the greater the need for more complex models that can handle multifactorial perturbations. The computational and collaborative tools are now available to retain the power of reductionist methods while encompassing the power of complex multifactorial experimental designs. A solution to this puzzle requires new types of animal models that more accurately mimic the complex structure of human populations simultaneously allowing control of genomes and environments.

Research involves long-range vision, gradual progress, and delayed gratification, and it is difficult to quantify the many losses that would be the consequence of failure to make discoveries through the use of animal models. Hence, these compromises are made between costs and benefits. It is usually faster, more efficient, and less costly to conduct studies using animal models rather than humans.

BUILDING MODELS AS A KEY TO PROGRESS

The phrase "animal model," first used widely in the 1960s, implicitly acknowledges the many fundamental differences between animals such as mice and our peculiar human species. Often human diseases cannot be fully replicated using other species, even chimpanzee. If a disease is hard to define in humans—autism, for example, slides across several diagnostic subcategories—then it will be hard to model in macaques or chimpanzees, let alone mice. Nonetheless, there are profound and compelling reasons to develop and refine animal models for as wide a variety of human diseases as possible, even those that might initially generate a cynical smile, such as mouse models for macular degeneration (mice have no macula or fovea) or developmental dyslexia (a subtle and uniquely human disorder affecting the ability to process and interpret text).

The phrase "animal model" is also used to indicate that the production of models is often an active process that involves an intense effort in selecting or modifying the genetics of a species or in devising treatments, which consistently produce valuable information and knowledge. Building a good animal model typically involve cycles of testing, modification, and refinement. The process may take years to refine. In the 20th century, technical advances were episodic, and animal models were introduced at a leisurely pace. For example, inbred strains of mice were initially generated by Clarence Little and colleagues in the late 1920s to demonstrate that differences in cancer susceptibility had a genetic basis. Little's first inbred strain was spontaneously prone to several types of cancer, whereas his second strain was not. The use of inbred strains diffused over a period of decades into other fields, in particular, immunology, developmental biology, neurology, behavioral genetics, and toxicology, but the underlying resources and models were not modified significantly.

NEW METHODS TO MAKE NEW MODELS New methods to generate models are being introduced at a rapid rate. The successful integration of exogenous genes into the oocytes of several inbred strains of mice in the early 1980s by Palmiter and Brinster dramatically accelerated the pace with which engineered mice could be generated. Hundreds of transgenic lines of mice are now available, including lines in which human genes are overexpressed. The Huntington's disease gene, *HTT*, and the β-amyloid precursor protein, *APP*, are two prominent examples of human genes that have been moved into mice to explore mechanisms of neurodegeneration.

Transgenic models were followed in the 1990s by the first wave of knockout mice, in which single genes were inactivated in all cells throughout life—what could be called the absolute knockout. The current trend, ca. the year 2000, is to introduce subtle and specific alterations in the expression of genes and their derivative proteins—what are called conditional knockouts. The effect of the knockout may be limited to a particular organ, tissue, cell type, or the knockout may be restricted to a particular stage of development.

It is now possible to imagine adding the equivalent of an expression "volume control" to each gene and to selectively control the settings of those controls on a cell-by-cell and stage-by-stage basis. This possibility is only a few years behind science fiction. Every year, researchers generate not only new models but also new methods to make models. Even the most active research groups find it challenging to track, let alone exploit, the profusion of molecular and cellular techniques. Technical advances in making models sometimes outpace the basic and clinical research they are intended to produce and serve. The technologies that are used to produce models now have an impact that is equivalent to major advances in instrumentation.

ALL MODELS ARE IMPERFECT Humans are a particularly difficult species to model. This fact leads to failures and misapplications, but it should spur further efforts rather than resignation. Human populations have uniquely human problems; the high prevalence of myopia, Alzheimer's disease, obesity, diabetes, asthma, and cancer is just a few unfortunate examples. Most of these problems are produced by a combination of genetic susceptibility factors and the effects of highly variable demographics, environments, and lifestyles.

Because of human diversity and environmental flexibility, some humans are not even particularly good models for other humans. Consider the well-known differences in alcohol metabolism and tolerance associated with aldehyde dehydrogenase gene variants (Han Chinese, for example, typically have low activity alleles and low ethanol tolerance), whose effects extend to social customs and population health. Dramatic individual differences in drug metabolism are associated with several cytochrome p450 gene variants. In some cases, genetic and environmentally induced variation makes the notion of the standard dose or treatment untenable. Recognition of this fact, coupled with advanced technology, drives an intense interest in individualized medicine. The difficulty of generating a good model or generalizing results from an animal to a human, or from one human to another, does not diminish the vital need for models—it simply emphasizes that multiple models are needed and that only a well-considered review of several animal models can provide sufficient grounds to begin the arduous, costly, and inherently risky process of testing new treatments in clinical trials.

Models rely on biological commonality. The fundamental basis for using animal models is that virtually all human disease is partly modulated by molecular and cellular interactions that are reasonably well conserved across a broad swath of the animal kingdom. There are of course species-specific exceptions, but this biological and genetic conservation often extends through the entire chordate phylum through to model organisms in other phylae and kingdoms, including *Drosophila*, nematode, plants, yeast, and bacteria.

Having full gene sequence data for many species has greatly enhanced the long-term ability to discover and exploit this biological commonality. New genomic data allow systematically testing the functions of genes, in isolation and in networks. With these rich comparative data, extrapolations can be made more confidently across species boundaries. The ocular disease aniridia type 2 is caused by mutations in the *PAX6* gene. A feature that has been highlighted by research in *Drosophila,* cephalopods, rodents, and humans is the general conservation of this transcription factor in modulating key aspects of eye development. Other aspects of *PAX6* are more variable, and the phenotypes naturally differ depending on the particular mutant allele of this gene and on the substantial variation between and within species.

Building up and outward from the genomic level to complex and contingent cellular networks that are closer to the disease process will remain challenging work for many years, but at least a list of the mammalian genetic vocabulary is being formed. Converting this list into a dictionary and encyclopedia of the mammalian genome is the next crucial phase that will make animal models much more powerful and useful.

CONSIDERATIONS OF COST, EFFICIENCY, AND NUMBERS OF ANIMALS Investigators attempt to maximize the impact of their research within the limits imposed by budget and expertise. Maximizing impact usually means conducting and interpreting a series of experiments that often require the use of many animals. The cost of acquiring, treating, and analyzing each case therefore is a significant part of the expense.

A key issue is the number of cases needed to give a compelling answer or an accurate estimate of the effect of treatment. One obvious and effective way to improve statistical power (the ability to detect a genuine biological signal) is to increase the number of cases that are studied within each group. The standard error of the sample mean is roughly proportional to the square root of the number of animals per group. A twofold reduction in experimental error requires approximately a fourfold increase in sample size.

Assuming that equally precise and equally relevant measurements can be obtained from a mouse, rat, rabbit, or dog, the statistical advantages of using a larger number of mice rather than a smaller number of dogs will be substantial (the cost ratio is roughly 1/30). Both assumptions will often be wrong—more accurate measurements can often be obtained from larger species. This is precisely why dogs have been the pre-eminent model used to study heart function, cardiovascular disease, and hypertension. It is not that dogs are inherently more like humans than mice or rats are, but that instrumentation used to study heart, kidney, and cardiovascular systems in humans was readily adaptable for use in animals of comparable size. This equipment was, therefore, relatively easy to modify to yield accurate data at a modest cost.

Guidelines of many scientific societies and funding agencies require that investigators use the "minimum number required to obtain *valid* results." This is a key statement formalized in the influential guide for the care and use of laboratory animals. The statement presupposes that researchers know in advance the effect size that they want to detect and that the variance structure and stability of the traits being measured is understood. A minimum number, however, is a recipe for truncated experimental design. ("Appropriate number" would be a wiser term than "minimum number.") By truncating a study to only include male rats at exactly 90 d of age, for example, numbers can effectively be minimized and investigators may be able to show a significant effect of a treatment with an α error rate of $p < 0.05$ with only two per group. To generate this significant result all that is needed is a lucky draw, a genuinely large effect, or an unintended confound (perhaps caging conditions varied). Should that information be published with an *n* of 4? Not at all. A statistically *significant* result is not necessarily a *valid* result. The actual trend in practice is to increase *n* to obtain better power, more precise estimates of effects, and better generality of conclusions.

Instead of striving for a minimum number, researchers should use a more complex and somewhat *ad hoc* procedure to determine the number of animals required to obtain valid results. The intended goal is usually to obtain results that have broad utility and some applicability to humans. To claim to have discovered a potentially important therapeutic effect of an estrogen treatment on the aging process in one inbred strain of mouse, for example, it should be almost mandatory to verify that difference in several other inbred and even outbred strains of mice. Differences that do not generalize across different strains of mice may interest mouse geneticists, but they are unlikely to interest a clinician treating patients. Ideally, similar results would also be demonstrated in another species before moving to clinical trials.

MOUSE MODELS IN BIOMEDICAL RESEARCH

Studies that exploit mice, many of which are referenced in other chapters and on an almost daily basis in the press, are designed ultimately to improve the diagnosis and treatment of human disease. There are inevitable limitations in relying on a single species that differs so much from humans in size, ecological niche, and reproductive strategy. However, mouse models have reached a high level of molecular and genetic sophistication.

Mice presage the achievements that can be expected with other species of mammals—and perhaps of the human species—over the next several decades. For example, the ability to inactivate a gene by homologous recombination (knockout technology) was introduced in mice in the early 1990s by Mario Cappechi and Oliver Smithies and successfully adapted to rats with a 12-yr lag. Many thousands of knockout lines are now in widespread use as models of human diseases and as test beds of gene function. This chapter does not review the burgeoning technical repertoire used to generate genetically engineered strains of mice, but focuses on several concepts and strategies surrounding the generation and use of mouse models.

SIZE AS A FACTOR IN ANIMAL MODELS
Mice are the smallest mammals commonly used in biomedical research. Adult body weight of various species and subspecies ranges from 10 to 30 g, roughly 1/3000 the size of humans. This scaling applies even to an organ such as brain that is considered unusually large in humans; the brains of both mice and humans comprise roughly 2% of total body mass, and in terms of neuron numbers mice are actually proportionally brainier than humans (approx 75 million vs 100 billion neurons). Like humans, mice have significant body size sexual dimorphism; males typically weigh 30–50% more than females.

The main advantage of small size is that a set of 8–10 animals can be maintained in good health in a shoebox-sized cage. Current practice is to maintain 4–5 adults/cage (an anthropomorphic standard for which there is no scientific support). Small size is also associated with particularly rapid development and rapid aging. Gestation in mice is typically 19 d. Mice do not open their eyes until 8–10 d of age, but they develop rapidly and can be weaned after 3 wk of age. Females often produce their first litters at 60–70 d. A full generation therefore typically requires about 3 mo, and up to four generations can be produced per year. Mice are usually fertile for a year or less, and life-span typically ranges from 600 to 800 d. Thus, the biomedical research community has easy access to a mammal in which size, length of the life cycle, and breeding costs are already optimized. These factors have contributed to rapid progress in generating useful mouse models for human disease.

Methods initially perfected in large species such as cats and dogs have been miniaturized to the point that it is now practical in many cases to exploit smaller species such as mice. This shift is driven not by ambiguous ethical gradations that may distinguish small from large mammals, but primarily by greatly improved prospects of generating useful results at a lower cost using instruments and methods specifically geared for studying small mammals. Almost equally accurate results will often be generated from mice as from humans and other large mammals. The main inducement to use mice is not always lower animal costs and higher numbers of research subjects (the mouse/rat cost ratio is only 1/2) but rather the enormous variety of genetically engineered and selected lines of mice.

In some cases there are hard limits to measurement precision that can be obtained using small animals. A case in point is the resolution limits of structural and functional MRI data sets. MRI imaging resolution in any species is not expected of much less than 10 μ because of water diffusion. The proportional in-plane resolution in the mouse brain will be roughly 1/15 that of humans (the cube root of the weight ratio), and a 50-μ resolution in mouse is equivalent in anatomical terms to a 700-μ resolution in human. This resolution limit is counterbalanced, however, by the ability to image many more mice that have been subjected to well-defined manipulations. Again, the inevitable tradeoff is evident between increased measurement precision in large animals vs increased precision and generality made possible using larger numbers of small animals.

INBREEDING AND ITS CONSEQUENCES
A hallmark of most mouse models is that they usually rely on a particular inbred stock or strain. Most transgenic mice, knockouts, and spontaneous mutations are bred onto inbred stocks such as C57BL/6, FVB, and 129 strains. Inbred strains make it possible to perpetuate a mouse model essentially as a permanent clone. An inbred strain can be considered a sexually reproducing "clone" of a single genome in which the only residual variation is that required to perpetuate both males and females.

An important distinction needs to be made between isogenic and monozygotic human twins and two inbred mice of the same sex. Identical twins have the same allelic diversity of other humans—they will often have two different alleles (the maternal and paternal allele) at genes and markers distributed across their entire genome. In contrast, inbred mice have been generated in a way that has eliminated nearly all allelic variation.

The problem with using inbred strains as models or as genetic "hosts" for specific engineered gene variants is that inbred strains are very odd types of mammals. There is almost nothing like an inbred strain in the wild (cheetahs and other species that have gone through severe population bottlenecks may come close). Human populations are not inbred to any significant extent; the inbreeding coefficients even in human populations such as Hutterites are low (<0.04) by the standards of mouse genetics (>0.5).

Production of an inbred strain requires just over 20 generations of consecutive matings between sibling males and females. Generating an inbred strain of mouse is therefore a 7–8 yr effort that is often not successful. Inbreeding greatly diminishes reproductive fitness; the deleterious effects of recessive alleles are exposed fully, and natural selection often expresses its disapproval. But in the relatively mild laboratory environment, 50–80% of incipient inbred strains reach the finish line, each permanently archiving a unique combination of gene variants inherited from the original source population as well as a small load of spontaneous mutations acquired and fixed during inbreeding itself.

The complete lack of heterozygous loci in inbred strains has the advantage of making perpetuation of a defined genome and strain feasible almost indefinitely, but the cost is that these strains are idiosyncratic and highly variable in how they respond to all kinds of exogenous factors. This fact can be viewed in a positive light—variation among strains is a great source material for genetic studies—but it also means that the effects of knockouts and mutations will typically be highly dependent on the genetic background (strain of mouse) on which a mutation is placed by breeding. The effects of a mutation when present on a C57BL/6J background cannot be generalized with much confidence to be similar to those of the same mutation on a 129X1/SvJ background.

There is really nothing like a "normal" mouse; wild-type means that a single gene is in its putative normal or wild-type state. In other words, the mouse happens to be wild type at a single one of approx 25,000 genes. C57BL/6J is not a wild-type mouse—it is an inbred strain that contains hundreds of recessive alleles and frank mutations that have been locked into its genome. Even nominally "wild-type" strains such as CD-1 that are bred with specific avoidance of sibling matings are clearly not wild type; these mice are albinos and are often completely blind.

When a pair of different inbred strains is bred to each other, they produce a filial 1 (F1) generation of offspring. The F1 progeny are still isogenic; males and females are genetically identical, just like their inbred parents. Unlike their parents, however, these F1 mice are heterozygous at all genes that differ between the original pair of parental strains. F1 animals, therefore, retain the advantage of being isogenic but also have the advantage of being much more similar to truly wild populations of mammals, including humans. A study of a knockout on a single F1 hybrid background is analogous to a study of a disease in a single human, and there is a compelling need to evaluate gene function in a broad sense and in the context of diverse genomes and environments.

STRATEGIES FOR MAKING MOUSE MODELS From a genetic perspective, human populations are inherently complex, an outcrossed population in which millions of common polymorphisms are simultaneously segregating and assorting according to Mendel's laws. Humans are also complex in terms of the highly variable environmental factors to which we are subjected, beginning with the formation of oocytes several decades before our own conception.

Mouse geneticists have intentionally constructed mice with simple genomes (fully inbred), and researchers retain tight control over most key environmental factors (diet, pathogen exposure, social structure, temperature, and so on). The reason to make mouse models with a structure diametrically opposite to the human condition is that this structure allows powerful experimental advantages. For example, a single point mutation or a single gene knockout can be introduced onto the fixed genetic "background" of an inbred strain. Similarly, the genome can be untouched and one facet of the environment be varied. Differences in phenotypes between control mice and experimental mice can therefore be confidently attributed to effects of genetic or environmental factors.

The reductionist approach using such models has been effective in revealing causes and effects. The statistics of single-factor experiments are simple, and a conventional *t*-test will usually give nearly optimal power to reject the null hypothesis. But the downside of reductionist models is precisely that they do not attempt to model the real-world genetic and environmental complexity of human populations. This problem has led to a serious critique not just of individual animal models (e.g., those used in cancer biology) but of the whole effort to generate animal models, even to study drug toxicology.

GENERAL MODELS AND INTEGRATING ACROSS SCALES Biomedical researchers are beginning to face major challenges in integrating data across scales, from single base pairs to social structure. It is also important to integrate data across systems, departments, and institutional boundaries—for example, to consider complex interactions between the immune system, neuroendocrine responses, metabolic networks, and cardiovascular performance. Integration across scale and systems is difficult and inefficient because of the inherently fractured and specialized nature of biomedical research. Few researchers gain mastery in a single field, let alone two or more, and generalists lose in the funding and publication competition with specialists. Most models necessarily reflect the highly honed specialty of researchers and are often of use only in a narrow field of application.

There are solutions to this problem, but they are unfortunately more latent than real. The foremost solution is the common use of reference panels of inbred or isogenic mice that have broad utility in many areas of research. Usually a model is considered to be a single entity—a single genetically modified mouse, such as a particular knockout line or a single inbred strain with a tendency to develop lymphomas. But a whole panel of inbred strains of mice, rather than an individual strain, can also be considered a model with which to systematically explore variation in many traits and in many environments. In this case, researchers rely on the range of variation that has been intentionally or inadvertently captured in the reference panel. Human populations in clinical research often consists of what are essentially reference panels—for example, the Framingham cohort and the very well studied panel of 60 large families that form the core of the CEPH Family Panel used throughout the 1990s in gene mapping experiments.

To clarify this distinction between single strain-single gene models and panels of strains, consider two contrasting approaches to studying the genetics of obesity using single mouse models or a reference population.

Approach 1 To analyze phenotypes associated with a spontaneous or induced mutation in a specific gene that leads to marked obesity in mice, a single line on a single genetic background (e.g., a new mutant allele of the leptin receptor on the background of strain DBA/2J) is generated, optimized, and studied. The homozygous knockout is compared with the heterozygote and the wild-type strain (−/−, −/+, and +/+). The phenotypic differences across these three classes may provide exquisite biochemical detail and high power. However, results may not be easily generalizable to other strains of mice such as C57BL/6 or 129X1/Sv, let alone to other species and to human populations. Because the model is unique, data generated are not easily aggregated and integrated using this novel line with data from other experiments and models. Integration will be at a comparatively high level: do the overall conclusions agree or not with those of other studies? The simple solution to the first problem of generality is to make a habit of studying monogenic manipulations on a set of different genetic backgrounds. This is quite easy in mice, because changing the background may simply involve one or two generation breeding experiment (an outcross of the mutation to a different wild-type strain).

Approach 2 The interest in the genetics of obesity continues, but now an entire reference panel of 30 or more genetically and phenotypically diverse strains of mice rather than the three classes of a Mendelian mutation is used. For example, variation in fat pad mass or leptin receptor protein level in hypothalamus across this panel could be assayed. Variation in this measurement across the panel is the "experimental" signal used for two types of subsequent analyses: (1) gene mapping studies of the chromosomal regions that contribute some fraction of the variation detected across the strains, and (2) association studies of variation in fat pad mass with hundreds of other phenotypes that have already been acquired in this same panel under similar and different conditions. Results of hundreds of experiments can be pooled and integrated for the simple reason that the same genetic individuals—members of the reference panel—are being used by multiple research communities. For example, data on fat pad mass could be compared with pre-existing data for the same strains on variation in blood pressure or activity levels. Networks of phenotypes can readily be explored that covary in the same way that clinical researchers search for patterns of comorbidity among diseases. The price for this integrated approach is obvious: there is more phenotyping to contend with, and the variation of interest does not have an immediate genetic cause. The mapping studies may suggest that three or more different chromosomal regions contribute to differences in phenotypes. Getting to the point of understanding the biochemical basis of a variant phenotype is still comparatively difficult.

There are several types of reference panels that share the attribute that their constituent strains are a stable resource. A major project of this type, the Collaborative Cross, involves interbreeding eight mouse strains to produce a set of about 1000 derivative strains, each with a unique but fixed set of allelic variants, phenotypes, and disease susceptibilities. Several smaller reference panels of this type typically consist of 8–80 strains of mice. For example, the BXD panel of recombinant inbred strains was made 30 yr ago by combining the genomes of two strains (C57BL/6J and DBA/2J) that have both been almost fully sequenced. A multiplicity of phenotype and genotype data from these BXD strains can be exploited in genetic mapping studies and can also be used in phenotype association studies to test the consistency, strength, specificity, and coherence of associations between an amazing variety of traits (see www.genenetwork.org for an example of this integrative approach).

HUMANIZING MICE Imagine a line of mice genetically engineered to biochemically resemble a human (as much as possible, given the massive scaling differences and biometric consequences). Transgenic mice in which human genes are inserted into the mouse genome represent the first step in this direction; it is now possible to extend this idea to groups of genes or even whole organs.

There has been substantial progress in generating new types of mice in which the endogenous immune system has been genetically extirpated. These mice can be engrafted with human hematopoietic stem cells that mature into lymphocytes and T- and B-cell subpopulations. Such humanized mice will be especially valuable in studying host–pathogen interactions in ways that would not otherwise be possible. Similar techniques are being developed to make mice that incorporate human liver and breast tissues, and this trend is expected to continue as more control is gained over tissue differentiation in vivo and in vitro. This process will inevitably have its own set of problems, but there will be inexorable progress in generating more faithful and useful models that can be used to study basic mechanisms and test the safety and efficacy of new treatments.

There is a risk (highlighted by Clifton Leaf) that researchers enamored with their sophisticated animal models may fail to promptly consider clinical applications or may be sidetracked into marginally relevant areas with little short-term payoff. Yet, strong counterbalancing incentives provided by funding agencies, pharmaceutical companies, and research institutions drive researchers to translate their results into effective clinical practice. In fact, these incentives can be so compelling that investigators may leap from research results to clinical tests without the delay imposed by an intermediate analysis of other model organisms to test generality and species specificity.

CONCLUSION

In light of costs and benefits and the urgent need for rapid advances, animal models are an essential component of biomedical research. Computer simulations, cell-based assays, and human association studies are all critical components of research, but they cannot substitute for the rigorous mechanistic insight into cause and effects that can be gained from expanded use of more sophisticated and general animal models. A failure to exploit these models to improve quality of life and to provide effective compassionate care would be negligent.

There will be a constant tension between what is regarded as uniquely human characteristics vs common denominators shared with other species. The major challenge in using animal models is to generalize results with reasonable fidelity to humans. To get to this point will often require higher numbers of cases because more variables need to be includeed—both sexes, several ages, several genotypes, and perhaps even several environmental conditions and several species. Achieving such goals may involve a balanced analysis of several model organisms, each with its own unique experimental and practical advantages.

ACKNOWLEDGMENTS

My thanks to Kathryn Graehl for critical reading and editing of this work. Supported in part by grants from NIAAA (INIA program), NIDA, NIMH and NIAAA (Human Brain Project), NCRR (Mouse BIRN), and NCI (Mouse Models of Human Cancer Consortium).

SELECTED REFERENCES

Biobank. University of Manchester. Manchester, England (www.biobank.ac.uk). Accessed May 11, 2005.

Brenner S. Nature's gift to science. Nobel Lecture 2002; pp. 274–282. (www.nobel.se/medicine/laureates/2002/brenner-lecture.pdf). Accessed Jan. 14, 2006.

Chesler EJ, Wang J, Williams RW, Manly KF. Web QTL: Rapid exploratory analysis of gene expression and genetic networks for brain and behavior. Nat Neurosci 2004; 7:485–486.

Crick F, Koch C. The unconscious homunculus. In: Metzinger T, ed. The Neuronal Correlates of Consciousness. Cambridge, MA: MIT Press, 2000; pp. 103–110.

deCODE Genetics. Reykjavik, Iceland (www.decodegenetics.com). Accessed May 11, 2005.

Gudrais E. Chimpanzees and the law. Harv Mag 2003;105:21, 22.

Kuperwasser C, Chavarria T, Wu M, et al. Reconstruction of functionally normal and malignant human breast tissues in mice. Proc Natl Acad Sci USA 2004;101:4966–4971.

Leaf C. Why we're losing the war on cancer. Fortune 2004;149:76–97.

Little CC. The role of heredity in determining the incidence and growth of cancer. Am J Cancer 1931;15:2780–2789.

Lusis AJ, West D, Davis C. Animal models of complex genetic disease. In: King RA, Rotter JI, Motulsky AG, eds. The Genetic Basis of Common Disease, 2nd ed. New York: Oxford University Press, 2002; pp. 65–86.

Nagy A, Gertsenstein M, Vintersten K, Behringer R. Manipulating the Mouse Embryo: A Laboratory Manual, 3rd ed. Cold Spring Harbor, NY: Cold Spring Harbor Laboratory Press, 2003.

National Academy Press: Guide for the Care and Use of Laboratory Animals. Washington, DC: National Academy Press, 1996.

Paired Box Gene 6; PAX6. OMIM. Johns Hopkins University. Baltimore, Maryland (www.ncbi.nlm.nih.gov/entrez/dispomim.cgi?id=607108). Accessed May 11, 2005.

Pauling L, Itano HA. Sickle cell anemia: a molecular disease. Science 1949;110:543–548.

Quiring R, Walldorf U, Kloter U, Gerhing WJ. Homology of the eyeless gene in Drosophila to the small eye gene in mice and anirdia in humans. Science 1994;2655:785–789.

Rader K. The mouse's tale: standardized animals in the culture and practice of technoscience. Cabinet Mag 2001;4. www.cabinet magazine. org/issues/4/themousestale.php). Accessed Jan. 14, 2006.

Ryan TM, Townes TM, Reilly MP, et al. Human sickle hemoglobin in transgenic mice. Science 1990;247:566–568.

Silver LM. Mouse Genetics. Concepts and Applications. New York: Oxford University Press, 1995.

Threadgill DW, Hunter KW, Williams RW. Genetic dissection of complex and quantitative traits: from fantasy to reality via a community effort. Mamm Genome 2002;13:175–178.

Vogel G. Scientists dream of 1001 complex mice. Science 2003;301: 456, 457.

Williams RJ. Biochemical Individuality. New York: John Wiley & Sons, 1998.

Zerhouni E. The NIH roadmap. Science 2003;302:63.

9 Ethical, Legal, and Social Implications

MARCIA VAN RIPER

SUMMARY

This chapter provides an overview of some of the complex ethical, legal, and social issues associated with advances in genomics and molecular medicine, such as equity in access to genetic information and services, use of genetic information in nonhealth-related settings, and genetic discrimination. It is hoped that this discussion will stimulate future discussions about these and other issues that are just beginning to emerge in the exciting, ever-changing world of genomic health care. Discussions such as these are critical to the development of appropriate policies and legislation.

Key Words: Discrimination; ethics; genetics; genetic information; genome; pharmacogenomics.

INTRODUCTION

Clinical practice has been dramatically altered by advances in genomics and molecular medicine, such as the sequencing of the human genome. Although it will probably be at least 10 yr before one's entire genome will be sequenced for $1000 or less, there have been important advances in the application of genomic information to the prevention, diagnosis, and treatment of human disease. Some of these advances include the use of preimplantation genetic diagnosis to help families affected by devastating genetic conditions have unaffected children; the use of genotyping to stratify patients according to their risk of specific diseases, such as long-QT syndrome; the use of gene-expression profiling to assess prognosis and guide treatment decisions for women with breast cancer; and the use of pharmacogenomics to tailor medications and dosages for individual genotypes.

Although advances such as these are promising and may ultimately transform the model of population-based risk assessment and empirical treatment into a predictive individualized model based on the molecular classification of disease and targeted treatment, they also have the potential to complicate the web of ethical, legal, and social issues already associated with advances in genomics and molecular medicine. This chapter provides an overview of the ethical, legal, and social issues connected with advances in genomics and molecular medicine.

GENETIC INFORMATION: CHANGES IN ACCESS AND USE

The term "genetic information" has been used in a variety of ways. Commonly used to indicate the information obtained from a specific genetic test, it may also be used to refer to information about a specific genetic condition, or information about a person's entire genome. Regardless of which definition is used, the term genetic information tends to elicit a wide variety of emotions, including excitement, wonder, relief, fear, sadness, and anger.

CHANGES IN ACCESS

Access to Genetic Information Through Genetic Professionals Previously, the primary way to gain access to genetic information was through interactions with genetic professionals (geneticists, genetic counselors, and nurses with expertise in genetics). Typically, genetic professionals follow a genetic services paradigm that includes the construction of a family pedigree, a risk assessment, education about the genetic component of specific conditions, psychosocial assessment and counseling, a discussion of testing and management options, and support with decision making. For many conditions, no treatments exist, so management options may be limited to surveillance and risk-reducing strategies. If genetic testing is available, genetic professionals usually provide both pre- and post-test counseling to give the individual or family who is considering genetic testing a chance to discuss possible ethical, legal, and social implications (ELSI) of testing. It also gives the genetic professional a chance to anticipate possible negative consequences of testing. If it appears that the individual or family might have difficulty dealing with the test results, additional counseling, and support can be provided.

Access to Genetic Information Through Other Sources There are a variety of ways to gain access to genetic information. Genetic services, especially genetic testing, are becoming increasingly available in mainstream health care. In addition, advances in technology and mass communication have made it possible for many people to access genetic information in their homes. The Internet is rapidly becoming a major source of genetic information. Although many individuals are using web-based resources to expand their understanding of specific genetic conditions, others are using Internet chat rooms and discussion boards to help in their decision making about genetic testing and management options, and some are receiving ongoing information and support through websites devoted to specific conditions. Moreover, some individuals and families are becoming aware of and gaining access to genetic testing through companies that offer direct-to-consumer marketing.

From: *Principles of Molecular Medicine, Second Edition*
Edited by: M. S. Runge and C. Patterson © Humana Press, Inc., Totowa, NJ

Ethical, Legal, and Social Issues Associated With Changes in Access Changes in access to genetic information increase the possibility that individuals and families from diverse backgrounds will be able to gain access to genetic information, but these changes also increase the possibility of ethical, legal, and social issues. For example, if an African-American woman with a strong family history of breast cancer is offered BRCA1/2 testing, she can give informed consent only after (1) she receives full disclosure of pertinent information concerning the test and (2) she fully understands the risks, benefits, and limitations of the test. If she undergoes the testing in mainstream health care, this is less likely to occur because many physicians in mainstream health care lack the time and expertise necessary to adequately counsel their patients about BRCA1/2 testing. In addition, the information she receives may not be clearly understandable or culturally sensitive. Also, depending on her socioeconomic status, she may not have the financial resources or insurance coverage needed to undergo testing. Concerns about cost, confidentiality, and insurance discrimination may prevent her from being tested.

In a study about BRCA1/2 testing in the community setting, 82% of the 646 women who underwent testing recalled discussing and reviewing the consent with their primary care provider. However, the time spent on this (median time spent on counseling and informed consent was 30 min, range was from 1 to 240 min) was much less than is usually devoted to this activity in specialty clinics and research programs. Almost 13% of the women did not recall discussing the consent form. Concerning how they became aware of their test results, 57% received their results during an office visit, 39% received them by telephone, 3% got their results in the mail, and 2% did not answer the question. Three of those who received their results in the mail had variants of uncertain significance. Whereas most of the women (67%) reported that the testing was paid for by their health insurance or through research funds, 25% paid for it themselves. The remaining women either had insurance claims pending or they did not report a source of payment. None of the women reported increased premiums or loss of health or life insurance because of undergoing the testing. These findings need to be viewed with caution because it had been less than 2 mo since they received their test results.

As with access to genetic information through physicians in mainstream health care, a number of ethical, legal, and social issues are associated with access to genetic information through the Internet. The first concern is that the information provided on these websites may be incorrect or misleading. Next, there are concerns about privacy and confidentiality, especially if the sharing of personal information is a prerequisite to gaining access to a website. Also certain websites can be used to purchase medications, dietary supplements, and genetic tests without the supervision of a health-care provider.

Findings from a study about direct-to-consumer sales of genetic services on the Internet suggest that most of the websites offered genetics services such as paternity testing, identity testing, and DNA banking. Only 14 out the 105 websites reviewed offered health-related tests. Although some of these tests were conventional genetic tests (hemochromotosis and cystic fibrosis), others related to nutrition, behavior, and aging. The authors of this study concluded that the availability of direct-to-consumer health-related genetics tests creates the potential for inadequate decision making prior to testing, a misunderstanding of test results, and access to genetic tests of questionable clinical value.

GeneWatch UK, a nonprofit group that monitors developments in genetic technologies noted a number of problems with the approach taken by one company that offers to provide products (lotions and other skin-care products) and services (guidance on training methods and nutrition requirements) that are designed to match an individual's genetic profile. According to GeneWatch UK, (1) the company's claims are misleading, (2) the company does not adequately inform their customers about possible risks associated with the testing, (3) the company plans to keep the DNA samples and link them to personal genetic information and lifestyle information as long as the customer continues to be a subscriber, (4) the customer's genetic information may ultimately be patented without their knowledge, and (5) the customer may experience negative consequences, such as financial burden because of the high cost of products that may not be necessary. Their analysis would suggest that individuals who use this source to gain access to their genetic information may experience a lack of informed consent, a violation of their right not to know, loss of privacy, workplace and insurance discrimination, confidentiality issues, and unnecessary financial burden.

CHANGES IN USE

Use of Genetic Information to Improve Health and Well-Being Initially, the primary use of genetic information was to help individuals and families affected by genetic conditions face the associated ongoing challenges. Once genetic testing became available for select conditions, possible uses for genetic information increased dramatically. For example, expectant couples can use the genetic information that they acquire through pre- and postaminocentesis counseling to help them prepare for the birth of a child with Down syndrome or the termination of an affected pregnancy. New parents can use the genetic information they receive following their child's positive newborn screen for phenylketonuria to start their child on a special formula known to prevent the mental retardation commonly associated with phenylketonuria. Individuals found to carry the gene for Huntington disease (HD) can use genetic information in their decision making about reproduction, as well as their decision making about how and where they want to live the rest of their life. Before the availability of genetic testing for familial adenomatous polyposis, children in families with a history of familial adenomatous polyposis were usually started on close surveillance, which comprised annual sigmoidoscopies, starting at around age 10. Because genetic testing is available, results of the test can be used to determine which children need this type of close surveillance.

With the development of risk-reducing strategies and treatments for select genetic conditions, possible uses of genetic information to improve health and well-being have increased again. For example, as data came to light indicating that an individual's short-term risk of developing a second breast cancer is substantially affected by whether she carries one of the BRCA mutations associated with hereditary breast and ovarian cancer, newly diagnosed breast cancer patients are increasingly being asked to consider undergoing BRCA1/2 testing before they make decisions about their treatment options. This way, they can use the results of their genetic test to help in decision making about possible treatment options. Women who test positive and choose to undergo a bilateral mastectomy rather than a breast-conserving procedure can avoid radiation treatment and possibly a second surgery. For some, an even more important use of their test results is to help their offspring, by making them aware of any increased risk.

Abbreviations

II. CARDIOLOGY

4E-BP1	4E-binding protein 1
AAA	abdominal aortic aneurysms
ABCA1	ATP binding cassette transporter A1
AC	adenylate cyclase
ACE	angiotensin-converting enzyme
ACS	acute coronary syndrome
ACTH	adrenocorticotropic hormone
ADP	adenosine diphosphate
AGT	angiotensinogen
Ang-I	angiotensin I
Ang-II	angiotensin II
APA	aldosterone-producing adrenocortical adenoma
Apo A-I	apolipoprotein A-I
Apo B	apolipoprotein B
ARH	autosomal-recessive hypercholesterolemia
ARVD	arrhythmogenic right ventricular dysplasia
ATPase	adenosine triphosphatase
β-MHC	β-myosin heavy chain
CABG	coronary artery bypass surgery
CAD	coronary artery disease
cAMP	w/e (cyclic adenosine monophosphate)
cbEGF	calcium-binding epidermal growth factor-like
CETP	cholesterol ester transfer protein
cGMP	cyclic guanosine monophosphate
CGRP	calcitonin gene-related peptide
CHD	coronary heart disease
CK	creatine kinase
cMyBPC	cardiac myosin binding protein C
CRP	C-reactive protein
CsA	cyclosporine A
cTnT	cardiac troponin T
CVD	cardiovascular disease
DCM	dilated cardiomyopathy
DGS	DiGeorge syndrome
DMD	Duchenne muscular dystrophy
EAD	early after depolarization
E-C	excitation-contraction
ECM	extracellular matrix
eEF2K	eukaryotic elongation factor-2 kinase
EGF	epidermal growth factor
eIF	eukaryotic initiation factor
ENaC	epithelial sodium channels
eNOS	endothelial nitric oxide synthase
EP	electrophysiology
EPCs	endothelial progenitor cells
ERK	extracellular signal-regulated kinase
ET-1	endothelin-1
FBN1	fibrillin-1 gene
FDB	familial defective apolipoprotein B
FH	familial hypercholesterolemia
FISH	fluorescence *in situ* hybridization
Gi	G inhibitory
GPCR	guanine nucleotide protein coupled receptor
GRA	glucocorticoid-remediable hyperaldosteronism
GSK-3	glycogen synthase kinase-3
HCM	hypertrophic cardiomyopathy
HDL	high-density lipoprotein
HMG CoA	3-Hydroxy-3-methyl-glutaryl coenzyme A
ICAM-1	intercellular adhesion molecule-1
ICD	implantable cardiac defibrillator
IDL	intermediate density lipoproteins
IGF-1	insulin-like growth factor-1
ISA	intrinsic sympathomimetic activity
JNKs	c-Jun N-terminal kinases
KO	knockout
LCAT	lecithin cholesterol acyl transferase
LDL	low-density lipoprotein
LDLR-/-	low-density lipoprotein receptor deficient
LMWH	low-molecular-weight heparin
LV	left ventricular
LVAD	left-ventricular assist device
LVH	left-ventricular hypertrophy
MAP	mitogen-activated protein
MAPK	mitogen-activated protein kinase
MAS	marker-assisted selection
MCIP	muscle-enriched calcineurin inhibitory protein
MCP-1	monocyte chemotactic protein-1
MEK	mitogen-activated protein and extracellular signal-regulated kinases
MEN-2	multiple endocrine neoplasia 2
MFS	Marfan syndrome
MHC	myosin heavy chain
MI	myocardial infarction
MLP	muscle LIM protein
MMP	matrix metalloproteases
mTOR	mammalian target of rapamycin
NBD	nucleotide binding domains
NCEP	National Cholesterol Education Program
NFAT	nuclear factor of activated T cells
NHANES III	Third National Health and Nutrition Examination Survey
NO	nitric oxide
NOS	nitric oxide synthase
PAI-1	plasminogen-activator inhibitor

PCI	percutaneous coronary intervention		SNP	single-nucleotide polymorphism
PDK1	phosphoinositide-dependent protein kinase-1		SNPs	single-nucleotide polymorphisms
PI3-K	phosphoinositide 3-kinase		SP	substance P
PKA	protein kinase A		SR	sarcoplasmic reticulum
PKB	protein kinase B		SSRE	shear stress response element
PKC	protein kinase C		STAT	signal transducer and activator of transcription
PRKAG2	γ-2 regulatory subunit of AMP-activated protein kinase		STE	ST elevation
			SVAS	supravalvar aortic stenosis
PTEN	phosphatase and tensin homolog		TIMP	tissue inhibitors of MMP
PTX	pertussis toxin		TOF	Tetralogy of Fallot
QTL	quantitative trait loci		t-PA	tissue plasminogen activator
RyR	ryanodine receptor		u-PA	urokinase-type plasminogen activator
SCD	sudden cardiac death		VCAM-1	vascular cell adhesion molecule-1
SDH	succinate dehydrogenase		VCFS	Velo-cardio-facial syndrome
SHR	spontaneously hypertensive rat		VEGF	vascular endothelial growth factor
SIDS	sudden infant death syndrome		VHL	von Hippel-Lindau syndrome
SMC	smooth muscle cells		VLDL	very low-density lipoproteins

10 Congenital Heart Disease

Lazaros K. Kochilas and Alvin J. Chin

SUMMARY

Cardiogenesis is a complex process involving different cell types, such as muscle, endothelial, neural crest, and matrix cells. These cells follow a "protocol" that emerges through changes in gene expression induced by developmental and mechanical cues. Data from human genetics and animal mutants suggest that most congenital heart malformations are arise from gene alterations. The next challenge will be to unravel the sequence of molecular decisions that result in the formation of heart and blood vessels from the first embryonic tissue layers. This knowledge is expected to result in novel strategies for diagnosis, treatment or prevention of heart diseases.

Key Words: Cardiac development; congenital heart defects; endocardium; genes; mutations; myocardial cells; neural crest cells; transcription factors.

INTRODUCTION

The heart is the first organ to form and function during mammalian organogenesis. The formation of the heart and vasculature is an extremely complex process because of its multicomponent constituency, with the heart at its center and the vascular network at its periphery. A diversity of cell types including muscle, endothelial, neural crest, and matrix secretory cells have to follow a strictly coordinated "protocol" to build the normal system. Underlying the complexity at the macroscopic level is corresponding complexity at the molecular level. In the human cardiovascular system, thousands of genes are expressed in any given single cell. Although a significant proportion of these genes are devoted to maintenance of basic cellular function, a subset of them has more restricted expression (spatial and temporal) and contributes to the cardiovascular system's diversity of cell types. The development of the cardiovascular system as a whole is the end product of the changes in gene expression in response to developmental and mechanical cues that drive growth, pattern formation and differentiation. Cardiac malformations occur in 5–8 of 1000 live births, and worldwide approx 1 million infants are born annually with heart defects (20,000/yr in the United States). Sufficient progress has occurred in identifying, characterizing, and surgically repairing physiologically important congenital cardiac defects so that

From: *Principles of Molecular Medicine, Second Edition*
Edited by: M. S. Runge and C. Patterson © Humana Press, Inc., Totowa, NJ

85% of these infants can expect to survive to adulthood. However, congenital heart defects are the leading cause of death during the first 5 yr of life and are associated with significant morbidity in neonatal life and beyond. Because only the most severe structural malformations thwart management schemes, prevention and early *in utero* detection are the remaining strategies to reduce the impact of heart malformation on the health of infants and children; however, any preventive approach would depend largely on knowing the percentage of congenital heart defects that are genetic. For example, if most congenital heart anomalies result from intrauterine insults (infectious agents, toxins, nutritional factors, mechanical stress, and so on) to the embryo during the first 30 d of gestation, then a prevention strategy would be ineffective, and improving fetal imaging skills should be a focus of effort; because most pregnancies are already monitored by ultrasound at least once for accurate dating, perhaps adding a "cardiac surveillance" portion to the imaging protocol would suffice to increase the chance of prenatal identification. However, evidence suggests that most congenital heart malformations result from gene alterations.

Therefore, the scientific challenge is to unravel the sequence of molecular decisions that result in the construction of the heart and blood vessels from the first embryonic tissue layers. Understanding the development of the cardiovascular system in more detail will allow exploration of novel interventional strategies for treatment or prevention of disease. In vertebrates studied, the heterogeneity of phenotypes associated with even single-gene null mutations points to the importance of modifier genes, environmental factors, and genetic polymorphisms in determining the severity and type of congenital heart disease. It will be important to identify these "modifier genes" because they may partially explain the variability of defects in human conditions such as the DiGeorge syndrome (DGS), usually associated with a multigene deletion. Much of the variability in diseases caused by point mutations occurs from the generation of hypomorphic alleles of different strengths. It is also important to study the effects of environmental factors like toxins, nutrients, and alcohol that are similarly implicated in cardiac development.

More than 150 genes are involved in cardiovascular morphogenesis (Table 10-1), but how they function to form the heart and great vessels remains obscure. Both forward and reverse genetic approaches are being investigated, and a variety of organisms are being scrutinized because the underlying mechanisms of patterning appear to be widely shared among vertebrates. Among these the mouse has been the classic model for cardiac genetic studies because

Table 10-1
Genes Involved in Cardiovascular Development

Protein family function	Gene name	Organism	Expression sites and stages of involvement	Other family genes with potential role in cardiac development
1. Gene/protein expression *Transcription factors*				
NK	Nkx2.5	Human: Heterozygous mutations: ostium secundum type ASD, TOF, Ebstein's anomaly, AV conduction defects and "left ventricular noncompaction" Mouse: Nkx2.5$^{+/-}$: ostium secundum type ASD, AV conduction defects and vulnerability to arrhythmia Nkx2.5$^{-/-}$: embryonic lethal at E10-E11 from cardiac insufficiency; cardiac developmental arrest at the stage of looping; poor chamber differentiation and trabeculation pattern *Drosophila:* *tinman* mutant embryos lack heart or visceral muscles	Nkx2.5 is expressed in myocardial precursors (mouse, *Xenopus*, zebrafish) and is required for completion of cardiac looping morphogenesis.	Nkx2.3, Nkx2.6, Nkx2.7, and Nkx2.8 (various species) Bagpipe (*Drosophila*) Bax: Nkx3.1 (mouse)
	Tinman			
GATA	GATA-4	Human: Heterozygous GATA-4 missense mutations are associated with familial VSDs Mouse: GATA-4$^{-/-}$: embryonic lethal at E8.5-E10.5 with cardiac bifida and absent pericardial cavity *Drosophila:* Pnr mutant embryos have excess pericardial cells and deficient development of cardioblasts Zebrafish: Fau (GATA-5 mutants): cardiac bifida	GATA-4 is expressed in endocardium, endocardial cushions and myocardium except distal outflow tract (mouse) and is required for ventral migration and fusion of cardiac primordia.	GATA-5, GATA-6 (mouse): display distinct overlapping but distinct spatio-temporal expression patterns during cardiogenesis. GATA6 is dispensable for early cardiac development but may play a role in later cardiomyocyte differentiation.
	Pannier (pnr)		*pannier* is expressed in the dorsal mesoderm and required for cardial cell formation, while repressing a pericardial cell fate.	
	GATA-5			
FOG	Fog2	Human: Heterozygous FOG2 missense mutations were reported to be associated with congenital diapharagmatic hernia and lung hypoplasia, but no cardiac defects Mouse: Fog2$^{-/-}$: embryonic lethal at midgestation with various cardiac defects characterized by thin ventricular myocardium, endocardial cushion defects (common atrioventricular canal), conotruncal abnormalities and hypoplastic coronary arteries	Expressed throughout the myocardium and is important for the normal looping and septation of the heart (mouse).	

	U-shaped (ush) zfh-1	*Drosophila:* Ush mutants lack heart formation. Zfh-1 mutants form a heart tube that is specifically missing the even-skipped (eve) –expressing subset of pericardial cells	U-shaped promotes heart development, by maintaining *tinman* expression in the cardiogenic region. *zfh-1* is expressed in the early mesoderm and later in the forming heart.
T-BOX	T/Brachyury/ntl/ Xbra	*Mouse:* T−/−: randomization of cardiac looping and orientation *Zebrafish:* no tail−/− mutants have randomization of cardiac orientation *Xenopus:* Xbra overexpression or inactivation causes randomization of heart looping	Brachyury is not expressed in the vertebrate heart.	Tbx2/3 (human, mouse, chicken), Tbx4 (mouse) xEomes (Xenopus) Tbx18 (mouse, zebrafish)
	Dorsocross (Doc 1/2/3)	*Drosophila:* Combined mutants for *Doc1-3* lack cardioblasts	*Doc1-3* are expressed in distinct areas of the cardiogenic mesoderm and the dorsal vessel in *Drosophila.*
	Tbx1	*Human:* TBX1 is included in the DGCR, whose haploinsufficiency is associated with DiGeorge syndrome (DGS) *Mouse:* Tbx1+/−: truncus arteriosus, IAA, RAA, aberrant RSCA and other aortic arch defects Tbx1−/−: perinatally lethal and occasionally embryonic lethal at E13.5-E14.5; DGS-like features with a range of conotruncal and aortic arch defects including truncus arteriosus, IAA, aberrant RSCA, VSD, TOF, TOF/Pulmonary atresia and branch pulmonary stenosis Tbx1 transgenics with Tbx1 overexpression display also conotruncal and arch anomalies *Zebrafish:* vgo/tbx1−/−: bilateral arch anomalies	*Tbx1* is expressed in cardiac crescent, cardiac outflow tract, mesodermal core of pharyngeal arches (mouse). In zebrafish *tbx1* expression is found in sinus venosus, atrium, ventricle and outflow tract.
	Tbx5	*Human:* HOS-1 (Tbx5): Heterozygous mutations are associated with Holt–Oram syndrome (limb defects and range of cardiac abnormalities: AV block, failure of septa formation and HLHS, aortic stenosis, mitral valve prolapse, and TOF) *Mouse:* Tbx5+/−: 50–80% perinatal lethality; ASD, VSD, limb defects	Tbx5 is expressed in embryonic epicardium, myocardium, and atrioventricular tissue; endocardial expression is restricted only in left ventricle in mouse but bilaterally in human; it can act as cellular arrest signal during cardiogenesis and thereby modulates cardiac growth and development.

(Continued)

Table 10-1 (Continued)

Protein family function	Gene name	Organism	Expression sites and stages of involvement	Other family genes with potential role in cardiac development
		Tbx5−/−: embryonic lethal at E10.5; severely hypoplastic posterior cardiac segments, delayed looping, absent atrial septum, and atrioventricular cushions Zebrafish: *Heartstrings (tbx5)* mutants have hearts that initially form and function normally but later fail to loop and display progressive hypoplasia of ventricle and atrium		The *Tbx20 Drosophila* orthologs, *mid*, and *H-15*, are required for the functional diversification of cardioblasts and the expression of *tinman*-dependent terminal differentiation genes within the dorsal vessel.
	hr-T/tbx20	Zebrafish: *hr-T morphants*: have dysmorphic hearts	*tbx20* is expressed in cardiac precursors at the anterior lateral plate and later throughout the myocardium (zebrafish).	
	spt/tbx16/ XvegT	Zebrafish/*Xenopus*: *spt*−/−: randomization of left-right development and heart looping situs	*tbx16* is expressed in mesoderm (zebrafish).	
NFAT	*NFATc1/CNB1*, *NFATc2*, *NFATc3*, *NFATc4*	Mouse: *NFATc1*−/−: Embryologically lethal at E13.5-E17.5; cardiac failure secondary to abnormal semilunar valve formation.	Calcineurin/NFAT signaling functions sequentially from myocardium to endocardium and is required for repression of *VEGF* in the endocardium (mouse). This repression allows endocardial cells to transform into mesenchymal cells and initiate valve formation in vertebrates.	
FOX	*Foxc1, Foxc2*	Mouse: *Foxc1*−/−, *Foxc2*−/−, and *Foxc1*+/−; *Foxc2*+/−: perinatally lethal, various aortic arch defects (mostly fourth arch derivatives), and VSD.	*Foxc1* is expressed in the endothelial cells and mesenchyme of the branchial arches (mouse). *Foxc2* is also expressed in the valves and cardiac outflow tract (mouse).	
	FoxH1	Mouse: *FoxH1*−/−: embryonic lethal between E8.5-E10.5. Primitive heart tube is formed but fails to develop outflow tract and right ventricle, development arrests at looping stage, and cardiac failure occurs Zebrafish: *schmalspur (sur)* mutants have severe defects in all axial structures and randomization of heart looping	*FoxH1* is expressed initially in the lateral plate mesoderm and then is restricted to the heart (mouse). FoxH1 functionally interacts with Nkx2-5 and is essential for development of the anterior heart field and its derivatives.	
	Foxp1	Mouse: *Foxp1*−/−: embryonically lethal at E14.5; thin myocardium and severe cardiac outflow tract, septation and cushion defects	*Foxp1* is expressed in myocardium and endocardium (early stages up to E14.5).	
	Foxp4	*Foxp4*−/−: embryonically lethal at E12.5; cardiac bifida	*Foxp4* is expressed in ciliated epithelial cells.	
	Foxj1(Hfh4)	*Hfh4*−/−: perinatally lethal, failure to grow, situs inversus or heterotaxy with randomization of heart position		

72

Gene family	Gene	Phenotype	Expression	Notes
Homeotic genes	*Hoxa-3*−/−	Mouse: *Hoxa-3*−/−: die around the time of birth with various conotruncal anomalies, thymic and parathyroid agenesis reminiscent of the human DGS	Expressed in the mesenchyme and endothelial cells of the third and fourth pharyngeal arches	*hoxd-3*, *hoxa-4*, and *hoxd-4*: expressed at the early stages of heart formation in the chicken.
	Gax	Mouse: Forced expression of *Gax* inhibits cardiomyocyte proliferation and causes thin myocardium phenotype	*Gax* has a biphasic pattern of expression in cardiomyocytes (an early one from begin of cardiogenesis up to E12.5 and a late one within compact layer at E15.5)	*Mtsh 1*, *Mtsh2* (mouse) are expressed in mesenchyme of branchial arches. *tsh* (*Drosophila*)
SOX	*Sox4*	Mouse: *Sox4*−/−: embryonic lethal at E14; die of heart failure; abnormal formation of semilunar valves and persistent truncus arteriosus	Expressed in endocardial ridges	*Sox7/8/9/10/17/18* (Human, mouse, chick, *Drosophila*)
Myc	*c-myc*	Mouse: *c-myc*−/−: embryonic lethal between E9.5–E10.5; heart failure.	*c-myc* is expressed in myocardial cells.	
	N-myc	*N-myc*−/−: embryonic lethal at E10.5–12.5; poorly developed ventricular myocardium, VSD	*N-myc* is expressed only in compact myocardium.	
Jun proto-oncogenes (components of AP-1 transcription factors)	*c-Jun*	Mouse: *c-jun*−/−: embryonic lethal at E13 with TA, RAA, aortic arch anomalies, and thin right ventricle	The different AP-1 components including Jun proteins are expressed in a development- and tissue-specific manner in multiple tissues including the heart.	*c-jun* and *junD* are genetically redundant. Mice lacking both *jun* genes display cardiovascular and angiogenic defects during embryonic development.
Iroquois	*Irx4*	Mouse: *Irx4*−/−: Hypertrophic cardiomyopathy in the adult mouse	Expressed in ventricular myocardium and plays a critical role in establishing chamber-specific gene expression in the developing heart	*Irx1*, *Irx2*, and *Irx5* may partially compensate for loss of *Irx4* function in the heart
Prh Homeobox (Hex)	*Prh/Hhex* (*Hex*)	Mouse: *Hhex*−/−: right ventricular hypoplasia, thin myocardium Zebrafish: *Hhex* knock-down causes randomization of gastrointestinal chirality	Expressed in the anterior tip of the primitive streak in the mouse embryo, as well as in the endothelium throughout the developing vascular network and in the third pharyngeal pouch	
ras-GTPase-activating proteins (*ras-GAPs*).	*Nf1*	Human: Patients with neurofibromatosis 1 have increased incidence of certain congenital heart defects like pulmonic stenosis and coarctation. Also a case with multiple coronary aneurysms has been reported in a child with neurofibromatosis Mouse: *Nf1*−/−: embryonic lethal at E14; poor development of ventricular myocardium, VSD, PTA, abnormal atrioventricular valves	Neurofibromin (Nf)-1 modulates epithelial-mesenchymal transformation and proliferation in the developing heart by down-regulating ras activity. It is expressed in human atrial and ventricular tissue. In the mouse, *Nf1* is expressed ubiquitously but is developmentally regulated in the heart and neural crest derivatives.	Mutations in the related genes *TSC1*, *TSC2* are associated with tuberous sclerosis and cardiac rhabdomyomas in humans
Pax (Paired domain homeoboxes)	*Pax3*	Human: Heterozygous mutations are associated with Waardenburg's syndromes 1 and 3 (no cardiac defects); homozygous mutations are presumed to be early embryonic lethal.	Expressed in migratory neural crest cells	

(Continued)

Table 10-1 (Continued)

Protein family function	Gene name	Organism	Expression sites and stages of involvement	Other family genes with potential role in cardiac development
		Mouse: *Pax3*$^{+/-}$(*Splotch*$^{+/-}$): no cardiac defects, only skin pigmentation defects *Pax3*$^{-/-}$: embryonic lethal at E13.5, persistent truncus arteriosus, thin ventricular myocardium, VSD		
bHLH	dHAND (Hand2)	Mouse: *dHand*$^{-/-}$: embryonic lethal at E10.5; absence of heart looping, absent right ventricle	dHAND is predominantly expressed in the morphologically right ventricle and eHAND in the left ventricle (mouse).	Xenopus dHAND and eHAND are also expressed bilaterally in the lateral mesoderm but without any left-right asymmetry. No eHAND homologue was found in zebrafish.
	eHAND (Hand1)	*eHAND*$^{-/-}$: embryonic lethal at E8.5-9.5; heart development arrests at late cardiac crescent stage showing incomplete heart tube fusion and no observable contractions		
	Hey1/Hesr1	Mouse: *Hey1*$^{-/-}$;*Hey2*$^{-/-}$: embryonic lethal at E11.5 with hypoplastic trabeculae, single ventricle, impaired EMT in atrioventricular cushions and defects in blood vessel development	The Hesr genes are expressed in the cardiac crescent. At later stages Hesr1 is expressed in the atria, while Hesr2 is also expressed in the atria, but predominantly in the ventricles, aortic and pharyngeal arches.	Hesr1/Hey-1/HRT-1/CHF-1 and hesr2 are redundantly required to mediate Notch signaling in the developing cardiovascular system (mouse).
	Hesr2 (hairy and enhancer of split2)/Hey2/ HRT2/grl	*Hey2*$^{-/-}$: die perinatally from cardiac failure and display various cardiac malformations including ventricular septal defects, tetralogy of Fallot, dysplastic atrio-ventricular valves and cardiac hypertrophy Zebrafish: *grl*$^{-/-}$: abnormal arterial development with variable disruption of aorta segments that resembles coarctation of the aorta		
	MesP1 MesP2	Mouse: *MesP1*$^{-/-}$: embryonic lethal at E10.5 with cardiac bifida *MesP1*$^{-/-}$;*MesP2*$^{-/-}$: embryonic lethal at E9.5 with absent mesodermal layer and heart formation *MesP2*$^{-/-}$: perinatally lethal with skeletal anomalies but no heart defects	MesP1 is expressed in cardiac precursors in the primitive streak (mouse). MesP2 is expressed in early mesoderm but its expression is down-regulated after E7.0 (mouse).	The bHLH transcriptional repressor mSharp-1/mDEC2 is expressed in the mouse heart at E8.5 and remains active until at least E16.5
Bicoid-related homeobox genes	Pitx2a,b,c,d	Human: Rieger syndrome (*RIEG/Pit2a* heterozygous mutants): ocular, dental, umbilical cord abnormalities Mouse: *Pitx2*$^{-/-}$: deletion of all Pitx2 isoforms is embryologically lethal at E14.5 with multiple developmental abnormalities (ASD, complete AV canal, abnormal arterio-ventricular	Pitx2 isoforms are expressed initially in the left lateral plate mesoderm at E8-9; later are expressed bilaterally in the derivatives of the lateral plate mesoderm and only Pitx2c is expressed asymmetrically in the left side of most organ primordia (heart, lungs and gut). Pitx2c is also expressed asymmetrically in the ventral part of branchial arches and at the junction with the aortic sac	

Gene family	Gene	Phenotype (mutant)	Expression / Comments
		connections, abnormal cardiac positioning [but normal cardiac d-looping], hypoplastic RV, right lung isomerism, open ventral wall, eye abnormalities) *Pitx2c−/−*: lethal in neonatal age with abnormalities of the aortic arch patterning and the outflow tract	Myocardin and MRTFs physically associate with SRF and activate SMC-restricted transcription. *MRTF-A* is expressed by multiple cell lineages and is a potent transcriptional coactivator of some SRF-dependent genes.
nieuwkoid/dharma homeobox	*nieuwkoid/ dharma*	Zebrafish: *bozozok/dharma* mutants display independent randomization of heart and gut chirality	*dharma* is expressed in the dorsal blastoderm and is required at the blastula stages for formation of the embryonic shield and expression of multiple organizer-specific genes.
SAP domain nuclear proteins	*Myocardin Myocardin-related transcription factor (MRTF)-B*	Mouse: *Myocardin−/−*: embryonically lethal at 10.5 with severely impaired embryonic vasculogenesis but no evidence of cardiac defects *MRTF-B−/−*: homozygous mutant mice die between embryonic day (E)17.5 and postnatal day 1 from cardiac failure and display cardiac outflow tract defects (TA, Double outlet right ventricle, IAA and large VSDs)	Master gene regulator of many cardiac specific genes, which is diffusely expressed in myocardial tissue. *MRTF-B* is expressed in the premigratory neural crest, in rhombomeres 3 and 5, and in the neural crest-derived mesenchyme surrounding the aortic arch arteries.
Hop homeobox	*Hop*	Mouse: *Hop−/−*: two phenotypic classes characterized by an excess (hypertrophic myocardium in adult age) or deficiency of cardiac myocytes (thin myocardium and embryonic death during midgestation from heart failure). *Hop−/−* mutants display also conduction defects below the level of the AV node Zebrafish: Inhibition of Hop activity in zebrafish embryos likewise disrupts cardiac development and results in severely impaired cardiac function	Expressed in cardiac precursors and cardiac myocytes (mouse). Balances growth vs differentiation of ventricular myocytes.
Cited nuclear proteins (CBP/p300 -interacting transactivator with ED-rich tail)	*Cited2*	Mouse: *Cited2−/−*: embryonic lethal at E13.5-E16.5 with cardiac outflow tract defects (TOF, DORV, truncus arteriosus, right aortic arch), adrenal agenesis, abnormal cranial ganglia and exencephaly	Expressed in primitive streak in areas fated to become heart tissue and in the presomitic and lateral plate mesoderm.
ZFHX	*ZFHX1B/SIP1*	Human: *SIP1* mutations are associated with Hirshprung's disease and PDA	Expressed ubiquitously
SMAD	*SMAD1-8*	Mouse: *Smad4−/−*: display cardiac hypertrophy *Smad5−/−*: embryonic lethality between E9.5 and E11.5 with defects in heart looping and embryonic turning	*Smad4* is expressed specifically in cardiomyocytes. *Smad5* is ubiquitously expressed in the mouse and zebrafish embryo. *Smads* act as BMP receptors by transducing their signaling effects.

(Continued)

Table 10-1 (Continued)

Protein family function	Gene name	Organism	Expression sites and stages of involvement	Other family genes with potential role in cardiac development
MADS	Mef2c	Mouse: Mef2c−/−: Embryonic lethal at E9.5–10.5; absence of heart looping, lack of OFT and right ventricle, single LV fused directly to atrial chamber, lacking trabeculae and dissociated cardiomyocytes. Drosophila: D-mef-2 mutants fail to express contractile protein genes in all muscle lineages (heart, visceral and somatic muscles)	Essential for differentiation of muscle cell lineages (mouse, Drosophila)	Mef2α, Mef2b, Mef2d (mouse). SRF is expressed in cardiac and skeletal muscle cells and is implicated in the control of cardiac muscle gene expression (mouse)
ETS	Ets1, Ets2	Chicken: Targeting Ets1/2 mRNA by antisense oligonucleotides causes abnormal coronary vessels	ETS are important for the epithelial-mesenchymal transformation in the primary and secondary heart fields (chicken)	Xl-fli, Xsap 1 (Xenopus): Expressed in heart and branchial arches
	pointed	Drosophila: Pnt mutants have excess cardioblasts	Pnt is a key regulator of cardioblast and pericardial cell fates in the posterior segments of the heart, by promoting pericardial cell development and opposing cardioblast development (Drosophila).	
GLI superfamily	ZIC3	Human: ZIC3 mutations are associated with X-linked heterotaxy (HTX1) Mouse: Zic3−/−: embryonic lethal, heterotaxy	Expressed in mesoderm (mouse)	
	Gli1/2/3	Human: Gli3 mutations are associated with skeletal malformations syndromes (mostly polydactuly) and cancer Mouse: Gli2−/−;Gli3+/−: VACTER-like phenotype, PTA and heart looping defects	Expression of Gli1 is more restricted and transcriptionally regulated by Shh, Gli2/3 expression is broader and less dependent from Shh signaling (mouse).	
TEA domain (TEAD) family	Transcriptional enhancer factor (TEF-1/TEAD1)	Mouse: TEF-1−/−: embryonic lethal at E12; noncompaction, VSD	Expressed in myocardium	
AP-2	TFAP-2B	Human: Missense mutations cause Char syndrome with persistence of ductus arteriosus	Expressed in third, fourth, and sixth pharyngeal arches and later in ductus arteriosus	
LIM	Isl1	Mouse: Isl1−/−: display cardiac malformations with absent outflow tract and most of the atria	Expressed in cardiomyocytes in the secondary (anterior) cardiac field.	
ladybird (lb)	lbe (early) lbl (late)	Drosophila: lb−/−: display hypoplasia of cardiac precursors. Overexpression of both lbe and lbl reveals hyperplasia of heart progenitors	lb genes are expressed in clusters of about four cells per hemisegment in the developing heart region.	
Protein synthesis/modification Subtilisin-like	SPC1/Furin	Mouse:	Spcs induce endoproteolytic maturation of TGF-β-related molecules. Spc1 is expressed in the visceral endoderm	

Category	Gene	Phenotype	Comments
proprotein Convertases (SPCs)	SPC4/PACE4	*Fur*⁻/⁻: embryonic lethal at E10.5 with failure of cardiac primordial to fuse in the ventral midline or with formation of a short unlooped heart with reduced number of cardiomyocytes. *Spc4*⁻/⁻: embryological lethal at E13.5–E15.5 with situs ambiguous, congenital heart defects (PTA, VSD, common atrium, DORV), combined with left pulmonary isomerism or complex craniofacial malformations including cyclopia	and the cardiogenic mesoderm. *Spc4* is expressed in the definite endoderm and the left lateral plate.
SPT translation elongation factors	*Spt5*, *Spt6*	Zebrafish: *sk8/s30* (*Spt5*) mutants have similar phenotype with pandora. *Pandora* (*Spt6*) mutants have dysmorphic hearts, decreased number of ventricular myocytes and pericardial effusion	*Spt5* and 6 are both transcriptional elongation factors that interact with each other.
Chromatin modification HDACs	*Hdac1* ; *Hdac5*, *Hdac9*	Mouse: *Hdac1*⁻/⁻: embryonic lethal at E10.5. The mutant embryos are severely dysmorphic and growth restricted, so that the cardiac phenotype could not be assessed. Zebrafish: *hdac1* mutants have dysmorphic and hypoplastic hearts with absent atrio-ventricular valve. Mouse: *Hdac5*⁻/⁻ and *Hdac9*⁻/⁻: sensitize animals to hypertrophic stimuli	Several class I HDAC members (1, 2, 3, 8) are also expressed in cardiac tissue (mouse, zebrafish) but their particular role in cardiac development is still unknown. Several class II HDAC members (in particular HDAC5 and 9) are very strongly expressed in cardiomyocytes and postulated to inhibit post-mitotic cardiac growth and repress cardiac hypertrophy (human, mouse).
CREB-binding protein	CREBBP	Human: Haploinsufficiency of the *CREBBP* gene (16p13.3 deletion) has been associated with a severe form of Rubinstein-Taybi syndrome that includes mental retardation, skeletal abnormalities, accessory spleens, lung laterality defects and congenital cardiac defects (hypoplastic left heart, VSD).	*CREBBP* and its paralog *EP300* are ubiquitously expressed transcriptional coactivators and act as histone acetyl transferases (HATs). EP 300
p300/CBP transcriptional activators	p300	Mouse: *p300*⁻/⁻: mutant mice die between E9.5-E11.5 from cardiac failure associated with defects of cardiac muscle differentiation	Expressed ubiquitously from early developmental stages. *p300* and *CBP* play a critical role in cardiac hypertrophy that is dependent on their histone acetyltransferase activity.
Polycomb genes	*rae28*	Mouse: *rae28*⁻/⁻: die around the time of birth with conotruncal anomalies (tetralogy of Fallot and aortic stenosis), asplenia and abnormalities in the eyes, hard palate, and parathyroid glands	The gene contains DNA binding domains that belong in the chromatin-associated group of proteins.

(Continued)

Table 10-1 (Continued)

2. Intercellular signaling and signal transduction (signals, ligands and receptors)

a. Secreted factors

Protein family function	Gene name	Organism	Expression sites and stages of involvement	Other family genes with potential role in cardiac development
Hedgehog	Shh/syu	Mouse: Shh$^{-/-}$: alterations in cardiac looping, tetralogy of Fallot with pulmonary atresia Zebrafish: syu$^{-/-}$: absent dorsal aorta and axial vein	Expressed in endoderm of pharyngeal arches	
	Ihh	Mouse: Shh$^{-/-}$;Ihh$^{-/-}$: developmental arrest at somitogenesis with small, linear heart tube, open gut and cyclopia (identical phenotype with Smo$^{-/-}$)		
TGF-β	TGF-β2	Mouse: TGF-β2$^{-/-}$: die in perinatal period with malformations of the cardiac outflow tract, the AV canal region, the aortic arches and the semilunar valves	TGF-β-related signals (like Nodal, lefty, southpaw; Gdf1) specify in vertebrates the anteroposterior and left-right axes. TGF-β2 is expressed in the endocardium and the myocardium adjacent to the endocardial cushion tissue.	TGF-β1 is expressed in endothelial cells. TGF-β3 is expressed in endocardial cushions
	BMP-1/Tolloid like proteases (Tld): Tolloid-like 1 (Tll-1)	Mouse: Tll-1$^{-/-}$: embryonic lethal during midegestation with AV-canal type of VSD and abnormal semilunar valves	Tll-1 is expressed specifically in precardiac tissue and endocardium at E7.5-8.5 mouse embryos.	
	Bmp2	Mouse: Bmp2$^{-/-}$: Early embryonic lethal with amnion and chorion malformations and abnormal development of the heart in the exocoelomic cavity. No cardiac defects in heterozygotes Zebrafish: Swirl/bmp2b mutants display dorsoventral patterning defects but no cardiac abnormalities	Bmp2 is expressed in the AV junctional myocardium and valve tissue and interacts with TGF-α3 for the formation of endocardial cushions.	
	Bmp4	Mouse: Bmp4$^{+/-}$: No cardiac defects in heterozygotes. Bmp4$^{-/-}$: Early embryonic lethal. Cardiac specific ablation of Bmp4 is embryonic lethal at E13.5 with outflow tract defects including truncus arteriosus, and in combination with a hypomorphic allele causes common atrioventricular canal Drosophila: Dpp mutant embryos: heart and visceral mesoderm formation is abolished (as in tinman)	Bmp4 is expressed in the cardiac outflow tract (incl. truncus arteriosus) and the endocardial cushion ridges (mouse). It has also a developmentally regulated expression in zebrafish.	Dpp (decapentaplegic) is required along with the secreted signaling molecule, wingless (wg) to specify the heart in Drosophila.

78

Gene	Expression	Phenotype	Notes
Bmp5/6/7	Bmp5 is expressed in the developing myocardium; Bmp6 is expressed in the outflow tract and the atrioventricular cushions; Bmp7 is expressed in overlapping and adjacent sites with Bmp6, including the endocardial cushions. It is also expressed diffusely in axial and lateral mesoderm, gut endoderm and allantois.	Mouse: Bmp5−/−;Bmp7−/−: embryos die at E10.5 with absent endocardial cushions Bmp6−/−;Bmp7−/−: embryos die between E10.5 and E15.5 due to cardiac failure with delayed formation of the outflow tract endocardial cushions, defects in valve morphogenesis and chamber septation	
Bmp10	BMP-10 expression is restricted initially in the trabeculated part of the common ventricular chamber and the bulbus cordis, but after E12.5, additional expression is seen in the atrial wall (mouse)	Mouse: Bmp10−/−: embryologically lethal at E10.5 with hypoplastic ventricular wall	BMP-10 is important for the trabeculation and ventricular growth of the embryonic heart.
Nodal	Nodal is expressed in left lateral plate mesoderm and is required for formation of the primitive streak. It is indirectly implicated in laterality defects in human, mouse, chicken, and frog.	Mouse: Nodal−/−: die in gastrulation but compound heterozygotes between hypomorphic and null alleles (Nodalfl/) die at E14.5 and display abnormal cardiac looping, dextrocardia or mesocardia, TGA and VSDs. HNF3-β+/−; nodallacZ/+ double-heterozygous embryos display randomization of heart looping and left pulmonary isomerism.	Mutations of the zebrafish nodal related gene cyclops (ndr2) does not cause laterality defects.
southpaw nodal related gene		Zebrafish: southpaw morphants display severe disruption of early (cardiac jogging) and late (cardiac looping) aspects of cardiac left-right asymmetry.	
LEFTA / lefty1 (Ebaf)	Lefty1 is expressed asymmetrically in the left lateral plate in the mouse embryo.	Human: Mutations identified in patients with laterality defects similar to mouse lefty1−/−. Mouse: lefty1−/−: laterality defects described as left thoracic isomerism.	Lefty2 (LEFTB) is also asymmetrically expressed in the left lateral plate in the mouse embryo and seems to be controlled by lefty1.
Gdf-1/Vg-1	Gdf-1 is expressed bilaterally in intermediate and lateral plate mesoderm. Vg1 cell-signaling pathway plays a central role in left-right coordinator function in Xenopus.	Mouse: Gdf1−/−: spectrum of laterality defects, including visceral situs inversus, right pulmonary isomerism, and a range of cardiac anomalies incl. abnormalities of cardiac looping, transposition of great arteries, VSD, and atrio-ventricular canal.	
TGF-β antagonists — Chordin(Chrd)	Chrd is a secreted Bmp-binding protein that is expressed in the mouse node and its derivatives, notochord and pharyngeal endoderm (mouse). Chordin gene is first expressed on the dorsal side of the embryo (starting before gastrulation) (Zebrafish, Xenopus).	Mouse: Chrd−/−: die during mid-gestation or at time of birth with DGS phenotype incl. Truncus arteriosus, right aortic arch and aortic arch branching abnormalities. Zebrafish/Xenopus: Chordino(dino) mutants display randomization of heart looping	The role of other bmp inhibitors like noggin, follistatin, and Sog on cardiac development is unknown

(Continued)

79

Table 10-1 (Continued)

Protein family function	Gene name	Organism	Expression sites and stages of involvement	Other family genes with potential role in cardiac development
Early response gene growth factor	SIL	Mouse: $SIL^{-/-}$: embryonic lethal around E10.5 with axial midline defects and randomized cardiac looping	Ubiquitously expressed	
Neurotrophin growth factors	Nt3	Mouse: $Nt3^{-/-}$: perinatally lethal with severe cardiovascular abnormalities including atrial and ventricular septal defects, and tetralogy of Fallot	Essential for the survival and/or migration of cardiac neural crest	
Vegf	Vegf	Human: Certain VEGF haplotypes are associated with increased risk for cardiovascular defects in del22q11 individuals Mouse: VEGF isoforms associated with decreased VEGF expression display various aortic arch abnormalities. Transgenics overexpressing VEGF die at E12-E14 and display conotruncal anomalies (TOF, pulmonary hypoplasia), VSD and thin myocardium	Expressed in the endoderm of the pharyngeal arches, the aortic sac, cardiac outflow tract, and ventricular septum	
Erythropoietin	Epo	Mouse: $Epo^{-/-}$: embryonic lethal during midgestation from failure of erythropoiesis. The mutants display also ventricular hypoplasia, detachment of epicardium and abnormalities of the vascular network	Erythropoietin affects cardiomyocyte proliferation in a cell non-autonomous manner.	Similar results were found also in the erythropoietin receptor knockout mice.
Wnt/Wingless	Dvl2(Dsh2)	Mouse: $Dvl2^{-/-}$: 50% perinatally lethal (predominantly the males) DORV, TGA, PTA	Widely expressed in embryonic and adult tissues. Important for cardiac neural crest development	Wnt1/Wingless: Wnt antagonism initiates cardiogenesis in Drosophila, Xenopus laevis and chick. Wnt1 is expressed in subset of cardiac neural crest cells
EGF-CFC	CFC1/Cryptic	Human: Loss-of-function mutations are associated with heterotaxic phenotypes with a variety of congenital heart defects (d-TGA, DORV, Pulmonary atresia, complete AV canal, HLHS, ASD, VSD, PDA) Mouse: $cryptic^{-/-}$: right pulmonary isomerism, dextrocardia, malposition or transposition of the great arteries and DORV	Expressed at E7.5 in the precardiac and lateral plate mesoderm in the mouse; later is expressed in the cardiac inflow and outflow tract.	Cripto and oep act as co-receptors or presenting molecules in nodal signaling pathway.
Adapter proteins	CRKL	Human: Included within the DGCR Mouse:	Expressed in dorsal neural tube, dorsal root ganglia, some clearly defined some of the branchial arches and the front nasal mass.	

Category	Gene	Phenotype	Expression/Notes
Semaphorins		Crkol−/−: abnormalities of the cardiac outflow tract and the aortic arch arteries	
	Sema3A	Mouse: Sema3A−/−: perinatally lethal with selective hypertrophy of the right ventricle and right atrial dilation	Sema3A is expressed in cardiac tissue (rat)
	Sema3C	Sema3C−/−: perinatally lethal, interrupted aortic arch, and PTA.	Sema3C is expressed in migratory and postmigratory neural crest cells in the myocardium surrounding the outflow tract. Important for the migration of cardiac neural crest cells to the outflow tract
Ephrins	ephrinB2	Mouse: ephrinB2−/−: embryonic lethal before E11.5 with poorly organized vessels, deficient myocardial trabeculation, pericardial effusion and no cardiac looping Endocardial-specific ephrinB2 inactivation leads to similarly defective cardiac morphogenesis	EphrinB2 is expressed in arterial endothelial cells.
EGF Neuregulin and EGFR signaling	NRG1	Mouse: NRG1−/−: embryonic lethal during midgestation due to the aborted development of myocardial trabeculae in ventricular muscle (Long 2003)	NRG1 is expressed by pluripotent neural crest cells and endocardium.
	HRG	HRG−/−: embryonic lethal at E10.5 with thin myocardium, irregular heart beat	
	HB-EGF	HB-EGF−/−: die in neonatal age from heart failure secondary malformed semilunar and atrioventricular heart valves, and hypoplastic, poorly differentiated lungs (Meno 1998)	Heparin-binding epidermal growth factor (HB-EGF) and betacellulin (BTC) are activating ligands for EGF receptor (EGFR/ErbB1) and ErbB4. HB-EGF is expressed by endocardial cells lining the margins of cardiac valves. Tumor necrosis factor-alpha converting enzyme (TACE) activates EGFR by deriving soluble HB-EGF. Proper cardiac valvulogenesis is dependent on EGFR activation that is required to regulate BMP signaling in endocardial cushions.
	Betacellulin (BTC)	HB-EGF−/−; BTC−/−: similar defects as described above with more accelerated occurence of cardiac failure and death	Although BTC and TACE do not belong to the same family of genes they all act through activation of the EGFR signaling pathway and are bundled together in this context.
	TACE	TACE−/−: similar phenotype with defective valvulogenesis as above	
FGF	Fgf8	Zebrafish: acerebellar: homozygous mutants for fgf8 have dysmorphic hearts with reduced ventricular mass Mouse: Fgf8 homozygous hypomorphic alleles display looping abnormalities as well as various aortic arch defects, including outflow tract, intracardiac and aortic arch anomalies	Fgf8 is expressed in cardiac precursors and later in the ventricular tissue, ectoderm of first pharyngeal arch and core mesenchyme of more caudal pharyngeal arches (mouse) Fgf8 is required for induction and patterning of myocardial precursors Fgf8 is a left determinant in the mouse but in the chicken appears to be a right determinant. Fgf1, 2, 4, 7, 12, 13, 16 Fgf10 is expressed in pharyngeal mesodermal cells that contribute to the arterial pole of the heart.
Endothelins	ET-1	Mouse: ET-1−/−: conotruncal and aortic arch defects	Expressed in the neural crest-derived pharyngeal mesenchyme, as well as endoderm and ectoderm
Nonmembranous protein tyrosine phosphatases	PTPN11	Human: Defects in PTPN11 account for 50% of patients with Noonan's syndrome (which includes cardiovascular anomalies such as pulmonary	PTPN11 is widely expressed in both embryonic and adult tissues and encodes the nonmembranous protein tyrosine phosphatases SHP-2, which mediates signal transduction from numerous

(Continued)

Table 10-1 (Continued)

Protein family function	Gene name	Organism	Expression sites and stages of involvement	Other family genes with potential role in cardiac development
		stenosis and hypertrophic cardiomyopathy) and some cases with Leopard syndrome (multiple lentigines, congenital cardiac abnormalities mostly pulmonic stenosis, ocular hypertelorism, and retardation of growth) Mouse: Ptpn11$^{D61G/D61G}$: Homozygous mutants for the D61G mutation in the Ptpn11 gene are embryonic lethal at E13.5 (grossly edematous and hemorrhagic, have diffuse liver necrosis and severe cardiac defects). Heterozygous embryos exhibit cardiac defects (DORV, thin myocardium, thickened atrioventricular and outflow tract valves, growth failure, perturbed craniofacial development and a mild myeloproliferative disease	receptor tyrosine kinases. It is positively associated with pulmonic stenosis but negatively associated with hypertrophic cardiomyopathy, suggestive of a more critical role for *SHP-2* in valvulogenesis than cardiomyocyte proliferation	
MicroRNAs	microRNA-1-1 (miR-1-1)	Mouse: Excess *miR-1-1* in the developing heart leads to a decreased pool of proliferating ventricular cardiomyocytes	*miR-1-1* and *miR-1-2* are specifically expressed in cardiac and skeletal muscle precursor cells	During cardiogenesis *miR-1* genes titrate the effects of cardiac regulatory proteins to control the balance between differentiation and proliferation.
b. Receptors and Ligands				
Notch	Notch1	Human: *Notch 1* mutations cause a spectrum of developmental aortic valve anomalies and severe valve calcification in non-syndromic autosomal-dominant human pedigrees Mouse: Notch1$^{-/-}$: embryonic lethal with severe neuronal and somitic defects. In addition, Notch1$^{-/-}$ mutants show defects in angiogenic vascular remodeling in the embryo, yolk sac, and placenta. Endothelial-specific *Notch1* inactivation recapitulates the Notch1$^{-/-}$ phenotype	*Notch1* and *Notch2* are expressed in the outflow tracts and the epicardium, in specific cell populations that express *JAG1*. *Notch 1* transcripts are particularly enriched in the aortic valve.	Notch1 (*Xotch*) and *Serrate1* are expressed in overlapping patterns in the early heart field in *Xenopus*. Notch signaling suppresses cardiomyogenesis through *suppressor hairless*, *Su(H)* and this is essential for the correct specification of myocardial and nonmyocardial cell fates
	Notch2	Notch2$^{del1/del1}$: mutants die perinatally and display myocardial hypoplasia, edema, kidney and ocular vascular defects		
	Notch4	Notch4$^{-/-}$: No vascular phenotype Notch1$^{-/-}$; Notch4$^{-/-}$: More severe vascular phenotype than Notch1$^{-/-}$	*Notch4* is restricted to the vascular endothelium	
Dsl proteins	Dll1	Mouse: Dll1$^{-/-}$: situs ambiguous phenotype, including	*Dll1* encodes one of the four known mammalian DSL	

	Phenotype	Expression	Function
Jagged-1 (JAG-1)	randomization of the direction of heart looping and embryonic turning. Human: Mutations in JAG1 are associated with Alagille syndrome (AGS) and cardiac defects (TOF, VSD, ASD, PDA, PTA, pulmonary atresia, hypoplasia of the entire pulmonary vascular tree) Mouse: Jag1−/−: embryonic lethal at E10.5 from hemorrhage and exhibit defects in remodeling of the embryonic and yolk sac vasculature (Hamblet 2002) Jag1+/−; Notch2+/−: Phenotype reminiscent of human Alagille syndrome	proteins and acts as a ligand for the receptor Notch. Dll is expressed in the human embryonic heart (atria, ventricular endocardium, coronary arteries and epicardium). In the mouse embryo. Jag-1 has more global expression but comparable in the heart (atria, ventricles, outflow tracts, valve precursors) and the great arteries (pulmonary arteries, descending aorta and all pharyngeal and their vascular derivatives)	
Receptors of TGF-β-like ligands			
TBRII	Mouse: TBRII^{nullflox};Wnt1-Cre+/−: Neural crest specific TBRII inactivation is perinatally lethal with DGS phenotype including truncus arteriosus and abnormal aortic arch branching	All receptors are expressed diffusely in several issues during embryonic mouse development	TBRI,TBRII, TBRIII and ALK2 mediate TGF-β signaling and induce epithelial-mesenchymal transformation in the AV cushions
Endoglin	Human: Endoglin+/−: Hereditary hemorrhagic telangiectasia type 1 (HHT1) Endoglin−/−: embryonic lethal at E10.5 with diffuse vascular abnormalities, absence of cardiac cushions formation and pericardial effusion	Endoglin is expressed at high levels on endothelial cells of capillaries, veins, and arteries (human) as well as on mesenchymal stromal cells in several tissues (mouse)	
ALK1 (acvrl1)	Human: Heterozygous mutations are associated with primary pulmonary hypertension and hereditary hemorrhagic telangiectasia type 2 (HHT2) Mouse: ALK1+/−: Hereditary hemorrhagic telangiectasia type 2 (HHT2) Zebrafish: Vbg(acvrl1)−/−: dilated cranial vessels	ALK1 is expressed in endocardial cells (mouse, chicken)	
ALK2 (acvrl2)	Mouse: ALK2^{nullflox};Tie2-Cre+/−: Endothelial-specific ALK2 inactivation is embryonically lethal and leads to endocardial cushion defects ALK2;Wnt1-Cre+/−: Neural crest-specific ALK2 inactivation causes craniofacial anomalies and aortic arch abnormalities reminiscent of human DGS phenotype	ALK2 is expressed abundantly in endocardial cells of the outflow tract, ventricle, and AV cushion (mouse, chicken)	
ALK3 (BMPR1A)	ALK3^{nullflox};αMHC-Cre+/−: Cardiac-specific deletion of ALK3 is embryologically lethal around E15.5 with endocardial cushion defects and hypoplastic trabeculae	ALK3 is expressed ubiquitously in mouse embryonic tissues (with the exception of liver)	ALK3(BMPR1A) is required for mesodermal formation in vertebrates.

(Continued)

Table 10-1 (Continued)

Protein family function	Gene name	Organism	Expression sites and stages of involvement	Other family genes with potential role in cardiac development
		ALK3 null/flox cGATA6-Cre+/−: Targeted *Alk3* deletion in cardiomyocytes of the AV canal results in atrio-ventricular valve defects reminiscent of Ebstein's disease and WPW		
	ALK5	α*MHC-ALK5*: Transgenics with cardiac-specific ALK5 activation display arrest of looping morphogenesis and a linear, dilated and hypoplastic heart tube	ALK5 is expressed throughout the heart.	ALK5 is not involved in the endothelial–mesenchymal transformation of the endocardial cushions.
	ACVR2B (ActRIIB)	Human: ACVR2B mutations were only rarely found among cases of LR axis malformation Mouse: ActRIIB−/−: Lethal at birth; randomized heart position, malposition of the great arteries, atrial and ventricular septal defects; right pulmonary isomerism and splenic abnormalities, recapitulating the clinical features of the human asplenia syndrome.		The ActRIIB-mediated signaling pathway interacts with retinoic acid and plays a critical role in patterning both anteroposterior and left–right axes.
	BmpR2	Human: Mutations in *BMPR2* were found in patients with primary pulmonary hypertension (PPH1) Mouse: *BmpR2+/−*: susceptible to pulmonary vascular obstructive lung disease *BmpR2−/−*: die in utero at gastrulation but homozygous mice for a *BmpR2* hypomorphic allele die at midgestation with cardiovascular defects like truncus arteriosus with interrupted aortic arch and dysmorphic semilunar valves		BmpR2 is required for primitive streak formation.
EGFR family/	EGFR	Mouse: *Egfr−/−*: *EGFR* mutant and null mice have abnormal semilunar valves with thickened leaflets Zebrafish: Inhibition of zebrafish *EGFR* activity in vivo impeded blood flow via the outflow tract into the aorta and impeded circulation in the axial and intersegmental vessels by 80 hpf. Analysis of the heart showed that the heart chambers and pericardial sacs were dilated and the outflow tracts were narrowed Mouse:	*EGFR* is ubiquitously expressed during gastrulation, somitogenesis and later stages (zebrafish).	*ErbB4* expressed in cardiomyocytes
Neuregulin receptors			*ErbB2* expressed in cardiomyocytes	

Family	Gene/Receptor	Phenotype	Expression
ErbB2		ErbB2−/−: similar with HRG−/−; die at midgestation because of heart malformation. Conditional mutation of the ErbB2 in cardiomyocytes leads to dilated cardiomyopathy	
Erb3		ErbB3−/−: embryonic lethal at E13.5 with underdeveloped AV valves and mildly reduced myocardial thickness	ErbB3 expressed in endocardial cushion mesenchyme
Cysteine-Rich with EGF-Like Domains	CRELD1	Human: CRELD1 is deleted in the cytogenetic disorder 3p− syndrome that is associated with common atrioventricular canal ASD and VSD	CRELD1 is ubiquitously expressed in early development but later becomes more markedly expressed in the developing heart and branchial arches (chicken). Expression persists in adulthood in most tissues (human).
Neurotrophin receptors	trkC	Mouse: trkC−/−: mice lacking all trkC receptor isoforms die in the early postnatal period with severe cardiac defects such as atrial and ventricular septal defects, and valvular defects including pulmonic stenosis	Expressed in the outflow tract, the posterior wall of the aorta and the cardiac ganglia
Eph receptors tyrosine kinases	EphB2/B3	Mouse: ephB2−/−;ephB3−/−: similar phenotype with ephrinB2 mutants but even more severely affected vessel formation ephB4−/−: similar phenotype as ephB2−/−.	ephB2 is expressed in endocardiac cells and mesenchyme. ephB3 is expressed in all endothelial cells and aortic arches. ephB4 is specifically expressed in endothelial cells of all major veins.
Semaphorin A receptors: neuropilins	Np1	Mouse: Np1−/−: embryonic lethal at E12.5 with congenital heart defects like transposed great arteries, truncus arteriosus and arch anomalies most notable absent fourth and sixth aortic arches	Np1 is a receptor for class 3 semaphorins and for VEGF and is preferentially expressed in the endothelial cells of arteries. Np2 is similarly a receptor for class 3 semaphorins but is preferentially expressed in the endothelial cells of veins. Plexin A2 belongs to the plexins family of receptors for transmembrane semaphorins and is expressed in migratory and postmigratory cardiac neural crest cells.
Integrins	α4β1 integrin	Mouse: α4β1 integrin−/−: embryonic lethal at E12.5 with absent epicardium and hemorrhagic cardiac disease.	α4β1 integrin is expressed both in epicardial cells and cardiac outflow tract cells and appears to be essential for epicardium formation and maintenance
FGFR	DFGF-R2 (DFGRI)/ Heartless (Htl)	Drosophila: Htl mutants lack visceral mesoderm, heart, and the dorsal somatic muscles.	Htl is expressed in the embryonic mesoderm and is essential for cell migration and establishment of several mesodermal lineages into primordia for the heart, visceral and somatic muscles.
PDGFRα	PDGFRα	Mouse: PDGFRα−/−: conotruncal defects, thin myocardium, pericardial effusion	Expressed in cardiac neural crest cells

(Continued)

Table 10-1 *(Continued)*

Protein family function	Gene name	Organism	Expression sites and stages of involvement	Other family genes with potential role in cardiac development
Ig superfamily	*VCAM-1*	Mouse: *VCAM*−/−: most of them embryonic lethal between E10.5 and E12.5 with severe placental defects, absent epicardium, bloody pericardial effusion and reduced compact layer of ventricular myocardium and intraventricular septum.	Expressed in the epicardium and the underlying myocardium, as well as in the intraventricular septum	*Pecam-1* is expressed in the endothelium of the dorsal aorta and the ventricular and outflow tract endocardium (mouse).
Retinoid acid receptors	*RXR*	Mouse: *RXRα*−/−: embryonic lethal at E14.5 from heart failure as result of a thin walled myocardium	Retinoic acid and its metabolites are signals that trigger and modulate cardiac morphogenesis during vertebrate development. The mediators of response to retinoids are transcription factors and proteins of the nuclear hormone receptor superfamily (*RARs*, *RXRs*), that bind these ligands. *RXRs* are expressed in neural crest cells (mouse, chicken). *RARs* are expressed in neural crest and its derivatives, in endocardial cells and sites of ectomesodermal interaction.	There is considerable overlap and redundancy among the various RAR receptors, so the exact role of each one is difficult to be determined. Conoventricular and conoseptal hypoplasia type VSDs have been identified in compound heterozygotes for various RAR receptor isoforms in association with excessive cell death in the conoseptum.
	RAR(α1/β2, α/β2, αγ)		*RARα*−/− and *β*−/−: thin walled myocardium *RAR* inhibition of all isoforms (α, β, γ) impairs the formation of third, fourth, and sixth pharyngeal arches and their derivatives and is associated with conotruncal defects (interrupted aortic arch, truncus arteriosus, VSD, DORV).		
Angiopoietin	*Agpt1*	Mouse: *Agpt1*−/−: embryonic lethal at E12.5 with severe vascular anomalies reminiscent of those seen in embryos lacking *TIE2*. Mutant mice have abnormal ventricular endocardium with decreased trabeculations and collapsed atrial endothelial lining.	Expressed in myocardium wall surrounding the *TIE2* expressing endocardium	
Erythropoietin receptor	*EpoR*	Mouse: *EpoR*−/−: embryonic lethal during midgestation with similar phenotype as the *Epo*−/− mice	*EPOR* is expressed in the developing heart in a subset of cardiac tissues (endocardium, epicardium, pericardium and endocardial cushions) but not myocardium.	
Endothelin receptors	*ET_A*	Mouse: *ET_A*−/−: conotruncal and aortic arch defects	Similar expression pattern as *ET-1*	
ECE	*ECE-1*	Mouse: *ECE-1*−/−: conotruncal and aortic arch defects (Rebagliati 1998)	Expressed in the pharyngeal ectoderm and the aortic arch endothelium.	
	ECE-2	*ECE-1*−/−;*ECE-2*−/−: as above plus atrioventricular valve abnormalities	Expressed in the endocardial cushions	
Orphan nuclear receptors	*COUP-TFII* (*Nr2f2*)	Mouse: *COUP-TFII*−/−: embryonic lethal with defects in angiogenesis and heart development; the atria and sinus venosus fail to develop past the primitive tube stage.	*COUP-TFII* is expressed in mesoderm but only in sinoatrial region of the forming heart.	svp (Drosophila)
Phospatidyl-serine recptor	*Ptdsr*	Mouse: *Ptdsr*−/−: Ablation of *Ptdsr* function in knockout mice causes perinatal lethality from cardiac failure associated with cardiac defects such as VSDs, double-outlet right ventricle, and	Expressed in mesoderm but only in sinoatrial region of the forming heart.	

At the top (continuation of previous text):

hypoplasia of the pulmonary artery. They also display thymus hypoplasia, ocular lesions, hematopoietic defects, growth retardation as well as delay in terminal differentiation of the kidney, intestine, liver and lungs during embryogenesis

c. Channels			
Connexins	Cx40	Mouse:	Both Cx40 and 45 are expressed in the His bundles in mice. Cx43 is expressed in proepicardial and cardiac neural crest cells and is involved in the proper epithelial–mesenchymal transformation of the proepicardial cells and the development of cardiac neural crest cells.
		Cx40−/−: cardiac conduction abnormalities but not complete cardiac block	
	Cx43	Cx43−/−: lethal in neonatal period, conotruncal defects in the RVOT, coronary artery abnormalities	
	Cx45	Cx45−/−: Embryologically lethal at E10; heart failure, endocardial cushion defect, conduction block	
3. Cell structure and motility			
KIF	Kif3A	Mouse:	Expressed in nodal cilia and ubiquitously. Important for leftward nodal flow
		Kif3A−/−: embryonic lethal at E10.5; cardiovascular insufficiency, pericardial effusion, randomization of laterality in heart looping	
	Kif3B	Kif3B−/−: left-right randomization	
Axonemal dynein	DNAH11	Human:	Initially is expressed symmetrically in the node at embryonic day 7.5 but at embryonic day 8, a striking asymmetric expression pattern is observed in all three germ layers, suggesting roles in both the establishment and maintenance of left–right asymmetry.
	Lrdynein (lrd)/iv	Mutation in DNAH11 has been found in a patient with Kartagener syndrome.	
		Mouse:	
		lrd−/−: Homozygous mutants display randomized left-right development but no congenital heart defects (identical with iv/iv mutant mice)	
Smoothened	Smo	Mouse:	Smo acts epistatic to Ptc1 to mediate Shh and Ihh signaling in the early mouse embryo.
		Smo−/−: developmental arrest at somitogenesis with small, linear heart tube, open gut, and cyclopia	
Laminin	Laminin	Drosophila:	Expressed in extracellular mattrix
		laminin A deficient embryos:display twists and breaks of cardioblasts at late embryonic stages as a result of dissociation of the pericardial cells	
		Mouse:	
		laminin–α2−/−: display phenotype equivalent with muscular dystrophy; mutants die prematurely at 5 mo from unidentified cause	
Hyaluronidase synthase	Has2	Mouse:	Important for AV cushion transformation
		Has2−/−: embryonic lethal at E9.5 with abnormal formation of AV cushions and outflow tract, thin myocardium, pericardial edema	

(Continued)

Table 10-1 (Continued)

Protein family function	Gene name	Organism	Expression sites and stages of involvement	Other family genes with potential role in cardiac development
UDP-glucose dehydrogenase	UDP-GD	Zebrafish: jekyll: zebrafish mutants for UDP-GD have thin myocardium and hypoplastic endocardial cushions		
Perlecan (heparin–sulfate proteoglycan)	Perlecan	Mouse: Perlecan−/−: embryonic lethal at E10 or at birth; TGA, hyperplastic semilunar valves	Perlecan is present in the basal surface of myocardium and endocardium, as well as surrounding neural crest cells. It controls production of heparin–sulfate proteoglycan and is important for AV cushion transformation.	
Versican	Cspg2 (versican)	Mouse: Hdf (Cspg2 −/−): Embryonic lethal at E10.5; the future right ventricle and conotruncus of the single heart tube fail to form and the endocardial cushions are absent	Cspg2 gene controls expression of the chondroitin sulfate proteoglycan versican and is required for the successful development of the endocardial cushion swellings and the embryonic heart segments that give rise to the right ventricle and conotruncus.	
Fibulin	Fibulin-2	Mouse: Fibulin-2 −/−: No cardiac developmental abnormalities	Expressed in AV cushions	
Fibrillin	Fbn-1 Fbn-2	Human: Heterozygous mutations of Fbn1 and Fbn2 are associated with Marfan's phenotype		
Elastin	Elastin	Human: Haploinsufficiency of Ch7q11.23 that includes elastin is associated with Williams-Bueren syndrome (supravalvular aortic stenosis, elfin facies, hypercalcemia and mental retardation)	Expressed in endocardial cells	
Collagen	COL3A1	Human: Ehlers-Danlos syndrome type IV results from mutations in the COL3A1 gene, which encodes the polypeptides in type III collagen		
	Collagen6 α1/α2	Mouse: Specific alleles of the collagen genes associated with atrioventricular canal defects	Collagen VI genes are expressed in the AV canal tissue of embryonic mouse hearts and are included in the region of the human chromosome 21 that is considered critical for congenital heart defects.	
Vinculin	Vinculin	Mouse: Vinculin−/−: early embryonic lethal between E8-E10 with severely reduced and akinetic myocardial and endocardial structures	Ubiquitously expressed (mouse)	
4. Metabolism Folbp	Folbp1	Mouse: Folbp1−/−: embryonic lethal at E10, growth retardation, neural tube defects and aortic arch defects	Folbp1 is expressed in the mesenchyme of the pharyngeal arches. Phenotype was rescued by folate rich diet.	
RALDH	RALDH1,2	Mouse: RALDH2−/−: embryonic lethal at E10.5 with formation of an unlooped medial distended cavity and severe impairment of posterior	RALDH2 is expressed in the mesenchyme and the early heart epicardium	RALDH1 is coexpressed with Raldh2 in the early heart epicardium, and is later specifically expressed in developing heart valves.

chamber (atria and sinus venosus) development. The developing ventricular myocardium consists of a thick layer of loosely attached and prematurely differentiated cardiomyocytes. Mutant mice harboring a hypomorphic allele of *RALDH2* die perinatally and exhibit the features of the human DiGeorge syndrome (DGS) with heart outflow tract septation defects and selective defects of the posterior (third to sixth) branchial arches

ASD, atrial septal defect; VSD, ventricular septal defect; TOF, Tetralogy of Fallot; IAA, interrupted aortic arch; RAA, right aortic arch; TA, truncus arteriosus; AV canal, atrioventricular canal; DORV, Double outlet right ventricle; HLHS, hypoplastic left heart syndrome; DGS, DiGeorge syndrome; DGCR, DiGeorge critical region; RSCA, retroesophageal subclavian artery; bHLH, basic helix-loop-helix; Prh, proline-rich homeobox; Hex, hematopoietically expressed homeobox; TGF, transforming growth factor; FGF, fibroblast growth factor; EGF, epidermal growth factor; PDGF, platelet-derived growth factor; Bmp, Bone morphogenetic protein; VEGF, vascular endothelial growth factor; RALDH2, retinaldehyde dehydrogenase. *Prh, proline-rich homeobox is the new name for Hex, hematopoietically expressed homeobox.*

of its close phylogenetic relationship to humans and the similarities between the mouse and the human heart at the anatomic and physiological levels. The completion of sequencing of the mouse genome adds an additional advantage over other species for dissecting genetic pathways associated with congenital malformations.

However, murine cardiac development is difficult to observe in a serial fashion in vivo without new imaging techniques because of the relatively inaccessible embryo, and because most mouse embryos with severe cardiac malfunction die early *in utero*, complicating functional analysis. Systematic screens of the mouse genome for recessive mutations affecting morphogenesis of several organs have been initiated but are decidedly expensive. Experimentation with the chick *Gallus gallus*, whose embryonic material is easily accessible for physical manipulation from the earliest stages, has proven beneficial for some areas like the study of neural crest. The African clawed frog *Xenopus laevis* has been used mostly to study the inductive interactions in the establishment of polarity and tissue differentiation. The drawback of these vertebrates is the long generation time and the inapplicability of classic genetics. The teleost fish *Danio (formerly Brachydanio) rerio* (zebrafish) has emerged as a model system because of its prolific egg production, rapid (90 d) generation time, optically transparent embryo, and extremely rapid heart development (48 h). In addition the sequencing of the zebrafish genome is close to completion. Loss-of-function gene models have been successfully created in zebrafish with the use of morpholino-modified antisense oligonucleotides. In zebrafish embryos the cardiovascular system is functional at 24 h but not essential for survival of the early embryo, which obtains adequate oxygen by simple diffusion, and even mutant embryos with complete lack of circulation can survive for 3 d. This is an important advantage over the mammalian embryos, whose survival is dependent on an intact circulation, and allows the study of zebrafish mutants with cardiovascular defects, whose mammalian embryonic counterparts undergo rapid degeneration and absorption. Despite the advantages of the zebrafish system for mutational analysis, there are some aspects of cardiovascular construction, namely septation and pulmonary artery formation that must be studied in higher vertebrates. Finally, the fruit fly, *Drosophila melanogaster,* completes the panel of experimental models used in cardiogenomics. One of the most remarkable discoveries was of the gene needed in *Drosophila* to produce a heart. Finding this gene, named *"tinman"* after the Wizard of Oz character in need of a heart, led to the identification of the evolutionarily conserved, and previously unknown, class of homeodomain-containing *"NK"* genes, which are critical for cardiac muscle development in all animals. Orthologous relationships between *NK* and other cardiac gene regulatory networks in *Drosophila* and mouse have been identified, showing that control of cardiac formation is likely to have been conserved over 600×10^6 yr.

Information on the genetic and molecular bases of cardiovascular development, function, and disease that has accumulated from the combination of data from animal models and human genetic studies is leading to a redefinition of the pathophysiology of congenital heart diseases, and innovative diagnostic and prognostic tools are emerging. This chapter discusses the anatomic malformations, which comprise the majority of cases of human congenital heart disease, but specifically excludes heritable cardiomyopathies, long QT syndrome and Marfan syndrome, discussed in other chapters.

CLINICAL FEATURES

The majority of human newborns with hemodynamically significant heart defects present in the first 2 wk of life with one out of four physiological arrangements: obstruction to pulmonary arterial circulation, obstruction to systemic arterial circulation, inadequate mixing between pulmonary and systemic circulations, or pulmonary venous obstruction. Because of the two-connected-pumps-working-in-parallel construction of fetal cardiac circulation (Fig. 10-1, left panel), these four types of hemodynamic aberrations are well tolerated for a 40-wk gestation. An obstruction to the pulmonary or aortic outflow is reliably compensated by blood flow shifting to the contralateral side of the heart. Transposition of the great arteries with intact ventricular septum does not have hemodynamic consequences because it merely constitutes a different variety of two-connected-pumps-working-in-parallel configuration. Anomalous pulmonary venous connection with pulmonary venous obstruction does not substantially alter prenatal hemodynamics because minimal blood flows into the lungs *in utero*.

The four physiological derangements described earlier are unmasked when the circulation is acutely changed at birth to a two-unconnected-pumps-working-in-series arrangement, with lungs but without placenta (Fig. 10-1, right panel). The rapidity of presentation is critically dependent on the time-course of foramen closure or ductal closure or both. Impaired pulmonary flow manifests as cyanosis, whereas impaired systemic circulation manifests as "low output syndrome." Inadequate mixing between the pulmonary and systemic circulations also appears as cyanosis. Because of the interstitial edema, pulmonary venous obstruction manifests as tachypnea in addition to cyanosis. Although these four hemodynamic subsets account for virtually all cases of heart defects appearing in the first 2 wk of life, severe cases of the rare malformation "absent pulmonary valve syndrome," whose cardinal feature is ventilatory failure because of airway impingement by adjacent markedly dilated pulmonary arteries, may also present on the first day of life.

A few types of malformation are evident after 2 wk of age. Isolated large septation defects resulting in left-to-right shunt physiology typically do not present in the first 2 wk of age because the magnitude of the left-to-right shunt depends mostly on the pulmonary vascular resistance, the latter parameter falling to its adult value gradually over the first 6 mo. The uncommon condition of anomalous origin of the left coronary artery from the pulmonary artery, which results in gradual-onset myocardial ischemia, also manifests after the neonatal period because the reduction in perfusion of the left ventricle is closely linked to the fall in pulmonary vascular resistance. Finally, in some rare forms of congenital heart defects, a physiologically corrected but inherently abnormal organization of the cardiac segments has no immediate hemodynamic effects (L-TGA). However, at a much later point, the longevity of this arrangement is challenged by the long-term mechanical cues (e.g., pressure or volume overload) normally not destined for these anatomic structures, and heart failure frequently occurs.

DIAGNOSIS

Although the screening protocol includes physical examination, arterial blood gas, electrocardiogram, and chest roentgenogram, the principal tool for detailed characterization of morphology and hemodynamics in the human newborn is ultrasound imaging. With

and so on), mice carrying specific mutations of nonnull, i.e., hypomorphic alleles may be more illuminating, because they may mimic the human conditions more closely. "Conditional," such as tissue- or stage-specific, mutant lines will also become more common. Zebrafish labs will continue to analyze the zygotic recessive mutations affecting cardiovascular development. Cloning the genes affected in these mutants will be facilitated by the completion of sequencing of the organism's genome. However, the construction of additional genetic tools such as transgenic fluorescent-reporter zebrafish lines whose embryos fluoresce green when a structure or tissue of interest is first specified could serve as the starting reagent for large-scale "targeted" mutagenesis screens in this organism. In the current postgenomic era, with the complete genome sequences of several species (including human, mouse, and zebrafish) at hand, the challenge will be to understand the function of genes within the cardiovascular system. One of the most powerful methods available to assign function to a gene is to inactivate the gene by reverse genetic approaches. In this regard loss-of-function gene models have been successfully created in zebrafish with the use of antisense morpholino oligonucleotides that can specifically inhibit the translation of a specific gene. However, this method is suited only for early developmental stages with the additional drawback of nonspecific side effects. Recently, a new reverse genetic approach, hitherto utilized in plants, target induced local lesions in genomes is being applied to zebrafish to generate allelic series in individual genes of interest. In humans, positional cloning will continue to be employed for large families with single-gene disorders. Attempts to correlate particular amino acid substitutions with specific human cardiac malformations will afford further insight into the structure-function relationships of the relevant proteins, whether they are transcription factors, signals, or receptors.

SELECTED REFERENCES

Abu-Issa R, Smyth G, Smoak I, Yamamura K, Meyers EN. Fgf8 is required for pharyngeal arch and cardiovascular development in the mouse. Development 2002;129:4613–4625.

Bao ZZ, Bruneau BG, Seidman JG, Seidman CE, Cepko CL. Regulation of chamber-specific gene expression in the developing heart by Irx4. Science 1999;283:1161–1164.

Bartman T, Walsh EC, Wen KK, et al. Early myocardial function affects endocardial cushion development in zebrafish. PLoS Biol 2004;2:E129.

Basson CT, Bachinsky DR, Lin RC, et al. Mutations in human TBX5 cause limb and cardiac malformation in Holt-Oram syndrome. Nat Genet 1997;15:30–35.

Biben C, Weber R, Kesteven S, et al. Cardiac septal and valvular dysmorphogenesis in mice heterozygous for mutations in the homeobox gene Nkx2-5. Circ Res 2001;87(10):888–895.

Bisgrove BW, Essner JJ, Yost HJ. Multiple pathways in the midline regulate concordant brain, heart and gut left-right asymmetry. Development 2000;127:3567–3579.

Brown CB, Boyer AS, Runyan RB, Barnett JV. Requirement of type III TGF-beta receptor for endocardial cell transformation in the heart. Science 1999;283:2080–2082.

Brown CB, Feiner L, Lu MM, et al. PlexinA2 and semaphorin signaling during cardiac neural crest development. Development 2001;128: 3071–3080.

Bruneau BG, Nemer G, Schmitt JP, et al. A murine model of Holt-Oram syndrome defines roles of the T-box transcription factor Tbx5 in cardiogenesis and disease. Cell 2001;106:709–721.

Cai CL, Liang X, Shi Y, et al. Isl1 identifies a cardiac progenitor population that proliferates prior to differentiation and contributes a majority of cells to the heart. Dev Cell 2003;5:877–889.

Camenisch TD, Spicer AP, Brehm-Gibson T, et al. Disruption of hyaluronan synthase-2 abrogates normal cardiac morphogenesis and hyaluronan-mediated transformation of epithelium to mesenchyme. J Clin Invest 2000;106:349–360.

Carraway KL III. Involvement of the neuregulins and their receptors in cardiac and neural development. Bioessays 1996;18:263–266.

Chang CP, Neilson JR, Bayle JH, et al. A field of myocardial-endocardial NFAT signaling underlies heart valve morphogenesis. Cell 2004;118: 649–663.

Chang H, Zwijsen A, Vogel H, Huylebroeck D, Matzuk MM. Smad5 is essential for left-right asymmetry in mice. Dev Biol 2000;219:71–78.

Charron J, Malynn BA, Fisher P, et al. Embryonic lethality in mice homozygous for a targeted disruption of the N-myc gene. Genes Dev 1992;6: 2248–2257.

Chen F, Kook H, Milewski R, et al. Hop is an unusual homeobox gene that modulates cardiac development. Cell 2002;110:713–723.

Conway SJ, Henderson DJ, Kirby ML, Anderson RH, Copp AJ. Development of a lethal congenital heart defect in the splotch (Pax3) mutant mouse. Cardiovasc Res 1997;36:163–173.

de la Pompa JL, Timmerman LA, Takimoto H, et al. Role of the NF-ATc transcription factor in morphogenesis of cardiac valves and septum. Nature 1998;392:182–186.

Delot EC, Bahamonde ME, Zhao M, Lyons KM. BMP signaling is required for septation of the outflow tract of the mammalian heart. Development 2003;130:209–220.

Deng Z, Morse JH, Slager SL, et al. Familial primary pulmonary hypertension (gene PPH1) is caused by mutations in the bone morphogenetic protein receptor-II gene. Am J Hum Genet 2000;67:737–744.

Donovan J, Kordylewska A, Jan YN, Utset MF. Tetralogy of Fallot and other congenital heart defects in Hey2 mutant mice. Curr Biol 2002; 12:1605–1610.

Elliott DA, Kirk EP, Yeoh T, et al. Cardiac homeobox gene NKX2-5 mutations and congenital heart disease: associations with atrial septal defect and hypoplastic left heart syndrome. J Am Coll Cardiol 2003;41(11): 2072–2076.

Funke B, Epstein JA, Kochilas LK, et al. Mice overexpressing genes from the 22q11 region deleted in velo-cardio- facial syndrome/DiGeorge syndrome have middle and inner ear defects. Hum Mol Genet 2001; 10:2549–2556.

Gaio U, Schweickert A, Fischer A, et al. A role of the cryptic gene in the correct establishment of the left- right axis. Curr Biol 1999;9:1339–1342.

Gajewski K, Fossett N, Molkentin JD, Schulz RA. The zinc finger proteins Pannier and GATA4 function as cardiogenic factors in Drosophila. Development 1999;126:5679–5688.

Garg V, Kathirya IS, Barnes R, et al. GATA4 mutations cause human congenital heart defects and reveal an interaction with TBX5. Nature 2003;24:443–447

Gerety SS, Anderson DJ. Cardiovascular ephrinB2 function is essential for embryonic angiogenesis. Development 2002;129:1397–1410.

Gessler M, Knobeloch KP, Helisch A, et al. Mouse gridlock: no aortic coarctation or deficiency, but fatal cardiac defects in Hey2 −/− mice. Curr Biol 2002;12:1601–1604.

Ghyselinck NB, Wendling O, Messaddeq N, et al. Contribution of retinoic acid receptor beta isoforms to the formation of the conotruncal septum of the embryonic heart. Dev Biol 1998;198:303–318.

Goldmuntz E. Recent advances in understanding the genetic etiology of congenital heart disease. Curr Opin Pediatr 1999;11:437–443.

Goldmuntz E, Bamford R, Karkera JD, dela Cruz J, Roessler E, Muenke M. CFC1 mutations in patients with transposition of the great arteries and double-outlet right ventricle. Am J Hum Genet 2002;70: 776–780.

Hamblet NS, Lijam N, Ruiz-Lozano P, et al. Dishevelled 2 is essential for cardiac outflow tract development, somite segmentation and neural tube closure. Development 2002;129:5827–5838.

Hatcher CJ, Kim MS, Mah CS, et al. TBX5 transcription factor regulates cell proliferation during cardiogenesis. Dev Biol 2001;230:177–188.

Hornberger LK, Sanders SP, Rein AJ, Spevak PJ, Parness IA, Colan SD. Left heart obstructive lesions and left ventricular growth in the midtrimester fetus. A longitudinal study. Circulation 1995;92:1531–1538.

Hove JR, Koster RW, Forouhar AS, Acevedo-Bolton G, Fraser SE, Gharib M. Intracardiac fluid forces are an essential epigenetic factor for embryonic cardiogenesis. Nature 2003;421:172–177.

Iwamoto R, Yamazaki S, Asakura M, et al. Heparin-binding EGF-like growth factor and ErbB signaling is essential for heart function. Proc Natl Acad Sci USA 2003;100:3221–3226.

Izraeli S, Lowe LA, Bertness VL, et al. The SIL gene is required for mouse embryonic axial development and left- right specification. Nature 1999;399:691–694.

Jackson LF, Qiu TH, Sunnarborg SW, et al. Defective valvulogenesis in HB-EGF and TACE-null mice is associated with aberrant BMP signaling. EMBO J 2003;22:2704–2716.

Jerome LA, Papaioannou VE. DiGeorge syndrome phenotype in mice mutant for the T-box gene, Tbx1. Nat Genet 2001;27:286–291.

Kasahara H, Lee B, Schott JJ, et al. Loss of function and inhibitory effects of human CSX/NKX2.5 homeoprotein mutations associated with congenital heart disease. J Clin Invest 2000;106:299–308.

Keating M. Elastin and vascular disease. Trends Cardiovasc Med 1994; 4:202–206.

Kelly RG, Brown NA, Buckingham ME. The arterial pole of the mouse heart forms from Fgf10-expressing cells in pharyngeal mesoderm. Dev Cell 2001;1:435–440.

Kim RY, Robertson EJ, Solloway MJ. Bmp6 and Bmp7 are required for cushion formation and septation in the developing mouse heart. Dev Biol 2001;235:449–466.

King T, Beddington RS, Brown NA. The role of the brachyury gene in heart development and left-right specification in the mouse. Mech Dev 1998;79:29–37.

Kirby ML, Gale TF, Stewart DE. Neural crest cells contribute to normal aorticopulmonary septation. Science 1983;220:1059–1061.

Kitajima S, Takagi A, Inoue T, Saga Y. MesP1 and MesP2 are essential for the development of cardiac mesoderm. Development 2000;127: 3215–3226.

Kitamura K, Miura H, Miyagawa-Tomita S, et al. Mouse Pitx2 deficiency leads to anomalies of the ventral body wall, heart, extra- and periocular mesoderm and right pulmonary isomerism. Development 1999; 126:5749–5758.

Klinedinst SL, Bodmer R. Gata factor Pannier is required to establish competence for heart progenitor formation. Development 2003; 130:3027–3038.

Kuo CT, Morrisey EE, Anandappa R, et al. GATA4 transcription factor is required for ventral morphogenesis and heart tube formation. Genes Dev 1997;11:1048–1060.

Lai YT, Beason KB, Brames GP, et al. Activin receptor-like kinase 2 can mediate atrioventricular cushion transformation. Dev Biol 2000; 222:1–11.

Laugwitz KL, Moretti A, Lam J, et al. Postnatal isl1 + cardioblasts enter fully differentiated cardiomyocyte lineages. Nature 2005;433:647–653.

Li S, Zhou D, Lu MM, Morrisey EE. Advanced cardiac morphogenesis does not require heart tube fusion. Science 2004;305:1619–1622.

Liao J, Kochilas L, Nowotschin S, et al. Full spectrum of malformations in velo-cardio-facial syndrome/DiGeorge syndrome mouse models by altering Tbx1 dosage. Hum Mol Gen 2004;13(15):1–9.

Lin Q, Lu J, Yanagisawa H, et al. Requirement of the MADS-box transcription factor MEF2C for vascular development. Development 1998;125:4565–4574.

Lindsay EA, Botta A, Jurecic V, et al. Congenital heart disease in mice deficient for the DiGeorge syndrome region. Nature 1999;401:379–383.

Lindsay EA, Vitelli F, Su H, et al. Tbx1 haploinsufficieny in the DiGeorge syndrome region causes aortic arch defects in mice. Nature 2001; 410:97–101.

Liu C, Liu W, Lu MF, Brown NA, Martin JF. Regulation of left-right asymmetry by thresholds of Pitx2c activity. Development 2001;128: 2039–2048.

Meno C, Shimono A, Saijoh Y, et al. lefty-1 is required for left-right determination as a regulator of lefty-2 and nodal. Cell 1998;94:287–297.

Merscher S, Funke B, Epstein JA, et al. TBX1 is responsible for cardiovascular defects in velo-cardio-facial/DiGeorge syndrome. Cell 2001;104:619–629.

Meyers EN, Martin GR. Differences in left-right axis pathways in mouse and chick: functions of FGF8 and SHH. Science 1999;285:403–406.

Michelson AM, Gisselbrecht S, Zhou Y, Baek KH, Buff EM. Dual functions of the heartless fibroblast growth factor receptor in development of the Drosophila embryonic mesoderm. Dev Genet 1998;22:212–229.

Milewicz DM. Molecular genetics of Marfan syndrome and Ehlers-Danlos type IV. Curr Opin Cardiol 1998;13:198–204.

Molkentin JD, Lin Q, Duncan SA, Olson EN. Requirement of the transcription factor GATA4 for heart tube formation and ventral morphogenesis. Genes Dev 1997;11:1061–1072.

Nasevicius A, Ekker SC. Effective targeted gene "knockdown" in zebrafish. Nat Genet 2000;26:216–220.

Niederreither K, Vermot J, Messaddeq N, Schuhbaur B, Chambon P, Dolle P. Embryonic retinoic acid synthesis is essential for heart morphogenesis in the mouse. Development 2001;128:1019–1031.

Ranger AM, Grusby MJ, Hodge MR, et al. The transcription factor NF-ATc is essential for cardiac valve formation. Nature 1998;392:186–190.

Reaume AG, de Sousa PA, Kulkarni S, et al. Cardiac malformation in neonatal mice lacking connexin43. Science 1995;267:1831–1834.

Reifers F, Walsh EC, Leger S, Stainier DY, Brand M. Induction and differentiation of the zebrafish heart requires fibroblast growth factor 8 (fgf8/acerebellar). Development 2000;127:225–235.

Saga Y, Kitajima S, Miyagawa-Tomita S. Mesp1 expression is the earliest sign of cardiovascular development. Trends Cardiovasc Med 2000; 10:345–352.

Sakata Y, Kamei CN, Nakagami H, Bronson R, Liao JK, Chin MT. Ventricular septal defect and cardiomyopathy in mice lacking the transcription factor CHF1/Hey2. Proc Natl Acad Sci USA 2002;99: 16197–16202.

Satoda M, Zhao F, Diaz GA, et al. Mutations in TFAP2B cause Char syndrome, a familial form of patent ductus arteriosus. Nat Genet 2000; 25:42–46.

Schneider VA, Mercola M. Wnt antagonism initiates cardiogenesis in Xenopus laevis. Genes Dev 2001;15:304–315.

Sissman NJ, Lefkowitz RJ, Willerson JT. Incidence of congenital heart disease. JAMA 2001;285:2579–2580.

Srinivasan S, Hanes MA, Dickens T, et al. A mouse model for hereditary hemorrhagic telangiectasia (HHT) type 2. Hum Mol Genet 2003;12: 473–482.

Srivastava D. HAND proteins: molecular mediators of cardiac development and congenital heart disease. Trends Cardiovasc Med 1999;9:11–18.

Srivastava D, Olson EN. A genetic blueprint for cardiac development. Nature 2000;407:221–226.

Stainier DY, Fouquet B, Chen JN, et al. Mutations affecting the formation and function of the cardiovascular system in the zebrafish embryo. Development 1996;123:285–292.

Stalmans I, Lambrechts D, De Smet F, et al. VEGF: a modifier of the del22q11 (DiGeorge) syndrome? Nat Med 2003;9:173–182.

Sucov HM, Dyson E, Gumeringer CL, Price J, Chien KR, Evans RM. RXR alpha mutant mice establish a genetic basis for vitamin A signaling in heart morphogenesis. Genes Dev 1994;8:1007–1018.

Supp DM, Brueckner M, Kuehn MR, et al. Targeted deletion of the ATP binding domain of left-right dynein confirms its role in specifying development of left-right asymmetries. Development 1999;126: 5495–5504.

Tartaglia M, Kalidas K, Shaw A, et al. PTPN11 mutations in Noonan syndrome: molecular spectrum, genotype-phenotype correlation, and phenotypic heterogeneity. Am J Hum Genet 2002;70:1555–1563.

Tevosian SG, Deconinck AE, Tanaka M, et al. FOG-2, a cofactor for GATA transcription factors, is essential for heart morphogenesis and development of coronary vessels from epicardium. Cell 2000;101: 729–739.

Thomas T, Yamagishi H, Overbeek PA, Olson EN, Srivastava D. The bHLH factors, dHAND and eHAND, specify pulmonary and systemic cardiac ventricles independent of left-right sidedness. Dev Biol 1998;196:228–236.

Trembath RC. Mutations in the TGF-beta type 1 receptor, ALK1, in combined primary pulmonary hypertension and hereditary haemorrhagic telangiectasia, implies pathway specificity. J Heart Lung Transplant 2001;20:175.

Tsukui T, Capdevila J, Tamura K, et al. Multiple left-right asymmetry defects in Shh(–/–) mutant mice unveil a convergence of the shh and retinoic acid pathways in the control of Lefty-1. Proc Natl Acad Sci USA 1999;96:11,376–11,381.

Vermot J, Niederreither K, Garnier JM, Chambon P, Dolle P. Decreased embryonic retinoic acid synthesis results in a DiGeorge syndrome phenotype in newborn mice. Proc Natl Acad Sci USA 2003;100: 1763–1768.

von Both I, Silvestri C, Erdemir T, et al. Foxh1 is essential for development of the anterior heart field. Developmental Cell 2004;7(3): 331–345.

Wallace KN, Yusuff S, Sonntag JM, Chin AJ, Pack M. Zebrafish hhex regulates liver development and digestive organ chirality. Genesis 2001; 30:141–143.

Wang B, Weidenfeld J, Lu MM, et al. Foxp1 regulates cardiac outflow tract, endocardial cushion morphogenesis and myocyte proliferation and maturation. Development 2004;131(18):4477–4487.

Wendling O, Dennefeld C, Chambon P, Mark M. Retinoid signaling is essential for patterning the endoderm of the third and fourth pharyngeal arches. Development 2000;127:1553–1562.

Wienholds E, van Eeden F, Kosters M, et al. Efficient target-selected mutagenesis in zebrafish. Genome Res 2003;13:2700–2707.

Winnier GE, Kume T, Deng K, et al. Roles for the winged helix transcription factors MF1 and MFH1 in cardiovascular development revealed by nonallelic noncomplementation of null alleles. Dev Biol 1999; 213:418–431.

Xue Y, Gao X, Lindsell CE, et al. Embryonic lethality and vascular defects in mice lacking the Notch ligand Jagged1. Hum Mol Genet 1999;8: 723–730.

Ya J, Schilham MW, de Boer PA, Moorman AF, Clevers H, Lamers WH. Sox4-deficiency syndrome in mice is an animal model for common trunk. Circ Res 1998;83:986–994.

Yanagisawa H, Hammer RE, Richardson JA, et al. Disruption of ECE-1 and ECE-2 reveals a role for endothelin-converting enzyme-2 in murine cardiac development. J Clin Invest 2000;105:1373–1382.

Yanagisawa H, Hammer RE, Richardson JA, Williams SC, Clouthier DE, Yanagisawa M. Role of Endothelin-1/Endothelin-A receptor-mediated signaling pathway in the aortic arch patterning in mice. J Clin Invest 1998;102:22–33.

Yin Z, Haynie J, Yang X, et al. The essential role of Cited2, a negative regulator for HIF-1alpha, in heart development and neurulation. Proc Natl Acad Sci USA 2002;99:10,488–10,493.

11 Inherited Cardiomyopathies

CAROLYN Y. HO AND CHRISTINE E. SEIDMAN

SUMMARY

Genetics is an emerging field in cardiovascular medicine. Remarkably, less than 50 yr ago genetics was a nascent field of basic research with little apparent relevance to cardiovascular science or any other medical subspecialty. Yet today cardiovascular genetics is a discipline that fully integrates high technology laboratory investigation and clinical medicine. From this unusual hybrid have emerged discoveries that precisely identify cause in here-to-for "idiopathic" disorders, that provide fundamental insights into disease processes, and that delineate subtypes in well-defined pathologies. Insights from these discoveries uproot traditional anatomic classifications of disease and integrate cell physiology and molecular biochemistry into the study of pathology. For researchers, practitioners, and patients alike, cardiovascular genetics has a growing impact on the definition and diagnosis of disease, on explaining prognosis, and expanding treatments.

Key Words: Dilated cardiomyopathy; DNA; gene; genetic risk; hypertrophic cardiomyopathy; mutation; modes of inheritance; preclinical disease; sequence.

INTRODUCTION

Cardiomyopathies are disorders of the myocardium, which arise from a variety of etiologies and trigger pathways that may culminate in hypertrophic or dilated remodeling of the heart. The details of the cellular and molecular events that lead to compensatory forms of cardiac remodeling in response to a superimposed load remain largely unknown. In contrast, there have been greater advances in the study of primary cardiomyopathies, disorders of cardiac myocytes, which remodel the myocardium in the absence of other underlying pathology. Inherited gene defects are increasingly recognized as the most common cause of hypertrophic cardiomyopathy (HCM) and a frequent cause of dilated cardiomyopathy (DCM). Elucidating the molecular mechanisms leading from genetic mutation to the clinical expression of disease will have profound effects on the understanding of broader issues of basic myocyte structure and function, and influence the approach to disease management.

HYPERTROPHIC CARDIOMYOPATHY

CLINICAL ASPECTS HCM was first described over 100-yr-ago but the modern characterization dates to 1959. It has been traditionally typified by unexplained cardiac hypertrophy in a nondilated ventricle (Fig. 11-1). By definition, this refers to myocardial hypertrophy that occurs in the absence of any systemic or cardiac condition (such as hypertension or aortic stenosis) which may account for an increased load on the heart. The most common pattern of hypertrophy is asymmetric septal hypertrophy, but there is a significant variation in both the location and extent of left-ventricular hypertrophy (LVH) in affected individuals. The histopathological hallmarks of this condition are myocyte hypertrophy with myocardial disarray and fibrosis (Fig. 11-2). Genetic studies have defined HCM to be a disease of the sarcomere, caused by mutations in genes encoding different components of the contractile apparatus.

Clinical manifestations of HCM are diverse and its description has been largely shaped by available diagnostic tools. Traditionally the most obvious and easily characterized features of this condition have been emphasized: outflow tract obstruction and LVH. However, resting outflow tract obstruction occurs in only approx 25% of patients. A provocable gradient may be detected in other patients by administering medications or performing maneuvers that reduce afterload or preload or increase cardiac contractility.

EPIDEMIOLOGY The prevalence of unexplained LVH in the general population is estimated to be 1 in 500. Most of these cases are likely attributable to mutations in genes that encode sarcomere proteins, making HCM the most common genetic cardiovascular disorder. HCM is also the leading cause of sudden death among competitive athletes in the United States.

SYMPTOMS The clinical spectrum of HCM is diverse. Although some individuals experience no or minor symptoms and are diagnosed only in the course of family screening, others develop refractory symptoms of pulmonary congestion, progressing to end-stage heart failure that may require cardiac transplantation. In a small subset, sudden cardiac death (SCD) may be the presenting event.

Shortness of breath, particularly on exertion, is the most common symptom of HCM, occurring in about 90% of patients. Other manifestations include chest pain (approx 30%, often exertional), palpitations, orthostatic lightheadedness, presyncope and syncope (15–25%), orthopnea/paroxysmal nocturnal dyspnea, and fatigue. There is no close correlation between the degree of LVH or outflow tract obstruction and the severity of symptoms. Although often multifactorial in etiology, the occurrence of syncope may be a marker for increased risk of SCD, especially in younger individuals.

From: *Principles of Molecular Medicine, Second Edition*
Edited by: M. S. Runge and C. Patterson © Humana Press, Inc., Totowa, NJ

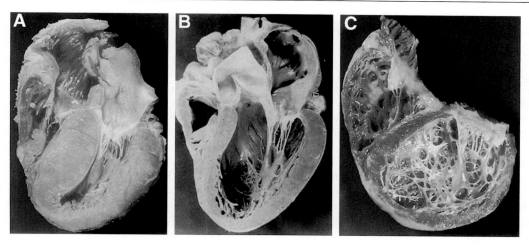

Figure 11-1 Gross pathological specimens of a heart with (**A**) hypertrophic cardiomyopathy (HCM) and (**C**) dilated cardiomyopathy (DCM). Note the marked increased in left-ventricular hypertrophy (HCM) and chamber dimensions (DCM) as compared with (**B**) the normal heart. (Please *see* color insert.)

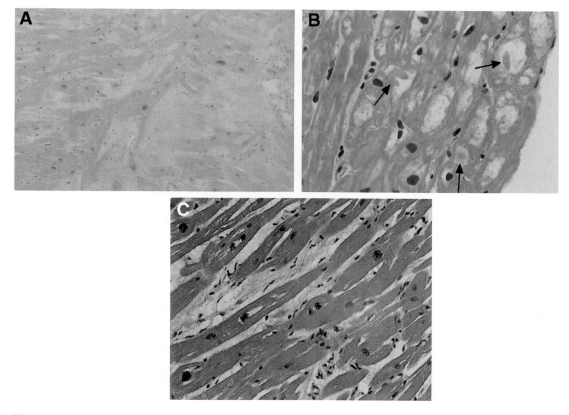

Figure 11-2 Histopathology of distinct human cardiomyopathies revealed by hematoxylin and eosin staining. (**A**) Hypertrophic cardiomyopathy specimen shows characteristic features of myocyte hypertrophy with myocardial disarray and fibrosis. (**B**) In contrast, histological specimens from patients with PRKAG2 mutations show myocytes with nonmembrane bound vacuoles (arrows) that stain for glycogen and amylopectin. Note mild amounts of fibrosis and absence of significant myocyte disarray. (From Arad M, Benson DW, Perez-Atayde AR, et al., 2002. Constitutively active AMP kinase mutations cause glycogen storage disease mimicking hypertrophic cardiomyopathy. J Clin Invest 2002;109:357–362. [Reproduced with permission of J Clin Invest.]) (**C**) Dilated cardiomyopathy caused by a phospholamban missense mutation shows myocyte enlargement without disarray and marked interstitial fibrosis. (From Science 2003;299:1410–1413.) (Please *see* color insert.)

PHYSICAL EXAMINATION Left ventricular (LV) systolic function is typically preserved; however, abnormal diastolic function has been well documented and may largely account for symptoms of pulmonary congestion and exercise intolerance. Diastolic dysfunction may be a fundamental manifestation of altered sarcomere function. It precedes the development of LVH in preliminary studies of individuals who have inherited a causal sarcomere gene mutation, but have not yet developed other typical features of disease. In addition to impaired contractile function, some individuals with HCM have altered blood pressure response to exercise, possibly related to abnormal vasomotor tone. This finding may indicate a worse prognosis with a higher risk for sudden death.

Typical findings on physical examination include a prominent LV apical impulse or lift, a fourth heart sound (S4), and a brisk, occasionally bifid carotid upstroke. If obstruction is present, there may be a harsh crescendo-decrescendo systolic murmur typically best heard at the apex and lower left sternal border, radiating to the axilla and base, but usually not to the neck. This murmur may reflect outflow tract obstruction as well as mitral regurgitation.

NATURAL HISTORY The natural history of HCM is highly variable, even among family members who have inherited the same causal mutation. HCM rarely presents in infancy or early childhood; development of LVH typically occurs in adolescence in conjunction with the pubertal growth spurt. The age of onset of hypertrophy may be determined to some extent by the specific nature of the underlying gene defect. Disease caused by mutations in the β-myosin heavy chain (β-MHC) gene is generally associated with phenotypically obvious disease with near-universal development of LVH by the second decade. In contrast, disease caused by mutations in the cardiac myosin binding protein C (cMyBPC) gene may not display clinically evident hypertrophy until the fourth or fifth decade of life. cMyBPC mutations have been associated with elderly onset HCM with initial clinical manifestations developing late in life.

Estimates of the annual mortality of HCM vary. Evaluation of populations drawn from specialized referral centers suggests a significant annual mortality rate of 4–6%. In contrast, community-based studies, which may be less susceptible to selection bias, suggest a more benign outcome with a projected annual mortality rate of 1–2%. HCM-specific causes of morbidity and mortality include SCD, progressive heart failure, atrial fibrillation, and heart failure, and stroke. Sudden death is the most feared complication of HCM and accurate estimation of an individual's risk for sudden death is a challenge. The risk for sudden death in the overall HCM population varies from 1 to 5% with about 10–20% of patients at highest risk. Less than 10–20% of patients progress to the "burnt-out" phase of HCM, marked by worsening symptomatic heart failure, LV systolic dysfunction, regression of LVH, and chamber dilatation. These patients may ultimately require cardiac transplantation for end-stage heart failure.

MANAGEMENT There are two major aspects to HCM management: alleviation of symptoms and assessment of the risk for SCD. Medical therapy is the cornerstone of treatment for symptomatic HCM and typically incorporates agents such as β-adrenergic and calcium channel antagonists to increase diastolic filling time, slow the heart rate, decrease contractility, and help normalize intracardiac filling pressures. For medically refractory patients with obstructive physiology, mechanical intervention to relieve outflow tract obstruction may be considered, including surgical septal myomectomy or catheterization-based alcohol septal ablation.

Clinical indicators of increased risk for sudden death include: a history of cardiac arrest or sustained ventricular tachycardia; significant nonsustained ventricular tachycardia on ambulatory monitoring; recurrent syncope; a hypotensive response to exercise in patients younger than 50 yr; massive LVH (>30–35 mm); and a family history of SCD or identification of a malignant genotype. However, estimation of an individual's risk is imprecise. If two or more risk factors are present, increased risk of SCD is present with an estimated annual mortality of 4–6%. Sudden death may be the

initial presenting symptom of HCM or occur in only mildly symptomatic patients. Although sudden death has been associated with vigorous physical activity and HCM is the leading cause of SCD in US competitive athletes, many episodes have occurred in the setting of only mild or no exercise. Implantation of a cardiovertor-defibrillator is effective in decreasing the risk of sudden death from lethal arrhythmias in appropriate individuals.

GENETIC ASPECTS The observation that HCM occurred in families defined it as a genetic cardiovascular disorder with Mendelian autosomal-dominant inheritance. Linkage analysis of large kindreds with HCM identified several disease loci on chromosomes 1, 11, 14, and 15. Positional cloning and candidate gene analysis identified discrete mutations in genes that encode for different elements of the contractile apparatus, including cardiac β-MHC, cardiac troponins T and I, cMyBPC, α-tropomyosin, actin, the essential and regulatory myosin light chains, and titin (Table 11-1). Thus, genetic studies established the paradigm of HCM as a disease of the sarcomere (Fig. 11-3).

The sarcomere is the functional unit of myocyte contraction. Proteins are organized into a latticework of thick (myosin heavy and light chains) and thin (actin, the troponin complex, and α-tropomyosin) filaments that interdigitate during muscle fiber shortening and lengthening. The detachment and attachment of actin and the myosin head serve as the molecular motor of contraction and relaxation. The hydrolysis of ATP provides fuel, and changes in intracellular Ca^{2+} concentration coordinate thick and thin filament interaction.

More than 300 individual mutations have been identified in 11 different components of the contractile apparatus. Types of mutations include missense mutations (resulting in amino acid substitution), nonsense mutations (resulting in premature termination of translation), short insertions and deletions, and alteration of splice donor or acceptor sites (resulting in altered transcripts). There is no significant founder effect in HCM as mutations tend to be "private"—unique from family to family with rare reappearances in unrelated kindreds. *De novo* or sporadic mutations are also well described.

Mutations in cardiac β-MHC, cMyBPC, and cardiac troponins T and I account for approx 80–90% of described HCM cases. Significant diversity exists in the clinical expression of these inherited gene defects. Although a handful of mutations have been described as characteristically "benign" or "malignant," heterogeneity of phenotype is the rule. Further identification of causal mutations and accurate description of genotype–phenotype correlations remain a work in progress, but the wide genetic and clinical spectrum of HCM make this challenging. As the ability to more precisely and sensitively assess phenotype improves, more accurate associations will emerge. Broad, recurring themes are outlined in Table 11-1. It remains unclear why some sarcomere mutations cause more severe disease than others and why individuals with the same mutation have a wide range of clinical features. Description of wider genetic and environmental factors that shape the expression of the underlying mutation is an active area of investigation.

Cardiac β-MHC Mutations Mutations in the cardiac β-MHC gene on chromosome 14 are thought to account for approx 40% of cases of HCM. This protein is organized into two functional domains: an amino terminal globular head that interacts with actin and a carboxyl terminal rod. The force of the power stroke is transduced through a hinge region connecting the rod and head domains. Most HCM-causing mutations are of the missense

Table 11-1
Mutations That Cause Hypertrophic Cardiomyopathy and General Phenotypic Correlations

	Gene	Designation	Chromosome	Frequency	Number of mutations	Phenotypic correlation
HCM-sarcomere proteins	β-myosin heavy chain	β-MHC	14q1	~30–40%	>80	Typically obvious disease with significant LVH; several severe phenotypes (end-stage heart failure and sudden death)
	Cardiac myosin binding protein C	cMyBPC	11q1	~30–40%	>50	Typically more mild disease, but severe phenotypes have been described; elderly onset HCM
	Cardiac troponin T	cTnT	1q3	approx 5%	>20	Typically mild LVH but increased association with sudden death
	Cardiac troponin I	cTnI	19p1	5%	>10	
	α-tropomyosin	α-TM	15q2	<5%	8	
	Myosin essential light chain	MLC-1	3p	Rare	2	Skeletal myopathy
	Myosin regulatory light chain	MLC-2	12q	Rare	8	Skeletal myopathy
	Actin		11q	Rare	5	
	Titin		2q3	Rare	1	
Inherited left ventricular hypertrophy	γ-subunit AMP kinase	PRKAG2	7q3	?	3	Glucose metabolism; preexcitation and conduction disease; catecholeminergic polymorphic ventricular tachycardia
	Lysosome associated membrane protein 2	LAMP2	X	?		
	Muscle LIM protein	CRP3	11p	?	3	

Adapted from J Mol Cell Cardiol 2001;33:655–670; Circulation 2001;104:2113–2116; Seidman JG, Seidman C. The genetic basis for cardiomyopathy: from mutation identification to mechanistic paradigms. Cell 2001;104:557–567; http://cardiogenomics.med.harvard.edu/project-detail?project_id=230, with permission from Elsevier.

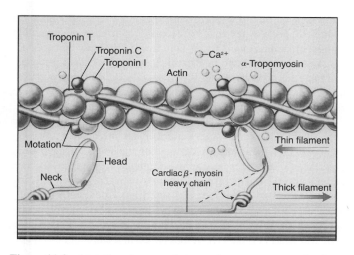

Figure 11-3 Mutations in genes that encode sarcomere proteins form the genetic basis of hypertrophic cardiomyopathy as well as some forms of dilated cardiomyopathy. (Reprinted with permission from N Engl J Med 2000; 343:1688–1696.)

variety and clustered within the globular head. The genetic basis of HCM was first described as missense mutation in this gene in which a single base pair is changed, resulting in the substitution of glutamine for arginine at residue 403.

Over 80 different β-MHC missense mutations have been reported in familial and sporadic disease. The phenotypic expression of these mutations tends to be fairly obvious with significant degrees of LVH apparent by late adolescence. Although heterogeneous, the clinical course of certain MHC mutations has been severe, associated with

a striking risk of sudden death or development of end-stage heart failure. The precise determinants of the relationship between prognosis and underlying gene mutation are likely multifactorial and poorly understood. Mutations that result in a change in the charge of the substituted amino acid appear to result in more severe disease, presumably owing to more dramatic effects on protein structure and function.

Cardiac Myosin Binding Protein C Missense, splice site, and deletion/insertion mutations in cMyBPC likely account for approx 30–40% of HCM cases. This large protein (1274 amino acids) is encoded on chromosome 11 and may function to provide structural support to the sarcomere and to modulate myosin ATPase activity in response to sympathetic stimulation. In a significant subset of individuals with cMyBPC mutations, the development of clinically apparent LVH is delayed until age 50 yr or older. Elderly onset HCM is associated with mutations in cMyBPC. Disease course is generally mild and not typically associated with attenuated survival, but there are reports of increased sudden death risk related to cMyBPC mutations.

Cardiac Troponin T Troponin T links the troponin complex to α-tropomyosin and, therefore, plays a central role in regulating contraction. The cardiac-specific isoform is encoded on chromosome 1. Approximately 5% of HCM is thought to be attributable to cardiac troponin T (cTnT) mutations. Traditionally, the clinical phenotype has been characterized by modest degrees of LVH but an increased risk of sudden death, although "benign" cTnT mutations are also described.

EXPERIMENTAL MODELS OF HCM Mutations in sarcomere proteins may alter actin–myosin crossbridge formation, intracellular calcium cycling, the energetics of force generation, or the transmission of force. However, the heterogeneity of HCM in the human population has challenged the dissection of the precise molecular mechanisms that lead from inherited gene defect to clinical phenotype.

To evaluate the consequences of specific mutations in a more precise and controlled manner, a variety of in vitro and in vivo experimental models of HCM have been developed. In vivo models are based on genetically modified animals in which β-MHC, cTnT, and cMyBPC mutations that cause human disease are introduced. The resultant animals develop a phenotype that recapitulates HCM phenotype, developing myocardial fibrosis, hypertrophy, and disarray in an age-dependent manner. Hemodynamic changes and abnormalities of diastolic function typically precede the development of LVH. Interrogation of these models remains a work in progress, but will allow further investigation into basic questions such as whether LVH is primary or secondary in response to either enhanced or impaired contractility; the influence of genetic background, modifier genes, the environment, and pharmacologic manipulation; and clarification of the early molecular events that lead to myocyte hypertrophy.

NEW PARADIGMS OF INHERITED CARDIAC HYPERTROPHY
HCM is caused by mutations in genes that encode elements of the contractile apparatus. Mutations have been described in nonsarcomere proteins that mimic the phenotype of HCM. Genetic studies of families and sporadic cases of unexplained LVH with conduction abnormalities (progressive atrioventricular block, atrial fibrillation, ventricular pre-excitation/Wolff–Parkinson–White syndrome) have identified a novel disease entity caused by mutations either in the γ-2 regulatory subunit (PRKAG2) of adenosine monophosphate-activated protein kinase, or in the lyosome-associated membrane protein 2 (LAMP2) gene both enzymes involved with glucose metabolism. Ventricular pre-excitation typically occurs early in life and is often symptomatic. Progressive conduction disease occurs with increasing age such that permanent pacemaker implantation was necessitated in 30% of affected individuals and helped serve as a discriminating feature from HCM caused by sarcomere mutations. Severe clinical outcomes were noted in a subset of patients with PRKAG2 and LAMP2 mutations, including progression to end-stage heart failure or transplantation and SCD.

Inherited LVH caused by PRKAG2 and LAMP2 mutations is a disease entity distinct from HCM caused by sarcomere protein mutations. Despite superficial similarities, this distinction is illustrated by the different morphologic appearances of these glycogen storage cardiomyopathies as compared with HCM. LVH in mutations caused by LAMP2 mutations is typically striking and concentric. Histopathologically, PRKAG2 and LAMP2 mutations do not display the myocardial disarray characteristic of HCM, but rather a relatively minor amount of fibrosis and prominent nonmembrane bound vacuoles that, if appropriately handled and stained, demonstrate glycogen and amylopectin accumulation. These histologic features are more consistent with other disorders of glycogen storage, such as Danon or Pompe disease. Different molecular signaling pathways are involved and therefore the clinical approach to individuals glycogen storage cardiomyopathies should not be predicated on management tenets of HCM.

Mutations in the muscle LIM protein (MLP) may also cause inherited LVH. This protein plays an essential role as a promoter of myogenesis and may also act as a cofactor in the regulation of muscle-specific gene expression in skeletal and cardiac muscle. Mice with a MLP gene knockout have been described to develop both a dilated and hypertrophic cardiac phenotype. Studies to analyze for mutations in the CRP3 gene (encoding MLP) in humans with hypertrophic heart disease revealed three novel missense mutations in three unrelated families.

DILATED CARDIOMYOPATHY

CLINICAL ASPECTS Heart failure is an important public health problem affecting 5 million patients in the United States. It is responsible for 1 million hospitalizations and 300,000 deaths annually. Pathologic remodeling of the heart resulting in increased chamber volume is termed DCM. Cardiac mass is increased because of enlargement of the chambers with only modest increase in ventricular wall thickness. Histopathologic changes may be relatively subtle with only minor myocyte hypertrophy, degeneration, and interstitial fibrosis.

DCM is a common cause of heart failure with a worldwide prevalence of about 36.5/100,000. Clinical manifestations may be somewhat protean, particularly in the early stages of disease. Characteristic symptoms include exertional dyspnea, fatigue, orthopnea, and lower extremity edema. Diagnosis is generally based on identifying increased cardiac dimensions and decreased contractile function. Exclusion of disorders that may cause cardiac dilation and dysfunction (coronary artery disease, alcohol abuse, thyroid disease, viral myocarditis, and infiltrative disorders such as hemochromatosis) generally leads to the diagnosis of "idiopathic" DCM; approx 25–30% are thought to have a genetic cause. The genetic basis of DCM is less specifically described than that of HCM. The clinical syndrome of DCM is also less distinctive than HCM, further challenging precise characterization.

There is significant variability in the clinical features of DCM because of single gene mutations. Age of onset ranges from early childhood to late adulthood, although most patients present during the fourth or fifth decades of life. Families may also manifest additional phenotypes that cosegregate with disease, including additional cardiac involvement (mitral valve prolapse and conduction system disease) and extracardiac conditions (sensorineuronal hearing loss and muscular dystrophies). These additional manifestations may be expressed in advance of DCM and therefore serve as supplemental measures to assign phenotypic status.

GENETIC ASPECTS The most common mode of inheritance of familial DCM is autosomal-dominant, but infrequent autosomal-recessive, X-linked, and mitochondrial transmission have been described (Table 11-2). Autosomal-dominant inheritance has been defined for a number of chromosomal loci and several specific genetic mutations have been characterized. Dominant mutations causing DCM may be associated with additional phenotypes as described above. Mutations that result in altered force generation and force transmission have been reported as a cause of autosomal-dominant DCM.

Missense mutations in β-MHC, α-tropomyosin, and an in-frame deletion of a lysine residue in cTnT have been identified as causes of autosomal-dominant DCM. Surprisingly, these mutations occur in sarcomere protein genes traditionally associated with causing HCM. The mechanisms by which mutations in the same gene lead to either a hypertrophic or dilated phenotype remain unclear. One speculation is that mutations associated with HCM may involve areas of the protein that are directly involved with generating energy or initiating the power stroke, resulting in impaired force generation, whereas mutations associated with DCM may result in impaired force transmission with subsequent cardiac enlargement and dysfunction.

Proper cardiac function also requires effective transmission of the force generated by the contractile apparatus to the extracellular

Table 11-2
Mutations That Cause Dilated Cardiomyopathy

	Gene	Inheritance	Chromosomal location	Associated phenotypes
Sarcomere proteins	β-myosin heavy chain	Autosomal-dominant	14q1	None
	Cardiac troponin T	Autosomal-dominant	1q3	None
	α-tropomyosin	Autosomal-dominant	15q22	None
	Actin	Autosomal-dominant	11q	None
Intermediate filament proteins/structural proteins	δ-sarcoglycan	Autosomal-dominant	5q33-34	None
	Desmin	Autosomal-dominant	2q35	Skeletal myopathy
	Desmoplakin	Autosomal-recessive	6p24	Wooly hair and keratoderma
	Plakoglobin	Autosomal-recessive	17q21	Arrhythmogenic right ventricular dysplasia, wooly hair, and keratoderma (Naxos syndrome)
Miscellaneous genes	Dystrophin	X-linked	Xp21	Muscular dystrophy
	Lamin A/C	Autosomal-dominant	1p1-q21	Conduction disease
	Tafazzin	X-linked	Xq28	Short stature and neutropenia (Barth syndrome)

Adapted from Schonberger J, Seidman CE. Many roads lead to a broken heart: the genetics of dilated cardiomyopathy. Am J Hum Genet 2001:69:249–260, with permission of The University of Chicago Press.

matrix. Filamentous proteins linking the sarcomere to the sarcolemma may assist in the propagation of force. Mutations in the portion of actin that participates in actin–cytoskeletal (rather than actin–myosin) interactions and mutations in the giant structural molecule, titin, have been implicated in causing isolated DCM. Intermediate-filament proteins, including desmin, connect actin to the dystrophin–sarcoglycan complex beneath the plasma membrane of all muscle cells. Mutations in desmin, dystrophin, and δ-sarcoglycan cause skeletal myopathies, some associated with myocardial involvement, as well as DCM with subclinical or no skeletal muscle involvement. The basis for the cardiac specificity of these mutations is unclear.

Rare syndromes with autosomal-recessive inheritance have been attributed to mutations in cellular adhesion molecules plakoglobin (associated with arrhythmogenic right ventricular dysplasia with palmoplantar keratosis and wooly hair—Naxos syndrome) and desmoplakin (similar phenotype with more prominent LV involvement). These molecules play critical roles at the junctions of desmosomes and adherens and therefore may participate in cell-to-cell force propagation. Sporadic or maternally inherited mutations in mitochondrial DNA can result in complex, multisystem phenotypes, including cardiac involvement with DCM.

Apart from disruption of the production or transmission of force, a separate paradigm of familial DCM has been suggested by the identification of a missense mutation in phospholamban as a cause of autosomal-dominant DCM. Phospholamban is a transmembrane sarcoplasmic phosphoprotein that regulates the Ca^{2+} ATPase pump, SERCA2a. This mutation may result in constitutive inhibition of SERCA2a via trapping of the phospholamban regulatory protein, protein kinase A. Therefore, alterations in myocyte Ca^{2+} homeostasis may be a primary trigger for the development of DCM.

The mechanisms by which other genetic mutations give rise to a DCM phenotype remain elusive. Mutations in tafazzin, an X chromosome-encoded acetyltransferase protein of unknown function, give rise to Barth syndrome, a triad of DCM, neutropenia, and 3-methylglutaconicaciduria. Dominant mutations in the nuclear envelope proteins, lamin, cause progressive conduction system disease with eventual development of DCM. Of note, distinct lamin A/C mutations can give rise to autosomal-dominant Emery–Dreyfus mus-

cular dystrophy, limb-girdle muscular dystrophy, and to familial partial lipodystrophy. Each of these clinical phenotypes may be associated with cardiac disease, predominantly DCM.

CONCLUSION

Unraveling the molecular and genetic basis of inherited cardiomyopathies will provide further insight into their fundamental pathophysiology, and to the mechanisms underlying more common forms of acquired dilated and hypertrophic heart disease. Screening of family members in DCM kindreds may identify individuals with asymptomatic LV dysfunction or dilatation. Early initiation of medical therapy at this stage improves symptoms, morbidity, and prognosis. More definitive treatment to interrupt the natural history of dilated and hypertrophic cardiomyopathies will be drawn from better mechanistic understanding of how inherited gene defects remodel the heart.

SELECTED REFERENCES

Arad M, Benson DW, Perez-Atayde AR, et al. Constitutively active AMP kinase mutations cause glycogen storage disease mimicking hypertrophic cardiomyopathy. J Clin Invest 2002;109:357–362.

Blanchard E, Seidman C, Seidman JG, LeWinter M, Maughan D. Altered crossbridge kinetics in the alphaMHC403/+ mouse model of familial hypertrophic cardiomyopathy. Circ Res 1999;84:475–483.

Bonne G, Carrier L, Richard P, Hainque B, Schwartz K. Familial hypertrophic cardiomyopathy: from mutations to functional defects. Circ Res 1998;83:580–593.

Braunwald E, Morrow AG, Cornell WP, Aygen MM, Hilbish TF. Idiopathic hypertrophic subaortic stenosis—clinical, hemodynamic and angiographic manifestations. Am J Med 1960;29:924–945.

Carrier L, Hengstenberg C, Beckmann JS, et al. Mapping of a novel gene for familial hypertrophic cardiomyopathy to chromosome 11. Nat Genet 1993;4:311–313.

Charron P, Carrier L, Dubourg O, et al. Penetrance of familial hypertrophic cardiomyopathy. Genet Couns 1997;8:107–114.

Charron P, Dubourg O, Desnos M, et al. Clinical features and prognostic implications of familial hypertrophic cardiomyopathy related to the cardiac myosin-binding protein C gene. Circulation 1998;97: 2230–2236.

Epstein ND, Cohn GM, Cyran F, Fananapazir L. Differences in clinical expression of hypertrophic cardiomyopathy associated with two distinct mutations in the beta-myosin heavy chain gene. A 908Leu–Val mutation and a 403Arg–Gln mutation. Circulation 1992;86:345–352.

Geier C, Perrot A, Ozcelik C, et al. Mutations in the human muscle LIM protein gene in families with hypertrophic cardiomyopathy. Circulation 2003;107:1390–1395.

Geisterfer-Lowrance AA, Christe M, Conner DA, et al. A mouse model of familial hypertrophic cardiomyopathy. Science 1996;272:731–734.

Geisterfer-Lowrance AA, Kass S, Tanigawa G, et al. A molecular basis for familial hypertrophic cardiomyopathy: A beta cardiac myosin heavy chain gene missense mutation. Cell 1990;62:999–1006.

Ho CY, Sweitzer NK, McDonough B, et al. Assessment of diastolic function with Doppler tissue imaging to predict genotype in preclinical hypertrophic cardiomyopathy. Circulation 2002;105:2992–2997.

Kamisago M, Sharma SD, DePalma SR, et al. Mutations in sarcomere protein genes as a cause of dilated cardiomyopathy. N Engl J Med 2000;343:1688–1696.

Klues HG, Schiffers A, Maron BJ. Phenotypic spectrum and patterns of left ventricular hypertrophy in hypertrophic cardimoypathy: morphologic observations and significance as assessed by two-dimensional echocardiography in 600 patients. J Am Coll Cardiol 1995; 26:1699–1708.

Marian AJ. Pathogenesis of diverse clinical and pathological phenotypes in hypertrophic cardiomyopathy. Lancet 2000;355:58–60.

Marian AJ, Roberts R. The molecular genetic basis for hypertrophic cardiomyopathy. J Mol Cell Cardiol 2001;33:655–670.

Maron BJ. Hypertrophic cardiomyopathy. Lancet 1997;350:127–133.

Maron BJ, Gardin JM, Flack JM, Gidding SS, Kurosaki TT, Bild DE. Prevalence of hypertrophic cardiomyopathy in a general population of young adults—echocardiographic analysis of 4111 subjects in the CARDIA study. Circulation 1995;92:785–789.

Moolman JC, Corfield VA, Posen B, et al. Sudden death due to troponin T mutations. J Am Coll Cardiol 1997;29:549–555.

Nagueh SF, Bachinski LL, Meyer D, et al. Tissue Doppler imaging consistently detects myocardial abnormalities in patients with hypertrophic cardiomyopathy and provides a novel means for an early diagnosis before and independently of hypertrophy. Circulation 2001;104:128–130.

Niimura H, Bachinski LL, Sangwatanaroj S, et al. Mutations in the gene for cardiac myosin-binding protein C and late-onset familial hypertrophic cardiomyopathy (see comments). N Engl J Med 1998;338:1248–1257.

Niimura H, Patton KK, McKenna WJ, et al. Sarcomere protein gene mutations in hypertrophic cardiomyopathy of the elderly. Circulation 2002;105:446–451.

Schmitt JP, Kamisago M, Asahi M, et al. Dilated cardiomyopathy and heart failure caused by a mutation in phospholamban. Science 2003;299:1410–1413.

Schonberger J, Seidman CE. Many roads lead to a broken heart: the genetics of dilated cardiomyopathy. Am J Hum Genet 2001;69: 249–260.

Seidman CE, Seidman JG. Hypertrophic cardiomyopathy. In: Scriver CR, Beaudet AL, Valle D, et al, eds. The Metabolic and Molecular Bases of Inherited Disease, 8th ed., vol. 4. New York: McGraw-Hill, 2000; pp. 5433–5452.

Seidman JG, Seidman C. The genetic basis for cardiomyopathy: from mutation identification to mechanistic paradigms. Cell 2001;104: 557–567.

Spirito P, Seidman CE, McKenna WJ, Maron BJ. The management of hypertrophic cardiomyopathy. N Engl J Med 1997;336:775–785.

Thierfelder L, MacRae C, Watkins H, et al. A familial hypertrophic cardiomyopathy locus maps to chromosome 15q2. Proc Natl Acad Sci USA 1993;90:6270–6274.

Tyska MJ, Hayes E, Giewat M, Seidman CE, Seidman JG, Warshaw DM. Single-molecule mechanics of R403Q cardiac myosin isolated from the mouse model of familial hypertrophic cardiomyopathy. Circ Res 2000;86:737–744.

Watkins H. Genetic clues to disease pathways in hypertrophic and dilated cardiomyopathies. Circulation 2003;107:1344–1346.

Watkins H, Anan R, Coviello DA, Spirito P, Seidman JG, Seidman CE. A de novo mutation in alpha-tropomyosin that causes hypertrophic cardiomyopathy. Circulation 1995;91:2302–2305.

Watkins H, Conner D, Thierfelder L, et al. Mutations in the cardiac myosin binding protein-C gene on chromosome 11 cause familial hypertrophic cardiomyopathy. Nat Genet 1995;11:434–437.

Watkins H, MacRae C, Thierfelder L, et al. A disease locus for familial hypertrophic cardiomyopathy maps to chromosome 1q3. Nat Genet 1993;3:333–337.

Watkins H, McKenna WJ, Thierfelder L, et al. Mutations in the genes for cardiac troponin T and alpha-tropomyosin in hypertrophic cardiomyopathy. N Engl J Med 1995;332:1058–1064.

Watkins H, Rosenzweig A, Hwang DS, et al. Characteristics and prognostic implications of myosin missense mutations in familial hypertrophic cardiomyopathy. N Engl J Med 1992;326:1108–1114.

Wigle ED, Sasson Z, Henderson MA, et al. Hypertrophic cardiomyopathy: The importance of the site and the extent of hypertrophy, a review. Prog Cardiovasc Dis 1985;28:1–83.

12 Heart Failure

Emerging Concepts in Excitation–Contraction Coupling and β-Adrenoceptor Coupling

CLIVE J. LEWIS, FEDERICA DEL MONTE, SIAN E. HARDING, AND ROGER J. HAJJAR

SUMMARY

The process that begins contraction in the heart is known as excitation–contraction (E–C) coupling because it couples electrical signals on the membrane of the cardiac cell to activation of the myofilament and cross-bridge cycling. The cardiac action potential is produced by the coordinated interaction of many ion channels, which transduce physiological signals within and between cardiomyocytes. These cardiomyocytes are further regulated by a number of receptors that control the strength of the contraction on a beat-to-beat basis and their morphology in a chronic fashion. In heart failure, a number of steps in E–C coupling become abnormal. In this chapter, we will examine the role of these abnormalities in the development of heart failure.

Key Words: β-receptor kinase; β-receptors; calcium; contractility; excitation contraction coupling; G proteins; L-type calcium channel; myofilaments; phospholamban; sarcoplasmic reticulum; sodium calcium exchanger.

INTRODUCTION

The understanding of cardiac excitation contraction coupling and β-adrenoreceptor signaling continues to evolve. Defects in the steps of excitation contraction coupling and β-adrenergic signaling have been identified in human and experimental models of heart failure. Abnormalities in ionic channels, transporters, kinases, and various signaling pathways collectively contribute to the "failing phenotype." β-adrenoceptors are widely expressed in human tissues and activated by neuronally released and circulating catecholamines. They are important mediators of the sympatho-adrenal axis regulating numerous physiological events, including relaxation of vascular smooth muscle, cardiac inotropy, chronotropy, and lusitropy. The traditional view of signal transduction is changing because of the emergence of concepts in the complexity of guanine nucleotide protein coupled receptor (GPCR)-effector coupling, an intracellular coupling.

From: *Principles of Molecular Medicine, Second Edition*
Edited by: M. S. Runge and C. Patterson © Humana Press, Inc., Totowa, NJ

EXCITATION–CONTRACTION COUPLING

On a beat-to-beat basis, depolarization of the cell membrane in cardiac myocytes leads to the opening of voltage gated L-type Ca^{2+} channels resulting in the influx of transsarcolemmal influx of Ca^{2+} into the cell (Fig. 12-1). These channels are in close proximity to the ryanodine receptors (RyRs), which are Ca^{2+} release channels located on the sarcoplasmic reticulum (SR). Ca^{2+} entering the cells through a single L-type Ca^{2+} channel induces the opening of one or a cluster of RyRs resulting in the local release of Ca^{2+} from the SR. During membrane depolarization, a large number of L-type Ca^{2+} channels are opened, resulting in a large release of Ca^{2+} from the RyRs, raising cytosolic Ca^{2+} from 0.1–0.2 to 2–10 μM.

A functional Ca^{2+} signaling and releasing unit has been characterized, namely the Ca^{2+} spark. Ca^{2+} sparks were first identified as the "elementary events" of spontaneous increases in intracellular $[Ca^{2+}]$, which were detected by laser scanning confocal microscopy and the fluorescent Ca^{2+} indicator fluo-3. Ca^{2+} sparks also can be produced by the triggering Ca^{2+} entered through the L-type Ca^{2+} channel during the E–C coupling process. Functionally, the Ca^{2+} sparks represent Ca^{2+} releases from the SR through the opening of the SR Ca^{2+} release channels/RyRs. Ca^{2+} sparks are produced by activation of 10–100 RyRs based on the ratio of the Ca^{2+} sparks' current and the single RyR channel current and because the morphology of Ca^{2+} sparks varies even within a single cell. Ca^{2+} sparks are depicted/measured by their morphology and the frequency of occurrence. The morphology information includes the sizes of Ca^{2+} sparks (amplitude, width, and duration), and the kinetics is described by the spark rising and decaying dynamics. The activity of individual RyRs and the number of the RyRs recruited during a spark play an important role in the spark morphology. Thus, the more active the Ca^{2+} release channels, the more Ca^{2+} would be released and consequently, increased size and more frequent occurrence of Ca^{2+} sparks would be observed. Therefore, direct modifications that change the RyRs activity or the modulators that regulate RyR activity will affect the size and frequency of Ca^{2+} sparks. SR Ca^{2+} content also regulates Ca^{2+} sparks because luminal (Ca^{2+}) plays a critical role in regulating RyR by increasing

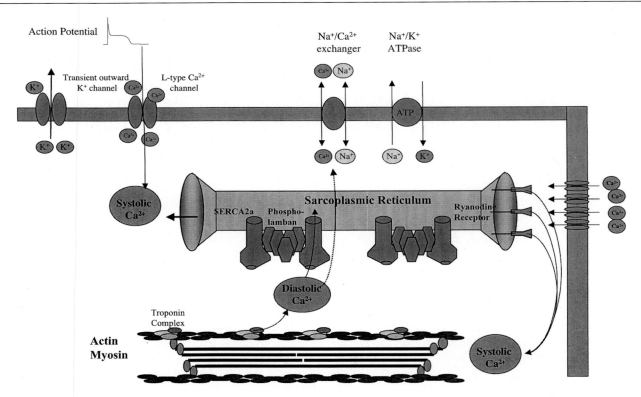

Figure 12-1 Depolarization of the membrane by the action potential leads to the opening of voltage gated L-type Ca^{2+} channels allowing the entry of a small amount of Ca^{2+} into the cell. Through a coupling mechanism between the L-type Ca^{2+} channel and the SR release channels (RyRs), a larger amount of Ca^{2+} is released activating the myofilaments leading to contraction. During relaxation, Ca^{2+} is reaccumulated back into the SR by the SERCA2a and extruded extracellularly by the sarcolemmal Na^+/Ca^{2+} exchanger.

the activity of the RyRs and by sensitizing the threshold of RyR for activation to the stimulus. The signaling between L-type Ca^{2+} channel and RyR Ca^{2+} sparks can be triggered by the Ca^{2+} influx through the L-type Ca^{2+} sparks during voltage pulses. Thus, the kinetics, fidelity, and stoichiometry of coupling between L-type Ca^{2+} channels and RyR play a critical role in determination of the signal transduction during the E–C coupling process. The distance of the cleft between the cell plasma membrane and the SR membrane, roughly 12 nm in normal cardiomyocytes, is critical for such coupling and signal transduction. Extension of the distance between them by pulling the plasma membrane under tight-seal condition decreases/abolishes the signaling reliability.

Relaxation occurs when calcium detaches from troponin C and is reaccumulated back into the SR by the cardiac isoform of the Ca^{2+} adenosine triphosphatase (ATPase) pump (SERCA2a) and extruded extracellularly by the sarcolemmal Na^+/Ca^{2+} exchanger. The contribution of each of these mechanisms for lowering cytosolic Ca^{2+} varies among species. In humans approx 75% of the Ca^{2+} is removed by SERCA2a and approx 25% by the Na^+/Ca^{2+} exchanger. SERCA2a transports Ca^{2+} back to the luminal space of the SR against a Ca^{2+} gradient by an energy dependent mechanism (one molecule of ATP is hydrolyzed for the transport of two molecules of Ca^{2+}), where it binds to a calcium buffering protein, calsequestrin.

The Ca^{2+} pumping activity of SERCA2a is regulated by phospholamban. In its unphosphorylated state, phospholamban inhibits the Ca^{2+} ATPase, whereas phosphorylation of phospholamban by cAMP-dependent protein kinase and by Ca^{2+}-calmodulin dependent protein kinase reverses this inhibition.

CALCIUM HANDLING IN HEART FAILURE

The myopathic heart exhibits abnormalities in the systolic and diastolic phases. Changes in diastolic function often appear earlier than systolic dysfunction. Compensated hypertrophy phenotypically demonstrates impaired relaxation parameters in the presence of normal or increased systolic function. The first report of abnormalities in calcium handling was made when calcium transients, recorded with the calcium indicator aequorin from trabeculae from myopathic human hearts removed at the time of cardiac transplantation, revealed a significantly prolonged calcium transient with an elevated end-diastolic intracellular calcium. This was corroborated by recordings in single isolated cardiomyocytes loaded with the fluorescent indicator Fura-2 from myopathic hearts. The calcium transients were characterized as having elevated diastolic calcium levels, decreased systolic Ca^{2+}, and a prolonged relaxation phase. Studies both in muscle strips and isolated cardiomyoctes found that systolic calcium concentration was decreased in the failing state whereas diastolic calcium concentrations were elevated. These differences were more accentuated at higher stimulation rates. Because intracellular calcium transients and calcium concentrations are regulated by the voltage-dependent Ca^{2+} channel, the SR ryanodine Ca^{2+} release channels, the SERCA2a/phospholamban complex, and the Na/Ca exchanger, several studies have focused on the relative changes in these proteins between myopathic and normal hearts.

Conflicting findings have been reported when calcium channels were measured with radioligand binding assays. One group reported an approx 20–30% reduction in mRNA and Bmax for dihydropyridine binding. However, two other groups found no difference in the

Beta Receptors in Cardiomyocytes

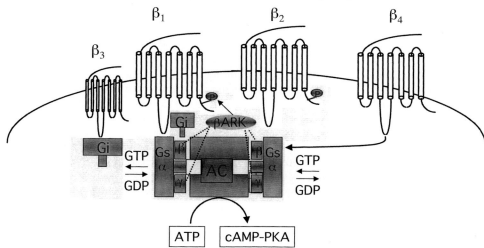

Figure 12-2 There are four β-adrenoceptor subtypes that modulate human myocardial function. β$_3$-adrenoceptor mediates cardiodepression mediated by the G$_i$ protein. "Putative" β$_4$-adrenoceptor causes cardiostimulant effects at concentrations 1000 times greater than those required to antagonize the cardiostimulant effects of catecholamines at β$_1$- and β$_2$-adreonceptors with high affinity.

number of calcium channels as measured with radioligand binding. Despite these conflicting reports it is appreciated that radioligand-binding assays can detect nascent channels and are only a surrogate marker of the number of active calcium channels.

Altered myocyte calcium handling might play an important role in the development of heart failure in humans. This hypothesis is consistent with alterations found in some of the key proteins involved in the uptake and release of calcium in myopathic hearts. Calcium is released from the SR through a calcium sensitive release channel, the RyR. RyR mRNA is reduced in both myopathic human hearts and animal models. Inconsistent reports on RyR protein levels in myopathic human myocardium have appeared in the literature. Some research has shown altered gating mechanisms and altered responses to ryanodine in myopathic human myocardium, whereas other studies have found normal basic properties. Thus, although gene expression of the RyR receptor might be unchanged, its gating behavior, i.e., activity, might be impaired in failing myocardium. Even though the number of receptors might not be changed in heart failure and hypertrophy, there is a defective coupling between the L-type calcium channel and the RyR. The molecular correlates of this uncoupling seem to be a hyperphosphorylation of the RyR.

HUMAN MYOCARDIAL FUNCTION IS MODULATED THROUGH FOUR β-ADRENOCEPTORS

β$_1$- and β$_2$-adrenoceptors coexist in human and rat myocytes with the β$_1$-adrenoceptor the predominant subtype, even in heart failure when the relative proportion of β$_2$-adrenoceptors increases (Fig. 12-2). The proportion of β$_2$-adrenoceptors is greatest in humans of all species studied. β$_1$- and β$_2$-adrenoceptors are pharmacologically and genetically distinct entities with only 71% amino acid identity in the transmembrane-spanning domains and 54% identity overall; however, they appear to have the same mechanism of signal transduction through G$_s$ and cAMP. Furthermore, epinephrine and norepinephrine are able to enhance contraction, relaxation, arrhythmia, and protein kinase A (PKA)-dependent phosphorylation of downstream regulatory proteins to

a similar extent through human β$_1$- and β$_2$-adrenoceptors, respectively, despite the difference in receptor number. To explain this, tighter coupling of the β$_2$-adrenoceptor to the Gs/adenylate cyclase (AC) pathway was proposed. Evidence suggests that β$_1$- and β$_2$-adrenoceptors have distinct physiological actions, coupled to distinct signal transduction pathways, and might occupy different spatial localization within the heart or within single cells (compartmentalization). In addition, β$_2$-adrenoceptors might exist in two active forms that couple in parallel to G$_s$ and G inhibitory (G$_i$), respectively.

In addition to β$_1$- and β$_2$-adrenoceptors, evidence is consistent with the involvement of four β-adrenoceptor subtypes in the modulation of human myocardial function. A third β-adrenoceptor has been cloned and found to mediate vasodilatation, adipocyte metabolism, and cardiodepression mediated by the G$_i$ protein. Pharmacological data also support existence of an atypical or novel β-adrenoceptor subtype, which mediates cardiostimulant effects including inotropy, chronotropy, and lusitropy and led to the proposal of the fourth cardiac β-adrenoceptor. "Putative" β$_4$-adrenoceptor pharmacology has been defined using nonconventional partial agonist β-adrenoceptor antagonists that cause cardiostimulant effects at concentrations 1000 times greater than those required to antagonize the cardiostimulant effects of catecholamines at β$_1$- and β$_2$-adrenoceptors with high affinity. These agents include clinically used β-adrenoceptor antagonists such as pindolol, alprenolol, oxprenolol, and bucindolol as well as the useful experimental agent CGP 12177A. This receptor phenotype differs from the "classic" described function of known GPCRs and might be explained by novel receptor states or conformations or receptor dimerization.

β$_1$- AND β$_2$-ADRENOCEPTOR COUPLING The coupling of β$_1$- and β$_2$-adrenoceptors to G proteins mediates the beneficial effects of catecholamines and is also involved in the pathophysiology of the heart, thus consideration of the emerging molecular mechanisms that can alter coupling of these subtypes is important. There has been much interest in single-nucleotide polymorphisms (SNPs) of GPCRs because they are thought to affect the responses to endogenous agonists and/or drugs and therefore alter the pathophysiology of disease states by altering G protein coupling and signaling.

The β_1-adrenoceptor gene is polymorphic with 18 SNPs of which seven lead to amino acid substitutions within the coding exon. Two loci have been studied closely: Glycine49Serine (A for G at nucleotide 145) and Glycine389Arginine (C for G at nucleotide position 1165). Expression studies have demonstrated that despite similar affinities for both agonists and antagonists, the 49Serine receptor variant was relatively resistant to agonist-promoted downregulation compared to the 49Glycine variant. The Glycine389Arginine polymorphism, however, in the cytoplasmic tail G_s coupling domain, affects coupling to AC. In expression studies, the 389Arginine variant demonstrated and approx 30-fold greater ability to couple to AC when activated by isoproterenol and approx twofold for the β_4-adrenoceptor agonist CGP 12177A. Several studies have investigated whether any clinical correlate of this pharmacogenetic effect can be demonstrated, but the lack of agreement means that no conclusions can be drawn. The 49Glycine variant does not appear more frequently in patients with heart failure but is associated with a greater mortality. In dilated cardiomyopathy patients, the 389Arginine variant was more frequent in those without ventricular tachycardia. Neither polymorphism appears associated with long QT syndrome or acute coronary syndrome but higher blood pressures were observed in subjects with at least one 389Arginine allele and the 389Arginine genotype in combination with a deletion mutant of the α_{2C}-adrenoceptor significantly increases the risk of heart failure in African Americans. In addition to the β_1-adrenoceptor, the β_2-adrenoceptor has several SNPs, the most interesting of which is Isoleucine164. This amino acid change results in decreased β_2-adrenoceptor activity via decreased G protein/AC coupling. For the Isoleucine164 variant there is a fivefold increased relative risk of mortality in patients with heart failure. Thus SNPs that affect G protein coupling and signaling might have important implications in understanding cardiac physiology, disease, and pharmacological therapy.

NON-CAMP DEPENDENT β_1-ADRENORECEPTOR COUPLING (DIRECT L-TYPE CA^{2+} CHANNEL COUPLING)   E–C coupling of the β_1-adrenoceptor via G_s/cAMP is well established, but the possibility of a membrane delimited, non-cAMP dependent mechanism exists involving activated $G_{\alpha s}$ directly interacting with the sarcolemmal L-type Ca^{2+} channel. Evidence for a non-cAMP dependent activation of Ca^{2+} channel comes from five lines of experiments:

1. $G_{\alpha s}$ reactivates Ca^{2+} channels that have run down in excised guinea-pig ventricular patches.
2. $G_{\alpha s}$ stimulates L-type Ca^{2+} channel activity after reconstitution in lipid bilayers.
3. Dihydropyridine and radio-labeled $G_{\alpha s}$ binding suggest that G proteins bind and activate purified Ca^{2+} channels.
4. Isoproterenol stimulated atrial myocytes demonstrate biphasic Ca^{2+} currents with the fast response (~5% total) resistant to phosphodiesterase inhibition by isobutyl methyl xanthine and $G_{\alpha s}$ activation by forskolin.
5. Incomplete blockade of β-AR responses by inhibitors of PKA.

However, there are some inconsistencies and the overall relevance of these findings under physiological conditions has been questioned.

Supportive evidence exists for a non-cAMP dependent activation of Ca^{2+} channel mechanism under physiological conditions in isolated, paced single rat ventricular cardiomyocytes overexpressing human sequence β_1-adrenoceptors. Increased basal, unstimulated myocyte contraction resulting from constitutive activity of overexpressed β_1-adrenoceptors (ability of a receptor to signal through a second messenger pathway and activation of downstream effectors in the absence of agonist) has been observed. The raised basal contraction could be returned to control levels by CGP 20712A acting as an inverse agonist. The constitutive activity appeared non-cAMP dependent because cAMP levels were not increased by β_1-overexpression and neither RpcAMPS (cAMP antagonist) nor carbachol (inhibits cAMP-mediated contraction) had a significant effect on contraction. However, the L-type Ca^{2+} channel current was significantly enhanced by β_1-overexpression supporting a direct membrane-delimited activation by $G_{\alpha s}$ of the constitutively active β_1-adrenoceptor.

Controversy remains over constitutive activity of the β_1-adrenoceptor. cAMP-dependent constitutive activity was observed in atria from transgenic mice and cell lines overexpressing β_1-adrenoceptors. However, no change was found in basal contraction amplitude or basal cAMP in myocytes from β_1/β_2 double knockout (KO) mice overexpressing β_1-adrenoceptors. Constitutive activity of the β_2-adrenoceptor has also been observed. In transgenic mice with approx 200-fold overexpression of the β_2-adrenoceptor, cardiac contractility and AC activity are raised to levels observed with maximal agonist stimulation in control. The constitutive activity could be reduced by the inverse agonist activity of ICI 188,551.

GPCRs are proposed to exist in equilibrium between two conformational states, an inactive form (R) and an active form (R*) that can interact with G proteins. Agonist binds to and stabilizes the R form resulting in a shift to the R* form that involves a conformational change allowing G protein activation by guanosine triphosphate binding. In the β-adrenoceptor overexpressing myocytes, the levels of R + R* are increased and sufficient to produce increased basal contraction (constitutive activity). Inverse agonism is thought to result from the antagonist binding to the inactive R form and shifting the equilibrium away from R* with a corresponding decrease in contraction and AC activity.

DIFFERENCES BETWEEN β_1- AND β_2-ADRENOCEPTOR COUPLING   Differences between β_1- and β_2-adrenoceptors emerged by studying chronic heart-specific overexpression of each subtype in transgenic mice. β_1-overexpressing mice have early mortality owing to the development of myocyte hypertrophy and myocardial fibrosis leading to heart failure despite unaltered cardiac function and basal AC activity. Proapoptotic effects mediated by activation of β_1-adrenoceptor signaling pathways might mediate this observation. Transgenic mice overexpressing β_2-adrenoceptors at a similar level did not show increased mortality or heart failure, although the explanation for this was unclear.

As opposed to the selective coupling of the β_2-adrenoceptor to G_s/AC in humans, a non-cAMP E–C mechanism has been suggested for mouse and rat heart. It was based on the observations that isoproterenol produced increases in contraction through β_2-adrenoceptors without changes in the speed of relaxation or phospholamban phosphorylation and that agents reducing cAMP-mediated effects did not affect contraction. The coupling of β_2-adrenoceptors to G_i was observed by the use of pertussis toxin (PTX) when cAMP-dependent E–C coupling was revealed. Interestingly, G_i activation

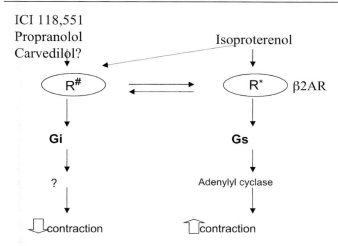

ICI 118,551
Propranolol
Carvedilol?

Isoproterenol

R#   R*   β2AR

Gi   Gs

?   Adenylyl cyclase

⬇contraction   ⬆contraction

Figure 12-3 Description of stimulus-trafficking in which different effects can be mediated by the same receptor acting though different G proteins, previously described for several GPCRs including β_2-adrenoceptors.

through β_2-adrenoceptors could oppose the proapoptotic effect of β_1-adrenoceptors through G_s. Mitogen-activated protein and phosphatidylinositol 3′-kinase pathways were identified as downstream mediators of β_2-/G_i signaling. The protection from early mortality owing to heart failure in β_2-overexpressing mice as opposed to β_1-overexpressing mice was linked to spontaneous upregulation of Gi (decreasing constitutive activity and hyperresponsiveness to catecholamines) and opposition of proapoptotic pathways. Subsequently β_2-adrenoceptors were observed to couple to both G_s and G_i resulting in activation of opposing signaling pathways.

Coupling of human β_2-adrenoceptors to G_i in failing ventricle has been confirmed. ICI 118,551 (selective β_2-adrenoceptor antagonist), at inverse agonist concentrations, produced a profound reduction of contraction in isolated ventricular myocytes from human heart, which could be prevented by treatment with PTX, indicating the involvement of G_i. The use of specific agonists/antagonists demonstrated G_i coupling to β_2- rather than β_1- or β_3-adrenoceptors. PTX-sensitive inverse agonist effects of ICI 118,551 have been observed in rat and rabbit by overexpressing human β_2-adrenoceptors or $G_{i\alpha2}$.

In failing human heart, β_2-adrenoceptors do not demonstrate constitutive activity and there is no "spare" β-adrenoceptor capacity, yet G_i is upregulated and there are dampened β_2-adrenoceptor responses. Thus a "stimulus-trafficking" modification has been proposed to the original theory of inverse agonism (Fig. 12-3). Stimulus trafficking describes the mechanism in which different effects can be mediated by the same receptor acting through different G-proteins; it has previously been described for several GPCRs including β_2-adrenoceptors. Binding of the inverse agonist is not to the inactive R form but to another active G_i-coupled form (R#), which occurs in parallel with the usual R*-G_s coupling. In nonfailing heart of mouse, rat or humans, total levels of β_2-adrenoceptor (R* + R#) and Gi levels are moderate with no effect on basal contraction. In failing heart, when G_i is upregulated, the G_i-R# form will shift the equilibrium away from R* resulting in the dampened contractile response to catecholamines observed in failing human heart. Inverse agonists bind to R# but because of the increased amount of G_i-R# in heart failure, a direct negative

inotropic effect of β-adrenoceptor antagonists is observed mediated by the β_2-adrenoceptor. In explaining the findings above, ICI 118,551 is an agonist through the G_i-R# but not the G_s-R* pathway. However, the downstream G_i linked targets for mediating the negative inotropic effect of ICI 118,551 have not been identified.

This negatively inotropic effect of ICI 118,551 has been observed for other β-adrenoceptor antagonists and is clearly important in human heart failure where they are used therapeutically to reduce mortality. The initial decrease in cardiac output during titration of β-adrenoceptor antagonists may, in addition to the removal of sympathetic tone, be owing to their direct negative inotropic effects.

COMPARTMENTALIZATION OF GPCR SIGNALING A large body of functional data supports the existence of subcellular compartmentalization of the cAMP/AC/PKA signaling pathway in heart. There appears to be a fixed and specific spatial relationship between components of cAMP generation, response mechanisms and degradation. Thus within a cardiac myocyte, not all cAMP gains access to all PKA and its downstream regulators, and only a limited amount of phosphodiesterases might degrade cAMP. Molecular mechanisms contributing to compartmentalization include localization of receptors, G proteins, and AC in caveolae within the sarcolemma; localization of PKA by A-kinase anchoring proteins resulting in scaffolding and inhibition of activity; localization of activated PKC isoforms, their downstream target substrates, and phosphodiesterase isoforms in caveolae; and compartmentalization of cAMP generation and phosphodiesterase degradation in sarcolemmal microdomains.

Evidence has highlighted compartmentalization of cAMP signaling in cardiac myocytes. In neonatal rat cardiac myocytes, specificity of signaling is guaranteed by tight localization of signaling events to the surface membrane. β-adrenoceptor stimulation generates multiple microdomains with increased concentrations of cAMP, but free diffusion of the second messenger is limited by the activity of phosphodiesterases and cannot transmit to nonsarcolemmal proteins. The possibility of compartmentalized cAMP signaling has also been investigated for the β_2-adrenoceptor in adult rat ventricular myocytes where contraction appeared dissociated from cAMP. L-type Ca^{2+} current and contraction to β_2- as well as β_1-adrenoceptor agonists was entirely abolished by the use of PKA inhibitors, suggesting functional compartmentalization of cAMP-dependent signaling.

Direct G protein activation of the L-type Ca^{2+} channel has also been suggested for β_2-adrenoceptor. However, a compartmentalized cAMP/PKA pathway mediating β_2-adrenoceptor signaling to the L-type Ca^{2+} channel seems more likely. In hippocampal neurons, the β_2-adrenoceptor appears to form a macromolecular signaling complex with the L-type Ca^{2+} channel, a G protein, AC, cAMP-dependent PKA and the counterbalancing phosphatase PP2A. This signaling complex ensures specific and rapid signaling. Moreover, β_2-adrenoceptors appear compartmentalized spatially, residing exclusively in caveolae isolated from quiescent rat cardiomyocytes allowing regulation of cAMP signaling in microdomains.

Further specificity of signaling might result from the selective coupling to different isoforms of AC. Nine mammalian isoforms of AC have been identified, of which types 5 and 6 are the predominant isoforms expressed in heart and are inhibited by multiple intracellular signaling pathways including G_i, PKA, PKC, and Ca^{2+}. In myocytes overexpressing AC6, a selective enhancement of β-adrenoceptor stimulated cAMP formation was observed with colocalization of β-adrenoceptor and AC in caveolar microdomains allowing rapid and specific signal transduction in cardiac myocytes. Whether selective AC isoform coupling occurs with different β-adrenoceptor subtypes is under investigation.

HOMO- AND HETERODIMERIZATION OF β_1- AND β_1-ADRENOCEPTORS

The classic GPCR model predicts that the stoichiometry of receptor, G protein and effector is 1/1/1; however, several studies have demonstrated that GPCRs exist as dimeric or oligomeric complexes. In addition to homodimers, heterodimers between members of the GPCR family exist. Homodimerization of both β_1-adrenoceptors and β_2-adrenoceptors has been observed in vitro and in vivo, and intermolecular interactions between receptors might have functional and structural implications for G protein-mediated signaling. The sixth transmembrane domain of the β_2-adrenoceptor appears to be involved in homodimerization because a peptide derived from this domain inhibits both dimerization and β-adrenoceptor G_s/AC coupling, indicating a functional role for dimerization. Agonist stimulation was also found to stabilize the homodimer, whereas inverse agonists favored the monomeric state, further suggesting that conversion between monomer and dimer forms might play a physiological role.

The coexistence of β_1- and β_2-adrenoceptor subtypes within a single myocyte raises the possibility of heterodimerization between these two receptors giving rise to potential novel pharmacology. Heterodimeriation of β_1- and β_2-adrenoceptors has been observed in cell lines and mouse cardiomyocytes cooverexpressing β_1- and β_2-adrenoceptors. β_1- and β_2-adrenoceptor colocalization has been demonstrated on the cell membrane surface together with novel functional properties. There was approx 1.5 log unit leftward shift in the concentration-response curve to isoproterenol of myocyte contraction when β_1- and β_2-adrenoceptors were coexpressed in myocytes from double β_1-/β_2-adrenoceptor KO mice. In addition, decreased affinity of known ligands was observed (K_d of CGP 20712A decreased approx 10-fold and the K_d of ICI 118,551 decreased approx 70-fold compared with each subtype expressed alone), suggesting that β_1- and β_2-adrenoceptors can form high-affinity heterodimers with a novel binding site and altered ligand binding properties. However, similar efficacy and potency of isoproterenol-stimulated cAMP production has been demonstrated when β_1- and β_2-adrenoceptors were expressed in cell lines alone or together when they were observed to form heterodimers. However, a unique functional property of β_1-/β_2-heterodimers was observed, with complete loss of the isoproterenol stimulation of ERK 1/2 mitogen-activated protein kinase activation, which is usually seen when β_2- (but not β_1-) adrenoceptors are expressed alone. Thus homo- and heterodimerization of β_1- and β_2-adrenoceptors alters G protein coupling and downstream signaling, although the functional basis of these interactions remains to be explored.

β_3-ADRENOCEPTOR COUPLING IN HUMAN HEART
The functional role and coupling mechanism for cardiac β_3-adrenoceptors remains unclear. β_3-adrenoceptors are pharmacologically characterized by four criteria:

1. Low affinity of classic β-adrenoceptor antagonists such as propranolol and nadolol.
2. Activation by selective β_3-adrenoceptor agonists BRL 37344, SR 58611A, and CL 316243.

3. Activation by nonconventional partial agonists CGP 12177A, cyanopindolol, and pindolol.
4. Blockade by selective β_3-adrenoceptors antagonists SR 59230A. Activation of recombinant β_3-adrenoceptors increases adenylyl cyclase activity by signaling via G_s.

β_3-adrenoceptor mRNA has been reported in human atrium and ventricle in addition to gastrointestinal and adipose tissue, and protein expression has been demonstrated in human heart. Nonetheless, little evidence suggests a cardiostimulant role for the β_3-adrenoceptor because cardiostimulant effects of selective β_3-adrenoceptor agonists have not been observed in human ventricle or atrium, or rat or ferret heart. β_3-adrenoceptor selective agonists BRL 37344 and SR 58611 increase L-type Ca^{2+} current 1.7- and 2.2-fold, respectively in human atrial myocytes by a nadolol-resistant mechanism and increased atrial inotropic and chronotropic response, but these effects are most likely mediated by activation of classic β_1- and β_2-adrenoceptors.

However, β_3-adrenoceptors also appear to couple to G_i and produce cardiodepression and action potential shortening in human ventricle with nanomolar potency. In addition, high concentrations of endogenous catecholamines were shown to elicit a nadolol-resistant cardiodepression. The cardiodepressant effect of β_3-adrenoceptor agonists was attenuated by pretreatment by PTX, suggesting mediation by coupling to G_i. The observation that the cardiodepressant effects were reduced by nitric oxide (NO)-antagonists led to the suggestion of a G_i/NO-dependent cyclic guanosine monophosphate signaling pathway mediating β_3-adrenoceptor negative inotropic effects in human ventricle. However, although NO-mediated β_3-adrenoceptor stimulation is present in human atrium, at least in nonfailing heart, it does not directly affect atrial contraction.

β_3-adrenoceptors are more resistant to desensitization than classic β_1- and β_2-adrenoceptors, and β_3-adrenoceptor expression appears increased in failing human ventricle. This suggests that in heart failure, the relative importance of β_3-adrenoceptors might be increased with impairment of contractility mediated by activation of β_3-adrenoceptors by high circulating concentrations of norepinephrine and coupling to a G_i/cyclic guanosine monophosphate/ NO signaling pathway.

However, the observation of cardiodepression by β_3-adrenoceptor selective agonists has not been confirmed in isolated human cardiac preparations by others. β_3-adrenoceptor selective agonists failed to cause cardiodepression in human atrium, and in failing ventricle in both whole trabeculae and isolated myocytes. Furthermore, the cardiodepressant effect of BRL 37344 was observed with nanomolar potency, whereas this compound has been observed to have micromolar potency at recombinant and adipocyte β_3-adrenoceptors. As described, negative inotropic effects of β-adrenoceptor antagonists have been demonstrated in failing human ventricle mediated primarily by a G_i-dependent interaction with the β_2-adrenoceptor. BRL 37344 has a similar affinity for the β_2- and β_3-adrenoceptor and produces positive inotropic effects in atrium mediated by β_1- and β_2-adrenoceptors. Thus in failing ventricle, the cardiodepressant effects of BRL 37344 could be mediated by β_2-adrenoceptor coupling to G_i. Clearly, the implication of β_3-adrenoceptor mediated cardiodepression is important, particularly in the context of heart failure, and further elucidation is required to address this controversy.

THE "PUTATIVE" β_4-ADRENOCEPTOR The β_4-adrenoceptor is of particular interest, because of its potential importance

blockade and stimulation. Naunyn Schmiedebergs Arch Pharmacol 1984;327:159–175.

Wenzel K, Felix S, Bauer D, et al. Novel variants in 3 kb of 5′UTR of the b1-adrenergic receptor gene (-93C4T, -210C4T, and -2146T4C): -21a6C homozygotes present in patients with idiopathic dilated cardiomyopathy and coronary heart disease. Hum Mutat 2000;16:534.

Wheeldon N, Mcdevitt D, Lipworth B. Cardiac Effects of the β_3-adrenoceptor agonist BRL 35135 in man. Br J Clin Pharmacol 1994;37:363–369.

White H, Maqbool A, McMahon A, et al. An evaluation of the beta-1 adrenergic receptor Arg389Gly polymorphism in individuals at risk of coronary events. A WOSCOPS substudy. Eur Heart J 2002;23: 1087–1092.

Wickman K, Clapham D. Ion channel regulation by G proteins. Physiol Rev. 1995;75:864–885.

Xamoterol in Severe Heart Failure Study Group. Xamoterol in severe heart failure. Lancet 1990;336:1–6.

Xiao R, Avdonin P, Zhou Y, et al. Coupling of beta2-adrenoceptor to Gi proteins and its physiological relevance in murine cardiac myocytes. Circ Res 1999;84:43–52.

Xiao R, Cheng H, Zhou Y, Kuschel M, Lakatta E. Recent advances in cardiac β_2-adrenergic signal transduction. Circ Res 1999;85:1092–1100.

Xiao R, Hohl C, Altschuld R, et al. β2-Adrenergic receptor-stimulated increase in cAMP in rat heart cells is not coupled to change in Ca^{2+} dynamics, contractility or phospholamban phosphorylation. J Biol Chem 1994;269:19,151–19,156.

Xiao R, Lakatta E. β1-Adrenoceptor stimulation and β2-adrenoceptor stimulation differ in their effects on contraction, cyotsolic Ca^{2+} and Ca^{2+} current in single rat ventricular cells. Circ Res 1993;73:286–300.

Xiao R. β-Adrenergic signalling in the heart: dual coupling of the β_2-adrenergic receptor to Gs and Gi proteins. Sci STKE 2001;104:RE15.

Yatani A, Brown A. Rapid beta-adrenergic modulation of cardiac calcium channel currents by a fast G protein pathway. Science 1989; 245:71–74.

Yatani A, Codina J, Imoto Y, Reeves J, Birnbaumer L, Brown A. A G protein directly regulates mammalian cardiac calcium channels. Science 1987;238:1288–1292.

Yatani A, Imoto Y, Codina J, Hamilton S, Brown A, Birnbaumer L. The stimulatory G protein of adenylyl cyclase, Gs, also stimulated dihydropyridine-sensititive Ca^{2+} channels. J Biol Chem 1988;263:9887–9895.

Zaccolo M, Pozzan T. Discrete microdomains with high concentration of cAMP in stimulated rat neonatal cardiac myocytes. Science 2002; 295(1):1711–1715.

Zhou Y, Cheng H, Bogdanov K, et al. Localized cAMP-dependent signalling mediates beta 2-adrenergic modulation of cardiac excitation-contraction coupling. Am J Physiol 1997;273:H1611–H1618.

Zhou Y, Yang D, Zhu W, et al. Spontaneous activation of beta(2)- but not beta(1)-adrenoceptors expressed in cardiac myocytes from beta(1)beta(2) double knockout mice. Mol Pharmacol 2000;58:887–894.

Zhu W, Yang D, Zhang S, et al. Heterodimerization of β_1- and β_2-adrenergic receptors in cardiac myocytes. Circulation 2002;106(Supp II):1124.

13 Aortic Diseases

SAUMYA DAS, JAMES L. JANUZZI, JR., AND ERIC M. ISSELBACHER

SUMMARY

Aneurysms are the most important disorder that affects the aorta. Aneurysms involving the abdominal aorta are typically associated with atherosclerosis, whereas those involving the thoracic aorta have many causes, including congenital abnormalities in the structure of the aortic wall. This chapter will discuss thoracic aortic aneurysms, such as Marfan syndrome, bicuspid aortic valve, and familial thoracic aortic aneurysm syndrome, and also abdominal aortic aneurysms.

Key Words: Aneurysm; aorta; bicuspid aortic valve; familial thoracic aortic aneurysm syndrome; Marfan syndrome.

INTRODUCTION

Although diseases of the aorta are significantly less common than those of the heart, because aortic disease can be life threatening, its diagnosis and treatment are clinically relevant. Aneurysms are the most important disorder that affect the aorta. Aneurysms involving the abdominal aorta are typically associated with atherosclerosis, whereas those involving the thoracic aorta have many causes, including congenital abnormalities in the structure of the aortic wall. Because aortic aneurysms typically do not produce symptoms until they are large, the diagnosis is often not made until a rupture or dissection occurs. However, mass population screening is not likely to be practical or cost effective. Therefore, the ability to identify genetic factors that could predict risk for aortic aneurysms would be a valuable guide screening and therapy in clinical practice.

THORACIC AORTIC ANEURYSMS

MARFAN SYNDROME Marfan syndrome (MFS) is the best-studied aortic disease regarding genetic basis and molecular mechanisms. The search for the causes of MFS exemplifies a systematic approach used to identify candidate genes and gain insight into the disorder's biology and pathophysiology.

MFS is a systemic disorder of connective tissue with protean manifestations, with the skeletal, ocular, and cardiovascular systems most often affected. The hallmark of MFS is abnormality of the medial layer of the aortic wall, characterized by fragmentation and disorganization of the elastic fibers, a generalized loss of elastin content, and deposition of amorphous matrix components. The mechanical properties of the aorta are primarily a function of the elastic fibers within the media, so loss or abnormalities of elastin could weaken the tensile strength of the aortic wall. Indeed, the most threatening consequence of MFS is dilatation of the aortic root and the ascending aorta, which, if untreated, can result in potentially fatal aortic dissection or rupture.

The syndrome is relatively uncommon, with a prevalence of one in 5000–10,000. Traditionally, the diagnosis has relied on a series of clinical criteria as outlined in the Ghent nosology, reflecting the pleiotropic manifestation of the disease: the phenotypes of the affected individuals form a continuum from the severe neonatal MFS to milder forms known by the acronym MASS (myopia, mitral valve prolapse, aortic dilatation without dissection, and skin and skeletal muscle abnormalities). The Ghent nosology was designed to account for varying presentations by defining highly specific major criteria with less specific minor criteria. A positive diagnosis requires a combination of major criteria in at least two organ systems and minor criteria in a third organ system.

The clustering of MFS in families is well recognized and classic genetic analysis has shown it to be autosomal-dominant with complete penetrance (but with pleiotropic manifestations). In exploring for the genetic cause of MFS, researchers first excluded certain candidate genes such as elastin. Then, in one affected family, positional cloning indicated that the mutation was localized to chromosome 15q21. Cloning and sequencing of the DNA in that region led to the identification of the *fibrillin (FBN)-1 gene*. Subsequently, FBN1 mutations were linked to the majority of the cases of MFS. In addition, a distinct gene on chromosome 3p24 was linked to another family with MFS.

The identification of the FBN1 prompted investigation into the role of FBN1, the protein product of the FBN1, in the development and homeostasis of the aortic wall. Studies undertaken to elucidate the basic structure of the fibrillin gene progressed on two fronts. Some investigators mapped the various mutations associated with MFS, attempting to correlate genotype and phenotype. Others examined the biology of fibrillin (and they are made up of microfibrils), trying to understand how specific abnormalities in protein structure may alter biology at the cellular, organ, and systemic level. Of the 337 mutations in the FBN1 reported in patients with MFS, 69 have been found in more than one unrelated individual, eight in three or more unrelated individuals, and only three mutations have been found in four of more unrelated individuals. Unfortunately, the difficulty expressing fibrillin and constituting microfibrils in vitro has hampered the correlation of structure and function. Consequently, only a few of these mutations have been tested experimentally.

From: *Principles of Molecular Medicine, Second Edition*
Edited by: M. S. Runge and C. Patterson © Humana Press, Inc., Totowa, NJ

The majority of FBN1 mutations in MFS are missense mutations that lead to substitution of one of six highly conserved cysteines. Cysteines are important in the formation of intramolecular disulfide bonds critical to protein folding, so substitution of any of these amino acids could disrupt fibrillin protein structure and, consequently, have deleterious effects on the global structure of microfibrils. Some of the other missense mutations are in the conserved calcium-binding motif. The binding of calcium by this motif may serve to rigidify the protein and perhaps even stabilize FBN1 against proteolytic degradation. Nevertheless, it remains unclear whether the primary consequence of the alteration in the structure of the fibrillin protein is an increased sensitivity to proteolysis, an altered protein–protein interaction, individual microfibril disarray, or overall disruption of the architecture of polymeric microfibrillin arrays owing to distortion in the individual monomeric fibrillin modules.

Most of the identified mutations do not seem to segregate with particular phenotypes. Indeed, even in classic MFS, there is a striking intrafamily variability. For example, family members sharing the same mutation can have clinical syndromes that vary widely in terms of the age of onset, the organ systems involved, and the severity of disease.

Nevertheless, a minority of mutations do produce more consistent phenotypes. For example, 20% of reported mutations are either nonsense mutations or have a frameshift resulting in a premature stop codon. Messenger RNAs containing these transcripts display a reduced concentration owing to a phenomenon called nonsense-mediated decay, and most of these manifest as a mild clinical phenotype. Indeed, none of these mutations has been reported to cause neonatal MFS, the most serious manifestation of the disease. Conversely, patients with the phenotype of neonatal MFS—who are diagnosed at birth and die primarily of heart failure from severe tricuspid and mitral regurgitation rather than aortic dissection—have mutations that cluster in exons 24–32. Another clinical phenotype, atypically severe MFS, which presents with early-onset cardiovascular complications with aortic dissection or need for aortic surgery before age 16, is also associated with mutations in exons 24–32, although these mutations are typically distinct from mutations found in neonatal and classic MFS.

Nonetheless meaningful conclusions about genotype–phenotype correlations have been difficult to draw. Without further detailed knowledge of the three-dimensional structure of fibrillin, its protein partners, and the biology of microfibrils, it would be hard to correlate mutations with clinical phenotypes. Furthermore, given that most mutations in FBN1 (apart from those seen in classic MFS) have been identified in only one affected individual or family, it would be hard to generalize genotype–phenotype correlations. Finally, MFS is likely only a small percentage of fibrillinopathies, because FBN1 mutations have been reported in Marfan-related aortic syndromes and disorders of skeletal system such as Weill-Marchesani syndrome. Further progress awaits characterization of these disorders and more knowledge of the role of microfibrils.

The histological hallmark of MFS is the disorganization and fragmentation of elastic fibers and a decrease in elastin content in the medial layer of the aorta. No comprehensive theory has emerged that explains how mutations in the FBN1 lead to this pathological hallmark. However, several major hypotheses have emerged. The first proposed mechanism is the dominant-negative model of pathogenesis. Microfibrils consist of polymers of the FBN1 protein. According to the dominant-negative model, mutant FBN1 proteins interfere with the assembly of wild-type FBN1—produced by the normal allele in heterozygotes—into microfibrils. This model is attractive from a theoretical standpoint because large polymers are especially sensitive to defects in monomeric components; in the case of fibrillin, mutations in the cysteine residues might affect not only intramolecular disulfide bonds but also intermolecular bonds that might be essential to the assembly of microfibrils.

Premature truncation codon mutations are associated with lower levels of mutant transcripts leading to decreased numbers of mutant fibrillin monomers. If the dominant-negative model were true, fewer mutant monomers should produce less interference with assembly of the remaining wild-type monomers, and hence a milder phenotype. Indeed, in one study the patient with the lowest proportion of mutant transcript (6%) had a clinically mild MASS phenotype, whereas another patient with higher levels of mutant transcript (16%) had the more severe classic MFS phenotype. However, this model may not alone be sufficient, as in one report patients with 2 and 7% mutant transcript levels both had severe manifestation of MFS.

Studies using cultured fibroblasts from MFS patients also seem to support the dominant-negative hypothesis. Using pulse-chase experiments with radioactive sulfur to label the cysteine-rich fibrillin proteins, the synthesis, secretion and aggregation of fibrillin molecules were studied. Fibroblast cell lines derived from patients with MFS (with a variety of mutations) showed only 35% expected fibrillin deposition (based on normal controls) in the extracellular matrix (ECM). Interestingly, three nonsense mutations with mutant transcripts proportions of 15–25% demonstrated ECM deposition rates of 7–25% of normal, whereas one nonsense mutation with a lower mutant transcript level of 6% showed ECM deposition of 54% normal, supporting a dominant-negative effect. A "threshold effect" may exist in which low levels of mutant transcript may be insufficient to disrupt the assembly of microfibrils from the wild-type fibrillin protein expressed from the wild-type allele, whereas higher levels of mutant proteins are able to exert their dominant-negative effect.

Finally, in a classic experiment, a mutant allele was expressed from an MFS patient in normal human and murine fibroblasts. There was substantially reduced ECM deposition of fibrillin in these cultures. Thus, even in the background of two normal alleles, the expression of the mutant monomer led to disruption of fibrillin deposition in the ECM.

The second proposed mechanism of the pathogenesis of MFS is an altered homeostasis of the microfibril. The elastic fibers within the aortic media consist of an amorphous core comprised primarily of cross-linked tropoelastin monomers surrounded by microfibrils. During development, microfibrils are found at the margins of maturing elastic fibers, leading to the hypothesis that microfibrils and FBN1 may play a crucial role in the deposition of elastic fibers during embryogenesis, and that the distortion in the architecture of elastic fibers seen in MFS thus reflects abnormal elastogenesis.

Mice with targeted mutations in the FBN1 were created to test this hypothesis, leading to a 10-fold reduction in the level of the mutant transcript. Heterozygous mice expressed very low levels of the mutant transcript and were morphologically and histologically indistinguishable from the wild-type mice. Homozygous mutant mice appeared normal at birth, but died shortly thereafter of vascular complications, with histologic analysis revealing thinning of the proximal aortic wall. Immunostaining showed substantial reduction in the amount of extracellular fibrillin, but a normal amount of elastin staining, suggesting that elastogenesis may proceed in a normal fashion even in the absence of normal development of microfibrils. The investigators hypothesized that microfibrils may be important in the homeostasis of the aortic wall, and in the absence of proper microfibril development, the aortic media is unable to sustain the hemodynamic stress to which it is subjected, eventually leading to aortic dilatation. The disruption of the elastic network may then be a secondary event.

Studies involving another mutant mouse model producing a five-fold reduction in gene expression support the concept. The homozygous mutant mice gradually develop severe kyphoscoliosis and die prematurely of Marfan-like vascular complications. Histological examination of these mice at birth shows normal vascular anatomy with a seemingly normal appearing elastin network in the aortic media. However, by 6 wk of age a sequence of events commences with focal calcification in the aortic elastic lamellae, progressing to intimal hyperplasia, monocytic infiltration, fragmentation of elastic lamellae, and eventually dilatation of the aortic wall.

An increase in fibrillin proteolysis is the third mechanism proposed of the pathogenesis of MFS. It is recognized that calcium binding to the calcium-binding epidermal growth factor-like (cbEGF) domains of fibrillin is essential for the proper assembly and integrity of the microfibrillar aggregates, and that calcium may protect wild-type fibrillin from proteolysis. Because FBN1 mutations reduce the calcium affinity of cbEGF motifs in vitro, investigators have hypothesized that mutations in the cbEGF domains might render the FBN1 aggregates more prone to proteolysis. Studies have been hampered by the difficulty of expressing full-length fibrillin in vitro, so most experiments have used fibrillin fragments. Nonetheless, these experiments have shown that certain FBN1 mutations increase protease susceptibility by exposing enzyme-specific cryptic cleavage sites for particular proteases. The clinical sequelae remain unclear. In one study, however, surgical thoracic aortic aneurysm specimens from patients with MFS did show increased immunofluorescence for certain matrix metalloproteinases (proteolytic enzymes), especially at the border of areas of cystic medial necrosis. Nonetheless, in contrast to the pathogenesis of abdominal aortic aneurysms (AAAs, discussed later), direct evidence linking proteases to the pathogenesis of MFS is lacking.

The pathogenesis of MFS thus remains unclear. It appears that all three mechanisms described may contribute to the ultimate disruption of the cellular and molecular architecture of the aortic wall's tunica media. A unified theory will require a better understanding of the dynamic biology of the microfibril, its interaction with other proteins, and its interaction with adjacent vascular smooth cells. Also unclear is the potential role of modifying genetic elements, which may be responsible for modulating the phenotypic expression of a particular MFS genotype.

BICUSPID AORTIC VALVE Bicuspid aortic valve is the most common congenital cardiac malformation, affecting 1–2% of the population. Bicuspid aortic valve is highly associated with other congenital aorta abnormalities, such as coarctation and patent ductus arteriosis. Bicuspid aortic valve is often associated with dilatation of the aortic root or ascending aorta and may progress to frank thoracic aortic aneurysms and aortic dissection. Consequently, despite its name, bicuspid aortic valve should be considered an abnormality of both the valve and aorta, rather than just the valve. Indeed, over time most individuals with a bicuspid aortic valve will develop complications—either valve dysfunction or aneurysm of the thoracic aorta—requiring surgical treatment.

The pathogenesis of the bicuspid aortic valve is not well understood. However, it seems likely that the abnormal aortic cusp formation during valvulogenesis is the result of a complex developmental process involving the ECM. During development the ECM provides scaffolding and cues that are critical in cellular migration and pattern formation. In the aorta, differentiation of the cushion mesenchymal cells into mature valve cells correlates with the expression of microfibrillar proteins fibrillin and fibulin. Genetic mutations that result in inadequate amounts of such proteins, or that disrupt the timing or function of such proteins, lead to abnormal valvulogenesis early in life, and perhaps a weakened aortic wall later in life, in turn resulting in aortic aneurysms and dissection. Although there does appear to be a familial risk, no single mutation resulting in the bicuspid aortic valve phenotype has been identified.

Research is focusing on transcriptional elements and signaling molecules that may alter the expression of the important ECM proteins. Mice deficient in endothelial nitric oxide synthase (eNOS) have a high incidence of congenital bicuspid aortic valves. In wild-type mice, the expression of endothelial nitric oxide synthase is noted in the myocardium as well as the endothelium during development, but is localized to the endothelium lining the valve at maturity, suggesting a role in valvulogenesis. Conversely, there was no difference in the diameter of the aortic lumen between the two groups.

Research has also concentrated on the etiology of the vascular complications associated with bicuspid aortic valve. The pathology of the aortic wall is likely the result of intrinsic defects in the ECM rather than a secondary consequence of valvular dysfunction. This is supported by the observation that dilatation of the ascending thoracic aorta can be found in young adults with a bicuspid aortic valve but without significant valvular stenosis or regurgitation. Similarly, even those with a bicuspid aortic valve who have undergone aortic valve replacement can develop ascending thoracic aortic aneurysms at a later date.

The thoracic aortic aneurysms associated with bicuspid aortic valve typically demonstrate accelerated degeneration of the aortic media. The histopathology in such cases is similar to that of patients with MFS who also have abnormal FBN1 content in their aortic wall.

FAMILIAL THORACIC AORTIC ANEURYSM SYNDROME In addition to the association of ascending thoracic aortic aneurysms with MFS and bicuspid aortic valve, some patients with such aneurysms and proven cystic medial degeneration have no other identifiable congenital abnormalities. Indeed, evidence suggests that many of these patients also have a genetic mutation that may account for cystic medial degeneration. Moreover, it is recognized that cases of thoracic aortic aneurysms in the absence of overt connective tissue disorders are often familial in nature and reflect a familial thoracic aortic aneurysm syndrome.

In an analysis of a large database of patients with thoracic aortic aneurysms, at least 19% of those without MFS had a family history of a thoracic aortic aneurysm. Most pedigrees suggested an autosomal-dominant mode of inheritance, although some suggested a recessive mode and possibly X-linked inheritance as well. Another series examined the families of 158 patients referred for surgical repair of thoracic aortic aneurysms or dissections and found that first-degree relatives of probands had a higher risk of thoracic aortic aneurysms compared with controls.

Investigation of the genetic basis for this syndrome is still in its infancy. Several genes have been implicated. A mutation on 3p24.2-25 has been identified that can cause both isolated and familial thoracic aortic aneurysms owing to cystic medial degeneration. However, despite a dominant pattern of inheritance, there is a marked variability in the expression and penetrance of the disorder, with some inheriting the gene but showing no manifestation. Two other studies of familial thoracic aortic aneurysm syndromes have mapped the mutations to at least two different chromosomal loci, but other families mapped to neither of these, suggesting genetic heterogeneity in addition to variable expression and penetrance.

ABDOMINAL AORTIC ANEURYSMS

Unlike the ascending thoracic aortic aneurysms discussed, abdominal aortic aneurysms (AAAs) are typically associated with aging and atherosclerosis. Gender plays a role; men are 10 times more likely than women to have an AAA of 4 cm or greater. However, women with an AAA have a significantly greater risk of rupture than men. It is also recognized that genes influence aneurysm formation. Those having a first-degree relative with an AAA have an increased risk of 13–32% compared with the 2–5% risk in the general population. In addition, those with familial aneurysms tend to be younger and have higher rates of rupture than those with sporadic aneurysms. However, no single gene defects for AAA have been identified, and pedigree analysis suggests that the increased risk is probably polygenic.

To clarify the genetic underpinnings and foster improvements in prevention and therapy, there has been intense investigation to elucidate the pathophysiology of AAA. Examination of human AAA tissue resected at surgery and experiments from explanted AAA tissue maintained in tissue culture have provided important clues. First, the pathologic hallmark seems to be destructive remodeling of the elastic media of the aortic wall, including progressive degradation of the fibrillar matrix proteins. Second, evidence of an infiltration of inflammatory cells exists, including B lymphocytes, T lymphocytes, and macrophages. Third, there is increased immunoreactivity for elastolytic matrix metalloproteases (MMP), particularly MMP-2, MMP-9, and MMP-12. Of these, MMP-9 is the most abundant elastase secreted by AAA human tissue explants in vitro and seems to be actively expressed by macrophages at the site of tissue damage in resected AAA tissue.

Of the animal models developed to study the specific roles of the various MMPs, one of the most durable is the elastase-induced rat or mouse model of AAA. In it, the infrarenal aorta is temporarily ligated proximally (just below the level of the renal artery) and distally at the level of the bifurcation. A catheter is introduced via an aortotomy at the distal site of ligation and the portion of the aorta between the two ligations is perfused with elastase for 5 min. The sutures are then removed and the aortic dimensions can be measured at various time-points. A moderate amount of aortic dilatation appears immediately after the perfusion. There is then no further increase in aortic diameter for the next 7 d. However, at 14 d, the aortas in the elastase infusion group were significantly dilated (compared with a heat-inactivated elastase control group) and reached aneurysmal proportions.

Light microscopy revealed minimal damage to the medial elastic lamellae for up to 7 d in both groups. By 14 d, however, the elastase-perfused aortas exhibited a dense inflammatory infiltrate along with extensive degradation of the elastin framework. In contrast, the aortas infused with inactive elastase appeared normal at 14 d. This supports a model in which the initial elastase infusion serves as an insult that evokes an inflammatory response leading to tissue destruction and elastolysis, and ultimately, aneurysmal dilatation of the aortic wall.

Work has focused on the molecular players immediately upstream of elastolysis, and hence may form reasonable targets for therapeutic intervention. As mentioned, the most obvious candidates were MMP-9, MMP-12, and MMP-2. Using the mouse model of elastase-induced aneurysmal dilatation, investigators found that the development of aneurysms in this model was temporally and spatially correlated with "chronic inflammation." Staining with antibodies seemed to indicate that these macrophages were the likely source of MMP-9. Furthermore, levels of MMP-9 and MMP-12 were both increased during development of elastase-induced AAA, and treatment of these animals with doxycycline, a nonselective MMP-inhibitor, led to a significant reduction in the size of the aneurysms. In a final set of elegant experiments, the authors attempted to uncover the role of various specific MMPs using mice with targeted disruption of the MMP-9 and MMP-12 genes. Elastase infusion resulted in a significantly smaller AAA size in MMP-9 knockout mice and in mice that had been bred to have combined deficiencies in MMP-9 and MMP-12. However, there was no reduction in AAA size in the MMP-12 knockout mice.

Examination of aortic tissue from these mice models revealed no suppression of the elastase-induced inflammatory response. Indeed, the MMP-9 knockout mice continued to display infiltration by macrophages and polymorphonuclear leukocytes, yet at 14 d the elastic lamellae remained well preserved. However, when the bone marrow of the MMP-9 knockout mice was reconstituted with wild-type bone marrow (i.e., not MMP-9 deficient), a significant increase in aortic diameter resulted. These experiments suggest that the signals to recruit the inflammatory response following exposure to elastase are not dependent on the presence of the MMPs examined. The expression of MMP-9 by the infiltrating macrophages appears to be crucial to elastolysis and the subsequent development of aortic aneurysms.

It is unclear what other agents may be involved in the MMP cascades that seem to underlie the development of aneurysms. For example, plasmin and plasminogen activators seem to be involved in the development of aneurysms in some mice models, and the overexpression of plasminogen-activator inhibitor (PAI-1) can suppress aneurysm formation in a rat model. Proteases such as plasmin/PA and elastases may be part of a cascade that leads to progressive activation of other proteases (such as MMP-9 from pro-MMP-9) much like the coagulation and complement cascade. Furthermore, protease inhibitors such as plasminogen-activator inhibitor and tissue inhibitors of MMP might act as checks to prevent rampant activation of the proteases. Disruptions or changes in the "balance of power" could alter the process in favor of proteases and hence elastolysis.

Despite the extensive progress in the understanding of the protease cascades that may be responsible for elastolysis, much less is known about the signals that initiate the inflammatory process in the wall of aortic aneurysms. There is a clear association between atherosclerosis and aneurysm formation, so atherosclerotic plaques (known to contain an inflammatory infiltrate) might be an "insult" to the arterial wall, akin to the exposure of mice aorta to elastase. A model of atherosclerosis and underlying endothelial cell dysfunction has emerged in the form of mice deficient in apo-E, which have accelerated atherosclerotic lesions. However, despite their extensive atherosclerotic lesions these mice do not develop AAA. Hence just the presence of atherosclerosis and the associated inflammation may not be sufficient to induce the formation of aneurysms. One possible explanation is that compensatory mechanisms in the vascular bed—such as the release of nitric oxide by endothelial cells—counteract some effects of inflammation.

Although endothelial cell-dependent relaxation of the vascular bed is mediated by nitric oxide, it appears that nitric oxide may have multiple other roles, including inhibition of smooth muscle cell proliferation, platelet aggregation/adhesion, and leukocyte activation. Perhaps removing this versatile signaling molecule in the presence of atherosclerotic plaque induces the formation of an aneurysm. This was accomplished experimentally by crossing e-NOS knockout and apo-E knockout mice to create mice deficient in both proteins. The "double knockout" mice were more hypertensive that control wild-type mice, and a significant proportion of these mice developed an AAA. The development of the AAA was not simply owing to hypertension, because lowering the blood pressure to levels seen in the control mice had no effect in reducing aneurysm development, suggesting that there may be a "multihit" mechanism for the development of AAA. Atherosclerotic lesions, such as those seen in the apo-E knockout mice, may serve as the initial insult leading to a chronic inflammatory state; meanwhile, the presence of preserved endothelial function mediated by nitric oxide may protect from the development of AAA. However, the addition of significant endothelial dysfunction (in this case the lack of the critical endothelial regulator nitric oxide) may be the second factor that accelerates the process of AAA formation.

SELECTED REFERENCES

Allaire E, Hasenstab D, Kenagy RD, et al. Prevention of aneurysm development and rupture by local overexpression of plasminogen activator inhibitor-1. Circulation 1998;98:249–255.

Aoyoma T, Francke U, Dietz HC, Furthmayr H. Quantitative differences in biosynthesis and extracellular deposition of fibrillin in cultured fibroblasts distinguish five groups of Marfan syndrome patients and suggest distinct pathogenetic mechanisms. J Clin Invest 1994;94:130–137.

Biddinger A, Rocklin M, Coselli J, Milewicz DM. Familial thoracic aortic dilatations and dissections: a case control study. J Vasc Surg 1997;25:506–511.

Booms T, Tiecke F, Rosenberg T, Hagemeier C, Robinson PN. Differential effects of FBN1 mutations on in vitro proteolysis of recombinant fibrillin-1 fragments. Hum Genet 2000;107:216–224.

Carmeliet P, Moons L, Lijnen R, et al. Urokinase-generated plasmin activates matrix metalloproteinases during aneurysm formation. Nat Genet 1997;17:439–444.

Chen J, Kuhlencordt PJ, Astern J, Gyurko R, Huang P. Hypertension does not account for the accelerated atherosclerosis and development of aneurysms in male apolipoprotein E/endothelial nitric oxide synthase double knockout mice. Circulation 2001;104:2391–2394.

Coady MA, Davis RR, Roberts M, et al. Familial patterns of thoracic aortic aneurysms. Arch Surg 1999;134:361–367.

Collod G, Babron M, Jondeau G, et al. A second locus for Marfan syndrome maps to chromosome 3p24.2-p25. Nat Genet 1994;8:264–268.

Curci JA, Liao S, Huffman MD, Shapiro SD, Thompson RW. Expression and localization of macrophage elastase in abdominal aortic aneurysms. J Clin Invest 1998;102:1900–1910.

Daugherty A, Cassis LA. Mechanisms of abdominal aortic aneurysm formation. Curr Atheroscler Rep 2002;4(3):222–227.

De Paepe A, Devereux RB, Dietz HC, Hennekam RC, Peyritz RE. Revised diagnostic criteria for the Marfan syndrome. Am J Med Genet 1996;62:417–426.

Dietz HC, Cutting GR, Pyeritz RE, et al. Marfan syndrome caused by a recurrent de novo missense mutation in the fibrillin gene. Nature 1991;352:337–339.

Dietz HC, McIntosh I, Sakai LY, et al. Four novel FBN 1 mutations: Significance for mutant transcript level and EGF-like domain calcium binding in the pathogenesis of Marfan syndrome. Genomics 1993;17: 468–475.

Eisenberg LM, Markwald RR. Molecular regulation of atrioventricular alvulospetal morphogenesis. Circ Res 1995;77:1–6.

Eldadah ZA, Brenn T, Furthmayr H, Dietz HC. Expression of a mutant human fibrillin allele upon a normal human or murine genetic background recapitulates a Marfan cellular phenotype. J Clin Invest 1995;95:874–880.

Fedak PWM, Verma S, David TE, Leask RL, Weisel RD, Butany J. Clinical and pathophysiological implications of a bicuspid aortic valve. Circulation 2002;106:900–904.

Freestone T, Turner RG, Coady A, et al. Inflammation and matrix metalloproteinases in the enlarging abdominal aortic aneurysm. Arterioscler Thromb Vasc Biol 1995;15:1145–1151.

Fukui D, Miyagawa S, Soeda J, Tanaka K, Urayama H, Kawasaki S. Overexpression of transforming growth factor beta1 in smooth muscle cells of human abdominal aortic aneurysm. Eur J Vasc Endovasc Surg 2003;25(6):540–545.

Kuhlencordt PJ, Gyurko R, Han F, et al. Accelerated atherosclerosis, aortic aneurysm formation, and ischemic heart disease in apolipoprotein E/endothelial nitric oxide synthase double-knockout mice. Circulation 2001;104(4):448–454.

Lee TC, Zhao YD, Courtman DW, et al. Abnormal aortic valve development in mice lacking endothelial nitric oxide synthase. Circulation 2000;101:2345–2348.

Loeys B, Nuytinck L, Delvaux I, De Bie S, De Paepe A. Genotype and phenotype analysis of 171 patients referred for molecular study of the fibrillin-1 gene FBN1 because of suspected Marfan syndrome. Arch Intern Med 2001;161:2447–2454.

Milewicz DM, Chen H, Park E-S, et al. Reduced penetrance and variable expressivity of familial thoracic aneurysms/dissections. Am J Cardiol 1998;82:474–479.

Miralles M, Wester W, Sicard GA, Thompson R, Reilly J. Indomethacin inhibits expansion of experimental aortic aneurysms via inhibition of the cox2 isoform of cyclooxygenase. J Vasc Surg 1999;29(5):884–893.

Nkomo VT, Enriquez-Sarano M, Ammash NM, et al. Bicuspid aortic valve associated with aortic dilatation. Arterioscler Thromb Vasc Biol 2002;23:351–356.

Pepe G, Giusti B, Atlanasio M, et al. A major involvement in the cardiovascular system in patients affected by Marfan syndrome: novel mutations in fibrillin 1 gene. J Mol Cell Cardiol 1997;29:1877–1884.

Pereira L, Andrikopoulds K, Tian J, et al. Targetting of the gene encoding fibrillin-1 recapitulates the vascular aspect of Marfan syndrome. Nat Genet 1997;17:218–222.

Pereira L, Lee SY, Gayraud B, et al. Pathogenetic sequence for aneurysm revealed in mice underexpressing fibrillin-1. Proc Natl Acad Sci USA 1999;96:3819–3823.

Pyeritz RE. The Marfan syndrome. Annu Rev Med 2000;51:481–510.

Pyo R, Lee JK, Shipley M, et al. Targeted gene disruption of metalloproteinase-9 suppresses development of experimental abdominal aortic aneurysms. J Clin Invest 2000;105:1641–1649.

Reinhardt DP, Ono RN, Notbohm H, Muller PK, Bachinger HP, Sakai LY. Mutations in calcium-binding epidermal growth factor modules render fibrillin-1 susceptible to proteolysis: a potential disease causing mechanism in Marfan syndrome. J Biol Chem 2000;275: 12,339–12,345.

Robinson PN, Booms P. The molecular pathogenesis of the Marfan syndrome. Cell Mol Life Sci 2001;58:1698–1707.

Robinson PN, Booms P, Katzke S, et al. Mutations of FBN1 and genotype-phenotype correlations in Marfan syndrome and related fibrillinopathies. Hum Mutat 2002;20:153–161.

Saito S, Zempo N, Yamashita A, Takenaka H, Fujioka K, Esato K. Matrix metalloproteinase expressions in arteriosclerotic aneurysmal disease. Vasc Endovascular Surg 2002;36(1):1–7.

Shah PK. Inflammation, metalloproteinases, and increased proteolysis: an emerging pathophysiological paradigm in aortic aneurysm. Circulation 1997;96:2115–2117.

Thompson RW, Holmes DR, Mertens RA, et al. Production and localization of 92-kilodalton gelatinase in abdominal aortic aneurysms: an elastolytic metalloproteinase expressed by aneurysm-infiltrating macrophages. J Clin Invest 1995;96:318–326.

Vaughan CJ, Casey M, He J, et al. Identification of a chromosome 11q23.2-q24 locus for familial aortic aneurysm disease, a genetically heterogeneous disorder. Circulation 2001;103:2469–2475.

14 Atherosclerotic Coronary Disease

ROBERT E. GERSZTEN AND ANTHONY ROSENZWEIG

SUMMARY

Atherosclerotic coronary artery disease is a complex biological process resulting in narrowing of the arterial vessels that supply the heart muscle with oxygen and nutrients. Despite major advances in the understanding of this process and its clinical management, it remains a major cause of morbidity and mortality throughout the world. In the United States, coronary artery disease accounts for about 500,000 deaths each year, of which about half are sudden. This chapter reviews the clinical presentation and treatment of this condition, focusing on advances and the biological insights they provide. Some of the leading hypotheses regarding the molecular mechanisms underlying this incompletely understood condition are considered.

Key Words: Angina; atherosclerosis; coronary artery disease; endothelial cells; genetic models; infarction; inflammation; ischemia; lipids; platelets; reperfusion; smooth muscle cells.

DEFINITION OF TERMS

The major complication of coronary artery disease (CAD) is myocardial injury and dysfunction from inadequate delivery of essential nutrients. Coronary obstruction can be severe before it limits blood flow, particularly under resting conditions, and thus this process can develop over years while remaining clinically silent. Inadequate blood flow that does not produce permanent myocardial cell damage is termed myocardial ischemia. Reduction or obstruction in flow sufficient in severity and duration to cause irreversible, clinically detectable myocardial damage is termed myocardial infarction (MI). Improved biochemical markers of myocyte injury with greater sensitivity and specificity (such as cardiac troponin isoforms) have made the detection of small amounts of myocardial injury feasible in a clinical setting. Detection of these markers identifies a subset of patients at higher risk for subsequent complications and increases the number of patients with diagnosable infarction who would previously have been considered to have suffered "only" an episode of ischemia. The clinical and biological spectrum from mild ischemia to substantial infarction appears to be a continuum rather than distinct categories.

The clinical symptoms associated with myocardial ischemia are termed angina pectoris. Many patients with coronary disease experience exertional symptoms in a consistent and predictable pattern termed chronic stable angina. A marked acceleration in the frequency, severity, or duration of angina, or a significant decrease in the level of exertion inducing angina, constitutes unstable angina and carries a substantial risk of progression to MI. Together unstable angina and MI comprise the acute or unstable coronary syndromes. The biological basis for the transition from no or chronic stable angina to an unstable coronary syndrome is the subject of intense investigation and has important clinical implications.

CLINICAL FEATURES

Elements contributing to the development of atherosclerotic lesions include genetic predisposition, elevated lipid levels, diabetes, tobacco smoking, and hypertension. Peripheral markers of inflammation such as C-reactive protein may provide independently informative risk stratification. Many of these clinical risk factors generally fit well with the prevailing inflammatory hypothesis of atherogenesis discussed next. However, a precise and comprehensive understanding of the pathophysiological mechanisms responsible remains elusive. Moreover, known factors do not fully account for individual or heritable risk of developing CAD.

Nevertheless, efforts to mitigate these now-established risk factors in combination with improvement in medical and surgical management have led to a significant decline in age-adjusted mortality rates for patients with cardiovascular disease over the past several decades. One of the major advances in management of MI has been the recognition of the importance of rapidly restoring reperfusion to the affected myocardium. The rapidity of reperfusion appears critical whether achieved through thrombolysis or catheter-based intervention. Though studies suggest a clinical advantage to the latter approach, logistical considerations and the availability of experienced interventionalists may sway the decision toward the former. Yet the increase in aggressive management of coronary disease has produced valuable clinical information, and in part through this experience, theories about the pathogenesis of the atherosclerotic plaque have also evolved. For example, serial angiographic studies show that often it is not the most angiographically severe lesions that become unstable clinically. Rather, nonobstructive lesions may progress rapidly to obstruction through plaque rupture and/or thrombosis. Thus the angiographic appearance of a lesion is a poor predictor of its clinical behavior. Lessons learned from clinical trials with lipid lowering agents are consistent with these observations. Although lipid reduction only modestly improves the angiographic severity of high-grade atherosclerotic lesions, it substantially reduces the risk of acute coronary events such as unstable angina or MI. In this sense, CAD is not simply a mechanical problem of luminal obstruction but also

From: *Principles of Molecular Medicine, Second Edition*
Edited by: M. S. Runge and C. Patterson © Humana Press, Inc., Totowa, NJ

a biological process, which increases the challenges and opportunities of managing such patients.

DIAGNOSIS AND MANAGEMENT

STABLE CORONARY DISEASE   The chest discomfort associated with ischemia is termed angina and is classically described as a substernal chest pressure brought on by exertion and relieved by rest. Radiation of this discomfort (to the arm or jaw) and associated symptoms such as dyspnea or diaphoresis are common. Other precipitants include emotional stress, cold weather, or even large meals. Comorbid diseases such as anemia, thyrotoxicosis, or infection should be considered as possible contributors. Angina most frequently results from epicardial coronary stenoses that impair coronary flow reserve. As it is decreased, stress-induced myocardial ischemia typically results in anginal chest discomfort. Angina often correlates with coronary stenoses of 70% of the luminal cross-section, whereas rest angina usually does not develop until stenoses are greater than 90%. Many patients with CAD have documented episodes of ischemia in the absence of anginal symptoms. The full implications and management of silent ischemia remain controversial.

Although the physical examination provides important insights into the status of the patient's cardiovascular system and general health, it can neither establish nor refute a diagnosis of CAD or angina. Further evaluation is useful for diagnosis in patients with suspected CAD and for prognosis in patients with known CAD. As with all clinical testing, a positive or negative result must be interpreted in the context of the prior probability that a diagnosis such as ischemic heart disease exists in the patient or population under study. Further testing is most useful when clinical evaluation places the prior probability of CAD in an intermediate level. If the prior probability of disease is extremely low, a positive test is most likely to be a false-positive and may precipitate a cascade of expensive, otherwise unnecessary and potentially harmful invasive testing. Conversely, if the prior probability is extremely high, a negative test is likely falsely negative and a positive test contributes little to the diagnosis. However, testing can be useful in patients with an intermediate probability of CAD, because a positive test may appropriately tip the balance toward invasive evaluation whereas a negative test may lower the likelihood of CAD sufficiently to obviate the associated risks. In patients with known CAD, exercise testing can provide a useful functional assessment and prognostic information.

Evocative testing is necessary because ischemia connotes a relative deficiency of blood flow that is usually not apparent at rest until stenoses become severe. In general, provocative approaches include exercise and pharmacological manipulations such as IV adenosine, dipyridamole, or dobutamine. The pharmacological approaches do not provide as much functional information as exercise-testing and generally should be reserved for patients who cannot exercise adequately. Clinical status (symptoms, blood pressure, and ECG) is monitored but is generally a more reliable indicator of ischemia with exercise than pharmacologic testing. Noninvasive assessment of myocardial perfusion is most commonly accomplished with radionuclide scintigraphy following the intravenous administration of a radioisotope such as thallium-201 or Technetium-99m. Such radionuclide scintigraphy improves the sensitivity and specificity of evocative testing. In addition, these techniques often allow differentiation between ischemic and infarcted zones. In the former, isotope uptake is reduced during initial stress but normalizes over time with isotope redistribution

(thallium) or reinjection (technetium). In contrast, in infarcted tissues, uptake is persistently diminished. Information about coronary flow can also be inferred from dynamic changes in systolic wall movement and thickening most commonly assessed by echocardiography. The sensitivity and specificity of stress echocardiography are similar to that of thallium stress testing. These imaging modalities increase the sensitivity, specificity and expense of evocative testing.

UNSTABLE CORONARY SYNDROMES   The hallmark of unstable coronary syndromes is rapidly progressive substernal chest pressure, often radiating to the jaw or left arm. The initial presentation, however, may be symptoms at rest. The discomfort of acute MI is qualitatively similar, though often more severe and prolonged. It is acute in onset and often associated with diaphoresis, dyspnea, and an impending sense of doom. Elderly and diabetic patients often have less typical symptoms. Underlying illnesses such as anemia or infection may precipitate the presentation of CAD. Acute infarction occurs in a minority of patients presenting with chest pain of presumed cardiac origin. Chest discomfort described as "pressure" or "burning" is most associated with acute infarction. Positional or pleuritic pain should prompt consideration of other etiologies. It should be noted that approx 25% of MIs are silent and associated with no or only mild and atypical symptoms. The prognosis of such silent infarctions appears similar to that of more classic presentations.

PHYSICAL EXAMINATION   Physical examination neither establishes nor excludes the diagnosis of acute MI or unstable angina. It does, however, provide critical clinical information of practical importance in patient management. Evaluation of the vital signs is particularly important in patients with chest pain. The heart rate is usually normal or slightly elevated, though infarctions involving the diaphragmatic portion of the heart are often accompanied by bradycardia and nausea. An irregular rhythm should raise the suspicion of ventricular ectopy or atrial fibrillation. Hypotension in the setting of chest pain may be secondary to pump failure and is a particularly ominous finding. Mild hypertension is more commonly found with acute onset of symptoms. Tachypnea may be secondary to evolving congestive heart failure.

The jugular venous pulsation is usually normal. An elevated measurement may denote chronically elevated right-sided filling pressures but should raise the possibility of right ventricular involvement. The diagnosis of right ventricular infarction may also be suggested by a paradoxical rise in venous pressure with inspiration, known as Kussmaul's sign.

Evaluation of the arterial pulse amplitude and duration provides important clues to possible valvular disease or associated noncoronary arterial disease. The pulse contour also reflects the patient's cardiac output. This evaluation may be confounded in elderly patients by noncompliant arteries in which the pulse amplitude may appear normal despite a significantly reduced cardiac output. The status of peripheral arteries and the quality of the lower extremity veins should be carefully assessed before consideration of interventions such as cardiac catheterization, angioplasty, intra-aortic balloon counterpulsation or bypass surgery.

The possible auscultatory findings in atherosclerotic heart disease are protean. An S4 heart sound is common. A third heart sound, however, reflects significant systolic impairment. Cardiac murmurs may be fixed or transient, emphasizing the importance of serial examination. Both stable and unstable symptoms may be precipitated or exacerbated by underlying valvular heart disease such as aortic stenosis. The murmur of papillary muscle dysfunction is often transient whereas mechanical complications such as ventricular septal defect may not occur until days into the hospital stay. A pericardial friction rub often occurs several days after infarction. Evaluation of the lungs centers on the presence of rales consistent with congestive heart failure. In the acute coronary syndromes (ACSs), pulmonary rales coupled with an S3 gallop is a poor prognostic sign.

LABORATORY EVALUATION   The classic ECG pattern of acute MI includes ST segment elevation in multiple leads reflecting a coronary distribution, followed by evolution of T-wave inversion and significant Q waves in these same leads, reflecting a Q-wave MI. However, patients with infarction can also present with ST segment depression or T-wave inversion alone without evolution of Q waves, termed non-Q wave-MI. The correlation of these ECG findings with pathological findings of transmural or subendocardial infarction is sufficiently imprecise to favor exclusive use of the ECG descriptors in clinical practice.

Serological markers of myocardial necrosis remain the cornerstone in establishing the diagnosis of MI. The serum creatine kinase (CK) and its myocardial-specific isozyme, CK-MB, are widely used. However, as previously noted, cardiac troponin isoforms have improved sensitivity and specificity compared with CK, and generally become abnormal by 6 h after injury facilitating more rapid risk stratification. The degree of elevation in all these markers correlates approximately with the amount of myocardium damaged but is influenced by other factors. Elevated levels of serum transaminase and lactate dehydrogenase with isoform reversal occur later after infarction. Measurement of these levels generally adds little to clinical management and should not be routinely employed in evaluation of acute chest pain. Panels of markers reflecting myocyte necrosis (Troponin), neurohormonal activation (brain natriuretic peptide), and inflammation (CRP) are being evaluated to see if together they provide more precise prognostic information.

MANAGEMENT   In approaching an individual patient, several goals must be considered simultaneously: prevention of disease progression, control of symptoms, and optimizing prognosis. Available tools include patient education and risk factor modification, pharmacological therapy, and mechanical interventions including surgical and catheter-based approaches. All these considerations must be integrated into a coherent clinical approach, which in practice is often influenced dramatically by the acuity of the patient's clinical presentation.

Patient education and behavior modification form the cornerstone of primary and secondary prevention. Aggressive risk factor modification, particularly reduction in serum lipids, can have a dramatic clinical impact even within a few years in populations with documented CAD. Randomized trials have documented angiographic regression of plaques, establishing that regression is possible in principle. However, even more intriguing is the observation that although the degree of regression has been modest, the improvement in clinical end points has been more dramatic. Reduction in serum lipids appears to have clinical benefits, which are only imperfectly reflected in the angiographic appearance of lesions. These clinical benefits can be realized during a relatively brief (2–3 yr) period of treatment, which underscores the importance of secondary prevention efforts. Although lifestyle modifications are emphasized as the first step in this process, it is often necessary to move to pharmacological lipid lowering therapies. The particular agent(s) employed is determined by the specifics of the patient's lipid profile.

Other therapies of proven clinical benefit in patients who have a history of MI include aspirin, β-blockade, and angiotensin-converting enzyme inhibitors, particularly in patients with a reduced left ventricular ejection fraction. These agents reduce the incidence of clinical cardiovascular events and mortality. For this reason, they should be considered in all patients after MI, even if they are asymptomatic. Medications that may be useful in the long-term treatment of coronary patients but have not been demonstrated to improve prognosis include calcium channel blockers and nitrates. In fact, in the setting of non-Q-wave infarction, the calcium channel blocker diltiazem had a deleterious effect on 1-yr survival in patients manifesting congestive heart failure during the initial hospitalization. These medications may help control anginal symptoms, hypertension, or arrhythmias, but should not be routinely prescribed independent of a specific indication because of the lack of proven outcome benefit.

Therapy for chronic stable angina includes pharmacological and mechanical interventions. The three classes of pharmacological agents primarily employed are β-blockers, calcium channel blockers, and nitrates. As noted, only the first has documented survival benefit in postinfarction patients but all three have been demonstrated to improve exercise tolerance and can reduce ischemic symptoms, both valid goals. Mechanical interventions encompass a variety of catheter-based approaches such as percutaneous transluminal angioplasty as well as coronary artery bypass surgery graft (CABG). CABG provides a survival benefit over medical therapy alone in patients with significant left main coronary disease or severe three-vessel coronary disease (particularly in the setting of compromised left ventricular function). In patients with one- or two-vessel coronary disease and mild symptoms, CABG does not confer a survival benefit. However, surgery eliminates or reduces anginal symptoms more effectively than medical therapy alone. Catheter-based interventions are also highly effective at reducing ischemic symptoms but have generally not been demonstrated to improve survival. Percutaneous coronary interventions (PCIs) have historically been plagued by a significant rate of restenosis. The advent of mechanical support (stents) has significantly reduced this rate. The development of stents that simultaneously mediate local release of pharmacological agents has had an even more dramatic reduction in restenosis. Although the indications for such interventions are undergoing evaluation, it is likely the number of such procedures will continue to grow.

Basic science findings have best been translated into therapy in relationship to platelet biology and evolving therapies for patients presenting with ACSs. In particular, efforts have centered on the abrogation of signaling triggered by the two major platelet agonists, adenosine diphosphate (ADP) and thrombin. Heparin, an indirect thrombin antagonist, works via activation of antithrombin 3, and is a mainstay of the medical regimen of all patients with ACSs. Comparative trials of the more specific low-molecular-weight heparin have demonstrated its superiority over unfractionated heparin in reducing cardiac events in ACS. Two direct thrombin inhibitors, hirudin, and bivalirudin, show trends toward benefit over heparin therapy alone in patients with ACS. The direct thrombin antagonist bivalirudin has also shown promise as an adjunctive therapy in patients undergoing percutaneous revascularization. However, owing to tremendous cost differences between low-molecular-weight heparin and direct thrombin inhibitors vs unfractionated heparin, these newer therapies have not gained widespread acceptance. Direct thrombin inhibitors are commonly used, though for anticoagulation of patients with heparin induced thrombocytopenia, a growing problem worldwide.

ADP receptor antagonists have become a mainstay of therapies for ACS and PCI. Clopidogrel in combination with aspirin confers a 20% reduction in cardiovascular death, MI or stroke compared with aspirin alone in both low- and high-risk patients with ACS. The benefit of treatment before PCI has also been seen with greater than 30% reduction in events even at 1 yr. Ongoing studies are also evaluating ADP receptor antagonism in primary prevention.

New strategies for profound inhibition of platelet activity at the injured coronary plaque have also focused on blockade of the platelet surface membrane glycoprotein IIbIIIa receptor, which binds circulating fibrinogen or von Willebrand factor and crosslinks platelets as the final common pathway to aggregation. Four agents directed against this receptor include chimeric monoclonal antibody fragments, peptide inhibitors, and nonpeptide mimetics. Multiple large scale placebo-controlled trials have evaluated approx 50,000 patients. Patients undergoing percutaneous interventions and high-risk patients with ACS appear to derive the greatest benefits. Benefits have been relatively uniform between the various classes of inhibition. Monoclonal antibody fragments may be most efficacious, potentially via their dual effects on platelet integins and the vitronectin receptor on the disrupted endothelium. Efforts to generate oral IIbIIIa antagonists for chronic therapeutic intervention have been unsuccessful likely because of partial agonist effects.

In acute MI, the immediate goal is restoration of adequate coronary flow as quickly as possible to minimize or avoid irreversible myocardial damage. Two general approaches are widely employed to achieve this goal: primary angioplasty and thrombolytic therapy. Additional clinical benefit exists from primary angioplasty if it can be accomplished quickly by experienced interventionalists. However, in many communities this is not practical and immediate administration of thrombolytic agents may be preferable. One study suggested that the benefits of angioplasty outweighed the potential disadvantages of the delays inherent in transferring patients to specialized centers, at least in some settings. Whether this approach is further validated and becomes generally accepted remains to be seen. Thrombolytic agents have not been beneficial in the treatment of unstable angina. However, therapy with heparin and aspirin—alone and in combination—reduces the rate of progression to frank infarction. Patients with unstable symptoms that cannot be controlled by heparin/aspirin and maximal anti-ischemic therapy should undergo early catheterization to define possible options for immediate mechanical intervention. The platelet glycoprotein IIb/IIIa receptor is a pivotal mediator of platelet aggregation as noted earlier. Platelet adhesion, the first step in the process of hemostasis, can be triggered by endothelial dysfunction or injury, resulting in interaction of platelets with the subendothelial matrix. Adhesion molecules of the vessel wall, along with clotting proteins such as fibrinogen, interact with platelet-membrane glycoproteins—of which integrins such as IIb/IIIa play a key role. Although some combination of these approaches appears likely to optimize early reperfusion, additional efforts are directed at determining whether adjunctive therapies can maximize myocardial salvage after reperfusion and lead to additional therapeutic benefit. Animal studies suggest this is, in principle, possible but these concepts have not been validated clinically.

GENETIC BASIS OF DISEASE

Atherosclerosis is a complex phenotype, which most commonly appears modulated by interactions between environmental factors and multiple genetic loci, only some of which have been

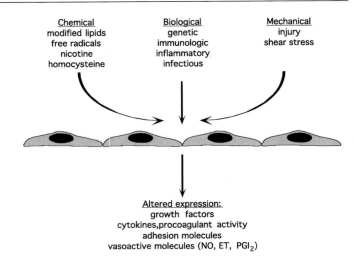

Figure 14-1   The central role of vascular endothelium. Many different stimuli may induce a similar repertoire of dysfunctional endothelial responses that ultimately contribute to clinical atherosclerosis. The endothelium provides a potential pathophysiologic link between well-established clinical risks factors such as hypercholesterolemia, cigarette smoking, or hypertension, and atherogenesis. The role of the endothelial effects of other agents such as homocysteine or viral infection as well as inflammatory cascades, remains more controversial. ET, endothelin-1; NO, nitric oxide; PGI$_2$, prostaglandin I$_2$.

identified. Genetic dyslipoproteinemias can substantially accelerate disease progression. Assessment of serum lipid levels should be included in the evaluation of all patients with CAD, thereby providing an initial screen for genetic dyslipoproteinemias as well. Similarly, understanding the genetic bases for other recognized clinical risk factors such as diabetes mellitus or hypertension has an important impact on the development and progression of CAD. Some studies have suggested an association between the deletional allele of the angiotensin converting enzyme gene and the risk of MI. However, this was not confirmed in a prospective study of a large cohort of US physicians. Elevated serum levels of homocysteine can result from genetic defects in specific metabolic enzymes and is independently associated with ischemic heart disease. The epidemiological relationship of CAD and markers of thrombosis such as fibrinogen levels are also being investigated. However, the genetic basis of most ischemic heart disease remains elusive. In part, this reflects the nature of most CAD seen clinically as a polygenic, quantitative trait. Experimental and statistical approaches to analysis of such traits have been developed and are being applied to a variety of CAD phenotypes. Ultimately, it is hoped that this approach can identify patients at risk, the likelihood of favorable responses to specific therapies, and unanticipated genes involved in disease pathogenesis. Although this represents an exciting approach to an important clinical problem, the impact of such approaches on clinical management remains to be validated. The conceptual and practical issues associated with such studies are addressed elsewhere in this text.

PATHOPHYSIOLOGY

MOLECULAR PATHOPHYSIOLOGY   Hypotheses concerning the molecular pathogenesis of ischemic heart disease seek to explain two related but distinct phenomena: the gradual development of obstructive atherosclerotic lesions responsible for stable angina and the rapid progression of these lesions to the ACSs.

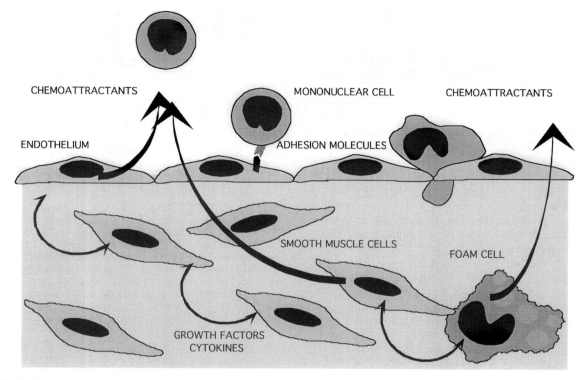

Figure 14-2 Leukocyte interactions with the vessel wall. An activated or dysfunctional endothelium may initiate a cascade of events that augment atherogenesis, including the recruitment of leukocytes through endothelial expression of cytokines and adhesion molecules, as well as alterations in smooth muscle cell function mediated by growth factors, cytokines, and vasoactive substances (indicated by arrows). Mononuclear cells and the foam cells they give rise to, as well as vascular smooth muscle cells, can also release growth factors and cytokines that further perpetuate this cycle.

It was first proposed that atherosclerotic lesions develop as a "response to injury" of the vascular endothelium, and much of the view of atherogenesis arises from these concepts. Subsequently this model has been modified to suggest that atherogenesis may begin with endothelial activation or dysfunction rather than actual injury or loss of the endothelium. Indeed, endothelial dysfunction may represent a common response to a wide variety of clinically relevant factors (Fig. 14-1), and the endothelium may represent a critical interface integrating these stimuli and modulating the behavior of circulating leukocytes and subintimal constituents of the vessel wall, such as smooth muscle cells (SMCs, Fig. 14-2). Activation of vascular endothelium may initiate a cascade of events leading to mononuclear leukocyte recruitment into the vessel wall with subsequent release of cytokines and growth factors contributing to SMC migration and proliferation, as well as abnormalities of extracellular matrix formation. Although this model is intuitively appealing and supported by a wealth of correlative studies, the precise molecular mechanisms involved in vivo are only incompletely understood. Even less well delineated are the mechanisms underlying the abrupt clinical change from stable angina (or no symptoms at all) to the unstable coronary syndromes. The anatomic correlate of this clinical transformation appears to be acute plaque rupture. Exposure of the atherosclerotic fatty core to the blood likely serves as a substrate for the propagation of clot and inflammation. Consistent with this model, pathological studies have emphasized the importance of a central lipid core in the process of plaque fissuring and confirmed the role of thrombosis in unstable angina and MI.

MURINE MODELS OF ATHEROSCLEROSIS   The understanding of atherogenesis and the ability to deduce causal relationships has been substantially advanced by the use of inbred murine models. Although most wild-type mouse strains appear resistant to atherosclerosis, certain strains—such as C57BL/6—develop lesions when placed on a high-cholesterol diet (often in combination with cholic acid). Studies in these mice have explored the role of specific mediators in atherogenesis and the genetic differences between atherogenesis-prone and resistant strains. However, lesions in this model do not progress beyond "fatty streaks." The advent of genetically manipulated murine models that recapitulate more of the morphological features of seen in advanced human atheroma has considerably enhanced such investigation.

The two most widely studied murine models of atherosclerosis are ApoE deficient (ApoE$^{-/-}$) and low-density lipoprotein receptor deficient (LDLR$^{-/-}$) mice. ApoE$^{-/-}$ mice fed a "Western" diet (21% fat by weight/40% by calories, 1.25% cholesterol) develop marked hyperlipidemia most consistent with Type III hyperlipidemia (rare in humans). On a standard chow diet, ApoE$^{-/-}$ mice develop fatty streaks lesions after approx 10 wk and these lesions progress, although the process is substantially accelerated on a Western diet. The complex plaques seen in this model are reminiscent of the human disease, although thrombosis is not generally described. LDLR$^{-/-}$ were initially developed as a model of familial hypercholesterolemia. In contrast to ApoE$^{-/-}$ mice, LDLR$^{-/-}$ mice do not develop significant atherosclerotic lesions on a normal chow diet, thus facilitating kinetic studies of atherogenesis. However, complex lesions are less common in LDLR$^{-/-}$ mice fed a Western diet and some investigators use supplemental, dietary cholic acid, which may have confounding pro-inflammatory effects. Both ApoE$^{-/-}$ and LDLR$^{-/-}$ models of atherosclerosis have been extensively characterized and although each has its potential advantages and advocates, results in both models have generally been concordant. Other models (e.g., transgenic overexpression of apoB100) provide important insights into the role of specific lipoproteins but have been less extensively characterized. In virtually all models of atherosclerosis, atheroma develops, preferentially in specific regions marked by disturbed flow and increased expression of pro-inflammatory endothelial cell effectors. In mice, these regions exhibit enhanced expression and increased activation of the family of transcription factors, nuclear factor-κB (NF-κB), which act as key regulators of the expression of genes modulating inflammation and survival.

The development of these models has enabled investigators to exploit the power of murine germline genetics to analyze the role of specific modifier loci as well as putative effectors in atherogenesis. By breeding atherogenic murine lines (e.g., ApoE$^{-/-}$ and LDLR$^{-/-}$) to different in-bred genetic backgrounds or mice engineered to lack or overexpress specific candidates, many useful insights into the role of these pathways in atherogenesis have been generated. However, these models do not generally recapitulate the biology of plaque rupture associated with unstable human lesions. A tacit hypothesis underlying much work in this field is that interventions that mitigate the overall burden of atherosclerosis also favorably modify the tendency to plaque rupture. This has been true clinically with some therapies such as statin treatment, which improve serum lipid profiles, inhibit lesion progression, and even more dramatically reduce the rate of unstable coronary syndromes. Nevertheless, the development of animal models that accurately reflect these processes—particularly in species amenable to genetic analysis—would further facilitate investigation into the biology of the unstable plaque and the events leading to ACSs.

ROLE OF LIPIDS   Autopsy studies have shown that fatty streaks frequently exist in the coronary arteries and aortae of teenagers. These lesions may constitute the earliest recognizable precursor of atherosclerotic plaques, although it is formally possible that they either do not progress or actually regress with time. The major lipid component of these lesions is oxidized LDL. In vitro experiments have shown that oxidized LDL stimulates the adherence of monocytes to vascular endothelium most likely through increased expression of endothelial adhesion molecules. Oxidized LDL also stimulates transcription and secretion of monocyte chemotactic protein (MCP)-1 by human aortic and SMCs in vitro. MCP-1 is a powerful chemoattractant for monocytes and memory T cells in vitro, which are the predominant leukocyte populations in atherosclerotic lesions. Lysophosphatidylcholine, which constitutes a significant fraction of oxidized LDL, is a chemoattractant for monocytes and also induces expression of the endothelial adhesion molecules vascular cell adhesion molecule (VCAM)-1 and intercellular adhesion molecule (ICAM)-1. In addition, oxidized LDL can stimulate platelet aggregation and promote procoagulant activity on the surface of macrophages by an increase in tissue thromboplastin activity and by stimulating the expression and secretion of tissue factor by monocytes or aortic endothelial cells. Finally, oxidized LDL may also contribute to the vasomotor dysfunction that can promote or exacerbate the atherosclerotic lesion. Therefore, in many patients with atherosclerosis, lipids (particularly oxidized lipids) likely constitute an early and persistent precipitant of endothelial activation and dysfunction.

SMOOTH MUSCLE CELLS   Abnormal growth of vascular SMCs is prominent in atherosclerosis. At least two phenotypes of the SMCs make up the vascular wall, based on examination of myosin filaments and details of the secretory protein apparatus. When cells are in a contractile phenotype, they respond to elements that promote vasoconstriction or vasodilation such as

Table 14-1
Cellular and Molecular Mediators of Atherosclerosis

Factor	Source	Target
Growth factors		
PDGF	EC, WBC	SMC
bFGF	EC, SMC, WBC	EC, SMC
M-CSF	EC	WBC
VEGF	SMC	
Cytokines		
IL-1	EC, SMC, WBC	EC, WBC, SMC
TNF-α	EC, SMC, WBC	EC, WBC, SMC
IFN-γ	WBC	EC, WBC, SMC
Chemokines (MCP-1)	EC, SMC, WBC	WBC
Vasoactive substances		
Nitric oxide	EC	SMC, WBC
Endothelin	EC	SMC
Prostaglandin	EC	SMC

bFGF, basic fibroblast growth factor; EC, endothelial cell; IFN, interferon; IL, interleukin; MCP, monocyte chemotactic protein; M-CSF, monocyte-colony stimulating factor; PDGF, platelet-derived growth factor; SMC, smooth muscle cells; TNF, tumor necrosis factor; VEGF, vascular and endothelial growth factor; WBC, white blood cells.

endothelin, angiotensin II, prostaglandin I2, or nitric oxide. A second synthetic phenotype has also been identified. In this state, SMC synthesize numerous growth factors and their receptors, cytokines, as well as matrix proteins. Multiple factors may be able to stimulate SMC proliferation and migration from the vessel media, through the internal elastic membrane. These activated SMCs, in turn, release substances that act in complex paracrine and autocrine manners, involving vascular endothelial and SMCs, as well as blood-borne elements such as white cells and platelets (Table 14-1 and Fig. 14-2). A particularly dramatic example of this process occurs after mechanical injury of the vessel during angioplasty, but a similar process may contribute to atherogenesis. A central issue in the investigation of atherogenesis is to define the source(s) of the critical factors that initiate and perpetuate the shift in SMC phenotype. Of note, a substantial advance in the management of CAD has been the development of coronary artery stents that release pharmacological agents, providing mechanical support and a local biological intervention, termed drug-eluting stents. Drug-eluting stents appear to dramatically reduce the rate of restenosis after coronary interventions. One of the preliminary successes of this approach has utilized stents that release rapamycin, an inhibitor of the signaling molecule mammalian target of rapamycin (mTOR). mTOR plays an important role transducing signals to growth and proliferation pathways in a wide variety of cell types, including SMCs. However, whether inhibition of mTOR and/or modulation of these signaling pathways underlies the clinical success seen with rapamycin eluting stents has not been demonstrated.

LEUKOCYTES   Because of their early and consistent association with atherosclerotic lesions, mononuclear cells appear to be central to atherogenesis. The mononuclear cells in atherosclerotic lesions are predominantly monocytes and lymphocytes of the memory T-cell phenotype (CD45 RO$^+$). Monocyte-derived foam cells are a major component of atheroma, comprising up to 60% of cells found in the necrotic lipid core, and 10–20% of cells in the fibrous cap. Recruitment of monocytes by activated endothelium marks an early event in atherosclerotic lesion formation. Mononuclear cells serve as the progenitors of foam cells and a

Lipoprotein	Density (g/mL)	Sources
Chylomicrons	< 0.98	Intestine
VLDL (Very Low-Density Lipoprotein)	0.98-1.006	Liver
IDL (Intermediate-Density Lipoprotein)	1.006-1.019	Catabolism of VLDL
LDL (Low-Density Lipoprotein)	1.019-1.063	Catabolism of IDL
HDL (High-Density Lipoprotein)	1.063-1.21	Liver, intestine, other

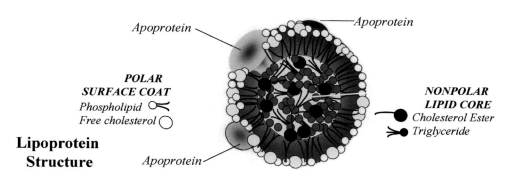

Figure 15-1 Lipoprotein classification and structure. Plasma lipoproteins can be divided into five density classes. The lightest density (chylmicrons and VLDL) are the most triglyceride-rich. LDL and HDL are cholesterol-rich. The general structure of a lipoprotein is shown in the lower half of the figure. More hydrophobic lipids are packaged on the inside of the lipoprotein whereas more polar lipids and the protein constituents are on the outside, where they can interact with the aqueous environments of blood and interstitial fluid.

hydrolyzed. After removal of their triglyceride, VLDL remnants (called IDL) can be further metabolized to LDL. VLDL serve as acceptors of cholesterol transferred from HDL, accounting in part for the inverse relation between HDL cholesterol and VLDL triglyceride. This transfer process is mediated by an enzyme called cholesterol ester transfer protein.

LOW-DENSITY LIPOPROTEINS   LDL are the major carriers of cholesterol in humans, responsible for supplying cholesterol to tissues with the highest sterol demands. LDL are also the lipoproteins most clearly implicated in causing atherogenic plaque formation. Circulating LDL levels can be increased in persons who consume large amounts of saturated fat and/or cholesterol. LDL levels are also elevated in those who have genetic defects that affect LDL receptor function (familial hypercholesterolemia [FH] and autosomal-recessive hypercholesterolemia [ARH]), the structure of LDL's apoprotein, apolipoprotein B-100 or who have polygenic disorders affecting LDL metabolism. When serum LDL exceed a threshold concentration, they traverse the endothelial wall and can become trapped in the arterial intima, where they may undergo oxidation or other biochemical modification, be taken up by macrophages, and stimulate atherogenesis. The association of total serum cholesterol with CHD is predominantly a reflection of the role of LDL.

HIGH-DENSITY LIPOPROTEINS   HDL are believed to function to protect tissues from the unwanted accumulation of cholesterol. They participate in a reverse cholesterol transport pathway in which peripheral tissues efflux cholesterol back to lipid-poor forms of HDL for return to the liver (Fig. 15-2). There, cholesterol can be secreted into the bile. The unesterified cholesterol from tissues that is transferred to HDL is esterified by the action of lecithin cholesterol acyl transferase (LCAT) and stored in the central core of HDL. This esterified cholesterol can be transferred back to lower density lipoproteins by the action of

cholesterol ester transfer protein or it may be removed at the liver by the action of a plasma membrane receptor called scavenger receptor B-1. A particularly effective reverse transport system is thought to explain, at least in part, why elevated HDL levels are associated with a reduced risk of developing CHD. Apolipoprotein (apo)-A-I is the major apoprotein of HDL, and its serum concentration also correlates inversely with the risk of CHD. Women have higher levels of HDL cholesterol than men and this may partly explain the lower incidence of CHD in premenopausal women. Exercise increases HDL levels, whereas obesity, hypertriglyceridemia, and smoking lower them.

CLINICAL FEATURES

In most individuals, alterations in serum lipoproteins produce no clinical manifestations until an atherosclerotic vascular event supervenes (e.g., a myocardial infarct, stroke, or peripheral vascular occlusion). Individuals with extremely elevated levels of serum triglycerides, because of VLDL, or chylomicron accumulation, or both, can develop pancreatitis. Such patients may first come to clinical attention because of an episode of pancreatitis or because their plasma is noted to be milky in appearance when routine blood tests are performed. Individuals with such marked triglyceride elevations (typically plasma triglyceride levels >1000 mg/dL) can also develop eruptive xanthomas, accumulations of lipid in the skin (Fig. 15-3). Individuals whose LDL levels are significantly elevated can also develop xanthomas, though these are typically located in either the Achilles tendon or extensor tendons of the hands. Individuals with accumulations of IDL can also develop xanthomas, which are classically of the tubero-eruptive or palmar type. Xanthelasmas, seen in individuals with elevated serum cholesterol levels, can often be detected in older individuals whose lipid levels are not dramatically increased. Individuals with some of the rare HDL disorders can

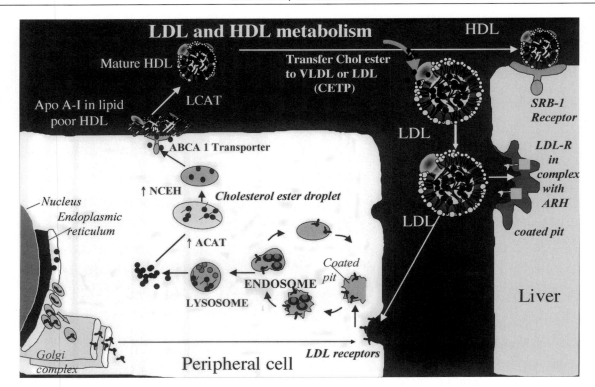

Figure 15-2 LDL and HDL metabolism. A schematized model of HDL and LDL metabolism. Cholesterol in a peripheral tissue cell, such as a macrophage, is initially stored in the cell as cholesterol ester. When stimulated by a lipid-poor HDL apoprotein A-I, the cell hydrolyzes the fatty acid from the cholesterol ester and the unesterified cholesterol is transported to the cell membrane. The action of the ABCA1 transporter results in the transfer of the free cholesterol to the apoprotein. Once bound to the apoprotein, the cholesterol is re-esterified by the action of LCAT creating the spherical HDL lipoprotein via storage of cholesterol ester in the core of the lipoprotein. HDL can then either donate this lipid back to LDL particles it encounters in the blood or travel to the liver in which its cholesterol ester content can be selectively removed by the action of scavenger receptor B-1. The cholesterol can be stored in the liver, reused for new lipoprotein synthesis, or excreted in the bile. Cholesterol that is transferred to LDL can be sent back to the periphery or the liver, in which LDL receptors bind and endocytose the particle. The action of the ARH gene product is important for LDL receptor activity in the liver. LDL originally derived from VLDL is secreted by the liver in a process not depicted in this slide.

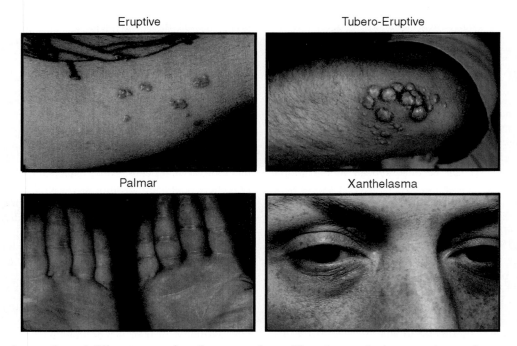

Figure 15-3 Xanthomas. Several different types of xanthomas are shown. The palmar and tubero-eruptive xanthomas are classically seen in patients with increased concentrations of IDL whereas the eruptive xanthomas are typically found in patients with massive serum triglyceride elevations resulting from excess chylomicrons and/or VLDL. (Please *see* color insert.)

present with corneal opacities, tendon xanthomas (deposits typically embedded in extensor tendons), or a peripheral neuropathy. Rarely, a lipid abnormality may be detected because of abnormal liver function tests caused by steatosis of the liver or by lipid accumulation in the eye (corneal arcus). With regular measurement of lipids in adults, standard practice in the United States, lipid disorders are most commonly detected by routine laboratory screening tests.

DIAGNOSIS

The diagnosis of a lipid disorder should be based on more than one measurement of serum lipids, because combined analytic and biologic variations in serum lipids range from 10 to 20%. The technology for measuring LDL levels directly has improved steadily, but in most laboratories, it remains a calculated value. To perform this calculation, the total and HDL cholesterol levels as well as the triglyceride value are measured. The LDL cholesterol concentration is then estimated using the following formula:

$$\text{LDL cholesterol} = \text{total cholesterol} - [\text{HDL cholesterol} + \text{triglyceride}/5]$$

The triglyceride/5 factor represents an estimate of VLDL cholesterol. The validity of this formula for estimating LDL cholesterol has been confirmed by ultracentrifugal measurement of lipoprotein levels and remains reasonably accurate as long as the total triglyceride is less than 400 mg/dL. To obtain an accurate calculation, patients must fast for at least 12 h to clear their blood of any chylomicrons, as these lipoproteins distort the triglyceride ratio on which the formula relies. If the triglyceride level is greater than 400 mg/dL, the LDL cholesterol must be determined by alternative methods. Apo B-100, present in both LDL and VLDL, can be measured directly to get an assessment of lower density lipoprotein particle numbers, but this is not routine in the United States. With increasing evidence for a greater atherogenicity of smaller, denser LDL particles, more sophisticated assessments of LDL number, and composition are being introduced into clinical practice in some regions of the world. Their place in the routine diagnostic evaluation of most patients remains controversial.

Before embarking on a treatment plan, conditions must be excluded that could cause hyperlipidemia secondarily. The most common clinical conditions that influence lipids levels are obesity, diabetes, and hypothyroidism. The latter two are best screened using a serum glucose (or Hgb A1-c) measurement and a thyrotropin stimulating hormone level, respectively. Many medications commonly cause a secondary hyperlipidemia, with antiretroviral therapy, estrogens, and glucocorticoids heading the list.

In the mid-1960s, a classifications scheme for lipid disorders was devised based on the phenotype of lipoprotein abnormalities. Because a better understanding of the genetics of these disorders has emerged that classification is rarely used. However, no unified classification of comparable simplicity has replaced it. Instead, the National Cholesterol Education Program (NCEP), Adult Treatment Panel III has promulgated a set of guidelines that are primarily aimed at targeting therapy in patients with elevated LDL levels or decreased HDL values. Table 15-1 summarizes the LDL-based treatment guidelines. Although the NCEP treatment targets for HDL and serum triglycerides are not as detailed as those for LDL values, HDL levels >40 mg/dL in men and 50 mg/dL in women are considered normal as is a serum triglyceride value <150 mg/dL.

Table 15-1
NCEP ATP III Treatment Guidelines

Risk factors	LDL treatment threshold	LDL treatment goal
<2 risk factors	>190	<160
>2 risk factors	>160	<130
10-yr risk <20%	10-yr risk <10% >130	
CHD or equivalent	10-yr risk 10–20% >130[a]	<100[a]
10-yr risk >20%		

[a]LDL between 100 and 129 is good, but not optimal.
LDL, low density lipoprotein; CHD, coronary heart disease.

GENETIC BASIS OF LIPID DISORDERS

Of the variety of genetic disorders of lipid metabolism, many do not primarily affect CHD risk and are not discussed here. The most important lipid disorders affecting coronary disease risk are those that increase the serum LDL level or reduce the HDL level. The most severely affected individuals often have a single gene defect responsible for their lipid disorder. Most hyperlipidemic patients, however, do not have a monogenic defect. Rather, they are most likely to have a polygenic disorder with a variable contribution from environmental factors (e.g., excessive saturated fat intake for high LDL levels; obesity or smoking for lower HDL levels). The application of the NCEP treatment guidelines does not require that a genetic diagnosis be made, as treatment is based on phenotype (lipid levels) and not genotype. Nevertheless, the identification of the causes of monogenic lipid disorders has been critical to the understanding of normal lipoprotein physiology. Several examples of monogenic LDL and HDL disorders illustrate key concepts in that understanding.

MONOGENIC LDL DISORDERS   The molecular basis of four monogenic disorders that primarily affect LDL levels has been characterized: FH, familial defective B (FDB), autosomal-recessive hypercholesterolemia (ARH) and PCSK9 mutations. As these disorders illustrate distinct mechanisms leading to elevated LDL levels, three of them will be described in greater detail.

Familial Hypercholesterolemia   FH is one of the most thoroughly studied and common genetic disorders; approx 1 in 500 individuals carry a mutation in one allele encoding the LDL receptor. These mutations results in defective clearance of LDL from the blood and a rise in serum total and LDL cholesterol levels. The elucidation of this defect and its associated cell biology led to insights into the homeostatic control of cholesterol metabolism that transformed the lipid field. Several hundred individual mutations in the LDL receptor have been identified. The gene, located on chromosome 19 and spanning 45 kb, has 18 exons that encode a mature protein of 839 amino acids. The inheritance of the disorder is autosomal-codominant. Heterozygous patients have LDL cholesterol levels in the 200–500 mg/dL range and the rare homozygous FH patient typically has an LDL cholesterol >500 mg/dL. Heterozygous patients commonly have tendon xanthomas and premature coronary artery disease, whereas these are universal in the untreated homozygous individual. Mutations in the LDL receptor have been described that affect multiple aspects of receptor biology, ranging from defective LDL binding to abnormal trafficking of the receptor to the plasma membrane. The effect of all of these mutations is to reduce LDL and IDL clearance from the blood, resulting in an enhanced conversion of IDL to LDL. The net result is markedly elevated LDL cholesterol levels in the plasma and a strong predisposition to early CHD if the disorder is not treated. FH heterozygotes typically respond well to 3-hydroxy-3-methyl-glutaryl coenzyme A (HMG CoA) reductase inhibitors (statins), though additional therapies may be needed to reach desirable LDL levels. FH homozygotes respond poorly to reductase inhibitors and inevitably develop early atherosclerotic vascular disease if LDL apheresis or liver transplantation is not performed.

Familial Defective Apo B FDB is an autosomal-codominant disorder caused by mutations near the carboxy terminus of apo B. apo B is a 4536 amino acid protein encoded by a gene on chromosome 2 that consists of 29 exons. The most commonly identified mutations in FDB affect an arginine at position 3500 that is either mutated to a glutamine or tryptophan. As most individuals with FDB are heterozygous for their mutation, and there is only one molecule of apo B per LDL particle, the LDL in the serum of these individuals is a mixture of normal LDL and FDB LDL. The LDL containing the defective apo B does not bind normally to the LDL receptor and is therefore cleared more slowly. The explanation for the lower receptor affinity of LDL carrying the FDB mutations is not known with certainty. There is evidence, however, of a molecular interaction between the arginine at 3500 and tryptophan at position 4369 that appears to be necessary for the adoption of an apo B conformation recognized by the LDL receptor. Patients with FDB have elevations in their LDL levels that fall within the range of those seen in FH heterozygotes, but the mean is generally lower than the mean in FH cohorts. There is considerable variability in both genetic populations, however, making generalizations about the diagnostic value of this measurement not very useful. Tendon xanthomas are common but not universal, and premature coronary artery disease is prevalent. Treatment with reductase inhibitors or other standard LDL lowering drugs is typically effective in FDB patients.

Autosomal-Recessive Hypercholesterolemia Studies of families in which LDL levels were inherited in an autosomal-recessive pattern led to a successful genetic linkage analysis that mapped the genetic defect in these families to the short arm of chromosome 1. Candidate gene sequencing led to the identification of mutations in a gene, designated ARH, comprising nine exons and eight introns. Patients diagnosed with ARH have been clinically similar to patients who are homozygous for LDL receptor mutations in that they have markedly elevated LDL cholesterol levels (typically >500 mg/dL), tendon xanthomas, and premature coronary atherosclerosis. The autosomal-recessive mode of inheritance is an important differentiating factor between ARH and FH, as is greater LDL receptor activity, measured in cultured fibroblasts taken from the patients. The defect in ARH patients appears to affect liver cholesterol metabolism disproportionately, and data indicate that the ARH gene product likely serves as an adaptor protein required for LDL receptor internalization via clathrin-coated pits. ARH patients do respond to HMG CoA reductase inhibitors, but this treatment is usually inadequate to control their markedly elevated LDL cholesterol levels, making them candidates for LDL apheresis.

MONOGENIC HDL DISORDERS Three distinct monogenic disorders that cause markedly reduced levels of HDL in the plasma by different mechanism are Tangier disease, LCAT deficiency, and apo A-I mutations.

Tangier Disease Tangier disease was first recognized in 1960 in a sibling pair living on Tangier Island in the Chesapeake Bay in Virginia. The dyad of enlarged, yellow-orange tonsils and little or no circulating HDL cholesterol are the classic findings. Cases have been identified in which the presenting symptom was a peripheral neuropathy. Patients may also have hepatosplenomegaly. Serum

LDL and total cholesterol levels are usually low, whereas serum triglyceride values are moderately elevated. Tangier disease is an autosomal-recessive disorder. The cause of Tangier disease was identified by several groups following mapping of the gene defect to chromosome 9. Candidate gene analysis in the appropriate genetic interval identified mutations in an ABC transporter as the cause. The transporter, called ATP binding cassette transporter A1 (ABCA1) is a full-sized ATP-binding cassette-containing protein that is predicted to span the plasma membrane 12 times (Fig. 15-4). ABCA1 is a 2261 amino acid protein encoded by a gene spanning 50 exons. Approx 50 mutations have been identified in the gene. ABCA1 mediates the efflux of cholesterol from cholesterol-enriched cells when stimulated by the major apoprotein of HDL, apo A-I (*see* Fig. 15-2). This activity is lost in Tangier patients and is reduced by approximately half in carriers of one abnormal ABCA1 allele. The mechanism of the movement of cholesterol from inside the cell to outside the cell has not been established. Individuals with Tangier disease and heterozygous carriers of ABCA1 mutations (a disorder called familial hypoalphalipoproteinemia) both appear to have increased risk of premature coronary disease. There is no specific therapy for this disorder.

Lecithin Cholesterol Acyltransferase Deficiency The esterification of free cholesterol in circulating lipoproteins is catalyzed by a plasma enzyme called LCAT. Two clinically separable syndromes result from a deficiency of LCAT. Fish eye disease is from a partial deficiency of LCAT, with patients presenting with dense corneal opacities and very low HDL cholesterol levels. Familial LCAT deficiency arises from a nearly complete absence of LCAT activity and produces a more severe syndrome characterized by corneal opacities, anemia, and proteinuric renal failure. The serum lipid and lipoprotein profile in the more severe disorder is characterized by normal or increased triglyceride levels, reduced LDL cholesterol values, and markedly diminished HDL levels. The gene encoding LCAT is located on chromosome 16 and consists of six exons. Cleavage of a signal peptide of 24 amino acids converts the pro-enzyme from a 440 amino acid precursor to the final 416 amino acid glycoprotein that circulates in the plasma. When unesterified cholesterol from tissues is transferred to HDL by passive diffusion or by ABCA1 mediated lipid transport, LCAT's activity esterifies the transferred cholesterol, trapping it in the HDL core (*see* Fig. 15-2). As cholesterol ester is more hydrophobic than unesterified cholesterol, it is energetically unfavorable for the cholesterol ester to transfer back to the cell of origin. These steps of cholesterol transfer and esterification are the initial events in the reverse cholesterol transport pathway whereby cholesterol is moved from peripheral tissues back to the liver. Apo A-I is the major activator of LCAT activity, accounting for the predominant effect of the enzyme deficiency on HDL levels. LCAT does, however, contribute to the esterification of cholesterol in lower density lipoproteins as well. Despite very low HDL levels, patients with either fish eye disease or familial LCAT deficiency do not seem to have a predilection for early coronary atherosclerosis. The small number of patients with the disease, some of whom have been found to have CHD, make it difficult to determine if the risk of coronary atherosclerosis is substantially altered by the enzyme deficiency. There is no specific treatment for LCAT deficiency. Corneal and kidney transplantation are performed in these patients to ameliorate their major clinical disabilities.

Apo A-I Mutations Apo A-I is the major structural protein of HDL. The gene encoding apo A-I is located on chromosome 11 and comprises four exons. Following cleavage of the signal and

ABCA1 Transporter

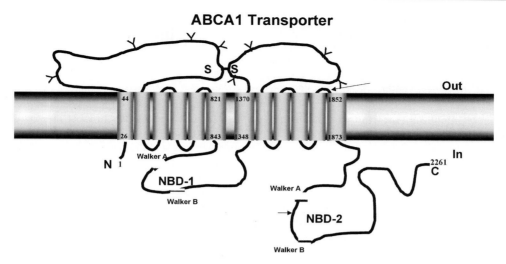

Figure 15-4   The ABCA1 transporter. The ABCA1 transporter is a full-sized 12-membrane spanning ATP-binding cassette protein. It is genetically altered in patients with Tangier disease, resulting in decreased cholesterol efflux from cells in response to apo stimulation. The ABCA1 transporter has two large loops positioned outside of the cell and the defining sequences of an ABC protein (Walker motifs in the nucleotide binding domains [NBD]) inside the cell. Approximately 50 mutations have been identified in the ABCA1 transporter, with most occurring either in the two large extracellular loops or in the NBD regions. The transporter has 2261 amino acids and the numbers on the graph indicate the approximate amino acid residue at each of the positions indicated.

prohormone sequences, a 243 amino acid mature protein is produced. The protein has multiple repeats of an amphipathic helical structure that enables it to interact with both lipid and aqueous environments. Mutations that cause profound alterations in apo A-I structure or expression have been reported, though they are extremely rare. Individuals carrying these mutations have virtually no circulating HDL and develop early CHD. Corneal opacities and xanthomas have been documented in many of these individuals. Most patients harboring these mutations are homozygous for the gene defect, usually as a result of consanguinity. Heterozygotes carrying these mutations commonly have half-normal HDL cholesterol levels, although cases with greater reductions in HDL levels have been reported, suggesting that some mutations may exert a dominant negative effect. As HDL typically contain four apo A molecules per particle (either four apo A-I or two A-I and two A-II proteins), a heterozygous individual carrying an expressed apo A-I mutant would have at least one mutant apo A-I on most HDL particles. The atherosclerosis of individuals with structural mutations in apo A-I appears to be more pronounced than that seen in the LCAT deficiency or Tangier disease patients. No specific therapy is available for this disorder, but aggressive LDL lipid-lowering therapy is justified.

SUMMARY OF GENETIC DISORDERS   The six LDL and HDL disorders described are illustrative of molecular genetic defects that contribute to abnormal lipid metabolism. These defects include the production of dysfunctional lipid uptake receptors (LDL receptor), post-receptor adaptor proteins (ARH), or lipid efflux transporters (Tangier disease and ABCA1); generation of abnormal apos that either lower (apo A-I mutations) or raise (FDB) lipoprotein levels; and synthesis of nonactive lipid modifying enzymes (LCAT). Many other monogenic disorders in lipid metabolism are due to mutations that affect proteins that fall into one of these classes.

MANAGEMENT

Aside from the rare patient at risk for hypertriglyceridemic pancreatitis, the goal for most hyperlipidemic patients is to reduce the risk of coronary morbidity and mortality. The approach to treatment

of hyperlipidemia outlined by the NCEP ATP III treatment panel is guided by an assessment of total CHD risk, not solely the lipid abnormality. For a given degree of LDL cholesterol elevation, the threshold for initiation of therapy decreases and the intensity of therapy increases with increasing CHD risk. Dietary modification, complemented by exercise and weight reduction, are combined with appropriate pharmacological therapy, when needed, to achieve the targets identified in the guidelines.

RISK ASSESSMENT AS A GUIDE TO SELECTION OF THERAPY   With benefit from treatment of hypercholesterolemia linked to the degree of pretreatment CHD risk, an assessment of that risk is imperative before deciding whom to treat, when to treat, and how aggressively to treat. The CHD risk assessment should be a comprehensive one, extending beyond lipid levels to include consideration of blood pressure, smoking, diabetes, family history of premature CHD, age, sex, and presence of established CHD or other atherosclerotic disease.

Treatment recommendations follow directly from the degree of estimated CHD risk. Dietary modification is the sole mode of therapy for patients at the lower end of the CHD risk spectrum, whereas pharmacologic measures are reserved for patients at higher risk or for those who fail dietary intervention. Studies showing benefits from HMG CoA reductase inhibitors in patients with LDL cholesterol levels less than 130 mg/dL may shift pharmacological treatment targets further downward.

DIETARY AND DRUG TREATMENT OF LIPID DISORDERS Reductions in total fat, saturated fat, partially hydrogenated unsaturated fatty acids, and dietary cholesterol are recommended for adults with elevated LDL cholesterol levels. Not only is it important to reduce total fat in the diet, but perhaps more critical is substituting foods that provide polyunsaturated and monounsaturated fats for those rich in saturated and trans-saturated fat. For patients with VLDL elevations, carbohydrate intake and alcohol use may be more important dietary factors to address than the cholesterol or saturated fat ingestion.

Weight loss (if obese), aerobic exercise, and smoking cessation can increase HDL and contribute to the dietary lowering of lower density lipoproteins and CHD risk. They also reduce CHD risk by decreasing blood pressure and glucose intolerance. When drug therapy is added to a lifestyle program, clinical trials have demonstrated significant reductions in the rate of atherosclerotic plaque progression, modest plaque regression, and declines in nonfatal and fatal cardiac events. In several studies, overall mortality has also been reduced.

HMG-Coa Reductase Inhibitors (The Statins)   Statins have become the first-line drug therapy for treatment of elevated LDL levels because of their effectiveness, patient acceptability, clinical outcomes data, and favorable safety record. They block the rate-limiting enzyme in cholesterol synthesis, HMG-CoA reductase. Serum LDL levels fall by 20–60%, depending on dose and preparation. HDL levels generally stay the same or increase slightly on statins. Statins also influence thrombotic and inflammatory mechanisms, effects whose importance remains to be elucidated.

Myalgias, with or without creatine kinase elevations, are the most common side effect of the class. Asymptomatic hepatocellular dysfunction manifested by an increase in serum levels of transaminases occur in approx 1% of patients taking the medications. Statins available in the United States and Canada are lovastatin, simvastatin, pravastatin, fluvastatin, atorvastatin, and rosuvastatin.

Niacin   Niacin is a B vitamin that must be used in megadoses to lower lipids. The precise mechanism of action is unknown, although a receptor for niacin was recently identified. Niacin, at doses of 1000 mg and higher, typically lowers LDL and VLDL levels, and raises HDL levels. It is the most effective HDL cholesterol-raising drug available. There are sufficient clinical trial data using niacin to conclude it is an effective anti-atherosclerotic agent, though there are no long-term, randomized prospective clinical trials establishing an overall mortality benefit with its use. Niacin's principal disadvantages include a litany of side effects, reflecting the large doses required. Niacin can exacerbate gout and diabetes, elevate liver enzymes, and produce rashes, nausea, and vomiting. It also triggers acute vasodilation that can result in flushing and even postural lightheadedness. Pretreatment with aspirin mitigates this reaction. Niacin is available in prescription and nonprescription formulations.

Cholesterol Absorption Inhibitors   Cholesterol absorption inhibitors block intestinal cholesterol absorption. The bulk agents (cholestyramine, colestipol, and colsevelam) interfere with micellar solubilization of cholesterol, whereas ezetimibe blocks an intracellular cholesterol transport pathway. LDL cholestrol reduction is typically 15–20% with these agents. Gastrointestinal side effects such as constipation, bloating, heartburn, and nausea are the major drawbacks to the use of the bulk agents. They are commonly used as an adjunct to statin therapy to achieve greater LDL reductions, or when statins are not tolerated.

Fibrates (Gemfibrozil and Fenofibrate)   These agents work by activating the peroxisome proliferation-activating receptor-α nuclear transcription factor, which decreases VLDL synthesis and enhances VLDL clearance. Thus, these drugs are primarily effective in the treatment of elevated triglyceride levels. They can be used in combination with statins to treat patients with combined VLDL and LDL disorders, but this therapy is associated with an increased likelihood of serious muscle breakdown leading to rhabdomyolytic renal failure. Side effects are rare but include abdominal discomfort.

CONCLUSION

Better understanding of the physiology and genetics of lipoprotein metabolism has resulted in better diagnostic and therapeutic interventions for patients with lipid disorders. Most patients with increased levels of LDL can be effectively treated with HMG CoA reductase inhibitors, either alone or in combination with niacin and/or cholesterol absorption inhibitors. Increased levels of VLDL are usually well managed by fibrate therapy, although weight loss and dietary changes are typically required to achieve optimal lipid targets. Disorders resulting in low HDL levels are still refractory to most interventions. Niacin therapy with moderate exercise can increase HDL values. Although this approach can lead to substantial rises in HDL levels, it is usually not effective in individuals who have a severe, monogenic disorder as the cause of their low HDL level. The growing understanding of the pathophysiology of atherosclerosis and progress in polygenic disorders is likely to lead to new therapies directed at non-lipid factors influencing CHD. Appropriate treatment of lipid disorders remains the cornerstone of any treatment program aimed at CHD prevention.

SELECTED REFERENCES

Boren J, Ekstrom U, Agren B, Nilsson-Ehle P, Innerarity TL. The molecular mechanism for the genetic disorder familial defective apolipoprotein B100. J Biol Chem 2001;276:9214–9218.

Brown MS, Goldstein JL. A receptor-mediated pathway for cholesterol homeostasis. Science 1986;232:34–47.

Brown BG, Zhao XQ, Chait A, et al. Simvastatin and niacin, antioxidant vitamins, or the combination for the prevention of coronary disease. N Engl J Med 2001;345(22):1583–1592.

Cohen JC, Kimmel M, Polanski A, Hobbs HH. Molecular mechanisms of autosomal-recessive hypercholesterolemia. Curr Opin Lipidol 2003;14:121–127.

Executive summary of the third report of the national cholesterol education program (NCEP) expert panel on detection, evaluation, and treatment of high blood cholesterol in adults (Adult Treatment Panel III). JAMA 2001;285:2486–2497.

Fitzgerald ML, Mendez AJ, Moore KJ, Andersson LP, Panjeton HA, Freeman MW. ATP-binding cassette transporter A1 contains an NH2-terminal signal anchor sequence that translocates the protein's first hydrophilic domain to the exoplasmic space. J Biol Chem 2001;276: 15,137–15,145.

Klein HG, Santamarina-Fojo S, Duverger N, et al. Fish eye syndrome: A molecular defect in the lecithin-cholesterol acyltransferase (LCAT) gene associated with normal alpha-LCAT-specific activity. Implications for classification and prognosis. J Clin Invest 1993;92:479–485.

Kuivenhoven JA, Pritchard H, Hill J, Frohlich J, Assmann G, Kastelein J. The molecular pathology of lecithin:cholesterol acyltransferase (LCAT) deficiency syndromes. J Lipid Res 1997;38:191–205.

Mensink RP, Katan MB. Effect of a diet enriched with monounsaturated or polyunsaturated fatty acids on levels of low-density and high-density lipoprotein cholesterol in healthy women and men. N Engl J Med 1989;321(7):436–441.

MRC/BHF Heart Protection Study of cholesterol lowering with simvastatin in 20,536 high-risk individuals: a randomised placebo-controlled trial. Lancet 2002;360:7–22.

Myant NB. Familial defective apolipoprotein B-100: a review, including some comparisons with familial hypercholesterolaemia. Atherosclerosis 1993;104:1–18.

Ordovas JM, Cassidy DK, Civeira F, Bisgaier CL, Schaefer EJ. Familial apolipoprotein A-I, C-III, and A-IV deficiency and premature atherosclerosis due to deletion of a gene complex on chromosome 11. J Biol Chem 1989;264:16,339–16,342.

Ridker PM, Hennekens CH, Buring JE, Rifai N. C-reactive protein and other markers of inflammation in the prediction of cardiovascular disease in women. N Engl J Med 2000;342:836–843.

Scandanavian Simvastatin Survival Study Group. Randomised trial of cholesterol lowering in 4444 patients with coronary heart diseases: The Scandanavian Simvastatin Survival Study (4S). Lancet 1994;344: 1383–1389.

Scriver CR, Beaudet AL, Sly WS, Valle D (eds). The Metabolic and Molecular Bases of Inherited Disease, 8th ed. New York: McGraw-Hill, 2001.

Singaraja RR, Brunham LR, Visscher H, Kastelein JJ, Hayden MR. Efflux and atherosclerosis. Arterioscler Thromb Vasc Biol 2003;23(8): 1322–1332.

Sorci-Thomas MG, Thomas MJ. The effects of altered apolipoprotein A-I structure on plasma HDL concentration. Trends Cardiovasc Med 2002;12:121–128.

Tunaru S, Kero J, Schaub A, et al. PUMA-G and HM74 are receptors for nicotinic acid and mediate its anti-lipolytic effect. Nat Med 2003;9:352–355.

16 Hypertension

Khurshed A. Katki and Donald J. DiPette

SUMMARY

Human hypertension is a complex disease. With the generation of animal models and techniques like genomics and proteomics, therapies for monogenic forms of hypertension are available. Our knowledge of essential hypertension and its therapy is restricted by its polygenic nature and the compounding interaction between genes and the environment. However, successful forays into the genetics of human hypertension should result in early intervention and more clinically and cost-effective therapies limiting the complications of this disease. Development of molecular profiles for essential hypertension and drug response genes to individualize therapy will potentially revolutionize the diagnosis and treatment of hypertension and its associated target organ diseases.

Key Words: Animal models; genetics; pharmacogenomics; rennin–angiotensin; salt sensitivity.

INTRODUCTION

Hypertension is a complex, multifactorial condition defined by a consistently elevated arterial blood pressure. If untreated, hypertension leads to morbidity and mortality primarily secondary to heart disease (congestive heart failure, coronary artery disease, and left-ventricular hypertrophy), renal failure, or stroke. As with many disease states, the molecular etiology of hypertension could originate with one gene (monogenic) or several genes (polygenic). Few cases of hypertension in humans have been shown to be monogenic. Because essential hypertension (i.e., hypertension not caused by a secondary etiology such as renal artery stenosis) is likely a complex, polygenic disease, a major task of hypertension research has been to elucidate its genetic basis. Owing to the complexity of the task, investigators have used multiple genetic strategies in the basic science and clinical research settings. In addition, essential hypertension is a multifactorial state involving interactions between genetic, environmental, and demographic factors. Essential hypertension is likely to result from an elaborate interaction between a network of major and minor genes that mediate the pathophysiological process of elevating blood pressure. In addition, susceptibility genes that modify an individual's response to environment, age, sex, body mass index, and probably other unknown factors compound these genetic interactions. Multiple epistatic effects within and between the causative and susceptibility

From: *Principles of Molecular Medicine, Second Edition*
Edited by: M. S. Runge and C. Patterson © Humana Press, Inc., Totowa, NJ

genes complicate this process. Thus, essential hypertension is a truly complex disease whose treatment and therapy depend not only on identifying candidate genes involved, but also on dissecting their interactions with other factors.

Advances in genomics and proteomics have provided powerful tools to study the genetics of multifactorial diseases like hypertension. However, with the exception of monogenic forms of hypertension such as familial hyperaldosteronism, Liddle's syndrome, and mutations in epithelial sodium channels (ENaC), little progress has been made in identifying the underlying genetics of essential hypertension. Thus, there is great difficulty in studying a pathophysiologically heterogeneous disease like hypertension that varies by renin status and sodium dependency, among other factors. This chapter focuses on some of the attempts to elucidate the underlying genetics and the molecular mechanism(s) that lead to the development and pathogenesis of hypertension.

ANIMAL MODELS USED TO STUDY THE GENETICS OF HYPERTENSION

Genetic animal models have been used to study the etiology of hypertension, mostly in the rat. Rats are used to study the genetics of hypertension because of their ease of handling and breeding and their low associated costs. However, because genetic manipulation is easier in the mouse than the rat, the use of the mouse model for hypertension research has increased. It is routinely possible to mutate, delete (knock-out), or add genes (knock-in) of interest in the mouse genome, and to couple these manipulations to the gain-or loss-of-structure and function. These strategies combined with newer methodologies to measure cardiovascular variables, especially in the mouse, have led to increased use of the mouse model to explore the genetics of hypertension.

IMPORTANCE AND USE OF RAT MODELS IN HYPERTENSION Genetic models of hypertension have been developed primarily in rats, but a number of species including dogs, rabbits, turkeys, and mice have been used. At least 18 genetic models of experimental hypertension exist in inbred rats (Table 16-1). The two most commonly studied strains of hypertensive rats are the spontaneously hypertensive rat (SHR) and the Dahl rats. The SHR and the stroke prone SHR are inbred strains that are mainly renin-independent. Both develop hypertension and target organ damage similar to that in human essential hypertension. The SHR is used to study the target organ complications of hypertension, to screen potential antihypertensive pharmacological agents and to investigate the genetics

Table 16-1
Genetic Models of Experimental Hypertension

Strain	Sub-strain(s)	Name	Associated phenotype	Blood pressure QTLs	Representative candidate genes/loci studied
CRDH		Cohen rosenthal diabetic hypertensive	NIDDM, high-blood pressure (176 ± 8 mmHg), fibrinoid necrosis in arteries and arterioles, smooth muscle, and vascular hyperplasia.	None	—
DSS/1		Dahl salt-sensitive	Sensitive to salt-induced hypertension	None	—
DSS/2		Dahl salt-sensitive	Sensitive to salt-induced hypertension	None	—
DSS/3		Dahl salt-sensitive	Sensitive to salt-induced hypertension	None	—
F344	F344/Crj F344/ NHsd F344/Pit	Fisher	Hypoxia-induced right-ventricular hypertrophy	Hypoxia-induced right-ventricular hypertrophy-1	Hirvh1
FH		Fawn hooded	Spontaneous hypertension. Altered serotonergic function, glomerular sclerosis and proteinuria	None	Genetic model of depression
FHH		Fawn hooded hypertensive	Systemic hypertension and proteinuria leading to premature renal failure and death.	Blood pressure QTLs 1, 2 and QTL cluster 14, 4255 SSLP markers	Bpfh1, Rf1, and Rf2
FHL/Eur		Fawn hooded low-blood pressure	Does not develop hypertension. Altered renal hemodynamics.	Blood pressure FH QTL2	Bpfh2, Rf3, Rf4, and Rf5
FHR		Fawn hooded hypertensive	Systemic hypertension and proteinuria, renal disease and hypertension under independent genetic control.		
GH		Genetically hypertensive rat	Inherited hypertension. Prevalence of cardiac hypertrophy and vascular disease. Levels of substance P in superior cervical ganglion, spinal cord, iris and trachea are twofold that of normal rats, and substance P containing sensory neurons are also elevated.	Blood pressure QTL7 on chromosome 6.	Renal α_2-adrenoreceptor
MHS		Milan hypertensive strain	High-blood pressure early in life, left-ventricular hypertrophy, renal atrophy, volume expansion and increased water intake, faster sodium transport	Blood Pressure QTLs on chromosomes 1,10,14, and 20	α-Adducin-1 gene, α_{1B}-adrenergic receptor, Na(+)/H(+) exchanger-3 gene.
SD-Tg (Ren2)27		Sprague-Dawley transgenic	Model for low-renin hypertension, susceptible to malignant hypertension, susceptible to cardio-vascular disease and cerebral haemorrhage.		Ren2 gene

Table 16-1 (Continued)

Strain	Sub-strain(s)	Name	Associated phenotype	Blood pressure QTLs	Representative candidate genes/loci studied
SHR		Spontaneously hypertensive rat	Polygenic hypertension, cardiovascular disease, increased peripheral vascular resistance, cardiac hypertrophy, increased neurogenic tone; environmental and dietary factors influence the degree of hypertension.	Blood pressure QTLs on chromosomes 1-6, 8-10, 11, 13, 16, and 19.	Bp16–23
SHRSP		Stroke prone SHR	Higher blood pressure than SHR, stroke is affected by genetic and environmental factors, excessive salt intake, cerebral hemorrhage or infarction in 82% of 100 d-old males and 58 % of 150 d-old females	Blood pressure QTLs on chromosomes 1–5,10, 18, and X. Sensitivity to stroke QTLs on chromosomes 1, 4, and 5.	Str1–3, Bp1–4, Bp13–15, Bp28, and Bp49.
SR		Sprague-Dawley rapp	No effect of a high-salt diet on development of hypertension, mild hydronephrosis, mutant form of cytochrome P450.	None	
SR/Jr		Salt-resistant rapp	Same as above	Blood pressure QTLs on chromosomes 1,8, 9,10,13, and 18	Bp12,24,25,30, 34,39,41.
SS		Sprague-Dawley	Develop salt-sensitive and fulminant hypertension, vascular and renal lesions.	Blood pressure QTLs on chromosomes 8,13,15,18.	Angiotensin, dopamine-1 and endothelin-3
SS/Jr		Salt-sensitive rapp	Endothelium-independent myogenic activation of gracilis arteries.	Blood pressure QTLs on chromosomes 1–3, 5,7,8–10,13,16–18	Angiotensin converting enzyme 1
WF		Wistar furth	Low-blood pressure, resistant to adrenal regeneration hypertension	None	Mammary carcinoma susceptibility genes 1–4

Bp, blood pressure; Bpfh, blood pressure fawn-hooded; FH, fawn hooded; Hirvh1, hypoxia-induced right-ventricular hypertrophy-1 gene; NIDDM, noninsulin-dependent diabetes mellitus; QTL, quantitative trait loci; Rf, renal failure; SHR, spontaneously hypertensive rat; Str, stroke.

potentially involved in high-blood pressure. At least three gene loci are thought to be involved in the earlier-mentioned process, one of which might be in close association with the *angiotensinogen* (*AGT*) gene. A similar multiple gene interaction is thought to be involved in human essential hypertension.

Genome wide scans using these models of hypertension are powerful tools yielding quantitative trait loci (QTL) on almost every rat chromosome. Whereas blood pressure QTLs have been confirmed on rat chromosomes 1, 2, 10, and 13, they have been suggested on each of the other rat chromosomes except chromosomes 6, 11, and 15. The use of consomic, congenic, and subcongenic rat strains have confirmed the above loci. Consomic strains incorporate a full chromosome of one strain onto a genetic background of a contrasting strain. Congenic strains incorporate only a part of the chromosome including the full length QTL segment of interest. Subcongenics incorporate only part of the QTL, the so-called region of interest. Consomic and congenic strains are constructed to confirm the physiological and phenotypic significance of a QTL, whereas subcongenic strains facilitate the progressive decrease in the QTL span to enable eventual detection of the "gene of interest" within that chromosomal region. A technique called marker-assisted selection has accelerated greatly congenic strain construction, because the progeny in the first backcross generation are expected to have a 50% genome-wide heterozygosity. However, heterozygosity among individual progeny follows a normal distribution with a mean of 50%. The marker-assisted selection strategy uses this normal distribution of heterozygosity to accelerate the production of congenic strains.

THE MOUSE AS A MODEL OF HYPERTENSION

Polygenic diseases like hypertension can be studied by two basic approaches: a phenotype-driven approach and a genotype-driven approach. In the former, using the phenotype of hypertension, the genes responsible for the phenotype are determined. This approach has the added potential to facilitate the discovery of unknown genes. Studies have revealed 10 QTLs on nine different chromosomes associated with blood pressure. Six different QTLs have been associated with salt-induced hypertension. These studies utilized a backcross between salt-sensitive C57BL/6J and salt-resistant A/J inbred mice fed 1% saline for 2 wk. Two of the three loci were found to affect hypertension by interacting with each other. Another major QTL was found on chromosome 15 by crossing BALB/cJ and CBA/CaJ. These results suggest that mapping QTLs in rodent models might guide the search for human blood pressure genes.

In the genotype-driven approach, a known gene is studied in an attempt to discover its function in the regulation of blood pressure commonly using transgenic techniques to overexpress a gene or, with the use of homologous recombination, to create a knockout or nonfunctional gene. Some studies highlighting the usefulness of the knockout technique to study blood pressure regulation are discussed later.

Evidence suggests that renal and nervous system mechanisms are responsible for some forms of hypertension. Some of the complex systems involved in blood pressure regulation such as the sympathetic nervous-catecholamine system, the renin–angiotensin system, the kallikrein–kinin system, the nitric oxide system, the prostaglandin system and the vasopressin system have been well studied. Several neuropeptides that are colocalized and released with norepinephrine or other neuropeptides are known to modulate blood pressure; the vasoconstrictor neuropeptide Y and the vasodilators calcitonin gene-related peptide (CGRP) and substance P (SP) are some of the best-studied examples. Knock-out mice devoid of the calcitonin/α-CGRP peptide or the neurokinin-1 receptor, the SP receptor, have provided valuable insight into the role that these neuropeptides play in blood pressure regulation. α-CGRP is responsible for approx 30% of basal coronary blood flow. The deoxycorticosterone-salt model of hypertension shows that deletion of the α-CGRP gene leads to a greater elevation in blood pressure and renders the heart and kidney more vulnerable to hypertension-induced end-organ damage. In addition, the deletion of the α-CGRP gene in the renal reduced-mass model of hypertension leads to an augmented role for SP to attenuate the elevated blood pressure. The increasing use of mutagenesis to construct new mouse models has been the latest molecular tool employed in an effort to study the various interactions of the genes involved in hypertension. The mutagenic agent N-ethyl-N-nitrosourea has been used in the large-scale generation of mutant mice. As new mouse models for hypertension are either generated or characterized, and as newer tools for genetic research in mouse models are developed, the understanding of human hypertension and the ability to treat, prevent, or cure it will increase accordingly.

HUMAN HYPERTENSION

Hypertension accounts for 6% of adult deaths worldwide although wide variability exists in the global occurrence. In the United States, the prevalence of hypertension is highest in the southeast. Various determinants of geographic variation in hypertension have been quantified, including obesity, fat and sodium intake, genetics, environment, and ancestry especially among African Americans. Data from the Third National Health and Nutrition Examination Survey show that in the United States the overall prevalence of hypertension is about 24% in persons 18 yr or older. Hypertension is slightly more common in men (24.7%) than women (23.4%), whereas the age-adjusted prevalence of hypertension was higher in non-Hispanic African Americans than non-Hispanic Caucasians and Mexican Americans (32.4, 23.3, and 22.6%, respectively). Hypertension is 8.5 times more prevalent in African Americans and is associated with a higher risk of target-organ damage than in Caucasians. In the past two decades, the level of awareness among Americans of their hypertensive condition has risen, although only slightly. Data from the Third National Health and Nutrition Examination Survey suggest that hypertension awareness was greatest among non-Hispanic African Americans (74%) and non-Hispanic Caucasians (70%) compared with Mexican Americans (54%).

Clinical trials have documented the benefits of lifestyle changes and appropriate pharmacological antihypertensive intervention in hypertension treatment. Among Hispanics, a rapidly growing heterogeneous ethnic group in the United States, there is a lower incidence of hypertension than that of the general population. Hypertension in Hispanics varies by gender and the country of origin; most data is limited to Hispanics of Mexican and Puerto Rican origin with limited data available on Cuban Americans.

GENETICS OF HUMAN HYPERTENSION

As mentioned, there is evidence of a genetic component of blood pressure levels and of several intermediate phenotypes associated with hypertension in humans. A common measure of familial aggregation of hypertension is the use of family history, which can also reveal undefined familial risk factors. Identifying families with a positive history of hypertension for genetic studies is of importance because these families should be more likely to have genes and behavioral habits that lead to hypertension. Gene–gene interaction as well as gene–environment interactions on blood pressure and the intermediate phenotypes controlling blood pressure can be studied in such families. Using linkage analysis, research suggests the presence of hypertensive genes at several locations over all the human chromosomes. Some of the consistent areas are the chromosomal arm 1q, 2p, 2q, 8p, 17q, and 18q. Other less consistent regions might still harbor important hypertension genes.

MONOGENIC FORMS OF HUMAN HYPERTENSION

Monogenic diseases are typically severe but rare with an allelic frequency of <1% in the population. They define new physiological paradigms and signaling pathways and help identify candidate genes that could play a more frequent role in polygenic diseases like essential hypertension, diabetes, and obesity. Some of the monogenic forms of hypertension include familial hyperaldosteronism, Liddle's syndrome, and mutations in ENaC. Aldosterone, the major circulating mineralocorticoid in humans, participates in blood volume regulation and sodium, and potassium hemostasis. It might also play a role in tissue fibrosis contributing to the target organ damage secondary to hypertension yet independent of the degree of blood pressure elevation. Familial forms of hyperaldosteronism include type I (glucocorticoid-remediable) and type II, which are discussed in the next section. Hyperaldosteronism is also seen in multiple endocrine neoplasia

(MEN). In 1966, the first cases of autosomal, type-I familial hyperaldosteronism, a dexamethasone-suppressible form of hyperaldosteronism, were reported. The genetic locus and mutation causing this disease have been identified. Aldosterone is synthesized exclusively in the zona glomerulosa of the adrenal gland in a series of six biosynthetic steps. The *CYP11B2* gene plays an important role in the synthesis of aldosterone; its product is capable of catalyzing three of the six steps in aldosterone synthesis: the 18-hydroxydehydrogenase, 18-hydroxylase, and the 1β-hydroxylase enzyme reactions. The *CYP11B2* gene is located on human chromosome 8q24.3-tel, in close proximity to the highly homologous *CYP11B1* gene whose protein product (1β-hydroxylase) catalyses the final step in cortisol synthesis. The defect in familial hyperaldosteronism type I involves a crossover of genetic material between the closely linked *CYP11B1* and *CYP11B2* genes. Fusion of the adrenocorticotropic hormone-responsive promoter of the former with the coding region of the latter, allows aldosterone synthesis to be controlled by adrenocorticotropic hormone, resulting in pathologically high levels of aldosterone and suppressibility of aldosterone to exogenous glucocorticoid administration. The lack of hypokalemia in many subjects with glucocorticoid-remediable aldosteronism has been related to a blunted aldosterone response to potassium. Primary aldosteronism is a disorder characterized by hypertension and in more severe forms hypokalemia, primarily because of an aldosterone-producing adrenocortical adenoma, removal of which led to some of the earliest cures of hypertension or to zona glomerulosa hyperplasia. Improved screening techniques, including a genetic screening test and the use of plasma aldosterone and plasma renin activity determinations, have led to this disease being recognized and treated with increasing accuracy and efficacy. The advent of laparoscopic adrenalectomy has greatly reduced the morbidity of surgical treatment of the adrenocortical adenoma form of this disease.

Hypertension is rarely (approx 0.05% of all hypertension) caused by a catecholamine secreting tumor or pheochromocytoma that is benign in most (approx 90%) of cases. Surgical resection cures approx 90% of cases, but if left undiagnosed or untreated, the tumor is invariably lethal causing cerebrovascular or cardiovascular complications from excess circulating catecholamines. Pheochromocytomas usually arise within the adrenal medulla, but develop occasionally in extra-adrenal sympathetic ganglia, sometimes also referred to as paragangliomas. Pheochromocytomas are also component features of some inherited cancer syndromes including MEN-2, von Hippel-Lindau syndrome (VHL), pheochromocytoma-paraganglioma syndrome and type 1 neurofibromatosis. Germline mutations in the VHL tumor suppressor gene cause VHL and germline mutations in the RET protooncogene cause MEN-2. Also, a subset of pheochromocytoma-only families segregates the germline VHL mutation but not the RET mutation. Germline mutations in three of the succinate dehydrogenase (mitochondrial complex II) subunits (SDHD, SDHB, and SDHC) cause susceptibility to head and neck paragangliomas. In addition, SDHD and SDHB mutations might cause susceptibility to familial and isolated pheochromocytoma with or without head and neck paragangliomas. The mechanisms by which succinate dehydrogenase subunit mutations predispose to pheochromocytoma have not been defined in detail but dysregulation of hypoxiaresponsive genes and impairment of mitochondria-mediated apoptosis have been suggested. Another putative mechanism involved in the initiation of pheochromocytoma is the binding of the VHL protein with fibronectin. It has been suggested that VHL protein binds directly to fibronectin thereby preventing the promotion of the fibronectin matrix assembly.

Another important monogenic form of hypertension is Liddle's syndrome, a rare autosomal-dominant disorder characterized by early onset of hypertension, excessive sodium retention, low plasma renin activity, and usually hypokalemia. Plasma levels of aldosterone are undetectable and mineralocorticoid receptor antagonism by spironolactone has no effect on blood pressure or serum potassium. Treatment includes ameloride therapy, which blocks sodium-reabsorption and potassium excretion by mineralocorticoid independent mechanisms. The defect in Liddle's syndrome results from a constitutive activation of ameloride sensitive ENaC on distal renal tubules, which causes excess sodium reabsorption. This channel is made up of at least three subunits normally regulated by aldosterone. Mutations of the cytoplasmic C-terminus of either β- or γ-subunits of ENaC cause Liddle's syndrome and have been localized on human chromosome 16. These mutations, mapped mainly to a proline-rich domain that promotes internalization and degradation of the ENaC molecules, lead to an increased cell surface expression of the ENaC molecule, which therefore explains a constitutive reabsorption of sodium accompanied by an increase in blood pressure. A mouse model for Liddle's syndrome has been generated by Cre-loxP mediated recombination, which mimics to an extent the human form of salt-sensitive hypertension. Under a high salt intake, the homozygous mice develop highblood pressure and hypokalemic metabolic alkalosis accompanied by cardiac and renal hypertrophy. Interestingly, like their wild type counterparts, both the homozygotes and the heterozygotes develop normally for the first 3 mo and have normal blood pressure, but already demonstrate increased sodium reabsorption in the distal colon and low plasma aldosterone, suggesting chronic hypervolemia. This model also establishes a causal relationship between dietary sodium intake, the expression of a gene in the kidney, and hypertension.

Sympathetic activation plays an important role in cardiovascular homeostasis. Regulation of cardiac and vascular function is mediated primarily or in part by β-adrenergic receptors. Stimulation of β-adrenoreceptors by catecholamines in disease states such as hypertension, congestive heart failure, and ischemic heart disease has many deleterious effects. Although three β-subtypes are known, and a fourth one is hypothesized, in the myocardium the predominant receptor subtypes are the β_1 and β_2. The long arm of human chromosome 5 contains a cluster of genes encoding the α_1- and β_2-adrenergic receptors and the dopamine receptor type 1A, all of which are involved in blood pressure regulation. The activation of β_1 and β_2 subtypes is linked to an increased cAMP formation (through interaction with stimulating guanine nucleotide binding protein) resulting in the activation of the cAMP-dependent protein kinase phosphorylation group of intracellular proteins that increase myocardial inotropy and chronotropy. β_2-adrenoreceptors play an important role in vascular function. Stimulation of β_2 receptors results in smooth muscle relaxation (i.e., vasodilation), which results in a reduction in systemic vascular resistance. Nonselective β-blockers (e.g., Propranolol) exert their antihypertensive effects mainly through cardiac and renal receptors. Second generation β-receptor antagonists such as metoprolol and atenolol, are β_1-selective and were developed in part to overcome the increased bronchoconstriction and peripheral vasoconstriction seen with β_2-blockade. Third generation β-blockers like labetolol and carvedilol are nonselective for β_1 and β_2 but also function as α-receptor antagonists, which overcome the increase in peripheral resistance caused by β_2-blockade. An increasing body of evidence suggests that three common β_2-polymorphisms and two common β_1-polymorphisms might play a role in the pathophysiology of cardiovascular disease including hypertension. Genetic variants of the β_2-receptor that decrease receptor number or enhance β_2-receptor downregulation (Gly16 and Gln27, respectively) appear to influence vascular tone and, thus, vascular reactivity and hypertension risk. However, conflicting reports on the studies of β_2-receptor codons 16 and 27 exist with differences in genetic background and linkage disequilibrium as possible reasons. In addition, a "gain of function" variant of the β_1-receptor, namely the Arg389 variant, also increases adrenergic tone and thereby the risk of hypertension. However, data demonstrating a role for the β_2-variant Ile164 in the pathophysiology of cardiac disease might be more convincing. Animal models and in vitro studies demonstrate that this mutation results in a loss of the receptor function. In clinical studies this mutation has an adverse impact on heart failure survival. In contrast, the β_1-Gly49 variant improves survival in heart failure, although no animal or in vitro data documents the functionality of this variant. Despite the presence of data implicating various β-receptor mutations in both hypertension and heart failure, little is known about the impact of these variants on the effectiveness of β-receptor blockade. Genetic background studies, specifically on the inherited patterns of β-receptor mutations, might help delineate patient subsets in whom β-blockade might be effective or ineffective. Thus, the potential to use genetic background screening to determine the effectiveness of potential β-blocker therapy remains an area for further investigation. Therefore, monogenic forms of hypertension although rare, play an important role in blood pressure regulation, and if left untreated, invariably lead to hypertension and debilitating secondary effects like renal failure, stroke, and even death.

POLYGENIC HYPERTENSION Essential hypertension results from the interaction of hereditary, environmental and demographic factors. These factors contribute to blood pressure variation even within an individual. It has been suggested that genetic factors account for about 40% of variation in blood pressure in human populations. The full expression of hypertension, therefore, is determined by the interaction of the various genes with each other and the environment resulting in a variety of phenotypes. Hence, essential hypertension does not follow the classic Mendelian rules of dominant or recessive inheritance. Several genes have been associated with blood pressure in general and more specifically with essential hypertension. One of the most systematically studied systems and their genetic components include the rennin-angiotensin-aldosterone system.

RENIN–ANGIOTENSIN SYSTEM AND ITS LINK TO HYPERTENSION The juxtaglomerular cells in the kidney synthesize renin, a single chain polypeptide, in response to macula densa signals of lowered cytosolic calcium, decreased renal arteriolar pressure, or increased renal α- or β-adrenergic nerve activity. Renin serves as a circulating enzyme for its substrate angiotensinogen (AGT) in the plasma to form a decapeptide called angiotensin (Ang)-I. Ang-I is further catabolized to an octapeptide Ang-II by the angiotensin-converting enzyme (ACE), which is endothelin bound and present in high concentration in the lung. Ang-II is a circulating vasopressor with various other functions such as sodium and volume retention secondary to stimulation of aldosterone release

from the adrenal glands. The *AGT* gene has the strongest evidence supporting its role in the development of human hypertension. Several studies in animals and humans support a link between *AGT* and hypertension. For example, in transgenic mice, the increased number of *AGT* alleles correlates directly to increasing blood pressure levels. Variants in the *AGT* gene generally correlate with higher circulating AGT levels, but there is no conclusive proof of the involvement of mutations of the *AGT* gene in the development of hypertension. Two well-known polymorphisms of the *AGT* gene, –6 A/G and the Thr235 alleles, are associated with hypertension in a variety of populations. Carriers of the A variant in the –6 position within the promoter region of the gene show a greater blood pressure response to sodium reduction, as do carriers of the Thr235 allele, which is also thought to be associated with the development of preeclampsia. Two main receptors of Ang-II, AT1 and AT2, have been defined with most known adverse effects of Ang-II being mediated via the former. Both AT1 and AT2 belong to the seven transmembrane class of G protein coupled receptor family. The genes for all the above peptides and enzymes have been investigated for their association to hypertension and salt sensitivity. There is also convincing evidence in humans linking the ACE locus to its plasma levels. However, the association of ACE variants to hypertension remains to be proved conclusively.

TYPE-II FAMILIAL HYPERALDOSTERONISM AND ITS ROLE IN HYPERTENSION As mentioned, familial hyperaldosteronism type II is characterized by an inheritance consistent with an autosomal-dominant pattern of autonomous aldosterone hypersecretion and is not suppressible by dexamethasone. Linkage analysis and direct mutation screening shows that this disorder is unrelated to genes for aldosterone synthase or the angiotensin II receptor but is polygenic in origin with a potential polymorphic locus on chromosome 7p22 region.

SALT SENSITIVITY AND HYPERTENSION The interaction between genetic variations and environmental factors such as salt intake (diet), stress, and physical activity can contribute to the development of essential hypertension. A genotype that responds to changes in its environment is broadly classified as sensitive whereas a phenotype that is not influenced by its environment is called insensitive. Various hemodynamic mechanisms regulate the heterogeneous relationship between salt and water intake and the resultant blood pressure levels within individuals, which can be broadly classified as salt-sensitive or salt-resistant. The rennin–angiotensin system plays a major role in sodium–water balance, which influences blood pressure. Hypertensive individuals with low plasma renin activity often exhibit a greater blood pressure response to sodium loading, and salt-sensitive hypertensive persons show a blunted rennin–angiotensin response when there is a shift from low to high sodium intake in the diet. Several genes in this system such as *AGT*, *ACE*, *AT1*-, and *AT2*- receptors have been investigated for their association with hypertension. A widely studied polymorphism of the ACE gene is the insertion/deletion in intron 16, with linkage evidence implicating the gene in hypertension risk. The I variant confers greater blood pressure increase associated with changes from low-salt to high-salt diet whereas the D variant is closely associated with microvascular and macrovascular sequelae of hypertension.

GENE POLYMORPHISMS AND PHARMACOGENOMICS IN HYPERTENSION Hypertensive persons are known to respond heterogeneously to antihypertensive drug therapy, probably reflecting factors such as differences in pharmacokinetic and pharmacodynamic properties of antihypertensive agents and differences in genetic response to various drug therapies. Pharmacogenetics, the study of genetic variations influencing the response to pharmacological agents, is an emerging field that mainly studies the gene–environment interaction. Genetic polymorphisms influence pharmacodynamic mechanisms of antihypertensive drug response. However, because most inter-individual variation in response to antihypertensive therapy remains unexplained, this is not a practical and clinically useful guide to select antihypertensive agents. Consequently, identifying and studying candidate genes that influence the pharmacodynamic determinants of blood pressure and the usage of genome wide scanning is the priority. The candidate gene approach has been studied, specifically the α-adducin gene and the genes within the rennin–angiotensin system. α-adducin is a heterodimeric, cytoskeletal protein involved in signal transduction. A Gly/Trp change at amino acid 460 (Trp460) at the human α-adducin locus was more frequent in 477 hypertensive patients than in 332 normotensive control subjects. Subsequently, heterozygotic patients with the Gly460Trp variant were shown to have a greater blood pressure reduction in response to diuretic therapy than did Gly460 homozygotes. These findings demonstrate that α-adducin polymorphisms might be useful in identifying a subset of salt-sensitive hypertensive patients who are more responsive to diuretic therapy. Further, studies such as those investigating the α-adducin gene demonstrate genes contributing to hypertension via a particular physiological mechanism (namely, increased renal sodium reabsorption and volume expansion) might serve as candidates to influence blood pressure response to antihypertensive therapy. Because the rennin–angiotensin-aldosterone system is directly related to sodium and volume homeostasis, genes encoding components of this system have been logical candidates for investigation to predict the blood pressure response to changes in dietary sodium and diuretic therapy. Because sex-specific effects of the ACE insertion/deletion polymorphism are present and appear to be mediated separately from effects on plasma renin activity or the generation of Ang-II, it has been hypothesized that local intrarenal and intraadrenal effects of this ACE polymorphism may differ between men and women.

With the sequencing of the human genome complete, pharmacogenomic studies that measure variations at a single gene locus as well as polygenic loci will improve the ability to predict individuals' responses to antihypertensive therapy. Current genome-wide search strategies to identify QTLs linking the blood pressure response to antihypertensive therapy are limited because they depend on the measurement of microsatellite markers in related family members. However, single-nucleotide polymorphism (SNP) measurements, which can be determined by microarray technology, have the potential to enable the discovery of novel genes influencing drug response by comparing haplotype frequencies between correlated individuals showing opposite extremes of distribution responses. SNPs are positions in the genome at which two alternative nucleotides occur at an appreciable frequency (>1%). As the most abundant form of polymorphism in the human genome, SNPs are estimated to occur about once in every 1000 bp. Thus there are more than three million SNPs per human genome (which consists of 3×10^9 bp). Importantly, DNA chips, which are synthesized oligonucleotides attached to a glass surface, facilitate the rapid genotyping of large numbers of SNPs in a reasonable time frame and cost. Such chips are commercially available to assess known mutations in the human cytochrome *P450* genes encoding the CYP2D6 and CYP2C19 enzymes, for example, which are responsible for metabolizing many commonly prescribed antihypertensive drugs. The P450 enzymes are well characterized with >150 different isoforms identified as products of >30 different *P450* genes. Two notable variants are the CYP2D2 and *N*-acetyltransferase 2 variants. CYP2D2 mutations lead to excessive β-blockade of alprenolol, bufarolol, carvedilol, metoprolol, propranolol, and timolol presumably resulting from reduced metabolism of these blockers. Carriers of the "rapid accelerator" *N*-acetyltransferase 2 polymorphism require a higher dose of the vasodilator hydralazine to control blood pressure. Thus, genotyping of participants might allow tailoring of antihypertensive drug therapy. Such measurements are a necessary step toward studying the interaction between environmental factors such as age, diet and other medications that influence antihypertensive drug response. This ability to accurately identify pathophysiological subgroups and reliably predict the blood pressure response in individually tailored therapies will lead to fewer adverse reactions and ultimately lowered therapeutic costs.

Human hypertension is a complex disease. With the exception of monogenic forms of hypertension, knowledge of essential hypertension and its therapy is severely restricted because of its polygenic nature and the compounding interaction between genes and the environment. With the use of the latest molecular technology of generating animal models, the sequencing of the human, mouse, and rat genomes, as well as the onset of the era of proteomics and genomics, this challenge might be overcome. Successful forays into the genetics of human hypertension should result in early intervention and more clinically and cost effective therapies that will limit complications of this common disease. The challenge for research is to develop "molecular profiles" of essential hypertension and drug response genes in order to develop individualized drug therapy. Drugs that are more specific for the molecular characteristics of individual patients should contribute to greater efficacy and reduced toxicity. With genetic screening of hypertensive patients as a possibility, and the availability of newer molecular techniques, there is the potential to revolutionize the way hypertension and its associated target organ diseases are diagnosed and treated.

SELECTED REFERENCES

Bader M, Peters J, Baltatu O, Muller DN, Luft FC. Tissue renin-angiotensin systems: new insights from experimental animal models in hypertension research. J Mol Med 2001;79(2–3):76–102.

Beckers A, Abs R, Willems PJ, et al. Aldosterone-secreting adrenal adenoma as part of multiple endocrine neoplasia type 1 (MEN1): loss of heterozygosity for polymorphic chromosome 11 deoxyribonucleic acid markers, including the MEN1 locus. J Clin Endocrinol Metab 1992;75(2):564–570.

Burt VL, Whelton P, Roccella EJ, et al. Prevalence of hypertension in the US adult population results from the Third National Health and Nutrition Examination Survey, 1988–1991. Hypertension 1995;25(3): 305–313.

Cardia SLR. Gene–environment interactions. In: Izzo JL, Black HR, eds. Hypertension Primer: Essentials of High Blood Pressure, 3rd ed. Baltimore: Lippincott Williams and Wilkins, 2002; pp. 221–224.

Conn JW. Primary aldosteronism, a new clinical syndrome. J Lab Clin Med 1995;45:3–17.

Conn JW, Knopf RF, Nesbit RM. Clinical characteristics of primary aldosteronism from an analysis of 145 cases. Am J Surg 1964;107: 159–172.

Cooper RS. Geographic patterns of hypertension: a global perspective. In: Izzo JL, Black HR, eds. Hypertension Primer: Essentials of High Blood

Pressure, 3rd ed. Baltimore: Lippincott Williams and Wilkins, 2002; pp. 231–233.

Cusi D, Barlassina C, Azzani T, et al. Polymorphisms of alpha-adducin and salt sensitivity in patients with essential hypertension. Lancet 1997;349(9062):1353–1357.

Doris PA. Hypertension genetics, single nucleotide polymorphisms, and the common disease: common variant hypothesis. Hypertension 2002; 39(2 Pt 2):323–331.

Ferdinand KC. Hypertension in blacks. In: Izzo JL, Black HR, eds. Hypertension Primer: Essentials of High Blood Pressure, 3rd ed. Baltimore: Lippincott Williams and Wilkins, 2002; pp. 264–266.

Hoffman MA, Ohh M, Yang H, Klco JM, Ivan M, Kaelin WG Jr. von Hippel-Lindau protein mutants linked to type 2C VHL disease preserve the ability to downregulate HIF. Hum Mol Genet 2001;10(10): 1019–1027.

Hrabe de Angelis MH, Flaswinkel H, Fuchs H, et al. Genome-wide, large-scale production of mutant mice by ENU mutagenesis. Nat Genet 2000;25(4):444–447.

Jackson RV, Lafferty A, Torpy DJ, Stratakis C. New genetic insights in familial hyperaldosteronism. Ann N Y Acad Sci 2002;970:77–88.

Jeunemaitre X, Soubrier F, Kotelevtsev YV, et al. Molecular basis of human hypertension: role of angiotensinogen. Cell 1992;71(1): 169–180.

Katki KA, Supowit SC, Li J, Wang DH, DiPette DJ. Subtotal nephrectomy-salt hypertension in a-CGRP knockout mice-role of substance P. 56th Annual Fall Conference and Scientific Sessions of the Council for High Blood Pressure Research of the American Heart Association September 25–28, 2002.

Kato N. Genetic analysis in human hypertension. Hypertens Res 2002; 25(3):319–327.

Kim HS, Krege JH, Kluckman KD, et al. Genetic control of blood pressure and the angiotensinogen locus. Proc Natl Acad Sci USA 1995; 92(7):2735–2739.

Kreutz R, Hubner N. Congenic rat strains are important tools for the genetic dissection of essential hypertension. Semin Nephrol 2002; 22(2):135–47.

Lifton RP, Dluhy RG, Powers M, et al. A chimaeric 11 beta-hydroxylase/aldosterone synthase gene causes glucocorticoid-remediable aldosteronism and human hypertension. Nature 1992;355(6357): 262–265.

Maher ER, Eng C. The pressure rises: update on the genetics of phaeochromocytoma. Hum Mol Genet 2002;11(20):2347–2354.

Manger WM, Gifford RW, Eisenhofer GF. Pathophysiology of pheochromocytoma. In: Izzo JL, Black HR, eds. Hypertension Primer: Essentials of High Blood Pressure, 3rd ed. Baltimore: Lippincott Williams and Wilkins, 2002, pp. 148–150.

McNamara DM, MacGowan GA, London B. Clinical importance of beta-adrenoceptor polymorphisms in cardiovascular disease. Am J Pharmacogenomics 2002;2(2):73–78.

Miller ER III. Geographic patterns of hypertension in the United States. In: Izzo JL, Black HR, eds. Hypertension Primer: Essentials of High Blood Pressure, 3rd ed. Baltimore: Lippincott Williams and Wilkins, 2002, pp. 233–235.

Nabel E. Genomic medicine: cardiovascular disease. N Engl J Med 2003; 349:60–72.

Nolan PM, Peters J, Strivens M, et al. A systematic, genome-wide, phenotype-driven mutagenesis programme for gene function studies in the mouse. Nat Genet 2000;25(4):440–443.

Pradervand S, Wang Q, Burnier M, et al. A mouse model for Liddle's syndrome. J Am Soc Nephrol 1999;10(12):2527–2533.

Rapp JP. Genetic analysis of inherited hypertension in the rat. Physiol Rev 2000;80(1):135–172.

Rossier BC, Pradervand S, Schild L, Hummler E. Epithelial sodium channel and the control of sodium balance: interaction between genetic and environmental factors. Annu Rev Physiol 2002;64:877–897.

Rubattu S, Struk B, Kreutz R, Volpe M, Lindpaintner K. Animal models of genetic hypertension: what can we learn for human hypertension? Clin Exp Pharm Physiol 1995;22(12):S386–S393.

Shimkets RA, Warnock DG, Bositis CM, et al. Liddle's syndrome: heritable human hypertension caused by mutations in the beta subunit of the epithelial sodium channel. Cell 1994;79(3):407–414.

Simon DB, Karet FE, Hamdan JM, DiPietro A, Sanjad SA, Lifton RP. Bartter's syndrome, hypokalaemic alkalosis with hypercalciuria, is caused by mutations in the Na-K-2Cl cotransporter *NKCC2*. Nat Genet 1996;13(2):183–188.

Stoll M, Jacob HJ. Genetic rat models of hypertension: relationship to human hypertension. Curr Hypertens Rep 2001;3(2):157–164.

Sugiyama F, Yagami K, Paigen B. Mouse models of blood pressure regulation and hypertension. Curr Hypertens Rep 2001;3(1):41–48.

Sutherland DJ, Ruse JL, Laidlaw JC. Hypertension, increased aldosterone secretion and low plasma renin activity relieved by dexamethasone. CMAJ 1966;95(22):1109–1119.

Tiret L, Rigat B, Visvikis S, et al. Evidence, from combined segregation and linkage analysis, that a variant of the angiotensin I-converting enzyme (ACE) gene controls plasma ACE levels. Am J Hum Genet 1992;51(1):197–205.

Turner ST, Schwartz GL, Chapman AB, Boerwinkle E. Use of gene markers to guide antihypertensive therapy. Curr Hypertens Rep 2001; 3(5): 410–415.

Vincent M, Samani NJ, Gauguier D, Thompson JR, Lathrop GM, Sassard J. A pharmacogenetic approach to blood pressure in Lyon hypertensive rats. A chromosome 2 locus influences the response to a calcium antagonist. J Clin Invest 1997;100(8):2000–2006.

Ward R. Familial aggregation and genetic epidemiology of blood pressure. In: Laragh JH, Brenner BM, eds. Hypertension: Pathophysiology, Diagnosis, and Management. New York, NY: Raven Press Limited, 1990, pp. 81–100.

Watson R, DiPette DJ. Experimental models of hypertension. In: Izzo JL, Black HR, eds. Hypertension Primer: Essentials of High Blood Pressure, 3rd ed. Baltimore: Lippincott Williams and Wilkins, 2002, pp. 120–122.

Wright FA, O'Connor DT, Roberts E, et al. Genome scan for blood pressure loci in mice. Hypertension 1999;34(4 Pt 1):625–630.

Yagil Y, Yagil C. Genetic models of hypertension in experimental animals. Exp Nephrol 2001;9(1):1–9.

17 Cardiac Hypertrophy

THOMAS FORCE AND JEFFERY D. MOLKENTIN

SUMMARY

Pathological cardiac hypertrophy develops in response to stresses, and can be concentric, eccentric, or both. An excess pressure load placed on the heart, for example, resulting from uncorrected hypertension or valvular disease, results in concentric hypertrophy. This hypertrophy is initially believed to be adaptive, normalizing systolic wall stress, though it is not clear that hypertrophy is necessary to maintain systolic function in the face of moderately elevated pressure loads. Eccentric hypertrophy results most often from volume loads such as those in valvular insufficiency. Finally, the hypertrophy that occurs in the remote noninfarcted myocardium, as part of the remodeling process following a myocardial infarction, may be both concentric and eccentric.

Key Words: Cardiac hypertrophy; concentric; eccentric; mechanical deformation; mTOR; NFAT; protein synthesis; reprogramming.

INTRODUCTION

Cells that are terminally differentiated, by definition, cannot undergo hyperplastic growth. Rather, normal growth of these cells, which include cardiomyocytes, is hypertrophic. This form of hypertrophy, termed physiological hypertrophy, is both concentric (characterized by addition of sarcomeres in parallel, leading to increased width of the myocyte) and eccentric (characterized by the addition of sarcomeres in series, leading to increased length of the myocyte). Pathological cardiac hypertrophy develops in response to stresses, and can be concentric, eccentric, or both. An excess pressure load placed on the heart, for example, resulting from uncorrected hypertension or valvular disease, results in concentric hypertrophy. This hypertrophy is initially believed to be adaptive, normalizing systolic wall stress, though it is not clear that hypertrophy is necessary to maintain systolic function in the face of moderately elevated pressure loads. Eccentric hypertrophy results most often from volume loads such as those in valvular insufficiency. Finally, the hypertrophy that occurs in the remote noninfarcted myocardium, as part of the remodeling process following a myocardial infarction (MI), may be both concentric and eccentric.

If the load placed on the heart is not normalized (such as via effective antihypertensive therapy), the heart may continue to hypertrophy, eventually leading to elevated filling pressures and the so-called diastolic heart failure. The hypertrophied heart may also begin to decompensate, leading to progressive dilatation, systolic dysfunction, and heart failure on that basis. Not surprisingly, left-ventricular hypertrophy is a significant risk factor for the development of heart failure, increasing the risk of this end point by 6- to 17-fold. Furthermore, within 5 yr of the first detection of left-ventricular hypertrophy, one-third of men and one-fourth of women are dead, usually from cardiac disease.

Given the importance of hypertrophy as a cardiac risk factor, investigators have begun to identify the molecular pathways that regulate the cardiac hypertrophic response in an attempt to identify novel pharmacological targets of potential clinical relevance. The focus of these investigations has been on the cell surface receptors for agonists that are believed to trigger the hypertrophic response, such as receptors for angiotensin (Ang)-II, endothelin (ET)-1, and α- and β-adrenergic agents, and therapies directed at the Ang-II receptor have been effective in regressing hypertrophy and in reducing cardiovascular end points even in patients with diabetes. However, given the vast number of agents that have been reported to induce hypertrophy (*see* below), and the increasing evidence that hypertrophy is multifactorial in origin, focus has shifted to intracellular signaling pathways that may function as final common pathways necessary for the hypertrophic response, irrespective of the inciting stimuli. With the rapid advances in the development of small molecule inhibitors of components of these pathways that can be used in vivo, it is essential to understand the signaling networks that regulate hypertrophic growth.

The hypertrophic response requires a dramatic reprograming of gene expression to upregulate gene products necessary for the growth of the cardiomyocyte. These include genes encoding contractile elements and proteins of the basic transcriptional and translational machinery that allow new protein production), and genes that encode proteins that remodel the extracellular matrix (e.g., matrix metalloproteases), allowing growth to proceed. Reprograming of gene expression occurs in response to specific growth signals that are generated from a multitude of sources and include soluble factors (growth factors and neurohormonal mediators), or biomechanical forces (stretch of the myocyte induced, for example, by an acute MI or an acute pressure load). To reprogram gene expression, these signals must be sensed at the cardiomyocyte membrane, and transmitted into the interior of the

From: *Principles of Molecular Medicine, Second Edition*
Edited by: M. S. Runge and C. Patterson © Humana Press, Inc., Totowa, NJ

cell, and eventually into the nucleus. This process is called signal transduction. This chapter introduces the field of signal transduction, specifically as it applies to hypertrophy of the heart, and describes how gene expression becomes reprogramed. Many growth factors trigger growth of cardiomyocytes, and an even larger number of signaling molecules mediate the growth response. The complexity of the field makes it impossible to cover all pathways involved in the hypertrophic response; two pathways are reviewed for which strong evidence exists implicating components of the pathway in both physiological and pathological hypertrophic responses: the calcineurin pathway and the phospho-inositide 3-kinase (PI3-K)/Akt pathway and its interactions with the mammalian target of rapamycin (mTOR) pathway, which has been implicated in cellular growth of a wide variety of species. In each case, the role of these pathways is evaluated in the rapidly growing field of mouse models of human disease. Finally, dysregulation of these pathways in the hearts of patients with advanced heart failure is reviewed, and potential targets for the treatment of heart failure are discussed.

STIMULI TRIGGERING THE HYPERTROPHIC RESPONSE

Two types of stimuli are thought to trigger the hypertrophic response, mechanical deformation of the membrane (cell stretch) and growth-promoting ligands binding to their cognate receptors in the myocyte cell membrane, though mechanical deformation activates ligand/receptor interactions as well.

MECHANICAL DEFORMATION Stretch of cardiomyocytes in culture leads to protein synthesis and a pattern of gene transcription that resembles the load-induced hypertrophic response in vivo. Stretch triggers these responses both via the direct activation of signaling molecules and by inducing the release of prohypertrophic agonists that appear to be of paramount importance in the maintenance of the response. The identity of the stretch "sensor" is not known. However, stretch may directly activate integrin signaling and stretch-activated ion channels, and either or both of these could be the sensor of membrane deformation. Heterotrimeric G proteins (Gq and Gi), which transduce signals from prohypertrophic factors released following stretch (see Humoral Factors), and possibly small G proteins, are activated so early after stretch that it is possible that these are also directly activated. One critical consequence of activation of these proximal mediators of the stretch response is an increase in cytosolic calcium concentration, necessary for activating calcineurin (discussed later). Only when the sensors are identified will the mechanisms be understood by which stretch activates cytosolic signaling pathways. In most biological response pathways, however, a stretch signal gradually accommodates so that the response is lost unless a new or greater stimulus is applied. Thus, additional factors are needed to maintain the response and to induce long-term hypertrophic growth, and these factors may be humoral.

HUMORAL FACTORS One of the central tenets of hypertrophic signaling is that membrane deformation induces the release of growth factors that act in an autocrine or paracrine fashion to amplify hypertrophic responses. Ang-II was reported to be released by stretched cardiomyocytes in culture, and autocrine/paracrine effects of Ang-II were reported to be, at least in part, responsible for the hypertrophic response of cardiomyocytes to cell stretch. Ang-II activates prohypertrophic signaling pathways via two mechanisms, one triggered directly by the receptor and its associated heterotrimeric G protein, Gq (see below), and the other triggered by transactivation of growth factor receptors with intrinsic tyrosine

kinase activity, most notably the epidermal growth factor receptor. Ang-II induces a cytosolic calcium transient (and production of reactive oxygen species) that activates a metalloprotease that releases heparin-binding epidermal growth factor-like growth factor. This then binds to its receptor, activating additional signaling pathways not directly activated by the Ang-II receptor. A second group of prohypertrophic factors released by mechanical stretch are the IL-6 family of cytokines, including cardiotrophin-1.

The insulin-like growth factor (IGF)-1 axis, including growth hormone, which acts in large part via inducing production of IGF-1, is the dominant regulator of normal postnatal growth of the mammalian heart, but IGF-1 may also play a role in pathological hypertrophy. In pathological states, IGF-1 is released in response to a variety of stimuli that induce remodeling including pressure overload and following MI. IGF-1 signaling is also activated in the remodeled hearts of patients with advanced heart failure.

Many of the prohypertrophic peptides, including Ang-II, ET-1, and α-adrenergic agents bind to receptors that are linked to heterotrimeric G proteins (i.e., consists of three subunits, α, β, and γ) of the Gq family. These G proteins convert receptor activation into mobilization of intracellular signaling pathways, and are the initial trigger for downstream events. Overexpression specifically in the heart of the α-subunit of Gq (the subunit that activates most of the signaling pathways downstream of receptors coupled to Gq) or of an activated mutant of αq led to cardiac hypertrophy. Expressing a peptide that inhibited Gq-dependent signaling significantly limits the hypertrophic response to pressure overload in vivo. Conditional inactivation of the gene encoding the α-subunit of Gq (and the related G_{11}) blunts the hypertrophic response. These studies confirm a critical role for Gq in hypertrophic signaling and in the hypertrophic response to pressure overload, and also support a central role for Gq-coupled receptors and their ligands in this process.

INTRACELLULAR SIGNALING PATHWAYS

There are two essential features of hypertrophic growth: reprograming of gene expression and protein synthesis. Each is regulated by a series of intracellular pathways activated by events at the membrane as described above. Each component is considered separately, though they are inextricably intertwined.

REPROGRAMMING OF GENE EXPRESSION To hypertrophy, the cardiomyocyte must upregulate the expression of a number of genes including those encoding components of the sarcomere and more specific growth-related and stress-induced genes. Other genes are downregulated as part of the response. Characteristic of the response is a re-establishment of a gene program that is often described as "embryonic" or "fetal" because several of the re-expressed genes are normally expressed in utero, but expression declines rapidly after birth. The genes induced by the hypertrophic response are often divided into three groups based on their time of expression: immediate early, intermediate, and late. Immediate early genes include the neurohormonal mediator, brain natriuretic peptide, and several stress-induced genes or genes involved in growth control. These include c-fos, c-jun, c-myc, egr-1, and heat shock protein 70. Intermediate response genes include atrial natriuretic peptide, angiotensinogen, and several sarcomeric components, β-myosin heavy chain (β-MHC) (and corresponding downregulation of α-MHC), myosin light chain-2, and skeletal α-actin (replacing cardiac α-actin). Late response genes include angiotensin converting enzyme and the Na/Ca exchanger.

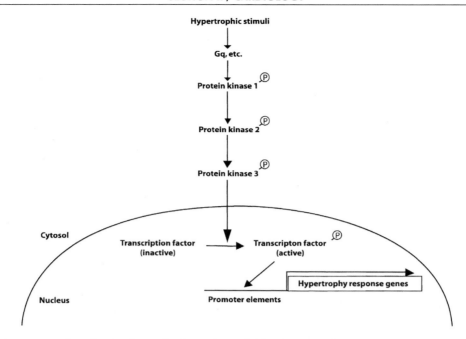

Figure 17-1   Schematic representation of a signal transduction pathway linking the cell surface receptor to nuclear events. Hypertrophic stimuli sensed at the membrane lead via a variety of signal transducers (e.g., Gq) to the activation of a protein kinase at the top of a multitiered cascade of protein kinases. This kinase phosphorylates kinase 2 in the cascade that in turn phosphorylates kinase 3. Kinase 3 then phosphorylates one or more transcription factors that bind to promoter elements in the regulatory regions of various "hypertrophic response genes" and activate gene expression. This multitiered cascade serves both to amplify the signal (one kinase molecule at each level activates many molecules at the next level) and to prevent the need for kinase 1 to translocate to the nucleus each time it is activated.

Reprograming of gene expression requires signal transmission from the cell membrane, in which the initiating stimulus is generated, to the nucleus. This is generally accomplished by linear cascades of proteins, most commonly protein kinases (but also the protein phosphatase calcineurin [*see* below]), phosphorylating and activating one another in sequence, culminating in the phosphorylation, and activation of one or more transcription factors (Fig. 17-1). The transcription factors then bind to promoter elements, specific DNA sequences, usually of approx 6–12 basepairs in length, within the promoters of genes. Thus each transcription factor usually targets several genes. The net result of the activation of the entire set of genes is the hypertrophic response. To illustrate how gene expression is reprogramed, the calcineurin-nuclear factor of activated T-cells (NFAT) signaling pathway, implicated as a key regulator of stress-induced hypertrophic growth, is used (Fig. 17-2). However, first the mouse models used to evaluate the role of signaling pathways in various disease states are reviewed and their advantages and disadvantages are examined.

Mouse Models of Cardiac Disease   Two basic models are employed: transgenic models and so-called "knockouts." Transgenics generally express a gene of interest specifically in the heart by expressing it under the control of a promoter that is only active in cardiac myocytes. The most commonly employed promoter is the α-MHC promoter. Expression from this promoter is constitutive. The gene of interest can encode the normal gene, a constitutively active mutant of the gene (e.g., a protein kinase that does not require activation by an upstream regulator), or a dominant inhibitory mutant of the gene (such a protein kinase that cannot be activated, interferes with the normal functioning of the pathway by binding to and sequestering upstream activators and downstream targets of the normal kinase). A number of different pathways have been implicated in regulating the hypertrophic response. However, many of these studies

relied exclusively on transgenic overexpression of a signaling molecule in the heart. Because the level of expression of the transgene is often many-fold higher than the level of the endogenous protein, producing nonphysiological levels of activation of normal downstream targets, caution in interpreting these studies is needed. In addition, gross overexpression of a transgene can lead to "cross talk" with other signaling pathways that are not normally regulated by that transgene. That said, many signaling pathways have fairly striking fidelity so that cross talk is often minimal and valuable information can be obtained using an overexpression approach. Transgenes have been expressed conditionally. That is, expression can be regulated by the investigator to occur at specific times. This approach may reduce the long-term adaptations that can occur with constitutive expression of a transgene.

The optimal proof of a role for a specific signaling factor in hypertrophic growth is that a specific molecule is sufficient to induce the hypertrophic response using a transgenic approach and that the molecule must also be demonstrated as necessary for the response. On rare occasions this can be accomplished with pharmacological inhibitors but usually it is done with strategies leading to deletion of a gene of interest (e.g., the complementary studies of the role of Gq in hypertrophic growth previously discussed). This is a much more difficult task because deleting a gene is technically much more demanding than creating a transgenic animal. In addition, the approach is often compounded by embryonic or neonatal lethality if the gene of interest serves essential functions in the organism. This problem has been addressed by an ingenious method (e.g., in the studies on Gq) employing transgenic (or adenovirus-mediated) expression of a viral protein, the Cre recombinase, expression of which can be induced at desired times in the life of the mouse. Cre then excises the target gene producing a so-called conditional knockout.

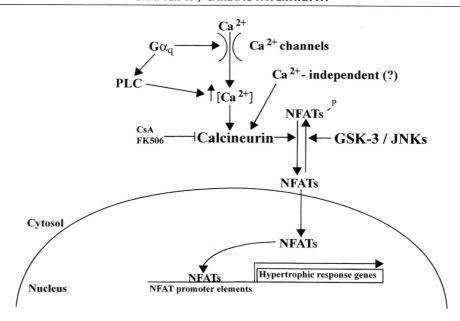

Figure 17-2 Schematic representation of the calcineurin/nuclear factor of activated T cells (NFAT) pathway. Diagram shows the possible sources of Ca^{2+} necessary for the activation of calcineurin and negative regulators of NFAT nuclear localization (GSK-3 and JNKs). The possible contribution of Ca^{2+}-independent inputs into calcineurin activation is also shown. *See* The Calcineurin-NFAT Signaling Pathway Reprograms Gene Expression for details.

Another problem with gene deletion strategies to study function of a gene is that many genes involved in hypertrophic signaling are members of multigene families and deletion of one is compensated for by the other family members. Crossing a mouse with one deleted gene with a second mouse with the other gene deleted can produce the desired knockout of all alleles within the family, but increases the likelihood of embryonic or neonatal lethality. Proving that a gene is necessary for a specific response, such as hypertrophy, remains an essential element in the evaluation of the role of a specific protein in that response.

The Calcineurin-NFAT Signaling Pathway Reprograms Gene Expression The calcineurin-NFAT pathway can serve to illustrate how gene expression is reprogramed. This pathway (Fig. 17-2) in a number of different models regulates hypertrophic growth. Calcineurin (also known as protein phosphatase 2B) is a calcium-calmodulin-activated protein phosphatase. It is uniquely activated by sustained elevations in intracellular calcium. Calcineurin specifically dephosphorylates proteins previously phosphorylated on serine or threonine residues. Calcineurin consists of a 59–63 kDa catalytic subunit referred to as calcineurin A, a 19 kDa calcium binding protein called calcineurin B, and the calcium binding protein calmodulin. Three mammalian calcineurin A catalytic genes have been identified (α, β, γ) that are highly homologous to one another. The calcineurin Aα and Aβ gene products are expressed in a ubiquitous pattern throughout the body, whereas calcineurin Aγ expression is more restricted.

Calcineurin catalytic activity is inhibited by the immunosuppressive drugs cyclosporine (Cs) A and FK506 through complexes with immunophilin protein. Thus, calcineurin plays a critical role in the regulation of T-cell reactivity and cytokine gene expression. Once activated, calcineurin directly dephosphorylates members of the NFAT family of transcription factors. When phosphorylated, NFATs are retained in the cytosol. Dephosphorylation by calcineurin exposes nuclear localization signals, promoting their translocation into the nucleus. Once in the nucleus, NFAT family members participate in the transcriptional induction of various immune response genes.

Calcineurin was identified as a hypertrophic signaling factor in the heart suggesting conservation in its function as a reactive signaling factor in multiple cell types. For example, overexpression of an activated form of calcineurin in the hearts of transgenic mice induced a profound hypertrophic response (two- to threefold increase in heart size) that rapidly progressed to dilated heart failure within 2–3 mo. These data demonstrated that calcineurin was sufficient to induce hypertrophy, and identified calcineurin as a potential causative factor associated with the transition to decompensation and heart failure. Investigation has focused on the evaluation of whether calcineurin is also necessary for the hypertrophic response to physiologically relevant stimuli. Hypertrophic agonists (e.g., phenylephrine, Ang-II, and ET-1) led to increased calcineurin enzymatic activity in cultured cardiomyocytes, and treatment of cultured neonatal cardiomyocytes with the calcineurin inhibitory agent CsA attenuated agonist-induced hypertrophy in vitro. Furthermore, calcineurin enzymatic activity and protein levels were upregulated in hearts from juvenile tropomodulin transgenic mice, a model of dilated heart failure. Similarly, increased cardiac calcineurin activity has been reported in hearts in which hypertrophy was induced by aortic banding, exercise, or salt feeding of salt-sensitive hypertensive rats. Other studies have examined the activity of calcineurin in samples from failing or hypertrophied human hearts. Analysis of hypertrophied human hearts or failing hearts because of ischemic or idiopathic dilated cardiomyopathy revealed a significant increase in calcineurin activity. Studies in patients with hypertrophic obstructive cardiomyopathy and aortic stenosis demonstrated a significant increase in cardiac calcineurin activity associated with a differentially processed form of the calcineurin catalytic subunit in the heart, presumably because of partial proteolysis. Collectively, these observations have demonstrated a link between cardiac hypertrophy and failure and the activation of a pivotal reactive signaling molecule in the heart, calcineurin.

Two approaches have been employed to determine whether calcineurin is necessary for the hypertrophic response in vivo, pharmacological inhibition with CsA or FK506 and gene targeting. Although CsA can attenuate agonist-induced cardiomyocyte hypertrophy in vitro, its effectiveness in vivo is somewhat more controversial, particularly when the hypertrophy is induced by pressure overload. Approximately 20 individual reports have shown that inhibition of calcineurin with either CsA or FK506 can antagonize cardiac hypertrophy and/or disease progression in a variety of rodent models. Thus, the majority of pharmacological animal studies support a role for calcineurin in the hypertrophic response, and the few negative accounts may reflect factors such as drug dosage, differences in the surgical preparations, sex, age, or type of animal model.

As with most pharmacological inhibitors, however, CsA and FK506 have targets other than calcineurin and inhibition of these targets, rather than calcineurin, could in theory account for the observed effects of the drugs on hypertrophy. To address the issue of specificity, targeted inhibition of calcineurin was achieved by creating a transgenic mouse overexpressing endogenous inhibitors of calcineurin. In one set of studies, the noncompetitive calcineurin inhibitory domains from the calcineurin interacting proteins, Cain/Cabin-1 and AKAP79, were expressed and in the other, muscle-enriched calcineurin inhibitory proteins MCIP1 and MCIP2 (DSCR1 and ZAKI-4) were expressed. Both models had reduced hypertrophy in response to pressure overload. In addition, transgenic mice expressing a dominant inhibitory mutant of calcineurin within the heart also demonstrated reduced cardiac hypertrophy to stress stimuli (aortic banding). Mice deleted for *calcineurinAβ* were generated and had reduced cardiac calcineurin activity that was associated with an impaired hypertrophic response to Ang-II infusion, isoproterenol infusion, or abdominal aortic constriction. These data extend the transgenic approaches discussed, and more specifically implicate the *calcineurinAβ* gene in regulating the hypertrophic response.

Calcineurin Targets Regulating the Hypertrophic Response The downstream transcriptional mechanisms whereby calcineurin might function in vivo remain largely uncharacterized. However, both NFAT and myocyte enhancer factor 2 transcriptional regulators are regulated by calcineurin (*see* Fig. 17-2), suggesting obvious candidates for genetic analysis in the heart. The NFAT family consists of five members, four of which (NFATc1-c4) are regulated by calcineurin. Calcineurin activation leads to dephosphorylation and nuclear translocation of NFATs where they activate gene expression. To identify the candidate downstream effectors of calcineurin that might mediate the hypertrophic response, *NFATc3* and *NFATc4* null mice were evaluated. Remarkably, *NFATc3* null mice, but not *NFATc4*, were determined to have impaired hypertrophy induced by activated calcineurin, abdominal aortic constriction, or Ang-II infusion. These data suggest that NFATc3 functions as a necessary transducer of calcineurin signaling in mediating the cardiac hypertrophic response. Collectively, analysis of multiple genetically-modified mouse models with altered calcineurin-NFAT signaling supports that calcineurin is an important regulator of the cardiac hypertrophic response. The calcineurin/NFAT pathway illustrates the paradigm of how a signal (increased cytosolic [Ca^{2+}]) generated in response to deformation of the membrane or to hypertrophic agonist binding to its receptor, activates one signaling

factor (calcineurin), which then dephosphorylates and activates a transcription factor (NFATc3) that, in turn, translocates to the nucleus, reprograms gene expression and, in so doing, regulates hypertrophic responses.

REGULATION OF PROTEIN SYNTHESIS The second key component of hypertrophic growth is the ability to dramatically upregulate protein synthetic capabilities. This is regulated by two complex, interacting pathways: the mTOR pathway, and the PI3-K pathway that, in addition to its role in regulating protein synthesis, also functions in reprograming gene expression. These pathways are essential in determination of cell, organ, and body size (i.e., normal growth) in species as diverse as *Drosophila* and humans. The pathways are also recruited in, and regulate the response to, pathological stress-induced hypertrophic growth (Fig. 17-3). Both the mTOR and PI3-K pathways regulate protein synthesis by modulating the activity of various translation factors, either initiating factors (that initiate the translation of mRNAs into proteins) or elongation factors (responsible for elongation of the polypeptide chain).

The mTOR Pathway mTOR is a protein kinase whose importance is suggested by its conservation in structure and function, throughout evolution, from yeast to human. Rapamycin, a specific inhibitor of mTOR, attenuates the hypertrophic response to pressure overload in mice, demonstrating the importance of mTOR in regulating hypertrophic growth in vivo. Although mTOR is absolutely critical in the regulation of protein synthesis, and studies employing rapamycin have identified specific targets of mTOR that regulate protein synthesis, the mechanisms regulating mTOR activity remain ill-defined. In brief, mTOR is activated when amino acids and energy supplies are plentiful (*see* Fig. 17-3). Teleologically this makes sense because protein translation is an enormous consumer of cell energy, so translation proceeding at times of amino acid or energy deprivation is undesirable. In addition, growth factors, including those leading to cardiac growth such as insulin and IGF-1, also activate mTOR probably via activation of PI3-K signaling.

One of mTOR's major targets is a protein, 4E-binding protein 1, which binds to and inactivates the eukaryotic initiation factor (eIF) 4E, preventing the initiation of translation. When activated, mTOR leads to the phosphorylation of 4E-binding protein 1, causing it to dissociate from eIF4E, thus allowing translation to proceed (*see* Fig. 17-3). A second target activated by mTOR, acting in cooperation with the PI3-K pathway, is the p70S6 kinase that phosphorylates the S6 protein of the small ribosomal subunit. p70S6K may regulate the translation of a specific set of mRNAs, the so-called 5′-TOP (tract of pyrimidines) mRNAs that encode ribosomal proteins. In addition, it may regulate one of the elongation factors, eEF2. The importance of p70S6K in cell and organ growth is illustrated by the marked reduction in cell, organ, and body size in mice deleted for even one of the two p70S6K genes. Furthermore, p70S6K is activated by pressure overload, and it is likely that the ability of rapamycin to block pressure overload hypertrophy is, in part, because of the inhibition of p70S6K activation by rapamycin.

The PI3-K Pathway The PI3-K pathway is also highly conserved throughout evolution (*see* Fig. 17-3). This pathway is remarkable because virtually every component has been shown in animal models in vivo to regulate cell and organ growth, including growth of the heart. The pathway is activated by most (if not all) of the agonists implicated in inducing cardiac hypertrophy including pressure overload. When activated, the PI3-K phosphorylates

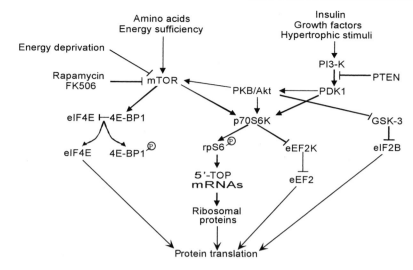

Figure 17-3 Schematic representation of the PI3-K and mTOR pathways. *See* the P13-K Pathway for details. rpS6, S6 ribosomal protein; eEF2K, the eukaryotic elongation factor 2 kinase that phosphorylates and inactivates eEF2 (eEF2K is inhibited by p70S6K).

the membrane phosholipid, phosphatidylinositol, at the 3′ position of the inositol ring, leading to the recruitment of the protein kinase, Akt (also known as protein kinase B [PKB]) to the cell membrane via interactions of a specific domain of PKB/Akt (the plekstrin homology domain) with the 3′-phosphorylated lipid. This brings PKB/Akt into proximity to its activator, the 3′-phosphoinositide-dependent protein kinase-1, which phosphorylates and activates PKB/Akt (in addition to the p70S6K discussed). PKB/Akt then plays a role in activating mTOR and, consequently, p70S6K and the protein translation machinery. Hence, it is probably not surprising that PI3-K, phosphoinositide-dependent protein kinase-1, and PKB/Akt all regulate cell and organ size, including size of the heart. One of the more striking cardiac-specific transgenic models is the mouse overexpressing PKB/Akt which has a markedly enlarged heart. Although activation of the translational machinery is probably an important mechanism driving the increased heart size in these mice, PKB/Akt also regulates transcription factors, either directly (e.g., members of the Forkhead family) or indirectly (via regulation of glycogen synthase kinase-3 [GSK-3]) that likely play a role in reprogramming gene expression in response to hypertrophic stress.

PKB/Akt regulates GSK-3, which also plays a role in regulating normal and pathological stress-induced growth of the heart. GSK-3β (and likely GSK-3α as well) is a negative regulator of cardiac growth. Transgenic animals expressing GSK-3β have dramatic reductions in normal cardiac growth and also have a markedly reduced hypertrophic response to pressure overload. Inhibition of GSK-3β, mediated by PKB/Akt, is necessary for the hypertrophic response to a number of agonists. GSK-3β-mediated inhibition of growth occurs via several mechanisms. For example, GSK-3β negatively regulates activity of the initiation factor, eIF2B. Thus inhibition of GSK-3β may be important for enhancing protein translation. However, GSK-3β also inhibits the activity of a number of transcription factors. Because several factors have been implicated in growth, including growth of the heart, GSK-3β may be particularly important in the reprograming of gene expression and relatively less important in regulating protein translation. This might make GSK-3β an attractive target for therapeutic intervention because

therapies targeting the translation machinery can be expected to have significant toxicity with long-term use. The GSK-3β targets include the NFATs, and thus GSK-3β acts in opposition to the calcineurin pathway (Fig. 17-2). Phosphorylation of NFATs by GSK-3β leads to exclusion of NFATs from the nucleus, preventing access to target genes. When the GSK-3β transgenic was bred with the calcineurin transgenic, hypertrophy was markedly reduced. Other known growth regulators negatively regulated by GSK-3β include c-Myc, GATA-4, β-catenin, and c-Jun.

The PI3-K pathway is negatively regulated by a phosphatase that dephosphorylates 3-phosphorylated phosphoinositides at the 3′ position called phosphatase and tensin homolog (PTEN) (*see* Fig. 17-3). Overexpression of a catalytically inactive mutant of PTEN in cultured cardiomyocytes led to cardiomyocyte hypertrophy. Furthermore, conditional inactivation of the PTEN gene in the heart also led to hypertrophy, further supporting a critical role for the PI3-K pathway in regulating cardiomyocyte growth. In summary, the consistency of the message from studies of multiple components of the PI3-K pathway has confirmed a role for this pathway in normal growth and in pathological stress-induced hypertrophic growth. This pathway, acting in concert with the mTOR pathway, is a dominant determinant of cell and organ size in mammals.

OTHER PATHWAYS INVOLVED IN GROWTH REGULATION   As suggested, a large number of signaling pathways have been implicated in the regulation of cardiomyocyte growth. However, either there are insufficient data to support a claim, or the data are too conflicting to make definitive statements concerning their role. This is probably most apparent from the literature on the role of stress-activated mitogen-activated protein (MAP) kinases in the hypertrophic response (Fig. 17-4). These kinases, the c-Jun N-terminal kinases (JNKs) and the p38-MAP kinases, have been exhaustively studied but there remains no consensus on their role, in large part owing to the lack of adequate pharmacological inhibitors that can be used in vivo. As a result, investigators have turned to gene-targeting approaches, but because both of these kinases are members of multigene families, studies have been complicated by functional redundancy, and crosses of knockouts have led to embryonic lethality. It is likely

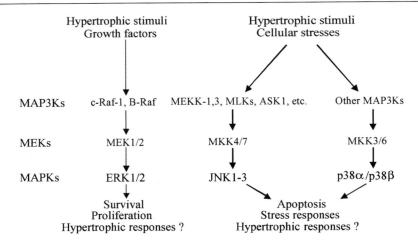

Figure 17-4 Schematic representation of the major MAPK pathways. The three-tiered kinase cascade consists of a MAP kinase kinase kinase (MAP3K) that phosphorylates and activates a MAP kinase kinase (also called MAPK and ERK kinase, MEK), that, in turn, phosphorylates the MAP kinases (MAPK), either the ERKs, JNKs, or p38-MAPKs.

that a definitive conclusion on the role of these kinases in hypertrophic growth awaits the availability of truly specific inhibitors of these kinases, or better yet, inhibitors of specific isoforms of these kinases, because there is evidence that different isoforms (and even different splice variants) may serve different functions within the cell. Assessment of the data suggests that the p38-MAP kinases may be more involved in the progression of heart failure, including remodeling of the matrix, and may play less of a role in hypertrophic growth. If confirmed, they may be attractive drug targets in the failing heart. Other work employing mice deleted for three of the four JNK1/JNK2 alleles suggests that the JNKs may reduce the hypertrophic response to pressure overload, in part by targeting NFATs much as GSK-3β does.

The extracellular signal-regulated kinases family (ERK) of MAP kinases (*see* Fig. 17-4) are also activated by hypertrophic stimuli. For studies of the role of the ERKs in hypertrophy, relatively specific inhibitors of the mitogen-activated protein kinase (MAPK) and ERK (MEKs) immediately upstream of the ERKs are available. Generally studies have found them to inhibit at least part of the hypertrophic response of cardiomyocytes in culture. Cardiac-specific overexpression of MEK1 (one of the immediate upstream activators of the ERKs) produced concentric cardiac hypertrophy, but unlike most other models, such as the calcineurin transgenic, the MEK1 transgenic animals did not progress to contractile failure. These data raised the concept of "beneficial" hypertrophy vs "detrimental" hypertrophy by clearly demonstrating that hypertrophy need not inexorably progress to heart failure, possibly because the ERKs (in contrast to many other prohypertrophic signaling molecules including calcineurin, the JNKs, and the p38-MAP kinases) are in many circumstances, cytoprotective. Of note, hypertrophy induced by overexpression of PI3-K also leads to hypertrophy without heart failure, and the PI3-K pathway, like the ERK pathway, is cytoprotective. These data suggest a potential approach to the treatment of patients with heart failure wherein pathways promoting progression of heart failure are inhibited whereas those prohypertrophic pathways that are also cytoprotective are stimulated.

The PI3-K and mTOR pathways are critical regulators of cell and organ growth via effects on the activity of several transcription factors regulating expression of hypertrophic response and on the general protein synthesis machinery. Calcineurin is another

important regulator that appears to act largely via effects on the NFAT family of transcription factors. Although other pathways have been implicated, data supporting an important role for these other pathways in physiological or pathological hypertrophy are not nearly as convincing. Thus it seems likely as drugs become available for the treatment of hypertrophic disorders, the initial focus will be on the components of the calcineurin and PI3-K/mTOR pathways. Whether long-term inhibition of these pathways, which regulate basic cellular responses of all cells in the body, will be tolerated is unknown. Alternative approaches, such as gene therapy, which can be delivered in an organ-specific (and even cell type-specific) manner, or organ-specific drug delivery may be necessary to target these pathways safely.

ALTERATIONS IN SIGNALING IN THE DISEASED HUMAN HEART

Discussion of the signaling profile of the hearts of experimental animals exposed to pressure overload raises two questions: How do the signaling alterations seen in the hearts of these animals compare with signaling alterations in the hearts of patients with hypertrophy or heart failure? Is there any evidence that abnormalities in these clinical scenarios are a cause of heart failure (as opposed to a consequence of the heart failure) and, therefore, will manipulating their activity alter the progression of disease?

One study has examined the signaling profile of hypertrophied hearts. Patients were scheduled to be transplant donors but for various reasons were not considered appropriate. Several had significant cardiac hypertrophy, allowing a comparison of the signaling profiles in those hearts vs normal hearts that were also rejected as donors. Of the signaling factors examined (calcineurin, ERK1/2, JNK, p38-MAP kinase, Akt, and GSK-3), the only factor consistently found to be activated in the hypertrophied hearts was calcineurin. Of note, patients with hypertrophy clearly had hypertension, but they were not suspected of having any cardiac disorder and in all cases, systolic function was not depressed. Therefore, clinically, they would be described as "compensated" hypertrophy. These data raised calcineurin as one potential therapeutic target in this phase of the disease.

In contrast to the limited data available on hearts with compensated hypertrophy, several studies have examined the signaling profile of hearts explanted from patients with advanced failure either going to transplant or undergoing left-ventricular assist device placement before transplant. These signaling factors were examined in at least one study: calcineurin, ERK1/2, JNKs, p38-MAP kinases, ERK5, the MAP kinase phosphatases (which inactivate the MAP kinases), Akt, GSK-3, and a signaling pathway activated by Ang-II and cytokines, the Janus kinase/signal transducer, and activator of transcription pathway. Where examined, calcineurin expression and activity were increased, though not to the same degree as in the hypertrophied hearts. Unfortunately, no clear consensus has emerged from the studies examining the MAP kinase pathways. The most consistent results appear to be for p38-MAP kinase activity, with three studies reporting activation of p38-MAP kinases in ischemic cardiomyopathy, and only one reporting inhibition. In contrast, in idiopathic cardiomyopathy, p38-MAPK activity has generally been reported to be decreased or unchanged; only one reported activation, although the magnitude of activation was very low. No consistent results have been reported for the JNKs and ERKs. Single reports examined the other factors. In these, ERK5 was inhibited and the MAP kinase phosphatases were activated. Akt was also found to be activated, irrespective of the etiology of the heart failure, and accordingly, its downstream target, GSK-3β, was inhibited. This profile suggested that the heart may be attempting to mount a hypertrophic response in the face of severe contractile dysfunction.

Thus, a signaling profile of the failing heart cannot be defined and it is unclear whether any signaling alterations cause or are consequential to the heart failure. It is unclear what if any effect manipulating these pathways would have on the progression of disease. Hearts that have been mechanically unloaded with left ventricular assist device show changes in activity of MAP kinases, with ERK1/2 and JNK activity decreasing and p38-MAP kinase activity increasing, concomitant with a decrease in cardiomyocyte size (i.e., regression of hypertrophy) and a decline in the rate of myocyte apoptosis. However, it is unclear if the regression of hypertrophy and reduction in apoptosis is because of the changes in activity of these MAP kinases.

Finally, the complexity of the heart failure signaling abnormalities and the changing activities of various pathways at various times in the progression of disease (as evidenced by the differences in signaling in the hypertrophied vs failing hearts) create uncertainty and lead to significant challenges for translational research. Patients with compensated hypertrophy vs advanced heart failure were at different ends of the pathophysiological spectrum of heart failure, and between these points, including the transition to and early progression of heart failure, very little data exists as to which pathways might be reasonable targets. It is likely, however, that interventions at different points in the progression of heart failure will have to focus on different targets, and it is not clear that these interventions will be equally or uniformly successful. Furthermore, the heterogeneity of signaling abnormalities, even among patients with the same clinical diagnosis, suggests that as has been proposed for cancer therapy directed at protein kinase pathways, therapy may need to be defined by the kinase "profile" of the individual patient rather than the clinical diagnosis. Otherwise, promising therapies may be discarded as ineffective because they were used in the wrong patients. Given the aggressive pursuit of inhibitors of these pathways by the pharmaceutical/biotechnology industry, the tools to be able to address these questions should be forthcoming.

SELECTED REFERENCES

Adams JW, Sakata Y, Davis MG, et al. Enhanced Gαq signaling: a common pathway mediates cardiac hypertrophy and apoptotic heart failure. Proc Natl Acad Sci USA 1998;95:10,140–10,145.

Ahkter SA, Luttrell LM, Rockman HA, Iaccarino G, Lefkowitz RJ, Koch WJ. Targeting the receptor-Gq interface to inhibit in vivo pressure overload myocardial hypertrophy. Science 1998;280:574–577.

Antos CL, McKinsey TA, Frey N, et al. Activated glycogen synthase kinase-3β suppresses cardiac hypertrophy in vivo. Proc Natl Acad Sci USA 2002;99:907–912.

Beals CR, Sheridan CM, Turck CW, Gardner P, Crabtree GR. Nuclear export of NF-ATc enhanced by glycogen synthase kinase-3. Science 1997;275:1930–1934.

Browne GJ, Proud CG. Regulation of peptide-chain elongation in mammalian cells. Eur J Biochem 2002;269:5360–5368.

Bueno OF, Wilkins BJ, De Windt LJ, Molkentin JD. Impairment of cardiac hypertrophy in CnAβ-deficient mice. Proc Natl Acad Sci USA 2002;99:9398–9403.

Bueno OF, De Windt LJ, Tymitz KM, et al. The MEK1-ERK1/2 signaling pathway promotes compensated cardiac hypertrophy in transgenic mice. EMBO J 2000;19:6341–6350.

Buttini M, Limonta S, Luyten M, Boddeke H. Distribution of calcineurin A isoenzyme mRNAs in rat thymus and kidney. Histochem J 1995; 27:291–299.

Cantley LC, Neel BG. New insights into tumor suppression: PTEN suppresses tumor formation by restraining the phosphoinositide 3-kinase/Akt pathway. Proc Natl Acad Sci USA 1999;96:4240–4245.

Chen WS, Xu PZ, Gottlob K, et al. Growth retardation and increased apoptosis in mice with homozygous deletion of the Akt1 gene. Genes Dev 2001;15:2203–2208.

Choukroun G, Hajjar R, Fry S, et al. Regulation of cardiac hypertrophy in vivo by the stress-activated protein kinases/c-Jun NH2-terminal kinases. J Clin Invest 1999;104:391–398.

Coghlan VM, Perrino BA, Howard M, et al. Association of protein kinase A and protein phosphatase 2B with a common anchoring protein. Science 1995;267:108–111.

Cohen P, Frame S. The renaissance of GSK-3. Nat Rev Mol Cell Biol 2001;10:769–776.

Communal C, Colucci WS, Remondino A, et al. Reciprocal modulation of mitogen-activated protein kinases and mitogen-activated protein kinase phosphatase 1 and 2 in failing human myocardium. J Card Fail 2002;8:86–91.

Cook SA, Sugden PH, Clerk A. Activation of c-Jun N-terminal kinases and p38-mitogen-activated protein kinases in human heart failure secondary to ischaemic heart disease. J Mol Cell Cardiol 1999; 31:1429–1431.

Cook SA, Matsui T, Li L, Rosenzweig A. Transcriptional effects of chronic Akt activation in the heart. J Biol Chem 2002;277: 22,528–22,533.

Crabtree GR. Generic signals and specific outcomes: Signaling through Ca2+, calcineurin, and NF-AT. Cell 1999;96:611–614.

Crackower MA, Oudit GY, Kozieradzki I, et al. Regulation of myocardial contractility and cell size by distinct PI3K-PTEN signaling pathways. Cell 2002;110:737–749.

Dahlof B, Devereux R, de Faire U, et al. The losartan intervention for endpoint reduction (LIFE) in hypertension study. Am J Hypertens 1997; 10:705–713.

Dahlof B, Devereux RB, Kjeldsen SE, et al. Cardiovascular morbidity and mortality in the losartan intervention for endpoint reduction in hypertension study (LIFE): a randomized trial against atenolol. Lancet 2002;359:995–1003.

Dancey J, Sausville EA. Issues and progress with protein kinase inhibitors for cancer treatment. Nat Rev Drug Discov 2003;2:296–313.

D'Angelo DD, Sakata Y, Lorenz JH, et al. Transgenic Gαq overexpression induced cardiac contractile failure in mice. Proc Natl Acad Sci USA 1997;94:8121–8126.

Daub H, Weiss FU, Wallasch C, Ullrich A. Role of transactivation of the EGF receptor in signaling by G-protein-coupled receptors. Nature 1996;379:557–560.

De Windt LJ, Lim HW, Bueno OF, et al. Targeted inhibition of calcineurin attenuates cardiac hypertrophy in vivo. Proc Natl Acad Sci USA 2001;98:3322–3327.

Deng L, Huang B, Qin D, Ganguly K, El-Sherif N. Calcineurin inhibition ameliorates structural, contractile, and electrophysiologic consequences of postinfarction remodeling. J Cardiovasc Electrophysiol 2001;12:1055–1061.

Dennis PB, Jaeschke A, Saitoh M, Fowler B, Kozma SC, Thomas G. Mammalian TOR: a homeostatic ATP sensor. Science 2001;294: 1102–1105.

Ding B, Price RL, Borg TK, Weinberg EO, Halloran PF, Lorell BH. Pressure overload induces severe hypertrophy in mice treated with cyclosporine, an inhibitor of calcineurin. Circ Res 1999;84:729–734.

Dolmetsch RE, Lewis RS, Goodnow CC, Healy JI. Differential activation of transcription factors induced by Ca2+ response amplitude and duration. Nature 1997;386:855–858.

Eguchi S, Dempsey PJ, Frank GD, Motley ED, Inagami T. Activation of MAPKs by angiotensin II in vascular smooth muscle cells. J Biol Chem 2001;276:7957–7962.

Eto Y, Yonekura K, Sonoda M, et al. Calcineurin is activated in rat hearts with physiological left ventricular hypertrophy induced by voluntary exercise training. Circulation 2000;101:2134–2137.

Fingar DC, Salama S, Tsou C, Harlow E, Blenis J. Mammalian cell size is controlled by mTOR and its downstream targets S6K1 and 4EBP1/eIF4E. Genes Dev 2002;16:1472–1487.

Flesch M, Margulies KB, Mochmann HC, Engel D, Sivasubramanian N, Mann DL. Differential regulation of mitogen-activated protein kinases in the failing human heart in response to mechanical unloading, Circulation 2001;104:2273–2276.

Force T, Michael A, Kilter H, Haq S. Stretch-activated pathways and left ventricular remodeling. J Card Fail 2002;8:S351–S358.

Frame S, Cohen P. GSK3 takes centre stage more than 20 years after its discovery. Biochem J 2001;359:1–16.

Fuentes JJ, Genesca L, Kingsbury TJ, et al. DSCR1, overexpressed in Down syndrome, is an inhibitor of calcineurin-mediated signaling pathways. Hum Mol Genet 2000;9:1681–1690.

Goldspink PH, McKinney RD, Kimball VA, Geenen DL, Buttrick PM. Angiotensin II induced cardiac hypertrophy in vivo is inhibited by cyclosporin A in adult rats. Mol Cell Biochem 2001;226:83–88.

Graef IA, Mermelstein PG, Stankunas K, et al. L-type calcium channels and GSK-3 regulate the activity of NF-ATc4 in hippocampal neurons. Nature 1999;401:703–708.

Gudi SRP, Lee AA, Clark CB, Frangos JA. Equibiaxial strain and strain rate stimulate early activation of G proteins in cardiac fibroblasts. Am J Physiol 1998;274:C1424–C1428.

Haq S, Choukroun G, Kang ZB, et al. Glycogen synthase kinase-3β is a negative regulator of cardiomyocyte hypertrophy. J Cell Biol 2000; 151:117–129.

Haq S, Choukroun G, Lim HW, et al. Differential activation of signal transduction pathways in human hearts with hypertrophy versus advanced heart failure. Circulation 2001;103:670–677.

Haq S, Michael A, Andreucci M, et al. Stabilization of β-catenin by a Wnt-independent mechanism regulates cardiomyocyte growth. Proc Nat Acad Sci USA 2003;100:4610–4515.

Hill JA, Karimi M, Kutschke W, et al. Cardiac hypertrophy is not a required compensatory response to short-term pressure overload. Circulation 2000;101:2863–2869.

Hill JA, Rothermel B, Yoo KD, et al. Targeted inhibition of calcineurin in pressure-overload cardiac hypertrophy. Preservation of systolic function. J Biol Chem 2002; 277:10,251–10,255.

Ho KK, Levy D, Kannel WB, Pinsky JL. The epidemiology of heart failure: The Framingham study. J Am Coll Cardiol 1993;22:6–13.

Hu H, Sachs F. Stretch-activated ion channels in the heart. J Mol Cell Cardiol 1997;29:1511–1523.

Jiang H, Xiong F, Kong S, Ogawa T, Kobayashi M, Liu JO. Distinct tissue and cellular distribution of two major isoforms of calcineurin. Mol Immunol 1997;34:663–669.

Kannel WB. Prevalence and natural history of electrocardiographic left ventricular hypertrophy. Am J Med 1983;75(Suppl 3A):4–11.

Keller RS, Shai S-Y, Babbitt CJ, et al. Disruption of integrin function in the murine myocardium leads to perinatal lethality, fibrosis, and abnormal cardiac performance. Am J Pathol 2001;158:1079–1090.

Kjeldsen SE, Dahlof B, Devereux RB, et al. Effects of losartan on cardiovascular morbidity and mortality in patients with isolated systolic hypertension and left ventricular hypertrophy: a losartan intervention for endpoint reduction (LIFE) substudy. JAMA 2002;288:1491–1498.

Klee CB, Ren H, Wang X. Regulation of the calmodulin-stimulated protein phosphatase, calcineurin. J Biol Chem 1998;273:13,367–13,370.

Kunisada K, Tone E, Fujio E, Matsui H, Yamauchi-Takihara K, Kishimoto T. Activation of gp130 transduces hypertrophic signals via STAT3 in cardiac myocytes. Circulation 1998;98:346–352.

Kyriakis JM, Avruch J. Sounding the alarm: protein kinase cascades activated by stress and inflammation. J Biol Chem 1996;271: 24,313–24,316.

Lai MM, Burnett PE, Wolosker H, Blackshaw S, Snyder SH. Cain, a novel physiologic protein inhibitor of calcineurin. J Biol Chem 1998;273: 18,325–18,331.

Lawlor MA, Mora A, Ashby PR, et al. Essential role of PDK1 in regulating cell size and development in mice. EMBO J 2002;21:3728–3738.

Lemke LE, Bloem LJ, Fouts R, Esterman M, Sandusky G, Vlahos CJ. Decreased p38 MAPK activity in end-stage failing human myocardium: p38 MAPK alpha is the predominant isoform expressed in human heart. J Mol Cell Cardiol 2001;33:1527–1534.

Levy D, Garrison RJ, Savage DD, Kannel WB, Castelli WP. Prognostic implications of echocardiographically determined left ventricular mass in the Framingham heart study. N Engl J Med 1990;322: 1561–1566.

Liao P, Georgakopoulos D, Kovacs A, et al. The in vivo role of p38 MAP kinases in cardiac remodeling and restrictive cardiomyopathy. Proc Nat Acad Sci USA 2001;98:12,283–12,288.

Lim HW, De Windt LJ, Mante J, et al. Reversal of cardiac hypertrophy in transgenic disease models by calcineurin inhibition. J Mol Cell Cardiol 2000;32:697–709.

Lim HW, De Windt LJ, Steinberg L, et al. Calcineurin expression, activation, and function in cardiac pressure-overload hypertrophy. Circulation 2000;101:2431–2437.

Lim HW, Molkentin JD. Calcineurin and human heart failure. Nat Med 1999;5:246, 247.

Lindholm LH, Ibsen H, Dahlof B, Devereux RB, Beevers G, de Faire U. Cardiovascular morbidity and mortality in patients with diabetes in the losartan intervention for endpoint reduction in hypertension study (LIFE): a randomized trial against atenolol. Lancet 2002;359: 1004–1010.

Lopéz-Rodríguez C, Aramburu J, Rakeman AS, Rao A. NFAT5, a constitutively nuclear NFAT protein that does not cooperate with Fos and Jun. Proc Natl Acad Sci USA 1999;96:7214–7219.

Luo Z, Shyu KG, Gualberto A, Walsh K. Calcineurin and cardiac hypertrophy. Nat Med 1998;10:1092, 1093.

Lupu F, Terwilliger JD, Lee K, Segre GV, Efstratiadis A. Roles of growth hormone and IGF-1 in mouse postnatal growth. Dev Biol 2001;229: 141–162.

MacKenna DA, Dolfi F, Vuori K, Ruoslahti E. ERK and JNK activation by mechanical stretch is integrin-dependent and matrix-specific in rat cardiac fibroblasts. J Clin Invest 1998;101:301–310.

Matsui T, Li L, Wu JC, et al. Phenotypic spectrum caused by transgenic overexpression of activated Akt in the heart. J Biol Chem 2002; 277:22,896–22,901.

McManus EJ, Alessi DR. TSC2: a complex tale of PKB-mediated S6K regulation. Nat Cell Biol 2002;4:E214–E216.

Meguro T, Hong C, Asai K, et al. Cyclosporine attenuates pressure-overload hypertrophy in mice while enhancing susceptibility to decompensation and heart failure. Circ Res 1999;84:735–740.

Mende U, Kagen A, Cohen A, Aramburu J, Schoen FJ, Neer EJ. Transient cardiac expression of constitutively active Gαq leads to hypertrophy and dilated cardiomyopathy by calcineurin-dependent and independent pathways. Proc Natl Acad Sci USA 1998;95:13,893–13,898.

Mervaala E, Muller DN, Park JK, et al. Cyclosporin A protects against angiotensin II-induced end-organ damage in double transgenic rats harboring human renin and angiotensinogen genes. Hypertension 2000;35:360–366.

Michael A, Haq S, Chen X, et al. Glycogen synthase kinase-3β regulates growth, calcium homeostasis, and diastolic function in the heart. J Biol Chem 2004;279:21,383–21,393.

Minamino T, Yujiri T, Terada N, et al. MEKK1 is essential for cardiac hypertrophy and dysfunction induced by Gq, Proc Nat Acad Sci USA 2002;99:3866–3871.

Molkentin JD, Dorn GW. Cytoplasmic signaling pathways that regulate cardiac hypertrophy. Annu Rev Physiol 2001;63:391–426.

Molkentin JD, Lu JR, Antos CL, et al. A calcineurin-dependent transcriptional pathway for cardiac hypertrophy. Cell 1998;93:215–228.

Montagne J, Stewart MJ, Stocker H, Hafen E, Kozma SC, Thomas G. Drosophila SK kinase: a regulator of cell size. Science 1999; 285: 2126–2129.

Morisco C, Seta K, Hardt SE, Lee Y, Vatner SF, Sadoshima J. Glycogen synthase kinase 3β regulates GATA4 in cardiac myocytes. J Biol Chem 2001;276:28,586–28,597.

Morisco C, Zebrowski D, Condorelli G, Tsichlis P, Vatner SF, Sadoshima J. The Akt-glycogen synthase kinase 3β pathway regulates transcription of atrial natriuretic factor induced by β-adrenergic receptor stimulation in cardiac myocytes. J Biol Chem 2000;275:14,466–14,475.

Müller JG, Nemoto S, Laser M, Carabello BA, Menick DR. Calcineurin inhibition and cardiac hypertrophy. Science 1998;282:1007.

Murat A, Pellieux C, Brunner HR, Pedrazzini T. Calcineurin blockade prevents cardiac mitogen-activated protein kinase activation and hypertrophy in renovascular hypertension. J Biol Chem 2000;275: 40, 867–40,873.

Murata M, Fukuda K, Ishida H, et al. Leukemia inhibitory factor, a potent cardiac hypertrophic cytokine. enhances L-type Ca2+ current and [Ca2+]i transient in cardiomyocytes. J Mol Cell Cardiol 1999;31: 237–245.

Muramatsu T, Giri PR, Higuchi S, Kincaid RL. Molecular cloning of a calmodulin-dependent phosphatase from murine testis: identification of a developmentally expressed nonneural isoenzyme. Proc Natl Acad Sci USA 1992;89:529–533.

Ng DC, Court NW, dos Remedios CG, Bogoyevitch MA. Activation of signal transducer and activator of transcription (STAT) pathways in failing human hearts. Cardiovasc Res 2003;57:333–338.

Oh H, Fujio Y, Kunisada K, et al. Activation of phosphatidylinositol 3-kinase through gp130 induces protein kinase B and p70 S6 kinase phosphorylation in cardiac myocytes. J Biol Chem 1998;273: 9703–9710.

Øie EB, Reidar OPF, Clausen H. Attramadal. Cyclosporin A inhibits cardiac hypertrophy and enhances cardiac dysfunction during postinfarction failure in rats. Am J Physiol Heart Circ Physiol 2000;278: 2115–2123.

Pap M, Cooper GM. Role of translation initiation factor 2B in control of cell survival by the phosphatidylinositol 3-kinase/Akt/glycogen synthase kinase-3beta signaling pathway. Mol Cell Biol 2002;22: 578–586.

Pete G, Fuller CR, Oldham JM, et al. Postnatal growth responses to insulin-like growth factor I in insulin receptor substrate-1-deficient mice. Endocrinology 1999;140:5478–5487.

Petrich BG, Molkentin JD, Wang Y. Temporal activation of c-Jun N-terminal kinase in adult transgenic heart via cre-loxP-mediated DNA recombination. FASEB J 2003;17:749–751.

Pham CG, Harpf AE, Keller RS, et al. Striated muscle-specific β1D-integrin and FAK are involved in cardiac myocyte hypertrophic response pathway. Am J Physiol 2000;279:H2916–H2926.

Prenzel N, Zwick E, Daub H, et al. EGF receptor transactivation by G-protein-coupled receptors requires metalloproteinase cleavage of proHB-EGF. Nature 1999;402:884–888.

Proud CG. Regulation of mammalian translation factors by nutrients. Eur J Biochem 2002;269:5338–5349.

Rao A, Luo C, Hogan PG. Transcription factors of the NFAT family: Regulation and function. Annu Rev Immunol 1997;15:707–747.

Ren J, Samson WK, Sowers JR. IGF-1 as a cardiac hormone: Physiological and pathophysiological implications in heart disease. J Mol Cell Cardiol 1999;31:2049–2061.

Ritter O, Hack S, Schuh K, et al. Calcineurin in human heart hypertrophy. Circulation 2002;105:2265–2269.

Rohde J, Heitman J, Cardenas ME. The TOR kinases link nutrient sensing to cell growth. J Biol Chem 2001;276:9583–9586.

Ross RS, Pham CG, Shai S-Y, et al. β1 integrins participate in the hypertrophic response of rat ventricular myocytes. Circ Res 1998;82: 1160–1172.

Rothermel B, Vega RB, Yang J, Wu H, Bassel-Duby R, Williams RS. A protein encoded within the Down syndrome critical region is enriched in striated muscles and inhibits calcineurin signaling. J Biol Chem 2000;275:8719–8725.

Rothermel BA, McKinsey TA, Vega RB, et al. Myocyte-enriched calcineurin-interacting protein, MCIP1, inhibits cardiac hypertrophy in vivo. Proc Natl Acad Sci USA 2001;98:3328–3333.

Ruwhof C, van der Laarse A. Mechanical stress-induced cardiac hypertrophy: mechanisms and signal transduction pathways. Cardiovasc Res 2000;47:23–37.

Sadoshima J, Izumo S. Mechanical stretch rapidly activates multiple signal transduction pathways in cardiac myocytes: potential involvement of an autocrine/paracrine mechanism. EMBO J 1993;12: 1681–1692.

Sadoshima J, Montagne O, Wang Q, et al. The MEKK1-JNK pathway plays a protective role in pressure overload but does not mediate cardiac hypertrophy. J Clin Invest 2002;110:271–279.

Sadoshima J, Xu Y, Slayter HS, Izumo S. Autocrine release of angiotensin II mediates stretch-induced hypertrophy of cardiac myocytes in vitro. Cell 1993;75:977–984.

Sakata Y, Hoit BD, Liggett SB, Walsh RA, Dorn, GW. Decompensation of pressure-overload hypertrophy in Gαq-overexpressing mice. Circulation 1998;97:1488–1495.

Sakata Y, Masuyama T, Yamamoto K, et al. Calcineurin inhibitor attenuates left ventricular hypertrophy, leading to prevention of heart failure in hypertensive rats. Circulation 2000;102:2269–2275.

Scanga SE, Ruel L, Binari RC, et al. The conserved PI3'K/PTEN/Akt signaling pathway regulates both cells size and survival in Drosophila. Oncogene 2000;19:3971–3977.

Schmelzle T, Hall MN. TOR, a central controller of cell growth. Cell 2000;103:253–262.

Schwartzbauer G, Robbins J. The tumor suppressor gene PTEN can regulate cardiac hypertrophy and survival. J Biol Chem 2001;276: 35,786–35,793.

Shima H, Pende M, Chen Y, Fumagalli S, Thomas G, Kozma SC. Disruption of the p70(s6k)/p85(s6k) gene reveals a small mouse phenotype and a new functional S6 kinase. EMBO J 1998;17:6649–6659.

Shimoyama M, Hayashi D, Takimoto E, et al. Calcineurin plays a critical role in pressure overload-induced cardiac hypertrophy. Circulation 1999;100:2449–2454.

Shimoyama M, Hayashi D, Zou Y, et al. Calcineurin inhibitor attenuates the development and induces the regression of cardiac hypertrophy in rats with salt-sensitive hypertension. Circulation 2000;102: 1996–2004.

Shioi T, Kang PM, Douglas PS, et al. The conserved phosphoinositide 3-kinase pathway determines heart size in mice. EMBO J 2000; 19:2537–2548.

Shioi T, McMullen JR, Kang PM, et al. Akt/Protein kinase B promotes organ growth in transgenic mice. Mol Cell Biol 2002;22:2799–2809.

Shioi T, McMullen JR, Tarnavski O, et al. Rapamycin attenuates load-induced hypertrophy in mice. Circulation 2003;107:1664–1670.

Shiojima I, Yefremashvili M, Luo Z, et al. Akt signaling mediates postnatal heart growth in response to insulin and nutritional status. J Biol Chem 2002;277:37,670–37,677.

Stocker H, Hafen E. Genetic control of cell size. Curr Opin Genet Dev 2000;10:529–535.

Subramanian A, Jones W, Gulick J, Wert S, Robbins J. Tissue-specific regulation of the alpha-myosin heavy chain gene promoter in transgenic mice. J Biol Chem 1991;266:24,613–24,620.

Sun L, Youn HD, Loh C, Stolow M, He W, Liu JO. Cabin 1, a negative regulator for calcineurin signaling in T lymphocytes. Immunity 1998; 8:703–711.

Sussman MA, Lim HW, Gude N, et al. Prevention of cardiac hypertrophy in mice by calcineurin inhibition. Science 1998;281:1690–1693.

Taigen T, De Windt LJ, Lim HW, Molkentin JD. Targeted inhibition of calcineurin prevents agonist-induced cardiomyocyte hypertrophy. Proc Natl Acad Sci USA 2000;97:1196–1201.

Takaishi T, Saito N, Kuno T, Tanaka C. Differential distribution of the mRNA encoding two isoforms of the catalytic subunit of calcineurin in the rat brain. Biochem Biophys Res Commun 1991;174:393–398.

Takeda Y, Yoneda T, Demura M, Usukura M, Mabuchi H. Calcineurin inhibition attenuates mineralocorticoid-induced cardiac hypertrophy. Circulation 2002;105:677–679.

Takeishi Y, Huang Q, Abe J, et al. Activation of mitogen-activated protein kinases and p90 ribosomal S6 kinase in failing human hearts with dilated cardiomyopathy. Cardiovasc Res 2002;53:131–136.

Tamemoto H, Kadowaki T, Tobe K, et al. Insulin resistance and growth retardation in mice lacking IRS-1. Nature 1994;372:182–186.

Ushio-Fukai M, Griendling KK, Becker PL, Hilenski L, Halleran S, Alexander RW. Epidermal growth factor receptor transactivation by angiotensin II requires reactive oxygen species in vascular smooth muscle cells. Arterioscler Thromb Vasc Biol 2001;21:489–495.

Vlahos CJ, McDowell SA, Clerk A. Kinases as therapeutic targets for heart failure. Nat Rev Drug Discov 2003;2:99–113.

Wang Z, Kutschke W, Richardson KE, Karimi M, Hill JA. Electrical remodeling in pressure-overload cardiac hypertrophy: Role of calcineurin. Circulation 2001;104:1657–1663.

Wang Z, Nolan B, Kutschke W, Hill JA. Na+-Ca2+ exchanger remodeling in pressure overload cardiac hypertrophy. J Biol Chem 2001;276:17,706–17,711.

Weinkove D, Leevers SJ. The genetic control of organ growth: Insights from Drosophila. Curr Opin Genet Dev 2000;10:75–80.

Wettschureck N, Rutten H, Zywietz A, et al. Absence of pressure overload induced myocardial hypertrophy after conditional inactivation of Gαq/Gα11 in cardiomyocytes. Nat Med 2001;7:1236–1240.

Wilkins BJ, De Windt LJ, Bueno OF, et al. Targeted disruption of NFATc3, but not NFATc4, reveals an intrinsic defect in calcineurin-mediated cardiac hypertrophic growth. Mol Cell Biol 2002;22: 7603–7613.

Woodgett JR. Judging a protein by more than its name: GSK-3. Sci STKE 2001;100:RE12.

Xia Y, McMillin JB, Lewis A, et al. Electrical stimulation of neonatal cardiac myocytes activates the NFAT3 and GATA4 pathways and up-regulates the adenylosuccinate synthetase 1 gene. J Biol Chem 2000;275:1855–1863.

Yang G, Meguro T, Hong C, et al. Cyclosporine reduces left ventricular mass with chronic aortic banding in mice, which could be due to apoptosis and fibrosis. J Mol Cell Cardiol 2001;33:1505–1514.

Yang J, Cron P, Thompson V, et al. Molecular mechanism for the regulation of protein kinase B/Akt by hydrophobic motif phosphorylation. Mol Cells 2002;9:1227–1240.

Youn TJ, Piao H, Kwon JS, et al. Effects of the calcineurin dependent signaling pathway inhibition by cyclosporin A on early and late cardiac remodeling following myocardial infarction. Eur J Heart Fail 2002; 4:713–718.

Zhang W, Kowal RC, Rusnak F, Sikkink RA, Olson EN, Victor RG. Failure of calcineurin inhibitors to prevent pressure-overload left ventricular hypertrophy in rats. Circ Res 1999;84:722–728.

Zhu W, Zou Y, Shiojima I, et al. Ca2+/calmodulin-dependent kinase II and calcineurin play critical roles in endothelin-1-induced cardiomyocyte hypertrophy. J Biol Chem 2000;275:15,239–15,245.

Zou Y, Hiroi Y, Uozumi H, et al. Calcineurin plays a critical role in the development of pressure overload-induced cardiac hypertrophy. Circulation 2001;104:97–101.

18 Arrhythmias

BARRY LONDON

SUMMARY

Ion channel mutations cause long QT syndrome, Brugada syndrome, conduction disorders, catecholinergic ventricular tachycardia, and some forms of familial atrial fibrillation and pre-excitation. Transgenic and gene-targeted mouse models of these disorders have further increased the understanding of links between ion channel mutations and these rare arrhythmia syndromes. Molecular genetics, pathophysiology, and implications of these findings are discussed later. It is important to realize, however, that the genetic basis of other inherited arrhythmic syndromes remains unclear, as does the role of genes that are not ion channels. In addition, the relationship of common genetic variants (polymorphisms) to arrhythmic risk is only beginning to be studied. This chapter highlights the avenues of future research that seem most likely to yield results.

Key Words: Arrhythmias; atrial fibrillation; Brugada syndrome; conduction disease; ion channel; long QT syndrome: Wolff-Parkinson-White syndrome (WPW).

INTRODUCTION

Modern experimental electrophysiology began with the explanation of the basis of the action potential in the squid giant axon, and clinical cardiac electrophysiology began with the development of electrocardiography. The fields progressed in two rather independent directions. The development of intracellular electrodes, the voltage clamp, and the single channel patch clamp revealed the subcellular events that underlie cardiac excitability and automaticity. Meanwhile, arrhythmia mapping, devices, and clinical trials defined the mechanisms that underlie human arrhythmias and assessed the efficacy of therapeutic interventions. The cloning and molecular biological analysis of ion channels has linked structure to function, and human genetic analysis has identified the genes and mutations responsible for rare inherited arrhythmia syndromes. Although the relation of single channel properties to the more common arrhythmias associated with ischemic and cardiomyopathic processes has lagged behind, molecular electrophysiology holds great promise as a unifying discipline in the age following the completion of the human genome project.

Ion channel mutations cause long QT syndrome, Brugada syndrome, conduction disorders, catecholinergic ventricular tachycardia, and some forms of familial atrial fibrillation and pre-excitation.

From: *Principles of Molecular Medicine, Second Edition*
Edited by: M. S. Runge and C. Patterson © Humana Press, Inc., Totowa, NJ

Transgenic and gene-targeted mouse models of these disorders have further increased the understanding of links between ion channel mutations and these rare arrhythmia syndromes. Molecular genetics, pathophysiology, and implications of these findings are discussed later. It is important to realize, however, that the genetic basis of other inherited arrhythmic syndromes remains unclear, as does the role of genes that are not ion channels. In addition, the relationship of common genetic variants (polymorphisms) to arrhythmic risk is only beginning to be studied. The avenues of future research that seem most likely to yield results are highlighted next.

INHERITED ARRHYTHMIA SYNDROMES

LONG QT SYNDROME

Clinical Presentation   The autosomal-dominant form of the rare long QT syndrome was first described in the early 1960s. Although the exact gene frequency is not known, it is one of the more common causes of sudden cardiac death among otherwise healthy adolescents and young adults (along with hypertrophic cardiomyopathy and myocarditis). It is characterized by syncope, unexplained seizures, and sudden death. Symptoms often begin near adolescence and are preceded by emotional events such as surprise and fear. The electrocardiographic manifestation of the disease is a prolonged QT interval and an abnormal T-wave morphology on the surface ECG, although the QT interval has considerable variability and some symptomatic affected individuals have QT intervals within the normal range (Fig. 18-1A). The most common arrhythmia is *torsade de pointes*, or polymorphic ventricular tachycardia with a rotating axis (Fig. 18-1B). The symptoms often respond to treatment with β-blockers, although some patients are refractory. The role of sympathectomy and timing of implantable cardiac defibrillator (ICD) therapy remain uncertain.

The autosomal-recessive long QT syndrome is associated with congenital deafness, and is extremely rare. The acquired long QT syndromes are caused by medications (particularly type-IA and type-III antiarrhythmics, certain antibiotics, and nonsedating antihistamines), ischemia, metabolic disorders, and neurological disorders. Acquired long QT syndrome is considerably more common than the autosomal-dominant and -recessive forms, and plays a major role in the design of novel pharmaceutical agents.

Molecular Basis of the Disease   QT prolongation results from action potential prolongation, and ion channel defects were therefore likely candidates. Positional cloning identified a number of K^+ channel and Na^+ channel mutations that cause the autosomal-dominant forms of this syndrome (Table 18-1). Of note, KvLQT1

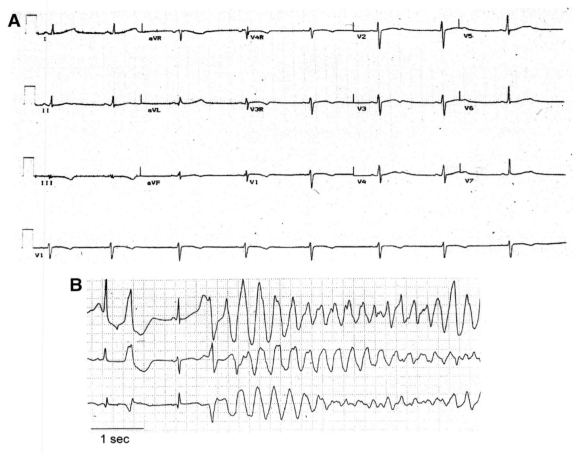

Figure 18-1 ECG manifestations of the long QT syndrome. (**A**) 12 Lead ECG of a child with the Romano-Ward autosomal-dominant long QT syndrome. (**B**) Lead II rhythm strip demonstrating *torsade de pointes*.

Table 18-1
Long QT Syndrome Loci

Locus	Protein	Gene	Pathophysiology	Chromosome
LQT1	KvLQT1	KCNQ1	$\downarrow I_{Ks}$	11p15.5
LQT2	HERG	KCNH2	$\downarrow I_{Kr}$	7q35-36
LQT3	Na$_v$1.5	SCN5A	$\uparrow I_{Na}$	3p21
LQT4	Ankyrin-B	Ank-B	?	4q25-27
LQT5	MinK/IsK	KCNE1	$\downarrow I_{Ks}$	21q21-22
LQT6	MiRP1	KCNE2	$\downarrow I_{Kr}$	21q21-22
LQT7	Kir2.1	KCNJ2	$\downarrow I_{K1}$	17q23

was first identified by the positional cloning at the LQT1 locus. Mutations of the K$^+$ channels KvLQT1 and HERG account for most cases, whereas Na$^+$ channel mutations are present in <5%. The ion channel mutations cause marked action potential prolongation, leading to reactivation of inward currents and triggered activity (Fig. 18-2). These early afterdepolarizations can then initiate re-entry and lead to syncope or sudden death.

Four K$^+$ channel α-subunits, with or without β-subunits, coassemble to form functional channels. Mutations of the K$^+$ channel α-subunit KvLQT1 (LQT1 locus) and the β-subunit IsK (minK; LQT5 locus) affect the slow component of the delayed rectifier K$^+$ current I_{Ks}, whereas mutations of the α-subunit HERG (LQT2 locus) and possibly the β-subunit MiRP1 (LQT6 locus)

affect the rapid component of the delayed rectifier K$^+$ current I_{Kr}. Some KvLQT1 and HERG mutations act solely through loss of function or haploinsufficiency, whereas others also contribute to the long QT syndrome via a dominant negative mechanism. In the latter cases, mutant subunits coassemble with wild-type subunits to form an abnormal or nonfunctional channel protein. It is also clear that many HERG mutations affect channel function by interfering with the trafficking of the channel to the cell membrane. Lower temperature and drugs such as E4031 rescue some of these mutants.

Patients with the autosomal-recessive or Jervell and Lange-Nielsen syndrome are homozygous for mutations in either KvLQT1 or minK. KvLQT1 and minK are expressed in the hair

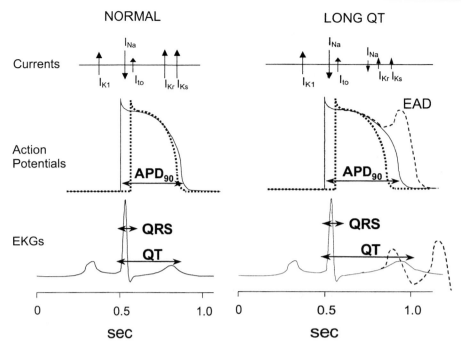

Figure 18-2 Ionic basis of the long QT syndrome. Schematic representation of transmembrane ionic currents (top), intracellular potentials (middle), and surface electrocardiograms (bottom) of a normal individual (left) contrasted with one having the long QT syndrome (right). For each individual, the shortest action potential (epicardial) is depicted by the dotted line and the longest (M-cell) by the solid line. Insufficient repolarizing K^+ currents (I_{Kr} or I_{Ks}) or a prolonged inward Na^+ current (I_{Na}) prolongs cellular action potential in different parts of the heart to different extents, leading to QT interval prolongation and T-wave broadening. The action potential prolongation can also lead to triggered activity (early afterdepolarizations) that can initiate runs of torsade (dashed line).

cells of the inner ear and play a key role in the production of endolymph, leading to congenital deafness in the recessive form. As expected, these patients have a more severe cardiac phenotype, and their parents are usually heterozygous for an ion channel mutation. In fact, the autosomal-dominant long QT syndrome can often be identified in each parent's family.

Mutations that interfere with inactivation of the cardiac Na^+ channel SCN5A cause long QT syndrome in families linked to the LQT3 locus on chromosome 3p21. Here, the Na^+ current fails to fully inactivate leading to a late inward current and action potential prolongation. Mutations in the ankyrin-B gene cause the rare LQT4 variant of long QT syndrome. Ankyrin-B interacts with a number of cardiac ion channels, receptors, and exchangers. The mechanisms that lead to QT prolongation and arrhythmias remain uncertain.

Sudden infant death syndrome (SIDS) is associated with QT prolongation. *De novo* and familial mutations in the long QT genes are responsible for some sudden infant death syndrome cases.

Some of the acquired forms of the long QT syndrome may also have a genetic basis. The pore region of HERG binds to a wide variety of drugs, and most pharmacological cases of the acquired long QT syndrome are caused by drugs that bind to HERG and decrease I_{Kr}. It is speculated that a decreased repolarization reserve in these individuals, possibly because of polymorphisms in other channel proteins, may lead to the increased susceptibility to certain K^+ channel blocking agents. In contrast, some mutations may cause drug-induced QT prolongation by directly affecting the blocking affinity of the drugs.

Andersen's syndrome is a congenital disorder associated with dysmorphic facial features, periodic paralysis, QT prolongation, and arrhythmias distinct from *torsade de pointes*. Mutations of the

inward rectifier channel Kir2.1 (*KCNJ2*) lead to a decrease in the current I_{K1} that controls the resting membrane potential of heart cells. It is debated whether Kir2.1 should be included with the other long QT genes.

Gene-Based Diagnosis The mapping of the long QT syndrome and the identification of the responsible genes allow prenatal and presymptomatic testing for patients with this disorder and their family members. The severity of the phenotype varies as a function of the mutation and the family. Some families have multiple cases of sudden death, whereas others with the same mutation do not. It is also clear that long QT mutations have variable penetrance, and that individuals carrying mutations often have normal QT intervals.

In the long QT syndrome, the clinical phenotype is related to genotype. Patients with KvLQT1 mutations are most likely to have symptoms associated with exertion, possibly related to the role of channel phosphorylation by β-adrenergic agonists. Patients with HERG mutations appear susceptible to emotional triggers, whereas SCN5A mutations lead to bradycardia with increased cardiac events at night. In addition, the ECG phenotype is correlated to genotype. KvLQT1 mutations are associated with short ST segments and broad-based T waves, HERG mutations with bifid T waves, and SCN5A mutations with late onset peaked/biphasic T waves.

Screening individuals for long QT mutations is technically difficult, owing to the large number of genes identified and the large size of the channels. In addition, mutations cannot be found in up to 40% of cases. In some of these, the mutations are probably in the parts of known genes that are not normally screened (introns, promoter regions). In others, mutations in other unidentified genes are probably present. As a result of these factors,

Table 18-2
Transgenic and Gene-Targeted Long QT Syndrome Mice

Protein	Gene	Mouse	Current	↑APD?	↑QTc?	Arrhythm	Reference
KvLQT1	*Kcnq1*	KO	I_{Ks}	No	No	ND	Lee MP, et al., 2000
KvLQT1	*Kcnq1*	KO	I_{Ks}	Yes	Yes	ND	Casimiro MC, et al., 2001
KvLQT1	*Kcnq1*	TG:DN	I_{Ks}	Yes	Yes	Brady	Demolombe S, et al., 2001
Merg1	*Kcnh2*	Merg1$^{+/-}$	I_{Kr}	Yes	Yes	Tachy	London B, 1998
Merg1b	*Kcnh2*	KO	I_{Kr}	ND	No	Brady	Lees-Miller JP, et al., 2003
Merg1	*Kcnh2*	TG:DN	I_{Kr}	Yes	No	ND	Babij P, et al., 1998
Na$_v$1.5	*Scn5a*	Targeted:ΔKPQ	I_{Na}	Yes	Yes	Tachy	Nuyens D, et al., 2001
Na$_v$1.5	*Scn5a*	KO	I_{Na}	No	No	Tachy, Brady	Papadatos GA, et al., 2002
Ankyrin-B	*Ank-B*	KO	I_{Na}	Yes	Rate related	Brady	Chauhan VS, 2000
MinK/IsK	*Kcne1*	KO	I_{Ks}	ND	Rate related	ND	Drici MD, et al., 1998
MinK/IsK	*Kcne1*	Targeted:LacZ	I_{Ks}	No	No	ND	Kupershmidt S, et al., 1999
K$_{ir}$2.1/IRK1	*Kcnj1*	KO	I_{K1}	Yes	Yes	ND	Zaritsky JJ, 2001
K$_{ir}$2.2/IRK2	*Kcnj2*	KO	I_{K1}	No	No	ND	Zaritsky JJ, 2001

TG, transgenic; KO, knockout; DN, dominant negative; ND, not done; APD, action potential duration; Tachy, tachyarrhythmias; Brady, bradyarrhythmias.

molecular diagnostic evaluation of long QT syndrome patients is only now becoming available.

Screening of newborns for QT prolongation also remains controversial. Without a reliable means to diagnose mutations, the number of false-positive ECGs would be prohibitive.

Gene-Based Treatment Knowledge of the underlying genetic cause allows for testing of gene-specific therapies. For example, sodium channel blockers such as mexilitine eliminate the late inward current in vitro and normalize QT intervals in patients. It remains to be seen whether such therapies will prevent arrhythmias and sudden death. The finding that some HERG trafficking mutations can be rescued by temperature and channel blocking agents also raises the possibility of specific pharmacological therapy.

Animal Models A number of transgenic and gene-targeted mouse models of long QT syndrome gene mutations have been engineered (Table 18-2). Deafness in homozygous minK knockout mice suggested a role for the genes encoding I_{Ks} in the Jervell and Lange-Nielsen syndrome. Similarly, prolongation of the action potential and QT intervals in ankyrin-B knockout mice enhanced its status as a candidate gene at the LQT4 locus. Despite these insights, the rapid heart rate (approx 600 beats/min) and low abundance of the repolarizing currents I_{Kr} and I_{Ks} in the adult mouse ventricle greatly complicate the interpretation of long QT-related arrhythmias in this model system.

Summary Great progress has been made in the clinical and genetic analysis of the long QT syndrome. The identification of ion channel mutations as the cause of the long QT syndrome has spurred much work in the structure–function relationships in cardiac ion channels. It has also led to significant advances in the understanding of cardiac electrophysiology and arrhythmias.

BRUGADA SYNDROME

Clinical Presentation Syncope, ventricular fibrillation, and sudden cardiac death have been reported in patients without overt structural heart disease in association with a right bundle branch block pattern and ST elevation (STE) in the right precordial leads of the ECG (Fig. 18-3A). This condition is known as the Brugada syndrome. Brugada syndrome is inherited in an autosomal-dominant manner, is diagnosed predominantly in men, and is rare in the United States. Arrhythmic sudden death is common, may be the first manifestation of disease, and is not prevented by antiarrhythmic

drug therapy (Fig. 18-3B). The surface ECG manifestations of the syndrome can transiently disappear in affected individuals, although the risk of arrhythmias may remain. This had led to the recommendation for ICD placement in symptomatic affected individuals and in asymptomatic individuals with a resting Brugada ECG pattern and inducible ventricular fibrillation during an invasive cardiac electrophysiology study.

The Brugada syndrome is rare in the United States, although the exact incidence is unknown. Sudden unexplained cardiac death is considerably more common in young southeastern Asian men, however, and has an incidence as high as 40/100,000 in northeast Thailand. At least some of the affected individuals have ECG findings similar to those seen in the Brugada syndrome, raising the possibility that it may be considerably more common in certain areas of the world. Another feature of the syndrome is male predominance. In a long-term follow-up in a series of 334 individuals with the Brugada ECG phenotype, most patients (67%) were male and an even greater percentage of the symptomatic patients were male (e.g., 86% of patients with aborted sudden death).

ECG abnormalities in Brugada syndrome are modulated by Na$^+$ channel blocking antiarrhythmic drugs. In particular, procainamide, flecainide, and ajmaline accentuate the STE on the ECG, and change the shape of the STE in the right precordial leads from saddleback to coved (the latter considered more diagnostic for the condition). This has led to the use of intravenous challenge with these medications to confirm Brugada syndrome in patients with suspicious ECGs and to diagnose the inherited form of the condition in asymptomatic relatives of affected individuals with near normal baseline ECGs. As the Brugada ECG pattern has become more recognized and screening with Na$^+$ channel blockers more prevalent, the apparent incidence of sudden death and malignant arrhythmias in affected individuals has fallen.

Invasive electrophysiology studies often demonstrate prolongation of the HV interval and easily inducible ventricular fibrillation during programmed stimulation in Brugada syndrome patients. Inducible ventricular arrhythmias during an electrophysiology study has a negative prognostic implication and should be used as an indication for ICD placement in asymptomatic individuals with a baseline abnormal ECG. Another study of 65 patients from 52 families with Brugada syndrome also demonstrated a less malignant phenotype in asymptomatic patients, but questioned the

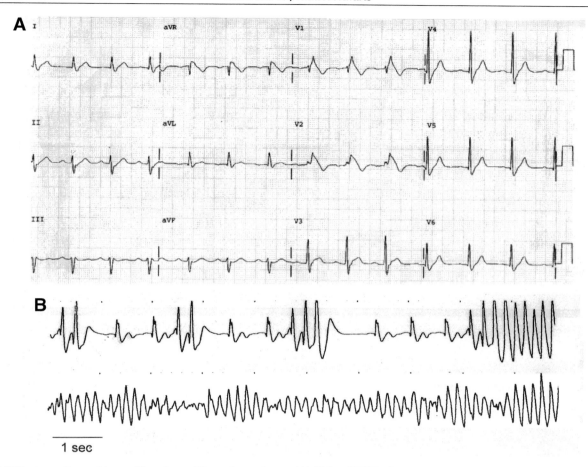

Figure 18-3 Electrocardiographic manifestations of Brugada syndrome. (**A**) 12 Lead ECG of an adult man with Brugada syndrome. (**B**) Telemetry strip demonstrating initiation of polymorphic ventricular tachycardia during syncopal spell prior to internal cardioverter-defibrillator shock.

utility of programmed electrical stimulation and drug testing with Na⁺ channel blockers. The response to Na⁺ channel blockers, originally reported as 100% sensitive, may also be unreliable in some families.

Molecular Basis of the Disease   Mutations of the cardiac Na⁺ channel SCN5A were initially identified in three small families with the Brugada syndrome. In one family, two missense mutations (R1232W in DIIIS1-S2 and T1620M in DIVS3-S4) resulted in a 10-mV rightward shift in the steady state inactivation curve of SCN5A and sped recovery from inactivation. In the other two families, single basepair deletions led to either a premature stop codon (ΔA1397 in DIIIS6) or a splice site mutation that likely truncated the channel (amino acid insertion in intron in DIS2-S3) and decreased the number of functional cardiac Na⁺ channels. Several dozen SCN5A mutations responsible for Brugada syndrome have been reported; most decrease inward Na⁺ current.

These Brugada syndrome SCN5A mutations differ from the SCN5A mutations that interfere with inactivation and cause the long QT syndrome in families linked to the LQT3 locus. Of interest, a family was identified that has characteristics of both long QT and Brugada syndromes resulting from a single SCN5A mutation. Similarly, flecainide (a Na⁺ channel blocker and proposed therapy for patients with the LQT3 form of LQTS) produces a Brugada syndrome ECG pattern in some individuals from LQT3 families.

ST segment elevation on the ECG reflects current flow in the heart during electrical systole, and most commonly reflects the injury current seen in the setting of a myocardial infarction. Several lines of evidence relate the STE in the Brugada syndrome to the presence of a prominent early repolarizing current, I_{to}, that leads to a spike and dome action potential in the epicardium of the right ventricle and the corresponding J wave on the ECG. Mutations of the cardiac Na⁺ channel SCN5A are thought to decrease the depolarizing inward Na⁺ current and lead to early repolarization in the right ventricular epicardium in which the transient outward K⁺ current (I_{to}) is large (Fig. 18-4). This causes a voltage gradient from endocardium to epicardium, STE on the ECG, and susceptibility to arrhythmias because of phase 2 reentry. The actions of the Na⁺ channel blocking agents procainamide, flecainide, and ajmaline to exacerbate the STE and unmask the ECG phenotype support this theory. Experiments using wedge preparations from dog hearts also show that decreased depolarizing Na⁺ current predisposes to loss of the action potential plateau (all-or-none repolarization) in the epicardium, prominent J waves, current flow from endocardium to epicardium with STE, and arrhythmias. In addition, I_{to} may be more prominent in males than in females, explaining the male predominance of the syndrome.

SCN5A mutations are found in <20% of patients with Brugada syndrome. A second Brugada syndrome locus was identified on chromosome 3p24 distinct from SCN5A by positional cloning in a large multigenerational family. In this family, conduction disease becomes more prominent with age, mitral regurgitation appears to be associated with the syndrome, and drug testing with intravenous

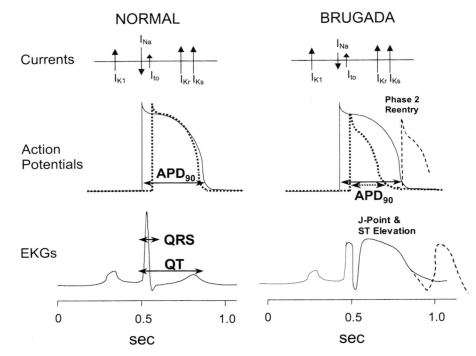

Figure 18-4 Ionic basis of the Brugada syndrome. Schematic representation of transmembrane ionic currents (top), intracellular potential (middle), and surface electrocardiogram (bottom) of a normal individual contrasted with one having Brugada syndrome. Insufficient depolarizing sodium (Na^+) current shortens the cellular action potential in the right ventricle leading to early repolarization of a part of the heart. This results in the potential for re-excitation of that cardiac muscle and the initiation of re-entry circuits.

procainamide is ineffective. In addition, other Brugada syndrome families have been identified that do not link to either of the chromosome 3 loci.

Gene-Based Diagnosis Patients with SCN5A mutations have longer PR intervals on surface ECG, longer HV intervals during electrophysiology study, and a greater increase in QRS duration during drug testing than those with no detectable SCN5A mutation. The efficacy of drug testing may also be gene or mutation dependent. It is unclear whether the male predominance in the syndrome is also gene dependent.

Summary Brugada syndrome is the second major arrhythmopathy that can result from ion channel mutations. Unlike long QT syndrome, the molecular basis for most cases remains uncertain. Elucidation of the remaining causes may uncover a new family of genes that interact with and modulate cardiac Na^+ channels.

PROGRESSIVE CARDIAC CONDUCTION DISEASE In addition to long QT and Brugada syndromes, SCN5A mutations cause progressive conduction system disease. Conduction disease has also been reported in LQT3 families and in Brugada families. Thus, Na^+ channel mutations can cause a spectrum of cardiac abnormalities that affect depolarization, repolarization, and conduction.

SHORT QT SYNDROME Families with an autosomal-dominant short QT syndrome and sudden cardiac death have been described. Of note, HERG mutations that abolish inward rectification and speed repolarization cause some of the cases. Thus, cardiac repolarization appears under tight control, with severe consequences resulting from either too little or too much HERG current.

FAMILIAL ATRIAL FIBRILLATION Atrial fibrillation usually occurs in elderly patients with hypertension, valvular disease, or ischemic heart disease, with atrial hypertension and stretch as the common underlying factor. A small fraction of cases are genetic, and loci on chromosomes 10q22-24 and 6q14-16 have

been identified. In addition, atrial fibrillation runs in a family with a mutation in KvLQT1 that eliminates rectification. It is not clear why ventricular repolarization is unaffected in this family. In any case, these findings show that K^+ channel mutations can cause a spectrum of disease states that span multiple cardiac chambers.

CATECHOLINERGIC VENTRICULAR TACHYCARDIA AND ARRHYTHMOGENIC RIGHT VENTRICULAR DYSPLASIA Mutations of the Ca^{2+} release channel of the sarcoplasmic reticulum cause increased Ca^{2+} release in the presence of β-agonists, leading to some cases of the autosomal-dominant arrhythmogenic right ventricular dysplasia (ARVD) and to the rare inherited adrenergically mediated ventricular tachycardias. Of note, the genes and mutations at the other six loci associated with the autosomal-dominant forms of ARVD remain unidentified. In general, gene identification is easier once the class of candidates has been identified. Mutations in the structural protein plakoglobin at 17q21 cause Naxos disease, an autosomal-recessive syndrome associated with wooly hair, palmoplantar keratoderma, and ARVD. A knockout mouse model of plakoglobin has a similar phenotype. It has been recently been shown that mutations in related genes cause some autosomal-dominant forms of ARVD.

WOLFF-PARKINSON-WHITE SYNDROME Bypass tract-mediated reentrant tachycardias (Wolff-Parkinson-White syndrome, WPW) result from abnormal connections between the atria and ventricles. Mutations of the gene that encodes the γ-2 regulatory subunit of AMP-activated protein kinase (PRKAG2) cause a rare inherited form of WPW syndrome associated with hypertrophic cardiomyopathy. Transgenic mice overexpressing a mutant form of PRKAG2 are pre-excited, but suggest that the gene mutation results in accumulation of glycogen. Thus, this condition appears to be a form of a storage disease, and is probably unrelated to the common forms of WPW.

THE GENETIC BASIS
OF COMMON ARRHYTHMIAS

SUDDEN DEATH IN HEART FAILURE

Clinical Presentation   Cardiac arrhythmias are responsible for >250,000 cases of sudden cardiac death each year in the United States, and only a small fraction of these are caused by the autosomal-dominant and autosomal-recessive inherited conditions described previously. Ventricular tachyarrhythmias accompany acute myocardial ischemia and infarction, occur postinfarction in the scarred ventricle, and are also common in myocarditis and idiopathic dilated cardiomyopathies. Re-entry through intraventricular electrical circuits is often documented by electrophysiological studies. Pharmacological treatment for these conditions remains limited, as sudden death can be the presenting symptom. Implantable cardioverter defibrillators are effective, but their use is limited by high cost and limitations to quality of life.

Molecular Basis of the Disease   Prolonged action potential duration and downregulation of the repolarizing K^+ currents I_{to} and I_{K1} are present in tissue and cardiac myocytes isolated from patients and animal models with heart failure. This delayed repolarization, along with enhanced dispersion of repolarization, may contribute to arrhythmias and sudden death. Mechanisms leading to arrhythmias may include triggered activity, such as early after depolarizations (resulting from recovery from inactivation of inward currents), and delayed afterdepolarizations (resulting from Ca^{2+} release from overloaded internal stores). In addition, re-entry leading to rotors and scroll waves may be enhanced by heterogeneities in ion channel distribution in the heart.

Polymorphisms that change protein function are widespread in genes that could affect cardiac rhythm, such as ion channels and β-adrenergic receptors. Although not proven, it is tempting to speculate that these subtle changes could predispose heart failure patients to arrhythmias. One such polymorphism in the cardiac Na^+ channel SCN5A, S1102Y, is relatively common in African Americans. This polymorphism is associated with an increased late sustained Na^+ current in vitro, mild QT prolongation in some families, and arrhythmias. Thus, it may be an important risk factor for arrhythmias in African Americans with heart disease. Caution is required in the interpretation of case–control association studies, however. As the authors note, "longitudinal studies will be required to confirm the predictive utility of Y1102."

Gene-Based Diagnosis and Treatment   Aside from ejection fraction, the search for clinical markers that predict sudden death in patients with systolic dysfunction has been disappointing. Large clinical trials have shown that ICD implantation improves survival in these patients. Based on the Multicenter Automated Defibrillator Implantation Trial II study, there are approx 3,000,000 patients in the United States who meet the indications for ICD placement along with approx 400,000 new ischemic cardiomyopathy cases each year. At $20,000 per ICD, the cost to the health-care system would exceed $8 billion each year. If genetic markers could be used to identify a subgroup of heart failure patients at high risk for arrhythmias, the impact on clinical care would be extremely high.

FUTURE DIRECTIONS: FROM ION CHANNEL TO ARRHYTHMIA

Many ion channels, pumps, and exchangers have been cloned and studied in vitro using isolated membranes, vesicles, *Xenopus* oocytes and cultured cells. These proteins form the basis of the currents that depolarize and repolarize the heart. A complete catalog of their identity, a model of their structure, and an understanding of the biophysical mechanisms by which they open, close, inactivate, interact, and distinguish between different ions has become reality. The roles of post-translational modification, trafficking, and individual genes in generating cardiac currents, the action potential, the ECG, and rare inherited arrhythmias are becoming understood. The relationship of these basic and clinical findings to the diagnosis and treatment of common arrhythmias remains in the future. Establishing this link is essential, however, if the molecular analysis of cardiac electrophysiology is to have maximal impact in the understanding and treatment of arrhythmias.

SELECTED REFERENCES

Abbott GW, Sesti F, Splawski I, et al. MiRP1 forms IKr potassium channels with HERG and is associated with cardiac arrhythmia. Cell 1999; 97:175–187.

Arad M, Moskowitz IP, Patel VV, et al. Transgenic mice overexpressing mutant PRKAG2 define the cause of Wolff-Parkinson-White syndrome in glycogen storage cardiomyopathy. Circulation 2003;107: 2850–2856.

Babij P, Askew GR, Nieuwenhuijsen B, et al. Inhibition of cardiac delayed rectifier K+ current by overexpression of the long-QT syndrome HERG G628S mutation in transgenic mice. Circ Res 1998;83: 668–678.

Bennett PB, Yazawa K, Makita N, George AL Jr. Molecular mechanism for an inherited cardiac arrhythmia. Nature 1995;376:683–685.

Bezzina CR, Rook MB, Wilde AA. Cardiac sodium channel and inherited arrhythmia syndromes. Cardiovasc Res 2001;49:257–271.

Bezzina C, Veldkamp MW, van Den Bert MP, et al. a single Na(+) channel mutation causing both long-QT and Brugada syndromes. Circ Res 1999;85:1206–1213.

Brugada P, Brugada J. Right bundle branch block, persistent ST segment elevation and sudden cardiac death: a distinct clinical and electrocardiographic syndrome. J Am Coll Cardiol 1992;20:1391–1396.

Brugada P, Brugada J. Further characterization of the syndrome of right bundle branch block, ST elevation, and sudden cardiac death. J Cardiovasc Electrophysiol 1997;8:325–331.

Brugada P, Brugada R, Brugada J, Geelen P. Use of the prophylactic implantable cardioverter defibrillator for patients with normal hearts. Am J Cardiol 1999;83:98D–100D.

Brugada J, Brugada R, Antzelevitch C, Towbin J, Nademanee K, Brugada P. Long-term follow-up of individuals with the electrocardiographic pattern of right bundle-branch block and ST-segment elevation in precordial leads V1 to V3. Circulation 2002;105:73–78.

Brugada R., Brugada J, Antzelevitch C, et al. Sodium channel blockers identify risk for sudden death in patients with ST-segment elevation and right bundle branch block but structurally normal hearts. Circulation 2000;101:510–515.

Brugada R., Hong K, Dumaine R, et al. Sudden death associated with short-QT syndrome linked to mutations in HERG. Circulation 2004; 109:30–35.

Brugada R, Tapscott T, Czernuszewicz GZ, et al. Identification of a genetic locus for familial atrial fibrillation. N Engl J Med 1997;336: 905–911.

Camm AJ, Janse MJ, Roden DM, Rosen MR, Cinca J, Cobbe SM. Congenital and acquired long QT syndrome. Eur Heart J 2000;21: 1232–1237.

Casimiro MC, Knollmann BC, Ebert SN, et al. Targeted disruption of the Kcnq1 gene produces a mouse model of Jervell and Lange-Nielsen syndrome. Proc Natl Acad Sci USA 2001;98: 2526–2531.

Chauhan VS, Tuvia S, Buhusi M, Bennett B, Grant AO. Abnormal cardiac Na+ channel properties and QT heart rate adaptation in neonatal AnkyrinB knockout mice. Circ Res 2000;86:441–447.

Chen Q, Kirsch GE, Zhang D, et al. Genetic basis and molecular mechanism for idiopathic ventricular fibrillation. Nature 1998;392:293–296.

Chen Y-H, Xu S-J, Bendahhou S, et al. KCNQ1 gain-of-function mutation in familial atrial fibrillation. Science 2003;299:251–254.

Demolombe S, Lande G, Charpentier F, et al. Transgenic mice overexpressing human KvLQT1 dominant-negative isoform, part I: Phenotypic characterization. Cardiovasc Res 2001;50:314–327.

Di Diego JM, Cordeiro JM, Goodrow RJ, et al. Ionic and cellular basis for the predominance of the Brugada syndrome phenotype in males. Circulation 2002;106:2004–2011.

Drici MD, Arrighi I, Chouabe C, et al. Involvement of IsK-associated K+ channel in heart rate control of repolarization in a murine engineered model of Jervell and Lange-Nielsen syndrome. Circ Res 1998;83:95–102.

Ellinor PT, Shin JT, Moore RK, Yoerger DM, McRae CA. Locus for atrial fibrillation maps to chromosome 6q14-16. Circulation 2003;107:2880–2883.

Ficker E, Obejero-Paz CA, Zhao S, Brown AM. The binding site for channel blockers that rescue misprocessed human long QT syndrome type 2 ether-a-go-go-related (HERG) mutations. J Biol Chem 2002;277:4989–4998.

Gaita F, Giustetto C, Bianchi F, et al. Short QT syndrome: a familial cause of sudden death. Circulation 2003;108:965–970.

Gollob MH, Green MS, Tang AS, et al. Identification of a gene responsible for familial Wolff-Parkinson-White syndrome. N Engl J Med 2001;344:1823–1831.

Hermida JS, Lemoine JL, Aoun FB, Jarry G, Rey JL, Quiret JC. Prevalence of the Brugada syndrome in an apparently healthy population. Am J Cardiol 2000;86:91–94.

Hille B. Ion Channels in Excitable Membranes, 2nd ed. Sunderland MA: Sinauer Associates, 1992.

Jervell A, Lange-Nielsen F. Congenital deaf-mutism, functional heart disease with prolongation of the Q-T interval and sudden death. Am Heart J 1957;54:59–68.

Keating MT, Sanguinetti MC. Molecular and cellular mechanisms of cardiac arrhythmias. Cell 2001;104:569–580.

Kupershmidt S, Yang T, Anderson ME, et al. Replacement by homologous recombination of the minK gene with lacZ reveals restriction of minK expression to the mouse cardiac conduction system. Circ Res 1999;84:146–152.

Laitinen PJ, Brown KM, Piippo K, et al. Mutations of the cardiac ryanodine receptor (RyR2) gene in familial polymorphic ventricular tachycardia. Circulation 2001;103:485–490.

Lee MP, Ravenel JD, Hu RJ, et al. Targeted disruption of the KvLQT1 gene causes deafness and gastric hyperplasia in mice. J Clin Invest 2000;106:1447–1455.

Lees-Miller JP, Guo J, Somers JR, et al. Selective knockout of mouse ERG1B potassium channel eliminates IKr in adult ventricular myocytes and elicits episodes of abrupt sinus bradycardia. Mol Cell Biol 2003;23:1856–1862.

London B, Pan X-H, Lewarchik CM, Lee JS. QT interval prolongation and arrhythmias in heterozygous Merg1-targeted mice. Circulation 1998;98:I56.

London B. Use of transgenic and gene-targeted mice to study K+ channel function in the cardiovascular system. In: Archer SA, Rusch JF, eds. Potassium Channels in Cardiovascular Biology. New York: Plenum Publishing, 2001: pp. 177–191.

Marban E. Cardiac channelopathies. Nature 2002;415:213–218.

Marx SO, Kurokawa J, Reiken S, et al. Requirement of a macromolecular signaling complex for β adrenergic receptor modulation of the KCNQ1-KCNE1 potassium channel. Science 2002;295:496–499.

McKoy G, Protonotarios N, Crosby A, et al. Identification of a deletion in plakoglobin in arrhythmogenic right ventricular cardiomyopathy with palmoplantar keratoderma and wooly hair (Naxos disease). Lancet 2000;355:2119–2124.

Mitcheson JS, Chen J, Lin M, Culberson C, Sanguinetti MC. A structural basis for drug-induced long-QT syndrome. Proc Natl Acad Sci USA 2000;97:12,329–12,333.

Mohler PJ, Schott J-J, Gramolini AO, et al. Ankyrin-B mutation causes type 4 long-QT cardiac arrhythmia and sudden cardiac death. Nature 2003;421:634–639.

Moss AJ, Zareba W, Hall WJ, et al. Prophylactic implantation of a defibrillator in patients with myocardial infarctions and reduced ejection fraction. N Engl J Med 2002;346:877–883.

Nademanee K. Sudden unexplained death syndrome in southeast Asia. Am J Cardiol 1997;79:10, 11.

Nuyens D, Stengl M, Dugarmaa S, et al. Abrupt rate accelerations or premature beats cause life-threatening arrhythmias in mice with long-QT3 syndrome. Nat Med 2001;7:1021–1027.

Papadatos GA, Wallerstein PMR, Head CEG, et al. Slowed conduction and ventricular tachycardia after targeted disruption of the cardiac sodium channel gene Scn5a. Proc Natl Acad Sci USA 2002;99:6210–6215.

Plaster NM, Tawil R, Tristani-Firouzi M, et al. Mutations in Kir2.1 cause the developmental and episodic electrical phenotypes of Andersen's syndrome. Cell 2001;105:511–519.

Priori SG, Napolitano C, Gasparini M, et al. Clinical and genetic heterogeneity of right bundle branch block and ST-segment elevation syndrome. A prospective evaluation of 52 families. Circulation 2000;102:2509–2515.

Priori SG, Napolitano C, Schwartz PJ, Bloise R, Crotti L, Ronchetti E. The elusive link between LQT3 and Brugada syndrome. The role of flecainide challenge. Circulation 2000;102:945–947.

Priori SG, Schwartz PJ, Napolitano C, et al. Risk stratification in the long-QT syndrome. N Engl J Med 2003;348:1866–1874.

Prystowsky EN, Klein GJ. Cardiac Arrhythmias: An Integrated Approach for the Clinician. New York: McGraw-Hill, 1996.

Rajamani S, Anderson CL. Anson BD, January CT. Pharmacological rescue of human K+ channel long-QT2 mutations: Human ether-a-go-go-related gene rescue without block. Circulation 2002;105:2830– 2835.

Romano C. Congenital cardiac arrhythmia. Lancet 1965;1:658, 659.

Sanguinetti MC, Curran ME, Spector PS, Keating KT. Spectrum of HERG K+-channel dysfunction in an inherited cardiac arrhythmia. Proc Natl Acad Sci USA 1996;93:2208–2212.

Schott J-J, Alshinawi C, Kyndt F, et al. Cardiac conduction defects associate with mutations in SCN5A. Nat Genet 1999;23:20, 21.

Schwartz PJ, Locati EH, Napolitano C, Priori SG. The long QT syndrome. In: Zipes DP, Jalife J, eds. Cardiac Electrophysiology: From Cell to Bedside, 2nd ed. Philadelphia: WB Saunders Co, 1995; pp. 788–811.

Schwartz PJ, Priori SG, Dumaine R, et al. A molecular link between the sudden infant death syndrome and the long-QT syndrome. N Engl J Med 2000;343:262–267.

Schwartz PJ, Priori SG, Spazzolini C, et al. Genotype-phenotype correlation in the long-QT syndrome. Gene-specific triggers for life-threatening arrhythmias. Circulation 2001;103:89–95.

Shirai N, Makita N, Sasaki K, et al. A mutant cardiac sodium channel with multiple biophysical defects associated with overlapping clinical features of Brugada syndrome and cardiac conduction disease. Cardiovasc Res 2002;53:348–354.

Smits JP, Eckard L, Probst V, et al. Genotype-phenotype relationship in Brugada syndrome: electrocardiographic features differentiate SCN5A-related patients from non-SCN5A-related patients. J Am Coll Cardiol 2002;40:350–356.

Splawski I, Timothy KW, Tateyama M, et al. Variant of SCN5A sodium channel implicated in risk of cardiac arrhythmia. Science 2002;297:1333–1336.

Tan HL, Bink-Boelkens MT, Bezzina CR, et al. A sodium-channel mutation causes isolated cardiac conduction disease. Nature 2001;409:1043–1047.

Tiso N, Stephan DA, Nava A, et al. Identification of mutations in the cardiac ryanodine receptor gene in families affected with arrhythmogenic right ventricular cardiomyopathy type 2 (ARVD2). Hum Mol Genet 2001;10:189–194.

Tomaselli GF, Marban E. Electrophysiological remodeling in hypertrophy and heart failure. Cardiovasc Res 1999;42:270–283.

Wang Q, Curran ME, Splawski I, et al. Positional cloning of a novel potassium channel gene: KVLQT1 mutations cause cardiac arrhythmias. Nat Genet 1996;12:17–23.

Ward OC. A new familial cardiac syndrome in children. J Ir Med Assoc 1964;54:103–106.

Wehrens XHT, Lehnart SE, Huang F, et al. FKBP12.6 deficiency and defective calcium release channel (ryanodine receptor) function linked to exercise-induced sudden cardiac death. Cell 2003;113:829–840.

Weiss R, Barmada MM, Nguyen T, et al. Clinical and molecular heterogeneity in the Brugada syndrome: A novel gene locus on chromosome 3. Circulation 2002;105:707–713.

Yan G-X, Antzelevitch C. Cellular basis for the Brugada syndrome and other mechanisms of arrhythmogenesis associated with ST-segment elevation. Circulation 1999;100:1660–1666.

Yang P, Kanki H, Drolet B, et al. Allelic variants in long-QT disease genes in patients with drug-associated torsades de pointes. Circulation 2002;105:1943–1948.

Zaritsky JJ, Redell JB, Tempel BL, Schwarz TL. The consequences of disrupting cardiac inwardly rectifying K+ current (IK1) as revealed by the targeted deletion of the murine Kir2.1 and Kir2.2 genes. J Physiol (London) 2001;533:697–710.

Zhang L, Timothy KW, Vincent GM, et al. Spectrum of ST-T-wave patterns and repolarization parameters in congenital long-QT syndrome. ECG findings identify genotypes. Circulation 2000;102:2849–2855.

Zhou Z, Gong Q, Epstein ML, January CT. HERG channel dysfunction in human long QT syndrome: Intracellular transport and functional defects. J Biol Chem 1999;273:21,061–21,066.

19 Genomics

CALUM A. MACRAE AND CHRISTOPHER J. O'DONNELL

SUMMARY

Genomics is the study of entire genomes and is now possible owing to the completion of the Human Genome Project. Genomic techniques are rapidly being exploited to discover susceptibility genes and to better understand the pathophysiology of cardiovascular diseases, both rare, Mendelian disorders, such as hypertrophic cardiomyopathy, and common complex disorders, such as myocardial infarction and atrial fibrillation. At present, the management of Mendelian disorders and of heritable complex disorders is grounded in a detailed family history and careful examination for signs and symptoms. Althought the application of genetic and genomic testing is limited in current clinical practice, a number of potential applications are anticipated in the nearterm future.

Key Words: Cardiomyopathy; family history; genetic association; genomics; genotype; heritability; mendelian disorders; mutation; myocardial infarction; pharmacogenomics; phenotype; single nucleotide polymorphism.

INTRODUCTION

Genomics has been proposed as the source of a revolution in medicine, although this revolution has yet to be realized in any practical sense. This is partly a reflection of the difficulties in applying the fundamental science to individuals or populations, but may also reflect intrinsic differences between the well-controlled context of the laboratory and the uncertainties of clinical medicine. This chapter discusses the general concepts of genomics, its immediate implications for human genetic studies, and the anticipated impact of genomics on the practice of cardiovascular medicine.

WHAT IS GENOMICS?

Genomics is in essence the study of entire genomes. It is made possible largely as a result of the success of the Human Genome Project, a multinational effort to sequence every base in a representative human genome. Although the Genome Project was successfully completed in 2003, final efforts to "finish" some sequences to the required level of accuracy continue. The technological advances spurred by this effort led not only to the comprehensive sequencing of the human genome, but also to the subsequent sequencing of a host of biologically and medically relevant organisms ranging from viruses to apes. Major efforts are now directed to identifying the variations between the genomes of individual humans, in the hope that these differences will characterize at a fundamental level the potential for developing disease, the prognosis of such disease, and the individual responses to drugs. The extent to which this promise will be realized remains the subject of intense debate, but it is clear that genomics will transform the study of biologic phenomena, irrespective of whether these phenomena are inherited.

The initial efforts to develop comprehensive catalogs of the most common genomic differences between individual humans, single nucleotide polymorphisms (SNPs), have revealed some of the fine structure of the human genome. It is now known that chromosomes are inherited as unique combinations of ancient building blocks of the order of only a few kilobases of DNA. These regions of low recombination, in which only a few different alleles might encompass all the variation that has ever existed, are interspersed with local regions of high recombination. This block structure allows much of a population's common variation to be captured by the typing of a relatively small proportion of the polymorphic sites, and will accelerate the advent of comprehensive genome mapping on a single "chip" or microarray. The intensive study of the basis for the noncontinuous nature of the genome will undoubtedly reveal other insights into human biology and disease.

Perhaps the most important and influential attributes of the discipline of genomics are its potential to study biological processes in a global and unbiased manner. For the first time, it is possible to study not just one gene, but rather all the genes and to relate variation in these genes directly to phenotype. The availability of complete sequence allows the expression levels of all the genes to be studied in parallel. Finally, it is feasible to understand in many ways how a genome functions, as a whole, using comparisons with the genomes of other organisms. This ability to define orthologous genes (both within coding sequences and beyond) also makes possible faithful modeling of human genetic diseases. Although far from complete, the success of this global strategy has heralded similar comprehensive approaches in whole tissues and organisms to the study of proteins (the proteome), metabolic pathways (metabolome), and noncoding RNA structure and function (the RNAome).

Genetic techniques have been applied to cardiovascular disease (CVD), and have been successful in dissecting the Mendelian disorders of lipids, cardiomyopathies, and arrhythmias. The comprehensive study of genes, and SNP expression, does not offer major theoretical advantages over conventional genetic markers, but will affect classic human genetics in several ways. First, the ready

From: *Principles of Molecular Medicine, Second Edition*
Edited by: M. S. Runge and C. Patterson © Humana Press, Inc., Totowa, NJ

Table 19-1
Basic Genomic Terminology

Allele	Any one of the sequence variants of a particular gene
Genome	The complete DNA sequence of an organism
Haplotype	A series of sequence variations that are linked together on a single chromosome
Introns and exons	Genes are initially transcribed as continuous sequences, but only some segments (the exons) of the resulting RNA molecules contain information that encodes the gene's protein product. The intervening regions between exons (the introns) are excised from the RNA and the exons are spliced together to form the final messenger RNA from which the protein is translated
Mutation	Any pathologic variation of the sequence from the reference state
Phenotype	The complete set of characteristics of an organism including morphology and function
Proteome	The complete repertoire of proteins encoded by a genome including post-translational modification
Single nucleotide polymorphism (SNP)	Most of the variation in DNA sequence between individual members of a population is the result of changes in single nucleotides
Transcription	The copying of a gene's RNA into DNA
Transcriptome	The complete repertoire of RNAs transcribed from a genome
Translation	The synthesis of a protein from the information encoded in a messenger RNA

availability of genomic data will ease the application of proven genetic strategies, allowing the relatively rapid identification and study of genes that were previously difficult or impossible to clone. The tools that the genomics revolution has spawned have already made mapping and mutation detection much faster and cheaper. Second, there is the potential that, if common alleles do cause common diseases, genomics will dramatically affect the mapping and cloning of common disease. Paradoxically the greatest legacy of genomics may be its role as a foundation for other "omics," ultimately influencing phenotyping more than genotyping.

GENOMICS FOR GENE DISCOVERY

In any disease, the presence of a major genetic effect has implications for molecular studies of the etiology of the disorder, and for the design and interpretation of studies of its diagnosis and management. These clinical inferences are often relevant long before the intricacies of the molecular pathways are understood. Studies of CVDs that are transmitted in a Mendelian fashion have identified rare variants in specific genes that can be proven, through empiric animal experimentation, to define the molecular basis of a number of relatively uncommon conditions—familial hypercholesterolemia, hypertrophic cardiomyopathy (HCM), and familial long QT syndrome. For the common, "complex" CVDs, such as myocardial infarction and congestive heart failure, that consist the leading cause of death and disability in developed nations, clear evidence exists for a modest underlying genetic basis. Completion of the sequence of the human genome has made possible extensive, and ultimately comprehensive, study of the associations with CVD of all common variants in all known genes. Dissection of the specific genetic variants underlying susceptibility to common CVDs is challenging and has met with modest success, due at least partly to the intrinsically smaller magnitude effects being studied, but it may also reflect the underlying limitations of the techniques. To place the clinical and molecular insights in context, Table 19-1 provides a background of vocabulary and techniques used in genetic analysis.

GENOMIC APPLICATIONS IN MENDELIAN DISEASES

Although cardiovascular disorders inherited in a Mendelian fashion account for a small proportion of the morbidity and mortality conferred by all CVDs, there have been significant successes in identifying genetic variants in many of the Mendelian disorders by use of classic genetic techniques. This section highlights the proven capabilities and limitations of Mendelian genetics and the potential pitfalls of simply extrapolating these techniques to the study of more complex disorders.

FAMILIAL AGGREGATION Although in some instances the genetic nature of a particular disorder is obvious, in many cases symptomatic individuals represent only a subset of those with the underlying trait. Large families with a clear family history of the disease may be the exception, even when a condition is highly heritable (Fig. 19-1). The expression of a phenotype may require additional genetic or environmental factors, or may vary stochastically. To gain an objective sense of how important genetic factors might be in a form of heart disease, systematic studies of familial aggregation and lineal transmission are necessary. Of the several ways of crudely estimating the degree of heritability, the most common is the simple sibling recurrence risk. Detailed assessment of the mode and magnitude of any heritable component requires more complex segregation analysis using multiple families. The genetic basis for HCM was obvious from simple inspection, but systemic analysis first suggested a large heritable contribution to dilated cardiomyopathy (DCM).

GENETIC LINKAGE Genetics has proven a powerful tool to define causal mechanisms in biology, not as a result of some unique property of DNA, but because of the magnitude of the underlying effect and the segregation of genes through families. In many situations in which disease genes have been cloned, the risk to first-degree relatives is several hundred times that in the general population. The theory behind proving causality using genetics parallels Koch's postulates in infection, another situation in which an abnormal genome is responsible for disease (Table 19-2). If

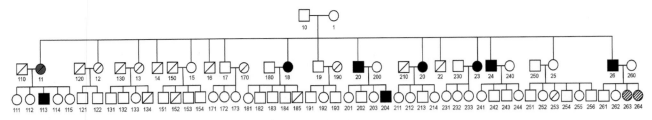

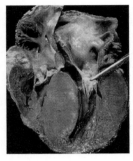

Figure 19-1 Hypertrophic cardiomyopathy: an archetypal monogenic cardiovascular disorder. Multiple alleles in multiple sarcomeric (and other) genes may cause this syndrome, characterized by unexplained left-ventricular hypertrophy and sudden death.

Table 19-2
Criteria for Defining a Causal Mutation: Discrimination From a Polymorphism

I The "mutation" should segregate perfectly with disease. The sequence anomaly must be present in all the affected individuals and absent from all the unaffected individuals. Ideally two independent means should be used to confirm that this is the case. The best statistical support for this segregation is a LOD or logarithm of the odds score (also used in anonymous mapping studies), which estimates the likelihood of random cosegregation as a function of the number of informative events.

II The "mutation" should not be present in a normal population. Rare polymorphisms may be overrepresented in any given large family. These polymorphisms may have functional significance, yet not be responsible for disease. For example, null alleles have been described for many genes including that encoding the cardiac beta myosin heavy chain, but when present in the heterozygous state may be of no import. It is necessary to screen a large normal population for any putative mutation to ensure that it is not simply an incidental polymorphism.

III The "mutation" should effect substantial change on the gene sequence. There should be indirect evidence that the mutation will have a biological effect. This may be obvious for some mutations that disrupt the sense of the entire coding sequence of the gene. Other mutations will have more subtle effects, changing only a single amino-acid residue. The confirmation of these substitutions as disease-causing may require additional studies, such as comparative sequence analyses (with the same gene in other species, or similar genes in the same species, to see if a particular residue is highly conserved), in vitro structure function analysis or in vivo genetic analyses.

IV The introduction of the "mutation" should be sufficient to cause disease. There should be direct evidence that the mutation has a biological effect. The ultimate proof of causality lies in the demonstration that the simple addition of the mutation is sufficient to recapitulate the disease. This is usually done in genetic model organisms, but the specific knock-in of a point mutation (the most common mutation calls in human disease) is rarely performed. Often a causal role is inferred from transgenic expression of a mutant gene or from knock-out of the gene. The demonstration of disease in association with a *de novo* mutation in humans is the logical equivalent.

there is a large genetic effect, given the way in which DNA is transmitted to the next generation, it is possible to define a segment of mutated DNA that when transmitted is sufficient to cause the phenotype in question. This specific segment of DNA can potentially be isolated and shown to be distinct from the normal sequence at that location. Finally, the mutated gene or its ortholog, if introduced into a normal organism, should be capable of causing the disease phenotype. Clearly the literal fulfillment of these criteria is not feasible in humans, but the methods of human molecular genetics combined with empiric testing in genetically modified model organisms, allow similar logic to be applied. Ultimately, the availability of comprehensive genomic information may allow these insights to be widely applied to traits with smaller heritable components, but this will require additional theoretical and technical advances.

If the DNA of family members can be screened for segments of the genomes that are consistently transmitted with the phenotype, then the causative gene can be mapped. The development of panels of informative markers, polymorphic between individuals, made such genetic linkage analyses possible. These anonymous markers allow individual DNA segments to be followed as they pass through a family, defining their relationship (or lack of relationship) with disease. Using a panel of markers that "scans" the entire genome, in even a single large family with a given genetic disease, it is possible to define a minimal location for the disease, and ultimately to identify the causal mutation. The passage, or segregation, of a phenotype through a single lineage is the hallmark of a genetic trait. Segregation also allows other features that track with this phenotype to be identified, informing the investigator about relationships between apparently unrelated clinical findings.

The imminent availability of SNP arrays, which enable an entire genome to be mapped at high density in a single experiment, will significantly change the utility of classic genetic approaches. The time required to map a disease locus will be dramatically reduced, the potential resolution of mapping will be increased, particularly if there are founder effects, and even the minimum size of family required to map a trait will be affected.

CLINICAL DIAGNOSIS AND GENETIC MAPPING It is impossible to separate human molecular genetics from clinical cardiological assessment. A minimal disease interval is defined in terms of recombinants, i.e., individuals whose phenotypes and genotypes are discordant because of inferred recombination between the marker and the disease-causing mutation. The definition of recombinant events is thus completely dependent on the clinical phenotype. Given the central role of phenotype in mapping and cloning a disease gene, it is conventional to adopt conservative criteria for assigning positive and negative affection status in human molecular genetics. It is much better to define an individual as unknown, than to attempt molecular studies with the wrong diagnosis. The need to exclude many equivocal family members has restricted positional cloning efforts to very large kindreds with highly penetrant forms of disease. The closer to the disease-causing mutation marker lies the fewer recombinants are evident, until ultimately the mutation itself should segregate perfectly with the phenotype. No matter how high the resolution of the genetic map, the size of any disease locus is likely to depend on the number of family members who can be definitively phenotyped.

Definitive phenotyping is even more challenging when the assumptions of a single gene disorder are not applicable. As the Human Genome Project is completed, phenotyping in many conditions remains largely unchanged. Mendelian genetics revealed that even a simple mode of genetic inheritance can result in complex phenotypic variation. In many ways the unbiased approaches of genomics may be most helpful in redefining not the resolution of genotyping but the resolution of phenotyping (*see* The Central Importance of Phenotypic Resolution).

POSITIONAL CLONING Once a minimal disease interval has been defined by genetic mapping, the techniques of positional cloning are used to identify all the genes within this interval and to screen these genes for mutations. The ability to grow, in yeast or bacterial artificial chromosomes, long segments of up to several hundred thousand basepairs of human DNA, allows large stretches of a human chromosome to be cloned in an overlapping set of such segments. This "contig" of human DNA clones can be manipulated and eventually sequenced to define the disease gene. Importantly the cloning of the mutated gene does not require any *a priori* assumptions regarding the mechanism of disease. This lack of dependence on previous hypotheses has resulted in the discovery of truly novel pathways, and is particularly powerful in complicated disorders with multiple manifestations (Fig. 19-2). The comprehensive genomic data from the completion of the Human Genome Project ensures that no matter how large the final disease locus, it is possible to rapidly identify the genes within the final interval. This has expedited the cloning of disease genes, and broadened the scope of positional cloning projects to include progressively smaller families with less penetrant diseases.

LOCUS AND ALLELIC HETEROGENEITY The ability to distinguish discrete pathological processes and to undertake genetic analysis of these phenotypes is limited by the resolution of current diagnostic techniques. Mutations in many different genes

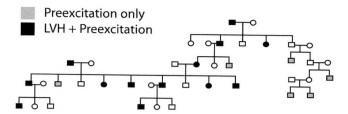

Figure 19-2 Mendelian conditions may have extremely pleiotropic manifestations. In families with AMP-activated protein kinase γ-2 mutations, affected family members may exhibit massive left ventricular thickening (not true hypertrophy), ventricular pre-excitation or atrioventricular block.

may give rise to very similar phenotypes, a phenomenon known as genetic heterogeneity. This situation is compounded by the fact that inherited cardiac conditions often result in premature mortality, so founder mutations are rare. For example, most HCM families with mutations in a specific sarcomeric contractile protein have a different mutation (so-called allelic heterogeneity). This degree of heterogeneity exists for most other Mendelian cardiac conditions. Importantly, subtle differences between the clinical manifestations of different mutated genes may not be detectable until genetic studies have been completed, and "pure" populations studied.

MODIFIERS OF SIMPLE TRAITS Any clinician who has cared for families with monogenic forms of CVD is likely to have been struck by the range of clinical manifestations seen in any single family, in which the primary genetic abnormality is identical in each affected individual (*see* Fig. 19-2). Although some of this variable expressivity represents the limited understanding of the phenotype itself, some variation is the result of modifier genes or of environmental factors. The discovery of such modifier loci or environmental agents is a major research focus.

The use of high-density SNP chips will allow investigators to identify the major locus in a single family and to genotype every family member across the entire genome, revealing other shared genomic regions that may be modifying the phenotype. If these modifiers can barely be discerned in the context of a simple disease caused by a single major gene, understanding the conditions in which multiple genes interact will be tremendously difficult.

GENOMIC APPLICATIONS IN COMMON, COMPLEX CVDS

HERITABILITY, DISEASE PHENOTYPES, AND QUANTITATIVE TRAITS Although there is generally no evidence for clearly dominant or recessive transmission of most common CVDs through families, there is compelling evidence for familial aggregation of risk factors for CVDs. For "qualitative" traits, such as myocardial infarction or stroke, evidence for familiality has been demonstrated by calculation of simple sibling recurrence risk ratios, or more sophisticated modeling of potential inheritance patterns. For "quantitative" traits such as low-density lipoprotein (LDL) cholesterol or systolic blood pressure, correlations among siblings or first-degree relatives can be calculated to estimate heritability, the proportion of variability in the quantitative trait that is attributable to shared genetic factors. Using these methods, a moderate (30–50%) degree of heritability has been demonstrated for several risk factors, including LDL cholesterol, systolic blood pressure, glucose levels, and body mass index, as well as quantitative subclinical vascular disease measures, such as carotid intima media thickness or coronary artery calcification.

GENETIC ASSOCIATION STUDIES Not all phenotypes segregate in large families and so other genetic techniques have been developed that do not use transmission probability, but rely on simple association of genotypes with phenotypes within a population. These studies are qualitatively different from linkage analyses, but have proliferated. The most commonly used association study design is the case–control study. Case–control genetic association studies have limitations. A primary and major potential problem is confounding bias from population stratification, which results in spurious association of a polymorphism with disease, simply because the disease and the unlinked sequence variant are found in the same population subgroup. This can be partly addressed by replicating the findings in large study cohorts drawn from genetically distinct populations. Another potentially important problem in multiple testing is the prior probability that any observed effect results from the specific polymorphism(s) studied is usually extremely low, resulting in an unacceptably high false-positive rate (through Bayesian inference). Confirmation associations in independent case–control studies provide increased support for the hypothesized genotype and phenotype association. However, because of these limitations, findings of associations in case–control studies are generally regarded as data that generate rather than confirm hypotheses.

Because segregation information is absent from these studies, it also is impossible to infer causality from the relationship between specific variants and a particular phenotype. If the genotype–phenotype association in question is not spurious, it may result from a functional variation within the candidate gene, but more commonly the association results from functional variation within a nearby or linked gene, in so-called linkage dysequilibrium with the tested polymorphism. These issues would partly be dealt with by using extended haplotypes of markers in large populations. Parallel evidence for a functional role of the putative variant is essential. These studies, which may use cell culture or model organisms, are possible much earlier because of the ready availability of detailed sequences for cognate genes in other genomes.

Family-based association studies are costly and difficult to conduct, but they offer distinct advantages over case–control designs. The conduct of family-based association tests such as transmission dysequilibrium testing in well phenotyped groups of nuclear families, such as trios of parents and an affected child, allows the study of transmission of alleles from parents to offspring, eliminating the possibility that population stratification may explain associations. Genetic association studies may be extremely difficult to interpret even when conducted in an exemplary fashion. Ideally, associations found from case–control studies can be confirmed in family-based association studies.

Association study designs may be used to analyze qualitative or quantitative traits. Large-scale screening studies of "complex" disease traits, such as myocardial infarction or congestive heart failure, have yielded interesting hypotheses regarding gene variants that may confer disease risk. However, very few genetic variants are strongly, consistently associated with a common CVD outcome in multiple studies, including family-based studies. Among the possible explanations, most common genetic variants may confer relatively small effects on a population-scale (thus, larger sample sizes may be needed) and important unmeasured environmental modifiers may play a substantial role but be substantially different in different populations. Further, clinically apparent disease traits, while heritable, may be heterogeneous. By contrast, quantitative preclinical disease phenotypes, such as decreased levels of high-density lipoprotein cholesterol, increased levels of hemostatic factors, or subclinical vascular disease, may represent more tractable measures for dissecting the role of specific genetic variants. Ideal quantitative phenotypes are heritable and strongly related to prospective risk for CVD. Some candidate gene variants have been consistently noted to explain a significant proportion of the interindividual variability of these "upstream" phenotypes, despite less consistent associations of the same variants with disease phenotypes. For example, although the angiotensin-converting enzyme deletion/insertion polymorphism is clearly associated with levels of serum angiotensin-converting enzyme, there are only modest associations of this polymorphism with blood pressure and inconsistent associations in dozens of studies with CVD outcomes such as coronary heart disease and congestive heart failure. Similarly, the *apolipoprotein E* polymorphism is clearly related to adverse lipid levels, but the totality of studies of associations with myocardial infarction has been less consistent in regards to the risk allele.

THE CENTRAL IMPORTANCE OF PHENOTYPIC RESOLUTION The precision and utility of a genotype–phenotype association is only as strong as the level of resolution of the underlying CVD phenotype, whether transmitted in a Mendelian fashion or via more complex inheritance patterns. Phenotypes defined by a heterogeneous collection of disease cases may obscure the real genotype–phenotype associations. For example, a collection of cases of congestive heart failure may include a diversity of etiologies, including HCM, DCM secondary to myocardial infarction, and DCM secondary to myocarditis. More refined phenotyping requires rigorous clinical evaluation and restriction of studies to fewer subjects with a homogeneous diagnosis. In some cases, current diagnostic criteria allow only limited phenotypic resolution, and further clinical refinement is necessary. Thus, a series of subjects with myocardial infarction may all be defined in a similarly restrictive manner using enzymatic, electrocardiographic, and angiographic criteria. However, further phenotype refinement may be necessary depending on underlying etiology of the atherothrombotic disease. Some subjects may suffer from familial hyperlipidemia, others from a strong genetic predisposition to arterial thrombosis, and still others from primary forms of arterial inflammation. It will be a challenge for future genomic studies to accurately resolve the substantial phenotypic heterogeneity underlying most disorders.

One potential response to this challenge arises from the ability to conduct massive analyses of gene expression and its responses. Microarrays are available that enable, in single experiments, characterization of the relative levels of expression of every gene in an organism (Fig. 19-3). These arrays will become available for humans, mouse, and other model organisms. Similarly unbiased efforts to characterize the quantitative dynamics of all expressed proteins (proteomics) and the totality of small molecules—lipid, carbohydrate, and metabolic substrate (metabolomics)—offers the potential to define phenotypes in multiple dimensions. The discovery of novel classes of regulatory (noncoding) RNAs have added (RNAomics) to this list. These approaches have been most successful in the study of clonal tissues such as neoplasms, but as investigators rigorously test the individual techniques in different situations their utility will be defined.

Although the statistical analysis and interpretation of the vast amounts of data from such experiments remains in its infancy, the implications of this technology are clear. No longer will it be

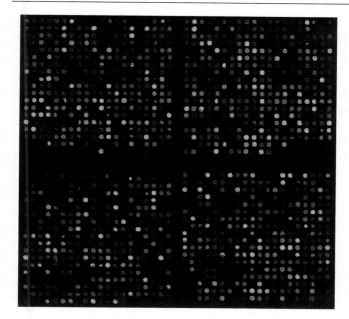

Table 19-3
Weblinks

- http://www.ncbi.nlm.nih.gov/
  The National Center for Biotechnology Information Home Page.
- http://www.ncbi.nlm.nih.gov/entrez/query.fcgi?db=OMIM Online
  Mendelian Inheritance in Man-an excellent manually annotated
  compendium of human inherited diseases and related information.
- http://genome.ucsc.edu/
  The UCSC Genome Browser is probably the most user friendly
  way to survey the human genome.
- http://www.ensembl.org/
  The ENSEMBL browser offers access to automatically annotated
  versions of multiple genomes.
- http://www.hapmap.org/cgi-perl/gbrowse/gbrowse/hapmap
  The home page for the human haplotype map-evolving rapidly.
- http://www.nhlbi.nih.gov/resources/pga/
  Home page for the NHLBI Programs in Genomic Applications.
- http://us.expasy.org/tools/
  A useful entry point for basic protein analyses.

Figure 19-3 Microarray. The use of high resolution printing techniques has enabled the generation of dense microarrays with many thousands of features. These allow the detection of enormous numbers of sequences in parallel in a single hybridization experiment, dramatically reducing the time and effort for mapping and expression studies.

adequate to characterize phenotypes in only one or two dimensions. Comprehensive characterization in multiple dimensions will be necessary. The potential to uncover heterogeneity, as has been seen in clonal lesions, is particularly exciting for geneticists studying common disorders, in which occult phenocopies (similar phenotypes resulting from other causes) may represent the single most destructive confounder of genetic approaches.

CURRENT CLINICAL APPLICATIONS

Genomic information is not yet of any utility in patient management in CVD. However, genomic principles and clinical genetics have the ability to inform patient care long before the genes for all inherited CVD have been cloned (Fig. 19-3). The application of clinical genetic principles in the diagnosis and management of inherited heart disease is outlined, and potential applications of genomics are described.

FAMILY-BASED DIAGNOSIS A definitive diagnosis of Mendelian disease in a first-degree relative dramatically changes the implications of any cardiovascular evaluation. Thus, minor ECG abnormalities are viewed differently in the context of a family history of HCM than without such history. In some cases the definitive diagnosis in a particular patient is only clear from the integrated evaluation of multiple individuals within the same family. This is increasingly recognized in families in which several "discrete" phenotypes, such as DCM and arrhythmogenic right ventricular cardiomyopathy, cosegregate. Only the complete evaluation of an entire kindred would allow these important features to be detected. The ethical implications of family-based diagnosis remain to be fully explored, but informed consent is critical if the data from multiple individuals are to be collected.

DIAGNOSIS

History The history often offers evidence that the presenting condition results from an inherited diathesis. Patients may have

had subtle evidence of disease, such as the cutaneous manifestations of a lipid disorder or a neural crest abnormality, from an early age. Functional limitations are often attributed to respiratory illnesses, but it is usually possible to discern other features of the underlying disease. Comparison of exercise capacity at various ages with that of peers is useful in the evaluation of symptoms such as dyspnea muscle pains or syncope. Other premature medical disorders may suggest specific conditions (*see* Online Mendelian Inheritance in Man weblink, Table 19-3).

A comprehensive family history is an integral part of every patient encounter, but is particularly important in the diagnosis and management of adult CVD in which the presenting symptoms may be sudden death. In addition to defining the basic structure of the family, it is vital to define in as much detail as possible any cardiac conditions (or even potential cardiac conditions) in first- or second-degree relatives. Once the basic family structure and an overview of any inherited traits is obtained, the symptoms, ages of onset, specific treatments (e.g., diuretics, pacemakers, ICDs, and surgery) and modes of death for every member of the nuclear family should be elicited. Specific enquiry regarding extracardiac phenotypes including skeletal or other myopathies, peripheral sensory or motor neuropathy, and premature diabetes or liver disease is recommended. Often a family history is not appreciated, simply because the potential connection between different phenotypes is not explicitly considered.

Other apparently unrelated disorders or events may represent *formes frustes* of the same primary abnormality. Probands will often be unaware of subtle distinctions between cardiac diseases, and many affected relatives of patients with one particular cardiovascular disorder may have been mislabeled with other cardiac conditions such as valvular heart disease or myocardial infarction. Thus, for example, atrial fibrillation in a young relative of a patient with cardiomyopathy is likely a manifestation of the same gene defect, and an unexplained motor vehicle accident may represent an undetected sudden death. The family history also allows some sense of the mode of inheritance to be obtained. A careful family history must also be a prominent feature in any follow-up visits. Patients often have gleaned additional family history from interactions with relatives because of the initial patient encounter. Indeed, empowering the patient to obtain such information should be a goal of this encounter.

Clinical Evaluation   The physical examination and subsequent clinical investigation of cardiac patients are also heavily influenced by the genetic basis of the major syndromes. The examination should look for general morphological abnormalities such as facial or other dysmorphism, midline defects, cutaneous anomalies, or the typical features of disorders such as myotonic dystrophy. Several forms of cardiomyopathy are associated with myopathy involving extraocular muscles, the limb girdles, or other muscle groups. Evidence of a skeletal myopathy may be subtle, such as a mild scoliosis or distorted pedal architecture. Finally, it is important to exclude tendon contractures, ataxia, peripheral neuropathy, or other neurological disorders. Many clinical diagnoses are, by definition, diagnoses of exclusion, and potentially reversible specific heart muscle diseases such as coronary artery disease, glycogen storage disorders, hemochromatosis, and dysthyroid heart disease should be formally eliminated.

Once appropriate permission has been obtained, objective data from other family members are extremely helpful. The direct examination of at-risk family members is often useful in making a diagnosis in equivocal cases. Pathognomonic components of the phenotype, including extracardiac features, may only be present in a subset of the family. Objective phenotypic assignment is especially helpful in inferring the mode of inheritance. Evidence of any mode of inheritance other than autosomal-dominant substantially changes the differential diagnosis in any CVD (*see* Online Mendelian Inheritance in Man weblink, Table 19-3). Mitochondrial patterns of inheritance usually occur in the context of left-ventricular hypertrophy or diabetes; X-linked and recessive syndromes are most often seen with DCM, but Freidereich's ataxia is also recessive. Progressive changes in the severity of a phenotype from one generation to the next, known as anticipation or reverse anticipation depending on the direction, are characteristic of triplet repeat expansion disorders such as myotonic dystrophy. The study of extended families offers a unique opportunity to investigate patient cohorts with remarkably homogeneous etiologies. In a family with a highly penetrant Mendelian disease an identical etiology may reasonably be inferred for each affected individual, and the key features of the specific disorder evaluated in exquisite detail. With the completion of the Human Genome Project, the potential is remarkable for molecular genetic analysis of even relatively small families, and referral to specialized centers for such studies should be considered.

Prognosis   The remarkable range of clinical outcomes, even within a single kindred, plagues the clinical management of both Mendelian and complex forms of CVD. In some families with cardiomyopathy, multiple members have died suddenly or required transplant, and in others the disease is little more than an incidental echocardiographic finding. Initial studies of the presentation, natural history, and clinical physiology of the cardiomyopathies were based on highly selected series from large national referral centers. Subsequent series from regional centers have attempted to redress the balance. However, the major biases implicit in studies of inherited disease have not been addressed in most instances. Without knowing the extent to which individuals (particularly phenotypic outliers) are related, or the contributions of specific families to the overall cohort, it is impossible to begin to interpret even simple studies.

The identification of the underlying gene defects led to the hope that molecular diagnostics would revolutionize risk stratification.

Preliminary work has suggested that specific mutations may be associated with high rates of adverse outcome, but these studies by necessity include multiple members from each family. Contradictory results have emerged from clinical and molecular studies. The extent of genetic heterogeneity, the large size of the genes involved, and the high rates of new mutation have slowed the arrival of genotype–phenotype studies based on serial probands. Understanding the distinctive contributions of the primary mutation, familial modifiers, and therapeutic interventions will require novel statistical methods for robustly extracting information from extended families.

In the absence of rigorous techniques to attribute risk to specific mutations, the effect of the mutation in different generations of the same family remains a reasonable (albeit imperfect) index of the likely natural history of the disease, and of the prognosis in an individual patient. Family members share not only the same causative mutation but also much of the genetic background, environment, and experiences. A complete family history and evaluation offers a sense of the range of expressivity of a particular genetic defect. It may be difficult to get any real overview of how a condition behaves in a small family, but in larger kindreds clear patterns of natural history sometimes emerge. It is usually possible to assess the penetrance, any major effects of gender and other features such as anticipation in larger families. These data are helpful in genetic counseling of potential parents.

The integration of imperfect data with similarly skewed results from heterogeneous clinical cohorts is unfortunately the current state of the art. Such data are susceptible to overinterpretation. Usually the disparate results between studies reflect the underlying etiologic heterogeneity of the study cohorts as much as any true biological differences. Large series of probands are being genotyped for several disorders, but the routine clinical use of genotyping will not be feasible until newer, less expensive sequencing methods are available. The rate of new mutations, and the fact that modifiers may significantly affect risk is also stimulating novel approaches to defining prognosis using proteomics or functional assays.

Another group of individuals who might benefit from screening are asymptomatic affected relatives. The risk of complications, including sudden death, is not clearly related to symptoms, and for both DCM and HCM there are available therapies, some of which are proven to reduce mortality. Systematic screening has been recommended for prognostic reasons in "at-risk" asymptomatic relatives of probands with DCM and HCM. It is possible to determine whether individuals have inherited the particular mutation segregating within the family if this is known, using lymphocyte-based DNA diagnostics. Although no objective data support any form of screening, if undertaken in specialist centers with appropriate counseling it is reasonable in the context of active research programs.

MANAGEMENT   The management of the inherited cardiovascular disorders has also proven difficult to study. Because the literature contains many equivocal or contradictory studies, consensus is often lacking. This absence of evidence-based strategies reflects the rarity of many of the conditions, aggregation of heterogeneous populations, and ultimately the failure to deal with familial confounders. In the face of these uncertainties, clinical decisions must be based on the available information, and as outlined earlier much of that information is likely to come from the patient's extended family. Management strategies must often be tailored to the family and their experiences with the disease. For example, despite the lack of support from randomized controlled trials, it is difficult not to implant an ICD in an affected young adult whose siblings have died suddenly from a familial disorder. A history of inherited disease is usually firmly embedded in the family psyche, and this may also require management approaches that extend beyond the individual patient. Family meetings and family counseling have a role, and involvement with a research group with long-term positive goals can be extremely helpful in engaging individuals who may have withdrawn from dealing with their disease.

POTENTIAL APPLICATIONS OF GENETIC TESTING IN COMPLEX DISORDERS

DIAGNOSTIC TESTING FOR PREVENTION

As mentioned, genetic tests of individual polymorphisms may have low predictive value for determining susceptibility for CVD. However, screening of a diverse spectrum of multiple genetic polymorphisms and gene/protein expression profiles may improve risk stratification for CVD by use of technologies to simultaneously assay numerous SNPs and/or gene expression profiles that may be associated with increased CVD risk. Multilocus genotyping assays are commercially available to interrogate SNPs or expression profiles of thousands of cardiovascular-related genes that may influence myocardial development and cardiac function. Simultaneous examination of many polymorphisms/expression profiles will provide a comprehensive assessment of genomic influences on CVD, which may not be highly predictive of disease, but is anticipated to provide useful information for dissecting genetic risk.

Formal validation will be needed, however, to determine accuracy and reliability before multilocus predictions of disease risk can be incorporated into routine clinical practice. Ultimately, the value of multilocus DNA tests will rest on the strength of evidence that individual genetic polymorphisms confer increased or decreased susceptibility to disease and/or are importantly modified by other genes or environmental factors. The value of coordinated patterns of gene expression related to disease will need to be distinguished from short-term fluctuations in expression resulting from circadian variations or from daily environmental influences such as diet or medication use.

Genetic testing is not used in routine clinical practice for primary or secondary CVD prevention. As more information about genetic and environmental determinants of complex diseases accumulates, the ability to diagnose and treat genetic risk will increasingly become an essential skill for cardiovascular clinicians and primary-care providers. Initial uses of such tests may involve their incorporation into current clinical practice for screening and decision making regarding lifestyle modification or preventive drug treatments, complementing the routine measurement of modifiable risk factors and risk factor scores, as advocated by consensus guidelines.

PHARMACOGENOMICS

The availability of comprehensive genomic data has led to exploration of the use of genetic information to predict the effects of specific medications. Much variation in drug responses is thought to be heritable, and in instances in which common pathways for drug metabolism are involved, several molecular mechanisms have been defined. For example, functional polymorphism in the cytochrome-*P450 2D6* gene is an important determinant of the active levels of drugs including codeine and azathioprine. The impact of such interindividual differences in drug absorption, metabolism, and excretion varies with the particular drug or combination of drugs. These polymorphisms may also have significant endogenous roles.

Genetic association studies, relating the incidence of individual candidate gene polymorphisms to particular outcomes, have proliferated in pharmacogenetics, as in the study of other complex traits. Although association studies may be the only method capable of unraveling population-wide genetic effects, these studies have proven difficult to reproduce and are of limited utility in defining causation. Locus resolution is often restricted, and ultimately even an important "disease gene" might be missed if it is represented by multiple uncommon alleles rather than a small number of common ancestral alleles. Because the principal target is known for many drugs, the application of association studies to pharmacogenetics has seemed more likely to succeed than in other settings. Suitable candidate genes are more readily defined, so the complexity of genome wide analyses is potentially reduced. However, even in this simplified context, significant limitations remain. Only a select proportion of the population is exposed to a given agent, and there may be a wide range of distinct responses, so that studies of sufficient power are impractical. The strategy is biased toward loci that have already been previously implicated in the drug's effect. Finally, many individuals take multiple drugs, which may confound the analyses. Theoretical and empiric evidence supports that to define the loci responsible for variation in the response to a drug and the interactions between these loci (the genetic architecture), classic segregation-based genetic techniques in model organisms will be necessary to complement human studies.

ETHICAL, LEGAL, AND SOCIAL ISSUES IN GENETIC TESTING

Potential issues that may arise when any form of genetic testing is being considered for general use, or in specific patients include ethical, legal, and social consequences of mapping and sequencing the human genome. As susceptibility testing for common CVDs becomes more widely available, and patients inquire about newly developed and emerging genetic tests, more responsibility for implementing, interpreting, and providing information about such testing will fall to cardiovascular specialists and physicians who may not be formally trained in genetics. To provide adequate genetic services, specialists and their care teams will need to develop strategies to communicate risk information and potential psychosocial consequences of genetic tests or testing to patients and family members, develop guidelines for obtaining informed consent and determining when genetic testing is appropriate, remain current with developments in genetics, provide patients with timely information, and become familiar with electronic and Internet resources. Optimal genetic services will include the active involvement of a board-certified genetic counselor.

CONCLUSION

Genomics, a direct result of the Human Genome Project, will allow complete characterization of variations between genomes of individual humans at the level of DNA, gene expression, and protein expression. The accelerating pace of genomic research is transforming the study of the biology of cardiovascular structure and function and the pathophysiology underlying CVD. The heralded promise of genomic medicine includes the potential for improved prediction of susceptibility to CVD and its prevention, risk stratification, and selection of optimal drug therapies. However, before genomic discoveries can be translated into clinical practice, there will need to be more detailed understanding of the complexities of genotype–phenotype associations for Mendelian disorders and complex CVDs. Revolutionary changes in the practice of cardiovascular medicine are likely to result as evidence accrues that genomic approaches confer net benefits for individual patients.

SELECTED REFERENCES

Allen J, Davey HM, Broadhurst D, et al. High-throughput classification of yeast mutants for functional genomics using metabolic footprinting. Nat Biotechnol 2003;21(6):692–696.

Ambros V. microRNAs: tiny regulators with great potential. Cell 2001; 107(7):823–826.

Bhattacharjee A, Richards WG, Staunton J, et al. Classification of human lung carcinomas by mRNA expression profiling reveals distinct adenocarcinoma subclasses. Proc Natl Acad Sci USA 2001;98(24): 13,790–13,795.

Cardon LR, Bell JI. Association study designs for complex diseases. Nat Rev Genet 2001;2(2):91–99.

Collins FS. Positional cloning moves from perditional to traditional. Nat Genet 1995;9(4):347–350.

Fox CS, Polak JF, Chazaro I, et al. Genetic and environmental contributions to atherosclerosis phenotypes in men and women: Heritability of carotid intima-media thickness in the Framingham Heart Study. Stroke 2003; 34(2):397–401.

Freimer N, Sabatti C. The human phenome project. Nat Genet 2003; 34(1):15–21.

Gabriel SB, Schaffner SF, Nguyen H, et al. The structure of haplotype blocks in the human genome. Science 2002;296(5576):2225–2229.

Jarcho JA, McKenna W, Pare JA, et al. Mapping a gene for familial hypertrophic cardiomyopathy to chromosome 14q1. N Engl J Med 1989;321(20):1372–1378.

Johnson GC, Esposito L, Barratt BJ, et al. Haplotype tagging for the identification of common disease genes. Nat Genet 2001;29(2):233–237.

Keating MT, Sanguinetti MC. Molecular and cellular mechanisms of cardiac arrhythmias. Cell 2001;104(4):569–580.

Kennedy GC, Matsuzaki H, Dong S, et al. Large-scale genotyping of complex DNA. Nat Biotechnol 2003;21(10):1233–1237.

Lander ES, Linton LM, Birren B, et al. Initial sequencing and analysis of the human genome. Nature 2001;409(6822):860–921.

Lander ES. The new genomics: global views of biology. Science 1996; 274(5287):536–539.

Lohmueller KE, Pearce CL, Pike M, et al. Meta-analysis of genetic association studies supports a contribution of common variants to susceptibility to common disease. Nat Genet 2003;33(2):177–182.

Marston SB, Hodgkinson JL. Cardiac and skeletal myopathies: can genotype explain phenotype? J Muscle Res Cell Motil 2001;22(1):1–4.

Michels VV, Moll PP, Miller FA, et al. The frequency of familial dilated cardiomyopathy in a series of patients with idiopathic dilated cardiomyopathy. N Engl J Med 1992;326(2):77–82.

Nora JJ, Lortscher RH, Spangler RD, et al. Genetic—epidemiologic study of early-onset ischemic heart disease. Circulation 1980;61(3): 503–508.

Ozaki K, Ohnishi Y, Lida A, et al. Functional SNPs in the lymphotoxin-alpha gene that are associated with susceptibility to myocardial infarction. Nat Genet 2002;32(4):650–654.

Peyser PA, Bielak LF, Chu JS, et al. Heritability of coronary artery calcium quantity measured by electron beam computed tomography in asymptomatic adults. Circulation 2002;106(3):304–308.

Risch NJ. Searching for genetic determinants in the new millennium. Nature 2000;405(6788):847–856.

Roden DM, George AL Jr. The genetic basis of variability in drug responses. Nat Rev Drug Discov 2002;1(1):37–44.

Rosenzweig A, Watkins H, Hwang DS, et al. Preclinical diagnosis of familial hypertrophic cardiomyopathy by genetic analysis of blood lymphocytes. N Engl J Med 1991;325(25):1753–1760.

Roses AD. Genome-based pharmacogenetics and the pharmaceutical industry. Nat Rev Drug Discov 2002;1(7):541–549.

Seidman JG, Seidman C. The genetic basis for cardiomyopathy: from mutation identification to mechanistic paradigms. Cell 2001;104(4): 557–567.

Smith DJ, Lusis AJ. The allelic structure of common disease. Hum Mol Genet 2002;11(20):2455–2461.

Spirito P, Seidman CE, McKenna WJ, et al. The management of hypertrophic cardiomyopathy. N Engl J Med 1997;336(11):775–785.

Terwilliger JD, Haghighi F, Hiekkalinna TS, et al. A bias-ed assessment of the use of SNPs in human complex traits. Curr Opin Genet Dev 2002;12(6):726–734.

Tiret L, Rigat B, Visvikis S, et al. Evidence, from combined segregation and linkage analysis, that a variant of the angiotensin I-converting enzyme (ACE) gene controls plasma ACE levels. Am J Hum Genet 1992;51(1):197–205.

Ureta-Vidal A, Ettwiller L, Birney E. Comparative genomics: Genome-wide analysis in metazoan eukaryotes. Nat Rev Genet 2003;4(4):251–262.

Warrington JA, Shah NA, Chen X, et al. New developments in high-throughput resequencing and variation detection using high density microarrays. Hum Mutat 2002;19(4):402–409.

Waterston RH, Lander ES, Sulston J. On the sequencing of the human genome. Proc Natl Acad Sci USA 2002;99(6):3712–3716.

Zhu H, Bilgin M, Snyder M. Proteomics. Annu Rev Biochem 2003;72: 783–812.

20 Cardiovascular Gene Therapy

David A. Dichek

SUMMARY

A variety of mono- and polygenic cardiovascular diseases are potentially treatable with gene therapy. Extensive animal studies and initial human trials have confirmed that genes with therapeutic effects within the cardiovascular system may be introduced in vivo. Nevertheless, practical concerns relating to the achievement of safe, efficient, and long-lasting gene therapy continue to dominate the field.

Key Words: Cardiovascular; Duchenne muscular dystrophy (DMD); familial hypercholesterolemia (FH); hypertrophic cardiomyopathy (HCM); LDL cholesterol; polygenic; urokinase-type plasminogen activator (u-PA).

INTRODUCTION

Elucidation of the genetic mechanisms that contribute to cardiovascular pathology has stimulated the development of gene therapy for cardiovascular disease. Gene therapy involves the introduction and expression of recombinant DNA with a goal of ameliorating or curing a disease condition. Gene therapy approaches have been developed to treat a variety of cardiovascular diseases and many of these approaches have shown promise in animal models of human diseases. Nevertheless, clinical trials of cardiovascular gene therapy are at an early stage, and the place of gene therapy as a treatment for cardiovascular disease remains uncertain. This chapter is devoted principally to a review of the theoretical basis, tools, and approaches to cardiovascular gene therapy, as established by in vitro and preclinical animal experiments. In addition, the status of clinical cardiovascular gene therapy trials is reviewed, and the likely future directions of the field are summarized.

CARDIOVASCULAR DISEASES POTENTIALLY AMENABLE TO GENE THERAPY

MONOGENIC DISEASES Cardiovascular diseases potentially amenable to gene therapy are summarized in Table 20-1. The potential of gene therapy is most obvious in the rare cases in which cardiovascular disease is caused by a single-gene defect. Specific examples of these monogenic cardiovascular diseases include the cardiomyopathy associated with Duchenne muscular dystrophy (DMD; MIM 31020), an X-linked genetic disease caused by a defect in the gene that encodes dystrophin (Chapter 70) and atherosclerotic disease resulting from homozygous familial

From: *Principles of Molecular Medicine, Second Edition*
Edited by: M. S. Runge and C. Patterson © Humana Press, Inc., Totowa, NJ

hypercholesterolemia (FH; MIN no. 14389), an autosomal-dominant disease with a gene dosage effect, caused by lowdensity lipoprotein (LDL) receptor deficiency (Chapter 15). Both DMD and homozygous FH are caused by absence of normal alleles (i.e., lack of one normal allele for DMD and lack of two normal alleles for homozygous FH). If heterozygotes are either asymptomatic (as in female carriers of DMD) or have a less severe form of the disease (as in FH), then homozygotes might be treated by the introduction of a normal allele. However, not all cardiovascular diseases arising from monogenic defects are clearly treatable by introduction of a normal allele. Hypertrophic cardiomyopathy (HCM), caused most often by dominant mutations in the genes encoding the β-myosin heavy chain, myosin-binding protein C, and troponin T (Chapter 11) cannot be treated with current gene therapy technology because the heterozygotes have a disease phenotype despite the presence of a normal allele. Gene therapy for this type of dominant mutation would require replacement or correction of the mutated allele, not simply addition of a normal allele. The technology for widespread gene replacement or correction in vivo does not yet exist.

POLYGENIC DISEASES Complex cardiovascular diseases such as atherosclerosis, thrombosis, heart failure, and hypertension have a polygenic basis and are also subject to significant modulation by environmental factors. Nevertheless, gene therapy approaches to polygenic cardiovascular diseases have been described, each of which is based on delivery of a normal allele of a single gene (Fig. 20-1). In each of these gene therapy approaches, delivery, and expression of the therapeutic gene are intended to stimulate metabolic pathways for which the therapeutic gene is rate-limiting. Stimulation of these pathways reverses the pathophysiology of the targeted disease. Thus, delivery of a single gene, such as antisense angiotensinogen, apolipoprotein (apo) A-I, or urokinase-type plasminogen activator (u-PA), may provide effective therapy for a complex disease process. This approach to gene therapy is similar to traditional pharmacotherapy, in which a therapeutic drug (e.g., a diuretic for essential hypertension, an angiotensin-converting enzyme inhibitor for heart failure, or coumadin for thromboembolic disease associated with atrial fibrillation) counteracts a disease process but does not correct the underlying cause.

Single-gene therapies for the polygenic diseases of atherosclerosis, thrombosis, heart failure, and hypertension have all shown promise in animal models. Gene therapy for atherosclerosis has focused primarily on manipulation of lipid metabolism. For example,

Table 20-1
Cardiovascular Diseases Potentially Amenable to Gene Therapy

Disease	Therapeutic genes[a]	Anticipated mechanism[b]	Results
Familial hypercholesterolemia (LDL receptor defective/absent)	LDL or VLDL receptor	LDL clearance	Ex vivo gene transfer in humans: 6–23% decrease in LDL cholesterol in three of five patients
			In vivo gene transfer in LDL receptor-deficient mice; correction of dyslipidemia
Dyslipidemia with no specific genetic defect	LDL receptor	LDL clearance	In vivo gene transfer into normal mice: decreased LDL cholesterol
	Apo A-I	Increase in HDL	In vivo gene transfer of apo A-I in atherosclerosis-prone mice: less atherosclerosis
Hypertension	Antisense to angiotensinogen or to β_2-adrenergic receptor	Vasodilation	Prolonged (>6 mo) blood pressure reduction in spontaneously hypertensive rats
Peripheral artery disease	VEGF	Angiogenesis	In vivo gene transfer in animal models of limb ischemia: increased vascularity and limb salvage
			In vivo gene transfer into patients with peripheral artery disease (in progress)
Occlusive arterial disease	Constitutively active retinoblastoma gene, hirudin, thymidine kinase, NO synthase	Cytostatic, cytotoxic, inhibition of smooth muscle cell proliferation	In vivo gene transfer into injured animal arteries: 35–70% reduction in neointimal formation
Thrombosis	Prostaglandin H synthase, t-PA, u-PA, thrombomodulin	Decreased thrombus formation, increased fibrinolysis	In vivo gene transfer in animal models of intravascular thrombosis: reduction in platelet deposition, fibrin accumulation, thrombus mass
Hypertrophic cardiomyopathy	Replacement of gene for mutated sarcomeric protein	Normalized sarcomere function	None; efficient in vivo gene correction currently technically unfeasible
Ischemic heart disease	VEGF, FGF	Angiogenesis	In vivo gene transfer in animal models of cardiac ischemia: increased vascularity, myocardial perfusion, and cardiac systolic function. Human trials in progress
Heart failure	Sarcoplasmic reticulum, calcium ATP-ase, β_2 adrenergic receptor	Improved calcium handling, increased contractility	In vivo gene transfer in animal models of heart failure: increased systolic function, decreased mortality

[a]Partial lists only.

[b]The anticipated mechanism has not always been experimentally verified in individual studies. ATPase, adenosine triphophatase; FGF, fibroblast growth factor; HDL, high-density lipoprotein; LDL, low-density lipoprotein; VEGF, vascular endothelial growth factor; VLDL, very low-density lipoprotein.

transfer of the gene that encodes the very low-density lipoprotein (VLDL) receptor that binds both LDL and VLDL significantly decreased plasma cholesterol and atherosclerosis in LDL receptor-deficient mice and gene transfer of apo A-I (the principal protein component of antiatherogenic high-density lipoprotein or HDL cholesterol), decreased atherosclerosis and promoted lesion regression in atherosclerosis-prone mice. Transfer of genes that encode either tissue-type plasminogen activator (t-PA) or u-PA into baboon endothelial cells decreased thrombus deposition in ex vivo arteriovenous shunts. Finally, myocardial transfer of the genes expressing either sarcoplasmic reticulum Ca^{2+}-adenosine triphosphatase (ATPase) or the β_2-adrenergic receptor improved cardiac function in animal models of heart failure. In each of these studies, overexpression of a single normal allele produced a therapeutic effect in an animal not known to have a specific genetic defect.

METHODS OF CARDIOVASCULAR GENE TRANSFER

To achieve delivery of a therapeutic gene product in vivo, three steps must occur: (1) recombinant DNA sequences must be introduced into the nucleus, (2) the DNA must be transcribed into RNA, and (3) the RNA must be translated into a functional protein. Steps 2 and 3 must occur in vivo; however, step 1, gene delivery, may be accomplished either "in vivo" or "ex vivo." In vivo gene transfer involves delivery of genetic material to cells within an intact animal (or human) tissue. Previously, ex vivo gene delivery involved removal of differentiated cells from the targeted tissue, gene transfer outside the organism, and reimplantation of the genetically modified cells into the tissue from which they were derived. However, the discovery that adult tissues may be colonized and possibly even regenerated by circulating or bone marrow-derived stem cells has opened the additional approach of stem cell removal, ex vivo gene transfer, and infusion of the genetically modified stem cells with targeting of the modified cells to a new location in a diseased tissue. Both in vivo and ex vivo gene therapy strategies have been used for cardiovascular gene therapy studies (Fig. 20-2).

EX VIVO GENE THERAPY In ex vivo gene therapy, cells are removed, maintained in culture, targeted with a therapeutic gene, and then reintroduced into the donor animal/patient. The role of the

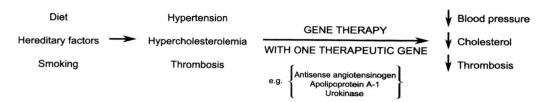

Figure 20-1 Gene therapy approaches to polygenic cardiovascular diseases. Environmental and hereditary factors are involved in the development of polygenic diseases such as hypertension, hypercholesterolemia, and thrombosis. Transfer of one therapeutic gene can potentially correct these polygenic diseases.

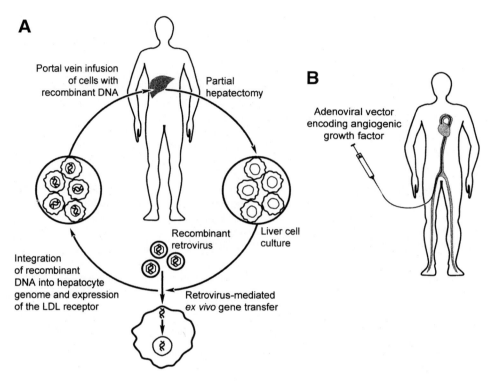

Figure 20-2 Methods for cardiovascular gene therapy. **(A)** Ex vivo gene transfer. This approach has been used to deliver the gene that encodes the low-density lipoprotein receptor to the liver in patients with FH. After partial hepatectomy, hepatocytes are transduced in vitro using a retrovirus vector, and recombinant DNA integrates into the hepatocyte genome. Finally, the transduced hepatocytes are reinfused via the portal vein. They exit the circulation and re-establish themselves within the liver. **(B)** In vivo gene transfer. A catheter is inserted into a peripheral artery and directed to the heart. This approach has been used to deliver genes that encode angiogenic growth factors, with the expectation that gene therapy will stimulate growth of collateral arteries and provide relief of myocardial ischemia.

reintroduced cells is primarily to deliver a recombinant gene product. The cells are usually not required to reconstitute a particular organ or tissue; therefore, the excised cells may be reimplanted in a location different from their site of excision. For example, hepatocytes harvested from one liver lobe and genetically modified ex vivo may be reinfused throughout the donor liver. Endothelial cells harvested from a donor vein or derived in vitro from progenitor cells harvested from the peripheral blood may be reimplanted as a luminal lining of an artery. Skeletal muscle cells or bone marrow stem cells might be harvested, genetically engineered to acquire biochemical features that are characteristic of cardiac myocytes, then reimplanted within the myocardium.

The primary advantages of ex vivo gene therapy are:

1. Gene delivery is performed under controlled, optimized conditions in which the efficiency of gene transfer into the targeted cells may be very high.

2. Gene delivery may be restricted to a specific cell type in which expression is optimized by careful design of a cell-type-specific transgene construct.

3. The potential for an immune response to the gene transfer vector is minimized by performing gene delivery in a setting remote from the host immune system (i.e., in a tissue culture dish).

The disadvantages of ex vivo gene transfer derive primarily from technical considerations:

1. Except in rare cases of monozygotic siblings, the requirements of histocompatibility mandate that the excised cells are reintroduced only into the donor individual. Thus, every animal (or human) receiving ex vivo gene therapy must undergo two invasive procedures: cell harvest and cell reintroduction.

2. Cell culture and ex vivo gene transfer must be performed under strict aseptic conditions to avoid the introduction of pathogenic microorganisms at the time of cell reimplantation.

3. The requirement that cells are removed and reinfused in ex vivo gene therapy imposes limitations on the type and number of cells that can be used. For cells to be removed for ex vivo genetic modification, they must be nonessential, and their removal and reimplantation must be practical. Thus, ex vivo cardiovascular gene therapy may be attempted with hepatocytes derived from partial hepatectomy and with endothelial and smooth muscle cells derived from excised, nonessential vessels. However, for cardiac gene therapy, the entire myocardium (or large sections of it) cannot be removed, engineered ex vivo, and reimplanted except as a brief, draconian procedure performed during cardiopulmonary bypass. Moreover, there is a limit to the number of cells that can be implanted en masse and survive after injection into the wall of a functioning heart.

IN VIVO GENE THERAPY   The advantages and disadvantages of in vivo gene therapy are essentially the reverse of those of ex vivo gene therapy. Advantages of in vivo gene therapy include:

1. Only one invasive procedure is required (i.e., injection of the gene vector).
2. Laborious and technically demanding steps of cell harvesting and reimplantation are eliminated.
3. Any cell within an intact tissue or organ is theoretically a target for in vivo gene therapy.

The disadvantages of in vivo gene therapy are:

1. Gene delivery may be technically difficult. Gene transfer may need to be performed within the myocardium or in the presence of flowing blood in a narrow end-artery supplying an ischemic territory. In clinical settings such as these, the gene transfer vector may be washed away or undesirable clinical consequences (ischemia, infarction) may intervene before successful gene delivery.
2. The target cells for in vivo gene delivery are likely to be a heterogeneous population. Moreover, these cells are exposed to vector only transiently. Optimization of gene transfer and expression is more difficult under these conditions than with ex vivo, isolated cells.
3. There is an obligatory exposure of the gene transfer vector to the immune system. This exposure may produce an immune response that causes rejection of the transduced cells or blocks gene delivery entirely if the recipient organism is already immune to the gene transfer vector. In its most severe form, immune responses to the vector can precipitate a systemic inflammatory syndrome leading to multiorgan failure and death.

Despite these disadvantages, the practical advantages of in vivo vs ex vivo gene transfer are overwhelming. For this reason, virtually all ongoing cardiovascular gene therapy trials employ an in vivo gene transfer approach.

VECTORS

In general, the uptake of foreign genetic material (unmodified DNA or RNA) by mammalian cells is an inefficient process. This inefficiency makes sense teleologically, as there is little advantage for a cell to allow its highly regulated and evolved genetic program to be altered at random by fragments of DNA and RNA that land on its surface. Although there are notable exceptions, to introduce genetic material into mammalian cells with reasonable efficiency, it has been necessary for investigators to associate the genetic material with a "vector" that can mediate entry, nuclear transport, and, in some cases, chromosomal integration. Gene therapy vectors belong to two general categories: nonviral vectors, which mediate gene transfer largely by physical means; and viral vectors, which make use of viral proteins and nucleic acid sequences to mediate efficient gene transfer and occasional chromosomal integration (Table 20-2).

NAKED DNA AND NONVIRAL VECTORS   Nonviral means of gene transfer include unmodified (naked) DNA, liposomes, and microparticle bombardment. The principal theoretical advantage of nonviral gene transfer is that the components can be prepared as standardized pharmaceutical reagents, which can maximize reproducibility and minimize toxicity. In some settings, nonviral gene transfer is quite effective. For example, muscle cells are particularly amenable to direct in vivo gene transfer with naked DNA. Promising preliminary clinical data has been reported from human trials using naked DNA injection into skeletal or cardiac muscle for cardiovascular gene therapy. However, the efficiency of gene transfer with nonviral vectors is low. In no case have naked DNA or other nonviral gene transfer approaches achieved long term, stable expression in the cardiovascular system nor have these approaches demonstrated unequivocal benefit in a clinical trial.

VIRAL VECTORS   Retroviral, adenoviral, adeno-associated viral, and lentiviral vectors are in use for cardiovascular gene therapy in animal models. These vectors differ regarding their ability to integrate into chromosomal DNA, their efficiency of gene transfer, their capacity for incorporating foreign DNA, and their safety profiles. Retroviral and lentiviral vectors can mediate integration of therapeutic DNA into the target cell chromosome, permitting long-term expression of transgenes and ensuring transmission of inserted DNA to the progeny of transduced cells. Adeno-associated viral vectors integrate into chromosomal DNA in some cases, but are also able to persist as functional episomal (i.e., extrachromosomal) genetic elements. Adenoviral vectors integrate at a very low frequency but may also persist for years as functional episomal elements. In general, retroviral and lentiviral vectors are inefficient mediators of gene transfer to the cells of the cardiovascular system. Adeno-associated virus is able to transfer genes to hepatocytes and muscle cells with reasonable efficiency but is an inefficient vector for gene transfer to endothelium. In contrast, adenoviral vectors achieve efficient gene transfer to most cell types (including skeletal and cardiac muscle cells, hepatocytes, endothelial, and smooth muscle cells) and are, therefore, widely used in both preclinical studies and early cardiovascular gene therapy trials. Nevertheless, the clinical use of adenovirus has been limited by toxicity, immunogenicity, and brevity of expression. Engineering of the adenoviral genome and capsid proteins to decrease toxicity and immunogenicity has shown great promise in improving the safety profile of adenoviral vectors and in extending the duration of adenovirus-mediated transgene expression.

CURRENT STATUS AND FUTURE DIRECTIONS

ATHEROSCLEROSIS RESULTING FROM DYSLIPIDEMIA

Because plasma LDL cholesterol is a genetically determined, major modifiable risk factor for the development and progression

Table 20-2
Major Advantages and Disadvantages of Available In Vivo Gene-Transfer Vectors

Method	Advantages	Disadvantages
Naked DNA	Favorable safety profile No integration into host genome[a] Permits large DNA inserts Easy to manipulate	Low efficiency
Liposomes	Favorable safety profile Wide range of target cells Permits large DNA inserts Commercially available	Low efficiency
Adenovirus	High efficiency Transduces nonreplicating cells No integration into host genome[a]	Derived from potential pathogen DNA insert size limited (<8 kb) except in helper-dependent vectors Direct toxicity Short duration of expression Inflammatory response Helper-dependent vectors difficult to produce
Retrovirus	Stable, long-term gene expression Probably safe in most clinical settings	Complex construction Low efficiency Potential reversion to replication competence Transduces replicating cells only Integration into host genome[a]; can cause insertional mutagenesis leading to malignancy
Adeno-associated virus	Long-term expression possible Parent virus is not a pathogen	DNA insert size limited (<5 kb) Less efficient than adenovirus, especially in vascular cells
Lentivirus	Stable, long-term expression Can transduce nondividing cells	Complex to produce Safety concerns regarding possible recombination with HIV Low efficiency

[a]Integration into the host genome might be favorable with respect to duration of expression; however, integration can also cause insertional mutagenesis.

of atherosclerotic cardiovascular disease, it is logical that gene therapy approaches for atherosclerosis have focused on lowering plasma LDL cholesterol. The first cardiovascular gene therapy trial, aimed at treatment of elevated plasma LDL cholesterol in patients with homozygous FH involved treatment of five FH patients with an ex vivo gene therapy strategy and revealed that the introduction of a normal LDL receptor allele was capable of increasing LDL catabolism and lowering LDL cholesterol in individual patients; however, in no case was LDL lowered to such an extent that any of the patients' cardiovascular disease risk was appreciably diminished. Moreover, the response of the patients was heterogeneous, with two of five showing no change in plasma LDL levels after gene therapy. The authors acknowledged that the inability to reconstitute more than a small fraction of the liver with genetically modified cells placed a severe limitation on this approach. The inefficiency of cell-based, ex vivo gene transfer forced them to forego further clinical trials and refocus their attention on achieving higher levels of hepatic gene transfer. This refocusing of attention eventually led to a clinical trial of in vivo adenovirus-mediated gene transfer for a metabolic disease. This trial, which appeared promising based on preclinical data, was terminated after a tragic death caused by a systemic inflammatory response to adenoviral vector infusion.

Other approaches to gene therapy for dyslipidemia that have shown promise in animal models include hepatic overexpression of the VLDL receptor to treat elevated LDL cholesterol and overexpression of apo A-I to raise plasma HDL levels. The rationale for the former approach is that the VLDL receptor can duplicate the function of the LDL receptor in removing atherogenic LDL particles from plasma. However, unlike the LDL receptor protein, which is a neoantigen and might therefore be immunogenic for patients with homozygous FH, the VLDL receptor protein is normally expressed by FH patients and should not be recognized as a neoantigen. The rationale for overexpression of apo A-I is that plasma HDL cholesterol is inversely correlated with atherosclerosis in humans; therefore, apo A-I expression leading to elevated plasma HDL might retard or reverse the progression of atherosclerosis. This rationale has received strong support in preclinical studies in which systemic infusion of adenoviral vectors expressing apo A-I have decreased atherosclerosis in animal models. Although expression of both the VLDL receptor and apo A-I appear powerful and feasible in animal models, these approaches generally require use of adenoviral vectors to achieve high levels of in vivo gene transfer to the liver. The unfavorable clinical experience with adenoviral gene transfer to the liver has therefore tempered enthusiasm for these approaches.

PERIPHERAL ARTERY DISEASE The identification and cloning of genes (such as vascular endothelial growth factor) that control the development and growth of blood vessels has inspired several investigators to propose gene therapy for limb ischemia because of peripheral artery disease. According to this paradigm, delivery of a gene encoding an angiogenic protein in or near an ischemic territory will stimulate the growth of blood vessels and relieve the ischemia. Several groups have reported preclinical data generated in animal models of limb ischemia that support the validity of this approach. Based on these data, trials of human gene therapy for limb ischemia have been initiated, using either naked DNA or adenoviral vectors encoding vascular endothelial growth factor. Initial results show that this therapy appears safe and promising. However, definitive results showing persistent clinical benefits have not been reported.

Arterial aneurysm formation has also been a target of preclinical gene therapy studies. Transfer of genes encoding protease inhibitors to the artery wall has decreased the incidence of aneurysm rupture in animal models. These results are promising; however, technical challenges in achieving efficient in vivo gene transfer to human arteries and the likely requirement for long-term gene expression to prevent rupture of human aneurysms has thus far precluded clinical trials of this therapy.

ISCHEMIC HEART DISEASE   Application of gene therapy to the treatment of ischemic heart disease has consisted primarily of efforts to stimulate growth of collateral vessels that bypass occluded or stenotic coronary arteries. These efforts are analogous to attempts (discussed earlier) to stimulate blood vessel growth in ischemic limbs. Again, studies in animal models of myocardial ischemia support the promise of a gene therapy approach. Clinical human gene therapy trials designed to promote myocardial angiogenesis, first reported in 1998, have been conducted using both plasmids and adenovirus, delivered either by direct myocardial injection during an open surgical procedure or by percutaneous catheter-based approaches. As with clinical studies of gene therapy for peripheral vascular disease, gene therapy trials for myocardial angiogenesis have shown that the therapy, as administered, appears safe. These trials have also suggested the presence of therapeutic effects, for example, improvements in myocardial perfusion scans, increased exercise tolerance, and decreased angina. Nevertheless, convincing evidence of patient benefit, obtained in an adequately powered, double blind, placebo-controlled trial, remains lacking. Larger trials, in progress, may provide this evidence.

Gene therapy approaches are also being developed with the goal of preventing myocardial damage during and after an ischemic episode. These approaches are based on the hypothesis that cardiomyocytes can be reprogrammed, by gene transfer, to resist both ischemia and postischemia reperfusion injury. Genes that have shown promise in animal models of ischemia/reperfusion include heme oxygenase, the antioxidants catalase and superoxide dismutase, and the protein kinase Akt. Challenges that must be met in extending these exciting findings to the clinic include achievement of efficient in vivo gene transfer to human myocardium and the need to accomplish gene delivery well in advance of a major ischemic episode. This latter consideration suggests that long-term, stable myocardial gene expression will be required in order for this approach to yield clinical benefit.

RESTENOSIS AFTER ANGIOPLASTY   Demonstration of successful in vivo gene transfer into injured mammalian arteries with both viral and nonviral gene transfer systems, along with the availability of animal models of local arterial injury, have stimulated several groups to develop and test gene therapy approaches to prevent restenosis after angioplasty. Transfer into injured arteries of cytotoxic genes (such as herpesvirus thymidine kinase) or cytostatic

genes (such as mutant, nonphosphorylatable retinoblastoma protein), decreased neointimal formation in animal models. Alternatively, transfer of "protective" genes, such as nitric oxide synthase, heme oxygenase, or hirudin, at the time of arterial injury also reduced neointimal formation. Other gene therapy approaches to the prevention of restenosis include expression of genes that block mitogenic signals, interfere with proteolysis (a process thought to play a major role in cell migration and remodeling), block matrix accumulation (e.g., by interfering with the action of transforming growth factor β_1), or maintain vascular smooth muscle cells in a contractile, nonproliferative state.

The overwhelming success of gene transfer in limiting neointimal formation in animal models has suggested that gene therapy to prevent restenosis would be the first human application of cardiovascular gene therapy. Indeed, restenosis is a reasonable target for gene therapy in that it is a focal disease, occurring at a location that is by definition accessible to percutaneous gene therapy approaches. However, gene therapy for restenosis was replaced by angiogenic gene therapy as the most clinically advanced cardiovascular gene therapy application. The reasons for the decline in interest in gene therapy for restenosis are instructive:

1. Alternative therapies, first metallic stents and then drug-eluting stents, have had a major impact on the incidence of restenosis. Gene therapy will always need to compete with other approaches and is most likely to be tried when effective therapies are lacking.

2. Local gene delivery in the human coronary circulation is far more challenging than in an isolated peripheral animal artery (Fig. 20-3). In contrast to animal experiments in which efficient gene therapy limits neointimal growth in a peripheral artery, it is unfeasible to isolate a human coronary artery lumen (maintaining both proximal and distal occlusion whereas preventing leakage via side branches) and maintain an elevated infusion pressure during 20 min of gene delivery. Although several local delivery catheters have been developed with the goal of optimizing gene delivery to the coronary artery wall, none appears able to achieve efficient, uniform vascular gene transfer while avoiding significant systemic vector release.

3. Direct vascular toxicity and proinflammatory effects of adenovirus (the most widely used vector for vascular gene transfer) may counteract the salutary effects of gene therapy.

Documentation of the proinflammatory effects of adenovirus when infused in the artery wall, a growing appreciation of the fundamental contribution of vascular wall inflammation to the pathogenesis of atherosclerosis, and the chilling effect of an adenovirus-related human death have moderated enthusiasm for restenosis gene therapy.

HEART FAILURE   For many years, patients with heart failure because of impaired systolic function had a dire prognosis and few therapeutic options. For this reason, gene therapy to improve systolic function could fill a significant, unmet clinical need. This unmet need has inspired investigators to develop gene therapy approaches to improve cardiac systolic function. These approaches have been tested in animals in which heart failure is induced by interventions such as experimental infarction or aortic banding. They have also been tested in the cardiomyopathic hamster, an animal model of congenital, genetically based cardiomyopathy such as that found in humans with muscular dystrophy or storage diseases such as Pompe's disease.

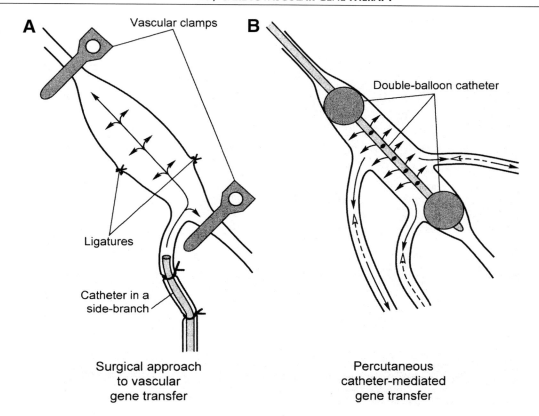

Figure 20-3 Methods for in vivo arterial gene transfer. (**A**) Surgical approach. Side branches are ligated and the target vessel segment is clamped proximally and distally. Infusion is performed under direct vision, and the vessel wall is maintained in a distended state by the infusion pressure. Systemic spread of the recombinant gene is limited. (**B**) Potential percutaneous approach. The recombinant gene is delivered through a double-balloon (or other local delivery) catheter. Systemic leakage via the side branches cannot be avoided, and distension cannot be maintained. In addition, collateral flow (dotted arrows) may enter the occluded artery and dilute or neutralize the vector solution. Gene delivery will likely be decreased and systemic exposure increased compared to the surgical approach. The use of double balloon catheters for arterial gene transfer has largely been via a surgical approach using direct vision and ligation of branch vessels as in (**A**).

Table 20-3
Hemodynamic Effects of SERCA2a Overexpression in Rat Hearts

Treatment	HR, beats/min	LVSP, mmHg	+ dP/dt, mmHg/s	– dP/dt, mmHg/s
Ad.βgal	442 ± 27	112 ± 24	5387 ± 818	-3748 ± 458
Ad.SERCA2a	440 ± 21	147 ± 22^a	7924 ± 1857^a	-6782 ± 971^a

[a]$p < 0.05$ compared to Ad.βgal. (Reproduced with permission from Miyamoto MI, del Monte F, Schmidt U, et al. Adenoviral gene transfer of SERCA2a improves left-ventricular function in aortic-banded rats in transition to heart failure. Proc Natl Acad Sci USA 2000;97:793–798. Copyright 2000 National Academy of Sciences.)

Measurements were made 7 d after in vivo gene transfer with a control adenovirus expressing β-galactosidase (Ad.βgal) or an adenovirus expressing SERCA2a (sarcoplasmic reticulum calcium ATPase); HR, heart rate; LVSP, left-ventricular systolic pressure; + dP/dt, maximal rate of rise of left-ventricular pressure (a measure of cardiac contractile function); – dP/dt, maximal rate of decline of left-ventricular pressure (a measure of the ability of the heart to relax after contraction).

Cardiomyocyte-directed gene therapy for systolic dysfunction has produced impressive results in animal models. Gene delivery to cardiomyocytes is most often accomplished by intracoronary infusion of adenoviral vectors, either in vivo or ex vivo. To optimize myocardial gene transfer, in some cases the aorta is cross-clamped and the vector is injected either within the left ventricle or into the aortic root. Although the aorta remains clamped, the vector recirculates through the coronary arteries and veins as the heart contracts, providing repeated opportunities for gene transfer vectors to leave the vasculature and enter a cardiomyocyte. Using this approach, alteration of cardiomyocyte calcium handling by overexpression of sarcoplasmic reticulum Ca^{2+} ATPase (Table 20-3)

or enhancement of β-adrenergic signaling either by overexpression of β_2-adrenergic receptors, expression of a dominant negative β-adrenergic receptor kinase (which interferes with downregulation of β-receptor signaling), or overexpression of adenylyl cyclase have all been effective in enhancing systolic function and decreasing progression to heart failure. Other animal studies reveal that myocardial gene transfer can inhibit the development of pressure-overload hypertrophy and prevent development of diastolic and systolic dysfunction.

Major challenges in applying gene therapy for heart failure to human disease include identification of a vector that will express a transgene in the heart for a prolonged period of time

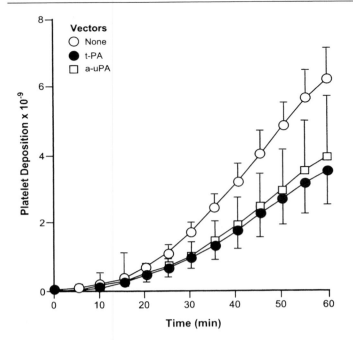

Figure 20-4   Gene therapy to prevent prosthetic graft thrombosis. Deposition of Indium-labeled platelets is measured on thrombi associated with synthetic vascular grafts. Grafts were seeded at equivalent densities with either untransduced endothelial cells or genetically engineered endothelial cells and exposed to flowing blood in a baboon ex vivo arteriovenous shunt. Data points are real-time measurements of platelet deposition, for untransduced endothelial cells (open circles; $n = 13$), endothelial cells transduced with a retroviral vector expressing human tissue plasminogen activator (t-PA; closed circles, $n = 8$), and a retroviral vector expressing a form of u-PA that is anchored to the cell membrane (a-uPA; $n = 5$). Bars represent standard error of the mean. (Reproduced with permission from Dichek et al., 1996.)

and verification that intracoronary vector infusion in humans is both safe and highly efficient in transducing cardiomyocytes. Reports of long-term transgene expression in animal hearts injected with adeno-associated viral and lentiviral vectors are encouraging. Nevertheless, a diseased heart in an octogenarian with a propensity to develop lethal arrhythmias is a far more challenging target for safe and effective gene transfer than the heart of an otherwise healthy laboratory animal. Finally, it is sobering to appreciate that certain medical interventions (such as phosphodiesterase inhibition) that have boosted systolic performance and improved patient well-being were ultimately linked with accelerated mortality. Gene therapy for systolic dysfunction will need to avoid this pitfall.

CARDIAC DYSRHYTHMIAS   Increased understanding of the molecular basis of cardiac conduction and identification of the genes that control the electrical events leading to depolarization and repolarization of cardiomyocytes has suggested that disorders of cardiac conduction might be treated by gene therapy. A seminal study in this area showed that gene transfer leading to expression, within porcine atrioventricular nodal cells, of a gene that inhibits β-adrenergic signaling significantly decreased the ventricular response to atrial fibrillation. A subsequent study demonstrated that expression in porcine myocardium of a gene that inhibits a specific cardiac potassium channel created a cellular "pacemaker" capable of depolarizing the ventricular myocardium. This biologically driven pacemaker could potentially substitute for dysfunctional

endogenous cardiac pacemaker tissue and prevent slow heart rates. These two studies reveal the potential for gene therapy to treat both tachyarrythmias (by increasing conduction block) or bradyarrythmias (by inducing spontaneous depolarizations). These are exciting findings; however, to be therapeutically useful, molecular electrophysiological approaches will need to rely on long-term, stable gene expression and will need to prove their value in comparison to well-established device and drug strategies for managing arrhythmias.

THROMBOSIS   Gene therapy for thrombosis initially focused on the thrombotic problems of intravascular prosthetic devices such as grafts and stents and on preventing thrombosis associated with angioplasty-induced arterial injury. Because intravascular prosthetic devices are acellular and cannot be targeted by in vivo gene transfer, an ex vivo, cell-based gene therapy strategy is obligatory. According to this strategy, endothelial cells are harvested from a superficial, nonessential vein and transduced with genes that express either t-PA or u-PA. These fibrinolytically "enhanced" cells are then seeded onto the surface of prosthetic devices before the devices are implanted. When the devices are implanted in vivo, increased expression of t-PA or u-PA could prevent device thrombosis. With this approach, overexpression of t-PA or u-PA from seeded endothelial cells decreased thrombus deposition onto a synthetic arteriovenous shunt placed in a baboon (Fig. 20-4). This antithrombotic effect was unaccompanied by evidence of systemic fibrinolysis, proving the concept that genetic manipulation of endothelial cells can decrease local thrombosis without creating a systemic fibrino(geno)lytic state. Although theoretically promising, these data are derived from very short-term experiments (1 h), whereas the clinical problem that they address (device thrombosis) may extend over years. The clinical utility of seeding vascular devices with genetically "enhanced" cells will depend on the availability of data showing that these cells or their progeny survive for prolonged periods of time after introduction in vivo. Progress relevant to this area includes the development of vectors capable of long-term in vivo transgene expression, such as adeno-associated virus and lentivirus, and the discovery that endothelial progenitor cells may be harvested from human peripheral blood and expanded ex vivo. These circulating progenitor cells could serve as a convenient source of endothelial cells that would be genetically modified and then used to line surfaces of intravascular prosthetic devices.

Other work on antithrombotic gene therapy has focused on decreasing thrombus formation in native arterial tissue. The rationale for this approach is that enhancement of the antithrombotic properties of the arterial surface will prevent the intravascular thrombotic events that precipitate myocardial infarctions and strokes. This approach could also be applied to venous tissue, to prevent venous thromboembolism. Antithrombotic gene therapy with a goal of preventing strokes and infarctions is supported by a large amount of clinical data showing efficacy of systemic antithrombotic and anticoagulant drugs such as aspirin, other platelet inhibitors, and coumadin. Because the efficacy of these systemically administered drugs is limited by systemic side effects, it is rational to replace them with targeted, local antithrombotic therapy that is limited to the artery or venous wall. Using this strategy, antithrombotic therapy would be delivered to the site of disease, and systemic side effects would be minimized.

The feasibility of antithrombotic gene therapy has been demonstrated in animal models of nondenuding arterial injury and in models of balloon injury. In the latter case, the clinical application

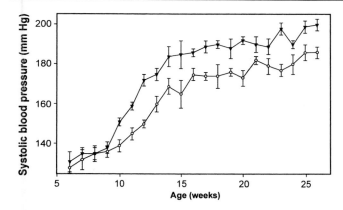

Figure 20-5   Gene therapy for hypertension. Spontaneously hypertensive rats (5-d-old) were given a single intracardiac injection of an adeno-associated viral vector expressing either sense angiotensinogen (triangles; $n = 6$–10) or antisense angiotensinogen (circles; $n = 8$–15). Systolic blood pressure was measured weekly. $p < 0.001$ between treatments and between times by two-way ANOVA. (Reproduced with permission from Kimura et al., 2001.)

of this technique would involve arterial gene transfer after angioplasty or surgical endarterectomy and would substitute antithrombotic gene therapy for the systemic antithrombotic drug therapy that is administered. Thus, both t-PA and thrombomodulin gene transfer decreased thrombus formation in nondenuded animal arteries. Gene therapy with tissue factor pathway inhibitor and C-type natriuretic peptide decreased thrombus formation in injured animal arteries. In all cases adenoviral vectors were used, and the studies were all short term. Improved vectors are needed to explore the potential of these approaches to provide durable protection against intravascular thrombosis and its complications.

HYPERTENSION   Human hypertension is a lifelong disease treated with lifelong, often multiple-drug therapy. This therapy is usually effective; however it is expensive, tedious for patients, and often accompanied by side effects. Gene therapy for hypertension provides the exciting possibility that a common, lifelong disease could be more conveniently and effective treated by the transfer and expression of a single gene. The power of gene therapy and the potential that it might someday revolutionize medical care is perhaps most evident in the context of common diseases such as hypertension.

Preclinical studies in animal models of systemic hypertension have yielded promising results. Systemic gene therapy with genes expressing vasodilator proteins such as kallikrein, adrenomedullin, and nitric oxide synthase have been effective in lowering blood pressure in hypertensive animals for up to 12 wk. Other investigators have used viral vectors to express full-length antisense transcripts that decrease expression of molecules that contribute to elevated blood pressure. For example, an adeno-associated virus vector encoding antisense transcripts to angiotensinogen decreased blood pressure in spontaneously hypertensive rats for up to 6 mo (Fig. 20-5). Systemic, antisense-mediated inhibition of β_1 adrenergic receptor expression also produced an antihypertensive effect.

Phase one clinical trials of antihypertensive gene therapy may be near. As these trials are initiated, it will be important to address several issues:

1. The applicability of studies in specific animal models to the pathophysiology of hypertension in humans.

2. The requirement for long-term, stable expression and the potential need for repeated gene delivery.
3. The need to develop practical means for the adjustment or reversal of antihypertensive gene therapy, should the effect of the inserted gene prove detrimental over time.

CONCLUSION

A variety of mono- and polygenic cardiovascular diseases are potentially treatable with gene therapy. Extensive animal studies and initial human trials have confirmed that genes with therapeutic effects within the cardiovascular system may be introduced in vivo. Nevertheless, practical concerns relating to the achievement of safe, efficient, and long-lasting gene therapy continue to dominate the field. It might be said that the understanding of the genetic basis of cardiovascular disease has outpaced the development of genetic technologies to alter its natural history. To be therapeutically useful, gene transfer techniques must, in general, achieve high efficiency, prolonged gene expression, and tissue-specific targeting, whereas avoiding induction of destructive inflammatory and immune responses. Each of these goals represents a substantial technical challenge. In addition, as progress extends beyond the initial excitement of overcoming technical hurdles and beginning clinical trials, gene therapy must ultimately prove its safety, efficacy, and even its superiority in relation to more traditional therapeutic interventions. Only then will gene therapy gain acceptance as a treatment for cardiovascular disease.

SELECTED REFERENCES

Allaire E, Forough R, Clowes M, Starcher B, Clowes AW. Local overexpression of TIMP-1 prevents aortic aneurysm degeneration and rupture in a rat model. J Clin Invest 1998;102:1413–1420.

Baumgartner I, Pieczek A, Manor O, et al. Constitutive expression of phVEGF-165 after intramuscular gene transfer promotes collateral vessel development in patients with critical limb ischemia. Circulation 1998;97:1114–1123.

Chang MW, Barr E, Seltzer J, et al. Cytostatic gene therapy for vascular proliferative disorders with a constitutively active form of the retinoblastoma gene product. Science 1995;267:518–522.

Channon KM, Qian H, George SE. Nitric oxide synthase in atherosclerosis and vascular injury: Insights from experimental gene therapy. Arterioscler Thromb Vasc Biol 2000;20:1873–1881.

Dichek DA, Anderson J, Kelly AB, Hanson SR, Harker LA. Enhanced in vivo antithrombotic effects of endothelial cells expressing recombinant plasminogen activators transduced with retroviral vectors. Circulation 1996;93:301–309.

Donahue JK, Heldman AW, Fraser H, et al. Focal modification of electrical conduction in the heart by viral gene transfer. Nat Med 2000;6:1395–1398.

Gelband CH, Katovich MJ, Raizada MK. Current perspectives on the use of gene therapy for hypertension. Circ Res 2000;87:1118–1122.

Giordano FJ, Ping P, McKirnan MD, et al. Intracoronary gene transfer of fibroblast growth factor-5 increases blood flow and contractile function in an ischemic region of the heart. Nat Med 1996;2:534–539.

Grines CL, Watkins MW, Helmer G, et al. Angiogenic Gene Therapy (AGENT) trial in patients with stable angina pectoris. Circulation 2002;105:1291–1297.

Grossman M, Rader DJ, Muller DWM, et al. A pilot study of ex vivo gene therapy for homozygous familial hypercholesterolaemia. Nat Med 1995;1:1148–1154.

Hajjar RJ, del Monte F, Matsui T, Rosenzweig A. Prospects for gene therapy for heart failure. Circ Res 2000;86:616–621.

Isner JM. Myocardial gene therapy. Nature 2002;415:234–239.

Kawashiri Ma M, Rader DJ. Gene therapy for lipid disorders. Curr Control Trials Cardiovasc Med 2000;1:120–127.

Kibbe MR, Billiar TR, Tzeng E. Gene therapy for restenosis. Circ Res 2000;86:829–833.

Kim I-H, Jozkowicz A, Piedra PA, Oka K, Chan L. Lifetime correction of genetic deficiency in mice with a single injection of helper-dependent adenoviral vector. Proc Natl Acad Sci USA 2001;98:13,282–13,287.

Kimura B, Mohuczy D, Tang X, Phillips MI. Attenuation of hypertension and heart hypertrophy by adeno-associated virus delivering angiotensinogen antisense. Hypertension 2001;37:376–380.

Losordo DW, Vale PR, Hendel RC, et al. Phase 1/2 placebo-controlled, double-blind, dose-escalating trial of myocardial vascular endothelial growth factor 2 gene transfer by catheter delivery in patients with chronic myocardial ischemia. Circulation 2002;105:2012–2018.

Maurice JP, Hata JA, Shah AS, et al. Enhancement of cardiac function after adenoviral-mediated in vivo intracoronary beta2-adrenergic receptor gene delivery. J Clin Invest 1999;104:21–29.

Miake J, Marban E, Nuss HB. Biological pacemaker created by gene transfer. Nature 2002;419:132, 133.

Miyamoto MI, del Monte F, Schmidt U, et al. Adenoviral gene transfer of SERCA2a improves left-ventricular function in aortic-banded rats in transition to heart feailure. Proc Natl Acad Sci USA 2000;97:793–798.

Nabel EG, Plautz G, Nabel GJ. Site-specific gene expression in vivo by direct gene transfer into the arterial wall. Science 1990;249: 1285–1288.

Rade JJ, Schulick AH, Virmani R, Dichek DA. Local adenoviral-mediated expression of recombinant hirudin reduces neointimal formation after arterial injury. Nat Med 1996;2:293–298.

Rajagopalan S, Trachtenberg J, Mohler E, et al. Phase I study of direct administration of a replication deficient adenovirus vector containing the vascular endothelial growth factor cDNA (CI-1023) to patients with claudication. Am J Cardiol 2002;90:512–516.

Rios CD, Chu Y, Davidson BL, Heistad DD. Ten steps to gene therapy for cardiovascular diseases. J Lab Clin Med 1998;132:104–111.

Rosengart TK, Lee LY, Patel SR, et al. Angiogenesis gene therapy: Phase I assessment of direct intramyocardial administration of an adenovirus vector expressing VEGF121 cDNA to individuals with clinically significant severe coronary artery disease. Circulation 1999;100:468–474.

Shah AS, Lilly RE, Kypson AP, et al. Intracoronary adenovirus-mediated delivery and overexpression of the beta2-adrenergic receptor in the heart: Prospects for molecular ventricular assistance. Circulation 2000; 101:408–414.

Su H, Lu R, Kan YW. Adeno-associated viral vector-mediated vascular endothelial growth factor gene transfer induces neovascular formation in ischemic heart. Proc Natl Acad Sci USA 2000;97:13,801–13,806.

Tangirala RK, Tsukamoto K, Chun SH, Usher D, Puré E, Rader DJ. Regression of atherosclerosis induced by liver-directed gene transfer of apolipoprotein A-I in mice. Circulation 1999;100:1816–1822.

Varenne D, Gerard RD, Sinnaeve P, Gillijns H, Collen D, Janssens S. Percutaneous adenoviral gene transfer into porcine coronary arteries: Is catheter-based gene delivery adapted to coronary circulation? Hum Gene Ther 1999;10:1105–1115.

Waugh JM, Yuksel E, Li J, et al. Local overexpression of thrombomodulin for in vivo prevention of arterial thrombosis in a rabbit model. Circ Res 1999;84:84–92.

Zoldhelyi P, McNatt J, Shelat HS, Yamamoto Y, Chen Z-Q, Willerson JT. Thromboresistance of balloon-injured porcine carotid arteries after local gene transfer of human tissue factor pathway inhibitor. Circulation 2000;101:289–295.

Pulmonary Diseases

III

SECTION EDITORS:
RICHARD C. BOUCHER AND PEADAR G. NOONE

Abbreviations

III. PULMONARY DISEASES

5-HT	serotonin
α_1-AT	α_1-antitrypsin
α-SMA	α-smooth muscle actin
AAV	adeno-associated virus
ACCESS	a case-controlled etiological study of sarcoidosis
ACE	angiotensin-converting enzyme
Ad	adenovirus
ADAM	a disintigrin and metalloproteinase domain
AGII	angiotensin II
AIP	acute interstitial pneumonia
ALI	acute lung injury
AM	alveolar macrophage
APC	antigen-presenting cell
ARDS	acute respiratory distress syndrome
ASL	airway surface liquid
ATS	American Thoracic Society
ß(2)-AR	ß(2)-adrenoreceptor
BAL	bronchoalveolar lavage
BHR	bronchial hyperresponsiveness
BMPR2	bone morphogenic protein receptor type 2
CA	central apparatus
CACC	calcium-activated chloride channels
CAMP	Childhood Asthma Management Program
cAMP	cyclic adenosine monophosphate
CAR	coxsackie adenovirus receptor
CC	Clara cell
CCR	CC chemokine receptor
CF	cystic fibrosis
CFRD	cystic fibrosis-related diabetes
CFTR	cystic fibrosis transmembrane conductance regulator
CG	cathepsin G
COPD	chronic obstructive pulmonary disease
CPI	chronic pneumonitis of infancy
DA	dynein arm
DAG	diacylglycerol
DIC	disseminated intravascular coagulation
DIP	desquamating interstitial pneumonitis
ECM	extracellular matrix
ECMO	extracorporeal membrane oxygenation
ECP	eosinophil cationic protein
EGF	epidermal growth factor
EGFR	epidermal growth factor receptor
EMTU	epithelial-mesenchymal trophic unit
ENaC	epithelial sodium channel
eNOS	endothelial nitric oxide synthase
ERS	European Respiratory Society
ET-1	endothelin-1
F	fast
FEV_1	forced expiratory volume in the first second
FGF	fibroblast growth factor
GM-CSF	granulocyte macrophage-colony stimulating factor
GST	glutathione S-transferase
GSTM1	GST mu
HB-EGF	heparin-binding epidermal growth factor-like growth factor
HLA	human leukocyte-associated antigen
HNE	human neutrophil elastase
HSP-70	Heat Shock Protein-70
HSVtk	herpes simplex thymidine kinase
IC	intermediate-chain dyneins
ICAM	intercellular adhesion molecule
iCD23	intact CD23
IDA	inner dynein arm
IFN	interferon
IGF	insulin-like growth factor
IGF1	insulin-like growth factor 1
IIP	idiopathic interstitial pneumonia
IL	interleukin
ILD	interstitial lung disease
IP_3	inositol triphosphate
IPF	idiopathic pulmonary fibrosis
LC	light-chain dyneins
LFA1	leukocyte function associated antigen 1
LIP	lymphoid interstitial pneumonia
LPS	lipopolysaccharide
L–R	left–right
LTC_4	leukotriene C_4
M	medium
MAPK	mitogen-activated protein kinase
MBL	mannose-binding lectin
MCC	mucociliary clearance
MDC	macrophage-derived chemokine
MHC	major histocompatibility complex
MIP1α	macrophage inflammatory protein 1α
MMP	matrix metalloproteinase
NE	neutrophil elastase
NOS	nitric oxide synthase
NSIP	nonspecific interstitial pneumonia
ODA	outer dynein arm
PA	pulmonary artery
PAF	platelet-activating factor
PAI	plasminogen activator inhibitor
PAP	pulmonary alveolar proteinosis

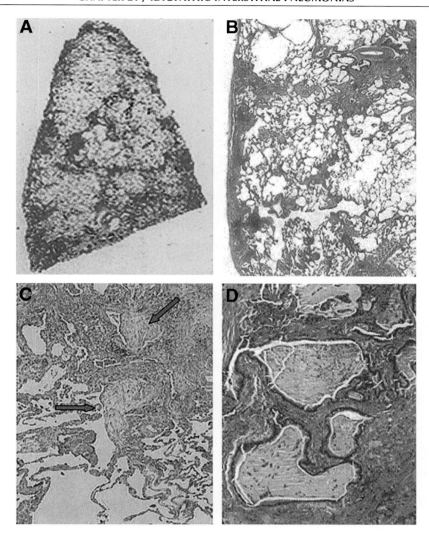

Figure 21-2 UIP pattern. These photomicrographs (H&E) of the pathological lesions appear to characterize the steps in progression of UIP. (**A**) Macroscopic view of lung biopsy showing that the lung injury is patchy and confined to the subpleural region. (**B**) Low magnification view shows marked fibrosis and cystic changes, with a striking subpleural distribution. Interstitial chronic inflammation is mild with a few lymphoid aggregates. (**C**) Multiple fibroblastic foci (arrows) of loose organizing connective tissue are the "leading edges" of the progressive fibrotic process. (**D**) Microscopic view of honeycombing. This process is irreversible.

are common in small to medium-sized pulmonary arterioles. The organizing phase shows loose organizing fibrosis, mostly within alveolar septa and type-II pneumocyte hyperplasia. There is widespread proliferation of fibroblasts and myofibroblasts, with minimal inflammatory infiltrate. The fibrotic changes are temporally homogeneous, and may be accompanied by the presence of hyaline membranes. With time, end-stage fibrosis develops and large cystic airspaces form. These cystic spaces are lined with alveolar epithelium, not bronchial epithelium as seen in the honeycombed spaces in UIP. The lungs may also progress to end-stage honeycomb fibrosis. However, if the patient survives, the lungs may resolve to normal.

LYMPHOID INTERSTITIAL PNEUMONIA Lymphoid interstitial pneumonia is characterized by a dense interstitial lymphoid infiltrate, including lymphocytes, plasma cells, and histiocytes with associated type-II cell hyperplasia and a mild increase in alveolar macrophages (Fig. 21-8). The alveolar septa are usually extensively infiltrated. Lymphoid follicles (follicles with germinal centers) are often present, usually in the distribution of

pulmonary lymphatics. Some architectural derangement (including honeycombing) and non-necrotizing granulomas may be seen. Intra-alveolar organization and macrophage accumulation may also be present, but only as minor components.

PATHOGENESIS OF LUNG FIBROSIS

Lung fibrosis is the final common pathway of a variety of insults to the lung including infectious, toxic, drug-induced, autoimmune, or traumatic injuries. The pathogenesis of lung fibrosis remains incompletely understood. However, there has been a major paradigm shift away from the prevailing theory that generalized inflammation progressed to widespread parenchymal fibrosis. The model emphasizing the role of inflammation may remain applicable to interstitial lung diseases that respond to anti-inflammatory agents (e.g., NSIP, hypersensitivity pneumonitis, and organizing pneumonia). However, the lack of a similar response to anti-inflammatory agents in patients with the UIP pattern provides strong evidence that inflammation does not play a critical role in the progressive and irreversible phase of this disease. In this context, there are two

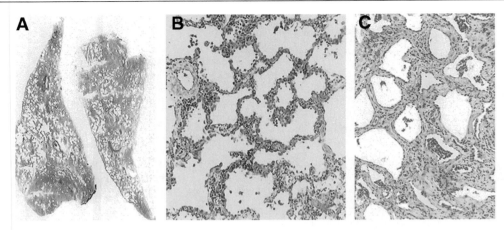

Figure 21-3 NSIP pattern. These photomicrographs (H&E) of the pathological lesions appear to characterize the steps in progression of NSIP. **(A)** Macroscopic view of lung biopsy showing that the lung is diffusely injured. **(B)** Early stage showing a cellular chronic interstitial inflammation (small lymphocytes and plasma cells)—this process appears to be reversible. **(C)** A later stage that shows diffuse thickening of the alveolar by fibrosis and mild interstitial inflammation. Alveolar pneumocyte hyperplasia is present. No fibroblastic foci are present.

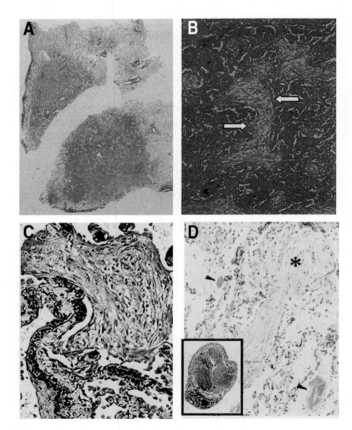

Figure 21-4 Organizing pneumonia pattern. These photomicrographs of the pathological lesions appear to characterize the steps in progression of organizing pneumonia. **(A)** Macroscopic view of lung biopsy showing that the process is patchy with normal lung adjacent to nodular areas of consolidation (H&E). **(B)** Low magnification view shows polypoid plugs of loose connective tissue within alveolar ducts and alveolar spaces (H&E). The connective tissue is all about the same age. **(C)** Higher magnification view shows a polypoid plug (pentachrome). The architecture of the lung is preserved. The connective tissue has a myxoid appearance owing to the abundant mucopolysaccharides and paucity of collagen. **(D)** Polypoid plugs of loose connective tissue within alveolar spaces (*) and dense collagen globules *(arrowheads)*. The insert shows an electron microscopic picture of a collagen globule. The structure of collagen globule is covered by

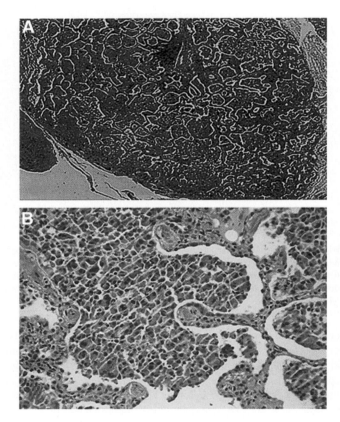

Figure 21-5 DIP pattern. These photomicrographs of the pathological lesions appear to characterize the steps in progression of DIP (H&E). **(A)** Low magnification view shows the alveolar spaces are diffusely involved by marked alveolar macrophage accumulation and there is mild interstitial thickening. **(B)** Higher magnification view shows the alveolar walls are mildly thickened by fibrous connective tissue and a few chronic inflammatory cells. The alveolar spaces are filled with macrophages.

Figure 21-4 *(Continued)* type-I alveolar epithelial cell. Collagen fibrils are densely arranged, and thin cytoplasm of fibroblasts is found between these fibrils. (Original magnification, ×5000.) (Reproduced with permission from Fukuda Y, Ishizaki M, Kudoh S, Kitaichi M, Yamanaka N. Localization of matrix metalloproteinases-1, -2, and -9 and tissue inhibitor of metalloproteinase-2 in interstitial lung diseases. Lab Invest 1998;78:687–698. Copyright Nature Publishing Group.)

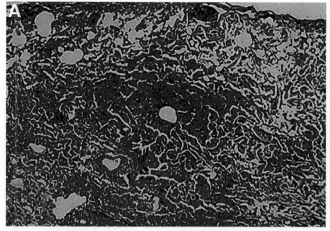

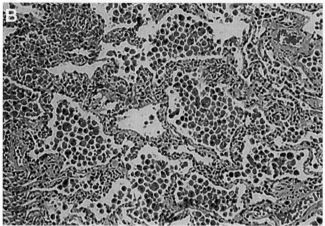

Figure 21-6 Respiratory bronchiolitis-associated interstitial lung disease pattern. These photomicrographs of the pathological lesions appear to characterize the steps in progression of respiratory bronchiolitis-associated interstitial lung disease (H&E). **(A)** Low magnification view shows bronchiolocentric consolidated process. Interstitial thickening confined to the peribronchiolar parenchyma. **(B)** A higher magnification view shows mild thickening of the wall of the respiratory bronchiole and adjacent alveolar walls. Faintly pigmented alveolar macrophages fill the lumen of respiratory bronchioles and the surrounding airspaces.

prominent schemes proposed for the development diffuse lung fibrosis: (1) an "inflammatory-fibrotic pathway" represented by most forms of ILD, in which there is an early, clearly distinguishable phase of inflammation, followed by a subsequent fibrotic phase, and (2) "epithelial damage and fibroblast activation pathway," represented by IPF.

THE INFLAMMATORY-FIBROTIC PATHWAY The normal host response to injury, regardless of the type of injury, is to evoke an inflammatory response that involves a complex set of interactions that appear to be tightly controlled in a time and context-dependent manner (Fig. 21-9). It appears that this initial inflammatory response to tissue injury (i.e., cell damage and disruption of normal structure) also sets into motion the repair responses. In most instances, the inflammation resolves naturally and the tissue returns to normal; the injured cells are replaced and the overall tissue structure is restored with minimal production of granulation tissue. In fact, in many of the apparently reversible interstitial lung disorders (e.g., NSIP and organizing pneumonia) the response to damage and inflammation

involves rapid re-epithelialization, fibrin formation, and the development of granulation tissue (i.e., a vascularized fibrotic response). As the epithelium repairs itself the granulation tissue resolves and the lung returns to a more normal structure and function. The bleomycin mouse model of lung injury is an example of this resolvable inflammatory and fibrotic reaction.

EPITHELIAL DAMAGE AND FIBROBLAST ACTIVATION PATHWAY The rationale for the theory that inflammation precedes fibrosis in UIP was the supposition that intra-alveolar macrophage-neutrophil accumulation (i.e., "alveolitis") was the earliest lesion in UIP. However, in UIP such intra-alveolar inflammation is rarely observed. Even in the thickened alveolar septa in UIP there is only a sparse inflammatory infiltrate. Moreover, in interstitial lung diseases (e.g., hypersensitivity pneumonitis, NSIP) in which inflammation is a prominent feature of early disease, fibroblastic foci are not seen and the extensive fibrotic pattern common in UIP does not develop. The agent(s) that incites this fibroproliferation remains unknown. Investigations have provided evidence that UIP may be the result of ongoing diffuse microscopic alveolar epithelial injury (in the absence of a prominent inflammatory response) and abnormal wound healing (Fig. 21-10).

Epithelial Injury and Failure of Re-Epithelialization An intact epithelial barrier is crucial to maintaining normal alveolar function (Fig. 21-10B). The epithelium plays a key role in the regulation of the inflammatory process in the lung. It is hypothesized that epithelial cells are not only the sites of initial injury in UIP, but also are major determinants of the repair process.

Following an injury in the normal repair process, the alveolar epithelium initiates wound healing to restore the integrity of this barrier. This rapid re-epithelialization of the denuded area, through epithelial cell migration, proliferation, and differentiation is critical to normal repair. Evidence shows that re-epithelialization may be mediated, in part, by adult stem cells.

Alveolar epithelial cell death is an early and consistent finding in UIP. In UIP, the alveolar epithelium shows a marked loss of or damage to type-I cells, hyperplasia of type-II cells, as well as altered expression of adhesion molecules and major histocompatibility complex antigens. The cause of the delayed or ineffective re-epithelialization in UIP is unknown and could result from loss of proliferative capacity, increased apoptosis, or ineffective migration of alveolar epithelial cells. Thus, delayed or ineffective re-epithelialization is a key trigger for recruiting, activating, and sustaining mesenchymal cells.

During wound healing, tissue injury causes disruption of blood vessels and extravasation of blood constituents into the wound. These constituents re-establish hemostasis and provide a provisional extracellular matrix for the repair process to begin. The epithelial cells must dissolve the fibrin barrier before migrating throughout the denuded wound surface. However, in patients with IPF, there is increased local procoagulant activity that may result from the dysfunctional alveolar epithelial cells. For example, tissue factor, a potent procoagulant factor, and plasminogen activator inhibitor-1 and -2 are both strongly expressed by alveolar epithelial cells in IPF. This procoagulant activity may impede epithelial cell movement through the extracellular matrix, prohibiting the repair process.

In areas where the basement membrane remains intact, type-II cells attempt to recover the epithelial surface as evidenced by their expression of a number of enzymes, cytokines, and growth factors. However, in UIP, the capacity of type-II alveolar cells to restore damaged type-I cells is seriously altered. Consequently, epithelial

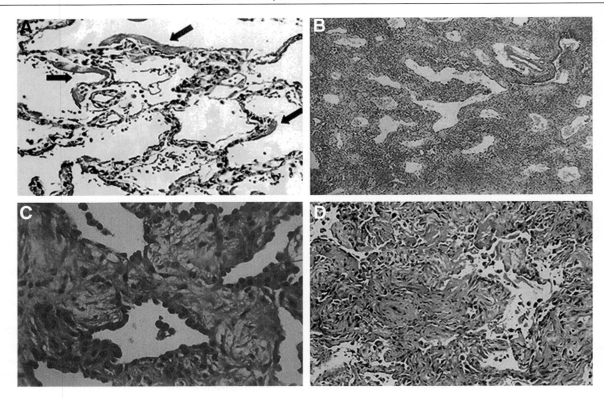

Figure 21-7   Diffuse alveolar damage (DAD) pattern. These photomicrographs of the pathological lesions appear to characterize the steps in progression of DAD in a patient with AIP (H&E). (**A**) The lung shows the early (exudative) stage with edema, diffuse alveolar wall injury, and hyaline membranes (arrows). (**B**) The lung shows diffuse alveolar wall thickening by proliferating connective tissue, type-II pneumocytes, and hyaline membranes. (**C**) A higher magnification view shows alveolar wall thickening by proliferating connective tissue and inflammation and prominent type-II pneumocyte proliferation. (**D**) The lung shows the organizing pattern of DAD with fibrosis in the alveolar septal walls consisting of a loose organizing type of connective tissue.

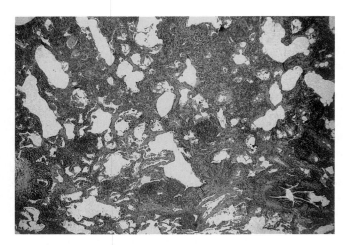

Figure 21-8   Lymphocytic interstitial pneumonia pattern. There is diffuse thickening of alveolar walls by a moderately severe infiltrate of lymphocytes and plasma cells.

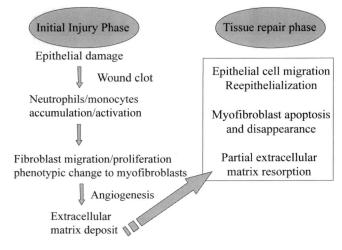

Figure 21-9   The normal wound healing model. (Adapted with permission from Selman M, King TE Jr, Pardo A. Idiopathic pulmonary fibrosis: Prevailing and evolving hypotheses about its pathogenesis and implications for therapy. Ann Intern Med 2001;134:136–151.)

cuboidalization, transitional reactive phenotypes, and alveolar collapse are observed. This failure to restore the alveolar epithelium and the disruption of the epithelial basement membrane allow fibroblast/myofibroblasts to migrate and proliferate in the alveolar space. This process leads to the deposition of intra-alveolar extracellular matrix.

Basement Membrane Disruption   The basement membrane is a complex structure of a variety of proteins that plays a

dynamic role in maintaining the integrity and differentiation of the overlying alveolar epithelium (*see* Fig. 21-10B). In addition to the alveolar epithelial cell injury, basement membrane disruption is also likely important in the pathogenesis of lung fibrosis. This physical disruption does not facilitate orderly repair of the damaged alveolar type-I epithelial cells. Instead, the damaged basement membrane allows migration of fibroblasts/myofibroblasts into the

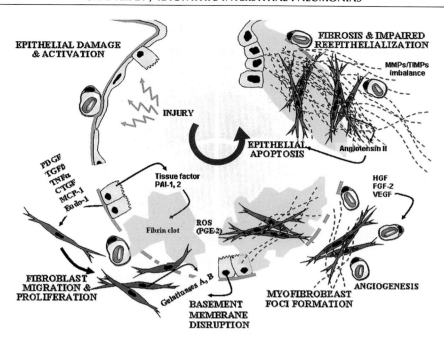

Figure 21-10 Hypothetical scheme of the key events leading to lung fibrosis in UIP. An unknown injury provokes multiple microinjuries that damage and activate alveolar epithelial cells (*top left*). A fibrin clot forms and serves as a provisional matrix for the migration and proliferation of reparative type-I alveolar epithelial cells. Neutrophils secrete proinflammatory mediators, reactive oxygen species, and metalloproteinases. Lymphocyte recruitment leads to the production of Th2-type cytokines, IL-4, and IL-13. Reepithelialization is delayed leading to a denuded, disrupted basement membrane. Alveolar epithelial cells secrete growth factors and induce migration and proliferation of fibroblasts and differentiation into myofibroblasts (*bottom left*). Subepithelial myofibroblasts and alveolar epithelial cells produce gelatinases that may increase basement membrane disruption and allow fibroblast-myofibroblast migration (*bottom right*). Fibroblasts migrate into the wound and produce extracellular matrix proteins and mediators such as angiotensin II, which may further promote alveolar epithelial cell apoptosis. Angiogenic factors may be elaborated, leading to the formation of nascent vasculature early in the disease process. Reciprocal communication between alveolar epithelial cells and mesenchymal cells results in a positive feedback loop that promotes ongoing fibrosis and destruction of alveolar architecture. Alveolar macrophages and epithelial cells secrete TGF-1, which promotes myofibroblast differentiation, increases ECM production, and inhibits apoptosis of fibroblasts/myofibroblasts. An imbalance between interstitial collagenases and tissue inhibitors of metalloproteinases provokes the progressive deposit of extracellular matrix (*top right*). Myofibroblasts produce angiotensinogen that as angiotensin II provokes alveolar epithelial cell death, further impairing reepithelialization. Signals responsible for myofibroblast apoptosis seem to be absent or delayed in UIP, increasing cell survival. As ECM deposition progresses, regression of blood vessels may occur. (*See* text for details about this process.) Endo-1, endothelin-1; CTGF, connective tissue growth factor; ECM, extracellular matrix; FGF-2, fibroblast growth factor-2; HGF, hepatocyte growth factor; MCP-1, monocyte chemoattractant protein-1; MMP, metalloproteinase; PAI, plasminogen activator inhibitor; PGE, prostaglandin E; PDGF, platelet-derived growth factor; ROS, reactive oxygen species; TGF-β, transforming growth factor-β; TIMP, tissue inhibitors of metalloproteinases; TNF-α, tumor necrosis factor-α; VEGF, vascular endothelial growth factor. (Adapted with permission from Selman M, King TE Jr, Pardo A. Idiopathic pulmonary fibrosis: Prevailing and evolving hypotheses about its pathogenesis and implications for therapy. Ann Intern Med 2001;134:136–151.)

alveolar spaces. Increasing evidence suggests that myofibroblasts themselves actually play a role in the degradation of basement membrane, thus facilitating their migration into the alveolar spaces. Gelatinases A and B, two members of the matrix metalloproteinases family that are produced by several lung cell types, degrade different components of the basement membrane, primarily type-IV collagen. In UIP, subepithelial myofibroblasts produce these gelatinases in some areas with denuded alveolar basement membranes.

Angiogenesis Evidence for the role of angiogenesis in the etiology of IPF remains limited and controversial (Fig. 21-10C). In contrast, although neovascularization is a prominent feature in organizing pneumonia, a usually reversible fibrogenic process, it is not a prominent feature of UIP. In fact, proangiogenic proteins have low levels of expression in fibroblastic foci in UIP compared with granulation tissue in organizing pneumonia. One study suggested that there is a net vascular ablation and redistribution of blood vessels in areas of interstitial thickening in UIP.

Myofibroblast Foci Evidence suggests that the earliest, and possibly the only, morphological changes associated with

subsequent progression to dense fibrosis in patients with UIP are the presence and extent of fibroblastic foci in the injured lung (Fig. 21-10D). Fibroblasts within these foci continually modify their interactions with the microenvironment. The extent of fibroblastic foci in UIP correlates with poor prognosis and survival.

Presumably, fibroblasts assume a migratory phenotype, followed by a proliferative phenotype, and finally a profibrotic phenotype during which they produce abundant extracellular matrix components. Most cells in the fibroblast foci are myofibroblasts: spindle-shaped cells aligned parallel to one another. The myofibroblasts in the UIP lesions are a synthetically active phenotype responsible for the connective tissue synthesis. They also appear to contribute to active contraction, which results in the distorted lung architecture characteristic of the UIP lesion. This is accompanied by imbalances in the production of matrix metalloproteinases and tissue inhibitors of metalloproteinases. In particular, TIMP-2 expression by the myofibroblasts in UIP appears to contribute to the irreversible structural remodeling in this disease. The UIP myofibroblasts have several additional features: they secrete angiotensin peptides that may induce apoptosis of adjacent alveolar epithelial cells;

there is diminished cyclooxygenase-2 expression/prostaglandin E2 synthesis; they express surface receptors such as CD40 typically associated with immune cells and are capable of producing a number of chemokines and cytokines.

GENETIC FACTORS IN LUNG FIBROSIS

Several findings support a potential genetic basis for the IIPs:

1. Familial pulmonary fibrosis, including its description in identical twins (some of whom have been separated geographically for many years), has been reported.
2. Alveolar inflammation has been identified in clinically unaffected family members of patients with familial pulmonary fibrosis. The significance of these findings remains unknown, but it is speculated that these unaffected family members might be at risk for the development of familial pulmonary fibrosis.
3. Pulmonary fibrosis appears in association with inherited disorders such as neurofibromatosis, Hermansky-Pudlak syndrome, tuberous sclerosis, Gaucher's disease, lymphangiomyomatosis, and the hypocalciuric hypercalcemia syndrome.
4. There is marked variation in response to profibrotic agents observed in humans despite similar levels of exposure (e.g., roentgenographically evident asbestosis occurs in only 25–50% of workers exposed to the highest cumulative dose of asbestos; hence, at least half of those heavily exposed to asbestos appear to be "resistant" to the fibrogenic effects of this dust).
5. Certain animal strains have a susceptibility to fibrotic agents, which suggests an inheritable predisposition.

FAMILIAL PULMONARY FIBROSIS   In Finland, it was estimated that the prevalence for familial pulmonary fibrosis was 5.9/million. The familial form explained 3.3–3.7% of all Finnish cases of IPF diagnosed according to the revised ATS/ERS international guidelines. Geographic clustering has been noted suggesting a recent founder effect in patients with familial pulmonary fibrosis. Familial cases of lung fibrosis account for 0.5–2.2% of all patients with IIPs, with a prevalence of 1.34 cases/10^6 population in the United Kingdom.

The clinical, roentgenographic, physiological, and morphological manifestations of familial pulmonary fibrosis are similar to the nonfamilial forms of lung fibrosis. Patients with familial pulmonary fibrosis presenting at a younger age usually appear to have more aggressive disease. However, the longest survivals have been seen in those presenting between the ages of 10 and 20 yr (this may have resulted from "lead time bias"—i.e., overestimation of survival duration owing to earlier detection). There may be a slight male predominance, and women tend to have a more favorable prognosis.

Familial pulmonary fibrosis has been associated with multiple pathological subsets of the IIPs: DIP, lymphocytic interstitial pneumonitis, and UIP. Mutations in the surfactant protein (SP)-C gene (*SFTPC*) are associated with familial desquamative and nonspecific interstitial pneumonitis and may cause type-II cellular injury (Fig. 21-11). The mutation was not seen in control chromosomes and thus is not likely to be a polymorphism. Electron microscopy of affected lung revealed alveolar type-II cell atypia, with numerous abnormal lamellar bodies. The authors hypothesized that the presence of two different pathological diagnoses in affected relatives sharing this mutation indicated that in this kindred, these diseases might represent pleiotropic manifestations of the same central

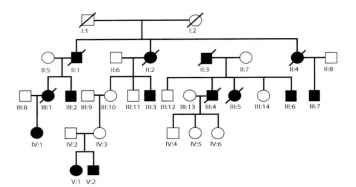

Figure 21-11   A mutation in surfactant protein C gene (*SFTPC*) caused familial pulmonary fibrosis (FPF). This kindred spans five generations, contains 97 total members, including 11 adults with FPF, including 6 with biopsy-proven usual interstitial pneumonitis, and 3 affected children (III : 5, V : 1,V : 2) with cellular nonspecific interstitial pneumonitis. (Reproduced with permission from Loyd JE. Pulmonary fibrosis in families. Am J Respir Cell Mol Biol 2003;29[3 Suppl]:S47–S50. Copyright American Thoracic Society.)

pathogenesis. Multiple heterozygous mutations in SP-C gene have been reported in association with children suffering from interstitial lung disease (DIP or NSIP), including familial and sporadic occurrences. In addition, a deficiency of SP-C has been described in a small kindred suffering from a poorly defined form of interstitial pneumonitis, despite no sequence variation in SP-C gene. It appears that the nature and biology of the SP-C mutation, amounts of production of the active SP-C peptide, the inheritance of other genetic modifiers or exposure to environmental factors may influence the variability in histopathological pattern among affected individuals. Taken together, these findings support a model in which misfolded proSP-C or SP-C protein can cause type-II alveolar cell injury that results in interstitial lung disease.

IMPLICATIONS OF THE PATHOGENETIC PATHWAYS OF LUNG FIBROSIS FOR THE TREATMENT OF LUNG FIBROSIS

Although the clinical course of IPF patients varies, their long-term survival is dismal, only 20–30% of IPF patients survive for 5 yr after their diagnosis. Individual patients may remain relatively stable (or experience very slow declines in lung function or progression of radiographic abnormalities) for an extended period of time (months to years) whereas others experience an accelerated phase with a rapid clinical decline and subsequent death (*see* Acute Exacerbation of IPF). Conventional management of IPF has been primarily based on the concept that suppressing inflammation would prevent progression to fibrosis. Clearly, this approach has failed; there is no effective treatment in use. Most therapeutic regimens have not targeted specific components of the epithelial damage/fibroblast activation pathway described earlier. It is hoped that as a result of better understanding of the natural history of IPF and the sequence of the pathogenic mechanisms (as well as of the plethora of biological events that control the fibrotic response), improved therapeutic strategies will be developed to improve patient outcome.

Because of the often poor responsiveness of IIP to corticosteroids, immunomodulatory agents have been tried with mixed results. Antifibrotic agents have been tried alone or in combination with corticosteroids in patients with UIP. A randomized control trial of interferon γ-1b and prednisolone compared with prednisolone alone failed to show an improvement in progression-free survival, pulmonary function, or the quality of life. There is increasing interest in these and other antifibrotic agents as the fibroproliferative nature of the pathophysiology is further defined.

ACUTE EXACERBATIONS OF IPF   It is increasingly apparent that "acute exacerbations" or an "accelerated phase of rapid clinical decline" characterizes the clinical course of IPF. These episodes are defined as acute worsening (occurring over <4 wk):

1. More dyspnea with same level of exertion.
2. Progressive hypoxemia.
3. New opacities on chest imaging studies.
4. Exclusion of infection or heart failure.

Occasionally, systemic symptoms such as fever, fatigue, and weight loss are present. In fact, rapid progression and hospitalization because of respiratory decompensation were both independent predictors of mortality in the subsequent 3 mo. Better understanding and management of these episodes appear critical to reducing the death rate in IPF.

ACKNOWLEDGMENT

The author thanks Thomas V. Colby and Jeffrey L. Myers for photomicrographs of the pathological lesions.

SELECTED REFERENCES

American Thoracic Society. Idiopathic pulmonary fibrosis: diagnosis and treatment. International consensus statement. American Thoracic Society (ATS) and the European Respiratory Society (ERS). Am J Respir Crit Care Med 2000;161:646–664.

American Thoracic Society/European Respiratory Society international multidisciplinary consensus classification of the idiopathic interstitial pneumonias. Am J Respir Crit Care Med 2002;165:277–304.

Baumgartner KB, Samet J, Stidley CA, Colby TV, Waldron JA, Collaborating Centers. Cigarette smoking: a risk factor for idiopathic pulmonary fibrosis. Am J Respir Crit Care Med 1997;155:242–248.

Burkhardt A. Alveolitis and collapse in the pathogenesis of pulmonary fibrosis. Am Rev Respir Dis 1989;140:513–524.

Chapman HA. Disorders of lung matrix remodeling. J Clin Invest 2004;113: 148–157.

Collard HR, Ryu JH, Douglas WW, et al. Combined corticosteroid and cyclophosphamide therapy does not alter survival in idiopathic pulmonary fibrosis. Chest 2004;125:2169–2174.

Coultas DB, Zumwalt RE, Black WC, Sobonya RE. The epidemiology of interstitial lung disease. Am J Respir Crit Care Med 1994; 150: 967–972.

Davies HR, Richeldi L, Walters EH. Immunomodulatory agents for idiopathic pulmonary fibrosis. Cochrane Database Syst Rev 2003(3):CD003134.

Flaherty KR, Colby TV, Travis WD, et al. Fibroblastic foci in usual interstitial pneumonia: idiopathic versus collagen vascular disease. Am J Respir Crit Care Med 2003;167:1410–1415.

Flaherty KR, Toews GB, Travis WD, et al. Clinical significance of histological classification of idiopathic interstitial pneumonia. Eur Respir J 2002;19:275–283.

Fukuda Y, Ishizaki M, Kudoh S, Kitaichi M, Yamanaka N. Localization of matrix metalloproteinases-1, -2, and -9 and tissue inhibitor of metalloproteinase-2 in interstitial lung diseases. Lab Invest 1998;78: 687–698.

Fukuda Y, Mochimaru H, Terasaki Y, Kawamoto M, Kudoh S. Mechanism of structural remodeling in pulmonary fibrosis. Chest 2001;120(1 Suppl):41S–43S.

Gauldie J, Kolb M, Sime PJ. A new direction in the pathogenesis of idiopathic pulmonary fibrosis? Respir Res 2002;3:1–3.

Henson PM. Possible roles for apoptosis and apoptotic cell recognition in inflammation and fibrosis. Am J Respir Cell Mol Biol 2003;29(3 Suppl):S70–S76.

Hunninghake G, Zimmerman MB, Schwartz DA, et al. Utility of lung biopsy for the diagnosis of idiopathic pulmonary fibrosis. Am J Respir Crit Care Med 2001;164:193–196.

Hunninghake GW, Lynch DA, Galvin JR, et al. Radiologic findings are strongly associated with a pathologic diagnosis of usual interstitial pneumonia. Chest 2003;124:1215–1223.

Johnston IDA, Prescott RJ, Chalmers JC, Rudd RM, Fibrosing Alveolitis Subcommittee of the Research Committee of the British Thoracic Society. British Thoracic Society study of cryptogenic fibrosing alveolitis: current presentation and initial management. Thorax 1997;52:38–44.

Kaminski N, Belperio JA, Bitterman PB, et al. Idiopathic Pulmonary Fibrosis. Proceedings of the 1st Annual Pittsburgh International Lung Conference. October 2002. Am J Respir Cell Mol Biol 2003;29 (3 Suppl):S1–S105.

Katzenstein ALA, Myers JL. Idiopathic pulmonary fibrosis. Clinical relevance of pathologic classification. Am J Respir Crit Care Med 1998;157:1301–1315.

Keane MP, Belperio JA, Moore TA, et al. Neutralization of the CXC chemokine, macrophage inflammatory protein-2, attenuates bleomycin-induced pulmonary fibrosis. J Immunol 1999;162:5511–5518.

King TE Jr. Idiopathic interstitial pneumonia. In: Schwarz MI, King TE Jr, eds. Interstitial Lung Diseases, 4th ed. Hamilton, Ontario, Canada: B.C. Decker, Inc., 2003; pp. 701–786.

King TE Jr, Schwarz MI, Brown K, et al. Idiopathic pulmonary fibrosis. Relationship between histopathologic features and mortality. Am J Respir Crit Care Med 2001;164:1025–1032.

Kuhn C III, Boldt J, King TE Jr, Crouch E, Vartio T, McDonald JA. An immunohistochemical study of architectural remodeling and connective tissue synthesis in pulmonary fibrosis. Am Rev Respir Dis 1989; 140:1693–1703.

Kuhn C III, McDonald JA. The roles of the myofibroblast in idiopathic pulmonary fibrosis: ultrastructural and immunohistochemical features of sites of active extracellular matrix synthesis. Am J Pathol 1991;138:1257–1265.

Lappi-Blanco E, Soini Y, Kinnula V, Paakko P. VEGF and bFGF are highly expressed in intraluminal fibromyxoid lesions in bronchiolitis obliterans organizing pneumonia. J Pathol 2002;196:220–227.

Loyd JE. Pulmonary fibrosis in families. Am J Respir Cell Mol Biol 2003;29(3 Suppl):S47–S50.

Nicholson AG, Fulford LG, Colby TV, Dubois RM, Hansell DM, Wells AU. The relationship between individual histologic features and disease progression in idiopathic pulmonary fibrosis. Am J Respir Crit Care Med 2002;166:173–177.

Raghu G, Brown KK, Bradford WZ, et al. A placebo-controlled trial of interferon gamma-1b in patients with idiopathic pulmonary fibrosis. N Engl J Med 2004;350:125–133.

Renzoni EA, Walsh DA, Salmon M, et al. Interstitial vascularity in fibrosing alveolitis. Am J Respir Crit Care Med 2003;167:438–443.

Richeldi L, Davies HR, Ferrara G, Franco F. Corticosteroids for idiopathic pulmonary fibrosis. Cochrane Database Syst Rev 2003(3):CD002880.

Selman M, King TE Jr, Pardo A. Idiopathic pulmonary fibrosis: prevailing and evolving hypotheses about its pathogenesis and implications for therapy. Ann Intern Med 2001;134:136–151.

Selman M, Ruiz V, Cabrera S, et al. TIMP-1, -2, -3, and -4 in idiopathic pulmonary fibrosis. A prevailing nondegradative lung microenvironment? Am J Physiol Lung Cell Mol Physiol 2000;279:L562–L574.

Thannickal VJ, Toews GB, White ES, Lynch JP 3rd, Martinez FJ. Mechanisms of pulmonary fibrosis. Annu Rev Med 2004;55:395–417.

Travis WD, King TE Jr, Bateman ED, et al. American Thoracic Society/ European Respiratory Society International Multidisciplinary Consensus Classification of the Idiopathic Interstitial Pneumonias. Am J Respir Crit Care Med 2002;165:277–304.

Uhal BD. Apoptosis in lung fibrosis and repair. Chest 2002;122(6 Suppl): 293S–298S.

22 Asthma

STEPHEN T. HOLGATE, GORDON DENT, AND MARK G. BUCKLEY

SUMMARY

Understanding of the molecular basis of asthma has progressed significantly in the last decade. The roles of immune recognition and effector cells in orchestrating airway inflammation have been developed, and a picture of how these cells—as well as structural cells within the airways—control long-term tissue remodeling is emerging, which provides a comprehensive view of the pathophysiological processes involved in the disease. Phenotypic changes in the asthmatic bronchial epithelium, and its interaction with other cells, have been identified which explain many features of asthma. Moreover, major steps have been taken in characterizing the genetic basis of the disease.

Key Words: ADAM33; cell–cell interactions; epithelium; fibroblasts; genetics; growth factor receptors; immunoglobulin E; inflammation; leukocytes; oxidants; remodeling.

INTRODUCTION

Asthma is often defined as a lung disease with three characteristics: reversible airway obstruction, bronchial hyperresponsiveness (BHR) to inhaled stimuli, and inflammation. The disease is generally a chronic condition that affects 5–7% of adults and up to 20% of children. However, the diagnosis of asthma is often difficult in children because of the high prevalence of virus-induced wheezing that may occur in the absence of asthma. The impact of asthma on any individual is highly dependent on the extent of control of the underlying disease process that can best be achieved by elimination of precipitating factors and effective use of drug therapy. Despite improved understanding of environmental factors underlying the origins and progression of chronic asthma and the availability of more effective drugs for its treatment, the prevalence of this disease and the numbers of hospitalizations and deaths attributed to the disease have been increasing, both in the developed and the developing world. At least some of these rising trends are based on lack of appropriate diagnosis and poor use of medication, in particular inadequate long-term treatment with antiinflammatory drugs. Nonetheless, the marked increases in frequency and severity of asthma serve to underscore the need for a better understanding of the molecular basis for the disease.

Perhaps the single most important conceptual "advance" in defining molecular mechanisms of asthma has been the recognition that it is an inflammatory disease. Evidence that inflammation is an important component of asthma was clear even in early descriptions of the cytopathology and histopathology of the disease. For example, analysis of sputum samples and airway tissue indicated that epithelial desquamation and airway eosinophilia were invariably present during acute attacks. However, the critical role of inflammation as a cause of the abnormal physiology was only firmly established in experimental models of the disease induced by nonallergic and allergic stimuli in which pathophysiology was closely linked to the development of an inflammatory response, and in bronchial biopsy and bronchoalveolar lavage (BAL) studies of asthmatic subjects under baseline conditions and during spontaneous or experimentally provoked exacerbations, in which evidence of abnormal airway function was again closely correlated with the presence of inflammatory cells and mediators.

In the context of airway obstruction, BHR and inflammation, morphological studies of asthma indicate that an overexuberant inflammatory response underpins much of the disordered airway function linked to disease expression, but certainly not all, especially in patients refractory to corticosteroids. Alteration in airway wall structure (sometimes referred to as remodeling) is also important through increased smooth muscle, matrix deposition, and increased vascular and neural networks. In addition, mucus hypersecretion is an important feature in chronic severe disease and in exacerbations.

The challenges that now confront researchers and clinicians are (1) defining the biochemical mechanisms responsible for asthmatic airway inflammation, and (2) determining the environmental and pharmacological means to more effectively inhibit inflammatory pathways or potentiate antiinflammatory ones. This chapter reviews prominent cellular and biochemical pathways responsible for airway immunity and inflammation. Defining these pathways has provided initial clues to the identity of genes activated during asthmatic disease.

MECHANISMS OF AIRWAY INFLAMMATION

The concept that inflammation leads to BHR and narrowing has led to a widening search for the types of inflammatory cells and mediators responsible for the cascade of events linking the initial stimulus to the final abnormality in airway function. Cell types implicated in the development of airway inflammation include immune cells (including mast cells, basophils, eosinophils, lymphocytes, neutrophils, and macrophages) as well as sentinel structural cells (including airway epithelial cells, vascular endothelial cells, and airway smooth muscle cells). Cell–cell interactions are

From: *Principles of Molecular Medicine, Second Edition*
Edited by: M. S. Runge and C. Patterson © Humana Press, Inc., Totowa, NJ

attributed to classes of mediators that include lipids, proteases, peptides, cytokines, and chemokines. It is not yet possible to integrate all of this information into a single model for the development of asthmatic airway inflammation. However, engagement of the allergic antibody IgE and the classification of T-cell responses to allergic and nonallergic stimuli that are inhaled into the airway have provided a useful framework. Using a scheme that was first developed in murine models of the immune response, T-cell dependent inflammation may be classified broadly into the T-helper 1 (Th1) and Th2 types. Th1 cytokines characteristically mediate delayed-type hypersensitivity involving interleukin (IL)-2, IL-12, interferon (IFN)-γ and tumor necrosis factor (TNF)-α, whereas Th2 responses promote B-cell-driven humoral immunity with coordinated upregulation of the cytokine gene cluster encoded on chromosome 5q$_{32-34}$ with secretion of IL-3, -4, -5, -6, -9, -13, and granulocyte/macrophage colony-stimulating factor (GM-CSF). Engagement of both B and T cells is critical to the evolution of asthma.

IMMUNE CELLS

B Lymphocytes   B lymphocytes, as the source of immunoglobulins, are crucial to any immune reaction. In the case of allergic reactions, such as those underlying the disease process of asthma, the function of allergen-specific B cells that differentiate into IgE-secreting plasma cells is of central importance.

Immunoglobulin E   Immunoglobulin E antibodies are secreted in response to parasitic infestations and in the course of allergic diseases. Although IgE antibodies account for just 0.002% of the immunoglobulin pool, they have considerable biological activity, because of their ability to sensitize mast cells and basophils to allergens by binding to cell surface receptors. Atopy, the predisposition of an individual to produce large amounts of IgE, is associated with an increased risk of developing allergic diseases such as allergic rhinitis, atopic dermatitis, and asthma. However, it must be acknowledged that in a minority of asthma patients, often with marked disease, it has proven difficult to demonstrate allergen sensitivity. Plasma cells secrete IgE and the synthesis of these antibodies is regulated by a variety of cytokines. IL-6 causes B cells to switch to the production of IgE class antibodies, and IgE synthesis is promoted by IL-4 and IL-13, products of Th2 cells, which are associated with allergic disease. In addition, IgE binding to its receptors on B cells provides a mechanism for feedback (*see* below).

Receptors for IgE fall into two main categories: those with high affinity and those with low affinity (Table 22-1). High affinity receptors (FcϵRI) on mast cells and basophils mediate many of the classical functions of IgE in type-I hypersensitivity reactions. These cells express an FcϵRI receptor made up of one α-, one β- and two γ-subunits ($\alpha\beta\gamma_2$), whereas antigen-presenting cells, such as dendritic cells and monocytes, express a truncated form lacking the β-subunit ($\alpha\gamma_2$). Immunoglobulin E binds to the extracellular portion of the α-subunit of FcϵRI. On receptor dimerization by multivalent antigen, the intracellular portion of the α-subunit becomes phosphorylated and associates with other components of the signaling cascade. The β-subunit, expressed selectively by mast cells and basophils (*see* Table 22-1), amplifies the signal intensity by enhancing γ-chain phosphorylation, and it is noteworthy that genetic studies have linked polymorphisms in the β-subunit to asthma (*see* Asthma as a Genetic Disease: DNA Markers and Molecular Genetics). Expression of high affinity IgE receptors on mast cells and basophils is upregulated by IgE binding without the need for receptor crosslinking by antigen. Thus, in the context of

Table 22-1
The Receptors for IgE

Receptor	FcϵRI	FcϵRII
Synonyms	High affinity IgE receptor	Low affinity IgE receptor CD23
Affinity constant	10^{10}–$10^9/M$	10^7–$10^6/M$
Gene family	Immunoglobulin supergene family	Lectin family
Regulation of expression	Increased by IgE binding	Increased by IL-4 and IL-13 IFN-α/γ can upregulate or downregulate
Cell expression	Mast cells ($\alpha\beta\gamma_2$) Basophils ($\alpha\beta\gamma_2$) Dendritic cells ($\alpha\gamma_2$) Monocytes ($\alpha\gamma_2$) Eosinophils ($\alpha\gamma_2$)	B lymphocytes T lymphocytes Dendritic cells Monocytes Eosinophils
Function	Release of inflammatory mediators, histamine and eicosanoids Antigen presentation	Regulation of IgE synthesis Proliferation and differentiation of B lymphocytes Antigen presentation

IFN, interferon; IL, interleukin.

an allergic environment characterized by increased IgE production, the capacity of mast cells and basophils to bind IgE, and therefore respond to allergens, is likely to be increased.

Dimerization of the FcϵRI on mast cells or basophils by multivalent allergen results in phosphorylation of tyrosine residues within the immunoreceptor tyrosine-based activation motifs of the β- and γ-subunits. These act as a scaffold for the assembly of a complex with cytoplasmic signaling molecules such as protein tyrosine kinase Syk. Many signaling events follow, including increases in inositol-1,4,5-trisphosphate and intracellular calcium ion concentration, culminating in the release of granule contents and generation of arachidonic acid metabolites. Many of these mediators, including histamine, leukotrienes, IL-4, and IL-13, are thought to be important contributors to the pathology of asthma.

Low affinity IgE receptors (FcϵRII, CD23) are expressed by a variety of cell types including B lymphocytes (*see* Table 22-1), and production of IgE itself is regulated by binding to its low affinity receptor. CD23 exists either as an intact, membrane-bound molecule (iCD23) or as soluble fragments (sCD23), the latter being the products of cleavage of iCD23 through a poorly understood sequence of proteolytic events. Membrane-bound iCD23 has a number of functions, including downregulation of B cell IgE synthesis in response to high local concentrations of IgE. In contrast, some sCD23 fragments, when bound to IgE, exert cytokine-like effects leading to increased IgE secretion from B cells and TNFα secretion from monocytes. Excessive formation of 29-, 33-, and 37-kDa sCD23 fragments has been implicated in the overproduction of IgE associated with allergic disease, and specific protease inhibitors targeting the proteolysis of iCD23 have exhibited inhibitory actions on IgE secretion that may prove beneficial in asthma.

An evaluation of the contribution of IgE to asthma pathophysiology has been made possible by clinical trials of a humanized recombinant antibody to IgE. The antibody employed bound solely to circulating IgE, sequestering it and reducing the amount available for binding to mast cells or basophils. Treatment of atopic asthmatic patients with this anti-IgE antibody was found to decrease exacerbations and symptom scores and enabled a reduction in corticosteroid usage. These trials support a central role for IgE in the pathogenesis of allergic asthma.

T Lymphocytes   In common with other allergic responses, asthmatic reactions depend on the outputs of allergen-specific T lymphocytes of the Th2 type. Activation of these cells leads to the production of Th2 cytokines, including IL-4, -5, and -13, which amplify the inflammatory response by contributing to further recruitment of Th2 cells and eosinophils.

T lymphocytes respond to numerous chemoattractants generated within the airways, including IL-16, lipid mediators, such as platelet-activating factor (PAF), and numerous chemokines. Of these, a small number attract Th2 cells selectively. The most important of these include agonists at the Th2/platelet CC chemokine receptor 4 (CCR4), such as macrophage-derived chemokine (MDC, CCL22) and thymus and activation-regulated chemokine (TARC, CCL17), as well as the mast cell-derived lipid mediator prostaglandin D_2 (PGD_2), which acts through the Th2/eosinophil/basophil-restricted receptor, chemo-kine receptor-homologous molecule expressed on Th2 cells (CRTHR). A further selective Th2 receptor, CCR8, which is activated by the mast cell-derived chemokine I-309 (CCL1) and also mediates chemotactic responses of monocytes and vascular endothelial cells, is under investigation.

Resident or transient T cells within the airways may act as a source of their own chemoattractants, as indicated by the dependence of IL-16 release from allergen-challenged mild asthmatic bronchial explants on the CD28/B7 T-cell costimulatory signals. The source of these factors in more severe disease remains open to question, however, because IL-16 makes little contribution to the T-cell chemotactic activity in moderate/severe asthmatic individuals' airway secretions. Moreover, the release of both IL-16 and IL-5 from allergen-stimulated moderate/severe asthmatic bronchial biopsies is independent of CD28/B7 costimulation. Although this might simply indicate the predominance of other costimulatory mechanisms in T cells within more severe asthmatic airways, it may also suggest that other cellular sources, such as the bronchial epithelium and eosinophils, may represent major sources of these cytokines in severe disease.

The role of IL-16 itself is the subject of extensive research. Although this cytokine had been considered primarily as a T-cell chemoattractant, studies have shown that it also acts to suppress the production of Th2 cytokines and may render T cells unresponsive to allergenic stimulation. The relative contributions of IL-16 and the selective Th2 chemoattractants, MDC, TARC, I-309, and PGD_2, might, therefore, prove important in determining the local outcome of recruitment of T cells to sites of inflammation in the airways.

Although Th1 and Th2 populations have been postulated to balance each other's responses, with Th1 cytokines suppressing Th2 cell differentiation and proliferation and vice versa, this model is not reflected in disease. Thus, IFN-γ-secreting Th1 cells do not suppress Th2-mediated inflammatory reactions in animal models of asthma but, rather, cause severe neutrophilic inflammation in addition to the Th2-driven eosinophilic inflammation. Similarly, in Th1-driven processes such as experimental autoimmune encephalomyelitis (a model of multiple sclerosis) and type-1 diabetes, the presence of Th2 cells exacerbates local inflammation rather than ameliorating it, as would be expected from the Th1/Th2

balance model. Both Th1 and Th2 inflammatory reactions are, however, suppressed by the cytokine synthesis inhibitor, IL-10, and the possible significance of this is indicated by the findings that spontaneous IL-10 generation is lowered in the airways of asthmatic individuals and that a polymorphism in the promoter region of the IL-10 gene is associated with elevated serum IgE levels and clinical history of asthma. The identification of IL-10-secreting regulatory T cell (Tr) and transforming growth factor (TGF)-β-secreting Th3 populations suggests mechanisms through which inflammatory reactions are suppressed at the specific sites in which these suppressive cells localize. The hypothesis that a deficiency of Tr cells may underlie heightened and persistent inflammation in diseases such as asthma is under investigation and may provide important information about the regulation of inflammatory reactions.

Mast Cells   Mast cells are pivotal not only to initiating acute bronchoconstriction in asthma through the release of autacoid mediators, but also contribute to ongoing cell recruitment in the chronic phases of the disease. Mast cells are distributed widely in the airways, being found in the smooth muscle layer, the *lamina propria*, between epithelial cells and in the epithelial lining fluid sampled by BAL. In asthma, there is a substantial increase in the mast cell population of the lungs, and measurements of mast cell mediators such as histamine and β-tryptase in BAL fluid indicate that these cells are active. Although various cell populations are increased in asthma, it is noteworthy that mast cells, but not T lymphocytes or eosinophils, are more numerous in the bronchial smooth muscle layer when compared to that of healthy controls.

Mast cells develop from bone marrow progenitors that enter the blood as immature cells and migrate into the tissues, maturing under the influence of locally generated cytokines (Fig. 22-1). The most important of these cytokines is stem cell factor (SCF), which is produced mainly by structural cells with which mast cells interact closely, such as epithelial cells, fibroblasts, endothelial cells and smooth muscle cells. SCF can be secreted and is a chemoattractant for mast cells. However, findings that, mice that secrete soluble SCF, but are homozygous for a mutation in the gene encoding the membrane-bound form of this cytokine (the Steel-Dickie allele [Sl^d]), are deficient in mast cells suggest that the SCF expressed on the cell membrane is more important for mast cell development. Other cytokines within the microenvironment, including T-lymphocyte-derived cytokines, influence mast cell development and thus mast cells obtained from different tissues produce a pattern of mediators and respond to activating stimuli in a manner that depends on their source.

The interaction of antigen with specific IgE is likely to be the most important trigger for mast cell activation in allergic disease. These cells express large numbers of high affinity receptors for IgE on their surfaces, and bind IgE circulating in the plasma. However, the binding of monomeric IgE molecules does not cause mediator release. Rather, mast cell activation occurs when multivalent antigen crosslinks receptor-bound IgE molecules, resulting in the secretion of the contents of their many cytoplasmic granules and the generation of newly synthesized PGD_2 and leukotriene C_4 (LTC_4). PGD_2 and LTC_4, together with mast cell-derived histamine, induce bronchial smooth muscle constriction and increase vascular permeability and thus make a major contribution to the edema and bronchoconstriction of the acute response to allergen inhalation.

In addition to these classical mediators of allergic reactions, mast cells produce an extensive repertoire of proinflammatory cytokines,

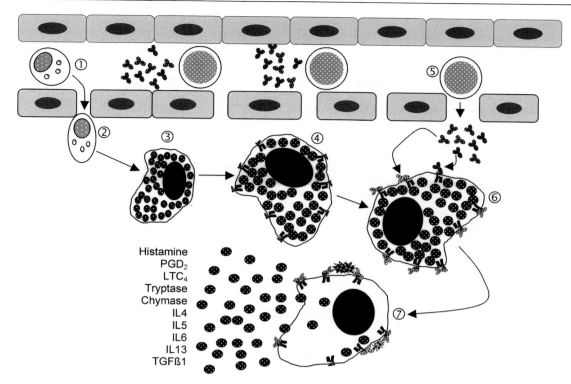

Figure 22-1 Mast cell progenitors leave the bone marrow and enter the circulation①. These progenitor cells migrate into the tissues in response to cytokines such as SCF, TGF-β, eotaxin, and RANTES②. Mast cells mature in the tissues and produce secretory granules③ and express high affinity IgE receptors④. IgE antibodies produced by B lymphocytes⑤ sensitize mast cells by binding to FcεRI receptors⑥. Crosslinking of FcεRI by multivalent allergen interacting with IgE results in mast cell degranulation and the secretion of mediators of inflammation and tissue remodeling⑦. IL, interleukin; LTC₄, leukotriene C₄; PGD₂, prostaglandin D₂; RANTES, regulated on activation normal T-cell expressed and secreted; SCF, stem cell factor; TGF-β₁, transforming growth factor-β₁.

including TNFα, IL-4, IL-5, IL-6, IL-8 (CXC chemokine ligand 8 [CXCL8]), IL-13, and GM-CSF. Mast cells generate these in substantial quantities and are unusual in that they store cytokines in their granules preformed and ready for rapid release. Of particular relevance to asthma, immunohistochemical studies have revealed that airway mast cells store IL-4, -5, and -13, cytokines associated with allergic-type immune responses, which promote processes such as IgE synthesis and eosinophil development.

Mast cells may also contribute to inflammation by means of their neutral proteases, tryptase and chymase, which are restricted to these cells. β-tryptase is found in the secretory granules of all mast cells and, as their most abundant product, has proved a valuable marker of mast cell activity. This enzyme has the capacity to regulate the behavior of a variety of cell types, inducing the release of IL-8 from endothelial cells and epithelial cells and secretion of both IL-6 and IL-8 by eosinophils. Injection of β-tryptase into the skin of guinea pigs or the peritoneum of mice results in the recruitment of inflammatory cells, whereas injection into the skin of guinea pigs provokes increased vascular leakage. These actions of β-tryptase require proteolytic activity, and one of the principal means by which cell behavior may be regulated by β-tryptase is thought to be through cleavage of the protease-activated receptor PAR2. This receptor is activated by certain proteases that cleave the N-terminal peptide at a specific site to generate a new amino-terminal, which functions as a tethered ligand that binds intramolecularly to the second extracellular loop of the receptor, resulting in the activation of intracellular signal transduction mechanisms. Of particular relevance to asthma, challenge of

sheep with inhaled tryptase causes bronchoconstriction and airway hyperresponsiveness. Furthermore, in animal models of asthma, low molecular weight inhibitors of β-tryptase protect against reductions in lung function provoked by inhalation of allergen. In addition to β-tryptase, mast cells produce two other forms of tryptase; α-tryptase, which is similar in sequence to α-tryptase, but secreted constitutively, and γ-tryptase, which is a transmembrane protein. γ-tryptase increases the expression of IL-13 by T lymphocytes, and in a mouse model this was found to promote airway hyperresponsiveness.

Chymase is produced in appreciable quantities only by a subset of mast cells most commonly found in submucosal and connective tissues. This enzyme activates IL-1β precursor and thus may play a proinflammatory role. As mentioned for tryptase, such a role is supported by animal studies in which injection of chymase into the skin of guinea pigs increases vascular leakage and injection into the peritoneum of mice causes inflammatory cell infiltration.

In addition to the inflammation that occurs in the asthmatic lung, structural changes take place, referred to collectively as airway remodeling (*see* Mechanisms of Airway Inflammation: Epithelial-Mesenchymal Communication in Asthma). Typical features of airway remodeling in asthma include thickening of the bronchial smooth muscle, subepithelial fibrosis, and epithelial cell metaplasia with increased formation of mucus-secreting goblet cells. Because mast cell numbers and mediator release are increased in fibrotic lung disorders, it seems likely that mast cells may be active contributors to airway remodeling in asthma. Mast cells produce considerable quantities of fibrogenic cytokines such as basic fibroblast growth factor (FGF) and TGF-β. Furthermore, mast cell proteases may have direct actions on structural cells to induce tissue remodeling. Thus, β-tryptase acts on multiple facets of fibroblast behavior, promoting fibroblast chemotaxis and proliferation, collagen deposition, and synthesis of basic FGF. Expression by dermal fibroblasts of α-smooth muscle actin (SMA) (an indicator of fibroblast to myofibroblast transformation) is increased by β-tryptase and this could be one mechanism promoting myofibroblast differentiation in the asthmatic airways. In addition, β-tryptase is a mitogen for both epithelial cells and airway smooth muscle cells and may thus promote remodeling. A cardinal feature of asthma is BHR, and application of this enzyme to isolated airway preparations causes hyperresponsiveness to histamine. Potential roles for chymase in remodeling processes are still under investigation, but it is known that chymase cleaves stromelysin (matrix metalloproteinase 3) to an active form and degrades human airway smooth muscle cell pericellular matrix. Most mast cells inhabiting the bronchial smooth muscle layer of asthmatic airways express chymase.

Thus, cell culture experiments (as summarized in Table 22-2) and animal models support a prominent role for mast cell mediators in reproducing key features of the pathophysiology of asthma. Although antihistamines are not effective in the treatment of asthma, a potential role for β-tryptase in the pathophysiology of asthma is supported by a trial in which a selective tryptase inhibitor protected against late phase bronchoconstriction after inhaled allergen challenge.

Granulocytes   Asthma is associated with an inflammation of the airways that is characterized by large numbers of granulocytes within both the tissues and the luminal space. Although an association of asthma with airway eosinophilia has been recognized for many years, the recognition that neutrophils may also be involved in some forms of severe asthma is more recent.

Eosinophils   Eosinophils are the characteristic infiltrating cells at sites of IgE-mediated immune reactions, including parasite infestation and allergy. Increased numbers of eosinophils are observed in the blood, sputum, BAL fluid, and submucosal tissues of allergic asthmatic subjects, with a broad relationship apparent between eosinophil numbers in the sputum and severity of disease. Increased numbers of eosinophil progenitor cells are also observed in the bone marrow of allergic asthmatics. Histological examination of asthmatic airways reveals both intact eosinophils and clusters of free eosinophil granules, indicating necrotic cytolysis, but little evidence of apoptotic eosinophils. It has been suggested that eosinophils are cleared from the mucosal tissues by migration into the lumen, in which the cells may undergo apoptosis or be eliminated through the mucociliary escalator.

The range of products released from activated or necrotic eosinophils indicates the potential for these cells to contribute to both the acute and chronic features of asthma. For example, LTC$_4$ is a potent bronchoconstrictor and mucous secretagogue, while reactive oxygen species (ROS, including superoxide anion radical and hydrogen peroxide) and basic granule proteins such as eosinophil cationic protein and eosinophil peroxidase act individually or in combination to injure respiratory epithelium. These so act along with eosinophil-derived cytokines such as IL-13 and TGF-β to stimulate fibroblast proliferation (*see* Mechanisms of Airway Inflammation: Epithelial-Mesenchymal Communication in Asthma), with consequences for tissue remodeling.

The abundant eosinophils in the airways may represent both mature cells recruited from the circulation and cells derived from IL-5-driven differentiation of progenitors within the lung. The

Table 22-2
Selected Cellular Targets for Mast Cell Mediators Likely to be of Importance in Asthma

Mediator(s)	*Cellular target*	*Action*
Immediate response		
Histamine,	Smooth muscle	Constriction
PGD$_2$, LTC$_4$	Endothelium	Increased permeability
Inflammatory responses		
IL-4, IL-13, TNFα	Endothelium	Upregulation of adhesion molecule expression
IL-4, IL-13	B lymphocytes	IgE production
IL-5	Eosinophils	Development and survival
β-tryptase	Endothelial cells	Vascular leakage, IL-8 production
	Eosinophils	IL-6 and IL-8 production
γ-tryptase	T lymphocytes	IL-13 production
Tissue remodeling		
Basic FGF	Fibroblasts	Proliferation
	Smooth muscle	
TGF-β	Fibroblasts	Production of extracellular matrix components
β-tryptase	Epithelium	Proliferation
	Smooth muscle	
	Fibroblasts	Proliferation, chemotaxis, synthesis of α-smooth actin, basic FGF and collagen

FGF, fibroblast growth factor; IL, interleukin; LTC$_4$, leukotriene C$_4$; PGD$_2$, prostaglandin D$_2$; TGF-β, transforming growth factor-β.

importance of the latter source of eosinophils in asthmatic airways remains to be established. In contrast, evidence supports a relationship between asthma and the expression in the airways of factors that attract and promote the survival of eosinophils. The importance of eosinophil recruitment in asthma has been called into question by the finding that the elimination of IL-5 by treatment of asthmatic subjects with an anti-IL-5 antibody leads to the reduction of blood and sputum eosinophils to negligible numbers without affecting the magnitude of early or late asthmatic reactions or airway responsiveness over a 30-d period. Because IL-5 is also required for the differentiation of lung precursors into eosinophils, it is unlikely that locally derived eosinophils account for the persistent asthmatic reactions, although mature tissue eosinophils do persist within asthmatic airways after anti-IL-5 treatment. The traditional view of eosinophil recruitment, secondary to the activation of resident inflammatory cells, being responsible for the late asthmatic reaction would appear to have been disproved. However, a contribution of resident eosinophils to the late reaction cannot be discounted. Furthermore, the role of eosinophils in the chronic tissue injury and remodeling underlying the pathology of asthma remains entirely open to investigation. It may be significant that eosinophils appear to play a distinct role in central pathological features such as subepithelial basement membrane thickening, even in severe, corticosteroid-resistant forms of asthma in which neutrophils form the predominant leukocyte type in airway exudates. Circumstantial evidence from the interactions of eosinophils with airway structural cells supports a role for eosinophils in these processes but experimental testing of the hypothesis is required to allow any conclusion to be made.

Eosinophils respond to a range of chemoattractants, including eotaxin (CC chemokine ligand 8 [CCL11]), regulated on activation,

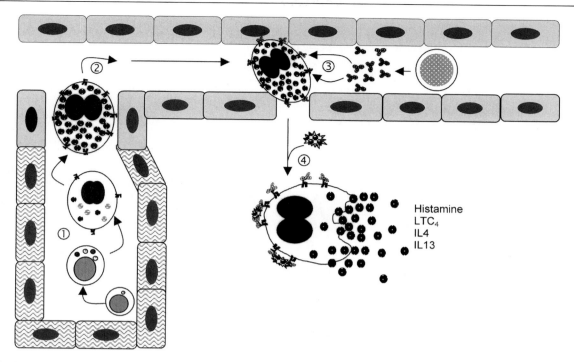

Figure 22-2 Basophils develop and mature within the bone marrow① before entering the circulation②. IgE antibodies produced by B lymphocytes bind to FcεRI on basophils, sensitizing them to allergens③. Crosslinking of the high affinity receptors by binding of multivalent allergens to IgE on the basophil surface causes secretion of granule contents and generation of mediators of allergic reactions ④. IL, interleukin; LTC_4, leukotriene C_4.

normal T cell expressed and secreted (RANTES; CCL5), IL-16, PAF, and PGD_2; they are also influenced by a range of survival factors, principally IL-3, IL-5, and GM-CSF. Sources of these factors include structural and resident inflammatory cells in the airways, such as the epithelium, fibroblasts, alveolar macrophages, mast cells and Th2 lymphocytes. In addition to attracting the cells into the airways and prolonging their survival, soluble factors in airway secretions can prime eosinophils for activation by secondary stimuli. For example, mediators, including PAF and CC chemokine receptor (CCR) 3 agonists such as eotaxin and RANTES, mobilize cytoplasmic lipid bodies, which are the subcellular structures in which the leukotriene-forming enzymes assemble to generate LTC_4 in eosinophils and basophils. This leads to greatly enhanced generation of LTC_4 in response to subsequent stimulation.

Basophils Investigations of the role of basophils in asthma pathogenesis were hampered for years by the lack of reagents for their reliable identification in tissue sections. Although basophils express highly sulfated proteoglycans in their secretory granules and may be stained with basic dyes such as toluidine blue and Alcian blue, and express high affinity IgE receptors on their cell surfaces that may be detected by immunohistochemistry, these are properties shared with the often more numerous mast cells. However, the advent of monoclonal antibodies specific for antigens unique to the secretory granules of basophils is now facilitating an assessment of their contribution to asthma. Basophils can be identified in the lungs of asthmatic patients, and are increased in number following inhaled allergen challenge, but they are much less numerous than other infiltrating cells such as eosinophils. However, an immunohistochemical study of the airways of patients who had died of asthma indicated the presence of much more substantial numbers of basophils, suggesting that basophils have a

greater role in fatal asthma. Findings of infiltration of large numbers of basophils into the nasal mucosa within an hour of allergen instillation indicate that, under some circumstances, basophils can be mobilized rapidly to the airways on allergen exposure.

Basophils develop from CD34+ bone marrow progenitors and mature before entering the peripheral blood (Fig. 22-2). They are comparatively rare leukocytes, typically comprising <1% of those circulating. Various cytokines contribute to basophil production and maturation, but chief among these is IL-3. Basophils express chemokine receptors CCR2 and CCR3 and may be recruited into the tissues by chemokines such as RANTES, monocyte chemotactic protein 1 and MCP3. They release mediators after stimulation with complement component C5a and bacterial formylated peptides but, in the context of asthma, activation is most likely to occur by IgE-dependent means. Basophils express FcεRI on their cell surface, and when this is crosslinked by IgE and multivalent allergen, secretion of mediators occurs. The responsiveness of basophils to activating stimuli can be increased by preincubation with "priming" cytokines such as IL-3, IL-5, GM-CSF or eotaxin, and thus basophils in an inflammatory environment may be more sensitive to activators. Basophil activation results in the secretion of histamine and LTC_4, both mediators of bronchoconstriction, and the release of considerable amounts of cytokines IL-4 and IL-13. These cytokines promote the generation of IgE antibodies and are associated with allergic reactions. It is noteworthy that while basophils produce IL-4 and IL-13, which are often thought of as Th2 cytokines, they do not generate Th1 cytokines such as IFN-γ or IL-2, or the more generally proinflammatory cytokines such as TNF-α, IL-1, or IL-6. Thus, basophil activation seems to favor the development of Th2 type responses associated with allergic reactions. Basophil-derived mediators are produced by other cell types

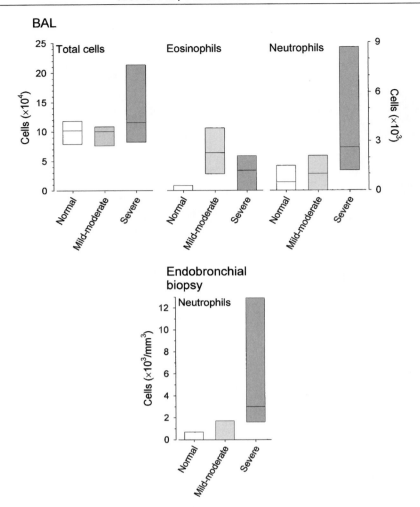

Figure 22-3   Inflammatory cells in BAL (upper panel) and endobronchial biopsies (lower panel) from normal individuals, mild/moderate asthmatic individuals requiring bronchodilator and inhaled glucocorticoids only, and severe asthmatic individuals treated with oral glucocorticoids for more than 5 yr. (Data are shown as median and interquartile range and are extracted from Wenzel SE, Szefler SJ, Leung DY, Sloan SI, Rex MD, Martin RJ. Bronchoscopic evaluation of severe asthma: persistent inflammation associated with high-dose glucocorticoids. Am J Respir Crit Care Med 1997;156:737–743.)

also, but it is possible that the antibodies specific for basophils could recognize novel mediators produced solely by basophils, and that the identification of their antigens may provide further insights into the nature of the contribution of basophils to asthma.

A number of therapies for asthma such as corticosteroids, leukotriene receptor antagonists and IgE sequestration using recombinant antibodies are likely to affect basophil function, but the extent to which actions on basophils underlies their clinical usefulness is unclear.

Neutrophils   An association between neutrophils and acute severe asthma has become apparent from the demonstration of neutrophilic inflammation in postmortem lung specimens from sudden-onset fatal asthma and status asthmaticus, as well as in sputum samples collected during acute asthma exacerbations. Exacerbations of asthma are due predominantly to infection of the lower airways by rhinoviruses and respiratory syncytial viruses, which promote the production of neutrophil chemoattractants by the respiratory epithelium and induce upregulation of epithelial intercellular adhesion molecule (ICAM) 1, a molecule that enables adhesion of neutrophils through binding of β_2 integrins.

A contribution of neutrophils to severe persistent asthma has been suggested, particularly in cases resistant to high-dose glucocorticoid treatment. This is based on bronchoscopic studies in which elevated neutrophil numbers were observed in BAL and endobronchial biopsies taken from severe persistent asthma patients treated with oral corticosteroids in comparison with healthy and bronchodilator-treated mildly/moderately asthmatic individuals (Fig. 22-3). Eosinophil numbers, in contrast, were elevated in steroid-free mildly/moderately asthmatic subjects but not in the corticosteroid-treated severe asthma patients. Similar findings have been reported in studies of induced sputum, in which neutrophil numbers were significantly raised in oral glucocorticoid- treated severe asthma subjects compared to bronchodilator-treated mildly asthmatic individuals. Although direct actions of glucocorticoids on cell survival have been demonstrated—with steroids enhancing neutrophil survival although hastening eosinophil apoptosis—other pathophysiological explanations for the differential cellular composition of the inflammatory exudates are possible. The neutrophil numbers in asthmatic airways are directly related to the concentrations of two major neutrophil chemoattractants—IL-8 and LTB_4—in the airway lining fluid and may, therefore, reflect a persistent secretion of these factors from the bronchial epithelium and alveolar macrophages, respectively.

Recruitment of Immune and Inflammatory Cells IL-4 has a number of actions that influence the development of airway inflammation. As noted, it is critical for the gene activation underlying differentiation of B cells into antibody-forming cells and consequent production of IgE and IgG isotypes. In the context of the scheme for Th2-type immune cell recruitment to the airway, IL-4 may also exert a separate but critical influence. In particular, IL-4-driven expression of vascular cell adhesion molecule 1 (VCAM1) on the endothelial cell surface might serve in the recruitment of inflammatory cells from the circulation (especially T cells and eosinophils bearing the $\alpha_4\beta_1$- and $\alpha_4\beta_7$-integrins). This possibility is supported by evidence of increased levels of immune cell IL-4 and endothelial cell VCAM1 in tissue from asthmatic subjects as well as inhibition of allergen-induced airway inflammation in animals lacking the IL-4 gene or treated with anti-VCAMl antibodies. The precise mechanism underlying the regulation of VCAM1 expression by IL-4 is uncertain, but it appears that it is not dependent on signal transducer and activator of transcription (STAT) 6-driven gene activation. Instead, IL-4 acts in concert with other cytokines (TNFα and IL-1). These cytokines are responsible for transcriptional activation of the VCAM1 gene through two adjacent nuclear factor-κB sites in the promoter region, whereas IL-4 stabilizes the resulting mRNA. This cytokine synergy results in exaggeration and prolongation of VCAM1 levels on the endothelial cell surface. Cytokine synergy may also reflect an important cell–cell interaction in which TNF-α (and in some cases IL-1) derived from mast cells and eosinophils acts in concert with IL-4 (and in some cases IL-13) derived from mast cells, eosinophils, Th2 cells and basophils to promote immune cell recruitment to the airway.

Other Mechanisms for Recruitment of Immune Cells In addition to IL-4 and TNFα effects on VCAM1, other events in endothelial cells and immune cells are also critical for full development of the Th2-type inflammatory response. For example, at least two other cell adhesion systems appear to be activated during allergen-triggered airway inflammation: (1) selectin binding to mucin-like molecules and (2) other cell adhesion molecules of the Ig supergene family that bind to integrin receptors. In the case of endothelial cells, allergen may trigger endothelial-leukocyte adhesion molecule 1 (ELAM1, CD62E, E-selectin) expression, which enables binding to a corresponding leukocyte sialyl-Lewis X carbohydrate ligand; and ICAM1 expression, which allows for binding to the leukocyte β_2-integrins leukocyte function associated antigen 1 (LFA1, $\alpha_L\beta_2$, CD11a/CD18) and Mac1 ($\alpha_M\beta_2$, CD11b/CD18). In addition to these cell adhesion systems for direct cell–cell contact, endothelial cells and immune cells also appear capable of generating a series of chemokines that may act over a greater distance to direct immune cell movement and activation in airway tissue. These three systems—selectin binding to mucin-like molecules, cell adhesion molecules binding to integrins and chemokine binding to G-protein-coupled receptors—may act in a specific combination to dictate the type of immune cells that enter or are retained in the airway tissue. These same systems also serve to control the activation status of immune cells acting, at least in some cases, through distinct signal transduction pathways.

Once inflammatory cells are recruited from the circulation, they are often directed toward the epithelial surface. It appears that epithelial cells (along with other parenchymal cells and resident immune cells) also possess at least two important mechanisms for influencing the movement of inflammatory cells after they arrive in the airway tissue: (1) concomitant activation of cell adhesion molecules on the epithelial cell surface that may interact with corresponding integrin receptors on the immune cell surface and (2) release of chemotactic factors that bind to specific receptors on the immune cell. In the case of airway epithelial cells, these systems appear to be more responsive to Th1-type cytokines, but there is evidence that they are also influenced by the level of TNF-α. Thus, even in the absence of a Th1-type response, expression by epithelial cells of cell adhesion molecules (especially ICAM1) and certain chemokines (from the CC- and CXC-chemokine families) is capable of supporting transepithelial migration and activation of immune cells.

Interestingly, there is no evidence of selectin or VCAM1 expression on airway epithelial cells (or fibroblasts and smooth muscle cells); thus, it is likely that these cell types present fewer ligands than do endothelial cells for directing leukocyte movement. The biological basis for this difference is not certain, but it makes sense; endothelial cells must be armed with ligands that slow down passing leukocytes (to allow tethering and triggering) and then select a specific leukocyte subset (to allow adhesion and transmigration) from the diverse circulating pool. This requires multiple specific molecular interactions. By contrast, parenchymal cells (epithelial cells, fibroblasts, and smooth muscle cells) come into contact with immune cells after selection and some degree of activation, so that they are required only to facilitate further leukocyte migration and retention. ICAM1 is well suited to mediate this process because nearly all immune cells constitutively express the β_2-integrins LFA1 or Mac1. In the case of T-cell traffic, the endothelial cells (and likely epithelial cells) also express a series of receptors (designated homing receptors or addressins) that serve to direct distinct subsets of lymphocytes to appropriate locations of lymphoid tissue. This type of cell adhesion (exemplified by some of the β_7-integrin interactions) is probably most important in maintaining a resident population of immune cells, but whether this system is also regulated during airway inflammation remains uncertain. The discovery that asthmatic airway smooth muscle secretes the mast cell chemoattractant IP10 might explain the increased numbers of mast cells in the smooth muscle layer that have been linked to heightened airway responsiveness.

EPITHELIAL-MESENCHYMAL COMMUNICATION IN ASTHMA Asthma is an inflammatory disorder of the airways involving T cells, mast cells and eosinophils characteristic of the Th-2 response. However, inflammation alone does not explain many of the features of this chronic and relapsing disease. Although atopy is an important risk factor for asthma, in the general population it only accounts for 40% of the attributable risk of having the disease. Eosinophils have been assumed to play a central role in disease pathogenesis; however, studies with an IL-5 blocking monoclonal antibody and recombinant human IL-12 have failed to reveal efficacy, despite markedly reducing circulating and airway eosinophil numbers (*see* Mechansisms of Airway Inflammation: Granulocyte Interactions With Airway Structural Cells). Thus, although being associated with asthma, atopy and airway eosinophilia would not seem to be critical requirements for disease expression. Genetic studies have also demonstrated that atopy and BHR have different patterns of inheritance. These findings imply that locally operating factors play an important role in

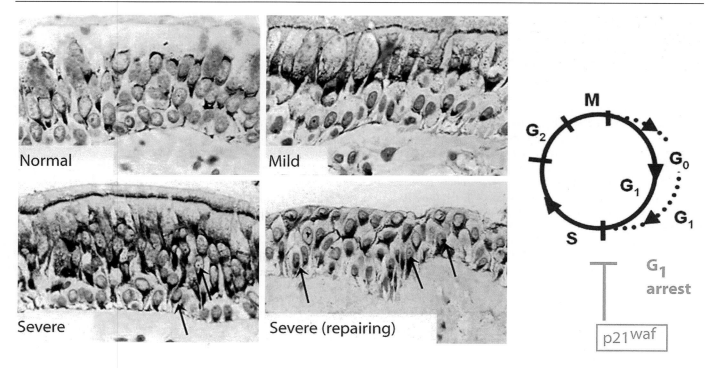

Figure 22-4   Increased expression of p21^{waf} in asthmatic epithelium in proportion to disease severity (left) and mechanisms of action of p21^{waf} in promoting cell cycle arrest. Note the nuclear localization of p21^{waf} in severe asthma.

predisposing individuals to asthma and provide an explanation for epidemiological evidence that identifies pollutant exposure, diet, and respiratory virus infection, which all increase oxidant stress in the airways, as important risk factors.

Morphometry has revealed that thickening of asthmatic airways accounts for a large component of BHR and is associated with resistance to corticosteroids. This failure of corticosteroids is reflected in the findings of the recent European Network for the Understanding Mechanisms of Severe Asthma (ENFUMOSA) study, which has revealed that these patients exhibit a greatly impaired quality of life, a component of fixed airway obstruction and have clear evidence of airway wall remodeling. In such patients, there is evidence of persistent matrix turnover with higher levels of cleaved tenascin C, matrix metalloproteinase 2 and collagen VI, indicating active tissue remodeling. Airway remodeling in adult asthma also provides an explanation of the accelerated decline in lung function observed over time. The Childhood Asthma Management Program (CAMP) study in children 5- to 11-yr-old showed that the beneficial effect of an inhaled corticosteroid on the postbronchodilator improvement in airway function observed during the first year of treatment was lost over the following 3 yr. This is best explained by airway remodeling that is insensitive to corticosteroids. A biopsy study has identified tissue remodeling as an early and consistent component of childhood asthma with fibroblast proliferation and collagen deposition in the subepithelial *lamina reticularis* being of greater diagnostic significance that tissue eosinophilia. Although remodeling had been considered secondary to long-standing inflammation, biopsy studies in young children have shown tissue restructuring up to 4 yr before the onset of symptoms, indicating processes that begin early in the development of asthma and occur in parallel with, or may be obligatory for, the establishment of persistent inflammation.

Epithelial Susceptibility to Injury and the Repair Phenotype in Asthma   The normal bronchial epithelium is a stratified structure consisting of a columnar layer supported by basal cells to serve as a physical and chemical barrier to the external environment. In asthma, the epithelium shows evidence of activation linked to structural damage and goblet cell metaplasia. Epithelial stress is seen in the form of widespread activation of the transcription factors NFκB, activator proteins (e.g., AP-1) and (STAT1), and by the increased expression of heat-shock proteins and the cyclin-dependent kinase inhibitor p21^{waf} (Fig. 22-4 *see below*). The altered epithelium also becomes an important source of autacoid mediators, chemokines and growth factors that sustain ongoing inflammation. To explain the disordered morphology and extent of activation, whether the asthmatic epithelium is more susceptible to injury and/or has an altered response to damage has been investigated.

Epithelial Susceptibility   Epithelial disruption is characteristically increased in the asthmatic bronchial epithelium. It has been proposed that this damage is artefactual; however, the finding of enhanced expression of the epidermal growth factor receptor (EGFR, HER-1, c-erbB1) and the epithelial isoform of CD44 indicate that injury has occurred in vivo. EGFR and CD44 expression in asthma increases with disease severity and is evident throughout the epithelium, suggesting that damage is widespread. Significantly, EGFR overexpression is insensitive to the action of corticosteroids

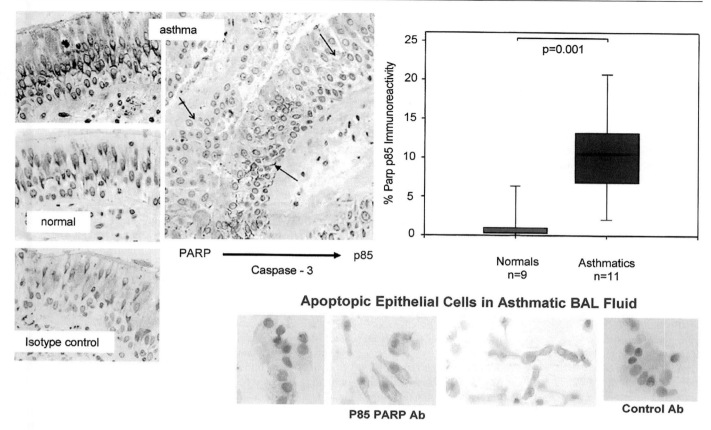

Figure 22-5 Increased immunostaining for the caspase-3 p85 cleavage product of poly ADP-ribose polymerase in asthmatic mucosal biopsies and BAL epithelial cells. (Please *see* color insert.)

and is positively correlated with the thickness of the *lamina reticularis*, linking epithelial injury to underlying remodeling. The extent of epithelial shedding in asthma is not observed in other inflammatory diseases, such as chronic obstructive pulmonary disease (COPD), in which the epithelium becomes multilayered owing to squamous metaplasia whereas the underlying *lamina reticularis* remains normal. Although these differences may reflect the quality of inflammation, airway eosinophilia is observed in the absence of asthma and neutrophils may dominate inflammation in severe asthma, as in COPD.

There also occurs increased epithelial expression of Fas and Fas ligand in patients who have died with asthma. In bronchial biopsies, there is markedly increased immunostaining of asthmatic columnar (but notably not basal) epithelial cells for p85, the caspase-3 cleavage product of polyADP polymerase, indicating that epithelial apoptosis is increased with disease (Fig. 22-5). Although such observational studies are able to identify differences between normal and asthmatic subjects, they are unable to determine whether the changes are a cause or consequence of inflammation. To address this, primary cultures of bronchial epithelial cells brushed from the airways of normal and asthmatic subjects have been established to compare responses under identical conditions in vitro. Although no difference in the rate of proliferation of these cultures under optimal growth conditions has been found, when rendered quiescent by growth factor depletion, those from asthmatic airways exhibit a significantly greater sensitivity to oxidant-induced apoptosis in the face of normal apoptotic response to the DNA and RNA synthesis inhibitor actinomycin D. This susceptibility to oxidants is unlikely to

be a secondary effect of airway inflammation, because it is preserved through several generations in vitro. Because epidemiological studies and limited investigations in primates have identified multiple interacting risk factors for asthma, including inhalant pollutants and diets low in antioxidants, the effect of environmental oxidants on a susceptible epithelium may provide a plausible triggering mechanism for the induction of epithelial activation and damage in asthma. Once initiated, the resulting inflammatory cell influx causes secondary damage through the production of endogenous ROS, resulting in chronic tissue injury and persistent inflammation. Consistent with this proposal, the epithelial expression of the neutrophil chemoattractants IL-8 and macrophage inflammatory protein 1 α (MIP1α) is increased in severe asthma, and their appearance correlates with increased EGFR expression as a marker of epithelial damage. Further in vitro studies have revealed that oxidant or epidermal growth factor (EGF) treatment of primary bronchial epithelial cells enhances MIP1α or IL-8 release, respectively. Thus, the susceptibility of the epithelial barrier to the action of different components of the inhaled environment may play a key role in determining the asthmatic phenotype.

Growth Arrest and Epithelial Repair In vitro studies point to a central role for activation of the EGFR in the restoration of the bronchial epithelium following injury because (1) EGF is a mitogen for bronchial epithelial cells; (2) mechanical damage induces rapid phosphorylation of the EGFR irrespective of the presence of exogenous ligand; and (3) wound closure is enhanced by EGF but not by the unrelated ligand keratinocyte growth factor (FGF7). Recognizing that EGF is a potent mitogen, the increase in epithelial EGFR in asthma is paradoxical because it is not matched by increased proliferation to replace columnar cells that have been shed and, in this way, contrasts with the hyperproliferative state of the epithelium seen in COPD. Although studies with primary cultures of normal and asthmatic bronchial epithelial cells have shown similar proliferation rates when maintained in medium supplemented with exogenous EGF, a potential mechanism for reduced EGFR-mediated proliferation in vivo emerges because the cyclin-dependent kinase inhibitor $p21^{waf}$ is overexpressed in basal, as well as columnar, epithelial cells in bronchial biopsies from patients with severe asthma (Fig. 22-4). In response to injury, $p21^{waf}$ acts as a checkpoint at the G1 to S-phase transition of the cell cycle, causing growth arrest to enable DNA repair to be completed before progression into S-phase or, in which damage is irreparable, to direct exit from the cell cycle and activate apoptosis. In this way, the decisions to survive or to enter into apoptosis are irrefutably linked. The EGFR ligands (EGF, TGF-β, amphiregulin, heparin-binding epidermal growth factor-like growth factor [HB-EGF], epiregulin and betacellulin) are pivotal determinants of the epithelial cell fate through their ability to act as survival factors that protect against proapoptotic stimuli and as mitogens that signal cell cycle progression. Although the ability of EGF to protect against oxidant-induced apoptosis in vitro has not been characterized, studies in animal models have shown that EGF can protect against smoke-induced tracheal injury in sheep.

As expression of $p21^{waf}$ is strongly induced by oxidant stress, the finding that asthmatic bronchial epithelial cells are more susceptible to oxidant injury provides one explanation for the high expression of $p21^{waf}$ in the asthmatic epithelium. However, $p21^{waf}$ is also induced by the antiproliferative growth factors TGF-β_1 and TGF-β_2, the levels of which are elevated in asthma, in COPD and in response to epithelial injury in vitro. The overall fate of the epithelium reflects the integration of survival and proliferation signals provided by EGF-like growth factors that activate mitogen-activated protein kinases (MAPK) and the counterbalancing proapoptotic and antiproliferative signals caused by injury and members of the TGF-β family. Although expression of EGF, TGF-β, and HB-EGF is unchanged in asthmatic bronchial epithelium relative to normal controls, markedly increased TGF-α production occurs in COPD. Thus in COPD, increased activation of the EGFR by EGF and analogous ligands protects against cigarette smoke-induced injury and overrides the antiproliferative effect of TGF-β, whereas in asthma an insufficiency of these ligands provides a unifying mechanism for increased epithelial susceptibility and impaired repair. This is supported by the finding of a marked decrease in epithelial immunostaining for phosphotyrosine (a global marker of tyrosine kinase activation) in the bronchial epithelium of mild asthma and the reported lack of MAPK activation. In contrast, in corticosteroid-refractory asthma, tyrosine kinase activity is markedly increased in relation to disease severity or treatment. Although the phosphorylated proteins within the asthmatic epithelium have not been identified, they are more likely to be linked to stress-induced changes than to proliferation because, in the bronchial epithelium of severe asthmatic subjects, $p21^{waf}$ is elevated whereas proliferating cell nuclear antigen remains low.

In asthma there is no increase in epithelial expression of the structurally related heregulin receptors HER2 (c-erbB2) or HER3 (c-erbB3), whereas in COPD both these receptors are overexpressed in parallel with the EGFR. As EGFR/EGFR homodimers are only weak activators of the MAPK pathway, this will further contribute to the inability of the asthmatic epithelium to counter antiproliferative

signals provided by the TGF-β. In contrast, EGFR:HER2 heterodimers are able to promote cell survival because of the presence of multiple binding sites for phosphatidylinositol 3-kinase on this receptor. Based on these findings, the duration of the epithelial repair may be prolonged in asthma resulting from an imbalance between proliferation and survival signals involving the EGFR/HER family and antiproliferative signals involving the TGF-β.

The Epithelial-Mesenchymal Trophic Unit

Epithelial-Mesenchymal Signaling High resolution computed tomography, postmortem and biopsy studies in chronic asthma have all revealed airway wall thickening. This involves deposition of interstitial collagens in the *lamina recticularis*, matrix deposition in the submucosa, smooth muscle hyperplasia and microvascular and neuronal proliferation (Fig. 22-6). Thickening of the *lamina reticularis* is diagnostic of this disease and, on the basis of measurements made in human airways and in a guinea pig model of chronic antigen exposure, it appears to reflect events linked to thickening of the entire airway wall. A layer of subepithelial mesenchymal cells has been described with features of myofibroblasts, the number of which was increased in asthma in proportion to the thickness of the reticular collagen layer. These cells correspond to an attenuated fibroblast sheath lying adjacent to the *lamina reticularis* and forming a network similar to hepatic stellate cells which, when activated by liver damage, are the key receptor cells responsible for fibrosis. Because the bronchial epithelium is in intimate contact with the attenuated fibroblast sheath, these two cellular layers are in a key position to coordinate responses to challenges from the inhaled environment into the deeper layers of the submucosa. Injury to epithelial monolayers in vitro results in increased release of fibroproliferative and fibrogenic growth factors including FGF2, insulin-like growth factor (IGF) 1, platelet-derived growth factor (PDGF), endothelin (ET)-1 and latent and active TGF-β_2. TGF-β, FGF2, and ET-1 are also increased in asthma, with TGF-β and FGF2 being encrypted in the extracellular matrix, as shown by their colocalization with the proteoglycans decorin and heparan sulfate, respectively. To further establish the relationship between EGFR signaling in the repair and remodeling processes, an EGFR-selective tyrosine kinase inhibitor has been used that suppresses epithelial repair in vitro with a resultant increase of release of TGF-β_2 by the damaged epithelial cells. This suggests parallel pathways operating in repairing epithelial cells, some of which direct efficient restitution and are regulated by EGFR, whereas others control profibrogenic growth factor production independently of the EGFR. In asthma, it seems likely that impaired epithelial proliferation causes the bronchial epithelium to spend longer in a repair phenotype, resulting in increased secretion of profibrogenic growth factors (Fig. 22-7).

Using a coculture model, there is direct evidence that epithelial injury causes myofibroblast activation. Thus, polyarginine (a surrogate for eosinophil basic proteins) or mechanical damage to confluent monolayers of bronchial epithelial cells grown on a collagen gel seeded with human myofibroblasts leads to enhanced proliferation and increased collagen gene expression owing to the combined effects of FGF2, IGF1, PDGF-BB, TGF-β, and ET-1. Furthermore, in mild–moderate asthma, inhaled corticosteroids reduce airway inflammation and levels of IGF1 and FGF2 but with minimal improvement in BHR and no effect on collagen deposition in the *lamina reticularis* or on TGF-β levels. Because corticosteroids reduce submucosal eosinophils by approx 80%, the persistently high TGF-β in BAL fluid most likely derives from the injured and repairing epithelium and associated matrix turnover rather than

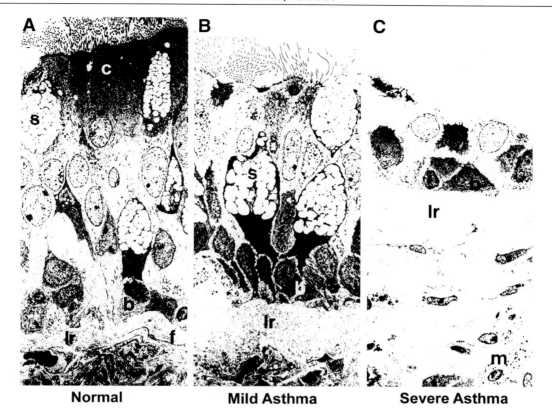

Figure 22-6   Transmission electron micrographs of airway epithelium in normal, mild asthma and severe asthma demonstrating disease-related thickening of the *lamina recticularis* and epithelial changes.

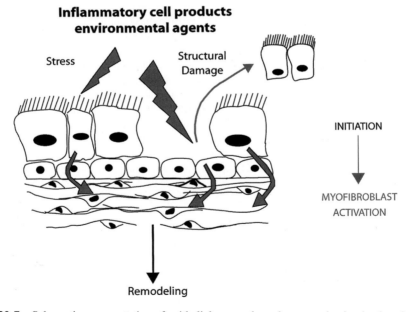

Figure 22-7   Schematic representation of epithelial-mesenchymal communication in chronic asthma.

from eosinophils. Both epithelial EGFR expression and TGF-β production are refractory to corticosteroids, and the combined effects of these signaling pathways on the epithelial-mesenchymal trophic unit (EMTU) could provide mechanisms for tissue remodeling and explain the incomplete resolution of lung function with inhaled corticosteroids observed in chronic asthma.

Communication between the epithelium and the subepithelial fibroblast sheath is reminiscent of the processes that drive physiological development of the airways during embryogenesis, in which the epithelium and mesenchyme act as a "trophic unit" to regulate airway growth and branching. Consequentially, it is proposed that the EMTU is reactivated in asthma to drive pathological

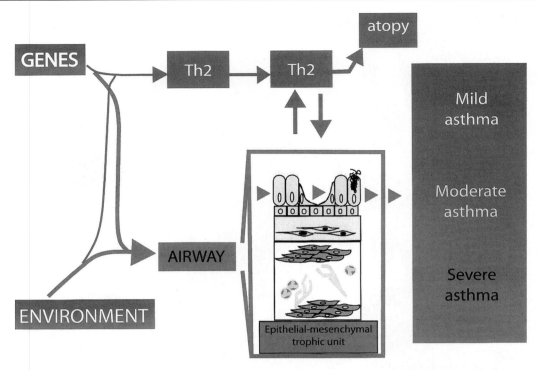

Figure 22-8 Schematic representation of the epithelial mesenchymal trophic unit and its relationship to Th2-related inflammation in asthma. Th, T-helper.

remodeling of the airways (Fig. 22-8). In subjects with asymptomatic BHR, longitudinal studies show that those who progress to asthma show parallel changes in inflammation and remodeling. Thickening of the *lamina reticularis* in bronchial biopsies from young children is also present several years before asthma becomes clinically manifest. During lung development, epithelial and mesenchymal growth is regulated, in part, by the balance of EGF and TGF-β signaling, as suggested also occurs in chronic asthma. In susceptible individuals, environmental factors may interact with EMTU in early life to initiate structural changes in the airways that may account for the decrease in lung function observed in young children who are susceptible to early wheezing and for the loss of corticosteroid responsiveness on baseline lung function observed in the CAMP study and related long-term studies investigating the disease-modifying effects of inhaled corticosteroids. This is supported by studies in nonhuman primates, in which intermittent exposure to ozone in the presence of allergen creates a phenotype resembling chronic asthma. Therefore, bronchial epithelial susceptibility seems either to precede or occur in parallel with factors predisposing to the Th2-mediated inflammation and is an absolute requirement to establish the microenvironment for inflammation to become persistent in the airways and for remodeling to occur.

Propagation of the Remodeling Responses by the EMTU
To study the mesenchymal cells that are involved in the remodeling responses in asthma, protocols have been established for their outgrowth from bronchial biopsies. These vimentin-positive fibroblasts can be grown readily from asthmatic mucosal biopsies and differ from those from normal airways in adopting stem cell characteristics, by proliferating rapidly in the absence of exogenous growth factors and in their ability to overcome contact inhibition in the presence of TGF-β_1 or TGF-β_2, enabling higher cell densities to be achieved. In this regard, TGF-β treatment in vitro also causes

submucosal fibroblasts to adopt a myofibroblast phenotype, as evinced by the induction of α-SMA, acquisition of contractile phenotype and synthesis of interstitial (repair) collagens. The relationship between myofibroblast activation and the underlying smooth muscle mass in asthma has yet to be studied. However, following allergen exposure, activation of the smooth muscle increases. In addition, mitogen treatment of asthmatic mucosal fibroblasts in vitro causes them to release both ET-1 and another vascular mitogen, vascular endothelial growth factor (VEGF). Thus, in addition to increased matrix deposition, activation of myofibroblasts contributes to smooth muscle and microvascular proliferation, which are both characteristic features of the remodeled asthmatic airway.

In a rabbit model of partial outflow obstruction in the bladder, TGF-β causes serosal thickening resulting from accumulation of myofibroblasts, which, over time, change phenotype into smooth muscle cells. In developing capillaries, endothelial cells and smooth muscle cells also share a common stem cell progenitor with vascular endothelial growth factor and PDGF acting as the key determinants of cell fate. Studies of normal and asthmatic airway (myo)fibroblasts reveal that these cells exhibit phenotypic plasticity, have some early features of smooth muscle (e.g., expression of the SM-22 protein) and can be further differentiated by TGF-β_1 and TGF-β_2 to express heavy chain myosin and α-SMA. This suggests that the cells have properties of both myofibroblasts and smooth muscle cells and are probably derived from a common (stem cell) progenitor. Thus, mediators released by the repairing bronchial epithelium provide a mechanism for myofibroblast activation to propagate and amplify airway remodeling. Such a mechanism would fit well with the findings on airway smooth muscle cultured from asthmatic airways.

GRANULOCYTE INTERACTIONS WITH AIRWAY STRUCTURAL CELLS The mechanisms through which eosinophils become activated are largely dependent on adhesion events, in

Eosinophil adhesion molecule	Counterligand
CD44	Hyaluronan
CD28	B7 (CD80/CD86)

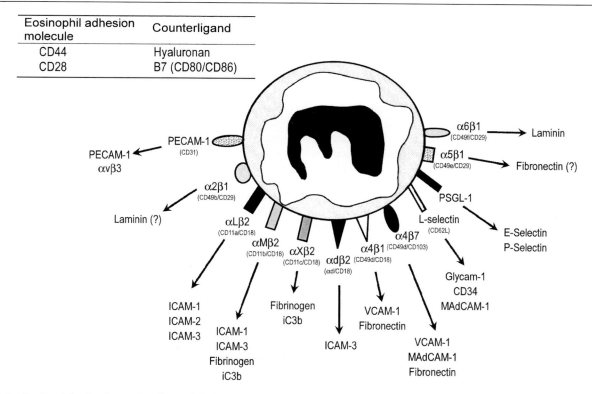

Figure 22-9 Eosinophil adhesion molecules and their counterligands. Inset: Recently identified eosinophil adhesion molecules. (Reproduced with permission from Giembycz MA, Lindsay MA. Pharmacology of the eosinophil. Pharmacol Rev 1999;51:213–340.)

which adhesion molecules on the cell's surface bind to counterligands on vascular endothelial cells, extracellular matrix, fibroblasts and epithelial cells (Fig. 22-9). For example, the release of IL-13 from eosinophils is dependent on ligation of CD28 by CD86 on adjacent eosinophils or by CD80 or CD86 on dendritic cells, macrophages or B lymphocytes. Similarly, TGF-β secretion from eosinophils is stimulated strongly by binding of cell-surface CD44 to the matrix glycosaminoglycan hyaluronan. Ligation of Mac1, which is responsible for eosinophil adhesion to bronchial epithelial cells through interaction with ICAM1, is a prerequisite for significant stimulation of ROS generation or degranulation; ligation of very late antigen 4 ($\alpha_4\beta_1$ integrin)—either by VCAM1 or by extracellular fibronectin—greatly enhances the production of ROS and LTC_4, the latter evinced by the ability of supernatants of VCAM1/PAF-stimulated eosinophils to provoke contraction of bronchial smooth muscle.

Lung fibroblasts represent a major source of the eosinophil chemoattractant, eotaxin, and also promote eosinophil survival through the release of GM-CSF. Because tissue-infiltrating eosinophils themselves represent a source of IL-13 and TGF-β, which potently and synergistically induce eotaxin release from fibroblasts, they have the potential to stimulate their own recruitment. This may provide a mechanism for amplified eosinophilic inflammation in airways in which fibroblast numbers and/or responsiveness are increased. Fibroblasts, whose synthesis of hyaluronan is upregulated by inflammatory cytokines such as IL-1β, provide a substrate for eosinophil adhesion through the ligation of eosinophil CD44, which promotes the secretion of TGF-β and may further amplify the production of eotaxin and, consequently, the recruitment of eosinophils. Adherence of eosinophils

to the fibroblast surface also occurs through β_1-integrin-dependent mechanisms that promote production of ROS and LTC_4, as well as release of granule proteins. Supernatants of activated eosinophils stimulate the proliferation of human lung fibroblasts, thereby providing a larger source of both hyaluronan and eotaxin.

The ability of eosinophils and neutrophils to activate the bronchial epithelium remains largely unexplored. Although neutrophil proteases are known to be highly potent mucous secretagogues, little is known about the actions of other leukocyte-derived products on the epithelium. In animal models, activated eosinophils and neutrophils promote the production of the bronchoconstrictor thromboxane A_2 by tracheal epithelium but this has not been confirmed in human cells. Eosinophil cationic protein stimulates epithelial secretion of IGF1, itself a stimulus for lung epithelial cell proliferation, whereas adherent eosinophils stimulate the release of secretory leukoprotease inhibitor from bronchial epithelial cell lines. The latter response may indicate a contribution of eosinophils to the suppression of acute inflammatory responses, with a shift toward chronic TGF-β-driven remodeling.

The airway epithelium is a major source of neutrophil chemoattractants, including IL-8 and growth-related oncogene α (CXCL1). Inflammatory activation of the epithelium would, therefore, be expected to promote neutrophil recruitment, although direct evidence of this is lacking. Neutrophils themselves are capable of causing epithelial detachment, via the action of serine proteases such as elastase and cathepsin G, and can stimulate epithelial IL-8 secretion via an action of defensins. Curiously, however, these neutrophil products are mutually antagonistic: defensins inhibit the cytotoxic actions of serine proteases whereas proteases inhibit the secretory response to defensins. It is difficult to deduce how these actions are balanced in vivo and to predict whether neutrophils primarily destroy or activate the airway epithelium.

ASTHMA AS A GENETIC DISEASE

POPULATION AND FAMILY STUDIES Evidence that genetic factors are important in common diseases often comes initially from studies comparing the frequency of disease among genetically related individuals with that in the general population. Accordingly, the evidence for a genetic component to the development of asthma includes (1) family studies indicating more frequent occurrence of asthma in first-degree relatives of asthmatic subjects; (2) familial aggregation patterns in which the rates of asthma were found to be significantly higher in those families with one or more asthmatic parent; and (3) studies showing that monozygotic twins are significantly more concordant for asthma than dizygotic twins. Reports during the past 50 yr have proposed both simple Mendelian and multifactorial models to explain the familial clustering of asthma (or allergy). These studies provided the general conclusion that the expression of asthma is likely to be heterogeneic and polygenic and to be the result of an interaction between genetic and environmental factors. Statistical analysis of data was often hampered by the absence of physiological criteria for a specific asthmatic phenotype, the difficulty in separating inheritance of the atopic predisposition from the inheritance of asthma, or the lack of controls for environmental factors. The development of phenotypic markers for asthma (or subtypes of asthma) has served to facilitate studies of its inheritance.

PHENOTYPIC INHERITANCE BHR is a common phenotypic marker of asthma, and family studies suggest that BHR is under genetic influence. In fact, concordance among identical twins is significantly greater for BHR than for asthma symptoms. In addition, BHR may be found in asymptomatic parents of asthmatic children without evidence of positive allergen skin tests or increased serum IgE, and the hyperresponsiveness is inherited in an autosomal-dominant pattern. Other studies have provided similar results, but some indicate that the trait may not be caused by segregation at a single autosomal locus.

The discovery of IgE and the observation that its levels may increase in association with atopic disease quickly placed IgE (and in particular its level of biosynthesis) as a candidate marker for atopy. Several observations indicate that the level of total serum IgE may correlate even better with the development of asthma than for atopy. These results suggested that asthma resulted from IgE-dependent mechanisms even in the absence of identifiable allergen sensitivity. A separate follow-up study confirmed the relationship between asthma and IgE levels and established a similar link between BHR and total serum IgE levels. Other investigators have confirmed these results and have added that an increase in circulating eosinophils may also be linked to the asthma phenotype. Genetic models for the inheritance of IgE levels were proposed in a series of population and family studies to support the existence of a relatively common recessive regulatory locus, with recessive homozygotes maintaining persistently high levels of IgE. In addition, a significant multifactorial background was detected.

DNA MARKERS AND MOLECULAR GENETICS By using markers for DNA polymorphisms, at least two genetic loci have been linked to atopy and possibly to asthma. Initial work defined a single dominantly inherited locus located on chromosome 11q13 controlling IgE hyperresponsiveness. The apparent discrepancy in mode of inheritance between results derived from segregation vs

linkage analysis may be related to the definition of phenotypes employed by the two types of studies. In the linkage studies, the definition of atopy was expanded to include asymptomatic subjects (identified by abnormal IgE responsiveness). Subsequent work on the 11q13-linked atopy "gene" suggested that it may be genetically linked to the site of the β-subunit of FcεRI and that a variation within this gene (Ile^{18}Leu) may be associated with atopy. These findings suggest that the FcεRI β-subunit is a candidate gene predisposing to atopy. The discovery that a single-nucleotide polymorphism (SNP) in the FcεR1-β gene produces a dysfunctional, alternatively spliced variant that is not transported to the cell surface provides a plausible explanation of how genetic variation in the IgE receptor can influence the expression of atopy. Additional work has linked markers for chromosome 5q31-33 with atopy (defined by total serum IgE) and BHR. The 5q31-33 site is near the genes for IL-4, IL-6, IL-9, and IL-13 (which are implicated in the control of IgE biosynthesis) as well as additional candidate genes encoding other cytokines, growth factors, and receptors (including the β$_2$ adrenoceptor). Fine mapping of this region is aimed at better definition of candidate genes linked to asthma.

Because antigen-dependent immune and inflammatory mechanisms participate prominently in the expression of the asthmatic phenotype, investigators have also attempted to establish linkage of asthma to loci within the major histocompatibility complex (MHC). The MHC/human leukocyte-associated antigen (HLA) class I (HLA-A, -B, and -C) and class II (HLA-DP, -DQ, and -DR) genes are among the most polymorphic human genes described, with more than 10 alleles defined for each locus. The nature of this polymorphism has been investigated extensively using serological reagents and nucleic acid typing probes. In some studies, significant HLA associations with asthma have been found, but in others there is no association between asthma and specific HLA alleles. It is likely that weak or conflicting associations are related to the heterogeneity of the phenotype and the possibility that a discrete abnormality may be restricted to a subset of asthmatic subjects. It appears likely that a particular sequence is necessary, but not sufficient, for responsiveness to a particular antigenic epitope, and that further genetic and environmental factors are required for the expression of specific immune responsiveness. Because considerable linkage disequilibrium exists between the MHC alleles and other putative candidate genes on chromosome 6p, such as TNF-α and TNF-β, it is highly likely that gene–gene as well as gene–environmental interaction in this chromosomal region explain the genetic associations with asthma.

NEWLY IDENTIFIED ASTHMA GENES There have been major breakthroughs in the discovery of novel asthma and atopy genes through positional cloning. A combination of microsatellite linkage and SNP association studies applied to populations enriched for asthma and allergy, followed by fine mapping and gene sequencing of segments of the human genome cloned into artificial bacterial chromosomes (contigs), has identified ADAM33, PHF11 (linked to IgE), and DPP10 (linked to T cell/chemokine responses) as entirely novel disease associated genes.

ADAM33 on chromosome 20p13 encodes a disintegrin and metalloprotease that is preferentially expressed by mesenchymal cells (Fig. 22-10). This Zn^{2+}-dependent metalloprotease has enzymatic properties to cleave a number of cell surface procytokines and their receptors, but whether the disease associated SNPs are related to this or another activity of the ADAM protein is not

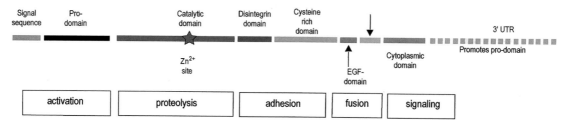

Figure 22-10 Schematic representation of the ADAM 33 gene and domain structure related to functions. EGF, epidermal growth factor; UTR, untranslated region.

known. PHF11 on chromosome 13q14 encodes a product containing two Pro-His-Asp zinc fingers that regulate transcription involved in IgE synthesis. DPP10 on chromosome 2q14 encodes a homologue of dipeptidyl peptidases with the property of cleaving terminal peptides from cytokines, chemokines and growth factors. Thus, it seems likely that ADAM33 is more closely involved in the BHR and remodeling aspects of asthma whereas PHF11 and DPP10 are more mechanistically linked to the allergic and inflammatory aspects of the disease.

CONCLUSION

Understanding and treating asthma depends on an appreciation of how inflammatory cells infiltrate the pulmonary airway and how the resulting infiltrate leads to characteristic pathological changes in airway tissue. In this context, investigators have pursued the regulatory controls over genes encoding critical components of the immune response to inhaled allergic and nonallergic stimuli. Initial evidence indicates that allergic and nonallergic asthma exhibit separate but overlapping cell–cell interactions orchestrated by immune cells and airway parenchymal cells.

SELECTED REFERENCES

Austen KF, Boyce JA. Mast cell lineage, development, and phenotypic regulation. Leuk Res 2001;25:511–518.

Brightling CE, Bradding P, Symon FA, Holgate ST, Wardlaw AJ, Pavord ID. Mast-cell infiltration of airway smooth muscle in asthma. N Engl J Med 2002;346:1699–1705.

Buckley MG, McEuen AR, Walls AF. The return of the basophil. Clin Exp Allergy 2002;32:8–10.

Conroy DM, Humbles AA, Rankin SM, et al. The role of the eosinophil-selective chemokine, eotaxin, in allergic and non-allergic airways inflammation. Mem Inst Oswaldo Cruz 1997;92(Suppl 2):183–191.

D'Amato G. Therapy of allergic bronchial asthma with omalizumab—an anti-IgE monoclonal antibody. Expert Opin Biol Ther 2003;3:371–376.

Falcone FH, Haas H, Gibbs BF. The human basophil: a new appreciation of its role in immune responses. Blood 2000;96:4028–4038.

Flood Page PT, Menzies-Gow AN, Kay AB, Robinson DS. Eosinophil's role remains uncertain as anti-interleukin-5 only partially depletes numbers in asthmatic airway. Am J Respir Crit Care Med 2003;167:199–204.

Hart PH. Regulation of the inflammatory response in asthma by mast cell products. Immunol Cell Biol 2001;79:149–153.

Horie S, Kita H. CD11b/CD18 (Mac-1) is required for degranulation of human eosinophils induced by human recombinant granulocyte-macrophage colony-stimulating factor and platelet-activating factor. J Immunol 1994;152:5457–5467.

Kepley CL, McFeeley PJ, Oliver JM, Lipscomb MF. Immunohistochemical detection of human basophils in postmortem cases of fatal asthma. Am J Respir Crit Care Med 2001;164:1053–1058.

Krishna MT, Chauhan A, Little L, et al. Inhibition of mast cell tryptase by inhaled APC 366 attenuates allergen-induced late-phase airway obstruction in asthma. J Allergy Clin Immunol 2001;107:1039–1045.

Levi-Schaffer F, Garbuzenko E, Rubin A, et al. Human eosinophils regulate human lung- and skin-derived fibroblast properties in vitro: a role for transforming growth factor beta (TGF-β). Proc Natl Acad Sci USA 1999;96:9660–9665.

Ono SJ. Molecular genetics of allergic diseases. Annu Rev Immunol 2000;18:347–366.

Powell RM, Hamilton LM, Holgate ST, Davies DE, Holloway JW. ADAM33: a novel therapeutic target for asthma. Expert Opin Ther Targets 2003;7:485–494.

Prussin C, Metcalfe DD. IgE, mast cells, basophils, and eosinophils. J Allergy Clin Immunol 2003;111(Suppl):S486–S494.

Reischl IG, Coward WR, Church MK. Molecular consequences of human mast cell activation following immunoglobulin E-high-affinity immunoglobulin E receptor (IgE-FcεRI) interaction. Biochem Pharmacol 1999;58:1841–1850.

Saini SS, MacGlashan D. How IgE upregulates the allergic response. Curr Opin Immunol 2002;14:694–697.

Siraganian RP. Mast cell signal transduction from the high-affinity IgE receptor. Curr Opin Immunol 2003;15:639–646.

Tsicopoulos A, Joseph M. The role of CD23 in allergic disease. Clin Exp Allergy 2000;30:602–605.

Yokota A, Kikutani H, Tanaka T, et al. Two species of human Fcε receptor II (FcεRII/CD23): tissue-specific and IL-4-specific regulation of gene expression. Cell 1988;55:611–618.

23 Pulmonary Emphysema

STEVEN D. SHAPIRO

SUMMARY

Chronic obstructive pulmonary disease (COPD) is a disease state characterized by airflow limitation that is not fully reversible caused by a noxious agent. COPD is the fourth leading cause of mortality and affects more than 16 million people in the United States, a number that has increased about 40% since 1982. As COPD and other cigarette-related diseases become epidemic worldwide, the biology of emphysema is clearly complex and poorly understood with limited translation into effective pharmacotherapy.

Key Words: Chronic obstructive pulmonary disease; cigarette; pulmonary emphysema.

INTRODUCTION

Chronic obstructive pulmonary disease (COPD) has been defined by the Global Initiative for Chronic Obstructive Lung Disease as a disease state characterized by airflow limitation that is not fully reversible caused by a noxious agent. The agent is almost uniformly long-term cigarette smoke exposure. COPD includes emphysema, an anatomically defined condition with destruction and enlargement of the lung distal to the terminal bronchioles; chronic bronchitis, a clinically defined condition with chronic cough and phlegm; and small airways disease, a condition related to narrowing of small bronchioles. COPD is only present if chronic airflow obstruction occurs; chronic bronchitis without chronic airflow obstruction is not included within COPD.

EPIDEMIOLOGY

CIGARETTE SMOKE EXPOSURE The death rate for COPD in the United States has also been increasing in contrast to falling death rates from heart and cerebrovascular diseases over the same interval. In 2001, for the first time ever, death rates for women exceeded those for men in the United States. Global burden of disease estimates suggest that COPD will rise from the sixth to the third most common cause of death worldwide by 2020.

Cigarette smoking is by far the most important risk factor for the development of COPD. Accelerated deterioration of ventilatory function is common among smokers; however, its magnitude is relatively small in most smokers. The relationship between amount of smoking and risk of COPD is unpredictable on an individual basis. Many persons with a high number of pack-years of smoking still have a normal or near-normal forced expiratory vol-

ume in the first second (FEV_1) whereas some individuals have a reduced FEV_1 with relatively modest smoking histories. Among smokers who have already sustained reductions in FEV_1, the consequences of continued smoking on ventilatory function are much more impressive than when all smokers are lumped together. The Lung Health Study found that among middle-aged smokers with an FEV_1 of 55–90% of predicted, differences of several hundred milliliter of FEV_1 developed within 5 yr between those who quit smoking and those who did not quit.

Although passive smoke exposure has been associated with reductions in pulmonary function, the importance of this risk factor in the development of the severe pulmonary function reductions in COPD remains uncertain. Although cigar and pipe smoking may also be associated with the development of COPD, the evidence supporting such associations is less compelling, likely related to the lower dose of inhaled tobacco byproducts during cigar and pipe smoking.

OTHER FACTORS The considerable overlap between subjects with asthma and COPD in airway responsiveness, airflow obstruction, and pulmonary symptoms led to the formulation of the Dutch hypothesis. It suggests that asthma, chronic bronchitis, and emphysema are variations of the same basic disease, which is modulated by environmental and genetic factors to produce these pathologically distinct entities. The alternative British hypothesis contends that asthma and COPD are fundamentally different diseases: asthma is viewed as largely an allergic phenomenon, whereas COPD results from smoking-related inflammation and damage. Determination of the validity of the Dutch hypothesis vs the British hypothesis awaits identification of the genetic predisposing factors for asthma and/or COPD, as well as the interactions between these postulated genetic factors and environmental risk factors.

Respiratory infections are important causes of COPD exacerbations; however, the association of both adult and childhood respiratory infections to the development and progression of COPD remains to be proven. Although several specific occupational dusts and fumes are likely risk factors for COPD, the magnitude of these effects appears to be substantially less important than the effect of cigarette smoking.

PATHOLOGICAL MECHANISMS IN COPD

Cigarette smoking leads to changes in the large airways, small airways, and lung parenchyma (Fig. 23-1). The effects of cigarette smoke exposure on different lung compartments is variable

From: *Principles of Molecular Medicine, Second Edition*
Edited by: M. S. Runge and C. Patterson © Humana Press, Inc., Totowa, NJ

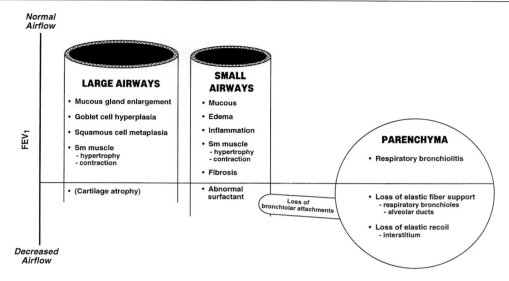

Figure 23-1 Pathological changes in relation to airflow in COPD. Changes observed in large airways (>2 mm), small airways (<2 mm), and lung parenchyma are depicted. Abnormalities above the line are associated with normal airflow (normal FEV_1), whereas those below the line are likely to cause decreased airflow (low FEV_1). Note, although controversial, most airway changes associated with excess material in the airway may not cause airflow obstruction. A unifying hypothesis for airflow obstruction involves loss of lung elastin resulting both in decreased small airway attachments and decreased parenchymal elastic recoil.

both within and between individuals, hence leading to disease heterogeneity within a given lung, and the contribution of the airways and lung parenchyma to airflow obstruction differs among individuals. Overall, small airway changes likely contribute to airflow obstruction initially, whereas emphysema predominates in advanced disease.

AIRWAY DISEASE

Large Airways The changes in the large airways, which include mucous gland enlargement and goblet cell hyperplasia, are responsible for chronic bronchitis. Epithelial cells undergo squamous metaplasia with loss of cilia. This not only predisposes to carcinogenesis, but impaired mucociliary clearance increases the risk of airway infections. Both bacterial and inflammatory host proteinases may promote airway remodeling further decreasing bacterial clearance. The serine proteinase neutrophil elastase (NE) also causes goblet cell degranulation and mucin production.

Small Airways (<2 MM) Changes that predispose to airway narrowing include goblet cell metaplasia, smooth muscle hypertrophy, excess mucus, edema, and inflammatory cellular infiltration. Reduced surfactant may increase surface tension at the air-tissue interface predisposing to airway narrowing or collapse. Emphysema, discussed next, appears to lead to airflow obstruction because the alveolar wall attachments that help maintain the patency of small airways by producing outward traction on their walls are decreased in number and the capacity of the attachments that do remain to develop traction is decreased. Airway remodeling with subepithelial fibrosis might be a critical factor in small airway narrowing. Little is known regarding mechanisms of airway fibrosis in COPD, but there are several potential mechanisms whereby a proteinase can predispose to fibrosis. This might seem counterintuitive because proteinases degrade matrix; however, the net effect on collagen depends on whether a particular proteinase can degrade collagen as well as other nonmatrix substrates. For example, matrix metalloproteinases (MMPs) degrade insulin-like growth factor (IGF) binding proteins releasing profibrotic insulin-like growth factor. Plasmin and other proteinases could release

and activate transforming growth factor-β. MMP-2 causes fibroblast proliferation. Thus, proteinases have multiple effects on cells and matrix that could result in net accumulation of collagen.

EMPHYSEMA Emphysema, characterized by destruction and enlargement of the gas-exchanging airspaces, that is, the respiratory bronchioles, alveolar ducts, and alveoli, characterized by obliteration and perforation of airspace walls with coalescence of airspaces into much larger ones than normal. The pathogenesis of emphysema can be dissected into at least four interrelated events: (1) chronic exposure to cigarette smoke leads to inflammatory cell recruitment within the lung's terminal airspaces; (2) these inflammatory cells release proteinases that damage the extracellular lung matrix; (3) cell death: loss of alveolar units must also encompass death to structural cells of the airspace (whether cell death is a cause or consequence matrix destruction is unknown); and (4) ineffective repair of the extracellular matrix and cellular constituents results in pulmonary emphysema.

Inflammation Synthesis of existing data regarding inflammatory cell response in human lungs following cigarette smoke exposure suggests the following sequence of events. Macrophages patrol the lower airspace under normal conditions. Cigarette smoke comes in contact with and activates lung epithelial cells and alveolar macrophages leading to cytokine/chemokine release followed by acute neutrophil recruitment, and subacute macrophage accumulation in the respiratory bronchioles and alveolar space. T cells (CD8+ > CD4+), and perhaps other inflammatory and immune cells, are also recruited. Concomitant cigarette smoke-induced loss of cilia in the airway epithelium predisposes to bacterial infection with neutrophilia. Cigarette smoke exposure might also directly impair immune cell function. Surprisingly, in end-stage lung disease, long after smoking cessation, there remains an exuberant inflammatory response suggesting that mechanisms of cigarette smoke-induced inflammation that initiate the disease differ from mechanisms that sustain inflammation after smoking cessation. Thus multiple interacting inflammatory cell types are present and likely contribute to the pathogenesis.

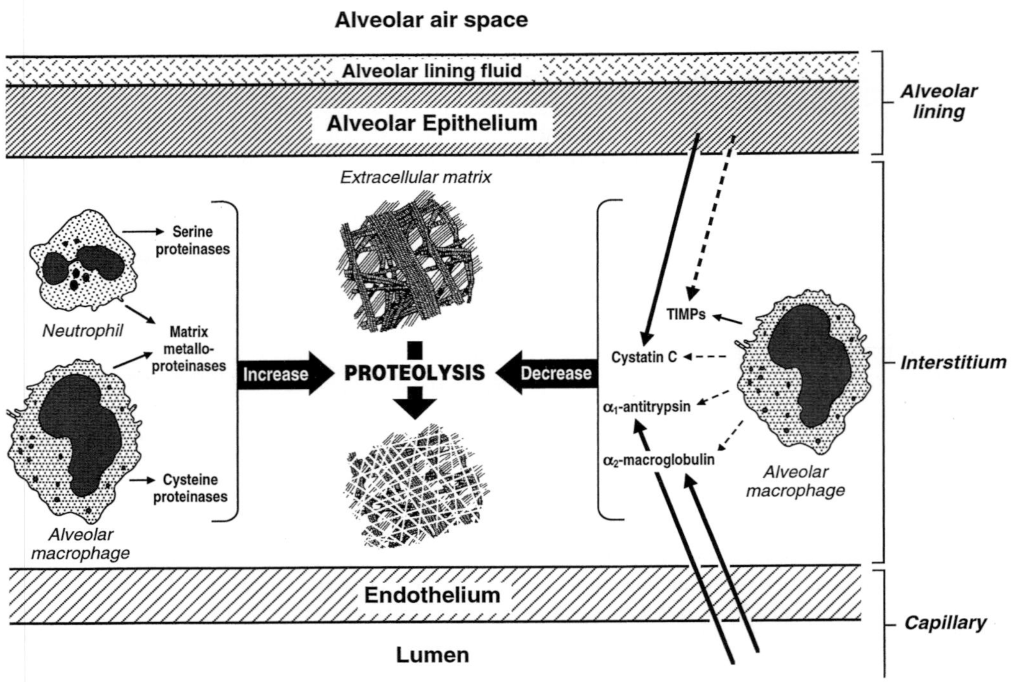

Alveolar air space

Figure 23-2 Proteinase–antiproteinase balance in the lung parenchyma determines the risk of proteolytic degradation of lung extracellular matrix. Proteinases released by neutrophils, macrophages, and perhaps resident cells have the capacity to degrade lung extracellular matrix components including elastin, thus predisposing to emphysema. Matrix proteolysis is limited by the presence of inhibitors to each class of proteinases. Some inhibitors are locally derived (TIMP, cystatin C) whereas others arrive via the bloodstream (α_1-AT, α_2-macroglobulin). The predominant sources are depicted by solid arrows; lesser sources are indicated by dashed arrows. (Adapted from Evans MD, Pryor WA. Cigarette smoking, emphysema, and damage to α_1-proteinase inhibitor. Am J Physiol 266 [Lung Cell Mol Physiol 10] 1994; L593–L611).

Proteinase–Antiproteinase Hypothesis In 1963, an association was reported of chronic airflow obstruction and emphysema with deficiency of serum α_1-antitrypsin (α_1-AT), the endogenous inhibitor of NE. In 1964 the first reproducible model of emphysema was described in experimental animals by injecting papain, a plant-derived proteinase, into the lungs via the trachea. Together these observations indicated that emphysema could be induced by proteolytic injury to the lung extracellular matrix, and eventually led to the proteinase–antiproteinase hypothesis of emphysema that has since been the prevailing concept of emphysema pathogenesis. Because only instillation of elastolytic enzymes caused the lesions, it is often called the elastase/antielastase hypothesis. However, there is evidence that collagen overexpression in transgenic mice is associated with airspace enlargement. Moreover, despite increased collagen accumulation in COPD, loss of alveolar units must also encompass collagen turnover.

According to the proteinase–antiproteinase hypothesis of emphysema, there is a steady or episodic release of proteolytic enzymes with elastolytic activity into the lung parenchyma (Fig. 23-2). Normally, plasma proteinase inhibitors, especially α_1-AT, permeate lung tissue and prevent proteolytic enzymes from digesting structural proteins of the lungs. Proteinase inhibitors synthesized locally in the lungs also contribute to the antiproteinase shield. Emphysema results from an augmentation of proteinase release in the lungs, a reduction in the antiproteinase defense within the lungs, or a combination of both increased proteinase burden and decreased proteinase inhibitory capacity. Accordingly, emphysema occurs when there is an imbalance between proteinases and antiproteinases in favor of proteinases.

From the study of proteinases in emphysema it has become appreciated that events controlling proteolytic injury to the extracellular matrix of the lung do not necessarily operate over the lungs as whole. Important events are tightly controlled and occur at or near the cell membrane of inflammatory cells. Thus, the proteinase–antiproteinase hypothesis has been modified to consider "imbalance" between proteinases and their inhibitors in compartments as small as the microenvironments immediately surrounding inflammatory cells.

Cigarette smoke exposure leads to a variety of changes in both airways and lung parenchyma that result in the syndrome termed COPD. A variety of proteinases participate in COPD with their major role being destruction of extracellular matrix, particularly elastin. However, proteinases also play a role in regulating inflammation through generation of chemokines and cytokines and by creating paths for cells through tissue barriers. NE is also a potent secretagogue. Thus, proteinases participate in multiple activities in several anatomic sites in the lung in the development of COPD.

Inflammatory Cells and Their Proteinases in the Lungs Defining the cells and proteinases responsible for destruction of lung extracellular matrix associated with cigarette smoking will be critical for development of appropriate proteinase inhibitors for application in COPD. For example, neutrophils are armed with a distinct set of serine proteinases and MMPs, whereas macrophages possess cysteine proteinases and the capacity to produce several MMPs. The profiles of proteinases differ between these inflammatory cell types, and regulation of proteinase expression is distinct. Neutrophils are short-lived and package active proteinases into

Table 23-1
Elastases Present in the Lung Parenchyma

Enzyme class	Enzyme	Molecular mass[a] (kDa)	Cell of origin	Matrix substrates other than elastin	Relative elastolytic activity, pH 7.5
Serine	Neutrophil elastase	27–31	Neutrophil (monocyte)	bm components[b]	100%
	Proteinase 3	28–34	Neutrophil (monocyte)	bm components[b]	40%
	Cathepsin G	27–32	Neutrophil (monocyte) (mast cell)	bm components[b]	20%
Matrix metalloproteinase	92 kDa gelatinase	92–95	Macrophage, neutrophil, eosinophil	Denatured collagens, types IV, V, and VII collagen	30%
	Metalloelastase	54	Macrophage	bm components[b]	35%
Cysteine	Cathepsin L	29	Macrophage	(Inactive at pH 7.5)	0%[c]
	Cathepsin S	28	Macrophage	(Unknown)	80%

Parentheses denote minor cellular sources.
[a]Denotes (pre)proenzyme forms.
[b]Basement membrane (bm) components include fibronectin, laminin, entactin, vitronectin, and type-IV collagen (nonhelical domains).
[c]These enzymes are significantly more potent than neutrophil elastase at pH 5.5.

granules ready for quick release, optimal for rapid egress from the vasculature and eradicating microorganisms. Macrophage metallo-proteinase expression, however, is highly regulated by inflammatory cytokines, matrix fragments, and other agents resulting in much slower release but sustained synthesis. Thus, macrophages appear to monitor and respond to their environment; properties that could allow for tissue remodeling and possibly control of other inflammatory events.

Neutrophils As noted, smoking causes lung retention of neutrophils, apparently by increasing adhesiveness of neutrophils and pulmonary microvascular endothelium, and possibly by increasing neutrophil stiffness so that the cells cannot deform enough to get through pulmonary capillaries normally. Neutrophils are thought to also become deformable and burrow through preformed holes in the basement membrane. Evidence for this is direct transmission electron microscopy visualization and the inability to prevent neutrophil migration through extracellular matrices with proteinase inhibitors. Bronchoalveolar lavage fluids from smokers contain more neutrophils than lavage fluids from nonsmokers, indicating that smoking leads to recruitment of neutrophils into lung tissue.

Neutrophil Serine Proteinases Serine proteinases are characterized by conserved His, Asp, and Ser residues that form a charge relay system that functions by transfer of electrons from the carboxyl group of Asp to the oxygen of Ser, which then becomes a powerful nucleophile able to attack the carbonyl carbon atom of the peptide bond of the substrate. Serine proteinases are synthesized as preproenzymes in the endoplasmic reticulum and processed by cleavage of the signal peptide (pre-) and removal of a dipeptide (pro-) by cathepsin C, and stored in granules as active packaged proteins. Distinct subsets of serine proteinases are expressed in a lineage-restricted manner in immune and inflammatory cells. Serine proteinases are also expressed in a developmentally specific manner. For example, NE, proteinase (PR) 3, and cathepsin G (CG) are major components of primary or azurophil granules that are formed during a specific stage during the development of myeloid cells. The fact that neutrophil serine proteinases have a pH optimum of about 7.4 suggests that these enzymes could damage lung tissue if liberated from the neutrophil. Also, active NE's and CG's concentration

on the outer face of their plasma membrane of activated neutrophils may help explain how these enzymes can function in the extracellular environment despite large excesses of α_1-AT and other inhibitors.

NE has activity against a broad range of extracellular matrix proteins including elastin (Table 23-1). Following the discovery of α_1-AT deficiency and the capacity of NE to cause emphysema in experimental animals, NE has been considered of primary importance in the pathogenesis of pulmonary emphysema. Further evidence supporting involvement of NE in this disease process includes: (1) the presence of human neutrophil elastase (HNE) and neutrophils in the lung tissue and bronchoalveolar lavage of patients with emphysema in some studies, (2) that smoking leads to an acute increase in a specific peptide released by HNE action on fibrinogen, and (3) that cigarette smoke can oxidize a methionine residue in the reactive center of α_1-AT, inactivating α_1-AT, and, thus, altering the NE: α_1-AT balance. Whether oxidative inactivation occurs in vivo is uncertain.

Gene targeting of NE has also demonstrated a role for NE in the development of emphysema. NE-deficient mice have been used to demonstrate a role for NE in killing Gram-negative bacteria. NE-mediated bacterial killing is related to proteolytic degradation of outer membrane proteins on the outer wall of Gram-negative bacteria. NE also degrades Gram-negative toxins. Application of NE null mutant mice to cigarette smoke exposure demonstrated 60% less airspace enlargement than wild-type mice. Many interactions between neutrophils/macrophages and NE or MMP-12 appear to explain that the deficiency of either protein significantly protects against emphysema in mouse models.

PR3 is approx 40% as potent as HNE against elastin. PR3 causes emphysema in experimental animals. This molecule has been identified as the autoantigen target of cytoplasmic-staining antipolymorphonuclear autoantibody in Wegener's granulomatosis. CG is stored in neutrophil primary granules and to a lesser degree in mast cells and a subset of peripheral blood monocytes. CG is chymotryptic, but also has matrix degrading activity with nearly 20% the elastolytic capacity of HNE. Moreover, CG increases elastolytic activity of HNE and may facilitate neutrophil penetration of epithelial and endothelial barriers by increasing their permeability.

Table 23-2
Proteinase Inhibitors Present in the Lung Parenchyma

Inhibitor	Molecular mass (kDa)	Cell of origin	Class of proteinases inhibited
α₂-macroglobulin	725	Hepatocyte, lung fibroblast, macrophage	Serine, metallo, cysteine
α₁-AT	52	Hepatocyte, macrophage	Serine[a]
SLPI	12	Large airway epithelial cell, type-II pneumocyte	Serine[b]
Elafin	12	Large airway epithelial cell	Serine
TIMP-1	27.5	Macrophages, resident lung parenchymal cell	Metallo
Cystatin C	13	Bronchial epithelial cell, macrophage	Cysteine

Parentheses denote minor cellular sources.
[a]α₁-AT has greater affinity for neutrophil elastase than for proteinase 3 and cathepsin G.
[b]SLPI does not inhibit neutrophil elastase.

Neutrophil metalloproteinases; neutrophils contain three MMPs (*see* below for general discussion of MMPs): the gelatinase B (MMP-9), neutrophil collagenase (MMP-8), and membrane-type metalloproteinases (MT6-MMP). In the neutrophil MMP-8 and MMP-9 are stored within specific granules. Neutrophil collagenase can degrade interstitial collagens, but is less active against other extracellular matrix components. MMP-9 is active against a number of substrates including denatured collagens (gelatins), basement membrane components, and elastin. MMP-9 is an important enzyme mediating vascular injury and aneurysm formation. MT6-MMP is a cell surface-bound MMP that has not been studied in detail.

Monocytes Monocytes resemble neutrophils in that they contain NE and CG in peroxidase-positive granules that are similar to the azurophil granules of neutrophils. These proteinases are synthesized by monocyte precursors in the bone marrow, and can be rapidly released by the circulating cell, perhaps for transvascular migration. Interestingly, expression of both of these serine proteinases is limited to a subset of "proinflammatory" monocytes (approx 15% of total) that appear to be those capable of tissue penetration. As monocytes differentiate into macrophages in tissues, they lose their NE and CG, but acquire the capacity to synthesize and secrete metalloproteinases.

Macrophages Alveolar macrophages are the most abundant defense cells in the lung under normal conditions and during states of chronic inflammation. Alveolar macrophages are prominent in the respiratory bronchioles of cigarette smokers where emphysematous changes first manifest. Because they are capable of producing factors that both promote destruction of extracellular matrix and protect against matrix destruction, macrophages may have a complex role in the pathogenesis of emphysema. Clearly, alveolar macrophages do have the capacity to degrade elastin by means of several different proteolytic enzymes (*see* Table 23-1).

Cysteine (Thiol) Proteinases Cysteine proteinases represent a large, diverse group of plant and animal enzymes with amino acid homology at the active site only. They are inhibited by cystatins, which are produced ubiquitously in local tissue environments (Table 23-2). Human alveolar macrophages produce the lysosomal thiol proteinases, cathepsins B, H, L, and S. These enzymes share similar sizes of 24–32 kDa and high mannose side chains (typical of proteins targeted for lysosomal accumulation).

Cathepsins B and H have little endopeptidase activity and may function to activate other proteins similar to interleukin converting enzyme. Cathepsins L and S have large active pockets with relatively indiscriminate substrate specificities that include elastin and other matrix components. These enzymes have an acidic pH optima but cathepsin S retains approx 25% of its elastolytic capacity at neutral pH (making it approximately equal to NE). Thus, these enzymes have the capacity to cause lung destruction if they are targeted to the cell surface or extracellular space (especially if macrophages can acidify their microenvironment). These properties are plausible but remain to be proven. Cathepsin L production is increased in smokers' alveolar macrophages.

Matrix Metalloproteinases MMPs comprise a family of matrix degrading enzymes thought to be essential for normal development and physiological tissue remodeling and repair. Abnormal expression of metalloproteinases has been implicated in many destructive processes, including tumor cell invasion and angiogenesis, arthritis, atherosclerosis, arterial aneurysms, and pulmonary emphysema. MMP family members generally share 40–50% identity at the amino acid level, and they possess common structural domains. MMPs are secreted as inactive proenzymes that are activated at the cell surface or within the extracellular space by proteolytic cleavage of the N-terminal domain. Catalytic activity depends on coordination of a zinc ion at the active site and is specifically inhibited by members of another gene family, called TIMPs for tissue inhibitors of MMPs (*see* Table 23-2). Optimal activity of MMPs is around pH 7.4. All MMPs except matrilysin have a carboxyl terminal hemopexin-like domain that is important for conferring substrate specificity and for TIMP binding. The gelatinases have an additional fibronectin-like domain that mediates their high-binding affinity to gelatins and elastin.

Individual members of the MMP family can be loosely divided into groups based on their matrix degrading capacity. As a whole, they are able to cleave all extracellular matrix components. The collagenases have the unique capacity to cleave native triple helical interstitial collagens but have a restricted substrate specificity. There are two gelatinases of MMP-2 (gelatinase A) and MMP-9 (gelatinase B), which differ in their cellular origin and regulation, but share the capacity to degrade gelatins (denatured collagens), type-IV collagen, elastin, and other matrix proteins. Stromelysins (MMP-3, -10, -11) have a broad spectrum of susceptible substrates, including most basement membrane components. Matrilysin

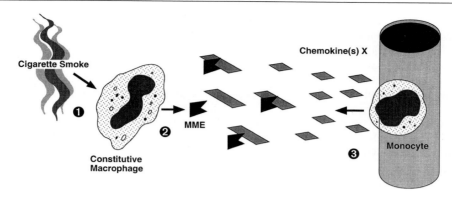

Figure 23-3 Mechanism of metalloelastase-mediated monocyte recruitment in response to cigarette smoke. Inhaled cigarette smoke induces constitutive lung macrophages to produce macrophage metalloelastase (MME). MME proteolytically generates a chemotactic gradient, presumably by cleaving a protein into a chemotactic fragment (chemokine[s] X) which attracts blood monocytes into the lung parenchyma.

(MMP-7), the smallest MMP (28 kDa as a proenzyme) has broad substrate specificity of stromelysin plus it has some elastase activity. Macrophage elastase (MMP-12) also has a potent broad substrate specificity that includes elastin. The newest members of the MMP family are MT-MMPs. MT1-MMP (MMP-14) activates MMP-2. MMPs are active against a variety of proteins besides extracellular matrix. They cleave and activate latent tumor necrosis factor-α, thereby regulating inflammation. MMPs degrade and inactivate α_1-AT, thus indirectly enhancing the activity of HNE. However, closely related cell surface ADAMs (a disintigrin and metalloproteinase domain), most notably ADAM-17, are thought to most efficiently "shed" active tumor necrosis factor-α.

Alveolar macrophages produce several MMPs including significant amounts of MMP-1, MMP-9, MMP-12, and smaller amounts of MMP-3 and MMP-7. Expression of these MMPs is highly regulated, and under quiescent conditions, such as in normal mature lung tissue, expression is limited. MMPs are induced and their production and activity are carefully controlled during normal repair and remodeling processes. With chronic inflammation, regulation of MMPs can go awry, and MMPs can be overexpressed and produced at inappropriate sites.

Because several MMPs are associated with COPD, manipulation of expression in mice has led to insights regarding potential roles of these enzymes in emphysema. Overexpression of a human collagenase (MMP-1) transgene driven by the haptoglobin reporter resulted in lung-specific expression in several independent founder lines of mice. These mice developed enlarged airspaces characteristic of emphysema. This was the first demonstration that an MMP could directly cause emphysema. Also, because MMP-1 is inactive against mature elastin, this result suggested that collagen degradation was sufficient to cause emphysema. However, it is not certain whether the alveolar pathology in these animals was owing to destruction of collagen in mature lung tissue or whether expression of the transgene during growth and development interfered with normal elastic fiber assembly, perhaps through destruction of the elastic fiber microfibrillar scaffold. However, sensitive techniques have shown that some of the founder lines do not express MMP-1 during early lung development.

Targeted mutations in genes of embryonic stem cells allow generation of strains of mice deficient in specific proteins. Strains of mice deficient in individual candidate elastases can be compared with each other and normal littermates with respect to their capacity to develop emphysema in response to cigarette smoke. Wild-type

mice, like humans, chronically exposed to cigarette smoke develop a macrophage predominant inflammatory infiltrate in the lungs, followed by airspace enlargement. In contrast to wild-type littermates, mice deficient in macrophage elastase (MMP-12) failed to recruit macrophages and did not develop pulmonary emphysema in response to cigarette smoke exposure. Whether human emphysema is also dependent on this single MMP is of course uncertain. Certainly this study demonstrates a critical role of macrophages in the development of emphysema and unmasks a proteinase-dependent mechanism of inflammatory cell recruitment that may have broader biological implications (Fig. 23-3).

Many cells in the lung have the capacity to produce MMPs. Eosinophils produce significant amounts of the MMP-9. T lymphocytes interacting with endothelial cell vascular cell adhesion molecule-1 are induced to express the MMP-2. Various resident lung cells can produce MMPs. Fibroblasts, for example, are a potential prominent source of MMP-1, MMP-2, MMP-3, and MT1-MMP. Type-II alveolar epithelial cells produce MMP-7 and perhaps other MMPs. Considering the variety of lung cells capable of producing MMPs, it seems plausible that MMPs participate in the lung destruction resulting in emphysema.

α_1-Antitrypsin Deficiency α_1-AT is a glycoprotein of 52 kDa synthesized primarily by the liver, consisting of a single polypeptide chain of 394 amino acids. Fully processed α_1-AT has three carbohydrate side chains that account for 12% of its molecular mass. The gene for α_1-AT is 12.2 kb located on chromosome 14 near the gene for α_1-antichymotrypsin, the inhibitor for CG, which like NE is contained in neutrophil azurophil granules. The α_1-AT gene has seven exons and six introns. Exons 4–7 code for the mature protein. The first two exons and a 5′ segment of exon three are encoded in the transcript expressed in macrophages, but not in hepatocytes. α_1-AT is an acute phase reactant. Plasma levels of α_1-AT rise with trauma, estrogen therapy, birth control pills, and pregnancy.

Proteolytic inhibition of NE and other serine proteinases by α_1-AT involves cleavage of the "strained" reactive open center of α_1-AT between methionine[358] and serine[359], resulting in an altered, "relaxed" α_1-AT conformation in complex with the proteinase. Formation of the complex renders the proteinase inactive and, because the complex is stable, inactivation is essentially permanent. α_1-AT inhibits many serine proteinases on a 1/1 molar basis; however, α_1-AT associates with NE much faster than with trypsin or other serine proteinases suggesting that inhibition of

NE is the primary function of α_1-AT. Because α_1-AT inhibits NE and other serine proteinases besides trypsin some authors prefer the designations α_1-proteinase inhibitor or α_1-antiproteinase, but the name α_1-AT is still commonly used for historic reasons. When α_1-AT is complexed with a proteinase, the complex binds to receptors (called serpin/enzyme complex receptors) on hepatocytes and monocytes.

α_1-AT is transmitted codominantly. Thus, the gene product from each parent is expressed in the offspring. A large number of α_1-AT alleles are known, but most involve a single amino acid change that does not alter expression of the protein or its function. The states produced by these different alleles are referred to as follows: normal, in which there is a normal serum concentration of functional α_1-AT; deficient, in which the serum α_1-AT is lower than normal; null, in which there is no measurable serum α_1-AT; and dysfunctional in which there is a normal serum concentration of α_1-AT, but it does not have the normal antiproteinase activity.

The nomenclature for the α_1-AT polymorphism uses letters to specify the allelic variants. The original letters were chosen to reflect electrophoretic mobility: F = fast; M = medium; S = slow; and Z = ultraslow. The normal phenotype, Pi M, exists in >90% of the population, with the MS and MZ phenotypes the next most common. The MS, MZ, and SS phenotypes, which are associated with modest deficiencies of α_1-AT (about half of the normal serum concentration), do not present an increased risk of emphysema, although there is an increased frequency of Pi MZ individuals in some COPD populations. Pi MS individuals may have an increased frequency of airway hyperreactivity. Because individuals with Pi SZ, who have an average of 37% of normal (1-AT serum concentration, rarely develop emphysema, serum levels >35% of normal are thought to be enough to provide protection.

As mentioned, cigarette smoke can oxidize a methionine residue in the reactive center of α_1-AT, inactivating its capacity as a proteinase inhibitor. The potential consequences of this reaction were demonstrated in a model in which dogs treated with chloramine-T, an agent that profoundly depresses α_1-AT functional activity, developed pulmonary emphysema. However, the initial studies in smokers that demonstrated oxidatively inactivated α_1-AT in the bronchoalveolar lavage fluid have not been corroborated.

Several α_1-AT phenotypes are associated with very low serum concentrations of α_1-AT. Of these, the Pi Z phenotype is by far the most common, accounting for >95% of such individuals. Pi Z individuals have approx 15% of the normal serum concentration of α_1-AT. The prevalence of the Pi Z phenotype in the United States is approx 1/3000 people. The Z allele is rare in Asians and African-Americans. The small number of other individuals with marked deficiency of α_1-AT have Pi SZ, Pi null–null, or Pi null–Z phenotypes.

Most Pi Z individuals eventually become symptomatic with COPD, resulting from emphysema, but there is considerable variation and some individuals reach advanced age with minimal symptoms. The wide variability in pulmonary function has been confirmed among Pi Z subjects with evidence for familial factors that segregated with deterioration in pulmonary function. Smoking has a marked effect on the age at which shortness of breath appears. On the average Pi Z smokers have symptoms by age 40, about 15 yr earlier than Pi Z nonsmokers.

The Pi Z phenotype is because of a point mutation involving a single nucleotide at codon 342 that results in coding for lysine instead of glutamic acid. This amino acid substitution alters the charge attraction between the amino acids at positions 342 and 290 present in the normal form of α_1-AT and prevents the formation of a fold in the molecule. This change in tertiary structure promotes dimerization of α_1-AT molecules. The dimerization leads to the aggregation of α_1-AT in the endoplasmic reticulum that impedes secretion of the protein from the cell and results in the low levels of α_1-AT in plasma and other body fluids The Z form of α_1-AT also has a rate of association with NE that is significantly slower than the association rate of normal α_1-AT with NE. Thus, the Pi Z phenotype leads to both a deficiency of α_1-AT protein and a form of α_1-AT that is less effective than normal α_1-AT as an inhibitor of NE.

The S variant of α_1-AT, which involves a single nucleotide alteration leading to substitution of glutamic acid[264] with a valine, does not accumulate in the liver. This protein is less stable, presumably resulting from loss of a salt bridge between the glutamic acid in position 264 and the lysine in position 387. The Pi null phenotype arises either because the α_1-AT gene is missing or there is a mutation in the α_1-AT gene that results in premature termination of the gene's transcription.

Cell Death Airspace enlargement with loss of alveolar units requires disappearance of both extracellular matrix and cells. Traditional theories suggest that inflammatory cell proteinases degrade lung extracellular matrix as the primary event with subsequent loss of cell anchoring leading to apoptosis. Studies suggest that endothelial and epithelial cell death could be the primary event (presumably with secretion of proteinases to dissolve the matrix). Whether these mechanisms play a role in human COPD is unknown; however, there is increased septal cell death associated with reduced lung expression of vascular endothelial growth factor and vascular endothelial growth factor receptor-2 (KDR/Flk-1) in human emphysematous lungs.

Repair Following injury, the ability of the adult lung to repair damaged alveoli appears limited. Whether the process of septation that is responsible for alveogenesis during lung development can be reinitiated is not clear. In animal models, treatment with all-trans retinoic acid resulted in limited but significant repair. Also, lung resection results in compensatory lung growth in the remaining lung in animal models. In addition to restoring cellularity following injury, it appears difficult for an adult to completely restore an appropriate extracellular matrix, particularly functional elastic fibers.

Lung Elastin The seminal observations about α_1-AT deficiency and production of emphysema in animals with elastolytic enzymes (and only with elastolytic enzymes) led to the concept that destruction of elastin in the lung parenchyma is key to the development of emphysema.

Elastin is the principal component of elastic fibers. Elastic fibers, which possess rubber-like reversible extensibility, come under tension, and provide elastic recoil throughout the respiratory cycle. In the lung parenchyma, elastic fibers loop around alveolar ducts, form rings at the mouths of the alveoli, and penetrate as wisps into the alveolar septae in which they are concentrated at bends and junctions.

Elastin is secreted as a soluble protein of 60–70 kDa called tropoelastin (Fig. 23-4). Tropoelastin molecules, encoded by a gene on chromosome 7 in the human, are deposited into the extracellular space and aligned on a "scaffold" of microfibrils that consists of a number of proteins, including fibrillins, microfibril associated proteins, and latent transforming growth factor-β

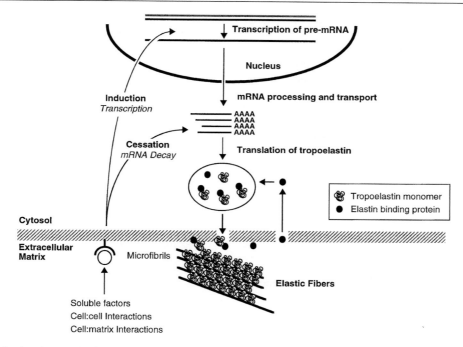

Figure 23-4 The synthesis of tropoelastin and assembly of the elastic fiber. Under the influence of extracellular and intracellular factors, tropoelastin pre-mRNA is transcribed within nucleus of the elastogenic cell. Differential splicing of tropoelastin pre-mRNA leads to different tropoelastin mRNAs and tropoelastin isoforms. After tropoelastin is secreted from the cell it associates with microfibrils adjacent to the cell surface. Uncertainty exists whether there is a carrier protein that facilitates the secretion of tropoelasin. Microfibrils are thought to be a scaffold on which tropoelastin monomers align. On the microfibril, most of the lysines in tropoelastin monomers are modified by lysyl oxidase to form covalent crosslinks (desmosines) between the monomers. The resultant polymer is elastin. (Courtesy of William C. Parks, PhD.)

binding proteins. In the extracellular space, lysyl oxidase modifies most of the lysine residues in tropoelastin monomers causing them to crosslink and form elastin, a highly insoluble, rubber-like polymer. The lysine-derived crosslinks in elastin are known as desmosines. Desmosines are unique to elastin, and therefore can be used to quantify elastin in tissues and as markers of elastin degradation in body fluids.

Elastin is resistant to many proteinases, most notably the collagenases that cleave interstitial collagens, but there are a number of enzymes that may come in contact with the lung that can degrade elastin (*see* Table 23-1). Under normal conditions, elastin synthesis in the lung begins in the late neonatal period, peaks during early postnatal development, continues to a much lesser degree through adolescence paralleling lung growth, and stops in adult life. There is some evidence that the tropoelastin gene always remains transcriptionally active but rapid mRNA degradation prevents expression of the protein. Multiple cell types are responsible for elastin synthesis in the lungs and associated structures. Lung elastin normally lasts a human life span, and there is virtually no elastin synthesis in the normal adult lung.

Although destruction of lung elastin appears to be necessary for the development of emphysema because of smoking, it remains unknown precisely how the breakdown of elastin translates into the deformity recognized as emphysema. Elastin depletion appears to be restricted to the sites of emphysema, rather than being a global deficiency of the lung that contains regions of emphysema. It has also been difficult to determine the capacity of the lung parenchyma to undergo repair after proteolytic injury. It is not known if normal elastic fibers can be properly formed in the lung after the period of growth and development. After an intratracheal injection of HNE into an experimental animal, there

is acute depletion of elastin followed by a burst of extracellular matrix synthesis so that over a few weeks the elastin content of the lungs returns to normal, although the lungs develop emphysema. However, the newly synthesized elastic fibers appear disorganized, similar to the elastic fibers in human emphysema. Studies of lung growth after pneumonectomy in adult rats indicate that elastin synthesis can be reinitiated in the adult lung and deposited at the sites at which elastin is normally produced during lung development. Nothing is known about the turnover of other extracellular matrix components in human lungs affected by COPD.

Collagen Collagen turnover in COPD is complex. Studies indicate increased collagen per unit volume of airspace wall in emphysematous lungs from smokers and in experimental animals subjected to chronic cigarette smoke inhalation. These findings suggest that the concept of emphysema formation as a purely destructive process may be in error. Although total collagen content is increased in emphysema, it appears logical that with loss of alveolar units, all local collagen must also be lost. Excessive collagen deposition, particularly in the small airways that might contribute to airflow obstruction, more than compensates for this loss.

CONCLUSION

As COPD and other cigarette-related diseases become epidemic worldwide, the biology of emphysema is clearly complex and poorly understood with limited translation into effective pharmacotherapy. This may change as critical questions are addressed regarding the pathogenetic mechanisms of COPD, including: what are the signals that initiate and perpetuate inflammation in the lungs during the development of emphysema associated with smoking? Inflammatory cells are the presumed source of injurious proteinases, but specifically which inflammatory cells are the culprits? Which proteolytic enzymes are involved in lung destruction, and how do they make contact with the lung extracllular matrix and maintain their catalytic activity in the presence of an abundance of proteinase inhibitors? Is it possible that resident cells of the lungs, such as fibroblasts, also contribute to alveolar septal destruction? Although elastin degradation may be central to emphysema, what is the role of other extracellular matrix components, particularly collagens, and what limits matrix repair? Use of genetic engineering, modern genetics, imaging, and bioinformatics among other techniques are being applied to understand the molecular basis of COPD.

SELECTED REFERENCES

Anthonisen NR, Connett JE, Kiley JP, et al. Effects of smoking intervention and the use of an inhaled anticholinergic bronchodilator on the rate of decline of FEV1. The Lung Health Study. JAMA 1994; 272:1497–1505.

Chapman H, Riese R, Shi G-P. Emerging roles for cysteine proteinases in tissue injury. Annu Rev Physiol 1997;59:63–88.

D'Armiento J, Dalal SS, Okada Y, Berg RA, Chada K. Collagenase expression in the lungs of transgenic mice causes pulmonary emphysema. Cell 1992;71:955–961.

Hautamaki RD, Kobayashi DK, Senior RM, Shapiro SD. Macrophage elastase is required for the development of emphysema induced by cigarette smoke in mice. Science 1997;277:2002–2004.

Kasahara Y, Tuder RM, Cool CD, Lynch DA, Flores SC, Voelkel NF. Inhibition of VEGF receptors causes lung cell apoptosis and emphysema. J Clin Invest 2000;106:1311–1319.

Mannino DM, Homa DM, Akinbami LJ, Ford ES, Redd SC. Chronic obstructive pulmonary disease surveillance—United States, 1971–2000. MMWR Surveill Summ 2000;51:1–16.

Massaro GD, Massaro D. Retinoic acid treatment abrogates elastase-induced pulmonary emphysema in rats. Nat Med 1997;6:675–677.

Mecham RP, Davis EC. Elastic fiber structure and assembly. In: Yurchenko P, Birk D, Mecham R, eds. Extracellular Matrix Assembly and Structure. San Diego: Academic Press, 1994; pp. 281–314.

Pauwels RA, Buist AS, Calverley PM, Jenkins CR, Hurd SS. Global strategy for the diagnosis, management, and prevention of chronic obstructive pulmonary disease. NHLBI/WHO Global Initiative for Chronic Obstructive Lung Disease (Gold) Workshop summary. Am J Respir Crit Care Med 2001;163:1256–1276.

Retamales I, Elliott WM, Meshi B, et al. Amplification of inflammation in emphysema and its association with latent adenoviral infection. Am J Respir Crit Care Med 2001;164:469–473.

Shapiro S. The macrophage in chronic obstruction pulmonary disease. Am J Respir Crit Care Med 2000;160(5 Pt 2):S29–S32.

Stockley RA. Proteases and antiproteases. Novartis Found Symp 2000; 234:189–199; discussion 199–204.

Silverman EK. Hereditary pulmonary emphysema. In: Rimoin DL, Connor M, Pyeritz RE, Korf BR, Emery AE, eds. Emery and Rimoin's Principles and Practice Of Medical Genetics. 4th ed., London: Churchill Livingstone, 2002.

Wright JL. Emphysema: Concepts under change—a pathologist's perspective. Mod Pathol 1995;8:873–880.

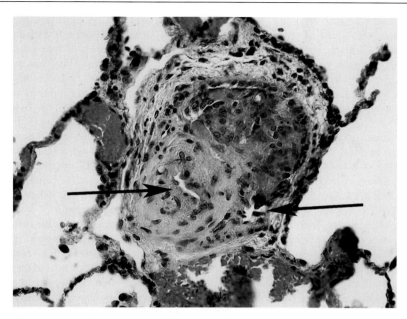

Figure 24-4 Plexiform lesion. The end-stage of pulmonary hypertension is associated with the formation of occlusive intimal lesions. Despite the often bizarre appearance of the lesions, adjacent lung tissue is generally normal, and distal blood vessels may also appear surprisingly unaffected. Clonal expansion of genetically abnormal endothelial cells may contribute to abnormal proliferation within the lesions, and chronic viral infection by human herpesvirus type VII may also be a predisposing factor to development of plexiform lesions. PAH, pulmonary arterial hypertension. (Please *see* color insert.)

individuals with chronically increased pulmonary blood flow. Immunostaining from lung biopsies demonstrates increased deposition of the glycoproteins tenascin C and fibronectin in the matrix. Association of tenascin C with proliferating SMCs has been demonstrated in animal models of pulmonary hypertension and in patients with congenital heart disease suggesting a facilitating role in promoting hyperplasia and hypertrophy. Also identified in humans and animal models of left-to-right shunt was an increase in elastase activity. Increased elastase activity can break down the extracellular matrix and release mitogens such as fibroblast growth factor 2 and basic growth factor. This is likely important in promoting the proliferation and migration of medial and adventitial cells.

HYPOXIA Acute hypoxia causes pulmonary vasoconstriction whereas chronic hypoxia additionally leads to vascular remodeling. The remodeling associated with chronic hypoxia is most pronounced in the medial layer of larger arteries in which hyperplasia and hypertrophy of SMCs occur and in small arteries and arterioles in which new smooth muscle is formed. Hypoxia increases shear stress, tension, and pressure all of which can initiate vascular remodeling. Whether hypoxia is a direct inducer of vessel remodeling or whether the stimulus to proliferate is related to the changes in shear stress resulting from vasoconstriction is unclear. In an animal model using unilateral banding of the main PA, hypoxia without flow did not lead to vascular remodeling or medial hypertrophy. This suggests that the effect of hypoxia on flow and shear stress is central to its induction of remodeling. Hypoxia has also been demonstrated to reduce the production and release of prostacyclin and NO while stimulating ET-1 release effectively tipping the balance in favor of vascular proliferation.

The extracellular matrix is a biologically active composition of collagen, elastin, and proteoglycans. Cells within the vessel and matrix can detect small changes, and disruption of the matrix in response to atherosclerosis and hypertension can stimulate vessel remodeling. Specific proteolytic enzymes, MMPs, regulate the composition and integrity of the extracellular matrix. Their expression is regulated by growth factors and cytokines; they are commonly upregulated in malignancies, closely correlating with a tumor's ability to metastasize. They are released by cells in the connective tissue particularly fibroblasts and myofibroblasts. MMP-2 and MMP-9 are two subtypes important in vascular smooth muscle cell (VSMC) activation and neointimal formation after balloon injury. Inhibitors of MMP-2 and MMP-9 decrease VSMC migration in primate arterial explants and overexpression of MMP-9 enhances VSMC migration in vitro. Secretion of MMPs by endothelial cells is an important step in angiogenesis. As endothelial cells migrate they secrete bursts of MMP-9 to degrade the basement membrane and allow cell transit. This ability to break down extracellular matrix to allow cells to migrate is critical for neovascularization.

Activated MMPs are not usually present in the quiescent adult pulmonary vessel. Hypoxia increases the activity of collagenolytic metalloproteinases, which results in the appearances of collagen breaks and fragments. The breaks in collagen allow migration of SMCs or fibroblasts from the media or adventitia and can lead to neointimal proliferation. Cleaved collagen fragments can also induce SMC and fibroblast proliferation. Extracts from the small peripheral pulmonary arteries of chronically hypoxic rats have an increase in collagenolytic activity relative to normoxic controls. This activity was most pronounced at 4 d and then again during recovery from hypoxia when resolution of vessel remodeling occurs. Inhibitors of MMPs can prevent hypoxia-induced pulmonary hypertension in rats, providing support for an important role of MMPs in pulmonary vascular remodeling.

ENDOTHELIN-1 ET-1 is a vasoactive peptide synthesized by the endothelium. It can bind receptors on both endothelial and SMCs although with different actions on each. ET-1 is a ligand for both the ET_A and ET_B receptors on the SMC and promotes vasoconstriction and proliferation. ET-1 also binds ET_B receptors on endothelial cells that promote the release of prostacyclin and NO. Elevated circulating levels of ET-1 are present in most forms of pulmonary hypertension suggesting a pathogenic role in its development or perpetuation. Elevated circulating levels of ET-1 are found in almost every type of vascular disease including atherosclerosis and vasculitis, however, suggesting that it is a nonspecific marker of vascular injury.

SEROTONIN 5-HT is a known mitogen for SMCs isolated from bovine and rat pulmonary arteries. The ability of 5-HT to remodel the pulmonary circulation has received great interest because of the development of pulmonary hypertension in individuals taking appetite suppressants that are known to interfere with the metabolism of 5-HT. Similar to ET-1, circulating 5-HT levels are elevated in most individuals with pulmonary hypertension. Treatments that increase 5-HT levels in rats exposed to long-term hypoxia worsen pulmonary hypertension, an effect that can be blocked by inhibitors of 5-HT uptake. In addition, mice that lack the 5-HT transporter required for the internalization of 5-HT develop less severe pulmonary remodeling when exposed to chronic hypoxia.

ANGIOTENSIN II Evidence that AGII plays a role in the development of pulmonary hypertension comes from experiments demonstrating induction of hypertrophy and hyperplasia in rat PA SMC in vitro. Expression of the angiotensin-converting enzyme (ACE) in the endothelial layer of small arteries and evidence of increased AGII binding to its receptor in the arterial walls of rats with hypoxia-induced pulmonary hypertension all support a role for AGII as a causative agent for the development of pulmonary hypertension. Additional evidence is provided by the ability of ACE inhibitors to attenuate pulmonary vascular remodeling.

CHRONIC LUNG DISEASE Pulmonary hypertension also develops in many forms of chronic lung disease including emphysema, interstitial lung disease, cystic fibrosis, and sickle cell disease. Pulmonary hypertension resulting from chronic lung disease is likely a different process than pulmonary hypertension arising from isolated involvement of the pulmonary vessels (like PPH, collagen vascular-associated pulmonary hypertension, and chronic increases in blood flow from congenital heart disease). Hypoxia, inflammation, and increases in flow/shear stress appear to be the initiating events. Inflammation in particular may play a role in the pulmonary hypertension associated with emphysema. Cigarette smoke impairs endothelial vasodilator function in vitro. Vascular remodeling similar to that seen in patients with hypoxia has been demonstrated in smokers with relatively preserved oxygenation. Whether the similarity is because of the like effects of cigaret smoking on shear stress or flow is not clear. It does suggest that direct injury to the pulmonary vessels from inflammation can occur independent of its impact on airways and lung parenchyma.

PULMONARY ARTERIAL HYPERTENSION AS A GENETIC DISEASE

The effect of mutations within the TGF-β superfamily of genes on the development and progression of pulmonary hypertension has received a great deal of attention. Of patients with PPH, approx 6% demonstrate an autosomal-dominant pattern of inheritance. In 2000, two separate groups identified germline mutations in the bone morphogenic protein receptor type 2 (BMPR2) that strongly correlated with the development of familial PPH. Additionally, mutations in the *Alk1* gene, a TGF-β type-I receptor, were also identified in families with hereditary hemorrhagic

telangectasia and PA hypertension. BMPR2 is a member of the TGF-β superfamily that transduces signals by binding to heterotrimeric complexes of type-I and -II receptors to activate serine/threonine kinases. This leads to the activation of intracellular messengers known as SMADs that act as transcriptional regulators. In PA SMC culled from the conduit PA of patients with PPH, it was demonstrated that TGF-β stimulated DNA incorporation and proliferation whereas it had a growth inhibitory effect on cells from normal controls. In addition, the normal antiproliferative effect of the secreted cytokine bone morphogenic protein 7, which is a ligand for BMPR2, was lost in cells from patients with PPH. However this loss of effectiveness was not seen in cells obtained from individuals with secondary pulmonary hypertension. In a mouse model, expression of a dominant negative BMPRII mutation in smooth muscle led to the development of pulmonary hypertension, providing strong support for the theory that mutations in this receptor can lead to PPH. Which intracellular signaling mechanisms are disrupted because of these mutations, the role of mutations in endothelium and other cell types, and how these mutations lead to pulmonary hypertension is not understood.

Epidemiological data also indicate that mutations in BMPR2 are present in the majority of individuals with sporadic (nonfamilial) forms of PPH. Mutations of the BMPR2 have also been identified in patients with veno-occlusive disease, a form of postcapillary pulmonary hypertension resulting from the obliteration of small pulmonary venules and veins. No clear defects in systemic vascular remodeling have been identified in these individuals suggesting some specificity of this pathway in regulating pulmonary vascular remodeling.

THERAPIES FOR PULMONARY HYPERTENSION

Attempts to treat pulmonary hypertension have adopted two general strategies: the use of specific blockers against mitogens (including calcium), which are known mediators of pulmonary hypertension, and attempts to increase the concentration and duration of action of the endothelial derived vasodilators, prostacyclin, and NO.

Calcium channel blockers such as nifedipine prevent the influx of calcium through the voltage-gated calcium (L-type channels) and are the first-line therapy in patients with pulmonary hypertension (Fig. 24-5). They can reverse vasoconstriction in some patients and blocking calcium entry may also have an antimitogenic function on SMCs. Unfortunately, in humans they are effective in only a minority of individuals with pulmonary hypertension. Elevated circulating levels of ET-1 are present in all forms of pulmonary hypertension. Bosantan, a nonspecific ET_A/ET_B blocker, has been approved for the treatment of PA hypertension. Although experimentally ACE inhibitors can attenuate the vascular remodeling associated with hypoxia-induced pulmonary hypertension, they are not used clinically because of their effects on systemic blood pressure.

NO is a potent vasodilator whose effect is mediated through the cyclic nucleotide cGMP. Intense scientific and pharmaceutical effort has investigated ways to augment NO's and cGMP's effects on the pulmonary circulation. Experimentally, gene therapy using adenovirus to overexpress eNOS has had some success in limiting pulmonary vascular remodeling. Technical barriers make it unsuitable for clinical use at this time, however. Nitroprusside and nitroglycerin are NO donors that can induce vasodilation even in the presence of an injured endothelium. Unfortunately, both can cause

Flow Diagram for Initiating PAH Therapy

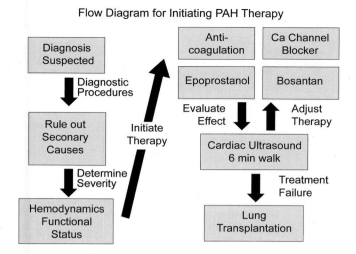

Figure 24-5 Flow diagram for initial therapeutic decision making in pulmonary arterial hypertension. Because of the complexity of caring for patients with pulmonary hypertension, initiation and maintenance of therapy should only be undertaken by a care team with extensive experience and adequate access to tertiary care services, including lung transplantation.

systemic hypotension making them less than ideal drugs to treat pulmonary hypertension. Inhaled NO has the advantage of acting locally in the pulmonary circulation because it is inactivated by hemoglobin long before reaching the systemic circulation. Toxicity of the gas as well as difficulties with delivery make this useful only in hospitalized patients particularly those awaiting lung transplant.

Another strategy to prolong the vasodilator and antiproliferative effects of NO is to prevent the degradation of cGMP. cGMP is generated when NO binds soluble guanylyl cyclase, which is central to the vasodilating and antimitogenic effects of NO. cGMP is hydrolyzed by PDE, a family of enzymes (numbering 20 and counting) that bind and inactivate cAMP and cGMP thus terminating their intracellular effects. Each PDE varies in location and specificity of substrate. PDE5 is primarily located in vascular smooth muscle and is specific for cGMP making it an attractive pharmacological target. Inhibitors of PDE5 such as zapronist and sildenafil prolong the half-life of cGMP and promote vascular relaxation. In cooperation with agents that increase NO availability such as inhaled NO or nitroglycerin, PDE5 inhibitors have a potent (and potentially dangerous) vasodilator effect. Clinical trials looking at the effect of PDE5 inhibitors on persistent pulmonary hypertension of the newborn and PPH are ongoing.

Intravenous prostacyclin is the drug of choice for individuals with PPH or scleroderma-associated pulmonary hypertension. Although prostacyclin is an effective vasodilator acutely, its ability to act as an anti-proliferative agent is central to its beneficial effect in pulmonary hypertension. Even patients who have no acute vasodilatory response to prostacyclin demonstrate improvement in pulmonary hemodynamics over 18 mo. Unfortunately, intravenous prostacyclin is expensive and the delivery system, which requires a central venous catheter, has many technical limitations. Inhaled and oral forms of prostacyclin are being studied as an alternative.

POTENTIAL NEW THERAPIES

The only approved therapies for PA hypertension are calcium channel blockers, intravenous prostacyclin, and the nonselective

ET-1 blocker bosantan. All act at least in part to reduce pulmonary vascular tone. New therapies specifically targeted at reversing the vascular remodeling associated with pulmonary hypertension are being investigated. Serine elastase inhibitors are an example of this strategy. Serine elastase activity is increased in animal models of pulmonary hypertension and is also elevated in humans with congenital heart disease. The increased activity leads to proteinase-dependent deposition of extracellular matrix proteins such as elastin, fibronectin, and tenascin C, which contributes to SMC proliferation. When given orally serine elastase inhibitors completely reversed the vascular lesions and normalized pulmonary pressures in an animal model of monocrotaline-induced pulmonary hypertension. This was associated with PA SMC apoptosis and loss of extracellular matrix, specifically elastin and tenascin C.

Inhibitors of the RhoA/Rho kinase pathway are also being considered as a treatment for pulmonary hypertension. RhoA GTPase mediates a number of cellular responses central to the development of pulmonary hypertension including activation of the contractile proteins, cell proliferation, and induction of gene expression. Animal models indicate a role for activation of the RhoA/Rho kinase pathway in both acute and chronic hypoxia. Acute administration of Rho kinase inhibitors attenuate acute hypoxic vasoconstriction in isolated mouse lungs whereas chronic administration decreases the degree of right ventricular hypertrophy and neomuscularization following 3 wk of hypoxia.

The HMG Co-A reductase inhibitors, (the statins) have replaced aspirin as the new wonder drug and look promising as a potential therapy for pulmonary hypertension. Statins have a potent antiproliferative effect on VSMCs, independent of cholesterol metabolism. They inhibit isoprenylation, which is required for the membrane localization and subsequent activation of small G proteins such as Ras and Rho, which are important intracellular messengers. In vitro, HMG Co-A reductase inhibitors not only block VSMC proliferation in response to serum but can also induce apoptosis. Already approved for the treatment of coronary artery disease they are being considered for clinical trials to treat PA hypertension.

CONCLUSION

PA hypertension results from the pathological elevation in pulmonary vascular resistance because of a combination of increased vascular tone and vessel wall remodeling. It is a heterogeneous disorder with the vascular phenotype dependent on the mechanism and severity of injury. With increasing duration and severity, pulmonary hypertension is associated with progressive vessel wall remodeling ultimately resulting in fixed, irreversible lesions. All three cell types within the vessel wall contribute to these vascular lesions through the combined effect of cell proliferation, cell migration, and matrix deposition. Therapies aim to restore vasodilator function while limiting mitogen-induced proliferation. New therapies need to reverse these vascular lesions by breaking down extracellular matrix and inducing controlled regression (apoptosis) within the vessel wall to provide the best chance to restore the pulmonary circulation to its natural low resistive state and reduce the morbidity and mortality associated with this disease.

SELECTED REFERENCES

Albert AP, Large WA. Store-operated Ca2+-permeable non-selective cation channels in smooth muscle cells. Cell Calcium 2003;33: 345–356.

Cowan KN, Heilbut A, Humpl T, Lam C, Ito S, Rabinovitch M. Complete reversal of fatal pulmonary hypertension in rats by a serine elastase inhibitor. Nat Med 2000;6:698–702.

Eddahibi S, Raffestin B, Hamon M, Adnot S. Is the serotonin transporter involved in the pathogenesis of pulmonary hypertension? J Lab Clin Med 2002;139:194–201.

Geraci MW, Gao B, Shepherd DC, et al. Pulmonary prostacyclin synthase overexpression in transgenic mice protects against development of hypoxic pulmonary hypertension. J Clin Invest 1999;103:1509–1515.

Gianetti J, Bevilacqua S, De Caterina R. Inhaled nitric oxide: more than a selective pulmonary vasodilator. Eur J Clin Invest 2002;32:628–635.

Hopkins N, McLoughlin P. The structural basis of pulmonary hypertension in chronic lung disease: remodelling, rarefaction or angiogenesis? J Anat 2002;201:335–348.

Jeffery TK, Wanstall JC. Pulmonary vascular remodeling: a target for therapeutic intervention in pulmonary hypertension. Pharmacol Ther 2001;92:1–20.

Lane KB, Machado RD, Pauciulo MW, et al. Heterozygous germline mutations in BMPR2, encoding a TGF-beta receptor, cause familial primary pulmonary hypertension. The International PPH Consortium. Nat Genet 2000;26:81–84.

Li S, Westwick J, Poll C. Transient receptor potential (TRP) channels as potential drug targets in respiratory disease. Cell Calcium 2003;33:551–558.

Loyd JE. Genetics and pulmonary hypertension. Chest 2002;122(6 Suppl):284S–286S.

Loyd JE, Parker B. Francis Lecture. Genetics and gene expression in pulmonary hypertension. Chest 2002;121(3 Suppl):46S–50S.

Mandegar M, Remillard CV, Yuan JX. Ion channels in pulmonary arterial hypertension. Prog Cardiovasc Dis 2002;45:81–114.

Mandegar M, Yuan JX. Role of K+ channels in pulmonary hypertension. Vascul Pharmacol 2002;38:25–33.

Nagaoka T, Morio Y, Casanova N, et al. Rho/Rho-kinase signaling mediates increased basal pulmonary vascular tone in chronically hypoxic rats. Am J Physiol Lung Cell Mol Physiol 2004;287(4):L665–L672.

Novotna J, Herget J. Possible role of matrix metalloproteinases in reconstruction of peripheral pulmonary arteries induced by hypoxia. Physiol Res 2002;51:323–334.

Pellicelli AM, Palmieri F, Cicalini S, Petrosillo N. Pathogenesis of HIV-related pulmonary hypertension. Ann NY Acad Sci 2001;946:82–94.

Rabinovitch M. Pathobiology of pulmonary hypertension. Extracellular matrix. Clin Chest Med 2001;22:433–449, viii. Review.

Rabinovitch M. Pulmonary hypertension: pathophysiology as a basis for clinical decision making. J Heart Lung Transplant 1999;18:1041–1053.

Rybalkin SD, Yan C, Bornfeldt KE, Beavo JA. Cyclic GMP phosphodiesterases and regulation of smooth muscle function. Circ Res 2003;93:280–291.

Stenmark KR, Bouchey D, Nemenoff R, Dempsey EC, Das M. Hypoxia-induced pulmonary vascular remodeling: contribution of the adventitial fibroblasts. Physiol Res 2000;49:503–517.

Stenmark KR, Gerasimovskaya E, Nemenoff RA, Das M. Hypoxic activation of adventitial fibroblasts: role in vascular remodeling. Chest 2002;122(6 Suppl):326S–334S.

Strange JW, Wharton J, Phillips PG, Wilkins MR. Recent insights into the pathogenesis and therapeutics of pulmonary hypertension. Clin Sci (Lond) 2002;102:253–268.

Sweeney M, Yuan JX. Hypoxic pulmonary vasoconstriction: role of voltage-gated potassium channels. Respir Res 2000;1:40–48.

Thomas AQ, Carneal J, Markin C, et al. Specific bone morphogenic protein receptor II mutations found in primary pulmonary hypertension cause different biochemical phenotypes in vitro. Chest 2002;121(3 Suppl):83S.

Thomas AQ, Gaddipati R, Newman JH, Loyd JE. Genetics of primary pulmonary hypertension. Clin Chest Med 2001;22:477–491, ix.

van den Driesche S, Mummery CL, Westermann CJ. Hereditary hemorrhagic telangiectasia: an update on transforming growth factor beta signaling in vasculogenesis and angiogenesis. Cardiovasc Res 2003;58:20–31.

Webb RC. Smooth muscle contraction and relaxation. Adv Physiol Educ 2003;27:201–206.

25 Acute Lung Injury

DAVID C. CHRISTIANI AND MICHELLE NG GONG

SUMMARY

The acute respiratory distress syndrome (ARDS)/acute lung injury is a major cause of morbidity and mortality throughout the world. ARDS is an acute syndrome of lung inflammation and increased permeability associated with severe hypoxia and bilateral infiltrates on chest radiographs with no evidence of left heart failure. This chapter reviews the evidence for genetic determinants in acute lung injury and ARDS with a focus on potential candidate gene polymorphism that may be important in the development and outcome of ARDS.

Key Words: Acute lung injury (ALI); acute respiratory distress syndrome (ARDS); angiotensin-converting enzyme (ACE); glutathnione-*S*-transferase (GST).

INTRODUCTION

The acute respiratory distress syndrome (ARDS)/acute lung injury (ALI) is a major cause of morbidity and mortality throughout the world. Annually approx 150,000 cases are reported in the United States with a reported mortality of 40–60%. The American-European Consensus Committee on ARDS defines ARDS as an acute syndrome of lung inflammation and increased permeability associated with severe hypoxia and bilateral infiltrates on chest radiographs with no evidence of left heart failure. Major risk factors for the development of ARDS have been described and include sepsis, trauma, pneumonia, burns, multiple transfusions, cardiopulmonary bypass, and pancreatitis. Other factors such as older age, chronic alcoholism, tobacco abuse, absence of diabetes, and greater severity of illness have also been found to contribute to the risk of developing ARDS. Despite the common occurrence of these risk factors, only a minority of patients with the acute injuries listed above develops ARDS. It is likely that given the same type and degree of insult, there are individual differences in susceptibility to developing ARDS.

Since the initial description of ARDS in 1967, research has focused on defining the pathogenesis, clinical presentation, course, and outcome of the syndrome. Initially, studies investigated the role of complement and endotoxin in lung injury. Then research concentrated more on the role of inflammation in the pathogenesis and course of ALI/ARDS. Additionally, clinical studies have evaluated variables that may influence the development and outcome of

ALI. Although many animal studies have been consistent, many human studies have reported conflicting results. Consequently, efforts to find clinical characteristics or biomarkers to predict, diagnose, or prognosticate outcomes in ARDS have been often disappointing. The understanding of why some patients develop and die from ARDS whereas others do not is incomplete. For example, although major risk factors for ARDS have been identified, most patients with these risk factors do not develop ARDS. Only approx 4% of patients with documented bacteremia and 41% of patients with sepsis syndrome develop ARDS.

Likewise, the search for molecular biomarkers in ARDS has been disappointing. Some studies have found increased plasma levels of tumor necrosis factor (TNF)-α to correlate with the development of ARDS and the severity and mortality in ALI. Other studies from different institutions did not detect the same association. Variable timing, sample type, and method of measurement may explain some of the conflicting results on cytokines in ARDS.

The role of genetic variability in the development and course of ALI had previously not been considered. However, discoveries about the genetic control and regulation of the innate immune defense and inflammatory response have raised the question of whether the multiple polymorphic alleles of genes that encode for cytokines and other mediators of inflammation may result in phenotypic differences in host inflammatory response. These differences may account for some of the heterogeneity in individual susceptibility to, and prognosis in, ARDS.

This chapter reviews the evidence for genetic determinants in ALI and ARDS with a focus on potential candidate gene polymorphism that may be important in the development and outcome of ARDS.

EVIDENCE FOR GENETIC DETERMINANTS OF ALI/ARDS

Almost all cases of ARDS/ALI occur as a complication of an initial injury such as sepsis, pneumonia, trauma, or aspiration. Whether a patient develops ARDS as a result of this initial injury depends partly on environmental factors such as comorbid diseases and treatment adequacy. Genetic variability is likely to affect development of ARDS in multiple aspects of this pathway (Fig. 25-1). There may be heritable determinants to the likelihood of developing ARDS after the initial injury. Alternatively, there may be variable genetic susceptibility to developing and manifesting the initial injury of sepsis or pneumonia. The likelihood by which a person with infection presents with shock may be genetically influenced.

From: *Principles of Molecular Medicine, Second Edition*
Edited by: M. S. Runge and C. Patterson © Humana Press, Inc., Totowa, NJ

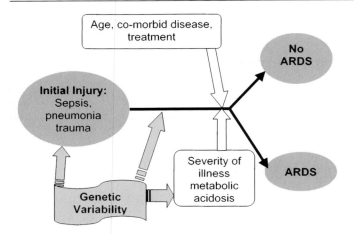

Figure 25-1 Genetic determinants in the development of ARDS. Genetic variability is likely to play a role in multiple aspects in the pathogenesis of ARDS from the susceptibility to developing the initial injury, to variable presentation of the injury (i.e., with or without shock) and ultimately to the likelihood of the progression from initial injury to ARDS.

Finally, genetic variability may influence outcome once ALI/ARDS develops.

Classic approaches to determining the genetic vs environmental contribution to diseases using twin, adoptees, or families to determine heritability are not feasible in ARDS. Workable criteria for a consistent diagnosis of ARDS were not available until 1988. The current definition of ARDS and ALI was proposed in 1994. Thus, it is likely that ARDS was underdiagnosed in the past. Additionally, the high mortality and older age of onset of ALI/ARDS limits the availability of affected family members for analysis. Thus, it is not surprising that there are no known family aggregates of ARDS. Nevertheless, intriguing studies indicate likely genetic determinants in ARDS.

There have been multiple reports of recurrent ARDS in some individuals. One report describes six patients with multiple episodes of biopsy-proven diffuse alveolar damage. The discovery of a group of patients prone to repeated lung injury raises the possibility of an inherent, possibly heritable, predisposition to ARDS. Because mortality in ARDS is high, it is not surprising that these cases of recurrent ARDS are rare. However, with mortality in ARDS improving, genetically susceptible patients may be more likely to survive their first bout of lung injury to develop another episode.

Although there are no family studies on ARDS, there are intriguing twin and adoption studies on serious infections and premature deaths. Genetic susceptibility to severe infection has important implications for ALI. Sepsis is the leading cause of ALI/ARDS and is associated with worse mortality than ALI secondary to other etiologies. Bacterial infection is found frequently in ARDS patients, with one autopsy study indicating a prevalence of 98%. Most ARDS fatalities result from refractory infection and sepsis, not from respiratory failure. Thus, it is likely that genetic polymorphisms that are important in developing severe infections may also be important in ALI.

In an epidemiological study of 218 pairs of Danish twins, a monozygotic twin whose cotwin died prematurely before the age of 60 had a significantly increased risk of dying prematurely. In another study involving 960 families with adopted children, the relative risk (RR) of dying prematurely from infections in an adopted individual is 5.81 (95% confidence interval [CI] 2.47–13.7) if one biological parent died before the age of 50 from infection. In contrast, if the adopted parent were to die prematurely of infection, the RR of dying from infection was 0.73 (95% CI 0.1–5.36) in the adoptee. These data suggest that premature death from infection has a stronger genetic than environmental component.

POTENTIAL CANDIDATE GENES IN ALI/ARDS

As a result of these studies, there have been some preliminary investigations into genetic susceptibility in sepsis and ALI. Although promising, these preliminary studies also demonstrate the difficulties involved in designing genetic studies on complex diseases like ALI/ARDS. A number of common genetic variants may have a role in ALI/ARDS because of their role in altering function (e.g., protein production or post-translational expression) in various pathophysiological steps that are important in the development of ALI/ARDS (Table 25-1). Some of these polymorphisms have been associated with variable protein levels or expression, but caution is advised in interpreting such associations. Plasma levels of protein are a crude assessment of the functional consequence of the polymorphism and a positive or negative association does not necessarily mean the polymorphism is the functional causative loci. Below is a brief evidence-based review of a few genes that can serve as potential candidates for investigation into the genetic susceptibility of ALI.

INFLAMMATORY/ANTI-INFLAMMATORY PATHWAY It is generally accepted that the development and evolution of ALI involves the activation of the inflammatory cascade. Instillation of inflammatory cytokines such as TNF-α and interleukin (IL)-6 in animals can result in histological changes identical to ARDS. In human studies, the results of these inflammatory cytokines in ALI have been inconsistent. Proinflammatory cytokines, such as TNF-α, IL-1, IL-6, IL-8, and anti-inflammatory modulators such as IL-10 and IL-1-receptor antagonists (IL-1ra) have featured prominently in studies of ALI, but there have been conflicting results on their role in predicting the development of or mortality in ALI. Potential reasons abound for the heterogeneous results from these studies of individual biomarkers in ALI. Given the complexity of the condition, it is unlikely that any particular mediator will dominate in the pathogenesis of ALI. Also, the cytokine profile may differ by the type of injury that predisposes an individual to ALI. Soluble intercellular adhesion molecule-1 and E-selectin concentrations are significantly higher in ARDS patients with sepsis than in trauma-related ARDS patients. Interest in the role of genetic variability in the development and course of ALI has grown. It is possible that multiple alleles of genes that encode for cytokines and other mediators of inflammation can result in phenotypic differences in host inflammatory response.

A number of candidate genes in the inflammatory/anti-inflammatory pathway may be important in the pathogenesis of ALI. Pre-B-cell colony enhancing factor (PBCEF) is a cytokine that have been previously found in sepsis to inhibit neutrophil apoptosis (Jia et al., 2004). Recently, the *PBCEF* gene was recently implicated in ALI (Ye, SQ et al., 2005). Increased expression of PBCEF was found in both animal models of ALI and in humans with ALI and increased PBCEF protein was found in the blood and serum of ALI patients. Two single-nucleotide polymorphisms (SNPs) were identified on the *PBCEF* gene, T-1001G and C-1543T. The *G* allele of

Table 25-1
Potential Candidate Genes for Risk or Clinical Course of ALI/ARDS

Potential role in ALI/ARDS	Candidate gene	Association with variable protein levels or function	Association with sepsis or ARDS
Inflammatory cytokines	PBCEF	Yes	Yes
	TNF-β	Variable	Variable
	TNF-B	Variable	Variable
	IL-6	Yes	Yes
Anti-inflammtory modulators	IL-1ra	Yes	Yes
	IL-10	Yes	Yes
Coagulation/Fibrinolysis pathway	PAI-1	Yes	No
Antioxidant	GST	Yes	No
Cell repair	HSP	Yes	No
Innate immunity	TLR-2	Yes	No
	TLR-4	Yes	Yes
	MBL	Yes	No
Lung function	SP-B	No	Yes
Fibrosis and inflammatory	TGF-β$_1$	Yes	No
Unclear	ACE	Yes	Yes

the T-1001G polymorphism and the GC haplotype was found to be associated with increased odds of developing ALI although no association with mortality in ALI was found.

TNF-α has often been studied in ALI. The –308 G to A transition polymorphism in the promoter region of *TNF-α* gene and the *Nco*I restriction fragment length polymorphism in intron 1 of the *TNF-α* gene are in linkage disequilibrium and have found to be associated with variable plasma levels of TNF-α and variable risk for sepsis and cerebral malaria in some but not all studies. We have found that the *–308A* allele of the *TNF-α* gene but not the *TNFB2* allele of the *TNF-α* gene was associated with the development of ARDS but only in the presence of a gene–environment interaction with whether the etiology for ARDS was directly pulmonary vs extrapulmonary. The *–308A* allele was significantly associated with increased mortality in ARDS (Gong et al., 2005).

Another potentially important candidate gene in ALI is *IL-6*. A SNP in position –174 in the promoter region of the *IL-6* gene on chromosome 7 has been identified. The *GG* genotype was found to be associated with increased plasma IL-6 levels although others have found higher IL-6 levels with the C allele. The *GG* genotype is associated with a twofold increased risk of culture positive sepsis in neonates, whereas in adults, there was no association to sepsis but the *GG* genotype was associated with survival in sepsis. The *variant C allele* was not associated with ARDS but it was found in lower frequency in nonsurviving critically ill individuals with and without ARDS.

Anti-inflammatory genes that are potentially important in ALI include *IL-10* and *IL-1ra*. Increased plasma levels of IL-10 correlate with severity of illness in pneumonia and mortality in sepsis and menningococcemia. A SNP in position –1082 is associated with increased IL-10 and increased severity of illness and risk of septic shock in patients with pneumonia. A functional penta-allelic polymorphism of *IL-1ra* consists of 86 basepair variable number of tandem repeats in intron 2. In vitro and in vivo studies have shown allele 2 of this polymorphism to be associated with increased IL-1ra. Allele 2 is associated with sepsis development and, along with polymorphisms of IL-1, with mortality in sepsis.

Other gene polymorphisms may be relevant in ALI but have not been associated with sepsis or lung injury. One example is NF-κβ, a regulatory protein for many of the proinflammatory cytokines such as TNF-α, IL-1, and IL-6. Because it serves as a gatekeeper to many inflammatory mediators and function, variability in the *NF-κβ* gene could be important in variable susceptibility to ALI. Although polymorphisms of the *NF-κβ* gene have been identified, none has been associated with functional variability, sepsis, or lung injury.

COAGULATION/FIBRINOLYSIS PATHWAY Interaction exists between the activation of the coagulation and fibrinolysis system and the inflammatory/anti-inflammatory pathway in sepsis and ARDS. Disseminated intravascular coagulation is a strong predictor of ARDS and mortality in sepsis. Commonly, microvascular thrombi are found in the lungs of patients with ARDS on autopsy and ARDS associated with disseminated intravascular coagulation has a high mortality rate.

Several polymorphisms of coagulation/fibrinolysis factors such as protein C and fibrinogen have been described in thrombotic diseases. Only one, the *plasminogen activator inhibitor (PAI)-1* gene, has been implicated in severe infectious disease. PAI-1 is an inhibitor of the fibrinolysis system in that it can complex with plasminogen activator compromising their ability to convert plasminogen to the active form, plasmin. Increased PAI-1 level is a good predictor for ARDS and mortality in ALI. A 4G/5G deletion/insertion polymorphism at position –675 in the promoter region of the *PAI-1* gene has been described, and is associated with increased serum PAI-1 levels and worse outcome in mennigococcal disease. It is possible that *PAI-1* polymorphism may be associated with risk of development and/or outcome in ARDS.

ANTIOXIDANT/CELL REPAIR A number of studies have found a possible imbalance between reactive oxygen species and antioxidants in the pathogenesis of ALI. The glutathione *S*-transferase (GST) are a family of enzymes that help regulate glutathione, a major cellular antioxidant. Several subtypes of GSTs include GST-α, GST-μ, GST-π, and GST-θ. Multiple polymorphisms of the GST enzymes have been found, some with demonstrated functional consequences. The genes for these subtypes have been implicated in the genetic susceptibility to lung cancer, chest abnormalities in rheumatoid arthritis, severe bronchial hyper-responsiveness in asthma, and chronic obstructive pulmonary disease (COPD). As yet, no clinical studies link the *GST* genes to sepsis or ALI.

Heat shock protein (HSP)-70 is the best-studied member of a group of intracellular stress proteins that protect against cell death from physiological stress like hyperthermia, environmental toxicants, or Gram-negative bacteria. HSP-70 limits lung injury in animal models of ALI. Peripheral blood monocytes from patients with ARDS had significantly lower expression of HSP-70 after hyperthermic stress compared with healthy controls with a positive correlation between HSP-70 inducibility and duration of mechanical ventilation.

Three genes encode for HSP-70 on chromosome 6. One, *HSP-70-2*, exhibits a biallelic *HSP-70-2 G/A Pst I* polymorphism that is associated with a lower expression of mRNA for *HSP-70* after stimulation. However, human studies have not demonstrated an association with sepsis or worse outcome in trauma. Another *Nco*I polymorphism on the *HSP70-Hom* gene was associated (but not significantly) with increased risk of ARDS (odds ratio 2.1, 95% CI 0.8–5.9) in one small ($N = 80$) study. Case–control studies of sepsis and ARDS/ALI are needed to evaluate the potential role of *HSP-70* gene polymorphisms, disease risk, and outcome.

INNATE IMMUNITY   As noted, sepsis and ALI are closely linked. Sepsis is a leading cause of ARDS and the leading cause of mortality in ARDS. Thus, it is possible that interindividual variation in host defense may also influence susceptibility to, and mortality in, ALI. To defend against infection, the innate immune system needs to be able to detect foreign pathogens, eliminate them rapidly before they can propagate or if needed, trigger a cascade of specific inflammatory response to contain and eradicate the organism. Thus, genes involved in innate immunity may be important in the pathogenesis of ALI.

A family of toll-like receptors (TLR) binds to bacterial constituents such as lipopolysaccharide and institutes the appropriate innate response. A SNP at *A-896G* in exon 4 of the *TLR-4* gene is associated with a replacement of an aspartic acid residue with glycine at amino acid 299 (*Asp299Gly*) and results in an alteration of the extracellular domain of the TLR-4. The variant allele of this polymorphism is associated with hyporesponsiveness to inhaled lipopolysaccharide. Although one study did not find any association with meningococcal disease, others found that the variant allele was associated with septic shock and Gram-negative infections. A SNP in TLR-2, *G2258A*, was associated with decreased response to bacterial peptides derived from *Borrelia burgdorferi* and *Treponema pallidum*. In one study, the variant allele was found in 2/22 (9%) of patients with Gram-positive septic shock compared with 0/69 (0%) of patients with other types of septic shock, although the sample size was too small for analysis. It is possible that polymorphism in *TLR-2* or *TLR-4* genes may play a role in susceptibility to ARDS/ALI.

Another potential candidate gene in ALI is the *mannose-binding lectin (MBL)* gene. MBL is a serum protein in the innate immune system that binds to polysaccharides on the surface of various bacteria and viruses, and facilitates opsonization and phagocytosis. SNPs have been identified on exons 1, 3 (known collectively as allele O) and in the promoter region of the *MBL* gene. The variant alleles of these polymorphisms are associated with lower serum levels of MBL. These variant alleles are associated with an increased risk of meningococcal disease, increased infections in children and patients with COPD and lupus, and greater severity of illness and worse outcomes in patients with cystic fibrosis. No studies of *MBL* variants in ARDS have been published.

OTHER POTENTIAL CANDIDATE GENES   A deletion polymorphism in the *angiotensin-converting enzyme (ACE)* gene, which is associated with higher ACE levels and activity, has been implicated in a number of diseases including myocardial infarction and hypertension. The biological role of *ACE* in sepsis and ALI is unclear. Most studies report *ACE* levels or activity to be low in ARDS. However, the high *ACE* producing *DD* genotype was found to be associated with severe meningococcal disease, ARDS, and increased mortality in ARDS. Further study is needed to confirm this finding.

After an acute injury, the lung often responds with evidence of fibrogenesis. Evidence of early pulmonary fibrosis in biopsy of ARDS patients has also been associated with a poorer outcome. Transforming growth factor (TGF)-β is likely to play a key role in the fibrinogenesis of the lung in ARDS. TGF-β is a cytokine produced in response to tissue injury. Its actions include the regulation and inhibition of inflammatory cytokines like TNF-β, IL-1, platelet-derived growth factors, and fibroblast growth factor; the induction of extracellular matrix deposition; the inhibition of protease degradation of the matrix; and the modulation of the expression of integrins to increase cellular adhesion to the matrix. Increased TGF-β mRNA has been found in the rat model of shock-induced ARDS. A SNP at position −509 in the promoter region of *TGF*-β$_1$ gene has been described that is associated with variable TGF-β levels. Polymorphisms in *TGF*-β$_1$ may be useful in predicting susceptibility to developing fibrosis, making them potential candidate genes for ALI.

Pulmonary surfactant is synthesized primarily by type-II alveolar cells and it has multiple important functions in the lung including lowering the surface tension on the alveolar surface and enhancing bacterial phagocytosis and chemotaxis of alveolar macrophages. One surfactant protein (SP), SP-B is predictive of ARDS development. Polymorphisms in the *SP-B* gene have been associated with ARDS in a few studies. In one small study, the frequency of an insertion/deletion variant polymorphism in intron 4 was 46.6% among 15 ARDS patients in contrast to 4.3% in the control group of normal blood donors ($p < 0.05$). An increased association has been found between the variant *SP-B* polymorphism and ARDS in women at risk for ARDS secondary to sepsis, aspiration, pneumonia, trauma, or massive transfusion after adjusting for age, race, and severity of illness. No association was found for the men, indicating possible gender modification of the risk conferred by the variant polymorphism of the *SP-B* gene. Another study found an association between the (1580C/T missense mutation in exon 4 of the *SP-B* gene and the development of ARDS especially in those patients with lung injury from predominantly direct pulmonary insults such as pneumonia. Another study on a different population of patients with community acquired pneumonia confirmed the association between the −1580 *C* allele and ARDS (Quasney et al., 2004).

ALI AS A COMPLEX DISORDER

Although there are likely to be genetic determinants in the development and evolution of ALI, elucidating these determinants will not be straightforward, because ALI is a complex disorder with complex genetic and exogenous determinants. The innate immune and inflammatory response, like many other mechanisms in physiology, involves a number of integrated biochemical and physiological systems that respond to and are modulated by environmental stimuli. To ensure stability and adaptability, the inflammatory response has both pro- and anti-inflammatory pathways with built-in redundancies, biofeedback loops for modulation, and counter-regulatory mechanisms. Although this system is under genetic regulation, it is likely to be controlled by multiple genes (genetic heterogeneity) with interaction between genes (gene–gene interaction) and between gene and exogenous stimuli such as infection, trauma, or other lung injuries (gene–environment interaction). The redundancies built into the system could result in a threshold effect in which the function of several genes needs to be affected before ALI will be manifested. Because of these multiple interactions, any single susceptibility gene in ALI will exhibit incomplete penetrance (i.e., not all individuals with the gene polymorphism will develop ALI). Epidemiologically, penetrance translates to RR, in which a highly penetrant gene corresponds to high RR of disease for the individual, whereas a low-penetrant gene confers a low to moderate RR of the disease.

The role of the environment is particularly critical in influencing the genetic determinants in a complex disorder like ALI. A predisposing injury is essential to its development. In two prospective studies on the development of ARDS, 78% of the ARDS cases developed after known conditions such as trauma, aspiration, sepsis, massive transfusion, drug overdose, near drowning, or pneumonia. In one of these studies, only 9% of the patients did not have a clearly recognized acute condition leading to ARDS. In addition, the type of injury affects the incidence of ARDS, the cytokine profile, and mortality. Thus, it is likely that any genetic determinants of ALI/ARDS will be modified by the type of injury that led to lung injury. Just as it is important to account for tobacco use in genetic studies of lung cancer and COPD, it is important to account for the type of injury that predisposes to lung injury in studies of populations at risk for ARDS/ALI.

Because of incomplete penetrance and interactions with other factors such as age, other genes and the environment, susceptibility genes for complex diseases like ALI may not determine the development and outcome of the disease. Rather, these gene polymorphisms, singly or in combination, will affect the probability of developing the syndrome after an injury. Traditionally, epidemiology has been concerned with discovering causal associations for diseases and disorders. Molecular epidemiology combines the use of molecular biological techniques such as modern genetics with epidemiology to identify and characterize disease in populations in the context of environmental exposures. In sorting out the genetic basis for lung injury, the discipline and tools of classic epidemiology will be important in study design and in accounting for multiple interactions and environmental influences.

CONCLUSION

The use of molecular epidemiology to better understand the genetic basis for ALI on a population level has important implications for research. This approach is an example of translational research in which significant findings in the laboratory are examined on a population level to determine their relative contribution to actual disease occurrences. There is also the potential for "backward" translation. Given the large number of molecules implicated in the pathogenesis of lung injury and the complex interactions between different molecular pathways, it is not always easy to discern in the laboratory which mechanism may be most important. The identification of a particular gene or genetic polymorphism that is important in a large population and the identification of environmental conditions in which genetic contribution is strongest can

help guide the molecular biologist to focus on the protein or molecular pathway with the greatest potential impact for the largest number of patients.

In addition, the identification of a group of patients who may be genetically at a higher risk for the development of ARDS under certain conditions has important implications for prevention and treatment. A goal of epidemiology is the identification of risk factors by which a population can be identified for future intervention. Although an individual's genetic susceptibility cannot be changed, the physician and the patient can alter other risk factors to decrease the overall risk of disease. In addition, the identification of individuals who are genetically susceptible to ARDS can pinpoint subgroups of patients who may most benefit from certain therapeutic modalities. Surfactant replacement therapy was not found to be beneficial in ARDS. However, it is possible that certain individuals with genetic susceptibility to ALI/ARDS because of a polymorphism in the *SP* genes may be more responsive to surfactant replacement because the lack of surfactant is more pivotal in the pathogenesis of their lung injury than other individuals with high or normal surfactant production. A better knowledge of the genetic predisposition to ALI could lead to individually tailored therapy.

Molecular epidemiological studies represent an exciting and novel approach to the study of ALI. It is not likely that a single susceptibility gene produces disease. Rather, susceptibility genes will be additional but important risk factors for determining the ultimate probability of disease. Although it will be undoubtedly challenging, the quest for genetic determinants in ALI holds great promise in helping clarify the risks and outcomes in this condition. Unlike other risk factors for ARDS, the nature of genetics allows for the prospective determination of individuals at high risk for the development of or mortality from ALI. This knowledge will be important in the design of future preventive and therapeutic trials.

ACKNOWLEDGMENTS

The above work is supported by Research Grants R01 HL60710 (D. Christiani), ES00002 (D. Christiani), and K23 HL67197 (M.N. Gong) from the National Institutes of Health.

SELECTED REFERENCES

Agnese DM, Calvano JE, Hahm SJ, et al. Human toll-like receptor 4 mutations but not CD14 polymorphisms are associated with an increased risk of gram-negative infections. J Infect Dis 2002;186(10): 1522–1525.

Arbour NC, Lorenz E, Schutte BC, et al. TLR-4 mutations are associated with endotoxin hyporesponsiveness in humans. Nat Genet 2000;25:187–191.

Ashbaugh DG, Bigelow DB, Petty TL, Levine BE. Acute respiratory distress in adults. Lancet 1967;2:319–323.

Bell RC, Coalson JJ, Smith JD, et al. Multiple organ system failure and infection in adult respiratory distress syndrome. Ann Intern Med 1983;99:293–298.

Bernard G, Artigas A, Brigham KL, et al., and the Consensus Committee. The American-European Consensus Conference on ARDS. Definitions, mechanisms, relevant outcomes and clinical trial coordinations. Am J Respir Crit Care Med 1994;149(3 Pt 1):818–824.

Parsons PE. Mediators and mechanisms of acute lung injury. Clin Chest Med 2000;21(3):467–476.

Bersten AD, Hunt T, Nicholas TE, Doyle IR. Elevated plasma surfactant protein-B predicts development of acute respiratory distress syndrome in patients with acute respiratory failure. Am J Respir Crit Care Med 2001;164(4):648–652.

Bone RC, Francis PB, Pierce AK. Intravascular coagulation associated with the adult respiratory distress syndrome. Am J Med 1976;61(5):585–589.

Border WA, Noble NA. Transforming growth factor β in tissue fibrosis. N Engl J Med 1994;331(19):1286–1292.

Brull DJ, Montgomery HE, Sanders J, et al. Interleukin-6 gene –174G>C and –572G>C promoter polymorphisms are strong predictors of plasma interleukin-6 levels after coronary artery bypass surgery. Arterioscler Thromb Vasc Biol 2001;21(9):1458–1463.

Brun-Buisson CJ, Bonnet F, Bergeret S, Lemaire F, Rapin M. Recurrent high-permeability pulmonary edema associated with diabetic ketoacidosis. Crit Care Med 1985;13(1):55, 56.

Cambien F, Poirier O, Lecerf L, et al. Deletion polymorphism in the gene for angiotensin-converting enzyme is a potent risk factor for myocardial infarction. Nature 1992;359:641–644.

Chevrolet JC, Guelpa G, Schifferli JA. Recurrent adult respiratory distress-like syndrome associated with propylthiouracil therapy. Eur Respir J 1991;4:899–901.

Clark JG, Milberg JA, Steinberg KP, Hudson LD. Type III procollagen peptide in the adult respiratory distress syndrome. Association of increased peptide levels in bronchoalveolar lavage fluid with increased risk for death. Ann Intern Med 1995;122(1):17–23.

Danis VA, Millington M, Hyland V, Grennan D. Cytokine production by normal human monocytes: Inter-subject variation and relationship to an IL-1 receptor antagonist gene polymorphism. Clin Exp Immunol 1995;99:303–310.

Dawson SJ, Wiman B, Hamsten A, Green F, Humphries S, Henney AM. The two allele sequences of a common polymorphism in the promoter of the plasminogen-activator inhibitor 1 gene respond differently to interleukin-1 in HepG2 cells. J Biol Chem 1993;268:10,739–10,745.

Deitch EA, Beck SC, Cruz NC, De Maio A. Induction of heat shock gene expression in colonic epithelial cells after incubation with *Escherichia coli* or endotoxin. Crit Care Med 1995;23:1371–1376.

Donnelly TJ, Meade P, Jagels M, et al. Cytokine, complement and endotoxin profiles associated with the development of adult respiratory distress syndrome after severe injury. Crit Care Med 1994;22:768–776.

Doyle IR, Bersten AD, Nicholas TE. Surfactant proteins-A and -B are elevated in plasma of patients with acute respiratory failure. Am J Respir Crit Care Med 1997;156(4 Pt 1):1217–1229.

Durand P, Bachelet M, Brunet F, et al. Inducibility of the 70 kD heat shock protein in peripheral blood monocytes is decreased in human acute respiratory distress syndrome and recovers over time. Am J Respir Crit Care Med 2000;161(1):286–292.

Entzian P, Huckstadt A, Kreipe H, Barth J. Determinations of serum concentrations of type III procollagen peptide in mechanically ventilated patients. Am Rev Respir Dis 1992;142:1079–1082.

Farjanel J, Hartmann DJ, Guidet B, Luquel L, Offenstadt G. Four markers of collagen metabolism as possible indicators of disease in the adult respiratory distress syndrome. Am Rev Respir Dis 1993;147:1091–1099.

Ferring M, Vincent JL. Is outcome from ARDS related to the severity of respiratory failure? Eur Respir J 1997;10:1297–1300.

Fishman D, Faulds G, Jeffery R, et al. The effect of novel polymorphisms in the interleukin-6 gene on IL-6 transcription and plasma IL-6 levels, and an association with systemic-onset juvenile chronic arthritis. J Clin Invest 1998;102:1369–1376.

Fourrier F, Chopin C, Goudemand J, et al. Septic shock, multiple organ failure and disseminated intravascular coagulation. Compared patterns of anti-thrombin III, protein C, and protein S deficiencies. Chest 1992;101:816–823.

Fourrier F, Chopin C, Wallaert B, Mazurier C, Mangalaboyi J, Durocher A. Compared evolution of plasma fibronectin and angiotensin-converting enzyme levels in septic ARDS. Chest 1985;87:191–195.

Fowler AA, Hamman RF, Good JT, et al. Adult respiratory distress syndrome: risk with common predispositions. Ann Intern Med 1983;98:593–597.

Fryer AA, Bianco A, Hepple M, Jones PW, Strange RC, Spiteri MA. Polymorphism at the glutathione S-transferase GSTP1 locus: a new marker for bronchial hyperresponsiveness and asthma. Am J Respir Crit Care Med 2000;161:1437–1442.

Gallagher PM, Lowe G, Fitzgerald T, et al. Association of *IL-10* polymorphism with severity of illness in community acquired pneumonia. Thorax 2003;58:154–156.

Gando S, Nakanishi Y, Tedo I. Cytokines and plasminogen activator inhibitor-1 in posttrauma disseminated intravascular coagulation: Relationship to multiple organ dysfunction syndrome. Crit Care Med 1995;23(11):1835–1842.

Garred P, Madsen HO, Halberg P, et al. Mannose-binding lectin polymorphisms and susceptibility to infection in systemic lupus erythematosus. Arthritis Rheum 1999;42:2145–2152.

Garred P, Pressler T, Madsen HO, et al. Association of mannose-binding lectin gene heterogeneity with severity of lung disease and survival in cystic fibrosis. J Clin Invest 1999;104:431–437.

Glynn P, Coakley R, Kilgallen I, Murphy N, O'Neill S. Circulating interleukin 6 and interleukin 10 in community acquired pneumonia. Thorax 1999;54:51–55.

Gong MN, Zhou W, Williams PL, et al. –308GA and TNFB polymorphisms in acute respiratory distress syndrome. Eur Respir J 2005;26:382–389.

Gong MN, Zhou W, Xu L, Miller D, Thompson BT, Christiani DC. Polymorphism in the surfactant protein-B gene, gender and the risk of direct pulmonary injury and ARDS. Chest 2004;125:203–211.

Gonzolez ER, Cole T, Grimes MM, Fink RA, Fowler AAI. Recurrent ARDS in a 39-year-old woman with migraine headaches. Chest 1998; 114:919–922.

Grainger DJ, Heathcote K, Chiano M, et al. Genetic control of the circulating concentration of transforming growth factor type β1. Hum Mol Genet 1999;8(1):93–97.

Harding D, Baines PB, Brull D, et al. Severity of meningococcal disease in children and the angiotensin-converting enzyme insertion/deletion polymorphism. Am J Respir Crit Care Med 2002;165:1103–1106.

Harding D, Dhamrait S, Millar A, et al. Is interleukin-6 –174 genotype associated with development of septicemia in preterm infants? Pediatrics 2003;112:800–803.

Headley AS, Tolley E, Meduri GU. Infections and the inflammatory response in acute respiratory distress syndrome. Chest 1997;111:1306–1321.

Hermans PW, Hibberd ML, Booy R, et al. 4G/5G promoter polymorphism in the plasminogen-activator-inhibitor-1 gene and outcome of meningococcal disease. Lancet 1999;354:556–560.

Hibberd ML, Sumiya M, Summerfield JA, Booy R, Levin M. Association of variants of the gene for mannose-binding lectin with susceptibility to meningococcal disease. Meningococcal Research Group. Lancet 1999;353:1049–1053.

Hierholzer C, Kalff JC, Omert L, et al. Interleukin-6 production in hemorrhagic shock is accompanied by neutrophil recruitment and lung injury. Am J Physiol 1998;275:L611–L621.

Hoffman R, Claypool W, Katyal S, Singh G, Rogers R, Dauber J. Augmentation of rat alveolar macrophage migration by surfactant protein. Am Rev Respir Dis 1987;135:1358–1362.

Hudson LD, Milberg JA, Anardi D, Maunder RJ. Clinical risks for development of the acute respiratory distress syndrome. Am J Respir Crit Care Med 1995;151:293–301.

Hulkkonen J, Pertovaara M, Antonen J, Pasternack A, Hurme M. Elevated interleukin-6 plasma levels are regulated by the promoter region polymorphism of the *IL6* gene in primary Sjogren's syndrome and correlate with clinical manifestation of the disease. Rheumatology 2001;40:656–661.

Hurme M, Santtila S. Il-1 receptor antagonist plasma levels are co-ordinately regulated by both IL-1ra and IL-1β genes. Eur J Immunol 1998;28:2598–2602.

Idell S. Coagulation, fibrinolysis and fibrin deposition in acute lung injury. Crit Care Med 2003;31(Suppl. 4):S213–S220.

Iribarren C, Jacobs DR, Jr, Sidney S, Gross MD, Eisner MD. Cigarette smoking, alcohol consumption, and risk of ARDS: a 15-year cohort study in a managed care setting. Chest 2000;117:163–168.

Ishii T, Matsuse T, Teramoto S, et al. Glutathione S-transferase P1 (GSTP1) polymorphism in patients with chronic obstructive pulmonary disease. Thorax 1999;54:693–696.

Jardin F, Fellahi JL, Beauchet A, Vieillard-Baron A, Loubieres Y, Page B. Improved prognosis of acute respiratory distress syndrome 15 years on. Intensive Care Med 1999;25:936–941.

Jia SH, Li Y, Parodo J, Kapus A, Fan L, Rotstein OD, Marshall JC. Pre-B cell colony-enhancing factor inhibits neutrophil apoptosis in experimental inflammation and clinical sepsis. J Clin Invest 2004;113:1318–1327.

Johnson J, Brigham KL, Jesmok G, Meyrick B. Morphologic changes in lungs of anesthetized sheep following intravenous infusion of recombinant tumor necrosis factor α. Am Rev Respir Dis 1991;144(1): 179–186.

Johnson AR, Coalson JJ, Ashton J, Larumbide M, Erdos EG. Neutral endopeptidase in serum samples from patients with adult respiratory distress syndrome. Comparison with angiotensin-converting enzyme. Am Rev Respir Dis 1985;132:1262–1267.

Kwiatkowski D, Hill A, Sambou I, et al. TNF concentration in fatal cerebral, non-fatal cerebral and uncomplicated Plasmodium falciparum malaria. Lancet 1990;336:1201–1204.

Lane DA, Grant PJ. Role of hemostatic gene polymorphisms in venous and arterial thrombotic disease. Blood 2000;95(5):1517–1532.

Lang JD, McArdle PJ, O'Reilly PJ, Matalon S. Oxidant-antioxidant balance in acute lung injury. Chest 2002;122(Suppl. 6):314S–320S.

Lin Z, Pearson C, Chinchilli V, et al. Polymorphisms of the human SP-A, SP-B, and SP-D genes: Association of SP-B Thr131Ile with ARDS. Clin Genet 2000;58:181–191.

Lindquist S. The heat shock response. Annu Rev Biochem 1986;55: 1151–1191.

Lipscombe RJ, Sumiya M, Hill AV, et al. High frequencies in African and non-African populations of independent mutations in the mannose-binding protein gene. Hum Mol Genet 1992;1:709–715 (Erratum in: Hum Mol Genet 1993 2(3):342).

Ma P, Chen D, Pan J, Du B. Genomic polymorphism within interleukin-1 family cytokines influences the outcome of septic patients. Crit Care Med 2002;30(5):1046–1050.

Madsen HO, Garred P, Kurtzhals JAL, et al. A new frequent allele is the missing link in the structural polymorphism of the human mannan-binding protein. Immunogenetics 1994;40:37–44.

Madsen HO, Garred P, Thiel S, et al. Interplay between promoter and structural gene variants control basal serum levels of mannan-binding protein. J Immunol 1995;155:3013–3020.

Majetschak M, Flohe S, Obertacke U, et al. Relation of a TNF gene polymorphism to severe sepsis in trauma patients. Ann Surg 1999;230(2): 207–214.

Marshall RP, Webb S, Hill MR, Humphries SE, Laurent GJ. Genetic polymorphisms associated with susceptibility and outcome in ARDS. Chest 2002;121(Suppl 3):68S–69S.

Marshall RP, Webb S, Bellingan GJ, et al. Angiotensin converting enzyme insertion/deletion polymorphism is associated with susceptibility and outcome in acute respiratory distress syndrome. Am J Respir Crit Care Med 2002;166:646–650.

Martin C, Papazian L, Payan MJ, et al. Pulmonary fibrosis correlates with outcome in adult respiratory distress syndrome: A study in mechanically ventilated patients. Chest 1995;107(1):196–200.

Mattey DL, Hassell AB, Dawes PT, et al. Influence of polymorphism in the manganese superoxide dismutase locus on disease outcome in rheumatoid arthritis: Evidence for interaction with glutathione S-transferase genes. Arthritis Rheum 2000;43(4):859–864.

Max M, Pison U, Floros J. Frequency of SP-B and SP-A1 gene polymorphism in the acute respiratory distress syndrome (ARDS). Appl Cardiopulm Pathophysiol 1996;6:111–118.

McGue M, Vaupel JW, Holm N, Harvald B. Longevity is moderately heritable in a sample of Danish twins born 1870–1880. J Gerontol 1993;48(6):B237–B244.

McKay CJ, Gallagher G, Brooks B, Imrie CW, Baxter JN. Increased monocyte cytokine production in association with systemic complications in acute pancreatitis. Br J Surg 1996;83:919–923.

McWilliams JE, Sanderson BJ, Harris EL, Richert-Boe KE, Henner WD. Glutathione S-transferase M1 (GSTM1) deficiency and lung cancer risk. Cancer Epidemiol Biomarkers Prev 1995;4(6):589–594.

Meduri GU, Tolley EA, Chrousos GP, Stentz F. Prolonged methylprednisolone treatment suppresses systemic inflammation in patients with unresolving acute respiratory distress syndrome: Evidence for inadequate endogenous glucocorticoid secretion and inflammation-induced immune cell resistance to glucocorticoids. Am J Respir Crit Care Med 2002;165:983–991.

Meduri GU, Headley S, Kohler G, et al. Persistent elevation of inflammatory cytokines predicts a poor outcome in ARDS. Chest 1995;107: 1062–1073.

Metnitz PG, Bartens C, Fischer M, et al. Antioxidant status in patients with acute respiratory distress syndrome. Intensive Care Med 1999; 25(2):180–185.

Milberg JA, Davis DR, Steinberg KP, Hudson LD. Improved survival of patients with acute respiratory distress syndrome (ARDS): 1983–1993. JAMA 1995;273(4):306–309.

Minambres E, Cemborain A, Sanchez-Velasco P, et al. Correlation between transcranial interleukin-6 gradient and outcome in patients with acute brain injury. Crit Care Med 2003;31(3):933–938.

Mira JP, Cariou A, Grall F, et al. Association of TNF2, a TNF-α promoter polymorphism, with septic shock susceptibility and mortality. JAMA 1999;282(6):561–568.

Montgomery AB, Stager MA, Carrico CH, Hudson LD. Causes of mortality in patients with the adult respiratory distress syndrome. Am Rev Respir Dis 1985;132:485–489.

Moss M, Bucher B, Moore FA, Moore EE, Parsons PE. The role of chronic alcohol abuse in the development of acute respiratory distress syndrome in adults. JAMA 1996;275(1):50–54.

Moss M, Gillespie MK, Ackerson L, Moore FA, Moore EE, Parsons PE. Endothelial cell activity varies in patients at risk for the adult respiratory distress syndrome. Crit Care Med 1996;24(11):1782–1786.

Moss M, Guidot DM, Steinberg KP, et al. Diabetic patients have a decreased incidence of acute respiratory distress syndrome. Crit Care Med 2000;28(7):2187–2192.

LaForce FM. Effect of alveolar lining material on phagocytotic and bactericidal activity of lung macrophages against Staphylococcus aureus. J Lab Clin Med 1976;88:691–699.

Lorenz E, Mira JP, Frees KL, Schwartz DA. Relevance of mutations in the TLR-4 receptor in patients with gram-negative septic shock. Arch Intern Med 2002;162:1028–1032.

Murray JF, Matthay MA, Luce JM, Flick MR. An expanded definition of the adult respiratory distress syndrome. Am Rev Respir Dis 1989; 138(3):720–723.

O'Neill SJ, Lesperance E, Klass DJ. Human lung lavage surfactant enhances staphylococcal phagocytosis by alveolar macrophages. Am Rev Respir Dis 1987;135:1358–1362.

Orfanos SE, Armaganidis A, Glynos C, et al. Pulmonary capillary endothelium-bound angiotensin-converting enzyme activity in acute lung injury. Circulation 2000;102(16):2011–2018.

Park WY, Goodman RB, Steinberg KP, et al. Cytokine balance in the lungs of patients with acute respiratory distress syndrome. Am J Respir Crit Care Med 2001;164(10 Part 1):1896–1903.

Parsons PE, Moore FA, Moore EE, Ikle DN, Henson PM, Worthen GS. Studies on the role of tumor necrosis factor in adult respiratory distress syndrome. Am Rev Respir Dis 1992;146:694–700.

Pittet JF, Mackersie RC, Martin TR, Matthay MA. Biological markers of acute lung injury: Prognostic and pathogenetic significance. Am J Respir Crit Care Med 1997;155(4):1187–1205.

Pociot F, Ronningen KS, Nerup J. Polymorphic analysis of the human MHC-linked heat shock protein 70 and HSP 70-HOM genes in insulin dependent diabetes mellitus. Scand J Immunol 1993;38(5):491–495.

Prabhakaran P, Ware LB, White KE, Cross MT, Matthay MA, Olman MA. Elevated levels of plasminogen activator inhibitor-1 in pulmonary edema fluid are associated with mortality in acute lung injury. Am J Physiol Lung Cell Mol Physiol 2003;285:L20–L28.

Quasney MW, Waterer GW, Dahmer MK, et al. Association between surfactant protein B + 1580 polymorphism and the risk of respiratory failure in adults with community-acquired pneumonia. Crit Care Med 2004;32:1115–1119.

Quinlan GJ, Lamb NJ, Tilley R, Evans TW, Gutteridge JM. Plasma hypoxanthine levels in ARDS: implications for oxidative stress, morbidity and mortality. Am J Respir Crit Care Med 1997;155(2): 479–484.

Read RC, Pullin J, Gregory S, et al. A functional polymorphism of toll-like receptor 4 is not associated with likelihood or severity of meningococcal disease. J Infect Dis 2001;184:640–642.

Rinaldo J, Christman JW. Mechanisms and mediators of the adult respiratory distress syndrome. Clin Chest Med 1990;11(4):621–632.

Rocco TR Jr, Reinert SE, Cioffi W, Harrington D, Buczko G, Simms HH. A 9-year, single-institution, retrospective review of death rate and prognostic factors in adult respiratory distress syndrome. Ann Surg 2001;233:414–422.

Russell JA. Genetics of coagulation factors in acute lung injury. Crit Care Med 2003;21(Suppl 4):S243–S247.

Savici D, Katzenstein AL. Diffuse alveolar damage and recurrent respiratory failure: report of 6 cases. Hum Pathol 2001;32(12):1398–1402.

Schaaf BM, Boehmke F, Esnaashari H, et al. Pneumococcal septic shock is associated with interleukin-10 –1082 gene promoter polymorphism. Am J Respir Crit Care Med 2003;168(4):476–480.

Schluter B, Raufhake C, Erren M, et al. Effect of the interleukin-6 promoter polymorphism (–174 G/C) on the incidence and outcome of sepsis. Crit Care Med 2002;30:32–37.

Schroder O, Schulte KM, Osterman P, Roher HD, Ekkernkamp A, Schulte KM. Heat shock protein 70 genotypes *HSPA1B* and *HSPA1L* influence cytokine concentrations and interfere with outcome after major injury. Crit Care Med 2003;31(1):73–79 (Erratum in: Crit Care Med 2003;31[4]1296).

Schroeder S, Borger N, Wrigge H, et al. A tumor necrosis factor gene polymorphism influences the inflammatory response after cardiac operation. Ann Thorac Surg 2003;75:534–537.

Schroeder S, Reck M, Hoeft A, Stuber E. Analysis of two human leukocyte antigen-linked polymorphic heat shock protein 70 genes in patients with severe sepsis. Crit Care Med 1999;27(7):1265–1270.

Shenkar R, Coulson WF, Abraham E. Anti-transforming growth factor-β monoclonal antibodies prevent lung injury in hemorrhaged mice. Am J Respir Cell Mol Biol 1994;11(3):351–357.

Sorensen TI, Nielsen GG, Andersen PK, Teasdale TW. Genetic and environmental influences on premature death in adult adoptees. N Engl J Med 1988;318(12):727–732.

Spragg RG, Lewis JF, Wurst W, et al. Treatment of acute respiratory distress syndrome with recombinant surfactant protein C surfactant. Am J Respir Crit Care Med 2003;167(11):1562–1566.

Steinberg KP, McHugh LG, Hudson LD. Causes of mortality in patients with adult respiratory distress syndrome. Am Rev Respir Dis 1993;147:A347.

Strange RC, Spiteri MA, Ramachandran S, Fryer AA. Glutathione-S-transferase family of enyzmes. Mutat Res 2001;482:21–26.

Stuber F, Petersen M, Bokelmann F, Schade U. A genomic polymorphism within the tumor necrosis factor locus influences plasma tumor necrosis factor-α concentrations and outcome of patients with severe sepsis. Crit Care Med 1996;24(3):381–384.

Stuber F, Udalova IA, Book M, et al. –308 Tumor necrosis factor (TNF) polymorphism is not associated with survival in severe sepsis and is unrelated to lipopolysaccharide inducibility of the human TNF promoter. J Inflamm 1996;46:42–50.

Suarez M, Krieger BP. Bronchoalveolar lavage in recurrent aspirin-induced adult respiratory distress syndrome. Chest 1986;90:452, 453.

Summerfield JA, Sumiya M, Levin M, Turner MW. Association of mutations in mannose binding protein gene with childhood infection in consecutive infection in consecutive hospital series. BMJ 1997;314:1229–1232.

Suzuki H, Matsui Y, Kashiwagi H. Interleukin-1 receptor antagonist gene polymorphism in Japanese patients with systemic lupus erythematosus. Arthritis Rheum 1997;40:389, 390.

Tang GJ, Huang SL, Yien HW, et al. Tumor necrosis factor gene polymorphism and septic shock in surgical infection. Crit Care Med 2003;28:1733–1736.

Turner DM, Williams DM, Sankaran D, Lazarus M, Sinnott PJ, Hutchinson IV. An investigation of polymorphism in interleukin-10 gene promoter. Eur J Immunogenet 1997;24(1):1–8.

Van der Poll Y, de Waal Malefyt R, Coyle SM, Lowry SF. Anti-inflammatory cytokine response during clinical sepsis and experimental endotoxemia: sequential measurements of plasma soluble interleukin-1 receptor type II, IL-10, and IL-13. J Infect Dis 1997;175:118–122.

Vervloet MG, Thijs LG, Hack CE. Derangements of coagulation and fibrinolysis in critically ill patients with sepsis and septic shock. Semin Thromb Hemost 1998;24(1):33–43.

Villar J, Edelson JD, Post M, Mullen JB, Slutsky AS. Induction of heat stress proteins is associated with decreased mortality in an animal model of acute lung injury. Am Rev Respir Dis 1993;147:177–181.

Villar J, Ribeiro SP, Mullen JB, Kuliszewski M, Post M, Slutsky AS. Induction of the heat shock response reduces mortality rate and organ damage in a sepsis-induced acute lung injury model. Crit Care Med 1994;22:914–921.

Ware LB, Matthay MA. The acute respiratory distress syndrome. N Engl J Med 2000;342(18):1334–1349.

Waterer GW, Quasney MW, Cantor RM, Wunderink RG. Septic shock and respiratory failure in community-acquired pneumonia have different TNF polymorphism associations. Am J Respir Crit Care Med 2001;163(7):1599–1604.

Westendorp RGJ, Hottenga JJ, Slagboom PE. Variation in plasminogen-activator–inhibitor-1 gene and risk of meningococcal septic shock. Lancet 1999;354:561–563.

Westendorp RG, Langermans JA, Huizinga TW, Verweij CL, Sturk A. Genetic influence on cytokine production and fatal meningococcal disease. Lancet 1997;329:170–173.

Westendorp R, Langermans J, Huizinga T, et al. Genetic influence on cytokine production and fatal meningococcal disease. Lancet 1997;349:170–173.

Wheeler AP, Bernard GR. Treating patients with severe sepsis. N Engl J Med 1999;340(3):207–214.

Yang IA, Seeney SL, Wolter JM, et al. Mannose-binding lectin gene polymorphism predicts hospital admissions for COPD infections. Genes Immun 2003;4(4):269–274.

Ye SQ, Simon BA, Maloney JP, et al. Pre-B-cell colony-enhancing factor as a potential novel biomarker in acute lung injury. Am J Respir Crit Care Med 2005;171:361–370.

Yost DA, Michalowski E. Adult respiratory distress syndrome complicating recurrent antepartum pyelonephritis. J Fam Pract 1990;31:81, 82.

Yoshida K, Ishigami T, Nakazawa I, et al. Association of essential hypertension in elderly Japanese with I/D polymorphism of the angiotensin-converting enzyme (ACE) gene. J Hum Genet 2000;45(5):294–298.

Zhang H, Slutsky AS, Vincent JL. Oxygen free radicals in ARDS, septic shock and organ dysfunction. Intensive Care Med 2000;26:474–476.

Zilberberg MD, Epstein SK. Acute lung injury in the medical ICU: Comorbid conditions, age, etiology and hospital outcome. Am J Respir Crit Care Med 1998;157(4 Pt 1):1159–1164.

26 Primary Ciliary Dyskinesia

PEADAR G. NOONE, MAIMOONA ZARIWALA, AND MICHAEL R. KNOWLES

SUMMARY

Mucociliary clearance is an important part of airway host defense. Abnormalities in this system may result in disease, for example, cystic fibrosis and primary ciliary dyskinesia (PCD). PCD reflects genetic-based abnormalities of airway ciliary structure, resulting in disease predominantly in the sinuses, middle ear, and lung. Although the biology of PCD has been known for decades, it is only recently that the genetics of the disease have begun to be elucidated. This chapter primarily focuses on the molecular basis of PCD, with a brief review of biology of ciliary structure/function, and the clinical aspects of the disease.

Key Words: Axonemes; bronchiectasis; cilia; dynein; mucus; mucociliary clearance; neonatal respiratory distress; nitric oxide; nontuberculous mycobacteria; obstructive pulmonary disease; otitis media; primary ciliary dyskinesia; *Pseudomonas aeruginosa*; sinusitis; situs inversus.

INTRODUCTION

Efficient airway defense is critical for protection of all lung surfaces, including the airways and distal alveolar surfaces, given the exposure of the lung to the potentially harmful contents of the outside atmosphere. Mucociliary clearance (MCC), which includes effective ciliary function, the integrated actions of airway epithelia to regulate surface liquid properties, and mucus secretion, is a key component of this defense system in the lung. Abnormalities in this defense system are reflected in the clinical expression of lung diseases. Cystic fibrosis (CF) is a prototype genetic disease of airway host defense that has been intensively studied, and the molecular basis of classic and nonclassic disease has largely been elucidated, though not completely. Abnormalities in the CF transmembrane regulator result in airway epithelial ion transport defects, and abnormal mucociliary/cough clearance, leading to chronic sinopulmonary disease and bronchiectasis as primary phenotypic manifestations. There is some phenotypic overlap of CF with another genetic disease of airway host defense, primary ciliary dyskinesia (PCD), although the latter has a completely different molecular and cell biological basis. PCD is a disease that reflects genetic abnormalities of airway ciliary structure and function, with a phenotype that reflects the anatomic distribution of ciliary organelles—i.e., otosinopulmonary disease and

From: *Principles of Molecular Medicine, Second Edition*
Edited by: M. S. Runge and C. Patterson © Humana Press, Inc., Totowa, NJ

female and male fertility problems. Although the ciliary ultrastructural and functional defects in PCD were described several decades ago, this disease's genetics have only begun to emerge. This chapter primarily focuses on the molecular basis of PCD, but first reviews ciliary structure and function and the clinical aspects of PCD.

PATHOGENESIS AND CLINICAL ASPECTS

The clinical presentation of PCD, a disease associated with defective ciliary structure and function with associated abnormalities in MCC, is predictable given the anatomic location and function of cilia in the human body. Ciliated epithelia are located in many tissues, including that of the embryo (nodal "monocilia," important for left–right [L–R] asymmetry), the ependyma of the brain, the middle ear and Eustachian tube, the conducting airways (including the sinuses), and the Fallopian tubes in females. The sperm tail in the male also has a structure and function analogous to that of the cilium. Thus, defective ciliary function results in clinical disease expressed predominantly in those tissues; *situs inversus* (resulting from abnormal monociliary function in early embryogenesis), otosinopulmonary disease, reduced female fertility, and male infertility.

CILIARY ULTRASTRUCTURE AND FUNCTION

Because the clinical phenotype is related directly to the location and function of cilia, it is worth considering normal ciliary ultrastructure and function before addressing the spectrum of disease associated with PCD. The molecular aspects of dyneins and related dynein genes are discussed later. Electron microscopic studies have led to significant insights into the structure of human cilia and similar structures. In addition, parallel studies in the flagellate protozoa, *Chlamydomonas*, have led to an increased understanding of the molecular and biochemical aspects of both normal and abnormal cilia structure and function, given the homology between the organelles of these primitive organisms and those of the human.

Cilia are projections of the cell membrane, with a "root system" made up of the ciliary necklace at the base of the cilium, and a ciliary rootlet and basal body embedded in the cell itself (Fig. 26-1). Adjacent cilia are functionally oriented in the same direction, as measured by the direction that the rootlets are facing, which has implications for overall mucociliary function in a synchronous, organized fashion—i.e., with all cilia beating in the same direction. The long axis of the ciliary shaft contains several microtubule-associated proteins (MAP, also termed axonemal proteins), the most obvious of which are dynein arms (DAs), arranged

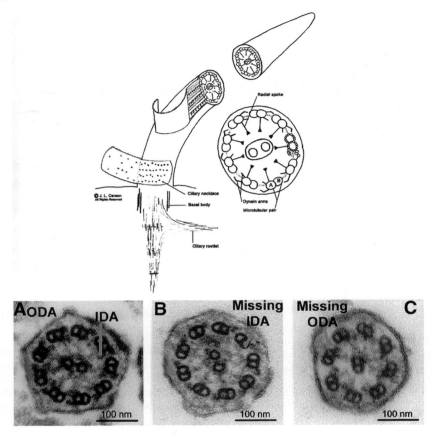

Figure 26-1 **Top panels:** Diagram of a longitudinal and cross-section of a cilium showing complex arrangement of axonemes and dyneins. The central complex and radial spokes are not labeled, but are clearly visible in both this diagram and the images in the bottom panel. (Image courtesy of Johnny Carson PhD, UNC Chapel Hill.) **Bottom panel:** (A) Cross-sectional electron micrograph images of human cilia from healthy control subject. (**B** and **C**) Two subjects with PCD. (**A**), Normal ODA and normal IDA visible. (**B**), Normal ODA, missing IDA. (**C**), Missing/stubby ODA, normal IDA. (Reproduced with permission from Johnny L. Carson.)

in pairs and in a configuration of nine outer microtubule pairs and a central pair (9 + 2 configuration) (*see* Fig. 26-1). Spokes radiate from the two central microtubules (the central apparatus [CA]) toward the peripheral microtubule doublets. The DAs (inner dynein arm [IDA] and outer dynein arm [ODA]) are spaced at 24-nm intervals along the length of one of the microtubule doublets (microtubule A), and are the "motor" proteins of cilium. Each cilium (5 μm long) contains approx 4000 DAs in pairs. Dynein utilizes ATP to effect conformational changes in the ciliary microtubules relative to each other, such that ciliary bending results.

The molecular aspects of DAs are discussed in detail later; however, a brief outline to illustrate the relationship between DA structure/function, and overall ciliary function is valuable at this stage. ODA structure appears less complicated than IDA structure. Electron microscopic techniques to visualize DAs in ciliary cross-sections from human epithelial specimens show that the ODA is easier to visualize in the normal and abnormal (missing, shortened) state than the IDA, which can be difficult to distinguish (*see* Fig. 26-1, bottom panel). The composition and arrangement of the IDA is complex, and varies along the flagellar axoneme (*see also* below, dynein structure/function). The IDA includes several subunits, termed light, intermediate, and heavy chains. From a functional standpoint, this structural difference between IDA and ODA appears to relate to the different role these structures play in

ciliary function. From a genetic standpoint, different genetic mutations lead to different "ciliary" phenotypes (abnormal ODA vs IDA vs "other"), although the clinical phenotype may be similar. Overall, ciliary beat consists of a power stroke, followed by a relaxation stroke, which makes biological sense when thinking about the swimming actions of protozoa, or the actions of cilia to propel mucus and inhaled "debris" proximally out of the respiratory tract in humans. Evidence from both mutant *Chlamydomonas* and humans with clinical disease, suggests that the ODA relates primarily to ciliary beat frequency and force, whereas IDA appears to relate more to ciliary bending patterns ("stiff"/"less supple"). For example, several mutant loci in the ODA in *Chlamydomonas* result in slow swimmers, and humans with abnormal ODA have reduced ciliary activity as compared with humans with abnormal IDA. However, *Chlamydomonas* with mutant inner DA systems exhibit reduced shear amplitude. High-speed video microscopy analyses of ciliary activity may further elucidate abnormal ODA and IDA, in terms of specific defects and their relationship with abnormal ciliary frequency/bending/"stiffness." Regulation of shear force is also required for effective ciliary beat, which involves rotational mechanisms between the CA, the radial spokes, and the outer axonemes. Mutant *Chlamydomonas* with defective CA show paralysis of flagellar beat, suggesting that this structure acts as a distributor for the regulation of dynein activity. Patients with PCD generally have visible ultrastructural and functional abnormalities in cilia that lead in vivo to abnormal MCC, loss of the protection afforded by this mechanical clearance system, and, thus, organ level expression of clinical disease manifested mainly in the ear, sinuses, and lung. However, occasionally patients may have structurally normal cilia; yet have a strong clinical "PCD phenotype." This suggests that there may be a spectrum of PCD; from that of "classic" disease with overt, defined ciliary abnormalities, to variant or nonclassic disease, with less easily defined ciliary ultrastructural defects.

Finally, one clinical observation in PCD relates to an unexpected role for another ciliary structure. "Monocilia" are ciliary structures similar to respiratory cilia but lacking a central doublet, which have an important role in early organ development in the embryo. When abnormal in PCD, defective monocilia are associated with another significant phenotypic marker of PCD, *situs inversus*.

ASSOCIATED CLINICAL DISEASE   The clinical spectrum of PCD has been well described for decades, although reviews continue to refine the phenotype. A neonatal respiratory syndrome, similar to transient tachypnea of the newborn, is a usual presenting feature of PCD, suggesting a link between effective ciliary function and the clearance of lung liquid in the neonatal period. Another striking phenotypic feature that may be detected at birth is *situs inversus* totalis (SI, known as Kartagener's syndrome when accompanied by PCD). Interestingly, SI is not genetically predetermined in patients with PCD, but occurs as a random phenomenon. Studies in a mouse model with abnormal situs suggest a role for nodal primary cilia (monocilia) in cell signaling in the formation of normal L–R asymmetry, such that defective monocilia structure and function lead to randomization of L–R asymmetry in affected animals. Monocilia are structurally different to epithelial cilia, for example, lacking a central doublet, and functionally beat in a rotatory manner, rather than the usual ciliary beat patterns. Thus, the normal rotatory action of monocilia initiates an asymmetric calcium signal at the left side of the node, and thus normal L–R asymmetry. In contrast, abnormalities of monociliary structure and rotatory beat (as occurs in PCD) lead to randomization of L–R cell signaling, and SI. Note that abnormalities in axonemal dynein also result in malfunction of monocilia. The combination of SI with any neonatal respiratory symptoms, or subsequent airway, sinus, or ear infections should prompt a diagnostic workup for PCD. In the vast majority of patients with *situs inversus* and PCD, the organs are a mirror image of normal, with no other structural or functional defects.

As patients with PCD grow older, several phenotypic markers feature prominently in the disease. A series from a large North American cohort of patients showed a phenotypic pattern consistent with earlier reports from Europe and Australia. Symptoms and signs of chronic airways infection, sinusitis, and otitis media are the cardinal features of the disease, and are responsible for the morbidity and mortality associated with PCD. Ear infections and "glue-ear" may be a prominent symptom in childhood, such that patients may be referred first to an otolaryngologist, who thus must retain a high degree of suspicion for the disease in the appropriate setting. Most patients and family members report a chronic cough as a prominent symptom. It appears that cough compensates for the lack of effective MCC in the disease and allows a degree of lung protection. Physiological data have shown that "effective" coughs may result in lung clearance almost equal to normal MCC over short time periods, even in PCD subjects with

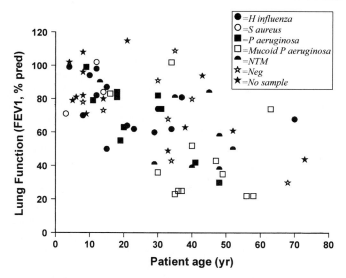

Figure 26-2   Lung function (forced expiratory volume in the first second [FEV$_1$]; % predicted) vs age in subjects with PCD ($n = 70$), plotted by the main organisms isolated in airway secretions (some subjects cultured more than one organism). Closed circles represent *H. influenza* ($n = 14$), open circles *S. aureus* ($n = 3$). Closed squares represent smooth *P. aeruginosa* ($n = 10$), open squares represent mucoid *P. aeruginosa* ($n = 12$, approx 35% of subjects, most over the age of 30 yr). Closed half circles represent nontuberculous mycobacteria ($n = 8$ [five of whom also cultured smooth *P. aeruginosa*]). Open stars represent subjects in whom sputum culture was negative for bacterial pathogens ($n = 8$), closed stars represent subjects in whom no sample was obtained ($n = 15$). Thirteen subjects had respiratory failure and an FEV$_1$ ≤ 40% predicted. (Adapted with permission from Noone PG, Leigh MW, Sannuti A, et al., 2004.)

no clearance at baseline. Clinical and radiographic evidence of bronchiectasis usually develops as the disease progresses. Comparisons with CF as a similar disease phenotype are useful, as PCD appears to run a milder course, presumably because of the different pathogenesis of the two diseases, CF being more complex. For example, there are overlaps in the microbiology of PCD airway secretions with CF. One study showed a variety of organisms in the sputum of patients with PCD (Fig. 26-2): *Haemophilus influenza, Staphylococcus aureus, Pseudomonas aeruginosa* (including mucoid *P. aeruginosa* in individuals over 30 yr of age) and nontuberculous mycobacteria, for example *Mycobacterium avium* complex and *M. abscessus*. The isolation of mucoid *P. aeruginosa* is interesting, as this organism has traditionally been associated with CF, even at a young age. Its isolation in a significant number of patients with PCD suggests that chronic failure of the mucociliary apparatus allows colonization/infection in the airways with this alginate (hence mucoid) secreting organism. Most patients with these organisms (especially mucoid *P. aeruginosa* and nontuberculous mycobacteria) in their airway secretions will be screened for CF, but with an appropriate phenotype, consideration should be given to screening for PCD also (*see* below, diagnostic workup).

Generally, PCD is a milder disease than CF, and cross-sectional studies of lung function across a wide age spectrum suggest that the loss of lung function over time is not as rapid as that of CF: approx 0.8%/yr loss of forced expiratory volume in the first second (FEV$_1$) in PCD vs approx 3.6%/yr loss of FEV$_1$ in CF. This likely relates to the complex pathogenesis of CF lung disease (loss of both mucociliary and cough clearance), as compared with the more discrete ciliary defect in MCC in PCD, in addition to the gastrointestinal, endocrine, and bone complications that occur in CF. However, data do suggest a negative impact of the disease on quality of life as PCD patients grow older. There are no generally devised and accepted "state-of-the-art" treatment protocols for PCD as a disease, other than to follow the general rules for that of non-PCD bronchiectasis. Thus, a therapeutic plan for PCD that is probably appropriate involves judicious use of pharmacological methods (e.g., bronchodilators, hypertonic saline, and "directed" antibiotics), and nonpharmacological methods (airway clearance, exercise). Not all drugs for use in CF have usage in other diseases such as PCD; for example, use of DNA-ase, a developed drug for use in CF may be less useful in non-CF bronchiectasis because of a different anatomic distribution of disease in non-CF bronchiectasis. As patients with PCD grow older, many develop more severe symptoms, and most develop digital clubbing. A significant percentage (up to 25% in one series) may develop respiratory failure as defined by hypoxemia, or an FEV_1 less than 40% predicted (*see* Fig. 26-2); a small proportion may eventually require lung transplantation.

Male infertility results from abnormal sperm tail function, whereas female fertility is more variable (some women being infertile, with others reporting a delay in conception following unprotected intercourse), presumably resulting from abnormal ciliary function in the Fallopian tube.

DIAGNOSIS The diagnosis of PCD requires a compatible clinical phenotype, in combination with laboratory studies demonstrating abnormal ciliary structure and/or function. The traditional approach is to search for ciliary ultrastructural defects (*see* Fig. 26-1). Samples of nasal ciliated epithelium can easily be obtained from the inferior turbinate using a plastic rhinoprobe and a nasoscope, without the need for local anesthesia, or invasive techniques. Analyses of ciliary cross-sections obtained from these nasal samples show structural abnormalities consisting of absent (or shortened) DAs in most patients with PCD. Defective ODA or IDA, or both, occur in more than 90% of patients with PCD, whereas a few patients may have other miscellaneous abnormalities, such as radial spoke defects, or "ciliary disorientation." Significant expertise is required in the technical aspects of producing high quality transmission electron micrographs, and in the interpretation of ciliary ultrastructure. For example, IDA defects may be more difficult to interpret than defects of the ODA, for reasons previously outlined. In addition, the IDA may look abnormal in non-PCD patients, presumably resulting from the nonspecific effects of inflammation and infection. Occasionally, patients with a strong phenotype (e.g., otosinopulmonary disease with *situs inversus*) have apparently normal looking cilia, which, given the complex structure of cilia, probably reflects abnormalities in structures not easily visible on electron microscopy, and may also relate to different genetic mutations encoding for structures other than dyneins, or for functional rather than structural abnormalities. A firm diagnosis is difficult to establish in such patients, and they may be labeled as having "nonclassic" disease, pending further advances in the molecular etiology of PCD in general.

From a functional standpoint, in vivo assessments may be determined using measures of nasal MCC (the saccharin test), or measures of lung MCC employing radio isotopic techniques. The significant limitation with the saccharin test is "noise" in the data

generated. Valid results of the test, for example, depend on voluntary suppression of swallow, head tilting, and other positional changes, which may be difficult for children and those with intractable cough. Measures of isotopic clearance from airway surfaces are more quantitative, although less available than other tests. Patients with PCD have no (or little) clearance of isotope from the lung when cough is suppressed. More rigorous techniques using high-speed video microscopy may provide better quantitation of ciliary beat frequency and patterns. Qualitative assessments of ciliary beat can define a dyskinetic beat pattern or immotility, and may provide an approximate, semi-quantitative assessment of "ciliary activity." Such methodology may yield false negatives, however, as some patients with PCD may have normal looking ciliary activity by this method.

Thus, structural assessments of cilia obtained from patients suspected of having PCD are the diagnostic "gold standards" for PCD. These studies of structure and adjunctive functional tests require the availability of significant expertise in terms of equipment and personnel, which may be prohibitive outside academic and research institutions. In addition, there is room for subjective error in diagnosing abnormalities in cilia structure, particularly that of the inner DA. As seen in the next section, nasal nitric oxide (NO) measures provide an additional noninvasive test that reliably helps diagnose PCD.

REGULATION OF CILIARY BEAT FREQUENCY AND THE ROLE OF NITRIC OXIDE: NASAL NO AS AN ADJUNCTIVE DIAGNOSTIC TEST Regulation of ciliary beat is complex, and several factors are involved, including intracellular calcium concentrations, cAMP, extracellular nucleotides such as ATP and UTP, and NO. Despite ciliary immotility in most patients with PCD, certain pharmacological agents that modulate ion transport as well as ciliary beat frequency (such as UTP), increase cough clearance in PCD, presumably acting via changes in airway surface liquid rheology rather than any direct actions on MCC. Ion transport appears normal in PCD, in contrast to the deranged sodium and chloride ion transport observed in CF airway epithelia.

Biological observations may lead to increased insights into the regulation of ciliary activity in vivo. Early observations of very low levels of nasal NO as measured in air from the upper respiratory tract in patients with PCD have been verified in larger datasets across a wide age and lung function spectrum, including pediatric and adult patients. There is a striking difference in the levels of NO produced in the upper airway of patients with PCD (very low levels) as compared with normal and disease controls (Fig. 26-3). There was no relationship between the levels of NO in PCD and the magnitude of lung disease as measured by FEV_1, or ciliary activity, or ciliary structural defect. Further, there was little overlap in nasal NO levels between PCD and disease controls such as CF, so that the test may prove to be a useful diagnostic tool.

The mechanism of the low NO in PCD remains elusive. Because NO has been linked to the upregulation of ciliary beat frequency, it is intriguing to speculate that low NO in PCD is related to the primary ciliary defect. NO is formed by the nitric oxide synthase (NOS) enzyme system, consisting of three NOS isoforms (NOS1, NOS2, and NOS3), in the presence of appropriate substrate (L-arginine and oxygen) and cofactors tetrahydrobiopterin. Of these, NOS3 appears to be the best candidate for involvement in ciliary beat regulation, because it is localized close to the base of cilia. NOS3 is activated in endothelium by stress; by analogy,

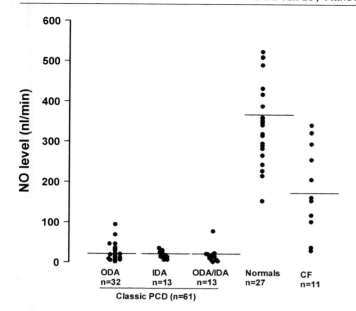

Figure 26-3 Nasal nitric oxide levels in subjects with PCD ($n = 61$ in total); $n = 16$ with both DA defective, $n = 32$ with ODA defective, and $n = 13$ with IDA defective. The data are compared with healthy controls ($n = 27$), and disease subjects with CF ($n = 11$). No differences were seen between any of the PCD subgroups, but significant differences were seen between PCD and healthy controls ($p = 0.0001$). Levels of nasal nitric oxide in CF were also different (higher) than PCD ($p = 0.0001$). (Adapted with permission from Noone PG, Leigh MW, Sannuti A, et al., 2004.)

the "stress" of ciliary bending may activate NOS3 via signaling mechanisms, and stimulate the production of NO, which in turn plays a role in regulation of ciliary beat in an autocrine or paracrine fashion. NOS3 is bound to caveolin-1 at the apical membrane of ciliated airway cells, in which it can be dissociated from this inhibitory binding and also activated by calmodulin and Ca^{2+}. In PCD, one hypothesis to explain low NO levels relates to reduced or absent ciliary "force" leading to reduced NOS3 activity, with a decrease in airway epithelial NO production. To more fully elucidate the role of NO in ciliary regulation, studies addressing NOS expression in PCD vs controls and physiological studies of ciliary beat and NO production in various normal and disease states are needed.

Thus, although a mechanistic explanation is lacking, reduced production of NO in the upper airway is a useful phenotypic marker of PCD that may serve as an adjunct "clinical" test in the diagnostic workup in PCD. From a research standpoint, low nasal NO levels in PCD may serve as a useful physiological marker of the deranged ciliary beat/NO axis.

MOLECULAR ASPECTS

As discussed, ciliary structure is complex, with many different structural components required for normal function. Thus, when addressing the genetics of PCD, research challenges include the appropriate selection of candidate genes for further study and prioritization of work. Because DA defects comprise the majority of ultrastructural defects in patients with PCD (or stated another way, PCD associated with DA defects is within the limits of diagnostic capability), it seems logical to start with a study of DA structure and function: that is, the ODA, the IDA, and then other "non-dynein" ciliary structures (e.g., radial spokes, central doublets).

Increased understanding of the structure and function of the various dyneins will augment knowledge of the relations between the various ciliary components and how mutations in different genes result in different "ciliary" phenotypes.

DYNEIN ARM STRUCTURE AND RELATED CANDIDATE GENES The axoneme is conserved phylogenetically, and the unicellular organism *Chlamydomonas* provides the opportunity to study the components of ciliary ultrastructure, and more specifically, DAs, radial spokes, and the CA (Fig. 26-4). Thus, there is a high degree of homology between structural components of *Chlamydomonas* and human cilia, and genes that encode for structural proteins. The 9 + 2 axoneme contains about 250 well-conserved polypeptides.

Dyneins are molecular "motors," with a mass of approx 1–2 MDa. Up to 15 different heavy chains have been identified. The ODA in *Chlamydomonas* possesses three dynein heavy chains, two intermediate chains, and at least eight light chains (*see* Fig. 26-4, top panel). Evidence suggests that mammalian ODA contain only two heavy chains. Several human homologs of *Chlamydomonas* ODA components are candidates for study in patients with PCD. Dynein heavy chain candidate genes are *DNAH5* (γ-heavy chain) and *DNAH9* (β-heavy chain), intermediate chain candidate genes are *DNAI1* (IC78) and *DNAI2* (IC69) and light chain candidate genes include LC1 (which is directly attached to heavy chain motor domain), *TCTEX2* (LC2) and LC4. Heavy and intermediate chains are good candidates with which to start, as these are likely to be defective in humans with missing or shortened ("stubby") ODA, evaluable using electron microscopic techniques, as shown by studies of patients with genetic mutations encoding for heavy or intermediate-chain dyneins (ICs) that show missing or stubby ODA.

The IDA appears to be different from the ODA, and is both structurally and functionally diverse (*see* Fig. 26-4, bottom panel). There are ICs, light-chain dyneins (LC), and heavy-chain dyneins, with different isoforms, with a very complex arrangement. Of several (approx 7–11) dynein heavy chain genes in the IDA, three have been identified (*DNAH1*, *DNAH3*, and *DNAH7*). To generate synchronous ciliary beat, the various IDA motors must coordinate with each other, with the ODA, the central pair and the radial spokes. Thus, elucidation of the many potential IDA defects that might relate to the expression of disease in humans presents significant challenges, particularly with reference to selection of candidate genes for testing in human disease models. Candidate genes for patients with PCD and IDA defects include *DNAH1*, *DNAH3*, and *DNAH7* (heavy chains), *hp28* and *TCTEL1* (light chain), and *DPCD*.

Candidate genes for patients with both ODA and IDA defects include *DNAI1* and *DNAI2* (intermediate chains), and also *DNAH3* and LC8, which are expressed by both IDA and ODA.

As discussed, other structural components of cilia also require attention because they may be structurally and functionally defective, leading to PCD. A pair of axonemes lies in the center of each cilium—the central pair—and appears to serve an anchoring function for the radial spokes, which themselves connect outward from the central pair to the peripheral doublets (*see* Fig. 26-4). Twenty-two polypeptides comprise the radial spoke and at least seven *Chlamydomonas* genes specifically affect the function of the flagellar radial spoke, with similar radial spoke defects observed in humans. The CA is made up of two single microtubules designated as C1 and C2. CA-associated structures

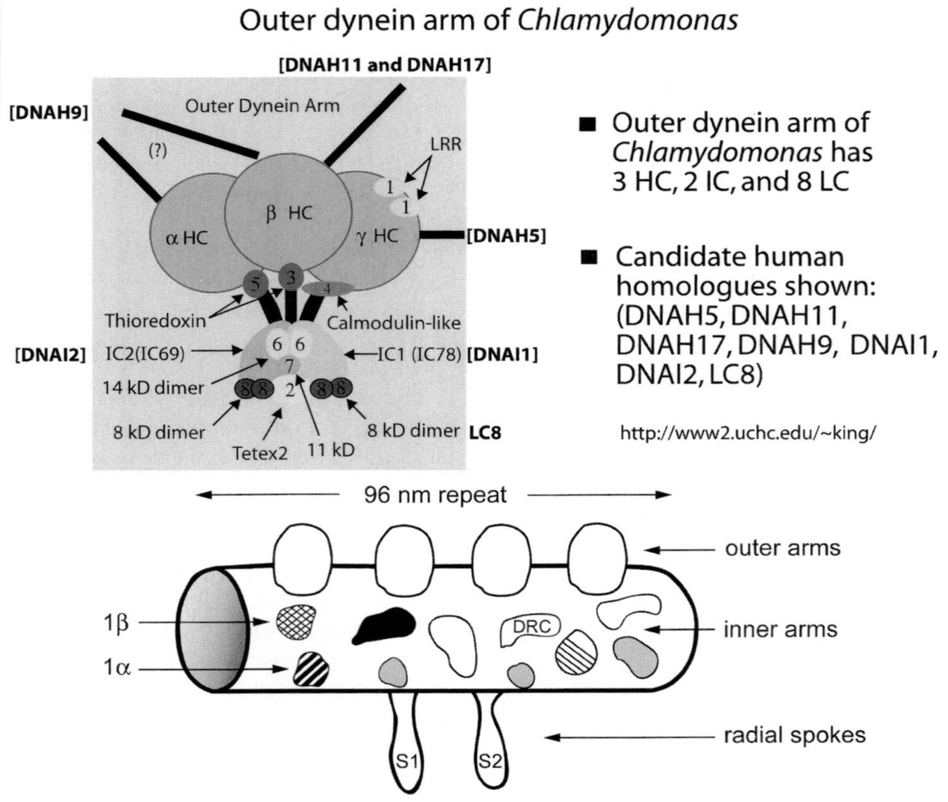

Outer dynein arm of *Chlamydomonas*

- Outer dynein arm of *Chlamydomonas* has 3 HC, 2 IC, and 8 LC

- Candidate human homologues shown: (DNAH5, DNAH11, DNAH17, DNAH9, DNAI1, DNAI2, LC8)

http://www2.uchc.edu/~king/

Figure 26-4   Top panel: ODA of *Chlamydomonas*. Human homologs are shown (DNAH5, DNAI1, DNAI2, DNAH9). (Adapted with permission from S.M. King http://www2.uchc.edu/~king/ .) **Bottom panel:** diagrammatic representation of the complexity of the arrangement of structures along one axoneme of the outer pair. Visible are the repeating nature of the structures (96 nm), the ODA on top, the radial spokes on the bottom, and the IDA represented by a complex "islands" of structures—the dynein heavy chains (DHC) 1α and 1β in a trilobed structure known as I1 IDA isoform, made up of dynein-heavy chains, three intermediate chains, and three light chains. DRC, dynein regulatory complex; located above the second radial spoke, S2. This illustration shows the complexity of the IDA particularly, and how different mutations in different structures result in IDA function, and thus ciliary abnormalities. (Adapted and reproduced with permission from Porter ME, Sale WS, 2000.)

include the central pair projections, the central pair bridging the two tubules and the central pair cap, which are attached to the distal or plus end of the microtubule. In *Chlamydomonas*, the CA includes 23 polypeptides ranging in molecular weight from 14 to 360 kDa. Ten of these polypeptides are unique to C1 and seven are unique to C2. CA ultimately regulates dynein-driven microtubule sliding in a pathway involving the radial spoke. CA agenesis was reported as causing clinical disease in three related patients with a strong phenotype for PCD. Thus, for patients who have no detectable DA defect, candidate genes include not only genes that encode ODA and IDA function, but also include genes that encode radial spoke proteins (*RSHL1*, *RSP3*, and *RSHL2*), and the CA (*PF15*, *SPAG6*, and *hPF20*).

Thus, the opportunity arises for the selection and testing of candidate genes derived from studies of *Chlamydomonas,* and studies in human disease, in which a well-defined PCD phenotype has been correlated to specific visible electron microscopic defects in ciliary structure.

GENETICS   PCD is inherited as an autosomal-recessive trait in most cases. Occasional reports suggest an autosomal-dominant inheritance. Digenic mode of inheritance (i.e., a genetic disease caused by interplay of a recessive mutation in two different genes that are functionally related) for PCD has not been seen, but it is

possible, as it occurs in other diseases. As might be predicted from the complexity of ciliary structure and function discussed, the disease is genetically heterogeneous at a ciliary structural level. Hence patients with PCD may resemble each other at a clinical phenotype level, whereas having a diverse array of ciliary abnormalities, and, thus, a completely different genetic basis for the same disease. This presents difficulties for categorization of patients, and identification of mutated genes. However, the emerging definition of ciliary ultrastructure in lower organisms and humans offers an excellent opportunity for the selection of candidate genes.

Although the disease appears to be relatively uncommon (at least in terms of a clear diagnosis), the prevalence is estimated to be approx 12,000–17,000 individuals in the United States, as extrapolated from radiographic surveys in Norway and Japan, based on the presence of dextrocardia, in association with clinical evidence of bronchiectasis. It might be hypothesized that PCD, or alternately, lung disease associated with genetic-based abnormalities in ciliary structure and function, is more common than generally appreciated. As the diagnosis may not be obvious or straightforward, especially in the absence of *situs inversus*, accurate numbers are not available. An added complication is the lack of a central registry for patients with PCD, though efforts are underway with a patient support group to establish such a registry.

Another dimension is the possibility of variant ("nonclassic") forms of PCD, manifested by a milder or intermediate phenotype, intermediate (or no) changes in ciliary ultrastructure, and with less severe functional derangements in ciliary beat. These patients may have "milder" mutations in genes associated with subtle defects in ciliary structure/function, but still be able to mount a partially effective MCC defense mechanism, in a manner analogous to the scenario that has emerged over the past decade with CF. Identification of the genetic mutations associated with "classic" PCD will enable further study of individuals suspected of having disease related to abnormal ciliary structure and function. For example, splice mutations on one allele might lead to partial protein function conferring a milder (than "classic") phenotype on that individual. Studies of the level of expression of mRNA from known mutated genes (e.g., splice mutations), performed using methodologies already tested in atypical CF (using e.g., nasal epithelial scrape samples), will likely offer the opportunity to expand such hypotheses and studies to other genes.

STRATEGIES FOR IDENTIFYING ASSOCIATED MUTATIONS Genome-wide linkage analysis is one approach to identify candidate loci putatively involved in PCD. This approach requires access to large numbers of families to yield meaningful data, and involves collection of sufficient numbers of DNA samples from affected patients and family members for significant results. More importantly, genetic heterogeneity presents a major challenge, because multiple genes are likely to be involved. For example, in a large study published in 2000, 61 families from Europe and North America were reviewed, and despite sophisticated analyses and biostatistics using 31 multiplex families (169 individuals, including 70 affected with PCD), no major locus for disease was found, although several potential loci on different chromosomes were described. However, the two genes identified as disease causing in PCD (*DNAI1* and *DNAH5*; *see* below) were not identified using this approach.

An alternate way to address the problem of genetic heterogeneity is to subgroup the patients into categories based on the ciliary ultrastructural defect. The categories would include clear-cut DA defects: specifically, in individual patients with an ODA defect alone, an IDA defect alone, either DA defective, or finally those with less common central pair/radial spoke defects. As indicated, this approach relies on high-quality electron microscopic images and rigorous analysis of adequate ciliary samples (ideally with more than one observer, at least one of whom is blinded to the identity of the subject), followed by careful segregation of multiple patients into categories depending on the ciliary ultrastructural defect. Once patients have been categorized as such, genetic testing can be targeted using a stepwise approach: those with ODA defects being tested (using genomic DNA) for known mutations in ODA genes (e.g., *DNAI1* and *DNAH5*), those with IDA defects for IDA mutations (e.g., *DNAH7*, *DPCD*), and other genes as the field advances and other candidate genes become known. If a genetic mutation is detected on one allele, full gene sequencing can be conducted to search for the novel mutation on the opposite allele. This strategy was successfully used to isolate mutations in *DNAI1* and *DNAH5*, which have now been established as disease-causing in PCD (*see* below). To "include" or "exclude" families of interest, testing for patterns of inheritability using intragenic polymorphisms may also be useful if parental/sibling DNA is available. If the mutation is not discovered in these initial tests, other techniques could be used, such as reverse transcription (RT)-PCR to check for the possible splice defects, or Southern blot analysis to check for the possible large rearrangements.

GENES TESTED TO BE DISEASE-CAUSING Two genes have been identified as causing PCD—*DNAI1* (an IC) and *DNAH5* (a heavy-chain dynein), both associated with defective ODA (http://www.gentest.org). Other genes have been tested in variable numbers of patients, and disease-causing mutations have not been found in patients with PCD, for example, *DNAH7*, *DNAH9*, *DNA12*, *LC8*, *hp28*, *LC4*, *SPAG6*, *hPF20*, *TCTEX2*, *HFH4/FoxJ1*, *DPCD*, and *POLL* (Table 26-1).

A defined mutation as the molecular basis for PCD was first reported in 1999. *DNAI1* (homologous to the *Chlamydomonas* IC IC78) gene was cloned as a candidate gene because it was found to be disrupted in an ODA-deficient mutant of *Chlamydomonas*. *DNAI1* (a 20 exon gene located on 9p13-p2) was tested in patients with defective ODA, and loss-of-function mutations were reported in one individual with PCD. One mutation was a 4-bp insertion in exon 5 (285′286insAATA), the other was a splice mutation in intron 1 (219 + 3insT now known as IVS1 + 2_3insT); both mutations result in a premature termination signal. Further reports of mutations in *DNAI1* in patients with PCD and ODA defects followed. Twelve mutant alleles of *DNAI1* have been found from six families tested, of which six mutant alleles harbored the "original" 219 + insT mutations. Two novel mutations were found in the same codon (568) in two other families. One was a missense mutation (W568S) and the other was a nonsense mutation (W568X). In the remaining families, all three carried the 219 + insT mutation on one allele, with novel mutations (G515S and a 12-bp deletion from codons 553 to 556) found on the opposite allele. Further genetic studies of *DNAI1* and PCD are ongoing at many centers. Other candidate genes have also been cloned by the group who cloned *DNAI1*, *DNAI2* (orthologous to *IC69* in *Chlamydomonas*), and *Hpf20* (orthologous to *pf20* in *Chlamydomonas*).

DNAH5 is another candidate gene located on chromosome 5p14-p15, which was cloned by a homozgygosity mapping strategy. This gene encodes a protein highly similar to *Chlamydomonas* γ-dynein heavy chain. Mutations in this gene have been identified in 8 patients from 25 tested families with PCD and ODA defects. One consanguineous family from the United States was homozygous for a splice site mutation in *DNAH5* (IVS74→−1G > C), which presumably leads to an inframe deletion of exon 75. This family with the splice mutation is of particular interest because it raises the possibility of measuring levels of gene expression in affected and unaffected (carrier) individuals, as compared with noncarriers. Homozygous disruption of the mouse *DNAH5* gene led to a PCD-like phenotype, and this mouse model may be useful to decipher the biochemical interaction of the *DNAH5* gene with other ciliary components.

OTHER CANDIDATE GENES Although the following genes have not been specifically associated with clinical expression of PCD, these candidates remain of interest for further investigation. For example, a deletion of DNA polymerase (Poll) was reported to cause a ciliary IDA defect in mice associated with hydrocephalus, *situs inversus*, chronic sinusitis, and male infertility. The mechanism(s) proposed might reflect the absence of the polymerase BRCT motif, which might be necessary for protein–protein interactions and ciliary formation, or transcription of genes necessary for cilia formation. Unexpectedly, work suggests that an alternative candidate gene (Dpcd) in the genomic region around the *Poll* might be the real gene of interest in the

Table 26-1
Candidate Genes for PCD

Ciliary ultrastructure	Chain type/structure	Gene (human)	Homolog	Chromosome (human)	Comments	Reference
ODA defect	Heavy	DNAH5	Chlamy.HC	5p14-p15	Mutations detected in PCD (eight families tested). Mouse KO yield hydrocephalus, *situs inversus*, sinusitis, immotile cilia with ODA defect	Olbrich H, Haffner K, Kispert A, et al., 2002; Ibanez-Tallon I, Gorokhave S, Heintz N, 2002.
		DNAH9 (DNELI)	S. urchin β-HC	17p12	No mutations detected in PCD (two families tested)	Bartoloni L, Blouin JL, Chung E, et al., 2001.
	Intermediate	DNAI1	Chlamy. IC78	9p21-p13	Mutations detected in PCD (six families tested)	Pennarun G, Escudier E, Chapelin C, et al, 1999; Zariwala M, Noone PG, Sannuti A, et al., 2001; Guichard C, Harricane MC, Lafitte JI, et al. 2001.
		DNAI2	Chlamy. IC69	17q25	No mutations detected in PCD (16 families tested)	Pennarun G, Chapelin C, Escudier E, et al., 2000; Bartoloni L, Mitchison H, Pazour G, et al., 2000. Benashski SE, Patel-King RS, King SM. 1999.
	Light	Seq. not available	Chlamy. LC1	Not available	The only light chain associated with motor domain of γ-HC. Not tested in PCD patients	Benashski SE, Patel-King RS, King SM. 1999.
		DNLC2A	Chlamy. LC2?	20q11.22	Not tested in PCD patients.	Benashski SE, Patel-King RS, King SM. 1999.
		DNAL4	Chlamy. LC4?	22q13.1	No mutation detected in 54 unrelated PCD patients	Gehrig C, Albrecht C, Duriaus-Sail G, et al., 2002.
		TCTE3 (TCTEX2)	Murine Tcte3 (Tctex2)	6q25-q27	No mutation detected in 36 PCD families	Neesen J, Dreckhahn JD, Tiede S, et al., 2002.
IDA defect	Heavy	DNAH3	Chlamy. HC	16p12	Sequence variant of unknown significance detected in PCD (six patients tested)	Blouin JL, Gehrig C, Jeganathan D, et al., 2001.
		DNAH7	Chlamy. HC	2q31-q33.2	No mutation detected in PCD (one patient tested)	Zhang YJ, O'Neal WK, Randell SH, et al., 2002.
	Intermediate	Seq. not available	Chlamy. IC140	Not available	IC140 is required for the assembly and docking of I1 complex to the doublet microtubule cargo	Perrone CA, Tritschler D, Taulman P, Bower R, Yoder BK, Porter ME., 2003.
		Seq. not available	Chlamy. IC138	Not available	Critical phosphoprotein required for the regulation of flagellar motility	Habermacher G, Sale WS., 1996.
	Light	hp28	Chlamy.LC p28	1p35.1	No mutation detected in 65 PCD families (four from UNC)	Gehrig C, Albrecht C, Duriaus-Sail G, et al., 2002. Pennarun G, Bridoux AM, Escudier E, Anselem S, Duriez B., 2001.
		TCTEL1	Chlamy. Tctex1	6p25.2-p25.3	Flagellar inner arm I1 dynein; attaches cargoes to dynein motor	DiBella LM, Benashski SE, Tedford HW, Harrison A, Patel-King RS, King SM., 2001.
Others		DPCD	Murine Dpcd	10q23	This gene resides in a close proximity of DNA POLL. No mutation detected in 51 PCD families	Zariwala M, O'Neal WK, Noone PG, Leigh MW, Knowles MR, Ostrowski LE., 2004.

		Gene	Homolog	Locus	Description	Reference
Both DAs defects	Heavy	DNAH3	Chlamy.HC	16p12	IDA protein, locus linked in PCD patients with ODA defect	Jeganathan D, Meeks M, Gehrig C, et al., 2001.
	Light	LC8	Chlamy.LC8	17q	Associates with ICs Chlamydomonas ODA, and also associates with IDA. No mutation detected in 58 PCD families	Bartoloni L, Mitchison H, Pazour G, et al., 2000. Benashski SE, Patel-King RS, King SM., 1999.
Other defects (normal DAs)	Heavy	DNAH1	Murine MDHC7	3p21.3	KO of this IDA dynein in mice yield reduced CBF; but no abnormal ultrastructure	Neesen J, Kirschner R, Ochs M, et al., 2001.
		DNAH11	Murine lrd, S. urchin β-HC	7p	One homozygous mutation in motor domain in PCD patient with 7 UPD	Bartoloni L, Blouin JL, Pan Y, et al., 2002.
	Radial spoke	RSHL1	Chlamy. RSP4 and RSP6, S. urchin p63	19q13.3	RSP 4 and RSP 6 make up a radial spoke head and important for regulation of DA activity and flagellar beating	Eriksson M, Ansved T, Anvret M, Carey N., 2001.
		RSP3 (AKAP)	Chlamy.RSP30	6q25.3	Located near the inner arm dynein, regulates flagellar motility	Gaillard AR, Diener DR, Rosenbaum JL, Sale WS., 2001
	Central apparatus genes	hPF20	Chlamy.PF20	2q34	No mutation detected in five PCD families	Pennarun G, Bridoux AM, Escudier E, et al., 2002.
		SPAG6	PF16	10p12.2	No mutation detected in 54 PCD patients	Blouin JL, Albrecht C, Gehrig C, et al., 2003.
		Seq. Not available	Chlamy.PF15, KLP1	Not available	Chlamydomonas mutants lacking central apparatus have paralyzed flagella; central apparatus important for motility	Smith EF, Lefebvre PA., 1997.
	Cilia absent	HFH4/FoxJ1	Mouse	17q22-q25	KO mice yield situs inversus and absence of cilia	Brody SL, Yan XH, Wuerffel MK, Song S, Shapiro S., 2000.
			Hfh4/FoxJ1		No mutation detected in eight PCD families	Maiti AK, Bartoloni L, Mitchison HM, et al., 2000.

clinical expression of a PCD phenotype. Moreover, subsequent studies have shown that another *Poll* knockout mouse (which did not knockout D*pcd*) did not exhibit a PCD phenotype. Supporting its relationship with ciliary function is the observation of increasing expression of DPCD during ciliogenesis. Although no mutations have been discovered in 51 unrelated PCD patients, *DPCD* remains a good candidate gene for patients with an IDA defect, especially in relation to splicing mutants, which have not been tested.

A human inner arm dynein-heavy chain (*DNAH7*; 12 kb in coding sequence) has also been cloned, using a proteomics approach. The entire coding region of *DNAH7* has been sequenced from overlapping segments of RT-PCR products from airway epithelial RNA from a PCD patient with missing IDA, and no disease-causing mutations have been identified. However, intragenic polymorphisms have been detected and are being used for further analysis.

Finally, a splice mutation in the gene encoding *p28*, a light chain of the IDA of *Chlamydomonas* axonemes, results in absent IDAs. No mutations in the human homologue (*hp28*) have been found to be associated with clinical PCD. Table 26-1 lists other candidate genes of interest with the associated references.

CONCLUSION

PCD is associated with significant morbidity from birth to adulthood. An increased understanding of the molecular pathophysiology of the structural and functional abnormalities in PCD will undoubtedly lead to an increased understanding of normal and abnormal physiology in the sinopulmonary and reproductive tracts. It will also lead to easier diagnosis through genetic testing, as well as open possibilities for targeted, novel treatments for PCD and other similar diseases. Identification of the genetic basis of "classic" PCD will also make it possible to identify less severe molecular abnormalities leading to milder disease phenotypes ("nonclassic" disease), and exploration of the hypothesis that less severe defects in cilia structure and function contribute to other airway and lung diseases. Recent exciting developments, to increase awareness of PCD from both a clinical and a research standpoint, include the formation of a patient advocacy and support group (www.pcdfoundation.org), and an NIH-funded consortium (http://rarediseasenetwork. epi.usf.edu/gdmcc/index.htm) of clinical research centers. This will allow large-scale efforts to increase the numbers of patients to receive an expert diagnostic workup (including research and genetic studies), as well as receive continuing care for their disease. Finally, therapeutic approaches will likely evolve to increase MCC in these patients with potentially conserved or "partially conserved" ciliary function.

ACKNOWLEDGMENTS

Elizabeth Godwin for editorial assistance, and the technical assistance of Susan Minnix RN and Rhonda Pace BS, and grants from the NIH (HL04225, HL34322, and RR00046).

SELECTED REFERENCES

Afzelius BA. A human syndrome caused by immotile cilia. Science 1976;193:317–319.

Afzelius BA. Electron microscopy of the sperm tail. J Biophys Biochem Cytol 1959;5:805–834.

Afzelius BA. Cilia-related diseases. J Pathol 2004;204:470–477.

Bartoloni L, Blouin JL, Pan Y, et al. Mutations in the DNAH11 (axonemal heavy chain dynein type 11) gene cause one form of situs inversus totalis and most likely primary ciliary dyskinesia. Proc Natl Acad Sci USA 2002;99(16):10,282–10,286.

Bartoloni L, Blouin JL, Chung E, et al. Axonemal beta heavy chain dynein DNAH9: cDNA sequence, genomic structure and investigation in its role in primary ciliary dyskinesia. Genomics 2001;72:21–33.

Bartoloni L, Mitchison H, Pazour G, et al. No deleterious mutations were found in three genes (HF4, LC8, IC2) on human chromosome 17q in patients with primary ciliary dyskinesia (abstract). Eur J Hum Genet 2000;8:484.

Benashski SE, Patel-King RS, King SM. Light chain 1 from the Chlamydomonas outer dynein arm is leucine rich repeat protein associated with the motor domain of the gamma heavy chain. Biochemistry 1999;38:7253–7264.

Bertocci B, De Smet A, Flatter E, et al. DNA polymerases mu and lambda are dispensable for IgG gene hypermutation. J Immunol 2002;168: 3702–3706.

Blouin JL, Albrecht C, Gehrig C, et al. Primary ciliary dyskinesia (Kartagener's syndrome): searching for genes in a highly heterogeneous disorder (abstract). Am J Hum Genet 2003;73(Suppl):2440.

Blouin JL, Gehrig C, Jeganathan D, et al. DNAH3: characterization of the full length gene and mutation search in patients with primary ciliary dyskinesia (abstract). Am J Hum Genet 2001;69:1081.

Blouin JL, Meeks M, Radhakrishna U, et al. Primary ciliary dyskinesia: a genome wide linkage analysis reveals extensive locus heterogeneity. Eur J Hum Genet 2003;8:109–118.

Boucher RC. Human airway ion transport (Pt 1). Am J Respir Crit Care Med 1994;150:271–281.

Boucher RC. Human airway ion transport (Pt 2). Am J Respir Crit Care Med 1994;150:581–593.

Bowman AB, Patel-King RS, Benashski SE, McCaffery JMl, Goldstein JS, King SM. Drosophila roadblock and Chlamydomonas LC7: a conserved family of dynein associated proteins involved in axonal transport, flagellar motility, and mitosis. J Cell Biol 1999;146: 165–180.

Braiman A, Ulzaner N, Priel Z. Enhancement of ciliary beat frequency is dominantly controlled by PKG and or PKA. In: Salathe M, Adler KB, Boucher RC, Satir P, eds. Cilia and Mucus: From Development to Respiratory Defense. New York: Marcell Dekker, 2001; pp. 67–80.

Brody SL, Yan XH, Wuerffel MK, Song S, Shapiro S. Ciliogenesis and left right axis defects in forkhead factor HFH-4 null mice. Am J Respir Cell Mol Biol 2000;23:45–51.

Brueckner M. Cilia propel the embryo in the right direction. Am J Med Genet 2001;101(4):339–344.

Bush A, Cole P, Hariri M, et al. Primary ciliary dyskinesia: diagnosis and standards of care. Eur Respir J 1998;12(4):982–988.

Camner P, Mossberg B, Afzelius BA. Evidence for congenitally nonfunctioning cilia in the tracheobronchial tract in two subjects. Am Rev Respir Dis 1975;112:807–809.

Camner P, Mossberg B, Afzelius BA. Measurements of tracheobronchial clearance in patients with immotile cilia syndrome and its value in differential diagnosis. Eur J Respir Dis 1983;64(Suppl 127):57–63.

Carson JL, Collier AM. Ciliary defects: cell biology and clinical perspectives. Adv Pediatr 1988;35:139–166.

Chilvers MA, Rutman A, O'Callaghan C. Ciliary beat pattern is associated with specific ultrastructural defects in primary ciliary dyskinesia. J Allergy Clin Immunol 2003;112(3):518–524.

Coren ME, Meeks M, Morrison I, Buchdahl RM, Bush A. Primary ciliary dyskinesia: age at diagnosis and symptom history. Acta Paediatr 2002;91(6):667–669.

Corey M, Edwards L, Levison H, Knowles M. Longitudinal analysis of pulmonary function decline in patients with cystic fibrosis. J Pediatr 1997;131:809–814.

Davis ME, Cai H, Drummond GR, Harrison DG. Shear stress regulates endothelial nitric oxide synthase expression through c-Src by divergent signaling pathways. Circ Res 2001;89(11):1073–1080.

DiBella LM, Benashski SE, Tedford HW, Harrison A, Patel-King RS, King SM. The Tctex1/Tctex2 class of dynein light chains: dimerization, differential expression, and interaction with the LC8 protein family. J Biol Chem 2001;276(17):14,366–14,373.

DiBella LM, King SM. Dynein motors of the Chlamydomonas flagellum. Int Rev Cytol 2001;210:227–268.

de Iongh RU, Rutland J. Ciliary defects in healthy subjects, bronchiectasis, and primary ciliary dyskinesia. Am J Respir Crit Care Med 1995;151(5):1559–1567.

Eliasson R, Mossberg B, Camner P, Afzelius BA. The immotile cilia syndrome: a congenital ciliary abnormality as an etiologic factor in chronic airways infection and male sterility. N Engl J Med 1977;297:1–6.

Ellerman A, Bisgaard H. Longitudinal study of lung function in a cohort of primary ciliary dyskinesia. Eur Respir J 1997;10(10):2376–2379.

El Zein L, Omran H, Bouvagnet P. Lateralization defects and ciliary dyskinesia: lessons from algae. Trends Genet 2003;19(3):162–167.

Eriksson M, Ansved T, Anvret M, Carey N. A mammalian radial spoke-head-like gene, RSHL1, at the myotonic dystrophy-1 locus. Biochem Biophys Res Commun 2001;281(4):835–841.

Escudier E, Couprie M, Duriez B, et al. Computer-assisted analysis helps detect inner dynein arm abnormalities. Am J Respir Crit Care Med 2002;166(9):1257–1262.

Fisher AB, Chien S, Barakat AI, Nerem RM. Endothelial cellular response to altered shear stress. Am J Physiol Lung Cell Mol Physiol 2001;281(3):L529–L533.

Gaillard AR, Diener DR, Rosenbaum JL, Sale WS. Flagellar radial spoke protein 3 is an A-kinase anchoring protein (AKAP). J Cell Biol 2001;153(2):443–448.

Gaston B, Drazen JM, Loscalzo J, Stamler JS. The biology of nitrogen oxides in the airways. Am J Respir Crit Care Med 1994;149(2 Pt 1):538–551.

Gehrig C, Albrecht C, Duriaus-Sail G, et al. Primary ciliary dyskinesia: Mutation analysis in dynein light chain genes mapping to chromosome 1 (HP28) and 22 (DNAL4). Paper presented at: European Human Genetics Conference 2002; May 25–28, 2002; Strasbourg, France.

Geremek M, Witt M. Primary ciliary dyskinesia: genes, candidate genes and chromosomal regions. J Appl Genet 2004;45:347–361.

Greenstone M, Rutman A, Dewar A, Mackay I, Cole PJ. Primary ciliary dyskinesia: cytological and clinical features. Q J Med 1988;67:405–430.

Guichard C, Harricane MC, Lafitte JJ, et al. Axonemal dynein intermediate-chain gene (DNAI1) mutations result in situs inversus and primary ciliary dyskinesia (Kartagener syndrome). Am J Hum Genet 2001;68(4):1030–1035.

Habermacher G, Sale WS. Regulation of flagellar dynein by an axonemal type-1 phosphatase in Chlamydomonas. J Cell Sci 1996; 109(Pt 7):1899–1907.

Hadfield PJ, Rowe-Jones JM, Bush A, Mackay IS. Treatment of otitis media with effusion in children with primary ciliary dyskinesia. Clin Otolaryngol 1997;22:302–306.

Halbert SA, Patton DL, Zarutskie PW, Soules MR. Function and structure of cilia in the fallopian tube of an infertile woman with Kartagener's syndrome. Hum Reprod 1997;12(1):55–58.

Holzmann D, Felix H. Neonatal respiratory distress syndrome—a sign of primary ciliary dyskinesia? Eur J Pediatr 2000;159(11):857–860.

Ibanez-Tallon I, Gorokhave S, Heintz N. Loss of function of axonemal dynein Mdnah5 causes primary ciliary dyskinesia and hydrocephalus. Hum Mol Genet 2002;11:715–721.

Jeganathan D, Meeks M, Gehrig C, et al. A genome wide scan reveals a putative novel locus for primary ciliary dyskinesia (abstract). Am J Hum Genet 2001;69:2015.

Kartagener M, Stucki P. Bronchiectasis with situs inversus. Arch Pediatr 1962;79:193–207.

Katsuhara K, Kawamoto S, Wakabayashi T, Belsky JL. Situs inversus totalis and Kartagener's syndrome in a Japanese population. Chest 1972;61:56–61.

Kispert A, Petry M, Olbrich H, et al. Genotype-phenotype correlations in PCD patients carrying DNAH5 mutations. Thorax 2003;58:552–554.

Knowles MR, Boucher RC. Mucus clearance as a primary innate defense mechanism for mammalian airways. J Clin Invest 2002;109:571–577.

Knowles MR, Durie PR. What is cystic fibrosis? N Engl J Med 2002;347(6):439–442.

Knowles MR, Friedman KJ, Silverman LM. Genetics, diagnosis and clinical phenotype. In: Yankaskas JR, Knowles MR, eds. Cystic Fibrosis in Adults. Philadelphia, PA: Lippincott-Raven, 1999:27–42.

Kobayashi Y, Watanabe M, Okada Y, et al. Hydrocephalus, situs inversus, chronic sinusitis, and male infertility in DNA polymerase lambda-deficient mice: possible implication for the pathogenesis of immotile cilia syndrome. Mol Cell Biol 2002;22(8):2769–2776.

LeDizet M, Piperno G. ida4-1, ida4-2, and ida4-3 are intron splicing mutations affecting the locus encoding p28, a light chain of Chlamydomonas axonemal inner dynein arms. Mol Biol Cell 1995;6(6):713–723.

Olbrich H, Haffner K, Kispert A, et al. Mutations in DNAH5 cause primary ciliary dyskinesia and randomization of left/right asymmetry. Nat Genet 2002;30(2):143, 144.

Maiti AK, Bartoloni L, Mitchison HM, et al. No deleterious mutations in the FOXJ1 (alias HFH-4) gene in patients with primary ciliary dyskinesia (PCD). Cytogenet Cell Genet 2000;90(1–2):119–122.

LeDizet M, Piperno G. The light chain p28 associates with a subset of inner dynein arm heavy chains in Chlamydomonas axonemes. Mol Biol Cell 1995;6(6):697–711.

McGrath J, Somlo S, Makova S, Tian X, Brueckner M. Two populations of node monocilia initiate left-right asymmetry in the mouse. Cell 2003;11:61–73.

McManus I, Mitchison H, Chung E, Stubbings G, Martin N. Primary ciliary dyskinesia (Siewert's/Kartagener's syndrome): respiratory symptoms and psycho-social impact. BioMed Central Pulmonary Medicine (serial online). November 27, 2003;3.

Meeks M, Bush A. Primary ciliary dyskinesia (PCD). Pediatr Pulmonol 2000;29(4):307–316.

Meeks M, Walne A, Spiden S, et al. A locus for primary ciliary dyskinesia maps to chromosome 19q. J Med Genet 2000;37(4):241–244.

Mickle JE, Cutting GR. Genotype-phenotype relationships in cystic fibrosis. Med Clin North Am 2000;84(3):597–607.

Munro NC, Currie DC, Lindsay KS, et al. Fertility in men with primary ciliary dyskinesia presenting with respiratory infection. Thorax 1994;49:684–687.

Narang I, Ersu R, Wilson NM, Bush A. Nitric oxide in chronic airway inflammation in children: Diagnostic use and pathophysiologic significance. Thorax 2002;57:586–589.

Narayan D, Krishnan SN, Upender M, et al. Unusual inheritance of primary ciliary dyskinesia (Kartagener's syndrome). J Med Genet 1994;31(6):493–496.

Neesen J, Dreckhahn JD, Tiede S, et al. Identification of the human ortholog of the t-complex-encoded protein TCTE3 and evaluation as a candidate gene for primary ciliary dyskinesia. Cytogenet Genome Res 2002;98:38–44.

Neesen J, Kirschner R, Ochs M, et al. Disruption of an inner arm dynein heavy chain gene results in asthenozoospermia and reduced ciliary beat frequency. Hum Mol Genet 2001;10(11):1117–1128.

Noone PG, Bali D, Carson JL, et al. Discordant organ laterality in monozygotic twins with primary ciliary dyskinesia. Am J Med Genet 1999;82(2):155–160.

Noone PG, Bennett WD, Regnis JA, et al. Effect of aerosolized uridine-5′-triphosphate on airway clearance with cough in patients with primary ciliary dyskinesia. Am J Respir Crit Care Med 1999;160(1):144–149.

Noone PG, Leigh MW, Sannuti A, et al. Primary ciliary dyskinesia: diagnostic and phenotypic features. Am J Respir Crit Care Med 2004;169(4):459–467.

Noone PG, Pue CA, Zhou Z, et al. Lung disease associated with the IVS8 5T allele of the CFTR gene. Am J Respir Crit Care Med 2000;162(5):1919–1924.

O'Donnell AE, Barker AE, Ilowite JS, Fick RB. Treatment of idiopathic bronchiectasis with aerosolized recombinant human DNase. Chest 1998;113:1329–1334.

Omoto CK, Gibbons IR, Kamiya R, Shingyoji C, Takahashi K, Witman GB. Rotation of the central pair microtubules in eukaryotic flagella. Mol Biol Cell 1999;10(1):1–4.

Omran H, Haffner K, Volkel A, et al. Homozygosity mapping of a gene locus for primary ciliary dyskinesia on chromosome 5p and identification of the heavy dynein chain DNAH5 as a candidate gene. Am J Respir Cell Mol Biol 2000;23(5):696–702.

Ostrowski LE, Blackburn K, Radde KM, et al. A proteomic analysis of human cilia: Identification of novel components. Mol Cell Proteomics 2002;1(6):451–465.

Pazour GJ, Agrin N, Walker BL, Witman GB. Identification of predicted human outer dynein arm genes: candidates for primary ciliary dyskinesia genes. J Med Genet 2006;43:62–73.

Pennarun G, Bridoux AM, Escudier E, Anselem S, Duriez B. The human HP28 and HFH4 genes: evaluation as candidate genes for primary ciliary dyskinesia. Am J Respir Crit Care Med 2001;163:A538.

Pennarun G, Bridoux AM, Escudier E, et al. Isolation and expression of human hPF20 gene orthologous to Chlamydomonas pf20. Am J Respir Cell Mol Biol 2002;26:362–370.

Pennarun G, Chapelin C, Escudier E, et al. The human dynein intermediate chain 2 gene (DNAI2): cloning mapping expression pattern and evaluation as a candidate for primary ciliary dyskinesia. Hum Genet 2000;107:642–649.

Pennarun G, Escudier E, Chapelin C, et al. Loss-of-function mutations in a human gene related to Chlamydomonas reinhardtii dynein IC78 result in primary ciliary dyskinesia. Am J Hum Genet 1999; 65(6): 1508–1519.

Perrone CA, Tritschler D, Taulman P, Bower R, Yoder BK, Porter ME. A novel dynein light intermediate chain colocalizes with the retrograde motor for intraflagellar transport at sites of axoneme assembly in chlamydomonas and mammalian cells. Mol Biol Cell 2003; 14(5): 2041–2056.

Piperno G, Mead K. Transport of a novel complex in the cytoplasmic matrix of Chlamydomonas flagella. Proc Natl Acad Sci USA 1997; 94(9):4457–4462.

Piperno G, Mead K, Henderson S. Inner dynein arms but not outer dynein arms require the activity of kinesin homologue protein KHP1(FLA10) to reach the distal part of flagella in Chlamydomonas. J Cell Biol 1996;133(2):371–379.

Razani B, Engelman JA, Wang XB, et al. Caveolin-1 null mice are viable but show evidence of hyperproliferative and vascular abnormalities. J Biol Chem 2001;276(41):38,121–38,138.

Regnis JA, Zeman KL, Noone PG, Knowles MR, Bennett WD. Prolonged airway retention of insoluble particles in cystic fibrosis versus primary ciliary dyskinesia. Exp Lung Res 2000;26(3):149–162.

Rossman CM, Forrest JB, Ruffin RE, Newhouse MT. Immotile cilia syndrome in persons with and without Kartagener's syndrome. Am Rev Respir Dis 1980;121:1011–1016.

Rossman CM, Lee RM, Forrest JB, Newhouse MT. Nasal ciliary ultrastructure and function in patients with primary ciliary dyskinesia compared with that in normal subjects and in subjects with various respiratory diseases. Am Rev Respir Dis 1984;129(1):161–167.

Rutland J, De Iong RU. Random ciliary orientation. N Engl J Med 1990;323:1681–1684.

Ruusa J, Svartengren M, Philipson K, Camner P. Tracheobronchial particle deposition and clearance in immotile cilia syndrome patients. J Aerosol Med 1993;6:89–98.

Sanderson MJ, Lansley AB, Evans JH. The regulation of airway ciliary beat frequency by intracellular calcium. In: Salathe M, Adler KB, Boucher RC, Satir P, eds. Cilia and Mucus: From Development to Respiratory Defense. New York: Marcel Dekker, 2001: pp. 39–58.

Sannuti A, Noone PG, Daines C, et al. Quantification of inner and outer dynein arms in primary ciliary dyskinesia (PCD). Am J Respir Crit Care Med 1999;159:A39.

Satir P. The cilium as a biological nanomachine. FASEB J 1999;13(Suppl 2):S235–S237.

Sisson JH, Carson JL. Bench to bedside: new findings in primary ciliary dyskinesia. Pulmonary and Critical Care Update [serial online] 2003;17:lesson 5. Available at www.chestnet.org/education/online/pccu/vol17/lessons5_6/index.php.

Smith EF, Lefebvre PA. The role of central apparatus components in flagellar motility and microtubule assembly. Cell Motil Cytoskeleton 1997;38(1):1–8.

Smith EF, Sale WS. Structural and functional reconstitution of inner dynein arms in Chlamydomonas flagellar axonemes. J Cell Biol 1992;117:573–581.

Stannard W, Rutman A, Walne A, O'Callaghan C. Central microtubular agenesis causing primary ciliary dyskinesia. Am J Respir Crit Care Med 2004;169:634–637.

Sturgess JM, Chao J, Turner JAP. Transposition of ciliary microtubules: Another cause of impaired motility. N Engl J Med 1980;303:318–322.

Sturgess JM, Chao J, Wong J, Aspin N, Turner JAP. Cilia with defective radial spokes: A cause of human respiratory disease. N Engl J Med 1979;300:53–56.

Supp DM, Witte DP, Potter SS, Brueckner M. Mutation of an axonemal dynein affects left-right asymmetry in inversus viscerum mice. Nature 1997;389:963–966.

Thai CH, Gambling TM, Carson JL. Freeze fracture study of airway epithelium from patients with primary ciliary dsykinesia. Thorax 2002;57:363–365.

Torgersen J. Situs inversus, asymmetry, and twinning. Am J Hum Genet 1950;2:361–370.

van der Baan S, Veerman AJ, Wulffraat N, Bezemer PD, Feenstra L. Primary ciliary dyskinesia: ciliary activity. Acta Otolaryngol 1986; 102(3–4):274–281.

Wanner A, Salathe M, O'Riordan TG. Mucociliary clearance in the airways: state of the art. Am J Respir Crit Care Med 1996;154:1868–1902.

Wills PJ, Wodehouse T, Corkery K, Mallon K, Wilson R, Cole PJ. Short term recombinant human DNase in bronchiectasis: effect on clinical state and in vitro sputum transportability. Am J Respir Crit Care Med 1996;154:413–417.

Witt M, Wang Y-F, Wang S, et al. Exclusion of chromosome 7 for Kartagener Syndrome but suggestion of linkage in families with other forms of primary ciliary dyskinesia. Am J Med Genet 1999; 64:313–318.

Wu H, Maciejewski MW, Marintchev A, Benashski SE, Mullen GP, King SM. Solution structure of a dynein motor domain associated light chain. Nat Struct Biol 2000;7:575–579.

Xue C, Botkin SJ, Johns RA. Localization of endothelial NOS at the basal microtubule membrane in ciliated epithelium of rat lung. J Histochem Cytochem 1996;44(5):463–471.

Zariwala M, O'Neal WK, Noone PG, Leigh MW, Knowles MR, Ostrowski LE. Investigation of the possible role of a novel gene, DPCD, in primary ciliary dykinesia. Am J Respir Cell Mol Biol 2004;30:1–7.

Zariwala M, Noone PG, Sannuti A, et al. Germline mutations in an intermediate chain dynein cause primary ciliary dyskinesia. Am J Respir Cell Mol Biol 2001;25(5):577–583.

Zhang YJ, O'Neal WK, Randell SH, et al. Identification of dynein heavy chain 7 as an inner arm component of human cilia that is synthesized but not assembled in a case of primary ciliary dyskinesia. J Biol Chem 2002;277(20):17,906–17,915.

27 Cystic Fibrosis

SCOTT H. DONALDSON AND RICHARD C. BOUCHER

SUMMARY

Cystic fibrosis is a genetic disease that affects multiple organ systems, yet leads to respiratory failure and premature death in most afflicted patients. Rapid advancements in our understanding of disease pathogenesis have occurred because of the cloning of the cystic fibrosis transmembrane conductance regulator gene. Recent work has shown that volume depletion of the periciliary fluid layer and mucus dehydration reduces mucus clearance and promotes the initiation and progression of CF lung disease. Therapies that correct dysregulated salt and water transport in the lung, either by correcting or bypassing the basic cystic fibrosis transmembrane conductance regulator defect, are now being developed and hold great promise.

Key Words: Airway surface liquid; bronchiectasis; Cftr; cystic; ENaC; fibrosis; ion transport; mucus clearance; mucociliary; *Pseudomonas*.

INTRODUCTION

In 1938, Anderson et al. first described "cystic fibrosis of the pancreas" as a distinct clinical entity. At that time, malnutrition resulting from insufficiency of the exocrine pancreas and overwhelming respiratory infection typically led to death within the first year of life. Subsequent observations began to lay the framework on which the understanding of the cystic fibrosis (CF) disease process has been built. Initially, it was recognized that multiple epithelial lined organs contained abnormally viscous mucus, whereas sweat from CF patients contained excessive amounts of salt. In the 1980s, multiple investigators described the altered epithelial ion transport processes that are characteristic of CF airways epithelia, raising the possibility that these abnormalities were fundamental to CF disease pathogenesis. Finally, the *cystic fibrosis transmembrane conductance regulator (CFTR)* gene was cloned in 1989 and was found to encode a cAMP-regulated plasma membrane polypeptide. From these seminal observations, our understanding of the CF disease process has evolved, although considerable controversy and competing hypotheses about aspects of the disease persist. As a result of this ongoing progress, clinical outcomes have continued to improve and novel therapies are being developed at an unprecedented rate. The predicted survival of patients with CF has increased to 34 yr of age, although further improvement in survival may require the development of new therapeutics. This chapter outlines the clinical

From: *Principles of Molecular Medicine, Second Edition*
Edited by: M. S. Runge and C. Patterson © Humana Press, Inc., Totowa, NJ

CF phenotype, describes the pathogenesis of CF lung disease, and suggests how new therapies may utilize the growing knowledge of CF pathogenesis to delay or prevent the development of this devastating disease.

CLINICAL DESCRIPTION OF A MULTISYSTEM DISEASE

Pulmonary disease accounts for considerable morbidity and greater than 90% of the mortality from CF. However, a broad spectrum of clinical manifestations is encountered in CF, stemming from epithelial dysfunction in multiple organ systems. The spectrum of disease manifestations greatly increases the complexity of care required by this population, mandating the establishment of specialized CF care centers in which accumulated expertise and experience has improved patient outcomes.

RESPIRATORY MANIFESTATIONS Newborns with CF have normal lung function and sterile, uninflamed airways. Early in life, however, persistent airway infection and inflammation develop as the result of impaired airway host defenses. The nature of this host defense deficit has been intensively studied and debated and is discussed later. CF lung disease progresses from subclinical infection and inflammation to overt symptoms (episodic or persistent cough, sputum) and airway obstruction (demonstrated by spirometry) in a highly variable fashion, but the disease process is usually evident during childhood. Overtime, periods of clinical worsening termed "exacerbations" can be identified, which require intensification of secretion clearance and antibiotic therapy aimed at the patient's airway microbial flora. Progressive lung destruction results from the relentless infectious/inflammatory process that is characteristic of CF airways, culminating in the pathological finding of bronchiectasis, obstructive lung disease, and ultimately respiratory failure and death in the majority of patients.

CF lung infections are caused by a typical group of pathogens. Early in life, viral infections are normal in frequency but may cause significantly more morbidity and may trigger the onset of persistent airway inflammation. *Haemophilus influenzae* is frequently encountered during childhood but rarely persists. *Staphylococcus aureus* and *Pseudomonas aeruginosa*, however, often occur early in life and generally persist, especially *P. aeruginosa*. Although these pathogens are also found in other clinical settings, and certainly in other causes of bronchiectasis, the frequency of *Pseudomonas* infection (80% of adults) and tendency to convert to the mucoid phenotype is particularly striking and suggests that the CF airway provides a unique environmental niche that favors this organism.

Similarly, the inability to clear *Pseudomonas* from the CF airway, despite the aggressive use of antibiotics and an intense host inflammatory response, defines the problem confronted by clinicians who treat CF lung disease. The persistence of *P. aeruginosa* likely reflects adaptation of this organism to the CF airway milieu and the development of bacterial mechanisms that allow evasion of secondary host defenses and therapeutic interventions. A number of other organisms are less commonly encountered in the CF lung, including *Stenotrophomonas maltophilia* and *Alcaligenes xylosoxidans*. Perhaps most notable, however, is the emergence of the *Burkholderia cepacia* complex as a group of pathogens with the capacity to lead to rapid clinical deterioration and frank sepsis ("cepacia syndrome"). Unfortunately, organisms in the *B. cepacia* complex are often resistant to most, if not all, known antibiotics and certain strains have proven to be highly transmissible between patients.

Other respiratory manifestations of CF are also encountered frequently. With increasing age, the incidence of pneumothorax and massive hemoptysis rises. Pneumothoraces (16–20% incidence in adult CF patients) result from the rupture of subpleural cysts. Hemoptysis is common and may occasionally be life-threatening (approx 5% incidence) in CF because the arterial circulation of bronchiectatic airways is often massively hypertrophied and vulnerable to erosion from mucosal ulcerations consequent to persistent intralumenal infection/inflammation. Less life-threatening but common respiratory tract manifestations include allergic bronchopulmonary aspergillosis (1–4% incidence), chronic sinusitis, and nasal polyposis.

EXTRAPULMONARY MANIFESTATIONS   The function of the exocrine pancreas is insufficient at birth or becomes so early in life in the majority of patients. Pancreatic insufficiency in CF results from the obstruction of pancreatic ducts with inspissated secretions and the subsequent autodigestion of pancreatic acinar regions. The inability to secrete pancreatic enzymes results in protein and fat malabsorption, causing steatorrhea. If unaddressed, persistent malabsorption leads to malnutrition, impaired growth, and fat-soluble vitamin deficiencies (vitamins A, D, E, and K). A small number of CFTR mutations are associated with retention of pancreatic sufficiency, however, and these patients typically are better nourished and typically have less severe respiratory phenotypes. Pancreatic sufficient patients are at risk for pancreatitis, however, which likely reflects the presence of residual exocrine tissue and opportunity for acute duct obstruction.

Endocrine pancreatic function is preserved in CF patients at birth, but may also be progressively lost overtime. The development of "cystic fibrosis-related diabetes" is age dependent, with the incidence peaking at 25% in 35–44 yr olds. Many more patients will have episodic hyperglycemia, especially during times of respiratory exacerbation. Of note, unrecognized or poorly controlled diabetes is thought to negatively impact nutrition and lung health and, therefore, must be screened for and managed carefully in these patients. Calorie restriction must be avoided to prevent worsening the patient's nutritional status, and insulin therapy is usually required to treat cystic fibrosis-related diabetes.

The CF intestinal tract epithelium has a limited ability to secrete chloride and water resulting from the absence of CFTR chloride channel function in the apical membrane of enterocytes lining the gut. As a result, patients may manifest both diarrhea from malabsorption and/or severe constipation and intestinal obstruction as the result of insufficient hydration of bulky, poorly digested intestinal contents. When terminal ileum obstruction occurs at birth (17% incidence), the resulting "meconium ileus" is nearly diagnostic of CF. A similar phenomenon occurring later in life is termed the "distal intestinal obstruction syndrome" (20% incidence). Rectal prolapse and gastroesophageal reflux are common in children with CF, and fibrosing colonopathy may occur in any patient treated with very high doses of pancreatic enzymes.

Focal biliary cirrhosis is an extremely common pathological finding in CF at autopsy, but produces clinically apparent disease in less than 5% of CF patients and is the cause of death in approx 2% of CF patients. Unlike many complications of CF, hepatic disease has a peak incidence during adolescence and a decreased prevalence in patients over age 20. Hepatic abnormalities can present as hepatosplenomegaly or as a persistent elevation of hepatic enzymes. Rarely, patients may present with esophageal varices and hemorrhage resulting from portal hypertension. Fatty liver is also common, and may improve with adequate nutrition. Finally, 10–30% of patients have dysfunctional gallbladders or gallstones.

More than 98% of men with CF are infertile because of azoospermia from vas deferens obstruction. The vas deferens may be absent at the time of birth, and its absence serves as a diagnostic clue pointing toward CF in situations of previously undiagnosed bronchiectasis. It appears that the male reproductive tract is the most sensitive organ to CFTR mutations, as a sizeable percentage of infertile men with congenital, bilateral absence of the vas deferens, who have no other demonstrable CF manifestations, have mild *CFTR* mutations. Interestingly, these mutations may be in gene regions that cause abnormal RNA splicing but produce normally functioning, though reduced amounts of CFTR protein. This syndrome explains that although 5% of normal CFTR message levels may be insufficient for male reproductive tract function, it is often sufficient to maintain normal pancreatic and respiratory tract function. This observation has important implications when considering therapies aimed at either delivering a normal *CFTR* gene ("gene therapy") or improving the processing/function of the existing, mutant CFTR protein. Importantly, female patients with CF maintain near normal fertility when factored for nutritional and respiratory status.

PATHOGENESIS OF CF LUNG DISEASE

The requirement to explain how CF lung disease results from *CFTR* gene mutations has spurred a great deal of research and a number of competing hypotheses. Fortunately, a more clear vision of CF disease pathogenesis is emerging as discussed in the following sections.

THE *CFTR* GENE AND PROTEIN   The *CFTR* gene was localized to a region on the long arm of chromosome 7 via positional cloning and consists of 250 kB of genomic DNA containing 27 exons. The *CFTR* gene encodes a 1480 amino acid protein, belonging to the adenosine triphosphate-binding casset family of transport proteins, which is typically targeted to the apical membrane of epithelial cells. The protein can be viewed as having two halves, each made up of six transmembrane domains and a nucleotide-binding domain, which are separated by a highly charged "R domain" containing multiple protein kinase A and protein kinase C phosphorylation sites. Nearly 1300 mutations have been reported, although the ΔF508 mutation accounts for 66% of mutant *CFTR* alleles. Because CF is an autosomal-recessive disorder, patients carry two mutant *CFTR* gene alleles, whereas parents are "carriers" with a normal *CFTR* gene and a single mutant *CFTR* allele and exhibit no clinical stigmata of the CF disease.

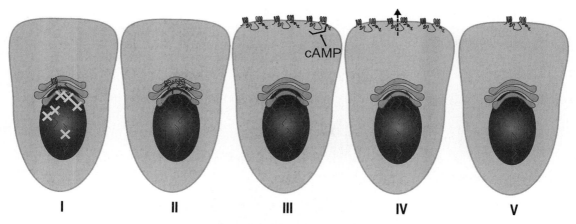

Figure 27-1   CFTR mutation classifications. Class I mutations result in the complete absence of CFTR protein production. Class II mutations cause protein misfolding, impaired cellular processing and retention in the endoplasmic reticulum. Class III mutations yield CFTR molecules that reach the plasma membrane but are resistant to activation by usual (e.g., cAMP) signaling pathways. Class IV mutations result in CFTR channels with reduced ionic conductivity. Class V mutations result in dramatically reduced quantity of normal CFTR protein.

CFTR mutations may be grouped into classes that reflect the mechanism by which loss of CFTR function occurs (Fig. 27-1). Class I mutations, including nonsense (i.e., stop mutation), frameshift and splice junction mutations generally result in the loss of protein production and complete absence of full length CFTR. Class II mutations reflect abnormal protein folding, and hence processing and targeting to the plasma membrane. This class of mutations includes the common ΔF508 mutation, in which misfolding prevents normal maturation and transport to the apical cell membrane. Class III mutations in the *CFTR* gene affect the regulation/activation of a mutant CFTR chloride channel that folds correctly and reaches the plasma membrane. Class IV mutations also reach the plasma membrane, but the mutant CFTR exhibits poor chloride conductance through the channel pore. Finally, class V *CFTR* mutations decrease the abundance of full-length CFTR mRNA and, hence, protein levels, and include mutations in the *CFTR* promoters and regions that influence mRNA splicing. These mutations may, however, permit the production of enough CFTR protein and function to yield a less severe disease phenotype. The concept of mutation classes carries therapeutic implications in that novel therapies are being developed to: (1) produce "read-through" of premature termination mutations (class I mutation; e.g., topical gentamicin); (2) promote movement of ΔF508 CFTR to the plasma membrane in which it may function adequately (class II mutation; e.g., 4-phenylbutyrate); and (3) activate mutant channels that reach the plasma membrane (class III/IV mutations; e.g., genistein).

CFTR AND EPITHELIAL TRANSPORT   Even prior to the cloning of the *CFTR* gene, it was recognized that a cAMP-stimulated chloride conductance was deficient in CF epithelia. Expression of the cloned *CFTR* gene in various heterologous systems demonstrated that *CFTR* itself encoded this missing chloride channel. Further, as the name implies, CFTR regulates other epithelial functions/ion channels, most notably the epithelial sodium channel (ENaC). Through a poorly defined mechanism, normal CFTR in airway epithelia provides a tonic inhibition of ENaC activity. In CF, therefore, ENaC activity is dysregulated and sodium hyperabsorption represents the dominant basal ion transport activity measured in many experimental systems, including the human nasal epithelium in vivo. CFTR may also regulate the

activity of calcium-activated chloride channels (CACC), as the activities of CACC and CFTR are reciprocally related in many epithelia.

A number of hypotheses have attempted to explain the development of CF lung disease via mechanisms that do not require CFTR channel function, including: (1) increased binding of *Pseudomonas* to CF airway surfaces resulting from observed alterations in glycosylation of membrane and/or secreted proteins; (2) persistent airway infection resulting from loss of CFTR-mediated epithelial phagocytosis of pseudomonas; and (3) intrinsic hyperinflammation of CF airways via an unexplained mechanism. Each of these hypotheses is not widely accepted resulting from conflicting experimental observations and the possibility that they may represent a secondary phenomena resulting from chronic airway infection/inflammation. More generally accepted are hypotheses that directly link CFTR malfunction to altered ion transport processes.

AIRWAY SURFACE LIQUID REGULATION IN NORMAL AND CF AIRWAYS   The liquid bathing airway surface is composed of two components, a periciliary gel (PGL) layer and a more viscous mucus layer that is positioned between the PGL and the airway lumen. This configuration allows the mucus layer to efficiently trap inhaled pathogens and particulates. The underlying PGL layer provides a physical environment in which cilia can beat freely and, thus, propel the mucus layer toward the mouth. The PGL also acts as a lubricant layer that prevents adhesion of the mucus layer to cell surfaces. Proper regulation of airway surface liquid (ASL) volume and the hydration of its component layers, therefore, are critical to the maintenance of mucus clearance. Whereas maintenance of PGL height is necessary to facilitate cilia motion, adequate hydration of the mucus layer is a key determinant of viscoelastic properties and transportability.

As ASL moves from distal airways toward the trachea, an enormous reduction in airway surface area occurs, necessitating active absorption of liquid across the airway to prevent obstruction of airway lumens. Conversely, there may be situations (e.g., exercise) or lung regions in which addition of liquid to ASL is necessary. The superficial epithelium lining airway surfaces regulates PGL height and mucus hydration through the coordinate regulation of Na⁺-mediated liquid absorption and Cl⁻-mediated liquid secretion.

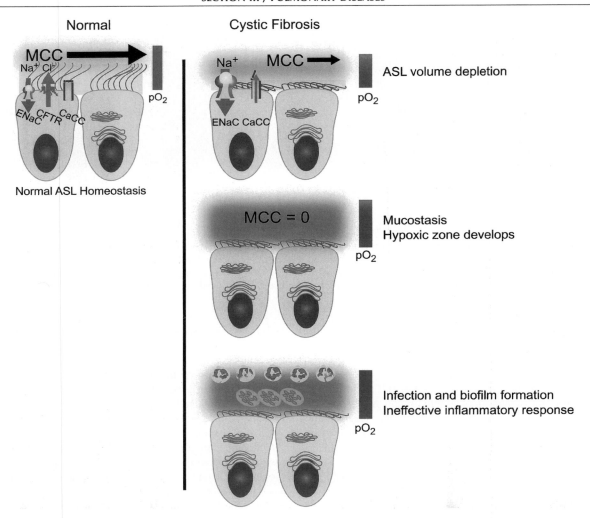

Figure 27-2 Pathogenesis of CF lung disease. (Upper left) Normal regulation of ASL volume requires the reciprocal regulation of CFTR and ENaC activities, which in turn supports normal MCC. (Upper right) In CF, absent CFTR and excessive ENaC activities result in depletion of ASL volume and concentration of airway mucus. (Middle right) Mucostasis ensues and is accompanied by the development of a hypoxic zone within mucus plaques. (Lower right) Finally, infection with typical CF pathogens, conversion to a biofilm mode of growth, and exuberant but ineffective inflammation results in clinically apparent CF lung disease. CaCC, calcium-activated chloride channels.

The absorption of airway liquid is accomplished via active sodium transport, with ENaC mediating the rate-limiting step in this process. Liquid secretion across the superficial epithelium is mediated, at least in part, by CFTR. Liquid may also be added to the PGL layer via bulk flow from converging distal lung units and by chloride/water secretion from submucosal glands (in part via CFTR). The relative contribution of each process is unclear but must vary between proximal airways, in which glands are present, and distal airway regions in which glands are not. As noted, CF epithelia hyperabsorb liquid resulting from dysregulation of ENaC and have lost the capacity to secrete liquid to restore ASL volume homeostasis on CF airway surfaces. As the result, the PGL layer is depleted and the mucus layer becomes concentrated and poorly transportable, thus impairing mucus clearance and predisposing the patient to airway infection.

The consequence of PGL depletion in CF is profound. First, absence of the PGL layer eliminates the low viscosity solution for cilia beat, and hence slows cilial-dependent mucus clearance, and also eliminates the lubricant activity that prevents the mucus layer from interacting with the cell surface. Second, mucins in the mucus layer become concentrated, greatly reducing the mesh diameter of the mucin network and increasing its adhesivity. The reduction in mesh size reduces bacterial motility, perhaps stimulating biofilm formation, and retards the ability of neutrophils to penetrate thickened mucus plaques to kill bacteria. Ultimately, the mucus layer becomes adherent to cell surfaces, making clearance via cough impossible as well. Adherent mucus plaques narrow and obstruct small airways and provide a nidus for infection. The cycle is then set for chronic infection, airway inflammation, mucin hypersecretion, and progressive airway obstruction and destruction. Importantly, restoration of PGL volume in CF cultures allows resumption of ciliary beating and mucus transport, giving hope that similar maneuvers will improve the CF condition in vivo.

In addition to the described changes in ASL volume homeostasis, an ASL compositional change in CF has been proposed by investigators. Initial reports of differences in ASL sodium and chloride concentrations between normal and CF subjects have largely been refuted by direct and indirect measures of ASL ionic composition (demonstrating isotonicity of ASL) using a variety of techniques and experimental systems. However, ASL may be

28 Gene Therapy for Lung Diseases

Jane C. Davies, Duncan M. Geddes, and Eric W.F.W. Alton

SUMMARY

Gene therapy is under development for a variety of lung disease, both those caused by single gene defects, such as cystic fibrosis and α_1-antitrypsin deficiency, and multifactorial diseases such as cancer, asthma, lung fibrosis, and ARDS. Both viral and nonviral approaches have been explored, the major limitation to the former being the inability to repeatedly administer, which renders this approach perhaps more applicable to conditions requiring single administration, such as cancer. Progress in development and clinical trials in each of these diseases is reviewed, together with some potential newer approaches for the future.

Key Words: α_1-antitrypsin deficiency; ARDS; asthma; cystic fibrosis; fibrosis; lung cancer; lung inflammation; lung transplantation; pulmonary edema.

INTRODUCTION

At first sight, given both the accessibility of the airways and the genetic basis of certain pulmonary diseases, the lung seems an ideal candidate for gene therapy. Several routes of access are available, including topical administration to the airway, intravascular administration, and direct injection. Two respiratory diseases, cystic fibrosis (CF) and α_1-antitrypsin (α_1-AT) deficiency, are common single gene disorders for which the genetic basis is known, and for which treatment strategies are not curative. These inherited diseases are the obvious initial target for gene therapy, but it has become clear that nongenetic and acquired diseases including cancer may also be amenable to this approach. Following early optimism, a wide range of barriers has emerged to gene expression in both the airway and alveolar region, some of which are of limiting success. The background to these barriers, methods being employed to overcome them, and the clinical progress in CF, α_1-AT deficiency, lung cancers, and a variety of other pulmonary diseases are discussed.

VECTORS FOR GENE TRANSFER IN LUNG DISEASE

Although naked DNA is capable of transfecting cells, low levels of efficiency have led investigators to explore the use of vectors, systems designed to transport the DNA into the cell. The majority of those in clinical trials have been based on either a recombinant virus or a nonviral system such as liposomes or polymers. Each approach has advantages and disadvantages (Thomas, 2003; Niidome, 2002); although a detailed discussion of each is outside the scope of this chapter.

From: *Principles of Molecular Medicine, Second Edition*
Edited by: M. S. Runge and C. Patterson © Humana Press, Inc., Totowa, NJ

VIRAL VECTORS Modified, replication-deficient adenoviruses (Ad) have been by far the most widely used of the viral vectors, despite the fact that their receptor (coxsackie adenovirus receptor) is not available from the apical side of the cell, but is situated basolaterally (Walters, 1999). Attempts to overcome this problem are discussed later. Adeno-associated virus (AAV) is a small replication-defective virus. In naturally acquired infection, which occurs in the presence of adenoviral coinfection, the AAV inserts into a specific site in the host genome, providing the potential advantage, therefore, of increased duration of transgene expression. However, this integration probably does not occur with the current generation of recombinant viruses (Snyder, 1999). In any case, opinion is divided as to whether this would be desirable, unless it could be targeted to a quiescent area of the genome rather than being random. An additional drawback is the small size of the virus, which makes insertion of the large pieces of cDNA, such as cystic fibrosis transmembrane conductance regulator (CFTR), problematic. Retroviruses also integrate, although this is not normally site-specific, but certain of these, such as lentiviruses have the added advantage of transfecting nondividing cells (Quinonez, 2002). The paramyxovirus, Sendai virus possesses several advantages, such as rapid penetration of mucus, binding to the cell surface via its apically situated receptor, sialic acid, and the capacity for cytoplasmic expression, which overcomes the potential of the nuclear membrane as a barrier. Based on these advantages, one group is exploring this virus as a vector for gene transfer in CF (Yonemitsu, 2000). A common drawback of all viral vectors is the host immune response. Recognition of viral proteins leads to both inflammation at the time of administration and to significantly reduced efficacy of any subsequent application, largely related to the development of neutralizing antibodies (Yei, 1994). Attempts to combat these mechanisms have included removal of various parts of the viral genome (Boucher, 1994) and the coadministration of anti-inflammatory or immunosuppressive agents (Chirmule, 1999; Kolb, 2001) although the safety of the latter approach remains to be confirmed. The requirement for repeated application will depend on which disease is being targeted. Clearly, for certain cancers, a single injection may suffice, and in fact, a strategy of transfecting cells in order to render them immunogenic and trigger cell killing is being utilized in some cancer trials (Tursz, 1996). In contrast, however, in a life-long disease such as CF, repeated application will almost certainly be required. In such a context, a viral vector may be inappropriate.

NONVIRAL VECTORS Many synthetic vectors are being explored for gene therapy; those used clinically have mainly been cationic liposomes or synthetic polymers. The full details of the mechanism by which the cationic liposome delivers DNA into the cell are incompletely understood, but the concepts have been well reviewed (Lee, 1996; Nishikawa, 2001). As much of the DNA delivered in this fashion fails to reach the nucleus, the system, at least theoretically, may be less efficient than some viral vectors. However, this does not appear to have been the case in clinical trials. More importantly, the relative lack of toxicity or immunogenicity is a major benefit. As discussed later, however, these approaches are not completely free from adverse effects. Nanoparticles, short pieces of DNA, are compact, small diameter particles, which may facilitate their transport through the nuclear pore. Addition of a receptor to mediate cellular uptake, serpin enzyme complex receptor, has shown promise with this approach in animal models (Ziady, 2002). Efficiency of nonviral gene transfer methods may be enhanced by a variety of adjunctive physical interventions including electroporation (Taylor, 2003; Sumner, 2003) or complexing the vector with magnetic particles and applying a magnetic field (Plank, 2003). There are clearly advantages and disadvantages to both the liposomal and the recombinant viral approaches. Future systems may be designed to incorporate the best of each.

ROUTES OF ADMINISTRATION

The route of administration depends on the desired cellular distribution and function of the therapeutic protein. Topical administration, directly onto the airway surface, would seem most appropriate for epithelial membrane-bound proteins such as CFTR, or proteins to be secreted into the airway, such as α_1-AT or cytokines. Such airway epithelial expression is likely to be most easily achieved by inhalation or nebulization, both of which have been extensively studied for delivery of nongene-based drugs. Some gene transfer studies have used bronchoscopic instillation. Although this could be impractical for diseases requiring repeated application such as CF, it may be useful for endobronchial tumors, in which direct visualization and targeted application would be of benefit. Localized injection, for example, into a tumor or pleural space may be highly appropriate for certain cancers, although limitations arise when only a small proportion of the tumor is accessible endobronchially, or when metastatic spread has already occurred. Intravascular injection may be appropriate to target the alveolar epithelium. For diseases such as α_1-AT deficiency or certain inflammatory diseases, in which the desired protein is secreted and circulates systemically, gene transfer to a distant organ, such as muscle or liver, which could serve as a "factory," is an attractive option.

BARRIERS TO GENE EXPRESSION IN THE AIRWAY

Limited success in early studies of gene transfer to the lung and airway led to the recognition of a wide range of barriers, both to cell entry and gene expression. An understanding of these mechanisms is beginning to lead to the rational design of either novel vectors, of adjunct therapies directed at the barrier itself, or of nondirected physical delivery methods. A series of barriers can be considered during the passage of a vector from outside the host through to the nucleus of the desired cell. With topical application to the lung, the vector must evade the mucociliary clearance system, penetrate the mucus barrier (which may be made more difficult by certain disease states, e.g., CF) (Stern, 1998) enter the cell through the glycocalyx and avoid lysosomal degradation to reach the nucleus, whereupon it must cross the nuclear membrane. Although the systemic approaches or local injection may help to overcome certain of these early barriers, the latter ones clearly still

pose a challenge. Additionally, for application by any route, the fact that both the vector and the DNA are composed of foreign material renders the complex potentially immunogenic. The vector, the DNA, or the expressed transgene product could trigger a host response, which could result in elimination of the applied complex, death of the expressing cell, or both. Details of the identified barriers in this journey and the methods being attempted to overcome these are described in detail.

CELL ENTRY: TOPICAL ADMINISTRATION

Reaching the Cell Surface   The conducting airways are lined with both ciliated and mucus-secreting epithelial cells, the major integrated function of these being the rapid removal of inhaled material (Houtmeyers, 1999). The mucus barrier also serves to prevent direct contact between inhaled particles and the cell surface, which in the case of airborne infection, for example, serves to limit the epithelial inflammatory response to pathogens. These successful host defense strategies are clearly potentially detrimental for topical gene transfer. In certain disease states this problem may be even more pronounced; for example, CF sputum, which is abnormal both in volume and composition, inhibits gene transfer by both viral and liposomal vectors (Stern, 1998; Perricone, 2000) as may pre-existing nonspecific inflammation at the airway surface (van Heekeren, 1998). Recognition of these barriers may lead to the pursuit of adjunctive therapies to increase efficacy, some such approaches such as the use of recombinant human DNase (Stern, 1998) or Nacystelyn (Ferrari, 2001) to reduce mucus viscosity, have shown promise in preclinical studies. Finally, several investigators have explored the use of either surfactant (Raczka, 1998) other low surface tension liquids (Weiss, 1999) or thixotropic agents (Seiler, 2002) to facilitate spreading of gene transfer vectors throughout the respiratory tract and increase contact time with the airway surface. These compounds may increase the distal airway and alveolar expression of therapeutic genes at the expense of more proximal airway expression, so the target area needs to be clearly identified before this approach could be considered applicable. The cell surface glycocalyx also inhibits entry; with one study demonstrating significantly enhanced Ad-mediated reporter gene expression after the removal of sialic acid with neuraminidase (Pickles, 2000).

Entering the Cell   Some vectors require a specific cell surface receptor in order to enter the cell. For example, although Ad naturally infects respiratory epithelia, the coxsackie adenovirus receptor to which it binds is not expressed on the apical cell surface. In vitro studies have demonstrated increased gene transfer after breakdown of intercellular tight junctions (Parsons, 1998), permitting access to basolaterally situated receptors, although the clinical applicability of such approaches remains to be determined as this could lead to potentially deleterious loss of epithelial integrity. Other groups are developing an interest in pseudotyping of viruses, adding a ligand specific for a cell surface receptor, in an attempt to increase efficiency (Romanczuk, 1991). With an alternative approach, the efficiency of both Ad and AAV has been increased by coprecipitation of these vectors with calcium phosphate, which appears to increase nonreceptor-mediated uptake via the apical cell surface, but may also aid endosomal release (Fasbender, 1998; Walters, 2000). One advantage of vectors such as Sendai virus is the direct cell entry via membrane fusion, which bypasses the endosome, allowing the virus to avoid degradation (Yonemitsu, 2000).

CELL ENTRY: SYSTEMIC ADMINISTRATION   Attempts have been made to circumvent barriers at the mucosal surface by delivering transgenes systemically. The intravenous route might make it possible to access the basolateral membrane of airway epithelial cells, characterized by a higher rate of endocytosis and an increased density of viral receptors. However, most studies have demonstrated that the cells transfected via the systemic circulation are pulmonary endothelial cells or alveolar epithelial cells (Griesenbach, 1998), with only a minority reporting airway epithelial cell transfection (Zhu, 1993; Koehler, 2001). This is likely to be related to a number of barriers including reticuloendothelial system clearance, escape from the vasculature, the interstitium, and the epithelial basement membrane. Various attempts to overcome these barriers have been reviewed (Fenske, 2001; Niidome, 2002).

CROSSING THE CYTOPLASM Once inside the cell, lysosomal breakdown (Zabner, 1995) and destruction by cytoplasmic DNases (Lechardeur, 1999) may further limit gene expression (Duan, 2000). Preliminary data with AAV suggest that the use of proteasome inhibitors may improve gene expression, and another group has demonstrated that specific sugar moieties conjugated to nonviral vectors may influence endosomal escape (Grosse, 2002). Alternative approaches include the addition of peptides to facilitate cytoskeletal transport, or the breakdown of cytoskeletal elements such as microtubules or microfilaments (Kitson, 1999).

ENTERING THE NUCLEUS In contrast to the situation with rapidly dividing cells, such as those grown in vitro, in nondividing or slowly dividing cells in vivo, the nuclear envelope successfully prevents the entry of foreign material into the nucleus. Molecules that need to enter, for example, transcription factors, do so through the nuclear pore complex, mediated by nuclear localizing sequences. This barrier is likely to be a major limiting step in successful gene transfer. In attempts to increase nuclear entry, investigators have explored the addition of a variety of moieties, for example, peptide sequences from the HIV TAT protein (Snyder, 2001) and novel nuclear localizing sequences (Munkonge, 1998). Alternatively, this barrier can be overcome completely by the use of vectors, which do not require nuclear entry for gene expression, such as Sendai virus or the development of cytoplasmic expression systems such as those incorporating T7 promoter and RNA polymerase (Brisson, 1999).

THE HOST IMMUNE RESPONSE The duration of gene transfer can be limited by a variety of mechanisms including transcriptional silencing of the promoter, or loss of the transfected cell, either naturally or via host defense recognition. Regarding the former, some progress has been reported with human polyubiquitin, UbC (Gill, 2001) or UbB promoters (Yew, 2001). Both innate and adaptive immune responses can limit the efficiency and duration of gene transfer, and may pose problems with all routes of administration, including production of a secreted protein at a distant site. Within the respiratory tract, alveolar macrophages can act either directly as phagocytes or indirectly as antigen presenting cells, resulting in fairly rapid clearance of a topically applied gene transfer vector (Worgall, 1997). Similarly, macrophages in the reticuloendothelial system can mediate clearance of a systemically applied vector (Plank, 1996). If vectors are not cleared by such innate immune mechanisms, the adaptive immune system has the potential to significantly impair gene transfer and expression. Both cell-mediated and humoral responses have been demonstrated with viral or synthetic vectors although the major problems in clinical trials have been encountered with viral vectors. Initiation of a cytotoxic T-lymphocyte response may result in killing of the transduced cells, thus effectively limiting the duration of transgene expression. Recognition of viral coat proteins and the production of neutralizing antibodies have created problems in some trials of repeated application of viral-mediated gene transfer (Yei, 1994), and naturally

acquired anti-Ad antibodies in the sputum of CF patients have been shown to inhibit transduction (Perricone, 2000). Selective deletions in the viral genome, and coadministration of agents to reduce the cytotoxic T-lymphocyte response (Chirmule, 1999), are showing some promise in increasing the duration of gene expression. However, this problem is not limited to viral vectors. The presence of unmethylated CpG motifs on plasmid DNA has been suggested as a cause for an observed inflammatory response with nonviral vectors (Schwartzt, 1997; Yew, 1999). Efforts are being aimed at either selectively methylating such motifs (although this can reduce expression levels) (McLachlan, 2000) or inhibiting the pathways through which they signal with agents such as chloroquine (Yew, 2000). Unlike the situation with viral vectors, cationic liposomes are equally effective on subsequent application (Hyde, 2000), which may render them more useful for diseases requiring repeated administration. Although apparently not a significant problem in clinical trials, the possibility of antibody production to previously unencountered transgene-derived protein also exists.

SPECIFIC LUNG DISEASES

CYSTIC FIBROSIS CF results from a variety of mutations in the gene encoding the CFTR protein, a cAMP-regulated chloride channel, leading to abnormal ion transport at the apical surface of epithelial cells (Welsh, 1993). Pulmonary disease dominates the clinical picture, leading to death in more than 90% of patients (Foundation, 1995). The hallmarks of CF lung disease are early, severe, and sustained neutrophil-mediated inflammation, and persistent infection (Armstrong, 1995). Conventional treatment for CF patients has advanced greatly, but at best, it slows the inevitable progression of lung damage. New approaches are therefore required.

Gene Therapy Although other organs are affected in CF, the lung is the major site of pathology, and thus has been the target in the majority of gene therapy trials. Topical gene delivery to the airway epithelium aims to normalize the functions of CFTR including ion transport. There are several unresolved questions with this approach, including (1) which types of cell should be transfected, (2) what degree of correction is required, and (3) how success should be measured. With respect to the cell type targeted, maximal CFTR expression in non-CF airways appears to be in the submucosal glands (Engelhardt, 1992), although clinically detectable disease begins in the distal small airways, in which expression in the surface epithelium is lower (Engelhardt, 1994). Topical application, for example via inhalation, is likely to target the surface epithelium, but is less likely to reach the deeper submucosal gland cells. Whether gene transfer to these cells will be necessary to elicit a clinical effect remains to be determined. Furthermore, surface epithelial cells are terminally differentiated (Warburton, 1998); loss of the transgene therefore occurs with the eventual death of the cell. Interest is focusing on identification of respiratory stem cells, gene transfer to which may have the potential to effect long-term CFTR expression in progeny cells. Regarding what degree of transfection is required; this is made more complex by the realization that different levels of expression may be required to restore the various functions of CFTR. For example, lower numbers of cells need to be corrected to restore chloride transport compared with those required for normalization of sodium absorption (Johnson, 1995), and differences have also been observed regarding the correction of glycoconjugate sulfation and ion transport (Zhang, 1998). Which function(s) of CFTR are most important and whether all identified functions (and perhaps as yet unrecognized ones) need to be corrected is an important question that remains to be resolved. However, based on genetic studies, it would seem that as little as 5–10% of wild-type levels of CFTR in each cell might be sufficient for a normal disease-free phenotype (Gan, 1995). The final issue is one of the assessment of success. Detection of either mRNA or CFTR protein provides evidence of gene expression but no confirmation of functional correction. Ion transport was the first function of CFTR identified, and is thought to be key in the disease pathophysiology. As such, it is the function most commonly assessed in both gene-based and pharmacological clinical studies. Ion transport is assessed most readily in vivo by measurement of transepithelial potential difference (PD), both at baseline and in response to a variety of drugs, including those that block the sodium channel, such as amiloride, and that stimulate chloride secretion (Knowles, 1981; Middleton, 1994). These measurements can be obtained in the airway via the bronchoscope (Alton, 1999), as well as from the nasal epithelium. Additional ex vivo techniques such as epifluorescence microscopy have also proved useful in some studies (Stern, 1995), and alternative functions of the protein, such as those involved in bacterial adherence (Alton, 1999), have also been utilized as end points.

Clinical Studies

Viral Vectors Many studies conducted in the nose and the lower airway, particularly those in the lower airway, have relied on molecular rather than functional evidence of gene expression. Expression has been transient, with variable dose responses. In one of the earliest studies, Ad/CFTR was administered to both the nose and lower airway bronchoscopically (Crystal, 1994). One of the highest dose patients became unwell with fever, hypoxia, and pulmonary infiltrates. The problem was attributed to vector-induced inflammation as no infective virus was detected. Significant local inflammatory reactions and the stimulation of neutralizing antibodies was a feature of the high-dose arm of another nasal study (Boucher, 1994), and flu-like symptoms and a cell-mediated immune response were seen at a high vector dose in a bronchoscopic study (Zuckerman, 1999). Interestingly, a study from France found no acute toxic effects at doses up to 5.4×10^8 plaque-forming units, and no increased inflammatory parameters or antiviral antibodies in bronchoalveolar lavage or serum (Bellon, 1997). Molecular analysis confirmed successful gene transfer, although no functional end points were employed. Attention has focused on the potential problems with repeated administration, with clinical trials addressing this issue in the nose and in the lower airway. In the nasal study, despite there being no detectable adverse effects, the ability of the Ad/CFTR to correct the abnormal chloride transport was reduced on subsequent application (Yei, 1994). In the lower airway study, Ad/CFTR was administered via an endobronchial spray in three doses over a 9-mo period to patients with CF, with bronchoscopic assessment 3 and 30 d after administration (Harvey, 1999). Almost 3 d after the first administration, vector-derived mRNA was detected in a dose-related manner, with those in the high-dose group expressing levels in the 5% of wild-type range, which has been demonstrated in vitro to be sufficient for phenotypic correction. Examination of distribution was unfortunately not possible, as the vector could not be identified with fluorescent *in situ* hybridization. mRNA levels were undetectable in all patients by d 30. The second administration resulted in some nondose-dependent expression, but the third administration produced no expression in any sample. Similarly to the study previously reported, these investigators detected no increase in serum neutralizing antibodies, although gene expression was not seen in patients with high preexisting levels of antibody. This study, therefore, confirms, that although repeated administration of adenoviral vectors appears safe, efficacy

is severely compromised, although the exact mechanism for this is uncertain. AAV-mediated *CFTR* transfer has been assessed in CF patients using preexisting antrostomies into the maxillary sinus for ease of administration and assessment (Wagner, 1998). Ten patients received escalating doses in an unblinded fashion with no significant inflammatory response. Molecular end points demonstrated gene transfer, with DNA detected up to 41 d after administration, but assessment of expression was difficult. Functional assessment with PD responses to isoprenaline and amiloride demonstrated some changes, although numbers were small. This group then performed a phase II study using a similar technique, which did not show significant changes in PD or time to sinusitis exacerbation, but in which there was some evidence of changes in inflammatory parameters (Wagner, 2002). Safety was confirmed in a phase I study in which AAV-*CFTR* was administered by nebulization to the lungs of mildly affected patients and the results of a multicenter placebo-controlled trial by the same group have been reported in abstract form (Moss, 2002). Forty-four patients from eight centers were recruited and small but significant changes in both lung function and inflammatory markers were described.

Nonviral Vectors Several early placebo-controlled clinical trials of liposome-mediated *CFTR* gene transfer to the nasal epithelium confirmed safety and demonstrated a degree of functional correction (Sorscher, 1994; Caplen, 1995; Gill, 1997; Porteous, 1997; Knowles, 1998). These studies led us to the first trial of liposome-mediated *CFTR* to the lower airway of patients with CF (Yonemitsu, 2000). Administration was well tolerated, but respiratory symptoms including mild chest tightness and cough were seen in both groups. This had not been observed with liposome alone in non-CF subjects (Chadwick, 1997), and may relate to the pulmonary inflammation present in the lungs of the CF patients. In addition, all patients in the treatment group reported mild influenza-like symptoms within the first 24 h. The reason for this was unclear, but it may relate to the presence of unmethylated CpG groups on the bacterially derived DNA. Importantly, these symptoms were not reported after nasal administration, which was included for comparison purposes, suggesting that for safety at least, the nasal epithelium may not be a good surrogate site for such trials. The major efficacy end point was lower airway PD. In neither group was there any change in the parameters of sodium absorption (baseline or amiloride response). The treatment group however demonstrated a significant response to perfusion with low chloride and isoprenaline, of approx 25% of non-CF values. Unlike the reported problems with readministration of adenoviral-mediated gene transfer, a study using DC-Chol/DOPE reported that repeated nasal administration was well tolerated and could be effective (Hyde, 2000).

α-1-ANTITRYPSIN DEFICIENCY Deficiency of α_1-AT, the principal endogenous antiprotease, leads to pulmonary emphysema and in some cases, liver disease. The disease is inherited in an autosomal-recessive fashion, with several mutations having been identified resulting in absent or severely low levels of circulating protein (Coakley, 2001). The principal action of α_1-AT in the lung is to counter the adverse effects of proteases such as neutrophil elastase in the distal conducting airways and alveoli. Therapy involves avoidance of damaging environmental triggers such as cigarette smoke, and symptomatic treatments. Plasma-derived α_1-AT can be administered intravenously, but is costly and has a short half-life necessitating frequent administration (Pierce, 1997). Its purification from human serum also raises the possibility of viral transmission. Gene therapy has, therefore, been considered as an alternative approach.

In contrast to the situation with CF, the secreted nature of the deficient protein makes expression at a distant site a possibility for exogenous gene transfer, and simplifies end point assays. The liver, as the natural site of synthesis, would seem the logical choice, and in vivo studies in animals have assessed several delivery systems and routes of administration including tail and portal vein injections, biliary infusion, and direct intrahepatic injection (Stecenko, 2003). Although successful, these initial studies reported inadequate levels of protein. AAV has also been used to transduce muscle, and one group has reported higher protein levels by implantation of genetically modified myoblasts in mice (Bou-Gharios, 1999). Another approach has been to transduce hematopoetic cells with a retrovirus encoding human α_1-AT, and reinfuse the bone marrow into mice (Saylors, 1998). A postulated advantage of this approach might be high expression of the transgene at sites of inflammation. The treated animals demonstrated extremely low levels of human protein at a 3-wk time-point, after which levels declined.

Several studies have assessed the feasibility of targeting the respiratory epithelium directly, in a fashion similar to that described for CF. In early studies on the cotton rat, adenoviral-mediated α_1-AT gene transfer via the trachea led to the detection of functional protein within epithelial cells for up to a week (Rosenfeld, 1991). Although the cells were capable of secreting the protein, the extracellular levels were once again too low to be therapeutically effective. Since then, studies demonstrating that airway epithelia can secrete the protein both apically and basolaterally provide encouraging evidence that the interstitium can be reached. In a study of aerosolized cationic liposome-mediated α_1-AT gene transfer to the rabbit lung, protein was demonstrated both in the airway and alveolar cells (Canonico, 1994).

The first clinical study of α_1-AT gene transfer has been reported (Brigham, 2000). Patients with α_1-AT deficiency received a single dose of cationic liposome-α_1-AT complex into one nostril, with the other nostril acting as a control. Protein was detected in nasal lavage fluid, with levels peaking at d 5 at approx one-third of normal values. This rise was not seen in fluid from the control nostril. In addition, levels of the proinflammatory cytokine, interleukin (IL)-8, were decreased in the treated nostril. Most interestingly this anti-inflammatory effect was not observed when intravenous-administered purified α_1-AT protein achieved levels within the normal range in nasal lavage, leading the authors to speculate that different routes of administration may lead to a variable response in different sites of expression. Future studies will address this issue and assess administration to the lower airway. One potential difficulty in later-phase studies will be the design of end points to assess clinical benefit in this disease, which progresses extremely slowly in nonsmoking patients.

CANCER In comparison to the two previous single gene disorders, cancer may seem a less obvious choice for gene therapy. Although cancer is fundamentally a disorder of genes, many mutations of different genes are usually necessary to produce disease. However, this is a rapidly growing field, with several approaches demonstrating some success.

Tumor Suppressor Gene Therapy Mutation of the tumor suppressor gene, *p53*, is one of the commonest findings in certain types of lung cancer (nonsmall cell) (Rom, 2000). Importantly, patients bearing mutations in *p53* on tumor cells are less likely to respond to treatment, either chemotherapy or radiotherapy. Early evidence that *p53* could be a useful therapeutic target came from in vitro studies (Fujiwara, 1994). Transduction with normal *p53*

rendered lung cancer cell lines more susceptible to apoptosis, an effect that was enhanced in the presence of the chemotherapeutic agent, cisplatin. Significantly, in animal models, a bystander effect has been observed, in which a subset of cells expressing the gene inhibits the growth of neighboring nontransfected cells.

Several viral-mediated clinical trials have been reported on patients with demonstrated *p53* mutations who were failing to respond to conventional treatment, although none of these has been controlled (Roth, 1996; Schuler, 1998; Swisher, 1999; Nemunaitis, 2000; Yen, 2000). The gene transfer agent has been administered locally into the tumor either via the bronchus or percutaneously under CT guidance. Side effects have been generally well tolerated, with some evidence of gene expression at high doses. Some studies have reported either stabilization or regression of growth in the injected tumors, with an absence of effect seen at uninjected sites. However, one multicenter study involving 25 patients with nonresectable tumors showed no evidence of benefit over conventional chemotherapy alone (Schuler, 2001).

Suicide Gene Therapy The basis of this approach is the transfer of a gene encoding an enzyme capable of converting a nontoxic to a toxic chemotherapeutic agent (Smythe, 2000). This limits the activity of the active drug to the site of gene expression and thus minimizes side effects. The most commonly used system has been the herpes simplex thymidine kinase (HSV*tk*) gene, which converts ganciclovir into a triphosphorylated derivative. This is incorporated into DNA in place of guanosine triphosphate and leads to inhibition of cell replication. Two major advantages of this approach are a significant bystander effect owing to local spread of toxic metabolites, and the stimulation of a local immune response. The approach is being utilized in trials of malignancies in many sites, including in patients with pleural mesothelioma (Sterman, 1998). With an adenoviral vector, intrapleural administration of HSV*tk* to 21 patients led to expression of transgene protein in just over 50%. Strong immune responses against Ad were initiated, although this was well tolerated. Partial regression of tumors has been reported in some patients.

Immunotherapy Immunogenetic therapy is based on the transfer of genes encoding molecules involved in the host immune response in an attempt to enhance immune recognition and destruction of tumor cells. Such genes include various cytokines, interferon (IFN)-γ, granulocyte-macrophage colony-stimulating factor, and heat shock proteins (Leroy, 1998). An alternative strategy has been to introduce a foreign gene, such as the bacterially derived β-*galactosidase*, in the hope that cells expressing this gene will be targeted for destruction. Two clinical trials examining feasibility demonstrated local tumor regression and the induction of strong antibody responses both to the adenoviral vector and the transgene (Tursz, 1996; Gahery-Segard, 1997). Other studies have administered vaccinia virus-mediated *IL-2* intrapleurally to patients with mesothelioma (Mukherjee, 2000). No clinical benefit has been shown despite increases in T-cell infiltrates. Preclinical studies are exploring the possibilities of using cytokine cocktails.

Oncolytic Adenovirus There are several replication-specific Ad, such as ONYX-015, which has a deletion in the E1B-55 kDa gene region that is required for inhibition of wild-type p53 function. Therefore, viral replication is prevented in cells with normal p53 function, but permitted in tumor cells with mutant p53, in which it leads to cell death, and a significant bystander effect (McCormick, 2000). This effect has been confirmed in preclinical studies (Bischoff, 1996; Heise, 1997), with the latter study showing synergy with conventional chemotherapeutic agents. One clinical study confirmed both safety and feasibility of intravenous-administered ONYX-015 in patients with end-stage metastatic lung cancers (Nemunaitis, 2001). Infusions were administered weekly with or without conventional chemotherapeutic agents. No dose-limiting toxicity was detected at doses up to 2×10^{13} particles, mild adverse events being fevers, rigors, and transient elevation of liver enzymes. All patients showed an increase in neutralizing antibody levels, and raised levels of circulating cytokines. Viral infection of tumor deposits was seen in one patient and at doses above 2×10^{12} circulating viral genome indicated replication. Replication-specific oncolytic viruses may therefore become a useful approach. Future studies may address the effects of transient immunosuppression, reduction in hepatic clearance of virus, and combination of this approach with cytotoxic drugs or therapeutic transgenes.

INFLAMMATORY AND MISCELLANEOUS DISEASES

Acute Lung Injury   Acute lung injury (ALI) (adult/acute respiratory distress syndrome) is the end result of a variety of insults, including severe sepsis, aspiration, trauma, near-drowning, and pancreatitis (Dennehy, 1999). The clinical hallmarks of ALI include impaired oxygenation, which is often poorly responsive to invasive ventilation and patchy infiltrates on chest X-ray in the absence of a raised pulmonary arterial wedge pressure or left atrial hypertension. Despite the improvements in intensive care management, which have led to a reduction in mortality, ALI carries a poor prognosis, particularly in children. No specific therapy exists, and management is largely supportive (Weinacker, 2001). The pathophysiology of ALI is a sequential process of immediate injury, exudative alveolar inflammation with edema and, finally, fibroproliferative repair (Dennehy, 1999). The recognition that the early stages of this process are characterized by generalized intravascular activation, endothelial damage and high levels of proinflammatory cytokines, has led to the development of novel gene and small molecule-based approaches to treatment. These have some theoretical advantages over the use of proteins, including the potential for cell specificity, the possibility of delivering intracellular proteins, duration of action, and possibly cost. Most approaches target either inflammation or oxidative stress, although other investigators have explored the potential for increasing fluid reabsorption and reducing pulmonary edema in this disease process.

Anti-Inflammatory Approaches   As with other inflammatory diseases, inflammation can be targeted either by antagonizing proinflammatory cytokines, or by increasing the levels or effects of anti-inflammatory cytokines. In the context of ALI, studies have been undertaken both with conventional gene transfer techniques, and with antisense oligonucleotides, which reduce translation to protein by specific binding to mRNA. Ad-mediated *tumor necrosis factor (TNF)-α receptor* gene transfer reduces septic shock in mice injected with lipopolysaccharide (LPS), and reduces pulmonary inflammation (Rogy, 1995). IM delivery of Ad/*IL-10*, a major anti-inflammatory cytokine, showed similar benefits, with a marked suppression of LPS-induced TNF-α and IL-6 production (Xing, 1997). Both *prostaglandin synthase* and *nitric oxide synthase* genes have demonstrated potential therapeutic benefit in animal models of ALI (Conary, 1994; von der Leyen, 1995). Antisense technology has also been used in this context: oligonucleotides against ICAM-1, a major intercellular adhesion molecule, reduced endotoxin-induced neutrophil influx to the lung (Kumasaka, 1996). Hyperoxia has been implicated in lung damage seen in both ALI and infant respiratory distress syndrome. The demonstration that this effect occurs via a mitogen-activated protein kinase, p38MAPK (which also mediates LPS and TNF-α induced damage) (Lee, 1994), has led to another

novel approach. This pathway is attenuated by CO, a byproduct of heme degradation catalyzed by hemoxygenase. Ad-expressing inducible *hemoxygenase, HO-1*, instilled intratracheally, increased the survival of rats with hyperoxic lung damage (Inoue, 2001).

Targeting Pulmonary Edema   In the healthy state, alveolar liquid is cleared by the basolaterally situated Na+,K+-ATPase, which is upregulated during the resolution phase of pulmonary edema (Factor, 2001), a recognized feature of ALI. A variety of vectors have been used to overexpress this ATPase in animal models of lung injury with pulmonary edema, with studies reporting both improved fluid clearance and enhanced survival (Factor, 2000; Stern, 2000). An alternative approach has been to increase activity of the epithelial sodium ion channel, ENaC, the levels and function of which are both upregulated by β(2)-adrenoreceptor (β[2]-AR) expression. β(2)-AR increased alveolar fluid clearance by more than 100% in a rat model (Dumasius, 2001), suggesting that this approach may be applicable in pulmonary edema clearance.

Asthma   Asthma is a disease of high prevalence characterized by type-2 T-helper lymphocyte-mediated inflammation (Lee, 2001) and airway hyperreactivity. Treatment with bronchodilators and anti-inflammatory agents is successful in treating wheeze, cough, and breathlessness in the vast majority of patients (Suissa, 2001). However, for the subgroup who does not respond, novel therapeutic approaches may be relevant. Following success in animal models with Th1-type cytokine protein therapy (IFN-γ [Lack, 1994] or IL-12 [Schwarze, 1998]), beneficial effects have been demonstrated with *IFN-γ* (Dow, 1999), *IL-4 receptor antagonist* (Zavorotinskaya, 2003), and *IL-12* (Hogan, 1998) gene transfer. Thus, in line with the multifactorial nature of the disease, many options are being explored for new gene therapies for asthma. Given the success of conventional treatment however, it is likely that such therapies may only be useful for a minority of patients who do not respond to standard regimes.

Fibrotic Lung Disease   Lung fibrosis can be idiopathic, part of a multisystem (e.g., autoimmune) disorder, or iatrogenic (following radiotherapy or drugs such as bleomycin [Fonseca, 1999]). The prognosis is often poor and available therapies are limited. A variety of growth factors, in particular transforming growth factor (TGF)-β are considered key in the progressive nature of the disease (Sime, 2001), leading to these molecules as targets for novel therapies. Both Smad7, a TGF-β antagonist (Nakao, 1999), and decorin, an endogenous proteoglycan with anti-TGF-β activities (Kolb, 2001) administered intratracheally to bleomycin-treated mice led to a significant reduction in fibrosis. Another group has demonstrated prevention of radiation-induced lung fibrosis and improved survival with liposome-mediated *manganese superoxide dismutase* (Epperly, 1998). The design of radiation-induced promoters (Scott, 2000) may help to limit sites of expression of therapeutic transgenes both in radiation-related fibrosis and lung cancers. Finally, a clinical study has shown dramatic success with IFN-γ 1β protein therapy, which in combination with prednisolone, led to improvements in pulmonary function and oxygen saturation (Ziesche, 1999); in contrast, the group treated with the corticosteroid alone deteriorated. This, and other reports suggesting a role for Fas-mediated alveolar cell apoptosis (Kuwano, 1999), may lead to new gene-based strategies for this disease.

Lung Transplantation   The major obstacle to organ transplantation programs worldwide remains the lack of sufficient donor organs. Medium to long-term success is, however, further limited both by acute ischemia-reperfusion injury, which is particularly problematic for lung transplantation (Mal, 1998), and by the host response leading to organ rejection (Ward, 2000). Given the short-age of available organs, strategies to attenuate these processes would be of major benefit. Organ transplantation theoretically creates a unique window of opportunity for gene therapy; in addition to administration to the host before removal of the organ, or the recipient after surgery, therapeutic genes could be administered to the organ ex vivo during the procedure. The feasibility of *Ad-β-gal* transfection either before procurement (via tracheostomy) or ex vivo after surgical removal has been demonstrated (Cassivi, 1999). At the critical time of reperfusion, significantly greater transgene levels were shown in lungs transfected via the tracheostomy than in those transfected ex vivo. Levels in other organs were virtually absent, confirming limitation to the lungs. However, another study using liposomes demonstrated that ex vivo transfection was superior to intravenous injection of donors prior to organ harvesting (Boasquevisque, 1999). Another concern may be the cold preservation of organs prior to transplantation, which adversely affects efficacy of gene transfer (Boasquevisque, 1998). The optimal route and timing of gene administration may therefore depend on the vector and the desired function and site of transgene expression.

Various mediators have been implicated in ischemia-reperfusion injury, including stimulated leukocytes and platelets, complement, proinflammatory cytokines, and oxidants (Mal, 1998). Attempts to combat this process with exogenous recombinant proteins have been limited, thought largely to be related to the inability to achieve and maintain high local levels. Gene transfer may therefore be a more useful approach. Ad/*hIL-10* was administered intravenously to rats 24 h before organ harvest (Itano, 2000). When assessed 24 h after isotransplantation, dose-dependent IL-10 expression was observed along with significant improvements in gas exchange and neutrophil sequestration when compared with controls (Ad-*LacZ*). In the higher dose group, myeloperoxidase and NO synthase were also decreased, suggesting that IL-10 may be of benefit in reducing injury at the time of reperfusion. Several groups have reported a reduction in rejection of donor lungs with a variety of methods. Lipid-mediated *Fas ligand* was administered retrogradely through the pulmonary venous system, prior to lung removal along (Schmid, 2000) with a single dose of cyclosporine. Compared with controls, the rats receiving *Fas*-transfected lungs had better d 5 gas exchange, and demonstrated significantly less histological evidence of acute rejection. Other groups have reported success with *TGF-β* both lipid-mediated ex vivo (Mora, 2000) and Ad IM into donor post-transplant (Suda, 2001). However, similarly to the situation with CF and α₁-AT deficiency, robust end point assays in lung transplantation trials will be complicated by the clinical heterogeneity of the patient groups studied.

FUTURE DIRECTIONS AND SUMMARY

The principle of gene therapy for lung disease has been proved, with clinical trials showing successful gene transfer in a variety of genetic and acquired disorders. The major problem is with low levels of efficiency, both in terms of cell entry and, for chronic diseases, duration, and the limitation by the host immune response of repeated application with viral vectors. Regarding efficiency, research is ongoing into both overcoming barriers to gene transfer and vector design, including viral pseudotyping and the development of newer generation cationic liposomes and synthetic vectors. Regarding long-term expression, approaches being investigated include manipulation of either the vector or the host to permit repeated administration, the use of integrating vectors, and attempts to identify and target respiratory epithelial progenitor cells. Focused efforts on these areas are

likely to lead to the development of successful gene therapy approaches in the near future for a number of respiratory diseases.

SELECTED REFERENCES

Alton EW, Stern M, Farley R, et al. Cationic lipid-mediated *CFTR* gene transfer to the lungs and nose of patients with cystic fibrosis: a double-blind placebo-controlled trial. Lancet 1999;353:947–954.

Armstrong DS, Grimwood K, Carzino R, Carlin JB, Olinsky A, Phelan PD. Lower respiratory infection and inflammation in infants with newly diagnosed cystic fibrosis. BMJ 1995;310:1571, 1572.

Bellon G, Michel-Calemard L, Thouvenot D, et al. Aerosol administration of a recombinant adenovirus expressing CFTR to cystic fibrosis patients: a phase I clinical trial. Hum Gene Ther 1997;8:15–25.

Bischoff JR, Kirn DH, Williams A, et al. An adenovirus mutant that replicates selectively in p53-deficient human tumor cells. Science 1996;274:373–376.

Boasquevisque CH, Mora BN, Bernstein M, et al. Ex vivo liposome-mediated gene transfer to lung isografts. J Thorac Cardiovasc Surg 1998;115:38–44.

Boasquevisque CH, Mora BN, Boglione M, et al. Liposome-mediated gene transfer in rat lung transplantation: a comparison between the in vivo and ex vivo approaches. J Thorac Cardiovasc Surg 1999;117:8–14.

Boucher RC, Knowles MR, Johnson LG, et al. Gene therapy for cystic fibrosis using E1-deleted adenovirus: a phase I trial in the nasal cavity. The University of North Carolina at Chapel Hill. Hum Gene Ther 1994;5:615–639.

Bou-Gharios G, Wells DJ, Lu QL, Morgan JE, Partridge T. Differential expression and secretion of alpha1 anti-trypsin between direct DNA injection and implantation of transfected myoblast. Gene Ther 1999;6:1021–1029.

Brigham KL, Lane KB, Meyrick B, et al. Transfection of nasal mucosa with a normal α₁-antitrypsin gene in α₁-antitrypsin-deficient subjects: comparison with protein therapy. Hum Gene Ther 2000;11:1023–1032.

Brisson M, He Y, Li S, Yang JP, Huang L. A novel T7 RNA polymerase autogene for efficient cytoplasmic expression of target genes. Gene Ther 1999;6:263–270.

Canonico AE, Conary JT, Meyrick BO, Brigham KL. Aerosol and intravenous transfection of human alpha 1-antitrypsin gene to lungs of rabbits. Am J Respir Cell Mol Biol 1994;10:24–29.

Caplen NJ, Alton EW, Middleton PG, et al. Liposome-mediated CFTR gene transfer to the nasal epithelium of patients with cystic fibrosis. Nat Med 1995;1:39–46.

Cassivi SD, Cardella JA, Fischer S, Liu M, Slutsky AS, Keshavjee S. Transtracheal gene transfection of donor lungs prior to organ procurement increases transgene levels at reperfusion and following transplantation. J Heart Lung Transplant 1999;18:1181–1188.

Chadwick SL, Kingston HD, Stern M, et al. Safety of a single aerosol administration of escalating doses of the cationic lipid GL-67/DOPE/DMPE-PEG₅₀₀₀ formulation to the lungs of normal volunteers. Gene Ther 1997;4:937–942.

Chirmule N, Truneh A, Haecker SE, et al. Repeated administration of adenoviral vectors in lungs of human CD4 transgenic mice treated with a nondepleting CD4 antibody. J Immunol 1999;163:448–455.

Coakley RJ, Taggart C, O'Neill S, McElvaney NG. Alpha 1-antitrypsin deficiency: biological answers to clinical questions. Am J Med Sci 2001;321:33–41.

Conary JT, Parker RE, Christman BW, et al. Protection of rabbit lungs from endotoxin injury by in vivo hyperexpression of the prostaglandin G/H synthase gene. J Clin Invest 1994;93:1834–1840.

Crystal RG, McElvaney NG, Rosenfeld MA, et al. Administration of an adenovirus containing the human CFTR cDNA to the respiratory tract of individuals with cystic fibrosis. Nat Genet 1994;8:42–51.

Koehler DR, Hannam V, Belcastro R, et al. Targeting transgene expression for cystic fibrosis gene therapy. Mol Ther 2001;4:58–65.

Dennehy KC, Bigatello LM. Pathophysiology of the acute respiratory distress syndrome. Int Anesthesiol Clin 1999;37:1–13.

Dow SW, Schwarze J, Heath TD, Potter TA, Gelfand EW. Systemic and local interferon gamma gene delivery to the lungs for treatment of allergen-induced airway hyperresponsiveness in mice. Hum Gene Ther 1999;10:1905–1914.

Duan D, Yue Y, Yan Z, Yang J, Engelhardt JF. Endosomal processing limits gene transfer to polarized airway epithelia by adeno-associated virus. J Clin Invest 2000;105:1573–1587.

Dumasius V, Sznajder JI, Azzam ZS, et al. Beta(2)-adrenergic receptor overexpression increases alveolar fluid clearance and responsiveness to endogenous catecholamines in rats. Circ Res 2001;89:907–914.

Engelhardt JF, Yankaskas JR, Ernst SA, et al. Submucosal glands are the predominant site of CFTR expression in the human bronchus. Nat Genet 1992;2:240–248.

Engelhardt JF, Zepeda M, Cohn JA, Yankaskas JR, Wilson JM. Expression of the cystic fibrosis gene in adult human lung. J Clin Invest 1994; 93:737–749.

Epperly M, Bray J, Kraeger S, et al. Prevention of late effects of irradiation lung damage by manganese superoxide dismutase gene therapy. Gene Ther 1998;5:196–208.

Factor P. Role and regulation of lung Na,K-ATPase. Cell Mol Biol 2001;47:347–361.

Factor P, Dumasius V, Saldias F, Brown LA, Sznajder JI. Adenovirus-mediated transfer of an Na+/K+-ATPase beta1 subunit gene improves alveolar fluid clearance and survival in hyperoxic rats. Hum Gene Ther 2000;11:2231–2242.

Fasbender A, Lee JH, Walters RW, Moninger TO, Zabner J, Welsh MJ. Incorporation of adenovirus in calcium phosphate precipitates enhances gene transfer to airway epithelia in vitro and in vivo. J Clin Invest 1998;102:184–193.

Fenske DB, MacLachlan I, Cullis PR. Long-circulating vectors for the systemic delivery of genes. Curr Opin Mol Ther 2001;3:153–158.

Ferrari S, Kitson C, Farley R, et al. Mucus altering agents as adjuncts for non-viral gene transfer to airway epithelium. Gene Ther 2001;8:1380–1386.

Fonseca C, Abraham D, Black CM. Lung fibrosis. Springer Semin Immunopathol 1999;21:453–474.

Fujiwara T, Grimm EA, Mukhopadhyay T, Zhang WW, Owen-Schaub LB, Roth JA. Induction of chemosensitivity in human lung cancer cells in vivo by adenovirus-mediated transfer of the wild-type p53 gene. Cancer Res 1994;54:2287–2291.

Gahery-Segard H, Molinier-Frenkel V, Le Boulaire C, et al. Phase I trial of recombinant adenovirus gene transfer in lung cancer: longitudinal study of the immune responses to transgene and viral products. J Clin Invest 1997;100:2218–2226.

Gan KH, Veeze HJ, van den Ouweland AM, et al. A cystic fibrosis mutation associated with mild lung disease. N Engl J Med 1995;333:95–99.

Griesenbach U, Chonn A, Cassady R, et al. Comparison between intratracheal and intravenous administration of liposome-DNA complexes for cystic fibrosis lung gene therapy. Gene Ther 1998;5:181–188.

Gill DR, Smyth SE, Goddard CA, et al. Increased persistence of lung gene expression using plasmids containing the ubiquitin C or elongation factor 1alpha promoter. Gene Ther 2001;8:1539–1546.

Gill DR, Southern KW, Mofford KA, et al. A placebo-controlled study of liposome-mediated gene transfer to the nasal epithelium of patients with cystic fibrosis. Gene Ther 1997;4:199–209.

Grosse S, Tremeau-Bravard A, Aron Y, Briand P, Fajac I. Intracellular rate-limiting steps of gene transfer using glycosylated polylysines in cystic fibrosis airway epithelial cells. Gene Ther 2002;9:1000–1007.

Harvey B-G, Leopold PL, Hackett NR, et al. Airway epithelial CFTR mRNA expression in cystic fibrosis patients after repetitive administration of a recombinant adenovirus. J Clin Invest 1999;104:1245–1255.

Heise C, Sampson-Johannes A, Williams A, McCormick F, Von Hoff DD, Kirn DH. ONYX-015, an E1B gene-attenuated adenovirus, causes tumor-specific cytolysis and antitumoral efficacy that can be augmented by standard chemotherapeutic agents. Nat Med 1997;3:639–645.

Hogan SP, Foster PS, Tan X, Ramsay AJ. Mucosal IL-12 gene delivery inhibits allergic airways disease and restores local antiviral immunity. Eur J Immunol 1998;28:413–423.

Houtmeyers E, Gosselink R, Gayan-Ramirez G, Decramer M. Regulation of mucociliary clearance in health and disease. Eur Respir J 1999;13:1177–1788.

Hyde SC, Southern KW, Gileadi U, et al. Repeat administration of DNA/liposomes to the nasal epithelium of patients with cystic fibrosis. Gene Ther 2000;7:1156–1165.

Inoue S, Suzuki M, Nagashima Y, et al. Transfer of heme oxygenase 1 cDNA by a replication-deficient adenovirus enhances interleukin 10 production from alveolar macrophages that attenuates lipopolysaccharide-induced acute lung injury in mice. Hum Gene Ther 2001;12:967–979.

Itano H, Zhang W, Ritter JH, McCarthy TJ, Mohanakumar T, Patterson GA. Adenovirus-mediated gene transfer of human interleukin 10 ameliorates reperfusion injury of rat lung isografts. J Thorac Cardiovasc Surg 2000;120:947–956.

Johnson LG, Boyles SE, Wilson J, Boucher RC. Normalization of raised sodium absorption and raised calcium-mediated chloride secretion by adenovirus-mediated expression of cystic fibrosis transmembrane conductance regulator in primary human cystic fibrosis airway epithelial cells. J Clin Invest 1995;95:1377–1382.

Kitson C, Angel B, Judd D, et al. The extra- and intracellular barriers to lipid and adenovirus-mediated pulmonary gene transfer in native sheep airway epithelium. Gene Ther 1999;6:534–546.

Knowles M, Gatzy J, Boucher R. Increased bioelectric potential difference across respiratory epithelia in cystic fibrosis. N Engl J Med 1981;305:1489–1495.

Knowles MR, Noone PG, Hohneker K, et al. A double-blind, placebo controlled, dose ranging study to evaluate the safety and biological efficacy of the lipid-DNA complex GR213487B in the nasal epithelium of adult patients with cystic fibrosis. Hum Gene Ther 1998;9:249–269.

Kolb M, Inman M, Margetts PJ, Galt T, Gauldie J. Budesonide enhances repeated gene transfer and expression in the lung with adenoviral vectors. Am J Respir Crit Care Med 2001;164:866–872.

Kolb M, Margetts PJ, Galt T, et al. Transient transgene expression of decorin in the lung reduces the fibrotic response to bleomycin. Am J Respir Crit Care Med 2001;163:770–777.

Kumasaka T, Quinlan WM, Doyle NA, et al. Role of the intercellular adhesion molecule-1 (ICAM-1) in endotoxin-induced pneumonia evaluated using ICAM-1 antisense oligonucleotides, anti-ICAM-1 monoclonal antibodies, and ICAM-1 mutant mice. J Clin Invest 1996;97:2362–2369.

Kuwano K, Hagimoto N, Kawasaki M, et al. Essential roles of the Fas–Fas ligand pathway in the development of pulmonary fibrosis. J Clin Invest 1999;104:13–19.

Lack G, Renz H, Saloga J, et al. Nebulized but not parenteral IFN-gamma decreases IgE production and normalizes airways function in a murine model of allergen sensitization. J Immunol 1994;152:2546–2554.

Lechardeur D, Sohn KJ, Haardt M, et al. Metabolic instability of plasmid DNA in the cytosol: a potential barrier to gene transfer. Gene Ther 1999;6:482–497.

Lee ER, Marshall J, Siegel CS, et al. Detailed analysis of structures and formulations of cationic lipids for efficient gene transfer to the lung. Hum Gene Ther 1996;7:1701–1717.

Lee JC, Laydon JT, McDonnell PC, et al. A protein kinase involved in the regulation of inflammatory cytokine biosynthesis. Nature 1994;372: 739–746.

Lee NA, Gelfand EW, Lee JJ. Pulmonary T cells and eosinophils: coconspirators or independent triggers of allergic respiratory pathology? J Allergy Clin Immunol 2001;107:945–957.

Leroy P, Slos P, Homann H, et al. Cancer immunotherapy by direct in vivo transfer of immunomodulatory genes. Res Immunol 1998;149:681–684.

Mal H, Dehoux M, Sleiman C, et al. Early release of proinflammatory cytokines after lung transplantation. Chest 2001;113:645–651.

McCormick F. Interactions between adenovirus proteins and the p53 pathway: the development of ONYX-015. Semin Cancer Biol 2000;10: 453–459.

McLachlan G, Stevenson BJ, Davidson DJ, Porteous DJ. Bacterial DNA is implicated in the inflammatory response to delivery of DNA/DOTAP to mouse lungs. Gene Ther 2000;7:384–392.

Middleton PG, Geddes DM, Alton EWFW. Protocols for in vivo measurement of the ion transport defects in cystic fibrosis nasal epithelium. Eur Respir J 1994;7:2050–2056.

Mora BN, Boasquevisque CH, Boglione M, et al. Transforming growth factor-beta1 gene transfer ameliorates acute lung allograft rejection. J Thorac Cardiovasc Surg 2000;119:913–920.

Moss RB, Aitken M, Clancy J, et al. A multi-centre, double-blind, placebo-controlled phase II study of aerosolised TGAAVCF in cystic fibrosis patients with mild lung disease. Pediatr Pulmonol 2002;(S24):250.

Mukherjee S, Haenel T, Himbeck R, et al. Replication-restricted vaccinia as a cytokine gene therapy vector in cancer: persistent transgene expression despite antibody generation. Cancer Gene Ther 2000;7:663–670.

Munkonge FM, Hillery E, Griesenbach U, Geddes DM. Alton EWFW. Isolation of a putative nuclear import DNA shuttle protein. Mol Biol Cell 1998;9:187A.

Nakao A, Fujii M, Matsumura R, et al. Transient gene transfer and expression of Smad7 prevents bleomycin-induced lung fibrosis in mice. J Clin Invest 1999;104:5–11.

Nemunaitis J, Cunningham C, Buchanan A, et al. Intravenous infusion of a replication-selective adenovirus (ONYX-015) in cancer patients: safety, feasibility and biological activity. Gene Ther 2001;8:746–759.

Nemunaitis J, Swisher SG, Timmons T, et al. Adenovirus-mediated p53 gene transfer in sequence with cisplatin to tumors of patients with non-small cell lung cancer. J Clin Oncol 2000;18:609–622.

Niidome T, Huang L. Gene therapy progress and prospects: nonviral vectors. Gene Ther 2002;9:1647–1652.

Nishikawa M, Huang L. Nonviral vectors in the new millennium: delivery barriers in gene transfer. Hum Gene Ther 2001;12:861–870.

Parsons DW, Grubb BR, Johnson LG, Boucher RC. Enhanced in vivo airway gene transfer via transient modification of host barrier properties with a surface-active agent. Hum Gene Ther 1998;9:2661–2672.

Patient Registry 1994 Annual Data Report. Bethesda, MD: Cystic Fibrosis Foundation, 1995.

Perricone MA, Rees DD, Sacks CR, Smith KA, Kaplan JM, St George JA. Inhibitory effect of cystic fibrosis sputum on adenovirus-mediated gene transfer in cultured epithelial cells. Hum Gene Ther 2000;11:1997–2008.

Pickles RJ, Fahrner JA, Petrella JM, Boucher RC, Bergelson JM. Retargeting the coxsackievirus and adenovirus receptor to the apical surface of polarized epithelial cells reveals the glycocalyx as a barrier to adenovirus-mediated gene transfer. J Virol 2000;74:6050–6057.

Pierce JA. Alpha1-antitrypsin augmentation therapy. Chest 1997;112:872–874.

Plank C, Mechtler K, Szoka FC Jr, Wagner E. Activation of the complement system by synthetic DNA complexes: A potential barrier for intravenous gene delivery. Hum Gene Ther 1996;7:1437–1446.

Plank C, Schillinger U, Scherer F, et al. The magnetofection method: Using magnetic force to enhance gene delivery. Biol Chem 2003;384:737–747.

Porteous DJ, Dorin JR, McLachlan G, et al. Evidence for safety and efficacy of DOTAP cationic liposome mediated CFTR gene transfer to the nasal epithelium of patients with cystic fibrosis. Gene Ther 1997;4:210–218.

Quinonez R, Sutton RE. Lentiviral vectors for gene delivery into cells. DNA Cell Biol 2002;21:937–951.

Raczka E, Kukowska-Latallo JF, Rymaszewski M, Chen C, Baker JR Jr. The effect of synthetic surfactant Exosurf on gene transfer in mouse lung in vivo. Gene Ther 1998;5:1333–1339.

Rogy MA, Auffenberg T, Espat NJ, et al. Human tumor necrosis factor receptor (p55) and interleukin 10 gene transfer in the mouse reduces mortality to lethal endotoxemia and also attenuates local inflammatory responses. J Exp Med 1995;181:2289–2293.

Rom WN, Hay JG, Lee TC, Jiang Y, Tchou-Wong K-M. Molecular and genetic aspects of lung cancer. Am J Respir Crit Care Med 2000;161:1355–1367.

Romanczuk H, Galer CE, Zabner J, Barsomian G, Wadsworth SC, O'Riordan CR. Modification of an adenoviral vector with biologically selected peptides: a novel strategy for gene delivery to cells of choice. Hum Gene Ther 1999;10:2615–2626.

Rosenfeld MA, Siegfried W, Yoshimura K, et al. Adenovirus-mediated transfer of a recombinant alpha 1-antitrypsin gene to the lung epithelium in vivo. Science 1991;252:431–434.

Roth JA, Nguyen D, Lawrence DD, et al. Retrovirus-mediated wild-type p53 gene transfer to tumors of patients with lung cancer. Nat Med 1996;2:985–991.

Saylors RL III, Wall DA. Expression of human alpha 1 antitrypsin in murine hematopoietic cells in vivo after retrovirus-mediated gene transfer. Mol Genet Metab 1998;63:198–204.

Schmid RA, Stammberger U, Hillinger S, et al. Fas ligand gene transfer combined with low dose cyclosporine A reduces acute lung allograft rejection. Transpl Int 2000;13(Suppl 1):S324–S328.

Schuler M, Herrmann R, De Greve JL, et al. Adenovirus-mediated wild-type p53 gene transfer in patients receiving chemotherapy for advanced non-small-cell lung cancer: results of a multicenter phase II study. J Clin Oncol 2001;19:1750–1758.

Schuler M, Rochlitz C, Horowitz JA, et al. A phase I study of adenovirus-mediated wild-type p53 gene transfer in patients with advanced non-small cell lung cancer. Hum Gene Ther 1998;9:2075–2082.

Schwarze J, Hamelmann E, Cieslewicz G, et al. Local treatment with IL-12 is an effective inhibitor of airway hyperresponsiveness and lung eosinophilia after airway challenge in sensitized mice. J Allergy Clin Immunol 1998;102:86–93.

Schwartz DA, Quinn TJ, Thorne PS, Sayeed S, Yi AK, Krieg AM. CpG motifs in bacterial DNA cause inflammation in the lower respiratory tract. J Clin Invest 1997;100:68–73.

Scott SD, Marples B, Hendry JH, et al. A radiation-controlled molecular switch for use in gene therapy of cancer. Gene Ther 2000;7:1121–1125.

Seiler MP, Luner P, Moninger TO, Karp PH, Keshavjee S, Zabner J. Thixotropic solutions enhance viral-mediated gene transfer to airway epithelia. Am J Respir Cell Mol Biol 2002;27:133–140.

Sime PJ, O'Reilly KM. Fibrosis of the lung and other tissues: new concepts in pathogenesis and treatment. Clin Immunol 2001;99:308–319.

Smythe WR. Prodrug/drug sensitivity gene therapy: current status. Curr Oncol Rep 2000;2:17–22.

Snyder RO. Adeno-associated virus-mediated gene delivery. J Gene Med 1999;1:166–175.

Snyder EL, Dowdy SF. Protein/peptide transduction domains: potential to deliver large DNA molecules into cells. Curr Opin Mol Ther 2001;3:147–152.

Sorscher EJ, Logan JJ, Frizzell RA, et al. Gene therapy for cystic fibrosis using cationic liposome mediated gene transfer: a phase I trial of safety and efficacy in the nasal airway. Hum Gene Ther 1994;5:1259–1277.

Stecenko AA, Brigham KL. Gene therapy progress and prospects: alpha-1 antitrypsin. Gene Ther 2003;10:95–99.

Sterman DH, Treat J, Litzky LA, et al. Adenovirus-mediated herpes simplex virus thymidine kinase/ganciclovir gene therapy in patients with localised malignancy: results of a phase I clinical trial in malignant mesothelioma. Hum Gene Ther 1998;9:1083–1092.

Stern M, Caplen NJ, Browning JE, et al. The effects of mucolytic agents on gene transfer across a CF sputum barrier in vitro. Gene Ther 1998;5:91–98.

Stern M, Munkonge FM, Caplen NJ, et al. Quantitative fluorescence measurements of chloride secretion in native airway epithelium from CF and non-CF subjects. Gene Ther 1995;2:766–774.

Stern M, Ulrich K, Robinson C, et al. Pretreatment with cationic lipid-mediated transfer of the Na+K+-ATPase pump in a mouse model in vivo augments resolution of high permeability pulmonary oedema. Gene Ther 2000;7:960–966.

Suda T, D'Ovidio F, Daddi N, Ritter JH, Mohanakumar T, Patterson GA. Recipient intramuscular gene transfer of active transforming growth factor-beta1 attenuates acute lung rejection. Ann Thorac Surg 2001;71:1651–1656.

Suissa S, Ernst P. Inhaled corticosteroids: impact on asthma morbidity and mortality. J Allergy Clin Immunol 2001;107:937–944.

Sumner SG, Pringle IA, Varathalingam A, Gill DR, Hyde SC. Use of electroporation to increase plasmid DNA transfer into epithelial cells of the respiratory tract. Mol Ther 2003;7:S67 (abstract).

Swisher SG, Roth JA, Nemunaitis J, et al. Adenovirus-mediated p53 gene transfer in advanced non-small cell lung cancer. J Natl Cancer Inst 1999;91:763–771.

Taylor W, Gokay KE, Capaccio C, Davis E, Glucksberg M, Dean DA. The effects of cyclic stretch on gene transfer in alveolar epithelial cells. Mol Ther 2003;7:542–549.

Thomas CE, Ehrhardt A, Kay MA. Progress and problems with the use of viral vectors for gene therapy. Nat Rev Genet 2003;4:346–358.

Tursz T, Cesne AL, Baldeyrou P, et al. Phase I study of a recombinant adenovirus-mediated gene transfer in lung cancer patients. J Natl Cancer Inst 1996;88:1857–1863.

van Heekeren A, Ferkol T, Tosi M. Effects of bronchopulmonary inflammation induced by Pseudomonas aeruginosa on gene transfer to airway epithelial cells in mice. Gene Ther 1998;5:345–351.

von der Leyen HE, Gibbons GH, Morishita R, et al. Gene therapy inhibiting neointimal vascular lesion: in vivo transfer of endothelial cell nitric oxide synthase gene. Proc Natl Acad Sci USA 1995;92: 1137–1141.

Wagner JA, Nepomuceno IB, Messner AH, et al. A phase II, double-blind, randomized, placebo-controlled clinical trial of tgAAVCF using maxillary sinus delivery in patients with cystic fibrosis with antrostomies. Hum Gene Ther 2002;13:1349–1359.

Wagner JA, Reynolds T, Moran ML, et al. Efficient and persistent gene transfer of AAV-CFTR in maxillary sinus. Lancet 1998;351:1702–1703.

Walters RW, Duan D, Engelhardt JF, Welsh MJ. Incorporation of adeno-associated virus in a calcium phosphate coprecipitate improves gene transfer to airway epithelia in vitro and in vivo. J Virol 2000;74:535–540.

Walters RW, Grunst T, Bergelson JM, Finberg RW, Welsh MJ, Zabner J. Basolateral localization of fiber receptors limits adenovirus infection from the apical surface of airway epithelia. J Biol Chem 1999;274: 10219–10226.

Warburton D, Wuenschell C, Flores-Delgado G, Anderson K. Commitment and differentiation of lung cell lineages. Biochem Cell Biol 1998; 76:971–995.

Ward S, Muller NL. Pulmonary complications following lung transplantation. Clin Radiol 2000;55:332–339.

Weinacker AB, Vaszar LT. Acute respiratory distress syndrome: physiology and new management strategies. Annu Rev Med 2001;52:221–237.

Weiss DJ, Strandjord TP, Liggitt D, Clark JG. Perflubron enhances adenovirus-mediated gene expression in lungs of transgenic mice with chronic alveolar filling. Hum Gene Ther 1999;10:2287–2293.

Welsh MJ, Smith AE. Molecular mechanisms of CFTR chloride channel dysfunction in cystic fibrosis. Cell 1993;73:1251–1254.

Worgall S, Leopold PL, Wolff G, Ferris B, Van Roijen N, Crystal RG. Role of alveolar macrophages in rapid elimination of adenovirus vectors administered to the epithelial surface of the respiratory tract. Hum Gene Ther 1997;8:1675–1684.

Xing Z, Ohkawara Y, Jordana M, Graham FL, Gauldie J. Adenoviral vector-mediated interleukin-10 expression in vivo: intramuscular gene transfer inhibits cytokine responses in endotoxemia. Gene Ther 1997;4: 140–149.

Yei S, Mittereder N, Tang K, O'Sullivan C, Trapnell BC. Adenovirus-mediated gene transfer for cystic fibrosis: quantitative evaluation of repeated in vivo vector administration to the lung. Gene Ther 1994;1: 192–200.

Yen N, Ioannides CG, Xu K, et al. Cellular and humoral immune responses to adenovirus and p53 protein antigens in patients following intratumoral injection of an adenovirus vector expressing wild-type P53 (Ad-p53). Cancer Gene Ther 2000;7:530–536.

Yew NS, Przybylska M, Ziegler RJ, Liu D, Cheng SH. High and sustained transgene expression in vivo from plasmid vectors containing a hybrid ubiquitin promoter. Mol Ther 2001;4:75–82.

Yew NS, Wang KX, Przybylska M, et al. Contribution of plasmid DNA to inflammation in the lung after administration of cationic lipid:pDNA complexes. Hum Gene Ther 1999;10:223–234.

Yew NS, Zhao H, Wu IH, et al. Reduced inflammatory response to plasmid DNA vectors by elimination and inhibition of immunostimulatory CpG motifs. Mol Ther 2000;1:255–262.

Yonemitsu Y, Kitson C, Ferrari S, et al. Efficient gene transfer to airway epithelium using recombinant Sendai virus. Nat Biotechnol 2000;18: 970–973.

Zabner J, Fasbender AJ, Moninger T, Poellinger KA, Welsh MJ. Cellular and molecular barriers to gene transfer by a cationic lipid. J Biol Chem 1995;270:18,997–19,007.

Zavorotinskaya T, Tomkinson A, Murphy JE. Treatment of experimental asthma by long-term gene therapy directed against IL-4 and IL-13. Mol Ther 2003;7:155–162.

Zhang Y, Jiang Q, Dudus L, Yankaskas JR, Engelhardt JF. Vector-specific profiles of two independent primary defects in cystic fibrosis airways. Hum Gene Ther 1998;20:635–648.

Zhu N, Liggitt D, Liu Y, Debs R. Systemic gene expression after intravenous DNA delivery into adult mice. Science 1993;261:209–211.

Ziady AG, Kelley TJ, Milliken E, Ferkol T, Davis PB. Functional evidence of CFTR gene transfer in nasal epithelium of cystic fibrosis mice in vivo following luminal application of DNA complexes targeted to the serpin-enzyme complex receptor. Mol Ther 2002;5:413–419.

Ziesche R, Hofbauer E, Wittmann K, Petkov V, Block LH. A preliminary study of long-term treatment with interferon gamma-1β and low-dose prednisolone in patients with idiopathic pulmonary fibrosis. N Engl J Med 1999;341:1264–1269.

Zuckerman JB, Robinson CB, McCoy KS, et al. A phase I study of adenovirus-mediated transfer of the human cystic fibrosis transmembrane regulator gene to a lung segment of individuals with cystic fibrosis. Hum Gene Ther 1999;10:2973–2985.

29 Sarcoidosis

KELLY D. CHASON AND STEPHEN L. TILLEY

SUMMARY

Sarcoidosis is a disease characterized by granulomatous inflammation in organs and tissues, which is believed to develop in genetically predisposed individuals following exposure to a triggering antigen. Although the etiology of sarcoidosis remains unproven, recent molecular investigations suggest that an immune response against mycobacterial and propionibacterial antigens may play a role in pathogensis. The immune response of sarcoidosis is characterized by a highly polarized Th1 cytokine profile elaborated by lymphocytes and macrophages within granulomas. Elucidation of the specific cytokine mediators of inflammation has led to better markers of disease activity as well as novel targets for new therapies.

Key Words: Antigen; etiology; genetics; granuloma; MHC; *Mycobacteria*; pathogenesis; *Propionibacteria*; sarcoidosis; treatment.

INTRODUCTION

Sarcoidosis is a systemic inflammatory disease characterized by granulomatous inflammation most commonly involving the intrathoracic lymph nodes and lung parenchyma, but with the capacity to involve almost any organ in a random, unpredictable fashion. Although it was previously proposed that sarcoidosis develops in genetically predisposed individuals following exposure to an immunogenic stimulus, significant insight has been gained into the genetic basis for this predisposition and the triggering agent(s). Cellular and molecular biology has improved the understanding of the immunopathogenesis of sarcoidosis, suggested better markers of disease activity, and fueled the development of more selective and potentially more potent therapies for this enigmatic disease.

IMMUNOPATHOGENESIS

ANTIGEN PRESENTATION Granuloma formation is thought to begin when poorly soluble antigenic material is either phagocytosed or internalized by receptor-mediated endocytosis by activated macrophages and dendritic cells. Endosomes containing antigen fuse with lysosomes and the antigenic proteins are broken down into peptide fragments, which are then loaded within the α-helices of human leukocyte-associated antigen (HLA) class II molecules. The resultant major histocompatibility complex (MHC)/peptide complexes are transported to the cell surface of these antigen presenting cells (APCs) where they are exposed for interaction with T-cell receptors (TCRs) present on antigen-specific T cells. Formation of this trimolecular complex (MHC/peptide/TCR) provides the first activation signal, whereas costimulatory molecules provide the additional signal necessary for T-cell activation. On activation, T cells produce cytokines and growth factors that drive the development of granulomas (Fig. 29-1).

PATHOLOGY The granulomatous inflammation of sarcoidosis is characterized by the accumulation of activated lymphocytes, macrophages, and dendritic cells in affected organs. Macrophages aggregate and differentiate into epithelioid histiocytes and multinucleated giant cells, whereas CD4+ T lymphocytes become interspersed within the developing granuloma. In additon, T lymphocytes, and to a lesser extent B lymphocytes, accumulate around the periphery of the granuloma, along with a rim of concentrically arranged fibroblasts.

The physical association of APCs and lymphocytes within the granuloma suggests that the inflammation of sarcoidosis is antigen driven. The oligoclonal expansion of T cells at sites of active disease provides direct evidence for this hypothesis. Perhaps the best example is the expansion of AV2S3 (Vα2.3)+ T cells in the bronchoalveolar lavage (BAL) fluid from HLA-DR17+ (DR*0301) Scandinavian patients with sarcoidosis. The oligoclonal expansion of other specific αβ+ T cells have also been found in the lung, skin, and blood, of other sarcoidosis patients.

CELLS AND CYTOKINES

Lymphocytes T-cell subsets in the BAL fluid of patients with sarcoidosis have been extensively characterized. Early in the disease CD4+ T cells predominate and release a highly polarized Th1 cytokine profile consisting of IL-2, interferon (IFN)-γ, and lymphotoxin. Interestingly, only alveolar T cells and not those of the peripheral blood secrete IL-2, further suggesting that interaction with APCs of the affected organ is required for their activation. Similar cytokine profiles are seen in other granulomatous disorders in which activation of cell-mediated immunity is triggered by microorganisms such as *Mycobacteria* and fungi.

B-cell activation also occurs in sarcoidosis. Many cases are associated with hypergammaglobulinemia, and immune complexes have been detected in a majority of patients. Although the contribution of the B-cell to disease pathogenesis is not as clear as that for the T-cell, it is speculated that a robust humoral immune response, like that typically seen in Lofgren's syndrome (acute sarcoidosis characterized by fever, hilar adenopathy, arthralgias,

From: *Principles of Molecular Medicine, Second Edition*
Edited by: M. S. Runge and C. Patterson © Humana Press, Inc., Totowa, NJ

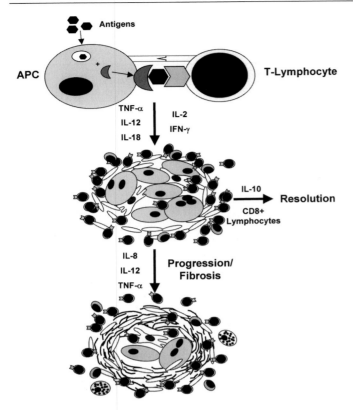

Figure 29-1 Development of granulomatous inflammation. APCs interact with CD4+ T lymphocytes by presenting antigenic peptides, bound to MHC molecules, to TCRs. When a costimulatory signal is also provided by CD40/CD28 binding, the T-cell becomes activated. Th-1 cytokines (IFN-γ, IL-12, IL-18) and TNF-α, released by activated lymphocytes and macrophages, promote the development of granulomas, which consist of clusters of epithelioid histiocytes (differentiated macrophages), dendritic cells, and T lymphocytes, and to a lesser extent B lymphocytes and fibroblasts. Granulomas may involute under the direction of anti-inflammatory cytokines (e.g., IL-10) or persist in the presence of a continued TNF-α stimulation and a Th-1 cytokine milieu. Fibrosis ensues as activated fibroblasts deposit collagen from the periphery of the granuloma to the center, under the direction of activation signals from macrophages and mast cells. (Please *see* color insert.)

and erythema nodosum), may contribute to antigen clearance and subsequent remission of disease.

Macrophages   Acting in concert with the T lymphocyte, the macrophage is another key player in disease pathogenesis. The alveolar macrophage pool expands in sarcoidosis, and these cells spontaneously release a number of proinflammatory cytokines that act with the T-cell-derived cytokines described above to drive the granulomatous inflammation. Alveolar macrophages obtained from patients with sarcoidosis spontaneously release IL-1, tumor necrosis factor (TNF)-α, macrophage inflammatory protein-1α, RANTES, IL-8, IL-12, and IL-18. IL-12 and IL-18 are thought to play a central role in disease pathogenesis by stimulating macrophage activation, IFN-γ production, and granuloma formation. In addition, IL-18 can enhance the cytotoxicity of natural killer cells and T cells.

Tumor Necrosis Factor   Perhaps the most studied cytokine produced during granulomatous inflammation is TNF-α. An increased release of TNF-α occurs from alveolar macrophages from patients with sarcoidosis, and release is significantly higher in patients with active vs inactive disease. Levels also correlate with

response to corticosteroid or immunosuppressive therapy. Perhaps the best evidence for the critical role of TNF-α in granuloma formation comes from in vivo experiments in which levels of this cytokine are reduced either genetically or pharmacologically. In mice deficient in TNF-α or mice treated with anti-TNF antibodies, granuloma formation in response to bacille Calmette-Guerin and *Mycobacterium tuberculosis* is significantly impaired. In humans treated with infliximab, a monoclonal antibody against TNF-α, tuberculous granulomas fail to develop and *M. tuberculosis* becomes disseminated throughout the body. Taken together, this evidence suggests that TNF-α may play a critical role in granuloma development in sarcoidosis, and provides rationale for trials of anti-TNF therapies for patients.

FIBROSIS   The course of sarcoidosis ranges from spontaneous remission to progressive, end-organ fibrosis. The course varies because granulomas may either involute or become encased by a dense band of activated fibroblasts capable of laying down collagen. Fibrosis proceeds from the periphery of the granuloma to the center, and unchecked, this fibrotic response can affect the normal physiology of the involved organ as well as result in irreversible organ destruction. Genetic factors clearly play a role in the propensity of an individual to develop disease remission or progression, and are described in detail next. At the cellular level, data suggests that maintenance of the granuloma may be controlled by IL-12, whereas resolution is associated with an influx of CD8+ lymphocytes and release of IL-10, a mediator known to suppress the inflammatory response. Interestingly, some of the same cytokines that promote the cellular immune response described above (e.g., IFN-γ) may also inhibit fibrosis.

Chronic disease is characterized by the continued production of IL-8, IL-12, and TNF-α. Although IL-8 is not seen in the BAL fluid of early disease, concentrations in patients with chronic disease approach levels seen in patients with idiopathic pulmonary fibrosis. IL-8 recruits neutrophils to the lung, and BAL neutrophilia distinguishes patients undergoing spontaneous remission from those with progressive disease. Thus, neutrophilic alveolitis in sarcoidosis may promote progression to fibrotic disease. Although the mechanisms by which IL-8 and neutrophils promote fibrosis in sarcoidois are incompletely understood, an association between increases in IL-8 and the fibrosis-promoting cytokine transforming growth factor (TGF)-β has been shown. TGF-β has been localized to macrophages within granulomas, a cell type critical for the induction of fibroblast proliferation and secretion of collagen within the lung. Similarly, mast cells contribute to fibrosis in granulomas through the release of fibroblast growth factors.

Although early sarcoidosis is clearly a Th1 polarized disease, it has been speculated that a shift to a Th2 cytokine production may contribute to the development of fibrosis. Th2 cytokines IL-4 and IL-13 can promote fibrosis by enhancing the production of collagen by fibroblasts. Such speculation is in part based on animal models showing that Th2-mediated granulomatous inflammation is more fibrotic than Th1-mediated models. However, human data confirming this paradigm in fibrotic sarcoidosis are lacking, and it is likely that profibrotic mediators such as TGF-β expressed in the lungs of patients with fibrotic disease influence fibrosis in a cytokine milieu unique to progressive sarcoidosis that is not necessarily confined to a prototypic Th1 or Th2 profile.

GENETICS

DISEASE SUSCEPTIBILITY GENES   A genetic basis for developing sarcoidosis has been suspected based on observations of familial clustering of disease and racial differences in disease prevalence. A case–controlled etiological study of sarcoidosis, involving more than 700 patients with sarcoidosis throughout the United States, revealed an approximately fivefold increase in relative risk of developing the disease in first-degree relatives. With advances in genomics technology, genome-wide microsatellite linkage analysis has been used to identify chromosomal regions that may contribute to the risk of sarcoidosis. Findings from these studies have revealed several areas of linkage suggesting that sarcoidosis is a "complex" genetic disease, with the resultant phenotype dependent on the interaction of multiple genes rather than a single mutation. The strongest linkage has been found on the short arm of chromosome 6 in the MHC region. These findings are consistent with other studies that have shown associations between specific MHC class II alleles and sarcoidosis, and provide further support that antigen presentation is involved in disease pathogenesis (Table 29-1). Some alleles associated with disease susceptibility include HLA DR 11,12,14,15, and 17. Several protective alleles have also been identified, with HLA DR1, DR4 being consistently protective across all ethnic populations evaluated. Interestingly, some of the proteins encoded by protective alleles share characteristic bulky, highly hydrophobic residues within a pocket of the HLADR complex antigen binding groove, while nonprotective alleles encode sequences with hydrophilic residues within this pocket. These observations of differences in avidity of antigen binding suggest one mechanistic explanation of how genotype may affect phenotype in sarcoidosis.

GENETIC DETERMINANTS OF DISEASE REMISSION VS PROGRESSION In addition to alleles conferring protection from or susceptibility to sarcoidosis, a genetic basis for remitting vs progressive disease has also been identified (*see* Table 29-1). In addition, some MHC haplotypes associated with resolving disease have been correlated with specific TCR repertoires also shown to predict remitting disease. T cells from patients carrying some of these protective alleles, such as the DRB1*0301 allele, have a tendency for diminished Th1 responses. Thus, a diminished capacity to produce a robust Th1 immune response may be an important requisite for remitting disease.

Many non-HLA candidate gene association studies have also been performed in sarcoidosis with variable degrees of reproducibility across populations. Table 29-1 summarizes some of the major associations. An excellent example of genotype–phenotype correlation emerging from one of these studies involves a mutation in the CC10 protein produced by clara cells. This protein is a counter-regulator of the inflammatory response, acting by several different mechanisms including the inhibition of IFN-γ, TNF-α, and IL-1β; and through inhibition of monocyte and fibroblast chemotaxis and phagocytosis. In sarcoidosis, increased levels of CC10 have been found in serum and BAL fluid from patients whose disease resolved compared with those whose disease progressed. An A to G substitution at position 38 (A38G) downstream from the transcription initiation site within the noncoding region of exon 1 correlates with reduced BAL fluid levels of CC10 and disease progression. Further studies such as these will begin to define the repertoire of mutations that collectively determine the phenotype of subgroups of patients with sarcoidosis.

ETIOLOGICAL TRIGGERS

Several lines of evidence, made possible by modern molecular genetic technology, support a pathophysiological construct in which granulomatous inflammation in sarcoidosis is antigen driven. Analysis of TCRs shows that the disease is neither a monoclonal proliferation of T cells, nor is it polyclonal as would be seen

Table 29-1
Candidate Genes in Sarcoidosis

Susceptibility genes	
MHC class I	HLA-B7, B8
MHC class II	HLA-DR 11,12,14,15,17
MHC class III	D6S1666 microsatellite marker locus
Chemokines	CCR5delta32 (32-bp deletion)
Cytokines	TNF–857 promoter polymorphism
Vitamin D receptor	*Bsm*I restriction site in intron 8
Protective genes	
Major histocompatibility complex	HLA-DR1, DR4
Chemokines	CCR2-64I (valine to isoleucine substitution)
NRAMP	CA repeat polymorphism in immediate 5′ region
Genes associated with disease remission	
MHC II	HLA-DR3, DR5, DQB1*0201, DRB1*0301
Cytokines	TNF–308 promoter polymorphism
Genes associated with disease progression	
MHC II	HLA-DR14, DR15, DQB1*0602
Clara cell	G38A exon 1 polymorphism
Other associated genes in some studies	
MHC II	HLA-DQ*0202
Angiotensin converting enzyme	267 bp insertion/deletion in intron 16
Antigen processing and presentation genes	TAP, HLA-DM, DO, LMP2, LMP7
Cytokines	IL-1α*137 + F13A*188

HLA, human leukocyte-associated antigen; IL, interleukin; MHC, major histocompatibility complex; NRAMP, natural resistance associated macrophage protein; TCR, T-cell receptor; TNF, tumor necrosis factor.

from nonspecific, diffuse immune activation. Rather, all characterizations of the T-cell response in sarcoidosis show an oligoclonal expansion of restricted T-cell clones, consistent with an antigen-driven process. Previously the putative antigen or antigens of sarcoidosis have remained elusive. Speculated environmental antigens such as pine pollen were not identified in large epidemiological investigations (a case–controlled etiological study of sarcoidosis).

The available data best supports microbial antigens as etiological triggers of sarcoidosis. A transmissible agent has long been suspected based on observations of localized disease outbreaks among individuals with close contact, increased rates of disease among health care workers, suspected transmission via organ transplantation, and sensitivity and specificity of the Kveim–Siltzbach reagent, in which an extract of tissue from sarcoid involved spleen elicits a cutaneous granulomatous reaction when administered subcutaneously to patients with sarcoidosis. This latter observation suggests that specific memory T cells are required for a positive test. Thus, sarcoid patients with a positive Kveim–Siltzbach reaction may already possess this T-cell repertoire resulting from previous exposure to or current colonization with the offending organism.

Although cultures from sarcoidosis tissue have only been reported to grow *Propionibacteria*, DNA from a number of different organisms has been amplified by polymerase chain reaction (PCR) from sarcoidosis tissue. Most of these studies have either been insufficiently robust or nonreproducible to seriously implicate these agents as putative pathogens. However, *Mycobacteria* and *Propionibacteria* have emerged as the most plausible candidates.

MYCOBACTERIA   Because of the clinical and pathophysiological similarities between sarcoidosis and tuberculosis (TB), extensive investigation for evidence of *Mycobacteria* in sarcoid tissue has been carried out. Although never consistently cultured from sarcoid granulomata, some studies have identified *Mycobacterial* DNA in these lesions. At least twenty PCR-based studies have examined the role of *Mycobacteria* in sarcoidosis (Table 29-2). These studies, with variable degrees of methodological strength, have yielded extremely variable results with mycobacterial DNA detected in 0–80% of cases. Mycobacterial catalase-peroxidase (mKatG) DNA and protein was found in 5/9 sarcoidosis patients in one study using a combination of molecular techniques including mass spectrometry, immunoblotting, and *in situ* hybridization. IgG antibodies to mKatG were detected in the sera of 12/25 patients. Detection of mKatG protein detergent/protease-treated sarcoidosis tissue suggests that poorly soluble protein aggregates containing mKatG may be the antigenic stimulus driving the granulomatous inflammation in a subset of patients with this disease.

PROPIONIBACTERIA   *Propionibacteria* are anaerobic, Gram-positive bacteria that reside in the skin of humans around hair follicles. Because of a thick cell wall as well as other factors, a commensal relationship with the human host is the norm. An enhanced immune response against these organisms is thought to contribute to the pathogenesis of acne. In somewhat similar fashion, some investigators have proposed that sarcoidosis is the result of an activated immune response against *Propionibacteria*. Colonization of the respiratory tract and intrathoracic lymph nodes by these bacteria, and the development of an immune response against them, may explain the predilection of this disease for the chest. Table 29-3 summarizes the molecular studies of *Propionibacteria* on human sarcoid tissue. In contrast to the molecular studies of *Mycobacteria*, *Propionibacteria* have been consistently detected in high percentages of sarcoid lymph nodes. Because studies with *Propionibacteria* represent one example of how molecular medicine is forwarding our understanding of disease pathogenesis, these studies are described below.

Cultures of Sarcoid Lymph Nodes   In 1978, Homma and colleagues investigated the bacterial growth (aerobic and anaerobic) from lymph nodes removed under aseptic conditions from patients with sarcoidosis. Although no aerobic bacteria were isolated, *Propionibacterium acnes* grew from approx 75% of the lymph nodes obtained from sarcoid patients (solid media: 28/40, liquid media: 31/40). No other bacteria or fungi grew in culture. In 1984, a second study with similar findings was published. Although *P. acnes* was cultured from 31/40 (77.5%) of sarcoid lymph nodes, only 38/180 (21%) of lymph nodes from control patients (cancer) grew the organism ($p < 0.001$). The percent positivity correlated strongly with the extent of granulomas within the cultured node. If greater than 75% of the node was involved with granulomatous inflammation, then 100% of cultures were positive. If 50–75% of the node was involved with granulomas, then 78% were positive. Nodes made up of less than 50% granulomas had a 67% positive culture rate. Despite these findings, *Propionibacteria* never emerged as a strong etiological candidate until the following molecular studies were reported.

Table 29-2
Molecular Studies of *Mycobacteria* in Sarcoidosis

Study	Year	Positive samples/ total samples
Gerdes et al.	1992	0/14
Thakker et al.	1992	2/20
Saboor et al.	1992	10/20
Bocart et al.	1992	2/22
Lisby et al.	1993	0/8;0/18
Fidler et al.	1993	7/16
Ghossein et al.	1994	0/10
Popper et al.	1994	2/15
El-Zaatari et al.	1996	8/9
Richter et al.	1996	2/24
Vokurka et al.	1997	0/15
Cannone et al.	1997	2/30
Popper et al.	1997	11/35
Wilsher et al.	1998	0/23
Ishige et al.	1999	3/15
Grosser et al.	1999	42/65
Ikonomopoulos et al.	1999	9/25
Li et al.	1999	16/20
Klemen et al.	2000	3/4
Gazouli et al.	2002	33/46
Eishi et al.	2002	5/118
Yamada et al.	2002	0/9

Table 29-3
Molecular Studies of *Propionibacteria* in Sarcoidosis

Study	Year	Positive samples / total samples
Ishige et al.	1999	15/15
Eishi et al.	2002	116/118
Yamada et al.	2002	8/9
Gazouli et al.	2002	20/46

Quantitative PCR   In 1999, Ishige and colleagues published their initial findings using quantitative PCR to look for mycobacterial and propionibacterial DNA in lymph nodes from patients with sarcoidosis. Tissue samples were obtained from 15 patients with sarcoidosis, 15 patients with TB, and 15 control lymph nodes (without metastases) from patients with gastric cancer undergoing surgery. DNA was extracted from all 45 tissue blocks and subjected to quantitative PCR using probes specific for *P. acnes*, *Propionibacterium granulosum*, and *M. tuberculosis*. As expected, TB DNA was amplified in 15/15 nodes from TB patients. Genomes of *P. acnes* were found in 12/15 nodes from sarcoid patients. The remaining three nodes in which *P. acnes* was undetectable were remarkable for the amplification of DNA from *P. granulosum*. Although 2/15 TB nodes and 3/15 control nodes showed some amplification of *P. acnes*, levels of amplification were just above the threshold of detection and the number of genomes was significantly lower than that seen in sarcoid nodes.

These findings were extended in a multicenter study involving two Japanese and three European centers involving 108 patients with sarcoidosis, 65 patients with TB, and 86 controls. Control nodes were obtained from patients with either nonspecific lymphadenitis or cancer patients with no evidence of nodal metastases.

With robust methodology using real-time (TaqMan) PCR with primers specific for *P. acnes*, *P. granulosum*, *M. tuberculosis*, *Mycobacterium avium*, *Escherichia coli* (negative control), and β-globin (positive control), these investigators found either *P. acnes* or *P. granulosum* in lymph nodes from 106/108 patients with sarcoidosis. *P. acnes* was detected more frequently than *P. granulosum*, similar to the previous pilot study. Amplification of *P. acnes* from TB and control nodes ranged from 0 to 60%, depending on the center and source of the nodal tissue. Importantly, total numbers of genomes of *P. acnes* was lower in TB and control nodes than in nodes from patients with sarcoidosis. The only other country in which *Propionibacteria* have been investigated by this methodology is Greece. In contrast to the universal presence of *Propionibacteria* (98%) in sarcoid lymph nodes from the multicenter study described above, a study with Greek patients found propionibacterial genomes in 44% of sarcoid nodes examined from 46 patients, with no amplification in control nodes.

In Situ **Hybridization** Evidence for *Propionibacteria* as a granulomatogenic stimulus of sarcoidosis was bolstered when the *in situ* localization of *P. acnes* in and around sarcoid granulomas was shown. With digoxigenin-labeled oligonucleotide probes specific for *P. acnes*, *in situ* hybridization was performed using catalyzed reporter deposition for signal amplification. Nine sarcoid lymph nodes and nine control nodes were examined. In all sarcoid nodes a signal was detected in epithelioid cells within granulomas and in mononuclear cells around granulomas. A similar signal was absent in control nodes, which included tuberculous granulomas. Although further characterization is necessary to confirm that these mononuclear cells with positive signal for *P. acnes* were indeed antigen-presenting cells, their location is highly suggestive. Moreover, this study, by showing *P. acnes* deep within the granuloma, refutes the hypothesis that findings by PCR represent contamination and suggests that *Propionibacteria* may indeed play an etiological role in sarcoidosis.

Animal Studies Animal studies with *Propionibacteria* show that granulomas develop in the lungs, lymph nodes, liver, and spleen following intravenous or intraperitoneal injection. Other features similar to sarcoidosis seen in mice following inoculation with these organisms include hilar adenopathy with nodal replacement by granulomatous inflammation, lymphopenia in the peripheral blood, and resistance to bacterial infection.

Taken together, these findings with *Propionibacteria* support what could be argued is one of the most attractive pathophysiological constructs for the immunopathogenesis of sarcoidosis. Propionibacterial DNA has been repeatedly and convincingly identified within granulomatous nodal tissue of large numbers of patients in Japan and Europe, DNA from this organism has been identified *in situ* within the granulomas on histological sections, and *Propionibacteria* are potent stimulators of granulomatous inflammation in animal models. Another interpretation of these findings, however, is that *Propionibacteria* propagate in nodal tissue of sarcoid patients resulting from an intrinsic immune defect in cell-mediated immunity, and that they may be associated with but not etiologically responsible for the development of disease.

MARKERS OF DISEASE ACTIVITY

PERIPHERAL LYMPHOPENIA One of the difficulties in managing patients with sarcoidosis is ascertaining the activity of disease at a given point in time. Peripheral lymphopenia is a simple marker of disease activity. The biological explanation for this phenomenon is that circulating lymphocytes are recruited to sites of active granulomatous inflammation, thus depleting the peripheral lymphocyte pool. As inflammation resolves with concomitant reductions in secreted cytokines and chemokines, as well as reduced adhesion molecule expression, a normal lymphocyte population is restored in the circulating blood.

ANGIOTENSIN-CONVERTING ENZYME Historically, the serum angiotensin-converting enzyme (ACE) was proposed and used as a serological marker of disease activity. Granulomas from some, but not all, patients secrete ACE, and levels can correlate with the activity of granulomatous inflammation. However, many patients with active sarcoidosis have normal ACE levels; therefore, this marker cannot be universally applied.

LYSOZYME Lysozyme is an antibacterial protein released from activated mononuclear phagocytes. Although it is nonspecific, levels of this enzyme are elevated in the serum of patients with sarcoidosis. Lysozyme levels have been shown to correlate with number of organs involved, radiographic stage, and are frequently elevated even in patients with normal ACE levels.

CYTOKINE MARKERS Following the identification of biological mediators present in sarcoidosis, several studies have been conducted regarding their potential use as markers of disease activity. Although levels of IFN-γ, IL-12, and IL-18 are indeed elevated in patients with sarcoidosis, there is considerable variability between individual patients as well as overlap with values observed in controls. Soluble forms of the TNF receptors are released into the BAL fluid and the bloodstream during active granulomatous inflammation. Elevated levels of soluble TNF-receptor II have been demonstrated in the serum of patients with active sarcoidosis, and these levels decrease in response to steroid therapy. Thus, serum levels of this soluble receptor may directly reflect the activation of macrophages within granulomas and may provide a novel serological marker of sarcoid inflammatory activity.

MECHANISMS OF THERAPY

With the remarkable progress in the understanding of the pathophysiology of sarcoidosis over the past decades, the mechanisms of action of the available therapies have become increasingly clear. Moreover, new, more selective, biologicals targeting some of the key mediators of disease have the potential to more potently suppress the inflammatory response of sarcoidosis with less toxicity than older agents.

CORTICOSTEROIDS Corticosteroids have been the mainstay of therapy for sarcoidosis since 1951, and their diverse actions on multiple cell types are responsible for their efficacy. Steroids enhance the expression of inhibitor κB, therefore reducing the amount of nuclear factor-κB available for translocation to the nucleus in which it can induce proinflammatory gene transcription. In part through this mechanism, steroids inhibit the expression of a number of proinflammatory cytokines important to granulomatous inflammation, including IL-2, IL-8, IL-12, IFN-γ, and TNF-α. In addition, they promote apoptois of activated T cells and reduce cellular activation. Despite these potent immunosuppressive effects, some studies suggest that long-term outcomes in sarcoidosis are only minimally affected by corticosteroid treatment. Moreover, although most patients appear to be at least somewhat steroid responsive, some have steroid refractory disease. Because of these issues and the well-known complications of long-term corticosteroid therapy, alternative agents are often necessary.

ANTIMALARIALS   Chloroquine and hydroxychloroquine have been used to treat sarcoidosis and are particularly efficacious for cutaneous and mucosal disease. These drugs interfere with MHC–peptide interactions by altering the intravesicular pH, and thus are thought to reduce the amount of presented antigen. They inhibit the degradation of proteins by acid hydrolases within lysosomes, and inhibit the assembly and transport of MHC–peptide complexes to the cell surface.

METHOTREXATE   Methotrexate interferes with purine metabolism and polyamine synthesis by inhibiting dihydrofolate reductase and transmethylation reactions. Low doses of methotrexate have anti-inflammatory properties by enhancing adenosine release from cells. Adenosine acts through G-protein coupled-cell surface receptors to produce a variety of effects including suppression of TNF, IL-6, IL-8, and reactive oxygen species release from macrophages, suppression of lymphocyte proliferation, and reduction in the expression of adhesion molecules important for lymphocyte trafficking.

TNF INHIBITORS   In light of the critical role of TNF in granuloma formation, drugs that inhibit TNF production or action have become attractive therapeutic options for sarcoidosis. Pentoxyfylline is a methylxanthine derivative that acts by inhibiting phosphodiesterase and thus raising intracellular cAMP. This drug inhibits TNF production by alveolar macrophages and inhibits IL-12 production by blood mononuclear cells. Unfortunately, because of gastrointestinal side effects, it remains difficult to achieve therapeutic doses of sufficient magnitude to suppress cytokine production in vivo.

Thalidomide also inhibits TNF production by mononuclear cells and has shown efficacy in cutaneous sarcoidosis. In addition to TNF inhibition, thalidomide also has suppressive effects on several other cytokines. However, thalidomide both suppresses and enhances IL-12 production depending on the experimental conditions, and its efficacy for granulomatous involvement of organs other than the skin is questionable. Finally, its use has been limited by important toxicities including teratogenicity and peripheral neuropathy.

Infliximab is a chimeric mouse/human monoclonal antibody that binds TNF-α, preventing its interaction with the TNF-receptor. Its efficacy in rheumatoid arthritis and Crohn's disease suggests that it may also be beneficial in sarcoidosis. Indeed, several case reports and small case series have reported impressive results in patients with sarcoidosis. Given the important role of TNF in immunity, it is not surprising that infliximab increases susceptibility to infection, and can lead to disseminated disease in patients with indolent TB masquerading as sarcoidosis. The efficacy and safety of infliximab for sarcoidosis is being evaluated in large, multicenter trials.

ANTIBIOTICS   Because accumulating data suggest that sarcoidosis may be caused by an exaggerated immune response against microbial peptides, antibiotics may have the potential to eradicate the triggering antigen. One small, uncontrolled study with minocycline for chronic, cutaneous sarcoidosis yielded impressive results with 83% of patients responding (67% complete remission of lesions, 16% partial remission). All patients with elevated ACE levels and lymphopenia at the onset of the trial showed normalization of ACE and resolution of lymphopenia with antibiotic therapy. Although bacterial killing may, in part, explain the efficacy of this intervention, tetracyclines have many anti-inflammatory properties that may contribute to the suppression of granulomatous inflammation in sarcoidosis. For example, tetracyclines inhibit chemotactic and phagocytic functions of leukocytes, block lymphocyte proliferation, and inhibit granuloma formation in vitro. Minocycline inhibits the proliferation of CD4+ T cells in response to TCR activation as well as the secretion of IL-2, IFN-γ, and TNF-α by them. Finally, minocycline inhibits TNF-α production by human keratinocytes. Although these results with mincocyline in cutaneous sarcoidosis are intriguing, larger, randomized clinical trials will be required to confirm the observations of this pilot study and to determine, if reproducible, the efficacy in other affected organs as well as in other diverse populations.

CONCLUSION

More effective treatment of sarcoidosis depends critically on a fundamental understanding of disease pathogenesis, at both the cellular and molecular levels. Significant strides have been made in the knowledge of the immunopathogenesis of sarcoidosis. Immunological studies have provided compelling evidence that an antigen is indeed driving the granulomatous inflammation of sarcoidosis, and molecular studies have revealed that components of an endogenous microbial organism may be one of the elusive antigens. The same technology that has made these studies possible can potentially be translated into a diagnostic test in hospital molecular genetics labs for the detection of putative antigens in individual patients.

In addition to an inciting antigen, the genetic make-up of the host appears to be a critical determinant not only for the initial development of an immunological response against the sarcoid antigen(s), but also for determining the course of disease. In this regard, the MHC region on the short arm of chromosome 6 has been most intensely investigated, and a number of genes in this area have been associated with risk and clinical course of disease. In a genome wide microsatellite linkage analysis to identify chromosomal regions contributing to the risk of sarcoidosis, the most prominent peak was found at the MHC. Candidate genes in this region include HLA genes, as well as immune response genes such as TNF-α.

The observation that TNF-α is critical for granulomatous inflammation has had important clinical translation. A serum assay that measures levels of the soluble receptor for TNF has been developed and may emerge as a sensitive marker of disease activity that can be used to follow the course of disease in the clinic. Anti-TNF therapies have been developed and early studies suggest that they may be the most potent suppressors of granulomatous inflammation available. If additional evidence continues to support a role for microbes as etiological triggers, then combination therapy with antibiotics aimed at eradicating the inciting organism, in combination with targeted immunosuppressive therapy to dampen an exuberant immune response, may offer patients a novel treatment approach with less toxicity and better efficacy than other options.

SELECTED REFERENCES

Abe C, Iwai K, Mikami R, Hosoda Y. Frequent isolation of Propionibacterium acnes from sarcoidosis lymph nodes. Zentralbl Bakteriol Mikrobiol Hyg [A] 1984;256(4):541–547.

Bachelez H, Senet P, Cadranel J, Kaoukhov A, Dubertret L. The use of tetracyclines for the treatment of sarcoidosis. Arch Dermatol 2001; 137:69–73.

Baughman RP, Keeton D, Lower EE. Relationship between interleukin-8 and neutrophils in the BAL fluid of sarcoidosis. Sarcoidosis 1994; 11:S217–S220.

Baughman RP, Lower EE. Infliximab for refractory sarcoidosis. Sarcoidosis Vasc Diffuse Lung Dis 2001;18:70–74.

Baughman RP, Lower EE, du Bois RM. Sarcoidosis. Lancet 2003;361: 1111–1118.

Baughman RP, Strohofer SA, Buchsbaum J, Lower EE. Release of tumor necrosis factor by alveolar macrophages of patients with sarcoidosis. J Lab Clin Med 1990;115:36–42.

Bocart D, Lecossier D, De Lassence A, Valeyre D, Battesti JP, Hance AJ. A search for mycobacterial DNA in granulomatous tissues from patients with sarcoidosis using the polymerase chain reaction. Am Rev Respir Dis 1992;145:1142–1148.

Cannone M, Vago L, Porini G, et al. Detection of mycobacterium tuberculosis DNA using nested polymerase chain reaction in lymph nodes with sarcoidosis, fixed in formalin and embedded in paraffin. Pathologica 1997;89:512–516.

du Bois RM, Goh N, McGrath D, Cullinan P. Is there a role for microorganisms in the pathogenesis of sarcoidosis? J Intern Med 2003;253: 4–17.

Duncan MR, Berman B. Gamma interferon is the lymphokine and beta interferon the monokine responsible for inhibition of fibroblast collagen production and late but not early fibroblast proliferation. J Exp Med 1985;162:516–527.

Eishi Y, Suga M, Ishige I, et al. Quantitative analysis of mycobacterial and propionibacterial DNA in lymph nodes of Japanese and European patients with sarcoidosis. J Clin Microbiol 2002;40:198–204.

el-Zaatari FA, Naser SA, Markesich DC, Kalter DC, Engstand L, Graham DY. Identification of Mycobacterium avium complex in sarcoidosis. J Clin Microbiol 1996;34:2240–2245.

Fidler HM, Rook GA, Johnson NM, McFadden J. Mycobacterium tuberculosis DNA in tissue affected by sarcoidosis. BMJ 1993;306:546–549.

Gazouli M, Ikonomopoulos J, Trigidou R, Foteinou M, Kittas C, Gorgoulis V. Assessment of mycobacterial, propionibacterial, and human herpesvirus 8 DNA in tissues of greek patients with sarcoidosis. J Clin Microbiol 2002;40:3060–3063.

Gerdes J, Richter E, Rusch-Gerdes S, et al. Mycobacterial nucleic acids in sarcoid lesions. Lancet 1992;339:1536, 1537.

Ghossein RA, Ross DG, Salomon RN, Rabson AR. A search for mycobacterial DNA in sarcoidosis using the polymerase chain reaction. Am J Clin Pathol 1994;101:733–737.

Grosser M, Luther T, Muller J, et al. Detection of M. tuberculosis DNA in sarcoidosis: correlation with T-cell response. Lab Invest 1999;79:775–784.

Grunewald J, Janson CH, Eklund A, et al. Restricted V alpha 2.3 gene usage by CD4+ T lymphocytes in bronchoalveolar lavage fluid from sarcoidosis patients correlates with HLA-DR3. Eur J Immunol 1992; 22:129–135.

Homma JY, Abe C, Chosa H, et al. Bacteriological investigation on biopsy specimens from patients with sarcoidosis. Jpn J Exp Med 1978;48: 251–255.

Hunninghake GW, Crystal RG. Pulmonary sarcoidosis: A disorder mediated by excess helper T-lymphocyte activity at sites of disease activity. N Engl J Med 1981;305:429–434.

Ikonomopoulos JA, Gorgoulis VG, Zacharatos PV, et al. Multiplex polymerase chain reaction for the detection of mycobacterial DNA in cases of tuberculosis and sarcoidosis. Mod Pathol 1999;12: 854–862.

Inoue Y, King TE Jr, Tinkle SS, Dockstader K, Newman LS. Human mast cell basic fibroblast growth factor in pulmonary fibrotic disorders. Am J Pathol 1996;149:2037–2054.

Ishige I, Usui Y, Takemura T, Eishi Y. Quantitative PCR of mycobacterial and propionibacterial DNA in lymph nodes of Japanese patients with sarcoidosis. Lancet 1999;354:120–123.

Kaneko H, Yamada H, Mizuno S, et al. Role of tumor necrosis factor-alpha in Mycobacterium-induced granuloma formation in tumor necrosis factor-alpha-deficient mice. Lab Invest 1999;79:379–386.

Katzenstein A-L. Katzenstein and Askin's surgical pathology of nonneoplastic lung disease. In: Livolsi V, ed. Major Problems in Pathology. Volume 13. Philadelphia, PA: W.B. Saunders, 1997; pp. 477.

Keane J, Gershon S, Wise RP, et al. Tuberculosis associated with infliximab, a tumor necrosis factor alpha-neutralizing agent. N Engl J Med 2001;345:1098–1104.

Klemen H, Husain AN, Cagle PT, Garrity ER, Popper HH. Mycobacterial DNA in recurrent sarcoidosis in the transplanted lung—a PCR-based study on four cases. Virchows Arch 2000;436:365–369.

Li N, Bajoghli A, Kubba A, Bhawan J. Identification of mycobacterial DNA in cutaneous lesions of sarcoidosis. J Cutan Pathol 1999;26: 271–278.

Limper AH, Colby TV, Sanders MS, Asakura S, Roche PC, DeRemee RA. Immunohistochemical localization of transforming growth factor-beta 1 in the nonnecrotizing granulomas of pulmonary sarcoidosis. Am J Respir Crit Care Med 1994;149:197–204.

Lisby G, Milman N, Jacobsen GK. Search for Mycobacterium paratuberculosis DNA in tissue from patients with sarcoidosis by enzymatic gene amplification. APMIS 1993;101:876–878.

Moller DR, Chen ES. Genetic basis of remitting sarcoidosis: triumph of the trimolecular complex? Am J Respir Cell Mol Biol 2002;27:391–395.

Moller DR, Forman JD, Liu MC, et al. Enhanced expression of IL-12 associated with Th1 cytokine profiles in active pulmonary sarcoidosis. J Immunol 1996;156:4952–4960.

Moller DR. Involvement of T cells and alterations in T cell receptors in sarcoidosis. Semin Respir Infect 1998;13:174–183.

Moller DR. Pulmonary fibrosis of sarcoidosis: new approaches, old ideas. Am J Respir Cell Mol Biol 2003;29:S37–S41.

Nakayama T, Hashimoto S, Amemiya E, Horie T. Elevation of plasma-soluble tumour necrosis factor receptors (TNF-R) in sarcoidosis. Clin Exp Immunol 1996;104:318–324.

Nishiwaki T, Yoneyama H, Eishi Y, et al. Indigenous pulmonary Propionibacterium acnes primes the host in the development of sarcoid-like pulmonary granulomatosis in mice. Am J Pathol 2004; 165:631–639.

Ohchi T, Shijubo N, Kawabata I, et al. Polymorphism of Clara cell 10-kD protein gene of sarcoidosis. Am J Respir Crit Care Med 2004; 169:180–186.

Ota M, Amakawa R, Uehira K, et al. Involvement of dendritic cells in sarcoidosis. Thorax 2004;59:408–413.

Pesci A, Bertorelli G, Gabrielli M, Olivieri D. Mast cells in fibrotic lung disorders. Chest 1993;103:989–996.

Pinkston P, Bitterman PB, Crystal RG. Spontaneous release of interleukin-2 by lung T lymphocytes in active pulmonary sarcoidosis. N Engl J Med 1983;308:793–800.

Popper HH, Klemen H, Hoefler G, Winter E. Presence of mycobacterial DNA in sarcoidosis. Hum Pathol 1997;28:796–800.

Popper HH, Winter E, Hofler G. DNA of Mycobacterium tuberculosis in formalin-fixed, paraffin-embedded tissue in tuberculosis and sarcoidosis detected by polymerase chain reaction. Am J Clin Pathol 1994;101:738–741.

Richter E, Greinert U, Kirsten D, et al. Assessment of mycobacterial DNA in cells and tissues of mycobacterial and sarcoid lesions. Am J Respir Crit Care Med 1996;153:375–380.

Robinson BW, McLemore TL, Crystal RG. Gamma interferon is spontaneously released by alveolar macrophages and lung T lymphocytes in patients with pulmonary sarcoidosis. J Clin Invest 1985;75:1488–1495.

Rybicki BA, Iannuzzi MC, Frederick MM, et al. Familial aggregation of sarcoidosis. A case-control etiologic study of sarcoidosis (ACCESS). Am J Respir Crit Care Med 2001;164:2085–2091.

Saboor SA, Johnson NM, McFadden J. Detection of mycobacterial DNA in sarcoidosis and tuberculosis with polymerase chain reaction. Lancet 1992;339:1012–1015.

Sato H, Grutters JC, Pantelidis P, et al. HLA-DQB1*0201: a marker for good prognosis in British and Dutch patients with sarcoidosis. Am J Respir Cell Mol Biol 2002;27:406–412.

Schurmann M, Reichel P, Muller-Myhsok B, Schlaak M, Muller-Quernheim J, Schwinger E. Results from a genome-wide search for predisposing genes in sarcoidosis. Am J Respir Crit Care Med 2001; 164:840–846.

Shigehara K, Shijubo N, Ohmichi M, et al. IL-12 and IL-18 are increased and stimulate IFN-gamma production in sarcoid lungs. J Immunol 2001;166:642–649.

Song Z, Marzilli L, Greenlee BM et al. Mycobacterial catalase-peroxidase is a tissue antigen and target of the adaptive immune response in systemic sarcoidosis. J Exp Med 2005;201:755–767.

Thakker B, Black M, Foulis AK. Mycobacterial nucleic acids in sarcoid lesions. Lancet 1992;339:1537.

Tomita H, Sato S, Matsuda R et al. Serum Lysozyme levels and clinical features of saroidosis. Lung 1999;177:161–167.

Vokurka M, Lecossier D, du Bois RM, et al. Absence of DNA from mycobacteria of the M. tuberculosis complex in sarcoidosis. Am J Respir Crit Care Med 1997;156:1000–1003.

Wilsher ML, Menzies RE, Croxson MC. Mycobacterium tuberculosis DNA in tissues affected by sarcoidosis. Thorax 1998;53: 871–874.

Yamada T, Eishi Y, Ikeda S, et al. In situ localization of Propionibacterium acnes DNA in lymph nodes from sarcoidosis patients by signal amplification with catalysed reporter deposition. J Pathol 2002;198: 541–547.

30 Disorders of Pulmonary Surfactant Homeostasis

JEFFREY A. WHITSETT, SUSAN E. WERT, AND BRUCE C. TRAPNELL

SUMMARY

Pulmonary surfactant is required for adaptation to air breathing after birth, reducing surface tension at the air–liquid interface in the alveolus to maintain lung volumes during the respiratory cycle. Disorders of pulmonary surfactant homeostasis are associated with acute and chronic respiratory disease in infants and adults. Mutations in the surfactant protein genes encoding SP-B and SP-C cause severe respiratory failure in infancy and chronic interstitial lung disease in older individuals.

Key Words: ABCA3 transporter; pulmonary alveolar proteinosis (PAP); pulmonary surfactant; *SFTPB*; surfactant proteins B (SP-B).

INTRODUCTION

Pulmonary surfactant is required for adaptation to air breathing after birth, reducing surface tension at the air–liquid interface in the alveolus to maintain lung volumes during the respiratory cycle. Pulmonary surfactant is a complex mixture of proteins and lipids whose synthesis, packaging, secretion, and catabolism are tightly controlled at transcriptional and post-transcriptional levels. It is well established that the lack of pulmonary surfactant causes respiratory distress syndrome (RDS) in preterm infants. Abnormalities in surfactant content, composition, and function are also associated with acute RDSs in older patients in a variety of clinical conditions associated with lung injury. As the genetic and cellular systems regulating surfactant homeostasis are increasingly understood, gene mutations, and abnormalities in the pathways mediating surfactant homeostasis are being implicated in the pathogenesis of both acute and chronic pulmonary disorders (Table 30-1). This chapter summarizes disorders of surfactant metabolism, including lung diseases caused by mutations in genes encoding surfactant proteins (SP)-B, -C the ABCA3 transport protein, and those related to abnormalities in granulocyte macrophage-colony stimulating factor (GM-CSF) signaling.

THE PULMONARY SURFACTANT SYSTEM Pulmonary surfactant is a lipid/protein complex that is synthesized by type-II epithelial cells lining the alveoli of the lungs (Fig. 30-1). Surfactant lipids, predominantly phosphatidylcholine, and SP-B and SP-C, are cotransported to lamellar bodies, the major intracellular storage organelle of pulmonary surfactant. Lamellar bodies are exocytosed into the airspace in response to stretch, β-adrenergic, and purinergic agonists. After exocytosis, lamellar bodies unravel and undergo a dramatic change in ultrastructural morphology, producing tubular myelin that represents the major extracellular pool of surfactant lipids from which mono- and multilayered films are formed. The lipid-rich films spread at the air–liquid interface in the alveoli and reduce surface tension, preventing alveolar collapse. Heavy (lamellar bodies and tubular myelin-rich forms) and light (lipid vesicles) can be isolated by differential centrifugation of lavage fluid obtained from the lung. The small aggregate fraction likely represents lipid remnants that are destined for uptake and reutilization or catabolism by type-II cells and alveolar macrophages (AMs). The large aggregate surfactant fraction is highly surface active. Surfactant pool sizes are relatively large at birth (50–100 mg/kg) and fall postnatally to adult levels of approx 5–10 mg/kg. Deficiency of pulmonary surfactant is associated with RDS in preterm infants, a common cause of infant morbidity and mortality. Intracellular and extracellular surfactant pool sizes are precisely maintained by the regulation of synthesis, secretion, reuptake, reutilization, and catabolism.

DISORDERS OF SP-B GENE *(SFTPB)*

SP-B is a 79 amino acid, amphipathic polypeptide that is produced by proteolytic processing of a 381 amino acid precursor as it is trafficked through the endoplasmic reticulum, Golgi apparatus, and multivesicular bodies, to the lamellar bodies in which the active peptide is stored. SP-B and SP-C are packaged together with surfactant lipids in the lamellar bodies and are secreted into the alveolus. The active 79 amino acid peptide is an amphipathic structure that interacts strongly with the choline and glycerol head groups of the surfactant phospholipids. SP-B is fusiogenic, creating extended lipid layers (monolayers and multilayers) that form highly stable films in the alveoli. SP-B enhances the spreading and stability of surfactant lipids and is critical for surfactant tension reduction during respiration. The importance of SP-B in pulmonary homeostasis was shown in SP-B gene knockout mice (*Sftpb⁻/⁻*) and in infants bearing mutations in the *SFTPB* gene. SP-B null mice and infants with mutations in *SFTPB* die of respiratory distress after birth. Marked ultrastructural abnormalities are observed in type-II epithelial cells in the lungs of SP-B-deficient mice, including the lack of lamellar bodies, accumulation of

From: *Principles of Molecular Medicine, Second Edition*
Edited by: M. S. Runge and C. Patterson © Humana Press, Inc., Totowa, NJ

Table 30-1
Disorders of Surfactant Homeostasis

Gene	Inheritance	Phenotype	Defect
ABCA3	Autosomal-recessive	RDS, ILD	Surfactant packaging
SFTPB	Autosomal-recessive	RDS	Surfactant packaging function
SFTPC	Autosomal-dominant	RDS, ILD	Surfactant function misfolded protein
GM-CSF	Not familial	PAP	Defect in alveolar macrophage

GM-CSF, granulocyte macrophage-colony stimulating factor; ILD, interstitial lung disease; PAP, pulmonary alveolar proteinosis; RDS, respiratory distress syndrome.

abnormal, large multivesicular bodies (lamellar body precursors), absence of tubular myelin, and lack of surfactant activity.

HEREDITARY SP-B DEFICIENCY Hereditary SP-B deficiency was first recognized in full-term infants dying from respiratory distress following birth. Since then, more than 75 infants in unrelated families have been identified with this disorder. Hereditary SP-B deficiency is an autosomal-recessive disease caused by mutations in the SFTPB gene that is located on human chromosome 2. More than 25 distinct mutations, including nonsense, missense, and stop codons have been identified. Mutations in the SFTPB gene results in either lack of SP-B mRNA with lack of protein production or the production of abnormal SP-B proproteins that result in misprocessed protein and lack of synthesis of the active SP-B protein. SP-B is required for the normal routing and packaging of surfactant lipids and SP-C in type-II epithelial cells of the lung. Thus, deletion of SP-B also results in the absence of SP-C in the airspaces. Mutations in SP-B generally cause lethal respiratory distress following birth. Several patients with partial defects in SP-B synthesis have been identified, their mutations causing severe chronic lung disease in infancy.

GENETICS Hereditary SP-B deficiency is a relatively rare, autosomal-recessive disorder; the carrier rate for mutations in SFTPB is estimated to be 1 in 600. A number of distinct mutations in the SP-B gene have been associated with hereditary SP-B deficiency. Mutation in exon 4 (termed the 121 insert) is the most common allele associated with this disorder, being detected in 50–60% of the affected individuals. Homozygous SFTPB 121 insert, and compound SFTPB 121 insert inherited in association with other SFTPB mutations have been detected. Although most mutations result in complete lack of SP-B protein in lung lavage, mutations in which alternative splicing results in production of some SP-B have been associated with chronic lung disease. Although mutations in SFTPB generally cause fatal respiratory distress after birth, haploinsufficiency has not been associated with a recognizable clinical disease in the few carriers studied. Heterozygous SP-B knockout mice are susceptible to lung injury and have subtle abnormalities in lung physiology at baseline, suggesting that partial reduction of SP-B may enhance susceptibility to pulmonary disease.

CLINICAL FINDINGS AND DIAGNOSIS IN HEREDITARY SP-B DEFICIENCY Human SP-B deficiency generally presents in full-term infants who develop respiratory distress after birth. In the most affected infants, grunting, retractions, and cyanosis are observed immediately after birth. Symptoms are generally observed before 12 h of age. History of affected family members and/or consanguinity has been associated with the disorder. Consistent with those of RDS in preterm infants, radiographic findings in full-term infants without other underlying causes of respiratory failure include diffuse alveolar infiltrates, alveolar collapse, reticular-granular infiltrates, and air bronchograms. Respiratory distress is progressive. In spite of oxygen and assisted ventilation, surfactant replacement, and/or extracorporeal membrane oxygenation, most infants die in the first weeks or months of life. Surfactant replacement is not effective, the infants generally having no or transient responses to therapy. Definitive diagnosis is made by identification of mutations in both alleles of the SFTPB gene. Lung histology is influenced by age and therapies that have been used to support the infant. Marked histological abnormalities are observed at autopsy or biopsy, with evidence of diffuse alveolar and bronchiolar damage, atelectasis, hyaline membrane interstitial thickening, type-II cell hyperplasia, accumulation of AMs, and proteins in the alveoli, often diagnosed as infantile desquamating interstitial pneumonitis (DIP) or congenital pulmonary alveolar proteinosis (PAP) (Fig. 30-2). Immunohistochemical staining for SP-B or pro-SP-B antibody results in lack of staining when SP-B mRNA is not produced (121 insert). Abnormal accumulation of mutant pro-SP-B or its processing intermediates has been observed in lungs of patients with mutations in which the abnormal proteins are produced and accumulate in either lung cells or within the airspace. Enzyme-linked immunosorbent assay and immunoblot analysis of lung secretions or lung tissue homogenates have been useful in screening for hereditary SP-B deficiency but may not be specific. The absence of SP-B in tracheal aspirates indicates an increased likelihood of the disorder but is not diagnostic. Because SP-B is required for the processing and secretion of SP-C, most mutations in SP-B also cause misprocessing of pro-SP-C and accumulation of an abnormal pro-SP-C peptide in the alveoli that can be detected immunohistochemically or by Western blot analysis. Detection of this pro-SP-C fragment is relatively specific for human SP-B deficiency. Hereditary SP-B deficiency is generally fatal in the neonatal period and no effective therapies have been identified. A number of infants have undergone lung transplantation with prolongation and improvement of life.

DISORDERS OF THE SP-C GENE (SFTPC)

A single gene encoding SP-C (SFTPC) is located on human chromosome 8. SP-C RNA produces a 191 amino acid proprotein from which the active peptide is produced by proteolytic processing in type-II epithelial cells of the lung. The active SP-C peptide associated with surfactant in the airspaces is a 35 amino acid polypeptide expressed only in type-II epithelial cells in the alveoli of the lung. SP-C was initially isolated from surfactant lipid extracts that were used to treat RDS in replacement surfactant preparations, prepared from mammalian lung. Pro-SP-C is palmitoylated and cotrafficked with pro-SP-B through the endoplasmic reticulum and multivesicular bodies to the lamellar bodies of type-II epithelial cells. Proteolytic processing occurs during transit to lamellar bodies. The active SP-C peptide is associated with surfactant lipids, packaged in lamellar bodies and secreted into the alveolar space with the active SP-B peptide and lipids. SP-C inserts into phospholipid films and vesicles via an extremely hydrophobic, α-helical domain that interacts with the acyl groups of the surfactant lipids. The active SP-C peptide is palmitoylated via covalent linkage to cysteine residues near its amino terminus. SP-C disrupts acyl group packaging in lipids, enhances their

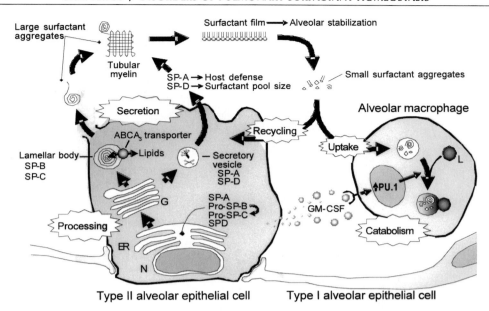

Figure 30-1 Pulmonary surfactant metabolism and homeostasis. The genes encoding surfactant protein (SP)-A, pro-SP-B, pro-SP-C, and SP-D are transcribed in the nucleus of alveolar type-II epithelial cells, translated into nascent polypeptides in the endoplasmic reticulum and processed in the Golgi network (processing). SP-B and SP-C are assembled into lamellar bodies along with surfactant phospholipids, the transport of which may be regulated by the ABCA3 transporter molecule, which is found in the limiting membrane of these organelles. SP-A and SP-D are secreted via nonlamellar body secretory vesicles. Following exocytosis of lamellar bodies and secretory vesicles into the alveolar surface liquid (secretion), lamellar bodies assemble into structures known as tubular myelin as well as large and small aggregate forms. Phospholipids from these extracellular structures move to form a continuous surfactant film that lines the alveolar spaces and airways with polar heads oriented toward the liquid and acyl chains toward the air. Surfactant large aggregate forms, extracellular lamellar bodies and tubular myelin, all have surface-active properties. Surfactant is inactivated by mechanical and biological processes and converted into the surface-inactive, small aggregate forms. Of surfactant small approx 70–80% aggregate forms are taken up by alveolar type-II cells, sorted to lysosomes and reutilized (recycling) or catabolized (not indicated). Alveolar macrophages internalize (uptake) and degrade the remaining small surfactant aggregates (catabolism). The latter process is critical for surfactant homeostasis and is dependent on granulocyte macrophage-colony stimulating factor, which acts via the transcription factor, PU.1, to stimulate catabolism of surfactant lipids and proteins as well as a number of other immune functions of alveolar macrophages.

spreading, and recruits lipids to the surface films to confer surfactant-like activity to purified surfactant lipids. Although SP-B and SP-C interact with lipids via distinct structures, both enhance surfactant activity and are active components of surfactant replacement preparations used clinically. Targeted disruption of the *SFTPC* gene in mice produces an unstable surfactant. In some strains of mice, deletion of SP-C causes severe interstitial lung disease, providing strong evidence for its importance in surfactant function and pulmonary homeostasis.

HEREDITARY SP-C DEFICIENCY Both lack of SP-C and mutations in the gene encoding SP-C *(SFTPC)* have been associated with acute and chronic lung disease in infants and adults. One family has been identified in which the mother and two daughters developed severe interstitial lung disease associated with the lack of production of SP-C, as assessed in lung lavage fluid, and by decreased immunostaining for pro-SP-C in lung biopsies. These findings are consistent with the observation that mice bearing a null allele for the *Sftpc* gene develop severe interstitial lung disease in the postnatal period. Mutations in the *SFTPC* gene cause both acute and chronic pulmonary disease in humans. *SFTPC* mutations also have presented with respiratory failure in the first days of life in full-term infants who develop unexplained respiratory distress, with clinical findings similar to those in SP-B deficiency. More commonly, mutations in *Sftpc* have been associated with chronic interstitial lung disease in infants, with histology being variably classified as chronic pneumonitis of infancy, nonspecific chronic interstitial pneumonitis, and DIP. In adults, the

disorder is classified as idiopathic pulmonary fibrosis, usual interstitial pneumonitis, nonspecific interstitial pneumonitis, or DIP. Although the age of onset and severity of the disease and pathological findings are highly variable, mutations in *SFTPC* are generally inherited in an autosomal-dominant manner, resulting in severe interstitial lung disease and susceptibility to acute respiratory failure following injury or infection. Variability in histopathological findings is likely related in part to distinct mutations, age, and environmental factors, and other genetic modifiers that influence the course of the disease and the pathology observed. A number of *SFTPC* alleles have been associated with severe pulmonary disease. An extended family bearing a dominantly inherited *SFTPC* gene was described in kindred of 16 individuals, most of whom developed severe interstitial lung disease. Chronic lung disease caused by *SFTPC* mutations manifests at various ages from childhood to adulthood. Dyspnea, clubbing, cyanosis, oxygen requirement, and pulmonary exacerbations following viral and other infections are common features of the disorder. Pathological findings include alveolar proteinosis, DIP, alveolar thickening, fibrosis, and mononuclear infiltration (*see* Fig. 30-2). Definitive diagnosis is made by identification of mutations in the *SFTPC* gene. A history of dominantly inherited idiopathic pulmonary fibrosis and RDS supports the likelihood of the diagnosis. However, *de novo* mutations in *SFTPC* appear to occur relatively frequently in this disorder. Immunostaining for pro-SP-C reveals intense staining of pro-SP-C or pro-SP-C peptides in type-II epithelial cells, likely representing accumulation of misfolded or

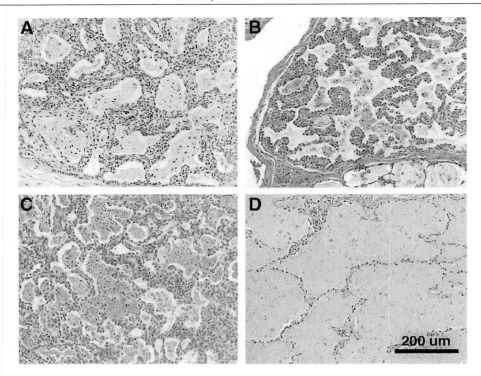

Figure 30-2   Histopathology of surfactant abnormalities found in the lungs of human patients with (**A**) mutations in the *SFTPB* gene, (**B**) mutations in the *SFTPC* gene, (**C**) mutations in the *ABCA3* gene, (**D**) and antibodies to granulocyte macrophage-colony stimulating factor. The histopathological findings in infants with mutations in the *SFTPB, SFTPC,* and *ABCA3* genes (panels A, B, and C, respectively) are remarkably similar, demonstrating varying degrees of interstitial thickening and muscularization of the alveolar septae, remodeling of the alveolar epithelium with type-II cell hyperplasia, as well as accumulation of eosinophilic, proteinaceous, granular material, and alveolar macrophages in the airspaces. However, histopathological findings in adults with antibodies to GM-CSF demonstrate thin-walled, expanded alveoli filled with very uniform, granular, eosinophilic material that is relatively devoid of macrophages. All tissue sections were stained with H&E. All panels are shown at the same magnification. Bar = 200 μm.

misprocessed pro-SP-C. The abnormal pro-SP-C protein interferes with the routing and processing of the pro-SP-C produced from the normal *SFTPC* allele. The pathogenesis of lung disease associated with mutations in *SFTPC* is not known with clarity. It is unclear whether the lack of the active SP-C peptide, pro-SP-C or cytotoxic effects of the accumulation of mutant pro-SP-C proteins contribute to the disease pathogenesis. Definitive therapies for *SFTPC* mutations have not been developed, and many of these patients develop severe respiratory disease. Lung transplantation has resulted in improved longevity and quality of life for some individuals with *SFTPC* mutations.

DISORDERS OF THE ABCA3 TRANSPORTER

Mutations in the ABCA3 transporter have been identified as a cause of acute RDS in term and newborn infants, and the cause of chronic interstitial lung disease in older individuals. ABCA3 is a 1704 amino acid, multiple transmembrane protein of the family of ABC transport proteins, of which the cystic fibrosis transmembrane regulator (CFTR) and the multiple drug resistance protein are members. Although the precise function of the ABCA3 transporter is unknown, its homologues are involved in lipid transport. ABCA3 is expressed in type-II epithelial cells of the lung, being detected at the limiting membranes of lamellar bodies in type-II epithelial cells (*see* Fig. 30-1). The structure of the ABCA3 transporter and its localization suggest its potential role in lipid transport to or from the lamellar bodies, implying its role in intracellular lipid homeostasis.

MUTATIONS IN *ABCA3*: CLINICAL FINDINGS   Mutations in the human *ABCA3* gene have been associated with fatal RDS in term newborn infants. The disorder is inherited in an autosomal-recessive manner. History of consanguinity and a family history of fatal neonatal respiratory distress support the likelihood of the disorder. Mutations have been found throughout the *ABCA3* gene. Like CFTR, ABCA3 is a relatively large multiple transmembrane protein. Like *CFTR*, mutations in *ABCA3* are likely to influence the levels of protein folding, routing, and trafficking to lamellar bodies, and its degradation or function. Although clinical findings in older individuals with the mutations in *ABCA3* are not fully clarified, chronic interstitial lung disease has been associated with the disorder and is under intense clinical study. Radiological findings are consistent with RDS in the newborn infants. Diffuse pulmonary opacification, reticular-granular infiltrates, and air bronchograms are observed. Infants present with grunting, retractions, and cyanosis in the first days of life, and rapidly develop respiratory failure that is refractory to ventilation, surfactant replacement, and extracorporeal membrane oxygenation. Alveolar proteinosis, and mixed AMs, alveolar wall thickening, and type-II cell hyperplasia, consistent with diagnosis of chronic pneumonitis of infancy and PAP, have been observed by microscopy at light and electron microscopic levels (*see* Fig. 30-2). Lamellar bodies are lacking or small, supporting the concept that the ABCA3 transporter affects surfactant lipid transport pathways. There are no known definitive therapies for lung disease caused by mutations in *ABCA3*. In spite of intensive care, affected individuals generally die from respiratory failure in the neonatal period. Clinical findings and disease progression in older individuals with *ABCA3* mutations are not known with certainty.

PULMONARY ALVEOLAR PROTEINOSIS

PAP is a rare disorder characterized by accumulation of lipoproteinaceous material within alveoli, a variable clinical course ranging from respiratory failure to spontaneous resolution and a predilection for secondary opportunistic infections. PAP occurs in three clinically and pathogenetically distinct forms: congenital, secondary, and acquired. Congenital PAP is a heterogeneous group of disorders arising from mutations in the genes encoding SP-B, SP-C, and the ABCA3 transporter as described earlier. Secondary PAP can occur in clinical contexts associated with either functional impairment or reduced numbers of AMs including some hematological malignancies, pharmacological immunosuppression, inhalation of inorganic dusts (e.g., silica) or toxic fumes, and in certain infections. Acquired PAP (also known as idiopathic, primary, or autoimmune PAP), initially described in 1958, has a prevalence of 0.37/100,000 individuals. It occurs primarily as a primary disorder of unknown etiology; however, findings strongly suggest that acquired PAP is an autoimmune disorder directed toward the cytokine, GM-CSF. The acquired form accounts for 90% of PAP in adults and is the focus of the remainder of this chapter.

CLINICAL FINDINGS AND DIAGNOSIS OF PAP   Acquired PAP usually presents in male smokers in the third decade, although it occurs without a gender bias in nonsmokers and also, albeit less commonly, in young children. Progressive exertional dyspnea of insidious onset and cough are typical (75%), whereas fever, chest pain, or hemoptysis also occur less commonly, especially if infection is also present. Significant pulmonary exposure is not a feature in most cases. The physical exam can be unremarkable or may show tachypnea, mild inspiratory crackles (50%), dyspnea (25%) and, infrequently, digital clubbing.

The plain chest radiograph reveals a patchy bilateral airspace disease often similar in appearance to pulmonary edema but without other radiographic signs of left heart failure. High-resolution CT shows patchy ground-glass opacifications with superimposed interlobular septal and intralobular thickening, which are typical but not diagnostic of PAP. Interestingly, the extent of the radiographic abnormalities can be disproportionately greater than expected based on the associated symptoms and physical findings. Routine laboratory tests are frequently within the normal range, however, serum lactate dehydrogenase can be elevated and may be a useful marker of disease severity or exacerbation. When abnormalities are present, pulmonary function tests reveal a restrictive ventilatory defect and a disproportionate, severe reduction of the diffusing capacity. Hypoxia can be significant and is caused by ventilation–perfusion mismatch and intrapulmonary shunt.

A diagnosis of PAP can be established by bronchoalveolar lavage in approx 75% of cases suspected resulting from clinical and radiographic findings. The bronchoalveolar lavage fluid is milky in appearance and forms waxy sediment on standing. Microscopically, it is acellular with relatively few inflammatory cells. AMs are abnormal in appearance ranging from small and monocyte-like to large foamy cells that are fragile and are destroyed during cytocentrifugation leaving large acellular eosinophilic bodies in a diffuse background of granular basophilic material. Both the proteinaceous material and AMs stain positively with periodic acid-Schiff reagent and SP immunohistochemical stains. Ultrastructural analysis reveals that the amorphous granular intra-alveolar material consists of surfactant. Open lung biopsy, the gold standard for diagnosis of PAP, reveals parenchymal architecture that is relatively preserved unless secondary infection is present. Alveoli are filled with granular material that is eosinophilic (*see* Fig. 30-2D) and stains strongly with periodic acid-Schiff reagent or by SP immunohistochemistry. A serological test has been developed for diagnosis of acquired PAP that is reported to have high sensitivity (100%) and specificity (98%).

The natural history of PAP typically is marked by persistent symptoms, which vary somewhat in intensity over time. Some individuals show spontaneous improvement (approx 8%) whereas others show progressive deterioration resulting in a 5-yr survival of 74.7 ± 8.1%. Most PAP deaths result directly from respiratory failure (approx 72%), whereas a smaller proportion are the result of uncontrolled infection (approx 20%). Secondary infections are common in PAP, unexpectedly owing to opportunistic pathogens such as *Nocardia* spp. The relatively frequent occurrence of extrapulmonary infections in PAP suggests a defect in systemic host defense.

PATHOGENESIS OF PAP   The initial description of PAP established that the material accumulating in alveoli in PAP was made up phospholipids, lesser amounts of proteins, and minimal carbohydrates. Subsequent studies suggested that this material was pulmonary surfactant but failed to determine if the alveolar filling abnormality was because of increased production, decreased clearance, or the expression of abnormal surfactant lipids or proteins. Ultrastructural, biochemical, and functional studies together with studies in genetically modified mice strongly support the concept that the alveolar material in PAP is, in fact, surfactant, which accumulates resulting from reduced clearance rather than overproduction. The association of acquired PAP with smoking suggests a possible etiological link, however the mechanism of this is unknown. A prolonged search over three decades to identify a presumed "irritant" (e.g., silica or an infectious agent) thought to stimulate increased surfactant production was fruitless. Notwithstanding, a number of AM abnormalities were identified, perhaps the most striking of which were large membrane-bound, surfactant-filled intracellular inclusion bodies that imparted a foamy appearance to the cells. Functional abnormalities were also noted including defects in chemotaxis, adhesion, phagocytosis, microbicidal activity, and phagolysosome fusion. The "overstuffed AM" theory was advanced to explain these findings, however, support for the theory was weakened by the finding that lung lavage fluid from PAP patients could recapitulate some of these abnormalities in normal AMs. Further, identification of an "immunoinhibitory" activity in the lungs and sera of these patients, which blocked mitogen-stimulated proliferation of normal monocytes, suggested a circulating factor might be involved in the pathogenesis of PAP.

ROLE OF GM-CSF IN MURINE PAP   An unexpected but important clue about the pathogenesis of PAP came in 1994 with the discovery that mice deficient in GM-CSF owing to gene ablation developed a pulmonary phenotype histologically similar to acquired PAP in humans. Before then, GM-CSF, a 23-kDa cytokine expressed similarly in humans and mice, was thought to primarily regulate growth of hematological cells in the bone marrow. However, the absence of gross baseline hematological disturbances in GM-CSF-deficient mice cast doubt on this belief. In contrast, development of PAP in these mice established a critical role for GM-CSF in the lung. Biochemically, histologically, and ultrastructurally, the alveolar material in murine PAP was similar to that derived from the lungs of human individuals with acquired PAP. Biochemical and molecular biological studies of these mice established that the disruption in surfactant homeostasis was not because of a decrease in production of surfactant. Rather, it was owing to a decrease in surfactant clearance secondary to decreased catabolism of both surfactant lipids and SP by AMs. Despite this catabolic defect, uptake of both surfactant lipids and proteins by AMs is not impaired, which accounts for the large foamy appearance of these cells that is characteristic of PAP.

A series of studies established that GM-CSF maintains surfactant homeostasis by regulation of surfactant catabolism by AMs. Double transgenic mice carrying an ablated GM-CSF gene and a transgene that expressed GM-CSF specifically in the lungs failed to develop PAP, thus demonstrating the lung as the site of action of GM-CSF. However, this study did not identify the precise cellular target of GM-CSF: did the critical regulation of surfactant homeostasis by GM-CSF involve AMs or alveolar type-II epithelial cells? This question was answered using another murine model of PAP caused by GM-CSF receptor gene ablation. Transplantation of bone marrow from mice with normal GM-CSF common β-chain receptor ($R_\beta c$) expression into GM $R_\beta c^{-/-}$ mice resulted in resolution of defective surfactant metabolism in PAP. Because in the recipient mice, only the AMs derived from the donor mice, but not alveolar type-II epithelial cells were responsive to GM-CSF; these results demonstrated that AMs were the principal therapeutic target of GM-CSF replacement.

The discovery that GM-CSF- and GM-CSF $R_\beta c$-deficient mice develop PAP prompted a re-evaluation of the pathogenesis of human-acquired PAP as a disorder of GM-CSF deficiency. No genetic mutations in either GM-CSF or its receptor have been identified in adult individuals with acquired PAP. Furthermore, the levels of immunoreactive GM-CSF are increased in PAP, not decreased as would be predicted based on the mouse findings.

AUTOIMMUNE ANTI-GM-CSF AUTOANTIBODIES A critical observation was made by researchers linking the pathogenesis of human-acquired PAP to GM-CSF through a series of experiments that re-examined the "immunoinhibitory" activity present in these patients. PAP lung lavage fluid, but not that of normals, inhibited GM-CSF-dependent proliferation of TF-1 cells and competitively inhibited binding of GM-CSF to cellular GM-CSF receptors or an anti-GM-CSF monoclonal antibody. This group subsequently identified the inhibitory activity in acquired PAP to be a neutralizing anti-GM-CSF antibody of the immunoglobulin G isotype class. The antibody is present in all cases of acquired PAP but not in cases of congenital or secondary PAP, other lung disorders or normal controls. Anti-GM-CSF autoantibodies are polyclonal, present at very high levels in blood and lungs, and bind GM-CSF with very high affinity. Importantly, they eliminate GM-CSF bioactivity from the lungs; the neutralizing capacity exceeds the GM-CSF concentrations by up to 20,000-fold. Thus, although GM-CSF itself is not absent in the lungs in acquired PAP, it is biologically inactivated by the neutralizing anti-GM-CSF autoantibody.

GM-CSF AND TERMINAL DIFFERENTIATION OF AM The clinical laboratory abnormalities of AMs in acquired PAP prompted detailed studies in GM-CSF deficient mice ($GM^{-/-}$). AMs from $GM^{-/-}$ mice had numerous abnormalities including defects in cell adhesion, cell-surface pathogen recognition receptor expression, nonspecific and receptor-mediated phagocytosis, superoxide production, microbial killing, and proinflammatory cytokine secretion. These diverse abnormalities suggested that pulmonary GM-CSF deficiency may cause a maturational defect in AMs. Strong support for this hypothesis came from the observation that the presence and level of pulmonary GM-CSF regulates

the presence and level of PU.1 in AMs. PU.1 is a transcription factor known to stimulate proliferation and differentiation of myeloid progenitors and is required for production of macrophages. The maturational defect hypothesis was further strongly supported by the observation that retroviral-mediated replacement of PU.1 in cultured AMs from GM-CSF-deficient mice restored all of the abnormalities described above and corrected abnormalities in catabolism of surfactant lipids and protein. Together, these data demonstrated that GM-CSF, via PU.1, stimulated the terminal differentiation of murine AMs in the lungs. These studies have established that GM-CSF, via PU.1, regulates surfactant homeostasis as well as several mechanisms of AM-mediated innate immunity in the murine lung (Fig. 30-3). The striking similarities in PAP histopathology, AM morphology, and parallels in macrophage dysfunction in murine and human PAP suggest a common pathogenic mechanism: elimination of pulmonary GM-CSF signaling causes incomplete maturation and dysfunction of AMs.

IMPLICATIONS OF PULMONARY GM-CSF FOR MECHANISMS OF LUNG HOST DEFENSE As the pulmonary resident of the mononuclear phagocyte system, the AM plays a central role in lung host defense. Thus, dysfunction of these cells because of the absence of pulmonary GM-CSF signaling might be expected to impair lung host defense. Consistent with this concept, GM-CSF deficient mice have increased susceptibility to pulmonary infection by group B *Streptococcus*, and *Pneumocystis carinii* (after CD4$^+$-depletion) and had severely impaired pulmonary clearance of bacterial, fungal, and viral pathogens. Patients with acquired PAP have increased susceptibility to microbial lung infections, suggesting a defect in lung host defense. Based on the strong similarities in murine and human PAP, it is tempting to speculate that the presence of autoimmune anti-GM-CSF antibody may impair AM-mediated lung host defense mechanisms in humans, too. However, further studies are required to determine if this is true.

THERAPY OF PAP Treatment of PAP depends on the clinical context. Congenital PAP is treated by supportive care, although lung transplantation has been reported. Secondary PAP generally resolves with treatment of the underlying condition, for example, chemotherapy for hematological malignancy. The standard of care for acquired PAP is whole lung lavage. Although not documented in prospective, randomized trials, whole lung lavage improves clinical, physiological, and radiographic findings and improves survival in acquired PAP (5-yr survival: 94 ±2% with lavage vs 85 ±5% without lavage; $n = 146$, $p = 0.04$). In patients requiring repeated lavage, the median duration of clinical benefit from lavage has been reported to be 15 mo.

Several experimental therapeutic trials of GM-CSF administration in patients with acquired PAP have been or are being conducted. One trial evaluated subcutaneous GM-CSF in 14 PAP patients, and found an overall response rate of 43% with an improvement. An ongoing study in the United States is also evaluating subcutaneous GM-CSF therapy in acquired PAP. In Japan, a network of investigators is evaluating aerosolized GM-CSF in acquired PAP. Although early results from these trials are encouraging, no firm conclusions can be drawn regarding the effectiveness of GM-CSF therapy for acquired PAP. Interestingly, however, a decrease in pulmonary anti-GM-CSF antibody levels in association with clinical improvement has suggested that "desensitization" to GM-CSF may be involved. Other experimental therapeutic approaches under current consideration include plasmapheresis, immune globulin, and agents to decrease B-lymphocyte antibody production.

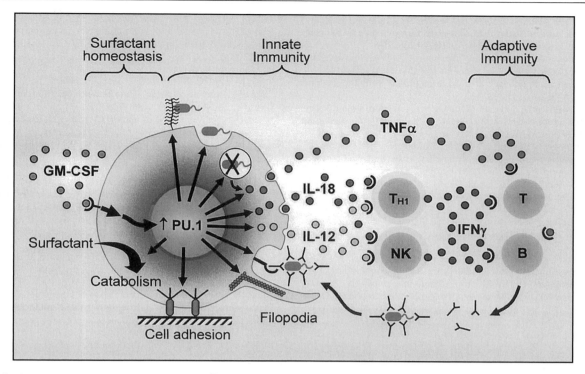

Figure 30-3 Model illustrating role of granulocyte macrophage-colony stimulating factor in modulation of murine alveolar macrophage function. Pulmonary GM-CSF stimulates PU.1 levels in alveolar macrophages in the lung. Alveolar macrophages from GM-CSF knockout mice have a number of functional abnormalities including defects in cell adhesion, surfactant catabolism, expression of microbial pathogen-associated molecular pattern receptors (e.g., Toll-like receptors, mannose receptor), phagocytosis of bacteria, fungi and virus, intracellular killing of bacteria (independent of uptake), pathogen-stimulated secretion of cytokines (tumor necrosis factor-α, IL-12, IL-18), Fc receptor-mediated phagocytosis, and SP and lipid uptake/degradation. Cytoskeletal organization is abnormal and may in part account for defects in phagocytosis. The inability of alveolar macrophages to release IL-12/IL-18 severely impairs the interferon (IFN)-γ response to pulmonary infection, thus impairing an important molecular connection between innate and adaptive immunity in the lung. Retroviral vector-mediated constitutive expression of PU.1 in AMs from GM$^{-/-}$ mice corrects all of these defects, suggesting that GM-CSF stimulates terminal differentiation of alveolar macrophages through the global transcription factor PU.1.

CONCLUSION

Disorders of pulmonary surfactant homeostasis are associated with acute and chronic respiratory disease in infants and adults. Mutations in the SP genes encoding SP-B and SP-C cause severe respiratory failure in infancy and chronic interstitial lung disease in older individuals. Mutations in the ABCA3 transport protein disrupt lamellar body function and surfactant function to cause acute and chronic lung disease with histological features similar to those associated with mutation in the SP genes. Mutations in SFTPB, SFTPC, and ABCA3 disrupt surfactant function and cellular homeostasis in the respiratory epithelium. In contrast, alveolar proteinosis, associated with accumulation of normal SP and lipids, is a disorder of surfactant catabolism by AMs.

SELECTED REFERENCES

Amin RS, Wert SE, Baughman RP, et al. Surfactant protein deficiency in familial interstitial lung disease. J Pediatr 2001;139:85–92.

Anderson KL, Smith KA, Conners K, McKercher SR, Maki RA, Torbett BE. Myeloid development is selectively disrupted in PU.1 null mice. Blood 1998;91:3702–3710.

Andriole MT, Ballas M, Wilson GL. The association of nocardiosis and pulmonary alveolar proteinosis: a case study. Ann Intern Med 1963; 60:266–275.

Asamoto H, Kitaichi M, Nishimura K, Itoh H, Izumi T. Primary pulmonary alveolar proteinosis—clinical observation of 68 patients in Japan (in Japanese). Nihon Kyobu Shikkan Gakkai Zasshi 1995;33:835–845.

Avery ME, Mead J. Surface properties in relation to atelectasis and hyaline membrane disease. Am J Dis Child 1959;97:517–523.

Ballard PL, Nogee LM, Beers MF, et al. Partial deficiency of surfactant protein B in an infant with chronic lung disease. Pediatrics 1995;96:1046–1052.

Ben-Dov I, Kishinevski Y, Roznman J, et al. Pulmonary alveolar proteinosis in Israel: Ethnic clustering. Isr Med Assoc J 1999;1:75–78.

Berclaz PY, Shibata Y, Whitsett JA, Trapnell BC. GM-CSF, via PU.1, regulates alveolar macrophage Fcgamma R-mediated phagocytosis and the IL-18/IFN-gamma-mediated molecular connection between innate and adaptive immunity in the lung. Blood 2002;100:4193–4200.

Bonfield TL, Russell D, Burgess S, Malur A, Kavuru MS, Thomassen MJ. Autoantibodies against granulocyte macrophage colony-stimulating factor are diagnostic for pulmonary alveolar proteinosis. Am J Respir Cell Mol Biol 2002;27:481–486.

Buechner HA, Ansari A. Acute silico-proteinosis: a new pathologic variant of acute silicosis in sandblasters, characterized by histologic features resembling alveolar proteinosis. Dis Chest 1969;55:274–278.

Carraway MS, Ghio AJ, Carter JD, Piantadosi CA. Detection of granulocyte-macrophage colony-stimulating factor in patients with pulmonary alveolar proteinosis. Am J Respir Crit Care Med 2000;161: 1294–1299.

Celada A, Borras FE, Soler C, et al. The transcription factor PU.1 is involved in macrophage proliferation. J Exp Med 1996;184:61–69.

Clark JC, Wert SE, Bachurski CJ, et al. Targeted disruption of the surfactant protein B gene disrupts surfactant homeostasis, causing respiratory failure in newborn mice. Proc Natl Acad Sci USA 1995;92:7794–7798.

Cole FS, Hamvas A, Rubinstein P, et al. Population-based estimates of surfactant protein B deficiency. Pediatrics 2000;105:538–541.

Cordonnier C, Fleury-Feith J, Escudier E, Atassi K, Bernaudin JF. Secondary alveolar proteinosis is a reversible cause of respiratory failure in leukemic patients. Am J Respir Crit Care Med 1994;149:788–794.

Dean M, Rzhetsky A, Allikmets R. The human ATP-binding cassette (ABC) transporter superfamily. Genome Res 2001;11:1156–1166.

deMello DE, Lin Z. Pulmonary alveolar proteinosis: a review. Pediatr Pathol Mol Med 2001;20:413–432.

Dranoff G, Crawford AD, Sadelain M, et al. Involvement of granulocyte-macrophage colony-stimulating factor in pulmonary homeostasis. Science 1994;264:713–716.

Dunbar AE III, Wert SE, Ikegami M, et al. Prolonged survival in hereditary surfactant protein B (SP-B) deficiency associated with a novel splicing mutation. Pediatr Res 2000;48:275–282.

Glasser SW, Burhans MS, Korfhagen TR, et al. Altered stability of pulmonary surfactant in SP-C-deficient mice. Proc Natl Acad Sci USA 2001;98:6366–6371.

Glasser SW, Detmer EA, Ikegami M, Na CL, Stahlman MT, Whitsett JA. Pneumonitis and emphysema in sp-C gene targeted mice. J Biol Chem 2003;278:14,291–14,298.

Glasser SW, Korfhagen TR, Weaver TE, et al. cDNA, deduced polypeptide structure and chromosomal assignment of human pulmonary surfactant proteolipid, SPL(pVal). J Biol Chem 1988;263:9–12.

Golde DW. Alveolar proteinosis and the overfed macrophage. Chest 1979;76:119, 120.

Golde DW, Territo M, Finley TN, Cline MJ. Defective lung macrophages in pulmonary alveolar proteinosis. Ann Intern Med 1976;85:304–309.

Hamvas A, Nogee LM, Mallory GB Jr, et al. Lung transplantation for treatment of infants with surfactant protein B deficiency. J Pediatr 1997;130:231–239.

Harris JO. Pulmonary alveolar proteinosis: abnormal in vitro function of alveolar macrophages. Chest 1979;76:156–159.

Huffman JA, Hull WM, Dranoff G, Mulligan RC, Whitsett JA. Pulmonary epithelial cell expression of GM-CSF corrects the alveolar proteinosis in GM-CSF-deficient mice. J Clin Invest 1996;97:649–655.

Ikegami M, Ueda T, Hull W, et al. Surfactant metabolism in transgenic mice after granulocyte macrophage-colony stimulating factor ablation. Am J Physiol 1996;270:L650–L658.

Jobe AH, Ikegami M. Surfactant metabolism. Clin Perinatol 1993;20:683–696.

Johansson J, Curstedt T. Molecular structures and interactions of pulmonary surfactant components. Eur J Biochem 1997;244:675–693.

Kavuru MS, Sullivan EJ, Piccin R, Thomassen MJ, Stoller JK. Exogenous granulocyte-macrophage colony-stimulating factor administration for pulmonary alveolar proteinosis. Am J Respir Crit Care Med 2000;161:1143–1148.

Kitamura T, Tanaka N, Watanabe J, et al. Idiopathic pulmonary alveolar proteinosis as an autoimmune disease with neutralizing antibody against granulocyte/macrophage colony-stimulating factor. J Exp Med 1999;190:875–880.

Kitamura T, Uchida K, Tanaka N, et al. Serological diagnosis of idiopathic pulmonary alveolar proteinosis. Am J Respir Crit Care Med 2000;162:658–662.

Klein JM, Thompson MW, Snyder JM, et al. Transient surfactant protein B deficiency in a term infant with severe respiratory failure. J Pediatr 1998;132:244–248.

Ladeb S, Fleury-Feith J, Escudier E, Tran Van Nhieu J, Bernaudin JF, Cordonnier C. Secondary alveolar proteinosis in cancer patients. Support Care Cancer 1996;4:420–426.

Lee KN, Levin DL, Webb WR, Chen D, Storto ML, Golden JA. Pulmonary alveolar proteinosis: high-resolution CT, chest radiographic, and functional correlations. Chest 1997;111:989–995.

LeVine AM, Reed JA, Kurak KE, Cianciolo E, Whitsett JA. GM-CSF-deficient mice are susceptible to pulmonary group B streptococcal infection. J Clin Invest 1999;103:563–569.

Lloberas J, Soler C, Celada A. The key role of PU.1/SPI-1 in B cells, myeloid cells and macrophages. Immunol Today 1999;20:184–189.

Muller-Quernheim J, Schopf RE, Benes P, Schulz V, Ferlinz R. A macrophage-suppressing 40-kD protein in a case of pulmonary alveolar proteinosis. Klin Wochenschr 1987;65:893–897.

Mulugeta S, Gray JM, Notarfrancesco KL, et al. Identification of LBM180, a lamellar body limiting membrane protein of alveolar type II cells, as the ABC transporter protein ABCA3. J Biol Chem 2002;277:22,147–22,155.

Nishinakamura R, Nakayama N, Hirabayashi Y, et al. Mice deficient for the IL-3/GM-CSF/IL-5 beta c receptor exhibit lung pathology and impaired immune response, while beta IL3 receptor-deficient mice are normal. Immunity 1995;2:211–222.

Nogee LM. Alterations in SP-B and SP-C expression in neonatal lung disease. Annu Rev Physiol 2004;66:601–623.

Nogee LM, Wert SE, Proffit SA, Hull WM, Whitsett JA. Allelic heterogeneity in hereditary surfactant protein B (SP-B) deficiency. Am J Respir Crit Care Med 2000;161:973–981.

Nogee LM, Dunbar AE III, Wert SE, Askin F, Hamvas A, Whitsett JA. A mutation in the surfactant protein C gene associated with familial interstitial lung disease. N Engl J Med 2001;344:573–579.

Nogee LM, Garnier G, Dietz HC, et al. A mutation in the surfactant protein B gene responsible for fatal neonatal respiratory disease in multiple kindreds. J Clin Invest 1994;93:1860–1863.

Oerlemans WG, Jansen EN, Prevo RL, Eijsvogel MM. Primary cerebellar nocardiosis and alveolar proteinosis. Acta Neurol Scand 1998;97:138–141.

Paine R III, Morris SB, Jin H, et al. Impaired functional activity of alveolar macrophages from GM-CSF-deficient mice. Am J Physiol 2001;281:L1210–L1218.

Prakash UB, Barham SS, Carpenter HA, Dines DE, Marsh HM. Pulmonary alveolar phospholipoproteinosis: Experience with 34 cases and a review. Mayo Clin Proc 1987;62:499–518.

Preger L. Pulmonary alveolar proteinosis. Radiology 1969;92:1291–1295.

Ramirez-Rivera J, Schultz RB, Dutton RE. Pulmonary alveolar proteinosis: a new technique and rational for treatment. Arch Intern Med 1963;112:173–185.

Robb L, Drinkwater CC, Metcalf D, et al. Hematopoietic and lung abnormalities in mice with a null mutation of the common beta subunit of the receptors for granulocyte-macrophage colony-stimulating factor and interleukins 3 and 5. Proc Natl Acad Sci USA 1995;92:9565–9569.

Rosen SG, Castleman B, Liebow AA. Pulmonary alveolar proteinosis. N Engl J Med 1958;258:1123–1142.

Ruben FL, Talamo TS. Secondary pulmonary alveolar proteinosis occurring in two patients with acquired immune deficiency syndrome. Am J Med 1986;80:1187–1190.

Schoch OD, Schanz U, Koller M, et al. BAL findings in a patient with pulmonary alveolar proteinosis successfully treated with GM-CSF. Thorax 2002;57:277–280.

Scott EW, Simon MC, Anastasi J, Singh H. Requirement of transcription factor PU.1 in the development of multiple hematopoietic lineages. Science 1994;265:1573–1577.

Selecky PA, Wasserman K, Benfield JR, Lippmann M. The clinical and physiological effect of whole-lung lavage in pulmonary alveolar proteinosis: a ten-year experience. Ann Thorac Surg 1977;24:451–461.

Seymour JF, Presneill JJ. Pulmonary alveolar proteinosis: progress in the first 44 years. Am J Respir Crit Care Med 2002;166:215–235.

Seymour JF, Presneill JJ, Schoch OD, et al. Therapeutic efficacy of granulocyte-macrophage colony-stimulating factor in patients with idiopathic acquired alveolar proteinosis. Am J Respir Crit Care Med 2001;163:524–531.

Shibata Y, Berclaz P-Y, Chroneos Z, Yoshida H, Whitsett JA, Trapnell BC. GM-CSF regulates alveolar macrophage differentiation and innate immunity in the lung through PU.1. Immunity 2001;15:557–567.

Shulenin S, Nogee LM, Annilo T, Wert SE, Whitsett JA, Dean M. ABCA3 gene mutations in newborns with fatal surfactant deficiency. N Engl J Med 2004;350:1296–1303.

Stanley E, Lieschke GJ, Grail D, et al. Granulocyte/macrophage colony-stimulating factor-deficient mice show no major perturbation of hematopoiesis but develop a characteristic pulmonary pathology. Proc Natl Acad Sci USA 1994;91:5592–5596.

Stratton JA, Sieger L, Wasserman K. The immunoinhibitory activities of the lung lavage materials and sera from patients with pulmonary alveolar proteinosis (PAP). J Clin Lab Immunol 1981;5:81–86.

Thomas AQ, Lane K, Phillips J III, et al. Heterozygosity for a surfactant protein C gene mutation associated with usual interstitial pneumonitis and cellular nonspecific interstitial pneumonitis in one kindred. Am J Respir Crit Care Med 2002;165:1322–1328.

Tokieda K, Iwamoto HS, Bachurski C, et al. Surfactant protein-B-deficient mice are susceptible to hyperoxic lung injury. Am J Respir Cell Mol Biol 1999;21:463–472.

Trapnell BC, Whitsett JA. GM-CSF regulates pulmonary surfactant homeostasis and alveolar macrophage-mediated innate host defense. Annu Rev Physiol 2002;64:775–802.

Trapnell BC, Whitsett JA, Nakata K. Pulmonary alveolar proteinosis. N Engl J Med 2003;349:2527–2539.

Tredano M, Griese M, Brasch F, et al. Mutation of *SFTPC* in infantile pulmonary alveolar proteinosis with or without fibrosing lung disease. Am J Med Genet 2004;126A:18–26.

Tredano M, Griese M, de Blic J, et al. Analysis of 40 sporadic or familial neonatal and pediatric cases with severe unexplained respiratory distress: relationship to *SFTPB*. Am J Med Genet 2003;119A:324–339.

Uchida K, Nakata K, Trapnell BC, et al. High-affinity autoantibodies specifically eliminate granulocyte-macrophage colony-stimulating factor activity in the lungs of patients with idiopathic pulmonary alveolar proteinosis Blood 2004;103:1089–1098.

Vorbroker DK, Profitt SA, Nogee LM, Whitsett JA. Aberrant processing of surfactant protein C (SP-C) in hereditary SP-B deficiency. Am J Physiol 1995;268:L647–L656.

Wang BM, Stern EJ, Schmidt RA, Pierson DJ. Diagnosing pulmonary alveolar proteinosis: a review and an update. Chest 1997;111:460–466.

Wasserman K, Masson GR. Pulmonary alveolar proteinosis. In: Murray JF, Nadel JA, eds. Textbook of Respiratory Medicine. Philadelphia: Saunders, 1994; pp. 1933–1946.

Weaver TE, Conkright JJ. Functions of surfactant proteins B and C. Annu Rev Physiol 2001;63:555–578.

Whitsett JA, Weaver TE. Hydrophobic surfactant proteins in lung function and disease. N Engl J Med 2002;347:2141–2148.

Whitsett JA, Ohning BL, Ross G, et al. Hydrophobic surfactant-associated protein in whole lung surfactant and its importance for biophysical activity in lung surfactant extracts used for replacement therapy. Pediatr Res 1986;20:460–467.

Wright JR, Clements JA. Metabolism and turnover of lung surfactant. Am Rev Respir Dis 1987;136:426–444.

Yamano G, Funahashi H, Kawanami O, et al. ABCA3 is a lamellar body membrane protein in human lung alveolar type II cells. FEBS Lett 2001;508:221–225.

Yoshida M, Ikegami M, Reed JA, Chroneos ZC, Whitsett JA. GM-CSF regulates surfactant protein-A and lipid catabolism by alveolar macrophages. Am J Physiol 2001;280:L379–L386.

Yusen RD, Cohen AH, Hamvas A. Normal lung function in subjects heterozygous for surfactant protein-B deficiency. Am J Respir Crit Care Med 1999;159:411–414.

ENDOCRINOLOGY | IV

SECTION EDITOR:
MICHAEL J. MCPHAUL

31 Mechanisms of Hormone Action

STEPHEN R. HAMMES, CAROL A. LANGE, AND MICHAEL J. MCPHAUL

SUMMARY

The completion of the human genome sequence has permitted the identification of additional signaling molecules of many different classes. The impact of this new information on the understanding of the pathophysiology of disease is already evidenced in terms of the ability to predict specific receptors or pathways that might harbor mutations in different disorders. Selected examples of such mutations are cited this chapter, and the reader is referred to other chapters in this section for detailed discussions of these disorders. Although written from a perspective that is grounded in endocrinology, the concepts regarding the receptor classes and signaling pathways are generally applicable to all areas of biology and medicine.

Key Words: Amino acids; cytokines; hormone; nuclear receptor; phosphotyrosine phosphatases; peptides; proteins; steroids; transmembrane domain receptors.

INTRODUCTION

Hormones provide a form of communication between different cells and from one organ to another. The dramatic effects of hormones on physiological functions such as growth and metabolism have promoted studies to elucidate their sources of production, sites of action, and how they are controlled. Because hormones exert their effects by binding to specific receptors, studies defining their mechanisms of action have also provided important paradigms for how receptors activate intracellular signaling cascades that lead to altered cellular responses.

Endocrine disorders ultimately involve abnormalities of hormone production or action. Etiologies of a relatively large number of these diseases with well-defined genetic bases have been identified. Numerous examples exist of mutations in genes that encode hormones, their receptors, second messenger signaling pathways, and of the factors that transduce hormone signals. This chapter reviews basic principles of hormone signaling through their receptors. A remarkable expansion of knowledge in this area has included information about the structures and many of the signal transduction networks for membrane receptors. In addition, numerous members of the nuclear receptor (NR) family have been cloned, revealing an unexpectedly complex family of proteins that serve as direct regulators of gene expression. Because of the breadth of knowledge available, this chapter is not comprehensive, but introduces the major classes of receptors and the mechanisms by which their signals are transduced. The completion of the human genome sequence has permitted the identification of additional signaling molecules of many different classes. The impact of this new information on the understanding of the pathophysiology of disease is already evidenced in terms of the ability to predict specific receptors or pathways that might harbor mutations in different disorders.

CLASSIFICATION OF HORMONES AND RECEPTORS

Hormones can be divided generally into three major classes:

1. Derivatives of amino acids (e.g., dopamine and catecholamines).
2. Peptides and proteins (e.g., thyrotropin-releasing hormone [TRH] or insulin).
3. Derivatives of steroids (e.g., estrogen or cortisol).

Amino acid derivatives and peptide hormones predominantly interact with membrane receptors on the cell surface, whereas the steroid hormones act by crossing the plasma membrane to interact with intracellular receptors.

As described later, membrane receptors can be divided into several distinct classes. After binding hormones, these receptors activate a complex array of second messenger signaling pathways that often involve cascades of kinases. NRs, such as the glucocorticoid or progesterone receptors (PRs), bind hormones in the cytoplasm before translocation into the nucleus (Fig. 31-1). Other receptors in this family, such as the thyroid hormone receptor, bind hormone in the nucleus without a separate hormone-induced translocation step. In the nucleus, these receptors interact with DNA target sites to either stimulate or repress the expression of specific genes.

Regardless of the class of receptors, certain principles apply to hormone–receptor interactions. Hormones bind to receptors with high affinity and specificity to allow appropriate physiological responses. Most receptors bind hormones with affinity constants that approach the circulating levels of hormones (usually $<10^{-9} M$) to allow responses over a dynamic range of physiologically relevant changes in hormone levels. Receptor numbers vary greatly in different target tissues, providing one of the major determinants of specific cellular responses to widely circulating hormones. For

From: *Principles of Molecular Medicine, Second Edition*
Edited by: M. S. Runge and C. Patterson © Humana Press, Inc., Totowa, NJ

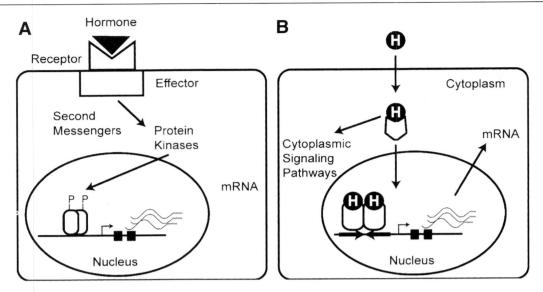

Figure 31-1 Membrane and NRs mediate hormone action. A membrane receptor is shown at the left and a nuclear receptor is shown to the right. **(A)** Hormones and growth factors bind with high affinity to the extracellular domain of the receptors. Membrane receptors modulate intracellular signaling pathways, which typically include cascades of protein kinases. These kinases act on many different cellular targets, including other receptors, ion channels, the cytoskeleton, metabolic pathways, and transcription factors. **(B)** NRs reside within the cytoplasm or the nucleus before hormone binding. Hormones traverse the plasma membrane and induce nuclear translocation and receptor activation. The activated receptors act as TFs to alter levels of gene expression. (Redrawn after Jameson JL. Principles or hormone action. Oxford Textbook of Medicine, 1996. Reprinted with permission from Oxford University Press.)

example, luteinizing hormone (LH) receptors are located almost exclusively in the gonads. In contrast, insulin receptors are widely distributed, reflecting the need for insulin-induced metabolic responses in most tissues.

Receptor specificity is a reflection of differential affinities of the receptor for structurally related molecules. Although structurally similar, LH, follicle-stimulating hormone (FSH), and thyroid-stimulating hormone (TSH) are highly selective for their individual receptors. Similarly, steroids such as progesterone, estrogen, and glucocorticoid exhibit no physiologically significant cross-reactivity among their receptors. There are important exceptions to these examples of specificity. Parathyroid hormone (PTH) and parathyroid hormone-related peptide appear to share a common receptor. Insulin, insulin-like growth factor (IGF)-I, and IGF-II cross-react to some degree with their respective receptors. This latter circumstance might explain why some malignancies that overproduce IGF-II can cause hypoglycemia because of inappropriate stimulation of insulin receptors by IGF-II.

FEEDBACK REGULATION IN ENDOCRINE AXES

Feedback regulatory systems are pervasive in the field of endocrinology. Each of the major hypothalamic–pituitary hormone axes is governed by negative feedback, which serves to maintain hormone levels within a narrow range. The principle of feedback control is represented by the example of the hypothalamic-pituitary-thyroid axis (Fig. 31-2). TRH stimulates TSH secretion from the pituitary. TSH stimulates the synthesis and secretion of thyroid hormones thyroxine (T4) and triiodothyronine (T3), which in turn suppresses the production of hypothalamic TRH and pituitary TSH. A typical regulatory loop therefore has both positive (TRH, TSH) and negative (T4, T3) components, providing exquisite control over hormone levels and action.

In addition to classic endocrine feedback loops in which hormones are produced by one gland and act on different tissues, a variety of local regulatory systems have also been characterized (Fig. 31-3). These autocrine and paracrine systems are used commonly during development and by most growth factors. Local control of growth factor production and action helps to restrict their sites of action. For example, circulating levels of activin are relatively low, but local production in the gonads and pituitary might permit localized biological effects without a requirement for systemic exposure to high levels of hormone. In many cases, the distinction between endocrine and paracrine actions might become blurred. For example, IGF-I appears to act both as a true hormone and a paracrine factor. In the liver, growth hormone (GH) increases production of circulating IGF-I. However, in most other tissues, the production of IGF-I is also regulated locally.

The clinical practice of endocrinology is intimately linked to these principles of feedback control systems and hormone action. With these concepts, it is often possible to localize whether a disorder is caused by hormone excess or deficiency, or by an abnormality in tissue sensitivity to hormone action. Advances in molecular genetics are allowing these diagnostic algorithms to expand by another dimension. In addition to measuring hormone levels, it is possible to test for enzyme deficiencies by identifying mutations in affected genes (e.g., 21-hydroxylase), or to predict genetic risk in inherited syndromes such as the multiple endocrine neoplasia (MEN) syndromes.

MEMBRANE RECEPTORS

Receptors on cell surfaces provide an essential component of communication with extracellular ligands. These membrane receptors fall into three general classes based on their structure and mechanisms of signal transduction: (1) the single transmembrane domain receptors; (2) the seven transmembrane domain

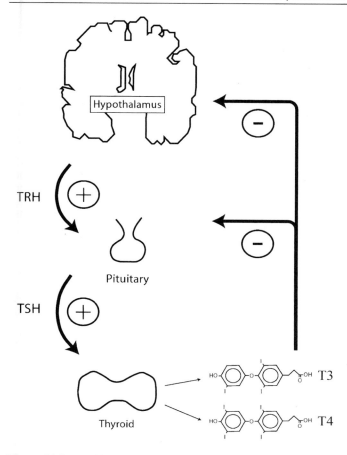

Figure 31-2 Positive and negative feedback regulation by hormones. The hypothalamic-pituitary-thyroid axis provides a prototypical example of feedback regulatory pathways in the endocrine system. Hypothalamic TRH stimulates TSH secretion by the pituitary gland. TSH stimulates the biosynthesis and secretion of thyroid hormones (T4 and T3) from the thyroid gland. Thyroid hormones feed back to inhibit the production of TRH and TSH. Because the pituitary integrates both positive and negative regulation, it establishes a set-point for TSH and consequently, thyroid hormone levels. (Redrawn after Jameson JL. Principles or hormone action. Oxford Textbook of Medicine, 1996. Reprinted with permission from Oxford University Press.)

receptors; and (3) the four transmembrane domain receptors. The latter class functions as neurotransmitter-gated ion channels and will not be described in this chapter.

SINGLE TRANSMEMBRANE DOMAIN RECEPTORS

TYROSINE KINASE RECEPTORS The tyrosine kinase family of membrane receptors (RTKs) consists of cell surface single transmembrane domain molecules that contain intrinsic tyrosine kinase activities. These receptors can be classified into several different subfamilies, including the (1) insulin/IGF; (2) epidermal growth factor (EGF)/neu/HER2; (3) platelet-derived growth factor (PDGF)/CSF1/vascular endothelial growth factor; and (4) GDNF/Ret classes. With the exception of the insulin/IGF receptor subfamily, whose members are constitutively expressed on the cell surface as dimers, the RTKs require ligand-activated dimerization to initiate signaling. The ligand binding domains are located in the amino-terminal extracellular region, where as the tyrosine kinase domains are located in the carboxyl-terminal cytoplasmic region (Fig. 31-4). Ligand binding induces stable dimerization of receptor

monomers. Each monomer transphosphorylates its partner within the activation loop of the kinase domain, resulting in receptor activation. Once activated, tyrosine residues in the cytoplasmic domains are autophosphorylated by the intrinsic tyrosine kinase. These phosphorylated tyrosine residues then serve as targets for multiple intracellular scaffolding and signaling molecules, recruiting them to the plasma membrane to form a membrane signaling complex that mediates a variety of signaling responses. The specificity of the signaling response of an individual RTK therefore depends on its location within the target cells as well as the milieu of phosphotyrosine binding molecules and other signaling proteins within the target cell.

Many different phosphotyrosine-binding molecules bind to RTKs. These proteins usually contain either a src-homology domain 2 (SH2) or a phosphotyrosine binding (PTB) domain (Table 31-1). In addition to PTBs, the formation of membrane signaling complexes is achieved through the use of multiple specific interaction domains. For example, Pleckstrin homology (PH) and FYVE domains bind to phospholipids within the internal plasma membrane, thus retaining proteins at the cell surface. Protein–protein interactions are mediated by src-homology 3 (SH3) and WW domains that recognize and bind to proline-rich regions, where as PDZ domains recognize and bind to hydrophobic C-terminal domain residues.

An example of a RTK recruiting a signaling complex to the inner cell surface is the activation of protein kinase B (PKB, or Akt) (Fig. 31-4A). Ligand binding to a RTK such as PDGF receptor leads to dimerization and autophosphorylation of tyrosine residues in the receptor carboxyl-terminal tails. Phosphatidylinositol-3-kinase (PI3K) then binds to these phosphotyrosines through SH2 domains, leading to activation of PI3K and subsequent PI3K-mediated phosphorylation of membrane-bound PIP2 to form PIP3. PIP3 in the membrane promotes localization of 3-phosphoinositol-dependent kinase (PDK1) and PKB to the inner plasma membrane through interactions with PH domains. Once together at the membrane, PDK1 phosphorylates and activates PKB, which then promotes multiple signals within the target cell. Similarly, phospholipase C (PLC)-γ binds to phosphorylated RTKs, such as the EGF and PDGF receptors through SH2 domains, where as binding to membrane phospholipids through PH domains. This leads to its phosphorylation and activation by the receptor kinase. PLCγ then converts PIP2 to inositol 1,4,5-trisphosphate (IP_3) and diacylglycerol, which promotes calcium mobilization and phosphokinase C (PKC) activation, respectively (Fig. 31-4B).

In addition to directly recruiting signaling molecules to the membrane receptor complex, phosphorylated RTKs can bind to scaffolding proteins that in turn bring signaling molecules to the membrane. For example, Shc binds to phosphorylated receptors through PTB domains, leading to RTK-mediated phosphorylation of Shc. The adaptor, growth factor receptor-binding protein 2 (Grb-2), then binds to phosphorylated Shc through an SH2 domain, followed by association of the guanine nucleotide exchange protein Sos, which then activates membrane bound Ras. Ras is a member of a large family of small guanine nucleotide binding proteins (G proteins) that act as "molecular switches." When bound to GDP, Ras proteins remain inactive and are thus unable to bind to downstream signaling "effector" molecules. Guanine nucleotide exchange factors, such as Sos, induce the exchange of GDP for GTP, thereby stimulating a conformational change that allows Ras to bind to one or more kinases from the Raf or, mitogen-activated extracellular reponse kinase kinase

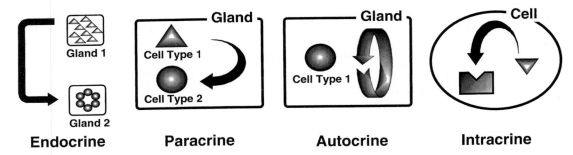

Figure 31-3 Hormones and growth factors can act at a distance or locally. Endocrine action often refers to hormones that are selected from one gland and enter the circulation to act on a different target gland. Paracrine action involves hormones or growth factors that are produced by one cell but act locally on an adjacent cell. In autocrine action, a growth factor acts on the same cell from which it is produced. Intracrine action suggests that some hormones act on intracellular receptors in the same cells in which they are produced. (Redrawn after Jameson JL. Principles of hormone action. Oxford Textbook of Medicine, 1996. Reprinted with permission from Oxford University Press.)

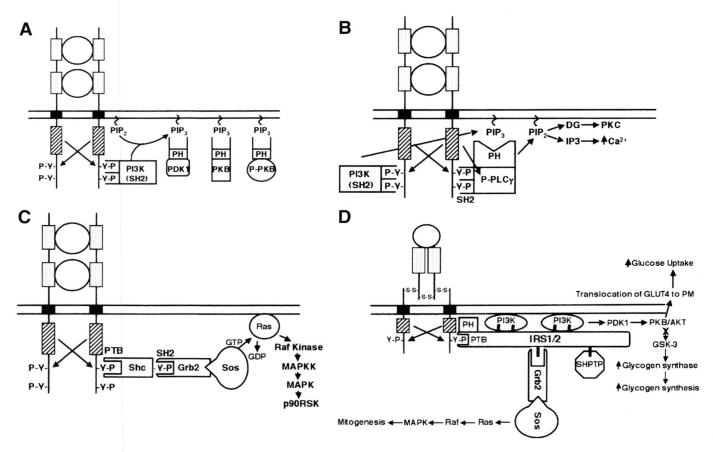

Figure 31-4 Activated RTKs recruit signaling complexes to the inner plasma membrane in many different ways. **(A)** Two ligands (circle) bind two receptors, leading to dimerization and phosphorylation of cytoplasmic tyrosine residues by the receptor's intrinsic tyrosine kinase. Phosphatidylinositol-3-kinase (PI3K) then binds to the phosphorylated tyrosines through its SH2 domains to bring it in close proximity to the membrane, where it mediates the conversion of PIP2 to PIP3. Phosphoinositide-dependent kinase (PDK) and phosphokinase B (PKB, also known as Akt) are then recruited to the membrane through binding to PIP3 through their Pleckstrin-homology (PH) domains, where PDK phosphorylates and activates PKB. **(B)** Phospholipase C (PLCγ) binds phosphorylated receptor and the inner cell membrane through src-homology 2 (SH2) and PH domains, respectively, where it is itself phosphorylated and activated by the receptor tyrosine kinase. PLCγ then mediates the conversion of PIP2 to diacylglycerol (DG) and inositol 1,4,5-trisphosphate (IP$_3$), which activate phosphokinase C (PKC) and calcium mobilization, respectively. **(C)** The scaffolding protein Shc binds to phosphorylated receptor through its PTB domain, in which it is phosphorylated by the receptor kinase. The Grb-2/Sos complex then binds to phosphorylated Shc through an SH2 domain in Grb-2, bringing Sos in close proximately to membrane-bound Ras. Sos mediates the exchange of GTP for GDPon Ras, which in turn activates the mitogen-activated protein kinase (MAPK) cascade. **(D)** Constitutively dimerized insulin/IGF receptors are activated by single ligands, leading to phosphorylation of cytoplasmic tyrosines. Insulin-related substrate (IRS) proteins then bind to the receptor and the inner plasma membrane through PTB and PH domains, respectively, where they are phosphorylated at many sites by the receptor tyrosine kinase. Multiple scaffolding and signaling molecules then bind to phosphorylated IRS proteins, leading to activation of a myriad of signaling pathways.

Table 31-1
Protein Interaction Domains

Domain	Target
PTB	Phosphotyrosine with amino-terminal specific sequences (NPXY)
SH2	Phosphotyrosine with carboxyl-terminal specific sequences (YXX(L/I)X)
SH3	Proline-rich (PXXP)
WW	Proline-rich (PXPX)
PH	Phosphoinositols (PIP2, IP$_3$)
FYVE	Phosphoinositols (PtdIns-3-P)
PDZ	C-terminal hydrophobic residues

Intracellular signaling complexes rely on multiple signaling modules. Phosphotyrosine binding (PTB) and src-homology 2 (SH2) domains interact with sequences containing phosphotyrosine residues in either the carboxyl-terminal or amino-terminal positions, respectively (L/I, hydrophobic amino acid; X, any amino acid). Src-homology 3 (SH3) and tryptophan-conserved (WW) domains bind to proline-rich sequences as indicated. Pleckstrin-homology (PH) and FYVE domains recognize phospholipids. Finally, PDZ domains interact with hydrophobic carboxyl-terminal residues.

(MEKK) families. For example, the interaction of GTP-bound Ras with the Ser/Thr protein kinase, Raf-1, acts to bring Raf-1 to the membrane, in which it is phosphorylated and activated. Raf-1 then mediates the direct phosphorylation and activation of MEK/ERK kinases, MEK1, and MEK2. MEKs 1 and 2 in turn activate MAPKs p42 and p44 by dual phosphorylation on threonine and tyrosine residues. The activation of three kinases within a cascade (Raf-1/MEK/MAPK) is collectively termed a "MAPK module." Because several isoforms exist for each kinase family member within the three-kinase cascade, many MAPK modules are possible. The specificity of MAPK modules is determined by interaction with scaffold proteins, which bind two or more components within the module and provide subcellular localization, organization, and insulation from other modules. Finally, to turn off the signal, a family of GTP-ase activating proteins (Ras-GAPs) then induce the intrinsic guanosine 5′-triphosphatase (GTPase) activity of Ras, returning it to its GDP- associated "off" conformation (Fig. 31-4C).

As a final example of RTK-mediated signaling, activation of other tyrosine kinase receptors (RTKs), including the insulin or IGF receptors, leads to insulin-related substrate (IRS) binding through PTB domains. IRS is then phosphorylated by the receptor, allowing multiple phosphotyrosine binding proteins to interact with the signaling complex, including PI3K and Grb-2 and activation of Ras and MAPK modules (Fig. 31-4D).

RTK activity is tightly regulated by a number of distinct mechanisms that have been identified as effecting control of the activity of specific receptors. These include inhibition of RTK activity (by phosphorylation or by association with specific inhibitory proteins), dephosphorylation by protein tyrosine phosphatases, and the internalization and degradation of activated receptors. Mutations in RTKs are infrequently associated with diseases. For example, homozygous mutations in several regions of the insulin receptor have been associated with leprechaunism, characterized by severe growth retardation and death in infancy (Chapter 32). Heterozygous mutations in the insulin receptor have been associated with the less severe Type A insulin resistance or Rabson-Mendenhall syndrome, both of which are characterized by marked insulin

resistance, acanthosis nigricans, hyperandrogenism, and polycystic ovarian syndrome. However, RTK overexpression occurs in a wide variety of epithelial cancers and is indicative of a poor prognosis.

Another fascinating series of RTK mutations leading to disease occurs with the RET proto-oncogene, a tyrosine kinase receptor. Activating mutations of the RET protein have been associated with MEN type 2A, an autosomal-dominant disorder characterized by a high incidence of medullary thyroid cancer and pheochromocytoma. Other activating mutations of RET have been associated with familiar medullary thyroid carcinoma. In contrast, inactivating mutations in the RET protein have been related to Hirchsprung's disease, a congenital malformation characterized by aganglionosis of the gastrointestinal tract.

CYTOKINE RECEPTOR FAMILY

Cytokines include traditional hormones, such as growth hormone and erythropoietin, as well as colony-stimulating factors and interleukins. In several cases, such as the interleukins, a variety of different endocrine, neural, hepatic, and hematopoietic systems are targets of the cytokines. The cytokine receptor family includes receptors for a broad range of molecules. Members of this family are single transmembrane receptors with extracellular ligand binding and intracellular domains (Fig. 31-5). In contrast to the RTKs, the cytoplasmic domains of this class of receptors do not possess intrinsic kinase activity. Moreover, although functional receptors many contain only a single type of subunit (e.g., GH, prolactin, erythropoietin, leptin), others consist of several subunits, some of which are shared among different cytokine receptors. The formation of oligomeric complexes (homodimeric, in the case of the growth hormone receptor [GHR] for example; heteromeric, in the case of most others) is required for the high affinity binding of ligand and the propagation of intracellular signals. Mutations within the receptor or ligand that interfere with the formation of these active multimers will attenuate or abrogate the generation of the intracellular signal. For example, Pegvisomant®, a mutant GH molecule that interferes with the ability of the GHR to dimerize, has been used to treat individuals with excess GH secretion and acromegaly. In addition, some members of this receptor family secrete soluble forms of the receptor that can bind circulating ligands. In the case of the GH receptor, the extracellular domain is shed into the circulation and functions as a GH binding protein.

The mechanism of cytokine-induced signal transduction was poorly understood for many years in view of the lack of intrinsic enzyme activity in the cytoplasmic domain of these receptors. Subsequent studies established that members of the cytokine receptor family signal by the activation of Janus kinases (JAKs) (see Fig. 31-5). The JAK family members, which include JAK1, JAK2, JAK3, and Tyk2, are cytoplasmic protein tyrosine kinases that associate with the cytoplasmic domain of cytokine receptors through conserved receptor motifs. The activated JAKs phosphorylate tyrosines in the cytoplasmic domain of the cytokine receptors, which creates binding sites for signal transduction molecules that contain SH2 domains. In addition, the JAKs transmit intracellular signals by phosphorylating a family of latent transcription factors (TFs) called the signal transducers and activators of transcription (STAT) proteins. It is likely that each specific receptor elicits responses from a constellation of kinases and STAT proteins. There also appear to be alternate pathways by which STAT proteins can be activated and considerable "cross talk" between these and other signaling pathways. Finally, the duration of the

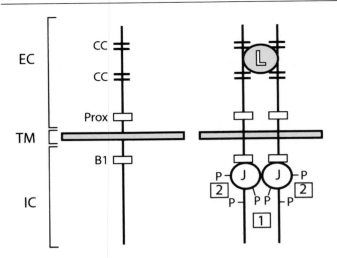

Figure 31-5 Signaling by the cytokine receptor family. Members of the cytokine receptor family are single transmembrane (TM) receptors that share conserved motifs within their extracellular (EC) and intracellular (IC) domains. In general, type-I cytokine receptors, such as the GH receptor, have conserved pairs of cysteine residues within their extracellular domains and a conserved WSXWS motif in the region adjacent to the transmembrane segment (Prox). A conserved element (PXP; box 1,"B1") forms a motif important to the recruitment of intracellular signaling molecules (left panel). The binding of ligand (L) results in the dimerization of the receptor, the recruitment of Janus-activated kinases (JAKs), and the phosphorylation of specific residues on the adjacent JAK molecules and on the receptor (labeled 1 and 2). These events are critical to the docking and phosphorylation of the STAT proteins. J is JAK and L is ligand.

signal transduced by the activated JAKs can be modulated by STAT-mediated induction of a class of proteins that serve to inhibit the activity of the JAKs. These suppressors of cytokine signaling (SOCS) proteins inhibit cytokine signaling by a number of mechanisms, including binding to the JAKs or the receptors to inhibit the activation of the JAKs or to the STATs to inhibit the binding STATS to the cytokine receptors.

Endocrine diseases associated with mutations of cytokine receptors include alterations in GH signaling (Chapter 34). Patients with familial GH resistance or Laron-type dwarfism have proportionate short stature associated with elevated plasma GH levels and do not respond to exogenous treatment with GH. In most cases, the syndrome is inherited in an autosomal-recessive fashion, and patients lack functional GH receptors secondary to gene deletions or point mutations in the receptor. The GH receptor from some patients with this syndrome has a point mutation in the extracellular domain that results in a small reduction in receptor affinity, but which abrogates the ability of the receptor to dimerize, thus demonstrating the importance of receptor dimerization in signal transduction. In a selected group of children with idiopathic short stature, approximately one-third had mutations in the GH receptor that affected the level of receptor expression or its affinity for GH.

SERINE–THREONINE KINASE RECEPTOR FAMILY
Although some receptors function as tyrosine kinases, others contain intrinsic serine/threonine kinase activity. These serine/threonine kinase receptors mediate signaling by members of the transforming growth factor (TGF)-β superfamily, which consists of a large number of multifunctional signaling proteins that play important roles in a myriad of processes, including inflammation, cellular proliferation,

and tissue development. Members of this superfamily include TGF-β proteins (regulators of cellular proliferation), activins (activators of FSH), bone morphogenetic proteins, or BMPs (inducers of bone and cartilage formation), and anti-Müllerian hormone (dedifferentiates the Müllerian duct system in males).

Although the TGF-β ligand superfamily is extraordinarily large and diverse, the serine/threonine kinases make up a relatively small family of transmembrane receptors made up of two subunits defined as type I and II receptors. The type I receptors are similar in structure to the type II receptors, and both contain serine-threonine kinase domains. Unlike the type II receptors; however, the type I receptors do not have the ability to bind ligand. In mammals, only five type II receptors and seven type I receptors have been identified for ligands belonging to the TGF-β superfamily. Ligands bind to cell surface type II receptors as homo- or heterodimers. This high-affinity interaction allows the recruitment of type I receptors to the ligand-receptor complex, resulting in a heteromeric complex consisting of two type I and two type II receptors. The type II receptor contains constitutive serine-threonine kinase activity that phosphorylates the type I receptor on serine and threonine residues on its recruitment to the cell surface. The type I receptor subsequently phosphorylates downstream signaling molecules, including members of the Smad family of TFs. Eight different Smad proteins have been identified and fall into three distinct classes: the receptor activated Smads (R-Smads) (Smads 1, 2, 3, 5, and 8), which are phosphorylated by the type I receptors, the common mediator Smad (Smad 4), which associates with the activated R-Smads as an obligate heterodimeric partner, and the inhibitory Smads (I-Smads) (Smads 6 and 7), which compete with the R-Smads for interaction with the type I receptors and act to antagonize TGF and BMP signaling. Activation of R-Smads results in the localization of the complexes to the nucleus and the binding of the Smad complexes to target genes within the genome. Smads act to both directly regulate transcription and modulate transcription mediated by a number of different transcription factors (TFs), including c-Jun, c-Fos, and the coactivator p300.

Mutations in Smad proteins have been associated with human carcinomas. For example, pancreatic and colon carcinoma cells often contain deletions in the Smad 4 gene. Alterations in other components of the TGF-β signaling cascade have also been linked to human disease. This is exemplified by male patients with mutations in the gene encoding the Müllerian-inhibiting substance or in the receptor that binds this ligand. Such men exhibit normal virilization of their internal and external genitalia, but retain Müllerian structures (Chapter 41).

PHOSPHOTYROSINE PHOSPHATASE FAMILY Years of research have led to the definition of the importance of protein phosphorylation in mediating multiple signaling pathways. Additional studies have demonstrated that dephosphorylation of proteins is an equally important regulatory process. More than 100 phosphotyrosine phosphatases (PTPs) have been identified. This family can be divided into three groups: tyrosine specific phosphatases, which are intracellular integral membrane proteins; dual specific phosphatases, which dephosphorylate serine and threonine residues in addition to tyrosines; and low molecular weight tyrosine phosphatases.

Prototypical membrane-bound tyrosine specific PTPs are PTPα and CD45. These proteins contain an extracellular ligand binding domain, a single transmembrane domain, and 1-2 cytoplasmic phophotyrosine phosphatase domains. CD45 is a positive regulator of T-cell activation, where, as PTPα appears to be a negative regulator of insulin signaling. Typical intracellular PTPs include PTP1B and SRC-homology 2-domain phosphatase-2 (SHP-2). These proteins contain a single catalytic domain with variable amino- or carboxyl-terminal extensions that often contain SH2 domains. Examples of dual-specific PTPs include MAPK phosphatases, as well as the cdc25 and PTEN phosphatases.

PTPs have been associated with many important physiological processes. For example, the intracellular phosphatase SHP-1 is a negative regulator of cytokine signaling, and mice with disruptions in the SHP-1 gene have sustained tyrosine phosphorylation of multiple signaling molecules with enhanced cellular proliferation. In addition, the dual-specific PTEN phosphatase appears to be a tumor suppressor that is mutated in multiple cancers, including brain, prostate, and breast tumors. The intracellular phosphatase PTP1B is a negative regulator of insulin signaling, and some evidence suggests that increased PTP1B activity might contribute to the insulin resistance seen in type-II diabetes mellitus. In support of this hypothesis, mice with disruptions in the PTP1B gene display increased insulin sensitivity and are resistant to obesity. Furthermore, PTP1B inhibitors lower blood glucose levels in ob/ob mice.

GUANYLYL CYCLASE RECEPTOR FAMILY The guanylyl cyclases (GCs) are enzymes that play important roles in many physiological processes of the cardiovascular, renal, and reproductive systems. The GCs are expressed in both soluble and particulate forms, with the latter serving in part as receptors for natriuretic peptides (NPs). Soluble GCs are discussed later. The particulate GCs generally consist of four domains: a variable extracellular peptide binding domain, a transmembrane domain, a relatively well-conserved intracellular kinase homology domain (KHD), and an intracellular GC catalytic domain. The KHD region appears to serve as an inhibitor of constitutive GC activity. Peptide binding to the extracellular domain results in a conformational change in the KHD region that allows it to bind to ATP. ATP binding in turn leads to activation of the intrinsic GC activity. Treatment with the drug amiloride prevents ATP binding to the KHD region and renders receptors unresponsive to ligand, emphasizing the importance of ATP binding for normal receptor function.

The particulate GC family consists of seven members, GC-A through GC-G, that are expressed on cell surfaces as homodimers or homo-oligomers. GC-A and GC-B bind to and are activated by NPs such as ANP (atrial), BNP (brain), and C-type. GC-C is expressed primarily in the small intestine, binds heat-stable enterotoxin and endogenous ligands, such as guanylin. GC-D is expressed in a subset of olfactory sensory neurons and might serve a role in olfaction. Two GC receptors, GC-E and GC-F, are expressed in the cones and rods of the retina, and mediate the restoration of levels of cGMP and calcium within the retina following excitation by light. Further, GC-E and GC-F are modulated by the GC activating proteins, which respond to intracellular calcium concentrations. GC-G is present in a number of tissues, particularly intestine, muscle, and lung. Activation of these receptors by the binding of peptide ligand or by other modulators, such enterotoxin or guanylin, leads to an increase in the intracellular concentrations of cGMP. These changes of intracellular cGMP lead to modulation of the activities of cGMP modulated protein kinases, cGMP-responsive phosphodiesterases, and cGMP-regulated ion channels.

The NPs are vasoactive hormones that play important roles in regulating blood pressure and cardiovascular homeostasis. ANP and BNP are expressed in the heart, and their secretion is stimulated by atrial stretching or increased pressure. They function to increase fluid and electrolyte excretion, inhibit vasoconstriction, increase glomerular filtration rate, and antagonize the renin-angiontensin system by inhibiting synthesis and release of renin and aldosterone.

Interestingly, alterations in GC receptor expression or activity have been associated with the control of important physiological processes. Animals with salt-sensitive hypertension appear to be less responsive to ANP, whereas disruption of the GC-A receptor gene in mice results in salt-resistant hypertension. In addition, ANP and BNP expression are markedly elevated in patients with congestive heart failure, and serve as sensitive markers for this condition. Mutations of the GC-E receptor protein and other components of cGMP-signaling pathways have been identified in patients with specific forms of inherited retinal dystrophies.

THE SEVEN-TRANSMEMBRANE DOMAIN RECEPTORS
The seven-transmembrane domain (7TM) family of receptors is the largest family of membrane receptors, containing >800 members that respond to a myriad of different ligands, including light, catecholamines (e.g., dopamine, epinephrine, and norepinephrine), amino acids (e.g., glutamate), peptide hormones (e.g., LH, FSH, TSH, TRH, and PTH), elements (e.g., calcium), odors, and proteases (e.g., thrombin). These receptors are characterized by a conserved 7TM configuration, with an extracellular amino-terminal domain and a carboxyl terminal cytoplasmic domain. The amino-terminal domain appears to mediate membrane targeting of the receptor, and, along with the hydrophobic domains, ligand binding and receptor dimerization. The cytoplasmic domain appears to interact with signaling and shutoff molecules located at or near the internal plasma membrane.

The 7TM receptors are also called G protein-coupled receptors (GPCRs), because G proteins mediate most of the signals induced by these receptors (Fig. 31-6). Three G proteins, Gα, Gβ, and Gγ form an inactive heterotrimeric complex at the inner plasma membrane. Agonist binding to a GPCR alters the receptor's conformation, allowing association of the receptor's cytoplasmic surfaces with the G proteins. This interaction leads to dissociation of the heterotrimeric G protein complex into separate Gα and Gβγ signaling molecules. The Gα family consists of at least 16 members that signal in a complex array of pathways (Table 31-2). Two of the best-characterized subfamilies are the Gα$_s$ and Gα$_i$ proteins, which stimulate or inhibit adenylyl cyclase, respectively. The resultant changes in intracellular cAMP concentrations mediated by these two proteins in turn promotes several secondary responses, including activation of protein kinase A (PKA). Gα subunits are activated by association with a ligand-bound GPCR, which leads to the exchange of GTP in place of GDP on the Gα subunit. The Gα subunit is structurally related to the Ras family of small G proteins; in yeast, Ras functions to stimulate yeast adenylyl cyclase and is functionally equivalent to Gα$_s$ in mammalian cells. Similar to Ras, hydrolysis of GTP to GDP by intrinsic GTPase activity then inactivates the Gα subunit. This cycle continues until the Gα subunit re-complexes with Gβγ. Gβγ subunits signal as heterodimers to mediate a number of signals, including modulation of adenylyl cyclase activity and activation of MAPK and phospholipase C-β.

The desensitization, or shutoff, of GPCRs also plays an important role in regulating GPCR-mediated signaling. Shutoff is achieved through several complex steps (Table 31-3). First, heterologous

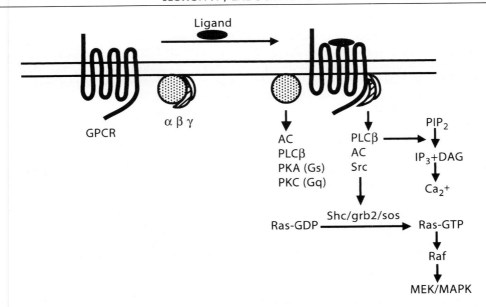

Figure 31-6 Agonist binding to a GPCR alters the receptor's conformation to promote association of the receptor with the G proteins. This interaction leads to dissociation of the heterotrimeric G protein complex into separate Gα and Gβγ signaling molecules. The resultant dissociated Gα and Gβγ subunits then mediate a number of signaling pathways, including modulation of adenylyl cyclase activity and activation of phospholipase C-γ (PLCγ), PKC, and Src. Signaling is shut off by the mechanisms listed in Table 31-3.

Table 31-2
G Proteins and Their Effectors

G protein	Expression	Effectors
$G\alpha_s$	Ubiquitous	Increase AC, Ca^{2+} channel activity;
$G\alpha_{olf}$	Olfactory	activate c-Src tyrosine kinases
$G\alpha_{t1}$	Rods	Increase cGMP
$G\alpha_{t2}$	Cones	phoshodiesterase activity
$G\alpha_{gust}$	Taste cells	Increase phosphodiesterase activity
$G\alpha_{i1}$	Neural > other tissues	Decrease AC; increase potassium
$G\alpha_{i2}$	Ubiquitous	channel activity; activate c-Src
$G\alpha_{i3}$	Other tissues > neural	tyrosine kinases
$G\alpha_o$	Neuroendocrine	Decrease potassium channel
$G\alpha_z$	Neural, platelets	activity; activate Rap1GAP1
$G\alpha_q$	Ubiquitous	Increase PLC-β1, PKC;
$G\alpha_{11}$	Ubiquitous	activate LARGRhoGEF
$G\alpha_{14}$	Liver, lung, kidney	
$G\alpha_{15/16}$	Blood cells	
$G\alpha_{12/13}$	Ubiquitous	Activate Rho proteins
$G\beta\gamma$	Ubiquitous	Increase AC, PLC, GIRK channels, MAPK, PI3K; inhibit $G\alpha_I$

The expression patterns and effectors of 15 subtypes of Gα subunits and Gβγ are shown. AC, adenylyl cyclase; cGMP, cyclic GMP; GAP, GTPase activating protein; GEF, guanine nucleotide exchange factor; PLC, phospholipase C; PKC, phosphokinase C; GIRK, G protein-regulated inwardly rectifying potassium channel; MAPK, mitogen-activated protein kinase; PI3K, phosphatidylinositol 3-kinase.

shutoff is mediated by PKA or PKC-induced phosphorylation of serine and threonine residues on the GPCR cytoplasmic tail, which leads to G protein uncoupling and formation of the inactive G protein heterotrimer. In addition, the cytoplasmic regions of GPCRs can be phosphorylated by G protein receptor kinases (GRKs). GRK-mediated phosphorylation can by itself lead to G protein uncoupling; however, GRK-phosphorylated GPCRs are also targets for arrestin binding, a process that further uncouples the receptor from G proteins. Arrestins in turn can mediate GPCR

internalization, often through clathrin-coated pits, to further shut off GPCR-mediated signaling. Depending on the GPCR, receptors are then either targeted to lysosomes for degradation, ubiquinated by intracellular factors, or dephosphorylated and returned to the cell surface in a process known as resensitization. Finally, GPCR shutoff is regulated by regulator of G protein signaling (RGS) proteins that function as GAPs to promote the conversion of GTP to GDP and Gα subunit shutoff. The extent of each of these mechanisms in regulating shutoff depends on the individual receptor as

Table 31-3
Mechanisms of GPCR Shutoff

Type of shutoff	Mediators	Mechanism
Second messenger	PKA, PKC	Phosphorylation of GPCR, uncoupling of G proteins
GRK/Arrestin-mediated	GRK 1-6 Visual and cone arrestins, β-arrestins 1 and 2, arrestins D and E	Phosphorylation of GPCR by GRK, arrestin binding to GPCR, GPCR Internalization, G protein uncoupling
Trafficking	Arrestins, clathrin, adaptin, caveolae	Internalization, lysosomal targeting, ubiquitinylation
RGS Proteins	>25 isoforms	GTPase activating proteins (GAPs)

Shutoff of GPCR-induced signaling is mediated by several different mechanisms. Receptors can be phosphorylated by second messengers (PKA and PKC). Alternatively, GPCRs can be phosphorylated by G protein-receptor kinases (GRKs), followed by arrestin binding and receptor internalization and trafficking. Finally, intrinsic GTPase activity in the Gα subunit can be accelerated through interactions with regulator of G protein signaling (RGS) molecules.

well as the levels of the many GRK, arrestin, and RGS isoforms expressed in the target cell.

Many disease states have been associated with mutations in either G proteins or GPCRs. For example, patients with McCune-Albright syndrome have somatic mutations in the $G\alpha_s$ subunit that render it constitutively activated. Many of these mutations disrupt the intrinsic GTPase activity of the $G\alpha_s$ subunit, thus resulting in a $G\alpha_s$ protein that is resistant to inhibition by RGS proteins. Individuals with McCune-Albright syndrome have abnormalities that would be expected from overstimulation of $G\alpha_s$-coupled receptors, including precocious puberty (LH receptor), thyroid tumors (TSH receptor), adrenal hyperplasia (adrenocorticotropic hormone receptor), growth-hormone secreting pituitary adenomas (growth hormone-releasing hormone receptor), café au lait spots (melanocyte-stimulating hormone receptor), and polyostotic fibrous dysplasia (PTH receptor). In contrast, patients with inactivating mutations in $G\alpha_s$ suffer from a complex array of syndromes known as pseudohypoparathyroidism. The clinical and biochemical phenotype of pseudohypoparathyroidism, which is inherited in an autosomal-dominant fashion, varies depending on the parent from which the mutated gene was inherited, ranging from hypocalcemia to the syndrome of Albright's hereditary osteodystrophy. Many of the abnormalities associated with pseudohypoparathyroidism appear to be related to PTH resistance; however, resistance to other hormones that signal through $G\alpha_s$ have been reported as well.

Diseases stemming from mutations in the GPCRs themselves are numerous; for example:

1. Inactivating mutations in the calcium sensor receptor that reduce the ability of the parathyroid glands to appropriately respond to serum calcium levels, resulting in increased PTH production, hypercalcemia, and hypophosphatemia. Heterozygotic mutations lead to the benign syndrome of familial hypocalciuric hypercalcemia, whereas homozygous mutations lead to neonatal severe hyperparathyroidism.

2. Activating mutations in the LH receptor in males that lead to precocious puberty and Leydig cell hyperplasia, whereas inactivating mutations lead to XY pseudohermaphroditism and Leydig cell hypoplasia.

3. Somatic activating mutations in the TSH receptor that result in hyperfunctioning thyroid nodules, and even thyroid cancer. Inactivating mutations have been associated with nonimmune hypothyroidism.

4. Inactivating mutations in the vasopressin receptor that result in accelerated receptor desensitization and internalization. These mutations are associated with nephrogenic diabetes insipidus, or vasopressin resistance.

INTRACELLULAR SIGNALING PATHWAYS

As described, membrane receptors represent a critical cellular link to the extracellular environment. Within the cell, an intricate set of signaling pathways communicate receptor responses to other receptors, as well as to the cytoplasmic and nuclear compartments. For the most part, these signaling pathways consist of enzyme cascades, although there are exceptions, including gases such as nitric oxide (NO), lipids, and TFs (such as the STAT proteins). In many cases, receptors activate multiple signaling cascades. It appears that the use of combinations of pathways provides an important mechanism for generating specific cellular responses. Another characteristic of signal transduction pathways is the potential for "crosstalk" in which one pathway might activate or inhibit another pathway. Again, this generates the potential for diverse responses. In the next section, specific examples are provided for some of the better-studied signaling pathways central to endocrine responses.

p21RAS AND MITOGEN-ACTIVATED PROTEIN KINASES

Because growth factors induce a variety of cellular responses, including proliferation, there has been great interest in delineating the pathways that mediate growth factor responses. Tremendous progress has occurred in the elucidation of numerous cytoplasmic and nuclear kinases involved in growth responses. The number of different kinases is enormous, and they have been estimated to account for as many as 5–10% of transcribed genes. The family of MAPKs includes the extracellular signal-regulated kinases (ERKs), stress-activated protein kinases (SAPKs) or c-Jun N-terminal protein kinases, p38-kinases, and ERK5 (Fig. 31-7). As noted, tyrosine phosphorylation of growth factor receptors, such as EGF, creates a binding site for a variety of adaptor proteins. One adaptor,

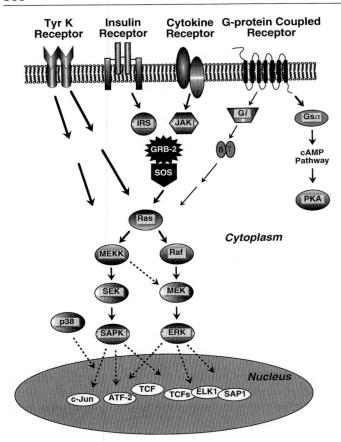

Figure 31-7   Signal transduction cascades. Most cells express a wide variety of different growth factor receptors. Each of these receptors can activate an array of signaling pathways, not all of which are shown. Tyrosine kinases induce the binding of src-homology 2 (SH2) domain proteins, such as Grb-2. Grb-2 binds to guanine nucleotide exchange factors, such as son of sevenless (SOS). This pathway can also be activated by the insulin receptor through insulin-related substrate (IRS) or by cytokine receptors through JAKs. Although Gsα-coupled receptors act primarily through the camp pathway, they can also activate mitogen-activated kinases (MAPK) through their β- and γ-subunits. This figure emphasizes that different receptors can activate the ras pathway along with one or more downstream kinase cascades. Ras activates several downstream kinases in a cell type-specific manner. The preferential activation of a particular MAPK module, such as activation of the ERK rather than the SAPK pathway, provides a mechanism for specific responses. Many cellular targets, including these kinases and a variety of transcription factors, are involved in cellular growth responses.

Grb-2, binds to tyrosine-phosphorylated proteins through its central SH2 domain. Grb-2 contains flanking SH3 domains that recruit proline- rich guanine nucleotide exchange factors, such as SOS (Drosophila son of sevenless). After growth factor treatment (e.g., EGF), the Grb-2–SOS complex associates with the tyrosine-phosphorylated receptor, which leads to the activation of p21ras and induction of downstream kinases.

The signal transduction pathways downstream of growth factor receptors involve a complex interplay of parallel, diverging, and converging pathways. The Ras proteins link growth factor receptor activation to protein phosphorylation and gene regulation through cascades of protein kinases. Induction of MAPKs requires dual phosphorylation on threonine and tyrosine residues by dual specificity MEKs. Several different protein kinases are capable of

functioning as MEKKs, including Raf-1 (*see* Fig. 31-7). In some cell types, the SAPKs and p38 kinases are activated by cellular stresses, including specific stimuli such as tumor necrosis factor (TNF)-α, ultraviolet (UV) irradiation, or genotoxic alkylating chemicals. The mechanisms by which one particular MAPK module is activated in response to a particular stimulus might depend on which combinations of kinases are present as well as interactions among various signaling cascades and specific scaffold molecules that bind to and organize the kinases participating in a particular MAPK module.

TFs (e.g., c-Jun, c-Fos, activating transcription factor [ATF]-2, Elk-1) are one of the targets of MAPK cascades and provide an important mechanism for altering patterns of gene expression in response to extracellular signals. Phosphorylation of such TFs can alter interactions with transcriptional partners, change DNA binding affinity for a particular DNA sequence, or affect the activation surfaces that interact with the basal transcription apparatus. As an example, c-Jun is phosphorylated by several different kinases, including ERKs and SAPKs. Amino-terminal phosphorylation of c-Jun by the SAPKs enhances transactivation function, whereas phosphorylation of c-Jun near its DNA binding domain enhances DNA binding.

As with many hormone regulatory systems, negative feedback is critical for dampening signal transduction systems once they have been activated. Because most of these pathways involve reversible protein phosphorylation, protein phosphatases provide a mechanism for temporally modulating specific signals. There might be as many as 1000 distinct protein phosphatase genes. The physiological importance of these phosphatases is exemplified by the ability of SV40 small t antigen to exert its cellular transforming effects by inhibiting protein phosphatase 2A, with consequent induction of MEK and ERK activity in the cell. Various growth factors induce phosphatases differentially. This might explain, in part, why treatment with one growth factor can result in sustained activation of ERK, whereas another factor causes transient stimulation of the kinase. Differences in the duration of signaling result in part through differential activation of G proteins in the Ras family. For example, rapid transient ERK activation is mediated by Ras coupling to Raf-1, whereas prolonged ERK activation involves an alternate small G protein family member known as Rap1, which couples to B-Raf in order to activate ERK. Additionally, signal strength and duration is translated into differential biological responses by altering the phosphorylation state, and thus the protein stability of short-lived TFs that are ERK substrates. Multisite, sequential phosphorylation of immediate early gene products, such as c-jun, c-fos, and c-myc, in response to sustained ERK activation stabilizes these molecules, resulting in their prolonged transcriptional activation, leading to increased cell proliferation.

CALCIUM SIGNALING   Many cellular responses involve alterations in intracellular calcium concentration as a mechanism for transmitting signals. There are two main pathways that initiate Ca^{2+} signaling. In excitable cells, the activities of voltage-dependent Ca^{2+} channels result in alterations of intracellular Ca^{2+} concentration. In nonexcitable cells, the slow inositol pathway (IP_3) predominates, initiated either by receptor tyrosine kinases or by GPCRs of the seven transmembrane domain class. These receptors stimulate the hydrolysis of the membrane lipid phosphatidylinositol 4,5-bisphosphate by phospholipase C, leading to the production of diacylglycerol and IP_3. IP_3 binds to one of the

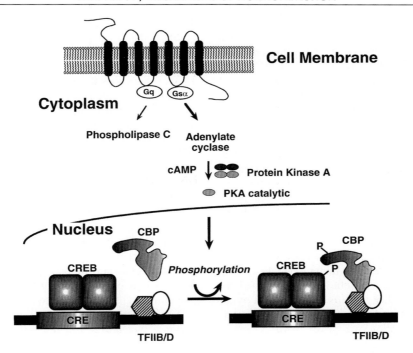

Figure 31-8   cAMP stimulation of transcriptional responses. GPCRs provide a major pathway for the generation of cAMP by adenylate cyclase. Increased cAMP levels within the cell cause dissociation of the tetrameric protein kinase A (PKA) holoenzyme leading to the release of the active catalytic subunit of PKA. The active catalytic subunit is translocated to the nucleus, in which it phosphorylates transcription factor (TF) CREB, which binds as a homodimer to specific cAMP response elements (CREs) on target genes. The phosphorylation of CREB induces the binding of the coactivator, CREB-binding protein (CBP), which is also a substrate for phosphorylation. These transcription factors act by interacting with basal TFs such as TFIIB and TFIID. Several other kinases might phosphorylate CREB, including the calcium-regulated kinases.

members of the InsP3R family of integral endoplasmic reticulum (ER) membrane proteins, activating it as a Ca^{2+} channel to liberate stored Ca^{2+} from the ER lumen into the cytoplasm. The effects modulated by such changes in free intracellular Ca^{2+} are transient, owing to the actions of intracellular calcium binding proteins and pumps that serve to rapidly lower the concentration of free calcium. Such rises in intracellular calcium concentration regulate numerous processes by binding to intermediary proteins, such as calmodulin (CaM), which serves as an intracellular sensor of calcium concentration. CaM binds to a number of enzymes (CaM-dependent protein kinases), protein phosphatases, ion channels, phosphodiesterases, and adenylate cyclases to modify their activities.

cAMP-DEPENDENT SIGNALING   Alterations in intracellular cAMP concentration represent an important mechanism by which extracellular signals are transduced to regulate cellular function. cAMP is synthesized by nine members of the adenylate cyclase family from ATP. These membrane-associated enzymes are composed of conserved membrane-spanning and cytoplasmic catalytic domains and are regulated by the binding of hormones and drugs to GPCRs to modulate the levels of intracellular cAMP. cAMP levels can be further modulated by the effects of other influences, including processes intrinsic to the cell, such as the cell cycle, and the actions of members of the phosphodiesterase family. This large family of enzymes includes members grouped into 11 different protein families that serve to hydrolyze either cAMP and/or cGMP.

Many of the pleiotropic array of cellular effects of cAMP are mediated by PKA, which acts on a number of cellular substrates, including enzymes, the cytoskeleton, and TFs. The effects of cAMP are mediated by its intracellular receptor PKA, which is made up of

two distinct subunits (regulatory [R] and catalytic [C]) in a tetrameric holoenzyme complex (R_2C_2). The regulatory subunits (RI and RII) contain two cAMP-binding domains at their carboxyl termini that regulate the assembly and activity of the complex. After the binding of cAMP, the holoenzyme dissociates into an R_2 dimer and two free active catalytic kinase subunits (C), which phosphorylate cytoplasmic and nuclear target proteins (Fig. 31-8). An additional complicating factor is that the effects of cAMP in the cell might not be uniformly distributed. Instead, proteins such as the A-kinase anchoring proteins might lead to a gradient of cAMP activation, even within different regions of individual cells.

Specific TFs are important targets of the PKA pathway. These include the CREBs and ATFs that are members of the bZIP class of TFs. Posttranslational modification of CREB by phosphorylation at specific serine residues induces conformational changes that alter the affinity of CREB for coactivator proteins, such as CREB-binding protein (CBP) or the TATA box-binding protein coactivator TAFII 110. CBP is thought to form a bridge between CREB and the basal transcription apparatus (Fig. 31-8). CBP also interacts with other bZIP proteins, such as c-Jun and c-Fos, other TFs, including c-Myb, as well as specific kinases. In addition to a clear role in cAMP signaling, CBP has also been implicated in mitogenic signaling and functions as a transcriptional coactivator with intrinsic histone-acetylase and ubiquitin ligase activities; both enzyme activities play key roles in transcription. Consistent with its role in multiple cell signaling pathways and transcriptional regulation, mutations of CBP cause Rubinstein-Taybi syndrome, which is associated with mental retardation, multiple congenital anomalies, and predisposition to malignancy. The bZIP dimerization structure of the CREB and ATF proteins provides the basis for numerous combinations of different members of this family. The closely related cAMP response element modulator gene product can act as a dominant negative regulator of CREB transcriptional activity, either by forming inactive heterodimers with CREB or by binding to the CRE as a component of an inactive complex.

Several other DNA regulatory elements and TFs are capable of stimulating gene transcription in response to increased cAMP and PKA activation. The TF, activator protein 2, also functions in basal, phorbol ester, and cAMP-mediated transcriptional induction. The CAAT enhancer binding protein (C/EBP) induces transcription of the adipocyte protein 2 gene promoter and stearoyl acyl CoA desaturase through a region that is also regulated by cAMP through PKA. cAMP-responsive regions of several genes appear to overlap with binding sites for NRs, some of which might also transduce cAMP effects.

Despite the range of effects mediated by these pathways, some effects of cyclic AMP could not be reproduced by the effects of activated PKA, suggesting that cAMP might regulate cellular processes by distinct mechanisms. Cyclic nucleotide gated ion channels have been identified that are directly modulated by the binding of cAMP to a ligand binding pocket on the cytoplasmic surface of the channel. In addition, two novel cAMP receptors, Epac1 and Epac2 (exchange protein directly activated by cAMP; also called cAMP-GEFI and cAMP-GEFII), have been identified. EpacI and II are guanine nucleotide exchange factors that activate the small G proteins Rap1 and Rap2 following the binding of cAMP.

cGMP-DEPENDENT SIGNALING In addition to the GCs that are structural components of membrane receptors (above), a smaller number of soluble GCs (also referred to as NO-sensitive GCs) have been identified. Two different α and two different β-subunits have been identified: α1, α2, β1, and β2. The active complexes are heteromeric, consisting of one α and one β-subunit. Each subunit consists of carboxyl terminal GC catalytic domains, which are conserved compared to the peptide receptor GCs. The amino termini of these proteins are less conserved and encode the segment responsible for coordinating a heme prosthetic group. This heme prosthetic group serves as the NO sensor and is responsible for the modulation of GC activity in response to changes in the intracellular concentration of NO. The NO is produced locally by members of the NO synthase family of enzymes, or pharmacologically, by agents such as nitroglycerine. As with members of the GC receptor family, the cellular effects of cGMP are mediated by effects on the activities of cGMP-dependent protein kinases, cyclic nucleotide-regulated ion channels, and cGMP-regulated cyclic nucleotide phosphodiesterases. Members of the phosphodiesterase family can further serve to modulate levels of cGMP; Sildenafil enhances the effect of NO in the regulation of vascular smooth muscle tone by inhibiting phosphodiesterase type 5.

NF-κB/REL FAMILY OF TRANSCRIPTION FACTORS

NF-κB was originally identified as a protein in nuclear extracts of B cells that bound to the enhancer element of the κ light chain gene. This binding activity was demonstrated to be present in the cell in a "latent" fashion, which could be rapidly activated in the presence of protein synthesis inhibitors by a variety of stimuli, including TNF, lipopolysaccharide, interleukin-1, phorbol esters, growth factors, and UV irradiation. The basis for the rapid and protein synthesis-independent nature of NF-κB activation was found to reflect the association of the active binding moiety with

an inhibitory subunit, IκB. The dissociation of IκB from NF-κB results in the rapid appearance and translocation of NF-κB DNA binding activity to the nucleus. The active form of NF-κB was found to be dimeric, exerting its effects by binding to specific target sequences with the genome to regulate gene expression.

Subsequent studies have considerably complicated this scenario. Five members of the NF-κB/Rel protein family have been identified, each with substantial sequence homology in what is termed the Rel homology domain. This segment is located at the amino terminus of each protein and contains elements critical for interaction with the inhibitory IκB proteins, dimerization, and DNA binding. Members of this protein family function as dimers, which may consist of identical or nonidentical subunits. In their inactive state, dimers of the NF-κB/Rel proteins are associated with monomers of the IκBα or IκBβ proteins. NF-κB activation is mediated by the IκB (IKK) complex, made up of catalytic components (IKKα and IKKβ) and a regulatory subunit (IKKγ or NEMO). Following stimulation by a number of important effectors, the IKK complex phosphorylates IκB on specific residues, promoting its ubiquitination and degradation.

NF-κB activation is central to the regulation of immune response, owing to its role in the regulation of a host of cytokines and chemokines. It has become clear that NF-κB activation plays an important role in the regulation of apoptosis. Indeed, in some systems, activation of NF-κB has been demonstrated to antagonize the effects of chemotherapy and radiation in inducing apoptosis. Such findings have led to attempts to sensitize tumors to the actions of chemotherapy and radiation by blocking the activation of NF-κB. In addition to diseases in which abnormalities of NF-κB expression occur, defects of the NF-κB signaling pathways have been identified. Incontinentia pigmenti is a rare X-linked-dominant disorder that affects ectodermal tissues resulting in abnormal skin pigmentation, retinal detachment, anodontia, alopecia, nail dystrophy and central nervous system defects. Over 90% of IP carrier females have a recurrent multiexon deletion of the IKKγ gene, which is required to activate the NF-κB pathway. In IP, mutations in IKKγ lead to the complete loss of NF-κB activation creating a susceptibility to cellular apoptosis in response to TNF-α. Although females, hemizygous as a result of X-chromosome inactivation, survive, this condition is lethal for males.

CELL-CYCLE REGULATORY SIGNAL TRANSDUCTION PATHWAYS Phosphorylation plays an essential regulatory role in the cell cycle, and a large array of cyclin-dependent kinases (CDKs) has been identified (Chapter 4). The regulatory subunits of the CDKs, known as cyclins, form complexes with their catalytic partners to function as heterodimeric holoenzymes that phosphorylate specific proteins, including the tumor suppressor protein pRb (Chapter 4). Phosphorylation of pRb blocks its critical inhibitory function, allowing cell-cycle progression and differentiation to occur. Several proteins capable of binding cyclins and inhibiting CDK activity have been identified and are referred to as CDKIs. The CDKIs inhibit cell-cycle progression and inhibit tumor formation. Translocation of the cyclin D1 gene has been associated with certain cases of hyperparathyroidism (Chapter 36), and actually led to the identification of cyclin D1 in humans. In these cases, a somatic inversion of chromosome 11 brings cyclin D1 under the control of the PTH promoter. Consequently, cyclin D1 is overexpressed in the parathyroid cell and results in cellular proliferation. The proliferative and transforming effects of cyclin D1 are independent of its ability to activate cyclin-dependent protein kinases, but instead require its interaction with the CEBP/β TF, in which cyclin D1 relieves the transcriptional repressive activity of CEBP/β at multiple gene promoters.

NUCLEAR RECEPTORS

Nuclear Receptor Action   The NR superfamily consists of structurally related proteins that are important modulators of gene expression in eukaryotes. The structures of the different family members are widely distributed in many species and are highly conserved, particularly in the segments encoding the DNA-binding domain (DBD) and ligand-binding domain (LBD) of the receptor proteins.

In humans, 48 different members of this family have been identified, based on sequence analysis of the human genome. In some circumstances, the NRs mediate the physiological actions of small cell-permeable hormones, such as the sex steroids (estrogen, testosterone, and progesterone), cortisol, aldosterone, thyroid hormone, and vitamin D, as well as retinoids that are derived from dietary vitamin A. In other instances, no ligand has been identified. These receptors might not require the binding of a ligand for functional activation and as a group are referred to as "orphan" NRs.

Structure and Classification of Nuclear Receptors   From the first analyses of NR structure and function, it was apparent that these proteins were organized in a modular fashion. The DBD, made up of two centrally located "zinc fingers," is the most highly conserved segment (Fig. 31-9). The structure of this segment has been well characterized using site-directed mutagenesis, X-ray crystallography, and nuclear magnetic resonance studies. Residues at the carboxyl terminal base of the first zinc finger are principal determinants of DNA binding specificity, where, as adjacent sequences at the base of the second zinc finger are critical to the formation of the dimerization interface. The DBDs of NRs that bind as monomers differ slightly in carboxyl terminal extensions of the DBD that contribute to the DNA binding by this element. Regions carboxy-terminal to the DBD specify sequences that localize the protein to the nucleus.

Other functionally important segments of the NRs have been delineated. For members that bind ligand, the LBD is located in the carboxyl terminus of the receptor. In addition to its role in ligand binding, this region contains several overlapping domains, including regions required for dimerization of the receptor and for transcriptional activation and repression. The structures of the LBDs of a number of NR family members have been solved by X-ray crystallography. These studies demonstrate that ligand binding induces important conformational changes that underlie the changes of activity of the NR in the regulation of gene activity. The amino-terminal segments of the NRs are the most variable and the least well characterized. In some cases, it contains additional transcription-activating domains and serves as a "docking site" for interactions with other proteins.

NRs can be classified by several different schemes. One useful method employs the mechanisms by which these molecules recognize DNA (*see* Fig. 31-10). The classic steroid receptors share a similar DBD and bind to DNA sequences similar to the inverted palindromic sequence depicted. This group includes receptors for glucocorticoids, mineralocorticoids, progesterone, and androgens. The steroid receptors have been particularly well characterized and exist in the cell complexed with proteins of the heat shock family in the absence of ligand. Following the binding of ligand, the receptors dissociate from the heat shock proteins, translocate to the nucleus, and bind monomers to target DNA sequences within or adjacent to responsive genes.

Other NRs differ in the manner that they bind to target DNA sequences. The diverse patterns of recognition include the binding as monomer, heterodimers, and homodimers (*see* Fig. 31-10). The retinoid X receptors (RXRs) serve as heterodimeric partners for several different NRs, including retinoic acid receptors (RARs), thyroid hormone receptors, vitamin D receptor (VDR), and peroxisome proliferator-activating receptors (PPARs). The heterodimers typically bind to hormone response elements (HREs) that are arranged as direct repeats rather than in a palindromic manner. The spacing between these half-sites, and variations in some of the contextual bases, provide specificity to different receptors, providing a partial explanation for how so many different receptors can share a common binding motif but elicit distinct cellular responses.

A number of members of the NR family were identified on the basis of sequence homology to the DBDs of characterized members of the NR family (e.g., the steroid receptors). This cloning exercise yielded cDNAs encoding proteins with structural similarities to the NRs (e.g., with the LBDs and DBDs), but for which no ligand had been defined. With time, ligands for several of these 'orphan' receptors have been identified. For example, the RXRs were initially classified as orphan receptors, but are known to bind 9-cis retinoic acid. The PPARs bind a variety of eicosanoids, as well as thiazolidinediones that are used to treat noninsulin-dependent diabetes. It remains to be determined whether ligands exist for all orphan members of the NR family. It appears likely that some members might not bind ligand, and instead might be constitutively active or regulated by other mechanisms, such as phosphorylation.

In addition to the diversity in types of receptor the NR family, in several cases receptor isoforms encoded by different genes provide an additional level of control. For example, there are two separate genes for TRs, two ERs, three for all-trans RARs, and three RXRs. In addition, many of these genes generate multiple receptor subtypes by virtue of alternate mRNA splicing or alternate promoter or initiator methionine usage. The function of individual isoforms has been defined in only a small number of instances, but in the case of the PR, the A- and B-isoforms have physiologically distinct roles. Receptor subtype expression is highly regulated during development, and there is striking tissue-specific expression of various NR isoforms in adult organs. Therefore, like the peptide hormone receptors, tissue responsiveness to the hormone signal is regulated at its most fundamental level by selective expression of the NR in responsive tissues.

Nuclear Receptor Function and the Modulation of Gene Expression   NRs interact with specific DNA sequences that are frequently located within or adjacent to promoter regions of regulated genes. After the receptor binds to DNA, it is positioned to interact with other TFs to alter rates of gene transcription. Considerable progress has been made toward defining the mechanism(s) by which NRs modulate these effects. Several of the NRs physically interact with the basal TF, TFIIB. Using in vitro transcription analysis, the NRs have been shown to facilitate the rate of assembly and stabilize basal TFs in the preinitiation complex that forms at the sites of transcriptional initiation.

An additional level of transcriptional control occurs through NR interactions with "coactivator" or "corepressor" proteins, which in turn interact with proteins of the basal TF complex. Several of these proteins have been identified on the basis of their ability to interact with NRs, using biochemical techniques or genetic screens in yeast. In general, coactivators recruit proteins that result

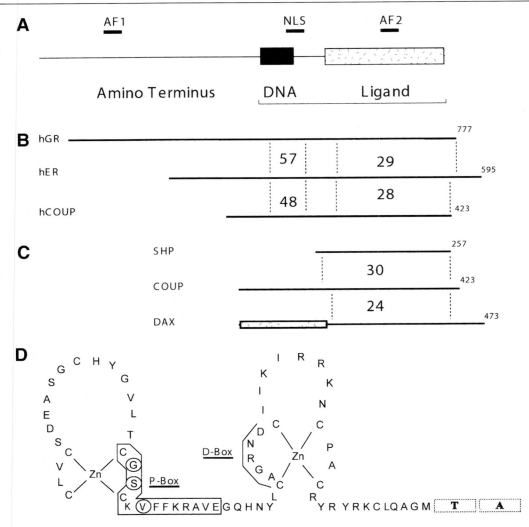

Figure 31-9 Modular structure of the NR family. Members of the NR family contain segments that are conserved to varying degrees among the family members. **(A)** A schematic structure of a prototypic NR is shown. The conserved ligand binding and DNA binding domains are indicated (hatched and filled rectangles, respectively). The relative positions of the activating functions (AF)-1 and -2 within the amino terminus and carboxyl terminus of the receptor proteins are shown. Sequences responsible for the nuclear localization of these proteins have been localized to the carboxyl terminal end of the DNA-binding domain. **(B)** Although the relative positions of the individual domains are in most instances maintained, the degree of sequence conservation varies widely. Members of the nuclear receptor family exhibit the highest degree of conservation when the amino acid sequences of the DNA binding domains of the receptor proteins are compared. Lesser degrees of homology are evident between the sequences that are made up of the LBDs of the receptors. In the example shown, the predicted amino acid sequences of three different members of the nuclear receptor family are compared. The degree of relatedness is shown for each of the two receptors when aligned with the predicted amino acid sequence of the human glucocorticoid receptor. The amino-terminal segments of the receptors differ considerably in size and sequence. The extent of homology is <15% when the amino termini of the receptor proteins are compared. **(C)** In some members of the nuclear receptor family, differences are evident even in the fundamental organization of the receptor proteins. The COUP-TF protein exhibits a structure similar to that of the other nuclear receptor protein, with a small amino terminus, a DNA binding domain comprised of two zinc fingers, and a segment corresponding to the ligand binding domains of the steroid receptors (COUP-TF is an orphan receptor). By contrast, although the amino acid sequence of the orphan nuclear receptor, DAX-1, predicts a segment homologous to the LBD of other nuclear receptors, the amino terminal segment is composed of distinctive segments that mediate the binding of this nuclear receptor to DNA (stippled box). SHP, short heterodimer partner, while in which as encoding segments similar to the ligand-binding domains of other nuclear receptors, lacks segments that mediate its binding to DNA. **(D)** Schematic organization of the human glucocorticoid receptor DNA binding domain. The zinc ions serve as nucleation centers for the two "zinc finger" modules of the DNA binding domain. The regions identified by mutagenesis studies as being important for receptor dimerization (D-box) and for target gene specificity (P-box) are indicated. In some members of the nuclear receptor family, carboxyl terminal extensions (CTE) of the DNA binding domain are important determinants of the high affinity binding of the receptor proteins to its DNA targets (the T- and A-boxes). (Reprinted with permission from Zoppi S, Young M, McPhaul MJ. Regulation of gene expression by the nuclear receptor family. Genetics of Steroid Biosynthesis and Function, Mason, JI, ed., Harwood Academic Publisher, 2002, pp. 376–403.)

in a more active chromatin configuration, and are associated with increases in transcription. By contrast, corepressors enable the recruitment of proteins that result in the compacting of chromatin and lowering of the transcriptional activity of genes.

In parallel with such studies, other investigators used biochemical fractionation methods to isolate the protein complexes that associate with ligand-bound forms of the NRs, such as the thyroid receptor and VDR. These studies led to the characterization of

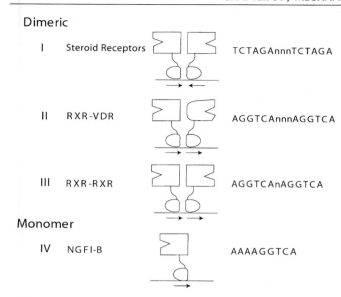

Figure 31-10 Schematic representations of the different mechanisms by which members of the nuclear receptor family recognize DNA. In many instances, members of the steroid receptor family (Class I) bind to sequences similar to the inverted palindromic sequence shown at right. In this type of recognition sequence, a three-nucleotide "spacer" (nnn) separates the individual half sites. Nuclear receptors (NRs) with nonsteroidal ligands (Class II) bind to DNA in association with the obligate heteromerization partner, retinoid X receptor (RXR). Depending on the receptor (e.g., vitamin D receptor, thyroid hormone receptor, peroxisome proliferator-activated receptor, or retinoic acid receptor) the spacing between the two individual half sites is distinct. Class III NRs bind as homodimers to their target sequences. Some members of the nuclear receptor family (Class IV) bind to their target DNA sequences as monomers. In these instances, nucleotide residues adjacent to the core response element form a critical component of the recognized sequence. (Reprinted with permission from Zoppi S, Young M, McPhaul MJ. Regulation of gene expression by the nuclear receptor family. Genetics of Steroid Biosynthesis and Function, Masson, JI, ed., Harwood Academic Publisher, 2002, pp. 376–403.)

large multiprotein complexes such as the thyroid receptor-associated proteins (TRAPs) and vitamin D receptor-interacting proteins (DRIPs). Subsequent analyses demonstrated that these protein complexes share considerable relationship to one another and to other multiprotein assemblies that interact with other transcriptional activators (e.g., ARC). Furthermore, each of these complexes shares considerable similarity to the transcriptional regulator complex, Mediator, which was originally defined genetically and biochemically in yeast.

These considerations led to the emergence of the puzzling dichotomy of transcriptional regulation by NRs. On one hand was the participation of nuclear coregulators, such as the coactivators and corepressors. However, biochemical and genetic studies suggested the importance of complexes such as the DRIP and TRAP complexes. This apparent duality has been partially reconciled by the demonstration that components of both types of complexes can be demonstrated at the sites of transcriptional regulation at different times following stimulation with hormone. These observations suggest that the complement of proteins that can be detected at important regulatory sites within a regulated gene are dynamic and might differ substantially at different times following the addition of hormone. The complement of such proteins that is present in different cell types might help explain the differential effects of ligands in different tissues.

Nongenomic Functions of Nuclear Receptors Exploration of the mechanisms by which members of the NR family modulate the transcription of responsive genes is ongoing. In general, these effects require sufficient time (e.g., hours) for the effects on the transcription of responsive genes to be exerted. In other circumstances, the timing of the observed effect is so rapid regarded to be inconsistent with regulation at the transcriptional level. These transcription-independent steroid responses are often termed "nongenomic," and in many cases appear to be mediated by interactions between classic NRs and membrane signaling molecules. Examples include estrogen-induced activation of the MAPK cascade and endothelial NO synthase activity in breast and endothelial cells, respectively; estrogen and androgen-mediated protection from apoptosis in bone cells; and progesterone- and testosterone-induced maturation of oocytes.

Although distinct in terms of mechanism, these two types of effect are not mutually exclusive. For example, growth factor signaling pathways alter the function of some NRs, such as the ER and PR. Such influences might exert important effects on the growth or gene expression patterns of cells in response to specific classes of ligand. For example, direct phosphorylation of ER or PR by MAPK can lead to responses to very low concentrations of steroid hormone ligands at hormone-responsive elements containing gene promoters, whereas activation of MAPKs by ER or PR might regulate genes targeted by Ets factors that are primarily phosphorylated and activated by MAPK family members.

Antagonism of Nuclear Receptor Function The reproductive NRs are notable owing to the existence of clinically important receptor antagonists. RU-486 binds with high affinity to the PR LBD (it also binds the glucocorticoid receptor) in such a manner that the ligand-receptor complex recruits corepressors, blocking its transcriptional activating properties. In like fashion, although ICI 164, 382, Tamoxifen and Raloxifene are bound in the ligand-binding cavity of the ERα, they cause the ER to adopt conformations that cause the recruitment of molecules that do not permit full transcriptional activation of estrogen-regulated genes. The conformation of the ER differs when bound to these different ligands, accounting for the recruitment of differential complements of corepressors and coactivators, and their activities as "pure" or selective ER modulators. The development of specific receptor antagonists for these and other members of the NR family is an active area of investigation (Table 31-4). The definition of functionally critical surfaces and the demonstration that the binding of small molecules to these surfaces (such as peptides) results in selective decreases in receptor function suggests that reagents to modulate the activity of many members of the NR might be possible.

Physiological Effects of Nuclear Receptors Members of the NR family serve important roles in development, cell differentiation, metabolism, and reproduction. Examples of these functions are described briefly to illustrate how NRs affect physiology.

The glucocorticoid receptor mediates the widespread effects of cortisol on blood pressure, blood glucose levels and insulin action, neuropsychiatric status, diurnal variation in body temperature, and immune responses. The closely related mineralocorticoid receptor binds aldosterone and regulates the renal handling of potassium and sodium.

The sex steroid receptors determine the phenotypic appearance of secondary sexual characteristics and control the production of oocytes and sperm. The androgens testosterone and 5α-dihydrotestosterone both bind to a single high-affinity receptor protein, the androgen receptor. In many systems, testosterone exhibits lower activity as

Table 31-4
Ligands and Antagonists for NRs

Receptor	Ligand	Antagonists
Glucocorticoid subfamily		
GR	Cortisol	RU-486
PR	Progesterone	RU-486
MR	Aldosterone, cortisol	Spironolactone
AR	Dihydrotestosterone	Flutamide, cyproterone
ER/TR subfamily		
ER	Estrogen	Tamoxifen, clomiphene, ICI 164,384
TR	Triiodothyronine (T3)	None
VDR	1,25-Dihydroxyvitamin D	None
RAR	All-*trans* retinoic acid	Ro 41-5253
RXR	9-*cis* Retinoic acid	None
PPARγ	Prostaglandin J_2, Thiazolidinedione	None

PR, progesterone receptor; GR, glucocorticoid receptor; MR, mineralocorticoid receptor; AR, androgen receptor; ER, estrogen receptor; TR, thyroid hormone receptor; VDR, vitamin D receptor; RAR, retinoic acid receptor; RXR, 9-*cis* retinoic receptor; PPAR, peroxisome proliferator activated receptor.

Table 31-5
Disorders Caused by Mutations in NRs

Receptor	Disorder	Mechanism	Inheritance
Androgen receptor	Androgen insensitivity	Loss-of-function: premature termination, DBD and LBD missense mutations	X-linked
	Prostate cancer	Gain-of-function: point mutations	Somatic
Estrogen receptor	Estrogen resistance	Loss-of-function: missense mutations, deletions	Autosomal-recessive
	Breast cancer	Gain-of-function: Missense mutations	Somatic
Glucocorticoid receptor	Glucocorticoid resistance	Loss-of-function: premature termination, DBD and LBD missense mutations	Autosomal-dominant
Thyroid hormone receptor β	Resistance to thyroid hormone	Loss-of-function: LBD missense mutations	Autosomal-dominant
Vitamin D receptor	Vitamin D-resistant rickets	Loss-of-function: DBD and LBD missense mutations	Autosomal-recessive
Retinoic acid receptor	Promyelocytic leukemia	Gain-of-function: fusion protein lacking RAR DBD	Somatic translocation
HFN4	MODY	Loss-of-function:	Autosomal-dominant
PPARγ	Obesity	missense	
Mineralocorticoid receptor	Hypertension	Gain-of-function: missense mutation	Autosomal-dominant
	Type I pseudo hypo aldosteronism	Loss-of-function: missense mutations	Autosomal-dominant

RAR, retinoic acid receptor.

an androgen, compared to DHT, presumably on the basis of a slightly lower affinity and stability of binding to the AR. Thus, the conversion of T to the more active metabolite DHT, by one of the two 5α-reductase isoenzymes, represents a mechanism by which tissue- or cell type- specific variations in androgenic effects can be modulated.

In the examples earlier, the physiological pathways regulated by the receptors were defined before the receptors were isolated and characterized. This is not true for many members of the NR family; the recognition of the biological importance of many members of this family has awaited the definition of phenotypes in humans and in animal models of disease. For example, steroidogenic factor (SF)-1 is an orphan receptor that was originally identified on the basis of its role in modulating the expression of genes encoding the steroidogenic cytochromes P450. Although these studies demonstrated that SF-1 is selectively expressed in the adrenal gland and in reproductive tissues, it was not until the targeted disruption of SF-1 was accomplished in the mouse that the critical role of this protein in the development of the adrenals and gonads was recognized. The subsequent identification of human patients with SF1 mutations has demonstrated the relevance of these findings in the mouse to humans.

NRs play a prominent role in human disease, many of which are described in detail in subsequent chapters (Table 31-5). Although the most well defined disorders are those of resistance to nuclear hormone action (loss-of-function mutations), an increasing number of diseases have been traced to alteration of structure that leads to an activation of the receptor protein.

SELECTED REFERENCES

Alberti L, Carniti C, Miranda C, Roccato E, Pierotti MA. RET and NTRK1 proto-oncogenes in human diseases. J Cell Physiol 2003;195:168–186.

Clapham DE. Calcium signaling. Cell 1995;80:259–268.

Cobb MH, Goldsmith EJ. How MAP kinases are regulated. J Biol Chem 1995;270:14,843–14,846.

Escriva H, Bertrand S, Laudet V. The evolution of the nuclear receptor superfamily. Essays Biochem 2004;40:11–26.

Ferguson SS, Barak LS, Zhang J, Caron MG. G-protein-coupled receptor regulation: role of G-protein-coupled receptor kinases and arrestins. Can J Physiol Pharmacol 1996;74:1095–1110.

Ghosh A, Greenberg ME. Calcium signaling in neurons: molecular mechanisms and cellular consequences. Science 1995;268:239–247.

Glass CK, Rose DW, Rosenfeld MG. Nuclear receptor coactivators. Curr Opin Cell Biol 1997;9:222–232.

Heldin CH. Dimerization of cell surface receptors in signal transduction. Cell 1995;80:213–223.

Hunter T. Protein kinases and phosphatases: the yin and yang of protein phosphorylation and signaling. Cell 1995;80:225–236.

Ihle JN. STATs: signal transducers and activators of transcription. Cell 1996;84:331–334.

Josso N, di Clemente N. Serine/threonine kinase receptors and ligands. Curr Opin Genet Dev 1997;7:371–377.

Jameson JL. Principles or hormone action. Oxford Textbook of Medicine, 1996. Oxford University Press, Oxford, UK.

Karin M. The regulation of AP-1 activity by mitogen-activated protein kinases. J Biol Chem 1995;270:16,483–16,486.

Kishimoto T, Taga T, Akira S. Cytokine signal transduction. Cell 1994;76:253–262.

Lamb J, Ramaswamy S, Ford HL, et al. A mechanism of cyclin D1 action encoded in the patterns of gene expression in human cancer. Cell 2003;114:323–334.

Mangelsdorf DJ, Thummel C, Beato M, et al. The nuclear receptor superfamily: the second decade. Cell 1995;83:835–839.

Marshall MS. Ras target proteins in eukaryotic cells. FASEB J 1995;9:1311–1318.

Massague J, Weis-Garcia F. Serine/threonine kinase receptors: mediators of transforming growth factor beta family signals. Cancer Surv 1996;27:41–64.

Piek E, Heldin CH, Ten Dijke P. Specificity, diversity, and regulation in TGF-beta superfamily signaling. FASEB J 1999;13:2105–2124.

Pierce KL, Premont RT, Lefkowitz RJ. Seven-transmembrane receptors. Nat Rev Mol Cell Biol 2002;3:639–650.

Rosenfeld RG, Buckway CK. Growth hormone insensitivity syndromes: lessons learned and opportunities missed. Horm Res 2001;55(Suppl 2): 36–39.

Saltiel AR, Pessin JE. Insulin signaling pathways in time and space. Trends Cell Biol 2002;12:65–71.

Schlessinger J. Cell signaling by receptor tyrosine kinases. Cell 2000;103:211–225.

Spiegel AM. Defects in G protein-coupled signal transduction in human disease. Annu Rev Physiol 1996;58:143–170.

Tremblay J, Desjardins R, Hum D, Gutkowska J, Hamet P. Biochemistry and physiology of the natriuretic peptide receptor guanylyl cyclases. Mol Cell Biochem 2002;230:31–47.

Wilks AF, Oates AC. The JAK/STAT pathway. Cancer Surv 1996;27: 139–163.

Woodgett JR, Avruch J, Kyriakis J. The stress activated protein kinase pathway. Cancer Surv 1996;27:127–138.

Zhang ZY. Protein tyrosine phosphatases: prospects for therapeutics. Curr Opin Chem Biol 2001;5:416–423.

32 Diabetes Mellitus

WILLIAM L. LOWE, JR.

SUMMARY

Diabetes mellitus is characterized by fasting and postprandial hyperglycemia. Type 1 diabetes occurs secondary to autoimmune destruction of the insulin-secreting pancreatic β-cells, whereas type 2 diabetes results from a deficiency of insulin action secondary to a combination of insulin resistance and relative β-cell dysfunction. Familial clustering of type 1 and 2 diabetes has suggested a genetic contribution to the etiology of the diseases, but monozygotic twin and other studies have indicated that environmental factors also contribute to their etiology. Although relatively rare monogenic forms of diabetes have been described, type 1 and 2 diabetes are, in general, complex, polygenic diseases.

Key Words: Autoimmunity; genetics; insulin; major histocompatibility complex; maturity onset diabetes of the young; mitochondria; peroxisome proliferator-activated receptor-γ; sulfonylurea receptor; type 1 diabetes; type 2 diabetes; Wolfram syndrome.

INTRODUCTION

Diabetes mellitus affects approx 5% of the general population with its prevalence varying among ethnic groups and geographic regions. Two types of diabetes, type 1 and 2, account for approx 10 and 90% of diabetes cases, respectively. Although these two disorders share a common phenotype, fasting and postprandial hyperglycemia, their etiology is distinct. Type 1 diabetes is characterized by pancreatic β-cell deficiency with a resulting absolute deficiency of insulin. The β-cell deficiency is most commonly secondary to autoimmune-mediated destruction. Type 2 diabetes, in contrast, is characterized by a deficiency of insulin action resulting from a combination of insulin resistance and relative β-cell dysfunction that is manifest as inadequate insulin secretion in the face of insulin resistance and hyperglycemia.

The familial clustering of both type 1 and 2 diabetes has long suggested a genetic contribution to the etiology of the diseases. In the case of type 1 diabetes, the concordance rate among monozygotic twins is 30–40% compared with a concordance rate of 5–10% among dizygotic twins. The risk of type 1 diabetes for siblings of an affected individual is approx 6%, whereas the risk in the general population is approx 0.4%. Although these data are consistent with a genetic contribution to the etiology of the disease, the lack of 100% concordance in monozygotic twins suggests that environmental factors make a significant contribution to

From: *Principles of Molecular Medicine, Second Edition*
Edited by: M. S. Runge and C. Patterson © Humana Press, Inc., Totowa, NJ

the disease pathogenesis. These environmental factors are not clearly defined, but some studies suggest that certain viral infections or early childhood diet may affect the risk of type 1 diabetes. Prenatal exposure to rubella is a clear risk factor, as 20% of children with the congenital rubella syndrome develop type 1 diabetes. Other potential risk factors for which there are conflicting or unconfirmed data include enterovirus infections and early introduction of either cow's milk protein, cereal, or gluten into the diet. Familial clustering of disease is much more apparent in type 2 diabetes. The concordance rate among monozygotic twins is 50–90%, whereas approx 40% of siblings and 30% of offspring of affected individuals develop either type 2 diabetes or impaired glucose tolerance. Again, these data are consistent with a significant genetic contribution to the development of type 2 diabetes but suggest that environmental influences are also important.

With the advent of molecular genetics, significant progress has been made in defining the genetics of rare, monogenic forms of diabetes as well as more typical type 1 and 2 diabetes. Progress is reflected in the classification of diabetes, which includes diagnostic categories of genetic defects in β-cell function and insulin action. This chapter describes the advances in the genetics of both type 1 and 2 diabetes, as well as monogenic forms of diabetes.

GENETICS OF TYPE 1 DIABETES MELLITUS

Type 1 diabetes often presents abruptly with marked hyperglycemia, polyuria, and ketoacidosis, which occur as a result of insulin deficiency. This dramatic presentation suggested initially that type 1 diabetes was the result of an acute event, but with an improved understanding of the pathogenesis of the disease, it is clear that disease onset is a chronic process that can be divided into a series of stages. As discussed next, individuals have a genetic predisposition for diabetes. In certain of these individuals, an autoimmune process is initiated, presumably in response to some environmental exposure. There is then a period of active autoimmunity characterized by the presence of autoantibodies and progressive β-cell destruction but with maintenance of normal blood sugars and glucose tolerance. With sufficient β-cell destruction, impaired glucose tolerance, which is typically not clinically evident, ultimately diabetes develops. Depending on the rate of decline of β-cell function, older patients may be presumed to have type 2 diabetes mellitus because of residual insulin secretion, albeit not sufficient insulin secretion to maintain euglycemia. As destruction of the residual β-cells continues, a new stress, for example, infection, often results in the acute presentation of diabetes.

Ultimately, absolute insulin dependence develops because of total or near-total β-cell destruction.

The autoimmune-mediated destruction of pancreatic β-cells is characterized by two features, autoantibodies and insulitis. Autoantibodies present in type 1 diabetes mellitus are directed against a variety of β-cell antigens, including insulin, glutamic acid decarboxylase (GAD65 and 67), and a catalytically inactive member of the transmembrane protein tyrosine phosphatase family (IA-2). Although the presence of two or more of these antibodies is predictive of progression to diabetes in relatives of affected individuals, they likely play little role in the immune-mediated destruction of the islets cells. Insulitis is characterized by inflammatory infiltrates in the islets consisting primarily of CD8+ cells but also of CD4+ cells, B-cells, macrophages, and natural killer cells. The cause of type 1 diabetes mellitus, and thus, the trigger for the autoimmune process, is complex and involves both a genetic predisposition and environmental factors.

Type 1 diabetes does not follow a simple Mendelian pattern of inheritance. As demonstrated by studies in identical twins, there is not 100% concordance between a susceptible genotype and disease presence. Presumably the penetrance of the disease genes is influenced by environmental factors. Moreover, studies in mice and humans clearly demonstrate that the disease is polygenic, suggesting that a sufficient complement of genes must be inherited to confer susceptibility to diabetes. Two approaches have been used to define genes that predispose to type 1 diabetes-identifying candidate genes by comparing the frequency of alleles of specific genes in diabetic and control populations (case–control or association studies) and genome scanning to identify chromosomal loci linked with disease susceptibility. Given the autoimmune etiology of type 1 diabetes, the major histocompatibility (MHC) locus or human leukocyte antigen (HLA) region was examined initially as a candidate susceptibility locus. Association studies identified this region as a potential susceptibility locus, and this was confirmed in subsequent linkage studies. This locus is referred to as *IDDM1*. One measure of the degree of familial clustering of a disease is to determine λ_s, which is the ratio of the disease risk in siblings of affected individuals compared with the risk of the disease in the general population. For type 1 diabetes, the λ_s is 15, whereas the λ_s for *IDDM1* is estimated to be 3.4, suggesting that *IDDM1* accounts for 45–50% of the familial aggregation of the disease.

The MHC is located on the short arm of chromosome 6 (6p21) and encodes proteins involved in the regulation of the immune process. The MHC consists of three major regions, A, B, and C, that encode class-I genes, and the D region that encodes class-II genes. The class-I molecules, which are expressed on most cell types, are highly polymorphic and present peptide fragments of endogenous antigens to cytotoxic CD8+ cytotoxic T-lymphocytes. The class-II molecules are expressed on a more limited subset of cells, which are primarily antigen-presenting cells (macrophages, dendritic cells, B-cells, and activated T-cells). Class-II molecules present foreign processed antigen to CD4+ helper T-cells and are, thus, involved in initiating the immune response. Class-II molecules consist of an α- and β-chain that are encoded by different genes. There are three major classes of class-II genes, the DP, DQ, and DR genes. The β- but not the α-chain in the DR molecules is polymorphic, whereas both the α- and β-chains are polymorphic in DQ and DP molecules. Indeed, 17, 30, and 177 different alleles encoding the DQ-α- and -β-chain and DR-β-chain, respectively, have been described.

Initially an association between class-I alleles and type 1 diabetes was demonstrated, but it is clear that class-II molecules are most important in conferring risk. The original association with class-I molecules was likely because of the nonrandom association of class-I alleles with the class-II alleles (linkage disequilibrium). Moreover, linkage disequilibrium of the DQ and DR alleles has created extended haplotypes (the presence of several genetic variants on the same chromosome) that modulate risk. Some of these class-II alleles predict susceptibility to type 1 diabetes, whereas others either confer protection or are neutral. As noted, the risk of type 1 diabetes in the sibling of an affected individual is 6%, but, if the sibling has inherited the same HLA haplotypes as their affected sibling, their risk of type 1 diabetes is 20%. The HLA alleles DR4 and DR3 are strongly associated with diabetes. Linkage disequilibrium between DR* and DQ* contributes to this association. The major determinants of risk in this region are the DRB1 and DQB1 loci, although other loci in the HLA region may modulate risk. Among type 1 diabetic subjects, 95% have either the DRB1*0301-DQB1*0201 or the DRB1*04-DQB1*0302 haplotype. The contribution of both the DRB1 and DQB1 loci to disease risk is illustrated by the ability of different DRB1*04 alleles on the same haplotype to modify the risk conferred by DQ8 (DQA1*0301-DQB1*0302). The DRB1*0401, *0402, and *0405 alleles are associated with high susceptibility, DRB1*0404 with moderate susceptibility, and DRB1*0403 with protection. In addition to alleles conferring risk, several HLA alleles conferring protection from diabetes have been identified. The best known of these is DQB1*0602. The haplotype DQA1*0102-DQB1*0602 is present in 20% of Europeans and North Americans but in less than 1% of children with diabetes. Although the mechanism by which different HLA molecules affect diabetes susceptibility is still being elucidated, it is likely that changes in peptide binding sites of different class-II molecules alter the specificity of the immune response to foreign or self-antigens by affecting the binding affinity of different peptide antigens for the class-II molecules. Because of the strong and extended linkage disequilibrium present in the HLA region, it has not been possible to determine whether other genes in this region, many of which affect antigen presentation and immunoregulation, also have an effect on disease susceptibility.

A second susceptibility locus, the insulin gene locus on chromosome 11p15.5, was identified using both a candidate gene approach and linkage analyses. Among the polymorphisms in this region is the variable number of tandem repeats (VNTR) locus in the 5′-flanking region of the insulin gene. The VNTR consists of tandem repeats of a 14–15 bp core sequence. Three different alleles have been identified. The class-I allele contains 30–60 repeats, and homozygosity for this allele is associated with a two to fivefold increased risk of type 1 diabetes. The class-III allele contains 141–209 repeats and has a dominant protective effect. The class-II allele has approx 80 repeats but is rare, and its association with disease susceptibility has not been defined. The impact of *IDDM2* on susceptibility to type 1 diabetes is modest. The λ_s for *IDDM2* is 1.2, and it accounts for 10% of the familial clustering of type 1 diabetes.

As defined by linkage analyses, *IDDM2* is located within a 50-kbp region of chromosome 11 that contains the genes encoding tyrosine hydroxylase, insulin, and insulin-like growth factor II. Multiple polymorphisms are present within this region, but an extensive series of genetic analyses mapped the *IDDM2* susceptibility locus to the VNTR in the 5′-flanking region of the insulin gene, suggesting that the variable number of repeats in some manner confers susceptibility to disease, perhaps because of effects on insulin gene expression. In vitro studies using the VNTR in reporter gene constructs have demonstrated that the VNTR modulates insulin gene expression, although conflicting data were obtained. In vivo studies have demonstrated that the class-III allele is associated with decreased pancreatic insulin gene expression compared with transcription from the class-I allele. A mechanism by which the VNTR could affect disease susceptibility via its effects on pancreatic expression of the insulin gene was not obvious. Subsequent studies, however, examined effects of the VNTR on pre- and postnatal expression of the insulin gene in the human thymus. Interestingly, the class-III allele is associated with an approx 2.5-fold increase in insulin gene expression in the thymus compared with the class-I allele. Similarly, increased levels of proinsulin are present in thymi from class-III/I heterozygotes compared with class-I/I homozygotes. Increased expression of insulin in the thymus might facilitate tolerance to insulin by promoting deletion of insulin-specific T-lymphocytes, and, thus, provide protection from type 1 diabetes.

Because IDDM1 and IDDM2 account for only approx 50% of the familial clustering of type 1 diabetes, additional genes must be involved. Two other susceptibility loci that have been identified based on association studies are CTLA4, which encodes cytotoxic T-lymphocyte-associated 4, and PTPN22, which encodes lymphoid-specific phosphatase (LYP). Susceptibility to type 1 diabetes was mapped to a 6.1 kb 3′ region of CTLA4 that appears to modulate alternative splicing of CTLA-4 mRNA. CTLA-4 downregulates T-cell activation. The susceptibility allele results in decreased formation of a soluble isoform of CTLA-4. Although not confirmed in humans, the soluble isoform appears to be a more potent regulator of T-cell inhibition. Interestingly, this same susceptibility allele also confers an increased risk of Grave's disease and autoimmune hypothyroidism. LYP also inhibits T-cell activation. A single nucleotide polymorphism (SNP) in PTPN22 that results in substitution of tryptophan for arginine at codon 620 is present with increased frequency in subjects with type 1 diabetes compared with the general population. The Trp[620] variant alters the association of LYP with intracellular signaling molecules and, presumably, its ability to regulate T-cell activation. Like CTLA-4, the PTPN22 variant is associated with other autoimmune diseases, including Grave's disease, rheumatoid arthritis, and systemic lupus erythematosis.

Another approach to identify type 1 diabetes susceptibility genes is genome scans using DNA from sibling pairs affected by type 1 diabetes. The aim of genome scans using affected sib pairs is to scan the entire genome with a collection of genetic markers, calculate the degree of allele sharing at each marker or locus, and identify those chromosomal loci in which allele sharing by the affected siblings occurs with greater frequency than expected, based on the frequency of the allele in the population. Increased sharing of alleles at a specific locus suggests that a gene(s) within that chromosomal locus contributes to the pathogenesis of the disease. Multiple genome scans have been performed resulting in the identification of many potential type 1 diabetes susceptibility loci (Table 32-1). Unfortunately, many of the findings have not been replicated in the different genome scans. Possible reasons for this are many. None of these potential loci has an effect approaching the magnitude of IDDM1. Rather, they likely confer a modest increase in susceptibility similar to that conferred by IDDM2. To demonstrate linkage of loci with a modest effect on disease susceptibility requires a large number of subjects. Most studies have lacked sufficient subjects to reliably demonstrate linkage of the different loci to type 1 diabetes. Indeed, despite clear association

of the IDDM2 locus with type 1 diabetes and a clear biological explanation for this association, linkage of IDDM2 to type 1 diabetes has not been reliably demonstrated by genome scans. Similarly, the PTPN22 locus on chromosome 1p13 has not been identified by genome scans. Analysis of a merged data set that contained 1435 families with 1636 affected sib pairs was recently reported. These data provided continued support for the contribution of IDDM1 and IDDM2 to disease susceptibility and identified eight additional non-HLA-linked loci that confer susceptibility. Three of these loci, 2q31-q33 (IDDM7 and IDDM12), 10p14-q11 (IDDM10), and 16q22-q24 provided significant evidence of linkage. There were six additional regions that exhibited somewhat weaker evidence for linkage, including 6q21 (IDDM15), 3p13-p14, 9q33-q34, 12q14-q12, 16p12-q11.1, and 19p13.3-p13.2. Unfortunately, except for IDDM2 (insulin gene) and IDDM12 (CTLA4), the specific genetic variants within these loci conferring disease susceptibility have not been identified. Other potential susceptibility loci with little support for linkage were IDDM4, IDDM6, IDDM9, IDDM11, IDDM16, IDDM17, and IDDM18. Thus, these loci either do not harbor susceptibility genes or have a very small effect that is difficult to detect.

Definition of the genetic etiology of type 1 diabetes will have several clinical implications. Most affected individuals are identified subsequent to the onset of diabetes when nearly complete β-cell destruction has occurred. A relatively limited subset of individuals at risk for developing type 1 diabetes can be identified before disease onset based on a family history of type 1 diabetes and the presence of antibodies directed against islet cells. Not all such individuals develop type 1 diabetes, however, and the risk of developing diabetes in these individuals is defined by the degree of loss of first phase insulin secretion during an intravenous glucose tolerance test. This loss of first phase insulin secretion occurs secondary to β-cell destruction and indicates activity of the autoimmune process. Because a significant decrease in first phase insulin secretion indicates that marked β-cell destruction has already occurred, if susceptible individuals can be identified earlier, based on their complement of susceptibility genes, and screening can be extended beyond those with a positive family history, it may be possible to intervene earlier, before the onset of β-cell destruction and, thus, have a much greater impact on delaying or preventing the onset of type 1 diabetes. Second, as the pathways that are responsible for initiating the autoimmune process are identified, new therapies designed to interfere specifically with these pathways and prevent β-cell destruction can be developed. These therapies will likely be more efficacious in preventing the onset of diabetes.

GENETICS OF WOLFRAM SYNDROME

Wolfram and Wagener described a syndrome consisting of diabetes mellitus and optic atrophy in 1938. Since then, the clinical spectrum and genetic basis of the syndrome have been described. Wolfram Syndrome is inherited in an autosomal-recessive fashion. Early onset (generally age <15 yr) of diabetes and optic atrophy are necessary for the diagnosis. The recognition of additional manifestations of the disease resulted in the acronym DIDMOAD (diabetes insipidus, diabetes mellitus, optic atrophy, and deafness). Wolfram Syndrome is a progressive neurodegenerative disease. Additional neurological features present in some affected individuals include psychiatric illness, urinary tract atrophy, peripheral neuropathy, ataxia, dementia, and mental retardation. Consistent with its neurodegenerative nature, MRI studies have revealed atrophy of the optic nerves and neurodegeneration in the lateral

Table 32-1
Susceptibility Loci for Type 1 Diabetes Mellitus

Susceptibility locus	Chromosome	Linked markers	Candidate genes
IDDM1	6p21	HLADR/DQ	HLA-DRB1, HLA-DQB1
IDDM2	11p15.5	Insulin VNTR	Insulin
IDDM3	15q26	D15S107	
IDDM4	11q13	D11S987, D11S1337	Low-density lipoprotein receptor related protein 5
IDDM5	6q25-q27	D6S476, D6S473, ESR	
IDDM6	18q21	D18S64, D18S487	
IDDM7	2q31-q33	D2S152, D2S1391	
IDDM8	6q25-q27	D6S446, D6S281, D6S264	
IDDM9	3q22-q25	D3S1279, D3S1303	CD80, CD86
IDDM10	10p11-q11	D10S191, D10S220	Glutamic acid decarboxylase 2
IDDM11	14q24.3-q31	D14S67	
IDDM12	2q33	D2S72	Cytotoxic T-lymphocyte-associated antigen-4
IDDM13	2q34	D2S164	
IDDM15	6q21	D6S283, D6S434, D6S1580	
IDDM16	14q32.3	IGH	IgG heavy chain locus
IDDM17	10q25	D10S554	
IDDM18	5q33-q34	IL12B 3′-UTR	IL-12 p40 gene
	Xp13-p11	DXS1068	Forkhead box P3
	16q22-q24	D16S504	
	19p13.3-p13.2	INSR	
	12q14-q12	D12S375	
	3p13-p14	D3S1261	
	16p12-q11.1	D16S3131	
	9q33-q34	D9S260	

HLA, human leukocyte antigen; IL, interleukin; VNTR, variable number of tandem repeats. Adapted with permission from Onengut-Gumuscu S, Concannon P. Mapping genes for autoimmunity in humans: type 1 diabetes as a model. Immunol Rev 2002;190:182–194. Redondo MJ, Eisenbarth GS. Genetic control of autoimmunity in type I diabetes and associated disorders. Diabetologia 2002;45:605–622. Concannon P, Erlich HA, Julier C, et al. Type 1 diabetes: Evidence for susceptibility loci from four genome-wide linkage scans in 1435 multiplex families. Diabetes 2005;54:2995–3001.

geniculate nucleus, basis pontis, and hypothalamic nuclei, including the paraventricular and supraoptic nuclei.

Diabetes mellitus is typically, although not invariably, the initial manifestation of the disease, with the mean of age of onset being 6–8 yr in one study. The mean age of optic atrophy was 11 yr, whereas diabetes insipidus and deafness presented in the second decade of life. Affected individuals are insulin deficient, with pathological specimens demonstrating islet atrophy with loss of β-cells, but relative sparing of the α- and δ-cells. Unlike type 1 diabetes, no HLA association or evidence for autoimmunity has been identified. Interestingly, for reasons that are unclear, microvascular complications are relatively unusual and, when present, develop more slowly than is typical in type 1 diabetes.

Linkage studies localized the gene responsible for Wolfram Syndrome to the short arm of chromosome 4 (4p16.3). Subsequently, the responsible gene, WFS1, was identified. WFS1 consists of 8 exons spanning 33.4 kbp of DNA and is expressed in a variety of tissues, including adult human heart, brain, lung, pancreas, and placenta. WFS1 encodes a novel approx 100-kDa protein, wolframin, which is predicted to have nine transmembrane domains. Wolframin is an integral membrane glycoprotein that is located primarily in the endoplasmic reticulum and is associated with ion channel activity. It likely serves either as a calcium channel or as a regulator of calcium channel activity. In the pancreas, wolframin is present in β-cells and, to a much lesser extent, α-cells. Mutations in WFS1 have been demonstrated in 90% of patients with Wolfram Syndrome, with the majority of patients being compound heterozygotes. Linkage to chromosome 4p16.3 was excluded in three families and linkage to a second locus, 4q22-q24, was established. The disease gene at this locus awaits identification.

GENETICS OF TYPE 2 DIABETES MELLITUS

Type 2 diabetes mellitus is a heterogeneous disorder that develops in response to both genetic and environmental factors (Fig. 32-1). In contrast to type 1 diabetes, type 2 diabetes is often diagnosed during routine screening by the detection of hyperglycemia or because of mild symptoms of hyperglycemia, for example, polyuria. Much like type 1 diabetes, individuals with type 2 diabetes pass through a series of phases before the onset of diabetes. Initially, plasma insulin levels are increased because of insulin resistance, but euglycemia is maintained. In the second phase, postprandial hyperglycemia is present despite persistent hyperinsulinemia. Finally, insulin secretion declines in the face of persistent insulin resistance, which results in diabetes. Thus, affected individuals demonstrate both insulin resistance, manifested as hyperinsulinemia and decreased insulin-stimulated glucose uptake into tissues, and abnormal β-cell function, manifested as altered glucose-induced insulin secretion. Obesity, via its effects on insulin sensitivity, also contributes to type 2 diabetes. Obesity, in turn, is affected by both energy expenditure and intake. Energy expenditure is dependent to

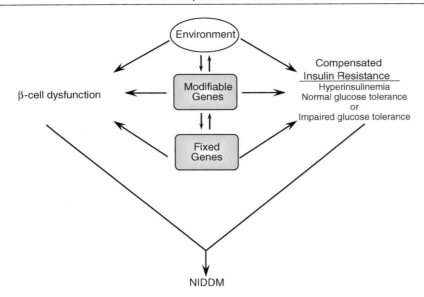

Figure 32-1 Schematic model of the etiology of type 2 diabetes mellitus. Type 2 diabetes is secondary to both insulin resistance and inadequate insulin secretion secondary to β-cell dysfunction. With sufficient β-cell function, euglycemia or impaired glucose tolerance is maintained in the presence of insulin resistance at the expense of hyperinsulinemia (compensated insulin resistance). With concomitant β-cell dysfunction, however, inadequate insulin secretion to compensate for the insulin resistance results in the onset of type 2 diabetes. Similarly, a primary defect in β-cell function may result in type 2 diabetes in the presence of some degree of insulin resistance. Both insulin resistance and β-cell dysfunction are influenced by genetic and environmental factors. Type 2 diabetes is multigenic, and its penetrance is secondary to the expression of several different genes, some of which are likely fixed and act independently of environmental factors. Other predisposing genes might be modifiable in that their expression or action is influenced by environmental factors. Interactions between genes are also likely to contribute to insulin resistance and β-cell dysfunction.

a large degree on resting metabolic rate, whereas energy intake is regulated by central nervous system and behavioral regulation of eating and satiety. All of the previously mentioned processes are in part heritable, but complex, and dependent on a variety of different gene products, each of which may have the potential to contribute to the genetic predisposition to type 2 diabetes.

Consistent with the heterogeneity of type 2 diabetes and the multiple contributing factors described, mathematical modeling has suggested that type 2 diabetes is a polygenic disease. Consequently, onset of the disease likely requires the simultaneous presence of a subset of genes that affect the above processes. Because different subsets of genes are probably sufficient to confer susceptibility to type 2 diabetes, susceptibility genes likely vary between, and possibly within, populations. Moreover, environmental factors that have not been fully defined contribute to the development of type 2 diabetes. Thus, disease susceptibility genes may be present in unaffected individuals because they lack a required complement of disease susceptibility genes or needed environmental factors to induce diabetes. This has and will continue to complicate attempts to define susceptibility genes for type 2 diabetes. An additional complication in defining the genetics of type 2 diabetes is its late onset. Typically, parents, especially affected parents who may have succumbed to the complications of diabetes, are not available for study, and offspring are unlikely to be affected. Thus, family studies of type 2 diabetes are difficult.

Despite the previously mentioned challenges, progress has been made in defining the genetics of late-onset type 2 diabetes. As with type 1 diabetes, the candidate gene approach and genome scanning have been used to identify genes that confer susceptibility to type 2 diabetes.

GENETICALLY DEFINED FORMS OF TYPE 2 DIABETES

Given the complexities of the genetics of type 2 diabetes, substantial effort has been applied using both candidate gene and positional cloning approaches to define the genetics of rare, but monogenic, forms of diabetes with the hope that this will provide insight into the genetics of type 2 diabetes.

Mitochondrial Diabetes Mellitus The role of mutations in mitochondrial DNA in disease etiology is becoming increasingly appreciated. Mitochondrial DNA is inherited maternally and encodes 13 polypeptide subunits involved in oxidative phosphorylation and the respiratory pathway, 22 transfer RNAs (tRNAs), and 2 ribosomal RNAs. Mitochondrial DNA is vulnerable to mutation because it is made up almost exclusively of coding sequences, lacks protection by histones, has inefficient repair mechanisms, and is exposed to reactive oxygen species produced during oxidative phosphorylation. Mitochondrial DNA undergoes mutation 5–10 times faster than nuclear DNA. The possibility that mitochondrial DNA mutations might contribute to the pathogenesis of diabetes mellitus was suggested by the association of diabetes with several mitochondrial diseases and by the maternal inheritance of mitochondrial DNA, given the slight preference for maternal transmission of type 2 diabetes.

Initially, a syndrome of diabetes mellitus and deafness caused by sensorineural hearing loss was identified in two pedigrees. In both, an A/G exchange at nucleotide 3243 in the mitochondrial tRNA$^{Leu(UUR)}$ gene was noted. This particular mutation was located within a mitochondrial DNA binding site for a protein that contributes to the termination of transcription at the boundary between the 16S ribosomal RNA and tRNA$^{Leu(UUR)}$ genes. Thus, this mutation alters both tRNA$^{Leu(UUR)}$ synthesis and mitochondrial protein stability. Interestingly, tRNA$^{Leu(UUR)}$ is a hot spot for mutations;

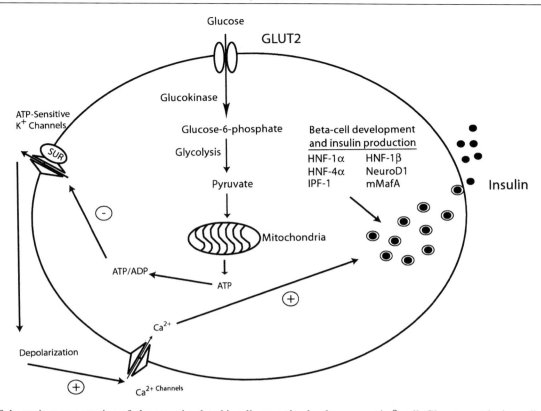

Figure 32-2 Schematic representation of glucose-stimulated insulin secretion by the pancreatic β-cell. Glucose uptake is mediated by GLUT2, and glucose is phosphorylated by glucokinase to generate glucose-6-phosphate. Metabolism of glucose-6-phosphate via glycolysis yields pyruvate, which enters the tricarboxylic acid cycle in the mitochondria to generate ATP. The generation of ATP increases the ATP/adenosine 5′ diphosphate ratio in the cytoplasm, which inhibits activity of the ATP-sensitive K$^+$ channel. The ATP-sensitive K$^+$ channel is a complex of the sulfonylurea receptor and an inward rectifying K$^+$-channel protein (KIR6.2). Inhibition of this channel results in membrane depolarization and opening of voltage-dependent Ca^{2+} channels. The resulting increase in the intracellular concentration of Ca^{2+} stimulates insulin secretion. β-cell development and insulin production are regulated by many factors, including several different transcription factors, some of which are listed.

11 disease-related mutations have been identified within this gene, 5 of which are associated with diabetes mellitus. The association of diabetes with point mutations and deletions in other mitochondrial genes has also been described.

Identification of these syndromes raised the question regarding the role of mitochondrial DNA mutations in the pathogenesis of diabetes mellitus. Of patients with type 1 and 2 diabetes mellitus, the A/G exchange in the tRNA$^{Leu(UUR)}$ gene is present in 0.5–1.5% of patients. If only those patients with a family history of diabetes are considered, the prevalence of the mutation is two to five times higher. Patients with the A/G exchange at nucleotide 3243 typically present with diabetes around age 35. Most also exhibit some degree of hearing loss because of reduced detection of high frequency tones. Detailed characterization of affected individuals and their siblings demonstrated that 48% presented with diabetes and deafness, 21% had diabetes alone, 15% had deafness alone, 3% had deafness associated with some neurological changes, and 13% had diabetes, deafness and the findings of the MELAS syndrome (mitochondrial myopathy, encephalopathy, lactic acidosis, and stroke-like episodes). The phenotypic variation presumably results from variable numbers of mitochondria containing normal compared with abnormal mitochondrial DNA (heteroplasmy) between tissues. Heteroplasmy results from unequal separation of mitochondrial populations during meiosis or mitosis and differential accumulation of subsequent mitochondrial mutations.

Although patients with mitochondrial DNA mutations were initially diagnosed as having either type 1 or 2 diabetes mellitus, there are differences between these patients and those with "typical" type 1 or 2 diabetes. Those diagnosed initially as having type 1 diabetes in general lack anti-islet cell antibodies and do not typically have a history of diabetic ketoacidosis, whereas those initially diagnosed as having type 2 diabetes tend to be leaner and more likely to be treated with insulin compared with general populations with type 2 diabetes. Subsequent studies to define the etiology of diabetes in patients with mitochondrial mutations demonstrated decreased insulin secretion in response to an oral glucose tolerance test, whereas measures of glucose utilization demonstrated essentially normal insulin sensitivity. The above findings suggest that the primary defect in patients with mitochondrial mutations is in the pancreatic β-cell. Oxidative phosphorylation and ATP generation play an important role in insulin secretion (Fig. 32-2), so mutations in β-cell mitochondrial DNA would likely interfere with insulin secretion because of insufficient ATP generation.

In patients with diabetes accompanied by hearing loss, a diagnosis of mitochondrial DNA mutations as the cause of the diabetes should be considered. Patients with these mutations should be advised that they will be much more likely to require insulin therapy because of the insulin deficiency that develops. Moreover, family members need to be carefully screened for both diabetes and evidence of sensorineural hearing. Frequently, the hearing loss develops

Table 32-2
MODY Genes

Condition	Gene	Chromosomal location	Function	Characteristics
MODY1	HNF4α	20q12-q13.1	Transcription factor	Onset in adolescence or early adulthood, microvascular complications frequent, rare cause of MODY
MODY2	Glucokinase	7p15.3-15.1	Glycolysis, glucose sensing	Onset at birth, mild hyperglycemia with minor deterioration with age, microvascular complications rare
MODY3	HNF1α	12q24.3	Transcription factor	Onset in adolescence or early adulthood, microvascular complications frequent, most common cause of MODY in most populations
MODY4	IPF1	13q12.1	Transcription factor	Onset in early adulthood, only one family described, homozygous mutation causes pancreatic agenesis
MODY5	HNF1β	17cenq21.3	Transcription factor	Onset in adolescence or early adulthood, rare cause of MODY, associated with renal cysts, proteinuria, renal failure and genital malformations
MODY6	NeuroD1	2q32	Transcription factor	Onset in adolescence or early adulthood, rare cause of MODY

HNF, hepatocyte nuclear factor; MODY, maturity onset diabetes of the young. Adapted with permission from Mitchell SMS, Frayling TM. The role of transcription factors in maturity-onset diabetes of the young. Mol Genet Metab 2002;77:35–43.

after the onset of diabetes, so those patients with diabetes need to be examined over time for hearing loss.

Maturity Onset Diabetes of the Young Maturity onset diabetes of the young (MODY) is a subtype of diabetes that is monogenic and provides a model for studying the molecular genetics of type 2 diabetes. MODY is characterized by an early age of onset of diabetes and an autosomal-dominant mode of inheritance that is based on the demonstration of a positive family history in three successive generations. Disease onset often occurs between ages 9 and 13 and typically, although not universally, occurs before age 25.

Characterization of MODY patients from different kindreds revealed phenotypic differences between patients suggesting heterogeneity, which molecular genetic analyses confirmed. Six variants of MODY, MODY1–6, have been characterized and are the result of mutations in different genes (Table 32-2). Initially, linkage to polymorphisms in the glucokinase gene on chromosome 7p was demonstrated in some patients, whereas in other patients analyses demonstrated linkage to markers on either chromosome 20q or 12q. Mutations in the glucokinase gene on chromosome 7p were shown to cause diabetes in kindreds with MODY2. Subsequent genetic analyses demonstrated that the kindred described as having MODY1 had a mutation in the hepatocyte nuclear factor (HNF)-4α gene on chromosome 20q, whereas kindreds with MODY3 had mutations in the HNF1α gene on chromosome 12q. As HNF-1β heterodimerizes with HNF-1α, it was examined as a candidate MODY gene. Mutations were identified, and HNF1β was designated as MODY5. Because of its role in kidney development and function, subjects with HNF-1β mutations frequently demonstrate nondiabetic renal disease, especially cystic renal disease, in addition to diabetes. Early onset diabetes was shown to segregate with heterozygous mutations in the insulin promoter factor (IPF)-1 gene in family members of a proband with pancreatic agenesis secondary to a homozygous frameshift mutation in the IPF1 gene. Thus, IPF1 was identified as MODY4. Two families in which mutations in NeuroD1, a helix–loop–helix transcription factor, cosegregate with diabetes have also been described. This has led to its designation as MODY6. Importantly, 10–20% of families meeting criteria

for MODY do not have mutations in any of the known MODY genes, suggesting that additional, unidentified MODY genes exist.

MODY genes play a critical role in pancreatic β-cell function and/or development. Glucokinase is a key enzyme in glucose metabolism in β-cells and hepatocytes which catalyzes the formation of glucose-6-phosphate from glucose and participates in glucose-sensing. It is important for linking glucose to insulin secretion. In patients with glucokinase mutations, the severity of enzyme impairment is correlated with the degree of hyperglycemia. Because of the decreased sensitivity of the β-cells to glucose in these patients, the dose–response curve for glucose-induced insulin secretion is shifted to the right, although increased insulin secretion is observed with increasing degrees of hyperglycemia. Whether altered glucose metabolism in hepatocytes contributes to the hyperglycemia is not known.

The genes responsible for MODY1 and 3–6 are transcription factors. HNF-4α is a transcription factor that is a member of the steroid/thyroid superfamily of nuclear receptors. Members of this receptor family are typically ligand-activated, but whether there is a ligand that activates HNF-4α is unknown. HNF-1α is a homeodomain transcription factor that functions as either a homodimer or heterodimer with the structurally related transcription factor HNF-1β. As their names imply, these factors are important for hepatic gene expression, but they are expressed in other tissues, including pancreatic islets. In pancreatic β-cells, HNF-1α and HNF-4α are part of an integrated network of transcription factors in which altered expression of one affects expression of the other. Although some of the identified mutations in HNF-1α and HNF-4α exert a dominant negative effect, the accumulated data suggest that MODY1 and 3 occur secondary to loss of a functional allele and a decreased level of active transcription factor (haploinsufficiency). In animal models, deficiency of HNF-1α directly or indirectly decreases expression of genes encoding proteins important for β-cell function, for example the pancreatic β-cell glucose transporter GLUT2, pyruvate kinase, and insulin, as well as genes encoding transcription factors important for pancreatic β-cell development and function, for example Pdx-1 (the mouse homologue

33 Pituitary Function and Neoplasia

SHLOMO MELMED

SUMMARY

The molecular pathogenesis of pituitary adenomas appears multifactorial. Clearly early proximal DNA-altering events might occur that may involve transcription factor dysregulation or hereditary mutations. Multiple promoting influences might subsequently impinge on the previously "initiated" cell and determine clonal expansion. These factors include disordered hypothalamic hormone receptor signaling, overstimulation by ectopic hypothalamic hormones, disordered paracrine growth factor action, disordered signal transduction, loss of negative feedback inhibition leading to pituitary hyperplasia, estrogen-mediated or paracrine angiogenesis, and loss of tumor suppressor activity. Once the cell has been transformed, its ultimate growth characteristics and neoplastic behavior appear to be determined by several genes acting relatively distally, including ras and nm23.

Key Words: Acromegaly; adrenocorticotropic hormone; corticotrophin-releasing hormone; Cushing's syndrome; gonadotropin-releasing hormone; hypothalamic; neoplasia; pituitary.

INTRODUCTION

The cell types of the mature adenohypophysis are derived embryologically from somatic ectoderm associated with Rathke's pouch. Highly specific trophic factors determine a precise temporal and spatial development of cells expressing unique gene products. The six hormones of the anterior pituitary gland are expressed by at least five distinct hormone-producing cell populations, including corticotrophs (pro-opiomelanocortin, POMC), somatotrophs (growth hormone, GH), lactotrophs (prolactin, PRL), thyrotrophs (thyroid-stimulating hormone, TSH), and gonadotrophs (follicle-stimulating hormone, FSH and luteinizing hormone, LH) (Table 33-1). Each of these cells is identified by specific assays of polypeptide gene expression, including single-cell mRNA, immuno-electron microscopy, and immunocytochemical assays. The temporal ontogeny of these gene products is initially adrenocorticotropic hormone (ACTH) and α-subunit. Distinct GH- and PRL-expressing cells follow and TSH, LH, and FSH are the final cell types to mature at 12 wk.

Each of the anterior pituitary trophic hormones is induced by a respective hypothalamic-releasing hormone, and their transcription is regulated by negative feedback inhibition of their respective target hormone (Table 33-2).

From: *Principles of Molecular Medicine, Second Edition*
Edited by: M. S. Runge and C. Patterson © Humana Press, Inc., Totowa, NJ

CORTICOTROPH CELLS

Corticotrophs constitute about 15–20% of the adenohypophyseal-cell population, and express strong granular cytoplasmic immunopositivity for ACTH and other POMC fragments.

Corticotrophin-releasing hormone (CRH) and glucocorticoids exert opposite effects on *POMC* gene transcription; CRH increases POMC mRNA and protein content through cAMP, whereas the glucocorticoid negative feedback effect is probably mediated through binding of the glucocorticoid receptor complex to *cis*-active POMC promoter sequences. Several enhancer elements have been identified on the *POMC* gene promoter. These appear to act synergistically in regulating POMC transcription. POMC transcription is also induced by β-adrenergic activation and insulin-induced hypoglycemia as well as by proinflammatory cytokines.

REGULATION OF ACTH

Ligand activation of the CRH receptor (Gs protein containing seven transmembrane domains) on the corticotroph stimulates ACTH synthesis and release. POMC transcriptional regulation is mediated by cAMP as well as indirectly by c-fos activation. Arginine vasopressin, physical stress, exercise, acute illness, and hypoglycemia all increase ACTH levels. Several cytokines mediating inflammatory and or immune responses, including tumor necrosis factor-α, interleukin (IL)-1, IL-6, and leukemia-inhibitory factor (LIF), also stimulate ACTH, whereas glucocorticoids and opiates inhibit ACTH transcription and release. This neuroimmune endocrine interface appears to occur both centrally and directly at the level of *POMC* gene expression. ACTH secretion is pulsatile, with an endogenous circadian rhythm associated with a parallel diurnal pattern of glucocorticoid secretion. Both ACTH and cortisol are higher in the early morning and decline at night.

Hypercortisolism might be caused by pituitary corticotroph adenomas (Cushing's disease) (70%) ectopic ACTH production (12%), cortisol-producing adrenal adenomas, carcinoma and hyperplasia (18%), and, rarely, ectopic CRH production. Iatrogenic hypercortisolism caused by prolonged administration of glucocorticoids produces a similar clinical syndrome.

ACTH-CELL ADENOMA Of all pituitary adenomas, approx 10–15% are ACTH producing tumors that are usually well-differentiated microadenomas. About 5% are silent corticotroph adenomas. Secretory granules in tumor cells immunostain positively for ACTH, β-endorphin, β-LPH, and N-terminal peptide. Although these adenomas exhibit unrestrained ACTH secretion with resultant

Table 33-1
Human Anterior Pituitary Hormone Gene Expression and Regulation

Cell	Fetal appearance (wk)	Hormone	Chromosomal gene locus	Protein	Size (kDa)	Amino acid number
Corticotroph	6	POMC	2p	Polypeptide	ACTH-4.5	266 (ACTH-39)
Somatotroph	8	GH	17q	Polypeptide	22	191
Lactotroph	12	PRL	6	Polypeptide	23	199
Thyrotroph	12	TSH	α-6q; β-1p	Glycoprotein α-, β-subunits	28	211
Gonadotroph	12	FSH, LH	β-11p, β-19q	Glycoprotein α-, β-subunits	34, 28.5	210, 204

Table 33-2
Regulation of Pituitary Hormone Secretion and Action

Hormones	Stimulators	Inhibitors	Peripheral receptor	Target	Trophic effects	Normal range
ACTH	CRH, AVP gp-130 cytokines	Glucocorticoids	GSTD	Adrenal	Steroid production	ACTH, 4–22 pg/L
GH	GHRH	Somatostatin, IGF-I, activins	Single transmembrane	Liver, other tissues	IGF-I production, growth induction, insulin antagonism	<0.5^a µg/L
PRL	Estrogen, TRH	Dopamine	Single transmembrane	Breast, other tissues	Milk production	M, <15; F, <20 µg/L
TSH	TRH	T_3, T_4, dopamine Somatostatin, glucocorticoids	GSTD	Thyroid	T_4	0.1–5 mU/L
FSH/LH	GnRH, estrogen	Estrogen, inhibin	GSTD	Ovary, testis	Sex steroid, follicle growth, germ cell maturation	M, 5–20 IU/L; F(basal), 5–20 IU/L

^{a}Integrated over 24 h.
GSTD, G_s protein coupled with seven transmembrane domains.
Adapted from Shimon I, Melmed S. In: Conn P, Melmed S, eds. Endocrinology, Totowa, NJ: Humana, 1996.

hypercortisolemia, they often retain suppressibility during high doses of administered glucocorticoids.

ECTOPIC ACTH SECRETION   ACTH production by small cell lung carcinomas and bronchial and thymic carcinoids might result in florid manifestations of Cushing's syndrome. The POMC mRNA transcript derived from nonpituitary ACTH-secreting tumors might be longer than the normal transcript or that detected in pituitary tumors. Corticotrophin-like intermediary peptide and β-melanocyte-stimulating hormone fragments might also be detected in ectopic tumors, indicating alternative POMC processing. Glucocorticoids do not suppress POMC mRNA expression in small cell lung cell lines, thus highlighting their unrestrained gene expression.

CUSHING'S SYNDROME   Patients typically present with truncal obesity, hirsutism (also associated with a "moon facies" and "buffalo hump"), cutaneous striae, muscle weakness, osteoporosis, acne, hypertension, depression, and ovarian dysfunction. Because hypercortisolemia is associated with insulin resistance, patients might also have impaired glucose tolerance. Ectopic Cushing's syndrome associated with small cell lung carcinoma is usually more acute with relatively rapid onset of hypertension, edema, hypokalemia, glucose intolerance, and hyperpigmentation. The most direct way to demonstrate ACTH hypersecretion of pituitary origin is by catheterization of the inferior petrosal venous sinuses. ACTH measurements in petrosal and peripheral venous plasma before and after CRH stimulation might document a central-to-peripheral venous gradient of ACTH concentrations.

ACTH hypersecretion by a corticotroph adenoma is usually suppressible by high doses of dexamethasone, whereas ectopic ACTH secretion persists despite high doses of dexamethasone. High-resolution pituitary MRI with gadolinium enhancement with a sensitivity of 2 mm is useful in determining the location of corticotroph adenomas. The treatment of choice is transsphenoidal adenomectomy, with a cure rate as high as 80% in experienced centers.

GROWTH HORMONE

Somatotrophs comprise more than 40% of pituitary cells and reveal intense cytoplasmic immunopositivity for GH. The GH genomic locus consists of five highly conserved genes, including human GH (exclusively expressed in somatotrophs), whereas the others are also expressed in placental tissue. Cis-elements within 300 bp of 5′ flanking DNA of the GH promoter mediate both pituitary-specific and hormone-specific signaling. These include Pit-1, a 33-kDa tissue-specific transcription factor, which binds to specific promoter sites on the *GH*, *PRL*, and *TSH*-β genes regulating their respective transcription. The tri-iodothyronine (T3) receptor might synergize with Pit-1 in stimulating GH transcription, although this effect might be species specific. Pit-1 also appears to be a determinant of growth hormone-releasing hormone (GHRH) receptor function, in as much as Pit-1 mutations might block GHRH-induced somatotroph proliferation.

Pulsatile GH secretion is associated with low or undetectable basal levels between peaks. Maximum GH secretory peaks occur within an hour of sleep onset. Somatostatin (SRIF) and GHRH interact to generate pulsatile GH release. GHRH stimulates GH synthesis and secretion, whereas SRIF, as well as the target hormone insulin-like growth factor (IGF)-I, inhibit GH secretion. GHRH signaling is mediated by cAMP, and several additional signals regulate *GH* gene expression, including glucocorticoids, IGF-I, activin, T3, and phorbol esters. The somatotroph expresses GH-secretory receptors, and ghrelin, a ligand for this receptor, is synthesized mainly in the gastrointestinal tract and induces GH by central mechanisms.

The GH receptor is expressed mainly in the liver and in other tissues. GH binding proteins are soluble short forms of the hepatic GH receptor and are identical to its cleaved extracellular domain. These proteins might prolong circulating GH half-life and might also competitively inhibit GH binding to peripheral surface receptors.

ACROMEGALY Of patients with acromegaly, >95% harbor a GH-secreting pituitary adenoma, two-thirds have pure GH-cell tumors, and the others have plurihormonal tumors, usually expressing PRL in addition to GH. Tumor-derived GH hypersecretion leading to acromegaly might be caused by excess GHRH or excess GH elaboration.

Ectopic acromegaly might be central as a result of excess GHRH production by functional hypothalamic tumors, or peripheral as a result of rare extrapituitary GH-secreting tumors (pancreas) and the more common tumors secreting GHRH (carcinoid, pancreas, small cell lung cancer). Patients with ectopic acromegaly exhibit normal (central) or elevated (peripheral) GHRH levels. Interestingly, somatotroph hyperplasia and ultimately true GH-cell adenomas might develop in these latter patients.

The clinical manifestations of acromegaly include acral enlargement and visceromegaly. Tongue, salivary glands, thyroid, heart, and soft organs all enlarge. Skeletal overgrowth leads to mandibular prognathism, frontal bossing, increased hand, foot and hat size, and wide incisor spacing. These features result in voice deepening, headaches, painful arthropathy and carpal tunnel syndrome, muscle weakness and fatigue, oily skin and hyperhidrosis, hypertension and left ventricular hypertrophy, and sleep apnea. Glucose intolerance because of insulin antagonism by GH commonly occurs. Overall mortality is increased in acromegaly because of an increased incidence of cardiovascular disorders, malignancy, and respiratory disease. Mortality rates correlate well with GH levels, and effective therapeutic suppression of GH might normalize mortality outcomes. Transsphenoidal adenoma resection is the indicated treatment for GH-secreting pituitary adenoma. Octreotide, a long-acting SRIF analog, significantly attenuates GH and IGF-I levels and blocks tumor growth in most patients; long-term administration of the long-acting octapeptide is also accompanied by marked clinical improvement. Pegvisomant, a GH receptor antagonist, prevents GH-receptor dimerization and normalized IGF-1 levels in >90% of patients. GH levels, albeit bioinactivated, are persistently elevated and long-term effects on tumor growth are still unclear.

PROLACTIN

The acidophilic lactotrophs contain PRL-immunostaining secretory granules and constitute 15% of adenohypophyseal cells. PRL is highly homologous to GH and placental lactogen, which might all have originally arisen from a common ancestral gene. The *PRL* gene has two lactotroph-specific transcription activation regions, a proximal promoter (−422 to +33) and a distal enhancer

element (−1831 to −1530), both containing specific binding sites for Pit-1. Dopamine, a potent inhibitor of PRL, acts through the D2 dopamine receptor to decrease intracellular cAMP and *PRL* gene transcription, synthesis, and release. Dopamine effects are mediated by the phosphoinositide–calcium pathway. Vasoactive intestinal polypeptide induces, whereas glucocorticoids and thyroid hormones suppress, PRL transcription and secretion. Estrogens and thyrotropin-releasing hormone (TRH) induce PRL transcription and secretion by either transactivating an estrogen-responsive PRL enhancer element or by inducing the phosphoinositide–protein kinase C pathway. The estrogen receptor might directly synergize with Pit-1 to induce PRL transcription.

Although PRL receptors are widely distributed, their hormonal regulation is tissue specific. High progesterone levels during pregnancy limit breast PRL receptor number, but early in lactation their numbers increase markedly. Prostatic PRL receptor levels are increased by testosterone and decreased by estrogens.

Prolactinomas are the most common hormone-secreting pituitary adenomas and, depending on their size, are classified as microprolactinomas (<10 mm, 90% of which affect women), or macroprolactinomas (>10 mm, 60% of which affect men). PRL serum levels >200 µg/L are usually associated with a prolactinoma. Hyperprolactinemia presents as hypogonadism with amenorrhea and galactorrhea in women, and impotence and infertility in men. Patients harboring macroadenomas are usually males, and their clinical presentation might be associated with local mass effect signs of headaches and visual field disturbances. Most patients are successfully treated with dopamine agonists whereas transsphenoidal surgery is reserved for drug-resistant tumors, which comprise approx 5–10% of patients.

THYROID-STIMULATING HORMONE

Thyrotrophs comprise 5% of the anterior pituitary cell population. TSH and the glycoproteins, LH, FSH, and human chorionic gonadotropin, are made up of two noncovalently linked subunits, a common α and a specific β. Although the α-subunit is expressed in pituitary thyrotrophs and gonadotrophs and in placental cells, cell-specific expression depends on different promoter regions. Tissue specificity is determined by the β-subunit despite their 75% structural homology. Both α- and β-subunit transcriptions are induced by TRH and inhibited by T3 and dopamine. TSH secretion is stimulated by TRH, whereas thyroid hormones, dopamine, SRIF, and glucocorticoids suppress TSH.

TSH-producing pituitary adenomas made up of <1% of pituitary tumors and secrete both TSH α- and β-subunits. The tumor-derived α-subunit is synthesized in excess of the β-subunit, a characteristic useful for differential diagnosis. TSH-secreting tumors fail to respond to thyroid hormone-negative feedback but are suppressed by SRIF. Clinical presentation usually includes hyperthyroidism and diffuse goiter, with elevated or inappropriately normal TSH levels in the presence of elevated thyroid hormones. Tumors are usually large and often invasive with commonly observed local mass effects. Transsphenoidal pituitary surgery is the preferred initial therapeutic approach, but surgical cure is elusive and most patients require adjuvant medical or radiation therapy. The SRIF analog, octreotide, suppresses TSH and might attenuate further tumor growth. Thyroid ablation to cure hyperthyroxinemia is not recommended because of the potential risk of pituitary tumor expansion as a result of disinhibition of the thyrotroph cells from negative feedback.

FOLLICLE-STIMULATING HORMONE AND LUTEINIZING HORMONE

Gonadotrophs comprise up to 10% of anterior pituitary cells and express both FSH and LH-β-subunits. Gonadotropin-releasing hormone (GnRH) induces the transcription of all three gonadotropin subunits, whereas estrogen attenuates their transcription, in part by inhibiting hypothalamic GnRH. However, estrogen might exert positive pituitary feedback and might actually increase LH-β mRNA under several physiological conditions. A gonadotroph-specific protein (SF-1) regulates pituitary α-subunit gene expression distinct from placental regulation of this gene.

GONADOTROPH CELL TUMORS Gonadotroph adenomas are among the most common pituitary adenomas. These "nonsecreting" or "incidental" adenomas are clinically nonfunctional because the gonadotropins and their subunits are either not released or are inefficiently secreted and usually do not produce a distinct clinical syndrome. These tumors result in elevated α- and FSH-β-subunit and, rarely, LH-β serum levels. Some adenomas secrete α-subunits but not intact FSH or LH. TRH administration usually induces secretion of gonadotropins or their subunits in patients harboring these nonfunctional adenomas, unlike the absent TRH response seen in normal subjects. Most nonsecreting adenomas immunostain positively for intact FSH and LH, or α-, FSH-β-, and LH-β-subunits. Excessive secretion of FSH or LH might occasionally downregulate the reproductive axis resulting in clinical hypogonadism. Mass effects, including optic chiasm pressure and other neurological symptoms, might be the initial symptoms of large gonadotroph tumors. Surgical excision is the most effective therapy and pharmacological agents are largely ineffective in shrinking these tumor masses.

ANTERIOR PITUITARY FAILURE

Hormone-specific anterior pituicytes are embryologically derived from a pluripotent precursor, and arise as a consequence of temporal and spatial control of homeodomain repressor and activator transcription factor expression. Mutations of early developmental genes (including *Rpx*, *Lhx3*, *Lhx4*, and *Pitx2*) pleiotropically affect adjacent midline structures, resulting in pituitary hypoplasia and multiple pituitary hormone deficits whereas mutations in genes determining specific pituitary lineages (including *Prop1*, *Pit1*, *Tpit*) are involved in single or combined pituitary hormone deficiencies with hypoplasia. Developmental *PROP-1* defects produce variable phenotypes. GH, PRL, and TSH expressing cells share a common developmental pathway, and *Pit-1* mutations can affect all three cell types. Ames dwarf (Prop1 df/df) and Pit-1 dw/dw mice display growth deficiency, hypothyroidism and infertility. Persistent transgenic murine pituitary Prop-1 expression results in delayed murine gonadotrope differentiation, persistent Rathke's cleft cysts, pituitary enlargement, and null cell nonsecreting pituitary adenomas. Several transgenic mice models expressing dysfunctional GH transcriptional regulation exhibit markedly attenuated or absent *GH* gene expression. For example, the Snell dwarf mouse has a *Pit-1* point mutation. In humans, sporadic and familial cases of *Pit-1* mutation exhibit varying degrees of combined GH, PRL, and TSH basal deficiency, or impaired reserve. Some of those patients might exhibit a hypoplastic pituitary gland (Tables 33-3 and 33-4). Autosomal-dominant or -recessive *Pit-1* mutations associated with this heterogeneous clinical syndrome include dysfunctional point mutations with defective bind-

Table 33-3
Pituitary Failure Associated With Pit-1 Mutations

Mutation	Clinical phenotype	Autosomal inheritance
DNA binding domain		
143Arg → Gln	Growth retardation	Recessive
158Ala → Pro	Hypothyroid; growth retardation	Recessive
172Arg → Stop	Hypothyroid	Recessive
271Arg → Trp	Growth retardation; impaired thyroid reserve	Dominant
135Phe → Cys	Growth retardation; hypothyroidism	Recessive
Activation domain		
24Pro → Leu	Growth retardation	Dominant

ing to pituitary gene promoters (e.g., 158 A to P), and dominant negative missense mutations (e.g., 271 Arg to Trp).

A missense mutation (77 Cys → Arg) in the GH molecule also leads to short stature. This mutant GH has weakened signal-transducing capacity, and might also function as a dominant negative inhibitor of wild-type GH.

PATHOGENESIS OF PITUITARY TUMORS

Each anterior pituitary cell type might give rise to monoclonal benign neoplasms that are hormonally functional or nonfunctional (Tables 33-5 and 33-6). Functional tumors are characterized by autonomous trophic hormone secretion, leading to clinical hormone excess syndromes, including hyperprolactinemia, acromegaly or Cushing's disease. Nonfunctioning pituitary adenomas secrete clinically inactive glycoprotein hormones or their free subunits. True pituitary carcinomas are extremely rare, and less than 40 cases have been unequivocally documented.

CLONAL ORIGIN OF PITUITARY ADENOMAS Complete resection of well-circumscribed pituitary adenomas often results in a cure of unrestrained or paradoxic hormone hypersecretion. This observation prompted the question regarding whether these tumors were clonal expansions of a single disordered cell. Disordered hypothalamic regulation would likely give rise to a generalized polyclonal cellular hyperplasia, as seen in patients harboring extrapituitary tumors elaborating hypothalamic-releasing hormones (e.g., GnRH, CRH). Alternatively, an intrinsic genetic defect within the pituitary would likely be associated with clonal proliferation.

Using X-chromosomal inactivation analysis of female patients heterozygous for sex-linked genes, several groups have confirmed the monoclonal origin of functional and nonfunctional pituitary tumors. When clonal analysis was performed on tumor DNA for hypoxanthine phosphoribosyl transferase or phosphoglycerate kinase in heterozygous patients with acromegaly, Cushing's disease, prolactinomas, and nonfunctioning tumors, a preferential loss of the inactive X-chromosome allele was observed after digestion with methylation-sensitive enzymes. These observations have prompted the quest for unraveling an intrinsic pituitary genetic defect resulting in either activation of a cell stimulator or inactivation of an inhibitor of cell proliferation.

HYPOTHALAMIC ORIGIN OF PITUITARY ADENOMAS Hypothalamic hormones regulate expression of the respective pituitary hormone genes by binding to specific cell surface receptors.

Table 33-4
Human Pituitary Transcription Factor Mutations

Factor	Hormone deficiency	Pituitary size	Associated phenotype
Early (pituitary commitment and progression)			
Hesx 1	Isolated GH: panhypopituitarism	Hypoplastic, hyperplastic	Septo-optic dysplasia
LHX 3	GH, TSH, PRL, LH, FSH	Hypoplastic	Rigid cervical spine
LHX 4	GH, TSH, ACTH	Hypoplastic	Chiari cerebellar deformity
PITX 2	GH	Hypoplastic	Reiger syndrome
Intermediate (pituitary patterning and cell type determination)			
Prop-1	GH, TSH, PRL	Hypoplastic	
	Later: FSH, LH, ACTH	Hyperplastic	
Late (cell type differentiation)			
Pit 1	GH, TSH, PRL	Hypoplastic	
T-Pit	ACTH	Hypoplastic	

Table 33-5
Classification of Pituitary Adenomas

Adenoma cell origin	Hormone product	Clinical syndrome
Lactotroph	PRL	Hypogonadism, galactorrhea[a]
Gonadotroph	RSH, LH, subunits	Silent or hypogonadism
Somatotroph	GH	Acromegaly, gigantism
Corticotroph	ACTH	Cushing's disease
Mixed growth hormone and prolactin cell	GH, PRL	Acromegaly, hypogonadism
Other plurihormonal cell	Any	
Acidophil stem cell	PRL, GH	Hypogonadism, acromegaly
Mammosomatotroph	PRL, GH	Hypogonadism, acromegaly
Thyrotroph	TSH	Hyperthyroidism
Null cell	None	Pituitary failure
Oncocytoma	None	Pituitary failure

[a]Females present with amenorrhea and infertility and males present with impotence or infertility.

Hormone-secreting tumors are listed in decreasing order of frequency. All tumors may cause local pressure effects, including visual disturbances, cranial nerve palsy, and headache.

In addition, these peptides might also induce DNA synthesis and enhanced mitotic activity in their target pituitary cells. Thus, mice expressing a GHRH transgene will exhibit somatotroph hyperplasia and ultimately adenoma. Patients harboring tumors elaborating ectopic GHRH or CRH might also present with GH-cell or ACTH-cell hyperplasia or adenomas, in addition to the hormone hypersecretory syndrome. Pituitary tumor-derived GHRH, SRIF, and TRH have been characterized by *in situ* or reverse transcriptase PCR techniques. These observations of intrapituitary peptide expression might imply a paracrine role for the hypothalamic peptides in pituitary tumorigenesis.

gsp MUTATIONS Peptide hormone signal transduction involves coupling of activated cell surface receptors with membrane G proteins, consisting of three polypeptides: an α-chain that binds to guanine nucleotide, and a β- and γ-chain. Ligand-induced activation of the receptor induces GTP binding, which causes a conformational change in G protein, releasing the α-subunit from βγ, allowing it to interact with target proteins. Hydrolysis of bound GTP to GDP by the intrinsic guanosine 5′-triphosphatase (GTPase) activity of the α-subunit terminates the ligand-induced signal (Fig. 33-1). GHRH, by binding to its somatotroph receptor coupled to G proteins, uses cAMP as a second messenger to stimulate GH secretion and somatotroph proliferation. A subset of GH-secreting pituitary tumors contains elevated intracellular cAMP levels and increased in vitro GH secretion, and is not responsive to further GHRH stimulation. Intratumoral adenylyl cyclase levels are constitutively enhanced approx 10-fold compared with levels in unaffected patients. The GHRH-independent induction of cAMP in these tumors could conceivably occur as a result of constitutive activation of GHRH receptor or the catalytic domain of adenylyl cyclase or the stimulatory subunit of G protein. Point mutations of Gsα were identified in approximately one-third of these tumors. These missense mutations occur either in Arg-201 (Arg → Cys or His) or in Gln-227 (Gln → Arg), in a region of the Gsα that is involved in GTP hydrolysis. Thus, these *gsp* mutations activate Gsα by inhibiting its intrinsic GTPase activity. In the cAMP-responsive somatotroph cells, therefore, conversion of Gs-α into an activating oncogene, *gsp*, might explain the pathogenesis of unrestrained cell proliferation and GH hypersecretion in these tumors. Gs-α activation also induces both the *Pit-1* promoter and serine phosphorylation of the cAMP response-protein (CREB) in acromegalic tissue, thus promoting somatotroph cell proliferation. In fact, CREB phosphorylation appears to be a universal finding in GH-cell adenomas, and is significantly lower in clinically silent gonadotroph cell adenomas.

Interestingly, the *gsp* mutation is detected at a negligible frequency in Japanese patients, implying a geographic selection for the mutation. No significant clinical phenotype is associated with *gsp* mutations, and ultimate tumor behavior and response to therapy is not altered in these patients. It would therefore appear that additional cAMP-associated signaling genes are involved in GH-cell tumorigenesis.

Ras MUTATIONS Transduction of intrapituitary hypothalamic, peripheral hormonal, and paracrine growth factor signals uses pathways other than those coupled to G proteins. The product of the proto-oncogene *ras* plays an important role in growth factor signal transduction. There are three functional *ras* genes, H-, N-, and K-*ras*, that encode a 21-kDa protein, p21ras. The guanine

Table 33-6
Gene Defects in Pituitary Tumors

Activating			Mechanism of overexpression/	
Gene	Protein	Tumor type	inactivation	Function/defect
Gsp	GNAS1	40% GH-secreting tumors McCune-Albright syndrome	Point mutation	Signal transduction/ Elevated cAMP
CREB	CREB	GH-secreting	Increased Ser-phosphorylated CREB	Dimerizes with Camp-response elements
PTTG	PTTG	All pituitary tumors	Unknown Estrogen?	Chromatid separation, regulates bFGF/disrupted cell cycle Chromsomal instability, mitogenesis, and angiogenesis
Hst	FGF4	Large prolactinomas	Unknown	Angiogenesis/overexpression Enhanced PRL transcription
H-ras	Ras	Metastatic pituitary carcinoma only	Point mutation, amplification	Signal transduction/stimulates tyrosine kinase pathway
FGFR	ptd-FGFR4	Prolactinomas	Truncated isoform	Cytoplasmic constitutive phosphorylation
Inactivating				
Gene	Protein			
Men1	Menin	Prolactinomas in familial MEN-1	11q13 loss of heterozygosity	Nuclear tumor suppressor/loss of function mutations
13q14	Rb?	Highly invasive tumors	13q14 loss of heterozygosity	Inconsistent Rb protein loss/disrupted cell cycle regulation Epigenetic defect
CDKN2A	pl6	All tumor types examined	Gene methylation leading to absent p16, allowing Rb phosphorylation and cell cycle progression	Cell cycle regulation/absent p16 protein leading to disrupted cell cycle regulation
CIP1/KIP1	p27	Transgenic mouse Models	Gene methylation leading to absent p27	Regulate multiple CDK enzymes including CDK4/6-cyclin Ds/absent p27 protein
GADD45γ		Adenoma	Unknown	Growth arrest after DNA damage

Modified from Melmed S, Kleinberg D. In: Larsen PR, Kronenberg HM, Melmed S, Polonsky KS, eds. Williams Textbook of Endocrinology, 10th ed. Philadelphia, PA: WB Saunders, 2003.

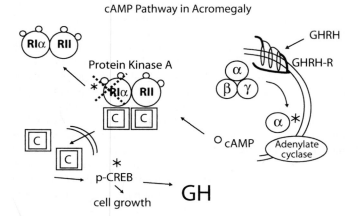

Figure 33-1 Cascade of events leading to GH gene regulation by activation of GHRH receptor and cAMP pathway. Lesions leading to acromegaly might occur at the level of GTPase, leading to elevated cAMP levels, PKA (Carney Complex) or at level of activated CREB. The genetic etiology of most sporadic GH-secreting tumors, however, remains elusive.

nucleotide-binding protein p21ras possesses intrinsic GTPase activity and is associated with the plasma membrane. Downstream ras signaling involves protein kinase cascades that transduce the incoming signal to the nucleus. Point mutations of the *ras* gene can convert it to a constitutively active oncogene that has been implicated in the development of a variety of tumors, and represents one of the most common mutations detected in human neoplasia. *Ras* gene mutations, however, occur rarely in pituitary tumors. Only a single invasive prolactinoma was found to harbor a missense *ras* mutation. Ras mutations were also detected in metastatic deposits of pituitary carcinomas, but not in the respective primary pituitary tumors. An activating transforming gene *(PTTG)* was isolated from rat and human pituitary tumors and is located on chromosome 5q33. These findings suggest that activation of ras is not an initial event in pituitary tumorigenesis; however, point mutations of *ras* might be important for the development or growth of metastases originating from rarely occurring pituitary carcinomas.

TUMOR SUPPRESSOR GENES Studies of the multiple endocrine neoplasia type (MEN) 1 gene locus surprisingly yielded evidence for tumor suppressor gene participation in pituitary tumorigenesis. Loss of heterozygosity (LOH) of chromosome 11q13 is present in hereditary pituitary tumors associated with MEN1, and in up to 20% of sporadically occurring pituitary adenomas, including GH-, PRL-, and ACTH-cell adenomas, as well as some nonfunctional tumors. Several of these tumors exhibiting 11q13 LOH concurrently were shown to harbor a gsp mutation, lending further credence to a multistep cause of pituitary tumors. The gene for MEN1 (menin) has been cloned; menin mutations in mice recapitulate the syndrome of parathyroid, pancreatic, and pituitary neoplasms. Sporadic pituitary tumors do not manifest menin mutations, even in the presence of chromosome II LOH.

The retinoblastoma susceptibility gene *(RB)* is inactivated in a variety of human tumors. Individuals with germline mutations on one *RB* allele have >90% chance of developing a childhood retinoblastoma. The *RB* gene maps to chromosome 13ql4, and LOH at this locus is seen in retinoblastoma cells. The *RB* gene product is a major determinant of cell cycle control and acts as a signal transducer interfacing the cell cycle with specific transcriptional activation. The RB protein is phosphorylated in a cell cycle-dependent manner, being maximal at the start of the S phase and low after mitosis and entry into G1, and its activity appears regulated by the state of phosphorylation. Loss of RB protein function deprives the cell of an important mechanism for restraining cell proliferation.

The role of the *RB* gene in pituitary tumor formation was initially suggested by observations made in transgenic mice, in which one allele of the *RB* gene was disrupted. Although homozygous RB mutations are lethal early in fetal life, mice heterozygous for the *RB* gene mutation are not predisposed to retinoblastoma, but interestingly demonstrate pituitary tumors at a high frequency. These tumors originate from the pars intermedia of the pituitary, and express POMC immunoreactive products. The wild-type *RB* allele is absent in these pituitary tumors, whereas the mutant allele is retained. Pituitary tumor tissue derived from these mice also expresses a truncated dysfunctional RB protein.

In benign human pituitary microadenomas, no LOH at the *RB* locus has been detected. However, in invasive pituitary macroadenomas and in pituitary carcinomas, allelic deletions at the RB locus were observed. Therefore, LOH at the *RB* locus is unlikely to be an initiating event in pituitary tumorigenesis, but rather *RB* or an associated tumor suppressor gene might play a role in progression of benign tumors to more invasive and malignant phenotypes. Because immunoreactive RB protein appears to be present in these tumors, it is likely that another tumor suppressor gene is located on chromosome 13 in close proximity to the *RB* locus and might be involved in pituitary tumor progression.

nM23, a nucleoside diphosphate kinase gene associated with suppression of breast cancer and melanoma metastases, is highly expressed in small noninvasive pituitary adenomas. Pituitary nM23 expression correlates inversely with cavernous sinus invasiveness and is markedly attenuated in large invasive tumors. Interestingly, although *p53* tumor suppressor gene mutations have been detected in a variety of human tumors, no *p53* mutation has been detected in a comprehensive screening of pituitary tumors.

INTRAPITUITARY PARACRINE GROWTH FACTORS

Several intrapituitary growth factors and cytokines are expressed in normal and tumorous tissue. Their paracrine or

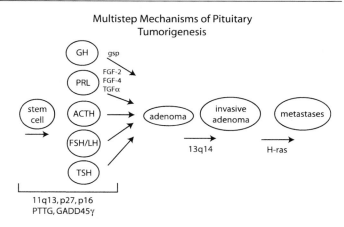

Multistep Mechanisms of Pituitary Tumorigenesis

Figure 33-2 Depiction of known molecular mutations associated with pituitary tumorigenesis. Both activating and inactivating mutations have been observed in the pathogenesis of experimental animal tumors, or in human tumors. True pituitary malignant transformation is exceedingly rare, and might reflect unique endocrine cell cycle control. Cellular origin of tumors, in decreasing order of frequency is gonadotroph (nonfunctioning), lactotroph, somatotroph, corticotroph, and thyrotroph.

autocrine regulation of specific pituitary function involves several trophic hormones either singly or in combination. These factors include epidermal growth factor, nerve growth factor, IGF-I, activin, and endothelin. Cytokines, including IL-6, IL-2, and LIF, also participate in paracrine regulation of trophic hormones. Although several in vitro and in vivo rat models have demonstrated growth factor-mediated pituitary mitogenesis, most of the information yielded from studies of human pituitary tumors is largely descriptive. The paucity of human tissue, as well as the failure of human pituitary cells to proliferate in vitro, has largely limited the subcellular regulatory studies required to establish a direct tumorigenic link for these growth factors.

The most compelling evidence in favor of a growth factor role in pituitary pathogenesis is that derived from studying the fibroblast growth factor (FGF) family. Basic FGF (bFGF) is abundantly expressed in the pituitary, regulates PRL and TSH secretion, and also might stimulate human pituitary cell mitogenesis in vitro. Interestingly, circulating bFGF, as well as bFGF autoantibodies, is detectable before pituitary tumor resection in patients with MEN1, and bFGF levels fall after surgery. These observations imply that at least in MEN1, the pituitary adenoma might be a source of this mitogen. FGF-4, which might behave as a transforming proto-oncogene is expressed in human prolactinomas and induces PRL transcription. *PTTG* pituitary tumor transforming gene was isolated by differential mRNA display of rat pituitary tumors and is abundantly expressed in human pituitary adenomas. Disrupted *PTTG* also blocks experimental pituitary tumor growth and PRL secretion. PTTG is the index mammalian securin protein, involved in regulating faithful sister chromatid separation. Overexpressed PTTG leads to cell cycle disruption and aneuploidy. A truncated FGF4 receptor is also mitogenic for pituitary tissue in vivo.

Other paracrine growth factors that have been implicated in pituitary tumorigenesis include epidermal growth factor, transforming growth factor-α and -β and IGF-I. The gp-130 family of cytokines, including IL-6 and LIF, are expressed in functional pituitary adenomas, regulate POMC transcription, and might be inhibitory for pituicyte mitogenesis.

Table 33-7
Protein Products and Chromosomal Loci Associated with Hereditary Pituitary Tumor Syndromes

| | Familial GH-secreting tumors | |
Syndrome	Protein product	Chromosomal loci
Multiple endocrine neoplasia type I	Menin	11q13
Carney complex	CNC1	17q24
	CNC2	2p16
McCune-Albright syndrome	Gsp	20q13
Isolated familial acromegaly	?	11q13

CONCLUSION

The molecular pathogenesis of pituitary adenomas appears multifactorial (Fig. 33-2). Clearly early proximal DNA-altering events might occur that might involve transcription factor dysregulation (e.g., Pit-1) or hereditary mutations (e.g., MEN, Carney complex) (Table 33-7). Multiple promoting influences might subsequently impinge on the previously "initiated" cell and determine clonal expansion. These factors include disordered hypothalamic hormone receptor signaling (e.g., gsp); overstimulation by ectopic (or paracrine?) hypothalamic hormones (e.g., GnRH, CRH); disordered paracrine growth factor action (e.g., FGF-4, bFGF); disordered signal transduction (e.g., CREB); loss of negative feedback inhibition leading to pituitary hyperplasia (e.g., hypothyroidism or hypogonadism); estrogen-mediated or paracrine angiogenesis (e.g., vascular endothelial growth factor); and loss of tumor suppressor activity (e.g., chromosomes 11 and 13). Once the cell has been transformed, its ultimate growth characteristics and neoplastic behavior appear to be determined by several genes acting relatively distally, including *ras* and *nm23*.

SELECTED REFERENCES

Alexander JM, Biller BM, Bikkal H, Zervas NT, Arnold A, Klibanski A. Clinically non-functioning pituitary tumors are monoclonal in origin. J Clin Invest 1990;86:336–340.

Bates AS, Farrell WE, Bicknell EJ, et al. Allelic deletion in pituitary adenomas reflects aggressive biological activity and has potential value as a prognostic marker. J Clin Endocrinol Metab 1997;82: 818–824.

Bertherat J, Chanson P, Montminy M. The cyclic adenosine 3'5'-monophosphate-responsive factor CREB is constitutively activated in human somatotroph adenomas. Mol Endocrinol 1995;9:777–783.

Biller B, Samuels M, Zagar A, et al. Sensitivity and specificity of six tests for the diagnosis of adult GH deficiency. J Clin Endocrinol Metab 2002;87:2067–2079.

Clayton RN, Boggild M, Bates AS, Bicknell J, Simpson D, Farrell W. Tumour suppressor genes in the pathogenesis of human pituitary tumours. Horm Res 1997;47:185–193.

Cohen LE, Wondisford FE, Salvatoni A, et al. A "hot spot" in the pit-1 gene responsible for combined pituitary hormone deficiency: clinical and molecular correlates. J Clin Endocrinol Metab 1995;80:679–684.

Cunha SR, Mayo KE. Ghrelin and growth hormone (GH) secretagogues potentiate GH-releasing hormone (GHRH)-induced cyclic adenosine 3',5'-monophosphate production in cells expression transfected GHRH and GH secretagogue receptors. Endocrinology 2002;143: 4570–4582.

Cushman LJ, Watkins-Chow DE, Brinkmeier ML, et al. Persistent Prop1 expression delays gonadotrope differentiation and enhances pituitary tumor susceptibility. Hum Mol Genet 2001;10:1141–1153.

Faglia G, Spada A. Genesis of pituitary adenomas: state of the art. J Neurooncol 2001;54:95–110.

Goffin V, Binart N, Touraine P, Kelly PA. Prolactin: the new biology of an old hormone. Annu Rev Physiol 2002;64:47–67.

Heaney AP, Horwitz GA, Wang Z, Singson R, Melmed S. Early involvement of estrogen-induced pituitary tumor transforming gene and fibroblast growth factor expression in prolactinoma pathogenesis. Nat Med 1999;5:1317–1321.

Herman V, Fagin J, Gonski R, Kovacs, Melmed S. Clonal orgin of pituitary andenomas. J Clin Endocrinol Metab 1990;71:1427–1433.

Herrington J, Carter-Su C. Signaling pathways activated by the growth hormone receptor. Trends Endocrinol Metab 2001;12:252–258.

Lamolet B, Pulichino AM, Lamonerie T, et al. A pituitary cell-restricted T Box factor, Tpit, activates POMC transcription in cooperation with Pitx homeoproteins. Cell 2001;104:849–859.

Levy A, Lightman S. Molecular defects in the pathogenesis of pituitary tumours. Front Neuroendocrinol 2003;24:94–127.

Liu J, Lin C, Gleiberman A, et al. Tbx 19, a tissue-selective regulator of POMC gene expression. Proc Natl Acad Sci USA 2001;98:8674–8679.

Melmed S (ed). The Pituitary. Cambridge, MA: Blackwell Science, 2002.

Melmed S, Ho K, Klibanski A, Reichlin S, Thorner M. Recent advances in pathogenesis, diagnosis and management of acromegaly. J Clin Endocrinol Metab 1995;80:3395–3402.

Nowakowski BE, Maurer RA. Multiple Pit-1 binding sites facilitate estrogen responsiveness of the prolactin gene. Mol Endocrinol 1994;8: 1742–1749.

Orth DN. Cushing's syndrome. N Engl J Med 1995;332:791–802.

Pei L, Melmed S, Scheithauer B, Kovacs K, Benedict WF, Prager D. Frequent loss of heterozygosity at the retinoblastoma susceptibility gene (RB) locus in aggressive pituitary tumors: evidence for a chromosome 13 tumor suppressor gene other than RB. Cancer Res 1995;55:1613–1616.

Shimon I, Melmed S. Genetic basis of endocrine disease: pituitary tumor pathogenesis. J Clin Endocrinol Metab 1997;82:1675–1681.

Zhang X, Horwitz G, Heaney T, et al. PTTG expression in pituitary adenomas: marker for functional tumor invasiveness. J Clin Endocrinol Metab 1999;84:761–767.

34 Growth Hormone Deficiency Disorders

Amy Potter and John A. Phillips, III

SUMMARY

Growth hormone (GH) is a multifunctional hormone produced in the pituitary that promotes postnatal growth of skeletal and soft tissues through a variety of effects. In addition to promoting growth of tissues, GH also exerts a variety of other biological effects, including lactogenic, diabetogenic, lipolytic, and protein anabolic effects, as well as sodium and water retention. The frequency of GH deficiency has been estimated at 1/4000–1/10,000 in various studies. Estimates of the proportion of GH-deficient cases having an affected parent, sib, or child range from 3 to 30% in different studies. This occurrence of familial clustering suggests that a significant proportion of cases might have a genetic basis. This chapter discusses the genetics and molecular pathophysiology of familial isolated growth hormone deficiency and combined pituitary hormone deficiency.

Key Words: Combined pituitary hormone deficiency; growth hormone; growth hormone releasing hormone receptor; isolated growth hormone deficiency; Laron syndrome; pituitary.

INTRODUCTION

Growth hormone (GH) is a multifunctional hormone produced in the pituitary that promotes postnatal growth of skeletal and soft tissues through a variety of effects. The GH gene, *GH1*, is part of a gene cluster that likely originated through duplication events during evolution (Fig. 34-1). Controversy remains about the relative contribution of direct and indirect actions of GH. The direct effects of GH have been demonstrated in many tissues and organs and growth hormone receptors (GHRs) have been documented in a number of cell types. However, a substantial amount of data indicates that a major portion of the effects of GH are mediated through the actions of GH-dependent insulin-like growth factor-1 (IGF-I). IGF-I is produced in many tissues, primarily the liver, and acts through its own receptor to enhance the proliferation and maturation of many tissues, including bone, cartilage, and skeletal muscle. In addition to promoting growth of tissues, GH also exerts a variety of other biological effects, including lactogenic, diabetogenic, lipolytic, and protein anabolic effects, as well as sodium and water retention.

At the cellular level, a single GH molecule binds two GHR molecules, causing them to dimerize (Chapter 31). Dimerization of the two GH-bound GHR molecules is thought to be necessary

From: *Principles of Molecular Medicine, Second Edition*
Edited by: M. S. Runge and C. Patterson © Humana Press, Inc., Totowa, NJ

for signal transduction, which is associated with the tyrosine kinase JAK-2. The diverse effects of GH might be mediated by a single type of GHR molecule that can possess different cytoplasmic domains or phosphorylation sites in different tissues. When activated by JAK-2, these differing cytoplasmic domains can lead to distinct phosphorylation pathways, one for growth effects and others for various metabolic effects. GHR is localized on the cell surface, and contains extracellular, transmembrane, and cytoplasmic domains (Fig. 34-2). The extracellular domain is cleaved, releasing the extracellular portion of GHR into the circulation as growth hormone-binding protein (GHBP). GHBP functions as a reservoir for GH in the plasma.

The frequency of GH deficiency (either isolated or concomitant with other pituitary hormone deficiencies) has been estimated at 1/4000–1/10,000 in various studies. Most cases are sporadic and assumed to arise from cerebral insults or defects that include cerebral edema, chromosomal anomalies, histiocytosis, infections, radiation, septo-optic dysplasia (SOD), trauma, or tumors affecting the hypothalamus or pituitary. MRI examinations detect hypothalamic or pituitary anomalies in approx 12% of patients who have isolated growth hormone deficiency (IGHD).

Estimates of the proportion of GH-deficient cases having an affected parent, sib, or child range from 3 to 30% in different studies. This occurrence of familial clustering suggests that a significant proportion of cases might have a genetic basis. The genetics and molecular pathophysiology of familial IGHD and combined pituitary hormone deficiency (CPHD) is discussed next. Table 34-1 shows an overview of the genetic disorders associated with GH deficiency or defective GH function.

CLINICAL FEATURES

Adequate amounts of GH are needed throughout childhood to maintain normal growth. Newborns with GH deficiency are usually of normal length and weight. Infants with CPHD might have signs of other pituitary hormone deficiencies, such as micropenis (gonadotropin deficiency) or fasting hypoglycemia (adrenocorticotropin deficiency, GH deficiency) in addition to their low linear growth, which becomes progressively retarded with age. In those with IGHD, skeletal maturation is usually delayed in proportion to their retardation in height. Truncal obesity, facial appearance younger than expected for chronological age, delayed secondary dentition, and high-pitched voice are often present. Puberty might be delayed until the late teens but normal fertility usually occurs.

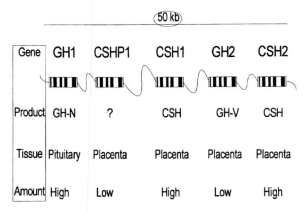

Figure 34-1 Schematic overview of the GH gene cluster, including the protein products and expression patterns of its component genes. *GH1* encodes the pituitary growth hormone; all of the other genes are expressed in the placenta. As the nomenclature of this gene cluster has been somewhat confusing, alternative names and abbreviations are given in parentheses where ever appropriate. *GH1*, the growth hormone gene; *GH-N*, the active form of growth hormone; *CSHP1*, chorionic somatomammotropin pseudogene 1 (CSHL1, chorionic somatomammotropin hormone like 1; CSL, chorionic somatomammotropin like); *CSH1*, chorionic somatomammotropin hormone 1 gene (CSA, chorionic somatomammotropin A); CSH, chorionic somatomammotropin hormone; *GH2*, growth hormone 2 gene; GH-V, growth hormone variant (produced only in the placenta); *CSH2*, chorionic somatomammotropin hormone 2 gene (CSB, chorionic somatomammotropin B). "?" denotes uncertainty concerning the presence or functionality of any protein product of this gene. Evidence suggests that most transcripts result in nonfunctional protein products, although some functional product might be present in low amounts.

Fine, wrinkled skin appearing similar to that of premature aging is seen in affected adults. Concomitant deficiency of other pituitary hormones—for example, luteinizing hormone (LH), follicle-stimulating hormone (FSH), thyroid-stimulating hormone (TSH), and adrenocorticotropic hormone (ACTH)—in addition to GH, is called panhypopituitary dwarfism or CPHD. With these additional hormone deficiencies, the retardation of growth and skeletal maturation is often more severe and spontaneous puberty might not occur.

Laron syndrome (*see* Laron Syndrome) is an autosomal-recessive disorder-caused by target organ resistance to the action of GH. Patients with Laron syndrome are similar in clinical appearance to those with severe IGHD. At the biochemical level, Laron syndrome subjects have low levels of IGF-I, despite increased circulating levels of GH. This contrasts with the low levels of both IGF-I and GH that are seen in GH deficiency. Patients with Laron syndrome do not respond to exogenous GH therapy, but replacement therapy with recombinant IGF-I (thus bypassing the dysfunctional GHR) is effective. Laron syndrome is caused by defects in GHR (*see* molecular pathology details in Laron Syndrome).

DIAGNOSIS

Although short stature, delayed growth velocity, and delayed skeletal maturation are all seen with GH deficiency, none of these signs is specific for this disorder. Patients should be evaluated for other systemic diseases causing growth failure (such as thyroid disease, occult renal disease, malabsorption syndromes, anemia, and others). IGF-I levels might be used as a screening test for GH deficiency. For patients with low IGF-I levels compared with age norms (or low-normal levels in a suggestive clinical setting), provocative

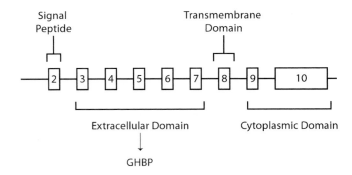

Figure 34-2 Structure of the coding region of the growth hormone receptor (GHR), demonstrating the signal peptide and extracellular, transmembrane, and cytoplasmic domains. Numbered boxes represent exons. GHR is cleaved by tumor necrosis factor-α converting enzyme (TACE, a metalloprotease) to form GHBP. In humans the cleavage site localizes to residues 240–247, close to the transmembrane domain.

testing to definitively prove GH deficiency is necessary. The most commonly used provocative tests include exercise, levodopa, insulin tolerance test, arginine, clonidine, and growth hormone releasing hormone (GHRH); typically, two tests are performed in combination, for example, insulin tolerance testing and arginine stimulation. Glucagon and propranolol have also been used for stimulation testing but are not commonly used currently. Inadequate GH peak responses (usually <7–10 ng/mL) differ from test to test. Patients whose stimulation tests confirm GH deficiency should undergo an MRI to rule out mass lesions or congenital anomalies (e.g., SOD) as the cause of the deficiency. Testing of the LH, FSH, TSH, and ACTH axes should be performed to identify any additional pituitary hormone deficiencies.

FAMILIAL ISOLATED GH DEFICIENCY

GENETIC BASIS AND MOLECULAR PATHOLOGY OF DISEASE Familial IGHD is associated with at least four Mendelian disorders. These include two forms that have autosomal-recessive inheritance (IGHD IA and IB), as well as autosomal-dominant (IGHD II) and X-linked (IGHD III) forms. A variety of molecular defects have been detected which cause these disorders (Table 34-2). These defects are reviewed on the basis of the type of inheritance (IGHD I–III) that they cause.

ISOLATED GROWTH HORMONE DEFICIENCY IA The most severe form of IGHD, called IGHD IA, has an autosomal-recessive mode of inheritance. Affected individuals occasionally have short lengths at birth and hypoglycemia in infancy, but uniformly develop severe dwarfism by 6 mo. In response to replacement therapy with exogenous GH, IGHD IA subjects have a strong initial anabolic and growth response that is frequently followed by the development of anti-GH antibodies in sufficient titer to block the response to GH replacement.

GH1 Gene Deletions Initially, all individuals with IGHD IA were homozygous for *GH1* gene deletions and developed anti-GH antibodies with treatment. Subsequently, additional patients with *GH1* gene deletions have been described who also have complete GH deficiency, but respond well to GH replacement. Thus, the clinical outcomes of subjects with the same molecular findings vary, making the presence of anti-GH antibodies an inconsistent finding in IGHD IA cases.

At a molecular level, Southern blot analysis showed deletions of approx 6.7, 7, or 7.6 kb, with most (~ 75%) being 6.7 kb. DNA

Table 34-1
Overview of Disorders Causing Growth Hormone Deficiency

Level of disorder	Type of deficiency	Gene involved	Inheritance	Defect
Pituitary	MPHD	POU1F1	R, DN	All cause defects in pituitary development with
		PROP1	R	varying degrees of pituitary hypoplasia
		HESX1	R	
	IGHD III	SOX3	X	Likely pituitary hypoplasia, syndrome includes mental retardation
Growth hormone releasing hormone receptor (GHRHR)	IGHD IB	GHRHR	R	Failure to respond to GHRH
Growth hormone	IGHD IA	GH1	R	Absent GH resulting from gene deletions, frameshifts, and nonsense mutations
	IGHD IB	GH1	R	Splicing defects
	IGHD II	GH1	DN	Splicing defects leading to defective processing/secretion of GH
	Biodefective growth hormone	GH1	?	Nonfunctional growth hormone molecule
Growth hormone receptor	Laron syndrome	GHR	R (most common), DN (rare)	Nonfunctional GHR causes resistance to growth hormone and deficiency of growth hormone effect

MPHD, multiple pituitary hormone deficiencies; IGHD, isolated growth hormone deficiency; R, recessive; DN, dominant negative; X, X-linked.

Table 34-2
Selected Mutations in the GH1 Genes of Subjects With IGHD

IGHD type	Location	Nucleotide change[a]	Effect of mutation	References
IA		Deletion	7.6-kb deletion of GH gene	Vnencak-Jones et al. (1990)
		Deletion	7-kb deletion of GH gene	Vnencak-Jones et al. (1990)
		Deletion	6.7-kb deletion of GH gene	Vnencak-Jones et al. (1990)
	Exon II	5536 del C	Frameshift after 17th aa of signal peptide	Duquesnoy et al. (1990)
	Exon II	5543 G → A	Stop codon after 19th aa of signal peptide	Cogan et al. (1993)
IB	Intron IV	6242 G → C	Donor splice site mutation, frameshift	Cogan et al. (1994)
	Intron IV	6242 G → T	Donor splice site mutation, frameshift	Miller-Davis et al. (1993)
	Intron IV	6246 G → C	Donor splice site mutation, frameshift	Abdul-Latif et al. (2000)
	Exon III	5938-39 del AG	Frameshift after 55th aa of mature GH	Igarashi et al. (1993)
II	Intron II	5863 A → T	Acceptor splice site mutation	Fofanova et al. (2003)
	Exon III	5865 G → T	Exon 3 skip	Takahashi et al. (2002)
	Exon III	5869 A → G	Exon splice enhancer mutation, exon 3 skip	Moseley et al. (2002)
	Intron III	5985 G → A	Donor splice site mutation, exon 3 skip	Cogan et al. (1995)
	Intron III	5985 G → C	Donor splice site mutation, exon 3 skip	Binder et al. (1995)
	Intron III	5986 T → C	Donor splice site mutation, exon 3 skip	Binder et al. (2001)
	Intron III	5989 G → C	Donor splice site mutation, exon 3 skip	Hayashi et al. (1999a)
	Intron III	5989 G → A	Donor splice site mutation, exon 3 skip	Kamijo et al. (1999)
	Intron III	5990 T → C	Donor splice site mutation, exon 3 skip	Cogan et al. (1994)
	Intron III	5990 T → G	Donor splice site mutation, exon 3 skip	Katsumata et al. (2001)
	Intron III	6012 G → A	Intron splice enhancer mutation, exon 3 skip	Cogan et al. (1997) McCarthy et al. (1998)
	Intron III	6012-29 del	Intron splice enhancer mutation, exon 3 skip	Cogan et al. (1997) McCarthy et al. (1998)
	Exon IV	6191 G → T	Val110Phe, possible altered protein folding	Binder et al. (2001)
	Exon V	6664 G → A	Arg183His, altered secretory granules	Deladoëy et al. (2001)

[a]Nucleotide numbering according to Chen EY, Liao Y, Smith DH, et al. The human growth hormone locus: nucleotide sequence, biology, and evolution. Genomics 1989;4:479–497.

GH, growth hormone; IGHD, isolated growth hormone deficiency.

sequence analysis of the fusion fragments associated with *GH1* gene deletions has shown that homologous recombination between sequences flanking the *GH1* gene causes these deletions (Fig. 34-3). *GH1* gene deletions are detected using PCR amplification of the homologous regions flanking the *GH1* gene and the fusion fragments associated with *GH1* gene deletions. Because the fusion fragments associated with 6.7-kb deletions differ in the size of fragments produced by certain restriction enzymes (*see Sma*I sites indicated by solid circle in Fig. 34-3), homozygosity or heterozygosity for these deletions can easily be detected by enzyme digestion of PCR

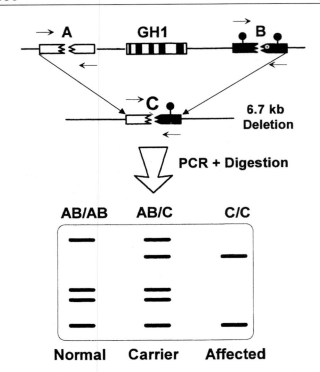

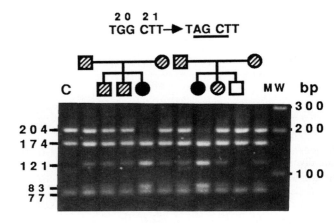

Figure 34-4 Detection of the GH G → A codon 20 (Trp → Stop) mutation by restriction enzyme digestion with *Alu*I and gel electrophoresis. Note when this mutation is present a new *Alu*I recognition site occurs and the normal 204 bp fragments are cleaved to 121 and 83 bp.

Figure 34-3 PCR amplification of homologous sequences flanking the GH1 gene. Flanking sequences are distinguished from GH-deletion fusion fragments by restriction enzyme digestion (•), shown above, and gel electrophoresis, shown below.

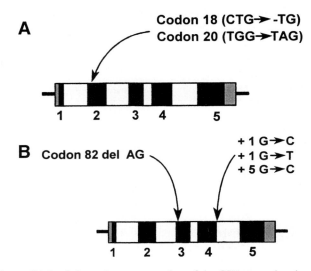

Figure 34-5 Schematic representation of the GH1 gene showing the locations of various isolated growth hormone deficiency (IGHD) IA (**A**) and IB (**B**) mutations. Shaded areas represent exons; clear areas represent introns. A +1 indicates position within the donor splice site.

products. A variety of studies suggest that 13–15% of subjects with severe IGHD (>–4.5 standard deviations [SD] in height) have *GH1* gene deletions. Frameshift and nonsense mutations have also been found in subjects with the IGHD IA phenotype, such that this disorder might best be described as complete GH deficiency as a result of *GH1* gene defects, rather than gene deletions alone.

GH1 Deletion and Frameshift Mutations   Two affected siblings diagnosed with IGHD IA have been reported who are compound heterozygotes for deletion and frameshift mutations of the *GH1* gene. Southern blot analysis showed the patients to be heterozygous for the 6.7 kb GH gene deletion. DNA sequence analysis of the retained *GH1* gene showed it had a cytosine deleted in the 18th codon of the prohormone sequence. This single-base deletion results in a frameshift within the signal peptide coding region that prevents the synthesis of any mature GH protein. These patients presented with severe growth failure, and after an initial growth response to treatment with exogenous GH, had high titers of anti-GH antibodies.

GH1 Nonsense Mutations   A G → A transition in codon 20 (Trp20Ter) of the *GH1* signal peptide has been reported in a consanguineous Turkish family with IGHD IA. This results in the termination of translation after residue 19 of the signal peptide and no production of mature GH. Patients homozygous for this mutation have no detectable GH and produce anti-GH antibodies in response to exogenous GH treatment. Interestingly, this mutation generates a new *Alu*I site that can be readily screened for by PCR amplification of the GH gene followed by *Alu*I digestion and gel electrophoresis (Fig. 34-4).

IGHD IB CAUSED BY GH1 MUTATIONS   Patients with IGHD IB are characterized by low, but detectable levels of GH, stature more than 2 SD below the mean for age and sex, autosomal-recessive inheritance, and a positive response and immunological

tolerance to treatment with exogenous GH. Some patients clinically diagnosed as IGHD IA because of an apparent lack of endogenous GH are actually type IB. In these patients, *GH1* gene defects result in mutant GH protein that cannot be effectively measured by radioimmunoassay. The presence of this protein might explain their good response to GH therapy and lack of anti-GH antibodies. Figure 34-5 shows selected *GH1* mutations causing IGHD IA and IB. IGHD IB is also caused by defects in the growth hormone releasing hormone receptor (*GHRHR*) gene. Lack of signaling through GHRHR leads to very low level or absent GH production.

GH1 Splicing Mutations   A G → C transversion in the first base of the donor splice site of intron 4 has been detected in a consanguineous Saudi Arabian family. The mutation causes the activation of a cryptic splice site 73 bases upstream of the exon 4 donor splice site. This altered splicing results in the loss of amino acids 103–126 of exon 4 and creates a frameshift that alters the amino acids encoded by exon 5. Such changes in the amino acids encoded by exons 4 and 5 affect the stability and biologic activity of the mutant GH protein, and bovine GH mutants also derange intracellular targeting of GH protein products to the secretory granule.

A G → T transversion has been identified at the same site in another consanguineous Saudi family. This G → T transversion had the same effect on splicing as the G → C transversion. Both of these mutations destroy an HphI site that enables their detection by restriction digestion of *GH1* gene PCR products followed by gel electrophoresis. Patients homozygous for these defects responded well to exogenous GH treatment and did not make anti-GH antibodies.

A G → C transversion of the fifth base of intron IV was identified in a highly consanguineous family diagnosed with IGHD I. This mutation created a new MaeII site that was used to screen all family members for the mutation. Reverse transcriptase-PCR analysis of GH mRNA transcripts from the lymphoblastoid cells of an affected patient demonstrated that the mutation destroyed the intron IV donor splice site and had the same overall effect on splicing as the +1G → C transversion previously described. Interestingly, heterozygous carriers of this mutation were later reported to have a higher frequency of short stature than homozygous wild type family members.

GH1 Deletions and Frameshifts An IGHD patient with severe growth retardation was found to have two GH gene defects. The first GH allele was a 6.7-kb deletion and the second had a 2-bp deletion in exon 3. This 2-bp deletion results in a frameshift within exon 3 and generates a premature stop codon at the position of amino acid residue 132 in exon 4. The patient had a positive response to GH replacement therapy and did not produce anti-GH antibodies, again suggesting that some GH-related protein was produced.

IGHD IB CAUSED BY GHRHR MUTATIONS The molecular basis for the "little" (lit) mouse phenotype, characterized by dwarfism and hypoplasia of the anterior pituitary gland, is a point mutation in the *GHRHR* gene that results in an Asp→Gly substitution at residue 60 (Asp60Gly). Anterior pituitaries of mutant mice showed spatially distinct proliferative zones of GH producing stem cells and mature somatotropes, each regulated by a different trophic factor. Subsequent studies have shown that the Asp60Gly mutant does not bind GHRH.

A nonsense mutation in the human *GHRHR* gene was found in two first cousins, a boy, and a girl, of a consanguineous Indian family with profound GH deficiency. Both the 3.5-yr-old girl and her 16-yr-old cousin showed poor growth since infancy and were extremely short. They were prepubertal with frontal bossing and predominantly truncal obesity. Although both failed to produce GH in response to standard provocative tests and to repetitive stimulation with GHRH, they responded to administration of exogenous GH. The affected individuals were homozygous for a G → T transversion at position 265 of their *GHRHR* genes, resulting in a premature termination mutation (Glu72Stop). Because both GH releasing peptide (a synthetic heptapeptide) and nonpeptidyl benzamines can stimulate GH release without involvement of the GHRH receptor, they might be useful in therapy of this disorder. Subsequently, the same *GHRHR* mutation was found in an isolate from the Indus valley of Pakistan. A splice mutation of the *GHRHR* gene was found in a large consanguineous kindred in Brazil. The mutation was a G → A transition at the +1 position of IVS1. A mutation that affects the PIT-1

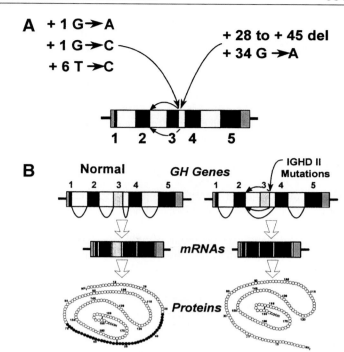

Figure 34-6 Schematic representation of **(A)** the GH1 gene showing the locations of various isolated growth hormone deficiency (IGHD) II mutations and **(B)** the mRNA splicing patterns of the normal growth hormone (GH) and IGHD II mutant GH genes. Note that the deleted amino acids corresponding to exon III are shaded in the normal peptide (left) and absent in the mutant peptide (right). Shaded areas represent exons; clear areas represent introns. A+ sign indicates position within the intron.

binding site in the *GHRHR* promoter (−124 A → C) and thereby decreases *GHRHR* expression has also been described.

IGHD II IGHD II has an autosomal-dominant mode of inheritance. Patients diagnosed with IGHD II have a single affected parent, vary in clinical severity between kindreds, and respond well to GH treatment. The majority of IGHD II patients with GH1 gene defects have mutations in intron 3 that alter splicing of GH transcripts, resulting in skipping of exon 3 (Fig. 34-6). The mechanism by which the mutant, truncated GH protein inactivates the normal GH protein appears to be related to altered intracellular processing of the GH protein product (*see* Dominant-Negative Mutations).

Dominant-Negative Mutations A T → C transition of the sixth base of the donor splice site of intron 3 was the first mutation associated with IGHD II. The mutation inactivates the intron 3 donor splice site causing deletion or skipping of exon 3 and loss of amino acids 32–71 from the corresponding mature GH protein products. All of the affected patients in this family were heterozygous for the intron 3 +6 T → C change and had low, but measurable, GH levels after provocative stimulation. Affected subjects responded well to treatment with exogenous GH without forming significant levels of anti-GH antibodies.

Many additional mutations causing altered splicing leading to IGHD II mutations have been identified (*see* Table 34-2). The intron 3 donor splice site appears to be a mutational "hot spot," with a recurring G → A transition at the first base of the donor splice site as well as other mutations. The G → A transition has been identified in nonrelated kindreds and is thought to arise because of the high mutation frequency of CpG dinucleotides. All of these donor splice site mutations cause exon 3 skipping in vitro.

Intron 3 mutations that alter splicing but do not occur within the consensus branch, donor, or acceptor sites have also been identified. One deletes 18 bp (del+28–45), and the second is a G → A transition of the 28th base of intron 3. Both of these mutations in vitro lead to exon 3 skipping. These mutations disrupt an intron splice enhancer sequence with the motif $G_2X_{1-4}G_3$, which normally regulates splicing. An exon 3 +5 A → G mutation has also been described that it disrupts an exon splice enhancer and causes partial or complete exon 3 skipping.

The mechanism for the autosomal-dominant inheritance pattern of these mutations was previously unknown, although it was hypothesized that the mutant protein somehow interfered with the function or secretion of the wild type protein translated from the normal allele. In 1999, it was demonstrated that *GH1* constructs with intron 3 donor splice site mutations (causing exon 3 skipping) caused significant inhibition of wild type GH secretion in neuroendocrine cell lines. In 2002, it was shown that a different mutation associated with IGHD II (R183H) was retained in cells after packaging into secretory granules for a longer period than wild type protein. Studies in mice transgenic for the intron 3 + 1 G → A mutation (Δexon3hGH) have clearly demonstrated that the mutated protein aggregates in the cytoplasm of the pituitary somatotropes. Few secretory vesicles were visible in these cells, and abnormal histology was seen. Mouse lines with the highest transgene copy numbers were most severely affected, with destruction not only of somatotropes but eventually other pituitary cell lines as well, leading to multiple pituitary hormone deficiencies.

In addition to the R183H mutation discussed earlier, other mutations causing IGHD II through amino acid changes rather than splicing changes have been found. Patients with IGHD II on the basis of an amino acid change tend to have a milder phenotype than those with splicing changes, but there is considerable interindividual variation. It is likely that these other missense mutations cause IGHD II by affecting protein packaging and/or secretion in a manner similar to that described for R183H.

IGHD III   IGHD III has an X-linked mode of inheritance, but distinct clinical findings in different families. Affected individuals in some kindreds have γ-globulinemia associated with their IGHD, but others do not, suggesting that contiguous gene defects of Xq21.3–q22 might occur in some cases. Interestingly, other cases of IGHD have an interstitial deletion of Xp22.3 or duplication of Xq13.3–q 21.2 suggesting that multiple loci might cause IGHD III.

SOX3, located on the X chromosome, is a member of the SRY-related high-mobility group box family of transcription factors. It has been associated with an X-linked syndrome of short stature, mental retardation, characteristic facies, and IGHD in one family. Analysis of the *SOX3* gene in that family showed an in-frame 33 bp duplication occurring within a poly-alanine tract. Mouse studies have shown that *SOX3* is widely expressed in the developing CNS and pituitary. Duplications of the X chromosome spanning the region Xq26.1–q27.3, which includes *SOX3*, have been associated with pituitary hypoplasia. This evidence suggests that overexpression of *SOX3* might lead to abnormalities of both the pituitary and other elements of the CNS; however, the exact mechanism remains to be confirmed.

BIODEFECTIVE GH

Treatment with exogenous human GH induced normal levels of IGF-I and a significant increase in growth rate in two unrelated boys with growth retardation, delayed bone ages, low levels of

IGF-I, and normal GH levels after stimulation. Although the family data did not support a specific mode of inheritance, a mutation resulting in a biologically ineffective GH molecule was speculated. A similar case confirmed a structural abnormality of the GH molecule: 60–90% of circulating GH was in the form of tetramers and dimers (normal, 14–39% in plasma) and the patients' GH polymers were abnormally resistant to conversion into monomers by urea.

Subsequently, a boy was reported who was short at birth (39 cm at 41 wk gestation) and at the age of 4.9 yr had a height that was –6.1 SD below the mean and a bone age of 2 yr. He had normal body proportions, with a prominent forehead and saddle nose. His IGF-I was 34 ng/mL (normal 35–293). Basal GH levels were 7–14 ng/mL and peak levels after insulin-induced hypoglycemia, arginine, and levodopa administration were 38, 15, and 35 ng/mL, respectively. Serum IGF-I was unchanged after 3 d of daily subcutaneous injections of 0.1 U of recombinant human GH/kg body weight (0.035 mg/kg). During prolonged treatment with GH (0.18 mg/kg/wk), his serum IGF-I was 200 ng/mL and his rate of linear growth increased to 6 cm/yr from 3.9 cm/yr before treatment. Assay of the bioactivity of his GH was below the normal range, and isoelectric focusing of his serum showed an abnormal GH peak in addition to a normal peak, whereas serum from his father and normal controls contained only one peak. The affected son was heterozygous for a C→T transition encoding an Arg→Cys substitution at codon 77 (Arg77Cys) of his GH1 gene. Inexplicably, his father, also heterozygous for this mutation, was of normal height, had a peak GH level of 23.7, and normal isoelectric focusing results. The same researchers have also reported a different mutation, Asp112Gly, in a 3-yr-old girl with short stature and high circulating GH levels as well as good response to exogenous GH therapy. This mutation is associated with GHR in a 1/1 ratio instead of 1/2, resulting in decreased intracellular signaling in vitro.

LARON SYNDROME: GROWTH HORMONE RESISTANCE

As mentioned, Laron syndrome is caused by defects in *GHR*. Most cases display autosomal-recessive inheritance, but at least two instances of autosomal-dominant (dominant negative) inheritance have been described.

AUTOSOMAL-RECESSIVE GH RESISTANCE   The first *GHR* mutations causing autosomal-recessive Laron syndrome were described in 1989, when both a partial *GHR* gene deletion and a missense mutation (Phe96Ser) in the extracellular portion of the receptor were discovered. Since then, many different mutations have been reported. The majority occurs in the extracellular portion of the receptor, causing the phenotype of Laron syndrome with normal-to-elevated GH levels, low-to-absent GHBP levels, and low IGF-I levels with poor growth. GHBP consists of the extracellular portions of *GHR* that have been proteolytically cleaved from the cell surface. Mutations that affect the extracellular portion of *GHR* lead to low GHBP levels. Such mutations are heterogeneous. For example, nine novel mutations were reported occurring in 13 unrelated patients: three were nonsense mutations, one caused a frameshift, two were splice site mutations, and three were missense mutations. All affected the extracellular domain of the receptor, and all 13 patients had undetectable GHBP. Exon 4 was also noted as a "hot spot" for mutations, with five out of the nine mutations occurring in exon 4.

Table 34-3
Selected Mutations in the POU1F1 Genes of Subjects with CPHD

Mode	Codon	Nucleotide change	Effect of mutation	References
AR		Deletion	Deletion of POU1F1 gene	Wit et al. (1989)
	135	T → G	Amino acid change (Phe → Cys)	Pelligrini et al. (1996)
	143	G → A	Amino acid change (Arg → Gln)	Ohta et al. (1992)
	158	G → C	Amino acid change (Ala → Pro)	Wit et al. (1989)
	172	C → T	Generates a stop codon	Tatsumi et al. (1992)
	230	G → A	Amino acid change (Lys → Glu)	Gat-Yablonski et al. (2002)
	239	T → C	Amino acid change (Pro → Ser)	Pernasetti et al. (1998)
	250	G → T	Generates a stop codon	Irie et al. (1995)
AD	24	C → T	Amino acid change (Pro → Leu)	Ohta et al. (1992)
	271	C → T	Amino acid change (Arg → Trp)	Radovick et al. (1992) Cohen et al. (1995)

AD, autosomal-dominant; AR, autosomal-recessive.

Mutations associated with elevated GHBP levels have also been reported. One patient with Laron syndrome had a marked elevated of GHBP. Investigation revealed a G → T transversion at exon 8 –1, causing skipping of exon 8 (which encodes the transmembrane domain) and a frameshift leading to a premature stop codon. The truncated protein is thus unable to be appropriately anchored in the cell membrane, and appears in the serum as GHBP. The patient was homozygous for the mutation, suggesting autosomal-recessive inheritance; the patient's mother was heterozygous for the mutation and of normal height with elevated serum GHBP levels.

DOMINANT-NEGATIVE GH RESISTANCE A patient with Laron syndrome and normal GHBP levels has been described. The patient and her mother had a heterozygous G → C transversion of the 3′ splice acceptor site before exon 9. This splice site mutation resulted in deletion of exon 9 with a frameshift and premature stop codon, resulting in reduction of the intracellular portion of the receptor to only seven amino acids. In vitro studies of this mutant showed that it was unable to initiate JAK/STAT signaling. Lack of the intracellular portion of the receptor would also be expected to reduce internalization and degradation of the receptor. The resulting accumulation of abnormal receptors on the cell surface would then competitively inhibit the normal receptor, accounting for the dominant negative phenotype. A mutation of the donor splice of intron 9 produced a truncated receptor structurally identical to that produced by the G → C transversion of the 3′ splice acceptor site prior to exon 9.

GHR DEFECTS IN IDIOPATHIC SHORT STATURE Idiopathic short stature (ISS) is the name given to short stature once systemic disorders and other known causes have been excluded. By definition, ISS patients have normal responses to GH stimulation testing. Some ISS patients might have low IGF-I and GHBP levels, and it has been theorized that at least some cases of ISS might be because of less severe or heterozygous mutations of *GHR*. Results of investigations suggest that *GHR* mutations account for a small but significant percentage of ISS cases.

FAMILIAL COMBINED PITUITARY HORMONE DEFICIENCY

GENETIC BASIS AND MOLECULAR PATHOPHYSIO-LOGY OF DISEASE Familial CPHD is characterized by deficiency of one or more of the other pituitary trophic hormones (ACTH, FSH, LH, or TSH) in addition to GH deficiency. Whereas the great majority of cases are sporadic, there are Mendelian forms

with autosomal-recessive, autosomal-dominant, or X-linked modes of inheritance. Mutations in several transcription factors, including *POU1F1* (also called *PIT1*), *PROP1*, and *HESX1* have been associated with CPHD in humans. *POU1F1* and *PROP1* are both members of the POU (for Pit-1, Oct-1, and Unc-86) homeodomain family of transcription factors and play an important role in pituitary development.

POU1F1 *POU1F1* (or *PIT1*) encodes a protein that binds to and transactivates promoters of the *GH1* and prolactin genes. It is required for differentiation and proliferation of somatotropes, lactotropes, and thyrotropes. At least 10 different *POU1F1* mutations have been found in humans in a subtype of CPHD associated with GH, prolactin, and TSH deficiency (Table 34-3).

Autosomal-Recessive *POU1F1* Mutations The first and second *POU1F1* mutations reported were found in two consanguineous Japanese families. One family had a C → T transition in codon 172 (Arg172Ter). Both parents were heterozygous and the affected child was homozygous for the mutation. In the second family, a missense mutation (Arg143Gln) was found. The patient was homozygous for this mutation, whereas the parents and two unaffected siblings were heterozygous. Both mutations occur in the POU-specific domain and are thought to affect binding of the POU1F1 protein to the DNA.

The third and fourth *POU1F1* mutations were found in two Dutch families who had postnatal growth failure with complete deficiencies of GH and prolactin, whereas the thyroxine (T4) levels were low or normal before or following GH replacement. Subjects in one family who had normal T4 levels were homozygous for a G → C substitution in codon 158 (Ala158Pro). This mutation interferes with formation of POU1F1 homodimers and dramatically reduces the altered POU1F1's ability to activate transcription. Subjects in the second family with low T4 levels had one deleted *POU1F1* gene and one *POU1F1* gene with the previous mutation. These cases emphasize the importance of determining prolactin levels and TSH responses to thyrotropin-releasing hormone (TRH) in evaluating CPHD. Because GH and TSH deficiency often occur together, finding a low prolactin level and absent TSH response should raise the question of a *POU1F1* gene defect.

A fifth *POU1F1* mutation was identified in a Thai patient with deficiency of GH, TSH, and prolactin. Both parents were healthy and heterozygous for a G → T transversion in codon 250 (Glu250Ter). The CPHD patient was homozygous for the mutation. This mutation resulted in complete loss of the POU-homeodomain that is necessary for DNA binding.

Table 34-4
Selected Mutations in the *PROP1* Genes of Subjects With CPHD

Mode	Codon	Nucleotide change	Effect of mutation	References
AR	101	Deletion	Two base pair deletion causes frameshift, premature stop at codon 109	Wu et al. (1998)
	117	T → A	Amino acid change (Phe → Ile)	Wu et al. (1998)
	120	C → T	Amino acid change (Arg → Cys)	Wu et al. (1998)

AR, autosomal-recessive.

A sixth *POU1F1* mutation has been reported in a consanguineous family of Tunisian descent. All four affected sibs were homozygous for a T → G transversion in codon 135 (Phe135Cys) in the POU-specific domain of *POU1F1*. The patients had pituitary hypoplasia and deficiencies of GH, TSH, and prolactin.

Autosomal-Dominant POU1F1 Mutations   The first dominant-negative mutation identified in the *POU1F1* gene was a G → T substitution in codon 271 (Arg271Trp). This mutation is located in the POU-homeodomain and does not affect binding of the mutant POU1F1 protein to DNA but functions as a dominant inhibitor of POU1F1 action by an unknown mechanism. Three unrelated patients have been reported to be heterozygous for this mutation. Two of the patients were evaluated as adults and had pituitary hypoplasia and deficiencies of GH, prolactin, and TSH. The third patient was identified at only 2 mo of age and had a normal pituitary and normal basal levels of TSH but a delayed TSH response in a TRH stimulation test. The authors suggest that, because POU1F1 might be necessary for anterior pituitary cell survival, the affected patient will develop hypoplasia and TSH deficiencies with age.

The second dominant-negative *POU1F1* gene mutation was a T → C transition in codon 24 (Pro24Leu). This proline residue resides within the major transactivating domain of *POU1F1* and is highly conserved in different species. The mechanism by which this mutation exerts its dominant-negative effect is also not known.

PROP1   Ames dwarf (df/df) mice have CPHD and hypocellular anterior pituitaries that lack somatotropes, lactotropes, thyrotropes, and GH transcripts. The genetic defect associated with the Ames dwarf phenotype has been found in the gene called Prophet of Pit-1 (*Prop-1*), which encodes a pituitary-specific homeodomain factor. Sequence analysis of the Prop-1 cDNA in the df/df mouse revealed a T → C transition in codon 83 that causes a Ser → Pro amino acid change in the first helix of its homeodomain. Although *Prop-1* is required for expression of *Pit-1*, the mechanism of its action remains uncertain.

Three human *PROP1* gene defects were found in studies of four families with familial autosomal-recessive CPHD (Table 34-4). In addition to the GH, prolactin, and TSH deficiency seen with *POU1F1* defects, *PROP1*-deficient subjects also have LH and FSH deficiency, which prevents the onset of spontaneous puberty. Family I had three affected sibs, all homozygous for a C → T transition in codon 120 of the *PROP1* gene (Arg120Cys). This Arg → Cys substitution in the third helix of the homeodomain greatly reduced the protein's DNA-binding and transactivating abilities. Families II and III had the same 2-bp AG deletion in codon 101 that causes a frameshift that results in a premature stop at codon 109. The truncated protein product had no DNA binding or transactivating abilities. The patient in family IV had two different *PROP1* gene mutations (compound heterozygosity). One allele had the 2-bp AG deletion described earlier and the second allele

had a T → A transversion (Phe117Ile) that resulted in greatly reduced DNA-binding and transactivating abilities.

Although the typical phenotype of *PROP1* mutations is panhypopituitary dwarfism with short stature occurring early in childhood, one patient has been described who reached a normal adult height without intervention. This patient had the expected hypogonadotropic hypogonadism with delayed puberty, and investigators theorized that the lack of estrogen allowed this female to continue growing until age 20, thus eventually reaching an adult height. The patient was deficient in GH, FSH, LH, prolactin, TSH, and ACTH.

HESX1   *HESX1* (mouse homologue, *Hesx1*) is a member of the paired-like homeobox gene class, which is important in the development of the pituitary gland as well as other midline brain structures in both the mouse and human. Mice homozygous null for *Hesx1* are severely affected, with reduced or absent eyes, olfactory placodes, and telencephalic derivatives. Rathke's pouch is absent in these mice and the anterior pituitary is small. Because these features are similar to the findings in the human syndrome of SOD, researchers sought mutations within the homologous human gene, *HESX1*. A homozygous C → T substitution at nucleotide position 478 (Arg53Cys) was demonstrated in two siblings with SOD and panhypopituitarism. Subsequently, the same group found that heterozygous *HESX1* mutations led to less severe phenotypes in humans (ranging from mild SOD with pituitary insufficiency, to CPHD without SOD, to IGHD).

TREATMENT

Recombinant GH is available worldwide and is administered by subcutaneous injection. To obtain an optimal outcome, children with GHD should be started on replacement therapy as soon as their diagnosis is established. The initial dosage of recombinant GH is based on body weight, but the exact amount used and the frequency of administration vary among protocols. The dosage increases with increasing body weight to a maximum during puberty and is usually discontinued by approx 17 yr.

Conditions that are treated with GH include those in which it has proven efficacy (and for which it is approved) and others in which its use has been reported but is not accepted as standard practice. Disorders in which GH treatment has been approved include the following: GHD (in isolation or associated with CPHD) in children and adults; Turner's syndrome; growth failure associated with chronic renal insufficiency in children; small for gestational-age children who have not caught up their linear growth by the age of 2; and the Prader–Willi syndrome; and ISS. The clinical responses of individuals with IGHD or CPHD to GH therapy varies depending on the severity and age at which, treatment is begun, recognition and response to treatment of associated deficiencies such as thyroid hormone deficiency, and whether treatment is complicated by the development of anti-GH antibodies. The outcome of

Turner's syndrome subjects varies with the severity of their short stature, chromosomal complement, and age at which treatment was begun. In Prader–Willi syndrome, improvements in body composition are an important outcome of treatment.

Additional disorders in which the use of GH has been reported but for which its efficacy is not accepted as standard practice include treatment of selected skeletal dysplasias such as achondroplasia, growth suppression secondary to exogenous steroids (as in chronic autoimmune diseases), and the Silver–Russell syndrome. There is, in general, insufficient data to establish the efficacy of GH replacement therapy in treating these disorders because of the limited number of subjects and lack of use of standardized protocols.

FUTURE DIRECTIONS

Several problems contribute to incomplete ascertainment of affected individuals, which in turn can result in less than optimal outcomes. Such problems include the spectrum of severity, lack of a single provocative test that is both very sensitive and specific, and lack of an assay to test for qualitative changes in endogenous GH. Improvements in techniques that address these problems could facilitate the detection of and improve the outcome for treated patients in the future.

A number of genetic defects in GH biosynthesis have been documented that prevent some affected individuals from secreting GH. These include defects that result in the synthesis of truncated GH molecules, lack of GHRH receptor function, and mutant GH products that have dominant-negative effects on the normal GH products that are present. In the future, agonists of GH secretion, for example, that complement the function of GHRH, might be found that can enhance release of the stored GH found in some of these cases. The efficacy of IGF-I in treating Laron dwarfism and IGHD IA patients who are resistant to exogenous GH because of anti-GH antibodies has been proven. Additional uses of IGF-I or perhaps isoforms of IGF-I that have prolonged half-lives might provide improved efficacy in the future.

Although potential applications of gene therapy to somatic cells are feasible, targeted and regulated expression that is pituitary specific remains impractical. Thus, potential applications of gene therapy to achieve appropriate hormonal regulation seem remote.

SELECTED REFERENCES

Abdul-Latif H, Leiberman E, Brown MR, et al. Growth hormone deficiency type IB caused by cryptic splicing of the GH-1 gene. J Pediatr Endocrinol Metab 2000;13:21–28.

Amselem S, Duquesnoy P, Attree O, et al. Laron dwarfism and mutations of the growth hormone-receptor gene. N Engl J Med 1989;321:989–995.

Arroyo A, Pernasetti F, Vasilyev VV, et al. A unique case of combined pituitary hormone deficiency caused by a PROP1 gene mutation (R120C) associated with normal height and absent puberty. Clin Endocrinol (Oxf) 2002;57:283–291.

Ayling RM, Ross R, Towner P, et al. A dominant-negative mutation of the growth hormone receptor causes familial short stature. Nat Genet 1997; 16:13, 14.

Binder G, Ranke MB. Screening for growth hormone (GH) gene splice-site mutations in sporadic cases with severe isolated GH deficiency using ectopic transcript analysis. J Clin Endocrinol Metab 1995;80: 1247–1252.

Binder G, Brown M, Parkas JS. Mechanisms responsible for dominant expression of human growth hormone gene mutations. J Clin Endocrinol Metab 1996;81:4047–4050.

Binder G, Keller E, Mix M, et al. Isolated GH deficiency with dominant inheritance: new mutations, new insights. J Clin Endocrinol Metab 2001; 86:3877–3881.

Chen EY, Liao Y, Smith DH, et al. The human growth hormone locus: nucleotide sequence, biology, and evolution. Genomics 1989;4:479–497.

Cogan JD, Phillips JA III, Sakati N, et al. Heterogeneous growth hormone (GH) gene mutations in familial GH deficiency. J Clin Endocrinol Metab 1993;76:1224–1228.

Cogan JD, Phillips JA III, Schenkman SS, et al. Familial growth hormone deficiency: a model of dominant and recessive mutations affecting a monomeric protein. J Clin Endocrinol Metab 1994;79:1261–1265.

Cogan JD, Prince MA, Lekhakula S, et al. A novel mechanism of aberrant pre-mRNA splicing in humans. Hum Mol Genet 1997;6:909–912.

Cogan JD, Ramel B, Lehto M, et al. A recurring dominant negative mutation causes autosomal dominant growth hormone deficiency—a clinical research center study. J Clin Endocrinol Metab 1995;80:3591–3595.

Cohen LE, Wondisford FE, Radovick S. Role of Pit-1 in the gene expression of growth hormone, prolactin, and thyrotropin. Endocrinol Metab Clin North Am 1996;25:523–540.

Cohen LE, Wondisford FE, Salvantoni A, et al. A hot spot in the Pit-1 gene responsible for combined pituitary hormone deficiency: clinical and molecular correlates. J Clin Endocrinol Metab 1995;80:679–684.

Dattani MT, Matrinez-Barbera JP, Thomas PQ, et al. Mutations in the homeobox gene HESX1/Hesx1 associated with septo-optic dysplasia in human and mouse. Nat Genet 1998;19:125–133.

Deladoëy J, Stocker P, Mullis PE. Autosomal dominant GH deficiency due to an Arg183His Gh-1 gene mutation: clinical and molecular evidence of impaired regulated GH secretion. J Clin Endocrinol Metab 2001;86:3941–3947.

Duquesnoy P, Amselem S, Gourmelen M, et al. A frameshift mutation causing isolated growth hormone deficiency type 1A. Am J Hum Genet 1990;47:A110.

Fofanova OV, Evgrafov OV, Polyakov AV, et al. A novel IVS2–2A→T splicing mutation in the GH-1 gene in familial isolated growth hormone deficiency type II in the spectrum of other splicing mutations in the Russian population. J Clin Endocrinol Metab 2003;88:820–826.

Gat-Yablonski G, Lazar L, Pertzelan A, et al. A novel mutation in PIT-1: phenotypic variability in familial combined pituitary hormone deficiencies. J Pediatr Endocrinol Metab 2002;15:325–330.

Gaylinn BD, Dealmeida VI, Lyons CE Jr, et al. The mutant growth hormone-releasing hormone (GHRH) receptor of the little mouse does not bind GHRH. Endocrinology 1999;140:5066–5074.

Goddard AD, Dowd P, Chernausek S, et al. Partial growth-hormone insensitivity: the role of growth-hormone receptor mutations in idiopathic short stature. J Pediatr 1997;131:S51–S55.

Godowski PJ, Leung DW, Meacham LR, et al. Characterization of the human growth hormone receptor gene and demonstration of a partial gene deletion in two patients with Laron-type dwarfism. Proc Natl Acad Sci USA 1989;86:8083–8087.

Hayashi Y, Kamijo T, Yamamoto M, et al. A novel mutation at the donor splice site of intron 3 of the GH-I gene in a patient with isolated growth hormone deficiency. Growth Horm IGF Res 1999a;9:434–437.

Hayashi Y, Yamamoto M, Ohmori S, et al. Inhibition of growth hormone (GH) secretion by a mutant GH-I gene product in neuroendocrine cells containing secretory granules: an implication for isolated GH deficiency inherited in an autosomal dominant manner. J Clin Endocrinol Metab 1999b;84:2134–2139.

Herington AC. New frontiers in the molecular mechanisms of growth hormone action. Mol Cell Endocrinol 1994;100:39–44.

Igarashi Y, Ogawa M, Kamijo T, et al. A new mutation causing inherited growth hormone deficiency: a compound heterozygote of a 6.7 kb deletion and two base deletion in the third exon of the GH-1 gene. Hum Mol Genet 1993;2:1073, 1074.

Iida K, Takahashi Y, Kaji H, et al. Growth hormone (GH) insensitivity syndrome with high serum GH-binding protein levels caused by a heterozygous splice site mutation of the GH receptor gene producing a lack of intracellular domain. J Clin Endocrinol Metab 1998;83:531–537.

Irie Y, Tatsumi K, Ogawa M, et al. A novel E250X mutation of the PIT1 gene in a patient with combined pituitary hormone deficiency. Endocrinol J 1995;42:351–354.

Kamijo T, Hayashi Y, Shimatsu A, et al. Mutations in intron 3 of GH-1 gene associated with isolated GH deficiency type II in three Japanese families. Clin Endocrinol (Oxf) 1999;51:355–360.

Katsumata N, Matsuo S, Sata N, et al. A novel and *de novo* splice-donor site mutation in intron 3 of the GH-1 gene in a patient with isolated growth hormone deficiency. Growth Horm IGF Res 2001;11:378–383.

Laumonnier F, Ronce N, Hamel BCJ, et al. Transcription factor SOX3 is involved in X-linked mental retardation with growth hormone deficiency. Am J Hum Genet 2002;71:1450–1455.

Leiberman E, Pesler D, Parvari R, et al. Short stature in carriers of recessive mutation causing familial isolated growth hormone deficiency. Am J Med Genet 2000;90:188–192.

Lin SC, Lin CR, Gukovsky I, et al. Molecular basis of the little mouse phenotype and implications for cell type-specific growth. Nature 1993;364:208–213.

Maheshwari H, Silverman BL, Dupuis J, et al. Dwarfism of Sindh: a novel form of familial isolated GH deficiency linked to the locus for the GH releasing hormone receptor. Program Abstr Endocr Soc Annu Meet 1996;OR46–2.

McCarthy EMS, Phillips JA III. Characterization of an intron splice enhancer that regulates alternative splicing of human GH pre-mRNA. Hum Mol Genet 1998;7:1491–1496.

McGuinness L, Magoulas C, Sesay AK, et al. Autosomal dominant growth hormone deficiency disrupts secretory vesicles in vitro and in vivo in transgenic mice. Endocrinology 2003;144:720–731.

Miller-Davis S, Phillips JA III, Milner RDG, et al. Detection of mutations in GH genes and transcripts by analysis of DNA from dried blood spots and mRNA from lymphoblastoid cells. Program Abstr Endocr Soc Annu Meet 1993;333.

Moseley CT, Mullis PE, Prince MA, et al. An exon splice enhancer mutation causes autosomal dominant GH deficiency. J Clin Endocrinol Metab 2002;87:847–852.

Neely EK, Rosenfeld RG. Use and abuse of human growth hormone. Annu Rev Med 1994;45:407–420.

Ohta K, Nobukuni Y, Mitsubuchi H, et al. Mutations in the Pit-1 gene in children with combined pituitary hormone deficiency. Biochem Biophys Res Comm 1992;189:851–855.

Olson LE, Dasen JS, Ju BG, et al. Paired-like repression/activation in pituitary development. Recent Prog Horm Res 2003;58:249–261.

Pelligrini-Bouiller I, Belicar P, Barlier A, et al. A new mutation of the gene encoding the transcription factor Pit-1 is responsible for combined pituitary hormone deficiency. J Clin Endocrinol Metab 1996;81:2790–2796.

Pemasetti F, Milner RDG, Al Ashwal AAZ, et al. Pro239Ser: a novel recessive mutation of the Pit-1 gene in seven middle eastern children with growth hormone, prolactin, and thyrotropin deficiency. J Clin Endocrinol Metab 1998;83:2079–2083.

Pfaffle RW, DiMattia GE, Parks JS, et al. Mutation of the POU-specific domain of Pit-1 and hypopituitarism without pituitary hypoplasia. Science 1992;257:1118–1121.

Pfaffle R, Kim C, Otten B, et al. Pit-1: clinical aspects. Horm Res 1996;45:25–28.

Phillips JA III. Inherited defects in growth hormone synthesis and action. In: Scriver CR, Beaudet AL, Sly WS, Valle D, eds. The Metabolic and Molecular Basis of Inherited Disease, 7th ed., vol. 3. New York: McGraw-Hill, 1995, pp. 3023–3044.

Phillips JA III, Cogan JD. Molecular basis of familial human growth hormone deficiency. J Clin Endocrinol Metab 1994;78:11–16.

Radovick S, Nation M, Du Y, et al. A mutation in the POU-homeodomain of Pit-1 responsible for combined pituitary hormone deficiency. Science 1992;257:1115–1118.

Ranke MB. Growth hormone therapy in children: when to stop? Horm Res 1995;43:122–125.

Rosen T, Johannsson G, Johansson JO, et al. Consequences of growth hormone deficiency in adults and the benefits and risks of recombinant human growth hormone treatment. Horm Res 1995;43:93–99.

Rosenfeld RG, Rosenbloom AL, Guevara-Aguirre J. Growth hormone (GH) insensitivity due to primary GH receptor deficiency. Endocr Rev 1994;15:369–390.

Salvatori R, Fan X, Mullis PE, et al. Decreased expression of the GHRH receptor gene due to a mutation in a Pit-1 binding site. Mol Endocrinol 2002;16:450–458.

Salvatori R, Hayashida CY, Aguiar-Oliveira MH, et al. Familial dwarfism due to a novel mutation of the growth hormone-releasing hormone receptor gene. J Clin Endocrinol Metab 1999;84:917–923.

Sanchez JE, Perera E, Baumbach L, et al. Growth hormone receptor mutations in children with idiopathic short stature. J Clin Endocrinol Metab 1998;83:4079–5083.

Silbergeld A, Dastot F, Klinger B, et al. Intronic mutation in the growth hormone (GH) receptor gene from a girl with Laron syndrome and extremely high serum GH binding protein: extended phenotypic study in a very large pedigree. J Pediatr Endocrinol Metab 1997;10:265–274.

Sobrier ML, Dastot F, Duquesnoy P, et al. Nine novel growth hormone receptor gene mutations in patients with Laron syndrome. J Clin Endocrinol Metab 1997;82:435–437.

Solomon NM, Nouri S, Warne GL, et al. Increased gene dosage at Xq26-q27 is associated with X-linked hypopituitarism. Genomics 2002;79:553–559.

Sornson MW, Wu W, Dasen JS, et al. Pituitary lineage determination by the Prophet of Pit-1 homeodomain factor defective in Ames dwarfism. Nature 1996;384:327–333.

Strasburger CJ. Implications of investigating the structure–function relationship of human growth hormone in clinical diagnosis and therapy. Horm Res 1994;41:113–120.

Strobl JS, Thomas MJ. Human growth hormone. Pharmacol Rev 1994;46:1–34.

Takahashi Y, Kaji H, Okimura Y, et al. Brief report: short stature caused by a mutant growth hormone. New Engl J Med 1996;334:432–436.

Takahashi Y, Shirono H, Arisaka O, et al. Biologically inactive growth hormone caused by an amino acid substitution. J Clin Invest 1997;100:1159–1165.

Tatsumi K, Miyai K, Notomi T, et al. Cretinism with combined pituitary hormone deficiency caused by a mutation in the PIT1 gene. Nat Genet 1992;1:56–58.

Thomas PQ, Dattani MT, Brickman JM, et al. Heterozygous HESX1 mutations associated with isolated congenital pituitary hypoplasia and septo-optic dysplasia. Hum Mol Genet 2001;10:39–45.

Vnencak-Jones CL, Phillips JA III, De-fen W. Use of polymerase chain reaction in detection of growth hormone gene deletions. J Clin Endocrinol Metab 1990;70:1550–1553.

Wajnrajch MP, Gertner JM, Harbison MD, et al. Nonsense mutation in the human growth hormone-releasing hormone receptor causes growth failure analogous to the little (lit) mouse. Nat Genet 1996;12:88–90.

Wit JM, Drayer NM, Jansen M, et al. Total deficiency of growth hormone and prolactin, and partial deficiency of thyroid stimulating hormone in two Dutch families: a new variant of hereditary pituitary deficiency. Horm Res 1989;32:170–177.

Wyatt DT, Mark D, Slyper A. Survey of growth hormone treatment practices by 251 pediatric endocrinologists. J Clin Endocrinol Metab 1995;80:3292–3297.

Wu W, Cogan JD, Pfaffle RW, et al. Mutations in PROP1 cause familial combined pituitary hormone deficiency. Nat Genet 1998;18:147–149.

Zhu YL, Conway-Campbell B, Waters MJ, et al. Prolonged retention after aggregation into secretory granules of human R183H-growth hormone (GH) a mutant that causes autosomal dominant GH deficiency type II. Endocrinology 2002;143:4243–4248.

35 Thyroid Disorders

PETER KOPP

SUMMARY

The thyroid is controlled by a classic hypothalamic-pituitary axis. The thyroid gland evolves from two distinct embryological structures. Thyroid disorders can broadly be divided into disorders of function or growth. The two alterations may occur independently or in combination. For example, in patients with Graves' disease, the thyroid is typically diffusely enlarged and secretes excessive amounts of thyroid hormone. This chapter gives an overview on the variety of defects affecting thyroid function and growth at all levels of the axis.

Key Words: Autoimmune thyroid disorders; Graves' disease; human chorionic gonadotropin; iodide; thyroid cancer; medullary thyroid cancer; multiple endocrine neoplasia type 2; pendred syndrome; thyroid disorders; thyrotropin-releasing hormone; thyroperoxidase.

INTRODUCTION

Insights into the molecular basis of numerous thyroid disorders have grown impressively. Careful clinical and biochemical phenotyping continues to be the essential first step in all attempts to unravel the underlying pathogenic mechanisms. Elucidation of the molecular basis has been enormously facilitated by the increasingly complete information on the human genome, growing knowledge about developmental processes, the complexity of signaling pathways, and mechanisms of hormone action. Aside from deepening the understanding of the mechanisms governing physiology and pathology of the hypothalamic-pituitary-thyroid axis, this increasingly dense knowledge has growing impact on diagnostic and therapeutic modalities.

THE HYPOTHALAMIC-PITUITARY-THYROID AXIS

The thyroid is controlled by a classic hypothalamic-pituitary axis (Fig. 35-1). The tripeptide thyrotropin-releasing hormone (TRH), synthesized in the paraventricular nucleus of the hypothalamus, stimulates the production and secretion of the glycoprotein thyrotropin (thyroid stimulating hormone [TSH]) in the pituitary. TSH in turn stimulates growth and function of thyroid follicular cells resulting in the production of the thyroid hormones thyroxine (T4) and triiododothyronine (T3) (Figs. 35-2 and 35-3). In the bloodstream, only a minute fraction of T4 and T3 is found as free

From: *Principles of Molecular Medicine, Second Edition*
Edited by: M. S. Runge and C. Patterson © Humana Press, Inc., Totowa, NJ

hormone whereas the majority is protein-bound to thyroxine-binding globulin (TBG), transthyretin (TTR), and albumin.

After uptake into peripheral cells, a process that is at least partially mediated by amino acid channels, T4 is either 5′-deiodinated by deiodinase I or II, a process that produces the more active T3, or it is modified into the inactive reverse triiododothyronine (rT3) by deiodination of the inner ring (*see* Fig. 35-3). At the cellular level, thyroid hormones have multiple effects on differentiation, growth, and metabolism. Thyroid hormone action is primarily mediated by nuclear receptors regulating gene transcription (Fig. 35-4). Albeit less well characterized, several nongenomic actions are a focus of growing interest. Negative regulation of the hypothalamic-pituitary-thyroid axis is exerted by T3, somatostatin and dopamine. At least in rodents, the transition from the fed to starved state is associated with a reduction in thyroid hormone levels, an adaptive response caused by a reduction in TRH and regulated by a decrease in leptin, a finding that emphasizes the intricate relationship between the thyroid axis and fuel homeostasis.

NORMAL DEVELOPMENT OF THE THYROID GLAND

The thyroid gland evolves from two distinct embryological structures. In humans, the thyroid *anlage* is first visible at embryonic day 20 (E20). It derives from the endodermal floor of the primitive pharynx and gives rise to thyroid follicular cells. These cells evolve into a diverticulum that expands caudally to form the thyroglossal duct. After rapid proliferation, they then expand laterally and by E30 the gland becomes bilobated. As the gland continues to descend and grow, the thyroglossal duct thins and elongates, eventually fragmenting and degenerating by E40. The ultimobranchial bodies, located in the fourth pharyngeal pouch, are of neural crest origin and, after undergoing a similar descent, differentiate into the parafollicular calcitonin-producing C cells. After migration and fusion of the two cell populations, thyroid follicular cells undergo further differentiation. This is marked by the expression of genes that are essential for thyroid hormone synthesis such as the TSH receptor, the sodium–iodide symporter (NIS), thyroperoxidase (TPO), and thyroglobulin (TG) (*see* Fig. 35-2). Thyroid hormone is detectable in the fetus at about gestational week 11.

OVERVIEW OF THYROID DISORDERS

Thyroid disorders can broadly be divided into disorders of function or growth. The two alterations may occur independently or in combination. For example, in patients with Graves' disease,

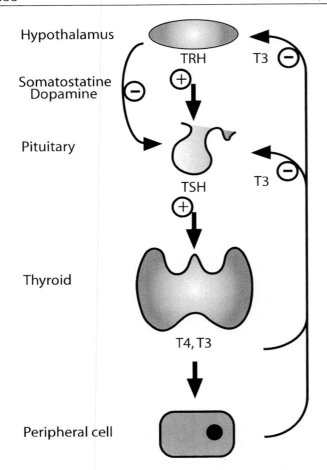

Figure 35-1 The hypothalamo-pituitary-thyroid axis. The hypothalamic thyrotropin-releasing hormone (TRH) enhances production and secretion of the pituitary hormone thyrotropin (TSH), which then stimulates thyroid hormone synthesis in follicular cells. Thyroid hormones act on multiple target genes in peripheral cells through nuclear receptors that regulate gene transcription. Triiododothyronine (T3) regulates TSH and TRH through a negative feedback mechanism. T4, thyroxine.

the thyroid is typically diffusely enlarged and secretes excessive amounts of thyroid hormone.

Disorders affecting thyroid function result either in hypothyroidism or in hyperthyroidism. Cardinal clinical characteristics are summarized in Table 35-1. Hypothyroidism is the most common disorder of thyroid function and most frequently caused by chronic autoimmune inflammation, Hashimoto's thyroiditis. The most frequent form of hyperthyroidism is Graves' disease, also an autoimmune disorder, followed by toxic multinodular goiters and toxic adenomas.

Congenital hypothyroidism affects approximately 1/3000–4000 infants. Screening programs introduced decades ago led to its early recognition and treatment, thus avoiding the disastrous consequences of thyroid hormone deficiency on brain development. In approximately 85% of all affected infants, congenital hypothyroidism is sporadic and associated with developmental defects referred to as thyroid dysgenesis. They include thyroid (hemi)agenesis, ectopic tissue and thyroid hypoplasia. Defects in one of the multiple steps required for normal hormone synthesis, dyshormonogenesis, account for approximately 10–15% of congenital hypothyroidism. Dyshormonogenesis is typically recessive and thus more common in families with consanguinity. Advances in molecular genetics led to

the characterization of numerous genes that are essential for normal development and hormone production of the hypothalamic-pituitary-thyroid axis. A wide spectrum of defects in these genes provide a molecular explanation for a subset of the sporadic and familial defects in pituitary and thyroid development, or TSH and thyroid hormone synthesis (Tables 35-2 to 35-4).

The transport of T4 is altered by a variety of defects in binding proteins (Table 35-5). Cellular uptake of thyroid hormones appears to be mediated by amino acid channels, and mutations in monocarboxylate transporter 8 (MCT8) lead to alterations in brain function and thyroid function tests (Table 35-6). Mutations in the nuclear thyroid hormone receptors (TR) may cause profound alterations in thyroid hormone action in the syndrome of resistance to thyroid hormones (RTH) (Table 35-7).

Abnormal growth of the thyroid may be associated with developmental malformations or hypoplasia, involutional changes associated with chronic inflammation, or goitrous enlargement. Goiters can be diffuse or nodular. The enlargement might be induced by chronic exogenous stimulation by TSH, for example because of iodine deficiency.

Worldwide, the most common cause of thyroid disorders is iodine deficiency. Insufficient iodine supply causes endemic goiter, the compensatory growth of the thyroid gland. If more severe, iodine deficiency can result in hypothyroidism and severe developmental retardation, endemic cretinism. Although eradicated in many parts of the world, iodine deficiency is still a major health problem affecting a substantial part of the world population.

Other causes for goitrous enlargement include stimulatory antibodies, or benign and malignant neoplasias. Benign thyroid nodules are common and found in >20% of individuals evaluated by ultrasonography. In contrast, thyroid cancers only account for approx 1% of malignancies. Although the molecular defects underlying the pathogenesis of thyroid nodules and adenomas as well as papillary, follicular, and anaplastic thyroid cancers are far from being completely understood, new insights have been obtained with the tools of molecular biology (Table 35-8). A majority of thyroid nodules are of monoclonal origin making somatic mutations in growth-controlling gene a likely cause for their development. Two large groups of genes have been implicated in uncontrolled cell proliferation and clonal expansion of mutated cells. Protooncogenes are activated through gain-of-function mutations in the regulatory or coding sequence thus creating the oncogene. This results in overexpression of the normal product or an abnormal form of the protein. Tumor suppressor genes control cell proliferation under normal conditions. Unrestrained growth of cells and thus formation of tumors can occur through loss-of-function of these genes. Among other important insights, the detection of certain molecular defects has modified diagnostic and therapeutic procedures. For example, mutations in the *RET* gene, which encodes the RET tyrosine kinase, are the molecular alterations found in medullary thyroid cancer (MTC) and the multiple endocrine neoplasia type 2 (MEN2) syndromes (Chapter 40). It is now possible to precisely detect carriers of the disease in early childhood and thus treat these patients accordingly.

This chapter gives an overview on the variety of defects affecting thyroid function and growth at all levels of the axis.

THYROTROPIN-RELEASING HORMONE DEFICIENCY

TRH is a hypothalamic tripeptide (Glu-His-Pro) generated from a large prohormone of 27 kDa. Besides its role as a stimulator

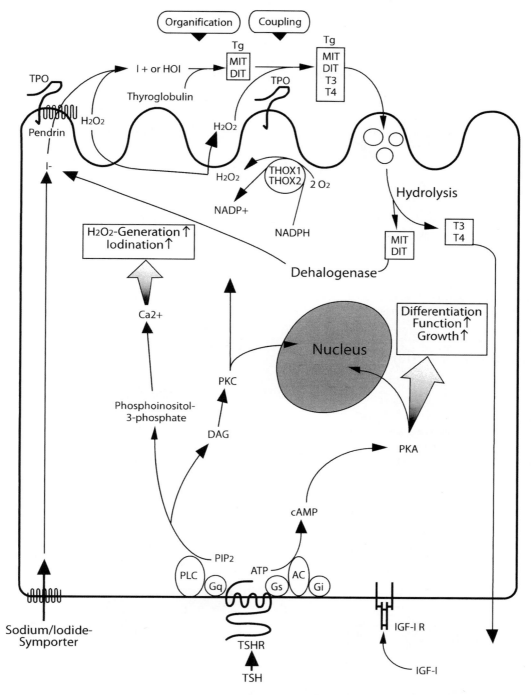

Figure 35-2 Thyroid hormone synthesis in a follicular cell. For details *see* text. AC, adenylyl cyclase; IGF-I, IGF-I R, insulin-like growth factor I (receptor); MIT, DIT, mono- and diiodotyrosine; PKA, protein kinase A; PKC, protein kinase C; PLC, phospholipase C; TG, thyroglobulin; TPO, thyroperoxidase.

of the pituitary gland in which it releases TSH and prolactin, TRH is a neurotransmitter in numerous areas of the brain and is also found in some peripheral organs.

A few patients with congenital hypothyroidism and isolated TRH deficiency without destructive hypothalamic lesions have been reported. The diagnosis of central hypothalamic hypothyroidism is made based on the constellation of low TSH and an increase thereof after administration of exogenous TRH. The molecular defect underlying these cases remains elusive and could affect synthesis or secretion of TRH. Targeted disruption of the TRH gene in mice led

to an overtly hypothyroid phenotype. Remarkably, the TSH levels were elevated in these mice but displayed diminished biological activity. Similar biochemical constellations with elevated TSH with reduced bioactivity have been found in some individuals with central hypothyroidism.

RESISTANCE TO TRH

Resistance to TRH in pituitary thyrotrophs was discovered in a boy with isolated central hypothyroidism. His T4 was decreased, the TSH was normal, and there was no increase of TSH and prolactin

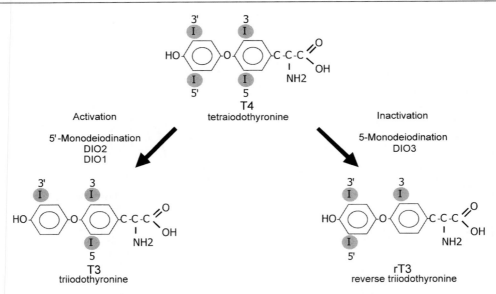

Figure 35-3 Structure of thyroxine (T4), triiododothyronine (T3) and reverse triiododothyronine (rT3). T4 is activated to T3 by deiodinase 1 and 2. T4 is inactivated into rT3 by deiodinase 3.

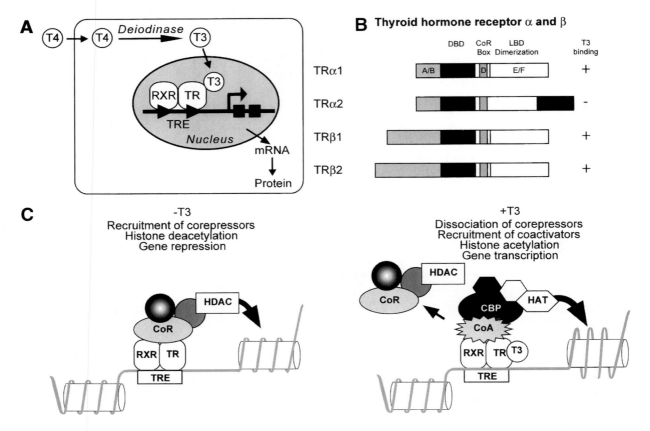

Figure 35-4 (**A**) Nuclear thyroid hormone action. Thyroxine (T4) enters the cell in which it is converted into triiododothyronine (T3) by 5′-monodeiodinases. In the nucleus, T3 interacts with thyroid hormone receptors. Thyroid hormone receptors bind to specific sequences, thyroid response elements (TRE) in the promoter regions of target genes in conjunction with other nuclear receptors such as the retinoid X receptor (RXR). (**B**) Schematic structure of the most abundant thyroid hormone receptor isoforms and their functional domains. The DNA binding domain consists of two zinc fingers. TRβ2 is most abundant in the pituitary gland in which it mediates negative regulation of thyrotropin (TSH). TRα2 does not bind T3; its exact physiological role is unknown. DBD, DNA binding domain; CoR box, interaction with corepressors; LBD, ligand binding domain; AF2, activation domain 2. (**C**) Model of thyroid hormone action on a positively regulated gene. In the absence of thyroid hormone, corepressors interact with thyroid hormone receptor homo- or heterodimers and silence transcription. Deacetylation of histones is associated with silenced transcription. Thyroid hormone relieves the interaction with corepressors and after binding of coactivators and factors of the basal transcription apparatus, gene expression is started, a process that involves chromatin remodeling through histone acetylation. RXR, retinoid X receptor; TR, thyroid hormone receptor; HDAC, histone deacetylase; CoR,Corepressor; CoA, Coactivator; CBP, CREB binding protein; HAT, histone acetyltransferase.

Table 35-1
Main Clinical and Biochemical Findings in Hyper- and Hypothyroidism

Hyperthyroidism	Hypothyroidism
Signs	
Hyperactivity	Lethargy
Tachycardia/Arrhythmia	Bradycardia
Hyperthermia	Cold intolerance
Increased perspiration	Dry skin
Hyperreflexia	Hyporeflexia
Muscle weakness	Myxedema
Tremor	Hoarseness
Weight loss	Weight gain
Eyelid retraction	
Exophthalmos (Graves' disease)	
Diffuse or nodular goiter	
Intrauterine/neonatal	
Mental retardation possible	Mental retardation
Advanced bone age	Neurological deficit
	Retarded bone age/growth
Symptoms	
Nervousness	Fatigue, sleepiness
Weakness	Depression
Palpitation	Constipation
Increased appetite	Decreased appetite
Irregular menses	Irregular menses
	Paresthesia
Laboratory	
(a) primary	
$T4 \Uparrow$, $T3 \Uparrow$, $TSH \Downarrow$	$T4 \Downarrow$, $T3 \Downarrow$, $TSH \Uparrow$
(b) central	
$T4 \Uparrow$, $T3 \Uparrow$, $TSH \Uparrow$	$T4 \Downarrow$, $T3 \Downarrow$, $TSH \Downarrow$

T3, triiododothyronine; T4, thyroxine; TSH, thyrotropin.

in response to TRH. Mutational analysis of the TRH receptor gene revealed compound heterozygous point mutations that inactivate the TRH receptor.

AUTONOMOUS PRODUCTION OF TSH

TSH is a heterodimeric glycoprotein hormone. It shares a common α-chain with the pituitary follicle-stimulating hormone (FSH) and luteinizing hormone (LH) as well as the placental hormone choriogonadotropin (CG). Each of these hormones has a unique β-chain. Two novel human glycoprotein hormone-like genes α2 (A2) and β5 (B5) have been cloned. The heterodimer formed by these subunits, referred to as thyrostimulin, activates the human TSH receptor, but not the LH and FSH receptors. Thyrostimulin is expressed in the pituitary and, given that TSH receptors are also found in a subset of anterior pituitary cells, it has been proposed that it may act as a paracrine hormone. Its physiological role and relevance remain, however, unresolved.

Hypersecretion of TSH by thyrotrope pituitary adenomas is a rare cause of hyperthyroidism. Biochemically, these patients are characterized by an inappropriate secretion of TSH and hyperthyroxinemia. Typically the secretion of free α subunit is excessive. Rarely, there is cosecretion of growth hormone. MRI and or CT-scan confirm the diagnosis. The molecular defect in the thyrotropes resulting in autonomous growth and function remains unclear. Clonal analysis using the X-inactivation technique in a very small number of tumors showed that they are of monoclonal origin suggesting that a somatic mutation or the loss of a tumor suppressor is at the onset of their development. Screening of several candidate genes (Gsα, Gqα, G11α, TRH receptor) in a small number of such tumors did not show alterations in these candidate genes. In a single TSHoma, a somatic mutation in the TRβ gene was identified (H435Y). This mutant TRβ has impaired T3 binding, and the T3-mediated negative regulation of the glycoprotein hormone α subunit and TSHβ genes is impaired suggesting that it may be responsible for the defect in negative regulation of TSH by thyroid hormone in the tumor.

Table 35-2
Hypothalamic and Pituitary Defects

Gene/protein	Phenotype	Molecular defect	Inheritance	Chromosome
TRH	Hypothalamic hypothyroidism	Unknown	AR	3q13.3-q21
TRH receptor	Pituitary hypothyroidism	Inactivating mutations	AR	8q23
	No increase of TSH and prolactin in response to TRH			
TSH	TSH-deficient hypothyroidism	Mutations in TSHβ-chain	AR	β-chain
	Prolactin increase to TRH			1p22
	TSH-secreting adenomas with hyperthyroidism	Unknown	Sporadic	
		TRβ mutation (1 case)		
POU1F1 (PIT1)	CPHD: GH, prolactin, TSH	Dominant negative or recessive mutations	AD, AR	3p11
PROP1	CPHD: GH, prolactin, TSH, LH, FSH, (ACTH)	Inactivating mutations	AR	5q
LHX3	CPHD: GH, prolactin, TSH, LH, FSH	Inactivating mutations	AR	9q34.3
	Rigid cervical spine			
LHX4	CPHD: GH, TSH, ACTH	Splice site mutation	AD	1q25
	Cerebellar and hindbrain defects	Haploinsufficiency?		
HESX1 (RPX)	CPHD with variable anterior pituitary hormone deficiencies	Homozygous or heterozygous point mutations	AR, AD	3p21.2-p21.1
	SOD			

ACTH, adrenocorticotropic hormone; AD, autosomal-dominant; AR, autosomal-recessive; CPHD, combined pituitary hormone deficiency; FSH, follicle-stimulating hormone; GH, growth hormone; LH, luteinizing hormone; SOD, septo-optic dysplasia; TRH, thyrotropin-releasing hormone; TSH, thyrotropin.

Table 35-3
Thyroid Hormone Synthesis Defects

Gene/protein	Phenotype	Molecular defect	Inheritance	Chromosome

TSH-receptor	Familial nonautoimmune hyperthyroidism
	Sporadic congenital nonautoimmune
	   hyperthyroidism
		Gain of function mutations in
		   extracellular and transmembrane
		   domain
			AD, Sporadic	14q31

	Toxic adenomas		SomaticAD	
	Hypersensitivity to hCG	Increased affinity for hCG		
	Euthyroid hyperthyrotropinemia Hypothyroidism	Partially or completely inactivating mutations	AR	
GNAS1/Gsα	Toxic adenoma	Somatic activating point mutations	Sporadic	20q.13.2
	McCune-Albright syndrome	Mosaicism for gain of function mutations	Sporadic	
	Pseudohypoparathyroidism Ia: Hypothyroidism, hypogonadism, AHO	Inactivating point mutations on maternal allele	AD	

NIS (SLC5A5)
   Sodium-iodide
   symporter
	Hypothyroidism with defective
	   iodide uptake
		Inactivating point mutations	AR	19p13.2-p12

Thyroperoxidase	Congenital hypothyroidism, goiter Iodide organification defect	Inactivating point mutations	AR	2p25

PDS (SLC26A4)	Pendred's syndrome:
	Sensoneurinal deafness,
	   goiter, partial organification defect
		Inactivating mutations,
		   small deletions
			AR	7q31

Thyroglobulin	Goiter with compensated or overt
	   hypothyroidism
	Classic endoplasmic reticulum storage
	   disease with retention of mutated protein
		Point mutations and splice
		   site mutations
			AR	8q24.2-q24.3

THOX2	Transient or permanent hypothyroidism Iodide organification defect because of deficient H_2O_2 generation	Monoallelic or biallelic mutations	Sporadic	15q15.3
Dehalogenase	Congenital hypothyroidism, goiter, loss of iodide through secretion of DIT, MIT	Point mutations	AR	6q25.1

AD, autosomal-dominant; AR, autosomal-recessive; DIT, diiodotyrosine, MIT, monoiodotyrosine; NIS, sodium-iodide symporter; TSH, thyrotropin.

Therapy consists in most cases in transsphenoidal removal of the pituitary adenoma. The somatostatin analog octreotide is useful in some patients unable to undergo surgery or with invasive tumors. Preoperatively, hyperthyroid patients should be controlled with thyreostatic drugs.

COMBINED PITUITARY HORMONE DEFICIENCY AND ISOLATED TSH DEFICIENCY

TSH deficiency may occur in the setting of panhypopituitarism, most commonly owing to a pituitary adenoma. Genetic defects in the development and function of the pituitary gland can result in various forms of combined pituitary hormone deficiency (CPHD) (Table 35-2). Patients with CPHD present with impaired production and secretion of one or several anterior pituitary hormones that may include TSH. Some patients also display midline malformations. Mutations in the TSHβ gene can result in isolated TSH deficiency. Therapy aims at substituting T4, and, if deficient, other hormones.

POU1F1 POU1F1 (traditionally referred to as PIT1) is a pituitary-specific transcription factor regulating the development of somatotropes, lactotropes, and thyrotropes as well as gene expression of growth hormone, prolactin and the β-subunit of TSH. It is a member of the POU family of transcription factors, an eponym that was created after the identification of the first three members of this group, Pit-1, Oct-1, and Unc-86. POU1F1 contains two

main functional domains, an activation domain and a DNA binding domain formed of a POU-specific and a homeodomain. The homeodomain is highly similar to the homeobox containing genes in Drosophila that control development of specific body segments, whereas the POU-domain is necessary for high affinity DNA binding. DNA sequences, which bind the transcription factor, are found in the promoters of the GH, prolactin, TSH-β, and POU1F1 genes. Several splice variants with variable activation domains have been reported and may define promoter specificity.

Mutations in the murine homolog Pit1 have been identified in the Snell and Jackson dwarf mice, which have deficiencies in GH, prolactin, and TSH. Patients with identical hormone deficiencies have mutations in the human homolog POU1F1. POU1F1 mutations can be inherited in an autosomal-dominant or -recessive manner. Recessive mutations alter the transactivation or DNA binding properties of the transcription factor. The dominant mutations bind to DNA, but impair transcription by the wild-type allele by altering dimerization and or interaction with other nuclear transcription factors.

A case of fetomaternal POU1F1 deficiency resulting from a heterozygous, dominant negative point mutation led to absolute fetal hypothyroidism in the fetus with dramatic delay in respiratory, cardiovascular, neurologic, and bone maturation. The absence of Pit-1 and the ensuing hypoprolactinemia in the mother resulted in puerperal alactogenesis. This case impressively illustrates the importance

Table 35-4
Developmental Defects

Gene/protein	Phenotype	Molecular defect	Inheritance	Chromosome
PAX8	Thyroid hypoplasia or ectopy Hypothyroidism	Point mutations (Haploinsufficiency?)	Sporadic AD	2q12-q14
TTF-1 (NKX2.1)	Mild hypothyroidism Respiratory distress Choreoathetosis Mental retardation	Chromosomal deletions and point mutations: Haploinsufficiency	Sporadic	14q13
TTF-2 (FOXE1)	Bamforth-Lazarus syndrome: Thyroid agenesis Cleft palate Choanal atresia Bifid epiglottis Spiky hair	Inactivating point mutations	AR	9q22

AD, autosomal-dominant; AR, autosomal-recessive; TTF, thyroid transcription factor.

Table 35-5
Binding Proteins Defects

Gene/protein	Phenotype	Molecular defect	Inheritance	Chromosome
TBG Thyroxine-binding globulin	Decreased total T4 levels, euthyroidism	Deletions, point mutations	X-linked recessive	Xq22.2
	Increased total T4 levels, euthyroidism	Gene amplification	Sporadic *de novo* germline mutations	
TTR Transthyretin	Hyperthyroxinemia Familial amyloidotic polyneuropathy	Point mutations	AD	18q11.2-q12.1
Albumin	Familial dysalbuminemic hyperthyroxinemia	Point mutations	AD	4q11-13
	Familial dysalbuminemic hypertriiodothyroninemia	Point mutations	AD	

AD, autosomal-dominant; T4, thyroxine.

Table 35-6
Other Genetic Defects Associated With Thyroid Dysfunction

Gene/protein	Phenotype	Molecular defect	Inheritance	Chromosome
MCT8 (SCL16A2)	Hemizygous males: Elevated T3 and TSH Severe mental retardation Spastic quadriplegia Rotary nystagmus Impaired gaze and hearing Heterozygous females: only thyroid function abnormalities	Deletions, point mutations	AR, sporadic	Xq13.2
Deiodinase 3	Consumptive hypothyroidism because of increased degradation of T4 and T3 in hemangiomas and other vascular tumors	Overexpression	Sporadic	14q32
KCNE3	Thyrotoxic periodic hypokalemic paralysis	Monoallelic point mutations	Sporadic?	11q13-q14

AR, autosomal-recessive; T3, triiododothyronine; T4, thyroxine; TSH, thyrotropin.

of POU1F1 in the control of different endocrine axes and the importance of prenatal thyroid hormone for fetal maturation.

PROP1 Characterization of the Ames dwarf mouse led to the cloning of the paired-like homeodomain factor Prop-1 (Prophet of pit1). PROP-1 is necessary for the expression of POU1F1 and is involved in ontogenesis, differentiation, and function of somatotropes, lactotropes, thyrotropes, and possibly gonadotropes. Inactivating mutations in the human *PROP-1* gene have been identified as a cause of an autosomal-recessive CPHD phenotype affecting these cell lineages. Of note, there is variability in the phenotypic expression among CPHD patients with PROP-1 mutations.

Table 35-7
Resistance to Thyroid Hormone

Gene/protein	Phenotype	Molecular defect	Inheritance	Chromosome
TRβ	Resistance to thyroid hormone. Goiter, variable degrees of hypo- and or hyperthyroidism	Heterozygous point mutations: Dominant negative activity of mutated allele One kindred with total deletion of coding region of TRβ locus	AD, sporadic AR	3p24.3
Unknown	Resistance to thyroid hormone without mutations in TRβ	Unknown	AD	unknown

AD, autosomal-dominant; AR, autosomal-recessive.

Table 35-8
Molecular Alterations in Benign and Malignant Thyroid Tumors

Gene	Chromosomal location	Lesion	Tumor
TSHR	14q31	Point mutations	Toxic adenoma Differentiated carcinoma
Gsα	20q13.2	Point mutations	Adenoma, toxic adenoma, differentiated carcinomas
B-RAF	7q34	Point mutations	PTC
RET/PTC	RET 10q11.2	Rearrangements RET/PTC1: paracentric inversion with H4 chromosome 10 RET/PTC2: reciprocal translocation with chromosome 17 with RIα PKA subunit RET/PTC3: intrachromosomal rearrangement with ELE1 gene	PTC
PAX8/PPARγ	PAX8 2q12-q14	Rearrangements t(2;3)(q13;p25)	FTC
RET	10q11.2	Point mutations	MEN, MTC
TRK	1q23-24	Intrachromosomal rearrangements	MNG, PTC
RAS	Hras 11p15.5 Kras 12p12.1 Nras 1p13.2	Point mutations	Adenoma, differentiated thyroid carcinoma
p53	17p13	Point mutations Deletion, Insertion	Differentiated carcinoma Anaplastic adenoma
Rb	13q14.1-14	mRNA variants	Differentiated carcinoma Anaplastic adenoma
p16 (MITS)	9p21	Deletion of coding region	Differentiated carcinomas cell lines
p21/WAF	6p21.2	Reduced expression	Differentiated and anaplastic carcinomas
MET	7q31	Overexpression	FTC
C-MYC	8q24.12-q24	Overexpression	Differentiated carcinoma
LOH	3p, 11q13 and multiple other loci	LOH	FTC
APC	5q21-q22	Autosomal-dominant inheritance with somatic second hit	PTC in Gardner syndrome
PTEN	10q23.31	Autosomal-dominant inheritance with somatic second hit	PTC in Cowden syndrome
PRKAR1A	17q23-q24	Autosomal-dominant inheritance with somatic second hit	FTC in Carney complex type 1

FTC, follicular thyroid carcinomas; LOH, loss of heterozygosity; PPAR, peroxisome proliferators-activated receptor; PTC, papillary thyroid carcinomas; Rb, retinoblastoma susceptibility gene.

LHX3 Recessive mutations in LHX3, a LIM homeodomain transcription factor, also cause CPHD of all anterior pituitary hormones with the exception of adrenocorticotrophic hormone. In addition, these patients have a rigid cervical spine and a limited ability to rotate the head. In Lhx3–/– mice, the primordium of the anterior pituitary is present, but with the exception of the corticotroph cells, there is no further growth and differentiation of the rostral part of the gland.

LHX4 Heterozygous mutations in the human LIM homeobox transcription factor LHX4 lead to an autosomal-dominant phenotype characterized by short stature, pituitary and cerebellar hindbrain defects, and abnormalities of the sella turcica.

HESX1 HESX1, also referred to as RPX, is a member of the paired-like class of homeobox transcription factors. Familial septo-optic dysplasia (SOD), a syndromic form of CPHD associated with optic nerve hypoplasia and agenesis of midline structures in the brain, can be caused by homozygous mutations in HESX1. A similar phenotype was observed in Hesx1–/– mice. Interestingly, a small proportion of the mice heterozygous for a Hesx1 null allele also had a milder form of SOD. This discovery prompted further screening of patients presenting with a wide spectrum of congenital pituitary dysfunctions. A subset of these patients was heterozygous for HESX1 mutations. Phenotypically, heterozygous HESX1 mutations result in various constellations of pituitary hormone deficiencies and the phenotype is variable among family members with the same mutation.

TSHβ MUTATIONS Congenital hypothyroidism caused by isolated hereditary TSH deficiency is a rare autosomal-recessive disease caused by mutations in the TSH β-chain. In these patients, TSH is unmeasurable or very low, and the administration of TRH does not result in a rise in serum TSH. The levels and the function of the other pituitary hormones are normal, including an adequate rise of prolactin in response to TRH. The first familial incidence was described in a Japanese family in two sisters with cretinism. Two other families from the same island were reported to harbor the same defect and it is thus likely that they originate from a common founder.

Several independently recurrent mutations have now been reported in 18 families that are, in part, of distinct ethnic origin. They include point mutations, frame shift mutations and a splice site mutation. The C105V/114X frameshift mutation destroys a disulfide bond essential for normal protein conformation and bioactivity, other mutations lead to disruption of heterodimer formation with the β-chain (e.g., G29R), and the reported splice site mutation results in skipping of exon 2.

AUTONOMOUS FUNCTION OF THE TSH RECEPTOR

TSH exerts its effects on thyroid follicular cells through the TSH receptor, a member of the G protein coupled seven transmembrane receptors. Together with the receptors for FSH and LH it forms a distinct subfamily defined by a large amino-terminal extracellular domain involved in binding of the hormone. The 744 amino acid receptor is encoded by a gene containing 10 exons and localized on chromosome 14q31. The TSH receptor is coupled to Gs and thus to the adenylyl cyclase cascade, which is the predominant signaling pathway for growth and function of the thyrocyte (*see* Fig. 35-2). It is, however, also coupled to Gq and activates the inositol phosphate pathway.

Mutations in several G protein coupled seven transmembrane receptors confer constitutive activation to these receptors, a mechanism characterizing an important pathophysiological entity. For example, they have been found in rhodopsin as a cause of retinitis pigmentosa, in the LH/CG receptor in male limited precocious puberty, and in the TSH receptor they cause hyperthyroidism. Point mutations in the Ca^{2+}-sensing receptor lead to autosomal-dominant hypocalcemia with hypercalcuric hypocalcemia, and in the parathyroid hormone receptor to metaphyseal chondrodysplasia.

ACTIVATING SOMATIC TSH RECEPTOR MUTATIONS IN TOXIC ADENOMAS AND THYROID CARCINOMAS

Somatic mutations in the TSH receptor are the main molecular cause of toxic adenomas. Functionally, these mutations increase basal cAMP levels; some of the mutants also activate the phospholipase C cascade. In contrast to activating mutations in other seven transmembrane receptors, there is a striking diversity in the affected residues that are scattered over almost the entire transmembrane domain of the TSH receptor.

Activating mutations in the TSH receptor have also been found in a small number of thyroid carcinomas with the unusual finding of increased hormone secretion. Remarkably, the mutations found in these tumors activate the cAMP cascade as well as the inositol triphosphate pathway. This supports the concept that concomitant activation of these two signaling cascades may promote transformation.

ACTIVATING GERMLINE TSH RECEPTOR MUTATIONS IN FAMILIAL NONAUTOIMMUNE HYPERTHYROIDISM

Activating mutations occurring in the germline give rise to familial nonautoimmune hyperthyroidism. Gain of function mutations are by definition dominant and one mutated allele is thus sufficient to result in disease. The subsequent activation of the adenylyl cyclase pathway increases function and growth of thyroid follicular cells resulting in hyperplasia and hyperthyroidism. The typical signs associated with autoimmune hyperthyroidism, i.e., exophthalmos, myxedema, stimulating autoantibodies, and lymphocytic infiltration of the thyroid gland are absent. Several families with nonautoimmune familial hyperthyroidism and documented TSH receptor mutation have been reported. The onset of hyperthyroidism may vary in carriers of the same mutation in a given kindred, suggesting that other factors such as genetic background and or iodine intake are modulating the phenotypic expression of the activated receptor.

ACTIVATING GERMLINE TSH RECEPTOR MUTATIONS IN NEONATAL NONAUTOIMMUNE HYPERTHYROIDISM

Congenital hyperthyroidism is usually caused by transplacental transfer of maternal antibodies in offspring of a mother with autoimmune thyroid disease. In this instance, the disease is transient and resolves within several weeks to months on clearance of the antibodies. However, a few cases show a persistent course with severe hyperthyroidism. *De novo* germline mutations in the TSH receptor have been found as cause of this unusual form of hyperthyroidism. The recognition of this entity of hyperthyroidism has clinical implications. In certain patients a more aggressive therapeutic approach (surgery, ablative radiotherapy) is indicated and, in families with nonautoimmune hyperthyroidism, molecular diagnostics allow an early diagnosis and treatment.

TSH RECEPTOR MUTATIONS CONFERRING HYPERSENSITIVITY TO HUMAN CHORIONIC GONADOTROPIN

A remarkable form of familial gestational hyperthyroidism is caused by a mutant TSH receptor displaying hypersensitivity to normal levels of human chorionic gonadotropin (hCG). The proband and her mother had a history of two miscarriages that were accompanied by hyperemesis. Subsequently, she had two pregnancies that were complicated by hyperthyroidism, severe nausea and vomiting. Analysis of the TSH receptor gene in the proband and her mother revealed a heterozygous point mutation resulting in the substitution of K183R in the extracellular domain of the TSH receptor. Functional studies in cells transfected with the mutated receptor documented hypersensitivity to hCG. Although the wild-type TSH receptor reacts only minimally to high doses of hCG, the K183R mutant is hypersensitive to hCG, although it is still 1000 times less responsive to hCG than the LH/CG receptor. The K183R mutant does not differ from the wild-type in terms of membrane expression, or basal and TSH stimulated cAMP accumulation. Aside from explaining the recurrent hyperthyroidism in these two patients, the K183R TSH receptor mutation is unique because the sensitivity is only increased for hCG but remains unaltered for the cognate ligand TSH. Reduction of ligand specificity by naturally occurring mutations is not limited to the TSH receptor. Heterozygous mutations in the FSH receptor permitting stimulation by hCG have been identified in women with pregnancy-associated ovarian hyperstimulation syndrome.

INSENSITIVITY TO TSH AND INACTIVATING MUTATIONS OF THE TSH RECEPTOR

TSH insensitivity results in a decrease in function and thus reduced synthesis and secretion of thyroid hormones and hypoplasia of the gland. Resistance to TSH may be caused by various molecular mechanisms, among them inactivating mutations in the TSH receptor that are partially or completely inactivating. The mode of inheritance is recessive and affected individuals are homozygous or compound heterozygous for inactivating mutations. Among these patients the phenotype encompasses a wide spectrum ranging from isolated TSH elevation to severe hypothyroidism, and there is a clear correlation between genotype and phenotype.

The first human case with TSH resistance resulting from a defect in the TSH receptor was documented in three sisters, offspring of unrelated parents, who were found to have normal peripheral thyroid hormone but high TSH levels, a constellation referred to as *euthyroid hyperthyrotropinemia*. Both parents only showed discrete TSH elevations. None of the family members had clinical signs of hypothyroidism. The three affected siblings were found to be compound heterozygous for mutations in the extracellular TSH-binding domain of the receptor (P162A and I167N). In vitro studies documented that the I167N mutation had almost no biological activity, whereas P162A displayed reduced activity. Euthyroid hyperthyrotropinemia resulting from mutations in the TSH receptor gene has subsequently been reported in several other families. More pronounced or complete inactivation of both TSH receptor alleles leads to mild or severe congenital hypothyroidism. Because of absent uptake of the radioisotope, scintigraphic studies often do not reveal any thyroid tissue. However, ultrasound of the neck reveals a normally located hypoplastic gland. Intriguingly, many of these patients have normal or elevated TG levels.

A loss of function mutation in the TSH receptor gene as a cause of TSH resistance was also discovered in the thoroughly studied hypothyroid *hyt/hyt* mouse. The phenotype of this inbred mouse strain is defined by congenital hypothyroidism, retarded growth, mild anemia, hearing loss, and infertility. The hypoplastic thyroids of these mutant mice are located in the proper position. Histologically, the thyroid follicular cells are developed, but incompletely differentiated, and the epithelial cells are not organized into structures recognizable as follicles.

The *hyt/hyt* mouse and patients with TSH-resistant congenital hypothyroidism with correctly located hypoplastic glands confirm that development and migration of the thyroid is independent of TSH stimulation. This is consistent with the observation that the genes for TPO, TG, and the TSH receptor are only expressed once the gland has reached its pretracheal location. Although early events of thyroid development are not dependent on TSH and its signaling pathway, this cascade is essential for complete differentiation, growth and function of thyroid follicular cells. These findings have

been corroborated in the TSH receptor knock-out mouse, or mice overexpressing a dominant negative cAMP response element binding protein (CREB) in the thyroid. These studies exemplify how careful phenotyping of several naturally occurring mutants and genetically modified mice provide fundamental insights into the molecular mechanisms controlling organogenesis, differentiation and function in vivo.

In other patients with sporadic or familial resistance to TSH, the TSH receptor gene was normal indicating locus heterogeneity owing to defects in other genes. Obvious candidate genes include genes encoding elements of the TSH-dependent signaling cascades or regulators of thyroid development and gene expression.

ACTIVATING AND INACTIVATING MUTATIONS IN GSA

Analogous to the mutations in the TSH receptor, gain of function mutations in the *GNAS1* gene encoding the α subunit of the stimulatory G protein (gsp mutations) lead to a constitutive activation of the cAMP pathway and subsequently to an increase of function and growth of cell types like the pituitary somatotropes or thyroid follicular cells.

In the thyroid, somatic gsp mutations have been found with variable frequencies in nontoxic and toxic adenomas, as well as in differentiated thyroid carcinomas. The most commonly affected amino acids are arginine 201 and glutamine 227. The ensuing substitutions (R201C or R201H; Q227R or Q227K) impair the hydrolysis of GTP to GDP, resulting in an ongoing activation of adenylyl cyclase. The same molecular defect is found as somatic mutation in 35–40% of somatotrope tumors in acromegalic patients.

Sporadic mutations in Gsα that occur early in development lead to the McCune-Albright syndrome. These patients are mosaic for the mutation and the clinical phenotype varies depending on its tissue distribution. The clinical manifestations include ovarian cysts that secrete sex steroids and cause precocious puberty, polyostotic fibrous dysplasia, café au lait skin pigmentation, GH-secreting pituitary adenomas, and hypersecreting autonomous thyroid nodules.

In pseudohypoparathyroidism type Ia, the affected subjects show resistance not only to parathyroid hormone, but also to TSH and gonadotropins, in combination with the features of Albright's hereditary osteodystrophy. The molecular cause is a reduction of expression of the stimulatory Gsα subunit by a variety of loss of function mutations. The disorder affects many cell types with the cardinal signs being stunted growth, obesity, skeletal abnormalities, and hypogonadism. At the level of the thyroid, it is typically associated with mild hypothyroidism. The GNAS1 gene is imprinted in a tissue-specific manner. Most tissues express both alleles, but the paternal allele is imprinted and thus inactivated in tissues displaying hormone resistance. In pseudohypoparathyroidism type Ia, the mutation disrupts the active maternal allele that subsequently results in a decrease in signaling and partial hormone resistance to the trophic hormone in tissues such as the proximal renal tubule, the thyroid and the gonads.

DEFECTIVE THYROID HORMONE SYNTHESIS

The major steps involved in thyroid hormone synthesis are summarized in Fig. 35-2. After active transport of iodide into the thyroid follicular cell by the NIS, iodide is brought to the apical pole of the cells oriented toward the follicular lumen. At the apical membrane, pendrin, probably in conjunction with one or several other unidentified channels, is involved in transport of iodide into the follicular lumen. TG is secreted by exocytosis into the follicular lumen. TPO, localized in the apical membrane, oxidizes iodide, and subsequently iodinates tyrosyl residues of the intrafollicular TG (organification or iodination) in the presence of hydrogen peroxide. Two elements of the NADPH-dependent H_2O_2-generating, system, THOX1, and THOX2, have been been identified. The iodotyrosines, mono- and diiodotyrosyl (MIT, DIT), are coupled to T4 or T3, a reaction that is also catalyzed by TPO (coupling). TG carrying T4, T3, and iodotyrosines is internalized into the follicular cell by fluid phase or receptor-mediated endocytosis and digested in lysosomes. Although the thyronines T4 and T3 are released into the bloodstream, MIT, and DIT are deiodinated by dehalogenase in the cell and the released iodide is recycled. A dehalogenase referred to as DEHAL1 has been cloned very recently. In patients with congenital hypothyroidism, defects have been identified at all major steps involved in hormonogenesis (Table 35-3).

DEFECTS OF IODIDE TRANSPORT   Normal iodide uptake at the basolateral membrane by the perchlorate-sensitive NIS is a rate-limiting step in thyroid hormone synthesis (*see* Fig. 35-2). Following the cloning of the *NIS* gene, several homozygous, or compound heterozygous mutations have been identified in individuals with hypothyroidism with iodine trapping defects. Most patients with iodide trapping defects have a diffuse or nodular goiter, little or no uptake of radioiodide, and a decreased saliva/serum radioiodine ratio. In children, the thyroid might be initially of normal size and often enlarges later in life.

The precise molecular mechanisms by which NIS mutations directly cause iodide transport defects have been identified in a subset of cases. The T354P mutation, an alteration found in several patients from Japan, causes NIS to lose its functional ability to transport iodide. In contrast, the functional defects of two other NIS mutations (Q267E, S515X) are the consequence of defective cellular trafficking and failure of the mutant proteins to reach the plasma membrane.

THYROPEROXIDASE   TPO is a glycosylated hemoprotein that catalyzes several essential reactions of thyroid hormone synthesis: oxidation of iodide, the iodination of tyrosine residues in TG and the coupling of iodinated tyrosines to generate T4 and T3 (*see* Fig. 35-2). TPO is the protein historically referred to as microsomal antigen in autoimmune thyroid disease. It is anchored in the membrane and has its catalytic site in the follicular lumen. The enzyme is closely related to myeloperoxidase and it is thought that they share a common ancestor; their chromosomal localizations are, however, distinct.

TPO defects are among the most frequent causes of inborn abnormalities of thyroid hormone synthesis. Because of the defective organification of iodide, these patients typically have a significant discharge of radioiodine after the administration of perchlorate. Mutations in the *TPO* gene have been reported in numerous families with a partial or total iodide organification defect. The overall incidence of congenital hypothyroidism is on average 1/3000, total iodide organification defect is thought to occur in approximately 1/66,000 of all infants with congenital hypothyroidism and almost all of these patients have homozygous or compound heterozygous mutations in the *TPO* gene.

PENDRED SYNDROME   Pendred syndrome is an autosomal-recessive disorder characterized by sensorineural deafness, goiter, and a positive perchlorate test. This disorder represents one of the most common forms of syndromic deafness, with an incidence estimated at 7.5–10/100,000 individuals. Although the classic presentation of the syndrome consists of the triad of deafness, goiter, and partial organification defect, the phenotypic expression of these components is

highly variable among families and even within the same family. Sensorineural hearing loss, in most instances profound prelingual deafness, is the hallmark of Pendred syndrome. More rarely, the hearing impairment manifests itself later in life as a progressive hearing loss. High resolution MRI of the inner ear reveals malformations of the vestibular aqueduct, endolymphatic duct, and endolymphatic sac in nearly 100% of individuals with a clinical diagnosis of Pendred syndrome. Goiter is the most variable component of the disorder, with some individuals developing very large goiters, whereas others present with minimal to no enlargement. Although many patients with Pendred syndrome are euthyroid, others have subclinical or overt hypothyroidism.

Pendred syndrome is caused by mutations in the *PDS* gene, now officially designated *SLC26A4*. It encodes pendrin, a member of the solute carrier family 26A, which contains several anion transporters and the motor protein prestin. Pendrin is predominantly expressed in the thyroid, inner ear, and the kidney. In thyroid follicular cells, pendrin is inserted into the apical membrane and functional studies suggest that it is involved in apical iodide efflux from thyrocytes. These observations are consistent with the clinical phenotype, which is characterized by impaired iodide organification. In the kidney, pendrin is thought to act as a chloride-bicarbonate exchanger in β-intercalated cells of the cortical collecting duct, a subpopulation of cells that mediate bicarbonate secretion. The critical role of pendrin in the inner ear has been corroborated by targeted disruption of the *Pds* gene in mice. *Pds*–/– mice develop early onset deafness and exhibit signs of vestibular dysfunction. In line with the enlargement of the endolymphatic system observed in human patients, analysis of the inner ear in these mice reveals dilated endolymphatic ducts and sacs beyond E15, presumably as a consequence of defects in anion and fluid transport.

During the last few years, more than 95 *PDS* gene mutations have been described, indicating marked allelic heterogeneity. The majority of *PDS* mutations are missense mutations and some of these mutants appear to be retained in the endoplasmic reticulum. A smaller number of mutations result in premature truncations or in alterations of splice donor or acceptor sites. Individuals with Pendred syndrome from consanguineous families are homozygous for *PDS* mutations, whereas sporadic cases typically harbor compound heterozygous mutations. Mutations in the *PDS* gene are not only found in patients with classic Pendred Syndrome, but also in individuals afflicted with familial enlarged vestibular aqueduct. The diagnosis of Pendred syndrome based on the clinical findings of deafness and goiter is not sufficient; it requires confirmation by imaging studies of the inner ear or/and molecular analysis of the *PDS* gene.

HYDROGEN PEROXIDE GENERATION H_2O_2 is an essential factor in the iodination and coupling reactions. Although the ability of follicular cells to produce H_2O_2 has been known for more than three decades, the enzyme system remains only partially characterized. Two NADPH oxidases, THOX1 and THOX2 (also called LNOX or DUOX) that are part of this system have been cloned. Structurally, these proteins contain seven putative transmembrane domains, four NADPH binding sites, 1 FAD binding site, and in line with the predicted regulation by calcium, an everted finger motif.

Heterozygous loss of function mutations in the *THOX2* gene result in mild transient congenital hypothyroidism. Biallelic THOX2 mutations are associated with a severe phenotype and confirm that H_2O_2 is essential for iodide organification. There are no reported mutations in THOX1.

Deficient H_2O_2 generation has been proposed to explain the phenotype in a few sporadic patients with euthyroid goiter and abnormal iodide organification, and a family with two siblings presenting with hypothyroidism, goiter, and an iodide organification defect. The molecular defect in these patients remains unknown.

THYROGLOBULIN   TG is produced by thyroid follicular cells and secreted into the follicular lumen. Some of its tyrosine residues are iodinated by TPO (organification/iodination), and the tyrosines MIT and DIT are subsequently coupled to form T3 and T4 (coupling). TG is therefore considered to be a thyroid hormone precursor. Besides its importance for hormone synthesis, it allows storage of iodine and thyroid hormone and thus to adapt to scarce iodine supply.

The monomer of TG is made up of a 19-amino acid signal peptide followed by 2749 residues containing 66 tyrosines. TG contains an average number of tyrosine residues, altogether 67, but only a minority of these residues localized in the carboxy- and amino-terminus are hormonogenic sites. Complete hydrolysis of iodinated TG yields only two to four molecules of the iodothyroxines T4 and T3. The mature protein is formed by two units in noncovalent linkage (19 S TG). Of the total weight, 10% are formed by carbohydrates, and glycosylation plays an important role in the structure of the protein. The TG monomer contains 20 glycosylation sites and extensive microheterogeneity has been reported in their use. The primary structure of the TG protein contains three regions with repetitive sequences with internal homology, and the carboxy-terminal part shares remarkable homology with acetylcholinesterase. This structure suggests the possibility of a convergent origin of the *TG* gene from two different ancestral DNA sequences.

The human *TG* gene is large, spans approximately 270 kb and contains 48 exons. The transcription of the *TG* gene is controlled by transcription factors such as thyroid transcription factor (TTF)-1 (NKX2.1), TTF-2 (FOXE1), and PAX 8. The full-length 8.5 kB mRNA sequence shows a 41-nucleotide 5′-untranslated segment preceding an open reading frame of 8307 bases and a 3′-untranslated segment ranging from 101 to 120 bp. There are numerous alternatively spliced RNA transcripts and the gene contains multiple polymorphisms, some of them silent, others with impact on the primary amino acid sequence.

Defects of TG synthesis or secretion have been studied in several animal strains and human patients. TG gene defects are inherited in an autosomal-recessive manner. The phenotype is typically characterized by goitrous enlargement of the thyroid. The metabolic status is variable and, depending on the severity of the defect, patients are hypothyroid, subclinically hypothyroid, or euthyroid. Unless treated with levothyroxine, goiters are often remarkably large and display continuous growth. Symptoms can result from compression of adjacent neck structures. The radioiodine uptake is elevated indicating an activation of the iodine concentration mechanism, because of chronic stimulation of TSH. In patients evaluated with a perchlorate discharge test, there is no increased release of radioiodine after administration of the competitor, indicating that the organification process itself is not affected. Serum TG levels can vary from low to low normal, and the presence of an abnormal TG level in a goitrous individual may suggest a defective TG synthesis. An abnormal TG synthesis may also be suggested by the presence of abnormal iodoproteins in the serum. Because there is no normal intrathyroidal TG, albumin as well as other proteins are iodinated, generating iodotyrosines and iodohistidines. This is, however, an unspecific sign and also found in endemic and sporadic goiters and thyroids affected by autoimmune Hashimoto's thyroiditis. Increased secretion of low-molecular weight iodinated material (>5%) in the

urine may also be helpful in establishing the diagnosis. Histological analysis often demonstrates scarce colloid, large follicular lumina, and cuboidal epithelial cells. In instances with-impaired TG export, TG-immunopositivity is found predominantly inside the cytoplasm. Although it is possible to diagnose TG defects at the molecular level, this is not a trivial task considering the large size of the gene; thus the data on molecular alterations are still relatively scarce. Further studies of patients with TG abnormalities may reveal a more detailed understanding of the structure-function relationship of TG.

The first models with abnormal TG to be studied in detail at the molecular level were the Afrikaander cattle and the Dutch goat. The Afrikaander cattle is characterized by large goiters and an euthyroid metabolic status. A recessive point mutation in exon 9 leads to a premature stop. Interestingly, alternative splicing allows rescuing the transcription to some degree by producing a misspliced 7.3-kb message missing exon 9, a mechanism referred to as *exon skipping*. The original reading frame is maintained in this transcript and it is translated into a functional protein missing the part encoded by exon 9. Both transcripts are, however, only present at low levels. The Dutch goat is goitrous as well and, provided that iodine intake is high, euthyroidism can be maintained. A nonsense mutation (Y296X) in exon 8 results in a truncated protein. The fact that the animal may remain euthyroid despite this truncation is indirect evidence that the amino-terminal part contains a major hormonogenic site.

Molecular analysis of several TG point mutations found in patients with congenital hypothyroidism and in the *cog/cog* mouse, which all present with goiters, reveal that at least some of these alterations result in a secretory defect and thus an endoplasmic reticulum storage disease. In contrast to these TG defects associated with goiter development, the recessive dwarf *rdw/rdw* rat displays a nongoitrous form of congenital primary hypothyroidism caused by a *Tg* gene mutation. The identification of a mutation in the *Tg* gene as a cause of nongoitrous hypothyroidism in the *rdw/rdw* rat challenges the previously held generalization that nongoitrous congenital hypothyroidism is caused by thyroid dysgenesis or defects in TSH-signaling.

It has been proposed that TG mutations may be associated with nonendemic simple goiter. These results await, however, further confirmation; the TG gene contains multiple polymorphisms, and in the absence of functional data it remains unclear whether these reported alterations are causally involved in the abnormal phenotype.

DEHALOGENASE DEFECT   After entering the follicular cell, TG is hydrolyzed and T4 and T3 are secreted into the blood (*see* Fig. 35-2). The iodotyrosines, MIT and DIT, which are much more abundant in the TG molecule than in T4 and T3, are deiodinated by an intrathyroidal dehalogenase and recycled for hormone synthesis. An intrathyroidal dehalogenase referred to as DEHAL1, which may exert this function, has been cloned. Very recently, mutations in *DEHAL1* have been reported in patients with a dehalogenase defect. In case of a defective dehalogenase system, MIT and DIT leak into the circulation and are excreted in the urine. This leads, especially if iodine is scarce, to a severe iodine loss and thus to hypothyroidism and goiter. Very recently, mutations in *DEHAL1* have been reported in patients with a dehalogenase defect.

Clinically, patients with a deiodinase defect present with congenital hypothyroidism and a goitrous gland. The diagnosis is established by administration of radiolabeled DIT. Normally, DIT will be deiodinated, whereas in the case of a defective dehalogenase, the majority will be secreted unaltered as DIT in the urine.

Furthermore, administration of iodide in sufficient amounts to compensate for the increased loss will reestablish a euthyroid metabolic state. The disorder is inherited in an autosomal-recessive fashion. Although only homozygotes are clinically affected, biochemical testing in heterozygotes demonstrates an increased secretion of labeled DIT in the urine. The clinical and biochemical phenotype of several kindreds have been studied in detail. The classic report traces the family history of an inbred kindred originating from the marriage of first cousins through 160 yr.

DEVELOPMENTAL THYROID DEFECTS ASSOCIATED WITH MUTATIONS IN TRANSCRIPTION FACTORS

In approximately 85% of all affected infants, congenital hypothyroidism is sporadic and associated with developmental defects referred to as thyroid dysgenesis. They include thyroid (hemi)agenesis, ectopic tissue, and thyroid hypoplasia.

Molecular defects only explain a minority of cases of thyroid dysgenesis (Table 35-4). It is likely that a further subset of patients with thyroid dysgenesis have defects in other transacting proteins or elements of the signaling pathways controlling growth and function. In other instances, thyroid dysgenesis might be a polygenic disease or have a multifactorial basis. With further characterization of the molecular basis of congenital hypothyroidism, genetic testing, and counseling may become increasingly important in the future.

PAX8

PAX8 is a paired domain thyroid-specific transcription factor responsible for thyroid development and for *TG* and *TPO* gene expression. PAX8 binds predominantly to the TPO promoter and with less affinity to the TG promoter.

Heterozygous mutations in PAX8 have been documented and characterized in sporadic and familial patients with thyroid hypoplasia or ectopy.

In humans, the biochemical and morphological phenotype may vary among patients with the same PAX8 mutation. Underlying mechanisms may include incomplete penetrance, a phenomenon associated with mutations in other *PAX* genes. Alternatively, the phenotypic expression might be modulated by modifier genes.

It is unclear why mutation of a single PAX8 allele is sufficient to result in congenital hypothyroidism in humans, a finding that contrasts with the observation that mice heterozygous for a disrupted *Pax8* gene do not display a pathological phenotype. Proposed mechanisms explaining that one mutated allele is sufficient to cause disease in humans include haploinsufficiency, allele-specific expression in the thyroid and, less likely, a dominant negative effect.

THYROID TRANSCRIPTION FACTOR-1 (TTF-1, NKX2.1) TTF-1 (NKX2.1, TITF-1, or thyroid specific enhancer-binding protein T/ebp), is a homeobox domain transcription factor of the NKX2 family involved in the development of the gland and in transcriptional control of the *TG, TPO,* and *TSH receptor* genes. It is expressed in the lung, forebrain, pituitary gland, and the thyroid. In the lung, TTF1 activates transcription of surfactant protein B.

Mice with targeted disruption of both *TTF1* alleles survive throughout gestation, but die at birth from respiratory failure. The lung is severely hypoplastic and consists of a sac-like structure without bronchioli, alveoli, or lung parenchyma. Both the thyroid gland and pituitary gland are completely absent, and the hypothalamus is severely malformed.

The observation of a newborn with severe respiratory distress, a normally located thyroid gland, elevated TSH levels and a het-erozygous deletion on chromosome 14q13 encompassing the *TTF1* locus suggested that haploinsufficiency for TTF1 could be associated with impaired lung maturation and thyroid function. Haploinsufficiency, i.e., inability of a single functional allele to maintain normal function, is a frequently observed pathogenetic mechanism associated with mutations in transcription factors. The detection of a similar heterozygous deletion of chromosome 14q12-13.3 in two female siblings with congenital thyroid dysfunction and recurrent acute respiratory distress gave further support to this concept. A few additional patients with hyperthyrotropinemia, neonatal respiratory distress, and ataxia associated with missense or frameshift mutations, or chromosomal deletions of the TTF-1 gene have been reported. The TSH levels were only mildly elevated and the thyroid was normal in size and position. The hallmark of this phenotype is the neurological deficit, which includes ataxia or choreoathetosis, truncal apraxia, and mental retardation, in combination with neonatal respiratory distress. Heterozygous TTF-1 mutations have also been identified as the molecular cause of hereditary chorea.

THYROID TRANSCRIPTION FACTOR-2 (TTF-2, FOXE1) TTF-2, official designation FOXE1, is a forkhead/winged-helix domain transcription factor activating the *TG* and the *TPO* gene promoters. Homozygosity for recessive mutations in TTF-2 results in a syndromic form of thyroid dysgenesis with the eponym Bamforth-Lazarus syndrome. This phenotype, first described in two brothers from a consanguineous family, includes thyroid agenesis, cleft palate, choanal atresia, bifid epiglottis, and spiky hair. Mice homozygous for a disrupted *Ttf2* gene die shortly after birth, and are profoundly hypothyroid. They exhibit either small lingual thyroid remnants or have complete thyroid agenesis, findings that support the important role of TTF-2 in thyroid development, and they also have cleft palates.

SERUM BINDING PROTEIN DEFECTS

Thyroid hormones circulate bound to plasma proteins, the three major proteins being TBG, TTR (formerly referred to as T4-binding prealbumin) and albumin. To a minor degree, α and β lipoproteins bind T4. Under physiological conditions, only 0.03% of T4 and 0.3% of T3 circulate as free hormone.

Abnormalities in transport proteins lead to a decrease or increase in total T4 or T3 levels; free hormone levels are within the normal range and patients are clinically euthyroid (Table 35-5). Failure to recognize these entities results in inappropriate treatment aimed at normalizing the thyroid hormone levels. TTR variants are of clinical importance because they are associated with various forms of amyloidosis.

THYROXIN-BINDING GLOBULIN TBG is an acidic glycoprotein with a single binding site for T4 or T3. The TBG concentration is low (1–2 mg/dL), but the protein has a high affinity for thyroid hormones (T4 > T3) and it carries approx 75–80% of the bound thyroid hormones. The mature protein contains 395 amino acids with four heterosaccharide chains with 5–9 sialic acids. Like corticosteroid-binding globulin it shows a high homology with the proteases α_1-antichymotrypsin and α_1-antitrypsin and it is a member of the serine protease inhibitor (serpin) family of proteins, although it is not a protease inhibitor. The carbohydrates play a minor role in T4 binding, but loss of carbohydrates decreases its stability and elevates the hepatic clearance rate. An increase in sialylation, for example, induced by estrogens, lowers the hepatic clearance and thus increases the TBG levels. Multiple other drugs increase or decrease TBG concentrations either by alteration of the synthesis rate and or the degree of sialylation. The single copy gene encoding TBG is localized on the X-chromosome (Xq11-q23).

TBG abnormalities are classified according to the levels of TBG into complete or partial deficiencies or TBG excess. Besides their biochemical classification, several TBG variants have been characterized at the molecular level. Complete TBG-deficiency is defined as absence of TBG in the serum of hemizygous (XY) individuals. The heterozygote females in these kindreds have TBG levels of about half the normal amount because random X-inactivation results on average in a 50% reduction of the protein. The prevalence of complete deficiency has been estimated at 1/15,000. Partial deficiency is the most common form of TBG deficiency. In white and mixed populations it is found with a frequency of 1/4000, roughly 50% of Australian Aborigines have an abnormal TBG (TBG-A), and a TBG migrating slowly on electrophoresis (TBG-S) is found in African and Pacific Islands populations. Some of these TBG-variants have a reduced affinity for T4 (TBG-A, TBG San Diego). In some variants, an accelerated rate of degradation is responsible for their low serum concentration. The identified mutations in the *TBG* gene that result in complete or partial deficiency consist of point mutations, deletions, frameshift mutations, and splice site mutations.

TBG excess is not as frequent as TBG deficiency with an incidence of approximately 1 in 25,000 births. TBG and T4 levels are elevated three- to fivefold in hemizygotes and two- to threefold in heterozygote females. The TBG increase is explained by overexpression of the protein because of gene amplification.

TRANSTHYRETIN   TTR is a homotetramer formed of subunits containing 127 amino acids and two T4 binding sites. Negative cooperativity allows only one site to be occupied at a given time. TTR has a substantially lower affinity for T4, but it is present in higher amounts than TBG (approx 25 mg/dL). TTR also binds retinol-binding protein and takes part in the transport of vitamin A. Binding of retinol does not influence T4 transport. The TTR gene contains four exons and is localized on chromosome 18. TTR is predominantly synthesized in the liver, but also in the plexus chorioideus. Although the exact role of TTR in the brain is not known, it has been postulated that T4 binds to TTR in the epithelial cells of the plexus chorioideus, is then secreted into the cerebrospinal fluid and subsequently distributed in the brain. More than 80 disease-causing mutations in TTR have been reported. Their impact on T4 affinity varies and may result in unchanged, increased or reduced affinity. Many of the point mutations have been related to distinct forms of amyloidosis. The inheritance is autosomal-dominant in most instances. Although the clinical manifestations vary, most have polyneuropathy, thus the eponym familial amyloidotic polyneuropathy, and amyloid depositions in the heart.

ALBUMIN   Albumin is a monomer of 69 kDa associated with the transport of various endogenous and exogenous hydrophobic compounds. Albumin has a relatively low affinity for T4 and T3, but because of its high concentration (approx 3.5 g/dL) it binds up to 10% of T4 and 30% of T3.

Familial dysalbuminemic hyperthyroxinemia is the most common cause of euthyroid hyperthyroxinemia. Familial dysalbuminemic hyperthyroxinemia is characterized by increased binding of T4 and thus elevated total T4, but normal free T4 levels. It is inherited in an autosomal-dominant manner. Studies of several families have led to the identification of two independently recurring point mutations in the albumin gene that lead to substitutions

of arginine at position 218 (R218H, R218P). Crystallographic analyses revealed that the two mutations result in conformational changes that favor binding of T4 on one of the four T4-binding sites on albumin.

In a family presenting with high serum total T3, but not T4, an albumin mutation L66P was identified. The L66P albumin leads thus to *familial dysalbuminemic hypertriiodothyroninemia* with an affinity for T3 that is approximately 40 times higher than wild-type albumin. In contrast, the affinity for T4 is barely changed.

UPTAKE OF THYROID HORMONE INTO CELLS

Cellular uptake of thyroid hormones appears to be mediated by amino acid channels. Point mutations and deletions in the X-chromosomal *MCT8* gene have been identified in several male patients presenting with elevated T3 and TSH levels and a remarkable neurological phenotype that includes severe mental retardation, spastic quadriplegia, rotary nystagmus, and impaired gaze, and hearing. In one instance, the disorder was found in several males of a consanguineous mating, in the other cases, it was sporadic. Heterozygous females have discrete thyroid hormone abnormalities, but no neurological alterations. The abnormal T3 elevation may be due to impaired uptake into cells such as neurons and resembles in many aspects to the phenotype in neurological cretinism. It remains unclear whether MCT8 transports other amino acid derivatives that could be involved in the development of the complex phenotype. The observations indicate, however, that the uptake of thyroid hormones is, at least in part, mediated by channels. Of note, studies have revealed that the Allan-Herndon-Dudley syndrome, a recognized cause of X-linked mental retardation with a wide spectrum of neurological alterations, is caused by mutations in MCT8.

PERIPHERAL MONODEIODINATION

In target tissues, T4 is metabolized into the more active compound T3 by intracellular 5′-monodeiodination or into the inactive metabolite rT3 by 5-monodeiodination (*see* Fig. 35-3). Because roughly 80% of T3 is generated by monodeiodination of T3, T4 is sometimes considered a prohormone. Monodeiodination of the outer and inner ring is catalyzed by three well-characterized deiodinases, which are unusual because they are selenoproteins. They contain the rare amino acid selenocysteine (Sec), which is encoded by UGA, a triplet that usually encodes a stop codon. The translation of the Sec codon requires specific stem loop sequences that are located in the 3′ untranslated region (SECIS element) of the mRNA.

Type 1 iodothyronine deiodinase (DIO1) primarily converts T4 to T3 and is sensitive to propylthiouracil. In humans, it is expressed in many tissues, including liver, kidney, thyroid, and pituitary. DIO2 deiodinates exclusively the outer ring. Its expression is abundant in the human pituitary, brain, thyroid, and skeletal muscle; high levels are found in the brown adipose tissue of rodents in which it plays an important role in adaptive thermogenesis. DIO3 is the major enzyme inactivating T4 and T3 (*see* Fig. 35-3). In addition to its expression in tissues such as the central nervous system and skin, DIO3 is particularly abundant in the placenta and regulates circulating fetal thyroid hormone concentrations during gestation.

Overexpression of DIO3 in infantile hemangiomas and other vascular tumors leads to *consumptive hypothyroidism* through inactivation of thyroid hormone at a rate that exceeds the maximal thyroid hormone synthesis.

THYROID HORMONE ACTION

Thyroid hormones exert their multiple cellular effects through nuclear TR, transcription factors that act by altering patterns of gene expression both as activators and repressors (*see* Fig. 35-4). The two TR genes, TRα and TRβ, cellular homologs of the viral erythroblastic leukemia oncogene v-erbA, were cloned based on their relationship to other members of the steroid receptor superfamily of nuclear receptors that share a characteristic modular domain structure with a central DNA binding domain and a carboxy-terminal ligand binding domain. In the TR, the carboxy-terminus of the receptor also contains nuclear localization signals, dimerization domains, and transactivation functions. The functional properties of the amino-terminal region of the receptor are less well characterized but seem also to be involved in transactivation.

The two TRs, TRα and TRβ, are encoded by separate genes located on chromosomes 17 and 3, respectively. Although they bind thyroid hormones with high affinity, TRα and TRβ differ in their developmental patterns of expression, tissue distribution and the patterns of splicing to create additional isoforms. The TR can bind as monomer or with greater affinity as homodimers and heterodimers, particularly with retinoid X receptors to thyroid hormone response elements (TREs) in specific target genes.

In most instances, unliganded TR represses transcription by recruiting corepressors, some of which have histone deacetylase activity (*see* Fig. 35-4C). Binding of T3 alters the conformation of the receptor resulting in release of the corepressor complex and recruitment of a coactivator complex that includes multiple histone acetyltransferases. The modification of histones is an important mechanism controlling chromatin structure and transcriptional events. Several TR-interacting coregulators act more directly on the basal transcriptional machinery suggesting that mechanisms independent of histone acetylation and deacetylation are also involved in TR action.

Although there is considerable heterogeneity in the TREs of different target genes, most TREs contain two or more "half sites" that correspond to the minimal recognition motif for a receptor monomer. The consensus TRE half-site consists of the DNA sequence AGGTCA. These half-sites can be arranged as a palindrome, a direct repeat spaced by four nucleotides, or as an inverted repeat, also called lap (an eponym created by inversion of *pal*indrome). Remarkably, TRs can bind to these TREs with different orientations as homodimers or heterodimers with cofactors, indicating flexibility in the determinants of the protein–protein interface. Receptor binding to these repeats is importantly influenced by neighboring nucleotides and by the spacing between the elements that provide one of the primary determinants of receptor specificity for different nuclear receptors like TRs, retinoid receptors and vitamin D receptors. Changes in gene transcription are reflected in alterations in mRNA levels followed by changes in protein biosynthesis. A large number of genes that respond to thyroid hormone have been identified.

The crystal structure of the rat TRα1 ligand-binding domain bound to T3 has been solved and permits a better understanding of structure-function relationship. Knowledge about the structure may also permit the design of novel agonists and antagonists that may have differential effects on TRs and of use in conditions such as hyperthyroidism, lipid disorders, and obesity.

Important insights into thyroid hormone action have been gained through systematic disruption of the TRα and TRβ genes

and isoforms, independently or in combination. More than ten mutant strains have been characterized. These studies reveal that TRβ is essential for the development of the inner ear, color vision, and liver function. TRα, abundantly expressed in the heart, is essential for normal cardiac function. Moreover, it is important for maintaining basal energy metabolism and regulating enchondral bone formation. Evaluation of the combined TR knock-out indicates that hypothyroidism is associated with more significant abnormalities than receptor deficiency. This supports that the unliganded receptors have a repressive function of physiological relevance. Knock-in experiments have also been successfully used to model the syndrome of RTH and continue to reveal fundamental insights into TR-mediated gene regulation. For example, mice heterozygous for a knock-in of a dominant negative mutation into the TRα1 gene display a phenotype with marked visceral adiposity and insulin resistance, increased TSH levels and minimally elevated T4 and T3 levels suggesting that TRα plays an important role in regulating both lipogenesis and lipolysis by modulating adrenergic activity.

Lastly, some thyroid hormone-mediated effects are rapid and not mediated by genomic actions. They involve effects on the cell membrane, mitochondria, and stimulation of signaling pathways. Of growing interest, these nongenomic effects await more thorough characterization.

RESISTANCE TO THYROID HORMONE

RTH was first recognized in 1967 in two sibs of a consanguineous marriage presenting with goiter, high levels of protein-bound iodine, deaf-mutism, delayed bone age, and stippled epiphyses, but without signs of hyperthyroidism. Abnormalities in thyroid hormone itself or its transport into tissues were excluded, and it was thus postulated that resistance in peripheral tissues was the explanation for the absence of signs and symptoms of thyrotoxicosis. Following the cloning of the TRs, linkage analysis demonstrated that TRβ is tightly linked to RTH, whereas no association could be demonstrated to TRα. The ultimate proof that a defect in the receptor is the cause of RTH was provided in 1989 by the demonstration of mutations in the TRβ gene, a finding that has been confirmed in multiple reports. RTH is a rare disorder, but because of growing awareness of its existence more than 400 familial and sporadic patients have been studied.

Biochemically, RTH is defined by elevated circulating levels of free thyroid hormones because of reduced target tissue responsiveness and normal, or elevated, levels of TSH. This "inappropriate" TSH elevation contrasts with the situation in hyperthyroidism, in which the pituitary secretion of TSH is suppressed. Patients with RTH typically present with goiter and signs of hypothyroidism in tissues expressing predominantly TRβ, but hyperthyroidism in organs with predominant TRα expression such as the heart. They can include short stature, delayed bone maturation, hyperactivity and learning disabilities, hearing defects and tachycardia. There is a striking clinical heterogeneity in patients with RTH, a phenomenon presumably caused by genetic background or nongenetic factors modulating thyroid hormone action.

With the exception of the first studied kindred, a single sibship harboring a deletion of the entire coding sequence of the entire TRβ gene and a recessive pattern of inheritance, RTH is most commonly caused by heterozygous mutations of the TRβ gene. They can be inherited in an autosomal-dominant manner or occur as *de novo* mutations. The mutant receptors act in a dominant negative fashion to block the activity of normal TRα and TRβ receptors. The mutations are clustered in three domains in the carboxy-terminal region of the receptor. Many mutations occur in CpG dinucleotide sequences, and consist in most cases of nucleotide substitutions that result in single amino acid substitutions. In a few cases, the mutations cause frameshifts, either altering the reading frame, or causing premature stop codons. No mutations have been found within the DNA binding domain or in the amino-terminus. In general, the mutations preserve some critical receptor functions such as dimerization and DNA binding, whereas inactivating other activities such as T3 binding and transcriptional activation.

The dominant negative activity of mutant TRs involves several mechanisms. Mutant TRs, which have lost their transcriptional activity, can block wild-type TR from binding to TREs. Given the decreased or impaired T3 binding, this will favor interactions with corepressors (see Fig. 35-4C). Some mutations may also have altered dimerization properties that may disrupt interaction with coactivators. These naturally occurring mutations continue to provide important insights into the mechanisms of thyroid hormone action, molecular mechanisms of dominant negative activity, and structure-function relationship of the TRs, which is now facilitated by the available crystal structure for TRα.

Several kindreds with a RTH phenotype without mutations in the TR and autosomal-dominant transmission of the disorder have been reported. It is likely that mutations in cofactors that are required for normal TR function are involved in the pathogenesis of RTH in these patients.

Somatic mutations in the TRs have been identified in a subset of thyroid cancers, a TSH-secreting pituitary adenoma, renal cell cancers, and hepatomas. Their exact role in the development of these neoplasias is unknown.

AUTOIMMUNE DISORDERS

Autoimmune thyroid disorders (AITD), Hashimoto thyroiditis and Graves' disease, are by far the most common diseases affecting the thyroid gland. They are characterized by an immune response to thyroidal antigens, infiltration by T cells and production of antibodies. In Graves' disease, thyroid-stimulating antibodies lead to activation of the TSH receptor and hyperthyroidism, a process involving mainly a Th2 cell response. In Hashimoto's thyroiditis, a predominantly Th1-mediated chronic inflammation leads to progressive destruction and hypothyroidism. Both disorders are found more frequently in women than in men (4–10/1), a difference that is most commonly explained by influences of sex steroids on immunoregulatory mechanisms. The incidence of Graves' disease in the general population has been estimated at 0.2–1%. Hashimoto's thyroiditis has been reported to occur in up to 3–4.5%, and approx 15% of elderly women have thyroid autoantibodies although there is not necessarily a clinical correlate.

Thought to be multifactorial, the AITD require a genetic predisposition in combination with environmental triggers. Epidemiological data support a strong genetic component in the development of AITD, further supported by twin studies. Graves' disease occurs in approximately 3–9% of dizygotic and 30–60% of monozygotic twins. For Hashimoto's thyroiditis, the concordance rate for monozygotic twins is approximately 40%, but very low for dizygotic twins. Of note, monozygotic twins are not identical in terms of their immune repertoire, which may explain that perfect concordance is absent. Genetic and molecular analyses have

allowed a partial understanding of the pathophysiological mechanisms underlying the two disorders, but their precise elucidation continues to form a major challenge.

As in other autoimmune diseases, associations have been established between the disease and the presence of certain human leukocyte antigens (HLA) constellations. Graves' disease is associated with HLA-DR3. However, most linkage studies have been negative. HLA correlations for Hashimoto's thyroiditis differ from the ones reported for Graves' disease and appear to include HLA-DR3, DR4, and DR5 haplotypes.

Candidate gene analyses aiming at investigating associations between variants in genes such as the TSH receptor, TPO, and the T-cell receptor with AITD have been negative. In contrast, the TG and cytotoxic T-lymphocyte antigen, four genes appear to be important susceptibility genes for AITD. Whole genome screens using AITD families identified several loci or genes with evidence for linkage to AITD (GD-1 on chromosome 14; GD-2 on chromosome 20; HT-2 on chromosome 12; Tab-1 on chromosome 2; the TG gene on chromosome 8). It also became apparent that gene–gene interactions occur between some of these genes. The identified loci show, in part, linkage to Graves' and Hashimoto's disease suggesting that certain genes underlie the development of AITD, but that additional genetic and or nongenetic factors are required for the expression of the specific phenotype.

ANTIBODIES AND AUTOIMMUNE THYROID DISEASE

Because stimulating autoantibodies against the TSH receptor (TSAb) are the cause of Graves' disease, their assessment can help establish the diagnosis. Most tests rely on measurement of the binding of these antibodies to the receptor but this test does not assess their bioactivity. Cloning of the TSH receptor led to the development of new bioassays that allow measurement of TSAb. They allow reliable distinction of TBAb; these blocking antibodies may also be present in other forms of AITD. For these new assay systems, the TSH receptor has been stably transfected into cell lines. Measurement of cAMP in response to a patient serum allows assessment of the presence and bioactivity of thyroid autoantibodies.

Molecular biology established that the microsomal antigen in autoimmune thyroiditis is in fact TPO. The epitopes within the TPO enzyme, which are the targets of autoantibodies, are still a matter of debate, however. Recombinant TPO can now also be produced for the assay of autoantibodies.

THYROTOXIC HYPOKALEMIC PERIODIC PARALYSIS

Periodic paralysis with hypokalemia can occur in patients with thyrotoxicosis. The clinical presentation is indistinguishable from familial hereditary hypokalemic paralysis without hyperthyroidism. Analysis of several genes encoding channels that are mutated in the familial form in patients with the thyrotoxic form led to the identification of a mutation in the KCNE3 potassium channel gene. No mutations could be found in other candidates such as the calcium channel CACN1AS or the sodium channel SCN4A.

THYROID CANCER

Thyroid cancers are relatively infrequent neoplasms and account for approx 0.6–1.6% of all malignancies. The incidence of thyroid cancer is 1–10/100,000 in most countries. In the United States, this results in approximately 20,000 new cases and 1200 deaths per year. Thyroid cancer is about three times more frequent in females. Remarkably, thyroid cancer has shown the highest increase in

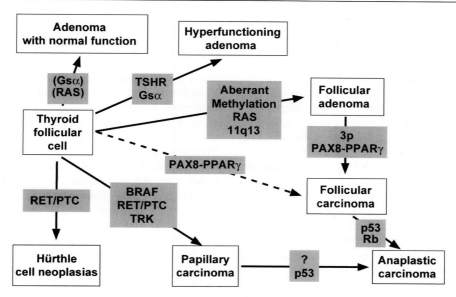

Figure 35-5 Molecular alterations involved in the pathogenesis of benign and malignant thyroid tumors. (Redrawn and modified after Fagin JA.)

cancer incidence (+4.3/100,000) during the 1992–2002 survey period of the Surveillance, Epidemiology, and End Results of the National cancer institute (http://seer.cancer.gov/).

Most thyroid malignancies are papillary thyroid carcinomas (PTC) or follicular thyroid carcinomas (FTC), both originating from follicular cells. PTC is by far the most common thyroid cancer (approximately 90%) in countries with sufficient iodine intake, FTC is comparatively uncommon. Their relative distribution is, however, variable and the incidence of FTC increases in regions with iodine deficiency. TG, only expressed in thyroid follicular cells, serves as an excellent tumor marker in patient follow-up. TG mRNA can be detected by reverse transcriptase PCR in serum samples and is being evaluated as a potential diagnostic tool for residual cancer. Besides the clinically relevant forms of PTC, occult PTC (<1 cm) are found in up to 36% of autopsies. The highly malignant anaplastic carcinoma (ATC) and several unusual variants of thyroid cancers (Hürthle cell carcinoma, insular thyroid carcinoma, primary squamous carcinoma, and lymphoma of the thyroid) are much rarer forms of thyroid malignancies. ATC is thought to arise from preexisting well-differentiated carcinomas in some cases. Hürthle cell carcinomas and insular carcinomas are both traditionally classified as variants of FTC, but are now considered to form distinct entities by many authors. This separate classification can be justified based on their greater tendency to recur and, particularly in the case of the insular carcinoma, a significantly compromised prognosis.

A major risk factor for the development of benign and malignant thyroid neoplasms is radiation. This has been recognized after use of external radiation for medical treatment of benign and malignant conditions in the neck and more dramatically after accidental releases of ionizing radiation from atomic explosions and accidents in nuclear facilities.

PTC, which presents with several distinct histological subtypes, may occur in the setting of some rare autosomal-dominant syndromes with disseminated neoplasias: familial adenomatous polyposis (Gardner's syndrome; APC gene mutations), as well as Cowden's syndrome (PTEN gene mutations), a condition characterized by multiple hamartomas with benign and malignant breast

tumors, gastrointestinal polyps, ovarian cysts and mucocutaneous papulae. The Carney complex, an autosomal-dominant disorder defined by cardiac myxomas, benign endocrine neoplasms and, more rarely, follicular cancers, is associated with activating mutations in the regulatory subunit 1A of the cAMP-dependent PKA (PRKAR1A). Nonsyndromic familial PTC has been reported repeatedly; in some instances the familial accumulation may, however, be the result of exposure to a shared risk factor than a familial disease in the strict sense. Familial aggregation of FTC seems to occur in families with dyshormonogenesis.

Several molecular mechanisms involved in the development of thyroid neoplasms have been elucidated during the last decade (Fig. 35-5; see Table 35-8). None of these markers has been used as a routine clinical test. New markers would be particularly desirable for the distinction of follicular adenomas and follicular carcinomas, two entities that cannot be discriminated by cytology.

CLONAL ANALYSIS Clonal analysis was performed in thyroid nodules, adenomas and cancers with the X-inactivation technique in females. Studies on clonality of thyroid neoplasms revealed that most thyroid nodules are monoclonal in origin, i.e., true adenomas. In multinodular goiters, polyclonal nodules coexist with nodules of monoclonal origin, and the latter may have distinct clonal origins in the same gland. As in the parathyroid gland, the diagnosis of a monoclonal lesion can often only be made with X-inactivation analysis because of marked histological heterogeneity even in monoclonal tissues. As expected, cancers are of monoclonal origin; the few reported exceptions are probably because of PTC with important amounts of stromal tissue.

Besides clonal analysis by means of the X-inactivation approach, loss of heterozygosity has been detected at multiple loci. Taken together, these results suggest that somatic mutations in growth-controlling genes or loss of tumor suppressors are involved in the development and or progression of most of these tumors.

GROWTH FACTORS AND ONCOGENES Studies on expression of growth factors and their receptors at the mRNA and protein level reported partially contradicting observations and it is difficult to draw definite conclusions concerning their exact role in the development of thyroid malignancies. Many of these proteins are abnormally expressed in benign and malignant thyroid tumors. In part, these alterations are secondary events because no structural abnormalities could be detected in the involved genes or the respective chromosomal location.

Amplification of the *MET* gene, encoding a heterodimeric tyrosine kinase whose ligand is the hepatic growth factor, has been reported in 70% of PTC and undifferentiated thyroid cancer, and in 25% of FTC; it was associated with aggressive clinical and histological phenotype. MET oncogene amplification has also been reported in a number of gastrointestinal, hepatocelllular, meningeal, and neuronal carcinomas. The abundance of transcripts for the transcription factor c-*myc* increases in less differentiated thyroid tumors and c-*myc* mRNA correlated negatively with that of the TSH receptor in one study.

Somatic mutations in oncogenes and or loss of tumor suppressors may result in loss of growth control and have been identified in several genes in benign and malignant thyroid tumors. Analogous to mutations in the α-subunit of Gs, mutations in the RAS oncogene can lead to a reduction of the guanosine 5′-triphosphatase activity resulting in continuous activation of the protein. Mutations in the three *RAS* genes, Ha-RAS, K-RAS, and N-RAS, which encode closely related 21-kDa proteins involved in signal transduction, have been found in numerous human tumors. The most frequently mutated codons are 12, 13, and 61 (corresponding to residue 227 of Gsα). Although mutations have been detected in both benign and malignant thyroid tumors in all three RAS genes, there is considerable variation in the reported prevalence of these mutations among several studies. The prevalence of activating mutations of all three RAS genes is higher in follicular adenomas and carcinomas than in PTC, suggesting that the different histological entities develop in response to distinct oncogenic pathways.

Somatic gsp mutations, activating mutations in the α subunit of the stimulatory G protein, occur in up to 38% of toxic adenomas (*see* above), but are relatively uncommon in PTC and FTC. Some of the amino acid substitutions at arginine 201 and glutamine 227, the most frequently involved residues, are rather unusual in differentiated carcinomas. As for other mutations in oncogenes, for example, RAS, the reported frequency is highly variable.

RET is a transmembrane tyrosine kinase for several ligands, among them glial cell-derived neurotropic growth factor, and is involved in neuronal differentiation. It is made up of five domains: a cadherin-like extracellular domain, a cysteine-rich domain involved in dimerization, a transmembrane domain and two intracellular tyrosine kinase domains. Normally, the RET protooncogene is not expressed in thyroid follicular cells but it is found in C-cells. Point mutations in the *RET* gene are at the onset of the MEN2 syndromes and familial medullary thyroid cancer (FMTC) (*see* FMTC and MEN2).

Rearrangements of the RET locus were detected after the observation of structural alterations in chromosome 10 in PTC and are referred to as RET/PTC rearrangements. There are several distinct types of translocations. A breakpoint in intron 11 upstream of the tyrosine kinase domains places different promoters upstream of the respective sequences. The tyrosine kinase domains are thereby under control of constitutive promoters resulting in continuous activity. RET/PTC1 is defined by a paracentric inversion of the long arm of chromosome 10 [inv(10)q11.2q21] recognized by the probe H4 (D10S170). RET/PTC2 is a recombination between chromosomes 10 and 17 [t(10;17)(q11.2;q23)] placing the R1α regulatory subunit of protein kinase A upstream of the

RET tyrosine kinase domains. The RET/PTC3 rearrangement puts the *ELE1* gene of chromosome 10, which is capable of transforming fibroblasts, adjacent to the tyrosine kinase sequences. RET/PTC rearrangements occur in approx 10–40% of all PTC. Some studies suggest a higher incidence of local invasion and distant metastases in PTC with RET/PTC rearrangements. RET rearrangements are particularly common in pediatric PTC; in children developing PTC as a consequence of the nuclear accident of Chernobyl, the incidence is even higher. PTC is frequently multicentric. Molecular analyses suggest that the tumor foci develop independently given that they often harbor distinct RET/PTC rearrangements. This could be explained by widespread DNA damage or, alternatively, genetic susceptibility, for example, associated with defects in DNA repair enzymes. Remarkably, RET/PTC rearrangements are not limited to PTC and are also found in Hürthle cell adenomas and carcinomas. This led to the reclassification of Hürthle cell tumors as variants of papillary carcinoma, a controversial concept.

The demonstration that RET/PTC1 rearrangement induces PTC in transgenic mice suggests that this rearrangement is an early event in their development. This is also supported by a high incidence of these rearrangements in occult PTC and the induction of RET/PTC1 rearrangements by irradiation of human fetal thyroid explants.

A second type of chimeric oncogene has been described in PTC. The TRK gene, encoding a receptor for the nerve growth factor, is placed under the control of several unrelated sequences through intrachromosomal rearrangements on chromosome 1q23-24: the TPR (tropomyosin) gene and a gene referred to as the TRK activating gene.

Recent studies have shown that B-RAF mutations are the most prevalent thyroid oncogene in papillary thyroid cancer. B-RAF is an intracellular serine-threonine kinase that is downstream of RAS. It is predominantly expressed in the thyroid, hematopoetic cells, neurons and the testis. Oncogenic mutations lead typically to a structural change that results in a catalytic activation. The B-RAF mutation T1796A is found in 40–70% of all papillary cancers. They are not found in other forms of well-differentiated thyroid carcinoma. Moreover, mutations in B-RAF, RET/PTC rearrangements and RAS mutations appear to be mutually exclusive. Remarkably, these oncogenes result in the activation of the same signaling cascade emphasizing its importance for tumorigenesis. PTC with B-RAF mutations have a more aggressive behavior and present frequently with extrathyroidal metastasis. Both RET and B-RAF are potential targets for kinase inhibitors, which may serve as new therapeutic modalities for well-differentiated thyroid cancer and MTC that are not curable with currently available treatments.

A fusion gene between the *PAX8* and the *peroxisome proliferators-activated receptor-γ* gene has been identified in a substantial number of follicular carcinomas. In contrast, it is relatively uncommon in follicular adenomas. Ongoing research is clarifying the oncogenic role of this fusion gene and its clinical utility in the distinction of follicular neoplasms.

The tumor suppressor genes that have been studied to some extent in thyroid malignancies are the retinoblastoma susceptibility gene (*Rb*) and the *p53* gene. *Rb* maps to chromosome 13q14 and encodes a 110-kDa protein. Rb is activated by cyclin-dependent kinases (CDK4/cyclinD) in the G1 phase and this induces the expression of genes required for DNA replication. During the cell cycle, Rb regulates the actions of several transcription factors like

E2F and cyclins. The suppressive effect on cell cycle progression and growth can be lost through heterozygous loss in a single Rb allele in the germline, associated with retinoblastomas and sarcomas, or somatic mutations found in several carcinomas. These mutations affect residues that can be phosphorylated or that are involved in protein–protein interactions. When studied at the genomic or protein level, no Rb abnormalities were found in thyroid carcinomas. This contrasts with a report on mRNA abnormalities in 55% of thyroid carcinomas and absent differences between differentiated carcinomas and ATCs. Of these latter tumors, 12% also harbored p53 mutations, a finding that was reported to be more prevalent in advanced disease.

P16, also called MTS1, is an inhibitor of CDK involved in the phosphorylation of Rb. The demonstration of homozygous deletions of P16, localized on chromosome 9p21, in two of three FTC and two of four PTC cell lines suggests that P16 might be an important tumor suppressor gene involved in the pathogenesis of thyroid malignancies. P16 abnormalities (mutations, deletions) occur in high frequency in adenocarcinomas of the pancreas.

The p53 gene plays an important role in the development and progression of several human cancers. It exerts its function as a tumor suppressor by arresting cells in the G_1 phase of the cell cycle, thus enabling repair of DNA damage. The p53 gene is localized on chromosome 17p13. Four monomers oligomerize to a tetramer. Germline mutations of p53 are found in the Li-Fraumeni syndrome, familial breast cancer (Chapter 74) and a wide variety of other human malignancies. As in other malignancies, mutations in p53 are also thought to be involved in the progression of thyroid carcinomas and to play a key element in the process of dedifferentiation. Although they are more frequently found in ATCs, they may even occur in some follicular adenomas and differentiated carcinomas.

MEDULLARY THYROID CANCER AND MULTIPLE ENDOCRINE NEOPLASIA

MEN, FMTC and MTC are more thoroughly reviewed in Chapter 40. MEN2A is an autosomal-dominant disease characterized by the association of MTC, parathyroid adenomas and pheochromocytoma. In MEN2B, parathyroid disease is absent, but patients additionally develop mucocutaneous ganglioneuromas, and some patients have a marfanoid habitus. FMTC is a familial cancer syndrome without other manifestations of the MEN complex.

Several mutations in the ret tyrosine kinase receptor have been identified as causes of MEN2A and FMTC. Most of these mutations affect conserved cysteines in the cysteine-rich domain thought to be involved in receptor dimerization and activation. In MEN2B, a mutation at position 918, substituting methionine–threonine, has been found in 95% of the patients.

Although genetic testing for the diagnosis of cancer predisposition remains controversial in many instances, the recognition of mutations in the *RET* gene as the cause of MEN2A and FMTC has profound clinical relevance. Before the availability of genetic testing, families with MEN2A and FMTC were evaluated on a regular basis by measuring calcitonin levels after stimulation with pentagastrin or calcium. This test was however hampered by a low specificity with the possibility of false-positive results and required repeated testing and a high compliance of the mostly asymptomatic family members. The possibility to identify gene carriers by mutational analysis allows identifying gene carriers accurately. Consequently, thyroidectomy can be performed in early childhood to prevent the development of MTC, which occurs

in approx 90% of affected patients. This procedure is thus associated with diagnostic accuracy, improved cure and lowered costs.

RECOMBINANT TSH AS A CLINICAL TOOL

After surgical procedures, patients with differentiated carcinomas of the thyroid are routinely evaluated by means of radioiodine scans and measurements of TG. To achieve a high sensitivity, these tests are traditionally performed after withdrawal of the suppressive treatment with T4 for several weeks to achieve an increase in TSH and thus a high uptake of radioiodine in residual tissue. Withdrawal of T4 leads to hypothyroidism and potentially to all the clinical problems associated with it. Moreover, the increase in TSH may lead to proliferation of residual tumor cells. To avoid these problems, exogenous TSH was successfully administered during uninterrupted treatment with T4 before performing radioiodine scans and TG measurements. These procedures have initially been performed with bovine TSH or human TSH from autopsies, sources that are no longer acceptable because of the possibility of anaphylactic reactions and the transmission of infectious disease (Jakob-Creutzfeld). After the cloning of the α- and β-subunits of human TSH, production of pure TSH in large quantities has been possible. Administration of recombinant human TSH is already used routinely in the follow-up of patients with differentiated thyroid cancer and may become a standard procedure. Recombinant TSH has also been applied successfully to stimulate uptake of radioiodine for the treatment of thyroid cancer or multinodular goiters.

GENETICALLY MODIFIED ANIMALS

Important new insights into the pathophysiological mechanisms controlling goiter and thyroid tumor formation have been gained with genetically modified mice, including a large number of transgenic models, knock-out and knock-in strains. These studies have allowed the confirmation of several paradigms in vivo. The characterization of the TG promoter easily achieves tissue-specific expression of transgenes in the thyroid. A first model expressed the chloramphenicol acetyltransferase to the thyroid; chloramphenicol acetyltransferase activity could be detected in thyroid tissue but not in any other tissue and assured that the *cis* regulatory elements present in the first 2000 bp of the promoter are sufficient for thyroid specific expression. Thyroid-specific expression of the large T antigen of SV40, one of the most potent known viral oncogenes, under control of the TG promoter resulted in rapidly growing undifferentiated goiters with progressive dedifferentiation with increasing age and loss of expression of thyroid specific genes. The loss of differentiation was accompanied by marked hypothyroidism. Most of these animals died early, primarily from tracheal compression. By targeted overexpression of the herpes virus thymidine kinase 1 gene using the TG promoter and treatment with the antiviral drug ganciclovir, thyroid follicular cells could be ablated selectively. Predicted by the property of the adenosine A2a receptor to be a constitutive activator of the adenylyl cyclase pathway, its overexpression under the control of the TG promoter resulted in severe hyperthyroidism, tachyarrhthmias, and premature deaths owing to congestive heart failure. These transgenic animals develop huge goiters that are initially diffuse but later develop nodules; they provide an interesting model for hyperthyroidism and formation of nodular goiters. The E7 oncogene of the human papillomavirus type 16 inactivates the tumor suppressor protein encoded by Rb. Transgenic mice expressing E7 under control of the TG promoter develop huge hyperplastic goiters with large follicles with well-differentiated follicular cells. The animals are euthyroid but show a higher radioiodine uptake suggesting a lowered hormonogenic activity. Overexpression of the RET/PTC1 oncogene in a transgenic model led to carcinomas comparable to human papillary cancers, indicating that the RET/PTC1 rearrangement can be the primary cause for development of thyroid papillary cancer. Disruption of CREB signaling by overexpression of a dominant negative CREB isoform results in a phenotype characterized by congenital hypothyroidism with a hypoplastic thyroid emphasizing the importance of the cAMP pathway for thyroid follicular cell growth and function.

Many of the knock-out models were mentioned above. Targeted disruption of the *Pax8*, *Ttf1*, and *Ttf2* genes revealed the essential role of these transcription factors in thyroid development. Pax8 –/– mice die shortly after weaning because of severe hypothyroidism. There are no detectable thyroid follicular cells after E12 indicating that Pax8 is required for the expansion of precursor cells. In contrast to humans, the heterozygous mice are normal. Ttf1 knock-out mice are not viable and have a complex phenotype that includes an absent thyroid, severe brain malformations (missing ventral forebrain and pituitary) and sac-like lung structures. Reminiscent of humans with haploinsufficiency for TTF1, heterozygous mice have elevated TSH levels and a neurological phenotype with impaired coordination. Mice homozygous for targeted disruption of Ttf2 have thyroid agenesis or a sublingual thyroid in combination with a cleft palate.

Deletion of transcription factors such as Hex and Eya1, as well as several members of the Hox family, results in complex phenotypes that not only affect the thyroid. Whether naturally occurring mutations in these genes are associated with developmental or functional thyroid defects is unknown.

Multiple mouse models have focused on the two TRs, TRα, and TRβ, and their isoforms. Disruption of these genes individually or in combination revealed the physiological role of the two receptors and their isoforms in various tissues. The combined knock-out for TRα and TRβ illustrated that the silencing of genes by TRs is of physiological importance. Lastly, several knock-in strains have been created in order to model RTH by introducing naturally occurring human mutations into TRβ or by introducing the corresponding mutation into TRα.

ACKNOWLEDGMENTS

I am indebted to Dr. J.L. Jameson, MD, PhD, for his mentoring and his many contributions to the previous version of this chapter. This work has, in part, been supported by grant 1R01DK63024-01 (NIH/NIDDK) and MAF D02FE-14 (Morris foundation) to P.K.

SELECTED REFERENCES

Bianco AC, Salvatore D, Gereben B, Berry MJ, Larsen PR. Biochemistry, cellular, and molecular biology, and physiological roles of the iodothyronine selenodeiodinases. Endocr Rev 2002;23:38–89.

Cohen LE, Radovick S. Molecular basis of combined pituitary hormone deficiencies. Endocr Rev 2002;23:431–442.

Dias Da Silva MR, Cerutti JM, Arnaldi LA, Maciel RM. A mutation in the KCNE3 potassium channel gene is associated with susceptibility to thyrotoxic hypokalemic periodic paralysis. J Clin Endocrinol Metab 2002;87:4881–4884.

Dohan O, De la Vieja A, Paroder V, et al. The sodium/iodide symporter (NIS): characterization, regulation, and medical significance. Endocr Rev 2003;24:48–77.

Dumitrescu AM, Liao XH, Best TB, Brockman K, Refetoff S. A novel syndrome combining thyroid and neurological abnormalities is associated with mutations in a monocarboxylate transporter gene. Am J Hum Genetics 2004;74:168–175.

Fagin J. Perspective: lessons learned from molecular genetic studies of thyroid cancer—insights into pathogenesis and tumor-specific therapeutic targets. Endocrinology 2002;143:2025–2028.

Fagin JA. How thyroid tumors start and why it matters: kinase mutants as targets for solid cancer pharmacotherapy. J Endocrinol 2004;183:249–256.

Friesema EC, Ganguly S, Abdalla A, Manning Fox JE, Halestrap AP, Visser TJ. Identification of monocarboxylate transporter 8 as a specific thyroid hormone transporter. J Biol Chem 2003;18:18.

Gillam MP, Kopp P. Genetic defects in thyroid hormone synthesis. Curr Opin Pediatr 2001;13:364–372.

Gillam MP, Kopp P. Genetic regulation of thyroid development. Curr Opin Pediatr 2001;13:358–363.

Jameson JL. Mechanisms of thyroid hormone action. In: DeGroot L, Jameson J, eds. Endocrinology. Philadelphia: WB Saunders, 2001; pp.1327–1344.

Krude H, Schutz B, Biebermann H, et al. Choreoathetosis, hypothyroidism, and pulmonary alterations due to human NKX2-1 haploinsufficiency. J Clin Invest 2002;109:475–480.

Liu YY, Schultz JJ, Brent GA. A thyroid hormone receptor alpha gene mutation (P398H) is associated with visceral adiposity and impaired catecholamine-stimulated lipolysis in mice. J Biol Chem 2003; 16:16.

Marians RC, Ng L, Blair HC, Unger P, Graves PN, Davies TF. Defining thyrotropin-dependent and -independent steps of thyroid hormone synthesis by using thyrotropin receptor-null mice. Proc Natl Acad Sci USA 2002;99:15,776–15,781.

Moreno JC, Bikker H, Kempers MJE, et al. Inactivating mutations in the gene for thyroid oxidase 2 (THOX2) and congenital hypothyroidism. N Engl J Med 2002;347:95–102.

O'Shea PJ, Williams GR. Insight into the physiological actions of thyroid hormone receptors from genetically modified mice. J Endocrinol 2002;175:553–570.

Pohlenz J, Dumitrescu A, Zundel D, et al. Partial deficiency of thyroid transcription factor 1 produces predominantly neurological defects in humans and mice. J Clin Invest 2002;109:469–473.

Postiglione MP, Parlato R, Rodriguez-Mallon A, et al. Role of the thyroid-stimulating hormone receptor signaling in development and differentiation of the thyroid gland. Proc Natl Acad Sci USA 2002;99: 15, 462–15,467.

Refetoff S, Dumont J, Vassart G. Thyroid disorders. In: Sriver CR, Beaudet AL, Sly WS, Valle D, Childs B, eds. The Metabolic and Molecular Bases of Inherited Disease. 8th ed., vol. 3. New York: McGraw-Hill, 2001, pp. 4029–4075.

Refetoff S, Weiss RE, Usala SJ. The syndromes of resistance to thyroid hormone. Endocr Rev, 1993;14:348–399.

Tomer Y. Genetic dissection of familial autoimmune thyroid diseases using whole genome screening. Autoimmun Rev 2002;1:198–204.

Vaidya B, Kendall-Taylor P, Pearce SH. The genetics of autoimmune thyroid disease. J Clin Endocrinol Metab 2002;87:5385–5397.

Wagner RL, Apriletti JW, McGrath ME, et al. A structural role for hormone in the thyroid hormone receptor. Nature 1995;378:690–697.

Weinstein LS, Yu S, Warner DR, Liu J. Endocrine manifestations of stimulatory G protein alpha-subunit mutations and the role of genomic imprinting. Endocr Rev 2001;22:675–705.

Yen PM. Molecular basis of resistance to thyroid hormone. Trends Endocrinol Metab 2003;14:327–333.

36 Disorders of the Parathyroid Gland

Andrew Arnold and Michael A. Levine

SUMMARY

The parathyroid glands play a crucial role in maintaining normal calcium homeostasis, primarily through their regulated secretion of parathyroid hormone. A variety of congenital and acquired causes of diminished parathyroid function exist, including developmental abnormalities and defective parathyroid hormone synthesis or release, and the genetic basis for many of these is known. Primary disorders of parathyroid hyperfunction, mostly owing to parathyroid gland tumors, can be familial or sporadic. Molecular pathogenetic insights into these disorders are substantial, and have been exploited for clinical management.

Key Words: Calcium receptor; cyclin D1; GCMB; HRPT2; hypoparathyroidism; hyperparathyroidism; MEN1; parathyroid; parathyroid adenoma; parathyroid carcinoma; PTH.

DEVELOPMENT AND GROWTH OF THE PARATHYROID GLANDS

The parathyroid glands first appear during the fifth week of gestation in human fetuses, which corresponds to day E11.5 in the mouse embryo. The inferior parathyroid glands and the thymus form as lateral evaginations of the third branchial pouches. As the thymus and parathyroid complex migrates caudally, the parathyroids become associated with the lower poles of the thyroid gland, thus resting below the superior parathyroid glands, which are derived from the fourth branchial pouch along with the ultimobranchial bodies. Errant migration can lead to considerable variability in the location of the parathyroid glands. Because of their more extensive repositioning during embryogenesis, the inferior parathyroids are more likely to assume an ectopic location than the superior parathyroids. Nearly all (84%) humans have four parathyroid glands, but the number of glands can vary from 1 to 12, and it is not unusual to find three (1–7%) or five (3–13%) parathyroid glands in normal individuals. Expression of the transcription factor encoded by the *GCMB* gene is critical for proper development of the parathyroids, because deletion of this gene results in the absence of the parathyroids in mice, and is associated with hypoparathyroidism in humans (*see* Familial Isolated Hypoparathyroidism).

The parathyroid glands grow to a total parenchymal weight of about 3 µg at a gestational age of 8 wk, to 300 µg by age 18 wk, and to 4 mg at birth. Mineralization of the fetal skeleton is facilitated by active calcium transport from mother to fetus across the placenta, utilizing a calcium pump in the basal membrane of the trophoblast that maintains a 1/1.4 (mother/fetus) calcium gradient throughout gestation. Parathyroid hormone (PTH) and PTH-related protein share in the regulation of the fetus' unique calcium and mineral metabolism, and both hormones are synthesized in the fetal parathyroids, with PTH-related protein also being produced in other fetal tissues (e.g., placenta and liver).

After birth parathyroid growth continues for three decades. Adult parathyroid tissue mass varies with sex, race, and overall nutritional status, and the combined weight of all parathyroid glands is approx 120 mg in normal adult males and 145 mg in females. Individual glands range in weight from 3 to 75 mg, with most glands weighing approx 35–55 mg.

Cell turnover in the adult parathyroid gland is approx 5%/yr, with cycling cells randomly distributed and without evidence for a separate stem cell population. As adult parathyroid cell number remains constant, the very slow rate of cell gain must be balanced by a correspondingly slow rate of cell loss, presumably occurring through apoptosis. How the remaining parathyroid cells are somehow triggered from G_0 to G_1 in order to maintain a stable cell number is unknown. Such a compensatory mitotic response typically occurs in endocrine cells under the control of the hypothalamus or the pituitary, but its occurrence in the parathyroid gland, for which no trophic hormone has been identified, suggests the existence of novel proliferative mechanisms. Under special circumstances, the rate of parathyroid cell proliferation can be increased. The parathyroid glands can enlarge greatly during states of chronic hypocalcemia, particularly during renal failure when hyperphosphatemia and low levels of calcitriol accompany hypocalcemia.

PTH STRUCTURE, BIOSYNTHESIS, AND SECRETION

The *PTH* gene is located on the short arm of chromosome 11. Its three exons encode mature PTH (84 amino acids), as well as its signal (25 amino acids) and "pro" (6 amino acids) peptides. The study of the structure and regulation of the *PTH* gene and the intricacies of PTH biosynthesis, post-translational processing, and intracellular targeting have led to the accrual of a body of information that is as complete as that for any other peptide hormone. In the sections that follow, these areas are briefly reviewed for purposes of introduction.

THE EXTRACELLULAR CALCIUM-SENSING RECEPTOR

Increases in the serum-ionized calcium inhibit the secretion of PTH. Conversely, reductions in serum-ionized calcium stimulate

From: *Principles of Molecular Medicine, Second Edition*
Edited by: M. S. Runge and C. Patterson © Humana Press, Inc., Totowa, NJ

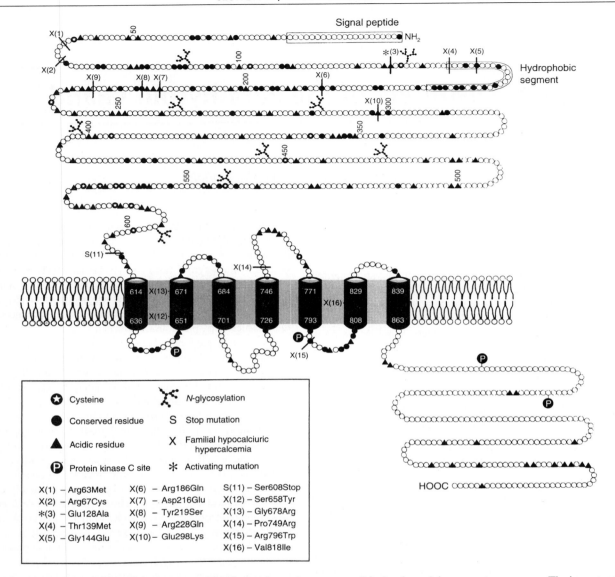

Figure 36-1 The structure of the calcium receptor. This figure shows the structure of the bovine calcium receptor or sensor. The important structural features are the seven putative transmembrane-spanning domains, the extracellular amino-terminal domain, and the cytoplasmic carboxyterminus. As can be seen from the key within the figure, both activating (causing hypoparathyroidism) and inactivating (causing familial hypocalciuric hypercalcemia) mutations can occur. (Reproduced with permission from Brown EM, Pollak M, Herbert SC. Molecular mechanisms underlying the sensing of extracellular Ca^{2+} by parathyroid and kidney cells. Eur J Endocrinol 1995;132:523–531. Copyright Society for the European Journal of Endocrinology 1995.)

the cascade of events that lead to the secretion of PTH. This inverse sigmoidal relationship between serum calcium and PTH secretion is precisely controlled, is the key physiological feature of the parathyroid gland, and accounts for the tight minute-to-minute regulation of PTH secretion and the strict maintenance of serum calcium. Parathyroid cells express on their surface a G protein coupled, seven transmembrane domain receptors with a large extracellular domain, encoded by the *CASR* gene on chromosome 3q. This receptor recognizes extracellular calcium in physiological concentrations and transduces signals through cytosolic calcium–inositol phosphate–phospholipase C intracellular pathways to regulate PTH release (Fig. 36-1). The calcium receptor is expressed in a restricted number of tissues (including the parathyroid gland, the thyroid C cell, the renal tubule, gastrointestinal tract, and the CNS).

TRANSCRIPTIONAL AND POST-TRANSCRIPTIONAL CONTROL *PTH* gene transcription is subject to both positive and negative regulation primarily through the combined regulatory effects of serum calcium concentration and of $1,25(OH)_2D$, the active form of vitamin D. Reductions in serum calcium and reductions in circulating $1,25(OH)_2D$ lead to activation of *PTH* gene transcription. Conversely, increases in serum calcium and in circulating $1,25(OH)_2D$ inhibit *PTH* gene transcription. These effects occur during a period of hours to days and are viewed as important in the long-term or tonic regulation of PTH secretion.

PTH BIOSYNTHESIS PTH synthesis requires translation of the PTH mRNA on ribosomes, entry of the nascent preproPTH into the cistern of the endoplasmic reticulum (ER), cleavage of the signal peptide cotranslationally by signal peptidase on the lumenal side of the ER, passage of the immature peptide through the lamellae of the Golgi apparatus, targeting of the peptide into the secretory granules of the regulated secretory pathway, and cleavage of the "pro" segment of the peptide, presumably within the Golgi compartment. In addition, the quantity of stored hormone within secretory granules appears to be subject to regulation through degradation of mature PTH within secretory granules or within phagolysosomes.

SHORT-TERM CONTROL OF SECRETION PTH secretion is regulated by the serum ionized calcium concentration. Changes in serum calcium concentration lead to immediate (minutes) and opposite changes in PTH secretion. The key features of this acute regulation appear to be those observed in other neuroendocrine peptide secretory systems (i.e., storage of preformed, completely processed hormone in dense core secretory granules, with secretory granule fusion to the cell membrane leading to immediate secretion) with one important difference: in most neuroendocrine cell types, fusion of secretory granules with the cell membrane is triggered by an increase in cytosolic calcium. The reverse is true in the parathyroid. The cellular mechanisms governing this inverse secretion-stimulus coupling in the parathyroid gland are incompletely understood.

HEREDITARY FORMS OF HYPOPARATHYROIDISM

The majority of patients with hypoparathyroidism have surgical or acquired autoimmune hypoparathyroidism. In contrast to these acquired forms of hypoparathyroidism, familial forms of congenital and acquired hypoparathyroidism have been described. These can be subdivided into familial syndromes in which hypoparathyroidism is accompanied by abnormalities in multiple other organ systems, and familial forms of hypoparathyroidism that are unaccompanied by other abnormalities.

FAMILIAL VARIETIES OF HYPOPARATHYROIDISM ASSOCIATED WITH MULTIPLE ORGAN SYSTEM ABNORMALITIES

These syndromes represent genetic syndromes associated with hypoparathyroidism, but given their multisystem abnormalities, it is intuitive that the parathyroid gland abnormalities are not intrinsic to defects within the parathyroid gland but are in some fashion secondary to other developmental or regulatory abnormalities.

HYPOPARATHYROIDISM ASSOCIATED WITH THE POLYGLANDULAR FAILURE SYNDROME Autoimmune hypoparathyroidism may occur alone or in association with additional features, including mucocutaneous candidiasis and adrenal insufficiency, as a component of the autoimmune polyglandular syndrome type 1 (APS-1). APS-1 may be sporadic or familial with an autosomal-recessive inheritance pattern. By contrast, the autoimmune polyglandular syndrome type 2 is characterized by adult-onset adrenal insufficiency associated with insulin-dependent diabetes mellitus and thyroid disease, and is thought to be polygenic with apparent autosomal-dominant inheritance. The APS-1 syndrome most commonly consists of the triad of hypoparathyroidism, adrenal insufficiency, and mucocutaneous candidiasis. The clinical onset of these disorders follows a predictable pattern, in which mucocutaneous candidiasis first appears at a mean age of 5 yr, followed by hypoparathyroidism at a mean age of 9 yr and adrenal insufficiency at a mean age of 14 yr. Patients may show only one or two of these features, and less than a year to decades may elapse between the diagnosis of one disease and the second in the same individual.

Some patients with APS-1 develop additional features. Alopecia occurs in approximately one-third of patients with the

highest incidence at ages 5–9 yr. It appears as hairless patches, and may proceed to complete baldness and lack of eye and body hair. Other features include keratoconjunctivitis, malabsorption and steatorrhea, gonadal failure, pernicious anemia, chronic active hepatitis, thyroid disease, and insulin-requiring diabetes mellitus. Enamel hypoplasia of teeth is also common, and appears to be unrelated to hypoparathyroidism. The presence of these additional defects in patients with APS-1 has led to the suggestion that a more inclusive term be used to describe the syndrome: "autoimmune polyendocrinopathy–candidiasis–ectodermal dystrophy." In cases that have been examined pathologically, complete parathyroid atrophy or destruction has been demonstrated. In some patients, treatment of hypoparathyroidism has been complicated by apparent vitamin D "resistance," possibly related to coexistent hepatic disease, steatorrhea, or both.

The autoimmune basis for the disorder is suggested by the findings of circulating autoantibodies directed against the parathyroid, thyroid, and adrenal glands in many patients, but the presence of organ-specific autoantibodies may not correlate well with the clinical findings. Some reports describe patients who have circulating autoantibodies that are directed against the parathyroid calcium-sensing receptor (CaR). These antibodies apparently behave as receptor activators and thereby decrease secretion of PTH (*see* Familial Isolated Hypoparathyroidism, autosomal-dominant hypocalcemia).

The APS-1 syndrome results from mutations in the *AIRE* (for autoimmune regulator) gene, and different geo-ethnic groups have unique *AIRE* mutations. The *AIRE* gene encodes a predicted 57.7-kDa protein that is expressed in thymus, lymph nodes, and fetal liver, and which contains motifs, including two plant homeodomain zinc fingers, that are suggestive of a role as a transcriptional regulator. Mutations in the *AIRE* gene are predicted to lead to truncated forms of the protein that lack at least one of the plant homeodomain zinc fingers, and which fail to localize to the cell nucleus.

THE DIGEORGE SYNDROME The DiGeorge syndrome (DGS) is the most frequent contiguous gene deletion syndrome in humans, occurring in approx 1 of 5000 live births. DGS is classified as a developmental field defect resulting from a defect in the development of the third and fourth branchial arches, which leads to thymic, parathyroid, and conotruncal cardiac defects. Because of thymic aplasia, T-cell-mediated immunity is impaired, and affected infants have an increased susceptibility to recurrent viral and fungal infections. Despite the emphasis on thymus dysgenesis in these syndromes, clinically significant immune defects occur in very few patients. The basic embryological defect is inadequate development of the facial neural crest tissues that results in maldevelopment of branchial pouch derivatives. Facial features associated with DGS include hypertelorism or telecanthus, short or hypoplastic philtrum, micrognathia, and low-set, posteriorly rotated ears. The most common cardiac defect is truncus arteriosus. The degrees of thymic hypoplasia and immune dysfunction also vary, and there is a tendency toward spontaneous remission. Last, there is variability in the degree of parathyroid hypoplasia and ensuing hypoparathyroidism, and in some cases hypoparathyroidism may be the principal or only feature of DGS. The presence of thymic hypoplasia or aplasia constitutes the "complete" form of DGS. Developmental field defects may have multiple causes and even multiple pathogenetic mechanisms, and DGS can arise in infants who were exposed *in utero* to retinoic acid, alcohol, or maternal diabetes mellitus.

Molecular mapping studies have demonstrated an association between the syndrome and deletions involving 22q11.2 (DGSI) in the great majority of patients with DGS. Many commercial laboratories offer genetic testing services that can identify these microdeletions in 22q11 by fluorescent *in situ* hybridization. Most cases of DGS are sporadic, but familial occurrence with apparent autosomal-dominant inheritance has been described. In these cases a heterozygous deletion of chromosomal region 22q11.2 is inherited from a mildly affected parent.

Analysis of the human DSG1 deleted region on chromosome 22q11.2 has defined a 250-kb minimal critical region that includes a variety of candidate genes, including a human homolog of a yeast gene, referred to as *UDFIL* that encodes a protein involved in the degradation of ubiquinated proteins. Deletion of the homologous region in the mouse (Df[16]1) causes a very similar disorder, and recently, mouse models that closely replicate the DGS have been generated through targeted ablation of genes within the DGS/ Df(16)1. Mice deficient in *Crkol*, a gene expressed in neural crest cells and which encodes an adapter protein implicated in response to growth factors and focal adhesion signaling, exhibit defects in multiple cranial and cardiac neural crest derivatives. A similar phenotype occurs in mice deficient in *Tbx1*, a transcription factor that is expressed in nonneural crest-derived cells of head mesenchyme, pharyngeal arches and pouches, and otic vesicles of the embryo. Haploinsufficiency of *TBX1*, the human homologue, has emerged as the likely explanation for the developmental defects of DGS1, including hypoplasia or aplasia of the parathyroid glands, as this gene is deleted in patients with DGS1. *TBX1* is a member of a family of transcription factors with more than 20 members identified in humans so far, and homologues in many other organisms. The discovery of the developmental role of *Tbx1* in the mouse prompted extensive searches for mutations of the *Tbx1* gene in patients with *del22q11* phenotype but without chromosomal deletion. These mutational analysis efforts culminated with the identification of five patients (three of whom were from the same family) carrying a *TBX1* gene. Most of these patients had a typical *del22q11DS*/DGS phenotype (including heart defects) but did not have learning disabilities. Hence, consistent with mouse genetic results, human *TBX1* mutation (presumably leading to haploinsufficiency, but this is not known yet) is sufficient to cause most of the abnormalities observed in *del22q11DS* or DGS.

The associated embryological defects that characterize the phenotype caused by loss of genes in the 22q11 region have been compiled to create the acronym "CATCH-22," which refers to cardiac anomalies, abnormal facies, thymic aplasia, cleft palate, and hypocalcemia with deletion at 22q. Because hypoparathyroidism in patients with DGS can be transient, with resolution during infancy, all infants with congenital hypoparathyroidism should be thoroughly evaluated for the genetic and physical defects associated with CATCH-22 syndrome, including evaluation of T-cell immunity.

Deletions at a second locus at 10p13, termed DGSII, have been found in some patients, but commercial molecular testing for the 10p13 microdeletion is not widely available. The genomic draft sequence of this region contains only one known gene, *BRUNOL3*, which is strongly expressed in the thymus during different developmental stages. Although *BRUNOL3* appears to be an important factor for thymus development, pathogenic mutations have not been found in DGS-like patients without chromosomal deletions.

HYPOPARATHYROIDISM ASSOCIATED WITH RENAL DYSGENESIS AND SENSORINEURAL HEARING LOSS

Hypoparathyroidism is also a variable component of Barakat syndrome, also termed the HDR syndrome because of the association of hypoparathyroidism with deafness and nephrosis. The HDR syndrome is associated with autosomal-dominant mutations in the *GATA3* gene located at 10p14 near the DGSII locus. Hypoparathyroidism also has been described in patients with rare familial syndromes that are associated with collateral developmental defects such as lymphedema, prolapsing mitral valve, brachytelephalangy, and nephropathy or microcephaly, beaked nose, and crognathia.

OTHER COMPLEX SYNDROMES ASSOCIATED WITH HYPOPARATHYROIDISM Hypoparathyroidism occurs in >50% of patients who have the Kenny–Caffey syndrome, an unusual syndrome characterized by short stature, osteosclerosis, basal ganglion calcifications, and ophthalmic defects. Studies indicate that the Kenny–Caffey syndrome is related to the Sanjad–Sakati syndrome, in which congenital hypoparathyroidism is associated with growth and mental retardation. Both of these autosomal-recessive disorders are linked to the same 2.6 cM region on chromosome 1q43-44, are allelic and are associated with defects in the *TBCE* gene, which encodes one of several chaperone proteins required for the proper folding of α-tubulin subunits and the formation of αβ-tubulin heterodimers. Cells from patients with these genetically related disorders show disturbances in subcellular organelles that require microtubules for membrane trafficking, such as the Golgi and late endosomal compartments. These findings provide evidence that the Sanjad–Sakati and Kenny–Caffey syndromes are chaperone diseases caused by a genetic defect in the tubulin assembly pathway, and establish a potential connection between tubulin physiology and the development of the parathyroid. Congenital hypoparathyroidism also occur as a feature of several generalized metabolic defects and in several mitochondrial neuromyopathies.

FAMILIAL ISOLATED HYPOPARATHYROIDISM

Isolated hypoparathyroidism may be sporadic or familial, with inheritance of PTH deficiency by autosomal-dominant, autosomal-recessive, or X-linked modes of transmission. The age at onset covers a broad range (1 mo to 30 yr), but the condition is most commonly diagnosed during childhood.

Isolated hypoparathyroidism has been associated with genetic defects that impair PTH synthesis (i.e., *PTH* gene defects) or secretion (i.e., *CASR* gene defects) as well as parathyroid gland development (e.g., *GCMB* gene defects). Defects in the *PTH* gene are an uncommon cause of hypoparathyroidism, with mutations reported in three families. One form of autosomal-dominant hypoparathyroidism has been attributed to a heterozygous mutation of the *PTH* gene consisting of a single base substitution (T → C) in exon 2. This mutation results in the substitution of arginine (CGT) for cysteine (TGT) in the leader sequence of preproPTH. The substitution of a charged amino acid in the midst of the hydrophobic core of the leader sequence inhibits processing of the mutant preproPTH molecule to proPTH by signal peptidase and is presumed to impair translocation of the mutant hormone and of the wild-type protein across the plasma membrane of the ER. Thus, this heterozygous mutation results in a dominant inhibitor phenotype that also prevents processing of the wild-type preproPTH molecule from the remaining normal *PTH* allele. This preproPTH mutation was the first signal peptide mutation reported to cause human disease; signal peptide mutations have subsequently been found in other molecules such as preprovasopressin (causing diabetes insipidus) and Factor X (causing a coagulopathy).

Mutations in the *PTH* gene are also the cause of autosomal-recessive hypoparathyroidism in two unrelated families. In one family, affected children were homozygous for a mutation in exon 2 that is predicted to disrupt normal processing of the preproPTH molecule. The mutant allele carries a T → C transition in the first base of codon 23 that results in the replacement of serine (TCG) by proline (CCG) at the –3 position of the signal peptide of preproPTH. This change is hypothesized to inhibit cleavage by signal peptidase at the normal position, and thereby lead to rapid degradation of the preproPTH protein in the rough ER. Affected patients who are homozygous for this allele present with symptomatic hypocalcemia within the first few weeks of life. In a second family, hypoparathyroidism occurred in members who were homozygous for a single base transversion (G → C) at the exon 2-intron 2 boundary. This mutation alters the invariant GT dinucleotide of the 5′ donor splice site that presumably affects annealing of the U1-snRNP recognition component of the nuclear RNA splicing enzyme. The use of a highly sensitive modification of reverse transcriptase-polymerase chain reaction allowed detection of very small amounts of preproPTH mRNA in cultured lymphoblasts from these patients, and revealed a PTH cDNA in affected subjects that was 90 bp shorter than the corresponding wild-type form. Nucleotide sequence analysis of the shortened cDNA revealed that exon 1 had been spliced to exon 3 in the mutant PTH mRNA, a process that resulted in the deletion of exon 2 from the mature transcript (i.e., exon skipping). The loss of exon 2 would eliminate both the initiation codon and the signal peptide sequence from the aberrant preproPTH mRNA, presumably explaining the molecular basis for autosomal-recessive hypoparathyroidism in this family.

Isolated hypoparathyroidism can also arise because of failure of the parathyroid glands to develop properly during embryogenesis. Homozygous mutations in the *GCMB* gene lead to congenital hypoparathyroidism because loss of this transcription factor results in failure of the parathyroid glands to develop (i.e., parathyroid agenesis) during embryogenesis. Mice and humans who are deficient in the transcription factor gcm2 (glial cell missing, 2) develop hypoparathyroidism but lack defects in other tissues derived from the neural crest or pharyngeal pouches. These data implicate the *GCMB* gene, located at chromosome 6p23-24, as a cause of autosomal-recessive parathyroid aplasia in humans, but the prevalence of *GCMB* gene mutations in IH remains unknown. An X-linked-recessive form of IH (OMIM 307700) has also been reported in two related multigeneration kindreds from Missouri, USA, and a deletion–insertion [del(X)(q27.1) inv ins (X;2)(q27.1;p25.3)] that could result in a position effect on *SOX3* expression has been identified in affected subjects.

Another mechanism underlying familial isolated hypoparathyroidism has been described. Heterozygous mutations in the gene encoding the CaR (*CASR*) that result in a *gain of function* have been identified in many subjects with autosomal-dominant hypocalcemia, a syndrome associated with low serum levels of PTH and relative hypercalciuria. In other cases, linkage of hypocalcemia to the chromosomal locus for the CaR (3q21-24) has provided indirect evidence for the involvement of this gene with familial hypoparathyroidism. Expression of mutant CaRs in

oocytes and mammalian cells leads to constitutive activation of the inositol phosphate signal transduction pathway. The host parathyroid cell, therefore, behaves as though it were being exposed to higher than normal concentration of extracellular calcium and appropriately fails to secrete PTH. Subsequent studies have identified similar activating mutations of the CaR gene in many patients with sporadic hypoparathyroidism. In both familial and sporadic cases, each affected propositus has demonstrated a unique mutation, suggesting that new mutations must sustain this disorder in the population. These results suggest that mutation of CaR gene may be the most common cause of genetic hypoparathyroidism.

The CaR is expressed in the parathyroid gland and the kidney, in which it appears to play an important role in regulating calcium reabsorption. Thus, gain-of-function mutations in the CaR are likely to account for the increased calcium clearance and relative hypercalciuria noted in patients with autosomal-dominant hypocalcemia. These patients may therefore be at increased risk of nephrocalcinosis or nephrolithiasis. By contrast, loss of function mutations of the CaR in patients with familial hypocalciuric hypercalcemia (FHH) (*see* FHH and Neonatal Severe Hyperparathyroidism) are associated with decreased calcium clearance and relative hypocalciuria.

FHH AND NEONATAL SEVERE HYPERPARATHYROIDISM

FHH, also called familial benign (hypocalciuric) hypercalcemia, is a disorder typically discovered incidentally on routine serum calcium screening. The hypercalcemia is usually mild (i.e., in the 10.5–12.0 mg/dL range), is lifelong, is generally not associated with the symptoms of hypercalcemia, and is associated with a reduction in the fractional urinary excretion of calcium. Historically, patients with FHH were confused with patients with typical sporadic parathyroid tumors, with the unfortunate consequence that affected patients underwent unnecessary partial parathyroidectomy, which would not alter the serum calcium, or equally unnecessary complete parathyroidectomy with the serious consequence of surgical hypoparathyroidism. Since the initial description of the syndrome in the 1970s, it has become clear that these patients manifest a form of biochemically defined primary hyperparathyroidism with slightly elevated or inappropriately normal serum PTH concentrations, that they have inappropriately efficient renal reabsorption of calcium, that the parathyroid glands have a defective ability to sense the hypercalcemia, and that multiple family members are typically involved, usually in an autosomal-dominant fashion.

Inherited inactivating mutations in the extracellular CaR (encoded by the *CASR* gene) are responsible for the features of FHH in most affected kindreds (*see* Fig. 36-1). The responsible mutations generally involve either the extracellular domain (presumably adversely influencing calcium binding to the receptor) or one of the transmembrane loops (presumably interfering with conformational changes that in turn lead to the activation of signal transduction pathways). In general, affected patients have been heterozygous for the mutant calcium receptor allele. Notably, infants have been described who have a potentially life-threatening syndrome, characterized by severe hypercalcemia (sometimes in the 20 mg/dL range) and, in contrast to typical FHH, prominent parathyroid hypercellularity. This syndrome has been referred to as neonatal severe hyperparathyroidism (NSHPT), and may occur within typical FHH kindreds. NSHPT can result from a germline double dose of a mutant, inactivated calcium receptor gene, often in the context of consanguineous parentage. Finally, germline heterozygosity for a calcium receptor gene bearing a specific missense mutation in the cytoplasmic tail was reported in familial parathyroid adenoma/hyperplasia with symptomatic hypercalcemia and hypercalciuria, suggesting a spectrum of possible phenotypic consequences of different germline CaR alterations.

In support of the concept that inactive mutant forms of the calcium receptor are responsible for these syndromes, expression in *Xenopus* oocytes of calcium receptors containing the same mutations as those encountered in humans results in impaired ability to sense extracellular calcium. Also, an FHH-like phenotype is found in mice in which a single *casr* allele has been inactivated, and a more severe phenotype similar to NSHPT is seen in mice in which both *casr* alleles have been disrupted. FHH families have been defined whose responsible genetic locus maps to the *CASR*'s 3q locus but no mutations are apparent in the gene's coding region. These findings suggest that mutations in the intronic or regulatory regions of the calcium receptor gene may explain additional kindreds. Mutations in other genes will undoubtedly be demonstrated in the future; for some families with FHH, the disease locus maps to locations distinct from 3q, namely 19p and 19q. It is presumed that the genes at these other loci encode other proteins that play a role in the calcium sensing machinery.

MOLECULAR GENETICS OF SPORADIC PARATHYROID GLAND NEOPLASIA

Primary hyperparathyroidism is caused by excessive secretion of PTH, resulting in hypercalcemia. Patients with primary hyperparathyroidism have both an excessive parathyroid cell mass and a resetting of the set point by which PTH secretion is tightly coupled to the parathyroid cell's ambient calcium level. In most (>80%) patients with primary hyperparathyroidism, a single benign parathyroid tumor (adenoma) is responsible, whereas multiple hypercellular glands are present in approx 15% (primary hyperplasia or "double adenomas"). Parathyroid carcinoma is rare, as is the ectopic secretion of PTH from nonparathyroid tumors. A comprehensive molecular pathophysiological description of parathyroid tumorigenesis will eventually need to fully explain the development of these types of tumors, as well as a variety of other special features such as the increased incidence of parathyroid tumors after exposure to neck irradiation and the disease's epidemiological weighting toward postmenopausal women. Detailed molecular understanding will likely yield information of diagnostic, prognostic, preventative, or therapeutic importance.

CLONALITY IN PARATHYROID TUMORIGENESIS The monoclonality or polyclonality of human tumors is an informative reflection of their underlying pathogenetic mechanism. Early data measuring isoforms of the X-chromosome-encoded protein G6PD in parathyroid adenomas in heterozygous women had indicated that apparently single parathyroid adenomas were polyclonal growths, likely to result solely from a generalized growth stimulus. These results, however, proved to be misleading, because modern molecular methods have now solidly established the monoclonality of typical parathyroid adenomas, both by X-chromosome inactivation analysis and by the direct demonstration of monoclonal genetic alterations in parathyroid adenomas (*see* below). Monoclonality highlights the concept that parathyroid adenomas are true neoplasms, consistent with clinical experience that surgical removal of the enlarged gland is generally curative. Neoplasia is a genetic disease, with most relevant DNA damage occurring somatically.

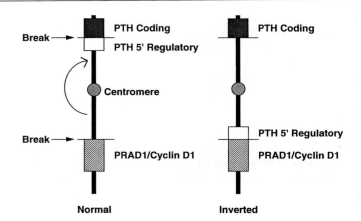

Figure 36-2 Schematic diagram illustrating the pericentromeric inversion of chromosome 11 deduced to have caused the observed rearrangement involving the *PTH* gene and the *PRAD1* gene in a subset of parathyroid adenomas. The tumor's other copy of chromosome 11, which contains an intact *PTH* gene, is not shown. (Reproduced with permission from Arnold A. Genetic basic of endocrine disease 5: molecular genetics of parathyroid gland neoplasia. J Clin Endocrinol Metab 1993;77: 1108–1112. Copyright 1993, The Endocrine Society.)

Monoclonality implies that the necessary accumulation of multiple mutations in a tumor progenitor cell occurs only rarely in a large population of cells within a tissue, conferring a selective growth advantage critical in tumor outgrowth or clonal evolution. The search for the specific oncogenes and tumor suppressor genes that are clonally activated or inactivated, respectively, in common sporadic parathyroid tumors is ongoing. Three notable successes and several important leads, described in the next section have emerged.

The clonal status of parathyroid tumors other than adenomas has also been investigated. As expected, parathyroid carcinomas are monoclonal. More surprisingly, however, a substantial percentage of parathyroid tumors in the setting of primary hyperplasia and severe secondary hyperparathyroidism of uremia are monoclonal, indicating that somatic mutations have given selected cells a growth advantage over their already hyperplastic neighbors. It is conceivable that the "conversion" from polyclonality to monoclonality may be a key factor in the increasing autonomy of PTH secretion that develops in many hemodialysis patients, making them refractory to conventional medical therapy. Future identification of the specific molecular culprits in such clonal outgrowths may lead to rational new therapy or preventive measures for this important clinical problem.

GENETIC DERANGEMENTS IN SPORADIC BENIGN PARATHYROID TUMORS

The Cyclin D1/PRAD1 Oncogene *Cyclin D1/PRAD1*, the only oncogene implicated in sporadic parathyroid neoplasia, was discovered by virtue of its proximity to a clonal chromosomal breakpoint in a subset of parathyroid adenomas. This chromosomal inversion causes overexpression of the *cyclin D1/PRAD1* gene by placing it in proximity to the strong tissue-specific enhancer of the *PTH* gene (Fig. 36-2). Cyclin D1 protein overexpression, resulting from gene rearrangement or other mechanisms, has been found in 20–40% of parathyroid adenomas. That such overexpression indeed causes parathyroid neoplasia has been experimentally validated by the demonstration of primary hyperparathyroidism in transgenic mice with parathyroid-targeted overexpression of cyclin D1. Cyclin D1 activation has also been incriminated in a variety of other human tumors, including B-cell lymphoma, breast, and esophageal cancers.

Cyclin D1/PRAD1 is recognized to have a crucial role in regulating progression through the G1 phase of the cell division cycle. To do so, the cyclin D1 protein is thought to act as an activating regulatory subunit for its partner cyclin-dependent kinase(s), cdk4 or cdk6. One action of active cdk4 or cdk6 may be phosphorylation of the retinoblastoma gene product pRB, moving the cell toward S phase, but this mechanism has not been established in parathyroid tissue.

TUMOR SUPPRESSOR GENES   Inactivation of both alleles of a tumor suppressor gene is typically necessary to adequately eliminate its antioncogenic product, and somatic deletion of a sometimes large stretch of DNA that includes the relevant gene is a common inactivating mechanism. Thus, identification of genomic regions that are clonally and nonrandomly lost in parathyroid adenomas can point to the locations of putative parathyroid tumor suppressor genes.

Of sporadic parathyroid adenomas, approx 25–35% contain allelic losses of chromosome 11 DNA, often (but not always) including the region containing the *MEN1* gene. This gene, responsible for familial multiple endocrine neoplasia type 1 (MEN1), was identified using positional cloning techniques (Chapter 39). Mutations in the affected individuals predict loss of function of the protein, indicating that *MEN1* is a tumor suppressor gene. The gene product, menin, is a 610-amino acid protein located in the nucleus, but the precise molecular mechanisms responsible for its tumor suppressor activity remain uncertain. In sporadic parathyroid tumors, not associated with familial MEN1, biallelic somatic mutations inactivating *MEN1* occur in 12–17%, or about half the tumors with allelic losses on 11q. It is not clear whether the tumor suppressor target in the remaining tumors with 11q loss is *MEN1* or a different gene in its vicinity. Mutation of another tumor suppressor gene, *HRPT2*, was identified as the cause of the rare autosomal-dominant hyperparathyroidism-jaw tumor (HPT-JT) syndrome, and somatic mutations in *HRPT2* have been reported in a few sporadic parathyroid adenomas. However, the rarity of these mutations stands in marked contrast to the high frequency of *HRPT2* mutations in parathyroid carcinoma (*see* Molecular Pathogenesis of Parathyroid Carcinoma). Finally, several other genomic regions of nonrandom clonal allelic loss in parathyroid adenomas highlight the locations of putative parathyroid tumor suppressor genes that remain unidentified, including 1p, 6q, 9p, and 15q. These data emphasize the molecular heterogeneity underlying parathyroid adenomatosis.

OTHER GENETIC ASPECTS   Some genes responsible for rare inherited predispositions to certain tumors have also proved important in more common, sporadic forms of the same tumors. The *MEN1* gene, as mentioned, is an example. The discovery of *RET* proto-oncogene germline mutation in MEN2a (Chapter 40) made this gene a candidate for involvement in nonfamilial hyperparathyroidism. However, studies have failed to document somatic *RET* mutations in sporadic parathyroid adenomas. Similarly, inactivating mutations of the extracellular CaR have been sought but not found in sporadic adenomas, although secondary changes in CaR expression may well be important in determining the tumors' altered sensitivity of PTH secretion to serum calcium. Finally, although the syndrome of familial isolated hyperparathyroidism can include phenotypic variants caused by germline mutations in *MEN1*, *CASR*, or *HRPT2*, additional genetic bases are likely to exist and, once identified, will be candidates for involvement in sporadic parathyroid tumors.

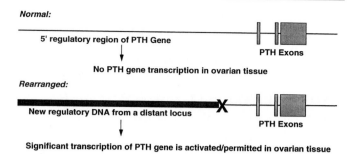

Figure 36-3   Molecular pathology of the ectopic production of PTH by an ovarian cancer. Schematic diagram of the normal *PTH* gene region (top) and the rearranged, amplified *PTH* gene region (bottom) in a PTH-secreting ovarian tumor. The bold "X" represents the breakpoint of the DNA rearrangement. (Reproduced with permission from Arnold A. Genetic basis of endocrine disease 5: molecular genetics of parathyroid gland neoplasia. J Clin Endocrinol Metab 1993;77:1108–1112.)

MOLECULAR PATHOGENESIS OF PARATHYROID CARCINOMA   Apart from distant metastasis and extensive local invasion, most histopathological features of parathyroid carcinoma can overlap with parathyroid adenoma. Molecular insights that distinguish between them are thus of potential diagnostic and therapeutic importance. Because parathyroid carcinoma is overrepresented in the rare hereditary HPT-JT syndrome, the *HRPT2* gene identified as responsible for this syndrome was examined as a candidate for involvement in sporadic parathyroid carcinoma. Inactivating mutations of *HRPT2* were found in the majority of parathyroid cancers, and because noncoding mutations would not have been detected in these analyses, *HRPT2* inactivation could be a factor in virtually all parathyroid cancers. Importantly, a subset of patients with apparently sporadic parathyroid carcinoma harbored unsuspected germline mutations of *HRPT2*, indicating that they may have HPT-JT or a phenotypic variant. The possibility of a familial disorder must be considered in any patient presenting with sporadic parathyroid carcinoma, and DNA diagnosis is being used for early diagnosis and treatment to prevent metastatic carcinoma in genetically susceptible family members.

Recurrent clonal alterations have been reported that strongly suggest the involvement and chromosomal locations of other genes important in malignant parathyroid neoplasia. For example, recurrent losses have highlighted a region on chromosome 13 as the site of at least one such tumor suppressor, still to be identified. Several additional locations of frequent clonal DNA losses or gains have been reported as well. Importantly, several genomic regions frequently lost in parathyroid adenomas, including 11q (location of *MEN1*), 6q, and 15q, are rarely if ever lost in carcinomas, suggesting that parathyroid carcinomas arise *de novo* rather than from preexisting adenomas. Cyclin D1 may be overexpressed in many parathyroid cancers but larger sample sizes are needed.

ECTOPIC SECRETION OF PTH

The ectopic secretion of PTH by nonparathyroid tumors is a rare cause of primary hyperparathyroidism. The molecular basis of ectopic PTH production in one such case, an ovarian carcinoma, was found to be a DNA rearrangement in the regulatory region of the tumor's *PTH* gene (Fig. 36-3). Similar detailed molecular pathology has not been described in other examples of human ectopic hormone excess, and might involve analogous DNA rearrangements or, alternatively, a change in the tumor tissue's characteristic DNA-binding proteins. Preliminary reports indicate that ectopic production of PTH in some neoplasms may be associated with expression of GCMB, which may induce transdifferentiation of neoplastic cells to a parathyroid cell-like phenotype.

SELECTED REFERENCES

Ahn TG, Antonarakis SE, Kronenberg HM, Igarashi T, Levine MA. Familial isolated hypoparathyroidism: a molecular genetic analysis of 8 families with 23 affected persons. Medicine 1986;65:73–81.

Arnold A. The cyclin D1/PRAD1 oncogene in human neoplasia. J Investig Med 1995;43:543–549.

Arnold A. Molecular basis of primary hyperparathyroidism. In: Bilezikian JP, Marcus R, Levine MA, eds. The Parathyroids, 2nd ed. San Diego, CA: Academic Press, 2001; pp. 331–347.

Arnold A, Horst SA, Gardella TJ, Baba H, Levine MA, Kronenberg HM. Mutation of the signal peptide-encoding region of the preproparathyroid hormone gene in familial isolated hypoparathyroidism. J Clin Invest 1990;86:1084–1087.

Baldini A. DiGeorge syndrome: an update. Curr Opin Cardiol 2004; 19:201–204.

Bowl MR, Nesbit MA, Harding B, et al. An interstitial deletion–insertion involving chromosomes 2p25.3 and Xq27.1, near SOX3, causes X-linked recessive hypoparathyroidism. J Clin Invest 2005;115:2822–2831.

Brown EM, Gamba G, Riccardi D, et al. Cloning and characterization of an extracellular Ca^{2+}-sensing receptor from bovine parathyroid. Nature 1993;366:575–580.

Carling T, Szabo E, Bai M, et al. Familial hypercalcemia and hypercalciuria caused by a novel mutation in the cytoplasmic tail of the calcium receptor. J Clin Endocrinol Metab 2000;85:2042–2047.

Carpten JD, Robbins CM, Villablanca A, et al. HRPT2, encoding parafibromin, is mutated in hyperparathyroidism-jaw tumor syndrome. Nat Genet 2002;32:676–680.

Chandrasekharappa SC, Guru SC, Manickam P, et al. Positional cloning of the gene for multiple endocrine neoplasia-type 1. Science 1997;276:404–407.

Chattopadhyay N, Mithal A, Brown EM. The calcium-sensing receptor: a window into the physiology and pathophysiology of mineral ion metabolism. Endocr Rev 1996;17:289–307.

Ding C, Buckingham B, Levine MA. Familial isolated hypoparathyroidism caused by a mutation in the gene for the transcription factor GCMB. J Clin Invest 2001;108:1215–1220.

Dotzenrath C, The BT, Farnebo F, et al. Allelic loss of the retinoblastoma tumor suppressor gene: a marker for aggressive parathyroid tumors? J Clin Endocrinol Metab 1996;81:3194–3196.

Gunther T, Chen ZF, Kim J, et al. Genetic ablation of parathyroid glands reveals another source of parathyroid hormone. Nature 2000;406: 199–203.

Hendy GN, D'Souza-Li L, Yang B, Canaff L, Cole DE. Mutations of the calcium-sensing receptor (CASR) in familial hypocalciuric hypercalcemia, neonatal severe hyperparathyroidism, and autosomal-dominant hypocalcemia. Hum Mutat 2000;16:281–296.

Krebs LJ, Shattuck TM, Arnold A. HRPT2 mutational analysis of typical sporadic parathyroid adenomas. J Clin Endocrinol Metab 2005;90: 5015–5017.

Kronenberg HM, Bringhurst FR, Segre GV, Potts JT Jr. Parathyroid hormone biosynthesis and metabolism. In: Bilezikian JP, Marcus R, Levine MA, eds. The Parathyroids, 2nd ed. San Diego, CA: Academic Press, 2001; pp. 17–30.

Motokura T, Bloom T, Kim HG, et al. A novel cyclin encoded by a bcl1-linked candidate oncogene. Nature 1991;350:512–515.

Parfitt AM. Parathyroid growth: normal and abnormal. In: Bilezikian JP, Marcus R, Levine MA, eds. The Parathyroids, 2nd edition. San Diego, CA: Academic Press, 2001; pp. 293–329.

Parkinson DB, Thakker RV. A donor splice site mutation in the parathyroid hormone gene is associated with autosomal-recessive hypoparathyroidism. Nat Genet 1992;1:149–153.

Pollak MR, Brown EM, Chou Y-HW, et al. Mutations in the human Ca^{2+}-sensing receptor gene cause familial hypocalciuric hypercalcemia and neonatal severe hyperparathyroidism. Cell 1993;75:1297–1303.

Pollak MR, Brown EM, Estep HL, et al. Autosomal-dominant hypocalcaemia caused by a Ca^{2+}-sensing receptor gene mutation. Nat Genet 1994;8:303–307.

Shattuck TM, Välimäki S, Obara T, et al. Somatic and germline mutations of the HRPT2 gene in sporadic parathyroid carcinoma. N Engl J Med 2003;349:1722–1729.

Sunthornthepvarakul T, Churesigaew S, Ngowngarmratana S. A novel mutation of the signal peptide of the preproparathyroid hormone gene associated with autosomal-recessive familial isolated hypoparathyroidism. J Clin Endocrinol Metab 1999;84:3792–3796.

Thakker RV. Molecular basis of PTH underexpression. In: Bilezikian JP, Raisz LG, Rodan GA, eds. Principles of Bone Biology, 2nd ed. San Diego, CA: Academic Press, 2002; pp. 1105–1116.

Van Esch H, Devriendt K. Transcription factor GATA3 and the human HDR syndrome. Cell Mol Life Sci 2001;58:1296–1300.

Yagi H, Furutani Y, Hamada H, et al. Role of TBX1 in human del22q11.2 syndrome. Lancet 2003;362:1366–1373.

Yamagishi H, Garg V, Matsuoka R, Thomas T, Srivastava D. A molecular pathway revealing a genetic basis for human cardiac and craniofacial defects. Science 1999;283:1158–1161.

37 Congenital Adrenal Hyperplasia

ROBERT C. WILSON AND MARIA I. NEW

SUMMARY

Congenital adrenal hyperplasia is a family of autosomal-recessive disorders caused by mutations that encode for enzymes involved in one of the various steps of adrenal steroid synthesis. This chapter discusses adrenal steroidogenesis, 21-hyroxylase deficiency, 11β-hydroxylase deficiency, 3β-hydroxysteroid dehydrogenase deficiency, 17α hydroxylase/17,20-lyase deficiency, lipoid congenital adrenal hyperplasia, and various treatments.

Key Words: Adrenal steroidogenesis; congenital adrenal hyperplasia (CAH); 3β-hydroxysteroid dehydrogenase deficiency; 11β-hydroxylase deficiency; 17α hydroxylase/17,20-lyase deficiency; 21-hydroxylase deficiency (21-OHD); lipoid congenital adrenal hyperplasia; salt wasting.

INTRODUCTION

Congenital adrenal hyperplasia (CAH) is a family of autosomal-recessive disorders caused by mutations that encode for enzymes involved in one of the various steps of adrenal steroid synthesis (Table 37-1). These defects result in the absence or the decreased synthesis of cortisol from its cholesterol precursor. The anterior pituitary secretes excess adrenocorticotropic hormone (ACTH) via feedback regulation by cortisol, which results in overstimulation of the adrenals and causes hyperplasia.

Symptoms owing to CAH can vary from mild to severe depending on the degree of the enzymatic defect. In the classical forms of CAH, defects in the cytochrome P450s 21-hydroxylase (21-OH) or 11β-hydroxylase (11β-OH) cause varying degrees of genital ambiguity in females owing to shunting of excess cortisol precursors to the androgen synthesis pathway (Fig. 37-1). Prenatal adrenal androgen excess causes virilization of female genitalia and postnatally results in advanced bone age and puberty in both females and males. Defects in androgen synthesis owing to defects in 3β-hydroxysteroid dehydrogenase (3β-HSD)/Δ^{5,4}-isomerase, in 17α-hydroxylase (17α-OH)/17,20-lyase, and in the steroidogenic acute regulatory protein (StAR) result in inadequate prenatal virilization of males and depressed puberty in both sexes. Less severe, nonclassical forms of CAH present postnatally as signs of androgen excess.

ADRENAL STEROIDOGENESIS

Aldosterone, cortisol (compound F) and testosterone are derived from cholesterol and utilize many of the same enzymes for their synthesis in the adrenal cortex (see Fig. 37-1). Therefore, defects in any of the enzymes that are common to the synthesis pathway of these hormones can result in the loss of a combination of some or all of their production.

Cortisol and aldosterone are synthesized in distinct zones of the adrenal cortex called the zona fasciculata and zona glomerulosa (ZG), respectively. Synthesis of these hormones is regulated by different mechanisms: cortisol synthesis is regulated by a negative feedback loop in which high serum levels of cortisol inhibit the release of ACTH from the pituitary, whereas low serum levels of cortisol stimulate the release of ACTH. This defines the hypothalamic–pituitary–adrenal axis (Fig. 37-2). Aldosterone, a hormone required for the regulation of sodium reabsorption across the tight epithelium of the renal distal tubule, controls fluid volume and is regulated by the renin-angiotensin system and by serum potassium. Angiotensin II (a potent vasoconstrictor) directly stimulates the secretion of aldosterone by the ZG when there is a reduction in renal perfusion resulting from an increase in plasma renin. Serum potassium also regulates the synthesis of aldosterone, though independently of volume status.

21-HYDROXYLASE DEFICIENCY

Over 90% of cases with classical CAH are because of 21-hydroxylase deficiency (21-OHD). There are three forms of this syndrome: classical salt wasting, classical simple virilizing, and nonclassical.

CLASSICAL SIMPLE VIRILIZING Fetal adrenocortical function begins in the third month of gestation. At this time, reduction or loss of 21-OH activity results in the buildup of 17α-hydroxyprogesterone (17-OHP). Because 17-OHP is a precursor of testosterone, elevated levels of 17-OHP are shunted to the androgen pathway, thus producing excess androgens. This excess adrenal androgen production coincides with the time of sexual development of the fetus and results in varying degrees of genital ambiguity in newborn females. In extreme cases, the urethra extends the full length of the phallus and cannot be distinguished from that of a normal male. In most cases, however, the excess androgens result in an enlarged clitoris with fusion of the labioscrotal folds; it can also result in a urogenital sinus. For these females, the internal genitalia are normal with normal development of ovaries and Müllerian structures.

Males affected with 21-OHD are born with normal genitalia. After birth, both females and males develop signs of androgen excess such as precocious development of pubic and axillary hair,

From: *Principles of Molecular Medicine, Second Edition*
Edited by: M. S. Runge and C. Patterson © Humana Press, Inc., Totowa, NJ

Table 37-1
The Forms of Adrenal Hyperplasia

Deficiency	Syndrome	Ambiguous genitalia	Postnatal virilization	Salt metabolism	Steroids increased	Steroids decreased	Chromosomal location
StAR	Lipoid hyperplasia	Males		No salt wasting	None	All	8p11.2
3β-Hydroxysteroid dehydrogenase	Classical	Males	Yes	Salt wasting	DHEA, 17-OH-pregnenolone	Aldo, T, cortisol	1p13.1
	Nonclassical	No	Yes	Normal	DHEA, 17-OH-pregnenolone	–	
17α-Hydroxylase	——	Males	No	Hypertension	DOC, cortico-sterone	Cortisol, T	10q24-25
21-Hydroxylase	Salt wasting	Females	Yes	Salt wasting	17-OHP, Δ^4-A	Aldo, cortisol	6p21.3
	Simple virilizing	Females	Yes	Normal	17-OHP, Δ^4-A	Cortisol	6p21.3
	Nonclassic	No	Yes	Normal	17-OHP, Δ^4-A	——	6p21.3
11β-Hydroxylase	Classical	Females	Yes	Hypertension	DOC, 11-deoxycortisol	Cortisol, ± aldo	8q21-22
	Nonclassical	No	Yes	Normal	11-deoxycortisol, ± DOC	——	8q21-22
Corticosterone methyl oxidase type II	Salt wasting	No	No	Salt wasting	18-OH-corticosterone	Aldo	8q21-22

Aldo, adosterone; T, testosterone; Δ^4-A, Δ^4-androstenedione; DHEA, dehydroepiandrosterone; DOC, 11-deoxycorticosterone; 17-OHP, 17α-hydroxyprogesterone

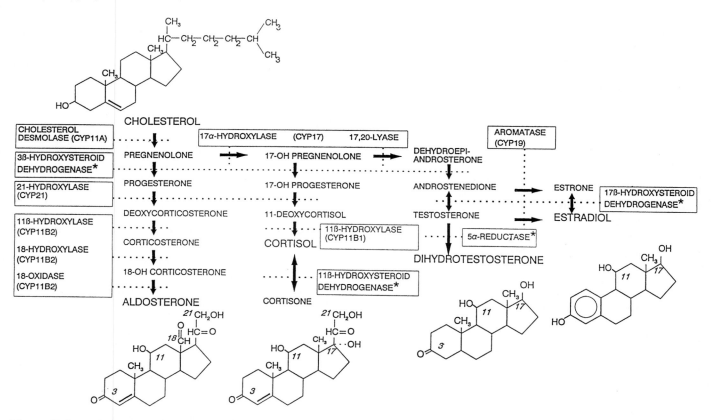

Figure 37-1 Pathways of steroid biosynthesis. Enzymatic activities catalyzing each bioconversion are enclosed in boxes. For activities mediated by specific P450 cytochromes, systematic names of the enzymes ("CYP" followed by number) are listed in parentheses. Other bioconversions (*) are mediated by different enzymes in various tissues. The planar structures of cholesterol, aldosterone, cortisol, dihydrotestosterone, and estradiol are placed near the corresponding labels.

acne, phallic enlargement, rapid growth, and musculoskeletal development. Though initial growth in these patients is rapid, because of premature epiphyseal fusion, potential height is reduced and short adult stature results. Diagnosis may be delayed in males,

as the genital ambiguity that leads to diagnosis at birth in females is absent in males. Even if diagnosis is not delayed and adrenal androgen excess is controlled, patients do not generally achieve their target height.

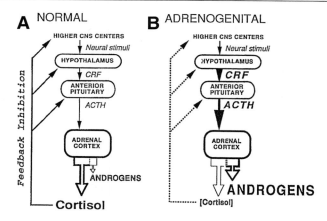

Figure 37-2 Feedback in the hypothalamic–pituitary–axis in (**A**) the normal individual and (**B**) the patient with classical CAH, formerly known as "adrenogenital syndrome."

CLASSICAL SALT WASTING Salt-wasting 21-OHD makes up approx 75% of cases with classical 21-OHD. Depending on the severity of the loss of 21-OH function, adrenal aldosterone secretion may not be sufficient for regulating sodium reabsorption by distal renal tubules. Patients with insufficient aldosterone can suffer from salt-wasting 21-OHD. These patients exhibit the same symptoms as those with simple virilizing 21-OHD but with the potential of adrenal crisis (azotemia, vascular collapse, shock, and death) because of renal salt wasting. Adrenal crisis can occur as early as 1–4 wk of life. Although salt-wasting 21-OHD females may be diagnosed at birth owing to ambiguous genitalia, affected males are at high risk of salt-wasting adrenal crisis because their normal genitalia do not make the condition obvious.

NONCLASSICAL Nonclassical 21-hydroxylase deficiency (NC21-OHD) may present at any time, in childhood, adolescence, or adulthood. Symptoms of NC21-OHD may include acne, premature development of pubic hair, advanced bone age, accelerated linear growth velocity, and as in classical 21-OHD, reduced adult stature owing to premature epiphyseal fusion. Symptoms have been observed to wax and wane.

Females affected with NC21-OHD are born with normal genitalia, though postnatal symptoms may include hirsutism, temporal baldness, severe cystic acne, delayed menarche, menstrual irregularities, and infertility. A subset of female patients with NC21-OHD develops polycystic ovaries.

Boys manifesting NC21-OHD may have early beard growth, acne, early growth spurt, premature pubic hair, and an enlarged phallus. Proportionately small testes as compared with the phallus is a reliable indication of adrenal androgen excess as opposed to testicular androgen excess. Adrenal androgen excess in men is not easily detectable and may only be manifested by short stature or oligozoospermia and diminished fertility.

A limited number of males and females who are affected with NC21-OHD remain asymptomatic, as discovered during family studies. However, biochemically such patients compare to affected individuals.

EPIDEMIOLOGY Newborn screening worldwide of nearly 6.5 million babies has demonstrated an overall incidence of 1:15,000 live births for the classical form of 21-OHD. However, in two isolates the frequency is much higher (Yup'ik Eskimos in Alaska, 1/282, and the inhabitants of La Réunion island in France, 1/2141). The incidence of classical CAH in either homogenous or heterogenous general populations is as high as 1/7500 live births (Brazil).

It has been suggested that NC21-OHD is the most common autosomal-recessive disorder. In some ethnic populations, the frequency of NC21-OHD is so high it is regarded to be the most frequent autosomal-recessive defect. The highest ethnic-specific disease frequency was found among Ashkenazi Jews at 1/27. Other ethnic-specific frequencies were found to be 1/53 for Hispanics, 1/63 for Yugoslavs, 1/100 in a heterogeneous New York City population, and 1/333 for Italians.

MOLECULAR GENETICS In 1977, molecular genetic studies of 21-OHD showed linkage with certain human leukocyte antigens (HLA), the human major histocompatibility complex, on the short arm of chromosome 6. For many years, HLA linkage was used for establishing the affected status in family studies. However, in some cases in which the parents shared the same HLA antigens, or if intra-HLA recombination occurred, HLA typing was not diagnostic.

The gene for 21-OH, cloned in 1984, is termed *CYP21*, following the nomenclature for cytochrome P450. Southern blot analysis determined that the *CYP21* gene was located within the serum complement component *C4*. This region of chromosome was duplicated, resulting in two isoforms of *C4* (*C4A* and *C4B*) and what initially looked like two isoforms of *CYP21*. Sequence analysis of the two *CYP21* genes revealed that one isoform contained a sequence that on translation resulted in a truncated nonfunctional protein, and it was therefore termed *CYP21P* for pseudogene. The nonfunctionality of *CYP21P* was confirmed in families without any hormonal abnormalities in which the CYP21P gene was completely missing.

CYP21 and *CYP21P* are 96–98% homologous (Fig. 37-3) and are arranged in tandem within C4A and C4B, separated by approx 30 kb. The duplication of the locus containing *CYP21* allows for misalignment of chromatids during meiosis, resulting in unequal crossing over. This results in a high frequency of deletions of the *CYP21* and *C4B* genes. Duplications also occur, but without any clinical consequence. Deletions of *CYP21* are found in approx 20% of the patients with classical 21-OHD.

CYP21 and *CYP21P* consist of 10 exons spanning approx 5 kb. Most of the 21-OHD patients carry mutations found in *CYP21P* (Fig. 37-4). The generally accepted mechanism by which these deleterious mutations are transferred to the active *CYP21* gene

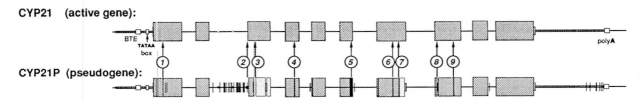

Figure 37-3 The two homologues: *CYP21* (the active gene) and *CYP21P* (the pseudogene). Noncorrespondent bases number less than 90 over a distance of 5.1 kb of DNA. Numbered are the pseudogene base changes frequently identified on mutant *CYP21* genes responsible for 21-OHD through an apparent process termed gene conversion. (1) Missense mutation Pro-30 to Leu. (2) Point mutation in intron 2 causes new acceptor 3′-site to be recognized by intron splicing mechanism. (3) Eight basepair deletion shifts the reading frame. (4) Missense mutation Ile-172 to Asn. (5) Cluster of three nonconservative amino acid substitutions. (6) Conservative amino acid substitution Val-281 to Leu. (7) Single-base T insert shifts reading frame. (8) Nonsense mutation Gln to TAG. (9) Radical amino acid substitution (Arg-356 to Trp). KEY: BTE, basic transcriptional element; large boxes/line spaces, exons/introns (to scale); light shading, out-of-frame coding; half-height open boxes, stop codons; vertical lines not numbered, neutral amino acid polymorphisms; half-height vertical lines, silent mutations.

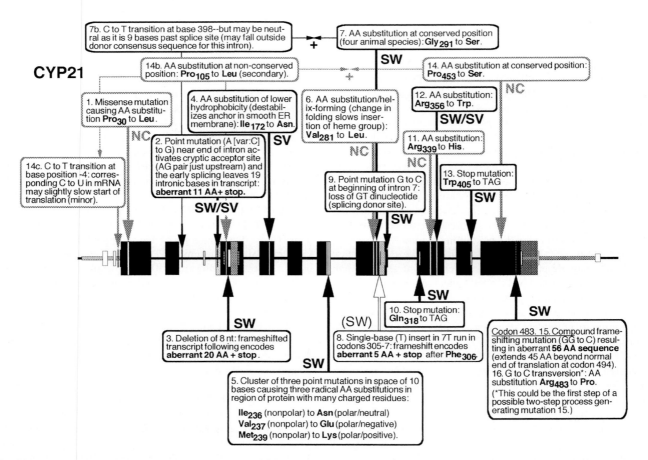

Figure 37-4 Mutations in the 21-hydroxylase gene (CYP21). CAH phenotypes: SW, salt wasting; SV, simple virilizing; NC, nonclassical.

from the homologous position in *CYP21P* is through gene conversion. Nine of these mutations can be transferred to the active *CYP21* gene. Four of these mutations result in truncated proteins owing to premature termination of translation and are associated with the salt-wasting phenotype: (1) a point mutation in the second intron near the 3′ splice site results in aberrant splicing of 13 nucleotides upstream of the normal splice site; (2) in the third exon, an eight base deletion can occur, resulting in nonsense amino acids and the occurrence of a stop codon 20 amino acids toward the carboxyterminus; (3) in exon 7, one T nucleotide can be inserted into a run of seven T nucleotides, resulting in a frameshift that produces five aberrant amino acids and premature termination; and (4) a

point mutation in exon 8 in codon 318 changes a glutamine to a stop codon. The five other mutations that can be transferred from *CYP21P* to *CYP21* result in amino acid substitutions.

1. A point mutation in exon 1 causes a substitution of proline by a leucine at codon 30 (P30L). This mutation had 30–60% of the activity of normal 21-OH when expressed in cell culture. The P30L mutation has been found to be associated with the nonclassical phenotype.
2. A point mutation in exon 4 causes a substitution of isoleucine by an asparagine at codon 172 (I172N) and is most often associated with the simple virilizing phenotype.

Table 37-2
Mutations Causing CAH

Exon/Intron	Mutation	NT/Mutation	AA	Phenotype
	30-kb deletion			SW
Ex 1	Missense	89 CΔT	P30L	NC
Int 2	Aberrant splicing of intron 2	656 A [or C] ΔG		SW, SV
Ex 3	Frameshift	Δ708–715	G110Δ8nt	SW
Ex 4	Missense	1001 TΔA	I172N	SV
Ex 6	Cluster	1382 TΔA 1385 TΔA 1391 TΔA	I236N, V237E, M239K	SW
Ex 7	Missense	1685 GΔT	V281L	NC
Int 7	Loss of splice donor site	1781 GΔC		SW
Ex 8	Nonsense	1996 CΔT	Q318X	SW
Ex 8	Missense	2060 GΔA	R339H	NC
Ex 8	Missense	2110 CΔT	R356W	SW
Ex 10	Missense	2580 CΔT	P453S	NC
Ex 10	Missense	2672 GΔC	R483P	SW

Ex, exon; Int, intron; Δ, deletion; SW, salt-wasting; SV, simple virilizing; NC, nonclassical; NT, nucleotide.

This mutation results in <2% of normal 21-OH activity in in vitro expression studies.

3. A cluster mutation in exon 6 resulting from the exchange of four nucleotides results in three amino acid substitutions and one polymorphism (the change codes for the original amino acid).

4. A point mutation in codon 281 substitutes a valine with a leucine (V281L). This mutation is associated with the nonclassical phenotype. Expression studies of the V281L mutation show 20-50% of normal 21-OH activity.

5. A point mutation in exon 8 results in the substitution of arginine with tryptophan (R356W). This mutation is associated with the salt-wasting phenotype.

Assignment of a phenotype to each of the individual mutation was done with patients that were either homozygous for the mutation or hemizygous for the mutation (the other allele had undergone a deletion). In addition to the nine mutations found in the pseudogene, several other mutations have been described in patients affected with 21-OHD. The most common mutations of *CYP21* are listed in Table 37-2, over 100 mutations in the CYP21 gene have been identified. A complete list of mutations may be viewed on the World Wide Web.

HORMONAL DIAGNOSIS Baseline serum concentrations of 17-OHP are diagnostic of classical 21-OHD. The best method for hormonal diagnosis of 21-OHD is comparing baseline serum 17-OHP concentration and serum 17-OHP concentrations following adrenal stimulation by administration of synthetic ACTH (Cortrosyn). In NC21-OHD diagnosis is made during the diurnal peak of cortisol production, as serum 17-OHP concentrations are elevated, though random basal serum concentrations may not differ from that of normal. Nomogram plots of baseline vs stimulated 17-OHP concentrations result in three distinguishable groups (Fig. 37-5): Patients with classical 21-OHD have the highest coordinates, followed by patients with NC21-OHD, followed by plots of heterozygotes and genetically unaffected individuals, which overlap and cannot be distinguished.

Newborn diagnostic screening for CAH has been instituted in approx 44 states (http://genes-r-us.uthscsa.edu). On day 2 or 3 of life, blood from a heel prick is spotted onto filter paper and is tested for 17-OHP levels by radioimmunoassay. In adults, NC21-OHD can also be screened by measuring morning salivary 17-OHP,

which correlates well with serum concentrations. It should be noted that serum 17-OHP may be elevated in premature infants and infants under stress, which can result in false positives.

PRENATAL DIAGNOSIS AND TREATMENT Prenatal diagnosis of 21-OHD has been performed for several decades. Originally, second trimester amniotic fluid was tested for elevated 17-OHP levels. However, in most cases when the fetus is a nonsalt waster, simple virilizer, or nonclassical, amnionic fluid 17-OHP levels are not elevated.

When HLA was found to be linked to 21-OHD, prenatal diagnoses using HLA serotyping of cultured fetal cells from amniocytes were performed. This procedure resulted in errors because of recombination or haplotype sharing between parents. Once mutations in CYP21 were identified, direct molecular analysis could be performed more accurately, and more effective prenatal diagnosis became possible. This technique requires fetal DNA derived from either cultured amniocytes or from cultured fetal cells obtained via chorionic villus sampling. Southern blot analysis is used to detect large gene deletions whereas allele-specific polymerase chain reaction is performed to detect the nine most common mutations. This technique allows for prenatal diagnosis within several days.

Prenatal treatment (Fig. 37-6) of female fetuses affected with 21-OHD can greatly reduce or prevent virilization of the external genitalia, avoiding the need for genital surgery and possible sex misassignment. To achieve this outcome, prenatal treatment must be initiated before the ninth week of gestation (ideally by the seventh week). Oral dexamethasone (20 μg/kg/d) is conventionally given in daily divided doses to mothers at-risk, without knowing the sex or affected status of the fetus. Dexamethasone is used because it crosses the placenta, crossing from maternal to fetal circulation, and thus suppresses fetal adrenal androgen secretion. Depending on which procedure is available, either chorionic villus sampling (10–12 wk of gestation) or amniocentesis (15–18 wk of gestation) is performed. Fetal cells are cultured for karyotyping and DNA analysis. If the fetus is male or the fetus is an unaffected female, prenatal treatment is terminated. Prenatal treatment is continued to term for affected female fetuses.

Maternal side effects owing to prenatal dexamethasone treatment can include mood changes, weight gain, pedal and leg edema, striae, elevated blood pressure, and general discomfort. However, the majority of these side effects disappear on discontinuation of treatment. Furthermore, owing to the proven benefits

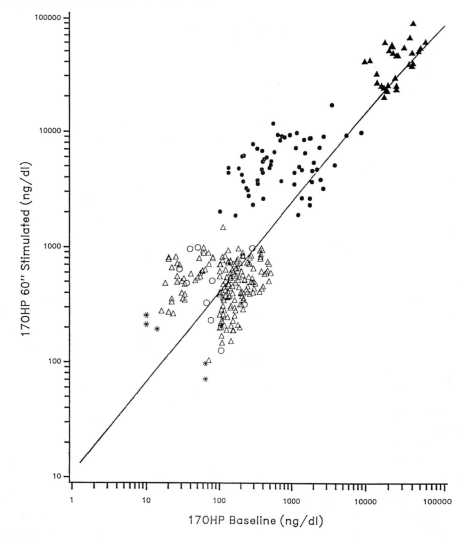

Figure 37-5 Nomogram relating baseline to ACTHstimulated serum concentrations of 17-hydroxyprogesterone. The scales are logarithmic. A regression line for all data points is shown. *, Genetically unaffected. Patients with: ▲, classical CAH; ●, nonclassical CAH. Heterozygotes for: Δ, classical CAH; ○, nonclassical CAH. (The data for this nomogram were collected from 1982–1991 at the Department of Pediatrics, The York Hospital, Cornell Medical Center, New York, NY 10021.)

of prenatal therapy, the majority of mothers, including those who developed side effects, reported that they would repeat therapy during a future pregnancy. In an ongoing study of over 600 pregnancies, in which over 300 received dexamethasone therapy, no enduring side effects have been reported in mothers and their offspring as compared to controls. In a different study, some patients have been followed in excess of 20 yr of age without reported side effects.

11B-HYDROXYLASE DEFICIENCY

Patients with 11β-hydroxylase deficiency (11β-OHD) are unable to convert 11-deoxycortisol (compound S) to cortisol. 11β-OHD is the second most common cause of CAH, representing 5–8% of all cases. The frequency of 11β-OHD is in the order of 1 in 100,000 births in Caucasians. As with 21-OHD, cases of mild, late-onset forms of 11β-OHD also have been reported.

As in 21-OHD, 11β-OHD results in shunting of excess 17-OHP to the androgen pathway, causing prenatal virilization of external genitalia in affected females at birth. Also, as in 21-OHD, both

males and females undergo premature virilization, resulting in precocious adrenarche and premature epiphyseal closure.

Patients with 11β-OHD also have a defective 17-deoxysteroid pathway. In 11β-OHD, 11-deoxycorticosterone (DOC) cannot be converted to corticosterone, which is eventually converted to aldosterone. In most cases, owing to their mineralocorticoid activity, elevated serum levels of DOC and its metabolites induce hypokalemia with metabolic alkalosis and hypertension. High levels of serum S and DOC, and their corresponding urinary tetrahydrometabolites, are diagnostic of 11β-OHD.

MOLECULAR GENETICS The genes that encode the two known isoforms of 11β-OH in humans are CYP11B1 and CYP11B2, located on chromosome 8, region q21-22, and separated by 30 kb. These isozymes have 93% identity between their amino acid sequences. CYP11B1 is highly expressed in all zones of the adrenal cortex and is regulated by ACTH. CYP11B2 is expressed in the ZG under the control of angiotensin II and potassium ion. Mutations in the CYP11B1 gene are responsible for 11β-OHD (Table 37-3).

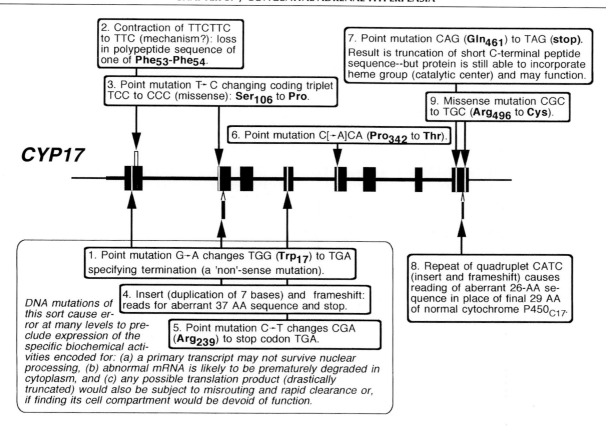

CYP17

2. Contraction of TTCTTC to TTC (mechanism?): loss in polypeptide sequence of one of **Phe$_{53}$-Phe$_{54}$**.

3. Point mutation T→C changing coding triplet TCC to CCC (missense): **Ser$_{106}$** to **Pro**.

6. Point mutation C[-A]CA (**Pro$_{342}$** to **Thr**).

7. Point mutation CAG (**Gln$_{461}$**) to TAG (**stop**). Result is truncation of short C-terminal peptide sequence--but protein is still able to incorporate heme group (catalytic center) and may function.

9. Missense mutation CGC to TGC (**Arg$_{496}$** to **Cys**).

1. Point mutation G→A changes TGG (**Trp$_{17}$**) to TGA specifying termination (a 'non'-sense mutation).

4. Insert (duplication of 7 bases) and frameshift: reads for aberrant 37 AA sequence and stop.

5. Point mutation C→T changes CGA (**Arg$_{239}$**) to stop codon TGA.

8. Repeat of quadruplet CATC (insert and frameshift) causes reading of aberrant 26-AA sequence in place of final 29 AA of normal cytochrome P450$_{C17}$.

DNA mutations of this sort cause error at many levels to preclude expression of the specific biochemical activities encoded for: (a) a primary transcript may not survive nuclear processing, (b) abnormal mRNA is likely to be prematurely degraded in cytoplasm, and (c) any possible translation product (drastically truncated) would also be subject to misrouting and rapid clearance or, if finding its cell compartment would be devoid of function.

Figure 37-9 Mutations in the 17α-hydroxylase/17,20-lyase deficiency gene (*CYP17*).

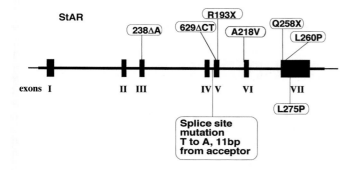

StAR

238ΔA   629ΔCT   R193X   A218V   Q258X   L260P   L275P

exons I   II   III   IV   V   VI   VII

Splice site mutation T to A, 11bp from acceptor

Figure 37-10 Mutations in the StAR gene.

adrenal androgens. Hydrocortisone (cortisol) is the most often used compound for replacement therapy in 21-OH, 11β-OH and 17α-OH deficiencies. Proper replacement therapy in 21-OHD and 11β-OHD ameliorates the effects of oversecretion of adrenal androgens, thus preventing further virilization, slowing accelerated growth and bone age advancement to a more normal rate, and allowing a normal onset of puberty. In 11β-OHD and 17α-OH deficiency, glucocorticoid treatment suppresses the oversecretion of DOC, leading to the remission of hypertension. Excessive glucocorticoid administration can cause cushingoid facies, growth retardation, and inhibition of epiphyseal maturation.

Hydrocortisone is the physiological hormone and therefore minimizes complications. Oral administration is the usual mode of treatment, conventionally given daily in divided doses. It is believed that divided doses better suppress the production of adrenal androgens.

Hydrocortisone given in two equally divided doses of 10–20 mg/m^2 daily is adequate for the otherwise healthy child. The dosage may have to be increased for a few days to two to three times that of the normal daily dosage during times of non-life-threatening illness or stress. Families are given injection kits of hydrocortisone (50 mg for young children; 100 mg for older patients) for times of emergency. Up to 5–10 times the daily dosage may be required during surgical procedures.

Patients who show a poor response to the standard dosage of hydrocortisone may have their dosage increased to 20–30 mg/m^2/d or their regimen may have to be changed to a synthetic hormone analog such as prednisone or dexamethasone. The use of these analogs requires critical dosage adjustment because they are more potent and longer acting.

Patients with salt-wasting CAH may also require mineralocorticoid replacement. A cortisol analog, 21-acetyloxy-9α-fluorohydrocortisone (Florinef: 9α-FF), is used for its potent mineralocorticoid activity. A combination of hydrocortisone and Florinef has proven effective in treatment of patients with salt-wasting 21-OHD.

In simple virilizing patients, it is common to find elevated PRA resulting from the interaction of the renin–angiotensin–aldosterone system and the hypothalamopituitary–adrenal axis. Florinef given in these cases reduces the plasma renin activity (PRA) which in turn further lowers ACTH levels and results in better control of androgens without increasing the glucocorticoid dose.

Patients with NC21-OHD and nonclassical 3β-HSD deficiency are treated with low doses of dexamethasone. Excess ovarian androgen production may have to be suppressed by the use of progestational and estrogenic agents, by suppression of the release of gonadotrophin. Other anti-androgen agents that may help include spironolactone and cyproterone acetate, and the androgen receptor blocker, flutamide. The aim of treatment in these patients is to minimize symptoms without giving rise to glucocorticoid side effects.

In LCAH, as all steroidogenic enzymes are normal, a substrate for steroidogenesis can be used for effective treatment of patients. Freely diffusable 20α-hydroxycholesterol is recommended, which must be implemented as a lifelong treatment plan. Successful continuing management of a patient for 18 yr was reported in 1985 using replacement glucocorticoids and mineralocorticoids in physiological doses, and estrogen replacement induced a pubertal growth spurt.

FUTURE DIRECTIONS

For many diseases reasonably well defined clinically, genetically, and molecularly, there remain a number of cases that demonstrate genotype–phenotype nonconcordance. In these cases, patients present with clinical signs that are not predicted by the genotype. Specifically, steroid 21-OH is being studied to elucidate the extent and reasons for discordance. As the mechanism for this phenomenon remains elusive, future studies should investigate the promoter and regulatory areas of the 21-OH gene. The surrounding genes may play a role in altering gene expression, though the different phenotypes of mutation-identical sibs casts doubt on this explanation. Activity of transcription factors, transport proteins, and other modifiers must also be studied.

ACKNOWLEDGMENT

We wish to express our appreciation to Brian Betensky for his editorial assistance in preparing this manuscript.

SELECTED REFERENCES

Bongiovanni AM. Congenital adrenal hyperplasia due to 3beta-hydroxysteroid dehydrogenase deficiency. In: New MI, Levine LS, eds. Adrenal Disease in Childhood, Pediatric and Adolescent Endocrinology, Volume 13. Basel: S Karger, 1984; pp. 72–82.

Forest MG, David M, Morel Y. Prenatal diagnosis and treatment of 21-hydroxylase deficiency. J Steroid Biochem Mol Biol 1993;45:75–82.

Kater CE, Biglieri EG. Disorders of steroid 17α-hydroxylase deficiency. Endocrinol Metab Clinic North Am 1994;23:341–357.

Cooper DN, Ball EV, Stenson PD. The human gene mutation database. University of Wales College of Medicine. http://www.hgmd.org/. June 23, 2004.

http://archive.uwcm.ac.uk/uwcm/mg/hgmd0.html2004
http://www.hgmd.org/2004

Lin D, Sugawara T, Strauss JF III, et al. The molecular basis of congenital lipoid adrenal hyperplasia. Pediatr Res 1995;37:545/93A.

Mornet E, Crete P, Kuttenn F, et al. Distribution of deletions and seven point mutations on CYP21B genes in three clinical forms of steroid 21-hydroxylase deficiency. Am J Hum Genet 1991;48:79–88.

New MI, Crawford C. Molecular genetics of steroid 21-hydroxylase deficiency. In: Wachtel S, ed. Molecular Genetics of Sex Determination. New York: Academic Press, 1994; pp. 399–438.

New MI, White PC. Genetic disorders of steroid metabolism. In: Thakker R, ed. Genetic and Molecular Biological Aspects of Endocrine Disease. London: Bailliere Tindall, 1995; pp. 525–554.

New MI, Wilson RC. Inaugural article: Steroid disorders in children: congenital adrenal hyperplasia and apparent mineralocorticoid excess. Proc Natl Acad Sci USA 1999;96:12,790–12,797.

New MI, Crawford C, Wilson RC. Genetic disorders of the adrenal gland. In: Rimoin DL, Connor JM, Pyeritz RE, eds. Principles and Practice of Medical Genetics, 3rd ed. New York: Churchill Livingstone, 1996; pp. 1441–1476.

New MI, Carlson A, Obeid J, et al. Update on prenatal diagnosis for congenital adrenal hyperplasia in 532 pregnancies. J Clin Endocrinol Metab 2001;86:5651–5657.

Pang S, Clark A. Congenital adrenal hyperplasia due to 21-hydroxylase deficiency: newborn screening and its relationship to the diagnosis and treatment of the disorder. Screening 1993;2:105–139.

Sparkes RS, Kilsak I, Miller WL. Regional mapping of genes encoding human steroidogenic enzymes: P450scc to 15q23-q24, adrenodoxin reductase to 17q24-q25; and P450c17 to 10q24-q25. DNA Cell Biol 1991;10:359–365.

Speiser PW, Dupont J, Zhu D, et al. Disease expression and molecular genotype in congenital adrenal hyperplasia due to 21-hydroxylase deficiency. J Clin Invest 1992;90:584–595.

Stocco DM, Clark BJ. Role of the steroidogenic acute regulatory protein (StAR) in steroidogenesis. Biochem Pharmacol 1996;51:197–295.

Wajnrajch JP, New MI. Defects of adrenal steroidogenesis. In: DeGroot LJ, Jameson JL, eds. Endocrinology, 4th ed. Philadelphia: Saunders, 2001; pp. 1721–1739.

White PC, Curnow KM, Pascoe L. Disorders of steroid 11beta-hydroxylase isozymes. Endocr Rev 1994;15:421–438.

White PC, Speiser PW. Congenital adrenal hyperplasia due to 21-hydroxylase deficiency. Endocr Rev 2000;21:245–291.

White PC, New MI, Dupont J. Structure of human steroid 21-hydroxylase genes. Proc Natl Acad Sci USA 1986;83:5111–5115.

Wilson RC, Mercado AB, Cheng KC, New MI. Steroid 21-hydroxylase deficiency: genotype may not predict phenotype. J Clin Endocrinol Metab 1995;80:2322–2329.

Yanase T, Simpson ER, Waterman MR. 17α-hydroxylase/17,20-lyase deficiency: from clinical investigation to molecular definition. Endocr Rev 1991;12:91–108.

Zerah M, Schram P, New MI. The diagnosis and treatment of nonclassical 3beta-HSD deficiency. Endocrinologist 1991;1:75–81.

38 Adrenal Diseases

RICHARD J. AUCHUS, WILLIAM E. RAINEY, AND KEITH L. PARKER

SUMMARY

The adrenal cortex play key roles in regulating intermediary metabolism, fluid and electrolyte balance, and the response to stress. Molecular analyses of specific disorders resulting from either the diminished or enhanced production/action of corticosteroids have led to the identification of a number of genes that play key roles in adrenal function and corticosteroid action. These genes provide potential targets for novel therapies that may revolutionize our approaches to these rare adrenal diseases. In addition, understanding the molecular causes of these diseases has provided important insights into basic adrenal functions that may translate into improved therapy of more common disorders such as hypertension and obesity.

Key Words: ACTH receptor; adrenocorticotrophic hormone (ACTH); adrenal cortex; glucocorticoids; glucocorticoid receptor; hypertension; mineralocorticoids; hypothalamic-pituitary-adrenal axis; mineralocorticoid receptor; stress; zonation.

INTRODUCTION

Thomas Addison first described the essential role of the adrenal glands for human survival in 1855, and Brown-Séquard confirmed this essential role in adrenalectomized experimental animals 1 yr later. Subsequent studies led to the concept that the basic function of the adrenal glands is to protect the organism against acute and chronic stress, popularized as the "fight-or-flight" response for the medulla and the "alarm" reaction for the cortex. Although the adrenal gland includes two functionally distinct compartments—the outer cortex that makes steroid hormones and the inner medulla that makes catecholamines—it is the cortical steroids that are essential for life. In contrast, disorders of both the adrenal cortex and the medulla cause disease states because of excess hormone production. This chapter reviews advances in understanding the molecular pathogenesis of genetic diseases associated with impaired production or action of adrenocortical steroids.

GENERALIZED GLUCOCORTICOID RESISTANCE

Generalized glucocorticoid resistance (GGR) is a rare disorder characterized by elevated circulating cortisol levels and the absence of most stigmata of glucocorticoid excess. Because glucocorticoids are crucial regulators of the central nervous system,

From: *Principles of Molecular Medicine, Second Edition*
Edited by: M. S. Runge and C. Patterson © Humana Press, Inc., Totowa, NJ

intermediary metabolism, cardiovascular function, inflammation, and immunity, a complete abrogation of glucocorticoid action in human beings presumably is incompatible with life, as is supported by the early postnatal death of knockout mice lacking the glucocorticoid receptor (GR) that mediates most actions of glucocorticoids. Thus, the described syndromes of GGR encompass partial glucocorticoid resistance resulting from GR defects.

CLINICAL FEATURES AND DIAGNOSIS Glucocorticoid production is tightly regulated by complex, reciprocal interactions among the hypothalamus, anterior pituitary, and adrenal cortex, collectively termed the hypothalamic–anterior pituitary–adrenal (HPA) axis (Fig. 38-1). A critical component of HPA function is negative feedback inhibition. Normally, glucocorticoids act via GR to diminish both the hypothalamic secretion of corticotropin-releasing hormone and the pituitary secretion of corticotropin (adrenocorticotropic hormone [ACTH]). The resulting decrease in ACTH secretion removes the major stimulus to glucocorticoid synthesis by the adrenal cortex, thereby permitting precise regulation of cortisol levels.

In the setting of partial loss of GR function, levels of cortisol that normally mediate feedback inhibition fail to suppress completely the HPA axis, which resets to a higher level because of compensatory increases in ACTH and cortisol secretion. Because the GR defect is partial, adequate compensation for the end-organ insensitivity apparently is achieved by the elevated concentration of cortisol in circulation; however, the excess ACTH secretion also stimulates the production of adrenal steroids with salt-retaining (e.g., corticosterone, deoxycorticosterone, cortisol) or androgenic (e.g., androstenedione and dehydroepiandrosterone) activities (*see* Fig. 38-1). Because the mineralocorticoid and androgen receptors are intact, GGR presents with symptoms and signs of mineralocorticoid excess (hypertension and hypokalemic alkalosis) and/or of hyperandrogenism (acne, hirsutism, male pattern baldness, menstrual irregularities, anovulation, and infertility). In children, the excessive secretion of adrenal androgens can cause sexual precocity. Finally, abnormal spermatogenesis and male infertility can result from effects of excess adrenal androgens on the regulation of pituitary gonadotropin secretion or from ACTH-induced growth of adrenal rests in the testes. These clinical manifestations are not observed in all patients with GGR, and the presentation may vary even within families.

The diagnosis of GGR is made by demonstrating a high cortisol production rate (high plasma total and free cortisol or elevated 24-h urinary free cortisol), resistance to dexamethasone suppression,

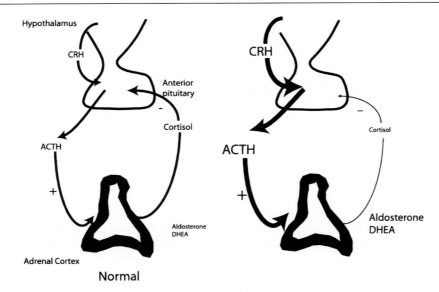

Figure 38-1 Dysregulation of corticosteroid production in glucocorticoid resistance syndromes. At left, normal feedback mechanisms allow precise regulation of corticotropin-releasing hormone, corticotropin (ACTH), and cortisol synthesis. In glucocorticoid resistance (right), partial insensitivity to cortisol feedback elevates the set-point for the hypothalamus, anterior pituitary, and adrenal cortex axis, reaching steady state at higher hormone production. As a consequence, mineralocorticoids (cortisol intermediates) and androgens (metabolites of adrenal DHEA-S) also accumulate. CRH, corticotropin-releasing hormone.

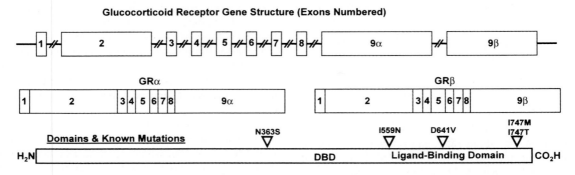

Figure 38-2 Structures of the gene, cDNA, and protein of the GRs are shown. The α- and β-isoforms are derived from alternative splicing of the last two exons. The ligand-binding domain and DNA-binding domain (DBD) of the GR-α protein are shown in protein structure, along with the location of four known mutations causing glucocorticoid resistance (arrowheads).

and preservation of the circadian and stress-induced patterns of glucocorticoid secretion, albeit at higher levels, without the stigmata of Cushing's syndrome.

GENETIC BASIS The cloning of the GR cDNA and gene permitted studies on the molecular mechanisms of glucocorticoid resistance (Fig. 38-2). The *GR* gene (officially designated *NR3C1*) is located on chromosome 5q31-32. Like most nuclear receptor proteins, GR has three main functional domains: an amino-terminal domain that includes residues important for transcriptional activation, the zinc-finger DNA-binding domain, and the carboxyl-terminal ligand-binding domain. Mutations that impair any of these functions may manifest clinically as GGR, and the molecular mechanism(s) by which these mutations impair receptor function may be complex and multifactorial.

Mutations within the ligand-binding domain (R477H, V571A, D641V, G679S, V729I, and I747M) decrease both affinity for glucocorticoids and agonist-induced transcriptional activation. A 4 bp deletion in a splice donor site of intron 6 reduces receptor number by 50%, presumably by decreasing the efficiency of RNA splicing, whereas other missense mutations reduce receptor number or function by effects exerted on the GR protein. Mutation I559N reduces receptor number by more than 50%, but this substitution also interferes with subcellular trafficking, perhaps because it is immediately adjacent to a nuclear localization motif. When tagged as a fusion with green-fluorescent protein, mutation I559N translocates to the nucleus more slowly than wild-type GR and only at high concentrations of agonist. Mutation I559N also interferes with agonist-induced nuclear translocation and transactivation by wild-type GR. These studies illustrate how a single GR mutation can impair its activity in multiple ways, including dominant negative effects on the function of the wild-type GR protein that yield clinical manifestations in heterozygotes. Of note, there is considerable heterogeneity in the phenotypes associated with various GR mutations and some family members with the identical mutation are clinically asymptomatic; these findings argue that genetic variations in other proteins may modulate GR function. Finally, no mutations in the gene for GR have been identified in some GGR subjects, again supporting the idea that proteins other

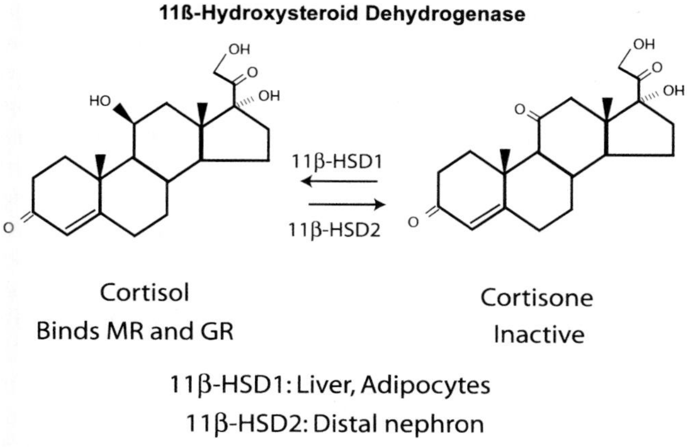

11ß-Hydroxysteroid Dehydrogenase

Cortisol
Binds MR and GR

Cortisone
Inactive

11β-HSD1: Liver, Adipocytes

11β-HSD2: Distal nephron

Figure 38-4   Role of the type-2 isozyme of 11β-hydroxysteroid dehydrogenase to protect the mineralocorticoid receptor. The structures of cortisol and cortisone are shown, as are the reactions catalyzed by the type-1 and -2 isozymes of 11β-hydroxysteroid dehydrogenase.

shows up to 53% of wild-type activity. These arginine substitutions are associated with progressively milder clinical phenotypes, although the correlation of activity with disease severity is not perfect. Interestingly, intrauterine growth retardation, a previously unrecognized manifestation of AME, is seen in most of the patients. Because 11β-HSD2 is highly expressed in the placenta, intrauterine growth retardation in AME patients has been attributed to the placental deficiency of the enzyme. One of the investigated kindreds did not harbor mutations of the *HSD11B2* gene, suggesting genetic heterogeneity for the disease.

CLINICAL MANAGEMENT   Patients with congenital AME respond to treatment with spironolactone (50–200 mg/d) and low-sodium diet. Treatment with the potent glucocorticoid dexamethasone may suppress cortisol levels sufficiently to control the hypertension, but care must be taken to avoid overreplacement. The hypokalemia also may respond to amiloride or triamterene. Early diagnosis and treatment are essential to avoid complications of hypertension.

FUTURE DIRECTIONS   The finding that patients with AME and mutations of the *HSD11B2* gene have intrauterine growth retardation correlates with the observation that low-birth weight infants are at increased risk for developing essential hypertension in later life. It is possible that genetic variations of 11β-HSD2 enzymatic activity have significant effects on fetal growth and on subsequent risk of hypertension. The *HSD11B2* gene thus may be one of the multiple genes that cause essential hypertension. However, an emerging link between 11β-HSD1 and obesity suggests that dysregulation of the cortisol-cortisone shuttle may cause other disease states. Fat contains 11β-HSD1 and targeted overexpression of this enzyme in adipocytes of transgenic mice is associated with increased adiposity, presumably because of increased local conversion of cortisone to active cortisol. Ongoing studies are examining whether alterations in *HSD11B1* are associated with conditions such as obesity and the metabolic syndrome in human beings.

GLUCOCORTICOID-REMEDIABLE ALDOSTERONISM

Glucocorticoid-remediable aldosteronism (GRA) was initially described as a familial syndrome of hypertension and hypokalemia

that responded clinically to treatment with glucocorticoids. Subsequent studies indicated that this autosomal-dominant disorder includes patients who do not have spontaneous hypokalemia and may occur in up to 1–3% of patients with primary aldosteronism.

CLINICAL FEATURES   Patients with GRA typically present with early-onset, moderate-to-severe hypertension. Although aldosterone production is increased, it is the 18-oxygenated cortisol derivatives in the urine and circulation that are characteristically elevated in patients with GRA. Earlier reports described patients with unprovoked hypokalemia, but subsequent studies have indicated that serum K$^+$ can often be in the normal range unless patients receive potassium-wasting diuretics. It also is appreciated that GRA is associated with a significant incidence of hemorrhagic strokes in affected family members, partly because of the early onset of hypertension, but also possibly related to direct effects of aldosterone on cerebral vasculature. Although the hypertension is often difficult to control with conventional agents, there is a distinct salutary response to glucocorticoids, hence the name GRA.

GENETIC BASIS   A critical component of normal adrenocortical function is the zone-specific expression of the two isozymes of steroid 11β-hydroxylase. CYP11B1 and CYP11B2 are encoded by highly homologous, tandemly duplicated genes on the long arm of chromosome 8 (8 q21-q22). GRA results from an unequal crossover that fuses the 5′-end of *CYP11B1*, including zone-specific regulatory sequences, with the 3′-end of *CYP11B2*, which encodes critical regions of the protein that determine the ability to catalyze the three separate reactions that convert 11-deoxycorticosterone to aldosterone. This chimeric gene causes the ectopic expression in the zona fasciculata of a protein that produces mineralocorticoids under ACTH stimulation, ultimately leading to mineralocorticoid excess and its attendant hypokalemia and hypertension. Furthermore, the ectopic fusion protein in the zona fasciculata also acts on cortisol to form the characteristic 18-oxygenated steroids. Site-directed mutagenesis studies show that amino acid substitutions V320A and/or N335D, the corresponding residues of CYP11B2, are sufficient to confer 18-oxygenase activity onto CYP11B1. Further studies also show that the location of the crossover is critical to determining the activity of the chimeric protein, which must contain most of the I-helix of CYP11B2 that starts near residue 295, to have aldosterone synthase activity.

CLINICAL MANAGEMENT   Because ACTH regulates steroid production by the zona fasciculata, administration of glucocorticoids will suppress ACTH and ameliorate the process. Traditionally, the potent glucocorticoid dexamethasone has been used in treatment. However, this logical therapy does not always normalize blood pressure, as the long-standing hypertension may induce secondary changes that do not respond to suppression of the synthesis of mineralocorticoids. Particularly in children, it is important to minimize the potential deleterious effects of glucocorticoid therapy. Thus, shorter-acting steroids such as cortisol and prednisone are sometimes preferred over dexamethasone, and careful titration of dose and monitoring for consequences of glucocorticoid excess (e.g., impaired linear growth) are essential.

As with AME, patients with GRA also can be treated with drugs that impair aldosterone action in the distal nephron, such as spironolactone, amiloride, and triamterene. Combination therapy with low doses of dexamethasone and moderate doses of spironolactone often allows good blood pressure control while minimizing glucocorticoid-related side effects.

FUTURE DIRECTIONS With the definition of the molecular basis of GRA, it is recognized that hypertension and hypokalemia are not always severe in this disorder. Further studies may identify modifier loci that affect the clinical severity of GRA, as well as other genes mutated in the rare GRA kindreds that do not harbor a chimeric *CYP11B1/CYP11B2* gene. The manifestations of GRA strikingly illustrate the essential role of zone-specific expression of the steroidogenic enzymes in normal adrenal function. However, little is understood about the mechanisms that determine zone-specific function. Subcapsular cells are capable of regenerating all three cortical zones, and one theory of zonation proposes that the subcapsular region contains adrenocortical progenitor cells that modulate their phenotype as they migrate centripetally from the zona glomerulosa to the zona fasciculata to the zona reticularis. There are no cell culture systems that accurately mimic the differential function of the zona glomerulosa vs the zona fasciculata, and the specific regulatory elements that confer zone-specific expression remain to be defined. Of note, advances in the use of relatively large DNA segments such as bacterial artificial chromosomes in transgenesis hold considerable promise for mapping the regulatory elements that specify zone-specific expression of *CYP11B1* and *CYP11B2* within the adrenal cortex.

CARNEY COMPLEX

Carney complex is a familial syndrome of multiple neoplasias (endocrine tumors and myxomas) and lentiginosis that is inherited in an autosomal-dominant manner. Although the existence of the complex was first suggested in 1985, combinations of several components of the syndrome and their familial occurrence had been reported earlier. Thus, the characteristic pathological findings of the adrenal glands (primary pigmented nodular adrenocortical disease [PPNAD])—multiple, small, pigmented, adrenocortical nodules, and internodular cortical atrophy—and a pituitary-independent, primary adrenal form of hypercortisolism were described in children and young adults with Cushing's syndrome as early as 1949. In the late 1970s, several familial cases of cutaneous and cardiac myxomas associated with lentigines (lentigo simplex) or ephelides and blue nevi of the skin and mucosae had been described under the acronyms, NAME (for nevi, atrial myxoma, myxoid neurofibromata, and ephelides) and LAMB (for lentigines, atrial myxoma, mucocutaneous myxoma, blue nevi) syndromes.

CLINICAL FEATURES Carney complex is manifested in children and young adults with at least two of the following: (1) PPNAD that can lead to Cushing's syndrome; (2) lentigines, ephelides, and blue nevi of the skin and mucosae; and (3) a variety of nonendocrine and endocrine tumors. The latter include myxomas of the skin, heart, breast, and other sites, psammomatous melanotic schwannomas, growth hormone-producing pituitary adenomas, testicular Sertoli cell tumors, and possibly other benign and malignant neoplasms, including tumors of the thyroid gland and ductal adenomas of the breast.

GENETIC BASIS Genes causing Carney complex were mapped by linkage analysis to chromosomes 2p16 and 17q22-24. The variant mapping to chromosome 17 apparently results from loss-of-function mutations of the type-1 regulatory subunit of cAMP-dependent protein kinase A (PKA, PPKAR1A). Mutations in *PPKAR1A* have been detected in approximately half of the patients with Carney complex, and also have been described in some sporadic endocrine tumors. Most mutations from Carney complex

kindreds introduce premature stop codons into the PPKAR1A mRNA, resulting in nonsense-mediated mRNA decay of the altered transcripts. Although the molecular basis for tumorigenesis in patients with PPKAR1A mutations has not been defined, most tumors show loss of heterozygosity at 17q22-24 owing to somatic loss of the wild-type *PPKAR1A* allele. Consequently, cells bearing only the inactive copy of the *PPKAR1A* gene have no functional regulatory subunit to downregulate the catalytic activity of cAMP-dependent PKA. Because PKA activity in adrenocortical cells increases steroidogenesis and cell growth, the formation of functional adrenal tumors when PPKAR1A is mutated and/or deleted is consistent with an important regulatory role for PPKAR1A to limit PKA stimulation. Furthermore, increased PKA activity can be demonstrated in tumors from Carney complex subjects bearing PPKAR1A mutations. The gene(s) responsible for the variant mapping to chromosome 2, as well as other genes potentially associated with Carney complex, remain to be defined.

CLINICAL MANAGEMENT Patients with the diagnosis of Carney complex require extensive and frequent monitoring for the detection and early treatment of the multiple tumors that are associated with this condition. Cardiac myxomas, if undiagnosed, can lead to sudden death, strokes, or peripheral embolization; thus, annual screening by echocardiography is recommended in patients with the complex and their families. If PPNAD is diagnosed, then bilateral adrenalectomy and lifelong replacement with glucocorticoid and mineralocorticoid is recommended.

FUTURE DIRECTIONS The lesions associated with Carney complex originate from cells of mesenchymal (myxomas) or neural crest origin (spotty skin pigmentation, endocrine tumors). These features suggest that the genetic defects leading to Carney complex are involved in early development, growth, and proliferation of the affected cells. Thus, candidate genes for cases not caused by PPKAR1A mutations include those involved in tumor suppression and the control of the cell cycle, as well as those with specific effects on the function and growth of mesenchymal cells, zona fasciculata cells, and melanocytes. Because there is considerable overlap between Carney complex and the familial lentiginosis syndromes (Peutz–Jeghers syndrome and others), it is expected that the Carney complex genes will contribute to the identification of the unknown genetic defects responsible for the various lentiginoses.

CONCLUSION

In addition to the diseases discussed here, the genes for a number of genetic conditions that affect adrenal function have been cloned. These include the genes for multiple endocrine neoplasia 2A and 2B (*RET* proto-oncogene) and Von Hippel–Lindau disease, which are associated with pheochromocytoma; the genes for other phakomatoses, such as neurofibromatosis -I and -II and tuberous sclerosis, which are associated with tumors of the adrenal medulla and sympathetic ganglia; and the gene for multiple endocrine neoplasia 1, which is associated with benign adrenal nodules. The gene responsible for the type-1 variant of polyglandular autoimmune endocrinopathy, which is characterized by the triad of autoimmune Addison's disease, hypoparathyroidism, and mucocutaneous candidiasis and also may include other endocrine defects, has been cloned and designated the autoimmune regulator. Although their roles in human adrenal disease have not yet been defined, additional genes that play important roles in adrenal development and physiology have been identified in transgenic and knockout mice. These genes include the transcriptional coregulator CITED2, Wnt4, and

Wilms' tumor-related 1. Because the era of molecular medicine continues, many exciting discoveries are expected in the understanding of normal physiology of the adrenal glands and the perturbations in various diseases.

SELECTED REFERENCES

Bonny O, Rossier BC. Disturbances of Na/K balance: pseudohypoaldosteronism revisited. J Am Soc Nephrol 2002;13:2399–2414.

Bray PJ, Cotton RG. Variations of the human glucocorticoid receptor gene (NR3C1): pathological and in vitro mutations and polymorphisms. Hum Mutat 2003;21:557–568.

Casey M, Vaughan CJ, He J, et al. Mutations in the protein kinase A R1alpha regulatory subunit cause familial cardiac myxomas and Carney complex. J Clin Invest 2000;106:R31–R38.

Chang SS, Grunder S, Hanukoglu A, et al. Mutations in subunits of the epithelial sodium channel cause salt wasting with hyperkalaemic acidosis, pseudohypoaldosteronism type 1. Nat Genet 1996;12:248–253.

Clark AJL, Weber A. Adrenocorticotropin insensitivity syndromes. Endocr Rev 1998;5:828–843.

Clipsham R, McCabe ER. DAX1 and its network partners: exploring complexity in development. Mol Genet Metab 2003;80:81–120.

Funder JW. Glucocorticoid and mineralocorticoid receptors: biology and clinical relevance. Annu Rev Med 1997;48:231–240.

Geller DS, Farhi A, Pinkerton N, et al. Activating mineralocorticoid receptor mutation in hypertension exacerbated by pregnancy. Science 2000;289:23–26.

Geller DS, Rodriguez-Soriano J, Vallo Boado A, et al. Mutations in the mineralocorticoid receptor gene cause autosomal dominant pseudohypoaldosteronism type I. Nat Genet 1998;19:279–281.

Hammer GD, Parker KL, Schimmer BP. Minireview: transcriptional regulation of adrenocortical development. Endocrinology 2005;146: 1018–1024.

Kino T, Chrousos GP Glucocorticoid and mineralocorticoid resistance syndromes. J Endocrinol 2001;169:437–445.

Kirschner LS, Carney JA, Pack SD, et al. Mutations of the gene encoding the protein kinase A type I-alpha regulatory subunit in patients with the Carney complex. Nat Genet 2000;26:89–92.

Malchoff CD, Malchoff DM. Glucocorticoid resistance and hypersensitivity. Endocrinol Metab Clin North Am 2005;34:315–326.

McMahon GT, Dluhy RG. Glucocorticoid-remediable aldosteronism. Cardiol Rev 2004;12:44–48.

Moneva MH, Gomez-Sanchez CE. Pathophysiology of adrenal hypertension. Semin Nephrol 2002;22:44–53.

Parker KL, Schimmer BP. Steroidogenic factor 1: a key determinant of endocrine development and function. Endocr Rev 1997;18:361–377.

Stratakis CA, Kirschner LS, Carney JA. Clinical and molecular features of the Carney complex: Diagnostic criteria and recommendations for patient evaluation. J Clin Endocrinol Metab 2001;86: 4041–4046.

Tulio-Pelet A, Salomon R, Hadj-Rabia S, et al. Mutant WD-repeat protein in Triple-A syndrome. Nat Genet 2000;26:332–335.

Wilson RC, Nimkarn S, New MI. Apparent mineralocorticoid excess. Trends Endocrinol Metab 2001;12:104–111.

39 Multiple Endocrine Neoplasia Type 1

RAJESH V. THAKKER

SUMMARY

Multiple endocrine neoplasia type 1 (MEN1) is characterized by the combined occurrence of tumors of the parathyroids, pancreatic islets, and anterior pituitary. In addition, some patients may also develop adrenal cortical, carcinoid, facial angiofibromas, collagenomas, and lipomatons tumors. MEN1 is inherited as an autosomal-dominant disorder and the gene causing MEN1 is located on chromosome 11q13. The MEN1 gene consists of 10 exons that encode a 610 amino acid protein, menin, which has a role in transcriptional regulation and genome stability. The mutations causing MEN1 are of diverse types and are scattered throughout the coding region. Mice deleted for a MEN1 allele develop endocrine tumors similar to those found in MEN1 patients. The availability of these mouse models for MEN1 will help to further elucidate the role of menin in regulating cell proliferation.

Key Words: Adrenal; carcinoid; lipoma; pancreatic islets; parathyroid; pituitary; tumors; tumor suppressor gene; Wermer's syndrome.

INTRODUCTION

Multiple endocrine neoplasia (MEN) is characterized by the occurrence of tumors involving two or more endocrine glands within a single patient. The disorder has previously been called multiple endocrine adenopathy or the pluriglandular syndrome. However, glandular hyperplasia and malignancy may also occur in some patients and the term "multiple endocrine neoplasia" is now preferred. There are two major forms of MEN referred to as type 1 and type 2, and each form is characterized by the development of tumors within specific endocrine glands (Table 39-1). Thus, the combined occurrence of tumors of the parathyroid glands, the pancreatic islet cells, and the anterior pituitary is characteristic of MEN1, which is also referred to as Wermer's syndrome. However, in MEN2, also called Sipple's syndrome, medullary thyroid carcinoma occurs in association with pheochromocytoma, and three clinical variants referred to as MEN2a, MEN2b, and medullary thyroid carcinoma only are recognized (*see* Table 39-1). Although MEN1 and MEN2 usually occur as distinct and separate syndromes as previously outlined, some patients occasionally develop tumors that are associated with both MEN1 and MEN. For example, patients suffering from islet cell tumors of the pancreas and pheochromocytomas, or from acromegaly and pheochromocytoma,

From: *Principles of Molecular Medicine, Second Edition*
Edited by: M. S. Runge and C. Patterson © Humana Press, Inc., Totowa, NJ

have been described and these patients may represent "overlap" syndromes. All these forms of MEN may either be inherited as autosomal-dominant syndromes, or they may occur sporadically, i.e., without a family history. However, the distinction between sporadic and familial cases may sometimes be difficult as in some sporadic cases the family history may be absent because the parent with the disease may have died before developing symptoms. This chapter discusses the main clinical features and molecular genetics of MEN1; MEN2 is reviewed in Chapter 40.

CLINICAL FEATURES

Parathyroid, pancreatic, and pituitary tumors constitute the major components of MEN1. In addition to these tumors, adrenocortical, carcinoid, facial angiofibromas, collagenomas, and lipomatous tumors may also occur in some patients.

PARATHYROID TUMORS Primary hyperparathyroidism is the most common feature of MEN1 and occurs in more than 95% of all MEN1 patients (Fig. 39-1). Patients may present with asymptomatic hypercalcemia, or nephrolithiasis, or osteitis fibrosa cystica, or vague symptoms associated with hypercalcemia, for example, polyuria, polydipsia, constipation, malaise, or occasionally with peptic ulcers. Biochemical investigations reveal hypercalcemia usually in association with raised circulating parathyroid hormone concentrations. The hypercalcemia is usually mild, and severe hypercalcemia resulting in crisis or parathyroid carcinoma are rare occurrences. Additional differences in the primary hyperparathyroidism of MEN1 patients from that in non-MEN1 patients include an earlier age of onset (20–25 yr vs 55 yr), and an equal male:female ratio (1/1 vs 1/3). Primary hyperparathyroidism in MEN1 patients is unusual before the age of 15 yr, and the age of conversion from being unaffected to affected has been observed to be between 20 and 21 yr in some individuals. No effective medical treatment for primary hyperparathyroidism is generally available and surgical removal of the abnormally overactive parathyroids is the definitive treatment. However, all four parathyroid glands are usually affected with multiple adenomas or hyperplasia, although this histological distinction may be difficult, and total parathyroidectomy has been proposed as a definitive treatment for primary hyperparathyroidism in MEN1, with the resultant lifelong hypocalcemia being treated with oral calcitriol (1,25 dihydroxy vitamin D_3). It is recommended that such total parathyroidectomy should be reserved for the symptomatic hypercalcemic patient with MEN1, and that the asymptomatic hypercalcemic MEN1 patient should not have parathyroid surgery

Table 39-1
The Multiple Endocrine Neoplasia (MEN) Syndromes

Type	Tumors	Biochemical features
MEN1	Parathyroids	Hypercalcemia and ↑PTH
	Pancreatic islets	
	Gastrinoma	↑Gastrin and ↑basal gastric acid output
	Insulinoma	Hypoglycemia and ↑insulin
	Glucagonoma	Glucose intolerance and ↑glucagon
	VIPoma	↑VIP and WDHA
	Ppoma	↑PP
	Pituitary (anterior)	
	Prolactinoma	Hyperprolactinemia
	GH-secreting	↑GH
	ACTH-secreting	Hypercortisolemia and ↑ATCH
	Nonfunctioning	Nil or α-subunit
	Associated tumors	
	Adrenocortical	Hypercortisolemia or primary hyperaldosteronism
	Carcinoid	↑5-HIAA
	Lipoma	Nil
MEN2a	Medullary thyroid carcinoma	Hypercalcitoninemia[a]
	Pheochromocytoma	↑Catecholamines
	Parathyroid	Hypercalcemia and ↑PTH
MEN2b	Medullary thyroid carcinoma	Hypercalcitoninemia
	Pheochromocytoma	↑Catecholamines
	Associated abnormalities	
	Mucosal neuromas	
	Marfanoid habitus	
	Medullated corneal nerve fibres	
	Megacolon	

[a]In some patients, basal serum calcitonin concentrations may be normal, but may show an abnormal rise at 1 and 5 min after stimulation with pentagastrin, 0.5 µg/kg.

Autosomal-dominant inheritance of the MEN syndromes has been established.

↑, increased; PTH, parathyroid hormone; VIP, vasoactive intestinal peptide; WDHA, watery diarrhea, hypokalemia, and achlorhydria; PP, pancreatic polypeptide; GH, growth hormone; ACTH, adrenocorticotrophin; 5-HIAA, 5-hydroxyindoleacetic acid; CgA, chromogranin A.

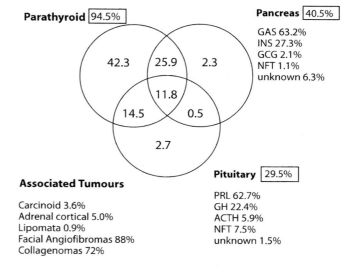

Figure 39-1 Schematic representation of the distribution of 384 multiple endocrine neoplasia type 1 tumors in 220 MEN1 patients. The proportions of patients in whom parathyroid, pancreatic, or pituitary tumors occurred are shown in the respective boxes; for example, 94.5% of patients had a parathyroid tumor. The Venn diagram indicates the proportions of patients with each combination of tumors, for example, 37.7% (25.9 + 11.8%) of patients had both a parathyroid and pancreatic tumor, whereas 2.3% of patients had a pancreatic tumor only. In addition to these tumors observed in one series, multiple facial angiofibromas were observed in 88% of 32 patients, and collagenomas in 72% of patients. The hormones secreted by each of these tumors are indicated: GAS, gastrin; INS, insulin; GCG, glucagon; NFT, nonfunctioning tumors; PRL, prolactin; GH, growth hormone; ACTH, adrenocorticotrophic hormone. Parathyroid tumors represent the most common form of MEN1 tumors and occur in approx 95% of patients, with pancreatic islet cell tumors occurring in approx 40% of patients, and anterior pituitary tumors occurring in approx 30% of patients. (Reproduced from Trump D, Farren B, Wooding C, et al. Clinical studies of multiple endocrine neoplasia type 1 [MEN1] in 220 patients. Q J Med 1996;89: 653–669, by permission of Oxford University Press.)

but have regular assessments for the onset of symptoms and complications, when total parathyroidectomy may be undertaken. However, all of these options should be discussed with the patient and an optimal course of management planned.

PANCREATIC TUMORS The incidence of pancreatic islet cell tumors in MEN1 patients varies from 30 to 80% in different series. The majority of these tumors produce excessive amounts of hormone, for example gastrin, insulin, glucagons, or vasoactive intestinal polypeptide (VIP), and are associated with distinct clinical syndromes.

Gastrinomas Gastrinomas, gastrin-secreting tumors, represent more than 50% of all pancreatic islet cell tumors (see Fig. 39-1) in MEN1 and approx 20% of patients with gastrinomas will have MEN1. Gastrinomas are the major cause of morbidity and mortality in MEN1 patients because of the recurrent severe multiple peptic ulcers that may perforate. The association of recurrent peptic ulceration, marked gastric acid production, and non-β-islet cell tumors of the pancreas is referred to as the Zollinger–Ellison syndrome. Additional prominent clinical features of this syndrome include diarrhea and steatorrhea. The diagnosis is established by demonstration of a raised fasting serum gastrin concentration in association with an increased basal gastric acid secretion. Medical treatment of MEN1 patients with the Zollinger–Ellison syndrome is directed to reducing basal acid output to less than 10 mmol/L, and this may be achieved by the parietal cell H+, K+-ATPase inhibitor, omeprazole. The ideal treatment for a nonmetastatic gastrinoma is surgical excision of the gastrinoma. However, in patients with MEN1 the gastrinomas are frequently multiple or extrapancreatic and the role of surgery has been controversial. For example, in one study, only 16% of MEN1 patients were free of disease immediately after surgery, and at 5 yr this had declined to 6%; the respective outcomes in non-MEN1 patients were better at 45 and 40%. The treatment of disseminated gastrinomas is difficult and hormonal therapy with octreotide, which is a human somatostatin analog, chemotherapy with streptozotocin and 5-fluoroaracil, hepatic artery embolization, and removal of all resectable tumor have all occasionally been successful.

Insulinoma Insulinomas are β-islet cell tumors that secrete insulin. They represent one-third of all pancreatic tumors in MEN1 patients (*see* Fig. 39-1). Insulinomas also occur in association with gastrinomas in 10% of MEN1 patients, and the two tumors may arise at different times. Insulinomas occur more often in MEN1 patients who are less than 40 yr, and many of these arise in individuals before the age of 20 yr, whereas in non-MEN1 patients insulinomas generally occur in those greater than 40 yr. Insulinomas may be the first manifestation of MEN1 in 10% of patients, and approx 4% of patients presenting with insulinoma have MEN1. Patients with an insulinoma present with hypoglycemic symptoms, which develop after a fast or exertion, and improve after glucose intake. Biochemical investigations reveal raised plasma insulin concentrations in association with hypoglycemia. Circulating concentrations of C-peptide and proinsulin, which are also raised, may be useful in establishing the diagnosis, as may an insulin suppression test. Medical treatment, consisting of frequent carbohydrate feeds and diazoxide, is not always successful and surgery is often required. Most insulinomas are multiple and small, preoperative localization with CT, celiac axis angiography and pre- or perioperative percutaneous transhepatic portal venous sampling is difficult, and success rates have varied. Surgical treatment, ranging from enucleation of a single tumor to a distal pancreatectomy or partial pancreatectomy, has been curative in some patients. Chemotherapy, which consists of streptozotocin or octreotide, is used for metastatic disease.

Glucagonoma　Glucagonomas, which are α-islet cell, glucagon-secreting pancreatic tumors, occur in less than 3% of MEN1 patients (*see* Fig. 39-1). The characteristic clinical manifestations of a skin rash (necrolytic migratory erytheyema), weight loss, anemia, and stomatitis may be absent and the presence of the tumor is indicated only by glucose intolerance and hyperglucagonemia. The tail of the pancreas is the most frequent site for glucagonomas; surgical removal is the treatment of choice. However, treatment may be difficult as 50% of patients have metastases at diagnosis. Medical treatment with octreotide or streptozotocin has been successful in some patients.

VIPoma　Patients with VIPomas, VIP-secreting pancreatic tumors, develop watery diarrhea, hypokalemia, and achlorhydria, referred to as the WDHA syndrome. This clinical syndrome has also been called the Verner–Morrison syndrome or the VIPoma syndrome. VIPomas have been reported in only a few MEN1 patients and the diagnosis is established by documenting a markedly raised plasma VIP concentration. Surgical management of VIPomas, which are mostly located in the tail of the pancreas, has been curative. However, in patients with unresectable tumor, treatment with streptozotocin, octreotide, corticosteroids, indomethicin, metoclopramide, and lithium carbonate has proved beneficial.

Ppoma　Ppomas, tumors that secrete pancreatic polypeptide (PP), are found in a large number of patients with MEN1. No pathological sequelae of excessive PP secretion are apparent and the clinical significance of PP is unknown, although the use of serum PP measurements has been suggested for the detection of pancreatic tumors in MEN1 patients.

PITUITARY TUMORS　The incidence of pituitary tumors in MEN1 patients varies from 15 to 90% in different series. Approximately 60% of MEN1 associated pituitary tumors secrete prolactin, less than 25% secrete growth hormone, 5% secrete adrenocorticotrophin, and the remainder appear to be nonfunctioning (*see* Fig. 39-1). Prolactinomas may be the first manifestation of MEN1 in less than 10% of patients, and somatotrophinomas occur more often in patients greater than 40 yr of age. Of patients with anterior pituitary tumors, less than 3% have MEN1. The clinical

manifestations depend on the size of the pituitary tumor and its product of secretion. Enlarging pituitary tumors may compress adjacent structures such as the optic chiasm or normal pituitary tissue and cause bitemporal hemianopia or hypopituitarism, respectively. The tumor size and extension are radiologically assessed by CT and nuclear MRI. Treatment of pituitary tumors in MEN1 patients is similar to that in non-MEN1 patients and consists of medical therapy or selective hypophysectomy by the transphenoidal approach if feasible, with radiotherapy being reserved for residual unresectable tumor.

ASSOCIATED TUMORS　Patients with MEN1 may have tumors involving glands other than the parathyroids, pancreas, and pituitary. Thus carcinoid, adrenocortical, facial angiofibromas, collagenomas, thyroid, and lipomatous tumors have been described in association with MEN1 (*see* Fig. 39-1).

Carcinoid Tumors　Carcinoid tumors, which occur in more than 3% of patients with MEN1 may be inherited as an autosomal-dominant trait in association with MEN1. The carcinoid tumor may be located in the bronchi, gastrointestinal tract, pancreas, or thymus. Bronchial carcinoids in MEN1 patients predominantly occur in women (M/F = 1/4), whereas thymic carcinoids predominantly occur in men, with cigarette smokers having a higher risk of developing tumors. Most patients are asymptomatic and do not suffer from the flushing attacks and dyspnea associated with the carcinoid syndrome, which usually develops after the tumor has metastasized to the liver. Octreotide has been successfully used to treat symptoms and may result in regression of gastric carcinoids.

Adrenocortical Tumors　The incidence of asymptomatic adrenocortical tumors in MEN1 patients has been reported to be as high as 40%. The majority of these tumors are nonfunctioning. However, functioning adrenocortical tumors in MEN1 patients have been documented to cause hypercortisolemia and Cushing's syndrome, and primary hyperaldosteronism, as in Conn's syndrome.

Lipomas　Lipomas may occur in more than 33% of patients, and are frequently multiple. In addition, pleural or retroperitoneal lipomas may also occur in patients with MEN1.

Thyroid Tumors　Thyroid tumors consisting of adenomas, colloid goiters, and carcinomas have been reported in more than 25% of MEN1 patients. However, the prevalence of thyroid disorders in the general population is high and it has been suggested that the association of thyroid abnormalities in MEN1 patients may be incidental and not significant.

Facial Angiofibromas and Collagenomas　Multiple facial angiofibromas, which are identical to those observed in patients with tuberous sclerosis, have been observed in 88% of MEN1 patients, and collagenomas have been reported in more than 70% of MEN1 patients.

GENETICS AND MEN1 MUTATIONS

The gene causing MEN1 was localized to chromosome 11q13 by genetic mapping studies that investigated MEN1 associated tumors for loss of heterozygosity (LOH) and by segregation studies in MEN1 families. The results of these studies, which were consistent with Knudson's model for tumor development, indicated that the MEN1 gene represented a putative tumor suppressor gene. Further genetic mapping studies defined a less than 300 kb region as the minimal critical segment that contained the MEN1 gene. Characterization of genes from this region led to the identification, in 1997, of the MEN1 gene, which consists of 10 exons with a 1830 bp coding region (Fig. 39-2) that encodes a novel 610 amino acid protein, referred to as "menin." Over 600 germline

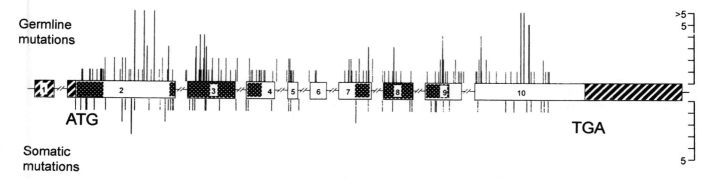

Figure 39-2 Schematic representation of the genomic organization of the multiple endocrine neoplasia type-1 gene illustrating germline and somatic mutations. The human MEN1 gene, located on chromosome 11q13, consists of 10 exons that span >9 kb of genomic DNA and encodes a 610 amino acid protein. The 1.83-kb coding region is organized into nine exons (exons 2–10) and eight introns (indicated by a line but not to scale). The sizes of the exons (boxes) range from 88 to 1312 bp and those of the introns range from 41 to 1564 bp. The start (ATG) and stop (TGA) sites in exons 2 and 10, respectively, are indicated. Exon 1, the 5′ part of exon 2 and 3′ part of exon 10 are untranslated (indicated by the hatched boxes). The locations of the three domains, which are formed by codons 1–40 (exon 2), 139–242 (exons 3 and 4), and 323–428 (exons 7–9), that interact with JunD are indicated by the stippled black boxes. The sites of the 623 germline mutations are indicated by the vertical lines above the gene and the sites of the 164 somatic mutations are represented below the gene. Mutations that have occurred more than four times (scale shown on the right) are indicated. (Reproduced by permission of the Society for Endocrinology. Pannet AAJ, Thakker RVT. Multiple endocrine neoplasia type1 [MEN1] gene. Endocr Relat Cancer 1996;6:449–473.)

mutations of the MEN1 gene have been identified, and most (>80%) of these are inactivating and consistent with its role as a tumor suppressor gene. These mutations are diverse in their types: approx 25% are nonsense mutations, approx 45% are frameshift deletions or insertions, approx 5% are in frame deletions or insertions, approx 5% are splice site mutations, and approx 15% are missense mutations (Fig. 39-3). More than 10% of the MEN1 mutations arise *de novo* and may be transmitted to subsequent generations. It is also important to note that 5–10% of MEN1 patients may not harbor mutations in the coding region of the MEN1 gene, and that these individuals may have mutations in the promoter or untranslated regions, which remain to be investigated. The mutations are not only diverse in their types but are also scattered throughout the 1830-bp coding region of the MEN1 gene (*see* Fig. 39-2) with no evidence for clustering as observed in MEN2 (*see* Chapter 40). Correlations between MEN1 mutations and the clinical manifestations of the disorder appear to be absent. This apparent lack of genotype–phenotype correlations, which contrasts with the situation in MEN2 (*see* Chapter 40), together with the wide diversity of mutations in the 1830 bp coding region of the MEN1 gene has made mutational analysis for diagnostic purposes in MEN1 time-consuming and expensive.

Tumors from MEN1 patients and non-MEN1 patients have been observed to harbor the germline mutation together with a somatic mutation or LOH involving chromosome 11q13, as expected from Knudson's model and the proposed role of the MEN1 gene as a tumor suppressor. The somatic mutations in tumors are scattered throughout the coding region (*see* Fig. 39-2) in a manner similar to that observed for the germline mutations. The 164 reported somatic mutations are also diverse in their types: approx 20% are nonsense mutations, approx 40% are frameshift deletions or insertions, approx 5% are inframe deletions or insertions, approx 5% are splice-site mutations, and approx 30% are missense mutations. Interestingly, somatic missense mutations have a significantly ($p < 0.001$) higher occurrence than germline missense mutations (*see* Fig. 39-3), although the reasons underlying this observation remain to be elucidated. Somatic MEN1 mutations also occur in sporadic (i.e., nonfamilial) tumors in patients

who do not have MEN1, and this is consistent with the Knudson hypothesis that predicts that mutations of a gene causing a hereditary cancer syndrome will also be involved in causing some nonhereditary forms of the cancer. Thus, MEN1 mutations have been reported in sporadic tumors of the parathyroids, pancreatic islet cells, anterior pituitary, and adrenal cortex (Fig. 39-4). Such MEN1 somatic mutations have also been observed in carcinoid tumors, lipomas, angiofibromas, and melanomas.

OTHER HEREDITARY ENDOCRINE TUMOR SYNDROMES AND GERMLINE MEN1 MUTATIONS

The role of the MEN1 gene in the etiology of other endocrine disorders in which either parathyroid or pituitary tumors occur as an isolated endocrinopathy has been investigated by mutational analysis. Germline MEN1 mutations have been reported in 16 families with isolated primary hyperparathyroidism. The sole occurrence of parathyroid tumors in these families is remarkable and the mechanisms that determine the altered phenotypic expressions of these mutations remain to be elucidated. Mutational analysis studies in another inherited isolated endocrine tumor syndrome, that of familial isolated acromegaly, have not detected abnormalities of the MEN1 gene, even though segregation analysis in one family indicated that the gene was likely to be located on chromosome 11q13. However, nonsense mutations have been detected in MEN1 families with the Burin or prolactinoma variant, which is characterized by a high occurrence of prolactinomas and a low occurrence of gastrinomas.

FUNCTION OF MEN1 PROTEIN (MENIN)

Initial analysis of the predicted amino acid sequence encoded by the MEN1 gene did not reveal homologies to any other proteins, sequence motifs, signal peptides, or consensus nuclear localization signal, and, thus, the putative function of the protein (menin) could not be deduced. However, studies based on immunofluorescence, Western blotting of subcellular fractions, and epitope tagging with enhanced green fluorescent protein, revealed that menin was located primarily in the nucleus. Furthermore, enhanced green

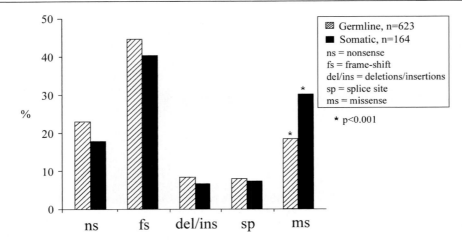

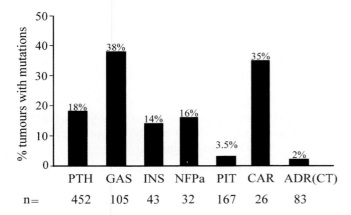

Figure 39-3 Frequency of germline and somatic multiple endocrine neoplasia type 1 mutations. A total of 623 germline mutations and 164 somatic mutations have been reported, and these are of diverse types, for example, nonsense, frameshifts, deletions, insertions, splice site, and missense mutations. The frequencies of each type of mutation in the germline and somatic group are similar with the exception of the missense mutations, which are found more frequently in tumors, i.e., the somatic group.

Figure 39-4 Frequencies of multiple endocrine neoplasia type-1 somatic mutations in nonfamilial (i.e., sporadic) tumors from non-MEN1 patients. The numbers (*n*) of tumors studied is indicated below for each group. Thus, MEN1 somatic mutations were observed in 18% of sporadic parathyroid tumors, 38% of gastrinomas (GAS), 14% of insulinomas (INS), 16% of nonfunctioning pancreatic islet cell tumors (NFPa), 3.5% of anterior pituitary (PIT) tumors, 35% of carcinoid tumors, and 2% of adrenocortical tumors (ADR[CT]). In addition, MEN1 somatic mutations have been observed in 57% of VIPomas (*n* = 7), 60% of glucagonomas (*n* = 5), 28% of lipomas (*n* = 7), 10% of angiofibromas (*n* = 19), and 2.5% of melanomas (*n* = 40) (data not shown).

fluorescent protein-tagged menin deletional constructs identified at least two independent nuclear localization signals (codons 479–497 and 588–608) that were located in the C-terminal quarter of the protein. Interestingly, the truncated MEN1 proteins that would result from the nonsense and frameshift mutations, if expressed, would lack at least one of these nuclear localization signals (*see* Fig. 39-2). Indeed menin is predominantly a nuclear protein in nondividing cells, but in dividing cells it is found in the cytoplasm. The function of menin remains to be elucidated but it does interact with a number of proteins involved in transcriptional regulation cell division, and genome stability. Thus, in transcriptional regulation, menin interacts with the activating protein-1, transcription factors JunD and C-jun, to suppress Jun mediated

transcriptional activation; members, for example, p50, p52, and p65, of the nuclear factor κB family of transcriptional regulators to repress nuclear factor κB mediated transcriptional activation; members of the Smad family, Smad3 and the Smad 1/5 complex, to inhibit the transforming growth factor-β and the bone morphogenetic protein-2 signaling pathways, respectively; and the mouse placental embryonic expression gene that encodes a homeobox containing protein. An interaction between menin and the nonmuscle myosin II-A heavy chain (NMHC II-A) indicates a role in cell division, as NMCH II-A may mediate alterations in cytokinesis and cell shape during cell division. A role for menin in controlling genome stability has been proposed because of its interactions with a subunit of replication protein (RPA2), which is a heterotrimeric protein required for DNA application, recombination, and repair; the tumor metastases suppressor NM23H1/nucleoside diphosphate kinase that induces GTPase activity; and the glial fibrillary acidic protein and vimentin, which are involved in the intermediate filament network. Thus, menin appears to have a large number of potential functions through interactions with proteins; whether these alter cell proliferation mechanisms independently or act via a single pathway remains to be elucidated.

MOUSE MODEL FOR MEN1

Mouse models for MEN1 have been generated through homologous recombination (i.e., knockout) of the mouse MEN1 gene. The mouse MEN1 gene consists of a 1833-bp open-reading frame that encodes a 611 amino acid protein. The mouse menin protein contains one more amino acid residue than the human menin, a glycine at 528. However, the mouse and human coding regions have 89 and 96% identities of the nucleotide and amino acid sequences, respectively, indicating a high degree of evolutionary conservation. One mouse knockout model for MEN1 was generated by introducing a floxed PGK-neomycin cassette into intron 2 and a third loxP site into intron 8, with the aim of deleting exons 3–8 in one allele. Heterozygous mice (+/–) developed parathyroid dysplasia and adenomas by 9 mo of age, pancreatic islet cell tumors that contained insulin by 9 mo of age, anterior pituitary tumors that contained prolactin by 16 mo of age, and adrenocortical carcinomas. The tumors, which had LOH at the MEN1 locus, were not associated with any serum biochemical abnormalities, such as hypercalcemia, or hypoglycemia, but those +/– mice developing pancreatic islet cell tumors or hyperplasia had elevated serum insulin concentrations. Thus, these heterozygous (+/–) mice provide a model for the human MEN1 disease. However, in another study, heterozygous mice (+/–) surprisingly died as embryos in late gestation, with some embryos developing omphaloceles. Two studies have reported that homozygous (–/–) mice die in utero at embryonic d 11.5–13.5. In one study these –/– mice were developmentally delayed and significantly smaller, and 20% of them developed craniofacial abnormalities. The craniofacial abnormalities were because of dysplasia of the membranous skull bones, and this developmental pathway involves the bone morphogenetic protein-2 signaling pathway. In another study, –/– mice were smaller in size, and developed extensive hemorrhage and edema. In addition, many of these –/– mice also had abnormalities of the neural tube, heart, and liver. Thus, many –/– mice had a failure of the closure of the neural tube, myocardial hypotrophy with a thin intraventricular septum, and decreased hepatic cellularity, which was associated with an altered organization and enhanced apoptosis. These results from the –/– mice reveal an important role for the MEN1 gene in the embryonic development of multiple organs.

FUTURE DIRECTIONS

Combined clinical and laboratory investigations of MEN1 patients will improve patient management and treatment, and also facilitate institution of a screening protocol. In addition, these advances will provide a better understanding of the role of these mutations in causing the endocrine tumors. One of the challenges remaining is the remarkable tissue specificity of the MEN1 tumors. The MEN1 gene is ubiquitously expressed from an early embryonic stage, and yet the tumors form principally in three endocrine glands. The availability of the mouse model may help to answer this question, and the availability of cellular models will help elucidate the role of menin in regulating cell proliferation via transcriptional regulation and genome stability.

ACKNOWLEDGMENTS

The author grateful to the Medical Research Council (MRC), UK for support; to B Harding for preparing the figures and to Miss Julie Allen for expert secretarial assistance.

SELECTED REFERENCES

Agarwal SK, Guru SC, Heppner C, et al. Menin interacts with the AP1 transcription factor JunD and represses JunD-activated transcription. Cell 1999;84:730–735.

Agarwal SK, Kester MB, Deblenko LV, et al. Germline mutations of the MEN1 gene in familial multiple endocrine neoplasia type 1 and related states. Hum Mol Genet 1997;6:1169–1175.

Bassett JH, Rashbass P, Harding B, Forbes SA, Pannett AA, Thakker RV. Studies of the murine homolog of the multiple endocrine neoplasia type 1 (MEN1) gene, MEN1. J Bone Miner Res 1999;14:3–10.

Bassett JHD, Forbes SA, Pannett AAJ, et al. Characterisation of mutations in patients with multiple endocrine neoplasia type 1 (MEN1). Am J Hum Genet 1998;62:232–244.

Bertolino P, Radovanovic I, Casse H, Aguzzi A, Wang Z-Q, Zhang C-X. Genetic ablation of the tumor suppressor menin causes lethality at mid-gestation with defects in multiple organs. Mech Dev 2003;120: 549–560.

Brandi ML, Gagel RF, Angeli A, et al. Guidelines for diagnosis and therapy of MEN type 1 and type 2. J Clin Endocrinol Metab 2001;86(12): 5658–5671.

Chandrasekharappa SC, Guru SC, Manickam P, et al. Positional cloning of the gene for multiple endocrine neoplasia-type 1. Science 1997;276: 404–407.

Chandrasekharappa SC, Teh BT. Functional studies of the MEN1 gene. J Med 2003;253:606–615.

Crabtree JS, Scacheri PC, Ward JM, et al. A mouse model of multiple endocrine neoplasia, type 1, develops multiple endocrine tumors. Proc Natl Acad Sci USA 2001;98:1118–1123.

Darling TN, Skarulis MC, Steinberg SM, Marx SJ, Spiegel AM, Turner M. Multiple facial angiofibromas and collagenomas in patients with multiple endocrine neoplasia type 1. Arch Dermatol 1997;133:853–861.

Guru SC, Goldsmith PK, Burns AL, et al. Menin, the product of the MEN1 gene, is a nuclear protein. Proc Natl Acad Sci USA 1998;95:1630–1634.

Heppner C, Bilimoria KY, Agarwal SK, et al. The tumour suppressor protein and inhibits NF-kappaB-mediated transactivation. Oncogene 2001;20(36):4917–4925.

Jensen RT. Management of the Zollinger-Ellison syndrome in patients with multiple endocrine neoplasia type 1. J Intern Med 1998;243:477–488.

Kaji H, Canaff L, Lebrun JJ, Goltzman D, Hendy GN. Inactivation of menin, a Smad3-interacting protein, blocks transforming growth factor type beta signalling. Proc Natl Acad Sci USA 2001;98(7):3837–2842.

Knudson AG. Antioncogenes and human cancer. Proc Natl Acad Sci USA 1993;90:10914–10921.

Larsson C, Skogseid B, Oberg K, Nakamura Y, Nordenskjold MC. Multiple endocrine neoplasia type I gene maps to chromosome 11 and is lost in insulinoma. Nature 1988;332:85–87.

Lemmens IH, Forsberg L, Pannett AA, et al. Menin interacts directly with the homeobox-containing protein Pem. Biochem Biophys Res Commun 2001;286:426–431.

Lopez-Egido J, Cunningham J, Berg M, Oberg K, Bongcam-Rudloff E, Gobl A. Menin's interaction with glial fibrillary acidic protein and vimentin suggests a role for the intermediate filament network in regulating menin activity. Exp Cell Res 2002;278:175–183.

Marx SJ. Multiple Endocrine Neoplasia Type 1. In: Vogelstein B, Kinzler KW, eds. Genetic Basis of Human Cancer, New York: McGraw Hill, 1998; pp. 489–506.

Norton JA, Fraker DL, Alexander R, et al. Surgery to cure the Zollinger-Ellison syndrome. N Engl J Med 1999;341:635–644.

Ohkura N, Kishi M, Tsukada T, Yamaguchi K. Menin. A gene product responsible for multiple endocrine neoplasia type 1, interacts with the putative tumor metastasis suppressor nm23. Biochem Biophys Res Commun 2001;282:1206–1210.

Olufenic SE, Green JS, Manikam P, et al. Common ancestral mutation in the MEN1 gene is likely responsible for the prolactinoma variant of MEN1 (MEN1 burin) in four kindreds from Newfoundland. Hum Mutat 1998;11:204–269.

Pannett AAJ, Kennedy AM, Turner JJO, et al. Multiple endocrine neoplasia type 1 (MEN1) germline mutations in familial isolated primary hyperparathyroidism. Clin Endocrinol (Oxf) 2003;58:639–646.

Pannett AAJ, Thakker RVT. Multiple endocrine neoplasia type 1 (MEN1) gene. Endocr Relat Cancer 1999;6:449–473.

Scacheri PC, Crabtree JS, Novotny EA, et al. Bidirectional transcriptional activity of PGK—neomycin and unexpected embryonic lethality in heterozygote chimeric knockout mice. Genesis 2001;30:259–263.

Skogseid B, Larsson C, Lindgren PG, et al. Clinical and genetic features of adrenocortical lesions in multiple endocrine neoplasia type 1. J Clin Endocrinol Metab 1992;75:76–81.

Skogseid B, Oberg K, Benson L, et al. A standardized meal stimulation test of the endocrine pancreas for early detection of pancreatic endocrine tumors in multiple endocrine neoplasia type 1 syndrome: five years experience. J Clin Endocrinol Metab 1987;64:1233–1240.

Sowa H, Kaji H, Canaff L, et al. Inactivation of menin, the product of multiple endocrine neoplasia type 1 gene, inhibits the commitment of multipotential mesenchymal stem cells into the osteoblast lineage. J Biol Chem 2003;23:21,058–21,069.

Stewart C, Parente F, Piehl F, et al. Characterisation of the mouse MEN1 gene and its expression during development. Oncogene 1998;17: 2485–2493.

Sukhodolets KE, Hickman AB, Agarwal SK, et al. The 32-kilodalton subunit of replication protein A interacts with menin, the product of the MEN1 tumour suppressor gene. Mol Cell Biol 2003;23:493–509.

Teh BT, Kytola S, Farnebo F, et al. Mutation analysis of the MEN1 gene in multiple endocrine neoplasia type 1, familial acromegaly and familial isolated hyperparathyroidism. J Clin Endocrinol Metab 1998;83: 2621–2626.

Teh BT, Zedenius J, Kytola S, et al. Thymic carcinoids in multiple endocrine neoplasia type 1. Ann Surg 1998;228:99–105.

Thakker RV. The molecular genetics of the multiple endocrine neoplasia syndromes. Clin Endocrinol (Oxf) 1993;39:1–14.

Thakker RV. Multiple Endocrine Neoplasia Type 1 (MEN1). In: DeGroot LJ, Besser GK, Burger HG, et al. eds. Endocrinology, Philadelphia: WB Saunders, 2000; 2815–2831.

The European Consortium on MEN1. Identification of the multiple endocrine neoplasia Type 1 (MEN1) gene. Hum Mol Genet 1997;6: 1177–1183.

Tomassetti P, Migliori M, Caletti GC, Fusaroli P, Corinaldesi R, Gullo L. Treatment of type II gastric carcinoid tumors with somatostatin analogues. N Engl J Med 2000;343:551–554.

Trump D, Farren B, Wooding C, et al. Clinical studies of multiple endocrine neoplasia type 1 (MEN1) in 220 patients. Q J Med 1996;89: 653–669.

Wolfe MM, Jensen RT. Zollinger-Ellison syndrome. Current concepts in diagnosis and management. N Engl J Med 1987;317:1200–1209.

Yaguchi H, Ohkura N, Tsukada K. Menin, the multiple endocrine neoplasia type 1 gene product, exhibits GTP-hydrolyzing activity in the presence of the tumor metastasis suppressor nm23. J Biol Chem 2002; 277:38,197–38,204.

Yamita W, Ikeo Y, Yamauchik K, Sakurai A, Hashizumek K. Suppression of insulin-induced AP-1 transactivation by menin accompanies inhibition of c-Fos induction. Int J Cancer 2003;103:738–744.

40 Multiple Endocrine Neoplasia Type 2

ROBERT F. GAGEL, SARAH SHEFELBINE, HIRONORI HAYASHI, AND GILBERT COTE

SUMMARY

Multiple endocrine neoplasia is a genetic endocrine tumor syndrome characterized by the presence of medullary thyroid carcinoma (MTC), pheochromocytoma, and hyperparathyroidism. There are two major variants. Multiple endocrine neoplasia (MEN) type 2A or Sipple syndrome has three clinical features: MTC, pheochromocytoma, and hyperparathyroidism; MEN2B has a different phenotype: MTC, pheochromocytoma, mucosal neuromas distributed throughout the mouth and gastrointestinal tract, and Marfanoid features including long thin arms and legs, an altered upper/lower body ratio, and pectus abnormalities. These clinical syndromes are caused by specific activating mutations of the RET tyrosine kinase receptor, important in neurological development of the gastrointestinal tract. MEN2 is one of a handful of genetic syndromes where the identification of a mutation leads to a specific action. Children with germline activating mutations of RET are treated in early childhood with a total thyroidectomy to prevent the development of metastatic MTC.

Key Words: Activating mutation; C cell; chromaffin cell; genetic testing; hereditary cancer; hyperparathyroidism; marfanoid features; medullary thyroid carcinoma; MEN2A; MEN2B; mucosal neuromas; multiple endocrine neoplasia type 2; parathyroid cell; pheochromocytoma; RET proto-oncogene; thyroid cancer; tyrosine kinase receptor.

INTRODUCTION

John Sipple first described components of the clinical syndrome that bears his name. Recognizing the association of thyroid cancer and bilateral pheochromocytomas in a patient at autopsy he reported this case with several others in a 1961 article. The type of thyroid carcinoma was more clearly defined and the clinical features of this syndrome, defined as multiple endocrine neoplasia (MEN) type 2, were separated from MEN1 (Table 40-1).

CLINICAL FEATURES

MEN2 consists of medullary thyroid carcinoma (MTC), pheochromocytoma, and hyperparathyroidism inherited as an autosomal-dominant trait. The nomenclature for this disease syndrome has evolved since its initial description; a classification system that reflects the clinical features and molecular causes is shown in

From: *Principles of Molecular Medicine, Second Edition*
Edited by: M. S. Runge and C. Patterson © Humana Press, Inc., Totowa, NJ

Table 40-1. The syndrome originally described by Sipple has been classified as MEN2A. MTC is found in nearly all gene carriers, pheochromocytoma in one-half, and hyperparathyroidism in 10–20%. Characteristics of all neoplastic components associated with MEN2 are bilaterality and multicentricity. This is especially important for MTC in which surgical cure is possible only by removal of all thyroid tissue.

There are three variants of MEN2A: familial medullary thyroid carcinoma (FMTC); MEN2A with cutaneous lichen amyloidosis (MEN2A/CLA); and MEN2A with Hirschsprung disease. MTC in FMTC is inherited as an autosomal-dominant trait without other features of MEN2A. The MTC associated with FMTC tends to be less aggressive and is most likely to be confused with sporadic MTC because other manifestations of MEN2A are not present, and many affected family members may be asymptomatic. A diagnosis of FMTC should be made only in large, multigenerational families because of the incomplete penetrance (50% or less) for other manifestations of MEN2A. The MEN2A/CLA variant, found in approx 18 kindreds worldwide, is the association of MEN2A with a characteristic pruritic skin lesion located over the central upper back. The clinical features, other than the skin lesion, are identical to classic MEN2A, although hyperparathyroidism may be less common. Finally, a handful of families have been described with MEN2A and Hirschsprung disease. The penetrance of the Hirschsprung phenotype is variable, ranging from complete penetration to a single affected member.

MEN2B is characterized by MTC and pheochromocytoma as well as a unique phenotype of marfanoid habitus and mucosal, oral and intestinal ganglioneuromatosis (see Table 40-1). This disorder is transmitted as an autosomal-dominant trait, although the majority of cases represent *de novo* mutations; the mutant allele is generally inherited from the father and the mutation is thought to occur during spermatogenesis. MTC associated with MEN2B is more aggressive than observed in MEN2A. Development of carcinoma during the first year of life is common and early death from metastatic MTC occurs in 30–40% of patients. The prognosis, however, is not universally poor. A number of multigeneration families suggest considerable variability in the outcome.

DIAGNOSIS

MEN2 is a clinical syndrome that affects multiple endocrine organs. MTC and pheochromocytoma are the most common causes of morbidity and death. Hyperparathyroidism and its associated

Table 40-1
The Multiple Endocrine Neoplasia Syndromes

Multiple endocrine neoplasia type 1
    Pituitary tumors
    Parathyroid neoplasia
    Islet cell neoplasia
Multiple endocrine neoplasia type 2
    Multiple endocrine neoplasia type 2A (MEN2A)
        Medullary thyroid carcinoma (100%)
        Pheochromocytoma (50%)
        Parathyroid neoplasia (10–20%)
    Variants of MEN2A
        Familial medullary thyroid carcinoma
        MEN2A with cutaneous lichen amyloidosis
        MEN2A with Hirschsprung disease
    Multiple endocrine neoplasia type 2B
        Medullary thyroid carcinoma (100%)
        Pheochromocytoma (50%)
        No parathyroid disease
        Marfanoid habitus (nearly 100%)
        Intestinal ganglioneuromatosis and mucosal neuromas
          (nearly 100%)

findings of hypercalcemia, nephrolithiasis, and bone loss are less commonly a clinical problem.

The C cell, the cell type comprising MTC, produces a small peptide hormone, calcitonin. In patients with MTC, serum calcitonin values are characteristically elevated and secretion may be stimulated 3- to 20-fold higher by intravenous pentagastrin, calcium, or by a combination of the two. Prospective studies utilizing provocative testing with pentagastrin or the combination of calcium and pentagastrin have been used successfully to identify MTC early in the course of the disease. Prospective pentagastrin screening and thyroidectomy has improved survival and quality of life in these kindreds, although not all children or young adults are cured utilizing this approach. As many as 10–15% of these patients have evidence of recurrent disease or elevated calcitonin values in long-term follow-up studies.

Pheochromocytoma occurs in approx 50% of family members with MEN2. These tumors cause palpitations, headaches, and attacks of nervousness early in the course of tumor development; hypertension is infrequently found in patients with small tumors or hyperplasia of the adrenal. In patients with large or bilateral tumors, hypertension and cardiac arrhythmias may occur. Before the recognition of this syndrome in 1961 it is estimated that one-half of the deaths in MEN2 kindreds occurred suddenly and were attributed to cardiac disease; many were likely related to pheochromocytoma. The goal of screening for pheochromocytoma in kindreds with MEN2 is to identify an adrenal tumor before it causes significant or life-threatening manifestations of catecholamine excess. One successful approach is the annual measurement of plasma or 12 or 24 h urine for catecholamines or metanephrines. Symptomatic patients frequently have an elevation of either plasma or urine catecholamines or metanephrines. MEN2-related pheochromocytomas are unique in that they preferentially produce disproportionate amounts of epinephrine and its metabolite metanephrine when compared with sporadic pheochromocytomas or those associated with von Hippel Lindau syndrome that produce predominately norepinephrine or normetanephrine. Patients with abnormal values should have imaging studies. CT

provides better definition of the adrenal medulla and is less expensive. MRI provides greater specificity if the adrenal medulla lights up on T2-weighted images.

The major diagnostic problems occur at the transition between normal and abnormal. Patients may have symptoms suggestive of pheochromocytoma with normal catecholamine measurements and imaging studies. In this situation the differentiation between intermittent abnormal catecholamine secretion and an anxiety disorder can be difficult. A trial of adrenergic blockade or inhibition of catecholamine synthesis with α-methyl tyrosine may help separate these two possibilities. If the patient is improved by pharmacological intervention and surgery is contemplated, the choice of which adrenal to remove may be difficult. Higher resolution CT scans using fine cuts through the adrenal glands permits localization in most cases; in others octreotide or met-iodobenzyl guanidine scanning may provide insight. Another alternative would be to continue the patient on adrenergic blockade or catecholamine synthesis inhibition until a pheochromocytoma can be clearly identified. Successful experience with long-term management of malignant pheochromocytoma, a much more challenging situation, suggests that this approach could be used safely in a compliant patient.

Earlier detection and improved surgical techniques have reduced the morbidity and mortality associated with pheochromocytoma to negligible levels. In fact, there is growing evidence that death from adrenal insufficiency may be a greater risk than death from pheochromocytoma; these concerns have led to a renewed interest and use of cortical sparing adrenalectomy, a technique in which the adrenal medulla is removed, leaving the cortex with intact vascularity.

GENETIC BASIS OF MEN2

MAPPING THE CAUSATIVE GENE The MEN2 gene was mapped to centromeric chromosome 10 in independent efforts in 1987. Subsequent work narrowed the region containing the MEN2 gene, leading to the identification of mutations of the *RET* proto-oncogene in 1993 (Fig. 40-1).

The *RET* proto-oncogene was first discovered in 1985 when a rearranged form of this gene was shown to cause transformation. The *RET* proto-oncogene encodes a tyrosine kinase receptor. A naturally occurring rearrangement was subsequently identified in 10–35% of papillary thyroid carcinomas (PTC) and named the PTC oncogene. Multiple different PTC variants exist, each resulting from a chromosome 10 rearrangement that places the tyrosine kinase domain of the *RET* proto-oncogene under the transcriptional control of another constitutively expressed gene. There is compelling evidence that the *RET* rearrangement causes transformation of the thyroid follicular cell in animal models of PTC.

The Glial Cell-Derived Neurotrophic FACTOR/RET/GFRA Receptor System A remarkable series of studies have defined a tyrosine kinase receptor signaling system important for the development of several components of the nervous system and normal kidney development. Individual components of this system include RET and a small protein ligand, glial cell-derived neurotrophic factor (GDNF), identified as a neuronal survival factor. The recognition that GDNF is a ligand for the RET tyrosine kinase receptor was not suspected until the mid-1990s when mice with *RET* or GDNF genes deleted were found to have nearly identical phenotypes, characterized by gastrointestinal neuronal features analogous to Hirschsprung disease, severe renal abnormalities, and developmental abnormalities of components of the

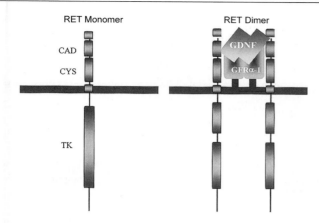

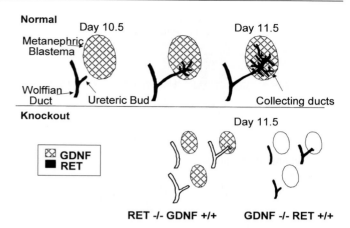

Figure 40-1 The RET tyrosine kinase receptor is a transmembrane receptor with a cadherin (CAD), cysteine-rich (CYS), and tyrosine kinase domain (TK). Interaction of GDNF, one of four ligands for RET, with the glial cell-derived neurotrophic factor receptor (GFRα-1) leads to dimerization of the receptor, autophosphorylation, and phosphorylation of downstream signaling substrates.

Figure 40-2 Schematic view showing mouse embryonic kidney development. The ureteric bud, derived from the Wolffian duct, normally migrates into the developing metanephric blastema to form the collecting system. In either *RET* (RET –/–) or *GDNF* (GDNF –/–) knockouts there is a defect in migration of the ureteric bud into the metanephric blastema resulting in a failure of normal kidney development. (Derived from information contained in work published by several authors: Schilling T, Burck J, Sinn HP, et al., 2001; Pichel JG, Shen L, Sheng HZ, et al., 1996; Moore MW, Klein RD, Farinas I, et al., 1996.)

sympathetic nervous system. Detailed studies in these animals showed gastrointestinal neuronal features analogous to those found in Hirschsprung disease with incomplete development of the enteric nervous system. There was also a complete lack of renal development in these animals. Components of the sympathetic nervous system, including the superior cervical ganglion, were also underdeveloped.

In an independent series of experiments, researchers discovered a receptor for GDNF, termed GDNF family receptor (GFR)-α and showed it to interact with the RET tyrosine kinase receptor. RET and GFRα-1, an extracellular protein tethered to the cell membrane by a glycosyl phosphatidylinositol linkage, together form a receptor for GDNF (*see* Fig. 40-1). Subsequent studies showed that targeted disruption of the mouse GFRα-1 gene causes a phenotype nearly indistinguishable from that observed for the mice in which GDNF and RET were deleted.

Additional work has defined a complex receptor system. The RET tyrosine kinase receptor forms the transmembrane backbone for each of these variants. The four ligands (GDNF, artemin [ARTN], persephin [PSPN], and neurturin [NRTN]) belong to the transforming growth factor-β superfamily and are collectively known as GDNF family ligands (GFL). The presence of seven cysteine residues characterize them as members of the cystine knot protein family. These ligands interact with RET and one of four GFRα proteins (GFRα-1, GFRα-2, GFRα-3, GFRα-4).

Perhaps more important than the components of the receptor system is the nature of the interaction between ligand and receptor system and how this interaction serves a developmental role. In a familiar theme of developmental biology, the ligand–receptor interaction serves to bring one tissue expressing the ligand into proximity with another expressing the receptor system. This interaction is perhaps best shown in the interactions between the ureteric bud and the metanephric blastema in kidney development. The ureteric bud (the developing renal ureteral collecting system) normally penetrates the metanephric blastema and branches to form the collecting system (Fig. 40-2). The peptide GDNF is expressed in the developing metanephric blastema and interacts with the RET receptor in the ureteric bud to promote branching of the ureteric bud into the developing kidney. In the absence of

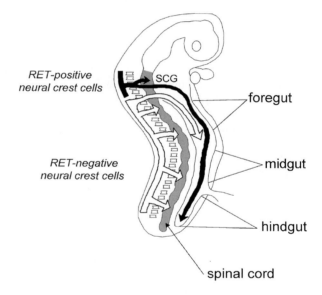

Figure 40-3 Migration of neural crest cells expressing the RET tyrosine kinase into the developing spinal cord and gastrointestinal tract. RET expressing cells form the superior cervical ganglion, parts of the dorsal root of the spinal cord, and the enteric neuronal plexus of the gastrointestinal tract.

either GDNF or RET there is a failure of this interaction, leading to an undeveloped, shrunken kidney.

Available facts suggest a similar pattern of interaction between RET and GDNF in the developing enteric neuronal system. Clearly, RET is expressed in neural crest cells associated with somites 1–5. These RET positive cells migrate into the spinal cord and into the developing gastrointestinal tract during embryonic life (Fig. 40-3). The finding of incomplete intestinal neuronal development in RET, GDNF, and GFRα-1 knockout mice, provides compelling evidence for an interaction between the ligand/receptor systems of importance in neuronal innervation of the intestine.

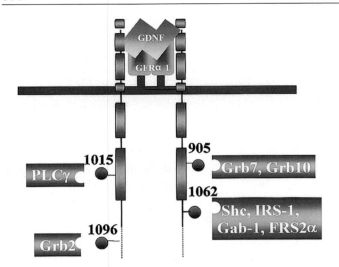

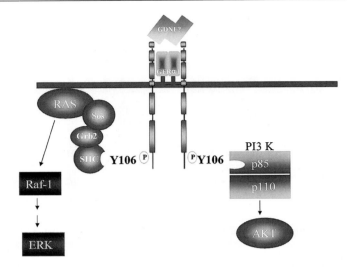

Figure 40-4   Diagram of the glial cell-derived neurotrophic factor/ RET/GDNF family receptor-α1 receptor system showing intracellular tyrosine phosphorylation sites at codons 905, 1015, 1062, and 1096 with known interacting signaling linkage proteins.

In the broader perspective these studies provide insight into an important neural crest development pathway. Studies of RET expression in developing embryos have shown RET expression in neural crest derived from somites one to five. Between day 9 and 10.5 there is migration of RET positive cells from the neural crest into the developing spinal cord and gastrointestinal tract (*see* Fig. 40-3). It is possible to envision a tropic effect of GDNF interaction with the RET/GFRα-1 receptor system to entice neural crest cells into their normal developmental location.

There is an evolving body of literature that GDNF, NRTN, ARTN, and PSPN function as survival factors. Indeed, GDNF was originally identified as a neurotrophic factor whose presence in a culture system prevented neuronal death. A substantial amount of data indicates that this receptor system functions in neurons and neuroendocrine cells to prevent apoptotic cell death. This is certainly evident in mice in which the GFL (GDNF, ATRN, PSPN, or NTRN), RET, or one of the four GFRα receptors have been deleted. In most of these single-gene deletion mice there are features that indicate a developmental loss of neurons at various developmental stages, arguing that this receptor system promotes neuronal survival. Postnatally, however, the receptor system appears to have a different set of functions that relate both to neuronal survival and specific neuronal function.

The interaction of one of the four GFLs with the RET/GFRα family receptor activates a complex cascade of signaling systems. There are at least four different tyrosine phosphorylation sites on RET that could mediate downstream signaling (Fig. 40-4). There is a general agreement that Tyr 1062 of RET activates both mitogen-activated protein kinase and phosphatidyl inositol-3-kinase pathways (Fig. 40-5). There is considerable evidence that tyrosine 1062 is necessary for the neoplastic transformation events found in MEN2. Substitution of another amino acid at codon diminishes the transformation efficiency of mutant RET.

MUTATIONS OF THE *RET* PROTO-ONCOGENE ASSOCIATED WITH MTC

The mutations of *RET* in MEN2 predominantly affect two domains within the RET tyrosine kinase receptor. Mutations of a cysteine-rich region of the extracellular domain are the most common mutations found in MEN2 and its

Figure 40-5   Transformation of the C cell by the mutant RET receptor requires phosphorylation of tyrosine 1062 and involves activation of at least two signaling pathways, PI 3 kinase and MAP kinase. There is evidence that glial cell-derived neurotrophic factor interaction with the RET/GDNF family receptor-α1 receptor system is not required for transformation caused by mutation of extracellular cysteine residues, but may be involved for mutations involving the tyrosine kinase domains.

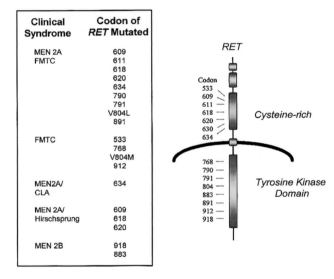

Clinical Syndrome	Codon of *RET* Mutated
MEN 2A FMTC	609 611 618 620 634 790 791 V804L 891
FMTC	533 768 V804M 912
MEN2A/ CLA	634
MEN 2A/ Hirschsprung	609 618 620
MEN 2B	918 883

Figure 40-6   Mutations of the *RET* proto-oncogene associated with hereditary medullary thyroid carcinoma. The most common mutations affect two regions of the RET tyrosine kinase. Mutations of an extracellular cysteine domain (codons 609, 611, 618, 620, 630, and 634), important for dimerization of the receptor, cause MEN2A and its variants. Mutations of the tyrosine kinase domain are found in MEN2B (codons 883 and 918) and a few families with FMTC (768, 804, 891, 912). Abbreviations: multiple endocrine neoplasia type 2A, MEN2A; familial medullary thyroid carcinoma, FMTC; MEN2A/cutaneous lichen amyloidosis, MEN2A/CLA; MEN2A/Hirschsprung disease variant, MEN2A/Hirschsprung; and multiple endocrine neoplasia type 2B, MEN2B.

variants (Fig. 40-6). Each of these mutations converts a conserved cysteine at codons 609, 611, 618, 620, 630, or 634 to another amino acid. Of all *RET* mutations, 75% affect codon 634 and a single mutation, cys634arg, accounts for >50% of all mutations associated with hereditary MTC. Genotype–phenotype correlation shows that a codon 634 mutation is most commonly associated with classic MEN2A or Sipple's syndrome. Mutations of the codons found in exon 10 (609, 611, 618, 620) are most commonly found in FMTC. Despite these correlative efforts, any of the extracellular cysteine mutations can be associated with MEN2A or FMTC, a point of importance in the clinical management of kindreds with these mutations. A clinician should not conclude that an individual with an exon 10 mutation will not develop a pheochromocytoma unless there are multiple generations within a family that have not developed pheochromocytoma. All patients with the MEN2A/CLA syndrome have codon 634 mutations. MEN2 can also be associated with mutations of codon 790, 791, V804L, and 891.

Germline mutations of the tyrosine kinase domain are found in MEN2B (codons 883 and 918) and FMTC (codons 768, V804M, and 912) (*see* Fig. 40-6). Of patients with MEN2B, 98% have the M918T substitution; a handful of MEN2B patients with the codon 883 mutation have been identified. The mutation in the remaining 1–2% has not been identified. In the handful of kindreds with the codon 533, 768, V804M, and 912 mutations the only clinical phenotype is familial MTC.

Additional evidence for the oncogenicity of these mutations came from studies in which expression of mutant *RET* proto-oncogene in NIH 3T3 cells caused transformation. These studies showed that codon 634 mutation resulted in dimerization of the RET tyrosine kinase receptor in the absence of its ligand, leading to autophosphorylation and phosphorylation of downstream proteins. Transfection of the *RET* cDNA containing the met918thr mutation also causes transformation, although dimerization of the receptor does not occur and a different set of substrate proteins are phosphorylated.

MUTATIONS OF THE *RET* PROTO-ONCOGENE ASSOCIATED WITH HIRSCHSPRUNG DISEASE   Two independent lines of analysis led to the identification of mutations of the *RET* proto-oncogene in patients with Hirschsprung disease. The identification of a chromosome 10 deletion in a child with Hirschsprung disease led to mapping studies in familial Hirschsprung disease that localized the causative gene to proximal chromosome 10q. Subsequent investigations identified inactivating and presumed activating mutations of the RET tyrosine kinase in Hirschsprung disease. Analysis of kindreds in which MEN2A and Hirschsprung disease cosegregate (*see* Table 40-1) have identified codon 609, 618, or 620 mutations of the *RET* proto-oncogene. Mutations of the endothelin-β receptor gene and its ligand, endothelin-3, have also been identified in Hirschsprung disease.

Mutation analysis is readily available from several commercial sources (www.genetests.org). Several techniques have been applied to detection of mutations including direct DNA sequencing and restriction analysis for specific mutations and denaturing gradient gel electrophoresis. Direct DNA sequencing has become the detection procedure of choice because it permits rapid sequencing of the seven exons known to be involved in MEN2. There are a few caveats. Genetic testing like most other forms of laboratory analysis will be associated with a small error rate caused by sample mix-up, contamination of the PCR reaction, failure of specific primers to amplify the mutant allele, or technician copying errors, collectively estimated in the range of 5%.

MUTATIONS OF THE *RET* PROTO-ONCOGENE IN SPORADIC MTC   Somatic met918thr mutations of the *RET* proto-oncogene have been identified in approx 25% of sporadic

MTCs. Evidence indicates that tumors with this particular mutation may pursue a more aggressive clinical course. It is important to consider *RET* proto-oncogene analysis in patients with apparent sporadic MTC because a compilation of available information indicates that 5–7% of patients with apparent sporadic MTC have germline mutations of the *RET* proto-oncogene.

MANAGEMENT/TREATMENT

MANAGEMENT OF MTC

Negative Genetic Test Results   The availability of reliable genetic testing makes it possible to identify gene carriers with near certainty. Children with negative test results can be excluded from further screening studies. It is important to *repeat* the analysis on more than one blood sample to be certain of the test results. This is especially true of individuals who have a normal *RET* analysis and will receive no further screening.

Positive Genetic Test Results   Clinical decision making based on *RET* proto-oncogene testing has evolved over the past several years. In an international conference focused on MEN there was consensus that genetic testing should form the basis for a decision for thyroidectomy. There was a general agreement that children with the highest risk mutations (codon 883, 918 associated with MEN2B) should have thyroidectomy performed shortly after birth. Those with high-risk codons (611, 618, 620, 630, 634, and 891) should be considered for thyroidectomy around the age of 5 yr, the earliest age at which metastasis has been identified in a child with one of these mutations. Others have argued for earlier thyroidectomy based on the finding of microscopic MTC (without evidence of metastasis) in younger children. In children with low-risk *RET* mutations (codons 790, 791, 768, 804, and 912), there are large kindreds in which there has never been a death caused by MTC. In these kindreds physicians are unwilling to recommend and parents are unwilling to accept a recommendation for early thyroidectomy. In patients with these mutations, thyroidectomy should be performed at some later age, perhaps between 10 and 15 yr of age. Some continue to perform pentagastrin or calcium testing for calcitonin and perform a thyroidectomy at the time of a positive test result. It is unclear whether earlier thyroidectomy would prevent the recurrences found in 15–20% of children thyroidectomized based on calcitonin testing in earlier series. A report of the European experience suggests that earlier thyroidectomy would be beneficial; in this large series metastasis to local lymph nodes was not observed until the mid-teenage years (although it is not clear how many lymph nodes were examined in each patient), suggesting earlier thyroidectomy may improve outcomes. At this point clinicians participating in the decision to perform early thyroidectomy should balance the risks and benefits of the procedure in each age group.

The completeness of thyroidectomy may be important. It is difficult to perform a total thyroidectomy without damage to blood vessels associated with the posterior capsule of the thyroid gland. Such damage can cause a higher incidence of hypoparathyroidism, a situation most surgeons choose to avoid. A few normal C cells in residual thyroid tissue attached to the posterior capsule may be of little concern in a 40- to 50-yr-old patient, but there is the real possibility that a few normal cells expressing a mutant RET kinase in a 5-yr-old child may transform over a several-decade period of follow-up. This concern has led some clinicians to recommend a total thyroidectomy including the posterior capsule, central lymph node dissection, and transplantation of parathyroid tissue to the nondominant arm. Whether this approach will improve the already excellent long-term cure rate for this disease is unclear, but seems worthy of investigation.

MANAGEMENT OF PHEOCHROMOCYTOMA The advent of genetic testing will have little impact on the management of pheochromocytoma in MEN2 other than to exclude 50% of family members with normal genetic tests from further screening. Patients with pheochromocytomas should have unilateral or bilateral adrenalectomy or a cortical sparing adrenalectomy, dependent on the specific clinical situation. Issues related to unilateral or bilateral adrenalectomy in this disease have been discussed in Chapter 38 and are not reviewed in this chapter. Patients with abnormal catecholamine secretion should have adrenal surgery performed prior to consideration of thyroidectomy.

MANAGEMENT OF HYPERPARATHYROIDISM Hyperparathyroidism occurs infrequently in children who have received prophylactic thyroidectomy for MTC. In one series there have been no cases of hyperparathyroidism in children who received thyroidectomy at a mean age of 13 yr with a mean follow-up period in excess of 20 yr. There is debate about the appropriate management of parathyroid neoplasia in older patients. Either subtotal parathyroidectomy or total parathyroidectomy with transplantation of parathyroid tissue to the nondominant forearm has been advocated.

FUTURE DIRECTIONS

Hereditary MTC is a rare disorder, but the specific molecular defect that causes this neoplastic syndrome provides a useful model in which to study strategies for inactivation of mutant RET tyrosine kinase activity. The fact that a single gene defect causes three different neoplastic manifestations makes it an interesting model for study. There are several small organic molecule tyrosine kinase inhibitors with activity against the RET kinase domain in phase I trials. The prolonged period during which transformation occurs makes MEN2 and hereditary MTC excellent models in which to assess the impact that prophylactic treatment with a drug designed to prevent RET activation would have on the natural history of the disease.

SELECTED REFERENCES

Airaksinen MS, Saarma M. The GDNF family: signalling, biological functions and therapeutic value. Nat Rev Neurosci 2002;3:383–394.

Angrist M, Bolk S, Thiel B, et al. Mutation analysis of the RET receptor tyrosine kinase in Hirschsprung's disease. Hum Mol Genet 1995;4:821–830.

Asai N, Iwashita T, Matsuyama M, et al. Mechanism of activation of the ret proto-oncogene by multiple endocrine neoplasia 2A mutations. Mol Cell Biol 1995;15:1613–1619.

Berndt I, Reuter M, Saller B, et al. A new hot spot for mutations in the ret protooncogene causing familial medullary thyroid carcinoma and multiple endocrine neoplasia type 2A. J Clin Endocrinol Metab 1998;83: 770–774.

Boccia LM, Green JS, Joyce C, et al. Mutation of RET codon 768 is associated with the FMTC phenotype. Clin Genet 1997;51:81–85.

Bolino A, Schuffenecker I, Luo Y, et al. RET mutations in exons 13 and 14 of FMTC patients. Oncogene 1995;10:2415–2419.

Borst MJ, Van Camp JM, Peacock ML, et al. Mutational analysis of multiple endocrine neoplasia type 2A associated with Hirschsprung's disease. Surgery 1995;117:386–391.

Brandi ML, Gagel RF, Angeli A, et al. Guidelines for diagnosis and therapy of MEN type 1 and type 2. J Clin Endocrinol Metab 2001;86:5658–5671.

Cance WG, Wells SA Jr. Multiple endocrine neoplasia type IIa. Curr Probl Surg 1985;22:1–56.

Carney JA, Go VL, Sizemore GW, et al. Alimentary-tract ganglioneuromatosis. A major component of the syndrome of multiple endocrine neoplasia, type 2b. N Engl J Med 1976;295:1287–1291.

Dang GT, Cote GJ, Schultz PN, et al. A codon 891 exon 15 RET protooncogene mutation in familial medullary thyroid carcinoma: A detection strategy. Mol Cell Probes 1999;13:77–79.

DeLellis RA, Wolfe HJ, Gagel RF, et al. Adrenal medullary hyperplasia. A morphometric analysis in patients with familial medullary thyroid carcinoma. Am J Pathol 1976;83:177–196.

Donis-Keller H, Dou S, Chi D, et al. Mutations in the RET proto-oncogene are associated with MEN2A and FMTC. Hum Mol Genet 1993;2:851–856.

Edery P, Lyonnet S, Mulligan LM, et al. Mutations of the RET protooncogene in Hirschsprung's disease. Nature 1994;367:378–380.

Eisenhofer G, Walther MM, Huynh TT, et al. Pheochromocytomas in von Hippel-Lindau syndrome and multiple endocrine neoplasia type 2 display distinct biochemical and clinical phenotypes. J Clin Endocrinol Metab 2001;86:1999–2008.

Eng C, Clayton D, Schuffenecker I, et al. The relationship between specific RET proto-oncogene mutations and disease phenotype in multiple endocrine neoplasia type 2. International RET mutation consortium analysis. JAMA 1996;276:1575–1579.

Farndon JR, Leight GS, Dilley WG, et al. Familial medullary thyroid carcinoma without associated endocrinopathies: a distinct clinical entity. Br J Surg 1986;73:278–281.

Gagel RF, Levy ML, Donovan DT, et al. Multiple endocrine neoplasia type 2a associated with cutaneous lichen amyloidosis. Ann Intern Med 1989;111:802–806.

Gagel RF, Marx S. Multiple endocrine neoplasia. In: Larsen PR, Kronenberg H, Melmed S, Polonsky KS, eds. Williams Textbook of Endocrinology. Philadelphia: WB Saunders, 2003:1717–1762.

Gagel RF, Tashjian AH Jr, Cummings T, et al. The clinical outcome of prospective screening for multiple endocrine neoplasia type 2a: an 18-year experience. N Engl J Med 1988;318:478–484.

Grieco M, Santoro M, Berlingieri MT, et al. PTC is a novel rearranged form of the ret proto-oncogene and is frequently detected in vivo in human thyroid papillary carcinomas. Cell 1990;60:557–563.

Hofstra RM, Fattoruso O, Quadro L, et al. A novel point mutation in the intracellular domain of the ret protooncogene in a family with medullary thyroid carcinoma. J Clin Endocrinol Metab 1997;82:4176–4178.

Hofstra RM, Landsvater RM, Ceccherini I, et al. A mutation in the RET proto-oncogene associated with multiple endocrine neoplasia type 2B and sporadic medullary thyroid carcinoma. Nature 1994;367:375–376.

Jhiang SM, Sagartz JE, Tong Q, et al. Targeted expression of the ret/PTC1 oncogene induces papillary thyroid carcinomas. Endocrinology 1996;137:375–378.

Jing S, Wen D, Yu Y, et al. GDNF-induced activation of the Ret protein tyrosine kinase is mediated by GDNFR-a, a novel receptor for GDNF. Cell 1996;85:1113–1124.

Kakudo K, Carney JA, Sizemore GW. Medullary carcinoma of thyroid. Biologic behavior of the sporadic and familial neoplasm. Cancer 1985;55:2818–2821.

Lee JE, Curley SA, Gagel RF, et al. Cortical-sparing adrenalectomy for patients with bilateral pheochromocytoma. Surgery 1996;120:1064–1071.

Lin LF, Doherty DH, Lile JD, et al. GDNF: a glial cell line-derived neurotrophic factor for midbrain dopaminergic neurons. Science 1993;260:1130–1132.

Mathew CG, Chin KS, Easton DF, et al. A linked genetic marker for multiple endocrine neoplasia type 2A on chromosome 10. Nature 1987;328:527–528.

Moore MW, Klein RD, Farinas I, et al. Renal and neuronal abnormalities in mice lacking GDNF. Nature 1996;382:76–79.

Mulligan LM, Eng C, Attie T, et al. Diverse phenotypes associated with exon 10 mutations of the RET proto-oncogene. Hum Mol Genet 1994;3:2163–2167.

Mulligan LM, Kwok JB, Healey CS, et al. Germ-line mutations of the RET proto-oncogene in multiple endocrine neoplasia type 2A. Nature 1993;363:458–460.

Nilsson O, Tisell LE, Jansson S, et al. Adrenal and extra-adrenal pheochromocytomas in a family with germline RET V804L mutation. JAMA 1999;281:1587, 1588.

Pachnis V, Mankoo B, Costantini F. Expresssion of the c-ret proto-oncogene during mouse embryogenesis. Development 1993;119:1005–1017.

Pichel JG, Shen L, Sheng HZ, et al. Defects in enteric innervation and kidney development in mice lacking GDNF. Nature 1996;382:73–76.

Romeo G, Ronchetto P, Luo Y, et al. Point mutations affecting the tyrosine kinase domain of the RET proto-oncogene in Hirschsprung's disease. Nature 1994;367:377, 378.

Sanchez M, Silos-Santiago I, Frisen J, et al. Newborn mice lacking GDNF display renal agenesis and absence of enteric neurons, but no deficits in midbrain dopaminergic neurons. Nature 1996;382:70–73.

Santoro M, Carlomagno F, Romano A, et al. Activation of RET as a dominant transforming gene by germline mutations of MEN2A and MEN2B. Science 1995;267:381–383.

Schilling T, Burck J, Sinn HP, et al. Prognostic value of codon 918 (ATG→ACG) RET proto-oncogene mutations in sporadic medullary thyroid carcinoma. Int J Cancer 2001;95:62–66.

Schuchardt A, D'Agati V, Larsson-Blomberg L, et al. Defects in the kidney and enteric nervous system of mice lacking the tyrosine kinase receptor Ret. Nature 1994;367:380–383.

Simpson NE, Kidd KK, Goodfellow PJ, et al. Assignment of multiple endocrine neoplasia type 2A to chromosome 10 by linkage. Nature 1987;328:528–530.

Sipple JH. The association of pheochromocytoma with carcinoma of the thyroid gland. Am J Med 1961;31:163–166.

Skinner MA, De Benedetti MK, Moley JF, et al. Medullary thyroid carcinoma in children with multiple endocrine neoplasia types 2A and 2B. J Pediatr Surg 1996;31:177–182.

Steiner AL, Goodman AD, Powers SR. Study of a kindred with pheochromocytoma, medullary carcinoma, hyperparathyroidism and Cushing's disease: Multiple endocrine neoplasia, type 2. Medicine 1968;47:371–409.

Takahashi M, Cooper GM. ret transforming gene encodes a fusion protein homologous to tyrosine kinases. Mol Cell Biol 1987;7:1378–1385.

Takahashi M, Ritz J, Cooper GM. Activation of a novel human transforming gene, ret, by DNA rearrangement. Cell 1985;42:581–588.

Trupp M, Arenas E, Falnzilber M, et al. Functional receptor for GDNF encoded by the c-ret proto-oncogene. Nature 1996;381:785–788.

Tsuzuki T, Takahashi M, Asai N, et al. Spatial and temporal expression of the *ret* proto-oncogene product in embryonic, infant and adult rat tissues. Oncogene 1995;10:191–198.

Vasen HFA, van der Feltz M, Raue F, et al. The natural course of multiple endocrine neoplasia type IIb: A study of 18 cases. Arch Intern Med 1992;152:1250–1252.

Verdy MB, Cadotte M, Schurch W, et al. A French Canadian family with multiple endocrine neoplasia type 2 syndromes. Henry Ford Hosp Med J 1984;32:251–253.

Wells SA Jr, Chi DD, Toshima K, et al. Predictive DNA testing and prophylactic thyroidectomy in patients at risk for multiple endocrine neoplasia type 2A. Ann Surg 1994;220:237–250.

Williams ED, Brown CL, Doniach I. Pathological and clinical findings in a series of 67 cases of medullary carcinoma of the thyroid. J Clin Pathol 1966;19:103–113.

Wohllk N, Cote GJ, Bugalho MMJ, et al. Relevance of RET proto-oncogene mutations in sporadic medullary thyroid carcinoma. J Clin Endocrinol Metab 1996;81:3740–3745.

Web site for localizing sites for genetic testing: www.genetests.org.

Zedenius J, Larsson C, Bergholm U, et al. Mutations of codon 918 in the RET proto-oncogene correlate to poor prognosis in sporadic medullary thyroid carcinomas. J Clin Endocrinol Metab 1995;80:3088–3090.

Zedenius J, Wallin G, Hamberger B, et al. Somatic and MEN2A de novo mutations identified in the RET proto-oncogene by screening of sporadic MTCs. Hum Mol Genet 1994;3:1259–1262.

41 Disorders of Sex Determination and Differentiation

CHARMIAN A. QUIGLEY

SUMMARY

Abnormalities of sex determination and differentiation comprise two major clinical groups: disorders of gonadal development (i.e., disorders of sex determination: sex reversal, true hermaphroditism), with secondary effects on genital development, and defects of genital development in the presence of normal gonads (disorders of sex differentiation: male and female "pseudohermaphroditism"). This chapter will review the embryology of normal sex determination and differentiation, the genetic basis of normal and abnormal sex determination and differentiation, and the approaches to diagnosis of disorders of sex determination and differentiation.

Key Words: Adrenogenital primordium; androgen insensitivity syndrome; congenital adrenal hyperplasia; gonadoblastoma; granulosa cell; hermaphroditism; labioscrotal fold; Leydig cell; Leydig cell hypoplasia; mosaicism; ovary determination; persistent Müllerian duct syndrome; primordial gonad; pseudohermaphroditism; Sertoli cell; sex differentiation; sex reversal; testis determination; theca cell; urogenital sinus.

INTRODUCTION

Sex determination and differentiation are distinct, consecutive processes that follow the establishment of chromosomal sex at the time of gamete fertilization, subsequently requiring the coordinated expression of a specific set (or sets) of genes in a strict spatiotemporal manner. The term *sex determination* (alternatively called *primary sex differentiation*) refers to the development of gonadal sex—a process that occurs at approx 6–7 wk gestation in the human male fetus, and approx 10–11 wk gestation in the female fetus. As generally used, the term *sex differentiation* refers to the processes downstream of gonadal development—those regulated by gonadal secretions or lack thereof (also called *secondary sex differentiation*). In essence, the genetic complement endowed at fertilization determines gonad type and the latter determines the pattern of differentiation of the internal genital ducts and external genitalia.

GENERAL CLINICAL FEATURES Abnormalities of sex determination and differentiation consists of two major clinical groups: disorders of gonadal development (i.e., disorders of sex determination: sex reversal, true hermaphroditism), with secondary effects on

genital development, and defects of genital development in the presence of normal gonads (disorders of sex differentiation: male and female pseudohermaphroditism). The disorders of sex determination and differentiation are summarized in Table 41-1. Approaches to diagnosis and management are discussed at the conclusion of the chapter.

Sex Reversal and True Hermaphroditism The terminology is sometimes confusing: sex reversal refers to the condition in which the individual's genetic sex opposes the gonadal (and therefore generally the phenotypic) sex. These are individuals with 46,XY karyotype who have no testes (in their place usually are streak gonads) and have a female (or ambiguous) phenotype, and those with 46,XX karyotype who have testes and varying degrees of genital masculinization. The archetypal and most common form of sex reversal is 46,XX maleness (approx 1 in 20,000 men has 46,XX karyotype). The phenotype of most 46,XX males is similar to that seen in Klinefelter syndrome (47,XXY): structurally normal (sometimes cryptorchid) testes are present and the internal and external genitalia are male. Testicular size and histology are normal in infancy. Pubertal virilization occurs to a greater or lesser degree, but like those with Klinefelter syndrome, affected postpubertal individuals have small testes and are azoospermic. Up to 20% of 46,XX males have subnormal masculinization, manifest by cryptorchidism, hypospadias or frank genital ambiguity. The testes have atrophic, hyalinized, seminiferous tubules and Leydig cell hyperplasia. The absence of spermatogenesis in 46,XX males may relate two factors, the presence of the extra X-chromosome, and the absence of Y-chromosomal genes involved in spermatogenesis. 46,XX males are taller than average for females, but shorter than 46,XY males, presumably because of absence of stature-determining genes located on Yq.

There are two main subtypes of 46,XX maleness (and 46,XX true hermaphroditism, described later)—XX^Y+ and XX^Y-. The majority of patients with complete 46,XX maleness are XX^Y+, resulting from translocation of all or part of the distal end of the Y-chromosome (Yp), containing the sex-determining region of the Y-chromosome *(SRY)*, to the short arm of an X-chromosome (Xp) during paternal gamete meiosis. In contrast, the majority of patients with 46,XX true hermaphroditism are XX^Y-. The molecular/ phenotypic inference from these findings is that the greater the amount of Y-chromosome material, the more complete the masculinization. Two specific hot spots for Yp-Xp recombination within areas of high X-Y sequence homology

From: *Principles of Molecular Medicine, Second Edition*
Edited by: M. S. Runge and C. Patterson © Humana Press, Inc., Totowa, NJ

Table 41-1
Genetic Disorders of Sex Determination and Differentiation

Disorders of sex determination (development of gonad discordant from karyotype)

46,XX sex reversal/true hermaphroditism (46,XX karyotype with testes or ovotestes)
XXY+ (SRY translocation to terminal Xp)
XXY− (probable mutation of downstream regulator of testis development)
46,XY sex reversal/true hermaphroditism (46,XY karyotype with ovaries, ovotestes or streak gonads)
SF1 deletion/mutation (homozygous, heterozygous)
WT1 deletion/mutation (heterozygous)
SRY deletion/mutation (Y-linked)
SOX9 mutation (heterozygous)
ATRX mutation (X-linked)
DHH mutation (homozygous)
Monosomy 9p (possible haploinsufficiency of DMRT1/2)
DSS (duplication)
WNT4 (duplication)

Disorders of sex differentiation (development of phenotype discordant from gonad)

46,XY pseudohermaphroditism (46,XY karyotype with testes and female or ambiguous internal or external genitalia)
Impaired testosterone production
LHCGR mutation (homozygous, compound heterozygous)
Defects of testosterone biosynthesis
StAR mutation/deletion (homozygous, compound heterozygous)
POR mutation (homozygous, heterozygous, compound heterozygous)
CYP11A mutation (heterozygous, compound heterozygous)
HSD3B2 mutation (homozygous, compound heterozygous)
CYP17 mutation (homozygous, compound heterozygous)
HSD17B3 mutation (homozygous, compound heterozygous)

Impaired androgen response
SRD5A2 deletion/mutation (homozygous, compound heterozygous)
AR gene deletion/mutation (hemizygous)

Impaired anti-Müllerian hormone production or action
AMH mutation (homozygous, compound heterozygous)
AMHR2 mutation (homozygous, compound heterozygous)

46,XX pseudohermaphroditism (46,XX karyotype with ovaries male or ambiguous internal or external genitalia)
Fetal androgen excess
Congenital adrenal hyperplasia
POR mutation (heterozygous, compound heterozygous, homozygous)
HSD3B2 mutation (homozygous, compound heterozygous)
CYP21 mutation (homozygous, compound heterozygous)
CYP11B1 mutation (homozygous, compound heterozygous)

Aromatase deficiency
CYP19 mutation (homozygous, compound heterozygous)
Disorders affecting Müllerian structures
HOXA13 mutation (heterozygous)
Mayer-Rokitansky-Kuster-Hauser syndrome (unknown etiology)

AMH, anti-Müllerian hormone; AMHR, anti-Müllerian hormone receptor; AR, androgen receptor; ATRX, α-thalassemia/mental retardation, X-linked gene; CG, chorionic gonadotropin; DHH, desert hedgehog; DSS, dosage-sensitive sex reversal; HOXA13, homeobox A 13; LH, luteinizing hormone; LHCGR, luteinizing hormone/chorionic gonadotropin receptor; POR, P450 oxidoreductase; SF1, steroidogenic factor 1; SOX, Sry-related homeobox gene; SRY, sec-determining region of the Y-chromosome; StAR, steroidogenic acute regulatory; WNT, wingless-type MMTV integration site family member; WT1, Wilms tumor 1.

have been reported to account for >50% of such recombination events. However, many 46,XX males have no definable genetic change and because approx 10% of 46,XX males with testes are completely negative for all Y-encoded sequences, it is likely that non Y sequences are responsible for testis determination in these cases. For example, female-to-male sex reversal has been found in association with duplication of the region of chromosome 17 containing the *SRY-related homeobox gene (SOX) 9*.

The converse of 46,XX maleness is complete gonadal dysgenesis in a 46,XY female (Swyer syndrome; XY gonadal dysgenesis),

however, it is much less common, occurring in only 1/100,000 females. Affected individuals have streak gonads with female internal and external genitalia, although significant phenotypic variation is found within affected families. Partial testicular dysgenesis is associated with genital development that essentially reflects the functional state of the gonads at the critical period of sex differentiation. Because of deficient estrogen production, breast development is poor and 46,XY females often present with delayed puberty or primary amenorrhea, accompanied by gonadotropin concentrations in the castrate range. Pubic hair is usually present. There is a high incidence of gonadal neoplasia (gonadoblastomas and germinomas). Probably because of the presence of Y-chromosomal stature-determining genes, affected women are of normal to tall stature compared with 46,XX females. Individuals with deletion of Yp (including the *SRY* gene) in addition to the general features described earlier, may have certain features of Turner syndrome such as lymphedema, likely because of haploinsufficiency of a gene or genes on Xp.

Male-to-female sex reversal has been reported in association with mutations of genes described in the following sections, including Wilms tumor 1 *(WT1), steroidogenic factor (SF) 1,* α*-thalassemia/mental retardation, X-linked gene (ATRX), SRY* and SRY homeobox-like gene 9 *(SOX9)* and also occurs in association with deletions of the region of chromosome 9 in which doublesex/ mab-related transcription factors *(DMRT1 and DMRT2)* reside, and with duplication of the chromosomal regions in which *dosage-sensitive sex reversal adrenal hypoplasia congenita locus on the X chromosome, gene 1 (DAX1;* X chromosome) and wingless-type MMTV integration site family *(WNT4;* chromosome 1) reside.

True hermaphroditism defines the condition in which, regardless of karyotype, there is coexistence of ovarian and testicular tissue in the same individual, either an ovary on one side and a testis on the other (~20% of patients), bilateral ovotestes (~30%) or one ovotestis and one testis or ovary (~50%). The testicular portions of the gonads are dysgenetic, with interstitial fibrosis and rare or absent spermatogonia, whereas the ovarian portions are histologically normal. Malignant degeneration of the gonad is reported in approx 5% of cases. Most affected invididuals have ambiguous genitalia, however, the phenotypic spectrum is broad: for example, a fully masculinized boy with bilaterally descended ovotestes has been reported. A hallmark, although not universal feature, is asymmetric genital development—Müllerian structures (that may include a full or hemiuterus) on one side and Wolffian structures on the other; a gonad-containing hemiscrotum on one side (more often the right) with a flat, empty labium majorum on the other. In general the pattern of development reflects the predominant functional nature of the gonad on the ipsilateral side. In association with an ovotestis, the internal genitalia may show elements of both Müllerian and Wolffian origin on the same side. The pattern of pubertal development reflects the function of the gonads and fertility is not uncommon.

Of affected individuals with true hermaphroditism, approx 70% have a 46,XX karyotype and some cases may represent a variant form of 46,XX maleness. Without thorough histological evaluation of the gonads it may be impossible to distinguish an undervirilized 46,XX male from a 46,XX true hermaphrodite. In addition, true hermaphroditism and complete sex reversal can coexist within the same family, so these disorders may be phenotypic variations of a certain genotype. The majority of patients with 46,XX true hermaphroditism are negative for any detectable Y-chromosomal sequences. About 20% of affected individuals have chromosomal mosaicism for 46,XX/46,XY or less commonly 46,XX/47,XXY; a small number of cases have a pure 46,XY karyotype and a few with 47,XXY karyotype have been reported. Although the molecular basis of this condition is unknown, genetic causes are implicated by the finding of familial cases of the disorder.

Pseudohermaphroditism Pseudohermaphroditism (either male [46,XY] or female [46,XX]) refers to conditions in which the karyotype and gonad are congruous, however, there is a discrepancy between the gonadal sex and the phenotypic sex: individuals with 46,XY karyotype and testes whose phenotype is female or ambiguous (e.g., disorders of androgen production or action) and those with 46,XX karyotype and ovaries whose phenotype is male or masculinized (e.g., disorders resulting in excess androgen production, such as congenital adrenal hyperplasia [CAH]). Individuals of either karyotypic sex with these disorders have phallic development that ranges from a diminutive clitoris in a 46,XY individual to a completely formed penis in a 46,XX individual; the labioscrotal region may be fully fused and rugose, or bifid and smooth; the internal structures may be mainly female-type (Müllerian, in the absence of anti-Müllerian hormone [AMH] action), mainly male-type (Wolffian, in the presence of local androgen action), or a combination of the two. The internal and external genital morphology essentially reflects fetal production of, and response to, androgens and AMH during the critical period of gestation.

OVERVIEW OF MOLECULAR PATHOPHYSIOLOGY

Because of the multiplicity of enzymes, hormones, receptors, and transcription factors involved, there are numerous opportunities for the usually well-coordinated processes of sex determination and differentiation to go awry. Some general principles are worth elucidating before delving into the specific disorders:

1. Hormones have no intrinsic action and must act through specific receptors. Thus hormone deficiencies are typically manifest by lack of function of the corresponding receptor. In general, steroid hormone deficiencies, resulting from defects of genes encoding the biosynthetic enzymes responsible for generation of the respective hormones, typically manifest only in the presence of two defective gene alleles and are inherited as autosomal-recessive traits.

2. Receptors that mediate hormone action comprise two broad categories. (1) Membrane-associated receptors act as transducers of the hormone signal. Binding of the hormone (typically a peptide) to the extracellular domain of such a receptor sets off an intracellular signal cascade in which a downstream factor or second messenger eventually influences gene transcription. (2) Intracellular receptors, such as those for the steroid and thyroid hormones, function as nuclear transcription factors themselves by entering the nucleus and binding directly with target genes to modify their transcription, usually in a ligand-dependent fashion. A subclass of the nuclear transcription factor family referred to as *orphan receptors* (e.g., DAX1) function in the absence of known ligand. In addition, other nonreceptor transcription factors of different classes and families also function in a ligand-independent manner (e.g., SRY, SOX9, WT1).

3. Defects of membrane-associated transducer-type receptors that mediate peptide hormone action, such as the luteinizing hormone/chorionic gonadotropin receptor (LHCGR), cause an increase or a decrease in the activity of the system, depending on whether the mutation is an activating or an inhibitory one. This is illustrated by the contrasting effects of mutations in the LHCGR: inhibitory mutations cause the syndrome of leydig cell hypoplasia (LCH, *see* LHCG Receptor), whereas activating mutations are associated with the syndrome of familial male precocious puberty (*see* Chapter 43). Defects of these receptors are expressed only in the presence of two defective gene alleles.

4. In the intracellular receptor system, absence of ligand or defective binding of ligand to the receptor translates to

absent or reduced activity of the ligand-dependent transcription factor; complete absence of a transcription factor (e.g., when the encoding gene is deleted) results complete loss of target gene transcription. Mutations of the DNA-binding regions of these receptors alter protein-DNA interactions between transcription factors and their target genes, potentially resulting in decreased, increased or sometimes promiscuous transcriptional activation, the latter resulting from loss of DNA-binding specificity. In the case of a heterozygous mutation, the abnormal protein produced from the mutant allele may interfere with the action of the normal protein produced from the wild-type allele of the gene—a "dominant negative" effect. In this situation, the mutant protein may block access of the normal factor to its target DNA, by forming inactive dimers that are unable to bind the target DNA sequence, or sequester other critical transcription factors because of disturbed protein–protein interactions. Defects in genes encoding nuclear transcription factors may manifest as dominant conditions, with dysfunction occurring in the presence of a single mutant allele (e.g., thyroid hormone receptor), or as recessive conditions in which both alleles must be mutated to cause disease (e.g., vitamin D receptor). Defects of this receptor class manifest clinically as hormone resistance syndromes, because hormone action is diminished in the presence of increased hormone levels.

EMBRYOLOGY OF NORMAL SEX DETERMINATION AND DIFFERENTIATION

Normal development of the gonads and genitalia has three major phases. First, in the earliest stages of gestation, the fetus develops a bipotential gonad, two sets of embryonic internal genitalia, and undifferentiated female-like external genitalia. The next step is the differentiation of the bipotential gonads into either ovaries or testes and the final phase is the differentiation and development of the internal and external genital primordia along male or female lines, depending on the nature of the hormonal products of the gonads (or lack thereof).

PHASE 1: DEVELOPMENT OF THE PRIMORDIAL STRUCTURES

GONADS At approx 5 wk of human gestation, the intermediate mesoderm in the area that will become the kidney, adrenal, and gonad condenses into distinct regions. As development progresses, the urogenital ridges form on the dorsal wall of the body cavity. The urogenital ridge consists of the mesonephros (the forebear of the primitive kidney) located laterally, and the genital ridge, which will become the primitive gonad, located medially. Development of the genital ridge is accompanied by thickening and proliferation of the coelomic epithelium, which penetrates the underlying mesenchyme to form the primitive sex cords. Blood vessels grow into the developing gonad from the mesonephros, subsequently developing in a sexually dimorphic manner. The primitive genital or gonadal ridges initially contain no germ cells. Between weeks 5 and 6 of gestation, primordial germ cells migrate from the endoderm of the yolk sac along the dorsal mesentery of the hindgut into the indifferent gonad, invading the developing primary sex cords. At this stage the gonad consists of an outer cortex and inner medulla, and no morphological difference between the gonads of male and female fetuses can be detected until approx 7

wk gestation, at which time testicular development begins in the male fetus.

INTERNAL GENITALIA Both the urinary and genital components of the urogenital system are derived, to a large extent, from the intermediate mesoderm, which becomes segmented into units termed nephrotomes. The lateral portions of the nephrotomes unite, forming a longitudinal duct on each side of the embryo, the mesonephric duct (later to become the Wolffian duct), by about week 4 of gestation. At approx 6 wk, the paramesonephric duct (to become the Müllerian duct) forms from the epithelium on the surface of the urogenital ridge, such that by 6 wk, both male and female fetuses are endowed with two sets of internal duct structures.

EXTERNAL GENITALIA Just as the gonads and internal genitalia are indistinguishable between the sexes for the first few weeks of life, so it is for the external genital primordia (Fig. 41-1). In the fourth week of gestation the external genitalia of both sexes are represented simply by a midline protuberance—the genital tubercle. By week 6 (still indifferent), two medial folds, the urethral folds, flank the urogenital groove and two larger folds, the labioscrotal folds, are present laterally.

PHASE 2: SEX DETERMINATION (DEVELOPMENT OF TESTIS OR OVARY)

TESTIS DEVELOPMENT Soon after the germ cells arrive, the gonad in the 46,XY fetus begins to differentiate; the first histologically discernible event in testis development is the appearance of primordial Sertoli cells, which differentiate from somatic cells of the coelomic epithelium at approx 7 wk gestation. The Sertoli cells proliferate, aggregate around the primitive germ cells and align into cord-like structures (medullary sex cords) that subsequently become the seminiferous tubules. The seclusion of germ cells within the tubules prevents meiosis and commits the germ cells to spermatogenic development. The prevention of meiosis may be the key event that directs gonadal development away from the ovarian pathway. This organizational process appears to be regulated by the Sertoli cells themselves. Germ cells are not required for this process, because morphological testis development occurs in their absence. About 1 wk later (approx 8 wk), steroidogenic Leydig cells differentiate from primitive interstitial cells of mesonephric origin, likely controlled by paracrine influences from Sertoli cells, possibly AMH. Another key event is the differentiation of peritubular myoid cells, thought to derive from the same interstitial cell lineage as Leydig cells. These myoepithelial cells are required for the development of the testis cords—the defining event in testicular organogenesis. Timing is critical as there is only a limited window during which these events can occur.

OVARY DEVELOPMENT In contrast with testis development, normal ovarian differentiation specifically requires the presence of germ cells. Without the germ cell seeding of the 46,XX gonadal primordium, the tissue degenerates into a nonfunctional, mainly fibrous "streak." Prior to week 10 of gestation the only histological feature that distinguishes an ovary is the absence of testicular features. Thereafter, ovarian structure becomes distinguishable, with the regression of the primary medullary sex cords, which are replaced by a vascular stroma. Secondary cortical sex cords that provide the supporting structure for the germ cells develop close to the surface of the gonad under the influence of the germ cell lineage. Within the sex cords the primary germ cells undergo vigorous mitotic replication to become oogonia; then the sex cords break up

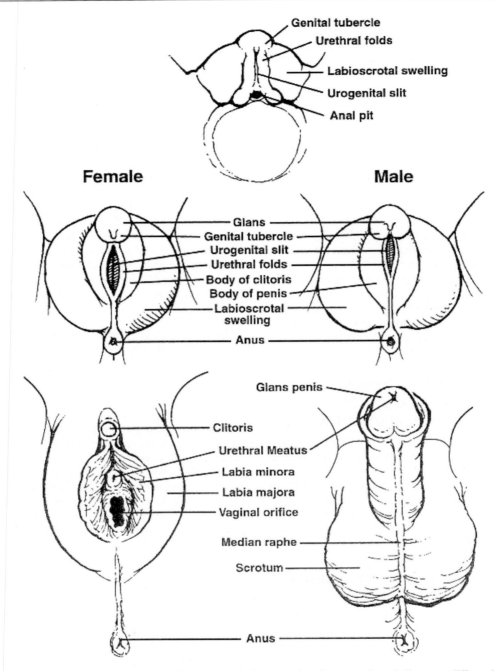

Figure 41-1   Differentiation of the external genitalia. (**Top**) At week 6 of gestation the external genitalia are undifferentiated, consisting of the midline genital tubercle, two medial urethral folds flanking the urogenital slit, and two larger labioscrotal swellings laterally. (**Left**) In the absence of androgen action the genital tubercle becomes the clitoris and the urogenital sinus remains patent. The vesicovaginal septum forms to separate the urethra from the vagina, located posteriorly. The urethral folds develop as the labia minora, whereas the labioscrotal folds enlarge slightly, remaining unfused, as the labia majora. (**Right**) In the male fetus in the presence of androgens (mainly DHT), the genital tubercle elongates to become the body of the penis, and the urethral folds fuse in the midline to form the penile urethra. The labioscrotal swellings fuse and enlarge to become the scrotum. These processes are completed approximately between weeks 8 and 12 of gestation.

into clusters, becoming the primordial follicles at about week 16. The primordial follicles contain the diploid (i.e., 46 chromosomes) primary oocytes, which after entering into the first stage of meiosis (reduction division) remain quiescent until puberty. Follicular (granulosa) cells arise from the same somatic cell lineage as Sertoli cells. Theca cells represent the ovarian counterpart of Leydig cells.

There is a notable difference in the chronology of testicular vs ovarian development, the process of testis formation being completed by 8 wk gestation, at which time the process of ovarian development has not yet begun. In fact, ovarian development is not completed until after most of the processes of phenotypic sex differentiation, described below, have occurred. This, and the fact that phenotypic development is normal even in complete absence of the ovary, highlights the lack of involvement of the ovary in the processes of normal female genital development.

PHASE 3: SEX DIFFERENTIATION (DEVELOPMENT OF MALE OR FEMALE GENITALIA)

INTERNAL GENITALIA: MALE   The primitive internal genital tracts are indistinguishable between the sexes until 7 wk gestation. From week 8 of gestation, hormonal secretions from the fetal testes induce masculinization of the internal genital structures in the 46,XY fetus. Initially the Wolffian ducts are stabilized (prevented from undergoing resorption) by the action (mainly local) of testosterone; between 9 and 13 wk gestation they undergo differentiation into the epididymides, vasa deferentia and seminal vesicles. Dihydrotestosterone (DHT) does not appear to mediate these processes, because the enzyme required for its production (5-α reductase 2) is not expressed in Wolffian tissues at the time of their differentiation. In parallel to the masculinization of the internal genitalia represented by Wolffian development, a process of "defeminization" of the redundant set of genital ducts occurs as the Müllerian ducts regress under the influence of locally acting AMH secreted by Sertoli cells. The Müllerian ducts are obliterated by week 11 of gestation, the only remnant of their existence in the male being the prostatic utricle. Absence of one testis results in retention of Müllerian structures and only limited Wolffian development on the ipsilateral side, indicating that the effects of AMH and testosterone are largely mediated in a paracrine fashion.

INTERNAL GENITALIA: FEMALE   In the absence of testicular secretions, as in the normal 46,XX fetus, the inverse set of genital tract developmental processes occurs. Without local androgen action, the Wolffian ducts regress. Meanwhile, absence of AMH allows the Müllerian ducts to develop. Their upper portions form the fallopian tubes; the lower sections fuse and differentiate as the uterus and upper part of the vagina. The lower portion of the vagina derives from the urogenital sinus (the ventral part of the embryonic mammalian cloaca formed by the growth of a fold dividing the cloaca where the gut and allantois meet), which remains patent in the absence of androgen action.

EXTERNAL GENITALIA: MALE   Under the influence of androgen action (primarily DHT), the genital tubercle elongates to form the body of the penis, and the urethral folds fuse ventrally from behind forward, to form the penile urethra. The labioscrotal folds grow toward each other, fusing in the midline to form the scrotum. DHT also induces the urogenital sinus to differentiate as the prostate, and inhibits the formation of the vesico-vaginal septum. These processes are completed by week 12 of gestation (Fig. 41-1). Between 12 and 24 wk gestation the testes migrate from their original lumbar location to the level of the internal inguinal ring above the scrotum. Descent of the testes through the inguinal ring and into the scrotum begins around week 28, and in most infants is completed by term.

EXTERNAL GENITALIA: FEMALE   In the absence of significant androgen action, such as in the normal female fetus, the genital tubercle elongates only slightly to form the clitoris (Fig. 41-1). The urogenital sinus remains open and the vesico-vaginal septum (a fold of tissue that separates the posterior wall of the bladder from the anterior wall of the vagina) forms, so that the urethra opens anteriorly and the vagina posteriorly. The vestibule of the urogenital sinus is bordered laterally by the urethral folds, which do not fuse and instead develop as the labia minora. Further lateral, the labioscrotal swellings enlarge somewhat but also remain unfused, forming the labia majora. There is minor fusion posteriorly, forming the posterior commissure, and anteriorly, producing the mons pubis. These events occur from about week 7–12 of gestation.

GENETIC BASIS OF NORMAL AND ABNORMAL SEX DETERMINATION AND DIFFERENTIATION

A complex interplay of genes, transcription factors, hormones, and receptors is required for normal sex determination and differentiation (Table 41-2). The primary event governing the path of morphological sex differentiation is the development of the gonad. In 1947 the elegant experiments of Jost determined that "maleness" was a state imposed on the fetus that would otherwise develop as a phenotypic female, leading to the theory that development of the ovary and female phenotype occur when the fetus is not exposed to the influences of specific "maleness-determining" genes. However, newer information, indicates that rather than being a passive, "default" process, female development likely also requires activation of specific, perhaps opposing, gene pathways. From these findings the concept has developed that sex determination represents the primordial "Battle of the Sexes"*—the dominance of one set of gonad-specific genes over another. The key event determining the winner of the battle appears to be whether the primordial germ cells that colonize the indifferent gonad enter meiosis. Testis cord development, under the influence of a number of *SOX* genes during a narrow developmental window, arrests the primordial germ cells in mitosis; in the absence of testis cord development, germ cells enter meiosis and ovarian development ensues. The genes involved in the regulation of sex determination and sex differentiation reside on both the sex chromosome and the autosomes. Based on studies of sex determination in other species it has been hypothesized that the mammalian sex chromosomes evolved from a homologous autosome pair.

The initial event in sex determination—the development of the primordial, bipotential gonad—depends on a network of interacting factors encoded by at least a dozen, and possibly scores of genes. Subsequent development of the testis or the ovary is exquisitely regulated by a team of cooperative transcriptional activators and repressors that selectively up- or downregulate the genes required for sex-specific gonadal differentiation.

BIPOTENTIAL GONAD AND PRIMORDIAL INTERNAL GENITAL DUCTS   There is a relationship between renal, adrenal, and gonadal cellular precursors that underlies both normal and abnormal development, because these tissues all arise from the same regions of the primitive mesoderm and coelomic epithelium known as *adrenogenital primordium*. The adrenal cortex derives from mesenchymal cells attached to the coelomic cavity lining adjacent to the urogenital ridge within the intermediate mesoderm; similarly, the steroid-producing cells of the gonads (Leydig and theca cells) differentiate from mesenchymal stem cells. The specific ontogeny of steroidogenic tissues has particular relevance for the understanding of the genetic regulation of gonadal development. Because these tissues have common cellular ancestors, it is not surprising that they share aspects of their genetic makeup. Thus the roles and responsibilities of a number of transcription factors involved in the early stages of renal, adrenal

---

*This term was coined by Blanche Capel and colleagues in "The Battle of the Sexes: Opposing Pathways in Sex Determination" in The Genetics and Biology of Sex Determination, Novartis Foundation Symposium 2002;244: pp. 187–202.

Table 41-2
Factors Involved in Sex Determination and Differentiation

Factors involved in primordial gonadal/reproductive tract formation

Gene name or pseudonyms	Human gene locus	Human protein name	Protein type	Genetic or cellular targets	Action	Effects of over- or under-expression
SF1[a] Ftzf1 Ad4BP NR5A1	9q33	SF1	Orphan nuclear receptor/zinc finger transcription factor	WT1, SRY, SOX9, DAX1, GnRHR, LHb, ACTHR, AMH, AMHR, StAR, P450scc, 21-OH'lase, 11b-OH'lase, oxytocin, SF1, others	Activates transcription of many genes in development of gonads, adrenals; regulates steroidogenesis. Synergizes with WT1; antagonizes DAX1. Dose dependent activity.	KO mice: no gonads or adrenals; retained Müllerian structures; abnormal hypothalamus. Haploinsufficient mice: reduced but not absent adrenal function. Homozygous human mutation: 46,XY sex reversal and adrenal hypoplasia. Heterozygous human mutation: 46,XX normal ovary, partial adrenal insufficiency.
WT1[a]	11p13	WT1	Zinc finger transcription factor; tumor repressor	DAX1, IGF-II, type 1 IGF receptor; PDGF-A, Pax2, WT1, SRY	Represses transcription; activates transcription of Sry. Dose dependent effects	XY homozygous deletion of WT1+KTS isoform: male-to-female sex reversal; XY homozygous deletion of WT1-KTS isoform: streak gonads in XX and XY. Human Denys-Drash syndrome: gonadal dysgenesis, congenital nephropathy, Wilms tumor.
Lim1 Lhx1	11p12-13	LIM1	Homeodomain transcription factor with 2 LIM domains (4 zinc fingers)	Not reported	Expressed at stage of primitive streak. Organizes development of anterior neural tissues	KO mice lack heads, kidneys and genital ridges.
Emx2[a]	10q26.1	EMX2	Homeodomain transcription factor	Wnt4, possibly Lim1	Similar to Lim1. Probably functions downstream of WT1	KO mice (XX or XY) lack kidneys, ureters, gonads and genital tracts and have brain defects. Human mutation causes schizencephaly; no urogenital phenotype reported.
Lhx9	1q31-32	LHX9	LIM homeodomain transcription factor, similar to LIM1	Binds SF1 promoter. May have additive effect with -KTS isoform of WT1 in activating SF1 expression	Drives formation of sex cords	XX and XY KO mice have gonadal agenesis.
CBX2 M33	17q25, near Sox9	M33	Transcription repressor	Possibly SRY	Mediates changes in chromatin structure	KO mice (XX or XY) have retarded development of gonadal ridges; XY mice have male-to-female sex reversal.
Wnt4[a]	1p35	WNT4	Cysteine-rich signaling molecule/secreted growth factor	Mesonephric mesenchyme	Directs Müllerian duct formation	XX and XY null mice have Müllerian agenesis (see "ovary" for details of human mutation).

406

Gene	Locus	Protein	Expression	Function	Mutations/Phenotype
c-Kit	4q12	Kit	Transmembrane tyrosine kinase receptor; protooncogene	Germ cell, hemopoetic and melanocyte precursors	Suppresses apoptosis, directs migration/ proliferation of stem cell populations	Mouse mutations: white coat color, sterility, anemia. Human mutation: piebaldism, mast cell luekemia.
Steel	12q22	Slf/KL	Ligand or c-Kit	Unknown	As for c-Kit	Mouse mutations: white coat color, sterility, anemia.

Factors involved in testis/male sex determination/differentiation[b]

Gene	Locus	Protein	Expression	Function	Mutations/Phenotype
SRY[a]	Yp11.3	SRY	HMG box-containing transcription factor	SF1, SOX9, CYP19, AMH	Bends DNA; may antagonize SOX3	XX mice expressing transgenic Sry female-to-male sex reversal. Human SRY mutations: 46,XY sex reversal. Translocation of SRY to X-chromosome: 46,XX female-to-male sex reversal or true hermaphroditism.
SOX9[a]	17q24-25	SOX9	HMG box-containing transcription factor of SRY family	Supporting cells of gonadal primordium	Stimulates differentiation of Sertoli cells	Odsex mice (deletion of regulatory locus upstream of Sox9): derepression of Sox9 expression in XX gonads → testis development.
ATRX[a] XH2 XNP	Xq13.3	ATRX	Helicase; transcription factor	Widespread expression early in mouse embryogenesis, more restricted expression later	Gene regulation at interphase and chromosomal segregation at mitosis	Human mutations cause α-thalassemia, mental retardation and genital anomalies → male-to-female sex reversal.
Dhh	12q13.1	DHH	Signaling molecule	Expressed only in testis	Involved in interactions between Sertoli cells and germ cells. May regulate mitosis and meiosis in male germ cells	Strain-specific effects: XY null mice have defective Leydig cell development and are feminized.
LHCGR[a]	2p21	LH/CG Receptor	G protein-coupled, 7-transmembrane peptide hormone receptor	Not applicable	Transduces LH signal to activate Gsα → cAMP. Required for Leydig cell testosterone production	Human mutation: Leydig cell hypoplasia → male pseudohermaphroditism. Mouse: normal sex differentiaition. Males and females infertile.
StAR[a]	8p11.2	StAR	Mitochondrial transport protein	Not applicable	Transports cholesterol to inner mitochondrial membrane	Human mutation: congenital lipoid adrenal hyperplasia and male pseudohermpahroditism.
SRD5A1[a] AR[a]	5p15 Xq11-12	5α-reductase2 AR	Mitochondrial enzyme Ligand-dependent nuclear receptor/transcription factor	Not applicable AMHR, ?CYP19	Converts testosterone → DHT Regulates transcription	Male pseudohermaphroditism. Mouse, rat: testicular feminization (Tfm). Human mutations: androgen insensitivity syndromes.
AMH[a]	19p13.2-13.3	AMH	Glycoprotein homodimer of TGFβ family	Not reported	Ligand for AMH-R	Persistent Müllerian duct syndrome.
AMHR[a]	12q13	Type II AMH receptor	Transmembrane serine/ threonine kinase receptor	Mesenchymal and epithelial cells of müllerian ducts	Mediates apoptosis of Mullerian duct	Persistent Müllerian duct syndrome.

(Continued)

Table 41-2 (Continued)

Gene name or pseudonyms	Human gene locus	Human protein name	Protein type	Genetic or cellular targets	Action	Effects of over- or under-expression
Factors involved in ovary/female sex determination/differentiation						
Wnt4[a]	1p35	WNT4	Cysteine-rich signaling molecule/secreted growth factor	Mesonephric mesenchyme	Directs initial Müllerian duct formation in both sexes; possible "anti-testis" factor in ovarian development	XX and XY null mice: Müllerian duct agenesis. Overexpression in XY: male-to-female sex reversal. Human: duplication of *WNT4* associated with 46,XY male-to-female sex reversal. Mutation in 46,XX: Müllerian regression, androgen excess.
FoxL2[a]	3q23	FOXL2	Transcription factor	Not reported	Expressed predominantly in ovary; earliest known marker of ovarian differentiation in mammals	Goat: deletion associated with XX sex reversal. Human mutation: 46,XX ovarian dysgenesis.
Fst	5q11.2	Follistatin	Glycosylated protein related to TGFβ family	Granulosa cells	Antagonizes action of activins and BMP15 in steroidogenesis; involved in Wnt4 signaling	Overexpression in XX mice: small ovaries with block in folliculogenesis; *Fst*-null XX mice: development of testis-like vasculature
Gdf9	Unknown	GDF9	Secreted growth factor member of TGFβ family	Ovarian somatic cells	Secreted by oocytes as paracrine factor required for ovarian somatic cell function	*Gdf9* null XX mice: block in oocyte differentiation
Bmp15 Gdf9b	Xp11.2	BMP15	Secreted growth factor member of TGFβ family	Granulosa cells	Paracrine stimulation of ovarian granulosa cell growth and proliferation; downregulates FSH receptor expression; antagonized by FST	XX KO mice: subfertile; homozygous mutation in XX sheep: premature ovarian failure; XX human heterozygous mutation: ovarian dysgenesis
Hoxa13[a]	7p15-p14.2	HOXA13	Homeodomain transcription factor	*Fgf8, Bmp7*	Involved in epithelial-mesenchymal interactions required for morphogenesis of terminal gut and urogenital tract, including Müllerian structures	Mouse: XX null will have hypoplasia of cervix and vagina. Human mutation: hand-foot-genital syndrome with uterine malformation in 46,XX
Factors with possible roles in either sex						
DAX1[a] Ahch NR0B1	Xp21	DAX1	Orphan nuclear receptor transcription factor	*Retinoic acid receptor, retinoid X receptor, StAR, P450scc, 3β-HSD, CYP17*	Antagonizes SF1; regulates testis cord organization. Dose-dependent effects.	Strain-specific defects in XY mice: overexpression → testis maldevelopment and sex reversal; homozygous deletion → adrenal hypoplasia, normal testes. Human mutations: adrenal hypoplasia congenital, hypothalamic hypogonadism

DMRT1/2	9p24.3	DMRT1 and DMRT2	Doublesex-MAB domain transcription factors	Not reported	Expressed only in genital ridge Dose-dependent effects on postnatal testis development	XY null mice have normal prenatal testis development, but abnormal postnatal testis differentiation. Human monosomy 9p: 46,XY testis maldevelopment; 46,XX primary hypogonadism
GATA4[a]	8p23.1-p22	GATA4	Zinc finger transcription factor	"*GATA*" motif on target genes; *AMH*; genes for steroidogenic enzymes	Expressed early in both ovary and testis	KO in mouse–embryonic lethal, no gonadal phenotype reported. Human mutation–cardiac defects; no gonadal phenotype reported
WNT7a	3p25	WNT7a	Signaling molecule	Mesenchymal and epithelial cells of Müllerian ducts	XY: involved in Müllerian duct regression; XX: stimulates development of Müllerian duct	XY null mice: retained Müllerian ducts; female *Wnt7a* deficient mice: defective, though not absent, development of oviducts and uterus

[a]Genes in which human mutations have been reported.

[b]Note: *see* Table 4 for enzymes of steroidogenesis.

A number of the genes listed have been implicated in gonadal/genital development only by studies in mice and defects have not been reported in humans.

ACTHR, adrenocorticotropic hormone receptor; AMH, anti-Müllerian hormone; AMHR, anti-Müllerian hormone receptor; AR, androgen receptor; ATRX, α-thalassemia/mental retardation, X-linked gene; BMP15, bone morphogenetic protein 15; CG, chorionic gonadotropin; DAX1, dosage-sensitive sex reversal-adrenal hypoplasia congenita locus on the X-chromosome, gene 1; DHH, desert hedgehog; DHT, dihydrotestosterone; DMRT1/2, Doublesex and MAB-3-Related Transcription Factors 1 and 2; FSH, follicle stimulating hormone; FST, follistatin; FOXL2, fork-head transcription factor 2; GDF, growth differentiation factor; GnRH-R, gonadotropin-releasing hormone receptor; HMG, high-mobility group; HOXA13, homeobox A 13; HSD, hydroxysteroid dehydrogenase; IGF, insulin-like growth factor; KO, knockout; KTS, lysine/threonine/serine; LH, luteinizing hormone; LHCGR, luteinizing hormone/chorionic gonadotropin receptor; LHX9, LIM homeobox gene 9; LIM, Lin-l1, Islet-1 and Mec-3; LIM1, LIM homeobox gene 1; PDGF, platelet-derived growth factor; SF1, steroidogenic factor 1; SOX, Sry-related homeobox gene; SRY, sex-determining region of the Y chromosome; StAR, steroidogenic acute regulatory protein; TGF-β, transforming growth factor-β; WNT, wingless-type MMTV integration site family member; WT1, Wilms tumor 1.

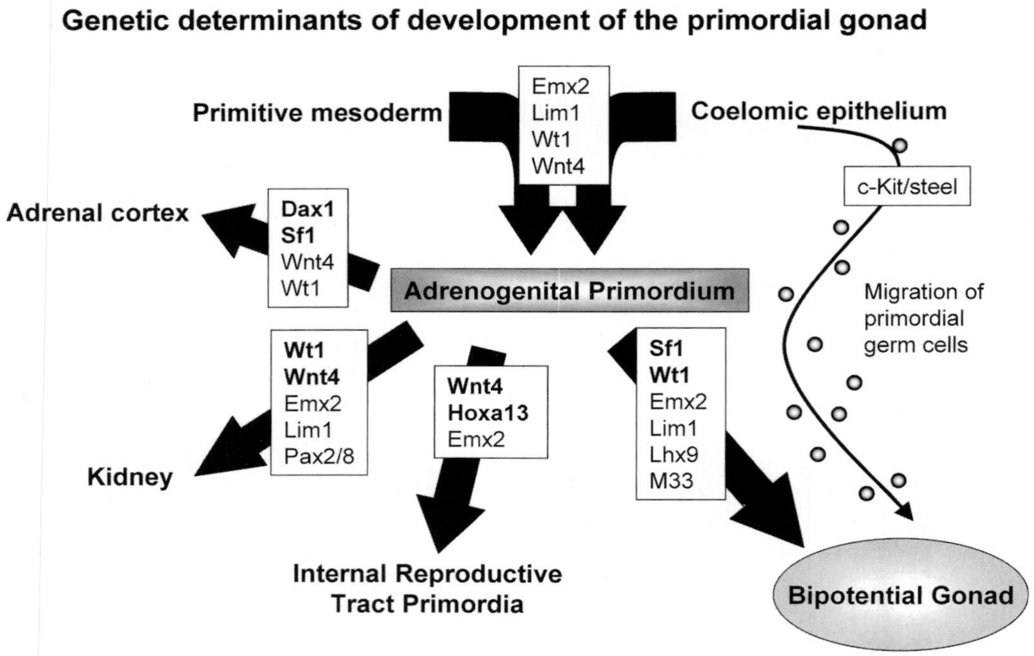

Genetic determinants of development of the primordial gonad

Figure 41-2   Genetic determinants of development of the primordial gonad. Transcription factors Emx2, Lim1, Wt1, and Wnt4 are required for development of the adrenogenital primordium, which forms following condensation of primitive mesoderm and coelomic epithelium. Thereafter, various combinations of transcription factors direct the fate of the undifferentiated primordial cells down one of a number of pathways to form the adrenal cortex, kidney, bipotential gonad and internal reproductive tract primordia. Factors highlighted in bold have been established to be involved in human development. Dax1, dosage-sensitive sex reversal-adrenal hypoplasia congenita locus on the X-chromosome, gene 1; Emx2, empty spiracles 2; Hoxa1, homeobox A1; Lhx9, LIM homeobox gene 9; Lim1, Lin-11, Islet-1, and Mec-3 homeobox gene 1; Sf1, steroidogenic factor 1; Wt1, Wilms tumor 1; Wnt4, wingless-type MMTV integration site family member 4.

and gonadal development overlap, when tissues are undifferentiated and the major developmental need of the organism is to increase cell mass. As development progresses, and populations of cells begin to differentiate along specific, irreversible paths, there is a requirement for a much more focused program of transcription factor action. This concept may help in the understanding of the diverse roles served by transcription factors such as SF1, WT1, and LIM (the acronym stands for Lin-11, Islet-1 and Mec-3—the three original members of the family) homeobox* gene 1 (LIM1), compared with the much more limited roles, expression, timing and cellular specificity of factors such as SRY and AMH.

Factors implicated in the early development of the bipotential gonadal and reproductive tract primordia on the basis of defects observed in humans include SF1, WT1, and WNT4. In addition, LIM1, empty spiracles 2 (EMX2), and LIM homeobox gene 9 (LHX9) are implicated in these processes on the basis of murine studies. Furthermore the ligand/receptor pair Steel/c-Kit is vital, at least in mice, to the process of germ cell migration from the yolk sac to the gonadal primordium in both sexes. Exact relationships between these factors and the precise timing and order of their expression remain to be determined; a hypothetical scheme for their potential roles in regulating the processes of early development of the reproductive tract is shown in Fig. 41-2. In the next section, descriptions of the molecular biology of individual factors and their molecular defects in humans, are provided. Additional genes postulated to be involved in these processes based on studies in nonhuman species are described briefly at the end of this section.

*The homeobox is the approx 180 bp sequence in the gene that encodes the approx 60 AA homeodomain of the respective protein.

Steroidogenic Factor 1 (SF1)

Normal Function   The orphan nuclear receptor transcription factor, SF1 (also referred to as adrenal 4-binding protein and officially termed nuclear receptor subfamily 5, group A, member 1) appears to be one of the earliest-acting and most critical factors in the primitive development of the reproductive tract. SF1 affects reproductive function at all three levels of the hypothalamic-pituitary-gonadal axis, as well as the adrenal gland, and subsequently regulates factors acting further down the pathway of gonadal/genital development in a male-specific fashion. Importantly, SF1 appears to act in a dose-dependent manner in both mice and humans.

The human *SF1* gene is located at chromosome 9q33, spans 30 kb of genomic DNA and contains seven exons including an initial noncoding exon. SF1 is a 461-amino acid (AA), 53-kDa protein containing two central DNA-binding zinc fingers (ZFs) typical of nuclear receptors, an activation domain and a C-terminal ligand-binding domain (for which no ligand has yet been identified, hence its designation as an "orphan" receptor). SF1 differs structurally from most nuclear receptors by lacking an N-terminal domain and differs functionally by binding as a monomer, rather than as the more usual dimer, to a nonpalindromic DNA sequence. Based on studies of human mutations, two regions of the protein appear particularly critical for function: the so-called P-box, located in the proximal portion of the first ZF, is responsible for interaction with the major groove of DNA; the A-box region downstream of the ZFs modulates monomeric binding to DNA.

In the mouse *Sf1* (also known as *FtzF1*, based on its similarity to the drosophila gene, fushi tarazu factor 1) is expressed in male

Emx2 may modulate their expression. In addition to developmental defects of the brain, *Emx2*-null mice lacked kidneys, ureters, gonads, and genital tracts. Degeneration of the Wolffian duct and mesonephric tubules was abnormally accelerated and Müllerian ducts did not form. These abnormalities imply a role for Emx2 in very early development of the renal, gonadal and internal genital primordia, probably at the stage of development of the mesonephros.

Lim Homeobox Gene 9 (LHX9)   *Lhx9*, encodes another member of the LIM family of transcription factors. Like Lim 1, Lhx9 also plays a role in primordial gonad development, evidenced by the finding of complete gonadal agenesis in *Lhx9*-null mice of both sexes, without apparent extra-gonadal defects (in contrast with the headless *Lim1*-null mutants). Gonadal agenesis appeared to result from failure of gonadal cell proliferation at about E12, rather than exaggeration of apoptosis. Lhx9 appears to be necessary for proliferation and invasion of the epithelial (somatic) cells of the genital ridge into the underlying mesenchyme and subsequent formation of sex cords—an essential step in formation of the gonads.

Lhx9 expression is detectable at E9.5 in epithelial and subjacent mesenchymal cells of the early gonadal ridge. Expression localizes to the interstitial region of the developing testis as morphological differentiation occurs, then disappears as epithelial cells differentiate into Sertoli cells and begin to express *Amh*. In the fetal ovary *Lhx9* is highly expressed in epithelial cords, then is downregulated as ovarian epithelial cells differentiate into granulosa cells. Thus it appears that *Lhx9* expression is inversely correlated with the degree of differentiation of mesenchymal cells of the gonad. In human embryos *LHX9* is expressed in the abdominal region of both sexes at the time of gonad formation. Human LHX9 mutations have not been reported, despite a careful search in at least one study in 27 patients with 46,XY gonadal agenesis or dysgenesis.

All *Lxh9*-null mice were phenotypically female. They had atrophic uteri, vagina, and oviducts indicating that Lhx9 is not required for development of the internal genital primordia. As would be expected in the situation of gonadal agenesis, the mice had high FSH concentrations and no detectable testosterone or estradiol.

A key role of Lhx9 may be in regulation of *Sf1* expression. Lhx9 binds directly to the *Sf1* promoter and may act synergistically with the –KTS isoform of Wt1 in activating *Sf1* expression. This regulatory interaction appears to be specific to the gonad, evidenced in *Lhx9*-null mice by the finding of normal adrenal *Sf1* expression despite absent expression in genital ridges.

NORMAL AND ABNORMAL TESTIS DETERMINATION

Male sex determination is synonymous with testis determination. Once development of the primordial gonadal and genital structures has occurred, the next steps diverge between the sexes. The process of testis development in the karyotypic male appears to be controlled by a switch-like mechanism that involves the crucial Y-chromosome-encoded transcription factor SRY, a related homodomain transcription factor, SOX9, and no doubt other genes and proteins that either regulate or are regulated by these factors. One of the earliest effects of *SRY* expression is the induction of somatic cell migration from the mesonephros into the XY gonad—a critical first step in preparation for development of testis cords. Subsequently, SOX9 directs the process of seminiferous tubule organization by Sertoli cells and regulates expression of the Sertoli cell glycoprotein AMH. AMH may in turn play a role in directing undifferentiated interstitial cells to develop as Leydig cells. Once testicular differentiation is established, other Y-encoded factors are required to maintain spermatogenesis. A number of other molecules have been identified as having involvement in testis development; however,

their exact positions in this pathway, their functions and the factors they regulate or by which they are regulated, remain to be elucidated. These include the +KTS isoform of WT1, the helicase enzyme ATRX, perhaps the intracellular signaling molecule, desert hedgehog (DHH) and gene(s) on chromosome 10q. Additional X-chromosomal sequences likely affect testis development, perhaps negatively, because the presence of one or more extra X-chromosomes (as found in Klinefelter syndrome and its variants) is associated with reduced testicular size.

There are many hypothetical schemes for the interactions of the ever-expanding coterie of transcription factors involved in testis determination, and no definitive model for this process exists. Analyses of humans with gonadal dysgenesis, mouse models and in vitro assays have revealed that testis determination results from a complex network of interacting transcription factors and target genes in a nonlinear web of upregulation or activation and downregulation or repression steps. A hypothetical model, based primarily on work in mice, is as follows:

1. Establishment of the gonadal primordium (multiple factors, described earlier).
2. Activation of Sry by Wt1 and Gata4.
3. Sry repression of Wnt4 and perhaps forkhead transcription factor 2 (Foxl2) thus.
4. Allowing Sf1 to.
5. Stimulate expression of Sox9 (possibly by interfering with binding of a repressor factor to the *Odsex* locus upstream of the *Sox9* gene) and perhaps Atrx, leading to.
6. Development of Sertoli cells followed by.
7. Wt1/Sf1/Sox9/Gata4-mediated induction of Amh expression.
8. Action of Amh via the Amh receptor(s) causing Müllerian duct regression.
9. Sf1-mediated stimulation of steroidogenic activity by fetal Leydig cells (Fig. 41-4).

There may be significant species differences in the processes of testis development, so although the mouse is generally a convenient model, differences between mice and humans must not be overlooked and the details of sex determination and differentiation that have been elucidated in rodents cannot necessarily be extrapolated to human development.

SRY-Related Homeobox (SOX) Genes   There is an ever-expanding family of DNA-binding, atypical transcription-regulating proteins related to each other by the presence of a central high mobility group (HMG) domain,* homologous (>60% AA identity) to the HMG domain of the founding member of the family, SRY. At least 20 *SOX* genes have been described, and a number of these appear to be involved in sex determination or have testis-specific expression, including *SRY* itself, *SOX9, SOX3, SOX30,* and perhaps *SOX8*. Only the most well characterized genes—*SRY* and *SOX9*—are discussed.

Sex-Determining Region Of The Y (SRY) Gene

Normal Function   The existence of a Y-chromosomal "maleness-determining" gene was postulated in the 1930s, and in the 1960s was designated the "testis-determining factor." Many candidates were proposed and rejected over the years, until 1990,

---

*The HMG domain is a 70–80 AA DNA-binding motif comprised mainly of hydrophobic and charged AAs, shared by a group of architectural proteins involved in DNA transcription, replication, recombination, and repair.

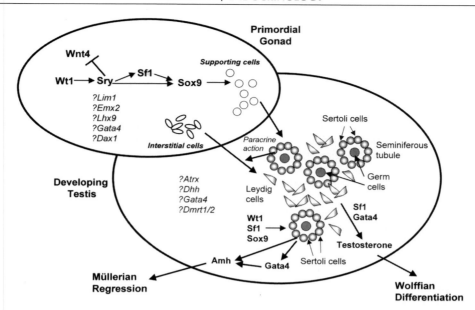

Figure 41-4 Hypothetical model of testis determination. The bipotential gonad of an XY fetus expresses the key testis-determining gene *Sry*, which is upregulated by Wt1 and Gata4. Sry represses the "anti-testis" gene, *Wnt4,* and perhaps *Foxl2* thus allowing Sf1 to stimulate *Sox9* expression leading to differentiation of supporting cells into Sertoli cells, the primary organizers of the seminiferous tubule. The seclusion of germ cells within the tubules prevents germ cell meiosis and commits them to spermatogenic development. Wt1, Sf1, Sox9, and Gata4 induce Sertoli cell expression of Amh, which, acting via its type 2 receptor, causes Müllerian duct regression. Under the influence of Sertoli cells, interstitial cells differentiate as Leydig cells, subsequently secreting testosterone under the drive of Sf1 and Gata4 inducing development of Wolffian structures. Other factors that have less well-defined roles include Lim1, Emx2, Lhx9, Dax1, Dhh, Atrx, and Dmrt1/2. AMH, anti-Müllerian hormone; ATRX, α-thalassemia/mental retardation, X-linked gene; DAX1, dosage-sensitive sex reversal-adrenal hypoplasia congenita locus on the X-chromosome, gene 1; DHH, desert hedgehog; DMRT1/2, Doublesex and MAB-3-Related Transcription factors 1 and 2; EMX2, empty spiracles 2; LHX9, LIM homeobox gene 9; LIM1, LIM homeobox gene 1; SF1, steroidogenic factor 1; SOX, Sry-related homeobox gene; SRY, sec-determining region of the Y-chromosome; WNT, wingless-type; MMTV integration site family member; WT1, Wilms tumor 1.

when the existence of such a gene was confirmed, with the discovery of *SRY*. Insertion of the mouse *Sry* gene into fertilized XX mouse eggs resulted in development of testes and male genitalia (female-to-male sex reversal). These seminal studies demonstrated that *Sry* was the key Y-chomosomal gene sufficient to induce maleness. However, replacement of the homeobox of *Sry* with that of *Sox3* or *Sox9* also results in sex reversal in XX mice, indicating that *Sox3* or *Sox9* can functionally replace *Sry* and elicit development of testis cords, male patterns of gene expression, and male genital development.

Human *SRY* is a 3.8-kb single-exon gene located just centromeric to the pseudoautosomal region of Yp (Yp11.3) that encodes a 204-AA (24 kDa) protein. Approximately the middle one-third of the protein (79 AAs) represents the HMG domain that endows SRY with its sequence specific DNA binding to a target nucleotide sequence. This region is the most critical to protein function and almost all human mutations are located here. Outside the HMG domain the remainder of the protein is poorly conserved among mammals.

The target genes of SRY are largely unknown, but may include those encoding AMH, SOX9, and the steroidogenic enzyme CYP11. Similarly, the exact mechanism of action and whether SRY has any direct transcriptional activating capacity, remain to be determined. Human SRY lacks a transcription activation domain (present in mouse), so it has been suggested that SRY function depends solely on the HMG domain and that it acts as an "architectural" transcription factor, by creating the spatial arrangement needed for the transcription "machinery" to work.

Expression of *Sry* occurs in fetal mouse gonad at the earliest stage of specific testis formation, being first detected at E10.5 in pre-Sertoli cells in the developing gonadal ridge, to which its

expression is limited, about 1 d before testicular morphology can be discerned. This finding suggests that these pre-Sertoli cells are integral to the process of testis development. Indeed, one of the primary events in testis development is induction of Sertoli cell differentiation. *Sry* expression peaks at E11.5 and declines once testicular development is established, at E12.5. *Sry* expression and Sertoli cell differentiation are followed by testis differentiation, manifest by Sertoli cell-regulated organization of seminiferous tubules and Leydig cell differentiation. In human testes *SRY* expression begins at approx 6 wk gestation, just prior to specific testis development. The fundamental role of SRY appears to be the upregulation of *SOX9* expression, which in turn stimulates development of the prime organizers of testicular architecture—the Sertoli cells. SRY may continue to act as a splicing factor in Sertoli cells and germ cells in the adult testis.

Despite its preeminent role in testis determination, other transcription factors appear to regulate *SRY* expression, including WT1. Furthermore other upstream and downstream factors must be activated or repressed to allow testis development to occur. Evidence for this conclusion includes the following:

1. *Sry* expression during mouse gonadogenesis; occurs during a very brief time window.
2. The majority of 46,XY females with gonadal dysgenesis have an intact *SRY* gene.
3. Some 46,XX males with testes are completely Y negative, indicating that non-Y sequences must be responsible for testis determination in these cases.

Clinical Features and Molecular Defects   The study of individuals with the syndromes of 46,XX maleness and 46,XY gonadal

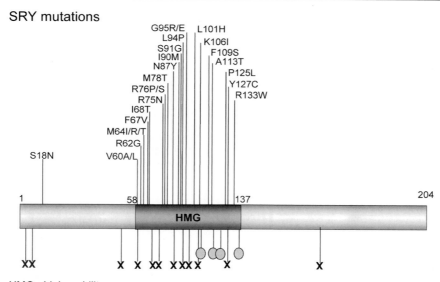

Figure 41-5   Mutations in human SRY.

dysgenesis was the catalyst for the eventual localization and characterization of the *SRY* gene. Of 46,XX males with unambiguous masculinization, >90% are *SRY* positive (this can be confirmed by PCR or fluorescent *in situ* hybridization analysis), whereas the converse holds for 46,XX males with genital ambiguity and 46,XX true hermaphrodites, of whom only a small number are *SRY* positive. Nonrandom inactivation of the X-chromosome carrying the translocated *SRY* is the postulated explanation for the presence of ovarian and testicular tissue in the same gonad in individuals with *SRY*-positive hermaphroditism. The coexistence of 46,XX complete maleness and 46,XX true hermaphroditism in a number of families may reflect variations in the pattern of inactivation of the *SRY*-bearing X-chromosome between affected individuals.

In parallel to the finding of *SRY* sequences in the majority of 46,XX males, it would be predicted that most sex-reversed 46,XY females would have *SRY* defects. However, in general this has not proven to be the case as mutations in *SRY* have been detected in only 15–20% of 46,XY sex-reversed individuals with complete or partial gonadal dysgenesis (more common in complete dysgenesis). Suggested explanations for this finding include the theoretical presence of mutations outside the HMG box, perhaps in sequences important for regulation of *SRY* expression, inactivating mutations in upstream regulators of *SRY*, mutations that induce constitutive activity in genes usually negatively regulated by SRY, or activating mutations in factors that suppress or interfere with SRY.

A variety of cytogenetic and molecular abnormalities have been reported in individuals with 46,XY sex reversal, including deletion of Yp, isolated deletion of *SRY*, nonsense mutations resulting in protein truncations, and at least 25 missense mutations within the *SRY* HMG box (Fig. 41-5). Only one missense mutation has been reported outside the HMG box, a serine to asparagine change in the N-terminal region. Most *SRY* mutations in 46,XY sex reversal produce nonconservative AA substitutions at highly conserved sites within the HMG domain. In vitro analysis of mutant SRY proteins reveals abnormal DNA binding and bending: some mutants bind DNA normally but less avidly, whereas others

bind with near-normal affinity but bend the DNA to a different angle. Less dramatic missense mutations cause partial, rather than complete, gonadal dysgenesis, as the mutant SRY protein likely retains some function. *SRY* mutations also have been reported in a few cases of 46,XY true hermaphroditism. One example was a postzygotic somatic mutation evidenced by the finding of both wild-type and mutant *SRY* alleles in gonadal DNA but only the wild-type *SRY* sequence in leukocyte DNA. There may be phenotypic variation between 46,XY individuals harboring the same *SRY* mutation, ranging from sex-reversed to unaffected, both within and between kindreds, perhaps because of variable penetrance or influences of the genetic background. The most severe *SRY* defects appear to arise *de novo*, whereas the milder defects are compatible with fertility and thereby transmission to offspring. Germline mosaicism for the *SRY* mutation may be associated with fertility in the fathers of affected individuals.

SRY Homeobox-Like Gene 9 (SOX9)

Normal Function   *Sox9*, like *Sry*, can induce testis formation when inserted into XX mouse embryos and appears to be equally as important as its brother *Sry*, in the process of testis development. The human *SRY* gene is located at 17q24-25, in a region termed sex reversal autosomal 1 and encodes a 509-AA protein with features of a transcription regulator—a DNA-binding HMG domain and two transcriptional activation domains, including a proline and glutamine-rich domain in its C-terminal region. In vitro deletion of this latter region destroys the transactivating function of the protein. Unlike *SRY*, *SOX9* displays strong sequence conservation throughout mammalian evolution. Furthermore, the sequence similarity between *SOX9* and *SRY* suggests a relationship between the two that may represent evolution from a dosage-dependent autosomal sex determination system to a dominant Y-chromosomal system.

Sox9 is initially expressed in the genital ridges of both sexes in mice at low levels and is subsequently downregulated in female genital ridges and upregulated in male genital ridges, its expression paralleling Sertoli cell differentiation, consistent with a role in testis determination. Based on the timing of expression and the

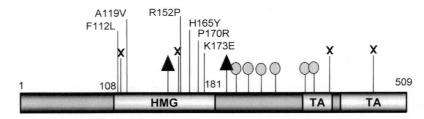

HMG = high mobility group; TA = transactivation. Mutations in 46,XY sex reversal are shown. Nonsense (stop) mutations are designated with 'X'; frameshift mutations are designated with ◯ ; splicing mutations are designated with ▲ .

Figure 41-6   Mutations in human SOX9.

presence of a potential binding site for Sry within its promoter, Sox9 appears to be acting just downstream of Sry and is likely a target gene for Sry. However, there is probably not an absolute requirement for Sry regulation of *Sox9*, because Sox9 can induce testis development in the absence of Sry. *Sox9* expression precedes that of *Amh* and Sox9 appears to play the pivotal role (in conjunction with Sf1, Wt1, and Gata4; Fig. 41-3B) in activating *Amh* expression, a role befitting a key maleness-determining factor. Sox9 may represent another "switch"-like mechanism, as it appears to act in a dominant fashion, similar to Sry. Indeed, Sox9 may be the pivotal maleness-determining factor, potentially displacing Sry in this role—a battle whose outcome is awaited.

Human *SOX9* expression is detectable in the testis at week 18 of gestation in the area of the rete testis and seminiferous tubules. In the adult, *SOX9* is expressed most strongly in the testis, pancreas, prostate, kidney, brain, and the skeleton and at low level in most other adult tissues.

Mice with heterozygous *Sox9* deletion had skeletal malformations equivalent to those seen in the human disease, campomelic dysplasia, and died soon after birth. However, the testes were normal in the male mutant mice in contrast to many human *SOX9* mutations, well known for causing male-to-female sex reversal in the heterozygous state, suggesting differences in SOX9/Sox9 function between mice and humans. Overexpression of *Sox9* in XX gonads is associated with testis development in *Odsex* mice, providing additional evidence for the importance of Sox9 in testis determination.

Clinical Features and Molecular Defects   *SOX9* was identified by cloning of a chromosomal translocation breakpoint from a sex-reversed patient with campomelic dysplasia, a rare syndrome featuring a distinctive form of skeletal malformation that causes severe limb bowing (campomelia), accompanied in approx 75% of affected 46,XY individuals by sex reversal (ovaries or streak gonads, and female internal and external genitalia). Affected 46,XX individuals have normal ovarian development, reflecting lack of involvement of SOX9 in this process. Death typically occurs in early childhood from respiratory compromise related to the skeletal dysplasia. A milder form of the condition, in which the limbs are not bowed is referred to as "acampomelic" campomelic dysplasia.

Heterozygous mutations in *SOX9* have been identified in 46,XY individuals with campomelic dysplasia and sex reversal (Fig. 41-6). In general *SOX9* mutations occur *de novo* and affect only one *SOX9* allele, although one case of compound heterozygosity has been reported. Most disease-causing mutations severely disrupt the protein (e.g., premature termination and frameshift mutations) and the phenotype appears to result from loss of function of the

transcription factor (haploinsufficiency). Affected sibling pairs with normal parents have been reported, as a consequence of gonadal mosaicism for the mutant gene. As with *SRY* mutations, variation in phenotype has been reported within the same family. For example, in one family with three children bearing a framsehift mutation, one 46,XY child had true hermaphroditism with ambiguous external genitalia, whereas a 46,XY sibling had sex reversal with bilateral ovaries and female genitalia. In patients with the milder "acampomelic" form, missense mutations resulting in AA substitutions within the HMG domain have been reported. The genital abnormalities are also milder than in those with complete *SOX9* inactivation, manifest in one such patient by a bifid scrotum, perineal hypospadias, and undescended right testis.

A number of patients with 46,XY autosomal-dominant sex reversal and campomelic dysplasia have chromosome 17 breakpoints at least 50–130 kb from the *SOX9* locus, suggesting the presence of other genes responsible for the same phenotype, or perhaps a disturbance of *SOX9* expression resulting from mutation of an upstream regulator. Positional cloning of the chromosome 17q breakpoint in one patient with sex reversal and "acampomelic" dysplasia identified a 3.5-kb complementary DNA that is expressed in testis but appears not to be translated. In addition, cases with chromosomal rearrangements involving 17q have been described most likely affecting regulatory elements upstream of *SOX9*.

Partial 46,XX female-to-male sex reversal has been reported in an infant with mosaicism for a chromosomal rearrangement resulting in duplication of *SOX9*. The child had severe penile/scrotal hypospadias, a small penis with descended palpable gonads in a bifid scrotum and absence of uterus on ultrasound. This finding suggests that an extra dose of *SOX9* is sufficient to initiate testis differentiation in the absence of *SRY* in humans as well as mice.

α-Thalassemia/Mental Retardation, X-Linked (ATRX)

Normal Function   α-Thalassemia/mental retardation, X-Linked (ATRX) (also known as X-linked helicase-2) is a helicase—an enzyme that catalyzes the unwinding of double-stranded nucleic acids—and is a member of a family of proteins involved in DNA recombination and repair, chromatin remodeling, chromosome segregation and regulation of transcription.

The large (>200 kb, 35 exon) *ATRX* gene is located at Xq13.3 (and is also on mouse X chromosome) and is subject to alternate splicing in different tissues. There is a homologous gene on the Y chromosome of marsupial mammals (not present in mouse or human) that is expressed specifically in the testis, giving additional weight to its role in male sex determination. The protein contains a nuclear localization signal and three ZFs in the N-terminal region; the C-terminal region contains six helicase domains and a glutamine rich sequence common in transcription factors. ATRX is thought to function by binding to DNA via the ZF region then opening the double helix with the helicase region in an ATPase-dependent manner. The protein is associated with pericentromeric chromatin during interphase and mitosis, suggesting that ATRX may act as part of a protein complex that modulates chromatin structure.

ATRX is expressed in a wide range of embryonic and adult human tissues, including developing brain and testis. Because of its X-chromosomal location, the gene undergoes X-inactivation in females to retain dosage equivalence with males. As a single active copy in normal females is not associated with testis development, although a single copy is adequate for testis development in males, ATRX likely functions downstream of a male-specific transcription factor such as SRY or SOX9, requiring activation by such a factor. Apart from the fact that human mutations are associated with sex reversal, little is known about the function of this protein in sex determination and differentiation, as comprehensive studies in mice are lacking.

Clinical Features and Molecular Defects The ATRX syndrome is an X-linked disorder characterized in 46,XY individuals by variable severity of α-thalassemia, psychomotor retardation, dysmorphic features, gonadal dysgenesis and undermasculinization. In sex-reversed patients the gonads are streaks, however, Müllerian ducts are absent, indicating that *AMH* expression, and therefore Sertoli cell development were retained during the critical period. Consequently, the critical period for *ATRX* expression appears to be after Sertoli cell development. Diverse mutations in the *ATRX* gene have been reported in individuals with the ATRX syndrome and several clinical variants of the syndrome reflect different mutations in the gene, including Smith-Fineman-Myers, α-thalassemia myelodysplasia and Juberg-Marsidi syndromes. There appear to be some genotype–phenotype correlations: mutations associated with sex reversal have mainly been those causing truncation of the protein with loss of the C-terminal region including the "P-element" (a 15-AA region homologous to that found in other transcriptionally active proteins) and the polyglutamine tract; mutations within a helicase domain are associated with severe mental retardation without thalassemia; and mutations that alter residues in carboxyl terminus outside the helicase domains result in the classic ATRX syndrome. As with other sex reversal disorders, phenotype may vary within a given family, likely reflecting influence of genetic background.

Desert Hedgehog (DHH)

Normal Function Desert hedgehog (Dhh) is a signaling molecule involved in interactions between Sertoli cells and germ cells whose primary role appears to be regulation of spermatogenesis. The 3-exon human *DHH* gene located at chromosome 12q13.1 encodes a 396-AA polypeptide.

In mice *Dhh* is expressed only in the testis and not in the ovary. Expression is initiated in Sertoli cell precursors shortly after activation of *Sry* expression, and persists to adulthood. This system appears to regulate mitosis and meiosis in male germ cells, its role varying at different stages of development. In the embryonic testis Dhh regulates germ cell proliferation and Leydig cell development, whereas in the postnatal testis it directs germ cell maturation. The receptor for Dhh, Patched2, is expressed on Leydig cells and peritubular cells, and one of the key roles of Dhh appears to be in the proper development of peritubular tissue. Consequently, the mechanism by which Dhh regulates germ cell development may be indirect, via other cell types, and may be secondary to the more general effects on organization of testicular structure.

In the initial murine studies, homozygous null male mice had small testes and were infertile because of lack of mature sperm. However, apart from the deficiency of germ cells, the testes were structurally and microscopically normal—including the Dhh-producing Sertoli cells themselves. In a subsequent study in mice from a different genetic background, more than 90% of null male mice were feminized. They had small, undescended, ectopically located testes and poor Leydig cell development with low serum testosterone, female external genitalia and a blind vagina. The latter study demonstrated requirement for Dhh for normal development of peritubular myoid cells and the basal lamina and subsequent well-organized development of seminiferous tubules. Thus *Dhh* may or may not be required for testicular organogenesis depending on genetic background (contrast the effect of a human *DHH* mutation described below) and there is phenotypic heterogeneity of the null mutation even within a single genetic background.

Clinical Features and Molecular Defects DHH is included within the section on testis determination primarily on the basis of a single 46,XY patient who had partial gonadal dysgenesis as a result of a homozygous mutation at the initiation codon in exon 1 of *DHH*, with predicted a failure of protein translation. The young woman, whose parents were first cousins, presented for evaluation of primary amenorrhea and had poor breast development, immature female external genitalia, a blind vagina, and a form of polyneuropathy. Laparoscopy revealed a testis on one side and a streak gonad on the other. Serum testosterone was low and FSH was elevated.

NORMAL AND ABNORMAL OVARY DETERMINATION

The factors directing ovarian development are less well characterized than those governing testis development. However, there is presumably an equally complex network of controls guiding this process, which likely requires action on two fronts: repression of autosomal testis-inducing genes such as *SOX9* (but not *SRY*, as this is absent from the normal XX embryo), and either derepression (removal of an inhibitory influence) or activation (direct stimulation) of ovary-inducing genes. Importantly, any factor that functions as a "testis inhibitor" must be expressed and active prior to the time that expression of autosomal testis-determining factors would otherwise occur. One such testis inhibitor likely resides on the X chromosome and is probably a dosage sensitive locus, expressed from both X chromosomes in females. A former candidate for this role was *DAX1,* based on the finding of streak ovaries in place of testes in individuals with duplication of the X-chromosomal region containing the gene. However, *DAX1* became less convincing as the "antitestis" gene when a female with homozygous *DAX1* deletion was reported. Current prime candidates for roles as testis inhibitors are Wnt4, follistatin and "*Odsex,*" a locus on chromosome 17 upstream of *Sox9* that may contain a gonad-specific *Sox9* regulatory sequence. No candidate for the role of a positive "ovary-determining factor" has been proposed; however, such a gene is probably also a dosage sensitive locus (therefore likely X chromosomal) required for germ cell survival in the ovarian milieu. This is suggested by the findings in individuals with Turner syndrome, who, in the absence of two functional copies of the X chromosome have ovarian regression because of early fetal demise of germ cells. It is therefore reasonable to speculate that initial ovarian differentiation occurs under the influence of a factor (or factors) expressed in the absence of the Y chromosome, and that subsequently, dosage-sensitive X chromosomal genes (required in double copy) are responsible for ovarian maintenance.

No clearly defined sequence of steps in the pathway of ovarian development has been established and this is likely a complex,

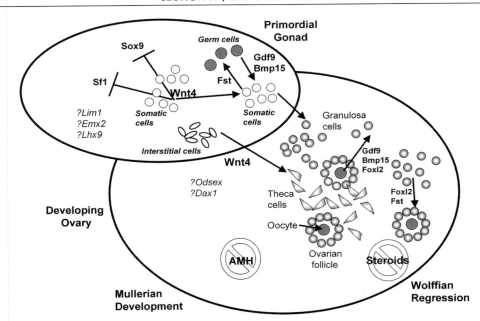

Figure 41-7 Hypothetical model of ovary determination. Wnt4 secreted by somatic cells increases expression of Fst, Dax1 and/or other factor(s) that antagonize Sf1 and repress Sox9 (perhaps by binding to the *Odsex* locus upstream of *Sox9*). Thus bipotential supporting cells do not differentiate as Sertoli cells, but instead as granulosa cells. Paracrine interactions between granulosa cells, secreting Foxl2 and Fst, and germ cells secreting Gdf9 and Bmp15, promote development of ovarian follicles. Wnt4 and Fst together inhibit activin-driven development of testicular (coelomic) vasculature, and Wnt4 inhibits differentiation of bipotential interstitial cells to Leydig cells. Because the XX fetal gonad does not produce sex steroids, the Wolffian ducts regress and external genitalia develop as female. Sertoli cells do not develop, therefore Amh is not produced, so Müllerian structures are maintained and subsequently differentiate under the influence of Hoxa13 and other factors. AMH, anti-Müllerian hormone; BMP15, bone morphogenetic protein 15; DAX1, dosage-sensitive sex reversal-adrenal hypoplasia congenita locus on the X-chromosome, gene 1; EMX2, empty spiracles 2; FOXL2, forkhead transcription factor 2; FST, follistatin; GDF, growth differentiation factor; Hoxa13, hoemobox A 13; LHX9, LIM homeobox gene 9; LIM1, LIM homeobox gene 1; SF1, steroidogenic factor 1; SOX, Sry-related homeobox gene; WNT, wingless-type MMTV integration site family member.

nonlinear, set of interconnected up- and downregulatory events. A speculative model, based on some of the known and hypothetical genetic events, mainly in mice, is as follows:

1. An unknown factor induces expression of Wnt4 by somatic cells.
2. Wnt4 increases expression of Dax1, Fst and/or other factor(s) that antagonize Sf1 and repress Sox9 (perhaps by binding to the *Odsex* locus).
3. Bipotential supporting cells do not differentiate as Sertoli cells, but instead as granulosa cells.
4. Paracrine interactions between granulosa cells, secreting Foxl2 and Fst, and germ cells secreting Gdf9 and bone morphogenetic protein 15 (Bmp15), promote development of ovarian follicles.
5. Wnt4 and Fst together inhibit activin-driven development of testicular (coelomic) vasculature.
6. Wnt4 inhibits differentiation of bipotential interstitial cells to Leydig cells.
7. The fetal gonad does not produce sex steroids, therefore the Wolffian ducts regress and external genitalia develop as female.
8. Because Sertoli cells do not develop, Amh is not produced.
9. Müllerian structures are maintained and subsequently differentiate under the influence of homeobox A 13 (Hoxa13) and other factors (Fig. 41-7).

Wingless-Type MMTV Integration Site Family Gene 4 (WNT4)

Normal Function *Wnt* genes belong to a family of protooncogenes with at least 16 known mammalian members

expressed in species ranging from Drosophila to man. These genes encode 38- to 43-kDa cysteine-rich glycoproteins with features typical of secreted growth factors (extracellular signaling molecules): a hydrophobic signal sequence and 21 conserved cysteines whose relative spacing is maintained. Transcription of *Wnt* genes appears to be developmentally regulated in a precise temporospatial manner. Interaction of Wnt factors with Frizzled receptors (members of the seven-transmembrane domain family) results in an intracellular signal cascade that in turn leads to transcriptional activation of target genes. By these interactions the Wnts regulate cell proliferation, morphology and fate. Members of this family are involved in sex determination and differentiation at various levels, including wingless-type MMTV integration site family gene 4 (WNT4) (ovary), WNT5A (external genitalia) and WNT7A (Müllerian duct regression, described later).

Wnt4 is required for the initial stages of Müllerian duct formation in both sexes in mice and appears to be required for normal ovarian development in females, making it a prime candidate for an "anti-testis" gene, interacting with Fst and perhaps Dax1 in this role (Wnt4 regulates expression of both factors). *Wnt4* expression is first detected in the mesonephric mesenchyme, which later forms the bipotential gonad, and is subsequently expressed in the indifferent gonads of both sexes. At the onset of sex-specific gonadal differentiation, *Wnt4* expression is downregulated in the male (probably by Sry/Sox9), but in the female is maintained within somatic cell lineages throughout fetal life. *Wnt4* is also strongly expressed in the mesenchyme underlying the Müllerian ducts, and in the adrenal cortex of both sexes, consistent with a role in regulation of steroidogenesis.

Homozygous *Wnt4*-null mice of both sexes had failure of differentiation of kidney mesenchyme and absence of Müllerian ducts in early gestation. Most striking were the specific effects in female mice, which had masculinization of the gonad and development of Wolffian ducts (the latter because of activation of gonadal steroidogenesis by Leydig cell precursors). Thus, Wnt4 acts in ovarian development by suppressing the differentiation of primordial interstitial cells into Leydig cells, thereby inhibiting testosterone synthesis and allowing female development to occur. Of note, the mice had no masculinization of the external genitalia, probably because testosterone was produced in insufficient quantities from the mutant gonads. Wnt4 further acts by stimulating *Fst* expression and these two factors act in concert to suppress/inhibit activin B, which would otherwise stimulate development of the testicular coelomic vasculature. The ovaries of the XX *Wnt4*-null mice had accelerated loss of oocytes to <10% of the number present in wild-type littermates, suggesting a role for Wnt4 in maintenance of the female germ cell line and oocyte development. The mice also had reduced gonadal *Dax1* expression, reflecting the role of Wnt4 as a regulator of *Dax1*. In complementary experiments overexpression of *Wnt4* in XY mice leads to reduction of testicular steroidogenesis secondary to reduction of Star, which in turn results from repression of Sf1 action by excess Wnt4.

Another member of this family, Wnt5a, is expressed in the genital tubercle and in the genital tract mesenchyme during embryogenesis and postnatally. Wnt5a mutant mice have a stunted genital tubercle and do not develop external genitalia.

Clinical Features and Molecular Defects   Mirroring the findings in mice, the phenotypic features of a 46,XX woman with a *WNT4* mutation included the absence of Müllerian structures (uterus and vagina) and signs of mild androgen excess, with a small vaginal introitus (no clitoromegaly) and acne. However, the extent of similarity between the mouse model and the naturally occurring human mutation is unknown, as no information was available regarding ovarian morphology. Additional evidence for the role of WNT4 in human sex determination comes from 46,XY patients with duplication of the region of 1p containing *WNT4* (1p35) who have varying degrees of undermasculinization ranging from cryptorchidism to sex reversal. One such patient who had fibrous gonads with rudimentary tubules, remnants of both Müllerian and Wolffian ducts, and ambiguous external genitalia was specifically demonstrated to have duplication of the *WNT4* gene, with overexpression of the protein.

Winged Helix/Forkhead Transcription Factor 2 (FOXL2)

Normal Function   Winged helix/forkhead transcription factor 2 (FOXL2) is implicated in the process of ovarian development by the finding of gonadal dysgenesis in some individuals with mutations of the gene and by the XX sex-reversed goat, which has a deletion in the chromosomal region containing the gene. The single-exon gene is located at human chromosome 3q23 and encodes a member of the winged helix/forkhead transcription factor family (there are at least 20 known human forkhead genes). These proteins contain a characteristic 100-AA DNA-binding domain and are involved in the development of tissues from all three germ layers. FOXL2 appears to be required for maintenance of ovarian follicles, which in turn is required for completion of ovarian development. In the absence of ovarian follicles the gonad regresses to become a fibrous streak; when follicles develop but undergo early atresia, premature ovarian failure ensues.

Foxl2 is highly conserved during evolution and abundantly expressed in the developing ovary of several species with different mechanisms of sex determination (mouse, chicken, and turtle); expression occurs around the time of sex determination and is sexually dimorphic, consistent with a conserved role of this factor in ovarian differentiation. *Foxl2* expression in developing mouse ovary begins at approximately E12.5 and continues into postnatal life; *Foxl2* is detectable in both somatic and germ cell populations in the developing ovary, and in granulosa cells and some oocytes in the adult ovary. Some *Foxl2* expression is also detectable in the developing oviducts. Inhibition of *Foxl2* expression by Sry has been proposed as one of the switch mechanisms that promotes testis development. Further understanding of the role of Foxl2 in ovarian determination awaits a knockout mouse model.

Clinical Features and Molecular Defects   Various mutations have been reported in *FOXL2* genes of a number of individuals with the blepharophimosis ptosis epicanthus inversus syndrome and premature ovarian failure. The mutations include frameshifts, premature termination, splicing defects, missence mutations and polyalanine expansion, and result in a form of gonadal dysgenesis that causes early ovarian regression.

Follistatin (FST)   Follistatin is a glycosylated single-chain protein functionally (but not structurally) linked to the transforming growth factor-β (TGF-β) superfamily of proteins. Secreted by granulosa cells, follistatin is an important regulator of cellular differentiation and secretion through its potent ability to bind and bioneutralize activin (a stimulator of FSH secretion with which it is colocalized in many tissue systems), and other members of the TGF-β superfamily.

The human *FST* gene is located at chromosome 5q11.2 and includes six exons that encode a 344-AA cysteine-rich protein. Exon 1 encodes a 29-AA signal peptide, whose cleavage results in isoforms of 288 and 215 AAs. The 288-AA protein is made up of a 63-AA N-terminal segment containing hydrophobic residues essential for activin binding, followed by 3 repeating 10-cysteine follistatin domains. Various 31- to 39-kDa follistatin isoforms are generated by alternative splicing, glycosylation, and proteolytic cleavage. Follistatin is highly conserved among species, with 97% AA homology between human and mouse.

Follistatin functions as a downstream component of signaling by WNT4, a key factor involved in repressing testis development. Because the presence of oogonia is critical for survival and maturation of the ovary, follistatin, which promotes survival of oocytes and maintenance of oogenesis, appears to be an important factor in normal ovarian development. Follistatin also antagonizes the action of activins and BMP15 on steroidogenesis in granulosa cells, probably via autocrine/paracrine mechanisms.

FST expression is tightly regulated during development and its promoter contains binding sites for several transcription factors. In the mouse, *Fst* mRNA can be detected in somatic cells of fetal ovaries from E11.5, declining after E14.5. *Fst* is not expressed in *Wnt4*-null mice, indicating that Wnt4 likely regulates its expression. *Fst*-null XX mice have aberrant development of the coelomic blood vessel, a hallmark of testicular organogenesis, as well as prenatal loss of germ cells in the ovarian cortex. Thus the coordinated actions of Wnt4 and Fst appear to be key to suppression of testis development via inhibition of activin-driven coelomic vessel development.

Human *FST* mRNA expression is detectable by Northern blot in nearly all tissues examined, with the highest expression in adult ovary, and in undifferentiated and partially differentiated granulosa cells, the pituitary, kidney, and fetal heart and liver. *FST* is not detectable in the human fetal testis. Human *FST* mutations have not yet been reported.

Transforming Growth Factor-β Family Members: Growth And Differentiation Factor 9 and Bone Morphogenetic Protein 15

The importance of the oocyte in directing the development and function of the ovary is illustrated by the oocyte-secreted factors, growth and differentiation factor 9 (GDF9) and bone morphogenetic protein 15 (BMP15), also referred to as growth differentiation factor 9b (GDF9b), two closely related members of the TGF-β superfamily. The development of an ovarian follicle requires a complex set of reciprocal interactions between the oocyte and granulosa cells for proper development of both cell types; granulosa cell function is not only crucial for oocyte growth but also to maintain follicular quiescence in vivo. The regulatory interactions between the oocyte and granulosa cell are largely orchestrated by the oocyte itself via paracrine factors such as GDF9 and BMP15/GDF9B, which may interact directly as heterodimers. These factors appear to play synergistic roles in development, survival, and function of oocytes and have key roles in granulosa cell development and folliculogenesis via paracrine oocyte-somatic cell interactions. In addition to interacting with one another, these factors also interact with other intra- and extraovarian factors, and both ligands use components of the same signaling pathway via transmembrane serine/threonine kinase receptors. Because fetal ovary differentiation is dependent on the presence of germ cells and their subsequent development as ovarian follicles, and GDF9 and BMP15 are required for these processes, it appears likely that both of these factors are involved in the normal development of the ovary, although their relative roles may differ among species.

Growth Differentiation Factor 9 (GDF9)

GDF9 is the first oocyte-derived growth factor required for ovarian somatic cell function in vivo. Gdf9 mRNA is expressed exclusively in oocytes in all species examined, but there appear to be important species differences in the timing of expression and roles of Gdf9/GDF9 between mice and other mammals. In the mouse ovary, Gdf9 is not expressed in primordial follicles but is expressed at all stages of follicular development thereafter in both neonatal and adult ovaries. Expression of Gdf9 mRNA begins slightly earlier than that of Bmp15/Gdf9b (discussed later), but Gdf9 does not appear to regulate Bmp15 because Gdf9-deficient mice continue to express Bmp15. Gdf9-deficient mice are infertile because of a block in oocyte differentiation and follicular development at the primary follicle stage. In human ovary, GDF9 mRNA and protein were not detected in primordial follicles but were abundantly expressed in oocytes (and were restricted to this cell type) of primary follicles. Understanding of the role of GDF9 in human ovarian development is hampered by lack of information regarding the human chromosomal locus of the gene, its expression during human fetal ovarian development, or naturally occurring mutations.

Bone Morphogenetic Protein 15 (BMP15)/Growth Differentiation Factor (GDF9b)

BMP15/GDF9b, another member of the TGF-β superfamily of extracellular signaling proteins, is the second oocyte-derived growth factor (after GDF9) that may be essential for ovarian function. The human BMP15 gene is located at Xp11.2 in a region of the X-chromosome conserved in human and mouse. However, there is relatively low AA sequence identity (76%) between the human and mouse proteins. BMP15 binds and activates two types of transmembrane serine/threonine kinase receptors, resulting in potent paracrine stimulation of ovarian granulosa cell growth and proliferation, accompanied by negative regulation of granulosa cell FSH receptor expression, resulting in downregulation of many FSH-responsive genes such

as StAR and P450SCC. Follistatin inhibits the biological activity of BMP15 (and other TGF-β members).

Mouse Bmp15 is expressed in oocytes at the one-layer primary follicle stage. Expression is similar to that of mouse Gdf9, to which Bmp15 is most closely related (52% identity at the AA level). Gdf9 expression is unaltered in Bmp15-null mice, implying lack of direct regulation of Gdf9 by Bmp15. Homozygous Bmp15 knockout female mice were subfertile, although not infertile, and their ovaries were often morphologically and histologically normal, suggesting that Bmp15 is less critical than Gdf9 for ovarian function because the Gdf9 knockout, being infertile, is more significantly impaired. In contrast, a homozygous naturally occurring Bmp15 missense mutation in sheep results in an early block in folliculogenesis and primary ovarian failure, highlighting species differences in the relative importance of these two related growth factors. In the human ovary, BMP15 is expressed after GDF9 in the oocytes of developing follicles; it is also detectable in pituitary gonadotropes.

Odsex

The Odsex locus is a region approx 1 mB upstream of the Sox9 gene on chromosome 17. Deletion of this region in XX mice resulted in male-pattern Sox9 expression and development of testes—female-to-male sex reversal. No specific gene has been identified within the region and it is hypothesized that instead the region may contain a gonad-specific regulatory sequence. It is proposed that when bound by a repressor factor, this sequence turns off Sox9 expression in the normal XX gonad. Absence of the sequence therefore results in aberrant Sox9 expression and testis development. One function of Sry in male development may be to inhibit the repressor of Sox9—a "double-repressor" mechanism of action.

OTHER FACTORS WITH PUTATIVE ROLES IN TESTIS AND/OR OVARY DETERMINATION

Dosage-Sensitive Sex Reversal-Adrenal Hypoplasia Congenita Locus on the X Chromosome, Gene 1 (DAX1)

Normal Function DAX1 (officially termed nuclear receptor subfamily 0, group B, member 1) is an orphan nuclear hormone receptor transcription factor that appears to function primarily as a transcriptional repressor. For some time DAX1 bore the title of main contender for the role of "antitestis" factor, until a role in testis development was demonstrated in a certain mouse strain and it was then touted as a "pro-testis" factor. Currently, the roles of DAX1 in the physiology of sex determination (as opposed to its roles in experimental mice) are unclear, as data regarding the impact of DAX1/Dax1 in testis and ovary development in mice vs humans are conflicting. Indeed, DAX1 may be the key example of a factor whose human physiological roles may not be deducible from murine experiments. Nevertheless, as reflected by its name, a role in sex determination and differentiation has long been postulated for DAX1 based on involvement of its chromosomal locus in human disease. In fact, DAX1 was initially discovered by cloning the region in Xp21 duplicated in a number of patients with 46,XY sex reversal, and deleted in patients with adrenal hypoplasia congenita (AHC).

The 5.0-kb, 2-exon DAX1 gene is located at Xp21.3-21.2 and encodes a 470-AA protein. The N-terminal region contains an unusual DNA-binding domain, comprising three repeats of a novel AA sequence (LxxLL), that has little homology with that of other nuclear receptors; the protein does not contain the typical central two-ZF DNA-binding domain. However, the ligand-binding domain has homology with another orphan nuclear receptor and with the retinoic acid and retinoid X receptors. The gene demonstrates a degree of evolutionary conservation, homologous sequences being detected in an X-linked pattern of distribution in many mammalian species, including mice. However, *Dax1* is autosomal rather than X-chromosomal in the tammar wallaby and the chicken, and does not have a sex-determining function in these species, suggesting that any sex determining role in placental mammals arose fairly recently in evolution. Furthermore, comparisons between mouse and human DAX1 show that specific domains of this transcription factor are evolving rapidly, perhaps explaining its different functions in mice vs humans and differing effects of DAX1 excess or deficiency in the different species.

There is strong expression of the homologous gene in the mouse (*Ahch*) in the first stages of gonadal and adrenal differentiation and in the developing hypothalamus and pituitary gonadotropes. Expression is downregulated at the time of overt differentiation of the testis, but persists in the developing ovary, suggestive of a role in ovarian development (although such a role remains hypothetical). There is significant overlap in the distribution of expression of *Dax1* and *Sf1* in numerous tissues, supporting the concept of linkage between these two transcription factors in regulation of development of steroidogenic tissues. The *Dax1* promoter contains binding sites for Sf1, and Sf1 regulates *Dax1* expression in vitro. Furthermore *Sf1*-disrupted mice lacked *Dax1* expression in the developing genital ridge in one study, although not in another. Wnt4 also may regulate *Dax1* expression, potentially explaining its increased expression in ovary vs testis. The physiology of Dax1 is complicated, because although Sf1 regulates *Dax1* expression, Dax1 inhibits Sf1-mediated transcription of other genes, suggesting a regulatory loop. Indeed, the fact that Dax1 blocks Sf1-mediated steroidogenesis seems to be inconsistent with its role as an important mediator of normal development of steroidogenic tissues. Hence, many aspects of Dax1 remain to be unraveled.

In human studies *DAX1* is expressed in Sertoli cells of the fetal testis by 16 wk gestation, in the adult testis and adrenal cortex, in the hypothalamus and pituitary gland, and at low level in adult ovary and liver. The expression of *DAX1* at all levels of the hypothalamic-pituitary-adrenal/gonadal axis supports its role in the coordinated development and regulation of the adrenal and reproductive systems. Because human *DAX1* is located in a region of Xp that normally undergoes X inactivation, single copy expression would be predicted for both males and females. However, differential regulation by sexually dimorphic factors such as WNT4 could help to explain differences in expression and function of DAX1 in male and female development.

Dax1 binds to target genes as a homodimer, likely acting as a competitive inhibitor of transcription at these sites. Indeed Dax1 has been demonstrated to repress *StAR* and *Cyp17* expression, to inhibit Sf1-mediated transactivation, thereby blocking steroidogenesis, and to antagonize the synergy between Sf1 and Wt1 in their upregulation of *Amh* expression; however, the latter appears to be via protein/protein interaction with Sf1, rather than an effect at the target gene. Sequences responsible for the suppressive function reside in the ligand-binding domain and in the N-terminal leucine repeat region of the protein. Although not yet described, a transcription activating function for Dax1 at other target sites is conceivable, much as has been described for Wt1, which has target-specific activation and repression activities.

Analysis of targeted disruption or transgenic overexpression of *Dax1* in mice highlights the importance of gene dosage and the genetic background on which such experimental changes are expressed. XY mice with *Dax1* deletion have normal testis development and masculinization (but have small testes and spermatogenetic defects) when the deletion is introduced into a normal mouse strain; in contrast, complete XY sex reversal (ovarian and phenotypic female development) occurs when the deletion is introduced into a strain of mice that carries a "weak" *Sry* gene (*M. domesticus poschiavinus*). Thus, depending on the genetic background in which it is acting, Dax1 could be interpreted as unnecessary for testis formation but required for postnatal spermatogenesis on one hand, or required for normal testis determination on the other. Findings are equally enigmatic in mice overexpressing *Dax1*: when these experiments were performed in the *poschiavinus* (weak *Sry*) strain, overexpression of *Dax1* resulted in XY sex reversal (just as deletion of the gene did), postulated to be because of antagonism of Sry. However, when the excess *Dax1* was expressed on the background of a normal *Sry* gene (*M. musculus*), only a transient delay in testis development was observed. Effects of mutation, homozygous deletion, or overexpression of *Dax1* in XX mice appear to be negligible, as such mice are fertile, giving no indication of a dosage effect on ovarian differentiation and challenging earlier speculation regarding the role of Dax1 as an ovary determinant.

Clinical Features and Molecular Defects *DAX1* has been implicated in two X-linked syndromes: dosage-sensitive sex (DSS) reversal and AHC/hypogonadotropic hypogonadism (HHG). The occurrence of sex reversal in the presence of two copies of sequences in the Xp21 region containing the *DAX1* gene led to the designation of this locus as the reversal region. Karyotypic males with this duplication have typical features of 46,XY sex reversal, with ovaries/streak gonads and a female phenotype. Individuals with deletion of this region have normal testes and male genitalia, although cryptorchidism and postnatal testicular dysfunction have been reported. These males have congenital hypoplasia of the adrenal glands and many die unexpectedly in early childhood of undiagnosed adrenal failure. Those who survive childhood also commonly have HHG resulting in failure of pubertal virilization. Deletion of *DAX1* has been reported in a number of patients with isolated AHC, whereas frameshift, premature termination, codon deletion and missense mutations have been found in *DAX1* genes of individuals with combined AHC/HHG, suggesting a possible dominant negative effect of a retained but structurally abnormal protein. Female carriers of AHC/HHG have no clear abnormality of either adrenal gland development or gonadotropin secretion; however, there have been some reports of menstrual irregularity and early menopause.

Doublesex and Mab-3-Related Transcription Factors 1 and 2 (DMRT1/2)

Normal Function Transcription factors related to the sexual regulatory factors Doublesex (in drosophila) and Mab3 (in earthworm) contain a conserved DNA-binding motif referred to as the "DM" (doublsex/mab) domain. Seven genes encoding such transcription factors, referred to as "*DM*" genes, have been discovered to date in humans and mice. DMRT1 and DMRT2 may have roles similar to SF1 and WT1, with functions as early regulators of primordial gonad formation, and later functions as testis-specific factors. The human genes encoding DMRT1 and 2 are both located at 9p24.3, <30 kb from the critical region for sex reversal on chromosome 9. The genes encode 226-AA peptides that share 80% identity in the 29-AA core region of the DM domain.

Gonad-specific expression is present in a number of species (mice, humans, chickens, amphibians, alligators, lizards, turtles, and fish). Given the different sex-determining switches in these groups, DMRT1 and DMRT2 are thought to represent an ancient, conserved component of the vertebrate sex-determining pathway, upstream of SRY. *Dmrt1* is expressed exclusively in the genital ridge of both XX and XY mouse embryos, before gonadal sex determination. In the early testis differentiation period *Dmrt1* then is upregulated in testes compared to ovaries. As testicular organogenesis proceeds, *Dmrt1* expression becomes restricted to the seminiferous tubules, in which it is expressed by both Sertoli cells and germ cells. Expression in Sertoli cells appears to be regulated by the transcription factors Sp1 and Sp3 and by the cell cycle regulator, Egr1. Expression is regulated by FSH in postnatal Sertoli cells and is testis-specific in human adults.

Male mice with homozygous deletion of *Dmrt1* had normal fetal testis development, but had severe defects in postnatal testis differentiation, resembling those associated with human deletions. Prior to postnatal day 7 the testes of the null mice appeared grossly normal. Thereafter, the testes were hypoplastic with disorganized seminiferous tubules, absent germ cells and fatty degeneration of Leydig cells. Notably, the gonadal tissue was not ovarian and there were no Müllerian duct-derived structures. Thus, the murine *Dmrt1* null phenotype is a postnatal failure of testis development, accompanied by germ cell death, rather than a prenatal failure of testis determination. No effect on gonadal development is seen in female mice.

Clinical Features and Molecular Defects   46,XY patients with monosomy for chromosome 9p have varying degrees of testicular maldevelopment (agonadism, streak gonad, hypoplasia) and ambiguous or female genitalia. In one patient with asymmetric gonadal development, a fallopian tube was present on the side of the absent gonad, as would be expected because of lack of ipsilateral *AMH* expression. One 46,XX patient also had primary hypogonadism, implicating the 9p region in ovarian as well as testicular development. This implies that genes in the 9p region (hypothesized, but not proven, to be *DMRT1 and DMRT2*) are necessary for formation of the bipotential gonad. However, there may be some functional compensation for lack of *Dmrt1* because XY null mice do not have sex reversal. Some patients have associated mental retardation and other congenital anomalies. Gonadoblastoma has been reported in one patient.

GATA4   GATA4 is a member of a group of structurally related DNA-binding transcription factors critical to the development of diverse tissues that control gene expression and differentiation in a variety of cell types. Members of this family contain one or two ZFs that recognize a consensus DNA sequence known as the "GATA" motif (i.e., the four nucleotides G, A, T, and A in this sequence) an important element in the promoters of many genes. With respect to sex determination, GATA4 may, like WT1 and SF1, have dual roles, being involved both in early development of the primordial gonad, and later in male-specific development.

Genes encoding many steroidogenic enzymes may be targets of GATA proteins as they contain the consensus GATA element within their 5′ regulatory regions, suggesting a role for GATA4 in regulation of steroidogenesis. For example, GATA4 has been demonstrated to regulate the *StAR* promoter in the ovary. GATA4 may act synergistically with SF1 through protein/protein interaction mediated by the GATA4 ZF region to regulate *Amh* expression, as there are binding sites for both factors adjacent to each other on the *Amh* promoter (Fig. 41-3B). The affinities of various GATA factors for specific promoters probably depend on interactions with cofactors and other more restricted transcription factors. For example, Leydig cells express factors known as "Friends of GATA" (FOG), which may play a role in tissue-specific effects.

In mice, *Gata4* is expressed from early stages of gonadal development (E11.5) in both sexes in the somatic cell population (later to become the Sertoli and granulosa cells), but not in the primordial germ cells. Abundant *Gata4* expression continues in Sertoli cells throughout embryonic testis development. During early ovarian development, *Gata4* mRNA and protein localize to the granulosa cells and are markedly downregulated shortly after the histological differentiation of the ovary on E13.5. This results in a sexually dimorphic pattern of greater *Gata4* expression in developing testes than ovaries. Reduced *Gata4* expression in the latter stages of ovary development coincides with the necessity for absence of Amh to allow normal Müllerian duct development in the female.

In the human testis, *GATA4* is expressed from early fetal life to adulthood. Like AMH, GATA4 represents an early marker of Sertoli cells, its expression peaking at 19–22 wk gestation (FSH and testosterone are also high during this period). Consistent with a role in regulation of steroidogenesis *GATA4* is also expressed in a number of human steroidogenic tissues such as Leydig cells during the fetal period and after puberty, the periods of most active androgen synthesis. Other tissues in which *GATA4* is expressed include fetal and postnatal granulosa cells, adult theca cells, fetal adrenal cortex, fetal germ cells and prepubertal spermatogonia (it is downregulated in these cells after puberty).

Targeted disruption of *Gata4* or *Fog2* in mice resulted in reduced *Sry* expression, failure of Sertoli cell differentiation and early failure of testis differentiation. Human GATA2 mutations are associated with cardiac defects but no gonadal phenotype has been reported.

NORMAL AND ABNORMAL MALE SEX DIFFERENTIATION
Once function of the testis is established, at approx 8 wk gestation, development of the male sexual phenotype is under the control of testicular secretions and the receptors that mediate their action. These include fetal LH, the LHCGR, steroidogenic enzymes involved in testosterone biosynthesis, steroid 5α-reductase 2 required for conversion of testosterone to DHT, the androgen receptor (AR), AMH and the type 2 anti-Müllerian hormone receptor (AMHR2).

Development of Wolffian structures requires testosterone, produced by steroidogenesis in testicular Leydig cells following activation of the cell surface LHCGR. During the first trimester of gestation the ligand for this receptor is probably chorionic gonadotropin (CG), produced in large quantity by the placenta. Subsequently, endogenous fetal LH is the primary ligand. The lack of dependence on fetal LH during male genital morphogenesis is evidenced by the normal penile structure of males with hypopituitarism; however, the subnormal penile size of these infants highlights the role of fetal LH/testosterone action in the penile growth that occurs in the third trimester. Sertoli cells may also help regulate Leydig cell steroidogenesis in a paracrine fashion. The outcome of this multistep process is a high local, and to a lesser extent systemic, concentration of testosterone.

Testosterone action is mediated by the AR, a nuclear receptor/transcription factor found in high concentration in the tissues of the Wolffian ducts (in which testosterone itself is the ligand) and external genitalia (in which the ligand is DHT). In the absence of high androgen concentration, as in the female or androgen-deficient fetus, there is insufficient activated AR to

A   Disorders of sex determination: true hermaphroditism

Disorders of sex differentiation: female pseudohermaphroditism

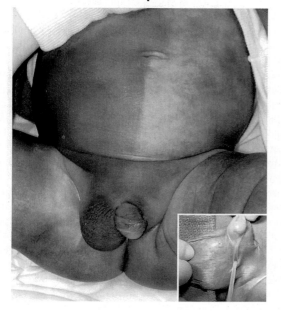

B

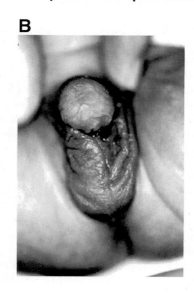

C   Disorders of sex differentiation: male pseudohermaphroditism of various degrees

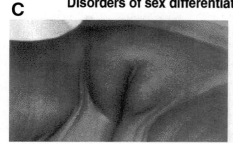
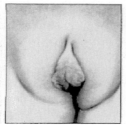
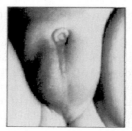
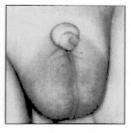

Figure 41-8 Clinical examples of disorders of sex determination and differentiation. **(A)** Disorders of sex determination: true hermaphroditism. This infant had 46,XX/46,XY mosaicism and normal male testosterone levels. Note the asymmetry of the labioscrotal folds and urethral orifice in a perineal location (inset). Internal genitalia mirrored the external asymmetry, with an ovary, Fallopian tube and hemiuterus on the left. The right scrotal fold contained an ovotestis. (Reproduced with permission from Karam JA, Baker LA. Images in clinical medicine. True hermaphroditism. N Engl J Med 2004;350[4]:394.). **(B)** Disorders of sex differentiation: female pseudohermaphroditism. This 46,XX child has significant virilization due to androgen excess resulting from 21-hydroxylase deficiency. Marked clitoromegaly and labioscrotal fusion are present. (Reproduced with permission from Pinhas-Hamiel O, Zalel Y, SmithE, Mazkereth R, Aviram A, Lipitz S Achiron R: Prenatal diagnosis of sex differentiation disorders: the role of fetal ultrasound. J Clin Endocrinol Metab 2002;87[10]:4547–4553. Copyright 2002 The Endocrine Society.) **(C)** Disorders of sex differentiation: male pseudohermaphroditism Left: 46,XY infant with androgen receptor mutation who subsequently showed significant penile enlargement in response to treatment with topical dihydrotestosterone gel. (Reproduced with permission from: Ong YC, Wong HB, Adaikan G, Yong EL. Directed pharmacological therapy of ambiguous genitalia due to an androgen receptor gene mutation. Lancet 1999; 354[9188]: 1444, 1445.) Right: These three individuals are 46,XY siblings with the same androgen receptor gene mutation who show significant phenotypic variability within a family. (Reproduced with permission from Holterhus PM, Sinnecker GH, Hiort O. Phenotypic diversity and testosterone-induced normalization of mutant L712F androgen receptor function in a kindred with androgen insensitivity. J Clin Endocrinol Metab 2000;85[9]:3245–3250.)

induce transcription of target genes required for stabilization and development of the Wolffian system and for masculinization of the external genitalia.

Müllerian duct regression is induced by the Sertoli cell glycoprotein hormone, AMH, mediated by AMHR2, a member of the serine/threonine kinase group of transmembrane proteins, localized in the mesenchyme surrounding the Müllerian ducts. AMH/AMHR2 action causes involution of Müllerian structures by apoptosis. What can be considered as perhaps the final phase of masculinization—testicular descent—is controlled in part by a Leydig cell secreted protein, insulin-like protein 3.

Male (46,XY) pseudohermaphroditism describes conditions in which an individual with male karyotype and normally formed testes has abnormal masculinization of the internal and/or external genitalia. In essence there are two major classes: defects of production or response to testosterone, and defects of production or response to AMH. The causes of male pseudohermaphroditism are summarized in Table 41-1. Clinical examples are provided in Fig. 41-8.

The genital phenotype in disorders of production and action of testosterone generally reflects the severity of the defect during fetal life. 46,XY individuals with profound deficiency of androgen production or action have fully female external genitalia. Those in whom some degree of androgen production and action is retained have a wide spectrum of genital phenotypes, ranging from minor degrees of posterior labial fusion and a clitoris-like phallus to ambiguous genitalia characterized by incomplete labioscrotal and urethral fusion to more significant masculinization with reasonable penile size accompanied by urethral hypospadias, penile chordee, and cryptorchidism. The testes may be located anywhere from the abdomen to the inguinal canals or the labioscrotal region. Internal genital structures range from feminized lower genital tracts with separate vaginal and urethral structures in cases in which there is minimal androgen action, to more masculinized structures such as a urogenital sinus with ectopic vaginal orifice, in milder cases in which a moderate degree of androgen action has occurred. The development of Wolffian duct structures (epididymis and vas deferens) is also variable, depending on the degree of local testosterone secretion/action in early gestation. The vaginal pouch is blind and Müllerian duct structures (uterus and fallopian tubes) are absent or diminutive because of the action of AMH secreted normally by the Sertoli cells.

An uncommon form of male pseudohermaphroditism occurs in conditions caused by failure of secretion or action of AMH. These males have normal testes and normal male external genitalia, but retain the Müllerian structures to varying degrees, sometimes including development of a complete uterus and fallopian tubes.

LHCG Receptor (LHCGR)

Normal Function   The LHCGR is a seven-transmembrane domain G protein-coupled receptor responsible for transducing the hormonal effects of LH and CG. It is required for male sex differentiation by its role in the early development of Leydig cells and in mediating Leydig cell steroidogenesis. The 60-kb, 11-exon LHCGR gene located at 2p21 is transcribed into a number of mRNA splice variants whose function is unclear. Exons 1–10 encode the major portion of the N-terminal extracellular domain, containing a leucine-rich repeat; exon 11 codes for a small part of the extracellular domain, as well as all seven transmembrane loops and the C-terminal intracellular region. The 85-95-kDa LHCGR has significant homology with the FSH and TSH receptors. Ligand binding induces increased intracellular production of cyclic AMP, the principal mediator of hormone action in this system.

Fetal Leydig cells in mice constitutively express LHCGR in the absence of hormone. In contrast, in mouse ovary LHCGR mRNA can be detected only on day 5 postnatally, after the onset of postnatal LH stimulation of gonadal function (detectable in granulosa, theca, interstitial, and luteal cells). No mouse model for LHCGR defects has been described.

Clinical Features and Molecular Defects   LCH is a rare (approx 1/1,000,000) autosomal-recessive cause of male pseudohermaphroditism in which Leydig cell differentiation and testosterone production are impaired because of absence or defective function of LHCGR on Leydig cell progenitors. In its severe form, patients present with female external genitalia and cryptorchid testes. Müllerian derivatives are absent, because Sertoli cells and therefore AMH production are normal. Although the genital phenotype is generally female, posterior labial fusion or a urogenital sinus may be present, and occasional patients with a small penis are reported, suggesting significant testosterone production in the first trimester. Because the testes remain quiescent, negligible development of either male or female secondary sexual characteristics

occurs at puberty, a feature that distinguishes this condition from the androgen insensitivity syndromes (AISs), in which high estrogen production at puberty typically produces ample breast development. Postpubertal individuals with LCH have slightly small testes due to hyalinization of the seminiferous tubules, interrupted spermatogenesis and absent or diminished Leydig cells, reflecting the requirement of LH for their development and survival.

The diagnosis of LCH should be suspected in a 46,XY infant with female or slightly masculinized external genitalia in the presence of low testosterone and high LH levels (Table 41-5). Unlike individuals with a testosterone biosynthetic defect, who also have low testosterone and high LH, there is no elevation of testosterone precursors and no increase in testosterone or its precursors in response to exogenous hCG administration. Failure of pubertal development in a phenotypic female with high LH and no measurable sex steroids would also suggest this diagnosis.

Diverse mutations in the LHCGR gene have been reported in patients with varying phenotypes of LCH. The mutations are not localized in any particular region of the gene and cause variable reductions of receptor activity. Most mutations are present in the homozygous or compound heterozygous state (i.e., both copies of the gene carry a mutation). Three phenotypically female 46,XY siblings with typical clinical findings of LCH and their 46,XX sister were homozygous for a nonsense mutation that predicts protein termination in the third cytosolic loop of the receptor. If the protein gets to the cell membrane (which it may not, if severely disturbed), it would be predicted to lack the sixth and seventh transmembrane domains and the intracellular domain, regions important for G protein-coupled signaling. The patient's 46,XX sister had late menarche at 20 yr of age, thereafter developed secondary amenorrhea, and had increased serum LH, suggesting that hapolinsufficiency for ovarian LHCGR may have impaired ovarian function. A similar mutation present in the compound heterozygous state in another pair of phenotypically female 46,XY siblings resulted in truncation within the 5th transmembrane domain. In this case not only was cAMP production impaired, but cell surface receptor expression was reduced, providing two reasons for lack of LH/CG action. A pair of affected 46,XY siblings born to consanguineous parents had a homozygous missense mutation resulting in an AA change in the 6th transmembrane domain of the receptor. Because the extracellular domain was intact the receptor had normal CG binding affinity, however, the ligand-bound state did not induce cAMP production, required for induction of steroidogenic enzyme activity.

Variability of the phenotype associated with LHCGR mutations is underscored by the report of a phenotypically male child with small penis whose testes were normally descended and whose serum LH was at the upper limit of normal. A missense mutation converted serine to tyrosine at position 616 in the seventh transmembrane domain. Surprisingly, in view of the normal masculinization, in vitro studies of the mutant receptor revealed absent LH binding and cAMP production. One possible explanation is that the receptor function *in utero* under the drive of maternal CG was adequate for normal first trimester Leydig cell function and testosterone secretion, but was inadequate in the presence of LH.

Proteins and Enzymes of Testosterone Biosynthesis Leydig cell testosterone production during the critical period from weeks 8 to 12 of male gestation is required for normal internal and external genital masculinization. Following LH/CG stimulation of Leydig cells, testosterone production requires the well-regulated

Table 41-5
Steroid Profiles in Disorders of Sex Differentiation

Enzyme/protein deficiency (Disorder)	Pregnenolone	Progesterone	17OH-Pregnenolone	17OH-Progesterone	Aldosterone	11-deoxy cortisol	DOC	Cortisol	DHEA	Androstenedione	Testosterone	DHT
LHCG Receptor (LCH)	N	N	N	N	N	N	N	N	N	N	↓↓	↓↓
StAR or P450scc (CLAH)	↓	↓	↓	↓	↓	↓	↓	↓	↓	↓	↓	↓
P450 oxidoreductase[a]	↑	↑↑	↑	↑↑	↓	↓	↑	↓	↑↑	↓	N or ↑	N or ↓
3β-hydroxysteroid dehydrogenase	↑↑	N or ↑	↑↑	N or ↑	↓	↓	↓	↓	↑↑	N or ↑	N or ↑[b]	N or ↓
17α-hydroxylase	↑	↑	↓	↓	↓	↓	↑	↓	↓	↓	↓	↓
17β-hydroxysteroid dehydrogenase	N	N	N	N	N	N	N	N	N or ↑	↑	↓	↓
21-hydroxylase	↑	↑	↑	↑↑↑	↓	↓	↓	↓	↑	↑	↑↑	N
11β-hydroxylase	N	N	N or ↑	N or ↑	↓	↑↑↑	↑	↓	↑	↑	↑	N
Aromatase	N	N	N	N	N	N	N	N	N	↑↑↑	↑↑↑	↑↑↑
5α-reductase	N	N	N	N	N	N	N	N	N	N	↑	↓
Androgen receptor (AIS)	N	N	N	N	N	N	N	N	N	N	N or ↑	N or ↑

[a]There is evidence for an alternate androgen production pathway during fetal life, resulting in prenatal virilization of affected females.

[b]Testosterone is likely low prenatally, increasing postnatally because of peripheral conversion by nontesticular 3β-HSD isozymes.

AIS, androgen insensitivity syndrome; CG, chorionic gonadotropin; CLAH, congenital lipoid adrenal hyperplasia; DHEA, dehydroepiandrosterone; DHT, dihydrotestosterone; DOC, 11-deoxycorticosterone; LCH, Leydig cell hypoplasia; LH, luteinizing hormone; LHCGR, luteinizing hormone/chronic gonadotropin receptor; N, normal.

develop polycystic changes and premature ovarian failure, accompanied by hypergonadotropic hypogonadism.

More than 30 distinct *StAR* mutations, present in the homozygous or compound heterozygous state, have been reported in over 50 patients with CLAH. Most *StAR* mutations are severe at the molecular level (e.g., frameshift mutations caused by small insertions or deletions, nonsense mutations leading to premature termination and splice site mutations), resulting in loss of translation or a severe protein truncation. One mutation common in Japanese and Korean patients (Q258X; 80% of affected alleles) that deletes the final 28 AAs of the StAR protein demonstrates the crucial biological role of the carboxyl terminus, as do missense mutations causing AA substitutions that cluster in exons 5–7 of the gene encoding AAs 169-275 in the carboxyl terminus. A specific mutation that converts arginine 182 to leucine is common in Palestinian Arabs (>70% of affected alleles). This mutation results in disordered protein folding that destroys protein function. Unlike other forms of CAH, heterozygotes have normal steroid responses to ACTH stimulation.

P450 Oxidoreductase (POR)

Normal Function P450 oxidoreductase (POR) is a flavoprotein (a protein containing the coenzyme flavin) that donates electrons to all P450 enzymes, including the steroidogenic enzymes cytochrome $P450_{17\alpha}$ (P450c17), mitochondrial cytochrome P450 steroid 21-hydroxylase (P450c21), and P450aromatase (P450arom) as well as those responsible for the metabolism of retinoic acid, drugs, fatty acids, and prostaglandins. POR may in fact be the sole electron donor for the whole P450 system, which plays an essential role in many developmental processes.

POR is located in the endoplasmic reticulum of steroidogenic cells bound in complex with its coenzymes flavin adenine dinucleotide (FAD) and flavin mononucleotide (FMN), and the cytochrome P450 proteins. POR binds nicotinamide adenine dinucleotide phosphate (NADPH), accepts a pair of hydrogens through its FAD moiety, then transfers them to its FMN moiety, finally passing them on one at a time from FMN to one of the cytochrome P450 enzymes, which then uses them in hydroxylation of its substrate(s). The human *POR* gene is located at 7q12 and encodes a 670-AA protein. The N-terminal region is required for anchoring the protein to the endoplasmic reticulum, ensuring proper spatial orientation with the P450 cytochromes and for binding the FMN molecule; the midportion of the protein contains two FAD-binding domains; and the carboxyl terminus contains the NADPH-binding domain. POR proteins from various species show high AA sequence homology, reflecting the importance of the enzyme throughout evolution.

Por is expressed extremely early in mice, at the two-cell stage of development, and knockout of the gene was embryonically lethal from approx E10 onward. No gonadal phenotype was reported, probably because the animals died before gonadogenesis could occur. Detailed ontogeny of human *POR* expression has not yet been reported.

Clinical Features and Molecular Defects Human *POR* gene mutations have been reported in a number of unrelated patients with ambiguous genitalia with or without a skeletal malformation disorder known as Antley-Bixler syndrome. Based on the patterns of disordered steroidogenesis, these cases were formerly thought to have an uncommon form of CAH with apparent combined deficiencies of 17α-hydroxlyase and 21-hydroxylase. Reported genital abnormalities include in females vaginal atresia, clitoromegaly, fusion of labia minora, and hypoplasia of labia

majora, and in males ambiguous external genitalia. Some patients die early, reportedly because of respiratory complications. *POR* mutations have generally been reported in the compound heterozygous state, most encoding single AA substitutions in the FAD-binding and NADPH-binding domains. Homozygous mutations associated with consanguinity and simple heterozygous missence mutations have also been reported. However, no human patient has been reported with two null alleles of the *POR* gene suggesting that complete POR deficiency is probably lethal. The mutant POR proteins containing AA substitutions had reduced capacity to oxidize NADPH and reduced catalytic efficiency in vitro. Proteins containing mutations detected in patients with the Antley-Bixler syndrome phenotype had disruption of both the 17α-hydroxylase and 17,20-lyase activities of $P450_{17\alpha}$. In contrast, the mutations detected in a female patient who presented with isolated amenorrhea in the presence of normal genitalia encoded milder AA substitutions that allowed the protein to retain some activity. Overall, the electron transfer properties of the mutant proteins correlated with phenotypes: the severely impaired enzyme was associated with genital and skeletal anomalies, whereas the more mildly dysfunctional enzyme resulted in disordered steroidogenesis without skeletal anomalies.

One striking aspect of the phenotype of affected 46,XX individuals is the combination of prenatal virilization with postnatal androgen deficiency. This is postulated to result from activation of an alternate androgen synthesis pathway in fetal life that does not function after birth, explaining why female virilization does not progress postnatally. Genitalia may be normal in males despite *POR* deficiency, suggesting adequate androgen production via either the typical or the alternate pathway. Transient maternal virilization has been reported during pregnancy in one case, presumably because of failure to aromatize fetal androgens resulting from reduced activity of P450 aromatase, which like other cytochromes P450, requires *POR* for full function.

Beyond the Antley–Bixler clinical syndrome, mild disorders of steroid synthesis are common, and could result from milder mutations in *POR*, which may be more common than is suggested by the low prevalence of Antley-Bixler syndrome. Although the relationship between *POR* mutations and the skeletal anomalies of patients with Antley-Bixler syndrome is unclear, it is of interest that developmental defects of the limb buds were also seen in *Por* knockout mice.

P450 Side-Chain Cleavage Enzyme (P450SCC)

Normal Function P450 side-chain cleavage enzyme (P450scc) is a mixed function oxidase located on the inner mitochondrial membrane in complex with adrenodoxin and adrenodoxin reductase. It is the first enzyme of steroidogenesis, catalyzing the conversion of cholesterol to pregnenolone in 3 distinct biochemical reactions: 20α-hydroxylation, 22-hydroxylation, and side-chain cleavage of the C20-C22 bond. Electrons are transferred from NADPH to adrenodoxin reductase, a membrane-bound flavoprotein cofactor, then to adrenodoxin, a soluble iron/sulfur protein, and finally to P450scc itself.

P450scc is encoded by the 20-kb, 9-exon *CYP11A* gene located at 15 q23-q24. *CYP11A* is expressed in steroidogenic tissues such as adrenal cortex, ovarian granulosa cells, testicular Leydig cells and placenta, and is also expressed in skin, heart and brain. Expression is enhanced by ACTH, gonadotropins, cAMP and SF1 (for which binding sites are located in the *CYP11A* promoter). There is also evidence for insulin-like growth factor (IGF-1)-mediated stimulation of *Cyp11a* expression in mouse Leydig cells. Expression patterns appear to be tissue- and species-specific, involving the use of alternate promoter sequences.

Mice with targeted disruption of the *Cyp11a1* gene were unable to make steroids, had markedly elevated ACTH and died shortly after birth. Male mice had small testes, epididymi and vas deferens, no prostate or seminal vesicles and feminized external genitalia. Similar to the findings reported in mice with *Star* deletions, the *Cyp11a1*-deleted mice had abnormal lipid deposits in the adrenals and testes, whereas the ovaries of the females were normal.

Clinical Features and Molecular Defects Mutations of *CYP11A* appear to be a much less frequent cause of CLAH than *StAR* defects, probably because total deficiency of this enzyme would completely abolish steroidogenesis, including placental steroidogenesis, causing fetal demise. The clinical phenotype of the 2 reported patients, both Japanese, represents a later-onset version of the clinical effects of *StAR* defects. A 46,XY phenotypic female with mild clitoromegaly presented with life-threatening adrenal insufficiency at 4 yr of age. She had low serum cortisol, with elevated ACTH and plasma renin activity. Her *CYP11A* gene had a heterozygous *de novo* in-frame 6-bp insertion in exon 4, resulting in insertion of two additional AAs into the protein, completely inactivating its enzymatic activity.

The second case involved a 9 mo-old 46,XX girl who presented primarily because of hyperpigmentation. Like the first patient her ACTH and plasma renin activity were markedly elevated, but adrenal steroid levels were normal. She had compound heterozygous mutations of *CYP11A:* a maternally inherited arginine 353 to tryptophan substitution caused marked reduction of P450scc activity, indicating that arginine 353 is crucial for P450scc activity; the second mutation created an alternative splice donor site that resulted in deletion of 61 nucleotides causing a frameshift and partial inactivation of the enzyme. The heterozygous nature of the patients' mutations was consistent with the partial preservation of adrenal steroidogenesis. As in the case of *StAR* mutations, the pathophysiology of the adrenal insufficiency in these cases appears to be progressive cellular damage caused by ACTH-stimulated accumulation of intracellular cholesterol. Thus, although homozygous absence of *CYP11A* is likely incompatible with term gestation, haploinsufficiency of *CYP11A* causes a late-presenting form of CLAH that can be explained by the same two-hit model of CLAH caused by STAR deficiency.

3β-*Hydroxysteroid Dehydrogenase (3βHSD)*

Normal Function The 3β-hydroxysteroid dehydrogenase (HSD)/Δ^5-Δ^4 isomerases (3β-HSD1 and 3β-HSD2) are two highly homologous, membrane-bound, noncytochrome, nicotinamide adenine dinucleotide (NAD)+-dependent, short chain alcohol dehydrogenase isozymes located in the endocplasmic reticulum and mitochondria. Both have two separate, sequential enzymatic activities—dehydrogenase activity and isomerase activity (conversion of Δ^5-steroids to Δ^4-steroids)—the net result of which is the conversion of 3β-hydroxy-Δ^5-steroids (pregnenolone, 17-hydroxypregnenolone, dehydroepiandrosterone [DHEA] and androstenediol) to the 3-keto-Δ^4-steroids (progesterone, 17α-hydroxyprogesterone [17-OHP], Δ^4-androstenedione and testosterone, respectively; Fig. 41-9). NAD phosphate, the product of the rate-limiting dehydrogenase reaction, induces a conformational change around the bound 3-oxo-Δ^5-steroid (the substrate for the second enzymatic step), to activate the isomerase reaction. This bifunctional

dimeric enzyme is therefore required for the biosynthesis of all classes of steroid hormones. Deficiency of 3β-HSD activity in steroidogenic tissues impairs both adrenal and gonadal (testicular and ovarian) steroidogenesis and is reported to be the second most common cause of CAH.

There are two highly homologous human genes encoding isoenzymes responsible for 3β-HSD activity—*HSD3B1* and *HSD3B2*, encoding 3β-HSD1 and 3β-HSD2, respectively. There is tight linkage between these genes, located at 1p13.1. *HSD3B1* is the predominant form expressed in placenta, liver, kidney, skin, mammary gland, and prostate. *HSD3B2* encodes the 371-AA 3β-HSD2 isoform expressed almost exclusively in the steroidogenic cells of the adrenals and gonads. The isozymes have 93.5% AA identity and have the same enzymatic activities but 3β-HSD2 has a somewhat lower affinity for its substrates. Specific AA residues are critical for the separate enzymatic activities: His261 for the dehydrogenase activity and Tyr263/264 for the isomerase activity. In bovine adrenocortical cells the enzyme colocalizes with P450scc at the inner mitochodrial membrane, suggesting a possible functional association between the two enzymes. 3β-HSD is detectable in human testicular interstitial cells from 8 wk gestation, consistent with the requirement for Leydig cell testosterone production critical for masculinization. In contrast, as might be expected because fetal ovarian steroid production is not required for female sex differentiation, 3β-HSD expression in ovary is not observed until 28 wk, at which time it is detected in theca and interstitial cells. Expression in the adrenal can be detected from approx 11 wk gestation, declining at midgestation and rising again in the third trimester. In cultured human adrenal cells 3β-HSD mRNA and protein levels are regulated by ACTH and angiotensin II. In mouse Leydig cells 3β-HSD expression is regulated by LH/CG. A putative SF1 binding site is present in the *HSD3B2* promoter, and promoter activity is enhanced by SF1.

Clinical Features and Molecular Defects Deficiency of human 3β-HSD2 impairs adrenal and gonadal steroidogenesis, resulting in variable deficiencies of all classes of steroids—glucorticoids, mineralocorticoids and gonadal steroids—causing CAH and disturbances of external genital development in both males (undermasculinization) and females (virilization).

Affected 46,XY individuals have impairment of internal and external genital masculinization resulting from inadequate fetal testosterone biosynthesis. Individuals with 46,XX karoytype may have mild virilization of the external genitalia presumed to result from ACTH-driven DHEA excess. In severe cases there is also salt-wasting adrenal insufficiency because of reduced synthesis of aldosterone and cortisol. Less severe "late-onset" cases present with more complete masculinization and without salt wasting, reflecting genetic heterogeneity.

Deficiency of 3β-HSD2 in karyotypic females is a less common form of 46,XX pseudohermaphroditism than 21-hydroxylase deficiency (described below), and may be associated with normal or mildly virilized genitalia (mild clitoromegaly with minor posterior labial fusion), not of sufficient severity to suggest genital ambiguity. Androgenization resulting in premature development of pubic and axillary hair and further clitoral enlargement may occur during childhood in response to exaggerated levels of the relatively weak androgen DHEA. Because of low estrogen production, there is no breast enlargement at puberty, either in 46,XX or 46,XY individuals.

The classic hormonal profile in 3β-HSD2 deficiency is markedly increased concentrations of the Δ^5-steroids (pregnenolone, 17-hydroxypregnenolone, and dehydroepiadrosterone) and their metabolites in the serum and urine. However, somewhat confusingly, Δ^4-steroids may also be increased, because of peripheral conversion of Δ^5-steroids to Δ^4-steroids resulting from 3β-HSD1 activity in peripheral tissues. Nevertheless, despite peripheral conversion, the ratio of Δ^5- to Δ^4-steroids and their metabolites is generally elevated. The peripheral Δ^5- to Δ^4-steroid conversion explains the paradoxic finding of ambiguous genitalia in conjunction with apparently normal δ^4-steroid levels in some of these patients. Although postnatal Δ^4-steroid concentrations may be normal, it is probable that testosterone was inadequate in the developing genitalia, and that specific activity of the testicular isozyme, 3β-HSD2, is required to generate adequately high androgen levels during embryogenesis.

More than 30 *HSD3B2* mutations have been identified in families with classic 3β-HSD deficiency. In contrast to mutations affecting StAR and P450scc, the majority have been homozygous missense mutations (associated with consanguinity), however, frameshift, nonsense, deletion and splicing mutations have also been reported. Compound heterozygosity has been reported in a number of classically affected patients, and minor manifestations of simple heterozygosity have been described, including mild overproduction of Δ^5-steroids and mild ovarian dysfunction. One affected female without genital ambiguity was homozygous for a nonsense mutation that produced a truncated protein of 169 AAs, compared with the usual 371 AAs. Compound heterozygosity for a missense mutation and an intronic mutation likely causing a splicing defect was found in another female with normal genitalia, whose affected brother had ambiguous genitalia.

In vitro studies reveal significantly reduced enzyme affinity and specific activity for its steroid substrates, and in some cases for the cofactor NAD+. The finding of a specific abnormality of NAD+ binding associated with substitution of aspartic acid for glycine at position 15 raises the speculation that this region may contribute to the NAD-binding domain of the enzyme. Although absence of salt losing in some undermasculinized males and some virilized females suggests that impairment of enzyme activity may differ between gonads and adrenals, the enzyme is similarly dysfunctional for either of its two main substrates, pregnenolone (adrenal) and DHEA (gonad) in vitro. Thus the absence of salt wasting in some individuals likely results from weak residual enzyme activity sufficient to prevent salt loss, but insufficient to produce the testosterone levels required for male sex differentiation. The clinical heterogeneity (i.e., salt-losing vs nonsalt losing; varying degrees of masculinization) is in part explained by the genetic heterogeneity. Not surprisingly, mutations that completely destroy enzyme activity are associated with a more severe syndrome than are those that allow retention of some enzyme function. No functional 3β-HSD2 is expressed in the adrenals or gonads of patients with the salt-wasting form. In general patients with nonsalt-wasting disease have up to 10% retained enzyme activity, typically associated with missense mutations. However, there is no clear correlation between the molecular defect, enzyme activity and clinical phenotype. Certain mutations appear to destabilize the protein, contributing further to the enzyme deficiency.

17α-Hydroxylase and 17,20-Lyase

Normal Function   A single enzyme, P450c17, catalyzes two consecutive oxidation reactions, the 17α-hydroxylase and 17,20-lyase (17,20-desmolase) reactions required for cortisol, androgen

and estrogen synthesis. P450$_{17\alpha}$ is encoded by *CYP17*, a 6.6-kb, 8-exon gene located on chromosome 10q24.3. The *CYP17* gene is similar to *CYP21* (encoding the 21-hydroxylase enzyme, described below), and the two may have originated from a common ancestral gene. The two genes have approx 30% homology, with some regions of higher and others of lower homology. The main difference is that *CYP17* has lost two exons present in *CYP21*.

The P450$_{17\alpha}$ complex anchored to the smooth endoplasmic reticulum of steroidogenic cells includes the cytochrome P450$_{17\alpha}$ enzyme itself, and a flavoprotein, POR (described above). P450$_{17\alpha}$ consists of an N-terminal membrane-attachment domain, a steroid-binding domain, a redox-interaction domain, and a heme-binding domain. P450$_{17\alpha}$ accepts electrons from NADPH via POR to catalyze its reactions. The 17α-hydroxylase reaction converts pregnenolone to 17-hydroxypregnenolone and progesterone to 17-hydroxyprogesterone (17-OHP), respectively (Fig. 41-9), the rate-limiting step in androgen biosynthesis. The 17,20-lyase reaction cleaves the C17,20 bond to convert the C21 steroid 17-hydroxypregnenolone to the C19 steroid DHEA and catalyzes the equivalent conversion of 17-OHP to Δ^4-androstenedione, although this latter reaction occurs much more slowly. DHEA and androstenedione are the major precursors of testosterone and estradiol respectively, although because of the enzyme's preference for Δ^5-steroids, most human sex steroids derive from DHEA. Specific AA residues are critical for either the 17α-hydroxylase or the 17,20-lyase activity. Serine phosphorylation of the enzyme increases lyase activity; dephosphorylation eliminates this activity. Other regulatory features may include variation in the ratio of POR to P450$_{17\alpha}$ itself, resulting in alteration of electron transfer to the enzyme.

P450$_{17\alpha}$ is present in human adrenal, testis and ovarian theca cells, but not in granulosa cells or placenta. *CYP17* expression begins between 41 and 44 d after conception in the human fetus, limited to the fetal adrenal zone. *CYP17* is upregulated by ACTH via cAMP and markedly by SF1 for which binding sites are located in the 5'-flanking region of the gene. SF1 regulation may be inhibited by DAX1. Expression is also regulated by the inhibin/activin system in the ovary. The ratio of 17α-hydroxylase to 17,20-lyase activity differs between adrenal and testis and is developmentally regulated at adrenarche, with an increase in the ratio of lyase to hydroxylase activity. The basis for the time- and tissue-specific differential regulation of the enzyme's two main activities is not fully understood.

Clinical Features and Molecular Defects   Deficiency of this enzyme is another fairly uncommon cause of male pseudohermaphroditism (but does not cause female pseudohermaphroditism), characterized by deficiency of either or both of this enzyme's 17α-hydroxylase and 17,20-lyase activities. Both enzymatic activities depend on correct steroid binding, but isolated lyase deficiency can occur in association with disturbances of the C-terminal region that normally interacts with POR. Because of fetal androgen deficiency, 46,XY individuals with 17α-hydroxylase deficiency in the adrenals and gonads have female or minimally masculinized external genitalia. In 46,XX individuals the external genitalia are normal; however, there is failure of breast, pubic and axillary hair development at puberty, because of deficiency of both adrenal androgens and ovarian estrogen (*see* Chapter 43). Deficiency of 17α-hydroxylase activity also impairs adrenal cortisol production, and the resultant compensatory ACTH hypersecretion stimulates synthesis of progesterone, 11-deoxycorticosterone (DOC), corticosterone, and 18-hydroxycorticosterone.

The excess of the latter 3 compounds causes salt and water retention, hypertension, and hypokalemia because of their mineralocorticoid activity. Renin activity is therefore suppressed and aldosterone production reduced. Despite impaired cortisol production, evidence of glucocorticoid deficiency is unusual, perhaps because corticosterone has weak glucocorticoid activity.

Isolated deficiency of gonadal 17,20-lyase activity prohibits synthesis of DHEA, Δ^4-androstenedione, testosterone and estradiol. Glucocorticoid and mineralocorticoid production are retained because the enzymatic defect is distal to these pathways. ACTH hyperstimulation in patients with 17α-hydroxylase deficiency results in elevated progesterone; those with isolated deficiency of 17,20-lyase activity of have elevated 17-OHP. hCG stimulation produces an increased ratio of 17-hydroxy-C_{21}-steroids (17-OHP and 17-hydroxypregnenolone) to C_{19}-steroids (DHEA and Δ^4-androstenedione).

A variety of *CYP17* defects have been described, either in a homozygous or compound heterozygous state. These include large deletions/insertions, small deletions and duplications, and single base mutations causing frame shifts, premature termination or AA substitutions. The approx 20 missense mutations are scattered throughout the gene, affecting residues in the membrane-attachment, steroid-binding, POR-interaction, and the heme-binding domains. Mutations in the steroid-binding domain cause combined complete or partial 17α-hydroxylase and 17,20-lyase deficiencies, whereas mutations in the POR-interaction domain cause less severe 17α-hydroxylase deficiency, but complete 17,20-lyase deficiency. A recreated mutant P450$_{17}$α, in which histidine at position 373 was replaced by leucine, failed to bind the heme moiety critical for catalytic activity. Other mutations are located distant from the critical heme-binding region or the active site, suggesting that the enzyme is sensitive to structural change.

Correlation between in vitro enxyme activity and clinical findings indicates that retention of approx 20% of normal 17,20-lyase activity is adequate for some degree of masculinization. One specific mutation, a 4-bp duplication that alters the reading frame of *CYP17*, was found in six Dutch families and six families of Canadian Mennonites, likely because of a founder mutation in the Dutch antecedents of the Mennonites. Individuals heterozygous for a *CYP17* mutation are clinically normal. However, ACTH stimulation may produce increased concentrations of 11-deoxycorticosterone, corticosterone, and 18-hydroxycorticosterone.

17β-*Hydroxysteroid Dehydrogenases (17β-HSD)*

Normal Function The 17β-hydroxysteroid dehydrogenases (17β-HSDs) (also known as 17β-ketosteroid reductases and as estradiol 17β-dehydrogenases) are NAD+/NADPH-dependent, membrane-bound noncytochrome enzymes. There are at least 11 17β-HSDs encoded by separate genes; only those related to gonadal steroidogenesis are discussed here. These enzymes catalyze the only reversible steps in the steroid biosynthetic pathway—interconversion of Δ^4-androstenedione↔testosterone, DHEA↔Δ^5-androstenediol and estrone↔estradiol by oxidation or reduction of C-18 and C-19 steroids (Fig. 41-9).

The nomenclature of this group of genes and enzymes is daunting: the type 1 enzyme, 17β-HSD I (estradiol-17β dehydrogenase II) is encoded by the *HSD17B1* (or *EDH17B2)* gene located at 17q 11-12. This locus contains two genes: the active gene is *h17β-HSDII; h17β-HSDI (EDH17BP1)*, is a pseudogene 89% homologous to the active gene. 17β-HSD I is the isozyme responsible for ovarian 17β-HSD activity. The type 2 isozyme, 17β-HSDII(2),

encoded by *HSD17B2*, is responsible for 17β-HSD activity in placenta and endometrium. The testicular (type 3) isozyme, 17β-HSDIII(3), responsible for the final step in testosterone synthesis, reduction of androstenedione to testosterone, is encoded by *HSD17B3 (EDH17B3)*, which shares only 23% sequence homology with the *HSD17B1* and two genes. The finding of small amounts of testosterone in patients with deficiency of the type 3 isozyme suggests that one of the other isozymes can also convert androstenedione to testosterone.

The 17β-HSDs are expressed in a tissue-specific fashion, some being expressed predominantly in estrogenic or androgenic tissues and others more widely, but are not expressed in the adrenals. In addition to ovary, testis and placenta, significant levels of *HSD17B* mRNAs are found in peripheral sites such as uterus, breast, prostate, and adipose tissue. The tissue-specific isozymes have differing specificity for either the oxidative or the reductive reaction. In peripheral locations, 17β-HSDs may play a role in regulating the levels of active androgens and estrogens, by utilizing either their oxidative or reductive functions. The testicular isozyme preferentially utilizes NADPH as its cofactor in reduction of androstendione to testosterone.

Clinical Features and Molecular Defects Deficiency of testicular17β-HSD 3 is the most common defect of androgen production, resulting in impaired testicular conversion of androstenedione to testosterone. 17β-HSD deficiency is inherited in an autosomal-recessive fashion and a number of extensive inbred Arab kindreds with numerous affected individuals have been reported. Although affected 46,XY individuals have female (or partially masculinized) external genitalia, their internal genitalia are well masculinized, with development of epididymis, vas deferens and seminal vesicles. This finding may be because of activity of 17β-HSD isozymes other than 17β-HSD3 converting testis-derived androstenedione to testosterone in the proximity of the Wolffian ducts. In contrast there is insufficient testosterone at the level of the external genital primordia to act as substrate for 5α-reductase conversion to DHT. Ratios of androstenedione to testosterone and estrone to estradiol are elevated in spermatic venous samples and there is impaired conversion of labeled Δ^4-androstenedione to testosterone by testicular tissue in vitro. This defect is restricted to the gonads - the site of expression of 17β-HSD3.

A striking feature of this disorder is the marked virilization that occurs at puberty. Affected 46,XY individuals develop a male body habitus with abundant body and facial hair, enlargement of the testes and penis to normal adult size, and pigmentation and rugation of the labioscrotal folds. Gynecomastia is variably present. Despite having been reared as females during childhood many affected individuals spontaneously adopt the male gender role, with apparently adequate sexual function, but with infertility. These clinical observations correlate with normalization of peripheral and spermatic vein testosterone levels. Part of this effect appears likely to be related to increased LH secretion and Leydig cell hyperplasia, because Δ^4-androstenedione levels remain markedly elevated, indicating persistent enzyme dysfunction. Peripheral testosterone production as a result of extragonadal 17β-HSD activity may also contribute. The phenotype and clinical course of individuals with 17β-HSD deficiency is similar to that of individuals with 5α-reductase deficiency (described below).

Although testosterone and androstenedione levels may vary among patients, the diagnosis of 17β-HSD3 deficiency is suggested by a 10- to 15-fold elevation of the ratios of Δ^4-androstenedione to testosterone and of estrone to estradiol in the perinatal period, following hCG stimulation in childhood, or after puberty. Because of a secondary increase in 3β-HSD activity, DHEA may be normal or mildly elevated. Glucocorticoid and mineralocorticoid synthesis remain normal because the enzymatic defect is confined to the gonads.

Homozygous or compound heterozygous *HSD17B3* mutations have been identified in >40 patients with 17β-HSD deficiency. The majority are missense mutations resulting in AA substitutions in various regions of the protein; splice site mutations are also common. Phenotypic variability among individuals with the same mutation is well described. Identical mutations have been found within kindreds from widely distant regions of the world, suggesting genetic founder effects. Specific mutations tend to segregate with certain ethnicities, so knowledge of the patient's ethnic background may be helpful in predicting the expected mutation. Like other autosomal-recessive disorders, rates of 17β-HSD deficiency are higher in populations with consanguinity. Compared with a rate of approx 1/140,000 in the Netherlands, Arabs in Gaza have a prevalence of 1/200–300. Homozygosity for a mutation that converts arginine 80 to glutamine was reported in 24 individuals from 9 such extended Arab families. This substitution impairs enzyme activity by increasing the NADPH cofactor binding constant 60-fold. One 46,XY phenotypic female had compound heterozygosity for two distinct AA substitutions and another had compound heterozygosity for a splice acceptor mutation and a missense mutation. When expressed in cultured mammalian cells in vitro the mutant enzymes displayed impaired enzyme activity.

Proteins and Enzymes of Androgen Action*

5α-Reductase

Normal Function The 5α-reductases are microsomal enzymes that catalyze the 5α-reduction of many C19 and C21 steroids, utilizing NADPH as a cofactor. There are two isozymes of 5α-reductase (they share approx 50% AA identity) encoded by separate genes, 5α-reductase 1 by *SRD5A1* at 5p15, and the enzyme important in the context of sexual differentiation, 5α-reductase 2, a 254-AA protein encoded by *SRD5A2* located at 2p23. The genes are structurally similar, with five coding exons each. 5α-reductase 2 mediates the conversion of testosterone to more potent androgen, DHT in androgenic target tissues.

The 5α-reductase isozymes have differential expression patterns: the type 1 isozyme is not detectable in the fetus, but is transiently expressed in newborn scalp and skin and postpubertal skin and is permanently expressed in the liver; the type 2 isozyme is expressed in the liver and in androgen target tissues, including the external genitalia, accessory sex organs, and prostate. It is expressed in the primordia of the prostate and external genitalia before their differentiation, but is not expressed in the Wolffian ducts untill after their differentiation, supporting the contention that testosterone rather than DHT is the critical androgen in this process. Expression is upregulated by androgens, as demonstrated by the marked increase in *SRD5A2* mRNA level in the prostate of castrate animals following testosterone administration. Expression appears to be regulated in the opposite fashion in the liver.

Clinical Features and Molecular Defects Deficiency of 5α-reductase 2 results in an autosomal-recessive form of male pseudohermaphroditism previously referred to as pseudovaginal

perineoscrotal hypospadias. Clusters of affected patients have been reported in consanguineous populations in the Dominican Republic, Pakistan, Lebanon and New Guinea. Deficiency of 5α-reductase 2 in the tissues of the fetal external genitalia and urogenital sinus results in inadequate local DHT concentrations. As in other forms of defective androgen production or action, there is subnormal masculinization of these structures. The genital phenotype varies widely among and even within affected kindreds, the most consistent findings being underdevelopment of the penis and prostate. Most patients have ambiguous external genitalia, with testes located in the inguinal region or a bifid scrotum, accompanied by a blind vaginal pouch or urogenital sinus. Because Sertoli cell AMH secretion is normal, Müllerian structures are absent. It is on the basis of these clinical findings, that the requirement for DHT in external genital masculinization was initially inferred. Because differentiation of the gonads and Wolffian ducts depends on high local concentrations of testosterone rather than DHT, the testes, epididymides, vasa deferentia, and seminal vesicles develop normally.

Reduced conversion of testosterone to DHT in target tissues results in a marked increase in testosterone: DHT ratio diagnostic of 5α-reductase 2 deficiency. In normal infants (2 wk–6 mo of age), the testosterone:DHT ratio is 4.8 ± 2.2 (mean ± standard deviation) following stimulation with hCG. Affected infants have markedly increased testosterone:DHT ratios, in the 20–60 range or higher. Serum LH may be mildly increased. 5α-reductase 2 deficiency can be differentiated endocrinologically from 17β-HSD deficiency (with which it shares phenotypic similarity) by the characteristically increased serum androstenedione in the latter condition.

One of the most intriguing and well-documented features of this disorder is the striking virilization, including increased muscularity and deepening of the voice, that occurs at puberty in many affected individuals. In addition, the testes often enlarge, descend and develop Leydig cell hyperplasia, although spermatogenesis is absent or severely impaired. LH is normal or elevated, and testosterone levels increase into the adult male range, whereas DHT remains disproportionately low, but measurable. The testosterone to DHT ratio may be in the range of 30–80 (compared with the normal ratio of approx 9–15 at this age). The pubertal virilization is thought to result from both the high testosterone concentrations and from increased conversion of testosterone to DHT by 5α-reductase 1 in liver and skin. Acne, facial hair, temporal hair recession, and prostatic enlargement do not develop, presumably because these events require higher concentrations of DHT. Gynecomastia does not develop because there is no increase in testicular estrogen production. Many affected individuals initially raised as females, change their gender role to male around the time of puberty.

At least 30 different mutations have been identified throughout the *SRD5A2* gene in affected families from >20 different ethnic groups, ranging from complete *SRD5A2* deletion in a New Guinea kindred, to single base mutations resulting in gene splicing defects, premature termination or AA substitutions (the majority). Deletions, premature termination codons and splice junction defects prevent expression of a functional enzyme. AA substitutions may produce an unstable enzyme or impair binding of testosterone and/or NADPH. Substitutions at the N- or C-terminal ends of the molecule are associated with defective testosterone binding, whereas reduced NADPH binding affinity occurs only with

---

*These proteins and their associated disorders are discussed in detail in Chapter 44.

C-terminal substitutions. Differences in enzyme stability and affinity for testosterone and NADPH among kindreds reflect the genetic heterogeneity of the enzyme defects, but there is little relationship between the severity of the mutation and phenotype.

Androgen Receptor (AR)

Normal Function The AR is a ligand-activated nuclear transcription factor that mediates the effects of androgens in induction of target gene transcription in androgen-dependent tissues. The 8-exon *AR* gene at Xq11-12 encodes a 110-kDa, 910–919 AA protein consisting of three major functional domains: N-terminal (transcription-regulating), DNA-binding (ZF) and steroid-binding. The AR is expressed in a wide array of genital and nongenital tissues, reflecting its role as a widespread transcription factor. Activation of AR by androgen binding results in interaction of the receptor/ligand complex as a homodimer with androgen response element DNA sequences in the promoter regions of target genes, to regulate their transcription. The exact targets of the AR in genital development remain to be determined, although the AMH receptor appears to be one of them. In external genital tissues, testosterone is converted by 5α-reductase 2 to DHT, which has greater affinity for the AR. Nevertheless, the same molecular events occur following interaction of either testosterone or DHT with AR. The female fetus bears the same AR as the male, thus it is primarily the available concentration of androgens that is the major determinant of genital masculinization. Because Chapter 44 is devoted exclusively to the molecular biology and physiology of the AR, discussion of this important factor in this chapter is limited.

Clinical Features and Molecular Defects Absence or defective function of the AR results in resistance to the effects of androgens, manifest clinically as AIS (previously referred to as testicular feminization), a heterogeneous condition thought to represent the single most common identifiable cause of male pseudohermaphroditism. Affected individuals have normal testicular function, but have variable defects of internal and external genital masculinization, associated with partial retention of Müllerian structures in some cases. In complete AIS (CAIS), which has a prevalence of approx 1/20,000 46,XY births, not only is the phenotype unequivocally female, the labia minora and majora and clitoris may be underdeveloped, suggesting involvement of low levels of androgen action in normal genital development in females.

Infants with CAIS fail to demonstrate the postnatal surge of LH and testosterone seen in normal male infants (and retained in those with partial AIS) and have blunted LH responses to exogenous gonadotropin-releasing hormone. This failure of the normal infantile "mini-puberty" may reflect lack of prenatal "priming" of the hypothalamus due to absence of hypothalamic AR. At puberty, LH, testosterone and DHT increase to supranormal levels and serum estrogen concentrations are also enhanced, as a result of LH-driven testicular estrogen secretion and peripheral aromatization of testosterone. AMH levels are also supranormal during the first year of life and at puberty, a finding that may help to differentiate AIS from intersex conditions caused by testicular dysgenesis, in which AMH is low. Pubertal development in CAIS is entirely female, accompanied by absence of pubic and axillary hair.

Infants with partial forms of AIS (PAIS) have widely varying degrees of genital masculinization and the clinical diagnosis is notoriously difficult, as hormonal profiles are often inconclusive.

The diagnosis of PAIS, should be suspected in a 46,XY infant with ambiguous genitalia if the classic elevations of LH and testosterone are present and if the responses of testosterone precursors, testosterone and DHT to exogenous hCG are normal or elevated. In contrast to those with CAIS, infants with PAIS have a vigorous "mini puberty" at approx 6–12 wk of age, as seen in normal male infants, with normal or supranormal LH and testosterone concentrations. Depending on the severity of the androgen resistance, varying degrees of virilization and/or feminization occur at puberty. The prevalence of PAIS is unknown. Demonstration of abnormal androgen binding in cultured genital skin fibroblasts or identification of a mutation in the AR gene of affected individuals confirms the diagnosis, but is generally impractical outside of research institutions. Furthermore, receptor levels in genital skin fibroblasts and androgen binding affinity often correlate poorly with the degree of masculinization and may be falsely negative if the defect falls outside the steroid-binding domain. In addition, in many cases of PAIS complete sequencing of the AR gene fails to reveal a mutation.

Over 300 distinct mutations have been reported in the *AR* genes of hundreds of unrelated individuals with various forms of AIS*. Like the clinical spectrum, the molecular defects are highly heterogeneous. Protein-disrupting defects such as complete and partial gene deletions (rare), small insertions and deletions of a few base pairs, splice junction mutations and premature termination codons, are found in patients with CAIS. Missense mutations causing AA substitutions, the most common mutational type, are found in both CAIS and PAIS. The majority of missense mutations are located in the exons encoding the steroid-binding domain, with all but a few of the remainder reported in the exons encoding the DNA-binding domain. Mutations within the steroid-binding domain cause variable defects of androgen binding—absent, reduced (affinity or capacity or both), or qualitatively abnormal (increased thermolability of binding, ligand dissociation or altered binding specificity). Mutations within the DNA-binding domain typically alter the affinity, capacity or specificity of AR binding to androgen response element DNA sequences, without significant effect on androgen binding. Whether the mutation affects DNA or androgen binding, the final common pathway of AR defects is reduction/loss of ability of the mutant receptor to regulate transcription of androgen-dependent target genes. The *AR* gene appears to be particularly mutation-prone, and approx 25% of mutations arise *de novo*. A few individuals have been identified as having more than one *AR* gene mutation.

Altlhough *AR* mutations can be demonstrated in almost all patients with CAIS, the same is not true for individuals with the clinical diagnosis of PAIS, of whom only approx 1/3 have a detectable alteration of the AR coding sequence. This may in part reflect inaccurate clinical differentiation between PAIS and other causes of male pseudohermaphroditism (e.g., 17α-hydroxylase deficiency) or may represent defects within noncoding regions of the *AR* gene or in cofactors required for normal AR action. Unfortunately, no genotype/phenotype correlation exists for *AR* mutations, and phenotype may differ widely among individuals with the same mutation, even within the same family (Fig. 41-8). Somatic mosaicism for both a mutant and a normal AR may account

---

* *see* www.mcgill.ca/androgendb.

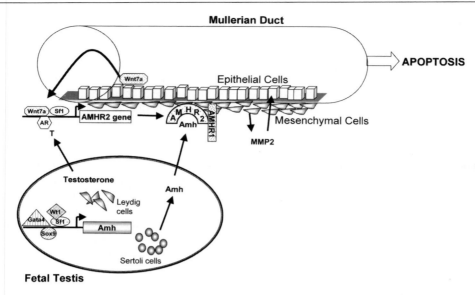

Figure 41-10   Interactions between Amh, its receptor and other transcription factors in induction of Müllerian regression during male embryogenesis. Within the fetal testis, a synergistic combination of transcription factors including Wt1, Sf1, Sox9, and GATA4, stimulates Sertoli cell production of Amh. Meanwhile, Leydig cells produce testosterone, under the stimulatory influence of Sf1 and other factors. The primitive Müllerian ducts consist of epithelial and mesenchmal elements. Epithelial cells secrete Wnt7a—an extracellular signaling molecule. Wnt7a interacts with Sf1 and the androgen receptor (activated by testosterone secreted by Legdig cells) to stimulate transcription of the Amh receptor (Amhr) gene and its expression by the mesenchymal cells surrounding the duct. Binding of Sertoli cell-derived amh to the amhr stimulates apoptosis of the Müllerian epithelium leading to obliteration of the duct lumen, progressing in a cranio-caudal direction down the duct, mediated by a paracrine "death factor" that may be a product of the activated Amhr. This process occurs during weeks 9–11 of human male gestation. Amh, anti-Müllerian hormone; Amhr, anti-Müllerian hormone receptor; AR, androgen receptor; MMP2, matrix metalloprotease 2; Sf1, steroidogenic factor 1; Sox9, Sry-related homeobox gene 9; Wnt7a, wingless-type MMTV integration site family member 7a; Wt1, Wilms tumor 1.

for phenotypic variability in some cases, and may have clinical relevance, because there may be a significant response to exogenous androgens in the cell populations carrying the normal AR. More complete analysis of AR mutations is provided in Chapter 44.

Mediators of Müllerian Duct Regression

Anti-Müllerian Hormone (AMH)

   Normal Function   Anti-Müllerian hormone (AMH or Müllerian inhibiting substance), produced by testicular Sertoli cells, is a member of the TGF-β family of growth factors that mediates regression of the Müllerian duct structures during normal male embryogenesis. The 5-exon, 2.75-kb *AMH* gene is located on human chromosome 19p13.3-13.2 and encodes a 560-AA glycoprotein that forms a 140-kDa homodimer.

   AMH is the first molecular marker after SRY specific for testis (Sertoli cell) differentiation, its expression in developing mouse testis beginning approx 2 d later than that of *Sry*, at approximately E13.5. *Amh* transcription appears to be initiated by Sox9 and subsequently upregulated by coordinated interactions at the *Amh* promoter between Sf1 and Sox9, Wt1, Gata4, and perhaps Dmrt1 (Fig. 41-3B). There is also some evidence suggesting upregulation of *Amh* expression by FSH and downregulation by androgens.

   The primary effect of AMH is to induce regression of Müllerian ducts during male sex differentiation (9–11 wk human gestation). These events occur in a paracrine fashion, with AMH secretion from one testis mediating only the regression of the ipsilateral Müllerian duct. Duct regression proceeds in a cranial-to-caudal direction associated with a cranial-to-caudal gradient of AMHR2 (discussed later). This is followed by a wave of apoptosis and accumulation of β-catenin, an adherens junction protein (a factor that mediates cell–cell adhesion) within peri-Müllerian mesenchymal cells. Müllerian epithelial apoptosis seems to be

mediated by an extracellular proteinase—matrix metalloproteinase 2—a downstream product of AMH/AMHR2 signalling that functions as a paracrine "death factor" (Fig. 41-10).

   AMH is produced by Sertoli cells not only during the critical period of sex differentiation, but also in late gestation, after birth, and even, albeit at a much reduced rate, in adulthood, suggesting that AMH may have physiological roles other than its control of Müllerian duct regression. After puberty, AMH production is downregulated by androgens (this feature is absent in individuals with androgen insensitivity). *AMH* is not expressed prenatally in the ovary. However, low amounts are released into the follicular fluid by mature granulosa cells postnatally and one postulated role of ovarian AMH is to inhibit recruitment of primordial follicles into the pool of growing follicles, via effects on granulosa and theca cells, not on the oocytes themselves. The net effect is to allow for enhanced oocyte maturation prior to selection for ovulation.

   As expected from the known function of this protein, male mice with homozygous deletion of *Amh* had normal male reproductive tracts, but also had uteri and oviducts. However, mice with mutations in the *Amh* promoter that affect the regulation of *Amh* transcription had variable phenotypes. Mutation at the Sf1 binding site was associated with reduced *Amh* expression, but expression that was nevertheless adequate to induce Müllerian regression. In contrast, male mice homozygous for a mutant Sox9 binding site did not initiate *Amh* transcription, resulting in complete retention of Müllerian ducts.

   Female mice overexpressing human *AMH* had no uteri or fallopian tubes and blind-ending vaginas. The ovaries were devoid of germ cells and underwent reorganization into seminiferous tubule-like structures after birth. Males were also abnormal, with under-virilized external genitalia and impaired Wolffian duct development associated with undescended testes notable for Leydig cell hypoplasia due to effects of excess AMH on Leydig cell development.

Clinical Features and Molecular Defects   Deficiency of AMH or abnormality of its receptor (described below) results in the persistent Müllerian duct syndromes (PMDS type 1 [AMH] and PMDS type 2 [AMHR2]), which are inherited in an autosomal-recessive, male-limited, pattern. Affected karyotypic males have normal male external genitalia, normal testicular histology and normal Wolffian duct differentiation, but have retained and differentiated Müllerian ducts and abnormalities of testicular descent. The typical case is that of a phenotypically normal male infant with unilateral ectopic testis and an inguinal hernia on the contralateral side. One testis descends into the scrotum and the ipsilateral fallopian tube and uterus follow it into the inguinal canal (*hernia uteri inguinalis*), bringing the contralateral testis along (transverse testicular ectopia). The Müllerian structures usually are detected only at the time of surgery for hernia repair. A less common clinical presentation is with bilateral cryptorchidism and inguinal hernias. In this situation the uterus is fixed in the pelvis and the testes are embedded in the broad ligament. These two clinical variants can occur within the same family. Serum testosterone is normal but AMH, which is readily measurable in the serum of normal males until puberty, is reduced. Because of the increased mobility of the testes, they are prone to torsion. In addition, there may be associated aplasia of the epididymis and upper part of the vas deferens. These problems, along with the often difficult task of attempting to relocate the testes, combine to impair fertility in most patients with PMDS.

Because the testes are invariably undescended in PMDS it has been proposed that AMH is involved in the process of human testicular descent. However, this speculation is tempered by the finding of variable AMH levels in boys with simple cryptorchidism and of normal gubernacular development in *Amh*-null mice. Testicular tumors have occasionally been reported.

Diverse *AMH* mutations have been identified in many patients with PMDS with low or undetectable serum AMH. Mutations tend to cluster in the exons encoding the N- and C-terminal regions of the protein (the carboxyl terminus is considered the biologically active region of the molecule) and are of various types including splicing mutations, nonsense mutations and missense mutations, which represent the majority. The fact that AMH molecules containing an AA substitution cannot be detected by standard enzyme-linked immunosorbent assay (ELISA) suggests that even a single AA substitution alters the structure of the protein enough to interfere with binding to the ELISA antibody. In the largest single study of 21 families, most patients were homozygous for *AMH* gene mutations, as the patients derived from consanguineous Arab or Mediterranean communities. About 40% of mutations have been reported in more than one family, but whether these represent a founder effect, or a mutational "hot spot" is not clear.

Anti-Müllerian Hormone Receptor Type 2 (AMHR2)

Normal Function   Anti-Müllerian hormone receptor, type 2 (AMHR2) is a membrane-bound serine/threonine kinase similar to those for TGF-β and activin. The 11-exon, 8-kb gene encoding human the 573-AA AMHR2 protein is located at 12q13. Exons 1–3 encode a short signal sequence and the extracellular domain of the receptor, exon 4 encodes most of the transmembrane domain, and exons 5–11 encode the intracellular serine/threonine kinase domains. AMH binding to AMHR2 in target tissues leads to phosphorylation of a TGF-β type I receptor and the resulting intracellular signal cascade that leads to target gene activation and eventually to apoptosis of Müllerian cells. Candidates for the role

of the specific type I receptor with which the type 2 receptor interacts include activin receptor-like kinase 2 (ALK2) and the bone morphogenetic protein receptor 1a, also known as ALK3.

Amhr2 is expressed in mesenchymal cells adjacent to the Müllerian ducts during mouse embryogenesis, consistent with the fact that the effects of Amh appear to be via changes in the mesenchyme surrounding the Müllerian ducts which in turn induces apoptosis of the Müllerian epithelium and duct regression. Amh causes regression of the cranial part of the Müllerian duct while it continues to grow caudally, associated with a cranial-to-caudal gradient of Amhr2 protein, followed by a wave of apoptosis spreading caudally along the Müllerian duct. *Amhr2* expression can also be detected in fetal Sertoli and Leydig cells and in fetal and adult granulosa cells. There is evidence that AMH action on Leydig cells causes downregulation of testosterone production. Like AMH itself, the receptor is also expressed postpubertally. Expression of both ligand and receptor in the same cells suggests an autocrine action. AMHR2 expression is enhanced by SF1 (which also regulates expression of AMH itself) and WNT7a and appears to be downregulated by the AR. The receptor may also be regulated by its ligand. Expression of the receptor in female Müllerian mesenchyme does not result in duct regression, because Amh is absent in females prenatally.

Male mice with homozygous deletion of *Amhr2* had a similar internal genital phenotype to those with *Amh* deletion: a complete set of male and female internal ducts. The phenotype of *Amh/Amhr2* double-knockout mutant males was indistinguishable from that of either single mutant.

Clinical Features and Molecular Defects   Apart from the fact that serum AMH concentrations are normal or high, the clinical phenotype of patients with *AMHR2* mutations (PMDS type 2) is indistinguishable from that of patients with AMH deficiency (PMDS type 1). Indeed, approx 1/2 of patients with the clinical findings of PMDS have mutations in the ligand and half in the receptor. The single most common mutation in the *AMHR2* gene is a 27-bp deletion in exon 10. Of the more than 20 different reported defects, others include nonsense mutations causing truncation of the receptor to varying degrees, and a variety of missense mutations causing AA substitutions in the extracellular or intracellular domain. As with *AMH* mutations, most *AMHR2* gene mutations are found in the homozygous state and about 1/3 are recurrent, having been reported in more than one family. In a minority of patients, no mutation of either the hormone or its receptor can be detected, and these cases may represent good candidates for analysis of the type 1 AMH receptor required for effective AMHR2 signaling.

Wingless-Type MMTV Integration Site Family Member 7a (WNT7a)

WNT7a is another member of the WNT glycoprotein growth factor/signaling molecule family (page 420) involved in regulation of cell fate and patterning. *Wnt7a* is expressed along the length of the Müllerian epithelium in mice of both sexes but appears to have differing roles in male vs female development. *Wnt7a* is expressed in Müllerian epithelial cells from E12.5-14.5, whereas *Amhr2* is expressed in the mesenchymal cells surrounding the Müllerian ducts at day 14.5. It is hypothesized that the Wnt7a signal from the epithelial cells regulates *Amhr2* expression in the adjacent mesenchyme (Fig. 41-10). *Wnt7a* expression declines following Müllerian duct regression in the male.

Male mice with homozygous deficiency of *Wnt7a* have retained Müllerian ducts, and do not express *Amhr2* in the mesenchyme of the Müllerian ducts. Thus, *Wnt7a* deficiency results in failure of *Amhr2* expression and therefore failure of Müllerian duct regression in males. In contrast, female *Wnt7a*-deficient mice have defective, though not absent, development of the oviducts and uterus. The human gene is expressed in placenta, kidney, testis, uterus, fetal lung, and fetal and adult brain but no human disease has been reported in association with this gene.

NORMAL AND ABNORMAL FEMALE SEX DIFFERENTIA-TION Beyond the fact that normal female external genital development requires no estrogen and minimal androgen, little is known about factors directly involved in female sex differentiation. Normal internal reproductive duct development requires persistence and differentiation of the Müllerian ducts into the uterus, upper vagina and fallopian tubes, and regression of the Wolffian ducts. Thus, AMH and testosterone action must be absent. The finding of familial disorders of reproductive tract development in females implies that genetic factors must indeed play a role in either stimulating Müllerian development, or inhibiting its repression. A small amount of information from murine and human studies of *HOX* genes has emerged.

Individuals with 46,XX pseudohermaphroditism develop ovaries but have varying degrees of masculinization of internal and external genital structures. There are far fewer known causes of virilization of a female fetus than there are of undermasculinization of a male fetus. Essentially, disorders of female sex differentiation represent the converse of male pseudohermaphroditism, in general resulting from prenatal exposure to excessive androgen concentrations. In addition to abnormal fetal androgen secretion, maternal androgen excess caused by androgen secreting tumors, drugs or medications with androgenic activity can result in masculinization of the female fetus. These latter problems are not discussed. Abnormalities of Müllerian or vaginal development, such as the Mayer-Rokitansky-Küster-Hauser (MRKH) syndrome, vaginal atresia and Müllerian agenesis, although technically not forms of pseudohermaphroditism because there is no masculinization, are nevertheless significant disorders of female sex differentiation and are also discussed briefly.

Disorders of Female Sex Differentiation Due to Excess Androgen Production The most common cause of excessive fetal androgen production in females is CAH due to deficiency of 21-hydroxylase, 11-hydroxylase, POR (discussed earlier), or 3β-HSD (discussed earlier). A much rarer cause of female pseudohermaphroditism is P450arom deficiency in which fetal virilization results from high levels of testosterone and androstenedione because of the inability of the placenta to convert these precursors to estrogens.

***21-Hydroxylase* (see *Chapter 37 for additional details*)**

Normal Function P450c21 catalyzes the hydroxylation of progesterone to DOC and 17-OHP to 11-deoxycortisol, using POR as a cofactor (Fig. 41-9). P450c21 is a 55-kDa protein encoded by the10-exon *CYP21* gene (*CYP21B or CYP21A2*) located at chromosome 6 p21.3 within approx 2 centimorgans of the human leukocyte antigen complex, with which it has tight linkage. There is a homologous pseudogene, designated *CYP21P* (or *CYP21A*), located nearby, that contains three deleterious mutations: an 8-basepair deletion in exon 3, a T insertion in exon 7, and a stop codon in exon 8.

Clinical Features and Molecular Defects Deficiency of P450c21 is the most common cause of CAH in both males and females. Inheritance is autosomal-recessive and the prevalence of the disorder ranges from 1/15,000 (some white populations) to 1/700 (Yupik Eskimo tribe). Hydroxylation is impaired in the zona

fasciculata of the adrenal glands, so that 17-OHP is not converted to 11-deoxycortisol, the immediate precursor of cortisol. Cortisol deficiency leads to a compensatory increase in ACTH secretion that in turn drives the adrenal gland, resulting in overproduction of cortisol precursors, particularly 17-OHP. These steroids are "shunted" down the remaining functional steroidogenic pathway, producing a surfeit of androgens (mainly testosterone) that result in virilization of 46,XX fetuses but have no untoward effect on the male fetus. In more than half of cases, 21-hydroxylase is also deficient in the zona glomerulosa and there is failure of conversion of progesterone to 11-DOC, resulting in deficiency of aldosterone. Shock or death may result from severe salt wasting and accompanying hypovolemia.

There are four major clinical forms of 21-hydroxylase deficiency: salt-wasting (approx 75% of cases), simple virilizing, non-classic late onset (also called attenuated or acquired), and cryptic (asymptomatic). Only the two most severe forms, those that produce genital ambiguity, are discussed. Female infants with the classic virilizing form of 21-hydroxylase deficiency have masculinization of the genitalia, ranging from limited clitoromegaly and posterior labial fusion in the milder cases, to intermediate phenotypes with labioscrotal fusion, a urogenital sinus and significant clitoral enlargement, to severely virilized genitalia that are indistinguishable from those of a cryptorchid male infant. The gonads are normal ovaries, and Müllerian duct derivatives develop normally, reflecting absence of AMH. Even in the most virilized infants, Wolffian development does not occur, perhaps because of differences in timing of adrenal vs gonadal androgen secretion. Untreated children have penile or clitoral enlargement, premature adrenarche, rapid linear growth and advanced skeletal maturation, ultimately leading to early epiphyseal closure and short stature.

The virilizing form of 21-hydroxylase deficiency is the most likely diagnosis in an infant with genital ambiguity in the presence of 46,XX karyotype and should be suspected in any partially virilized infant in whom gonads cannot be located, either by palpation or by ultrasonography. The presence of a uterus enhances the likelihood of this diagnosis. Increased serum concentrations of 17-OHP are invariably present in infants with enzyme deficiency severe enough to cause virilization; this is accompanied by hyponatremia and hyperkalemia in those with the salt-wasting form. An ACTH stimulation test is not necessary to make this diagnosis in a virilized female infant.

Molecular defects in *CYP21B* have been elucidated in a large number of patients with 21-hydroxylase deficiency. Many appear to have arisen as a result of recombination events between *CYP21B* and its homologous pseudogene, *CYP21P*, and cause either deletion of *CYP21* (approx 20% of salt-wasting cases), or transfer of mutations from the pseudogene to the functional gene. This process, termed "gene conversion," is suggested to account for the predominance of 21-hydroxylase deficiency over other forms of CAH. Single base mutations are also common. In a comprehensive study of 88 families the most common mutation was an A-G change in the second intron affecting mRNA splicing (26%); large deletions occurred in approx 21%; substitution of isoleucine 172 by asparagine was found in 16% and replacement of valine 281 by leucine in 11%. Homozygosity for severe mutations is present in approx 50% of those with classic salt-wasting disease and compound heterozygosity is also common. The clinical and enzymatic findings of such patients reflect the combined effect of mutations in each allele.

In vitro analysis of mutant 21-hydroxylase enzymes has been performed in a number of cases. A mutant containing threonine at position 428 in place of cysteine has complete loss of enzymatic activity and heme binding. Of note, cysteine 428 is invariant among all P450 enzymes and is thought to be the heme-binding site. Other AA substitutions depress enzyme activity to varying degrees. Weak correlations exist between enzyme activity (phenotype) and mutation (genotype).

11β-Hydroxylase

Normal Function There are two cytochrome P450 isozymes with 11β-hydroxylase activity involved in the latter steps of cortisol and aldosterone production. Regulated by ACTH, P450C11 (P450XIB1) catalyzes the final step in cortisol synthesis, 11β-hydroxylation of 11-deoxycortisol to cortisol in the zona fasciculata of the adrenal gland. The aldosterone synthase isozyme (P450AS, P450aldo, P450cmo, P450XIB2), regulated by the renin-angiotensin system, catalyzes the three-step conversion of 11-DOC to aldosterone (11-hydroxylation, 18-hydroxylation, 18-oxidation) in the zona glomerulosa. Both enzymes use POR as a cofactor. Two genes encode 93% homologous 479- to 503-AA enzymes: the 6.5-kb, 9-exon *CYP11B1* gene localized to 8q22 encodes P450C11; a contiguous gene, *CYP11B2*, located approx 40 kb away within the same chromosomal locus, encodes P450AS. *CYP11B1* and *CYP11B2* are structurally homologous to *CYP11A*, which encodes P450scc (discussed earlier), and the trio represent a subfamily within the P450 superfamily.

Clinical Features and Molecular Defects Deficiency of 11β-hydroxylase results in the second most common form of CAH, accounting for 5–8% of cases, depending on ethnic background. The condition occurs with relatively high frequency in consanguineous families in Saudi Arabia, and in Moroccan and Iranian Jews. Affected 46,XX infants present with variable genital virilization, similar to those with 21-hydroxylase deficiency, in the presence of normal ovaries and female internal genital structures. Some affected females have been so extremely virilized that they have been reared as males, the diagnosis delayed until puberty, when breast development and menses occurred. Driven by increased ACTH levels, 11-deoxycortisol is massively elevated and serum concentrations of 11-DOC, adrenal androgens and testosterone (by conversion from androstenedione) are also increased. The key clinical feature that distinguishes this condition from 21-hydoxylase deficiency is the presence of hypertension, induced by high concentrations of 11-DOC, whose mineralocorticoid activity causes sodium retention, variable hypokalemia and suppression of plasma renin activity. There is minimal correlation between the severity of the virilization and the hypertension. Precocious pseudopuberty and advanced skeletal maturation occur in untreated cases in both sexes.

Mutations in *CYP11B1* include frameshift mutations that delete the enzyme's heme-binding domain and a number of missense mutations. The majority of molecular defects are *de novo* point mutations clustered in exons 6–8 of the gene, suggesting that this region encodes residues critical for enzymatic activity. The relatively high frequency of mutations in this gene is suggested to result from its high number of CpG dinucleotides, a well-recognized mutational "hot spot" in the human genome, rather than from recombination between *CYP11B1* and *CYP11B2*, (as occurs between CYP21 and its adjacent pseudogene). Substitution of arginine by histidine at position 448 is the predominant defect in P450C11 in Moroccan Jews, suggesting a founder effect. This AA is highly conserved and thought to be required for heme binding, which is critical for enzymatic activity.

Aromatase

Normal Function P450arom is a cytochrome P450 enzyme located in the endoplasmic reticulum of estrogen-producing cells. Using POR (described above) as a cofactor, it catalyzes conversion of C19 steroids (androstenedione and testosterone) to C18 estrogens (estradiol, estrone, estriol). Androgens produced by the fetal adrenal gland, then desulfated and aromatized by the placenta are the major source of circulating estrogens during pregnancy. P450arom is encoded by *CYP19*, a 9-exon, 70-kb gene located at chromosome 15q21.1. P450arom is expressed in a wide variety of human tissues, ranging from the preimplantation blastocyst to the placenta, ovarian granulosa and luteal cells, testicular Sertoli and Leydig cells, adipose tissue, brain, muscle, and liver. Expression is regulated in part by the use of tissue-specific alternative promoters; however, the same protein is expressed in all tissues.

Clinical Features and Molecular Defects An apparently rare cause of female pseudohermaphroditism is the inability to convert fetal androgens to estrogens because of lack of placental P450arom activity as a result of mutations in the fetus. In two cases, the mothers developed progressive virilization in the latter part of pregnancy, associated with high androgen and low estrogen concentrations. Despite this, growth of the fetuses and placentas throughout gestation were normal. Following delivery maternal virilization resolved and in vitro assay of the placenta revealed negligible P450arom activity. Absence of maternal virilization in a third case suggested that some P450arom activity was retained.

The affected 46,XX infants had male-appearing or ambiguous external genitalia with marked clitoral enlargement, rugation and fusion of labioscrotal folds, and a single meatus at the base of the phallic structure. The virilization results from placental inability to aromatize DHEA, which is therefore converted to androstenedione and testosterone, leading to massive elevations of the latter. An affected 46,XY infant had normal masculinization.

The two affected 46,XX patients developed features of androgen excess at puberty, associated with ovarian cysts. Clitoral enlargement and facial acne were noted, the result of high adrenal androgens. In addition, the affected individuals had absence of breast development, attributed to deficiency of ovarian P450arom (and therefore low estrogens). Gonadotropins were modestly elevated, accompanied by high testosterone and low estradiol concentrations, which also resulted in delayed skeletal maturation and tall stature. There was also significant osteoporosis in the affected adult male.

The defects in these cases were inherited in an autosomal-recessive manner and there was known parental consanguinity in one case. In the first case, the affected girl was homozygous for a splice junction point mutation that resulted in translation of an abnormal peptide containing an extra 29 AAs. The mutant enzyme retained only a minimal level of activity in vitro. In the second case, the affected individual had compound heterozygosity for two single base mutations that introduced two separate AA substitutions into the enzyme: arginine 435 to cysteine and two residues downstream, cysteine 437 to tyrosine. The mutant enzymes had extremely low activity in the presence of the R435C substitution, and complete absence of activity with the C437Y defect. Cysteine 437 is very highly conserved, and is apparently involved in heme binding, hence the destructive effect of the mutation on enzyme function. In the final case, the mutation introduced a cysteine in place of the highly conserved residue arginine 375, located in a region of the protein that may be involved in anchoring the enzyme to the cell membrane. The mutant protein expressed in vitro had only 0.2% of the activity of wild-type P450arom. These cases, as well as the single reported case of an estrogen receptor mutation, and the evidence from estrogen receptor -deleted transgenic mice, indicate that contrary to longstanding belief, estrogens are not required for fetal survival.

Disorders of Female Sex Differentiation Affecting Müllerian Structures

Homeobox A 13 (HOXA13) and Related Genes

Normal Function   A member of the homeobox family of genes that encode the developmentally important homeodomain proteins, *homeobox A 13* (*HOXA13*) and related genes, play important roles in the morphogenesis of the terminal part of the gut and urogenital tract and are involved in Müllerian development. *HOXA13* is specifically discussed because in addition to urogenital abnormalities in *Hoxa13*-deficient mice, mutations affecting uterine development have been reported in humans. The human *HOXA13* gene is located within a cluster of at least 8 homeobox genes on chromosome 7, at 7p15-p14.2. Within the protein certain residues and AA motifs are strongly conserved in fish, amphibian, reptile, chicken, and marsupial and placental mammals.

In mice, *Hoxa13* is expressed early in the epithelial cells of tissues of the developing hindgut in a manner that suggests a fundamental role in the epithelial-mesenchymal interaction necessary for tail growth and posterior gut/genitourinary patterning. In the development of the embryonic mouse Müllerian tract *Hoxa9*, *Hoxa10*, *Hoxa11*, and *Hoxa13* are all expressed along the length of the paramesonephric duct. Later in development, expression of *Hoxa13* is localized to the cervical and vaginal tissues. After birth, a spatial *Hox* axis is established, corresponding to the postnatal differentiation of this organ system: *Hoxa9* is expressed in the fallopian tubes, *Hoxa10* in the uterus, *Hoxa11* in the uterus and cervix, and *Hoxa13* in the upper vagina. In the developing mouse genital tubercle, *Hoxa13* is essential for normal expression of *Fgf8* and *Bmp7* in the urethral plate epithelium.

Mice with the semidominant mutation "hypodactyly" (Hd) have a 90-bp deletion within the first exon of *Hoxa13*. Homozygous (Hd/Hd) female mice have profound hypoplasia of the cervix and vaginal cavity, in addition to absence of digits. In male mutant mice, hypospadias occurs as a result of the combined loss of *Fgf8* and *Bmp7* expression in the urethral plate epithelium, as well as the ectopic expression of *noggin* in the flanking mesenchyme. Complete deletion of *Hoxa13* causes more profound defects: *Hoxa13*(–/–) mutant fetuses have agenesis of the caudal portion of the Müllerian ducts, lack development of the presumptive urinary bladder and have premature stenosis of the umbilical arteries, which could account for the lethality of this mutation at midgestation.

Clinical Features and Molecular Defects   The hand-foot-uterus or hand-foot-genital syndrome is an autosomal-dominant disorder whose features include limb anomalies (short first metacarpals, small thumbs and great toes, short fifth fingers and fusion or delayed ossification of wrist bones) and disturbances of Müllerian fusion including a partially divided (bicornuate) or completely divided (didelphic) uterus; affected males have hypospadias of variable severity. Heterozygous mutations in *HOXA13* have been found in a number of families with this condition. Such mutations have generally been severe, causing protein truncation that likely eliminates the DNA-binding capacity of the protein. It is of interest that mutations in *HOXA13* have somewhat

similar effects to those of another, better characterized, homeobox gene – *SOX9* – which also causes defects in both skeletal and sexual development.

Mayer-Rokitansky-Kuster-Hauser Syndrome   (MRKH) Although individuals with the Mayer-Rokitansky-Kuster-Hauser (MRKH) clearly are phenotypic females, there is nevertheless a failure of female sex differentiation of the internal genitalia. Affected girls usually present in their teens with primary amenorrhea despite otherwise normal secondary sexual development. Examination reveals absence or severe hypoplasia of the vagina; uterine agenesis is usual, however, some uterine development (uni- or bicornuate uterus) or occasionally a normal uterus, may be present. The ovaries are normal. There appear to be 2 subtypes of the disorder—the typical (isolated) and atypical forms, frequency being approximately equal. The typical form is characterized by presence of symmetric muscular buds (Müllerian remnants) and normal fallopian tubes. The atypical form has asymmetric aplasia of one or both buds, with or without dysplasia of the fallopian tubes. The atypical form may have associated anomalies including renal defects (agenesis or ectopia in approx 30–50% of patients) and skeletal abnormalities (vertebral malformations; Klippel-Feil anomaly) of variable severity. Laparoscopy is required to distinguish the typical from the atypical form. The most severe form of the disorder, MURCS, includes M̲üllerian duct aplasia, r̲enal agenesis/ectopia, and c̲ervical s̲omite dysplasia (Klippel-Feil anomaly). Because of these associated anomalies, all girls and women with vaginal atresia should undergo skeletal radiographs and renal/ pelvic ultrasound.

The MRKH syndrome is thought to result from failure of fusion of the lower Müllerian ducts during early embryogenesis. Cases in which there is associated skeletal dysplasia may represent a mesodermal malformation spectrum. The MRKH syndrome occurs in 1 in 4000–5000 females and represents the cause of primary amenorrhea in 15% of cases. Most cases are sporadic, however, a genetic defect likely underlies familial cases (~5%), which have been reported in patterns consistent with sex-limited autosomal-dominant or autosomal-recessive inheritance. Although one study suggested a potential relationship between a heterozygous mutation in the gene encoding galactose-1-phosphate uridyl transferase and vaginal agenesis in about half of patients studied, the data were inconclusive and have not been formally confirmed.

APPROACHES TO DIAGNOSIS

Abnormalities of sex determination and differentiation in infancy require evaluation by an experienced team, including a pediatric endocrinologist, urologist, and geneticist. The principal aims of the diagnostic evaluation are to determine: (1) presence of potentially life-threatening adrenal steroid deficiencies and electrolyte derangements; (2) chromosomal sex; (3) type and functional status of the gonads; and (4) internal genital anatomy.

The history should determine the presence of similarly affected siblings and of consanguinity between parents or of ethnic background in which inbreeding is common (suggestive of autosomal-recessive conditions such steroidogenic enzyme defects and 5α-reductase 2 deficiency). A family history of sudden death in infancy, ambiguous genitalia, lack of pubertal development, amenorrhea or infertility may be found in some cases of CAH. A history in maternal relatives, of genital abnormalities, severe, persistent gynecomastia or infertility suggests an X-linked condition such as androgen insensitivity. Maternal virilization during pregnancy could suggest P450arom deficiency. Clinical examination,

production follows loss of germ cells. Androgen replacement is the treatment of choice for testosterone deficiency, whereas treatment of severe gynecomastia is surgical.

The phenotype of Klinefelter syndrome is mild compared to disorders involving an extra autosome, for example, trisomy 21 (Down syndrome). The reason is that the additional X chromosome in Klinefelter syndrome is inactivated, whereas the extra chromosome in Down syndrome or other autosomal aneuploidy syndromes remains active. Hence relatively few genes, namely those escaping X inactivation, have an increased functional dosage in Klinefelter syndrome. For this same reason, XXX females are usually normal. Individuals with greater numbers of X chromosomes, for example, 48,XXXY; 48,XXXX; 49,XXXXY; or 49, XXXXX karyotypes, often show more severe abnormalities such as mental retardation or skeletal malformations, even though all but one X chromosome is inactivated. The abnormalities are presumably caused by further increase in the dosage of genes that escape X inactivation. Similar phenotypes have been noted in men with severe Y aneuploidy, for example, 48,XYYY or 49,XYYYY karyotypes, suggesting that the culprit genes are present on both the X and Y chromosomes, for example, *SHOX*.

RING X MOSAICISM Turner syndrome variants involving mosaicism for a ring X chromosome, or 45,X/46,X,r(X) karyotype, are sometimes associated with severe abnormalities such as mental retardation and multiple congenital anomalies. In general, the severity of the phenotype inversely correlates with the size of the ring; larger rings tend to be associated with a milder phenotype. The explanation for the severe phenotypes associated with small rings might lie with X inactivation and dosage compensation. Some small ring X chromosomes either lack the XIC region or fail to express the XIST gene; these rings express some genes that are normally X inactivated. The severe phenotype is probably caused by functional disomy, or expression of both copies, of one or more X-linked genes.

DOSAGE-SENSITIVE SEX REVERSAL A few XY females have been reported with partial duplications of the short arm of the X chromosome that include band Xp21.1 (*see* Fig. 42-1). Because the duplicated X is not inactivated in the absence of a second complete X chromosome, sex reversal is caused by a twofold increase in expression of a gene or genes within the duplication. This locus has been designated dosage-sensitive sex reversal (DSS). Detailed mapping of partially overlapping duplications narrowed the DSS region to a small interval containing *NROB1*, which encodes a member of the nuclear hormone receptor superfamily. Loss-of-function mutations in *NROB1* cause congenital adrenal hypoplasia and hypogonadotropic hypogonadism. Overexpression of *NROB1* in transgenic mice causes XY sex reversal, confirming that *NROB1* is DSS.

EFFECTS OTHER THAN GENE DOSAGE

As mentioned, gonadal failure associated with Turner and Klinefelter syndrome may involve abnormal dosage of X-linked genes that escape inactivation. However, animal studies suggest that the presence of an unpaired X chromosome may cause germ cell apoptosis through a meiotic pachytene checkpoint mechanism. The effect is clearest for spermatogenesis, and explains the observation that men with balanced X-autosome translocations are almost invariably infertile. The presence of an analogous meiotic checkpoint during oogenesis is less certain. For example, gonadal function is usually normal in 47,XXX women. On the other hand, a meiotic checkpoint could explain why some X-autosome translocations are

associated with premature ovarian failure. In particular, women whose translocations break within a "critical region" of the X chromosome long arm, Xq13 to Xq26, often have primary or secondary amenorrhea. A number of these translocation breakpoints have been characterized in detail, and most do not appear to disrupt X-linked genes. Although not definitive, these data suggest that the ovarian failure associated with balanced X-autosome translocations is resulting from "nongenic" chromosomal effects such as interference with meiotic pairing or long-range perturbation of X inactivation.

SELECTED REFERENCES

Bardoni B, Zanaria E, Guioli S, et al. A dosage sensitive locus at chromosome Xp21 is involved in male to female sex reversal. Nat Genet 1994;7:497–501.

Binder G, Fritsch H, Schweizer R, Ranke MB. Radiological signs of Leri-Weill dyschondrosteosis in Turner syndrome. Horm Res 2001;55: 71–76.

Blaschke RJ, Rappold GA. SHOX in short stature syndromes. Horm Res 2001;55(Suppl 1):21–23.

Burgoyne PS, Baker TG. Meiotic pairing and gametogenic failure. Symp Soc Exp Biol 1984;38:349–362.

Carrel L, Cottle AA, Goglin KC, Willard HF. A first-generation X-inactivation profile of the human X chromosome. Proc Natl Acad Sci USA 1999;96:14,440–14,444.

Chandley AC, Cooke HJ. Human male fertility—Y-linked genes and spermatogenesis. Hum Mol Genet 1994;3:1449–1452.

Disteche CM. The great escape. Am J Hum Genet 1997;60:1312–1315.

Ford CE, Jones KW, Polani PE, De Almeida JC, Briggs JH. A sex-chromosome anomaly in a case of gonadal dysgenesis (Turner's syndrome). Lancet 1959;1:711–713.

Graves JA, Wakefield MJ, Toder R. The origin and evolution of the pseudoautosomal regions of human sex chromosomes. Hum Mol Genet 1998;7:1991–1996.

Hassold TJ. Chromosome abnormalities in human reproductive wastage. Trends Genet 1986;2:105–110.

Lahn BT, Page DC. Functional coherence of the human Y chromosome. Science 1997;278:675–680.

Lahn BT, Pearson NM, Jegalian K. The human Y chromosome, in the light of evolution. Nat Rev Genet 2001;2:207–216.

LeMaire-Adkins R, Radke K, Hunt PA. Lack of checkpoint control at the metaphase/anaphase transition: a mechanism of meiotic nondisjunction in mammalian females. J Cell Biol 1997;139:1611–1619.

Lippe B. Turner syndrome. Endocrinol Metab Clin North Am 1991;20: 121–152.

Lyon MF. X-chromosome inactivation. Curr Biol 1999;9:R235–R237.

Migeon BR, Luo S, Jani M, Jeppesen P. The severe phenotype of females with tiny ring X chromosomes is associated with inability of these chromosomes to undergo X inactivation. Am J Hum Genet 1994;55: 497–504.

Miyabara S, Sugihara H, Maehara N, et al. Significance of cardiovascular malformations in cystic hygroma: a new interpretation of the pathogenesis. Am J Med Genet 1989;34:489–501.

Page DC. Hypothesis: a Y-chromosomal gene causes gonadoblastoma in dysgenetic gonads. Development 1987;101(Suppl):151–155.

Pennington BF, Bender B, Puck M, Salbenblatt J, Robinson A. Learning disabilities in children with sex chromosome anomalies. Child Dev 1982;53:1182–1192.

Prueitt RL, Chen H, Barnes RI, Zinn AR. Most X;autosome translocations associated with premature ovarian failure do not interrupt X-linked genes. Cytogenet Genome Res 2002;97:32–38.

Reijo R, Lee TY, Salo P, et al. Diverse spermatogenic defects in humans caused by Y chromosome deletions encompassing a novel RNA-binding protein gene. Nat Genet 1995;10:383–393.

Ross JL, Scott C Jr, Marttila P, et al. Phenotypes associated with SHOX deficiency. J Clin Endocrinol Metab 2001;86:5674–5680.

Sinclair AH, Berta P, Palmer MS, et al. A gene from the human sex-determining region encodes a protein with homology to a conserved DNA-binding motif. Nature 1990;346:240–244.

Skuse DH, James RS, Bishop DV, et al. Evidence from Turner's syndrome of an imprinted X-linked locus affecting cognitive function. Nature 1997;387:705–708.

Swain A, Narvaez V, Burgoyne P, Camerino G, Lovell-Badge R. Dax1 antagonizes Sry action in mammalian sex determination. Nature 1998; 391:761–767.

Therman E, Laxova R, Susman B. The critical region on the human Xq. Hum Genet 1990;85:455–461.

Therman E, Sarto G. Inactivation center on the human X chromosome. In: Sandberg A, ed. Cytogenetics of the Mammalian X Chromosome, vol. 3A. New York: Alan R. Liss, 1983; pp. 315–325.

Tsuchiya K, Reijo R, Page DC, Disteche CM. Gonadoblastoma: molecular definition of the susceptibility region on the Y chromosome. Am J Hum Genet 1995;57:1400–1407.

Willard HF. X chromosome inactivation, XIST, and pursuit of the X-inactivation center. Cell 1996;86:5–7.

Zinn AR, Page DC, Fisher EM. Turner syndrome: the case of the missing sex chromosome. Trends Genet 1993;9:90–93.

43 Disorders of Pubertal Development

Tomonobu Hasegawa

SUMMARY

Puberty is the continuous maturation of growth and development to attain full sexual development and fertility by the hypothalamic–pituitary–gonadal axis and other complex endocrine systems. Although the physiology and molecular mechanism of normal puberty are not completely understood, we have made great progress in the management and treatment of disorders of pubertal development such as precocious puberty and delayed puberty. Moreover, the gene abnormalities of disorders of pubertal disorders have been elucidated one after another. This chapter mainly focuses clinical issues and single gene disorders of disorders of pubertal development.

Key Words: Congenital adrenal hyperplasia; constitutional delay of puberty; delayed puberty; familial male limited precocious puberty; hypergonadotropic hypogonadism; hypogonadotropic hypogonadism; Kallmann syndrome; Klinefelter syndrome; McCune–Albright syndrome; precocious puberty; premature pubarche; premature; puberty; thelarche; Turner syndrome.

INTRODUCTION

Puberty is the continuous maturation of growth and development to attain the full sexual development and fertility by the hypothalamic–pituitary–gonadal axis and other complex endocrine systems. It begins in late childhood and ends in early adulthood. At term, adolescence usually includes psychosocial changes during puberty. This chapter reviews the physiology of normal puberty and the pathophysiology of the disorders of pubertal development.

PHYSIOLOGY OF NORMAL PUBERTY

PHYSICAL CHANGES The physical changes of puberty span a continuum (Tabel 43-1). In girls, the first physical change of puberty is usually breast development (thelarche), although pubic hair growth (pubarche) may be first in a minority of instances. Breast development is followed by pubic hair, then axillary hair growth within 1–2 yr. On an average, menarche occurs 2 yr from the onset of breast development. In boys, the first physical change of puberty is always testicular enlargement. The formal measurement of testicular volume is possible using Prader orchidometer. Testicular volume of 4 mL represents the onset of puberty. Testicular enlargement is followed by penile enlargement and development of pubic hair. The development of axillary and facial hair, acne, and voice change occur in the later half of puberty. Adult testicular volumes and penile dimensions are generally achieved between the ages 14 and 18 yr.

The pubertal growth spurt shows other sexually dimorphic features. Prepubertal growth is similar in both genders; the growth velocity is highest during infancy and decreases to a nadir before the pubertal growth spurt. With respect to the pubertal growth spurt, the later onset of the pubertal growth spurt in boys leads to approx 2 yr difference in peak height velocity, and boys have greater magnitude of peak height velocity.

HORMONAL CHANGES Many dramatic hormonal changes occur during puberty. Two kinds of maturation play central roles. The first involves hypothalamic (gonadotropin releasing hormone; GnRH)–pituitary (gonadotropin)–gonadal axis and the second is the growth hormone (GH)-insulin-like growth factor (IGF)-1 axis. However, it should be emphasized that complex hormonal interactions characterize puberty.

Hypothalamic (GnRH)–Pituitary (Gonadotropin)–Gonadal Axis In the prepubertal stage, the hypothalamic-pituitary-gonadal axis is dormant. Hypothalamus and pituitary activity are thought to be suppressed by neuronal restraint pathways and negative feedback by minute amounts of gonadal steroid hormones. Such neuronal restraint pathways are poorly understood. The signals that control the onset of puberty are also poorly characterized. It appears that the mechanisms responsible for the onset of puberty are extremely complex and likely involve the integration of numerous different signals.

The onset of puberty is heralded by striking increases in luteinizing hormone (LH) secretion at night, manifested by an increase in amplitude and frequency of LH pulses. At least 1 yr before the clinical evidence of the onset of puberty, low serum concentrations of LH during sleep can be measured in serial serum samples obtained every 10–20 min. This sleep-entrained LH secretion is episodic owing to the pulsatile secretion of GnRH (GnRH pulse generator). By contrast, it is difficult to demonstrate the episodic secretion of follicle-stimulating hormone (FSH), as FSH clearance is slower than LH because of its higher sialic acid content. Gonadotropins are responsible for the maturation of the gonads. As pubertal maturation progresses, the amplitude and frequency of gonadotropin pulses increase during the day, in a pattern similar to that seen at night, until the final stage of sexual maturation is reached. In girls, the GnRH pulse generator ultimately establishes the regular cyclic variations of gonadotropins,

From: *Principles of Molecular Medicine, Second Edition*
Edited by: M. S. Runge and C. Patterson © Humana Press, Inc., Totowa, NJ

Table 43-1
"Tanner Stage" of Development in Secondary Sexual Characteristics

Boys: genital (penis) development
Stage 1 Prepubertal: testes, scrotum, and penis of about same size and proportion as in early childhood
Stage 2 Enlargement of scrotum and testes. Skin of scrotum reddens and changes in texture
Stage 3 Enlargement of penis, at first mainly in length. Further growth of testes and scrotum
Stage 4 Increased size of penis with growth in breadth and development of glans. Testes and scrotum larger; scrotal skin darkened
Stage 5 Genitalia adult in size and shape

Girls: breast development
Stage 1 Prepubertal: elevation of papilla only
Stage 2 Breast bud stage: elevation of breast and papilla as small mound. Enlargement of areola diameter
Stage 3 Further enlargement and elevation of breast and areola, with no separation of their contours
Stage 4 Projection of areola and papilla to form a secondary mound above level of breast
Stage 5 Mature stage: projection of papilla only, related to recession of areola to general contour of breast

Both sexes: pubic hair
Stage 1 Prepubertal: vellus over pubes is not further developed than over abdominal wall
Stage 2 Sparse growth of long, slightly pigmented, downy hair, straight or slightly curled, chiefly at base of penis or along labia
Stage 3 Considerably darker, coarser, and more curled hair. Hair spreads sparsely over junction of pubes
Stage 4 Hair now adult in type, but area covered is still considerably smaller than in adult. No spread to medial surface of thighs
Stage 5 Adult in quantity and type with distribution of horizontal (or classically "feminine" pattern)
Stage 6 Spread up linea alba (male-type pattern)

---

estrogen, and progesterone of the menstrual cycle. In boys, the same GnRH pulse generator establishes a pattern characterized by relatively constant levels of gonadotropins and testosterone, with minimal diurnal variation.

Undoubtedly, androgen is the principal effector of the physical changes of sexual maturation during puberty in boys, whereas estrogen drives the development of secondary sexual characteristics in girls. Several clinical observations support that estrogen is the main contributor to the process of skeletal maturation, growth spurt, and skeletal mineralization in both genders. First, effective suppression of the rapid skeletal maturation in boys with GnRH-independent precocious puberty requires inhibition of aromatase activity to reduce serum estradiol concentrations, in addition to the use of antiandrogens to interfere with androgen action. Second, patients with aromatase deficiency of both genders exhibit delayed skeletal maturation and have no pubertal growth spurts. Third, patients with complete androgen insensitivity (46,XY) exhibit pubertal growth spurts, suggesting that the growth spurt in boys is not mediated via the androgen receptor, but is instead controlled indirectly via the estrogen receptor, after the conversion of testosterone to estrogen.

GH-IGF-1 Axis The secretion of GH increases two- to three-fold during puberty. GH is produced by the somatotrophs of the anterior pituitary gland and its secretion is regulated mainly by the effects of GH-releasing hormone and somatostatin. Treatment of late pubertal boys with an estrogen receptor antagonist diminished GH secretion, suggesting the critical role of estrogen to increase GH secretion during puberty, even in boys. The mechanism by which estrogen enhances GH secretion is not completely understood.

The effect of GH is primarily through hepatic synthesis of IGF-1. During puberty, increased GH secretion leads to increased serum IGF-1 concentrations, which correlate better with pubertal Tanner stages than chronological age.

Adrenal Androgens Before puberty, the increased secretion of adrenal androgens (dehydroepiandrosterone [DHEA] and dehydroepiandrosterone-sulfate [DHEA-S]) by the zona reticularis ("adrenarche") occurs. Although an adrenal androgen-stimulating factor has been postulated to induce adrenarche, no such factor

has been identified. The physiological role of adrenarche has not been elucidated, although adrenal androgen may be functioning in development of scrotal and labial hair. Importantly, the timing of adrenarche and puberty are independent.

Leptin Leptin produced by adipose tissue has a key role in regulating the onset of puberty and/or pubertal development. In boys, serum leptin concentrations increase just before the onset of puberty and decrease after the initiation of puberty. In girls, serum leptin concentrations increase after the onset of puberty, remain stable in midpuberty, and further increase in late puberty. Judging from animal studies, leptin alone is insufficient to induce or promote puberty. However, individuals with congenital leptin deficiency or congenital leptin resistance resulting from mutations of the leptin (*LEP*) or leptin receptor (*LEPR*) genes exhibit hypogonadotropic hypogonadism. Leptin treatment to a 9-yr-old girl with congenital leptin deficiency induced an early pubertal pattern of LH response in GnRH stimulation tests.

THE PATHOPHYSIOLOGY OF DISORDERS OF PUBERTAL DEVELOPMENT

PRECOCIOUS PUBERTY Precocious puberty has been generally defined as the onset of pubertal development before the age of 8 yr in girls and before the age of 9 yr in boys. This definition is arbitrary; however, because of the variation in the age at which puberty begins among different ethnic groups (*see* Table 43-2). In 1999, the Lawson Wilkins Pediatric Endocrine Society proposed new guidelines not to evaluate girls with either breast or pubic hair development after the age of 7 yr in Caucasians and after the age of 6 yr in African Americans. This has not been universally accepted, as some authors believe that the definition of precocious puberty being pubertal development before the age of 8 yr in girls may identify girls with onset of puberty between 6 and 8 yr who may benefit from treatment.

Incomplete (or partial) precocious puberty is isolated manifestations of pubertal development without other signs of puberty such as premature thelarche and premature pubarche (described in Incomplete [or Partial] Precocious Puberty [Variation of Normal Puberty]).

Table 43-2
Mean Age (Years) at the Onset of Development of Breast,
Pubic Hair, and Menarche in Different Ethnic Groups

	Breast	Pubic hair	Menarche
Caucasian	10.3	10.5	12.7
African-American	9.5	9.5	12.1
Mexican-American	9.8	10.3	12.2

Classification Precocious puberty is classified as GnRH-dependent or GnRH-independent. GnRH-dependent precocious puberty is because of the early activation of the normal pubertal hypothalamic–pituitary–gonadal axis. GnRH-gonadotropin activates the gonads leading to increasing gonadal steroid hormone secretion and progressive sexual maturation. Conversely, GnRH-independent precocious puberty is not because of the early activation of normal puberty.

GnRH-dependent precocious puberty is sometimes called gonadotropin-dependent, central, or true precocious puberty. GnRH-independent precocious puberty is also called gonadotropin-independent, peripheral, or pseudoprecocious puberty. The terms "GnRH-dependent" and "GnRH-independent" are employed in this chapter. This terminology is preferred as GnRH is essential for the activation of the gonadotropin–gonadal axis in normal puberty. Furthermore, precocious puberty because of an intracranial human chorionic gonadotropin (hCG)-secreting tumor is definitely GnRH-independent, but gonadotropin dependent and central precocious puberty.

The second classification of precocious puberty is isosexual or heterosexual (contrasexual). "Heterosexual" refers to feminization in boys or virilization in girls. GnRH-dependent precocious puberty is always isosexual by definition, whereas GnRH-independent precocious can be either isosexual or heterosexual.

General Evaluation Evaluation of patients with early pubertal development should always begin with a detailed clinical history. The sequence of sexual developmental changes is most important in differentiating GnRH-dependent and GnRH-independent forms. History should focus on central nervous system (CNS) abnormalities (trauma, infection, neoplasia, irradiation, and so on). Growth charts are indispensable to discern a pattern of rapid linear growth. On physical examination in girls, determining whether maturation is isosexual or heterosexual is critical. In boys, testicular volume should be measured. Any pubertal development without testicular enlargement (less than 3 mL) suggests GnRH-independent precocious puberty. In both sexes, neurological abnormality that suggests CNS disorders should be assessed.

Diagnostic evaluation starts with the assessment of bone age and the measurements of serum gonadotropins, particularly LH. Advanced bone age indicates gonadal steroid hormone action. Sensitive immunometric assays for serum LH such as the immunochemiluminometric assay are widely available. Using such assays, serum LH concentrations are detectable in more than half of children with GnRH-dependent precocious puberty. A random LH more than 0.3 mIU/mL by immunochemiluminometric assay is highly suggestive of GnRH-dependence. By contrast, gonadotropins are undetectable in prepubertal children and children with GnRH-independent precocious puberty. Measurements of estradiol and testosterone should be obtained. Undetectable estradiol, however, does not exclude the absence of precocious puberty, as the detection limits of the current assays are not

Table 43-3
Causes of GnRH-Dependent Precocious Puberty

Idiopathic
CNS disorders
  CNS tumors
    Hypothalamic hamartoma, astrocytoma, ependymoma, cranio-pharyngioma, optic glioma, and others
  Other CNS lesions
    Static encephalopathy (a result of infection, neonatal asphyxia, hypoxia, severe head trauma, and others)
    Low-dose cranial radiation
    Hydrocephalus
    Arachnoid cyst
Maternal uniparental disomy for chromosome 14

Combined GnRH-dependent and GnRH-independent
  Treated congenital adrenal hyperplasia
  McCune–Albright syndrome, late
  Familial male limited precocious puberty, late
  Functional ovarian cyst, late

sufficiently sensitive. Serial measurements of serum LH concentration, usually every 10–20 min, during nocturnal sleep have greater diagnostic power than single random waking measurements. Pulsatile secretion of LH during nocturnal sleep is well illustrated in GnRH-dependent precocious puberty.

Measurement of both LH and FSH concentrations following a GnRH stimulation test is the standard to differentiate GnRH-dependent from GnRH-independent precocious puberty. LH predominance or a peak LH to FSH ratio >1.0 in the GnRH stimulation test is diagnostic for GnRH dependence in any assays. FSH predominance, however, can be present in the early phase of GnRH-dependent precocious puberty.

Once GnRH-dependent precocious puberty is confirmed, cranial CT and/or MRI is warranted for the CNS disorders (Table 43-3). Additional useful imaging studies are pelvic ultrasonography and MRI. Bilateral ovarian volume more than 2 mL together with large bilateral cysts (>9 mm) suggests GnRH-dependence. A uterine length more than 3.5 cm and a fundus to cervix ratio more than 1.0 indicate estrogen activity.

GnRH-Dependent Precocious Puberty GnRH-dependent precocious puberty is more than 10-fold more frequent in girls than boys, although the reason for this skewed sex ratio is not clear. GnRH-dependent precocious puberty is most often idiopathic in girls, whereas a CNS disorder is demonstrated in 25–75% of boys.

Clinically the sequence of sexual development is preserved. In girls, the first sign is breast development, followed by the appearance of pubic hair, axillary hair, and withdrawal bleeding. In boys, enlargement of testes is the first, although most children do not notice this change. This is followed by enlargement of the penis, the appearance of pubic hair, and facial acne. Erections and nocturnal emissions are not uncommon.

Causes Of cases of GnRH-dependent precocious puberty in girls, two-thirds are idiopathic (Table 43-3). The mechanism of the early activation of GnRH activity in this category is largely unknown.

CNS disorders are well-recognized causes of GnRH-dependent precocious puberty. Precocious puberty with any neurological signs and symptoms, including developmental delay, suggests GnRH-dependence.

Although less common, CNS tumors are important causes of precocious puberty, particularly in girls younger than 6 yr of age and boys of any age. CNS tumors causing GnRH-dependent precocious puberty are rarely malignant, and can be viewed as causing precocious puberty by one of two distinct mechanisms. First, tumors may act as ectopic GnRH pulse generators that have escaped the normal inhibitory influences exerted in the prepubertal period. Hypothalamic hamartoma is representative of this type of disorder and is the most common CNS lesion associated with precocious puberty. It is more frequently found in boys and the onset is usually before 3 yr of age in girls. The association of gelastic (laughing) episodes or seizures is classic, but rare. Hypothalamic hamartomas are visualized as iso-intense masses on MRI. Histologically, such hamartomas are benign congenital CNS malformations made up of disorganized but otherwise normal neuronal and glial elements. In other instances, tumors may interrupt the normal inhibitory pathways exerted in the prepubertal period. Astrocytomas, ependymomas, craniopharyngiomas, and optic gliomas have all been identified in such cases. The possibility, however, cannot be excluded that focal derangements of the cellular environment in the vicinity of GnRH neurons may be causally related to premature activation of the GnRH pulse generator.

Other CNS lesions are relatively common. Static encephalopathy is a result of infection, neonatal asphyxia, hypoxia, severe head trauma, and other causes during the neonatal period, infancy, or early childhood. These lesions can interrupt the normal tonic inhibitory pathways exerted in the prepubertal period. Cranial radiation has dose-dependent dual effects on hypothalamic–pituitary–gonadal axis. Low doses of cranial radiation (18–24 Gy) may cause precocious puberty. Low-dose cranial radiation has been widely used in the CNS prophylactic treatment of acute lymphoblastic leukemia and has been associated with a downward shift in the distribution of ages at pubertal onset and menarche in girls who have received such treatment. Precocious puberty in girls owing to prior low-dose cranial radiation is increasing in frequency. By contrast, precocious puberty is rare in boys treated in this manner. High doses of cranial radiation (more than 50 Gy to the hypothalamic-pituitary area) may cause gonadotropin deficiency.

The chance of finding CNS disorders in both sexes may be inversely proportional to the age of the child, with the greatest yield in children younger than 4-yr old. Routine MRI is less likely to have positive findings in girls whose pubertal development began after 6 yr of age. In contrast, in a series of 4000 children referred to the National Institutes of Health (NIH), one-third of the girls and more than 90% of the boys had identifiable CNS disorders visible on CT or MRI. This high prevalence of CNS disorders may be biased by the composition of the referral population.

Maternal uniparental disomy for chromosome 14 (UPD14) may cause GnRH-dependent precocious puberty and intrauterine growth retardation. GnRH-dependent precocious puberty in maternal UPD14 results from the loss of the functionally active paternally derived allele. Evidence for a maternal imprinting (paternal expressive) gene(s) on chromosome 14 includes the presence of GnRH-dependent precocious puberty and intrauterine growth retardation in cases with either maternal heterodisomy or isodisomy, and that paternal UPD14 results in a very different phenotype.

Treatment The most important but difficult issue is to determine when treatment is indicated. Treatment goals are to improve adult height and to prevent psychosocial problems, including age-inappropriate treatment. Natural history of GnRH-dependent precocious puberty is the early completion of physical growth and

sexual maturation. Despite early acceleration ahead of peers, early epiphyseal fusion usually leads to compromised adult height compared with genetic height potential. Major psychosocial problems are the disruption of familial, educational, and peer relationships, because adults may relate to these children in response to their sexual maturity rather than their chronological age. Some "adolescent" behavior may be exhibited, although sexual behavior such as increased fondling and masturbation are infrequent. Advanced sexual maturity may place these children at increased risk of being sexually abused. Thus, when compromised adult height is highly likely or any psychosocial problems occur, treatment is absolutely required. On the contrary, when compromised adult height is less likely and psychosocial problems do not occur, treatment should be postponed and the child closely observed. Not all children with GnRH-dependent precocious puberty require treatment. Very slowly progressing sexual precocity is possible and may not require treatment. This group can be characterized by the following: the onset age is near 8 yr in girls and 9 yr in boys, and the bone age is less than 2 yr advanced in comparison to chronological age.

The first choice of treatment is long-acting synthetic agonist analogues of GnRH (GnRHa). GnRHa induces "hypogonadism" by the continuous nonpulsatile GnRH action on the pituitary gonadotrophs. The first demonstrable endocrinological change effected by this treatment is reduction in basal and GnRH-stimulated LH and FSH. GnRHa treatment results in suppression of pubertal physical changes, a decrease in growth velocity, and the disappearance of psychosocial problems. The majority of treated girls experience no increase in breast development, and one-third show regression to an earlier Tanner stage. Effects on pubic hair are less predictable, although most children show either no progression or a minor degree of regression. When treated appropriately to prepubertal endocrinological status, the slowing of growth velocity is accompanied by slowing of bone age maturation. Preservation of or increase in adult height can be achieved. The length of time that treatment is continued depends on bone age and estimates of adult height in individual cases. The adult height by GnRHa treatment is higher than predicted height at the start of treatment, but lower than target height and predicted height at the end of treatment. Most studies suggest that the prognosis of adult height is better if bone ages are relatively young at the start of treatment, indicating the importance of early diagnosis and intervention. The combination of GH and GnRHa treatment may improve the prognosis of adult height more than GnRHa treatment alone. Clinical trials addressing this issue are ongoing.

Two major concerns have been raised regarding potential side effects of GnRHa treatment. First, GnRHa treatment may suppress the increase of bone mineral density (BMD), an important feature of normal puberty. Despite this, it has been reported that bone mineral density was not compromised in girls treated with GnRHa for GnRH-dependent precocious puberty who had completed treatment and had subsequently attained a bone age of greater than 14 yr. Second, some have questioned the reversibility of the suppression of pituitary–gonadal axis ("hypogonadism") following cessation of GnRHa treatment. The available data show that pubertal development resumed after withdrawal of treatment. Theoretically, fertility should not be hampered by such treatments, but longitudinal follow-up is necessary.

GnRH-Independent Precocious Puberty GnRH-independent precocious puberty is about one-fifth as common as

Table 43-4
Causes of GnRH-Independent Precocious Puberty

Boys and girls
Late onset congenital adrenal hyperplasia[a]
McCune–Albright syndrome
Peutz–Jeghers syndrome
Adrenal carcinoma associated with Cushing syndrome[a]
Primary hypothyroidism, prolonged and untreated
Iatrogenic

Boys
Testicular disorders
    Familial male limited precocious puberty
    Leydig cell adenoma
Human chorionic gonadotropin-secreting tumors
Androgen-secreting tumors

Girls
Ovarian disorders
    Granulosa cell tumors
    Functional ovarian cysts
Other estrogen-secreting tumors

[a]Isosexual in boys but heterosexual in girls.

Table 43-5
Prevalence of Clinical Features of MAS

Clinical findings	Prevalence (%)
Fibrous dysplasia	99
Café au lait spots	82
Gonadal abnormalities (boys and girls)	82
Boys: precocious puberty and/or abnormal testes on US or Leydig cell hyperplasia	77
Girls: precocious puberty	78
Thyroid abnormalities (total)	69
Hyperthyroidism	34
Abnormal gland on US only	34
Renal phosphate wasting	49
Growth hormone excess	18
Cushing's syndrome	7
Primary hyperparathyroidism	4
Idiopathic pancreatitis	4

GnRH-dependent forms. This form of precocious puberty is clinically characterized by sexual development of unusual sequence, no history of CNS abnormality, and no rapid linear growth. From an endocrine standpoint, GnRH-independent forms are characterized by increased production of gonadal steroid hormones in the absence of activation of the hypothalamic–pituitary axis (Table 43-4). GnRH-independent precocious puberty includes conditions that mimic the effect of pituitary gonadotropins on gonadal function, such as hCG from germ cell tumor.

Molecular mechanisms underlying two forms of GnRH-independent precocious puberty, McCune–Albright syndrome (MAS) and familial male limited precocious puberty (FMPP), are discussed later.

McCune–Albright Syndrome MAS originally was defined by the clinical triad of precocious puberty, polyostotic fibrous dysplasia of bone, and café au lait spots of skin. It was advocated that MAS' definition should be broader than the triad; fibrous dysplasia plus at least one of the typical hyperfunctioning endocrinopathies and/or café au lait spots. Reasons why a broadening of the definition has been proposed include that although MAS is rare, clinical manifestations vary individually and almost any combination of the clinical features (Table 43-5) is possible. Second, other hyperfunctioning endocrinopathies can be found in association with precocious puberty, including hyperthyroidism, GH excess, Cushing's syndrome, and so on. Third, clinical manifestations other than those within the triad are possible, such as liver dysfunction, idiopathic pancreatitis, and sudden death. Fourth, fibrous dysplasia is not rare and is the most common component of MAS. Fibrous dysplasia can involve a single skeletal site or multiple sites. Fifth, the clinical features of MAS may develop over time. Prevalence of the different clinical features of MAS in the NIH series is summarized in Table 43-5.

Precocious puberty in MAS is GnRH-independent, although the coexistence of GnRH-dependent and GnRH-independent forms is possible in longstanding cases. The prevalence of precocious puberty is less in boys, although that of gonadal abnormalities between boys and girls is similar. In affected girls, the first sign of sexual development is usually vaginal bleeding or spotting. A waxing and waning course of precocious puberty is not uncommon. Ultrasonography and/or MRI scan may reveal ovarian cysts.

The peculiar bone lesion of MAS is fibrous dysplasia. Fibrous dysplasia can occur in any bone, with the common locations being the skull base and proximal femurs. The clinical manifestations can be pain, limp, or pathological fractures. Alternatively, fibrous dysplasia in craniofacial bones can cause a painless lump or facial asymmetry. Radiographs show expansile lesions. Sarcomatous degeneration occurs rarely.

Café au lait spots are usually present at birth or shortly thereafter. These are large and irregular and have serrated outlines, called "coast-of-Maine." Common sites of café au lait spots are the forehead, the neck or upper back, the shoulder and upper arm, the lumbosacral region, and the buttocks, and often limited to half of the body.

Constitutive active mutations of the *GNAS1* gene have been identified in mosaic fashion (somatic mosaicism) in MAS (Fig. 43-1A,B). *GNAS1* encodes the α-subunit of the stimulatory G protein (Gsα), which regulates adenylate cyclase activity. G protein has a key role in intracellular signal transduction of G protein-coupled receptors (GPCR). In these membrane receptors, ligands bind GPCR, activating the adenylate cyclase system, the membrane-bound enzyme that catalyzes the formation of the intracellular second messenger, cAMP.

A heterozygous substitution was identified in exon 8 of the *GNAS1* gene, predicting the replacement of arginine by histidine or cysteine at position 201 of the mature Gsα protein. This substitution causes a marked decrease in the intrinsic GTPase activity of Gsα, prolonging the survival of the active conformation of GTP and resulting in constitutive activation of adenylate cyclase activity. The consequent increased production of cAMP explains the hyperfunctioning of multiple endocrine organs where GPCRs are expressed. Moreover, more mutant allele was expressed than wild type in tissues histologically most affected. This mutation was detected in bone as well as skin lesions.

This somatic mutation may occur very early in gestation leading to prenatal lethality, relatively early in gestation leading to typical MAS because of abnormal monoclonal cell population, or later in life leading to hyperfunction in single endocrine organ. Because these mutations arise somatically, MAS is not inherited.

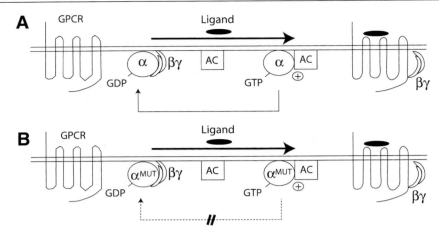

Figure 43-1   In each panel, the parallel horizontal lines are the plasma membrane with the extracellular space above and the intracellular space below. GPCR is G protein-coupled receptor and AC is adenylate cyclase. (**A**) GPCR in normal state. In the basal state, the G protein is a heterotrimer (α-, β-, and γ-subunits) with guanosine diphosphate (GDP) tightly bound to the α-subunit (Gsα). When ligand binds to the G protein-coupled receptor, the interaction with the G proteins leads to the dissociation of guanosine diphosphate, the binding of GTP, and the dissociation of the Gsα and the βγ-subunits. GTP-bound Gsα activates AC activity, inducing signal transduction. Under physiological conditions, the regulation of AC activity is transient and is terminated by the hydrolysis of the bound GTP by the intrinsic GTPase activity of Gsα. The Gsα-subunit with bound GDP reassociates to form the αβγ–heterotrimer. (**B**) GPCR in McCune–Albright syndrome (MAS). In MAS, constitutive active mutations of the *GNAS1* gene encoding Gsα have been identified in mosaic fashion. The mutated Gsα (αMUT) has a markedly reduced intrinsic GTPase activity. When ligand binds GPCR, activated GPCR induces the release of GDP, the binding of GTP, the activation of Gsα, its dissociation from the βγ-dimer, and the regulation of AC activity. Owing to the decreased intrinsic GTPase activity of the Gsα, activated Gsα is not inactivated efficiently, leading to constitutive induction of signal transduction.

For GnRH-independent precocious puberty in MAS, the use of an aromatase inhibitor is recommended. In boys, an aromatase inhibitor is frequently combined with an antiandrogen agent. Surgery is the mainstay for treatment of fibrous dysplasia. Bisphosphonate has been used to reduce pain, although no evidence is available to indicate whether such treatments can alter the natural history of fibrous dysplasia. Effective treatment for café au lait spots has not been described.

Familial Male-Limited Precocious Puberty   FMPP or familial testotoxicosis is an autosomal-dominant, male-limited form of GnRH-independent precocious puberty. Histologically, Leydig cell hyperplasia is evident. FMPP is caused by a heterozygous constitutive active mutation of the gene encoding luteinizing hormone/chorionic gonadotropin (CG) receptor (LHCGR).

FMPP is characterized by

1. GnRH-independent precocious puberty.
2. Male-limited autosomal-dominant inheritance.
3. The onset of puberty before 4 yr of age.

A family history of precocious puberty and/or short adult height in males is usually obtained. Sporadic cases have also been reported. Affected males present with progressive virilization by age 4 yr. The clinical hallmark is the relatively mild enlargement of the testes for the degree of virilization. Testosterone production in testes can occur autonomously with increased serum testosterone concentration. Typically, affected subjects have advanced bone maturation, leading to short adult height. Females carrying the same heterozygous mutation are not affected, because activation of both LH and FSH receptors is required for estrogen production in the ovarian follicle.

The molecular pathogenesis of FMPP has been traced to heterozygous constitutively active mutations within specific segments of the LHCGR gene. The LH/CG receptor is a member of the GPCR family. In vitro studies of such mutant receptors have demonstrated marked increase in cAMP production in the absence of ligand, consistent with GnRH-independent precocious puberty. Treatment aims to reduce testosterone production (in the testes) and androgen action (peripherally). Androgen receptor antagonists, aromatase inhibitors, inhibitors of 17, 20 lyase, or the combination of these agents have been employed.

Late-Onset Congenital Adrenal Hyperplasia   Congenital adrenal hyperplasia (CAH) is an autosomal-recessive disorder characterized by deficiencies of one of the enzymes critical to normal adrenal steroidogenesis (Chapter 37). In CAH, compensatory hypersecretion of adrenocorticotropic hormone (ACTH) stimulates the increased adrenal androgen. GnRH-independent precocious puberty can be induced by this increased adrenal androgen. Late onset (or nonclassic) CAH should be considered in any child with premature pubarche, especially in association with enlarged penis without testicular enlargement in boys (isosexual precocious puberty) and in association with clitoromegaly in girls (heterosexual precocious puberty). When untreated, rapid linear growth and advanced bone age are likely. Deficiency of 21-hydroxylase accounts for more than 90% of CAH, which is caused by homozygous or compound heterozygous CYP21A2 mutations. Deficiency of 11β-hydroxylase owing to homozygous or compound heterozygous CYP11B1 mutations is less frequent.

hCG-Secreting Tumor   hCG-secreting tumors, such as germinoma, hepatoblastoma, or pinealomas, may lead to GnRH-independent isosexual precocious puberty exclusively in boys. Girls with hCG-secreting tumors do not develop precocious puberty, just as girls with LHCGR mutation of FMPP do not. The intracranial pineal region is the common site for germinoma. Mediastinal germinoma producing hCG have been reported in Klinefelter syndrome (described in Klinefelter Syndrome). Precocious puberty caused by hCG secreting tumors is definitely GnRH-independent, as no hypothalamus-pituitary activation is evident. Because of the extensive structural homology of the β-subunits of hCG and LH, at high levels, hCG can stimulate the production of testosterone via activation of the LH/CG receptor in Leydig cells.

Hormone Production From Tumors in Ovary, Testis, or Adrenal Glands The most common clinical presentation of granulosa cell tumors of the ovary is GnRH-independent precocious puberty, as most can produce estrogen. Granulosa cell tumors are the most common type of ovarian tumors in children, although the etiology is unknown. Tumors are often associated with a large cyst or solid mass, which are easily visible on pelvic ultrasound. They are benign and noninvasive. Surgical resection is the treatment of choice.

Peutz–Jeghers syndrome is an autosomal-dominant disorder characterized by

1. Melanocytic macules of the lips, buccal mucosa, and digits.
2. Multiple gastrointestinal hamartomatous polyps.
3. An increased risk of various neoplasms.

Ovarian theca cell tumors in girls with this syndrome can cause GnRH-independent precocious puberty. Gynecomastia (GnRH-independent heterosexual precocious puberty) has been reported in boys with Peutz–Jeghers syndrome having a testicular sex-cord tumor with increased aromatase activity. The occurrence of ovarian tumors in girls, however, far exceeds that of testicular tumors in boys. A deletion of exons 4 and 5 and an inversion of exons 6 and 7 in an STK11 encoding a widely expressed serine/threonine kinase was found in a large family with Peutz–Jeghers syndrome. Other heterozygous mutations in STK11 have been identified in this disorder. The germline mutations in STK11 in conjunction with somatic mutations in a second allele have been proposed to cause neoplasms in this syndrome.

Leydig cell adenomas are associated with GnRH-independent precocious puberty in boys. In boys with Leydig cell adenomas, signs of isosexual precocious puberty typically appear between the ages of 5 and 9 yr, later than FMPP. The somatic mutation of LHCGR gene in these tumors has been reported. This mutation was proven to be constitutively active, analogous to those seen in FMPP, leading to GnRH-independent precocious puberty. Surgical resection of the tumor results in arrest of pubertal development.

Adrenal carcinoma associated with Cushing syndrome sometimes causes GnRH-independent precocious puberty, whereas adrenal adenoma rarely does. Adrenal carcinoma can produce adrenal androgen, leading to isosexual precocious puberty in boys, and heterosexual precocious puberty in girls. Serum concentrations of DHEA-S, DHEA, and androstenedione are usually elevated. Small adrenal carcinoma is curative by surgery, but larger ones may require additional treatments such as chemotherapy.

Incomplete (or Partial) Precocious Puberty (Variation of Normal Puberty)

PREMATURE THELARCHE Premature thelarche is an isolated breast development without other signs of puberty in girls that commonly occurs in the first 2 yr. Rapid linear growth and advanced bone age are absent. The natural course is spontaneous regression often within 18 mo or no additional change in breast size. Premature thelarche is typically associated with a degree of FSH secretion. If performed, a GnRH stimulation test usually reveals an FSH predominance response. Serum estradiol is undetectable. The prevalence of ovarian microcysts detected by ultrasonography is increased. The etiology of premature thelarche has

not been elucidated, although it has been attributed to an increased sensitivity of the breast tissue to estrogen. Careful follow-up for the appearance of other pubertal signs and linear growth is indicated. Premature thelarche can develop to GnRH-dependent precocious puberty in approx 10–15% of cases.

PREMATURE PUBARCHE Premature pubarche is the isolated development of pubic hair, which is usually a benign condition resulting from early adrenarche. A report of the characteristics of 171 subjects with premature pubarche included abnormalities of steroidogenesis (late-onset 21-hydroxylase deficiency, and so on) in 12% of patients as diagnosed by ACTH stimulation tests. Late-onset CAH should, therefore, be considered in any child with premature pubarche. Premature pubarche must be followed closely to monitor for developing GnRH-dependent precocious puberty. Some girls with premature pubarche may develop functional hyperandrogenism in the midteenage years associated with polycystic ovarian syndrome.

DELAYED PUBERTY
Delayed puberty is defined as the failure to mature sexually at an appropriate age. Both delayed onset of puberty and failure to complete pubertal development are considered as delayed puberty. In the United States, the ages of 12 or 13 yr in girls and 14 yr in boys serve as practical guidelines to determine the need for evaluation for delayed onset of puberty. In girls, if more than 5 yr have elapsed between the beginning of breast development and menarche, failure of complete pubertal development is considered. In boys, 3–4 yr are normal to complete pubertal development.

Classification Delayed puberty is classified as hypogonadotropic (or secondary) hypogonadism, hypergonadotropic (or primary) hypogonadism, and constitutional delay of puberty. Hypogonadotropic hypogonadism is failure of maturation of hypothalamic-pituitary axis, which is the stimulation signal for the gonads. Hypergonadotropic hypogonadism is the failure of gonads to respond to hypothalamic-pituitary stimulation. Constitutional delay of puberty is delayed maturation of hypothalamic-pituitary–gonadal axis (variation of normal puberty).

General Evaluation Evaluation of patients with delayed pubertal development begins with a detailed clinical history of the onset and pattern of puberty. Recording growth charts (heights and weights) throughout childhood is mandatory. Consistent growth delay (short stature) suggests constitutional delay of puberty. A history of CNS tumors and their treatment, ability to smell, hypopituitarisim, any medication causing hyperprolactinemia as well as general medical history is relevant in both genders. Past history should be focused on cryptorchidism, hypospadias, or micropenis in boys and coarctation of the aorta in girls. Family history is important such as growth, onset and patterns of puberty, infertility, and ability to smell. A family history of delayed onset of puberty suggests constitutional delay of puberty. Physical examination starts with measurements of height, weight, upper–lower segment ratio, and arm span. The evaluation of Tanner stage as well as pubertal development should be performed. In boys, testicular size must be measured. Careful general examination is important to determine whether any major or minor anomalies are present. Neurological examination including the ability to smell should be done routinely.

The initial diagnostic evaluation usually involves the assessment of bone age and measurements of basal serum LH, FSH, and gonadal steroid hormones (testosterone in boys and estradiol in girls). A bone age more than 13.5 yr in boys or 11.5 yr in girls suggests an active hypothalamic-pituitary axis. Very high concentrations of serum LH and FSH with low gonadal steroid hormones indicate hypergonadotropic hypogonadism. In such cases, a GnRH stimulation test is unnecessary as the hyper response in hypergonadotropic hypogonadism can be predicted by high basal gonadotropins. The difficult task is the differentiation between hypogonadotropic hypogonadism and constitutional delay of puberty. In prepubertal ages, neither basal gonadotropins nor gonadal steroid hormones can differentiate between the two. It should be noted that gonadotropin responses following GnRH stimulation are seldom helpful. GnRH stimulation tests yield overlapping responses that do not permit the differentiation of hypogonadotropic hypogonadism and constitutional delay of puberty. In boys, a hCG stimulation test may provoke a similar response in both hypogonadotropic hypogonadism and constitutional delay of puberty. Serial measurements of serum LH during nocturnal sleep may reveal pulsatile patterns suggestive of puberty, but this is not useful to differentiate hypogonadotropic hypogonadism from constitutional delay of puberty at prepubertal ages.

Once hypogonadotropic hypogonadism is confirmed, cranial CT and/or MRI is warranted for exclusion of CNS disorders (Table 43-6). MRI readily visualizes olfactory bulbs in healthy children even in neonates. Olfactometry or an intravenous olfactory stimulation test may be required to reveal hyposmia.

Hypogonadotropic Hypogonadism   Hypogonadotropic hypogonadism refers to the deficiency of pulsatile release of gonadotropins, which may result from a variety of hypothalamic and pituitary disorders. In the presence of a hypothalamic defect, or absence of GnRH-secreting neurons, failure of GnRH secretion results in a lack of stimulation of pituitary gonadotrophs. In contrast, pituitary disorders, such as tumors or hypophysitis, cause direct failure of pituitary gonadotropin secretion. In practice, it is not uncommon to encounter difficulty in determining whether the origin of hypogonadotropic hypogonadism is hypothalamic or pituitary.

Causes   No human GnRH deficiency owing to GNRH mutation has been reported, although a mouse *Gnrh* mutation (hpg mouse) exists (Table 43-6). Molecular analysis of the hpg mouse revealed a deletion in the hpg genome of at least 33.5 kb removing the two exons of the *Gnrh* gene. This deletion resulted in a transcriptionally active gene that leads to the synthesis of a truncated GnRH protein and a hypogonadotropic hypogonadism in homozygous state.

GnRH resistance owing to homozygous or compound heterozygous mutations in the GnRH receptor gene has been described in up to 20% of patients with "idiopathic" hypogonadotropic hypogonadism. The clinical features of GnRH receptor gene mutations are variable. Male patients may have prepubertal-sized or adult-sized testes. All female patients had primary amenorrhea, but showed no or Tanner stage III breast development. In one female patient, pulsatile administration of GnRH induced ovulation and allowed pregnancy. Kallmann's syndrome is discussed later.

One human LHβ deficiency resulting from LHB gene mutation has been reported. The affected individual had delayed puberty and arrested spermatogenesis. Laboratory data showed a high serum concentration of immunoreactive LH with low serum testosterone. A homozygous loss of function missense mutation Q54R was identified in the LHB gene. This mutation alters an

Table 43-6
Causes of Hypogonadotropic Hypogonadism

GnRH or GnRH receptor deficiency
  GnRH deficiency (GNRH mutation)[a]
  GnRH resistance (GNRHR mutation)
  Others
Kallmann's syndrome
  KAL1 mutation
  FGFR-1 mutation
  Others
Isolated gonadotropin deficiency
  LHβ deficiency
  FSHβ deficiency
  GPR54 deficiency[b]
  Others
Hypogonadotropic hypogonadism with other endocrine
  abnormalities due to single gene disorder
  PC1 deficiency
  α-subunit deficiency[a]
  Congenital leptin deficiency (LEP mutation)
  Congenital leptin resistance (LEPR mutation)
  DAX1 mutation
  Others
Congenital combined pituitary hormone deficiency
  HESX1 mutation
  LHX3 mutation
  LHX4 mutation
  PROP1 mutation
  EGR1 mutation[a]
  Others
Panhypopituitarism with invisible or thin pituitary stalk
CNS disorders
  Tumor
  Irradiation
  Surgery
  Anatomic defect
  Autoimmune disease
  Others
Functional gonadotropin deficiency
  Anorexia nervosa
  Excessive exercise
Chronic systemic illness
  Emotional stress
  Malnutrition
  Hyperprolactinemia
  Others

[a]No human mutations have been reported so far.
[b]The level of abnormality, hypothalamus or pituitary, is not fully understood.

amino acid that is conserved in all β-subunits of the glycoprotein hormones. CHO cells were transfected with cDNAs encoding α-glycoprotein subunit (GSU) and either the wild or mutant LHB to assess the biological effects of the mutation. When LH concentrations were measured in culture medium by radioimmunoassay and radioreceptor assay, LH concentrations in the medium by radioimmunoassay were higher in cells transfected with αGSU and mutant LHB cDNAs compared with those transfected with αGSU and wild LHB cDNAs. However, the mutant LH was undetectable by radioreceptor assay, indicating that the absence of biological activity of mutant LH was because of its inability to bind its receptor.

A small number of women have been reported to have FSHβ deficiency resulting from homozygous or compound heterozygous FSHB gene mutations, V61X/V61X and V61X/C51G. These women presented with delayed puberty and primary amenorrhea. Laboratory data showed an undetectable serum concentration of FSH and high LH. Exogenous FSH treatment resulted in follicular maturation, ovulation, and fertility. V61X caused a deletion of the C-terminus, including residues 90-110, that was essential for heterodimer formation. The C51G substitution mutates a residue that is part of a motif thought to be essential to the organization of the core of the protein. The functional effects of V61X and C51G were studied by coexpressing αGSU and mutant FSHB genes. Immunoradiometric assay of culture media showed undetectable concentrations of mutant FSH, consistent with patients's laboratory data. Two men have been reported to have a homozygous FSHB gene mutation, V61X/V61X or C82R/C82R, presenting with azoospermia. Other patients have been reported to have isolated gonadotropin deficiency. However, in most instances the LHB and FSHB gene analyses have not been reported.

Homozygous or compound heterozygous loss of function mutation of the GPR54 gene causes hypogonadotropic hypogonadism. GPR54 is a GPCR whose ligand is a 54 amino acid peptide derived from the KiSS1 protein. Affected subjects carried a homozygous deletion of 155 nucleotides encompassing the splicing acceptor site of intron 4-exon 5 junction and part of exon 5, homozygous L102P, homozygous L148S, or compound heterozygous R331X/X339R. The transfection of COS-7 cells with L148S, R331X, or X339R plus introduced stop codon after polyA tail showed decreased accumulation of inositol phosphate by ligand stimulation. The patient with R331X/X339R had attenuated secretion of endogenous GnRH. The Gpr54 knockout mice had isolated hypogonadotropic hypogonadism, but they showed responsiveness to both exogenous gonadotropins and GnRH and had normal levels of GnRH in hypothalamus. These studies established the central role for GPR54 in GnRH secretion.

Hypogonadotropic hypogonadism with other endocrine abnormalities resulting from single gene disorder has been reported, consistent with the complex interactions within the hypothalamic-pituitary–gonadal axis and other endocrine systems being absolutely required for normal puberty. For example, prohormone convertase (PC)-1 deficiency because of a PC1 gene mutation causes hypogonadotropic hypogonadism, obesity, and hypocortisolemia. Although PC1 regulates posttranslational modification of prohormones and neuropeptides, it has not been elucidated why PC1 deficiency causes hypogonadotropic hypogonadism. Individuals with congenital leptin deficiency or congenital leptin resistance because of LEP or LEPR gene mutation show hypogonadotropic hypogonadism associated with obesity. Male patients with X-linked adrenal hypoplasia congenita because of hemizygous DAX1 mutation exhibit primary adrenal insufficiency in infancy or early childhood and hypogonadotropic hypogonadism. Some studies have revealed that hypogonadotropic hypogonadism in DAX1 mutation represents defects at the pituitary gonadotrophs as well as the hypothalamus, consistent with the expression of DAX1 at both sites. No fertile male patient with hemizygous DAX1 mutation has been described following GnRH or gonadotropin treatment, suggesting critical roles of DAX1 for the process of spermatogenesis. Interestingly, delayed puberty has been described in one female with a heterozygous DAX1 mutation in one family, and hypogonadotropic hypogonadism without adrenal insufficiency has been

described in one female with a homozygous DAX1 mutation. Analysis of DAX1 gene in more than 100 patients with "idiopathic" hypogonadotropic hypogonadism failed to identify any mutations.

Patients with congenital combined pituitary hormone deficiency can have hypogonadotropic hypogonadism when the mutated genes regulate gonadotroph differentiation. Two children with homozygous HESX1 mutation with septo-optic dysplasia and congenital combined pituitary hormone deficiency have impaired gonadotropin secretion, although these children are prepubertal. Homozygous LHX3 mutations have been reported in patients with congenital combined pituitary hormone deficiency including hypogonadotropic hypogonadism. These patients have normal ACTH secretion and limited head rotation because of cervical spine rigidity. Heterozygous LHX4 mutation has been reported in familial combined pituitary hormone deficiency including hypogonadotropic hypogonadism. Patients with PROP1 mutation may develop hypogonadotropic hypogonadism, although the onset of hypogonadism varies. These patients have GH and thyroid-stimulating hormone deficiency in childhood and may develop progressive ACTH deficiency.

Panhypopituitarism with an invisible or thin pituitary stalk can produce hypogonadotropic hypogonadism. These patients usually have a history of complicated delivery as breech presentation or neonatal asphyxia. The invisible or thin pituitary stalk reflects its injury (transection) at birth or the primary abnormality of the stalk. Hypogonadotropic hypogonadism as well as GH, thyroid-stimulating hormone, and ACTH deficiency may gradually develop.

CNS disorders may cause hypogonadotropic hypogonadism by impairing hypothalamic or pituitary function. Sellar or suprasellar tumors (e.g., craniopharyngioma) commonly disturb the processes of pubertal development, causing either precocious puberty (as described earlier) or delayed puberty. Such tumors are often associated with other kinds of pituitary defects, of which GH deficiency is by far the most common.

Anorexia nervosa is notorious for causing functional gonadotropin deficiency in adolescent females. The prevalence of anorexia nervosa is definitely increasing in the United States and other industrialized countries. Anorexia nervosa is characterized by severe weight loss, a distorted body image, obsessive fear of obesity, and multiple endocrine abnormalities including functional gonadotropin deficiency. The recovery of most of endocrine abnormalities after weight gain suggests that endocrine abnormalities are secondary to weight loss. However, amenorrhea or infertility may persist for months to years after weight gain. Higher brain dysfunction in anorexia nervosa may hamper the complete recovery of functional gonadotropin deficiency.

Increasing evidence shows the link between excessive exercise and functional gonadotropin deficiency, especially in adolescent females. Long-distance runners, swimmers, ballet dancers, figure skaters, and gymnasts are well-known athletes who may develop amenorrhea. Excessive exercise itself or strict weight control can cause functional gonadotropin deficiency.

Hyperprolactinemia may cause functional gonadotropin deficiency. Hyperprolactinemia is because of pituitary prolactinoma, hypothyroidism, or drugs such as neuroleptics, antihypertensives, dopamine receptor antagonists, and antidepressants. Galactorrhea may or may not be present. The mechanism by which hyperprolactinemia causes functional gonadotropin deficiency is most likely multifactorial. Increased prolactin may inhibit GnRH secretion and/or decrease responsiveness of gonadotrophs to GnRH.

Treatment The goals of treatment of hypogonadotropic hypogonadism are to induce and maintain puberty and establish fertility. Gonadal steroid hormone replacement can induce and maintain puberty, testosterone in boys and estrogen in girls, when patients are at pubertal ages (about 13 yr in boys and 12–13 yr in girls). Gonadal steroid hormones should be gradually increased to an adult dosage to mimic normal pubertal development. In girls, cyclic therapy using estrogen and progesterone is necessary to establish regular withdrawal bleeding. Pulsatile GnRH treatment or the combination of gonadotropins is effective both to induce and maintain puberty and to establish fertility. It is uncertain whether prolonged gonadal steroid hormone replacement in male hypogonadotropic hypogonadism causes irreversible damage to spermatogenesis before the induction of the treatment to establish fertility. Treatment of underlying diseases should focus on CNS disorders and functional gonadotropin deficiency.

Kallmann's Syndrome Kallmann's syndrome is characterized by the association of hypogonadotropic hypogonadism and anosmia (or hyposmia). Hypogonadotropic hypogonadism is hypothalamic in origin, and anosmia (or hyposmia) results from agenesis or hypoplasia of the olfactory bulbs and tracts (*see* Etiology). Three modes of transmission have been described: X-linked (KAL1), autosomal-dominant (KAL2), and autosomal-recessive (KAL3). The prevalence of Kallmann's syndrome in boys is four times that in girls.

Clinical Features Typical clinical features of Kallmann's syndrome are delayed puberty and no or reduced sense of smell (often unrecognized by the patient). Boys with Kallmann's syndrome may have micropenis and/or bilateral or unilateral cryptorchidism in infancy. Both genders fail to develop puberty. Patients may have other clinical features depending on the mode of transmission. Renal agenesis is observed in up to 40% of KAL1, but not in KAL2. Synkinesia (mirror image movements) is associated principally with KAL1, but has also been observed in KAL2. Cleft lip/palate is present mostly in association with KAL2, but may also be seen in KAL1. MRI can clearly demonstrate the absence of olfactory bulbs and hypoplasia of the olfactory sulci, even in newborn infants. Olfactometry or the intravenous olfactory stimulation test is helpful to identify or confirm anosmia or hyposmia. In contrast to the delayed puberty caused by CNS tumors or constitutional delay of puberty, patients with Kallmann's syndrome usually have appropriate or tall stature for their age. Untreated adults and individuals of pubertal age commonly have eunuchoid proportions. Some subjects with KAL1 or fibroblast growth factor receptor (FGFR)-1 (*see* below) mutations manifest varying combinations of these features or do not have any of the clinical features. In the reported KAL2 families with FGFR-1 mutation, the prognosis of fertility was not compromised without treatment or by the combination of gonadotropins.

Etiology During embryogenesis, olfactory neurons and GnRH-secreting neurons originate in the olfactory placode in the nose and migrate into the CNS. The olfactory nerves associate with the terminal nerve and vomeronasal nerve to produce a bridge between the olfactory epithelium and the forebrain. The cells that will become GnRH-secreting neurons arise within the region of the olfactory placodes and migrate from the nasal epithelium, through the cribriform plate of the nose and then along the olfactory tract–forebrain axis to reach the preoptic and hypothalamic areas, where they differentiate to become the GnRH-secreting neurons. Given the developmental connection between GnRH-secreting and olfactory neurons, abnormalities in this developmental stage can cause Kallmann's syndrome.

An X-linked form of Kallmann's syndrome, KAL1, is caused by the deletion of or mutation of KAL1, which is located at Xp22.3. Examination of the expression of the KAL1 gene during embryogenesis demonstrates that it can be detected in various neuronal populations of the CNS, including cells of the olfactory bulbs. This gene partially escapes X inactivation and encodes a 680 amino acid protein, anosmin-1, an extracellular matrix component. An inactive homologous pseudogene, KALP, is located on the Y chromosome at Yq11. The derived amino acid sequence of KAL1 predicts a protein that contains a leader peptide with protease inhibitor domain that is followed by 4 fibronectin type III repeats; no transmembrane or anchoring regions are present. The protein, anosmin-1, is *N*-glycosylated, secreted in the cell culture medium, and localized at the cell surface. Several lines of evidence indicated that heparan-sulfate chains of proteoglycans are involved in the anosmin-1 to the cell surface. Anosmin-1 is thought to have a dual branch-promoting and guidance activity and is involved in the patterning of mitral and tufted cell axon collaterals to the olfactory cortex. Anosmin-1 may bind by means of a heparan sulfate proteoglycan to its cognate receptor or by other extracellular cues to induce axonal branching and axon misrouting. The role of KAL1 in events such as kidney formation and migration is obscure, although the expressed KAL1 in the Wolffian duct might be involved in renal development by interaction with the metanephric mesenchyme.

Heterozygous loss of function mutations in FGFR-1 have been identified in an autosomal dominant form of Kallmann's syndrome (KAL2). FGFR-1 is located at 8p11.2-p12 and encodes the FGFR-1; and its gain of function has been shown to cause craniosynostosis. Several lines of evidence suggest that KAL1 and FGFR-1 interact functionally to effect the normal migration of GnRH-secreting and olfactory neurons. Anomsin-1 may directly participate in FGF signaling through interactions with the FGFR-1. Notably, nonpenetrance of the disease in some mutation carriers can simulate autosomal-recessive transmission.

An autosomal-recessive form of Kallmann's syndrome (KAL3) also exists. The responsible gene for KAL3 has not been identified.

Constitutional Delay of Puberty (Variation of Normal Puberty) Constitutional delay of puberty is a common, benign condition that represents a variant of normal puberty. The time of onset of puberty is delayed compared with the general population, although the pattern of pubertal development is normal. Boys are referred for evaluation of this condition significantly more often than girls. Together with their delayed pubertal development, these children often have short stature, approximately two to three standard deviations below the mean, called constitutional delay of growth and puberty. The bone age is usually delayed 2–4 yr behind chronological age. These children demonstrate pubertal development that is more commensurate with their bone age than their chronological ages. Adult height and complete pubertal maturation are achieved significantly later, some young men reporting continued linear growth in their late teens or early twenties. Adult height is generally appropriate for the genetic background, but is commonly in the low normal range. The family history often reveals other individuals with suspected constitutional delay of puberty, most often in males. Constitutional delay of puberty usually does not require treatment.

Hypergonadotropic Hypogonadism Hypergonadotropic (or primary) hypogonadism is failure of the gonads to respond to hypothalamic–pituitary stimulation. Hypergonadotropic hypogonadism is associated with elevated serum concentration of

Table 43-7
Causes of Hypergonadotropic Hypogonadism

Chromosome abnormalities
  Klinefelter syndrome
  Turner syndrome
  Other sex chromosome abnormalities
  Autosomal chromosome abnormalities

Isolated gonadal dysgenesis
  Perrault syndrome
  Others

Gonadotropin resistance
  LH/CG resistance because of LHCGR mutation
  FSH resistance because of FSH resistance mutation
  LH and FSH resistance because of GNAS1 mutation
  (pseudohypoparathyroidism, type 1A)
  Others

Enzymatic defects in gonadal steroid hormone biosynthesis

Syndromes associated with hypergonadotropic hypogonadism

Gonadal destruction
  Vanishing
  Trauma
  Torsion
  Autoimmunity
  Surgery
  Chemotherapy
  Infections
  Radiation
  Others

Exposure to environmental estrogen *in utero* (boys)[a]

Unknown
  Galactosemia
  Others

[a]Proposed but not proved.

gonadotropins owing to the absence of the negative feedback effects of gonadal steroid hormones.

Causes The most common causes of hypergonadotropic hypogonadism are chromosome abnormalities such as Klinefelter syndrome, Turner syndrome and Down syndrome (Table 43-7). Why hypergonadotropic hypogonadism is common in chromosomal abnormalities is not completely understood, although pairing failure of homologous chromosomes in meiocytes is proposed to cause germ cell loss. Klinefelter syndrome and Turner syndrome are discussed later.

An uncommon form of hypergonadotropic hypogonadism is isolated gonadal dysgenesis. This condition appears to be genetically heterogeneous and both sporadic and familial cases have been reported. Affected patients having female external genitalia, either with 46,XX or 46,XY, typically present with no pubertal development. They do not have any other abnormalities such as short stature and minor anomalies.

One familial variant of isolated gonadal dysgenesis is Perrault syndrome, gonadal dysgenesis in 46,XX with sensorineural hearing loss. This syndrome is autosomal recessive with obligatory ovarian dysgenesis in 46,XX homozygotes and facultative sensorineural hearing loss in 46,XX and 46,XY homozygotes. The molecular defect has not been identified.

The receptors for the gonadotropins LH/CG and FSH are both members of the GPCR family. Selective defects in the gonadal response to gonadotropins have been traced in several pedigrees to mutations of the genes encoding the LH/CG and FSH receptors.

LH/CG resistance is resulting from loss of function mutations in the LHCGR gene. Male patients are classically associated with a form of male pseudohermaphroditism termed Leydig-cell hypoplasia, rather than being associated with delayed puberty. This disorder is characterized by female phenotype in the presence of a 46,XY karyotype, low serum concentration of testosterone, increased LH, and lack of testosterone secretion in response to a hCG stimulation test. Homozygous or compound heterozygous loss of function mutations in the LHCGR gene has been identified. The identification of a missense mutation of the LHCGR gene in a phenotypic male infant evaluated for a small but normally formed penis suggests that the range of altered phenotypes associated with LH/CG resistance because of loss of function mutations in the LHCGR gene may be broader than initially identified. A 46,XX subject with homozygous K354E was a phenotypically normal adult female with primary amenorrhea and cystic ovaries, suggesting that female patients with LH/CG resistance had some pubertal development, but impairment in the normal ovarian cycle.

Follicle-stimulating hormone resistance is caused by a loss of function mutation in the FSHR gene. A homozygous loss of function missense mutation in FSHR gene was found in Finnish female patients associated with 46,XX hypergonadotropic ovarian dysgenesis, which was originally classified as isolated gonadal dysgenesis. The disorder is common in this population (1:8300 females) and is inherited in an autosomal-recessive manner. Males homozygous for this mutation had a normal phenotype with variable degrees of spermatogenetic failure, but surprisingly, did not show azoospermia or absolute infertility.

LH and FSH resistance can be because of GNAS1 mutations (pseudohypoparathyroidism, type 1A [PHP1A]). GNAS1 encodes Gsα and displays imprinting (*see* precocious puberty, MAS in this chapter). Maternally inherited loss of function heterozygous mutation in GNAS1 causes PHP1A. PHP1A can be associated with resistance to multiple hormones, including hypergonadotropic hypogonadism. Patients with pseudohypoparathyroidism, type 1B (PHP1B) exhibit parathyroid hormone resistance, typically without other endocrine abnormalities. PHP1B is most likely caused by mutations in regulatory regions of the GNAS1 gene inherited from the mother that are predicted to interfere with the parent-specific methylation of GNAS1.

Other causes include enzymatic defects in gonadal steroid hormone biosynthesis, syndromes associated with hypergonadotropic hypogonadism, gonadal destruction, and unknown etiologies (*see* Table 43-7).

Treatment The goal of treatment of hypergonadotropic hypogonadism is to induce and maintain puberty. Gonadal steroid hormone replacement (*see* Treatment of Hypogonadotropic Hypogonadism) can induce and maintain puberty. Gonadal steroid hormone replacement therapy in Turner syndrome is more complex, requiring coordination of timing with respect to GH therapy to optimize adult height.

Unfortunately, other than sperm or egg donation, treatment to establish fertility in any hypergonadotropic hypogonadism is unsatisfactory. Some successful pregnancies have been reported, however, by testicular sperm extraction/microsurgical epididymal sperm aspiration combined with in vitro fertilization/intracytoplasmic sperm injection.

Klinefelter Syndrome The most common form of male hypergonadotropic hypogonadism is Klinefelter syndrome

(47,XXY karyotype), which occurs with a prevalence of 1:2500 adult males. Patients with Klinefelter syndrome may demonstrate a slowing or arrest of pubertal development as gonadal function declines after the age of puberty, although gonadal function remains relatively normal until that age. The hallmark of physical findings is small testes, and infertility is the rule. Subjects are relatively tall owing to the additional copy of the X-linked SHOX gene. Mean full-scale I.Q. is between 85 and 90. When a patient with Klinefelter syndrome develops precocious puberty, germinoma of the mediastinum is highly likely.

Turner Syndrome The most common form of female hypergonadotropic hypogonadism is Turner syndrome (45,X karyotype, typically), which occurs with an incidence of 1 in 2000 live-born females. Turner syndrome is a well-defined X chromosome abnormality characterized by short stature, Turner somatic stigmata, and hypergonadotropic hypogonadism. With respect to hypergonadotropic hypogonadism, adult patients usually have "streak" gonads consisting of fibrous tissue without germ cells. However, germ cells may be present in gonads in fetal life and infancy. Short stature is primarily ascribed to SHOX haploinsufficiency in addition to nonspecific growth disadvantage caused by chromosome imbalance. Turner somatic stigmata, either surface (webbed neck, high arched palate, ptosis, and so on) or visceral (coarctation of the aorta, horseshoe kidney, and so on), may be because of haploinsufficiency of postulated "lymphogenic gene(s)" on the short arm of X chromosome and nonspecific developmental disadvantage caused by chromosome imbalance.

GH treatment improves growth rates as well as adult height. Recommendations for diagnosis, treatment, and management of Turner syndrome have been published by the fifth international symposium on Turner syndrome.

SELECTED REFERENCES

Achermann JC, Gu WX, Kotlar TJ, et al. Mutational analysis of DAX1 in patients with hypogonadotropic hypogonadism or pubertal delay. J Clin Endocrinol Metab 1999;84:4497–4500.

Ahima RS, Dushay J, Flier SN, Prabakaran D, Flier JS. Leptin accelerates the onset of puberty in normal female mice. J Clin Invest 1997;99: 391–395.

Aittomäki K, Lucena JLD, Pakarinen P, et al. Mutation in the follicle-stimulating hormone receptor gene causes hereditary hypergonadotropic ovarian failure. Cell 1995;82:959–968

Balducci R, Boscherini B, Mangiantini A, Morellini, Toscano V. Isolated precocious pubarche: an approach. J Clin Endocrinol Metab 1994;79:582–589.

Beranova M, Oliveira LM, Bedecarrats GY, et al. Prevalence, phenotypic spectrum, and modes of inheritance of gonadotropin-releasing hormone receptor mutations in idiopathic hypogonadotropic hypogonadism. J Clin Endocrinol Metab 2001;86:1580–1588.

Chehab FF, Mounzih K, Lu R, Lim ME. Early onset of reproductive function in normal female mice treated with leptin. Science 1997;275: 88–90.

Clement K, Vaisse C, Lahlou N, et al. A mutation in the human leptin receptor gene causes obesity and pituitary dysfunction. Nature 1998; 392:398–401.

Counts DR, Pescovitz OH, Barnes MK, et al. Dissociation of adrenarche and gonadarche in precocious puberty and in isolated hypogonadotropic hypogonadism. J Clin Endocrinol Metab 1987;64:1174–1178.

Dattani MT, Martinez-Barbera JP, Thomas PQ, et al. Mutations in the homeobox gene HESX1/Hesx1 associated with aepto-optic dysplasia in human and nouse. Nat Genet 1998;19:125–133.

De Roux N, Genin E, Carel J-C, Matsuda F, Chaussain J-L, Milgrom E. Hypogonadotropic hypogonadism due to loss of function of the KiSS1-derived peptide receptor GPR54. Proc Natl Acad Sci USA 2003;100:10,972–10,976.

De Roux N, Young J, Misrahi M, et al. A family with hypogonadotropic hypogonadism and mutations in the gonadotropin-releasing hormone receptor. N Engl J Med 1997;337:1597–1602.

Dode C, Levilliers J, Dupont J-M, et al. Loss-of-function mutations in FGFR1 cause autosomal dominant Kallmann syndrome. Nat Genet 2003;33:463–465.

Dunkel L, Perheentupa J, Virtanen M, et al. Gonadotropin-releasing hormone test and human chronic gonadotropin test in the diagnosis of gonadotropin deficiency in prepubertal boys. J Pediatr 1985;107:388–392.

Farooqi IS, Jebb SA, Langmack G, et al. Effects of recombinant leptin therapy in a child with congenital leptin deficiency. N Engl J Med 1999;341:879–884.

Feuillan PP, Foster CM, Pescovitz OH, et al. Treatment of precocious puberty in the McCune-Albright syndrome with the aromatase inhibitor testolactone. N Engl J Med 1986;315:1115–1119.

Fokstuen S, Ginsburg C, Zachmann M, Schinzel A. Maternal uniparental disomy 14 as a cause of intrauterine growth retardation and early onset of puberty. J Pediatr 1999;134:689–695.

Heger S, Partsch CJ, Peter M, Blum WF, Kiess W, Sippell WG. Serum leptin levels in patients with progressive central precocious puberty. Pediatr Res 1999;46:71–75.

Heger S, Partsch CJ, Sippell WG. Long-term outcome after depot gonadotropin-releasing agonist treatment of central precocious puberty: Final height, body proportion, bone mineral density, and reproductive function. J Clin Endocrinol Metab 1999;84:4583–4590.

Hemminki A, Markie D, Tomlinson I, et al. A serine/threonine kinase gene defective in Peutz-Jeghers syndrome. Nature 1998;391:184–187.

Jackson RS, Creemers JW, Ohagi S, et al. Obesity and impaired prohormone processing associated with mutations on the human proormone convertase 1 gene. Nat Genet 1997;16:303–306.

Jenne DE, Reimann H, Nezu J, et al. Peutz-Jeghers syndrome is caused by mutations in a novel serine threonine kinase. Nat Genet 1988;18:38–43.

Kaplowitz PB, Oberfield SE. Reexamination of the age limit for defining when puberty is precocious in girls in the United States: implications for evaluation and treatment. Drug and Therapeutics and Executive Committees of the Lawson Wilkins Pediatric Endocrine Society. Pediatrics 1999;104:936–941.

Kawate N, Kletter GB, Wilson BE, Netzloff ML, Menon KMJ. Identification of constitutively activating mutation of the luteinizing hormone receptor in a family with male limited gonadotrophin independent precocious puberty (testotoxicosis). J Med Genet 1995;32: 553, 554.

Kosugi S, Van Dop C, Geffner ME, et al. Characterization of heterogeneous mutations causing constitutive activation of the luteinizing hormone receptor in familial male precocious puberty. Hum Mol Genet 1995;4:183–188.

Latronico AC, Anasti J, Arnhold IJP, et al. Testicular and ovarian resistance to luteinizing hormone caused by inactivating mutations of the luteinizing hormone. N Engl J Med 1996;334:507–512.

Laue L, Chan WY, Hsueh AJ, et al. Genetic heterogeneity of constitutively activating mutations of the human luteinizing hormone receptor in familial male-limited precocious puberty. Proc Natl Acad Sci USA 1995;92:1906–1910.

Laue L, Wu SM, Kudo M, et al. A nonsense mutation of the human luteinizing hormone receptor gene in Leydig cell hypoplasia. Hum Mol Genet 1995;4:1429–1433.

Layman LC, Cohen DP, Jin M, et al. Mutations in gonadotoropin-releasing hormone receptor gene cause hypogonadotropic hypogonadism. Nat Genet 1998;18:14, 15.

Laymen LC, Lee EJ, Peak DB, et al. Delayed puberty and hypogonadadism caused by mutations in the follicular-stimulating hormone β-subunit gene. New Engl J Med 1997;337:607–611.

Lazar L, Kauli R, Pertzelan A, Phillip M. Gonadotropin-suppressive therapy in girls with early and fast puberty affects the pace of puberty but not total pubertal growth or final height. J Clin Endocrinol Metab 2002;87:2090–2094.

Levine MA, Downs RW Jr, Moses AM, et al. Resistance to multiple hormones in patients with pseudohypoparathyroidism; association with deficient activity of guanine nucleotide regulatory protein. Am J Med 1983;74:545–556.

Liu G, Duranteau L, Carel J-C, Monroe J, Doyle DA, Shenker AS. Leydig-cell tumors caused by an activating mutation of the gene encoding the luteining hormone receptor. New Eng J Med 1999;341:1731–1736.

Liu J, Litman D, Rosenberg MJ, Yu S, Biesecker LG, Weinstein LS. A GNAS1 imprinting defect in pseudohypoparathyroidism type 1B. J Clin Invest 2000;106:1167–1174.

Mantzoros CS, Flier JS, Rogol AD. A longitudinal assessment of hormonal and physical alterations during normal puberty in boys. V. Rising leptin levels may signal the onset of puberty. J Clin Endocrinol Metab 1997; 82:1066–1070.

Matthews CH, Borgato S, Beck-Peccoz P, et al. Primary amenorrhoea and infertility due to a mutation in the β-subunit of follicle-stimulating hormone. Nat Genet 1993;5:83–86.

Merke DP, Tajima T, Baron J, Cutler GBJ. Hypogonadotropic hypogonadism in a female caused by an X-linked recessive mutation in the DAX1 gene. N Engl J Med 1999;340:1248–1252.

Nachtigall LB, Boepple PA, Pralong FP, Crowley WF Jr. Adult-onset idiopathic hypogonadotropic hypogonadism—a treatable form of male infertility. N Engl J Med 1997;336:410–415.

Neely EK, Bachrach LK, Hintz RL, et al. Bone mineral density during treatment of central precocious puberty. J Pediatr 1995;127:819–822.

Netchine I, Sobrier ML, Krude H, et al. Mutaions in LHX3 results in a new syndrome revealed by combined pituitary hormone deficiency. Nat Genet 2000;25:182–186.

Nishi Y, Hamamoto K, Kajiyama M, Kawamura I. The Perrault syndrome: clinical report and review. Am J Med Genet 1988;31:623–629.

Ogilvy-Stuart AL, Clayton PE, Shalet SM. Cranial irradiation and early puberty. J Clin Endocrinol Metab 1994;78:1282–1286.

Ozata M, Ozdemir IC, Licinio J. Human leptin deficiency caused by a missense mutation: multiple endocrine defects, decreased sympathetic tone, and immune system dysfunction indicate new targets for leptin action, greater central than peripheral resistance to the effects of leptin, and spontaneous correction of leptin-mediated defects. J Clin Endocrinol Metab 1999;84:3686–3695.

Patten JL, John DR, Valle D, et al. Mutation in the gene encoding the stimulatory protein of adenylate cyclase in Albright's hereditary osteodystrophy. New Engl J Med 1990;322:1412–1419.

Paul D, Conte FA, Grumbach MM, Kaplan SL. Long term effect of gonadotropin-releasing hormone agonists therapy on final and near-final height in 26 children with true precocious puberty treated at a median age of less than 5 years. J Clin Endocrinol Metab 1995;80:546–551.

Pescovitz OH, Hench KD, Barnes KM, Loriaux DL, Cutler GB Jr. Premature thelarche and central precocious puberty: the relationship between clinical presentation and gonadotropin response to luteinizing hormone-releasing hormone. J Clin Endocrinol Metab 1988;67:474–479.

Phillip M, Arbelle JE, Segev Y, Parvari R. Male hypogpnadism due to a mutation in the gene for the b-subunit of follicular-stimulating hormone. N Engl J Med 1998;338:1729–1732.

Rao E, Weiss B, Fukami M, et al. Pseudoautosomal deletions encompassing a novel homebox gene cause growth failure in idiopathic short stature and Turner syndrome. Nat Genet 1997;16:54–63.

Saenger P, Wikland KA, Conway GS, et al. Fifth international symposium on Turner syndrome. Recommendations for the diagnosis and management of Turner syndrome. J Clin Endocrinol Metab 2001;86:3061–3069.

Schwindinger WF, Francomano CA, Levine MA. Identification of a mutation in gene encoding the subunit of the stimulatory G protein of adenylyl cyclase in McCune-Albright syndrome. Proc Natl Acad Sci USA 1992;89:5152–5156.

Seminara SB, Seminara SB, Messager S, et al. The GPR54 gene as a regulator of puberty. New Engl J Med 2003:349;1614–1627.

Shenker A, Laue L, Kosui S, Merendino JJ Jr, Minegishi T, Cutler GB Jr. A constitutively activating mutation of the luteinizing hormone receptor in familial male precocious puberty. Nature 1993;365:652–654.

Smith EP, Boyd J, Frank GR, et al. Estrogen resistance caused by a mutation in the estrogen-receptor gene in a man. N Engl J Med 1994;331:1056–1061.

Tapanainen JS, Aittomaki K, Min J, Vaskivuo T, Huhtaniemi IT. Men homozygous for an inactivating mutation of the follicle-stimulating hormone (FSH) receptor gene present variable suppression of spermatogenesis and fertility. Nat Genet 1997;15:205, 206.

Tauber M, Berro B, Delagnes V, et al. Can some growth hormone (GH)-deficient children benefit from combined therapy with gonadotropin-releasing hormone analogs and GH? Results of a retrospective study. J Clin Endocrinol Metab 2003;88:1179–1183.

Weinstein LS, Shenker A, Gejm an PV, Merino MJ, Friedman E, Spiegel AM. Activating mutations of the stimulatory G protein in the McCune-Albright syndrome. N Engl J Med 1991;325:1688–1695.

Weiss J, Axelrod L, Whitcomb RW, Harris PE, Crowley WF, Jameson JL. Hypogonadism caused by a single amino acid substitution in the β subunit of luteinizing hormone. N Engl J Med 1992;326:179–183.

Wu T, Mendola P, Buck GM. Thinic differences in the presence of secondary sex characteristics and menarche among US girls: The Third National Health and Nutrition Exanimation Survey, 1988–1994. Pediatrics 2002;110:752–757.

Wu W, Cogan JD, Pfaffle RW, et al. Mutations in PROP1 cause familial combined pituitary hormone deficiency. Nat Genet 1998;18:147–149.

44 Defects of Androgen Action

Michael J. McPhaul

SUMMARY

The development of the male phenotype is a complex process that involves the active participation of genes involved at many levels, from those specifying gonadal differentiation to the androgen receptor (AR) itself. Defective virilization can be caused by defects anywhere along the pathway. Considering the clinical syndromes caused by known defects of genes such as steroid 5α-reductase II and the AR, the pathogenesis of a large proportion of defects in virilization remains unexplained. It is conceivable that some might represent defects in genes required for normal AR function or at steps beyond the site of action of the AR itself (e.g., coactivators, or defects in genes activated by the AR).

Key Words: Amino; androgen receptor (AR); 5α-dihydrotestosterone; 5α-reductase; Reifenstein's syndrome; sex-determining region Y; testosterone.

INTRODUCTION

Since 1935 it has been recognized that the principal androgen secreted by the testes is testosterone. Although testosterone is the most abundant circulating androgen, 5α-dihydrotestosterone is the predominant hormone found complexed to the androgen receptor (AR) in the nuclei of target cells, such as the prostate. This finding opened a new perspective on androgen physiology and focused attention on the 5α-reductase enzyme(s) that catalyze this conversion as potential modulators of androgen action in selected tissues. As described later, this inference has been confirmed by the recognition that some abnormalities of male sexual development can be traced to defects in the conversion of testosterone to 5α-dihydrotestosterone.

STRUCTURE AND FUNCTION OF THE AR

Abundant biochemical and genetic data demonstrated that the actions of androgen were mediated by a single receptor that was encoded on the X-chromosome, and that defects in this receptor protein, the AR, could result in a range of abnormalities of male phenotypic sexual development. The isolation of cDNAs encoding the AR revealed it to be a member of a large group of related transcription factors, the nuclear receptor family. This family includes members that are ligand responsive, such as the steroid, thyroid hormone, and retinoid receptors, and others that are thought to be constitutively active or modulated by other influences, such as

From: *Principles of Molecular Medicine, Second Edition*
Edited by: M. S. Runge and C. Patterson © Humana Press, Inc., Totowa, NJ

phosphorylation. All exhibit a modular structure (displayed for the AR in Fig. 44-1) consisting of a highly conserved DNA-binding domain, a less highly conserved carboxyl-terminal ligand-binding domain, and an amino-terminal segment that is poorly conserved between individual family members, both in terms of primary amino acid sequence, and length.

The DNA-binding domain is made up of two elements (termed "zinc fingers") that mediate the sequence-specific DNA binding of the AR. This segment is the most highly conserved region between members of this gene family. The carboxy-terminus is approx 250 amino acids long and encodes the portion of the protein that binds androgens with high affinity. The amino-terminus of the AR is somewhat atypical in that it contains three segments made up of repeated amino acids (one of repeated glutamine residues, one of repeated proline residues, and one of repeated glycine residues). Polymorphisms of these regions appear to have little effect on AR function in normal individuals, but expansions of the glutamine repeat have been implicated in the pathogenesis of spinal and bulbar muscular atrophy (SBMA, Kennedy's syndrome, *see* AR Mutations: Special Cases).

The nonligand-bound AR is thought to exist in the cell in association with a number of ancillary proteins, particularly members of the heat shock protein family. After the binding of hormone, the receptor dissociates from these proteins and binds to specific DNA sequences within or adjacent to androgen-responsive genes. This ligand-activated receptor interacts with components of the transcriptional apparatus to stimulate and stabilize active transcription complexes. In some models, the AR appears to modulate genes in a negative fashion or to alter mRNA stability, but these phenomena have been less well characterized.

AR DEFECTS

CLINICAL FEATURES   A spectrum of phenotypes can result from defects of AR function (Table 44-1). Patients completely unresponsive to the actions of androgen (referred to as complete testicular feminization or complete androgen insensitivity) have a 46,XY karyotype, but an external phenotype that is completely female in appearance, despite normal or elevated levels of circulating androgens. Owing to the secretion and action of Müllerian inhibitory substance by the functional testes present in these patients, the uterus and fallopian tubes are absent. Such individuals are usually raised as females and might first seek attention for evaluation of primary amenorrhea. Gonadectomy is often performed, because the intraabdominal testes show an increased rate

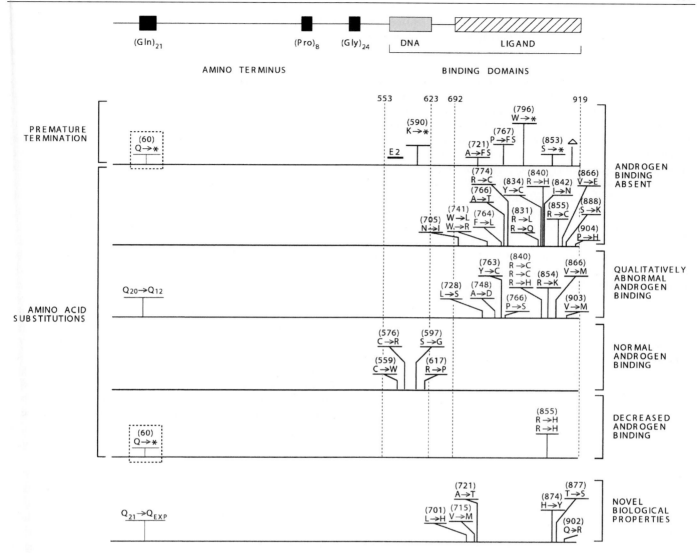

Figure 44-1 Mutations of the human AR that cause abnormalities of AR function (above). A schematic representation of the human AR is shown. The approximate boundaries of the DNA and LBDs are indicated, as are the locations of the repeated stretches of glutamine, proline, and glycine residues within the amino terminus (below). A selected grouping of mutations causing androgen resistance are grouped according to the type of genetic lesion (amino acid substitution or premature termination codon, left margin) or the effect that the mutation has receptor function (right margin). Also comprised in this figure are a selected number of mutations reported in literature that have been detected in prostate cancer specimens that appear to alter the binding characteristics and activities of the AR. The expansion of the glutamine repeat that causes spinal bulbar muscular atrophy is also represented. (Adapted from McPhaul MJ, Marcelli M, Zoppi S, Griffin JE, Wilson JD. Genetic basis of endocrine disease. J Clin Endocrinol Metab 1993;76[1]:17–23.)

Table 44-1
Phenotypes Associated With Defects in the Genes Encoding the Androgen Receptor and 5α-Reductase II

Gene	Syndrome	External genitalia	Wolffian duct derivatives	Müllerian duct derivatives
AR	Complete female feminization Complete androgen insensitivity	Completely female	Not virilized	Absent
	Incomplete testicular feminization	Predominantly female; some clitoromegaly, closure of the posterior fourchette	Usually partially virilized	Absent
	Reifenstein syndrome	Substantial phallic development, but with severe forms of hypospadias	Variable defects	Absent
	Under-virilized, fertile male	Male phenotype with small phallus	Male	Absent
	Infertile male	Male phenotype	Male	Absent
5α-Reductase II	5α-Reductase deficiency	Can be variable: ranging from female external genitalia at birth to a predominantly male phenotype with hypospadias	Normal male	Absent

of malignant tumor development. With estrogen replacement, these individuals often lead completely normal lives as women, although they are infertile. Partial androgen insensitivity encompasses a wide range of abnormalities of male phenotypic development. Affected individuals have phenotypes ranging from predominately female to minor defects of male development.

The term incomplete testicular feminization has been applied to individuals with nearly complete forms of androgen resistance who demonstrate only slight evidence of virilization (such as clitoromegaly). These patients are usually managed in a fashion similar to that of patients with complete testicular feminization.

Reifenstein's syndrome is a constellation of features that includes severe defects of male urogenital development (perineal or penoscrotal hypospadias) and gynecomastia. Reifenstein's syndrome represents a far more difficult challenge. As noted clinically, the developmental abnormalities are substantial and surgical correction of these defects often requires multiple separate surgical procedures. Such efforts are further hampered by the small size of the genitalia of affected children. After surgical correction, most individuals with this phenotype are raised as males, although many exhibit difficulty with gender identity.

At the mildly affected end of the spectrum, a small number of individuals have been described in which normal development of the external genitalia has occurred, but in which some degree of undervirilization is clinically evident. In some, this phenotype has been associated with azoospermia and infertility without undervirilization. In others, normal sperm density and fertility is identified in men with varying degrees of virilization. Patients with these phenotypes have been identified as having AR defects on the basis of a family history and abnormalities of in vitro ligand-binding assays of the AR. Although specific AR defects have been reported in association with these syndromes, it is not clear how frequently such phenotypes are caused by AR defects in the general population. Information derived from the analysis of groups of individuals with infertility would suggest that AR mutations can be identified in only a small subset of such patients.

An unusual variation of the undervirilized phenotype is that presented by patients with spinal and bulbar muscular atrophy (SBMA) (see Chapter 116). Patients with this syndrome have normal male development and normal male secondary sexual characteristics throughout much of their lives but develop signs of clinical androgen resistance beginning in middle age. Although these signs of androgen resistance are unmistakable (usually gynecomastia), the difficulties presented by the symptoms of anterior motor neuron degeneration pose a far more serious threat to the health of such patients and represent the usual cause of death in affected individuals. Interestingly, expansions of this same element have been identified in a subset of patients with infertility.

AR MUTATIONS AND DEFECTIVE AR FUNCTION

Molecular defects of the AR that cause the syndromes of androgen resistance have been studied by a number of groups. The causative mutations have been identified in more than 100 pedigrees and include all of the major clinical syndromes. A database listing the mutations causing androgen resistance is accessible through the internet.

Deletions or insertions of the AR gene occur with a frequency of approx 5–10% of patients with androgen resistance and range in size from single or multiple nucleotides to deletions of the entire gene. Because such mutations disturb the open reading frame of the AR, patients with this type of mutation do not express an intact receptor protein and, with few exceptions, lack detectable androgen

binding in their cells, and tissues. In addition, because the intact AR is not present in the tissues of such patients, AR function is absent and affected individuals always demonstrate the phenotype of complete androgen insensitivity (complete testicular feminization).

In contrast to the frequency of deletions and insertions in the AR gene, single nucleotide substitutions are much more frequent and account for the bulk of patients with androgen resistance as a result of AR mutations. In some cases, such substitutions result in large-scale alterations of receptor structure, as when they result in alterations of AR mRNA splicing or introduction of premature termination codons within the AR open reading frame. These instances, as with gene deletion or insertion mutations that interrupt the primary sequence of intact AR protein, are usually associated with a lack of detectable androgen binding in tissues and a phenotype of complete androgen insensitivity.

Single nucleotide substitutions that result in single amino acid changes within the AR protein are the most frequent type of mutation in the AR. These defects fall into two general categories: those within the DNA-binding domain and those that have been localized to the ligand-binding domain of the receptor. Unlike the other mutation categories previously described (deletions, insertions, premature termination), the effect of these substitutions on AR function can vary, and the entire spectrum of androgen-resistant phenotypes has been traced to single amino acid substitutions within the AR protein. In most instances, the principal effect of the amino acid substitution is on AR function and major effects on the level of AR abundance, as measured in patient fibroblasts, are uncommon.

Amino acid substitutions in the DNA-binding domain have little effect on the binding of ligand by the mutant receptor. Despite the capacity of these mutant ARs to bind ligand normally, receptor function is reduced after ligand stimulation, compared with the activity of the normal AR. This reduced function is caused by a decreased capacity of the mutant AR to bind to target sequences within responsive genes. In this category of mutation, the degree of impairment of receptor binding to DNA appears to have a direct relationship to the degree that receptor function is reduced. Similar conclusions hold true for larger alterations of receptor structure occurring within the DNA-binding domain that maintain the reading frame of the receptor (e.g., deletions of single amino acid residues within the DNA-binding domain or the single reported instance caused by in-frame deletion of exon 3).

Amino acid substitutions in the ligand-binding domain (LBD) can result in a variety of changes in the capacity of the AR to bind its ligand. In a surprisingly small proportion of cases, the amino acid replacement renders the receptor completely unable to bind ligand. Under these circumstances, it is presumed that as a result the alteration of the LBD structure the binding pocket is radically distorted. This conformational change blocks the capacity of the AR to bind its ligand and the mutant receptor is thus "locked" into an inactive conformation. This type of mutant AR is functionally equivalent to mutations that result in the synthesis of truncated forms of the AR, as even pharmacological doses of potent synthetic androgens are unable to restore receptor function in vivo or in functional assays performed in vitro.

Far more frequently, however, amino acid substitutions in the LBD lead to the synthesis of mutant ARs that exhibit the capacity to bind hormone, but with properties that are abnormal compared to the normal AR (e.g., bind ligand with a reduced affinity or stability). Although the exact type of ligand-binding abnormality differs depending on the nature and location of the amino acid substitution within the ligand-binding domain, it appears that the formation and

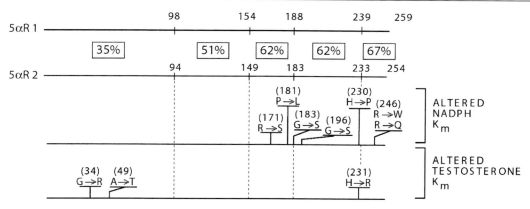

Figure 44-2 Comparison of the structure of human steroid 5α reductases I and II and mutations that alter the binding of testosterone and nicotin-amide adenine dinucleotide phosphate (above). Alignment of the predicted protein sequences of steroid 5α-reductase I (259 amino acids) and steroid 5α-reductase II (254 amino acids). The degree of sequence identity is shown for each of the five coding exons (boxed percentages) (below). Mutations identified within the coding sequence of the steroid 5α-reductase II gene in patients with 5α-reductase deficiency. Although more than 50 mutations been identified that cause 5α-reductase deficiency, a much smaller proportion have been analyzed biochemically. In this figure, only the mutations that cause alterations in the binding of testosterone or NADPH are indicated. Comprised in this figure is an amino acid substitution A49T that has been suggested to be associated with an increased risk of prostate cancer. (Drawn after Russell DW, Wilson JD. Steroid 5α-reductase: two genes/two enzymes. Annu Rev Biochem 1994;63:25–61.)

stability of the hormone-receptor complex is the final determinant of the degree of impairment of mutant AR function. In vitro studies of such mutant receptors demonstrate that the use of multiple high doses of physiological ligands (testosterone or dihydro-testosterone) or the use of potent nonmetabolizable androgen agonists can overcome the defective function of many mutant ARs of this type. In addition to its mechanistic implications, this finding might have substantial clinical implications as well, because it suggests that the pharmacological manipulation of many mutant ARs might be possible.

Studies have investigated the levels of expression and the function of normal and mutant ARs. In most circumstances the major effect of most mutations in the AR is not at the level of AR abundance, but at the level of AR function. This is not true in all cases, however, with the most obvious exceptions being mutations that result in truncation of the receptor protein (e.g., termination codons or alterations of mRNA splicing).

GENOTYPE–PHENOTYPE CORRELATIONS AND PHENOTYPIC MODIFIERS

The breadth of mutations that has been identified has permitted the recognition that the effect of an AR mutation depends on the extent to which AR expression and function are altered.

In considering the large number of identified mutations, there is generally good agreement in terms of the phenotype observed when the same mutation is identified in different pedigrees. This agreement is clearest in patients with complete forms of androgen insensitivity and a greater degree of variation is observed in patients with partial forms of androgen insensitivity. This is likely because at the time of sexual development, relatively small variations in AR levels or activity can have discernible effects on the degree of observed virilization. Two different mechanisms have been reported as potential modifiers of the phenotype in different individuals with the same genotype. The first, differences in the level of 5α-reductase activity, contributes to differences between patients with distinctive partial phenotypes of androgen insensitivity. The second mechanism, somatic mosaicism, could account for even larger variations in observed phenotype.

AR MUTATIONS—SPECIAL CASES

The androgen-resistance syndromes described are caused by mutations that impair receptor function to varying degrees. Two additional types of AR mutation have been identified that result in an alteration of AR responsiveness or an apparent "gain" of function.

The first example of a "gain of function" mutation in the AR is the genetic defect causing Kennedy's syndrome. This disease, also known as SBMA, is characterized by signs and symptoms caused by a progressive degeneration of spinal and bulbar motor muscles. These features are associated with clinical signs compatible with mild androgen insensitivity, which also appear in middle age. The pathogenesis of this extraordinary disease was traced to the expansion of a triplet nucleotide repeat (CAG) encoding a repeated sequence of glutamine residues within the amino-terminus of the receptor (see Fig. 44-1). The expansion of this glutamine repeat, the first of an increasing number of similar diseases that have also been traced to the expansion of trinu-cleotide repeats (Chapter 116), is thought to have two different effects on AR function. First, it is clear that the expansion of this segment of the AR diminishes the capacity of the AR to activate responsive genes after androgen stimulation. This diminished AR function can be demonstrated using a variety of functional assays and is presumably the cause of the subtle signs of androgen resistance observed in affected individuals. It is clear from the study of rare patients with complete deletions of the AR that the SBMA phenotype (progressive death of motor neurons in bulbar nuclei and in the spinal cord) is not caused by a simple lack of functional AR. Instead, this disease appears to be caused by a type of toxic "gain of function" that is caused by the expression of ARs containing the expanded glutamine repeats in specific cell types. Analogy to results obtained from the study of the Huntington disease gene (also caused by a glutamine repeat expansion) would suggest that the glutamine expansion might permit interaction of the mutant AR with intracellular targets in spinal motor neurons that somehow mediate the observed cell-type-specific toxicity. Alterations of axonal transport have been identified as one neuron-specific function that might contribute to the pathogenesis of this disorder.

Table 44-2
Distribution of 5α-Reductases I and II Expression in Rat and Human Tissues

	Rat		Human	
	Type I	Type II	Type I	Type II
Skin	—	—	+[*]	+[a†]
Testes	D[*]	1+[*]	ND[†]	
Epididymis	D[*e]	5+[*e]	ND[†]	+[b†],*
Vas deferens	D[*]	1+[*]	—	—
Seminal vesicle	D	1+[*]	ND[†]	+[†]
Ventral prostate	D[d*]	D[d*]		
Prostate			ND[†],*	+[c†],*
Ovary	2+[*]	ND[*]		
Adrenal	3+[*]	D[*]		
Brain	3+[*]	ND[*]		
Colon	3+[*]	D[*]		
Heart	ND[*]	ND[*]		
Intestine	3+[*]	D[*]		
Kidney	3+[*]	ND[*]		
Liver	4+[*]	ND[*]	+[†],*	+[†],*
Lung	2+[*]	ND[*]		
Muscle	ND[*]	ND[*]		
Spleen	D[*]	ND[*]		
Stomach	D[*]	ND[*]		
Pons	—	—	ND	+
Cerebral	—	—	ND	+
Hypothalmus	—	—	ND	+

[a]Histochemical studies indicate that the expression of 5α-reductase II is localized to the cells of the dermal papilla.

[b]Staining localized to epithelial cells in histochemical studies.

[c]Staining localized to basal epithelial and stroma cells.

[d]Type I is detected in basal epithelial cells and type II in stroma cells in in situ hybridization studies of the regenerating rat central prostate.

[e]Types I and II are localized to the epithelial cells using in situ hybridization.

Summary of studies measuring 5α-reductases I and II expression using measurements of the corresponding RNA (*) or protein (†) are derived from published studies of Russell and coworkers. The rating scales (1+ least, 5+ highest) used in summary are designed to convey a sense of the relative abundance of the 5α-reductase isozymes in the two species—rat and human—that have been studied most carefully. Because the rat and human have been conducted separately, they can only be compared with one another in a qualitative fashion. D is detectable (i.e., at the limits of detection). ND, is not detected; —, values not reported. In addition to the results tabulated here, the studies of Thigpen et al. clearly indicate that in the human substantial changes in abundance can be demonstrated in the expression of the types I and II isoenzymes in a tissue at different times in development.

The second type of AR mutation that causes a gain or alteration of receptor function is the mutations identified in human prostate cancer specimens. First recognized in the AR gene of a prostate tumor cell line, LNCaP, amino acid substitutions have been detected in a number of clinical prostate cancer specimens. Although a number of these mutations have been found, fewer have been completely studied concerning their effect on the ligand responsiveness of the mutated AR. In instances in which detailed studies have been performed, tests of receptor function using androgen-responsive reporter genes demonstrate that the mutant ARs can be stimulated by ligands that cannot ordinarily activate the normal AR. Such ligands include adrenal androgens and even compounds (such as hydroxyflutamide) that act to antagonize the function of the normal AR. Although it is not possible to conclude how important these mutant receptors are in the progression of prostate cancers toward the androgen-independent phenotype, the preponderance of analyses suggest that such mutations are found most frequently in advanced stage tumors, particularly in patients treated with AR antagonists, such as hydroxyflutamide.

5α-REDUCTASE DEFICIENCY

PHYSIOLOGICAL AND CLINICAL STUDIES   The observation that 5α-dihydrotestosterone was the principal hormone bound to the AR in the nuclei of target cells suggested the potential importance of 5α-reductase in androgen physiology. The subsequent identification of rare patients with specific defects of virilization that formed reduced quantities of 5α-reduced androgen metabolites emphasized the importance of this metabolic step. The normal virilization of other tissues, such as the epididymis in patients with clinical 5α-reductase deficiency, led to the concept that the action of testosterone was sufficient to effect the actions of androgen in selected tissues, but that the formation of 5α-dihydrotestosterone was crucial in others, such as the prostate. This dichotomy has not yet been completely explained at a mechanistic level.

CLINICAL PHENOTYPE   The clinical features of many infants with deficiencies of 5α-reductase are consistent with marked defects of androgen action (see Table 44-1). The external genitalia are characterized by a microphallus, severe hypospadias, and a bifid scrotum. A blind vaginal pouch is present and opens either directly onto the perineum or onto a urogenital sinus. Owing to the production of Müllerian inhibitory substance by the functional testes, no Müllerian structures are present. It is of interest that in association with the pubertal rise in testosterone levels, several changes may take place in the phenotype of affected individuals. The phallus enlarges and some male secondary sexual characteristics appear, such as changes in voice and muscle mass. Notably, this increase in testosterone has not been reported to result in acne, prostate growth, or male pattern baldness. It has also been reported that in some individuals, raised initially as females, gender identity may change after the pubertal rise in androgen levels. The ability to identify individuals with 5α-reductase II deficiency at the molecular level has permitted the recognition that this syndrome also includes individuals with less severely affected phenotypes.

5α-REDUCTASE STRUCTURE AND MECHANISM OF ACTION

Attempts to purify 5α-reductase using classic techniques of protein purification failed and its structure remained elusive until expression cloning in Xenopus oocytes was employed to isolate a cDNA encoding a steroid 5α-reductase from the rat prostate. This advance permitted a number of studies and resulted in the isolation of cDNAs encoding two related isozymes (Fig. 44-2) encoded by two distinct, related genes from humans and from all vertebrate species examined to date. Inspection of the structures of the cDNAs indicates substantial sequence divergence between the two isozymes, both within and between different species. Both enzymes are extremely hydrophobic and are thought to be imbedded in the nuclear membrane of cells, accounting for the failure of extensive efforts to purify the enzyme in an active form. Structural variations between the two isozymes confer substantial differences in their physical properties that have been exploited to develop compounds that inhibit one or the other isozyme preferentially.

Studies of the distribution of the two isozymes (Table 44-2) have demonstrated that the patterns of expression of these two proteins

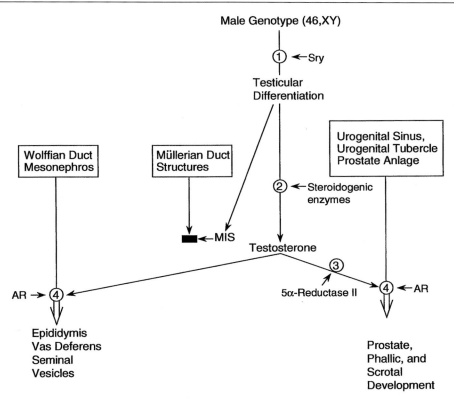

Figure 44-3 Schematic of the pathways controlling the development of the normal male phenotype. Male sexual development is a complex cascade of events that can be affected by lesions in a number of genes. Some, such as lesions in the AR or the sex-determining region Y gene, can cause disturbances of virilization of all androgen-responsive tissues. The effects of defects in other genes, however, (such as mutation of 5α-reductase II), are manifest only in selected tissues. It is likely that defects in other genes can contribute to defects of virilization, as a large proportion of subjects with abnormalities of male phenotypic development cannot be accounted for by defects in the genes most carefully studied to date, such as the AR and steroid 5α-reductase 2 genes.

differ, both in terms of tissue, cell type, and developmental stage. These disparities suggest substantially different physiological roles for the two enzymes.

GENETIC DEFECTS OF STEROID 5α-REDUCTASE II The genetic lesions causing clinical 5α-reductase deficiency have been identified in pedigrees from around the world. In all instances, when a genetic defect has been detected, it has been localized to the 5α-reductase II gene. Unlike the AR, the gene encoding 5α-reductase II is autosomal and each individual possesses two copies. For this reason, mutations causing clinical 5α-reductase deficiency are recessive and the inheritance of two defective 5α-reductase II gene alleles is required for the defects to be manifest. 5α-reductase II deficiency is infrequently caused by deletions or insertions in the gene. More often, defects in the gene are caused by mutations that result in premature termination of the protein or single amino acid substitutions within the open reading frame. Identification of the locations of these substitutions and determination of the physical properties of the mutant enzymes have permitted the identification of amino acid residues important for binding of steroid substrates and for the binding of nicotinamide adenine dinucleotide phosphate, a cofactor required for the reduction reaction. These studies have also identified sites that have been mutated repeated in apparently unrelated pedigrees. These regions are apparently more susceptible to mutation.

As a consequence of the recessive nature of clinical 5α-reductase II deficiency, it would be expected that the genetic basis of this rare trait would be traced most frequently to homozygosity for a single defec-

tive allele (e.g., consanguinity). Surprisingly, a high proportion of patients (approx 30%) have been found to be compound heterozygotes, suggesting either an unexpectedly high mutation rate of the 5α-reductase II gene or a high frequency of individuals in the general population that carry single defective alleles. This apparent paradox has not been resolved.

GENETIC DEFECTS OF STEROID 5α-REDUCTASE I An abnormal phenotype caused by a deficiency of 5α-reductase I in humans has not been described. The differential expression of steroid 5α-reductase I in selected tissues (*see* Table 44-2) suggests that specific phenotypes in humans that result from lesions in this gene or abnormalities of its expression might be identified in the future.

Because of the lack of mutations in the human population, the first insights into the nature of defects that might be expected in humans have come from experiments in mice in which steroid 5α-reductase I gene has been disrupted by homologous recombination. Male mice homozygous for this targeted null allele develop normally, both prenatally and postnatally. Unexpectedly, although female mice homozygous for this same null allele develop normally into adulthood, when pregnant, such mice fail to initiate parturition normally. Experiments in which different steroids were administered to these steroid 5α-reductase I-deficient mice suggested that the synthesis and action of 5α-reduced androgens were important elements of the normal parturition process in mice. Although the mechanisms and generality of these findings remain to be determined, such results suggest that

5α-reductase I might play important—and even unexpected—roles in human physiology as well.

ADDITIONAL LESSONS FROM MURINE MODELS   Based on the phenotypes of human patients with defects of 5α-reductase II, it was anticipated that defects of virilization would be observed in animals in which the 5α-reductase II gene had been disrupted. Surprisingly, male mice in which both 5α-reductase II genes had been inactivated showed no defects of external genitalia development and only modest reductions in the size of fully formed seminal vesicles and prostates. These findings have been attributed to the observation that in animals with disruptions of either the 5α-reductase II or both the 5-reductase I and II genes, testosterone levels in target tissues are dramatically elevated. These results support the concept that 5α-reductase serves to amplify weak androgenic signals in tissues in which androgen concentrations are limiting (Fig. 44-3).

ACKNOWLEDGMENT

The original work is in this chapter and was supported by NIH grants DK03892 and DK52678 and by grant I-1090 from the Robert A. Welch Foundation.

SELECTED REFERENCES

Boehmer AL, Brinkmann AO, Nijman RM, et al. Phenotypic variation in a family with partial androgen insensitivity syndrome explained by differences in 5alpha dihydrotestosterone availability. J Clin Endocrinol Metab 2001;86:1240–1246.

Boehmer AL, Brinkmann O, Bruggenwirth H, et al. Genotype versus phenotype in families with androgen insensitivity syndrome. J Clin Endocrinol Metab 2001;86:4151–4160.

Giovannucci E, Stampfer MJ, Krithivas K, et al. The CAG repeat within the androgen receptor gene and its relationship to prostate cancer. Proc Natl Acad Sci USA 1997;94:3320–3323.

Gottlieb B. Androgen Receptor Gene Mutation Data Base. The Lady Davis Institute for Medical Research, Sir Mortimer B.Davis-Jewish General Hospital. Montreal, Quebec, Canada. http://www.androgendb.mcgill.ca/. Accessed on March 29, 2006.

Hardy DO, Scher HI, Bogenreider T, et al. Androgen receptor CAG repeat lengths in prostate cancer: correlation with age of onset. J Clin Endocrinol Metab 1996;81:4400–4405.

Hiort O, Sinnecker GH, Holterhus PM, Nitsche EM, Kruse K. The clinical and molecular spectrum of androgen insensitivity syndromes. Am J Med Genet 1996;63:218–222.

Holterhus PM, Bruggenwirth HT, Brinkmann AO, Hiort O. Post-zygotic mutations and somatic mosaicism in androgen insensitivity syndrome. Trends Genet 2001;17:627, 628.

Holterhus PM, Bruggenwirth HT, Hiort O, et al. Mosaicism due to a somatic mutation of the androgen receptor gene determines phenotype in androgen insensitivity syndrome. J Clin Endocrinol Metab 1997;82:3584–3589.

Holterhus PM, Wiebel J, Sinnecker GH, et al. Clinical and molecular spectrum of somatic mosaicism in androgen insensitivity syndrome. Pediatr Res 1999;46(6):684–690. http://www.androgendb.mcgill.ca/. Accessed on March 29, 2006.

Imperato-McGinley J. 5 Alpha-reductase-2 deficiency. Curr Ther Endocrinol Metab 1997;6:384–387.

Lumbroso S, Lobaccaro JM, Vial C, et al. Molecular analysis of the androgen receptor gene in Kennedy's disease. Report of two families and review of the literature. Horm Res 1997;7:23–29.

Mahendroo MS, Cala KM, Hess DL, Russell DW. Unexpected virilization in male mice lacking steroid 5 alpha-reductase enzymes. Endocrinology 2001;142:652–662.

Mahendroo MS, Cala KM, Russell DW. 5α-Reduced androgens are required for parturition in mice. Mol Endocrinol 1996;10:380–392.

Mahendroo MS, Russell DW. Male and female isoenzymes of steroid 5alpha-reductase. Rev Reprod 1999;4:179–183.

Marcelli M, Zoppi S, Wilson CM, Griffin JE, McPhaul MJ. Amino acid substitutions in the hormone-binding domain of the human androgen receptor alter the stability of the hormone receptor complex. J Clin Invest 1994;94:1642–1650.

Quigley CA, DeBellis A, Marschke KB, El-awady MK, Wilson EM, French FS. Androgen receptor defects: historical, clinical, and molecular perspectives. Endocr Rev 1995;16:271–321.

Thigpen AE, Silver RI, Guileyardo JM, Casey ML, McConnell JD, Russell DW. Tissue distribution and ontogeny of steroid 5α-reductase isozyme expression. J Clin Invest 1993;92:903–910.

Wigley WC, Prihoda JS, Mowszowicz I, et al. Natural mutagenesis study of the human steroid 5 alpha-reductase 2 Isozyme. Biochemistry 1994;33:1265–1270.

Wilson JD, Griffin JE, Russell DW. Steroid 5α-reductase 2 deficiency. Endocr Rev 1993;14:77–93.

45 Molecular Endocrinology of the Testis

MARCO MARCELLI, GLENN R. CUNNINGHAM, JOSÉ M. GARCIA,
KIRK C. LO, AND DOLORES J. LAMB

SUMMARY

This chapter reviews genetically influenced causes of male hypogonadism. Acquired cases of hypergonadotropic hypogonadism and acquired forms of gonadotropin deficiency from functional causes or systemic diseases have not been included because they do not have a genetic etiology.

Key Words: Alström syndrome; Dystrophia myotonica 1 (DM1); hypergonadotropic; Kallmann syndrome (KS); Klinefelter syndrome; 46,XX; 46,XY; reproductive system; Smith–Lemli–Opitz syndrome (SLOS); testis.

INTRODUCTION

Two distinct functions of the male reproductive system are essential for the survival of human species. First is the continuous production, nourishment, and storage of male gametes (spermatozoa). The second function is synthesis and secretion of the androgenic hormones necessary for male sexual differentiation and function. The testis is controlled by signals from the hypothalamus-pituitary–gonadal (HPG) axis, in addition to local paracrine and autocrine signals to fulfil these functions.

MALE HYPOGONADISM

Disorders of testicular function result from abnormalities involving the endocrine (Leydig cells) and/or reproductive (germ cell maturation) compartments of the testis. Low testosterone (T) production in adult males is usually accompanied by decreased libido, abnormal secondary sexual characteristics, and infertility, as normal spermatogenesis requires normal production of testicular androgens (hypogonadism with undervirilization and infertility). However, there are situations in which hypogonadism is restricted to the germinal compartment (hypogonadism with infertility and normal virilization).

The serum level of gonadotropins indicates at what site within the HPG axis the defect is localized. In instances in which gonadal function is abnormal and the hypothalamic-pituitary (HP) structures are normal (hypergonadotropic or primary hypogonadism), gonadotropin levels are elevated. When the primary defect lies at the level of the HP structures (hypogonadotropic or secondary hypogonadism), gonadotropin levels are inappropriately normal or low. Depending on the serum level of gonadotropins, hypogonadism can be classified as hypergonadotropic or hypogonadotropic (if resulting from testicular or HP disorders, respectively) (Table 45-1) and eugonadotropic (if the abnormality lies only in the germinal cells and serum T levels are normal).

Both congenital and acquired forms of Leydig cell dysfunction have been described, and the clinical picture that results when T synthesis is impaired is different depending on whether androgen deficiency developed prenatally, before puberty, or after puberty (Table 45-2). If the developing fetus was not exposed to an adequate level of androgen because of testicular failure during fetal development, the infant manifests pseudohermaphroditisms, characterized by a large spectrum of potential abnormalities, including ambiguous genitalia, micropenism, and rudimentary testes. If reduced T production developed before puberty, but testicular function was normal during embryogenesis, androgen-related somatic changes normally observed at puberty are absent or incomplete and the patient develops an eunuchoid habitus because of failure of the epiphyses to close, and poor development of skeletal muscles and body hair. If reduced T production developed after puberty, the first symptom of the patient is impotence, whereas loss of secondary sexual characteristics may take several years to become complete.

Hypogonadism manifested by abnormal sperm production can be associated with normal virilization, because many infertile men produce a normal or only a minimally abnormal amount of T. However, in other cases infertility is associated with a reduced production of T and clinical signs of androgen deficiency (infertility from hypergonadotropic or hypogonadotropic disorders [*see* Table 45-1]). In such cases, infertility may be a direct consequence of the reduced T production.

HYPERGONADOTROPIC DISORDERS

Hypergonadotropic abnormalities of the testes are owing to primary testicular failure (*see* Table 45-1). They can be classified in two main groups: congenital or acquired disorders. Some genetic syndromes lead to primary hypogonadism as a result of chromosomal abnormalities, enzymatic defects, or receptor defects. Others are congenital multiorgan diseases with associated hypogonadism, and it is not always clear why patients affected by some

From: *Principles of Molecular Medicine, Second Edition*
Edited by: M. S. Runge and C. Patterson © Humana Press, Inc., Totowa, NJ

Table 45-1
Hypogonadotropic and Hypergonadotropic Disorders

(A) HYPERGONADOTROPIC DISORDERS	(B) HYPOGONADOTROPIC DISORDERS
Genetically inherited	**Genetically inherited**
Chromosomal abnormalities	**Associated with gonadotropin deficiency**
Klinefelter	GPR54 deficiency
	Kallmann syndrome
46,XX males	Fertile eunuch syndrome
46,XY pure gonadal dysgenesis	Hypogonadotropic hypogonadism from biologically
	inactive molecules of the hypothalamic–pituitary axis
Multi-organ diseases	
Alström syndrome	Hypogonadotropic hypogonadism from mutations of
Dysptrophia myotonica 1	genes causing combined pituitary hormone deficiencies
Dystrophia myotonica 2	Hypogonadotropic hypogonadism from mutations of
	genes associated with obesity
Cardiomyopathy with hypogonadotropic	
hypogonadism	Leptin and leptin receptor
Alopecia-mental retardation syndrome with	Prohormone convertase-1
convulsions and hypergonadotropic	
hypogonadism	
Insulin-resistant diabetes with acanthosis	
nigricans, hypogonadism, pigmentary	
retinopathy, deafness, and mental retardation	
Testicular regression syndrome (bilateral anorchia)	
Hypergonadotropic hypogonadism in autoimmune	
polyglandular syndromes I and II	
Receptor defects	**Associated with central nervous system disorders**
LH resistant testis	Prader–Lahart–Willi
Syndromes of androgen resistance	Laurence–Moon–Biedl
	Möbius
	Borjeson–Forssman–Lehman syndrome
	Leopard syndrome
	Rud's syndrome
	Loewe's syndrome
	Carpenter syndrome
Defects of steroidogenesis	**Associated with adrenal insufficiency**
7-dehydrocholesterol reductase deficiency	Adrenal hypoplasia congenita
(7-DHCR-D) or Smith–Lemli–Opitz syndrome	
Lipoid CAH	
3β-hydroxysteroid dehydrogenase 2 deficiency	
17α-hydroxylase 17,20-lyase (CYP17) deficiency	
17β-hydroxy steroid dehydrogenase deficiency	
Acquired	**Acquired**
Viral	**Associated with anatomic disorders**
Medications	Pituitary apoplexy
Trauma	Primary or metastatic tumors of pituitary or
	adjacent structures
Environmental	Infection
Autoimmunity	Infiltrative disorders (Hemochromatosis, sarcoidosis,
	histiocytosis, lymphocytic hypophysitis)
Ionizing radiations	Empty sella
	Functional
	Secondary to Cushing's syndrome
	to ethanol
	to exercise
	to empty sella
	to hyperprolactinemia
	Associated with systemic diseases
	AIDS
	Liver diseases
	Renal diseases
	Hemochromatosis
	Neurological diseases

7-DHCR-D, 7-dehydrocholesterol reductase deficiency; CAH, congenital adrenal hyperplasia; LH, luteinizing hormone.

Table 45-2
Manifestations of Leydig Cell Dysfunction

Prenatal leydig cell dysfunction:
  External genitalia: female, ambiguous; male, hypoplastic
  Wolffian ducts derivatives: absent—rudimentary
  Müllerian ducts derivatives: absent
  Gonads: Small—rudimentary testes, which can be located within
    the abdomen, inside the inguinal canal or in the scrotum
Prepubertal Leydig cells dysfunction:
  External genitalia: small penis <3–4 cm, small testis <5 mL,
    lack of rugal folds and pigmentation sin the scrotum
  Accessory sex organs: small prostate and seminal vesicles
  Hair growth: no development of terminal facial hair, no recession
    of scalp line, decreased body hair, female escutcheon
  Linear growth: eunuchoid skeletal proportions
  Bone development: delayed bone age, predisposition to
    osteoporosis
  Voice: voice remains high pitched
  Muscle mass: absent-reduced development of muscle mass
  Psyche: decreased libido
Postpubertal Leydig cell dysfunction:
  External genitalia: softening and decreased volume of the testes
  Psyche: decreased libido, sexual potency, and aggressivity
  Bone: predisposition to osteoporosis
  Hair growth: decreased growth and amount of facial, pubic,
    and axillary hair
  Spermatogenesis: impaired spermatogenesis
  Muscles: decreased muscle mass

---

of these disorders develop hypogonadism. Acquired diseases causing primary hypogonadism result from the direct exposure of the testis to a variety of exogenous toxic agents. Typical endocrine abnormalities in these patients consist of decreased to undetectable serum levels of T. Gonadotropins are elevated owing to the absence of negative feedback inhibition exerted by T.

HYPERGONADOTROPIC HYPOGONADISM CAUSED BY CHROMOSOMAL ABNORMALITIES

KLINEFELTER SYNDROME Klinefelter syndrome initially was described in 1942, when techniques to study serum hormone levels and chromosomal abnormalities were not available. Its frequency is approx 1/600 male newborn and approx 1/300 spontaneous abortions. Of males with this syndrome, 85% have a 47,XXY chromosomal pattern; however, 46,XY-47,XXY mosaicism is detected in approx 10% of the patients. Less frequently it is found in 46,XX males, or in individuals with Xq trisomy, X-autosome translocations, or poly-X's (48XXXY, 49XXXXY).

Prepubertal diagnosis is possible in the cases when microphallus or cryptorchidism is part of the prepubertal phenotype, when the testes are recognized to be unusually firm or when a karyotype is requested for other reasons. The onset of puberty usually occurs at a normal age, so features of undervirilization, gynecomastia, small testes, azoospermia, decreased muscular mass, and abnormal skeletal proportions resulting in an eunuchoid habitus are most often detected in the postpubertal patient. Small testicular size resulting from the loss of germ cells is a consistent clinical abnormality. In addition, progressive hyalinization and fibrosis of the seminiferous tubules result in an increased testicular consistency.

Mild mental retardation and personality disorders are identified more frequently in patients with Klinefelter syndrome than in the general population, and these abnormalities usually are more evident in the group of patients with polysomic-X conditions. Other conditions that have been detected with increased frequency in patients with Klinefelter syndrome include thyroid abnormalities, diabetes mellitus (DM), breast, and other types of cancer.

From a clinical standpoint, Klinefelter patients affected by 47XXY/46XY mosaicism manifest less serious phenotypic abnormalities, and these individuals can be fertile. However, other variants of this disease, including 48,XXXY, 48,XXYY, and 49,XXXXY individuals, are associated more frequently with cryptorchidism, growth retardation, mental deficiency, antisocial behavior, facial dysmorphism, and skeletal abnormalities.

The endocrine features of these patients show a typical evolution that becomes evident over a period of years. Usually, basal follicle-stimulating hormone (FSH), luteinizing hormone (LH), and T are normal before age 12; however, by age 14 LH and FSH are elevated. At these early states, serum T levels usually are within the normal range. When the patient has reached his middle 20s, however, primary gonadal failure becomes more evident, and T levels are low or low normal, despite elevated gonadotropins. If untreated, most patients become T deficient. Final diagnostic confirmation of this syndrome is obtained by analyzing the karyotype, and by detecting one of the many chromosomal abnormalities described earlier.

Genetic Basis The most common cause of Klinefelter syndrome is nondisjunction during the first or second meiotic division. The extra X chromosome can be of paternal or maternal origin with approximately the same frequency. Most maternal cases are associated with impaired disjunction during the first meiotic division, and maternal age is a factor in these cases. The percentage of XY sperm increases with increasing paternal age. A second possible mechanism, occurring in 3% of the cases, is nondisjunction after the first postzygotic mitosis. A third potential mechanism was described in an Italian family, in which the mother had a 46,XX/47,XXX mosaicism, possibly because of a nondisjunction event during her zygotic development, and three of her children were affected by the classic Klinefelter karyotype 47,XXY. The etiology of the 46XY/47,XXY mosaicism derives from nondisjunction events in mitosis during zygotic development. Patients with mosaicism have lesser degrees of gynecomastia and androgen deficiency. Normal testicular size has been described in some of these patients, especially when the normal stem cell line 46,XY is present in the testis. The additional sex chromosomes in patients with 48,XXYY karyotype derives from successive nondisjunction events in the first and second meiotic division in the father. In contrast, the additional X chromosomes in 49,XXXXY patients are maternally derived, and originate from sequential nondisjunction events in both the first and second meiotic divisions. These individuals usually have radioulnar synostosis, hypogonadism, and mental retardation, and they are at increased risk for congenital heart defects. Whether the Klinefelter phenotype requires the entire extra X chromosome to develop remains a question. One study of phenotype–karyotype correlations has associated the development of the Klinefelter phenotype with genes mapping to region Xq11–Xq22, but this observation was not confirmed by other investigators in a patient with a 47,X,del(X)(pter-p11),Y karyotype.

Treatment These patients' main complaints are the symptoms of hypogonadism, particularly gynecomastia, infertility and reduced libido, learning difficulties, and several psychosocial problems. Standard treatment is replacement with T, which should be started at puberty or when T deficiency is recognized.

Gynecomastia usually is unresponsive to treatment with T, and many patients require surgical reduction mammoplasty. Infertility is not improved by treatment with T. Most patients are azoospermic when they present with infertility. However, individuals with mosaic Klinefelter syndrome usually do have sperm in their ejaculate. Intracytoplasmic sperm injection (ICSI) has made fertilization of an egg with a single sperm possible. Many centers that offer assisted reproductive techniques can retrieve spermatids or spermatozoa from needle aspiration of the testes or from open testicular biopsies. Available data indicate that patients with non-obstructive azoospermia, obstructive azoospermia, or Klinefelter syndrome are at some increased risk of having sex chromosome aneuploidy. Nonetheless, the majority of spermatozoa or spermatids have a normal number of chromosomes. The testes of these individuals must have a few spermatogonia with a mosaic chromosomal pattern. Although reports have only a limited number of patients, fertilization rates are approx 50%, pregnancy rates approx 25%, and live births/couples are approx 10%. Because this disorder is associated with an increased risk of developing breast cancer (approx 20 times that for normal men), some authors have advocated yearly screening mammography, but it is not clear whether it would be useful. These individuals are at increased risk for having osteopenia or osteoporosis even when they have been treated with T replacement therapy. Therefore, it may be necessary to add calcium, vitamin D, and possibly a bisphosphonate to the treatment regimen if their bone mineral density indicates significant risk of fractures.

46,XX MALES A variant of the Klinefelter syndrome, the reported incidence of 46,XX varies from 1/9000–20,000 male newborns. Most cases are sporadic. The phenotype resembles that of Klinefelter patients. The major difference is short stature, because of the absence of Y sequences that are important for normal somatic growth, normal intellectual development, and normal skeletal proportions. The testes are small and firm, androgen production is compromised, and gynecomastia is common in adolescent patients. Germ cells are absent, and serum levels of gonadotropins are elevated. Affected individuals have male psychosexual identification.

These patients usually are referred to a physician to investigate typical phenotypic abnormalities that become evident after puberty. Some patients are referred at an earlier stage of their life, because at times this entity is associated with hypospadias, particularly in the subgroup of patients in which no Y sequences are detected. The identification of a 46,XX karyotype associated with a male phenotype and endocrine studies showing hypergonadotropic hypogonadism and infertility permit successful diagnosis.

Genetic Basis The presence of Y material containing *Sry* can be demonstrated in the X chromosome of approx 80% of these patients. This event is because of X–Y recombination occurring outside the pseudoautosomal segments in which X–Y pairing normally occurs, resulting in the transfer of *Sry* from the Y to the X chromosome. The consensus is that *Sry* translocated to the X chromosome is sufficient to trigger testicular differentiation and the development of a male phenotype. The remainder of these patients (approx 20%) does not carry any identifiable Y sequence and have larger incidence of ambiguous genitalia. No mechanism has been identified to account for the male phenotypic development observed in these patients. Possibilities include an activating mutation in an autosomal or X chromosomal gene normally induced by *Sry* in the cascade of events leading to the differentiation of the male gonad, and undetected mosaicism with a Y-bearing cell line.

The pathogenesis of infertility in these patients is probably due, as in Klinefelter syndrome, to the presence of two X chromosomes in the germ cells and to the lack of the long arm of the Y chromosome that contains the azoospermia factor (AZF) gene necessary for normal spermatogenesis. These individuals require regular follow up for possible long-term androgen replacement and counseling through a cooperative interdisciplinary approach.

46,XY PURE GONADAL DYSGENESIS 46,XY gonadal dysgenesis, of which complete and an incomplete forms have been described, occurs in sporadic and familial forms. At birth, patients with the complete form appear to have normal external female genitalia. At puberty they do not develop secondary sexual characteristics, do not menstruate, and have streak gonads. Laparotomy reveals bilateral streak gonads, atrophic fallopian tubes, and a rudimentary uterus with a narrow lumen. They are chromatin negative and have a 46,XY karyotype.

In the incomplete form of the disease, virilization of the phenotype depends on the degree of differentiation achieved by the gonads, which varies from streak gonads to dysgenetic testes, and on their residual capacity to produce T and anti-Müllerian hormone (AMH). In the incomplete form of the disease, virilization is never normal. Therefore, the characteristics of the internal and external genitalia of these patients are more ambiguous than in the complete form. The presence of spontaneous gynecomastia is associated with an estrogen secreting neoplasm, which in these patients is frequently the gonadoblastoma type. Unlikely 46,XX males, this entity is associated with normal stature resulting from the presence of most of the Y chromosome.

Diagnosis A form of primary hypogonadism, 46,XY pure gonadal dysgenesis is typically associated with increased level of gonadotropins. T levels are almost undetectable in patients with the complete form and decreased but detectable in patients with the incomplete form. The diagnosis should be suspected in individuals presenting with primary hypogonadism, a 46,XY karyotype, and with the phenotype and pattern of inheritance discussed.

Genetic Basis This disease is associated with a remarkable degree of genetic heterogeneity. It has been associated with abnormalities occurring in the Y-linked *Sry* gene, with an X-linked pattern of inheritance, and with a sex-limited autosomal-dominant inheritance. Defects of *Sry* (deletions of the *Sry* gene or point mutations), have been detected in approx 10–15% of the sporadic cases and in kindreds with the familial form. Other X-linked and autosomal genes that could be involved, most of which may play a role in the cascade of events leading to testicular differentiation, include DAX1, WT1, AMH, SF-1, WNT4, DMRT1, XH2, DSS and SOX-9 Defects occurring in these genes are discussed later. The association of this disease with alterations in the sequence of *Sry* and other autosomal or X-linked genes is leading to more sophisticated understanding of the complex cascade of events required for normal testicular differentiation. The eventsequence and precise mechanism of interaction among these factors are not completely clear and being investigated.

Treatment The sex of rearing should be based on the degree of genital ambiguity. When this critical dilemma has been properly addressed and skeletal growth is complete, the rudimentary gonads should be removed prophylactically, because they may undergo malignant degeneration. At this point T or estrogen replacement should be started to ensure the development of the secondary sexual characteristics, and the prevention of osteopenia.

HYPERGONADOTROPIC HYPOGONADISM FROM MULTI-ORGAN DISEASES

ALSTRÖM SYNDROME   This rare entity, described in 1959 by Alström, is characterized by autosomal-recessive inheritance, and multifactorial disorders including cone-rod retinal dystrophy, obesity, type-2 DM, acanthosis nigricans, sensorineural deafness, chronic nephropathy, and a late-onset cardiomyopathy. Phenotypic expression varies considerably, even within sibships. Although hypogonadism was not considered a feature of this disease in the initial description of Alström, subsequent articles have described its presence, which typically is reported in affected men, but not women. It is a primary form of hypogonadism, associated with low T and high gonadotropin levels. Alström syndrome usually is associated with normal secondary sexual characteristics, but the testes are small and demonstrate hyalinized tubules and thickening of the lamina propria. A few members of Alström kindreds have been fertile and produced normal offspring. Other metabolic and endocrine abnormalities described include hypothyroidism, growth hormone (GH) deficiency, hyperuricemia, and hyperlipidemia. The most frequent causes of death are hepatic dysfunction and congestive heart failure secondary to dilated cardiomyopathy. Unlike other multiorgan diseases, Alström is not associated with mental retardation.

Genetic Basis   The syndrome has been mapped to chromosome 2p13 as a result of linkage studies in French Acadian and Algerian families. The identification of the gene responsible for Alström syndrome was reported in 2002. This transcript, named *ALMS1*, was mutated in six of eight families studied by one group, and in all six families studied by another group. The function of the *AMLS1* gene is uncertain. It shares analogy with mucin genes and contains a large tandem-repeat domain comprising 34 imperfect repetitions of 47 amino acids that contain no cysteine residues; but unlike mucins, *AMLS1* does not have high serine and threonine content. *AMLS1* is ubiquitously expressed, and this could explain the disease's syndromic nature, as concomitant defective ALMS1 function in multiple tissues may cause the many phenotypes observed.

DYSTROPHIA MYOTONICA 1   Dystrophia myotonica 1 (DM1) is an autosomal-dominant disorder that expresses remarkable variability in its clinical manifestations. Although usually apparent in adulthood, a congenital form of DM1 characterized by neonatal hypotonia, motor, and mental retardation has also been described in a few cases. The muscular abnormalities consist of progressive weakness and atrophy of the facial, neck, and distal muscles of the extremities and by prolonged contraction with inability to relax. Other features include cataracts, cardiac arrhythmias, baldness, primary hypothyroidism, mental retardation, type-2 DM with insulin resistance, and primary testicular failure in up to 80% of these patients.

Hypogonadism in DM1 is a primary testicular disease as suggested by the presence of T levels ranging from modestly decreased to low normal and slightly elevated gonadotropins that "hyperrespond" in gonadotropin-releasing hormone (GnRH) stimulation tests. The disease duration and the degree of testicular atrophy correlate with T and free T levels, suggesting that hypogonadism tends to worsen with age. There is good correlation between the circulating levels of T and the clinical signs of androgen deficiency, which usually are mild. Patients may maintain normal facial and body hair growth, and normal libido. Testicular histology varies from normal to marked tubular atrophy, and/or peritubular hyalinization, with or without loss of the interstitial cells. Testicular size is frequently decreased in association with complete germinal cell destruction. Infertility is reported in as many as 44% of the cases.

Genetic Basis   DM1 is an autosomal-dominant disorder in which the primary genetic defect consists of an amplified trinucleotide (CTG) repeat in the three prime untranslated region of the dystrophia myotonica protein kinase (*DMPK*) gene, which has been mapped on chromosome 19q13.2-13.3. In the normal population, the CTG repeat length ranges from 5 to 30. Severity varies with the number of repeats; mild forms are associated with 50–80 repeats, whereas severe forms have up to 2000 or more copies. Amplification is because of parent-to-child transmission. Extreme amplifications occur almost exclusively in the offspring of affected women. This explains anticipation (increase in severity in successive generations) and that amplification is usually not transmitted through the male line. Myotonia has been reproduced in transgenic mice expressing a human actin gene containing 250 CTG repeats, demonstrating that the expression of CUG-repeat RNA has a deleterious gain-of-function independent of *DMPK*. Developments support a model in which nuclear accumulation of RNA from the expanded allele results in a transdominant effect on RNA processing by altering the function of CUG-binding proteins. A known CUG-binding protein with abnormal phosphorylation and nuclear/cytoplasmic distribution in DM1 cells is CUG-BP, a member of the CELF family of RNA-processing factors that regulates alternative splicing. Increased steady-state level of the splicing regulator, CUG-BP, is present in DM1 skeletal muscle, and this has been associated with abnormal splicing of proteins such as the insulin receptor (IR), resulting in predominant expression of the lower signaling nonmuscle isoform (IR-A). A similar mechanism was detected for abnormal splicing of CLC1, the main chloride channel in muscle, which results in a chloride channelopathy associated with membrane hyperexcitability in DM. Although these findings explain only two of the clinical manifestations of DM1 (i.e., insulin resistance and electrical myotonia), it is likely that the other clinical manifestations will be explained similarly. The mechanism causing hypergonadotropic hypogonadism/infertility in DM1 has not been elucidated, but likely consists in the abnormal splicing of one of the downstream effectors of gonadotropin signaling in the testes.

Treatment   Replacement therapy with T has been advocated for patient with low T to correct the hypogonadism, and to increase and maintain muscular size and strength.

DYSTROPHIA MYOTONICA 2   Molecular analysis of a subgroup of patients with clinical features similar to those of DM1 did not yield mutations in the three-prime untranslated region of *DMPK*. This finding was instrumental in the identification of a parallel disorder, called dystrophia myotonica 2 (DM2/proximal myotonic myopathy), characterized by expansion of a CCTG repeat located in intron 1 of the zinc finger protein 9, ZNF9. DM2 is a dominantly inherited disorder in which clinical features similar to those of DM1 include progressive weakness, myotonia, disease-specific muscle histology, cardiac arrhythmias, iridescent cataracts, male hypogonadism, insulin insensitivity, and hypogammaglobulinemia. Hypergonadotropic hypogonadism was present in most (17 of 26) of the men serologically tested for testicular function and was characterized by elevated FSH, low or low-normal T levels, and oligospermia. By analogy with the mechanism causing DM1, it is thought that intranuclear accumulation of RNA with the microsatellite CCUG may be responsible for the DM2's clinical manifestation by causing accumulation of a CUG-BP-like factor (possibly CUG-BP itself) followed by the abnormal splicing of a variety of proteins.

TESTICULAR REGRESSION SYNDROME (BILATERAL ANORCHIA) This syndrome is also known as congenital anorchia, testicular agenesis, or vanishing testicular syndrome. It is found in approx 1% of boys receiving surgery for bilateral cryptorchidism.

The phenotype detected in these patients correlates with the time of embryological development reached when testicular function became deficient. Individuals in which testicular function became abnormal before 8 wk of gestation develop female internal and external genitalia. Individuals developing abnormal testicular function between 8 and 10 wk of gestation develop an intermediate phenotype, with ambiguous genitalia and variable masculinization of the internal structures. Loss of testicular function after 10 wk of gestation is associated with the development of a normal male phenotype. In each instance, no histological or hormonal evidence for the presence of a functioning testis is available. Hormonal studies are compatible with primary gonadal failure, with high gonadotropin and low T level.

Diagnosis of this disorder should be suspected in patients with anorchia, in whom intra-abdominal gonads cannot be demonstrated by provocative testing or during explorative surgery.

The pathogenesis for the degeneration/disappearance of the testes is controversial as it could result from trauma, vascular insufficiency, or infection. Several sibships with multiple affected individuals have been reported. In one pedigree there was parental consanguinity, suggesting a possible autosomal-recessive transmission.

CARDIOMYOPATHY WITH HYPERGONADOTROPIC HYPOGONADISM Bilateral anorchia was originally reported by Malouf in 1985 in two sisters with congestive cardiomyopathy and ovarian dysgenesis. The association of cardiomyopathy and primary hypogonadism has also been described in male patients. In one case, it was described with mental retardation and cataracts, in another case with a distinctive type of collagenoma in the male members of the family. In the latter kindred, the authors described an autosomal-dominant mode of inheritance.

ALOPECIA-MENTAL RETARDATION SYNDROME WITH CONVULSIONS AND HYPERGONADOTROPIC HYPOGONADISM The initial report of this syndrome was of two brothers who had total alopecia and no scalp hair, eyelashes, or eyebrows at birth. During their first month, they developed tonic-clonic convulsions, which disappeared after age 4. Later in life, they still had alopecia of the scalp but normal eyebrows, and slight mental retardation. Their serum FSH levels were elevated, consistent with hypergonadotropic hypogonadism. Because it is difficult to identify hypergonadotropic hypogonadism before puberty, other similar cases described in prepubescent children may represent the same entity. The genetic basis is not known and may represent a new autosomal-recessive condition.

INSULIN-RESISTANT DIABETES WITH ACANTHOSIS NIGRICANS, HYPOGONADISM, PIGMENTARY RETINOPATHY, DEAFNESS, AND MENTAL RETARDATION This syndrome was initially described by Edwards et al. in 1976 in three males who had small testes, subvirilization, and gynecomastia in association with mental retardation, deafness, retinitis pigmentosa, acanthosis nigricans, and disturbance of glucose metabolism and hyperinsulinism. Siblings with a similar syndrome were subsequently described by Boor et al. in 1993. This syndrome has some general similarities with Alström syndrome, from which it is differentiated by the presence of mental retardation and the absence of renal insufficiency.

HYPERGONADOTROPIC HYPOGONADISM IN AUTO-IMMUNE POLYGLANDULAR SYNDROMES I AND II Male hypergonadotropic hypogonadism is a minor manifestation of autoimmune polyglandular syndromes I and II. The main manifestations of autoimmune polyglandular syndrome I, which usually emerge with high penetrance during the initial 15 yr of life, comprise mucocutaneous candidiasis, hypoparathyrodism, and Addison's disease. The type-II form of the disease appears with lower penetrance in the ensuing years, up to the fifth decade. Hypogonadism has been described in up to 60 and 14% of affected females and males, respectively. Patients affected by the disease show an autosomal-recessive pattern of inheritance. The disorder has a high prevalence in Finland, Sardinia, and consanguineous Iranian Jewish families. The gene responsible for this disease was localized to the short arm of chromosome 21 and identified as *AIRE*. It encodes a DNA-binding protein expressed predominantly in the thymus and in lymphoid tissues. The mechanism through which *AIRE* causes disease is unknown. Main and minor manifestations become evident over a spectrum of several years. Therefore, it is recommended to screen these patients for the development of organ-specific antibodies, abnormal calcium and phosphorus levels, thyroid and liver function tests, and plasma vitamin B12 levels to allow the early detection of new disorders before overt symptoms and signs develop. Steroid producing cell autoantibodies have been positive in all patients with hypogonadism in which they were investigated.

Hypogonadism is associated with autoimmune polyglandular syndrome II in approx 4% of the cases. Although this syndrome aggregates in families, there is no clearly discernible pattern of inheritance. Multiple genetic loci, with human leukocyte antigen having the strongest effect, and environmental factors determine susceptibility.

HYPERGONADOTROPIC HYPOGONADISM FROM RECEPTOR DEFECTS

LH-RESISTANT TESTIS (LEYDIG CELL HYPOPLASIA) It is intuitive that mutations in gonadotropin or gonadotropin receptor genes are rare conditions because they severely affect fertility. However, sporadic mutations have been detected in all gonadotropin subunit genes and their related receptor genes, because heterozygous mutations do not affect fertility. Rarely, homozygous or compound heterozygous mutations have been identified, and the phenotypes of these patients have significantly contributed to the understanding of reproductive biology. Leydig cell hypoplasia is a rare condition associated with homozygous or compound heterozygous inactivating mutations of the LH receptor gene. In 46,XY individuals it is associated with primary testicular failure and a spectrum of phenotypic abnormalities of the internal and external genitalia. It is inherited as an autosomal-recessive disorder. In male patients the main clinical features of this syndrome are ambiguous external genitalia, ranging from extreme forms that present as 46,XY females, usually associated with complete inactivation of the LH receptor gene, to milder forms, usually associated with residual function of the LH receptor, in which phallic development is observed. The internal genitalia consist of a blind ending, rudimentary vagina, owing to the absence of Müllerian derivatives, because of normal production of AMH, and the presence of Wolffian duct-derived structures. The overall phenotype of the complete form is similar to that of complete androgen insensitivity, but no feminization occurs at puberty because there is no production of testicular androgen, which serves as substrate for peripheral aromatization. Complete receptor inactivation is associated with male pseudohermaphroditism but, with incomplete inactivation, the phenotype is that of poor genital masculinization, ranging from micropenis to hypospadias. The histological features of the testis are drastic reduction in the number of Leydig cells and limited germ cell maturation.

Although virilization of the external genitalia is limited in these patients, Wolffian duct-derived structures, such as the vas deferens and the epididymis, have undergone normal embryological development in some cases. This implies that during fetal development these patients' Leydig cells are able to produce androgens despite the inactivating mutations of the LH receptor, suggesting that during early fetal development Leydig cell maturation and androgen production may be independent of LH/human chorionic gonadotropin (hCG) stimulation. Mice with a targeted disruption of the LH receptor have been characterized. Interestingly their phenotype at birth is indistinguishable from wild type of heterozygous littermates, providing conclusive evidence of a phenomenon previously described; rodent fetal testes are able to produce sufficient amounts of T for male differentiation in the absence of gonadotropin stimulation.

Inactivating mutations of the LH receptor have been also described in females, in which the syndrome has a more benign phenotype: primary amenorrhea in the background of normally developed primary and secondary sexual characteristics, a small uterus, normal-sized vagina with hyposecretory function and thin walls and decreased bone mass, indicating osteoporosis resulting from hypoestrogenism. Ovarian histology shows all stages of follicular development, indicating normal FSH function, but, in agreement with lack of LH activity, no preovulatory follicles, or corpora lutea.

Diagnosis These patients manifest a resistance to LH, shown by the elevated level of LH and low level of T. FSH is normal in most cases, and abnormally elevated in a minority of patients. T precursors such as dehydroepiandrosterone (DHEA), 17α-progesterone, progesterone, and androstenedione are low compared to normal males. The GnRH challenge test is associated with an LH "hyperresponse" and with only marginal FSH increase. T is usually completely unresponsive to hCG stimulation.

A clinical picture of abnormal virilization associated with low T and T precursors in the presence of high LH is virtually diagnostic of this syndrome. Alternatives to consider in the differential diagnosis are androgen resistance because of defects in the androgen receptor, type-2 5α-reductase deficiency, and defects of T biosynthesis. Each defect should be differentiated based on the clinical phenotype and hormonal data.

Genetic Basis The association of Leydig cell hypoplasia with an abnormal binding activity of the LH receptor and with the endocrine features described led to the identification of LH receptor mutations in affected patients. Several inactivating mutations of the LH receptor have been identified. Usually mutations associated with major structural abnormalities (i.e., truncation, missense mutations, or insertions causing premature truncation of the sequence) are associated with complete inactivation of receptor function. However, missense mutations are found in patients affected by partial and complete phenotypes.

Molecular Pathophysiology Mutations in the coding sequence of the LH receptor can affect any of the functions of this molecule, including LH binding, G protein activation with subsequent production of cAMP, posttranslational modifications, or postsynthesis transport. Because many mutations have been identified, a comparison is possible between the phenotype of these patients and the residual activity of their LH receptor established by in vitro functional analysis. Mutations associated with complete obliteration of receptor activity, such as Cys343Ser (in the extracellular domain), Cys543Arg (in the fifth transmembrane domain), Ala593Pro (in the sixth transmembrane domain), and those causing premature truncation, are associated with pseudohermaphroditism. In contrast mutations with minimal residual activity, such as Cys131Arg (in the extracellular domain), are associated with micropenis and hypospadias, whereas those with an even more subtle abnormality, such as Ser616Tyr and Ile625Lys (both in the seventh transmembrane domain), are associated with micropenis, the more subtle phenotypic abnormality detected in these patients. Analysis of this mutant receptor showed a low number of hCG-binding sites with normal high affinity, but lack of cAMP production.

Treatment Androgen or estrogen replacement therapy is indicated depending on gender selection. The final choice of how these patients should be raised depends on the same criteria established for patients with other forms of male pseudohermaphroditism. The intra-abdominal gonads should be surgically removed at diagnosis to prevent neoplastic degeneration. It is usually recommended that pediatric patients affected by micropenis should receive a course of T treatment to normalize the size of the phallus.

Inactivating Mutations of the FSH Receptor Gene Few mutations have so far been identified in the FSH receptor gene, which may indicate that the resulting phenotype is subtle and escapes identification, or that a selection mechanism prevents inheritance of FSH receptor mutations based on a strong dominant negative effect on fertility. A population-based study on ovarian dysgenesis has identified the only known inactivating mutation of the FSH receptor. In women, this mutation is associated with ovarian dysgenesis and primary or early-onset secondary amenorrhea with high levels of serum gonadotropins. In contrast, men with the same mutation have normal virilization, normal circulating T, normal or modestly elevated LH, elevated FSH, low inhibin B, and low testicular volume. Although none of these individuals had azoospermia, all of them had some abnormality of their semen analysis, ranging from severe or moderate oligospermia to normal sperm concentration with low volume. Of the five individuals identified two had two children each. Functional analysis of the FSH receptor resulting from this mutation showed near normal binding affinity, but reduced plasma membrane expression, and no activity at the postreceptor level. Hence FSH signaling contributes to testicular size and to the quality of the ejaculate, but it is not essential to male puberty, or to the onset of spermatogenesis. Male FSH receptor null mice produced in the laboratory essentially represent a phenocopy of the patients described earlier.

SYNDROMES OF ANDROGEN RESISTANCE Hypogonadism because of androgen receptor defects is associated with a spectrum of clinical phenotypes, from 46,XY women with the syndrome of complete testicular feminization to phenotypically normal men affected by infertility. The clinical features, endocrinology, biochemistry, and molecular biology of these syndromes are discussed in Chapter 44.

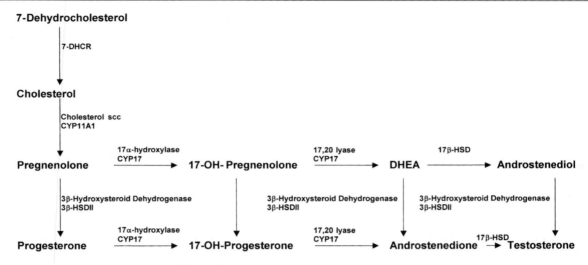

Figure 45-1   Pathway of testosterone synthesis.

HYPERGONADOTROPIC HYPOGONADISM FROM DEFECTS IN T SYNTHESIS IN 46,XY INDIVIDUALS

Several enzymatic steps are necessary for the formation of cholesterol, the common precursor of all steroid hormones. After cholesterol is formed, the StAR (steroidogenic acute regulatory protein) and five well-characterized additional enzymatic steps lead to its conversion to T (Fig. 45-1). A syndrome associated with hypergonadotropic hypogonadism has been described in patients affected by 7-dehydrocholesterol reductase deficiency (7-DHCR-D), the enzyme responsible for the final step leading to cholesterol biosynthesis. Genetic diseases associated with impaired activity of each of the five remaining enzymes and of the StAR also have been described. Because normal production of T by the developing testis is critical for development of the normal male sexual phenotype, abnormalities of these proteins are associated, in 46,XY individuals, with different degrees of male pseudohermaphroditism. Four of these proteins (P450scc, 3β-hydroxy-steroid-dehydrogenase, 17α-hydroxylase, and the StAR) are involved in both cortisol and T biosynthesis. Hence their abnormalities cause a combination of male pseudohermaphroditism and hypoadrenalism. Some of these abnormalities are partial, some become clinically evident only at puberty.

7-DEHYDROCHOLESTEROL REDUCTASE DEFICIENCY OR SMITH–LEMLI–OPITZ SYNDROME   Smith–Lemli–Opitz syndrome (SLOS) is an autosomal-recessive malformation syndrome characterized by mental and growth retardation, ambiguous genitalia, and congenital anomalies like microcephaly, cleft palate, and cutaneous second and third toe syndactyly. From biochemical testing, the disease incidence was estimated at 1 in 40,000–60,000. SLOS is caused by a defect in 7-dehydrocholesterol reductase (7-DHCR), the final enzyme in the pathway leading to cholesterol biosynthesis. Affected individuals usually have low plasma cholesterol levels, and invariably have elevated levels of cholesterol precursors including 7-DHCR. Mildly affected individuals may have only subtle dysmorphic features and learning and behavioral disabilities. Cholesterol is important in cell membranes, serves as the precursor for steroid hormones and bile acids, and is a major component of myelin. Cholesterol is covalently bound to the embryonic signaling protein sonic hedgehog (Shh) in a step necessary for the autoprocessing of the precursor to its active form; this

critical maturation step occurs at about gestational d 0–7 in humans. Thus, defective signaling of Shh early during development may be a reason why these patients present with several congenital abnormalities. Urogenital anomalies are frequent and are most easily recognized in males. Because of easily recognizable genital abnormalities, males are more likely than females to be evaluated for the diagnosis of SLOS. Many 46,XY individuals with severe manifestations of SLOS have undermasculinization of the external genitalia. This results in female external genitalia in up to 20–25% of 46,XY patients with SLOS described. Because the enzymatic abnormality leading to this disease causes inadequate synthesis of the main precursor to all steroid hormones, a major impairment in the level of C21 and C19 steroids would be expected. Although case reports of adrenal insufficiency with biochemical stigmata of impaired aldosterone production have been reported, this type of presentation is unusual. Further, despite the documented inability to synthesize adequate T in some cases, other patients had normal gonadal function. The HP function seems to be normal in most of these patients. A global mechanism explaining the impaired masculinization of these patients has not been identified and additional hypotheses not completely verified include the presence of concomitant androgen receptor insensitivity, or of 5α reductase 2 deficiency.

CONGENITAL LIPOID ADRENAL HYPERPLASIA   The first step in steroidogenesis is the conversion of cholesterol to pregnenolone by the mitochondrial enzyme, P450scc (CYP11A). Pituitary hormones such as adrenocorticotrophic hormone (ACTH) and gonadotropins induce steroidogenesis by interacting with their receptors and changing intracellular cAMP concentrations in the target cells, which induces p450scc activity in two ways. The acute phase, which occurs within seconds to minutes, involves enhanced mobilization and delivery of cholesterol from the outer mitochondrial membrane into the inner mitochondrial membrane to the steroidogenic complex through phosphorylation of pre-existing and rapid synthesis of new StAR. The chronic phase, which requires hours to days, involves increased transcription of the genes implicated in steroidogenesis, including CYP11A. In the absence of StAR, up to 14% of maximal StAR-induced steroidogenesis can persist as StAR-independent steroidogenesis.

Lipoid congenital adrenal hyperplasia (CAH) is a rare autosomal-recessive defect associated with genetic abnormalities of the StAR, in which synthesis of all steroid hormones (estrogens, glucocorticoids, mineralocorticoids, and androgens) is impaired. The responsible gene is located on chromosome 8q24.3. The disease is more prevalent in the far east, where it is the second most common form of CAH.

Many newborn patients with this disease are hyperpigmented, have female external genitalia irrespective of karyotype, suffer a severe form of salt-losing CAH, and accumulate lipids in the gonads and adrenals, causing gross enlargement of these organs. Interestingly, the time of presentation of these abnormalities is not uniform. For instance, adrenal insufficiency may not present until years after birth, whereas hypogonadism usually is severe at birth in males but does not manifest until after puberty in some females. The most likely explanation for this phenomenon is that the disease has a dual mechanism of presentation. The first, which takes place beginning at the time of embryological development, is related to loss of StAR-dependent steroidogenesis. The second, which requires time to develop, consists in progressive engorgement of steroid-producing cells with lipid droplets that ultimately cause cytopathic changes and deterioration of StAR-independent steroidogenic capacity. Male infants with this syndrome present with male pseudohermaphroditism, characterized by female external genitalia with a blind ending hypoplastic vagina, absent uterus and fallopian tubes, hypoplastic Wolffian derivatives, and cryptorchid testes. No virilization is observed at puberty. Heterozygous parents of affected siblings develop normally. The condition is fatal in infancy in two-thirds of the cases.

This disease should be suspected at birth in patients with a salt-losing crisis and the phenotype discussed earlier. Typical enlargement of the adrenals and testes, visible with MRI or CT aids diagnosis. Usually serum cortisol, aldosterone, and T are undetectable; ACTH, FSH, and LH are elevated; and no response is evident following stimulation with ACTH or β-hCG. At puberty a minimal degree of virilization can occur in 46,XY individuals.

Genetic Basis　This disease had previously been ascribed to defects of the P450$_{scc}$ system (CYP11A1), which consists of the cholesterol side-chain cleavage enzyme, and of two electron transfer proteins, termed adrenodoxin reductase and adrenodoxin. This conclusion was based on hormonal studies of affected patients who were unable to produce adrenal and gonadal steroids, and on the inability of mitochondria from affected tissues to convert cholesterol to pregnenelone. A role for P450$_{scc}$ has been excluded in molecular studies of affected individuals, in which abnormalities in the coding sequence of this gene have never been detected. In addition, P450$_{scc}$, adrenodoxin reductase and adrenodoxin genes are normally transcribed and translated in the steroidogenic tissue of affected individuals, suggesting that the lesion responsible for lipoid CAH was located elsewhere. When the role of the StAR became clear, this factor appeared immediately to be the candidate gene responsible for lipoid CAH. Molecular analysis of the StAR confirmed that this factor has a central role in the etiology of lipoid CAH. Mutations affecting both alleles of the StAR gene have been detected in 95% of affected patients. Most families have homozygous mutations; fewer subjects are compound heterozygotes. Interestingly, individuals of Caucasian descent have a large array of different genetic abnormalities, consisting of missense, nonsense, and splice-site mutations, whereas predominant mutations have been detected in patients of Japanese or Arab descent. There is an association between residual StAR activity and time of presentation of certain symptoms. For instance, a compound heterozygous patient presenting with mutations A218V and L275P, each of which maintains approx 20% of StAR activity, survived 4 mo

without hormonal replacement. Another compound heterozygous subject carrying mutations M225P (with 43% of activity) and Q258X (totally inactive), survived for 10 mo without therapy. The importance of these mutations in the etiology of lipoid CAH has been demonstrated by showing that StAR cDNAs carrying these mutations lack the ability to promote pregnenolone synthesis in transfected cells and by the presence of a phenotype similar to the human disease in mice with targeted inactivation of the StAR.

Therapy　Glucocorticoid and mineralocorticoid replacement is the first therapeutic step for these patients. Given the sexual phenotype, most patients are raised as females. Prophylactic orchidectomy followed by estrogen replacement should be performed to prevent the neoplastic degeneration of the retained gonads and to avoid any possible virilization at puberty.

Late-Onset Congenital Lipoid Adrenal Hyperplasia From Heterozygous Mutations in the Cholesterol Side-Chain Cleavage Enzyme (P450scc)　Because P450scc is needed for placental biosynthesis of progesterone, required to maintain pregnancy, it is assumed that inactivating mutations of this enzyme are not compatible with survival. In agreement with this idea, the only identified mutations of P450scc are heterozygous in-frame insertions of Gly and Asp between Asp271 and Val272. The patient was a 4-yr-old 46,XY individual, with atypical features of classic congenital lipoid adrenal hyperplasia consisting in a 4-yr survival without hormonal replacement, before experiencing life-threatening adrenal insufficiency, lack of hypertrophy of the adrenal glands on CT, and some degree of genital virilization, consisting in clitoromegaly. The mutation was found in multiple cell types, but neither parent carried it, suggesting that it arose *de novo* during meiosis. In vitro analysis of the resulting cDNA was associated with total inhibition of enzymatic activity, whereas cotransfection of wild type and mutant cDNAs showed that the mutation did not exert a dominant negative effect. The authors proposed that P450scc haploinsufficiency results in subnormal responses to ACTH, so that continuous ACTH stimulation leads to slow accumulation of adrenal cholesterol, eventually causing cellular damage and a late-onset form of congenital lipoid adrenal hyperplasia explainable with the same two-hit model that has been postulated for congenital lipoid adrenal hyperplasia caused by StAR deficiency, as described earlier.

3β-HYDROXYSTEROID DEHYDROGENASE 2 DEFICIENCY

3β-hydroxysteroid dehydrogenase (HSD) regulates the conversion of Δ^5-3β-hydroxysteroids (pregnenolone, 17-OH pregnenolone, DHEA, and androstenediol) into the corresponding Δ^4-3-ketosteroids (progesterone, 17-OH-progesterone, androstenedione, and T, respectively). Absent or reduced activity of this enzyme is potentially associated with impaired formation of all steroid hormone classes including progesterone, mineralocorticoids, glucocorticoids, androgens, and estrogens. Two isoenzymes with 3β-HSD activity have been cloned, and have been designated type-I and type-II 3β-HSD. Their structural organization consists of four exons and three introns, which are included in a genomic DNA fragment of approx 7.8 kb. The type-I 3β-HSD mRNA is transcribed in the breast, placenta, skin, and, to a much lower degree, in the gonads. The type-II isoenzyme is transcribed exclusively in the adrenals, testis, and ovary. Inactivating mutations of type-II 3β-HSD are responsible for the syndrome.

There is heterogeneity in the clinical presentation of 46,XY individuals affected by this disease. The two major clinical features are incomplete virilization and salt wasting. The degree of salt wasting ranges from life threatening to inapparent. Similarly, virilization defects can range from the development of genital ambiguities (including hypospadias, micropenis, and presence of a blind ending vagina), to, rarely, the development of normal external genitalia. In most instances, the Wolffian ducts derivatives develop normally, suggesting that although the prenatal testes were capable of some androgen production, even though the quantities were insufficient to permit normal development of the sexual phenotype. The Müllerian duct derivatives involute normally, indicating normal production of AMH by the Sertoli cells. At puberty these patients have typical hypergonadotropic hypogonadism with high gonadotropin and low T. The endocrine abnormalities are associated with spermatogenic arrest and phenotypic features of undervirilization. No correlation has been made between the degree of salt wasting and impairment of male sexual differentiation, suggesting that 3β-HSD mutations can affect the different steroidogenic pathways differentially.

The diagnosis of this disorder should be suspected in patients presenting with adrenal and gonadal insufficiency. An elevated ratio of Δ^5- to Δ^4-steroids and significant increase in plasma ACTH levels are characteristic of this disorder; however, the interpretation of the endocrine data can be complicated by the increased level of some Δ^4 steroids, including serum 17-OH-progesterone and Δ^4-androstenedione, and urinary pregnanetriol. This is because of the presence of two 3β-HSD enzymes, of which only type II is mutated.

Genetic Basis   This disease is transmitted as an autosomal-recessive character, and the gene is located in the region p11-p13 of chromosome 1. The identification of two isoenzymes with the same activity and with a different pattern of expression may explain the normal to elevated serum level of some Δ^4-3-ketosteroids in the patient population with 3β-HSD deficiency. Because the disease causes salt wasting and ambiguous genitalia, it would be expected that the type-II isoenzyme (exclusively transcribed in the adrenals and gonads) is the mutated gene and the type-I isoenzyme (transcribed in the periphery) would maintain its activity and be responsible for the residual conversion of Δ^5-3β-hydroxysteroids to Δ^4-3-ketosteroids. Indeed, the molecular abnormalities causing clinical 3β-HSD deficiency have been localized exclusively to the type-II isoenzyme. Additionally it is expected that mutations do not affect the type-I isoenzyme because it regulates progesterone production in the placenta, and lack of placental progesterone production would not be compatible with fetal survival. Numerous mutations in the coding region of the 3β-HSD gene have been identified by sequence analysis, including missense, nonsense, and frameshift mutations, have been detected in homozygous and compound heterozygous patients. Their functional characterization has helped define the functionally important regions of the 3β-HSD gene.

Molecular Pathophysiology   A reproducible correlation exists between the impairment of the enzymatic activity caused by each mutation and the patients' clinical abnormalities. This is particularly true regarding the presence of salt-wasting forms of the disease in which no residual enzymatic activity is detected. Molecular analysis of the 3β-HSD gene of these patients has shown the presence of nonsense mutations (causing the synthesis of prematurely truncated proteins) and missense mutations (causing the replacement of critical amino acids). Mutations causing salt wasting are frequently localized in exon 4. One of the few patients of this group with minimal residual enzymatic activity (0.1–0.3%) was a compound heterozygous carrying two missense mutations (Leu108Trp and Pro186Leu). The presence of such low

level of activity is most likely inadequate to prevent the development of salt wasting.

In patients with nonsalt-wasting forms of the disease, there is residual 3β-HSD activity ranging from 1 to 10%, a level that appears to permit enough mineralocorticoid synthesis to prevent salt wasting. Interestingly, in patients with this milder form of the disease there has not been description of premature stop codons, which are expected to completely abolish 3β-HSD activity, but only of missense or splicing mutations. The mutated amino acid residues are conserved in all members of the vertebrate 3β-HSD isoenzymes described.

Therapy   Therapy involves replacement with glucocorticoids and, if required, mineralocorticoids. Sufficient androgens should be given early in life to correct the microphallus and allow surgical treatment of hypospadias. Normal replacement doses should be given at the time of puberty.

17α-HYDROXYLASE 17,20-LYASE DEFICIENCY   Two important steps of the steroidogenic pathway are regulated by the enzyme 17α-hydroxylase 17,20-lyase (CYP17). The first reaction consists in the 17α-hydroxylation of pregnenolone and progesterone into 17α-hydroxypregnenolone and 17α-hydroxyprogesterone. These C_{21} steroids undergo cleavage of the C-17,20 carbon bond via the 17,20-lyase reaction during the second step, to yield the C_{19}-steroids DHEA and androstenedione.

More than 140 cases with 17α-hydroxylase/17,20-lyase deficiency have been reported; most are affected by the complete and a minority by the partial form of the disease. Also, a number of patients with isolated 17,20-lyase deficiency (ILD) have been described.

Clinical Features   Of the enzymatic activities catalyzed by CYP17, 17α-hydroxylase is critical for the production of both glucocorticoid and sex steroids, whereas 17,20-lyase, is critical for the production of sex steroids only. In theory defects of CYP17 activity could occur as isolated deficiencies of 17α-hydroxylase or 17,20-lyase or as combined 17α-hydroxylase/17,20-lyase deficiency. In practice, only cases with complete or partial 17α-hydroxylase/17,20-lyase deficiency have been described, whereas ILD has been only recently accepted as an independent entity.

In the complete form of CYP17 deficiency, the deficient production of cortisol is associated with a compensatory overproduction of ACTH, which stimulates the synthesis of large amounts of corticosterone, usually found at concentrations 50- to 100-fold higher than normal, and 11-deoxycorticosterone (DOC) and 18-hydroxycorticosterone. Although corticosterone and DOC have a lower affinity to the glucocorticoid receptor than cortisol, their activity is sufficient to prevent the development of overt adrenal insufficiency. As a result of the increased production of corticosterone, DOC and 18-hydroxycorticosterone, affected patients develop retention of water and salt, hypokalemic alkalosis, and hypertension. Suppression of renin and of aldosterone production is usually a feature; however, a few individuals with normal or elevated aldosterone have been reported in the Japanese literature. Deficient production of sex steroids is associated in these patients with hypogonadism and a compensatory overproduction of gonadotropins. Because normal levels of T are necessary during fetal life for the development of the normal male sexual phenotype, affected patients manifest a range of abnormalities of the external genitalia, from an apparent female phenotype with a blind ending vagina to hypospadias or micropenis. The Wolffian derivatives can be hypoplastic or normal, the Müllerian derivatives are normally involuted, and hypoplastic testes may be located intra-abdominally, in the inguinal canal, or in the scrotum. Usually, patients with some form of virilization are thought to have partial deficiency of CYP17 activity. There is lack of correlation between the severity of hypertension and hypokalemia and that of hypogonadism, suggesting that the various mutations of CYP17 can affect formation of C_{21} or C_{19} compounds in different ways.

Patients with ILD do not have hypertension and hypokalemia because adrenal 17α-hydroxylase is normal, and there is adequate production of cortisol. However, in view of 17,20-lyase deficiency, sex steroid production is decreased to a minimum. In 46,XY individuals, this leads to pseudohermaphroditism, intra-abdominal testes, and lack of pubertal development.

Diagnosis   CYP17 deficiency should be considered in every 46,XY patient with a family history of pseudohermaphroditism that suggests an autosomal-recessive inheritance. It is usually recognized in young adults with hypertension, hypokalemia, and ambiguous genitalia. The diagnosis of 17α-hydroxylase deficiency can be confirmed by demonstrating increased serum concentrations of pregnenolone, progesterone, corticosterone, DOC, and 18-hydroxycorticosterone, associated with increased urinary excretion of their respective glucuronidated metabolites. Plasma renin activity, serum cortisol, and aldosterone are usually suppressed and ACTH is elevated. Affected males have low T and elevated gonadotropins. The response to hGC and ACTH stimulation tests are impaired. This steroid pattern applies to patients with combined CYP17 deficiency. In patients with ILD clinical symptoms are usually limited to the sexual phenotype. An important feature of this latter group of patients is the presence of normal serum level of cortisol and DOC and of their urinary metabolites. However, because of the presence of 17,20-lyase deficiency, these patients have increased serum levels of progesterone, 17-OH-progesterone and 17-OH-pregnenolone, increased urinary levels of pregnanetriolone, and decreased serum levels of T and of its precursors.

Genetic Basis   The human $P450_c17$ gene (CYP17) is a single copy gene, located on chromosome 10q24-25. It consists of eight exons and seven introns spanning 6569 bases. Full length cDNA clones have been isolated from adrenal and testicular sources, and have the same nucleotide sequence. When the cDNA clones encoding this enzyme were expressed in cultured cells, the expressed protein displayed both 17α-hydroxylase and 17,20-lyase activities. The molecular and functional analyses of several mutations of the CYP17 gene show that the genetic lesions of 17α-hydroxylase deficiency are random events and that there are not structural features of the gene predisposing to specific abnormalities. Functional analyses of mutations from patients affected by the complete form of CYP17 deficiency show that most impair both 17α-hydroxylase and 17,20-lyase activities, further demonstrating that this gene encodes a protein possessing both enzymatic activities. Only a limited number of mutations have been reported more than once and were detected in unrelated individuals of Guamaian and German-Dutch descent, indicating that this disorder is genetically heterogeneous, unless associated with a specific ethnic group.

Molecular Pathophysiology   The description of the molecular defects and functional abnormalities affecting patients with the complete and incomplete forms of CYP17 deficiency and ILD has elucidated several aspects of this disease. Activation of CYP17 involves a chain of actions including proper anchorage of the enzyme onto the microsomal membrane, heme binding, substrate binding, transfer of electrons from NADPH-cytochrome P-450 oxidoreductase, and O_2 binding. Mutations specifically affecting heme, substrate binding, and electron transferring have been identified.

Combined CYP17 Deficiency   Numerous mutations resulting in loss of both 17α-hydroxylase and 17-20-lyase activity have been identified in the CYP17 gene. Premature termination codons resulting from nonsense mutations or from other abnormalities of the open reading frame (including deletions or insertions of DNA) lead to truncated forms of the protein, which, by being deprived of the C-terminal heme-binding domain, becomes functionally inactive. Complete loss of enzymatic function in three patients with missense mutations has identified residues Ser_{106}, His_{373} and Arg_{440} as critical for the accomplishment of both 17α-hydroxylase and 17-20-lyase activities. Of note is the speculation that the mutation occurring in amino acid residue 106 may affect substrate binding, whereas the two other mutations (His_{373} and Arg_{440}) affect heme binding.

Partial Combined CYP17 Deficiency   Partial deficiency of 17α-hydroxylase and 17-20-lyase has been studied in two patients. One of these patients was a boy with ambiguous genitalia, carrying two different CYP17 mutant alleles: one resulting in an $Arg_{239}Stop$ nonsense mutation and the other causing a $Pro_{342}Thr$ missense mutation. The residual activity of these two alleles was, respectively, 0 and 20% of normal. These data, together with the functional analysis of a 46,XY female with homozygous premature termination codons (with residual functional activity of 0%) and of her normally virilized heterozygous father (thought to have a residual functional activity of 50%), have been useful to understand the amount of 17α-hydroxylase activity necessary for the development of the male sexual phenotype. Because the boy with ambiguous genitalia had a residual activity of 20% and the normally virilized individual described earlier was thought to have a residual activity of 50%, it would appear that the threshold activity necessary to change the sexual phenotype from female to ambiguous male is between 0 and 20%, and to change from ambiguous to normal is between 20 and 50%.

Isolated 17,20-Lyase Deficiency (ILD)   The existence of this syndrome was initially in doubt, because molecular genetics studies in one of the first patients described demonstrated that his mutation was responsible for loss of both 17α-hydroxylase and 17-20 lyase activities. However, the report of two 46,XY Brazilian hermaphrodites with a hormonal picture characterized by normal amounts of 17-hydroxysteroids and severely reduced sex steroids and C_{19} precursors, led to conclusive evidence that this syndrome does exist. Abnormalities in the interaction of CYP17 with redox partner proteins P450-oxydoreductase and cytochrome-b_5 form the biochemical basis for the syndrome of ILD. The unifying mechanism causing ILD consists in the neutralization of positive charges in the redox partner binding site, which results in inhibition of electron transferring from NADPH cytochrome P450 oxidoreductase. In support of this hypothesis, mutagenesis of several positively charged residues of the redox partner binding site, such as Arg347His (or Arg346Ala in the rat sequence), Arg358Gln, Lys89Asn, and Arg449Ala, is associated with selective loss of 17,20 lyase activity.

Treatment consists in replacement with cortisol, which accomplishes suppression of ACTH followed by the normalization of DOC, corticosterone, and 18-hydroxycorticosterone, and by the normalization of renin and aldosterone levels. Adult 46,XY individuals reared as females require estrogen replacement and removal of the abdominal gonads to prevent their malignant

Table 45-3
Features of Isoenzymes With 17β-HSD Activity

Type	17β-HSD deficiency	Size/No. amino acids	No. exons	Chromosome localization	Tissue localization	Cellular localization	Preferred substrate	Preferred cofactor	Catalytic preference
1	Normal	327	6	17q21	Ovaries, placenta	Cytosol	Estrone, estradiol	NADPH	Reduction
2	Normal	387	5	16q24	Endometrium, placenta, liver	Microsomes	androgens, estrogens	NAD+	Oxidation
3	Mutated	310	11	9q22	Testis	Microsomes	androgens, estrogens	NADPH	Reduction
4	Normal	736	24	5q2	ubiquitous	Peroxisomes	estrogens	NAD+	Oxidation
5	Normal	323	9	10p14,15					Reduction
6	Normal	341	9	10p11.2			Estrogens, androgens		
7	Normal			6p21.3	Ovaries, testes, kidney		Estradiol, testosterone and dihydro-testosterone		

HSD, hydroxysteroid dehydrogenase.

degeneration. Adult 46,XY individuals raised as males require androgen replacement, surgical correction of their external genitalia, and, if necessary, orchidopexy.

17β-HSD DEFICIENCY The enzyme 17β-HSD catalyzes the conversion of androstenedione, DHEA, and estrone into T, androstenediol, and estradiol, respectively. As such, it converts two weak precursors, androstenedione and estrone, into two potent hormones, T and estradiol, that, on interacting with high affinity with their receptors, induce their biological effects. The reaction catalyzed by 17β-HSD is reversible. The reduction of the 17 keto group is thought to occur mainly in the testis and ovary, in which it is required for the synthesis of T and estradiol. The oxidation reaction, thought to occur in several peripheral tissues, is important for the inactivation of these two hormones.

Seven different isoenzymes with 17β-HSD activity have been isolated and designated 1 through 5 and 7 through 8 according to the chronological order of their identification. They have different biochemical features, and are expressed in different tissues (Table 45-3). Interestingly, isoenzymes 1 and 3 favor the reduction reaction, whereas types 2 and 4 favor the oxidation reaction. Isoenzymes 2 and 4 have ubiquitous tissue distribution, whereas isoenzymes 1 and 3 are expressed in a more selective way. The mRNA of the type-1 isoenzyme is present in the ovary and placenta, whereas the type-3 mRNA has been detected almost exclusively in the testis. Mutations of type-3 isoenzyme have been associated with 17β-HSD deficiency.

Clinical Features A significant number of patients with classic 17β-HSD deficiency have been reported. The prevalence of the syndrome is particularly elevated in the Gaza strip, in which it is estimated that 1 in 100–150 individuals is affected. The pattern of inheritance is autosomal-recessive. At birth these patients present with female external genitalia, absent Müllerian and normal Wolffian duct derivatives, and undescended testes. Based on this phenotype, gender assignment is female in almost every case. At puberty certain aspects virilize (developing a deep voice, large phallus, and various degrees of body and facial hair) and other aspects feminize (developing variable degree of gynecomastia). Some of these individuals have undergone a change in gender role behavior in parallel with the virilization occurring at the time of

puberty. Impaired 17β-HSD activity explains the abnormal virilization of the external genitalia at birth, the elevated serum level of androstenedione and decreased T, and the enhancement of pituitary gonadotropin production. A milder form of late-onset 17β-HSD deficiency has been identified in three adult patients with gynecomastia and hypogonadism in a study of 48 subjects with idiopathic pubertal gynecomastia. However, DNA sequence analysis of the coding sequence of type-3 17β-HSD has not yielded any abnormality in these patients.

Endocrine Features and Diagnosis The diagnosis should be considered in 46,XY patients presenting with pseudohermaphroditism inherited with an autosomal-recessive pattern. Plasma androstenedione, estrone, and gonadotropins levels are elevated, whereas T and dihydroT are decreased or in the low normal range. Steroid hormone metabolism has been studied in the testes of several affected subjects, and the conversion of androstenedione to T was consistently abnormal. However, other authors have found that the oxidative reaction catalyzed by 17β-HSD was normal in cultured fibroblasts obtained from one patient.

Most of these patients are diagnosed at puberty, when they are referred for failure to menstruate, or because they develop a mixed pattern of virilization and feminization. The diagnosis of 17β-HSD deficiency is more challenging in the newborn. However, the correct interpretation of the endocrine data, and use of dynamic endocrine tests such as the hCG stimulation tests should permit the diagnosis of this disorder in any age group.

Genetic Basis Because of its biochemical characteristics and tissue distribution, type-3 17β-HSD was considered to be a good candidate to cause the clinical abnormalities of 17β-HSD deficiency. Subsequent analysis has identified mutations of this gene in families with the typical phenotypic, endocrine, and genetic features of the syndrome. The mutations detected included missense mutations, splice junction abnormalities, and a small deletion resulting in a frameshift. Patients with the syndrome were most frequently homozygous, but heterozygous, and compound heterozygous have been described as well. The mutation Arg80Gln has been detected in three unrelated families, including a member of the large kindred from the Gaza strip and two Brazilian families. Considering the high incidence of 17β-HSD deficiency in the Gaza strip, screening programs for this mutation may be worthwhile there to detect heterozygosity or for prenatal diagnosis. The real frequency of this mutation in the entire Arab population of the Gaza strip could be very high, considering that homozygous females are asymptomatic, have normal internal and external genitalia, undergo normal sexual development, and have unimpaired fertility.

Molecular Pathophysiology Many of the mutations described have been recreated in vitro and their activity studied in transfected cells. Some are completely inactivating. However, in agreement with biochemical studies performed in the cultured genital skin fibroblasts, mutation Arg80Gln retains a small amount of activity. Detailed analysis of the enzymatic activity of this mutant has revealed a 100-fold decreased affinity for the cofactor NADPH, localizing at least a portion of the NADPH-binding domain to the region surrounding residue 80. These developments in the molecular biology of 17β-HSD deficiency have permitted understanding of why these patients undergo virilization at the time of puberty. The consensus is that androstenedione, produced by the testes in supraphysiological concentrations at puberty, provides the substrate for the extraglandular production of T by one of the other 17β-HSDs that are not impaired in this disorder. However, some clinical features of 17β-HSD deficiency are not completely explained. For instance, it is not clear why the embryonic structures of the developing male genitalia respond to the hormonal abnormalities created by 17β-HSD deficiency in a different way. In this disorder the Wolffian derivatives undergo almost normal virilization during embryogenesis, whereas the external genitalia do not virilize at all, suggesting the presence of an alternative pathway for T biosynthesis *in utero*.

Treatment Patients who are not diagnosed at birth are usually raised as female, and treatment consists of gonadectomy followed by estrogen replacement at the time of expected puberty. When the diagnosis is correctly identified in early infancy and gender reassignment is possible, the patients should receive T treatment at pediatric doses and genitoplasty early in infancy and be replaced with adult doses of T at the time of expected puberty. The basic enzymatic defect persists, and impaired spermatogenesis is present during adulthood.

TYPE-2 5α-REDUCTASE DEFICIENCY The enzyme 5α-reductase is involved in the conversion of T into his powerful 5α reduced metabolites dihydroT. Two isoenzymes have been isolated that share this enzymatic activity, and have been designated types-1 and 2 5α-reductase. The clinical syndrome is associated with mutations of the type-2 isoenzyme (Chapter 44).

HYPOGONADOTROPIC DISORDERS

Several congenital and acquired disorders (*see* Table 45-1) account for hypogonadotrpic hypogonadism (HH). Their common denominator consists in the impaired production of GnRH or of gonadotropins by the hypothalamus and/or pituitary gland. This, in turn results in failure to stimulate the correct production of gonadal steroids, and in a spectrum of clinical manifestations that vary, depending on whether the abnormality developed before birth, before puberty, or after puberty (*see* Table 45-2).

HYPOGONADOTROPIC DISORDERS ASSOCIATED WITH ISOLATED GONADOTROPIN DEFICIENCY

GPR54 DEFICIENCY In primates, the HPG axis is active during neonatal life. It is followed by a period of dormancy during childhood, and it is again triggered to function at puberty. Mechanisms regulating the period of dormancy during childhood, and the awakening at puberty have been unclear. However, knowledge of the central mechanisms regulating sexual maturation at puberty has significantly improved. Based on the clinical observation that patients with HH have partial or complete absence of LH pulsation, and normal responsiveness to physiological replacement with exogenous GnRH, it was established that the defect of endogenous GnRH lies at the level of its synthesis, secretion or activity. Thus, linkage analysis of affected families, and identification of candidate genes has permitted the identification by two groups of GPR54 as a new gene regulating pubertal development. GPR54, a G protein-coupled receptor for a ligand called kisspeptin-metastin, is expressed in the human brain, pituitary gland, and placenta, and was found to have mutations in 4 of 113 cases of HH. Conclusive evidence that GPR54 is part of the pathway triggering pubertal development came from the characterization of the phenotype of a Gpr54$^{-/-}$ mouse. In this mouse, beside lack of pubertal development both in males and females, no significant differences were found between normal and mutant mice in the concentration of GnRH in hypothalamic extracts, and normal ability to synthesize FSH and LH at the level of the pituitary gland. Because both patient and mice with this genetic defect were able to respond to exogenous GnRH with an appropriate, or in the case of a patient, increased release of LH, GPR54 may regulate the release of GnRH at the level of the hypothalamus. The mechanism is still unknown, however, the discovery of GPR34 opens a large number of avenues to further understand the mechanism of how puberty is triggered. For instance, future investigations on potential abnormalities in the biosynthesis/release of the ligand kisspeptin-metastin or on the signaling pathway activated by its interaction with GPR34, have the possibility to uncover new mechanisms of how puberty is triggered and further causes of hypogonadotropic hypogonadism.

KALLMANN SYNDROME The first description of Kallmann syndrome (KS) dates to 1856 by Maestre de San Juan, but it was not until the original description by Kallmann in 1944 that the disease was recognized as an inherited entity. It is found in 1/10,000 newborn males, and in 1/50,000 newborn females, and occurs in both sporadic and familial forms. Sporadic cases are more frequent than familial cases. Owing to its predominance in the male sex, it was initially thought that KS is an X-linked disorder. However, there is convincing evidence that additional forms exist that demonstrate autosomal-recessive and autosomal-dominant forms of transmission. In agreement with this heterogeneous inheritance, abnormal genes have been detected in the X chromosome (*KAL1*) and, in patients with the autosomal-dominant form, in chromosome 8 (*KAL2*). *KAL1* (anosmin-1) and *KAL2* (fibroblast growth factor receptor-1 [FGFR-1]) have been located in the Xp22.3 and 8p11.2-p12 regions, respectively. The gene responsible for the autosomal-recessive form of KS (*KAL3*) has not been identified.

Embryology of the LH-RH Neurons Molecular events associated with the migration of the GnRH-secreting neurons during embryogenesis are intimately connected with the pathogenesis of KS. These neurons originate in the epithelium of the olfactory placode, from where they migrate into the brain by the twelfth week of gestation along the pathway of the developing olfactory tract, represented by the olfactory, terminalis, and vomeronasal nerves. The GnRH neurons enter the brain through the nervus terminalis and vomeronasal, and then course into the septal-preoptic area and the hypothalamus. The normal migration of the GnRH neurons depends on genes located in Xp22.3, the same area of the X chromosome that is deleted in patients with the X-linked form of KS. This was demonstrated in a fetus with KS and a deletion of Xp22.3, in whom GnRH expressing neurons were not found in the hypothalamus, but were instead identified beneath the forebrain, within the dural layers of the meninges and on the cribriform plate. When the migration is completed, there are fewer GnRH neurons in the brain (~1500), than there were in the nose at the beginning of this process, probably because many cells die or differentiate into other cell types during migration. Only after reaching their final destination do the GnRH-containing neurons acquire the capacity to secrete GnRH.

Clinical Features and Diagnosis Individuals affected by KS can sometimes be recognized before puberty because of the presence of microphallus and/or cryptorchidism, heralding fetal T deficiency. Others are recognized at puberty when they present with delayed appearance of the secondary sex characteristics and gynecomastia or for the development of eunuchoid features. Abnormalities observed in KS other than those related to hypogonadism include hyposmia, anosmia, cleft lip, or cleft palate. Other symptoms occasionally described are sensory neural deafness, ocular motor abnormalities, abnormal spatial visual attention, mirror movements of the hands (bimanual synkinesia), cerebellar dysfunctions, congenital cardiac abnormalities, choanal atresia, cleft palate or lips (more commonly seen in the autosomal-recessive form), pes cavus deformity, and unilateral or, in some cases, bilateral renal aplasia. Mental retardation has been described, however, the genotype analysis of these patients showed large deletions on Xp22.3 that extended beyond the Kallmann locus. On the contrary, patients with mutations restricted to the Kallmann locus tend to have normal intellectual function. Regarding the prevalence of anosmia, one of the cardinal symptoms of KS, it was reported that no patient of molecularly confirmed X-linked KS has intact smell although not every patient is aware of it and that tests may be needed for its detection. In contrast, others have reported that anosmia is not present in every patient, and in some large series this feature is absent in up to 50–60% of the cases. Affected females usually have partial or complete anosmia. Some KS patient also manifest other diseases, like chondrodysplasia puntata, ichthyosis, short stature, ocular albinism, and mental retardation, which are associated with large chromosomal deletions, usually of the distal short arm of the X chromosome.

Hypogonadism is due in KS to reduced secretion of GnRH by the hypothalamus; many KS individuals have adequate response of LH and FSH after sufficient priming of the pituitary with exogenous GnRH, although in some cases inadequate responses of LH and FSH to the administration of GnRH and of T to hCG have been shown. Subjects with documented X-linked KS usually have apulsatile LH secretion, whereas those with autosomal-modes of inheritance demonstrate more variably abnormal GnRH-induced LH pulses. The decreased secretion of GnRH results in an abnormal secretory pattern of LH pulses, ranging from decreased or absent amplitude to diminished frequency. In the complete form of GnRH deficiency, LH and FSH deficiency is severe, and no evidence of sexual maturation is evident. In the incomplete form, (known as the fertile eunuch syndrome), there is both normal FSH and low LH, or partial defects in both, with some degree of germ cell maturation. Laboratory tests reveal low serum FSH and LH level, and low T. However, a large degree of heterogeneity in the

serum levels of FSH and LH can be observed. On MRI, bilateral agenesis of the olfactory bulbs or sulci can be seen in greater than 50% of the cases.

The diagnosis is suggested by the typical clinical picture and laboratory tests that demonstrate hypogonadotropic hypogonadism. The most challenging differential diagnosis is with delayed puberty. Important criteria are to show the presence of anosmia or hyposmia, any other associated congenital defect or positive family history for KS. However, the separation of these two entities may require a prolonged period of observation, detailed laboratory investigations, and MRI scans of the head. Testicular biopsies of males show decreased number of germ cells and a spermatogenic state at the primary spermatocyte stage. Leydig cells are not histologically identifiable. Urine gonadotropins have been reported as low in some patients tested. Early diagnosis is important because treatment with chorionic gonadotropin can correct cryptorchidism and establish fertility probably in an age-dependent manner.

Genetic Basis and Molecular Pathophysiogy Using positional cloning techniques, two independent groups isolated the gene for KS (*KAL1*) that is located at the Xp22.3 interval. Evidence that this gene is responsible for KS came from the observation that in some affected patients it contained extensive deletions, or point mutations. The presence of a highly conserved *KAL1* homologue in the Y chromosome has somehow delayed the development of mutations scanning strategies, however, point mutations within the 14 exons of the gene have been detected in a number of patients. In a series of 101 patients with idiopathic hypogonadotropic hypogonadism, 59 had true KS (hypogonadotropic hypogonadism and anosmia/hyposmia), whereas, in the remaining 42, no anosmia was evident. Of the 59 KS patients, 21 were familial and 38 were sporadic cases. Mutations in the coding sequence of *KAL1* were identified in only three familial cases (14%) and four of the sporadic cases (11%) suggesting that confirmed mutations in the coding sequence of the *KAL1* gene occur in the minority of KS cases, and that most cases of KS are caused by other defects. Sequence analysis of the *KAL1* gene product, the extracellular matrix protein called anosmin-1, has provided interesting insights into the pathogenesis of KS. Anosmin-1 is 680 amino acids long and seems to play a key role in the migration of GnRH neurons and olfactory nerves to the hypothalamus. Owing to the lack of a transmembrane domain or a phosphatidyl inositol anchorage site, it is thought to be an extracellular matrix molecule. Of two important motifs in the search for homologies, the first is a four-disulfide core domain found in a number of proteins with protease inhibitory activity that is located in the N-terminal part of the molecule. The second is a region of similarity with the fibronectin type III repeat, found in numerous adhesion molecules involved in axon to axon interaction or in neuronal migration. Based on these sequence homologies, anosmin-1 may represent an extracellular matrix factor that possesses both antiprotease and adhesion (or antiadhesion) functions. This protein may play a critical role in the migration process involving the olfactory and GnRH neurons during embryogenesis. Its absence or abnormal function in KS may help to explain the double clinical defect (hypogonadism, anosmia) observed in many of these patients. In addition, abnormalities of anosmin-1 could also explain some of the other, less frequent, manifestations of the disease. RNA *in situ* hybridization studies have demonstrated *KAL1* mRNA expression in the Purkinje cells of the cerebellum, the nucleus of the oculomotor nerve, the mesonephros and facial mesenchyme, which correlates with the presence in some KS patients of cerebellar dysfunction, eye movement defects, unilateral renal aplasia, and cleft palate.

The *KAL1* gene does not explain the autosomal-type of inheritance in some KS patients. Loss-of-function mutations in the FGFR-1 gene, located in chromosome 8p11.2-11.1, has been described in cases with the autosomal-dominant form of KS (*KAL2*). In four familial cases and eight sporadic cases, heterozygous mutations of FGFR-1 were detected: one nonsense mutation, two frameshift mutations, two donor splice-site mutations, and seven missense mutations. FGF signaling is involved in a variety of developmental processes, including organogenesis. Interactions between FGF, the FGF receptor and heparan sulfate proteoglycans are necessary for the induction of receptor dimerization and autophosphorylation of intracellular tyrosine residues that may stimulate tyrosine-kinase activity in the receptor, or serve as docking sites for downstream signaling molecules. The mutations in FGFR-1 could hinder the formation of functional receptor dimers interfering with the normal development of the olfactory bulb. It is also possible that, in subjects with KAL-1 mutations, anosmin-1 is involved in FGF signaling by binding to heparan sulfate proteoglycans that are essential for FGFR-1 dimerization, and that the higher prevalence of the disease in males is because of gender difference in anosmin-1 dosage, because KAL1 partially escapes X inactivation. Based on this, it would be expected that the higher production of anosmin-1 in females maintains FGFR-1 signaling also in conditions of haploinsufficiency. In agreement with this hypothesis, in four of the five families in whom FGFR-1 mutations were detected, the abnormality was transmitted by an asymptomatic mother.

HH FROM BIOLOGICALLY INACTIVE MEMBERS OF THE HP AXIS

Abnormalities occurring in the sequences of the genes encoding GnRH, the GnRH receptor (GnRHR), LH or FSH have the potential to explain some cases of idiopathic HH or infertility in males. As discussed later, individuals with mutations of all these genes, except GnRH, have been described in patients. These mutations are rare, because they severely affect fertility. However, because heterozygous mutations of these genes do not affect fertility, occasional homozygous or compounded heterozygous have been detected, and have elucidated the functions of the two gonadotropins in conditions in which the activity of one of them has been selectively eliminated. Unlike the gonadotropin receptor genes in which mutations causing both loss- or gain-of-function have been identified, mutations occurring in the genes of the HP axis are invariably inactivating.

GnRH GENE MUTATIONS Evidence supporting the possibility that mutations of the GnRH gene are associated with hypogonadotropic hypogonadism is illustrated by the hpg mouse, an animal model with hypogonadism and infertility because of a deletion of the GnRH gene. In this animal model, reintroduction of a wild type GnRH gene restores a normal phenotype and reproductive functions. Despite a significant number of studies, no mutations in the sequence of the GnRH gene have been detected in humans so far.

GnRH RECEPTOR MUTATIONS The GnRHR gene is located in chromosome 4q21.2. It consists of three exons and encodes a heptahelical transmembrane G protein-coupled receptor. On binding GnRH, GnRHR activates phospholipase C, which then causes intracellular accumulation of inositol triphosphate,

mobilization of calcium, and eventually release of LH and FSH. Mutations of GnRHR represent the first identified autosomal-recessive cause of HH. Prevalence is 17 and 40% among all sporadic and autosomal-recessive cases of HH, respectively. Identified mutations associate with a broad spectrum of phenotypes, ranging from the mild abnormalities seen in the fertile eunuch syndrome, to severe cases of complete GnRH resistance. Regardless of the phenotypic impairment, all these patients have normosmia. Male patients display small testes and micropenis, whereas cryptorchidism is observed in some cases. T, LH, and FSH levels are usually low, although in patients affected by the syndrome's incomplete form, the concentration of these hormones can be within the normal range. Studies using GnRH stimulation have confirmed that many of these patients have the incomplete form of the syndrome, as only 25% failed to respond to a single IV injection of 100 µg. Similar conclusions can be reached in patients tested with pulsatile administration of GnRH; lack of any response was observed in 50%, whereas the remaining exhibited loss of spontaneous LH pulsatility or reduced amplitude of LH peaks with normal frequency. Most affected patients are compound heterozygotes, and mutations in Q106R and R262Q represent hot spots identified in unrelated pedigrees. Homozygosity is usually associated with a more severely affected phenotype. Expression of mutated receptors in heterologous cells has shown either GnRH-binding defects, or decreased activation of phospholipase C. In many cases the mutated receptors maintained some activity, and this explains the lack, in some patients, of a typical phenotype.

MUTATIONS IN THE CODING SEQUENCE OF GONADOTROPIN SUBUNIT GENES Four glycoprotein hormones are known, LH, FSH, hCG, and thyroid-stimulating hormone (TSH). They are composed of a common α-subunit and a specific β-subunit, which undergo coupling through noncovalent interactions. Subsequently, each dimer undergoes post-translational modifications consisting in glycosylation at a variety of sites. FSH is essential in males to stimulate Sertoli cell function and spermatogenesis, whereas LH induces T production by the Leydig cells.

No germ-line mutation in the common α-subunit gene has been identified. Only one somatic mutation has been detected in this protein in a patient affected by a carcinoma. The resulting mutated common α-subunit was unable to couple with the β-subunit of the other glycoprotein hormones. The fact that no human germ-line mutations of the common α-subunit have been detected probably implies that they are lethal, as they would prevent the formation of all glycoprotein hormones and of the vital functions mediated by some of them.

MUTATIONS OF THE β-SUBUNIT OF THE LH GENE In males, only one case of hypogonadism with infertility has been associated with mutations of the LH gene. The propositus of this study was a 17-yr-old patient with a hormonal profile showing low T, high immunoreactive LH, and normal FSH. A testicular biopsy revealed arrest of spermatogenesis, and the absence of Leydig cells. When this patient was treated with exogenous hCG, a normal increase in T secretion occurred, which was in contrast with the initial diagnosis of primary hypogonadism. Subsequently, the LH of this patient was found to be devoid of biological activity using a dispersed Leydig cell bioassay, suggesting the production of an immunologically active but biologically inactive LH molecule. Sequence analysis of the coding sequence of the LH gene revealed the patient to be homozygous for a missense mutation, Q to R at amino acid residue 54. Functional experiments have shown that this mutation impairs the ability of the resulting LH to bind and activate its receptor. This study was extended to other members of the family, including three maternal uncles and the mother of the propositus, and has elucidated how heterozygous carriers of both sexes manifest clinically. The mother, an obligate heterozygote, underwent normal puberty and was fertile. The three heterozygous maternal uncles underwent normal puberty, reported normal libido and sexual performance, and had a normal physical examination. However, their serum T concentration was low on several occasions, and at the time of the study they were childless. Therefore, given the limited nature of the pedigree, it would appear that heterozygous mutations of the LH gene do not present with important clinical abnormalities in the female sex, but may be associated with infertility in males.

Although mutations of the LH gene causing hypogonadism and infertility have only been detected in one male patient, the description of this case report has permitted a better understanding of the physiological role played by LH during the embryological development of the male sexual phenotype. The proband of this study was born with normal masculinization of his genitalia and with descended testes. Thus, LH may not be critical for normal male sexual development, and during embryogenesis adequate amounts of androgens from the adrenals or the testes are produced, probably under the stimulation of placental hCG. Pituitary LH starts having a role in regulating testicular function only after birth, which explains why this patient was born with a normal phenotype, but failed subsequently to produce the T necessary to induce pubertal development.

Variants of the β-Subunit of the LH Gene   A relatively common variant of the β-subunit of the LH gene was identified as a consequence of anomalous LH assay results that employed a variety of monoclonal antibodies to detect LH in serum in a normally cycling woman who had two children. One of the antibodies, raised against an epitope present only in the intact LH dimer, failed to detect any LH-related immunoreactivity in this woman. Sequence analysis identified a genetic variant (V-LH) of the gene consisting of two missense mutations in the same allele: W8R and I15T. This V-LH allele has been found in Japan, in 28% of the normal Finnish population, 28.3% of Australian aborigines, and >10% of Northern Europeans. Consequences of these two mutations are that I15T introduces an additional glycosylation signal, whereas W8R is responsible for the lack of immunoreactivity of V-LH to the specific antibody described earlier. The V-LH form is more active than wt-LH, but has a shorter half-life of 26 vs 48 min. Interestingly, eight point mutations have been identified in the promoter of the V-LH allele, which account for an increased transcription/synthesis of the gene. Thus, the decreased half-life of the V-LH allele is somehow compensated by increased synthesis. Although this allele has been related to recurrent spontaneous abortions, menstrual irregularities, and polycystic ovarian disease in females, in males it has been associated with a delay in the progression of puberty in boys and with increased prevalence in elderly men of low T and high LH concentrations.

MUTATIONS OF THE β-SUBUNIT OF THE HCG GENE
Of the six hCG β-subunit genes present in the human genome, only number five is highly expressed. Sequence analysis of this gene has identified a V79M mutation in 4.2% of the general population. This polymorphism has been detected only in the heterozygous form. This mutated β-subunit of the hCG gene is less likely to associate with the common α-subunit, however the activity of the

resulting dimer is normal. The fact that this polymorphism was present only as a heterozygous character implies that it is probably lethal when present in both alleles.

MUTATIONS OF THE β-SUBUNIT OF THE FSH GENE
Mutations in the sequence of the β-subunit of the FSH gene have been reported in women with a phenotype characterized by primary amenorrhea, absence of thelarche, and infertility. Replacement with exogenous FSH induced follicular maturation, ovulation, and pregnancy. In view of its central role in spermatogenesis but not steroidogenesis, infertility would be the abnormality expected to be associated with inactivating FSH mutations in males. In agreement with this, all patients described were referred initially for work up of azoospermia. The first patient presented with azoospermia, normal puberty, absent FSH, normal LH and T, and had a C82R mutation (not studied in vitro). The second patient had delayed puberty, and endocrine studies showed undetectable FSH, low T, and elevated LH in addition to azoospermia. Similarly to one of the females described, he was found to have a 2 bp deletion in codon 61. The first patient was treated without success with exogenous FSH, suggesting that his azoospermia potentially was caused by unidentified abnormalities. Based on the expected phenotype of FSH deficiency, it is not clear why the second patient presented with Leydig cell hypofunction. The possibility that FSH may be required also for steroidogenesis is a possibility, however, because other models of FSH inactivation (such as inactivating mutations of the FSH receptor) and the other patient with a mutation the β-subunit of the FSH gene did not have abnormalities in testicular androgen synthesis. Additional cases need to be identified to better understand the role of FSH action in males.

HYPOGONADOTROPIC HYPOGONADISM FROM MUTATIONS OF GENES CAUSING COMBINED PITUITARY HORMONE DEFICIENCIES

Abnormalities of transcription factors required for ontogenesis of the pituitary gland can cause HH with or without deficiencies of other pituitary hormones. Pituitary transcription factors associated with combined pituitary hormone deficiency have been described and include the PROP1, HESX1, and LHX3 genes. Patients with anomalies of these genes are affected by variable forms of hypopituitarism presenting with a clinical spectrum ranging from GH deficiency to panhypopituitarism. Usually ACTH secretion is spared.

HESX1 mutations are associated with septo-optic dysplasia. The clinical manifestations are clearly present when both alleles are affected; however, heterozygous mutations of this gene have been described in association with milder forms of hypopituitarism. Functional analysis of HESX1 genes mutagenized to incorporate the mutations detected in patients was performed in heterologous cells and showed altered DNA-binding activity of this transcription factor.

Mutations of LHX3 are associated with hypopituitarism and a form of rigid cervical spine that prevents dissociation of head and trunk movements. Pituitary hypoplasia is usually present, and detectable by MRI. The mutations described prevent the transcriptional activity of this homeobox gene by inhibiting its DNA-binding ability.

PROP-1-deficient patients have an autosomal-recessive form of GH, TSH, prolactin, and gonadotropin deficiency. From a molecular point of view, PROP-1 fails to work as a transcription factor in response to missense mutations or deletions of the coding sequence. PROP-1 expression in the developing pituitary gland is necessary for the expression of PIT1, another important transcription factor for pituitary development. However, unlike patients with inactive PROP-1, PIT1 deficiency is associated with lack of GH, prolactin and TSH, but not of LH and FSH secretion.

HYPOGONADOTROPIC HYPOGONADISM FROM MUTATIONS OF GENES ASSOCIATED WITH OBESITY

LEPTIN AND LEPTIN RECEPTOR   Mutations of the leptin and leptin receptor genes are associated with morbid obesity, insulin resistance, hyperphagia, and hypogonadotropic hypogonadism. Although these mutations are extremely rare, they have been instrumental in clarifying the role played by leptin and leptin-R in controlling food intake. Interestingly, patients with mutations of the leptin gene have been treated with recombinant leptin and this therapy has achieved not only weight normalization, but also induction of puberty. Although these data clearly describe a central role for the leptin–leptin receptor axis in the induction/progression of puberty, it is not clear whether leptin has a direct action on hypothalamic structures regulating pubertal development, or if it sensitizes the hypothalamus to the action of other neuropeptides.

PROHORMONE CONVERTASE-1 (PC1)   Prohormone convertase-1 (PC1) is an endopeptidase required for the post-translational modification of hormones required for the normal initiation/maintenance of puberty. A patient with a compound heterozygous lesion of the PC1 gene has been described with a clinical presentation consisting of extreme obesity, HH, adrenal insufficiency and hypoinsulinemia. Interestingly, the levels of precursor hormones such as proinsulin and POMC were elevated, suggesting that lack of PC1 activity is associated with an inability to correctly process prohormones into the final, active product. HH would therefore be the consequence of a defective processing of hormones or neuropeptides involved in the development of normal HP anatomy and physiology.

HYPOGONADOTROPIC HYPOGONADISM ASSOCIATED WITH CENTRAL NERVOUS SYSTEM DISORDERS

Several congenital syndromes exist in which central nervous system disorders are associated with hypogonadotropic hypogonadism (Table 45-4). One hypothesis is that these disorders may be the consequence of a spectrum of congenital abnormalities simultaneously disrupting the neuronal pathways for the GnRH neurons in the hypothalamus and normal CNS development. The identities and function of the gene(s) responsible for this group of syndromes are unknown.

PRADER–WILLI SYNDROME   Prader–Willi syndrome (PWS) is an unusual condition occurring in 1 of every 10,000–25,000 newborns. It is generally sporadic, although families with more than one case have been described. At least four genetic abnormalities are associated with PWS, and each of them leads to a common mechanism of disease consisting in silencing the expression of paternal genes consists between 15q11-q13. The most common genetic abnormality described in 70–75% of PSW patients is a large deletion of 15q11-q13, which is paternal in origin. An alternative mechanism observed in 25% of the cases consists of maternal uniparental disomy. Under these circumstances the presence of a second structurally normal maternal chromosome 15 does not complement the missing paternal chromosome, and the

Table 45-4
Syndromes Associated With Central Nervous System Disorders

Syndrome	Clinical and genetic features
Prader–Willi	See text
Möbious	See text
Laurence-Moon-Biedl	See text
Börjeson-Forssman-Lehman	X-linked mental retardation (XLMR) syndrome, mapped to Xq26-27. Associated with ptosis, hypotonia, mental retardation, hypogonadism
LEOPARD	Lentigenes, ECG conduction defects, ocular hypertelorism, pulmonic stenosis, retarded growth, deafness, hypogonadism
Rud's	Mental retardation, epilepsy, hypogonadism, ichthyosis
Loewe's	XLMR syndrome mapped to Xq26. Associated with cataracts, renal tubular acidosis, hypogonadism, hypotonia mental retardation.
Carpenter's	Obesity, acrocephaly, craniosynostosis, agenesis of the hands and feet

result consists in production of the same PWS phenotype observed in the case of large deletions of paternal origin. Of PWS patients, 5% inherit a copy of chromosome 15 from each parent, but they have abnormal DNA methylation and gene expression throughout the imprinted 15q11-q13 region. Finally, a few rare cases have a balanced translocation in 15q11-q13. The described mechanism of disease suggests that the maternally inherited PWS gene(s) are silent and only the paternally inherited PWS gene(s) are expressed. Because a parallel clinical condition known as the Angelman syndrome has been described in which the segment of DNA between 15q11-q13 is only paternal, both maternal and paternal contributions of chromosome 15q11-q13 are required for normal development. This pattern of inheritance—when expression of a gene depends on whether it is inherited from the mother or the father—is called genomic imprinting. The mechanism of imprinting is uncertain, but it may involve DNA methylation.

Clinical Features   The PWS phenotype is characterized by muscular hypotonia, infantile feeding problems or failure to thrive, childhood obesity associated with insatiable appetite, carbohydrate intolerance/type 2 DM, short stature, mental deficiency, infantile hypotonia, small hands and feet, a characteristic face, and hypogonadism. The latter is present in 95% of the cases, is mostly because of GnRH deficiency, and is associated with cryptorchidism, micropenis, and scrotal hypoplasia. Some of these patients have undergone testicular biopsy, and the microscopic picture consisted in few germ cells, thickening of the tubular basement membrane, and presence of Leydig cells. Puberty is generally delayed, and in some individuals it never occurs. Premature puberty has been described in two cases. Pubertal growth spurt and bone maturation are also compromised in PWS. GH secretion is impaired, partly resulting from a reduced level of circulating sex steroids, and partly resulting from an intrinsic depression of GH level. The responses of serum gonadotropin concentrations to a single GnRH bolus are usually attenuated, however long-term treatment with clomiphene or GnRH may stimulate gonadotropin secretion. These observations suggest the possibility that in PWS gonadal function is impaired in part by a hypothalamic defect preventing normal production of GnRH, and in part to primary testicular dysgenesis and poor spermatogenesis.

Genetic Basis   Several of the genes in the PWS deletion region are subject to genomic imprinting *(SNRPN, ZNF127, IPW, PAR1, PAR5, PW71,* and *NECDIN)*. This explains that the PWS phenotype only results when the paternally contributed PWS region is absent. However, the precise cause of PWS is unknown. The only identified protein products are those for the *SNRPN* and *ZNF127* genes. *SNRPN* is a small ribonuclear protein involved in alternative mRNA splicing; gene expression occurs only in the paternally inherited chromosome and is primarily in brain and heart.

No abnormal gene product associated with PWS has been identified. Considering the role played by SNRPN in mRNA splicing and the complex phenotype of PWS, one is tempted to speculate that a malfunctioning SNRPN contributes to PWS by altering the expression of several different and unrelated genes. A mouse model of PWS has been developed with a large deletion that includes the SNRPN region and the PWS "imprinting center" and shows a phenotype similar to infants with PWS.

These and other molecular biology techniques may lead to a better understanding of PWS and the mechanisms of genomic imprinting.

Whether any of these genes is directly involved in the phenotype of PWS is under investigation.

Treatment   Treatments are carried on throughout the life of these patients, beginning at birth when they receive enteric gastric tube feeding because of their feeding difficulties. It is important to prevent excessive weight gain, because this is associated with increased risk of type 2 DM and of cardiovascular diseases. GH replacement has a positive effect on linear growth, which appears to be sustained for up to 4 and 5 yr. Patients should undergo correction of their cryptorchidism to prevent future development of testicular neoplasia. Whether sex steroids replaced is appropriate for these patients is controversial. It would be desirable to promote development of the secondary sexual characteristics and bone mass; however, these patients are also known for behavioral problems such as temper tantrums and violent outbursts. The general consensus is that low replacement doses of T should be offered, and if aggressiveness increases, T treatment should be discontinued.

LAURENCE–MOON–BIEDL SYNDROME   This syndrome has traditionally included the association of retinitis pigmentosa, obesity, mental retardation, polydactyly, spastic paraparesis, and hypogonadism. Two syndromes with different manifestations are recognized. The Laurence–Moon syndrome, associated frequently with spastic paraparesis and rarely with polydactyly, and the Bardet–Biedl syndrome, with frequent occurrence of dystrophic extremities and renal disease, and rare neurological manifestations. Hypogonadism is present in both syndromes, manifesting as microphallus, hypospadias and undescended testes. There is disagreement on the origin of testicular failure as cases of both primary and secondary hypogonadism have been reported. The disease is transmitted as an autosomal-recessive character, as indicated by a consanguinity rate of 48% among parents of affected patients in one series, and by a male to female ratio of 47/41 by combining two large studies.

MÖBIOUS SYNDROME   Möbious syndrome, also known as congenital oculofacial paralysis, is associated with multiple cranial nerve paralyses (III, IV, V, IX, X, XII) mental retardation, gait disturbances, peripheral neuropathy, and hypogonadism.

Gonadotropin deficiency has been documented in several patients; however, considering the normal gonadotropin response to GnRH, GnRH deficiency is likely to constitute the primary defect. It is transmitted as an autosomal-dominant trait, although sporadic cases have also been described. The clinical characteristics of other syndromes belonging to this group of diseases are summarized in Table 45-4.

HYPOGONADOTROPIC HYPOGONADISM ASSOCIATED WITH ADRENAL INSUFFICIENCY

ADRENAL HYPOPLASIA CONGENITA   Adrenal hypoplasia congenita (AHC) is a rare congenital disorder, in which HH is associated with adrenal insufficiency. The AHC gene was cloned from the dosage-sensitive sex reversal region of the human chromosome Xp, which when duplicated produces feminization of 46,XY individuals. The gene contains two exons, and encodes a protein known as DAX-1 (DSS-AHC critical region of the X chromosome, gene 1). The AHC gene is located in Xp21, in close proximity to genes associated with mental retardation, Duchenne muscular dystrophy, and glycerol kinase deficiency. Thus, AHC is frequently associated with Duchenne muscular dystrophy, glycerol kinase deficiency, or mental retardation.

Clinical Features   AHC usually presents with symptoms of adrenal insufficiency early in infancy or childhood, because of an inappropriate development of the adrenal glands. This presentation may be confused with CAH. However, unlike CAH patients, AHC is associated with lack of hyperandrogenism, and absent response to exogenous corticotropin. At birth, the testes are undescended in up to 50% of infants with AHC. However, failure to develop secondary sexual characteristics at puberty is the typical presentation. Heterogeneity in the clinical presentation represents another feature of this syndrome. For example, in some individuals adrenal insufficiency becomes apparent only during adulthood, and in others HH may be only partial. Additionally, in some pedigrees the same mutation has manifested itself with a large spectrum of phenotypes, ranging from adrenal insufficiency to HH, or absence of a distinctive phenotype.

Genetic Basis   DAX-1, a new member of the nuclear hormone receptor superfamily, is deleted in AHC deletion patients, and point-mutated in AHC nondeletion patients. It is a putative transcriptional silencer, whose endogenous ligand has not been identified. It is essential for the development of the pituitary gonadotrophs and adrenal cortex, and it inhibits the transcription of SF-1. It regulates gonadotropin secretion both at the hypothalamic and pituitary level. Dynamic tests of affected individuals indicate defective GnRH production and pulsatile secretion of LH. Based on studies performed at different ages in affected individuals, the effects of DAX-1 on gonadotropin secretion are detectable only after puberty. More than 80 mutations of the DAX-1 gene have been identified in affected individuals, and they consist in frameshift, nonsense, and missense mutations, most of which are located in the COOH-terminal region of the molecule. Sequence analysis of the DAX-1 gene also has been performed in 100 males with HH of unknown etiology, but no mutations were detected suggesting that in the general population affected by HH, DAX-1 abnormalities are uncommon, unless the subject is affected by concomitant adrenal insufficiency. Targeted inactivation of the DAX-1 mouse analog (Ahch) has been performed, and the resulting normal phenotype in female mice indicates that unlike initial speculations DAX-1 is not an ovary-determining gene. Interestingly,

meiosis; they progress to the dictyotene stage of the first meiotic prophase in which they remain arrested until they are ovulated. Oocytes that do not enter meiosis undergo apoptosis. Formation of primordial follicles (Fig. 46-1A) begins at approx 16 wk gestation and is complete by 6 mo after birth.

Other factors might also play a role in follicle formation. Involvement of gonadotropins or other pituitary factors in the process of follicle formation is suggested by the poorly organized rete ovarii and inefficient follicle formation in monkeys that were hypophysectomized *in utero*. The Booroola Merino and Inverdale strains of sheep, studied because of their increased rate of multiple gestations, have delayed, or defective follicle formation. Homozygotes for the Booroola mutation FecB^B show delayed follicular formation and growth, whereas homozygotes for the Inverdale mutation FecX^I show a total failure of development past the primary stage. The FecB gene has been identified as the type-I receptor for bone morphogenic protein (BMPRIB). FecX has been localized to a region that contains BMP15, also known as growth and differentiation factor (GDF)-9B. It is not clear what role these factors play in human folliculogenesis.

INITIAL RECRUITMENT AND EARLY FOLLICLE GROWTH
Primordial follicles (*see* Fig. 46-1A) can begin further development at any time after their formation, or they might remain dormant for more than 50 yr. As a primordial follicle begins to mature, the granulosa cells become cuboidal and divide to form several layers around the oocyte (Fig. 46-1B). The zona pellucida, a glycoprotein layer around the oocyte that is formed by both granulosa cells and the oocyte, appears as the granulosa cells differentiate. A distinct theca layer begins to condense around the follicle and becomes vascularized. Because the theca is separated from the avascular granulosa by a basement membrane, access of serum proteins to the granulosa and oocyte is functionally limited. As both the granulosa and theca cells continue to divide and the oocyte increases in size, a fluid collection known as the antrum develops within the granulosa layer. Follicular fluid is a transudate from the thecal vasculature, but also contains proteins secreted by granulosa cells, many of which are paracrine factors important for continued follicular development.

How primordial follicles are maintained in a relatively static condition for decades and then induced to grow and differentiate is poorly understood. Primordial follicles do not demonstrate differentiated function, suggesting that these follicles or the surrounding stroma either express suppressors, or fail to express activators, of the genes that initiate follicular development. When small portions of ovary are removed and grown in organ culture, most of the primordial follicles begin growth all at once. This suggests that when primordial follicles are within the ovary, there is suppression of their activation that is not present in the organ culture environment.

It has been hypothesized that interaction of oocytes and granulosa factors might play a role in initiating follicle growth. Two factors that might be involved in this process are c-kit and GDF-9. In the mouse, GDF-9 and the closely related GDF9B are expressed in oocytes at the primary through preovulatory follicle stages, and are necessary for follicular development past the early secondary stage. Female mice deficient in GDF-9 are infertile and resistant to gonadotropin stimulation, despite the expression of gonadotropin receptors in their ovaries. Granulosa cells secrete kit ligand and the c-kit receptor is expressed by oocytes. When cultured ovarian fragments are treated with kit ligand, there is increased primordial follicle activation. GDF-9 treatment enhances kit ligand expression in

granulosa cells, but kit ligand treatment inhibits oocyte expression of GDF-9 and GDF-9B (also known as BMP-15). Some investigators have hypothesized that complex negative and positive feedback loops regulate oocyte–granulosa interactions and that the balance of these factors is what ultimately controls the initiation of follicle growth. Experiments with reconstituted follicles incorporating granulosa or oocytes missing various factors implicate the oocytes as playing a critical role in upregulating expression of granulosa-derived factors that continue the process of follicle development.

Suppression of growth might be as important a factor in controlling folliculogenesis as active initiation of growth. A candidate suppressor of granulosa cell differentiated function is the product of the Wilms' tumor gene, WT1, a zinc-finger transcription factor. In rodents, high levels of WT1 are expressed in the gonadal ridge and in the granulosa cells of primordial follicles and lower levels in primary and early secondary follicles, but minimal levels in more developed follicles. WT1 represses the expression of inhibin-α, insulin-like growth factor (IGF)-II, IGF-I receptor, early growth response gene 1, PAX-2, platelet-derived growth factor (PDGF)-A, colony stimulating factor 1, and TGF-α. By suppressing the expression of growth and differentiation genes, WT1 might act on early follicles as a "stasis factor," and as the level of WT1 falls, the rate of follicular development increases. Further studies should elucidate the regulation of WT1 expression, as well as the interaction of WT1 with other genes involved in follicular development. Though positive and negative regulators of growth and development might have a role in initial follicle development, why one follicle grows and another nearby follicle remains dormant is still a mystery.

DYNAMICS OF FOLLICLE GROWTH   Once entering the growing pool, most growing follicles progress to the antral stage, at which point they inevitably undergo atresia. After puberty, a small number of the antral follicles can be rescued by gonadotropins to continue growth, and normally one Graafian follicle is formed each month in preparation for ovulation. Antral follicles (2–5 mm in diameter) develop into Graafian follicles in only 14 d during the follicular phase of the menstrual cycle, although more than 85 d are needed for late secondary follicles to grow into preovulatory follicles. In addition, it has been estimated that more than 120 d are needed for primary follicles to grow into the secondary stage and even longer for the development of primordial follicles into primary follicles. Thus, several menstrual cycles are required for progression through the early stages of follicle development. Follicles are exposed to multiple cycles of gonadotropin fluctuations through their development. The role of cyclic, rather than tonic, gonadotropins has not been investigated in early follicle development.

Early follicular growth can occur in the absence of gonadotropin stimulation, as evidenced by the presence of preantral follicles in the ovaries of anencephalic infants as well as in gonadotropin-deficient patients. Although larger antral follicles are clearly dependent on gonadotropin for further mitosis and differentiation as well as protection from apoptosis, several in vitro studies of rodent follicles have suggested a role for follicle-stimulating hormone (FSH) in earlier follicle development as well, perhaps in conjunction with activin or other factors. Many factors such as IGF-1, TGF-β, Müllerian inhibitory substance, bone morphogenic proteins, keratinocyte growth factor, fibroblast growth factors FGFs, hepatocyte growth factor, and vascular endothelial growth factor VEGF have been proposed to affect preantral follicle growth and development (Table 46-2). The exact roles of the

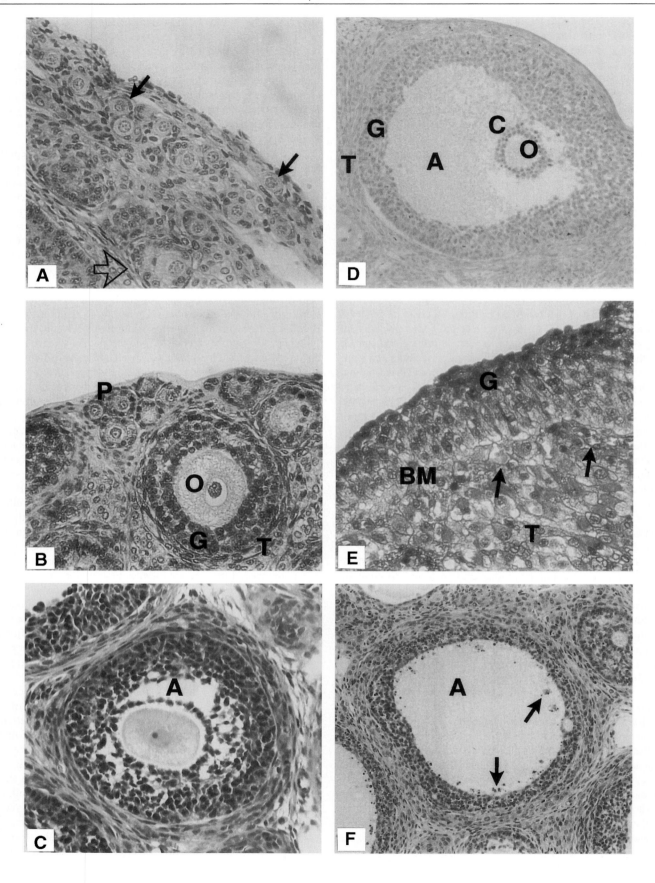

Table 46-2
Growth Factor Actions

Growth factor	Action
Tyrosine kinase receptors	
Insulin/IGF-I/IGF-II	Possibly increase early follicle growth; enhance gonadotropin-stimulated steroidogenesis; enhance LHR expression
Epidermal growth factor-TGF-α	Stimulate GC proliferation; inhibit FSHR(GC); and LHR(thecal cell) expression; inhibit steroidogenesis and inhibin secretion
FGF	Stimulate GC proliferation; inhibit TC steroidogenesis; stimulate angiogenesis
SCF	Germ cell migration, proliferation and survival; oocyte growth?; meiosis inhibition?
PDGF	Enhance TC proliferation; inhibit TC steroidogenesis
VEGF	Stimulate angiogenesis
Nerve growth factor	Possible role in early follicle development
Keratinocyte growth factor	GC mitogen; suppress apoptosis
Hepatocyte growth factor	GC mitogen
Serine–threonine kinase receptors	
inhibin[a]	Augment thecal steroidogenesis
activin	Augment progesterone production; enhance FSH action
MIS	Promote meiosis, follicle growth
TGF-β	Follicle growth; inhibit thecal $P450_{c17}$; inhibit differentiation
GDF-9[a]	Initiation of follicle development?
7-TM G protein linked receptors	
Gonadotropin-releasing hormone	Promote meiosis; promote apopotosis
Vasoactive inhibitory protein	Early follicle growth and differentiation
Pituitary adenylate cyclase-activating protein	Early follicle growth and differentiation
Cytokines	
IFN-γ	Decrease granulosa steroidogenesis; promote apoptosis
TNF-α	Decrease granulosa steroidogenesis; induce LIF/IL-1 expression
IL-1	Increase prostaglandins; decrease progesterone; prevent premature follicle rupture?
IL-2	Suppress ovulation; augment progesterone production
IL-6/IL-11/OSM/LIF	Promote germ cell survival; suppress FSH action

[a]Inhibin and GDF-9 are included with the serine–threonine kinases because of homology. Their receptors have not yet been described. FGF, fibroblast growth factor; FSH, follicle-stimulating hormone; FSHR, follicle-stimulating hormone receptor; GC, granulosa cell; GDF, growth and differentiation factor; IFN, interferon; IGF, insulin-like growth factor; IL, interleukin; LHR, luteinizing hormone receptor; LIF, leukemia-inhibitory factor; MIS, Müllerian inhibitory substance; $P450_{c17}$, 7a-hydroxylase/17,20-lyase; PDGF, platelet-derived growth factor; SCF, stem cell factor; TC, theca cell; TGF, transforming growth factor; VEGF, vascular endothelial growth factor.

specific factors are not clearly established. There is considerable functional overlap between the different factors and possibly interaction of their signal transduction pathways. In this area the redundancies of function make it difficult to establish a role for each factor in follicle development, because no one factor is indispensable. Functional genomics and proteomics might help clarify the complex interactions of growth factors and their downstream signaling in early follicle development.

THE OVARIAN CYCLE   The pulsatile secretion of FSH and luteinizing hormone (LH), which begins at puberty initiates the cyclic ovarian function that results in the menstrual cycle. Cyclic gonadotropins lead to the maturation of a single dominant follicle per ovulatory cycle, its ovulation and transformation into a corpus luteum, and then the regression of the corpus luteum in the absence of pregnancy. The ovarian cycle is normally 26–30 d in length and has been classically divided into a follicular phase and a luteal phase, each of roughly 14 d, separated by ovulation at midcycle (Fig. 46-2). For reference, the first day of menstrual bleeding is designated cycle day 1. The follicular phase, which begins with the onset of menses, is characterized by the selection of one member of a cohort of developing early antral follicles to become the dominant follicle. This follicle becomes the largest follicle in either ovary, reaching a diameter of 20 mm or more before ovulation, and it secretes increasing amounts of estrogen. The dominant follicle can be identified by vaginal sonography by cycle day 6 and it has established an estrogen-dominant follicular

Figure 46-1   (**A**) Primordial follicles just below the epithelium of the ovary (dark arrows) with clusters of transitional and primary follicles (open arrow). (**B**) Primary follicles (P) and a secondary follicle with an oocyte (O) surrounded by granulose cells (G) with an external theca layer (T). (**C**) A slightly larger follicle that is beginning to develop an antrum (A). (**D**) A maturing Graafian follicle, with a large antrum (A), a cumulus (C) surrounding the oocyte (O), with well-developed granulose and theca layers. (**E**) Higher magnification of the follicular wall of a preovulatory follicle. The granulose layer is separated from the thickened theca layer by the basement membrane (B). Just beneath the basement membrane, a rich vascular network (dark arrows) is developing. (**F**) An atretic follicle, with cellular debris or apoptotic bodies (dark arrows) visible in the antrum.

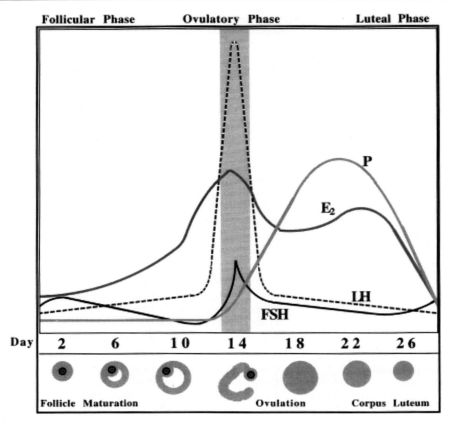

Figure 46-2 The serum levels of estrogen (E), progesterone (P), follicle-stimulating hormone (FSH) and luteinizing hormone (LH) throughout the follicular and luteal phases of the ovarian cycle. (Modified from Carr BR. The ovary, in Textbook of Reproductive Medicine.)

microenvironment by cycle day 8. The luteal phase, which begins at the time of ovulation, is characterized by the organization of the corpus luteum from the remaining granulosa and theca cells of the dominant follicle. The corpus luteum produces the large quantities of progesterone necessary to sustain an early pregnancy.

FOLLICULAR STEROIDOGENESIS Only healthy, dominant follicles produce significant quantities of estrogen. Follicular steroidogenesis requires the cooperation of both granulosa and theca cells and the stimulation of these cells by FSH and LH, respectively. FSH and LH are heterodimeric glycoprotein hormones produced by the pituitary. They share a similar α-subunit but contain distinct but related β-subunits. The receptors for FSH and LH are also distinct but homologous proteins, each of which is a member of a family of receptors that have seven membrane-spanning regions and transmits its signal by activating a guanosine triphosphatase designated Gs (Fig. 46-3). Binding of gonadotropin to its receptor thereby activates adenylate cyclase and increases generation of cAMP, an activator of the protein kinase A pathway of signal transduction. Although the role of FSH and luteinizing hormone receptors in steroidogenesis is well established, LH has been suggested to have additional functions resulting from the activation of the phosphoinositol or protein kinase C pathways, perhaps through AKT.

Because all of the enzymes required for estrogen synthesis from cholesterol are not present in significant quantities in either the granulosa or theca alone, both cell types must participate in this process. Theca cells, which have receptors for LH but not FSH, respond to LH stimulation by producing the enzymes P450 cholesterol side chain cleavage (P450scc) and 17α-hydroxylase/17,20-lyase (P450$_{c17}$), as well as cholesterol transport proteins. Cholesterol is

metabolized to pregnenolone by P450$_{scc}$ and then to dehydroepiandrosterone (DHEA) by P450$_{c17}$ (*see* Fig. 46-3). DHEA is converted to androstenedione by the action of hydroxysteroid dehydrogenase 3β-(HSD). Androstenedione diffuses out of the theca cell, across the follicular basement membrane, and into granulosa cells, in which it is converted into estradiol through the action of the enzymes P450 aromatase and 17β-hydroxysteroid dehydrogenase. Both of these enzymes are upregulated by FSH. This cooperation in estrogen biosynthesis between theca and granulosa cells has been termed the two-cell model of ovarian steroidogenesis.

FOLLICULAR SELECTION AND DOMINANCE In a spontaneous cycle, usually only one follicle is selected to become dominant and eventually ovulate, whereas the remaining antral follicles undergo atresia. How a follicle escapes the fate of atresia and assumes dominance is not well understood. The understanding of this process has been considerably enhanced by observing the results of ovulation-induction treatment in infertile women. Such therapies work by increasing circulating FSH, of either exogenous or endogenous origin, and thereby often result in multiple dominant follicles in a single cycle. Greater than normal FSH levels appear to "rescue" follicles in a developing cohort that might otherwise have undergone atresia, lending credence to the concept that FSH plays a critical role in this process. In a natural ovulatory cycle, circulating FSH begins to rise at the end of the luteal phase, in association with decreasing serum levels of estrogen and inhibin, a granulosa-derived protein that inhibits pituitary FSH release. This FSH increase advances the growth of the leading cohort of follicles. By cycle day 6, the estrogen and inhibin secreted by these growing follicles lead in turn to a decrease in

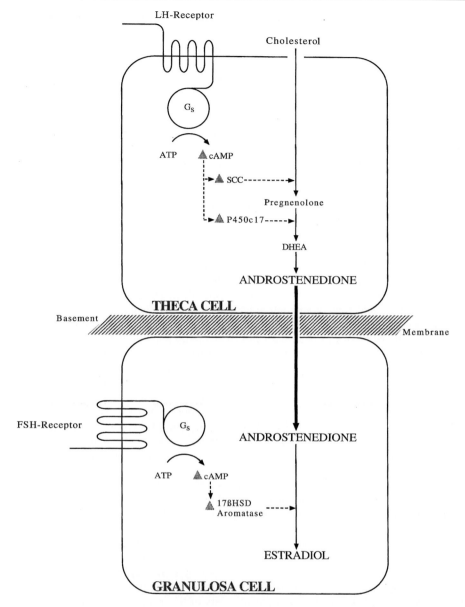

Figure 46-3   The cooperation of the granulosa and the theca cells in the production of estrogen from cholesterol.

serum FSH (*see* Fig. 46-3), which coincides with a slowing of growth and the eventual atresia of the nondominant follicles. The role of FSH in preventing follicular atresia is supported by studies of granulosa cell apoptosis in vitro.

FSH stimulates granulosa cell expression of several proteins that could function in a positive feedback loop to promote development of the dominant follicle. Foremost of these is the LHR. The induction of LH responsiveness in the granulosa is critical to allow the dominant follicle to ovulate in response to the midcycle LH surge and subsequently to develop into a corpus luteum. It also might allow intracellular cAMP levels to be maintained in the face of declining FSH stimulation. FSH also induces granulosa cells to increase production of other proteins that modulate follicular function. An example is inhibin, which acts on the theca to augment androstenedione biosynthesis as well as on the pituitary to decrease FSH output, thereby slowing the development of nondominant cohort follicles.

The exact process of selection of the dominant follicle from its cohort of recruited follicles is unknown. Research into this question has focused on the regulation of luteinizing hormone receptors, the process of angiogenesis in growing follicles, the role of cytokines and growth factors in the synergistic regulation of follicle growth and steroidogenesis, and the regulation of aromatase by steroid metabolites. The role of the balance in intracellular second messenger pathways and receptor crosstalk is also being investigated.

Numerous putative autocrine and paracrine ovarian regulatory factors have been investigated. Much information has accumulated on the action of such factors on ovarian tissues in vitro (*see* Table 46-2), and clearly such proteins have a role in modulating gametogenesis and steroidogenesis. However, the ability of a factor to elicit a response in an isolated in vitro system does not necessarily imply that it can elicit the same response in a dynamic organism with multiple modulatory influences. The role of individual factors in vivo has been technically more difficult to establish, because many of these factors exist in families with multiple receptors and ligands that can potentially compensate for another factor rendered inactive. Genetic knockout techniques, though helpful, can also produce systemic effects that prevent the demonstration of a clear ovarian role of the nonfunctional gene. Targeted transgenic studies in which the alteration of gene expression can be limited both developmentally and anatomically will likely aid in clarifying the intraovarian role of many substances. The difficulties encountered in identifying the roles of each ovarian paracrine factor suggest that the redundancy in the reproductive system has evolutionary significance in that it reduces the dependence of the reproductive process on any single gene product.

FOLLICULAR ATRESIA   Once a primordial follicle leaves the quiescent state and enters the growth phase, it must progress inevitably to either ovulation or loss through atresia. The vast majority of ovarian follicles are lost through atresia. Atresia can occur at any stage of follicle development, but the early antral stage appears to be particularly susceptible. Atresia of antral follicles has been well studied in several animal models and involves granulosa cell apoptosis. Apoptosis thus plays a major role during folliculogenesis and dominant follicle selection, in addition to its role in the reduction of oocyte number in the fetal ovary. Apoptosis is usually associated with degradation of chromosomal DNA into oligonucleosomal fragments by the activation of a Ca^{2+}/Mg^{2+}-dependent endonuclease.

The regulation of susceptibility to and prevention of apoptosis is dependent on the developmental stage of the follicle. Many factors can prevent apoptosis of preovulatory follicles, such as IL-1, fibroblast growth factors, epidermal growth factor and IGFs. But these factors are less able to protect smaller antral follicles or preantral follicles. FSH is the most potent antiapoptotic factor for the smaller antral follicles, but does not prevent apoptosis in follicles prior to the antral stage. By contrast activation of the cGMP pathway does prevent induced apoptosis in preantral follicles. The varying ability of growth factors, cytokines and hormones to block apoptosis at different developmental stages might play an important role in folliculogenesis and in limiting the number of follicles ovulated per cycle. For instance, the dependence of small antral follicles on FSH for development and survival provides an important bottleneck in folliculogenesis. There is a marked increase in the rate of follicle atresia in this group of follicles just as FSH becomes the most potent survival factor. Thus follicles at this stage are exquisitely sensitive to fluctuations of FSH during the menstrual cycle.

A number of molecules have been implicated as intracellular mediators of apoptosis in granulosa cells. Members of the Bcl-2 family of apoptosis regulatory proteins, which includes Bcl-2, Mcl, Bax, Bcl-x-long, and Bcl-x-short, are expressed by granulosa cells of humans and other species. Granulosa cell expression of Bax mRNA was decreased by gonadotropin treatment and increased in serum-free follicle culture, but Bcl-2 expression was unaffected. The tumor suppressor p53, which can promote apoptosis, was localized to granulosa cells only in atretic follicles, and its expression was increased in serum-free follicle culture and decreased by treatment with gonadotropins. Caspases are also present in granulosa cells. Inhibitors of caspases can block apoptosis in granulosa cells and oocytes. Studies of the regulation of mediators of apoptosis are ongoing and are beginning to be performed in primates. These studies might prove invaluable in understanding the role of apoptosis in human folliculogenesis and in preventing abnormally high rates of follicle loss to apoptosis.

OVULATION   As the dominant follicle matures, it produces increasing amounts of estrogen, thereby effecting positive feedback on the pituitary gonadotrophs to produce the midcycle gonadotropin surge. The LH surge begins about 36 h and peaks about 10 h before ovulation; it triggers the major events of ovulation, including resumption of meiosis, cumulus expansion, cumulus-oocyte expulsion, and luteinization. The underlying regulation of these seemingly independent events has been studied intensively by those interested in both fertility control and infertility treatment. The duration of the LH surge is critical in triggering the events of ovulation; in primates, LH levels must be maintained for 18–24 h for oocyte maturation to occur, but for 34–48 h for optimal granulosa luteinization and corpus luteum function. Surge levels of LH are also necessary for the expression of prostaglandin-related genes in the rodent ovary.

In the developing follicle, resumption of meiosis is inhibited by a communication between the cumulus cells and the oocyte. In vitro, meiosis resumes in oocytes from antral follicles if the cumulus is removed or in response to cAMP. Atretic follicles of some species might exhibit meiosis briefly, as the granulosa cells lose function. Follicular fluid and granulosa cell-conditioned media both can inhibit meiosis of oocytes in vitro. These findings have led to the suggestion that granulosa cells produce an oocyte maturation inhibitor (OMI) under gonadotropin regulation. The identity of OMI has remained elusive. Hypoxanthine, a purine derivative, can inhibit meiosis in vitro and has been suggested to be the physiological OMI. Other candidate OMIs include inhibin and Müllerian inhibitory substance. Alternatively, the inhibition of meiosis might be a result of the functional relationship between the granulosa and the oocyte, and maturation might follow its physical disruption. This issue has not been resolved.

During the process of ovulation, the cumulus–oocyte complex loses its connection to the mural granulosa cells and probably briefly floats freely in the follicular fluid. At this time the follicular circumference is expanding, but the intrafollicular pressure does not increase. For the oocyte to be ovulated and reach the fallopian tube, it must pass through the mural granulosa layer, the follicular basement membrane, the theca layer, the ovarian stroma, and the surface epithelium of the ovary. This process is simplified because the enlarging follicle migrates (or expands) to the periphery of the ovary, adjacent to the surface epithelium.

Prostaglandins of the E and F series are elevated in follicular fluid before ovulation; and in rats prostaglandin synthetase is regulated by LH. The exact function of prostaglandins in ovulation is not known, but high doses of prostaglandin synthetase inhibitors interfere with ovulation in humans.

The process of ovulation has been compared with the inflammatory response of wound healing. As in wound healing, plasminogen activators (PA) play a role in the tissue remodeling that occurs during ovulation and formation of the corpus luteum. The regulation of the PA system at the time of ovulation has been characterized in the rat. Tissue plasminogen activator (tPA) is secreted by rat granulosa cells and produced but not secreted by the theca. Production of both tPA and an inhibitor, called plasminogen activator inhibitor (PAI), are stimulated by the gonadotropin surge; but PAI mRNA expression peaks approx 6 h after rats are given human chorionic gonadotropin (hCG) as a surrogate LH surge, whereas tPA expression does not peak until 12 h after hCG; thus, the inhibitor is likely present before the production of the activator. Before ovulation, tPA mRNA and protein are expressed at high levels by the granulosa, whereas PAI is expressed strongly by the preovulatory theca and surrounding interstitium. After hCG, follicles enlarge rapidly and protrude from the ovarian surface. At 12 h after hCG, thecal expression of PAI in the portion of the follicle closest to the ovarian surface is lower than in the rest of the follicle. Granulosa expression of tPA in this region is greater than in the rest of the follicle. This temporal and spatial differential expression of tPA and its inhibitor could allow plasmin, which is generated from plasminogen from both serum and follicular fluid, to thereby activate collagenases only at the site of the stigma, in which the cumulus–oocyte complex escapes from the follicle. The localized follicular expression of interstitial and type-IV collagenases and their inhibitors also appears to be regulated by LH.

Experimental disruption of the components of the PA system by several methods decreases the efficiency of ovulation, but seldom results in complete ovulatory suppression. Transgenic mice lacking either tPA or urokinase (uPA) gene function are fertile and have no obvious reproductive phenotype. Animals derived from these lines and lacking both functional genes have impaired wound healing. Although they are still fertile, early studies suggest that they ovulate at a decreased rate. The lack of clear inhibition of ovulation in the absence of PAs suggests that, as with follicle growth, the process of ovulation is also governed by redundant regulatory systems.

THE LUTEAL TRANSITION   After the release of the oocyte, the follicle begins its transition to the corpus luteum, the endocrine organ of pregnancy. The factors regulating this metamorphosis are not entirely understood, but the quality of luteal function is correlated with the adequacy of the follicular phase of the cycle. Studies of human granulosa and luteal cells cultured in vitro implicate the absolute level of intracellular cAMP in driving the cellular events of luteinization. The relatively lower levels of cAMP generated by FSH induce cell growth and replication, but the higher levels generated in response to LH lead to cessation of cell division and increased steroidogenesis. This cAMP effect might be augmented by other second messenger pathways activated by LH. A 43-kDa cAMP response-element binding protein is expressed in growing primate follicles, but not in corpora lutea, and correlates with expression of proliferating cell nuclear antigen. Differential expression of cAMP response-element binding protein might be another mechanism by which cAMP can exert different responses in the same tissue at different times.

Another key step in the formation of the corpus luteum is angiogenesis, the growth of numerous small vessels into the previously avascular granulosa. vascular endothelial growth factor, which stimulates proliferation of capillary endothelial cells, is expressed by human granulosa-luteal cells under positive regulation by LH. Other angiogenic factors, including basic fibroblast growth factor and PDGF, might also be involved in this process. Vascularization allows the granulosa direct access to serum-derived growth factors and hormones, as well as to low-density lipoprotein cholesterol used as a precursor for progesterone synthesis.

Progesterone, the principal product of the corpus luteum, is necessary both to prepare the uterine endometrium for implantation and to maintain early gestation. The LH surge induces large increases in granulosa cell steroid acute regulatory protein, $P450_{scc}$, and 3β-HSD expression, which lead to more efficient synthesis of progesterone. The human corpus luteum, unlike that of some other mammals, continues to secrete estrogen in addition to progesterone, particularly during the midluteal phase (*see* Fig. 46-3). The human corpus luteum

is also distinctive, in that 17-hydroxy-progesterone is not a substrate for the lyase function of $P450_{c17}$, as it is in many other species. Therefore the metabolism of pregnenolone either to progesterone by 3β-HSD or to androstenedione (an estrogen precursor) by $P450_{c17}$ is a key branch point in luteal steroid production and the regulation of these enzymes could be a critical determinant of luteal steroid products.

LUTEAL REGRESSION   In the absence of pregnancy, the corpus luteum begins to degenerate spontaneously after 2 wk. Luteal regression is classically described in two phases: functional regression and structural regression. Functional regression involves decreased production of progesterone and decreased expression of steroidogenic enzymes. Structural regression is more prolonged and involves apoptosis. Both spontaneous and experimentally induced luteal regression are associated with morphological apoptosis or oligonucleosomal DNA fragmentation. Although prostaglandins have been implicated in spontaneous luteal regression in nonprimate species, the mediators of luteolysis in primates have not been definitively identified. Macrophages, lymphocytes, and their secretory products (cytokines), as well as prostaglandins, might also play a role. Macrophages and lymphocytes invade the corpus luteum and become more numerous as the corpus luteum ages. Cytokines, including interferon-γ of lymphocyte origin and TNF-α of macrophage origin, decrease steroidogenesis by luteal cells from human, rat, and cow. Fas antigen has been localized to the human corpus luteum, suggesting its involvement in luteal regression. Regulators of functional and structural luteolysis might be different in the primate as the role of the corpus luteum is different in mammals with a menstrual cycle. The human corpus luteum exists for 2 wk in a nonpregnant cycle. Rodent corpora lutea secrete progesterone for less than a day before the next estrous cycle begins. Ongoing studies in primates are likely to shed more light on the regulators of luteal regression in humans.

OVARIAN SENESCENCE   Menopause refers to the permanent cessation of menses. Ovarian function generally follows a gradual decline, with cyclical bleeding becoming increasingly irregular. Only approx 10% of women experience an abrupt natural cessation of menses. Women might ovulate during the menopausal transition, but bleeding during this interval is often the result of fluctuations in estrogen levels not related to ovulation and luteal demise. Therefore, a patient's memory of the timing of her last menstrual period might not be an accurate estimation of the cessation of ovulatory function. Several prospective studies of ovarian function during the menopausal transition are under way and should provide more information about ovulatory function and menopause.

Primordial follicles are believed to enter the growth phase at a relatively constant rate and are gradually depleted over time. There is excellent evidence; however, that their rate of loss increases as menopause approaches. This accelerated loss, predicted to begin on the average at age 38 yr, is associated with a decrease in inhibin and an increase in FSH serum levels. It has also been demonstrated that some women experience wide fluctuations in estrogen levels for several years leading up to the menopause. It is not understood why the rate of follicular loss increases at this age, but it might be dependent on the mass of the declining primordial follicle pool. Ongoing studies of unilaterally ovariectomized women, who have a decreased follicle pool, might shed light on this question.

Studies of reproductive senescence in transgenic mice have provided some interesting insights into the role of the follicle pool. Mice with mutations that result in a smaller initial pool of primordial follicles have earlier senescence. Mice that have slower entry of primordial follicles to the growing pool do not always have delayed reproductive senescence and might even have POF. However, mice that have mutations or deletions that result in defective apoptosis in the ovary do have a delay in the timing of ovarian failure. Those with alterations in antiapoptotic molecules, like Bcl-2 have earlier ovarian failure. Functional studies of interruption of the apoptosis pathway in the ovaries of primates are ongoing and might reveal important information on the role of apoptosis in the maintenance and protection of the primordial pool of follicles that will have direct relevance for humans.

CONCLUSION   Human ovarian tissue has been difficult to obtain for regulatory studies of folliculogenesis, luteinization, and luteolysis, and significant differences exist between humans and nonprimate animal models. For this reason, primate models continue to be important in the study of these processes. However, the use of new technologies, which allow the evaluation of smaller amounts of tissue, and the development of cell lines and long-term tissue culture techniques, are allowing more in-depth studies of human tissues involving the regulation of follicular growth and atresia, ovulation, luteinization, and steroidogenesis.

OVARIAN DYSFUNCTION

DISORDERS OF INCREASED OVARIAN FUNCTION

McCune–Albright Syndrome   McCune–Albright syndrome (MAS), or polyostotic fibrous dysplasia, is caused by a postzygotic mutation in the GNAS1 gene encoding the α-subunit of $G_s\alpha$, a G protein that stimulates adenylate cyclase. The resulting sporadic activation of G protein-linked processes throughout the body leads to diverse manifestations, including bony lesions, café-au-lait skin lesions, and endocrine dysfunction. In the ovary, the activating mutation of the adenylate cyclase system leads to the premature development of relatively normal-appearing follicles, which include a thecal component and can secrete estrogen, independent of gonadotropin stimulation. As a result, half of girls affected with MAS exhibit signs of isosexual precocity, often presenting with vaginal bleeding. Follicles grow and produce estrogen in the absence of FSH stimulation. Often progesterone is produced as the follicles enlarge, suggesting that premature luteinization and LH-like effects are stimulated. Because there is no LH surge, the follicles do not ovulate but regress, thus explaining the relapsing and remitting manifestations of precocity in MAS girls and irregular cycles in women. Both bilateral and unilateral ovarian involvement has been reported. Normal pregnancies have been reported in adult women with MAS who had developed isosexual precocity in childhood, but infertility and subfertility are also common. Infertility might result as a direct effect on the ovary or because of dyssynchronous hormonal stimulation of the endometrium reducing the likelihood of implantation. Long-term evaluation of larger numbers of these patients is needed to accurately evaluate their fertility potential. It is possible that some cases of idiopathic gonadotropin-independent sexual precocity might be localized manifestations of mutations similar to that in MAS, but this has not been demonstrated.

Granulosa Cell Tumors   Granulosa cell tumors represent 5–10% of all ovarian neoplasms and can be divided into two types, juvenile and adult, on the basis of histology and age of occurrence. Juvenile tumors are diagnosed in the first three decades of life, whereas adult-type tumors often present after menopause. About 5% of all granulosa cell tumors are diagnosed before the normal age of puberty. These tumors are generally multicystic and only rarely malignant. When these tumors occur prepubertally, approx 80% produce sufficient estrogen to result in isosexual precocity; they account for about 10% of isosexual precocity in girls. Some of these tumors also produce inhibin, indicative of differentiated granulosa cell function. Serum inhibin levels are often used in surveillance for tumor recurrence.

Many investigators have evaluated possible genes involved in granulosa cell growth and apoptosis as culprits in the evolution of granulosa cell tumors. Most studies have not differentiated between the two types possibly limiting the ability to interpret their data. It seems reasonable that juvenile and adult tumors are different enough to have different etiologies. Juvenile tumors are well differentiated and occur early when FSH levels are low. Adult tumors peak after menopause, a time when FSH levels are often very elevated. Several studies have searched for activating mutations of the follicle-stimulating hormone receptor (FSHR) or Gs_α-subunit in juvenile granulosa cell tumors, but no mutation has been identified. Mutations of the growth-inhibiting WT1 gene have been associated with juvenile granulosa cell tumors. Some syndromes involving abnormal tissue growth, such as Proteus Syndrome or Ollier Disease have also been associated with juvenile granulosa cell tumors. In rats, selective activation of the estrogen receptor-β has been associated with granulosa cell tumors, but estrogen receptor-β mutations have not been described in humans, although estrogen receptor-β expression is noted to be high in adult granulosa cell tumors.

In the adult-type granulosa cell tumor, mutations have been identified in the G_i-subunit of regulatory G proteins, although the physiological significance of these mutations has not been established. It is uncertain why the inability to turn off a normally transcribed stimulatory signal, as with the G_i mutation previously described, should be manifested as tumor in later life, whereas the uncontrolled activation of the same signal, in MAS, is manifested as a relatively normal-appearing follicle earlier in life. Further studies are necessary to elucidate the regulatory events involved in the stimulation of follicular growth by cAMP. Further studies of juvenile and adult granulosa cell tumors will likely yield important new information regarding both granulosa tumorigenesis and normal follicle developmental regulation.

Multifollicular Ovulation   Twin and higher-order multiple gestations have long been a source of general curiosity and scientific interest. Monozygotic twinning results from the division of a single zygote after fertilization and is believed to be primarily related to zygote factors, with possible contributions from uterine and implantation factors. The incidence of monozygotic twinning has been relatively constant over time and among diverse ethnic groups. By contrast, the incidence of dizygotic twinning, which results from the separate fertilization of two ovulated eggs, varies among ethnic groups and has fluctuated over time. Although the study of genetically identical monozygotic twins has been of great interest because of the ability to examine the effect of different environments on the same genetic background, ovarian physiologists are understandably more interested in dizygotic twinning as a resource to evaluate the mechanisms determining the ovulatory quota. In every species a relatively constant number of oocytes are released each cycle, the ovulatory quota. This results in the distinct average litter sizes of a species or strain. In humans, usually only a single fertilizable egg is produced per cycle, though this control can be overridden by agents that increase gonadotropin stimulation of the ovary.

Variations in the incidence of dizygotic twinning fueled discussion of the possibility of the underlying molecular mechanisms involved. Dizygotic twins have been noted to occur with a frequency as high as one in eight pregnancies in some African populations and as low as 1 in 400 in some Pacific Rim countries. The incidence of twinning varies over the reproductive life span, with a higher frequency noted in the later reproductive years. Twinning also occurs with a high frequency within some families. Pharmaceutical agents to induce and augment spontaneous ovulation are associated with increased rates of multifollicular ovulation and multifetal pregnancy. One of these, clomiphene citrate, acts as a partial estrogen antagonist, thereby decreasing the negative feedback of estrogen on pituitary FSH secretion. This increase in FSH secretion presumably promotes ovulation by rescuing some recruited follicles that would otherwise have undergone atresia. Injections of FSH, as either human menopausal gonadotropins or purified or recombinant FSH, similarly stimulate development of increased numbers of follicles. The ability to induce superovulation pharmacologically and produce large numbers of mature oocytes in a single cycle has been critical in the development of in vitro fertilization and other assisted reproductive technologies. The introduction of these therapies for the infertile couple has fueled the study of the control of follicular growth, selection, dominance, and atresia.

Is there a molecular explanation for the increased ovulatory quota in families or population clusters with high rates of twinning? Mothers of twins have been studied in search of hormonal differences that could result from a genetic mutation and would be reflected in increased FSH action on the ovary. Some studies have shown higher levels of both estrogen and FSH in the follicular phase in mothers of twins, whereas inhibin levels might be either normal or elevated. Examination of familial twin clusters has revealed no mutations in the FSH-β, gonadotropin-releasing hormone (GnRH), GnRH receptor, inhibin-α, PPARγ, peroxisome proliferators-activated receptor (PPAR)γ, LH-β, and FSHR genes. No other mutation has been found in humans that could account for the apparent increased gonadotropin activity and enhanced follicular survival.

Further understanding of the molecular basis of the ovulatory quota has resulted from genetic studies of two strains of sheep with large litter size, the Booroola Merino and the Inverdale. The Booroola gene mutation, designated FecB^B, is autosomal and is associated with an increased number of ovulations in the heterozygous state and a further increase in the homozygote. The altered physiology results in maturation of larger numbers of follicles of a smaller size, with no net difference in total granulosa cell mass compared with wild-type Booroolas. Serum FSH is slightly elevated, but no other abnormalities in the hypothalamic-pituitary-ovarian axis are detectable. The Inverdale mutation, FecX^I, is X-linked. FecX^I heterozygotes, like FecB^B heterozygotes and homozygotes, show an increased number of antral follicles, but homozygotes display failure of ovarian development and have streak gonads.

FecB was identified as BMPRIB and FecX as GDF9B/BMP15. Though linkage analysis of the Australian twins cohorts has ruled out BMPRIB association with twinning in this population, these studies have increased interest in the role of the BMP family in follicle regulation. Further findings in this field are anticipated.

Hyperreactio Luteinalis Hyperstimulation of follicle development is a well-recognized side effect of treatment with exogenous gonadotropins. The hyperstimulation syndrome consists of greatly enlarged ovaries that are extremely fragile, ascites, depleted intravascular volume, and even pulmonary effusion. The "leaky capillaries" that are the culprit of the shifts in intravascular volume are thought to result from ovarian derived vasoactive factors secreted after the LH surge. Rare spontaneous cases of hyperstimulation that occur well after ovulation, during the first trimester of pregnancy have also been described. This condition is known as hyperreactio luteinalis and is usually associated with pregnancies with extremely high hCG levels, such as molar pregnancy or multiple gestations. It was thought that the elevated hCG could cross-react with the FSHR and activate it, though this explanation was controversial. Mutations in the FSHR have been described that result in hyperreactio luteinalis even with normal first trimester levels of hCG. Studies of binding and activation of the mutant receptors demonstrate that as little as 10 IU/mL concentration of hCG can activate the mutant receptors, whereas the wild-type receptor is minimally activated by 10,000 IU/mL hCG. The kinetics of FSH binding and activation of the receptors is not substantially different between the mutant receptors and wild-type controls. The described families had normal fertility, emphasizing normal FSH action in stimulating follicle development. Symptoms are only present in early gestation when hCG is present in high enough levels to cause hyperstimulation. Surprisingly, the mutations are not in the extracellular binding domain of the receptor, but in the serpentine portion in the cell membrane. It is hypothesized that the mutations allow a more relaxed configuration of this large transmembrane receptor that allows the low-affinity hCG binding to stabilize the receptor in its active form, thus resulting in the abnormal activation of the FSHR during pregnancy.

DISORDERS OF DIMINISHED OVARIAN FUNCTION

A number of disorders lead to diminished ovarian function. The spectrum of ovarian phenotypes of these disorders, which can include lack of estrogen production, menstrual acyclicity, and infertility, often overlaps, leading to confusion both in classifying these disorders and in determining their molecular basis. Diminished ovarian function is traditionally classified by its time of onset relative to menarche, but many disorders might have their origin in fetal life or childhood and remain unrecognized until clinical presentation when a girl fails to exhibit estrogen-induced secondary sexual characteristics at the time of expected puberty. A developmental approach to the classification of diminished ovarian function might be more helpful in understanding and recognizing these naturally occurring functional ovarian defects.

Ovarian Dysgenesis Absolute ovarian failure can result from improper ovarian development during embryogenesis. As discussed, ovarian development depends on complex interactions between germ cells and components of the gonadal ridge, and interference with either component will result in ovarian dysgenesis, with fibrous streaks devoid of germ cells replacing the ovaries. Patients with streak ovaries are sexually infantile and generally have elevated serum gonadotropins by the time of expected puberty, because they lack normal negative feedback from ovarian estrogen and inhibin.

The most common cause of gonadal dysgenesis is Turner's syndrome, or monosomy X (Chapter 42). The lack of a second X chromosome results in streak gonads and numerous characteristic somatic features, including shield chest, widely spaced nipples, and lymphatic abnormalities. In Turner's syndrome, germ cells apparently migrate normally to the ovaries, but primordial follicles are not formed efficiently and germ cells are lost. Gonadal dysgenesis in girls with Turner's syndrome could potentially result from a defect at any of the stages of follicle formation, including the entry of oocytes into meiosis and the association of oocytes with granulosa cells.

Gonadal dysgenesis also occurs in women with two apparently normal X chromosomes. Several disorders that include craniofacial abnormalities are associated with ovarian dysgenesis, including an interstitial deletion of chromosome 2q found in a girl with ovarian dysgenesis, mental retardation, craniofacial abnormalities, and cardiac defects. Deletions of chromosome 3q have also been associated with gonadal dysgenesis and ovarian failure. Large chromosomal deletions might interfere with the process of pairing in meiosis, resulting in early germ cell loss. However, gonadal dysgenesis also occurs with apparently normal karyotypes. In Denys–Drash syndrome, a mutation in the WT1 gene is associated with renal malformations, Wilms' tumor, and gonadal dysgenesis. Most cases of this syndrome are in genetic males, but a few have been reported in genetic females.

Sensorineural deafness and blepharophimosis have also been associated with lack of ovarian function. Blepharophimosis ptosis epicanthus inversus syndrome is caused by mutations in the forkhead transcription factor gene FOXL2 (3q23) and is characterized by eyelid and ocular muscle abnormalities in combination with lack of ovarian function. As further understanding is gained of the regulation of patterning in development, other genes with unexpected roles in ovarian failure might be discovered.

Failure of Ovarian Function   In another group of disorders, the ovaries might be formed normally but still not function adequately. This might result from deficiency of specific factors regulating the initiation of follicle growth, such as GDF-9. Alternatively, normally formed but unresponsive ovaries have been shown to result from mutations affecting gonadotropin function.

An FSHR mutation was identified among a group of Finnish women selected because of primary or early secondary amenorrhea. Initial study of these women suggested a recessive pattern of inheritance, and linkage analysis of multiplex families mapped the trait to chromosome 2p, the known location of the FSHR gene. Sequencing the FSHR gene in affected individuals revealed a mutation in exon 7, which encodes a portion of the extracellular domain of the receptor. In expression studies, this mutant receptor was unable to stimulate cAMP production in response to FSH. Further analysis of the receptor in the expression system demonstrated apparently normal ligand binding affinity but extremely low levels of receptor expression. The authors concluded that the recessive disorder leading to amenorrhea resulted from either abnormal FSHR trafficking or increased receptor degradation.

Though LHR defects have long been recognized as a cause of testicular Leydig cell hypoplasia, an inactivating mutation of LHR was associated with anovulation in a woman who apparently exhibited secondary sexual characteristics at puberty but had a small uterus and never had regular cyclic menses. Three of her sisters were XY pseudohermaphrodites with normal female external genitalia and absent Leydig cells on gonadal histology. The LHR in all four of these patients contained a homozygous mutation that created a stop codon in the third intracellular loop, resulting in a nonfunctional receptor. The index patient's history demonstrates that LHR function is not essential for estrogen production in quantities sufficient for breast development, despite being necessary for ovulation and luteinization.

There are also isolated reports of mutations associated with gonadotropin subunit defects. Hypergonadotropic hypogonadism

has been reported in a woman with a homozygous mutation in the FSH-β gene that results in an FSH molecule unable to bind to its receptor. Her fertility was restored with exogenous FSH treatment. In contrast to female heterozygotes with the FSHR mutation described earlier, which often have large families, this patient's mother, an obligate heterozygote, was subfertile and had ovulatory dysfunction. It is possible that the presence of a defective FSH molecule interfered with the function of the normal protein, thereby reducing the efficiency of follicle growth and ovulation.

Defects in the enzymes necessary for estrogen biosynthesis can also result in sexual infantilism, but ovarian stimulation and in vitro fertilization have been performed successfully in some patients with estrogen deficiency, indicating that estrogen is not necessary for human preovulatory follicle development though it might play a role in oocyte maturation.

Premature Ovarian Failure   POF, also called premature menopause, is clinically defined as the loss of ovarian function before the age of 35 yr despite adequate gonadotropin stimulation. Generally this term is applied to women who have undergone normal pubertal sexual maturation and have experienced some degree of cyclic ovarian function. Premature ovarian senescence can result from either an abnormally small initial endowment of primordial germ cells or increased germ cell loss with time.

A number of X-linked conditions are associated with POF. Although Turner's syndrome usually results in severe early germ cell loss and gonadal dysgenesis, some germ cell survival can occur in ovaries of women with X-chromosome mosaicism or partial deletions, allowing for short-lived ovarian function including normal puberty and even, rarely, fertility. Two X-chromosome loci have been linked to POF by the study of translocations in affected families: POF1, at Xq26–q28, and POF2, at Xq13.3–q21.1. The specific genes at these loci responsible for this phenotype have not been identified though a mutation in a human homolog of the Drosophila "diaphanous" gene has been associated with POF2. It has also been hypothesized that the break points of the X chromosome in this critical region cause aberrations in pairing or X inactivation during folliculogenesis that might result in apoptosis at meiotic checkpoints.

Another X-chromosome locus that might be associated with ovarian senescence is the fragile X gene, fragile X mental retardation protein, which maps to Xq28. The fragile X syndrome is caused by a lack of fragile X mental retardation protein protein resulting from an amplification of CCG triplet nucleotide repeats within the promoter region of this gene. Males with fragile X syndrome exhibit mental retardation, facial dysmorphism, and macroorchidism. Female fragile X carriers show an increased rate of premature menopause and an increased rate of dizygotic twinning, which might be an epiphenomenon of the increase in gonadotropins as ovarian senescence approaches. It is unclear how these observations are related to the fragile X genotype. Although fragile X mental retardation protein might play a role in germ cell proliferation in the testis, its role in the ovary has not been demonstrated. If it affects the efficiency of primordial follicle formation, a mutation at this locus might lead to a decrease in the overall follicular complement and, thus, an earlier cessation of cyclic ovarian function.

Any defect that decreases the efficiency of formation of primary follicles, resulting in a smaller starting pool of follicles, could potentially lead to POF, even if follicles were depleted at a normal rate. Increased atresia of oocytes in primordial follicles in the fetus or of small follicles at a later time could also lead to POF. Dysregulation of the complex mechanisms that regulate ovarian apoptosis could be a factor, although no such defects have been demonstrated in women. However, studies in mice that block the function of pro-apoptotic molecules have delayed reproductive senescence. Further studies of familial POF clusters might reveal defects in factors regulating cell–cell interaction, cell growth, or apoptosis.

Progressive Ovarian Damage   Galactosemia is an autosomal-recessive metabolic disorder characterized by a deficiency of galactose-1-phosphate uridylyltransferase, leading to an inability to metabolize galactose and the accumulation of potentially toxic galactose-1-phosphate in tissues. Treatment with dietary galactose restriction improves or prevents the development of abnormalities of the liver, kidney, eye, and central nervous system. Ovarian failure develops over several years in association with follicular depletion. The time of its onset is variable and might depend on the age of institution of dietary treatment. Both primary amenorrhea and rare pregnancies have been observed. The gonadotropins produced by these women are biologically active, despite the fact that galactose is present in the carbohydrate moiety of normal gonadotropins. The gonadotropin receptors are probably also normal, because ovulation can occur and testicular function in males with galactosemia is normal. The molecular basis for the accelerated depletion of ovarian follicles in galactosemia is unknown.

Autoimmune disorders might also cause progressive ovarian damage and lead to POF. POF might occur as an isolated autoimmune endocrinopathy, or it might be associated with other known autoimmune diseases of the endocrine system, including Hashimoto's thyroiditis, insulin-deficient diabetes, and Addison's disease. Histological examination of the ovaries in women with autoimmune POF often reveals a lymphoplasmacytic infiltrate involving growing but not primordial follicles. Abnormal ovarian monocytes and fibroblasts have been reported, as well as altered serum cytokine profiles. Although antiovarian antibodies have been described in some cases of POF, they are not consistently directed against any single antigen. Of interest, preliminary studies have suggested that the fragile-X-related gene product might be an autoantigen within the ovary. Ovarian failure often follows a relapsing and remitting course and pregnancies can occur, occasionally after prolonged absence of ovarian function. It is hoped that ongoing longitudinal studies of these patients will provide more information about the etiology and most effective treatment for this frustrating and unpredictable condition.

POLYCYSTIC OVARY SYNDROME   In 1935 Stein and Leventhal published a case series describing women with enlarged ovaries containing many cysts. These women tended to be amenorrheic, hirsute, obese, and infertile. When they underwent resection of part of each ovary (wedge resection) many patients experienced a restoration of menstrual cyclicity. Because that landmark report, the polycystic ovarian syndrome (PCOS) has been a constant arena of study for reproductive biologists and gynecologists. With the discovery of the long-term effects of hyperandrogenemia and hyperinsulinemia on the health of these women, and the emergence of Syndrome X, the study of PCOS has entertained more widespread interest.

Despite decades of study and an enhanced understanding of the complexity of this syndrome, the etiologies of these phenomena remain elusive. Though it appears to be a heritable condition, it is also likely to be mulifactorial in nature. Susceptibility loci might include genes involved in steroid production and metabolism, insulin signaling, and regulation of folliculogenesis.

PCOS defined in the clinical setting as chronic anovulation in association with clinical and/or biochemical evidence of ovarian hyperandrogenism. The condition affects an estimated 5–10% of reproductive age women and is a common cause of secondary amenorrhea. In addition to menstrual irregularities and androgen excess, women with PCOS frequently present with insulin resistance and are at risk for type-II diabetes. They also can express features of metabolic cardiovascular syndrome including central adiposity, obesity, lipid abnormalities, and hypertension, though a thin PCOS phenotype has also been described. It has been suggested that psychological symptoms might also be a feature of PCOS.

Proposed etiologies of PCOS have included fundamental alteration of steroid biosynthesis, insulin resistance secondary to a postreceptor defect, intrinsic alteration of the hypothalamic pituitary drive, and abnormal control of follicular apoptosis resulting in persistent follicles. None of these hypotheses alone explains all of the sequelae associated with PCOS.

The Polycystic Ovary   There has been a dichotomy in the criteria for diagnosing PCOS in the United States and Europe. In Europe the typical sonographic appearance of greater than eight small subcapsular cysts along with increased stromal density has been considered sufficient for the diagnosis of PCOS. However, in the United States, biochemical evidence of hyperandrogenism and irregular menses are often the criteria used to assign the diagnosis of PCOS without regard to the ovarian morphology. This can lead to confusion when comparing studies using different definitions, and careful attention to the inclusion criteria is thus required when evaluating the literature regarding PCOS.

Cystic ovaries have been reported in up to 20% of normal women with regular menstrual cycles, but nevertheless are a key feature of PCOS. Ovaries of PCOS women contain twice the number of follicles as control ovaries from cycling women. Though these follicles have an elevated estrogen to androgen ration, they are not atretic as would be expected in control ovaries. This had led to the consideration that there is an abnormality in apoptotic regulation of these follicles. Granulosa cells from these follicles have a reduced number of FSHRs compared with follicles from control ovaries, suggesting a reduced ability to respond to FSH stimulation. However, when granulosa cells from polycystic ovary cysts are grown in culture, FSHR expression can be stimulated and aromatase induced. Women with PCOS are often extremely sensitive to ovarian stimulation with exogenous gonadotropins. The number of small antral follicles at the beginning of an ovulation induction cycle is a risk factor for the ovarian hyperstimulation syndrome.

Women who undergo a reduction in ovarian mass through unilateral oophorectomy, Stein and Leventhal's original wedge resection, or the more modern "ovarian drilling" with laser or electrocautery often will have resumption of menstrual cycles and even restoration of fertility for a time. Traditionally it was thought that the ovarian reductive procedures worked because of a reduction in the androgen-producing ovarian stroma, however, more thought is being given to the effects of the follicles themselves. When women with PCOS approach menopausal age, they undergo the same reduction in the follicle pool as normal women. Some investigators have reported increased menstrual regularity and a reduction in serum LH and androgen levels as PCOS women approach the perimenopause.

Hyperandrogenism Hyperandrogenism is a hallmark of PCOS. Elevated testosterone is generally thought to result from excessive androstenedione produced by the ovarian theca. In vitro, theca from PCOS ovaries produces more androstenedione than theca from normal ovaries. Acne and hirsuitism result from the increased presence of C19 steroids that can be metabolized to dihydrotestosterone at the level of the hair follicle. Androstenedione can also be metabolized to estrogens in the peripheral tissues. This results in a tonic level of estrogen that can be in the midfollicular range. Tonic estrogen unopposed by progesterone is a major risk factor for endometrial hyperplasia and cancer.

The elevated androgens also result in down-regulation of sex hormone binding globulin. Reduction of sex hormone binding globulin results in a reduction in bound testosterone and increased relative free testosterone. Elevated androgens are thought to play a role in the adverse health effects described in PCOS women, such as increased cardiovascular and small vessel disease. However, these effects might also be indirect and related more to the elevated low-density lipoprotein cholesterol and decreased antioxidants seen in polycystic ovary women. Oral contraceptives are effective in modulating many of the effects of PCOS, not just in protecting the uterus from hyperplasia. Oral contraceptive use increases sex hormone binding globulin, thus resulting in a reduction of the "free testosterone," even in rare cases when total testosterone remains elevated. Whether early and consistent OCP use in the treatment of PCOS can diminish the long-term adverse health effects seen in PCOS has not yet been established.

Hypothalamic/Pituitary Inputs A key characteristic of PCOS is altered gonadotropin secretion. Classically, LH levels are elevated but FSH levels are in the normal range, though the elevated LH/FSH ratio is no longer necessary or sufficient to make the diagnosis of PCOS. The classic description of the "vicious cycle" of altered hypothalamic/pituitary/ovarian axis feedback involves the conversion of ovarian androstenedione to estrogen in the peripheral compartment. The resulting tonic estrogen levels enhance pituitary LH secretion, whereas suppressing FSH secretion. Elevated LH continues the cycle by stimulating excessive thecal androgen production. Though increased LH pulse frequency and amplitude have been demonstrated by many investigators, LH drive in PCOS might be less responsive to suppression by exogenous sex steroids and there might also be reduced sensitivity to endogenous steroid feedback, particularly progesterone.

Attention has been given to neurotransmitters mediating GnRH activation. Opiodergic and dopaminergic regulation are thought to be intact in women with PCOS. However, γ-amino-butyric acid (GABA) is elevated in the cerebrospinal fluid of women with PCOS compared with ovulatory controls. It has been suggested that either GABA could be acting in an excitatory fashion and stimulating GnRH neurons or the increased GABAergic tone functions as a compensatory response restraining GnRH. In animal models, GABA is excitatory to GnRH neurons when acting through the GABA A receptor. Further studies are warranted to clarify the role of the GABAergic system in PCOS.

The Insulin Connection Insulin resistance is commonly found in women with PCOS and it has been estimated that approx 10–15% of women with PCOS will develop diabetes. Hyperinsulinemia is observed in both lean and obese women with PCOS and is because of increased insulin secretion in response to peripheral insulin resistance. The insulin resistance is thought to result from a postreceptor defect because receptor number and binding affinity have been reported to be normal. Though the metabolic action of insulin is altered in PCOS, some investigators have reported that the mitogenic effects of insulin are intact.

There are insulin receptors in the ovary as well as IGFI and IGFII receptors present. IGFs are also produced in the ovary and are thought to be autocrine and paracrine factors involved in follicle development and steroid production. The IGF binding protein family is also present in ovarian follicles and might affect growth factor availability as well as have independent regulatory functions. Insulin and insulin-like growth factor increase FSH-stimulated steroid enzyme expression in both granulosa and theca cells in tissue or organ culture. There is an increase in ovarian stroma in women with PCOS, and it is hypothesized that the elevated insulin levels acting either through the insulin receptors or the IGF receptors results in increased growth of the stroma/theca of the polycystic ovary. Insulin and IGFs enhance the production of androstenedione from ovarian theca. Furthermore, when insulin-sensitizing agents are given to women with PCOS, not only do serum insulin levels fall, but androgen levels are also reduced.

The relationship between insulin, androgens, and ovarian function is, without question, complex. Women with insulin resistance and type II diabetes do not necessarily exhibit reproductive impairment. Further, women with cystic ovaries and/or hyperandrogenism are often reproductively "normal" and do not display insulin resistance. Women with PCOS who have undergone surgical ovarian reduction often experience a reduction in androgen levels and a restoration of ovarian cyclicity without a compensatory correction in insulin action. Interestingly, women with PCOS often begin to ovulate in response to insulin sensitizing agents such as metformin or activators of PPARγ. Unlike surgical intervention, which has no demonstrated effect on insulin, reduction of serum insulin levels has the effect of reducing androgens in PCOS. Yet not all women with PCOS exhibit insulin resistance. In obese women with PCOS and insulin resistance, weight loss can result in reduced serum insulin and androgen levels as well as return of ovulation and fertility. Yet, thin women can have PCOS and insulin resistance and changes in weight seem to have no effect on them.

These issues emphasize the syndromic nature of PCOS and point toward multifactorial etiologies (involving hypothalamic, steroidogenic, intraovarian, and metabolic factors) that result in a final common pathway of hyperandrogenic anovulation.

PCOS Genetics It is generally agreed that PCOS has a genetic component, but the mode of inheritance is not well understood, hampered in part by an unidentified male phenotype. Several studies have investigated relationships with different genes and the PCOS phenotype. One investigated 37 candidate genes involved in steroidogenesis, insulin action, gonadotropin regulation, and obesity to characterize candidate genes implicated in the etiology of PCOS. Of these, follistatin and CPY11A (P450 side-chain cleavage) were revealed as potential as markers. Although the relationship of CYP11A was not significant following statistical adjustment, other studies have indicated its potential as a marker for altered androgen secretion characteristic of PCOS.

The variable number tandem repeats in the insulin gene might represent a susceptibility locus for PCOS, though the statistical analysis has been questioned. A polymorphism in the D3 dopamine receptor was found with increased frequency in hyperandrogenic, dysovulatory Hispanic women, and was associated with resistance to ovulation induction with clomiphene. However, this correlation was not confirmed in a larger population of Caucasian women.

Polymorphisms in the IL-6 gene promoter are more common in women with hyperandrogenism. In general, there has been no universal genetic marker identified for PCOS.

PCOS is clearly more than a reproductive disorder. It is characterized by multiple endocrine and metabolic derangements that can lead to chronic, negative health effects in afflicted women. Further understanding of its etiology is necessary so that improved screening, prevention, and treatment interventions can be developed to improve the overall health of women with PCOS.

CONCLUSION

The mechanisms that direct germ cells in the yolk sac to migrate to the gonadal ridge and become enclosed in a follicular apparatus, and then direct these follicles to grow in controlled cohorts during 50 yr or more, are far from being completely identified. More is known about the effects of gonadotropins and growth factors on cohorts of follicles recruited to the final steps of preovulatory development, but the exact molecular mechanisms governing dominance, ovulation, and luteinization also remain to be clarified. Tissue remodeling is clearly of prime importance in the cycling ovary, but it is apparently regulated by multiple redundant systems. The importance of normal ovarian function to the overall health of women is becoming more appreciated. The systemic consequences of prolonged hypoestrogenemia in untreated gonadal failure or of the hyperandrogenism of PCOS emphasize the role of the ovary in long-term women's health issues. As knowledge of the processes involved in normal folliculogenesis advance, a more precise picture of the myriad causes of ovarian dysfunction will become apparent.

SELECTED REFERENCES

Aittomaki K, Lucena JL, Pakarinen P, et al. Mutation in the follicle-stimulating hormone receptor gene causes hereditary hypergonadotropic ovarian failure. Cell 1995;82:959–968.

Barbieri RL, Smith S, Ryan KJ. The role of hyperinsulinemia in the pathogenesis of ovarian hyperandrogenism. Fertil Steril 1988;50:197–212.

Bolivar J, Guelman S, Iglesias C, Ortiz M, Valdivia MM. The fragile-X-related gene FXR1 is a human autoantigen processed during apoptosis. J Biol Chem 1998;273(27):17,122–17,127.

Cataldo NA, Dumesic DA, Goldsmith PC, Jaffe RB. Immunolocalization of Fas and Fas ligand in the ovaries of women with polycystic ovary syndrome: relationship to apoptosis. Hum Reprod 2000;15:1889–1897.

Chandrasekher YA, Hutchison JS, Zelinski-Wooten MB, Hess DL, Wolf DP, Stouffer RL. Initiation of periovulatory events in primate follicles using recombinant and native human luteinizing hormone to mimic the midcycle gonadotropin surge. J Clin Endocrinol Metab 1994;79:298–306.

Daniels TL, Berga SL. Resistance of gonadotropin releasing hormone to drive sexsteroid-induced suppression in hyperandrogenic anovulation. J Clin Endocrinol Metab 1997;82:4179–4183.

Donovan PJ. Growth factor regulation of mouse primordial germ cell development. Curr Top Dev Biol 1994;29:189–225.

Dunaif A, Thomas A. Current concepts in the polycystic ovary syndrome. Annu Rev Med 2001;52:401–419.

Ehrmann DA, Barnew RB, Rosenfield RL, Cavaghan MK, Imperial J. Prevalence of impaired glucose tolerance and diabetes in women with polycystic ovary syndrome. Diabetes Care 1999;22:141–146.

Faddy MJ, Gosden RG. A mathematical model of follicle dynamics in the human ovary. Hum Reprod 1995;10:770–775.

Franks S, Gharani N, McCarthy M. Genetics and infertility II: candidate genes in polycystic ovary syndrome. Hum Reprod Update 2001;7:405–410.

Gharani N, Waterworth DM, Batty S, et al. Association of the steroid synthesis gene CYP11a with polycystic ovary syndrome and hyperandrogenism. Hum Mol Genet 1997;6:397–402.

Gilling-Smith C, Story H, Rogers V, Franks S. Evidence for a primary abnormality of the cal cell steroidogenesis in the polycystic ovary syndrome. Clin Endocrinol (Oxf) 1997;47:9309.

Gulyas BJ, Hodgen GD, Tullner WW, Ross GT. Effects of fetal or maternal hypophysectomy on endocrine organs and body weight in infant rhesus monkeys (Macaca mulatta): with particular emphasis on oogenesis. Biol Reprod 1977;16:216–227.

Hirshfield AN. Development of follicles in the mammalian ovary. Int Rev Cytol 1991;124:43–101.

Hoek A, van Kasteren Y, de Haan-Meulman M, Hooijkaas H, Schoemaker J, Drexhage HA. Analysis of peripheral blood lymphocyte subsets, NK cells, and delayed type hypersensitivity skin test in patients with premature ovarian failure. Am J Reprod Immunol 1995;33:495–502.

Homburg R, Amsterdam A. Polycystic ovary syndrome-loss of the apoptotic mechanism in the ovarian follicles? J Endocrinol Invest 1998;9:552–557.

Horie K, Fujita J, Takakura K, et al. The expression of c-kit protein in human adult and fetal tissues. Hum Reprod 1993;8:1955–1962.

Hsu SY, Hsueh AJW. Tissue-specific Bcl-2 protein partners in apoptosis: an ovarian paradigm. Physiol Rev 2000;80(2):593–614.

Kaiser UB. The pathogenesis of the ovarian hyperstimulation syndrome. N Engl J Med 2003;349:729–732.

Kaufman FR, Donnell GN, Roe TF, Kogut MD. Gonadal function in patients with galactosaemia. J Inherit Metab Dis 1986;9:140–146.

Knochenhauer ES, Key TJ, Kahsar-Miller M, et al. Prevalence of polycystic ovary syndrome in unselected black and white women of the southeastern United States: a prospective study. J Clin Endocrinol Metab 1998;83:3078–3082.

Kol S, Adashi EY. Intraovarian factors regulating ovarian function. Curr Opin Obstet Gynecol 1995;7:209–213.

Latronico AC, Anasti J, Arnhold IJ, et al. Brief report: testicular and ovarian resistance to luteinizing hormone caused by inactivating mutations of the luteinizing hormone-receptor gene. N Engl J Med 1996;334:507–512.

Legro RS. The genetics of polycystic ovary syndrome. Am J Med 1995;98:9S–16S.

Legro RS, Kunselman AR, Dodson WC, Dunaif A. Prevalence and predictors of risk for type 2 diabetes mellitus an impaired glucose tolerance in polycystic ovary syndrome: a prospective, controlled study in 254 affected women. J Clin Endocrinol Metab 1999;84:165–169.

Lemieux S, Lewis GF, Ben-Chetrit A, Steiner G, Greenblatt EM. Correction of hyperandrogenemia by laparoscopic ovarian cautery in women with polycystic ovary syndrome is not accompanied by improved insulin sensitivity or lipid-lipoprotein levels. J Clin Endocrinol Metab 1999;11:4278–4282.

Leonardsson G, Peng XR, Liu K, et al. Ovulation efficiency is reduced in mice that lack plasminogen activator gene function: functional redundancy among physiological plasminogen activators. Proc Natl Acad Sci USA 1995;92:12,446–12,450.

Leondires MP, Berga SL. Role of GnRH drive in the pathophysiology of polycystic ovary syndrome. J Endocrinol Invest 1998;21:476–485.

Leung PC, Steele GL. Intracellular signaling in the gonads. Endocr Rev 1992;13:476–498.

Loucks TL, Talbott EO, McHugh K, Keelan M, et al. Do polycystic appearing ovaries affect the risk of cardiovascular disease among women with polycystic ovary syndrome? Fertil Steril 2000;74:547–552.

Luoh SW, Bain PA, Plakiewicz RD, et al. Zfx mutation results in small animal size and reduced germ cell number in male and female mice. Development 1997;124:2275–2284.

Lyons J, Landis CA, Harsh G, et al. Two G protein oncogenes in human endocrine tumors. Science 1990;249:655–659.

Matthews CH, Borgato S, Beck-Peccoz P, et al. Primary amenorrhoea and infertility due to a mutation in the beta-subunit of follicle-stimulating hormone. Nat Genet 1993;5:83–86.

McGee EA, Hsueh AJ. Initial and cyclic recruitment of ovarian follicles. Endocr Rev 2000;21(2):200–214.

McGee EA, Hsu SY, Kaipia A, Hsueh AJ. Cell death and survival during ovarian follicle development. Mol Cell Endocrinol 1998;140(1,2):15–18.

McGrath SA, Esquela AF, Lee SJ. Oocyte-specific expression of growth/differentiation factor-9. Mol Endocrinol 1995;9:131–136.

McNatty KP, Smith P, Hudson NL, et al. Development of the sheep ovary during fetal and early neonatal life and the effect of fecundity genes. J Reprod Fertil Suppl 1995;49:123–135.

Morales A, Laughlin G, Butzow T, Maheshwari H, Baumann G, Yen SSC. Insulin, somatotropic, and luteinizing hormone axes in lean and obese women with polycystic ovary syndrome: common and distinct features. J Clin Endocrinol Metab 1996;81:2854–2864.

Nelson VL, Qin KN, Rosenfield RL, et al. The biochemical basis for increased testosterone production in theca cells propagated from patients with polycystic ovary syndrome. J Clin Endocrinol Metab 2001;86:5925–5933.

Polson DW, Wadsworth J, Adams J, Franks S. Polycystic ovaries: a common finding in normal women. Lancet 1988;I:870–872.

Rabinovici J, Blankstein J, Goldman B, et al. In vitro fertilization and primary embryonic cleavage are possible in 17 alpha-hydroxylase deficiency despite extremely low intrafollicular 17 beta-estradiol. J Clin Endocrinol Metab 1989;68:693–697.

Richards JS. Hormonal control of gene expression in the ovary. Endocr Rev 1994;15:725–751.

Santoro N. Mechanisms of premature ovarian failure. Ann Endocrinol (Paris) 2003;64(2):87–92.

Smits G, Olatunbosun O, Delbaere A, et al. Brief Report Ovarian hyperstimulation syndrome due to a mutation in the follicle stimulating hormone receptor. N Engl J Med 2003;349:760–766.

Somers JP, Benyo DF, Little-Ihrig L, Zeleznik AJ. Luteinization in primates is accompanied by loss of a 43-kilodalton adenosine 3′,5′ monophosphate response element-binding protein isoform. Endocrinology 1995;136:4762–4768.

Stein IF, Leventhal ML. Amenorrhea associated with bilateral polycystic ovaries. Am J Obstet Gynecol 1935;29:181–191.

Talbot JA, Bicknell EJ, Rajkhowa M, Krook A, O'Rahilly S, Clayton RN. Molecular scanning of the insulin receptor gene in women with polycystic ovarian syndrome. J Clin Endocrinol Metab 1996;81:1979–1983.

Tsafriri A. Ovulation as a tissue remodelling process. Proteolysis and cumulus expansion. Adv Exp Med Biol 1995;377:121–140.

Urbanek M, Legro RS, Driscoll DA, et al. Thirty-seven candidate genes for polycystic ovary syndrome: strongest evidence for linkage with follistattin. Proc Natl Acad Sci USA 1999;96:8573–8578.

van der Meer M, Hompes PGA, de Boer JAM, et al. Cohort size rather than follicle stimulating hormone threshold concentration determines ovarian sensitivity in polycystic ovary syndrome. J Clin Endocrinol Metab 1998;83:423–426.

Vasseur C, Rodien P, Beau I, et al. A chorionic gonadotropin sensitive mutation in the follicle stimulating hormone receptor as a cause of familial gestational spontaneous ovarian hyperstimulation syndrome. N Engl J Med 2003;349:753–759.

Waterworth DM, Bennett ST, Gharani N, et al. Linkage and association of insulin gene VNTR regulatory polymorphism with polycystic ovary syndrome. Lancet 1997;349:986–990.

Weinstein LS, Shenker A, Gejman PV, Merino MJ, Friedman E, Spiegel AM. Activating mutations of the stimulatory G protein in the McCune-Albright syndrome. N Engl J Med 1991;325:1688–1695.

Wild RA. Metabolic aspects of polycystic ovary syndrome. Semin Reprod Endocrinol 1997;15:105–110.

Young RH, Scully RE. Endocrine tumors of the ovary. Curr Top Pathol 1992;85:113–164.

Zhang LH, Rodriguez H, Ohno S, Miller WL. Serine phosphorylation of human P450c17 increases 17,20-lyase activity: implications for adrenarche and the polycystic ovary syndrome. Proc Natl Acad Sci USA 1995;92:10,619–10,623.

METABOLIC DISORDERS

V

SECTION EDITOR:
SAMUEL KLEIN

Abbreviations

V. METABOLIC DISORDERS

αARs	α-adrenergic receptors
Akt	protein kinase B
apo AIV	Apolipoprotein AIV
βARs	β-adrenergic receptors
BAT	brown adipose tissue
C/EBP	CCAAT/enhancer binding proteins
CCK	cholecystokinin
cPLA$_2$	cytosolic phospholipase A$_2$
DAG	diacylglycerol
EC	endothelial cell
FFA	free fatty acid
GI	gastrointestinal
GLP-1	Glucagon-like peptide-1
GSK3β	glycogen synthase kinase 3-β
HSL	hormone-sensitive lipase
IGF-1	insulin-like-growth factor
IRS	insulin-receptor substrate
IRS-1	insulin receptor substrate 1
MAFbx	muscle atrophy F-box protein or atrogin-1
MHC	myosin heavy chain
mtDNA	mitochondrial DNA
mTOR	mammalian target of rapamycin
MuRF1	muscle ring finger protein 1
NF-κB	nuclear factor κ B
NFAT	nuclear factor of activated T cells
OLETF	otsuka long-evans tokushima fatty
PCr	creatine phosphate
PDE	phosphodiesterase
PDK-1	3′-phosphoinositide-dependent protein kinase-1
PI-3 kinase	phosphatidyl inositol-3 kinase
PI-3	phosphoinositide-3
PKA	protein kinase A
PKC	protein kinase C
PPARγ	peroxisome proliferator-activated receptor-γ
PTEN	phosphatase and tension homolog detected on chromosome 10
PYY	peptide YY
ROS	reactive oxygen species
SHIP	SH2-containing inositol-5-phosphatase
SNS	sympathetic nervous system
SREBP	sterol regulatory element binding protein
T2DM	type 2 diabetes
TNF	tumor-necrosis factor
Ub	ubiquitin
UCP	uncoupling protein
WAT	white adipose tissue

47 Gastrointestinal Regulation of Food Intake

PATRICK TSO AND MIN LIU

SUMMARY

The gastrointestinal tract regulates food intake by sending and receiving signals from the brain both through humoral and neural pathways. This system works efficiently because body weight remains remarkably constant over time despite the slight tendency to gain weight as some individual's age. Ghrelin, a peptide secreted by the stomach, promotes food intake and is located ideally to monitor the volume of food and liquid ingested. Cholecystokinin is released by enteroendocrine cells of the duodenum postprandially and plays an important role in the secretion of pancreatic enzymes and the contraction of the gallbladder to release bile into the duodenum to aid digestion and nutrient absorption. Additionally, cholecystokinin is a satiety signal that appears to play a role in the regulation of food intake. Apolipoprotein AIV (apo AIV) might be an important signal in regulating food intake and the absorption of fat. It appears to participate in the packaging and secretion of chylomicrons. Apo AIV probably works peripherally and centrally to inhibit food intake. When nutrients reach the lower small intestine, they stimulate the secretion of peptide YY (PYY), glucagon-like peptide-1, and potentially other signals as well. Their function is to simultaneously reduce food intake and gastric emptying.

Glucagon-like peptide-1 and PYY might work directly on inhibiting food intake or indirectly by boosting the production of apo AIV, which is true for PYY. Contrary to long-standing beliefs, secretion of these peptides occurs early after food ingestion, thereby slowing gastric emptying and allowing for slower delivery of food to the small intestine for digestion and absorption. Understanding how this highly integrated system works might provide solutions to the obesity epidemic in affluent countries.

Key Words: Apolipoprotein AIV; cholecystokinin; gastrointestinal; ghrelin; glucagon-like peptide-1; peptide YY.

INTRODUCTION

The amount and type of food consumed by most individuals varies from meal to meal. Emotions, social pressures, time of day, convenience, exercise, and cost are a few of the many factors that determine what and how much people eat. Interestingly, despite so many interacting variables, our body weight remains remarkably stable and varies little over long periods. Because changes in body weight depend on both caloric intake and energy expenditure, maintenance of body weight implies that intake is equal to energy consumption, helping to achieve a constant body weight. This chapter integrates the functions of selected gastrointestinal (GI) peptides that regulate food intake to present a cohesive view of how food intake is physiologically regulated by the GI tract.

To understand the regulation of food intake, it is important to appreciate the many signals that are involved in initiating hunger and in terminating eating. "*Satiety*" is defined as "*sufficiency, or satisfaction, as full gratification of appetite or thirst, with abolition of the desire to ingest food or liquid*." Satiety signals are distinct from the longer-acting adiposity signals. Adiposity signals, leptin and insulin, are mostly involved in the long-term regulation of food intake and energy metabolism as dictated by energy needs and the amount of energy stores (adipose tissue) in the body. In contrast, satiety signals are released by the GI tract resulting from the ingestion of food, participate in the digestive process, and provide signals to the nervous system that influence behavior. A primary purpose of these signals is to match "the capacity of the GI tract to process the ingested food" to "food intake," thereby ensuring that the GI tract is functioning optimally without being overwhelmed. This chapter discusses these signals from the proximal to the distal GI tract. The effects of the cephalic phase (the sight and smell of food) and its involvement in food intake regulation are not included.

GHRELIN

PRODUCTION Ghrelin is the ligand for stimulating the release of growth hormone from the pituitary through a G protein coupled receptor. It is a peptide of 28 amino acids in which the serine 3 residue is n-octanoylated. The O-n-octanoylation at serine 3 is essential to all of ghrelin's activity. Ghrelin secretion is induced by fasting and inhibited by refeeding or the ingestion of alcohol. Daily peripheral administration of ghrelin results in body weight gain in both mice and rats. Ghrelin is made from specific cells in the stomach and present most abundantly in the fundus of the stomach. Additionally, ghrelin is made by the small intestine.

PHYSIOLOGICAL FUNCTIONS Administration of peripheral or central ghrelin stimulates food intake as well as gastric acid secretion. Plasma ghrelin levels increase before each meal and fall to a nadir 1 h following the cessation of a meal. This finding is consistent with ghrelin's hypothesized role to stimulate food intake. Plasma ghrelin levels of subjects participating in a diet-induced weight reduction program rose following intervention consistent with increased appetite and tendency to regain lost weight. Ghrelin levels have also been investigated following gastric bypass surgery.

From: *Principles of Molecular Medicine, Second Edition*
Edited by: M. S. Runge and C. Patterson © Humana Press, Inc., Totowa, NJ

For instance, a reduction in circulating ghrelin levels among patients following gastric bypass is observed compared to their presurgery levels, consistent with the tendency of gastric bypass patients to eat less and therefore lose weight. Contrary to these studies, others have reported circulating ghrelin levels to increase following gastric bypass surgery. Reasons for these differences are unclear but might be related to the extent and/or exact site of surgical intervention.

In a clinical study of 24 patients having short bowel syndrome, circulating ghrelin was found to decrease. This decrease was proposed to result from tissue mass reduction in these patients and their subsequent inability to secrete ghrelin. In two separate studies, patients with Prader–Willi syndrome were found to have very high circulating levels of ghrelin, which is consistent with their enormous appetites and massive obesity. The circulating level of ghrelin is decreased in obese subjects and an inverse relationship exists between percentage of body fat and the circulating fasting ghrelin concentration.

How endogenous ghrelin secretion is turned on or off is not understood, nor is the function of endogenous ghrelin. However, a picture is emerging based on exogenous ghrelin, which appears to be an important hormone in initiating food intake, consistent with the observation that endocrine cells that secrete ghrelin are present in the stomach while other meal-related stimuli are active (such as gastric distension). With fasting or restriction of food intake, ghrelin secretion is high, so concern to induce eating. Following ingestion of food, its role in inducing food intake has been accomplished and so the secretion of ghrelin is markedly reduced. Patients with Prader–Willi syndrome probably have a genetic dysregulation of ghrelin secretion that causes them to behave differently from other obese humans who have an inverse relationship between percentage of body fat and plasma ghrelin. Although this hypothesis is compelling, it is based only on observed correlations.

CHOLECYSTOKININ

PRODUCTION   Cholecystokinin (CCK) is a hormone secreted by the enteroendocrine cells in the upper small intestine in response to the presence of amino acids and fatty acids in the lumen.

PHYSIOLOGICAL FUNCTIONS   The proposal that CCK plays a role in the regulation of food intake came from the demonstration that intraperitoneal administration of CCK caused satiety in rats. Exogenous CCK is also a satiety factor in man. Compared with a saline infusion, the infusion of the C-terminal octapeptide of CCK (CCK-8) suppresses liquid food intake without obvious outward side effects. CCK-8 also decreases solid food intake in man.

The satiety effect of CCK has been further characterized in animal models. In rodents, the inhibitory effect of CCK on food intake involves the vagus nerve, as abdominal vagotomy attenuates its satiety effect. Chemical denervation of the intestinal sensory nerves by capsaicin treatment also significantly reduces peripheral CCK-induced satiety. Further, convincing evidence exists that satiety caused by peripheral CCK administration involves CCK_A receptors in the periphery.

Despite evidence from both animals and humans demonstrating that exogenous CCK helps regulate food intake, this possible physiological role of endogenous CCK has been challenged because of the relatively small change that occurs in its circulating level following a meal. That is, the changes in the circulating level of CCK during a meal are significantly below the level of circulating CCK needed to achieve satiety by exogenously administered CCK. Nonetheless,

endogenous secreted CCK plays a role in the regulation of food intake based on experiments involving the CCK receptor antagonist, devazepide. In both primates (rhesus monkeys) and rats, a blockade of the CCK type A receptor by devazepide increases food intake. That endogenous CCK plays a role in the regulation of food intake has been further supported by studies using Otsuka Long-Evans Tokushima Fatty rats. These obese and diabetic rats have a defective CCK_A receptor. Otsuka Long-Evans Tokushima Fatty rats, having disordered food intake, consume a larger meal size than wild-type rats. Chronic ingestion of larger meal size increases daily food intake resulting in obesity when extended over a long interval.

Evidence suggests that CCK does not act alone, but instead interacts synergistically with other signals to regulate food intake. For instance, while subthreshold doses of either CCK-8 or leptin alone do not affect food intake, together they significantly reduce the intake of food. The combined action of CCK and leptin is mediated peripherally involving capsaicin-sensitive sensory fibers. Reduction in food intake is mediated by the coadministration of CCK and leptin is mediated by both the peripheral action of CCK and a central action of leptin. Reduction in food intake by exogenously administered CCK is significantly smaller in animals fed a diet high in fat over a long period. Further, reduction of gastric emptying by CCK is also attenuated in animals fed a high-fat diet over a substantial time. Thus, it is possible that the blunted response to CCK in animals chronically fed a diet high in fat might contribute to the dysregulation of food intake and thus account for associated obesity.

APOLIPOPROTEIN AIV

PRODUCTION   Apolipoprotein AIV (apo AIV) is a protein secreted by the enterocytes of the small intestine. The small intestine's production of apo AIV is regulated physiologically, decreasing with fasting and increasing with lipid feeding. Both mono- and polyunsaturated fatty acids stimulate the secretion of apo AIV by the small intestine to the same degree. Furthermore, bile diversion significantly reduces apo AIV synthesis by the intestinal mucosa. Thus, intact enterohepatic circulation is necessary for maintaining normal basal secretion of apo AIV by the gut. In vivo studies show that the synthesis and secretion of apo AIV by the GI tract are also regulated by peptides secreted by the lower small intestine, one candidate being peptide YY (PYY). PYY is secreted by the endocrine cells in the lower intestine in response to lipid absorption, which in turn stimulates the production and secretion of apo AIV by the jejunum. Unlike the stimulation of apo AIV production by lipid absorption in the jejunum, stimulation of apo AIV production by PYY is posttranscriptional, i.e., there is increased synthesis without a change in the mRNA level.

PHYSIOLOGICAL FUNCTIONS   Evidence suggests that Apo AIV regulates food intake. The first report of apo AIV as a satiety factor investigated rats with intravenous cannulas, who were fasted for 24 h and then infused intravenously with either saline, fasting lymph (lymph collected from fasting animals), or chylous lymph (lymph collected from animals actively absorbing fat). Food intake was then monitored. Animals receiving lymph from fasted rats consumed food comparable to animals that received saline. However, animals administered intravenous intestinal lymph from rats actively absorbing lipid had profound inhibition of food intake. These data suggested the presence of an active component(s) in chylous lymph that inhibits food intake, which was demonstrated to be apo AIV. Intravenous administration of 200 µg of apo AIV (a physiological dose) inhibited food intake to the same degree as chylous lymph in 24-h food-deprived rats. This unique function had not been previously ascribed to apo AIV. Moreover, it is not a function that is shared by apo AI. Hence apo AIV might be a circulating signal released by the small intestine in response to fat feeding and responsible for the anorectic effect associated with the ingestion of lipids.

Circulating apo AIV might affect the brain. Administration of apo AIV into the third ventricle of the brain in animals inhibited food intake in a dose-dependent manner. Further, the removal of apo AIV from the cerebrospinal fluid by using apo AIV antibodies caused rats to eat during the middle part of the light phase, a time when they normally do not eat. Hence, evidence exists that apo AIV can act centrally to reduce food intake.

Apo AIV inhibits gastric acid secretion and gastric motility. Two studies found food intake to be significantly inhibited by a physiological dose of apo AIV. The action of apo AIV is not limited to its central action as apo AIV administered peripherally inhibits gastric motility.

Both apo AIV mRNA and apo AIV protein are present in the rat hypothalamus. Hypothalamic apo AIV appears to be highly regulated as it decreases with fasting and increases with the infusion of lipid into the stomach. Thus, hypothalamic apo AIV appears to change in synchrony with serum apo AIV, and both are significantly higher in *ad libitum*-fed than in food-deprived rats. That hypothalamic apo AIV is involved in regulating food intake is further supported by the observation that administration of AIV antiserum into the third ventricle of *ad libitum*-fed rats significantly reduces hypothalamic apo AIV mRNA. Additionally, it results in animals consuming food at a time when they normally do not eat (during the middle of the light cycle). Neither administration of apolipoprotein AI antiserum nor nonbinding normal goat serum influenced food intake.

If endogenous apo AIV participates in the regulation of food intake, then apo AIV knockout animals would be expected to become obese from consuming excess food. To test this hypothesis, the growth, feeding behavior, and fat absorption of apo AIV knockout mice were measured; all were reported as normal. However, male mice showed increased food intake following an 18 h fast. Preliminary data indicate the apo AIV knockout mice gained excess weight over a period of weeks when fed a diet high in fat (40% butterfat) relative to wild-type controls. Using the lymph-fistula mouse model, apo AIV knockout mice adequately digest, absorb, and transport a modest lipid load into lymph. However, when lipid load is increased, these animals have delayed formation and secretion of chylomicrons by the intestinal mucosa. The importance of apo AIV in the normal formation and secretion of chylomicrons has been studied. Air bubble surfactometry and drop volume tensiometry were used to study the involvement of apo AIV in chylomicron assembly; apo AIV plays an important role in stabilizing the surface of expanding chylomicrons intracellularly. Also, overexpression of apo AIV in newborn swine intestinal epithelial cells greatly enhances intestinal fat absorption by promoting chylomicron formation and secretion. Thus, in addition to its role in inhibiting food intake, apo AIV also plays an important role in the formation and secretion of chylomicrons.

The regulation of jejunal apo AIV synthesis and secretion by PYY has potential physiologic significance. The distal intestine plays an important role in the control of upper GI function, especially the stomach. Nutrients, including lipids, when delivered to the ileum cause a slowing of gastric emptying, decreased intestinal motility and transit, and decreased pancreatic secretion. The presence of nutrients in the ileum also inhibits food intake. The mechanism responsible for producing these effects has been collectively termed the "ileal brake" and is believed to relate to the release of one or more peptide hormones from the distal intestine. PYY is an obvious candidate for this inhibitory effect on food intake because it is secreted from the distal intestine when lipid is infused. Such effects have traditionally been considered operative only during the abnormal delivery of undigested nutrients to the distal gut, such as would occur in the malabsorptive state. The upper small intestine is considered the primary site for the absorption of fat and the lower small intestine is thought to absorb fat only when fat malabsorption occurs in the upper small intestine, but this idea has been challenged. In both rats and dogs, nutrients frequently reach the distal gut soon after the ingestion of lipids even under normal conditions because of rapid gastric emptying during the early phases of food ingestion. Consequently, it appears that a much greater length of intestine is involved in the absorption of lipid and conditions, than previously recognized. Thus, the "ileal brake" might play an important role in the normal control of gut function and the control of lipid absorption. Once the homeostatic "ileal brake" phenomenon begins, the upper small intestine is unquestionably the primary site for the absorption of fat. It is tempting to speculate that apo AIV might contribute to the "ileal brake" phenomenon because PYY is a potent stimulant of apo AIV formation and secretion by the jejunum.

GLP-1 AND PYY

PRODUCTION   Glucagon-like peptide-1 (GLP-1) is synthesized by endocrine cells located in the ileum and colon. It is secreted in response to nutrient ingestion and plays multiple roles in metabolic homeostasis following nutrient absorption.

Initial studies of GLP-1 biological activity utilized the full length N-terminal extended forms of GLP-1 (1–37 and 1–36[amide]), which have low biological activity. Later, it was recognized that removal of the first six amino acids resulted in a shorter version of the GLP-1 molecule with substantially greater biological activity. GLP-1 is rapidly degraded in the blood by dipeptidyl peptidase. PYY is a peptide secreted by the same endocrine cells in the ileum that secrete GLP-1. The release of PYY by these enteroendocrine cells is stimulated by the presence of nutrients in the ileum including carbohydrates and fat.

PHYSIOLOGICAL FUNCTIONS   GLP-1 (7-36) amide, when administered centrally, causes profound reduction in food intake. In healthy human subjects, intravenous infusion of graded doses of synthetic human GLP-1 resulted in a dose-dependent reduction in food intake. These normal human subjects reported less hunger and early satiety during the period of GLP-1 infusion.

However, humans infused intravenously with GLP-1 showed a marked reduction in gastric emptying and only an insignificant effect on food intake was observed. Central administration of GLP-1 produced conditioned taste aversion in rodents. Unlike leptin, central administration of GLP-1 resulted in aversive side effects. Additional experiments are warranted to interpret this apparent discrepancy in the function of GLP-1 as a satiety factor against its role as a taste aversive factor. The aversive and caloric effects of GLP-1 might be caused by differential activation of distinct receptor populations in the brain, providing the answer.

Peripheral injection of PYY (3–36) in rats significantly inhibits food intake, and this action is probably mediated through the Y2 receptor as PYY failed to inhibit food intake in Y2 receptor null mice. Electrophysiological recordings show that PYY inhibits electrical activity of hypothalamic neuropeptide neurons, thus resulting in the activation of hypothalamic pro-opiomelanocortin neurons. Infusion of physiological doses of PYY decreased appetite and food intake significantly.

Both PYY and GLP-1 hormones are released when the ileum is exposed to nutrients. These hormones are thought to slow gastric emptying and gastric acid secretion. Their major digestive function is to prevent the lower small intestine from becoming overwhelmed by newly ingested nutrients. Thus, they complement apo AIV in regulating the amount of food consumed as well as the amount of food emptied by the stomach. Because PYY stimulates jejunal apo AIV synthesis and secretion and this action is mediated through the vagus nerve, it is possible that PYY's role in the regulation of food intake is mediated partly or totally through apo AIV. However, it is unclear whether GLP-1 affects apo AIV synthesis in the gut.

SELECTED REFERENCES

Barrachina MD, Martinez V, Wang L, Wei JY, Tache Y. Synergistic interaction between leptin and cholecystokin to reduce short-term food intake in lean mice. Proc Natl Acad Sci USA 1997;94: 10,455–10,460.

Batterham RL, Cowley MA, Small CJ, et al. Gut hormone PYY(3-36) physiologically inhibits food intake. Nature 2002;418:650–654.

Covasa M, Ritter RC. Adaptation to high-fat diet reduces inhibition of gastric emptying by CCK and intestinal oleate. Am J Physiol 2000; 278:R166–R170.

Covasa M, Ritter RC. Reduced sensitivity to the satiation effect of intestinal oleate in rats adapted to high-fat diet. Am J Physiol 1999; 277:R279–R285.

Cummings DE, Clement K, Purnell JQ, et al. Elevated plasma ghrelin levels in Prader Willi syndrome. Nat Med 2002;8:643, 644.

Cummings DE, Purnell JQ, Frayo RS, Schmidova K, Wisse BE, Weigle DS. A preprandial rise in plasma ghrelin levels suggests a role in meal initiation in humans. Diabetes 2001;50:1714–1719.

Date Y, Kojima M, Hosoda H, et al. Ghrelin, a novel growth hormone-releasing acylated peptide is synthesized in a distinct endocrine cell type in the gastrointestinal tracts of rats and humans. Endocrinology 2000;141:4255–4261.

Date Y, Nakazato M, Murakami N, Kojima M, Kangawa K, Matsukura S. Ghrelin acts in the central nervous system to stimulate gastric acid secretion. Biochem Biophys Res Commun 2001;280:904–907.

DelParigi A, Tschop M, Heiman ML, et al. High circulating ghrelin: a potential cause for hyperphagia and obesity in Prader-Willi syndrome. J Clin Endocrinol Metab 2002;87:5461–5464.

Fujimoto K, Cardelli JA, Tso P. Increased apolipoprotein A-IV in rat mesenteric lymph after lipid meal acts as a physiological signal for satiation. Am J Physiol 1992;262:G1002–G1006.

Fukagawa K, Gou HM, Wolf R, Tso P. Circadian rhythm of serum and lymph apolipoprotein AIV in ad libitum-fed and fasted rats. Am J Physiol 1994;267:R1385–R1390.

Geloneze B, Tambascia MA, Pilla VF, Geloneze SR, Repetto EM, Pareja JC. Ghrelin: a gut-brain hormone effect of gastric bypass surgery. Obes Surg 2003;13:17–22.

Gibbs J, Young RC, Smith GP. Cholecystokinin elicits satiety in rats with open gastric fistulas. Nature 1973;245:323–325.

Glatzle J, Kalogeris TJ, Zittel TT, Guerrini S, Tso P, Raybould HE. Chylomicron components mediate intestinal lipid-induced inhibition of gastric motor function. Am J Physiol 2002;282:G86–G91.

Grider JR. Role of cholecystokinin in the regulation of gastrointestinal motility. J Nutr 1994;124:1334S–1339S.

Gutzwiller JP, Goke B, Drewe J, et al. Glucagon-like peptide-1: a potent regulator of food intake in humans. Gut 1999;44:81–86.

Hayashi H, Nutting DF, Fujimoto K, Cardelli JA, Black D, Tso P. Transport of lipid and apolipoproteins A-I and A-IV in intestinal lymph of the rat. J Lipid Res 1990;31:1613–1625.

Hewson G, Leighton GE, Hill RG, Hughes J. The cholecystokinin receptor antagonist L364,718 increases food intake in the rat by attenuation of the action of endogenous cholecystokinin. Br J Pharmacol 1988;93:79–84.

Holdstock C, Engstrom BE, Ohrvall M, Lind L, Sundbom M, Karlsson FA. Ghrelin and adipose tissue regulatory peptides: effect of gastric bypass surgery in obese humans. J Clin Endocrinol Metab 2003; 88:2999–3002.

Kalogeris TJ, Qin X, Chey WY, Tso P. PYY stimulates synthesis and secretion of intestinal apolipoprotein AIV without affecting mRNA expression. Am J Physiol 1998;275:G668–G674.

Kinzig KP, D'Alessio DA, Seeley RJ. The diverse roles of specific GLP-1 receptors in the control of food intake and the response to visceral illness. J Neurosci 2002;22:10,470–10,476.

Kissileff HR, Pi-Sunyer FX, Thornton J, Smith GP. C-terminal octapeptide of cholecystokinin decreases food intake in man. Am J Clin Nutr 1981;34:154–160.

Kojima M, Hosoda H, Date Y, Nakazato M, Matsuo H, Kangawa K. Ghrelin is a growth-hormone-releasing acylated peptide from stomach. Nature 1999;402:656–660.

Kratz M, Wahrburg U, von Eckardstein A, Ezeh B, Assmann G, Kronenberg F. Dietary mono- and polyunsaturated fatty acids similarly increase plasma apolipoprotein A-IV concentrations in healthy men and women. J Nutr 2003;133:1821–1825.

Krsek M, Rosicka M, Haluzik M, et al. Plasma ghrelin levels in patients with short bowel syndrome. Endocr Res 2002;28:27–33.

Liddle RA. Regulation of cholecystokinin secretion in humans. J Gastroenterol 2000;35:181–187.

Lin HC, Zhao XT, Wang L. Fat absorption is not complete by midgut but is dependent on load of fat. Am J Physiol 1996;271:G62–G67.

Liu M, Doi T, Shen L, et al. Intestinal satiety protein apolipoprotein AIV is synthesized and regulated in rat hypothalamus. Am J Physiol 2001;280:R1382–R1387.

Long SJ, Sutton JA, Amaee WB, et al. No effect of glucagon-like peptide-1 on short-term satiety and energy intake in man. Br J Nutr 1999;81: 273–279.

Lu S, Yao Y, Meng S, Cheng X, Black DD. Overexpression of apolipoprotein A-IV enhances lipid transport in newborn swine intestinal epithelial cells. J Biol Chem 2002;277:31,929–31,937.

MacLean DB. Abrogation of peripheral cholecystokinin-satiety in the capsaicin treated rat. Regul Pept 1985;11:321–333.

Matson CA, Reid DF, Cannon TA, Ritter RC. Cholecystokinin and leptin act synergistically to reduce body weight. Am J Physiol 2000;278: R882–R890.

Moran TH, Amegloio PJ, Peyton HJ, Schwartz GJ, McHugh PR. Blockade of type A, but not type B, CCK receptors postpones satiety in rhesus monkeys. Am J Physiol 1993;265:R620–R624.

Moran TH, Katz LF, Plata-Salaman CR, Schwartz GJ. Disordered food intake and obesity in rats lacking cholecystokinin A receptors. Am J Physiol 1998;274:R618–R625.

Okumura T, Fukagawa K, Tso P, Taylor IL, Pappas TN. Apolipoprotein A-IV acts in the brain to inhibit gastric emptying in the rat. Am J Physiol 1996;270:G49–G53.

Reidelberger RD, Heimann D, Kelsey L, Hulce M. Effects of peripheral CCK receptor blockade on feeding responses to duodenal nutrient infusions in rats. Am J Physiol 2003;284:R389–R398.

Reidelberger RD, Solomon TE. Comparative effects of CCK-8 on feeding, sham feeding, and exocrine pancreatic secretion in rats. Am J Physiol 1986;251:R97–R105.

Rodriguez MD, Kalogeris TJ, Wang XL, Wolf R, Tso P. Rapid synthesis and secretion of intestinal apolipoprotein A-IV after gastric fat loading in rats. Am J Physiol 1997;272:R1170–R1177.

Schwartz MW, Woods SC, Porte D Jr, Seeley RJ, Baskin DG. Central nervous system control of food intake. Nature 2000;404:661–671.

Smith GP, Gibbs J. Gut peptides and postprandial satiety. Fed Proc 1984;43:2889–2892.

Spiller RC, Trotman IF, Adrian TE, Bloom SR, Misiewicz JJ, Silk DB. Further characterization of the "ileal brake" reflex in man – effect of the ileal infusion of partial digests of fat, protein, and starch on jejunal motility and release of neurotensin, enteroglucagon, and peptide YY. Gut 1998;29:1042–1051.

Spiller RC, Trotman IF, Higgins BE, et al. The ileal brake-inhibition of jejunal motility after ileal fat perfusion in man. Gut 1984;25:365–374.

Stacher G, Steinringer H, Schmierer G, Schneider C, Winklehner S. Cholecystokinin octapeptide decreases intake of solid food in man. Peptides 1982;3:133–136.

Tang-Christensen M, Larsen PJ, Goke R, et al. Central administration of GLP-1-(7-36) amide inhibits food and water intake in rats. Am J Physiol 1996;271:R848–R856.

Thiele TE, Van Dijk G, Campfield LA, et al. Central infusion of GLP-1, but not leptin, produces conditioned taste aversions in rats. Am J Physiol 1997;272:R726–R730.

Tohno H, Sarr MG, DiMagno EP. Intraileal carbohydrate regulates canine postprandial pancreaticobiliary secretion and upper gut motility. Gastroenterology 1995;109:1977–1985.

Tschop M, Smiley DL, Heiman ML. Ghrelin induces adiposity in rodents. Nature 2000;407:908–913.

Tschop M, Weyer C, Tataranni PA, Devanarayan V, Ravussin E, Heiman ML. Circulating ghrelin levels are decreased in human obesity. Diabetes 2001;50:707–709.

Turton MD, O'Shea D, Gunn I, et al. A role for glucagon-like peptide-1 in the central regulation of feeding. Nature 1996;379:69–72.

Weinberg RB, Cook VR, DeLozier JA, Shelness GS. Dynamic interfacial properties of human apolipoprotein A-IV and B-17 at the air/water and oil/water interface. J Lipid Res 2000;41:1419–1427.

Weinstock PH, Bisgaier CL, Hayek T, et al. Decreased HDL cholesterol levels but normal lipid absorption, growth, and feeding behavior in apolipoprotein A-IV knockout mice. J Lipid Res 1997;38:1782–1794.

Wren AM, Small CJ, Abbott CR, et al. Ghrelin causes hyperphagia and obesity in rats. Diabetes 2001;50:2540–2547.

Wren AM, Small CJ, Ward HL, et al. The novel hypothalamic ghrelin stimulates food intake and growth hormone secretion. Endocrinology 2000;141:4325–4328.

48 Cellular Regulation of Lipolysis

Allan Green

SUMMARY

Lipolysis is the pathway by which adipocyte triglycerides are hydrolyzed and mobilized as free fatty acids, during periods when energy expenditure exceeds caloric intake. Hormone-sensitive lipase is the major enzyme involved in regulation of lipolysis. Numerous hormones acutely regulate lipolysis, but the most physiologically important are insulin (inhibitory) and catecholamines (stimulatory). Hormone-sensitive lipase is activated by phosphorylation in response to stimulatory hormones through a cAMP-mediated cascade. Conversely, insulin and other hormones that inhibit lipolysis decrease phosphorylation of hormone-sensitive lipase. Lipolysis can also be regulated over the longer term by changes in gene expression in response to growth hormone, cytokines, insulin, and glucose.

Key Words: Adipose tissue; adipocytes; fat metabolism; free fatty acids; glycerol; hormone-sensitive lipase; lipid metabolism; lipolysis; perilipin; triglyceride.

INTRODUCTION

In humans and other mammals, energy is stored primarily as glycogen in skeletal muscle and liver, and as triglyceride in adipose tissue. An average adult stores only about 1500 calories as glycogen, but even a fairly lean adult can store more than 100,000 calories as triglyceride. Glycogen and triglyceride, therefore, serve to maintain energy requirements between meals and during short bursts of exercise (primarily glycogen) and during longer periods of food deprivation or during prolonged exercise (primarily triglyceride).

When required, triglyceride is mobilized from adipose tissue by a highly regulated process known as lipolysis. Lipolysis proceeds in a stepwise fashion to release three molecules of free fatty acid (FFA) and one molecule of glycerol from each triglyceride molecule. FFA and glycerol are released into the interstitial space, and eventually into the circulation. Glycerol is metabolized primarily in the liver, but FFA are oxidized by most tissues. Indeed many tissues will oxidize FFA in preference to glucose; a mechanism known at the glucose–fatty acid cycle, hence "sparing" glucose during a prolonged fast for those tissues that have an absolute requirement for glucose, such as the brain, kidney medulla, and erythrocytes.

Circulating FFA concentrations are determined mostly by the rate of adipose tissue lipolysis. Although FFA are an excellent oxidative substrate for energy-requiring processes, they are also extremely toxic. At higher concentrations FFA can have adverse effects on membrane function, and are cardiotoxic. It is thought that high circulating FFA is a major contributor to life-threatening ventricular arrhythmia during an acute myocardial infarction. At lower concentrations FFA induce insulin resistance, increase hepatic glucose output and have adverse effects on pancreatic β-cell function. Evidence suggests that excess adipose tissue lipolysis and consequent elevations in FFA are central to the insulin resistance of obesity, and a key factor in development of type-2 diabetes. For these reasons, it is essential that lipolysis is a tightly regulated process, to supply FFA only when needed for oxidation in other tissues.

STORAGE OF TRIGLYCERIDES White adipose tissue accounts for the majority of triglyceride storage in adult humans. White adipocytes are the primary cell within the white adipose tissue, with the remaining cells (blood vessels, connective tissue, and so on) collectively known as the stromal-vascular cells. Within white adipocytes, insoluble triglyceride is stored as a single droplet that occupies most of the cell. A small rim of cytoplasm, containing the nucleus, mitochondria, and other cellular components, surrounds the triglyceride droplet. Adipocytes are almost spherical, but a small "bulge" can often be observed on one side of the cell, which contains the nucleus. The triglyceride droplet is coated with a variety of proteins, including perilipins and lipotransins; some of which are involved in regulation of lipolysis (*see* Perilipins).

EXPERIMENTAL MODEL SYSTEMS Adipocyte lipolysis results in release of both fatty acids and glycerol. Fatty acids can be re-esterified back to triglyceride. By contrast, adipocytes cannot reutilize glycerol, because they do not express glycerol kinase. For this reason, in vitro studies of lipolysis are almost always performed by measuring the rate of glycerol release, rather than fatty acids. Glycerol can be readily assayed using a variety of enzymic and colorimetric techniques.

Lipolysis has been studied in a variety of whole tissue, isolated cell, and tissue culture systems. Each technique has advantages and disadvantages. Early studies, performed with whole fat pads or minced tissue, led to the widespread use of the rat epididymal fat pad, which was originally used because it is very thin and therefore metabolites, oxygen, and carbon dioxide readily diffuse in and out of the tissue. In 1964, a method was developed for isolation of adipocytes from rat epididymal fat pads by collagenase

From: *Principles of Molecular Medicine, Second Edition*
Edited by: M. S. Runge and C. Patterson © Humana Press, Inc., Totowa, NJ

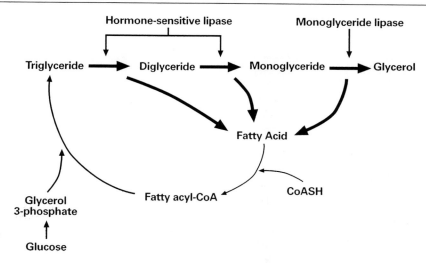

Figure 48-1 Pathways for lipolysis and re-esterification in adipocytes. Triglyceride is hydrolyzed sequentially to diglyceride, monoglyceride, and glycerol, by the actions of hormone-sensitive lipase and monoglyceride lipase. Adipocytes release both glycerol and FFAs, but a portion of the latter can be re-esterified to triglyceride. The glycerol backbone is derived through glycolysis from glucose, rather than glycerol, because adipocytes do not express glycerol kinase.

digestion. In this technique, pieces of adipose tissue are incubated with crude bacterial collagenase, which liberates the adipocytes. This method is particularly convenient because on low-speed centrifugation these cells float to the top of the tube, whereas other cells sediment to the bottom. Slight variations of this technique have been used for studies of adipocyte metabolism for more than 40 yr. The technique has been modified to allow primary culture of these cells, so that they can be studied in vitro for up to a week or more. The collagenase digestion technique can be used to study adipocytes from different anatomic sites, including adipose tissue from human subjects obtained during surgery, liposuction, or biopsy.

Several cell lines can be maintained in tissue culture and then treated with various agents in vitro to induce their differentiation into adipocytes. The most widely used have been the 3T3-L1 and 3T3-F442A cells, originally derived from mouse fibroblasts. Such cells have the advantage that they can be experimentally manipulated and passaged in vitro before differentiation. Major disadvantages are that they are heteroploid, transformed cell lines that may or may not be representative of true adipocytes. However, these cells have been extremely useful for studies of adipocyte differentiation.

Another technique based on isolation of preadipocytes from human adipose tissue allows these cells to be maintained in tissue culture, and then induced to differentiate in vitro using methods similar to those used in the 3T3-L1 cells. Several promising findings have been reported using this technique.

PATHWAY OF LIPOLYSIS AND RE-ESTERIFICATION A triglyceride molecule consists of a glycerol backbone to which is esterified three long-chain fatty acids. Triglycerides are hydrolyzed sequentially, primarily by two enzymes (Fig. 48-1). An enzyme known as hormone-sensitive lipase (HSL) is responsible for removing two of the three fatty acids. That is, HSL hydrolyzes both triglycerides and diglycerides. The rate-limiting step for lipolysis is removal of the first fatty acid by HSL and, as the name implies, multiple hormones and other agonists alter the activity of this enzyme. A second enzyme, monoglyceride lipase, is responsible for hydrolysis of the third fatty acid to liberate free glycerol, and has little or no ability to hydrolyze either triglyceride or diglyceride.

A portion of the fatty acids released from adipocytes can be re-esterified to triglyceride. This process of lipolysis and re-esterification can form a so-called substrate cycle between triglyceride, fatty acids, and back to triglyceride. In this re-esterification process, the source of the glycerol backbone is glycerol 3-phosphate derived from glucose, rather than glycerol itself, because adipocytes do not express glycerol kinase.

REGULATION OF THE RATE OF LIPOLYSIS

Mechanisms for regulation of the rate of lipolysis can be broadly categorized into two classes. First, there are mechanisms by which the rate of triglyceride breakdown can be varied dramatically over the short term, i.e., seconds to minutes. Second, overall rates of lipolysis can be regulated on a more long-term basis, altering total triglyceride breakdown over hours, days, or longer.

SHORT-TERM REGULATION OF LIPOLYSIS A number of hormones can readily stimulate lipolysis in adipocytes in vitro by a factor of 10- to 20-fold, or more. These stimulatory hormones include the catecholamines, adrenocorticotropic hormone, glucagon, vasoactive intestinal peptide, thyroid stimulating hormone, and the natriuretic peptides. Conversely, lipolysis can be inhibited by a variety of agents, including adenosine, E-series prostaglandins, catecholamines acting at α_2-adrenergic receptors, dopamine, adenosine receptor agonists, nicotinic acid, and insulin. However, the only hormones with a generally accepted role in short-term regulation of lipolysis in humans are the catecholamines and insulin.

The majority of the hormones that stimulate or inhibit lipolysis do so through a cyclic adenosine 5′-monophosphate (AMP)-dependent mechanism, as illustrated in Fig. 48-2. Most of these hormones alter cellular cyclic AMP concentrations through classical G protein-coupled mechanisms. The receptors involved are typical G protein-coupled receptors, consisting of seven transmembrane domains, with the N-terminal sequence outside the cell, and the C-terminus forming a cytoplasmic tail. Stimulatory receptors activate the stimulatory G protein known as G_s, whereas receptors that inhibit lipolysis activate the inhibitory G protein, G_i. These in turn either activate or inhibit adenylyl cyclase, which produces cyclic

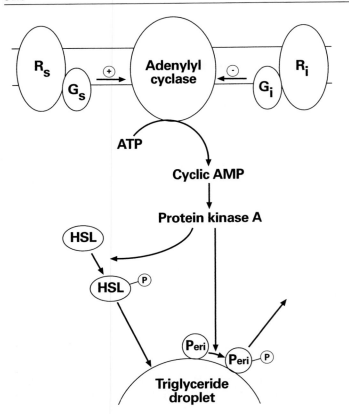

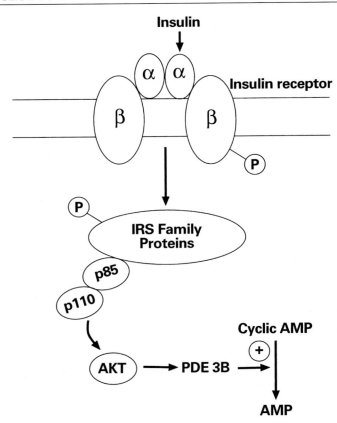

Figure 48-2 G protein-coupled receptor regulation of lipolysis. Stimulatory receptors (e.g., β-adrenergic receptors) couple through activation of G_s to increase cyclic AMP concentrations, activate PKA and phosphorylate both hormone-sensitive lipase and perilipin (Peri). The phosphorylated perilipin migrates away from the triglyceride droplet, hence increasing the accessibility of the lipid droplet to phosphorylated HSL, which migrates to the droplet, hence increasing the rate of lipolysis. Conversely, inhibitory receptors (e.g., A_1-adenosine receptors) couple through G_i to inhibition of cyclase, which decreases cyclic AMP concentrations, eventually leading to inhibition of lipolysis. P, phosphate ion.

Figure 48-3 Mechanism by which insulin inhibits lipolysis. Insulin binds to the α-subunit of the insulin receptor, which induces autophosphorylation of the β-subunit. This results in tyrosine phosphorylation of various members of the insulin receptor substrate family, which binds and activates PI-3 kinase. This results in activation of Akt, leading to activation of phosphodiesterase-3B. PDE3B activation results in hydrolysis of cyclic AMP, leading to inhibition of lipolysis. P, phosphate ion.

AMP from the substrate, ATP. Cyclic AMP activates protein kinase A (PKA), which phosphorylates and activates HSL.

Stimulation of Lipolysis Catecholamines are the major class of hormones that activate lipolysis in adipose tissue. They activate lipolysis through typical β-adrenergic receptors. Adipocytes express $β_1$- and $β_2$-adrenergic receptors, similar to those found in other tissues. However, adipocytes also express a third, atypical form, the $β_3$-adrenergic receptors. These $β_3$-adrenergic receptors are expressed predominantly in brown adipose tissue, but to a smaller degree in white adipocytes.

The natriuretic family of peptides is best known for its involvement in blood pressure regulation. Receptors for atrial, brain, and C-type natriuretic peptides have been reported on rodent adipocytes, and these peptides stimulate lipolysis in human (but not rodent) adipocytes, both in vivo and in vitro. The second messenger responsible for this effect is cyclic guanosine 5′-monophopshate (GMP), rather than cyclic AMP. However, the physiological significance of this is not known. There are numerous other receptors on adipocytes, which, when activated, can stimulate lipolysis. Again, the physiological relevance of these receptors is not clear.

Inhibition of Lipolysis There are a number of G protein-coupled receptors that inhibit lipolysis by decreasing cyclic AMP concentrations. Many of these are members of the G protein-coupled receptor family, with the seven transmembrane domain structure described earlier. The best described in this class are A_1-adenosine and $α_2$-adrenergic receptors. In addition, E-series prostaglandins are potent inhibitors of adenylyl cyclase and lipolysis in adipocytes (in contrast to most tissues, in which these prostaglandins increase cyclic AMP concentrations). Catecholamines can inhibit lipolysis by acting at $α_2$-adrenergic receptors. Finally, nicotinic acid is a potent pharmacological inhibitor of lipolysis. Although it is well established that nicotinic acid inhibits lipolysis through a G protein-coupled mechanism, the receptor to which it binds has not yet been identified.

Physiologically, there can be little doubt that insulin is the most important hormonal inhibitor of lipolysis. In the fed state, circulating insulin is sufficient to maximally suppress adipocyte lipolysis. The mechanism by which insulin inhibits lipolysis differs from that of the G protein-coupled receptors. Most of the metabolic actions of insulin (stimulation of glucose transport, glycogen synthesis, fatty acid synthesis, and so on), including inhibition of lipolysis, involve activation of an enzyme, phosphatidyl inositol-3 kinase (PI-3 kinase). PI-3 kinase activation arises from a complex signaling pathway, starting with insulin binding to its receptor (Fig. 48-3). The insulin receptor is a tetrameric glycoprotein, consisting of two α-subunits and two β-subunits, joined by disulfide bonds. The α-subunits possess cysteine-rich regions, which bind insulin. Insulin binding to the α-subunit results in activation of a tyrosine kinase activity in the β-subunits, resulting in autophosphorylation and activation of the receptor. Once phosphorylated, the insulin receptor tyrosine phosphorylates several intracellular substrates including insulin receptor substrate (IRS)-1, IRS-2, IRS-3, and IRS-4 and products of the shc gene. Phosphorylated substrates of the insulin receptor then bind and regulate a number of effector molecules that contain so-called SH2 (src-homology 2) domains, and hence initiate intracellular cascades of phosphorylations and dephosphorylations that lead to the various metabolic and mitogenic actions of insulin. One of these is the enzyme PI-3 kinase, which seems to be central to the metabolic actions of insulin. PI-3 kinase is made up of a p110 catalytic subunit, and a p85 regulatory subunit. Activation of PI-3 kinase results from dissociation of these two subunits.

Activation of PI-3 kinase results in various events, including activation of a low Km, cyclic GMP-inhibitable phosphodiesterase called phosphodiesterase-3B. This activation may be mediated through protein kinase B (also known as Akt). This increased phosphodiesterase activity lowers cyclic AMP concentrations, leading to a decrease in the activity of HSL, as described later.

Autocrine/Paracrine Regulation of Lipolysis Adipose tissue has traditionally been viewed as an inert tissue whose main function was to store energy in the form of triglyceride and release energy in the form of FFAs. Although this is clearly a major function, it has become clear that adipose tissue produces many hormones, cytokines, and metabolites that can have profound effects throughout the body. Such hormones include leptin, resistin, angiotensinogen, tumor necrosis factor (TNF)-α, insulin-like growth factor I, adiponectin, adenosine, and prostaglandins. Many of these hormones are secreted into the bloodstream, but some appear to act primarily in an autocrine or paracrine fashion. Isolated adipocytes release sufficient adenosine that, in the absence of any other added agent, the rate of lipolysis is almost fully suppressed. Addition of adenosine deaminase (which converts adenosine to the much less active inosine) to suspensions of rat adipocytes stimulates lipolysis to a similar extent as does isoproterenol, suggesting that endogenous adenosine can have a profound effect on adipocyte lipolysis. Similarly, E-series prostaglandins likely have an autocrine role in regulation of lipolysis.

TNF-α, expressed in adipose tissue, and at higher levels in adipocytes from obese subjects, is thought to have an important role in the etiology of insulin resistance in obesity. However, TNF-α circulates at extremely low concentrations in both lean and obese subjects, raising the possibility that the more important effect of adipocyte-derived TNF-α is within the adipose tissue itself. TNF-α increases the rate of lipolysis (see Cytokines) and hence this is likely an example of autocrine or paracrine regulation.

G Proteins in Regulation of Lipolysis Adipocytes express various G proteins at high concentrations. Hormones that stimulate adenylyl cyclase do so by activating G_s. Adipocytes express two forms of $G_s\alpha$, of approx 47 and 43 kDa. These isoforms arise from alternative splicing of mRNA from a single gene. As in other tissues, G_s can be ADP-ribosylated and activated by treatment of the cells with cholera toxin. The subsequent increase in cyclic AMP dramatically increases the rate of lipolysis.

A_1-adenosine receptors, and others that inhibit adenylyl cyclase, are also classical G protein-coupled receptors. Effects of these inhibitory agonists are blocked by pertussis toxin, known to ADP

ribosylate and inactivate at least six G protein α-subunits. Each of these has in common a cysteine residue located four amino acids from the C-terminus, which is the site for toxin-catalyzed ADP-ribosylation. These pertussis toxin-sensitive G proteins include at least two forms of G_o, and three subtypes of G_i: G_i1, G_i2, and G_i3. The only pertussis toxin substrates detectable in adipocytes are the α-subunits of G_i1, G_i2, and G_i3. These isoforms are products of separate genes, but are highly homologous and of a similar size (40–41 kDa). The question of which isoform of G_i is/are responsible for inhibition of adenylyl cyclase has not been resolved. In vitro evidence using recombinant G proteins has demonstrated that each is capable of inhibiting adenylyl cyclase, but whether each is involved in vivo is unknown.

Adenylyl Cyclase Adenylyl cyclase is central to the action of the majority of hormones and neurotransmitters that both stimulate and inhibit lipolysis. The notable exception is likely insulin, as described earlier. Adenylyl cyclase catalyzes the conversion of ATP to cyclic AMP, the archetypal, and first recognized cellular second messenger.

The classical mechanism by which agonists activate and inhibit lipolysis is that adenylyl cyclase is activated by $G_s\alpha$, and inhibited by $G_i\alpha$. Through such a mechanism, hormones that stimulate cyclase, and hence lipolysis, do so by activating G_s to liberate $G_s\alpha$. Conversely, hormones that inhibit lipolysis do so by activating G_i, thus liberating $G_i\alpha$, which inhibits cyclase and hence lowers cyclic AMP and inhibits lipolysis.

At least nine isoforms of adenylyl cyclase have been cloned. These are large, membrane-bound proteins. All of the cloned isoforms are stimulated by $G_s\alpha$. Therefore, the classical view of stimulation of lipolysis by lipolytic hormones such as epinephrine is probably correct, although perhaps not complete. However, the various isoforms of adenylyl cyclase vary markedly in their response to $G_i\alpha$, with some being insensitive to inhibition. Conversely, some are activated by G protein β/γ-subunits, which would be liberated by activation of either G_s or G_i (as well as other G proteins). Furthermore, certain adenylyl cyclases are activated by Ca^{2+}/calmodulin, whereas others are inhibited by Ca^{2+}, in a calmodulin-independent manner. Adipocytes express most, or perhaps all of these isoforms. Differences in the expression of these adenylyl cyclase isoforms may be part of the explanation for very different responses of adipocytes from different anatomic sites to lipolytic and antilipolytic stimuli. However, the physiological significance of the complexity of adenylyl cyclase regulation has not been established.

Protein Kinase A Acute activation of lipolysis by cyclic AMP is mediated through activation of PKA, also known as A-kinase. PKA is a heterotetrameric protein, consisting of two regulatory and two catalytic subunits. The regulatory subunits serve to maintain PKA in an inactive state, and binding of cyclic AMP to these regulatory subunits results in dissociation and hence activation of the enzyme. PKA also has various isoforms, including at least two forms of the regulatory subunit and three isoforms of the catalytic subunit. The function of this enzyme is to phosphorylate appropriate substrates within the cell on activation by cyclic AMP. In adipocytes, the major proteins phosphorylated in response to PKA are HSL and perilipin.

Hormone-Sensitive Lipase HSL is a soluble enzyme of approx 84 kDa. The human enzyme has 775 amino acid residues. The activity of HSL is markedly increased by phosphorylation, and deactivated by dephosphorylation. In addition to its role in adipose tissue lipolysis, it is thought that HSL serves as the neutral cholesterol ester hydrolase activity important in steroidogenesis. Consistent with this, HSL is expressed abundantly in adipose tissue and steroidogenic tissues, and to a much smaller degree in heart and skeletal muscle.

An intriguing recent finding is that mice with targeted disruption of the HSL gene are phenotypically not unlike normal mice. The greatest abnormalities are in steroidogenesis, consistent with the putative role of this enzyme in hydrolysis of neutral cholesterol esters. Triglyceride lipase activity both in vivo and in vitro is blunted, but not absent. These findings suggest that there are one or more other HSL(s) yet to be identified.

HSL is a cytoplasmic protein. On activation, for example by a catecholamine, the cascade of events described earlier results in activation of PKA, which phosphorylates HSL. Activation and inactivation of HSL results from phosphorylation and dephosphorylation of a single serine residue, Ser-563 in the rat sequence. This has been termed the regulatory site, and the surrounding sequence is typical of a PKA substrate. A second serine residue, only two amino acids away from the regulatory site (Ser-565) can also be phosphorylated. This is termed the basal site because its phosphorylation does not appear to be influenced by hormones. From in vitro studies it appears that phosphorylation of site 2 prevents phosphorylation of site 1, suggesting a regulatory role. Phosphorylation of HSL results in its translocation from the cytoplasm to the lipid droplet, in which it hydrolyzes triglyceride.

Perilipins   In the "basal" state, the lipid droplet within the adipocyte is coated with several proteins, including the perilipins, which are important in hormonal regulation of adipocyte lipolysis. These perilipins (perilipin A and perilipin B) coat the lipid droplet, and impair access of HSL to the triglyceride. The two forms present in adipocytes arise through alternative splicing of mRNA from a single gene, and perilipin A is the prevalent form in adipocytes. Studies with perilipin knockout mice have demonstrated that adipocytes from perilipin deficient animals have elevated basal lipolysis, but dramatically blunted response to lipolytic agonists.

Like HSL, perilipins are phosphorylated in response to increased cyclic AMP levels, and this phosphorylation results in their translocation to the cytoplasm, resulting in increased access of HSL to the lipid droplet.

LONG-TERM REGULATION OF LIPOLYSIS   The mechanisms described earlier are likely important in short-term, minute-to-minute regulation of lipolysis. Much less is known of mechanisms that regulate lipolysis on a more long-term basis. However, it is known that lipolysis can be regulated chronically by a number of mechanisms. For example, expression of HSL decreases in obese subjects after weight loss, and fasting increases expression of this enzyme. Aging and obesity are both associated with long-term alterations in adipose tissue lipolysis. Various hormones, and especially cytokines, chronically alter the rate of lipolysis. Such alterations are increasingly recognized as important in development of insulin resistance, which may be at least partly secondary to excess fatty acid release from adipose tissue and subsequent effects on skeletal muscle and liver metabolism.

Growth Hormone   Growth hormone can increase the rate of adipocyte lipolysis. Depending on the experimental system studied, this effect depends on concomitant treatment with a glucocorticoid, usually dexamethasone. The growth hormone-induced increase in lipolysis is slow to develop, on the order of hours. The mechanism is related to redistribution of G_i from the membrane to an intracellular compartment, hence decreasing its ability to inhibit adenylyl cyclase. However, details of the mechanism by which growth hormone causes this redistribution of G_i are not known.

Cytokines   Various cytokines increase the rate of adipocyte lipolysis, especially TNF-α and IL-6. These cytokines are produced by adipocytes, and so this may be an example of autocrine or paracrine regulation of lipolysis. TNF-α is known to be overexpressed in the adipose tissue of obese humans, and this adipocyte-derived TNF-α is likely involved in the insulin resistance of obesity. TNF-α has direct effects on insulin signaling, but also increases the rate of adipocyte lipolysis. The resulting increase in circulating FFAs may be more important in development of insulin resistance than the direct effect on the insulin signaling cascade.

Details of the mechanism by which TNF-α increases the rate of adipocyte lipolysis are unknown. However, activation of the TNF receptor is required. This leads to activation of two mitogen-activated protein kinases, known as extracellular signal-regulated kinases 1 and 2. Activation of the transcription factor, nuclear factor (NF)-κB, is also thought to be necessary for the lipolytic effect of TNF-α. NF-κB is a ubiquitously expressed transcription factor central to the inflammatory response. Therefore its involvement in the lipolytic effect of TNF-α may partially explain the relationship between chronic inflammation and insulin resistance. Exactly how activation of NF-κB relates to lipolysis is unknown, but two mechanisms have been proposed. One is that a decrease in the cellular concentration of perilipin allows for higher rates of lipolysis, because perilipin normally limits the access of HSL to the triglyceride droplet. A second is that TNF-α chronically decreases the cellular concentration of the various isoforms of G_i, which may release tonic inhibition of adenylyl cyclase, thus chronically increasing the rate of lipolysis.

Insulin and Glucose   Insulin is the most important acute inhibitor of lipolysis. However, prolonged incubation of adipocytes with insulin (several hours) actually increases the rate of lipolysis. Furthermore, this stimulatory effect of insulin is dependent on glucose. Neither glucose nor insulin alone causes this chronic stimulatory effect. Rather, the combination of high glucose and high insulin increases both basal and isoproterenol-stimulated rates of lipolysis, possibly from increased expression of HSL. Whether this is because of the insulin or the glucose is unknown. Each can regulate the expression of many genes, but it is possible that the insulin increases lipolysis primarily by increasing the rate of glucose uptake into the cell, and it is the glucose that increases expression of HSL and hence lipolysis. This effect likely contributes to the well-documented phenomenon of "glucose toxicity" that worsens insulin resistance in hyperglycemic subjects. In this scenario, hyperglycemia would contribute to excess lipolysis, and hence excess circulating FFA. The elevated FFA would then impair insulin action, further exacerbating the hyperglycemia.

CONCLUSION

Adipocyte lipolysis can be stimulated and inhibited by numerous mechanisms, involving a variety of hormones, neurotransmitters, and cytokines. The mechanisms of action of many of these agents at the cellular and molecular levels are becoming well understood. However, the physiological significance of many of these systems has not been determined. The major physiologically significant hormones in humans are insulin and the catecholamines. The increased rate of lipolysis during fasting is primarily because of a decline in circulating insulin concentrations and insulin resistance, and a slight increase in circulating catecholamines and

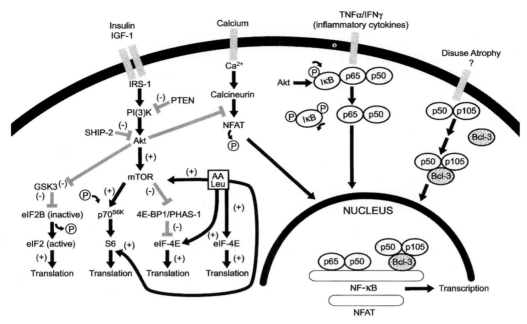

Figure 50-2   Intracellular signaling pathways that are potentially involved in muscle atrophy and hypertrophy associated with various clinical conditions. → indicates activation; ⊣ or ⊢ indicates inhibition. Adapted from Nader GA et al. (2002), Bodine SC et al. (2001), Goberdhan DC et al. (1999), Rommel C et al. (2001), Dupont-Versteegden EE et al. (2002), Guttridge DC et al. (2000), and Hunter RB et al. (2002).

PROTEIN TRANSLATION AND SIGNALING PATHWAYS

Several other factors and signaling pathways appear to be involved in muscle atrophy and hypertrophy. Insulin and insulin-like-growth factor (IGF-1) bind to a similar membrane receptor and initiate a signaling cascade that enhances protein translation. IGF-1 expression in muscle is increased with resistance exercise training and IGF-1 overexpressing transgenic mice have skeletal muscles that are twice as large as those from wild-type mice. Circulating IGF-1 levels and muscle IGF-1 mRNA expression decline with advancing age and likely contribute to sarcopenia. Direct injection of IGF-1 into muscle following immobilization conserves muscle protein and reduces the severity of muscle atrophy. Insulin and IGF-1 bind to a membrane receptor and cause a conformational change in the receptor tyrosine kinase. This results in transphosphorylation and secondary phosphorylation of the insulin receptor substrate (IRS-1), which in turn activates phosphatidyl-inositol-3 (PI-3) kinase. Evidence suggests that the PI-3 kinase/protein kinase B (Akt) pathway (Fig. 50-2) is involved in mediating skeletal muscle hypertrophy and atrophy. Phosphatidyl-inositol-3,4,5-triphosphate, a membrane-binding site for the serine/threonine kinase Akt, is initially activated by PI-3 kinase. Following activation by 3′-phosphoinositide-dependent protein kinase-1 (PDK-1), Akt mediates phosphorylation of several substrates involved in protein synthesis, gene transcription, and cell proliferation. The active form of Akt (Akt-1) regulates skeletal muscle hypertrophy in vitro and in vivo systems. Deletion of Akt-2 activity has been associated with a diabetic phenotype and possible impairments in glucose transport, another condition often associated with advancing age. The lipid-binding site on the Akt molecule is regulated by at least two factors: SH2-containing inositol-5-phosphatase (SHIP) 1-3; and phosphatase and tension homolog detected on chromosome 10 (PTEN) (*see* Fig. 50-2).

Overexpression of phosphatidylinositol-3,4,5-triphosphate dephosphorylates SHIP1-3 and PTEN and results in decreased cell size and inhibition of hypertrophy.

Signals downstream from PI-3 kinase and Akt are involved in skeletal muscle hypertrophy and atrophy. Inhibition of the Akt target mTOR (mammalian target of rapamycin) blocks phosphorylation of downstream targets p70^{S6} kinase (p70^{S6K}) and 4E-binding protein 1/phosphorylated heat- and acid-stable protein-1 (Fig. 50-2), and prevents hypertrophy. Moreover, another substrate of Akt/mTOR, glycogen synthase kinase 3β (GSK3β) (Fig. 50-2), has also been implicated as a mediator of hypertrophy. Akt phosphorylation inactivates GSK3β, which induces hypertrophy in skeletal myotubes. Evidence suggests that cytosolic phospholipase A$_2$ (cPLA$_2$) is a negative regulator of the IGF-1 pathway, and cPLA$_2$ knockout mice have cardiac and skeletal muscle cells that are 20–25% larger than wild-type mice. Many cellular regulators of muscle hypertrophy and atrophy have been identified and these might also play a role in sarcopenia.

Other pathways that may potentially be involved in sarcopenia include the calcineurin-NFAT (nuclear factor of activated T cells) pathway, β-adrenergic signaling, and the NF-κB pathway. Calcineurin is activated by an increase in intracellular calcium (Ca^{2+}) and calmodulin concentrations, in which it can dephosphorylate members of the NFAT family, specifically the NFATc1 isoform. NFAT then translocates to the nucleus and mediates gene transcription (Fig. 50-2). Disuse atrophy has been associated with increased calcineurin and NFAT translocation to the nucleus. When slow-twitch muscle calcineurin activity was inhibited by cyclosporin A, the muscle began to express fast-twitch proteins and properties. This suggests that activation of the calcineurin-NFAT pathway might contribute to the induction of slow fiber type genes resulting in a slow oxidative phenotype. Because advancing age is associated with selective type II fiber atrophy, the role that this pathway plays in sarcopenia is not clear.

β_2 adrenergic agonists also appear to block skeletal muscle atrophy and induce hypertrophy. The cyclic adenosine monophosphate system involvement via Gα3 activation or the PI-3 kinase/Akt via Gβ/γ protein activation appears to be involved in β-2 mediated hypertrophy. Furthermore, the NF-κB transcription factor (p65/p50) inhibits skeletal muscle differentiation through the expression of cyclin D1 and is activated by tumor necrosis factor (TNF) and interferon (IFN)-γ, two cytokines associated with cachexia and other inflammatory diseases (Fig. 50-2). TNF also appears to inhibit myogenesis through decreased differentiation in MHC and protein levels of MyoD. However, NF-κB may also be activated during disuse atrophy by factors other than cytokines. This disuse activation appears to involve factors p50, Bcl-3, and c-Rel and might be associated with an upregulation of survival genes (Fig. 50-2).

MITOCHONDRIAL DYSFUNCTION

Mitochondrial DNA (mtDNA) is a 16-kb circular genome that encodes 22 tRNAs, 2 rRNAs, and 13 polypeptides involved in the electron transport chain. Mitochondria provide the majority of energy (ATP) used for muscle contraction as well as many other metabolic functions. Mitochondrial protein synthesis is regulated at multiple levels. Approximately 15% of mitochondrial respiratory chain proteins are encoded by mtDNA, whereas the others are encoded by nuclear DNA. Muscle mitochondrial protein synthesis rate is reduced in middle-aged adults. Similarly, mitochondrial oxidative enzyme activities, electron transport chain function, ATP, and creatine phosphate (PCr) concentrations decline with advancing age. These findings suggest that impairments in mitochondrial function may contribute to reduced muscle endurance and aerobic capacity frequently found in the elderly.

MITOCHONDRIAL DNA ALTERATIONS

The association between declines in mitochondrial enzyme activity and protein synthesis, and sarcopenia are not clear, but might be associated with alterations in mtDNA. This theory of aging is based on the hypothesis that chemical alterations to mtDNA occur and accumulate throughout life. The mitochondrion is the site of cellular respiration and oxidative metabolism. Estimates indicate that approx 2% of the oxygen consumed is converted to superoxide free radicals in the electron transport process. MtDNA may be particularly susceptible to oxidative damage because it is in close physical proximity to ROS generated during electron transport. Also, mtDNA is not protected by histones and it has a poor repair efficiency. Oxidative damage to mtDNA bases occurs 10–20 times more than in nuclear DNA. The polymerase chain reaction technique has been used to detect low-abundance alterations/mutations/deletions in mtDNA sequences that are associated with advancing age. Whether alterations in muscle mtDNA provide the basis for the pathogenesis for sarcopenia is under investigation.

"Common" mtDNA deletions are defined as deletions that are common among different animals or tissues. Initial investigations of mtDNA alterations identified an age-related "common deletion:" an increase in a specific 4977-bp mtDNA deletion mutation. It extended from nucleotides 8483–13,459 of the mitochondrial genome and was flanked by a 13-bp direct repeat. This deletion was determined to be associated with aging when it was found in older individuals but not in infants or fetal tissue. Although it is not clear if this "common deletion" causes sarcopenia, it may be

involved because the highest levels of this deletion were found in older nerve and muscle tissues. Additional examinations have also identified other mtDNA deletions. Moreover, it was determined that multiple mtDNA deletions were common, they were not limited to specific areas of the genome, and they did not extend to or appear to be distributed in an uneven, mosaic pattern throughout the muscle fiber. The mechanisms for mtDNA deletions are unclear; however, multiple hypotheses have been proposed.

A relationship between deletion mutations and an abnormal phenotype of the muscle fiber has been observed, suggesting physiological significance of mtDNA abnormalities. These deletions were associated with electron transport chain-deficient areas of the fiber and a decreased fiber cross-sectional area. Moreover, this phenotype was associated with fiber breakage which may also suggest a susceptibility to muscle damage with aging.

Other mtDNA modifications have been reported. Nucleotide modifications, specifically oxidized modifications, in the mtDNA increase with aging in a variety of species as well. One modification in particular, 8-hydroxydeoxyguanosine (8-OH-dG), increases with age in various tissues, including muscle, in humans as well as other species. Nucleotide point mutations in the mtDNA, although rare, have also been reported to be associated with aging. However, the estimated frequency of mtDNA point mutations appears to be low (0.1–2.4%) with advancing age and their physiological significance in sarcopenia is not clear.

OTHER POTENTIAL CONTRIBUTORS TO SARCOPENIA

Other endocrine and inflammatory factors appear to alter muscle protein synthetic and proteolytic pathways, and might contribute to sarcopenia. Glucocorticoids activate catabolic responses by increasing mRNA expression of Ub and Ub-subunits. Insulin is involved in both muscle proteolysis and protein synthesis. Insulin is generally thought to inhibit muscle proteolysis. Conversely, it appears that there is a minimum level of insulin required for protein synthesis, specifically following exercise. Excess thyroid hormone T_3 levels induce muscle proteolysis. The inflammatory cytokines TNFα, IL-1, and IL-6 activate muscle proteolysis. Muscle TNFα protein and mRNA levels are elevated in physically frail elders and inversely correlated with the rate of muscle protein synthesis. Resistance exercise training reduced muscle TNFα levels and increased the rate of muscle protein synthesis in frail elders. TNFα may interfere with the pretranslational assembly of muscle protein; stimulate inducible nitric oxide expression through NF-κB activation, thereby increasing oxidative damage to the muscle, increase Ub conjugation of proteins, and induce muscle cell death through apoptosis or necrosis.

CONCLUSION

Several molecular mechanisms for muscle atrophy and hypertrophy have been identified. However, it is not known whether these pathways contribute to the pathogenesis of muscle wasting (sarcopenia) with advancing age, and what are the most effective interventions (hormone, nutrient, muscular activity, and pharmacological) to suppress muscle proteolysis and activate protein synthesis. Exercise training and augmenting muscle IGF-1 expression increase muscle protein synthesis and mass in senescent muscle. Pharmacological interventions that inhibit TNFα, SHIP-2, GSK3β, or proteasome activity, or activate Akt, mTOR, or p70^{S6k} need to be tested for efficacy in senescent muscle.

ACKNOWLEDGMENTS

The authors were supported by National Institutes of Health grants DK54163, DK49393, DK59531, DK56341, RR00954, RR00036, and training grant DK07120.

SELECTED REFERENCES

Aiken J, Bua E, Cao Z, et al. Mitochondrial DNA deletion mutations and sarcopenia. Ann N Y Acad Sci USA 2002;959:412–423.

Balagopal P, Rooyackers OE, Adey DB, Ades PA, Nair KS. Effects of aging on in vivo synthesis of skeletal muscle myosin heavy-chain and sarcoplasmic protein in humans. Am J Physiol 1997;273:E790–E800.

Balagopal P, Schimke JC, Ades P, Adey D, Nair KS. Age effect on transcript levels and synthesis rate of muscle MHC and response to resistance exercise. Am J Physiol Endocrinol Metab 2001;280:E203–E208.

Baumgartner RN, Stauber PM, McHugh D, Koehler KM, Garry PJ. Cross-sectional age differences in body composition in persons 60+ years of age. J Gerontol A Biol Sci Med Sci 1995;50:M307–M316.

Bodine SC, Latres E, Baumhueter S, et al. Identification of ubiquitin ligases required for skeletal muscle atrophy. Science 2001;294:1704–1708.

Bodine SC, Stitt TN, Gonzalez M, et al. Akt/mTOR pathway is a crucial regulator of skeletal muscle hypertrophy and can prevent muscle atrophy in vivo. Nat Cell Biol 2001;3:1014–1019.

Boffoli D, Scacco SC, Vergari R, Solarino G, Santacroce G, Papa S. Decline with age of the respiratory chain activity in human skeletal muscle. Biochim Biophys Acta 1994;1226:73–82.

Campbell MJ, McComas AJ, Petito F. Physiological changes in ageing muscles. J Neurol Neurosurg Psychiatry 1973;36:174–182.

Cao Z, Wanagat J, McKiernan SH, Aiken JM. Mitochondrial DNA deletion mutations are concomitant with ragged red regions of individual, aged muscle fibers: analysis by laser-capture microdissection. Nucleic Acids Res 2001;29:4502–4508.

Carlson BM, Faulkner JA. The regeneration of noninnervated muscle grafts and marcaine-treated muscles in young and old rats. J Gerontol A Biol Sci Med Sci 1996;51:B43–B49.

Chakravarthy MV, Davis BS, Booth FW. IGF-I restores satellite cell proliferative potential in immobilized old skeletal muscle. J Appl Physiol 2000;89:1365–1379.

Chance B, Sies H, Boveris A. Hydroperoxide metabolism in mammalian organs. Physiol Rev 1979;59:527–605.

Chin ER, Olson EN, Richardson JA, et al. A calcineurin-dependent transcriptional pathway controls skeletal muscle fiber type. Genes Dev 1998;12:2499–2509.

Cho H, Mu J, Kim JK, et al. Insulin resistance and a diabetes mellitus-like syndrome in mice lacking the protein kinase Akt2 (PKB beta). Science 2001;292:1728–1731.

Cohn SH, Vartsky D, Yasumura S, et al. Compartmental body composition based on total-body nitrogen, potassium, and calcium. Am J Physiol 1980;239:E524–E530.

Coux O, Tanaka K, Goldberg AL. Structure and functions of the 20S and 26S proteasomes. Annu Rev Biochem 1996;65:801–847.

Crespo P, Xu N, Simonds WF, Gutkind JS. Ras-dependent activation of MAP kinase pathway mediated by G-protein beta gamma subunits. Nature 1994;369:418–420.

Decary S, Mouly V, Hamida CB, Sautet A, Barbet JP, Butler-Browne GS. Replicative potential and telomere length in human skeletal muscle: implications for satellite cell-mediated gene therapy. Hum Gene Ther 1997;8:1429–1438.

DeVol DL, Rotwein P, Sadow JL, Novakofski J, Bechtel PJ. Activation of insulin-like growth factor gene expression during work-induced skeletal muscle growth. Am J Physiol 1990;259:E89–E95.

Dupont-Versteegden EE, Knox M, Gurley CM, Houle JD, Peterson CA. Maintenance of muscle mass is not dependent on the calcineurin-NFAT pathway. Am J Physiol Cell Physiol 2002;282:C1387–C1395.

Ferrington DA, Krainev AG, Bigelow DJ. Altered turnover of calcium regulatory proteins of the sarcoplasmic reticulum in aged skeletal muscle. J Biol Chem 1998;273:5885–5891.

Fleming JE, Miquel J, Cottrell SF, Yengoyan LS, Economos AC. Is cell aging caused by respiration-dependent injury to the mitochondrial genome? Gerontology 1982;28:44–53.

Fluckey JD, Vary TC, Jefferson LS, Evans WJ, Farrell PA. Insulin stimulation of protein synthesis in rat skeletal muscle following resistance exercise is maintained with advancing age. J Gerontol A Biol Sci Med Sci 1996;51:B323–B330.

Gibson MC, Schultz E. Age-related differences in absolute numbers of skeletal muscle satellite cells. Muscle Nerve 1983;6:574–580.

Glass DJ. Signalling pathways that mediate skeletal muscle hypertrophy and atrophy. Nat Cell Biol 2003;5:87–90.

Goberdhan DC, Paricio N, Goodman EC, Mlodzik M, Wilson C. Drosophila tumor suppressor PTEN controls cell size and number by antagonizing the Chico/PI3-kinase signaling pathway. Genes Dev 1999;13:3244–3258.

Greenlund LJ, Nair KS. Sarcopenia-consequences, mechanisms, and potential therapies. Mech Ageing Dev 2003;124:287–299.

Greiwe JS, Cheng B, Rubin DC, Yarasheski KE, Semenkovich CF. Resistance exercise decreases skeletal muscle tumor necrosis factor alpha in frail elderly humans. FASEB J 2001;15:475–482.

Guttridge DC, Mayo MW, Madrid LV, Wang CY, Baldwin AS Jr. NF-kappaB-induced loss of MyoD messenger RNA: Possible role in muscle decay and cachexia. Science 2000;289:2363–2366.

Haq S, Kilter H, Michael A, et al. Deletion of cytosolic phospholipase A(2) promotes striated muscle growth. Nat Med 2003;9:944–951.

Hasten DL, Pak-Loduca J, Obert KA, Yarasheski KE. Resistance exercise acutely increases MHC and mixed muscle protein synthesis rates in 78–84 and 23–32 yr olds. Am J Physiol Endocrinol Metab 2000;278: E620–E626.

Hinkle RT, Hodge KM, Cody DB, Sheldon RJ, Kobilka BK, Isfort RJ. Skeletal muscle hypertrophy and anti-atrophy effects of clenbuterol are mediated by the beta2-adrenergic receptor. Muscle Nerve 2002;25: 729–734.

Hunter RB, Stevenson E, Koncarevic A, Mitchell-Felton H, Essig DA, Kandarian SC. Activation of an alternative NF-kappaB pathway in skeletal muscle during disuse atrophy. FASEB J 2002;16:529–538.

Jagoe RT, Goldberg AL. What do we really know about the ubiquitin-proteasome pathway in muscle atrophy? Curr Opin Clin Nutr Metab Care 2001;4:183–190.

Kimball SR, Farrell PA, Jefferson LS. Invited review: role of insulin in translational control of protein synthesis in skeletal muscle by amino acids or exercise. J Appl Physiol 2002;93:1168–1180.

Kopsidas G, Kovalenko SA, Heffernan DR, et al. Tissue mitochondrial DNA changes. A stochastic system. Ann N Y Acad Sci 2000;908:226–243.

Lecker SH, Goldberg AL. Slowing muscle atrophy: putting the brakes on protein breakdown. J Physiol 2002;545:729.

Lee CM, Weindruch R, Aiken JM. Age-associated alterations of the mitochondrial genome. Free Radic Biol Med 1997;22:1259–1269.

Lexell J, Taylor CC, Sjostrom M. What is the cause of the ageing atrophy? Total number, size and proportion of different fiber types studied in whole vastus lateralis muscle from 15- to 83-year-old men. J Neurol Sci 1988;84:275–294.

Li YP, Lecker SH, Chen Y, Waddell ID, Goldberg AL, Reid MB. TNF-alpha increases ubiquitin-conjugating activity in skeletal muscle by up-regulating UbcH2/E220k. FASEB J 2003;17:1048–1057.

Lindle RS, Metter EJ, Lynch NA, et al. Age and gender comparisons of muscle strength in 654 women and men aged 20–93 yr. J Appl Physiol 1997;83:1581–1587.

McKenzie D, Bua E, McKiernan S, Cao Z, Aiken JM. Mitochondrial DNA deletion mutations: a causal role in sarcopenia. Eur J Biochem 2002;269:2010–2015.

Melov S, Shoffner JM, Kaufman A, Wallace DC. Marked increase in the number and variety of mitochondrial DNA rearrangements in aging human skeletal muscle. Nucleic Acids Res 1995;23:4122–4126.

Mitch WE, Goldberg AL. Mechanisms of muscle wasting. The role of the ubiquitin-proteasome pathway. N Engl J Med 1996;335:1897–1905.

Morley JE, Baumgartner RN, Roubenoff R, Mayer J, Nair KS. Sarcopenia. J Lab Clin Med 2001;137:231–243.

Musaro A, McCullagh K, Paul A, et al. Localized Igf-1 transgene expression sustains hypertrophy and regeneration in senescent skeletal muscle. Nat Genet 2001;27:195–200.

Nader GA, Hornberger TA, Esser KA. Translational control: implications for skeletal muscle hypertrophy. Clin Orthop 2002:S178–S187.

Proctor DN, Balagopal P, Nair KS. Age-related sarcopenia in humans is associated with reduced synthetic rates of specific muscle proteins. J Nutr 1998;128:351S–355S.

Richter C, Park JW, Ames BN. Normal oxidative damage to mitochondrial and nuclear DNA is extensive. Proc Natl Acad Sci USA 1988;85: 6465–6467.

Rommel C, Bodine SC, Clarke BA, et al. Mediation of IGF-1-induced skeletal myotube hypertrophy by PI(3)K/Akt/mTOR and PI(3)K/Akt/ GSK3 pathways. Nat Cell Biol 2001;3:1009–1013.

Rooyackers OE, Adey DB, Ades PA, Nair KS. Effect of age on in vivo rates of mitochondrial protein synthesis in human skeletal muscle. Proc Natl Acad Sci USA 1996;93:15,364–15,369.

Roth SM, Martel GF, Ivey FM, et al. Skeletal muscle satellite cell characteristics in young and older men and women after heavy resistance strength training. J Gerontol A Biol Sci Med Sci 2001;56: B240–B247.

Solomon V, Baracos V, Sarraf P, Goldberg AL. Rates of ubiquitin conjugation increase when muscles atrophy, largely through activation of the N-end rule pathway. Proc Natl Acad Sci USA 1998;95: 12,602–12,607.

United States Census Bureau. Projections of the total resident population by 5-year age groups and sex with special age categories: Middle series, 2006–2010. Information and Research Services Internet Staff (Population Division), Washington, D.C. 2000.

Vandervoot AA, Symons TB. Functional and metabolic consequences of sarcopenia. Can J Appl Physiol 2001;26:90–101.

Volpi E, Sheffield-Moore M, Rasmussen BB, Wolfe RR. Basal muscle amino acid kinetics and protein synthesis in healthy young and older men. JAMA 2001;286:1206–1212.

Wallace DC. Mitochondrial diseases in man and mouse. Science 1999; 283:1482–1488.

Wang Y, Michikawa Y, Mallidis C, et al. Muscle-specific mutations accumulate with aging in critical human mtDNA control sites for replication. Proc Natl Acad Sci USA 2001;98:4022–4027.

Yarasheski KE, Zachwieja JJ, Bier DM. Acute effects of resistance exercise on muscle protein synthesis rate in young and elderly men and women. Am J Physiol 1993;265:E210–E214.

Yarasheski KE, Zachwieja JJ, Campbell JA, Bier DM. Effect of growth hormone and resistance exercise on muscle growth and strength in older men. Am J Physiol 1995;268:E268–E276.

51 Adipose Tissue Development and Metabolism

SHEILA COLLINS, YUSHI BAI, AND JACQUES ROBIDOUX

SUMMARY

Excess body fat is associated with many medical complications and obesity has become a major health problem in the United States and most other industrialized countries. The existence of adipose tissue as a specialized organ reflects the mechanism developed by organisms over time to cope with irregular and unpredictable supplies of nutrients. This ability to store fat was probably a survival feature of *Homo sapiens*; however, excess body fat has become a major heath problem. This chapter will briefly examine development and metabolic functions of adipose tissue and how these processes are regulated.

Key Words: Adipose tissue; β-adrenergic receptors; brown adipose tissue; peroxisome proliferator-activated receptor-γ; triglyceride; white adipose tissue.

INTRODUCTION

The existence of adipose tissue as a specialized organ reflects the mechanism developed by organisms over time to cope with irregular and unpredictable supplies of nutrients. The ability to store fuel as body fat was particularly important in omnivorous mammals, and was probably a key survival feature of *Homo sapiens*. However, excess body fat is associated with many medical complications and obesity has become a major health problem in the United States and most other industrialized countries.

The mechanism(s) responsible for the link between obesity and metabolic diseases, such as insulin resistance and diabetes, is not completely known but is likely to involve abnormalities in free fatty acid metabolism. In general, the rate of fatty acid release into the systemic circulation is greater in obese than lean persons. In addition, an ever-increasing array of adipose tissue-derived cytokines and endocrine factors has been identified with suspected actions on insulin sensitivity and the cardiovascular system. In contrast, extreme deficiencies in body fat, such as lipodystrophy, also cause metabolic abnormalities including insulin resistance and diabetes. Therefore, it is important to understand the development and metabolic functions of adipose tissue and how these processes are regulated.

From: *Principles of Molecular Medicine, Second Edition*
Edited by: M. S. Runge and C. Patterson © Humana Press, Inc., Totowa, NJ

ADIPOSE TISSUE: CELL TYPES AND DEPOTS

Adipose tissue has been classified into two major types based on gross appearance, cell type-specific gene expression, and predominant type of adipocytes: white adipose tissue (WAT) and brown adipose tissue (BAT). WAT is named for its white/yellowish color. It contains adipocytes with a single large lipid inclusion (termed "unilocular"), resulting in displacement of the cytoplasm and the nucleus into a thin rim surrounding the lipid droplet. However, even among WAT depots there can be significant differences in metabolic and hormonal sensitivity.

BAT is named for its "brown" color, which is derived from a rich blood supply and an enormous number of mitochondria per cell. In overall appearance, the adipocytes in BAT are smaller than white adipocytes and are characterized by numerous small lipid inclusions (termed multilocular). Although recognized anatomically as a special organ structure, in the early 1960s the true function of BAT was realized when it was proposed to be thermogenic. Since then, substantial work has shown that BAT is uniquely capable of responding to various environmental stimuli to generate heat from stored metabolic energy. In response to sympathetic nervous system (SNS) activation, BAT undergoes an orchestrated hyperplastic and hypertrophic expansion, increased blood flow, and recruitment of lipid and carbohydrate fuels for oxidative metabolism. A unique and critical element of this thermogenic mechanism for dissipation of the proton gradient in brown fat mitochondria is owing to a brown fat specific mitochondrial uncoupling protein, also called "thermogenin." This mitochondrial protein, termed uncoupling protein 1, allows controlled proton leakage across the mitochondrial inner membrane that generates heat at the expense of respiration-coupled ATP production. The uncoupling activity in brown fat mitochondria is "activated" by free fatty acids that are released as a result of catecholamine-stimulated lipolysis.

BAT is most abundant in newborn mammals and is principally involved in heat production. In the human fetus, BAT is located in the dorsal cervical, axillary, suprailiac, and perirenal regions. With increasing age and size, true homogeneous BAT depots disappear. This is also true for large mammals such as dogs and nonhuman primates. However, brown adipocytes can also be found within white fat depots in the adult of all these species, particularly in the intra-abdominal and intrathoracic areas, but relatively rarely in the subcutaneous depot. In the common small laboratory animals, such as mice and rats, BAT is prominent in the interscapular and axillary areas from birth through adulthood. In fact, in newborn rodents BAT is the only adipose tissue, and it is only with suckling of the lipid-rich milk that WAT depots begin to appear. In addition, brown adipocytes are present within WAT depots, such as the perigonadal, perirenal, and mesenteric fat of adult rodents. Cold challenge or treatment with certain thermogenic agents further provokes the elaboration of brown adipocytes in laboratory animals; patients with pheochromocytoma possess large amounts of BAT owing to chronic catecholamine stimulation.

ADIPOGENESIS: PREADIPOCYTE COMMITMENT AND DIFFERENTIATION

Understanding the fundamental factors that send cells along an irreversible program of highly specialized gene expression to form a specific tissue type requires the study of pluripotent cells. The adipogenic cell lines created in the 1970s provided the technical basis to permit isolation of adipocyte-specific genes and identify their regulatory factors. Many key transcription factors that promote adipogenesis have been identified. They include the family of CCAAT/enhancer binding proteins (C/EBP), peroxisome proliferator-activated receptor-γ (PPARγ) and the sterol regulatory element binding protein family. The expression of the C/EBPs and PPARγ2 genes occurs in a cascade-like fashion during adipocyte commitment and differentiation. Data from studies conducted in cell culture models and in genetically modified animals show that agents or manipulations that interfere with the expression of these factors can inhibit adipocyte differentiation, or result in an incomplete state of differentiation.

PPARγ2, which is expressed at high levels in adipose tissue, is particularly important for adipocyte differentiation. Failure to express PPARγ2 prevents adipogenesis, and providing PPARγ2 to PPARγ-deficient cells fully restores their capacity for differentiation.

In addition to PPARγ2, C/EBPα is required to express the full complement of genes that define the mature adipocyte phenotype. The relative importance of C/EBPα in regulating adipocyte differentiation may be different in brown and white adipocytes. C/EBPα–/– mice, in which vital hepatic expression of C/EBPα was preserved, had intact interscapular BAT, but no evidence of WAT in any depot. This observation demonstrated a clear molecular distinction between the developmental fates of white and brown adipocytes.

ROLE OF THE SYMPATHETIC NERVOUS SYSTEM AND β-ADRENERGIC RECEPTORS IN LIPOLYSIS

The amount of triglyceride stored in adipose tissue reflects the cumulative sum over time of the differences between energy intake and expenditure. The net efflux of nonesterified fatty acids from adipose tissue fluctuates between periods of relative stimulation (e.g., after an overnight fast or during a bout of exercise) and relative suppression (e.g., after a meal). Both WAT and BAT are innervated by the SNS. However, because sympathetic innervations are more abundant in BAT than in WAT, neural-derived norepinephrine is presumed to play a greater role in BAT, whereas catecholamines derived from the circulation play a relatively greater role in WAT. However, there can also be significant levels of norepinephrine in the immediate vicinity of the nerve terminals in WAT.

The role of the SNS in the control of lipolysis includes the α-adrenergic receptors (αARs) and β-adrenergic receptors (βARs) as the recipients of these catecholamine signals. They are members

of the large family of G protein-coupled receptors that are integral membrane proteins of the plasma membrane. There are three subtypes of βARs (β_1AR, β_2AR, and β_3AR), all of which are expressed in white and brown adipocytes. However, the relative proportions of these subtypes vary between species, fat depots, and metabolic status. For example, rodent species possess abundant levels of the β_3AR and lesser amounts of the two other subtypes, whereas the reverse is true in humans, although there is clearly a need to examine intra-abdominal depots in normal humans more carefully.

The control of lipolysis (Fig. 51-1) by the βARs is principally initiated by the sequential activation of adenylyl cyclase and cAMP-dependent protein kinase, ultimately culminating in the phosphorylation of hormone sensitive lipase and perilipin A. In addition to the β-adrenergic stimulation of lipolysis, catecholamines can also be antilipolytic themselves through their interaction with the α_2ARs and its resulting inhibition of cAMP production. The balance between the relative amounts of the βAR and α_2AR can thus determine the relative efficacy of catecholamines for triglyceride hydrolysis. In that respect, there is some evidence from experimental studies in animals and humans that a shift to a higher α_2/β ratio can contribute to net lipid storage. The lipases and lipid droplet binding proteins that control triglyceride hydrolysis are targets of the signaling cascades initiated by the adrenergic receptors. However, there are likely to be additional, unidentified, lipases and lipid droplet scaffolding proteins with regulatory roles (e.g., the S3-12 protein).

ADIPOCYTE-DERIVED CYTOKINES

Until the mid-1990s, adipose tissue was generally regarded to be a passive storage depot for excess caloric intake. The discovery of leptin as an adipose-derived hormone that informs on the status of energy reserves has provided a new perspective on adipose tissue biology. In the ensuing years there has also been a deeper appreciation that a large number of cytokines and growth factors are secreted from adipose tissue. One of the molecules isolated independently by several groups that have received intense investigation is now commonly referred to as adiponectin. There is excitement over the possibility that it might be an important player in the regulation of insulin sensitivity in other tissues such as skeletal muscle and liver. Plasma levels of adiponectin are reduced in obese persons and patients with type-2 diabetes or coronary artery disease.

Markers of inflammation are also increased in obese humans and many animal models. For example, mRNA levels of tumor necrosis factor-α and interleukin-6 are elevated in human adipose tissue. Similarly, monocyte chemoattractant protein 1 mRNA is overexpressed in the adipose tissue of genetically obese mice compared with wild type littermates. Although it was presumed these molecules were solely produced by the adipocyte, studies utilizing transcriptional profiling by microarray have added a new dimension to this issue. In one approach, a comparison among preadipocytes, adipocytes, and macrophages for common patterns of gene expression showed that the preadipocyte profile is much closer to the macrophage than to the adipocyte profile. In another study, profiled transcript expression in perigonadal adipose tissue suggested that the percentage of cells expressing the macrophage marker F4/80 significantly and positively correlated with both adipocyte size and body mass. This has raised the question regarding the relative contribution of the adipose tissue vs the macrophage as a source of these inflammatory mediators (Fig. 51-2). Irrespective

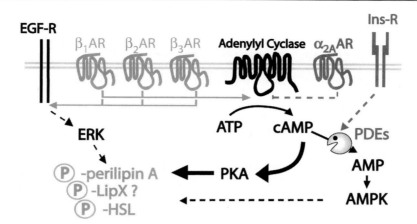

Figure 51-1 Positive and negative control of lipolysis through the actions of catecholamines and insulin. The three β-adrenoceptor (βAR) subtypes respond to the catecholamines, epinephrine, and norepinephrine by increasing cAMP levels, which in turn can activate the cAMP-dependent protein kinase (PKA). Targets of PKA include hormone sensitive lipase (HSL), perilipins and perhaps additional lipases (LipX). Each βAR can also activate ERK MAP kinase by different mechanisms, but each involves recruitment of a tyrosine kinase growth factor receptor such as EGF-R. ERK contributes to lipolysis but its targets are still under investigation. Catecholamines also activate the α$_2$-adrenoceptor (α$_{2A}$AR) to inhibit adenylyl cyclase activity and lower overall cAMP levels. Insulin through its receptor (Ins-R) also acts to oppose the stimulating effects of cAMP in part by increasing the activity of phosphodiesterases (PDEs), a by-product of which is AMP, which could activate AMP kinase. (Note: Re: LipX?—adipose triglyceride lipate [V6*ATGL*] was recently discovered as a key BAR-regulated lipase in fat [Zimmerman, 2004].)

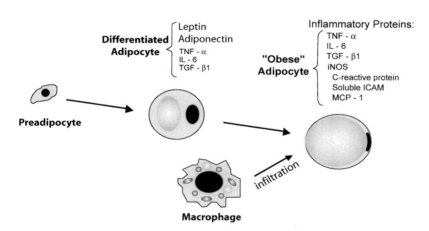

Figure 51-2 Proposed functions of adipocytes in different metabolic states. In the early differentiated stage, adipocytes secrete large amounts of hormones with insulin-sensitizing properties, and small amounts of cytokines. In the obese state, large lipid-filled adipocytes continue to produce leptin, but significantly less adiponectin. There is significant macrophage infiltration that together with adipocytes secretes enhanced amounts of proinflammatory cytokines.

of whether the macrophage existing in adipose tissue under the condition of obesity is owing to preadipocyte conversion or recruitment, it might still contribute to a proinflammatory milieu within adipose tissue. Moreover, once set into motion, this situation could perpetuate a vicious cycle of ever more macrophage recruitment, production of inflammatory cytokines, and impairment of adipocyte function.

CONCLUSION

The knowledge of adipocytes has advanced from being considered an inert storage depot for excess energy to a member of the endocrine system. Advances in modern molecular biology are revising previously well-established biochemical events in adipocytes, such as catecholamine stimulation of lipolysis and thermogenesis. Continued progress in adipocyte biology will provide a better understanding of the role of fat cells in the pathogenesis and pathophysiology of metabolic disorders.

SELECTED REFERENCES

Arita Y, Kihara S, Ouchi N, et al. Paradoxical decrease of an adipose-specific protein, adiponectin, in obesity. Biochem Biophys Res Commun 1999;257:79–83.

Ball EG, Jungas RL. On the action of hormones which accelerate the rate of oxygen consumption and fatty acid release in rat adipose tissue in vitro. Proc Natl Acad Sci USA 1961;47:932–941.

Ballard K, Malmfors T, Rosell S, et al. Adrenergic innervation and vascular patterns in canine adipose tissue. Microvasc Res 1974;8(2):164–171.

Bamshad M, Aoki VT, Adkison MG, et al. Central nervous system origins of the sympathetic nervous system outflow to white adipose tissue. Am J Physiol 1998;275:R291–R299.

Bastard JP, Jardel C, Bruckert E, et al. Elevated levels of interleukin 6 are reduced in serum and subcutaneous adipose tissue of obese women after weight loss. J Clin Endocrinol Metab 2000;85(9): 3338–3342.

Belfrage P, Fredrikson G, Nilsson NO, et al. Regulation of adipose tissue lipolysis: phosphorylation of hormones sensitive lipase in intact rat adipocytes. FEBS Lett 1980;111(1):120–124.

Bukowiecki L, Collet A, Follea N, Guay G, Jahjah L. Brown adipose tissue hyperplasia: a fundamental mechanism of adaptation to a cold and hyperphagia. Am J Physiol 1982;242:E353–E359.

Cannon B, Hedin A, Nedergaard J. Exclusive occurrence of thermogenin antigen in brown adipose tissue. FEBS Lett 1982;150:129–132.

Charriere G, Cousin B, Arnaud E, et al. Preadipocyte conversion to macrophage. Evidence of plasticity. J Biol Chem 2003;278(11): 9850–9855.

Cinti S. The Adipose Organ. Milano, Italy: Editrice Kurtis, 1999.

Clifford GM, Londos C, Kraemer FB, et al. Translocation of hormone-sensitive lipase and perilipin upon lipolytic stimulation of rat adipocytes. J Biol Chem 2000;275(7):5011–5015.

Collins S, Surwit RS. The β-adrenergic receptors and the control of adipose tissue metabolism and thermogenesis. Recent progress in hormone research. A R Means 2001;56:309–328.

Collins S, Daniel KW, Rohlfs EM, et al. Impaired expression and functional activity of the β_3- and β_1-adrenergic receptors in adipose tissue of congenitally obese (C57BL/6J ob/ob) mice. Mol Endocrinol 1994;8(4):518–527.

Coppack SW, Frayn KN, Humphreys SM, et al. Arteriovenous differences across human adipose and forearm tissues after overnight fast. Metabolism 1990;39(4):384–390.

Dixon TM, Daniel KW, Farmer SR, Collins S. CAATT/enhancer binding protein- is required for transcription of the β_3AR gene during adipogenesis. J Biol Chem 2001;276:722–728.

Emorine LJ, Marullo S, Briend-Sutren MM, et al. Molecular characterization of the human beta 3-adrenergic receptor. Science 1989;245: 1118–1121.

Galitzky J, Reverte M, Carpene C, et al. Beta 3-adrenoceptors in dog adipose tissue: studies on their involvement in the lipomobilizing effect of catecholamines. J Pharmacol Exp Ther 1993;266(1):358–366.

Géloën A, Collet AJ, Bukowiecki LJ. Role of sympathetic innervation in brown adipocyte proliferation. Am J Physiol 1992;263:R1176–R1181.

Girardier L. The regulation of the biological furnace of warm-blooded animals. Experientia 1977;33:1121–1131.

Granneman JG, Lahners KN, Chaudhry A, et al. Molecular cloning and expression of the rat β_3-adrenergic receptor. Mol Pharmacol 1991;40:895–899.

Gregoire FM. Adipocyte differentiation: from fibroblast to endocrine cell. Exp Biol Med (Maywood) 2001;226(11):997–1002.

Hamm JK, el Jack AK, Pilch PF, Farmer SR. Role of PPAR gamma in regulating adipocyte differentiation and insulin-response glucose uptake. Ann N Y Acad Sci 1999;892:134–145.

Hara T, Fujiwara H, Shoji T, Mimura T, Nakao H, Fujimoto S. Decreased plasma adiponectin levels in young obese males. J Atheroscler Thromb 2003;10(4):234–238.

Hodgetts V, Coppack SW, Frayn KN, et al. Factors controlling fat mobilization from human subcutaneous adipose tissue during exercise. J Appl Physiol 1991;71(2):445–451.

Honnor RC, Dhillon GS, Londos C, et al. cAMP-dependent protein kinase and lipolysis in rat adipocytes. I. Cell preparation, manipulation, and predictability in behavior. J Biol Chem 1985;260:15,122–15,129.

Horowitz JF, Coppack SC, Paramore D, Cryer PE, Klein S. Effect of short-term fasting on lipid kinetics in lean and obese women. Am J Physiol Endocrinol Metab 1999;276:E278–E284.

Hotamisligil GS, Shargill NS, Spiegelman BM. Adipose expression of tumor necrosis factor-alpha: direct role in obesity-linked insulin resistance. Science 1993;259(5091):87–91.

Hu E, Liang P, Spiegelman BM. AdipoQ is a novel adipose-specific gene dysregulated in obesity. J Biol Chem 1996;271:10,697–10,703.

Hull D, Segall MM. Distinction of brown from white adipose tissue. Nature 1966;212(61):469–472.

Jensen MD. Lipolysis: contribution from regional fat. Annu Rev Nutr 1997;17:127–139.

Kawamura M, Jensen DF, Wancewicz EV, et al. Hormone-sensitive lipase in differentiated 3T3-L1 cells and its activation by cyclic AMP-dependent protein kinase. Proc Natl Acad Sci USA 1981;78(2):732–736.

Kern PA, Saghizadeh M, Ong JM, Bosch RJ, Deem R, Simsolo RB. The expression of tumor necrosis factor in human adipose tissue. Regulation by obesity, weight loss, and relationship to lipoprotein lipase. J Clin Invest 1995;95(5):2111–2119.

Kliewer SA, Forman BM, Blumberg B, et al. Differential expression and activation of a family of murine peroxisome proliferator-activated receptors. Proc Natl Acad Sci USA 1994;91(15):7355–7359.

Kortelainen M-L, Pelletier G, Ricquier D, Bukowiecki LJ. Immunohistochemical detection of human brown adipose tissue uncoupling protein in an autopsy series. J Histotchem Cytochem 1993;41:759–764.

Koutnikova H, Cock TA, Watanabe M, et al. Compensation by the muscle limits the metabolic consequences of lipodystrophy in PPAR gamma hypomorphic mice. Proc Natl Acad Sci USA 2003;100(24): 14,457–14,462.

Kratchmarova I, Kalume DE, Blagoey B, et al. A proteomic approach for identification of secreted proteins during the differentiation of 3T3-L1 preadipocytes to adipocytes. Mol Cell Proteomics 2002;1(3): 213–222.

Lafontan M, Berlan M. Fat cell α_2-adrenoceptors: the regulation of fat cell function and lipolysis. Endocrine Review 1995;16(6):716–738.

Lafontan M, Berlan M. Fat cell adrenergic receptors and the control of white and brown fat cell function. J Lipid Res 1993;34:1057–1091.

Lean ME, James WP, Jennings G, Trayhurn P. Brown adipose tissue in patients with phaeochromocytoma. Int J Obes 1986;10(3):219–227.

Linhart HG, Ishimura-Oka K, DeMayo F, et al. C/EBPalpha is required for differentiation of white, but not brown, adipose tissue. Proc Natl Acad Sci USA 2001;98(22):12,532–12,537.

Merklin RJ. Growth and distribution of human fetal brown fat. Anat Rec 1974;178(3):637–645.

Nahmias C, Blin N, Elalouf JM, et al. Molecular characterization of the mouse β_3-adrenergic receptor: relationship with the atypical receptor of adipocytes. EMBO J 1991;10:3721–3727.

Nakano Y, Tobe T, Choi-Miura NH, et al. Isolation and characterization of GBP28, a novel gelatin-binding protein purified from human plasma. J Biochem (Tokyo) 1996;120:803–812.

Pajvani UB, Scherer PE. Adiponectin: systemic contributor to insulin sensitivity. Curr Diab Rep 2003;3(3):207–213.

Reitman ML, Arioglu E, Gavrilova O, Taylor SI. Lipoatrophy revisited. Trends Endocrinol Metab 2000;10:410–416.

Ren D, Collingwood TN, Rebar EJ, Wolffe AP, Camp HS. PPAR gamma knockdown by engineered transcription factors: exogenous PPAR gamma2 but not PPAR gamma1 reactivates adipogenesis. Genes Dev 2002;16(1):27–32.

Ricquier D, Bouillaud F. Mitochondrial uncoupling proteins: from mitochondria to the regulation of energy balance. J Physiol 2000;529:3–10.

Robidoux J, Martin TL, Collin S. Beta-adrenergic receptors and regulation of energy expenditure: a family affair. Annu Rev Pharmacol Toxicol 2004; 44:297–323.

Rohlfs EM, Daniel KW, Premont RT, et al. Regulation of the uncoupling protein gene (Ucp) by β_1, β_2, β_3-adrenergic receptor subtypes in immortalized brown adipose cell lines. J Biol Chem 1995;270(5): 10,723–10,732.

Rosen ED, Hsu CH, Wang X, et al. C/EBP-alpha induces adipogenesis through PPARgamma: a unified pathway. Genes Dev 2002;16:22–26.

Rosen ED, Sarraf P, Troy AE, et al. PPAR gamma is required for the differentiation of adipose tissue in vivo and in vitro. Mol Cell 1999; 4(4):611–617.

Rosen ED, Walkey CJ, Puigserver P, Spiegelman BM. Transcriptional regulation of adipogenesis. Genes Dev 2000;14(11):1293–1307.

Rosenbaum M, Leibel R, Hirsch J, et al. Obesity. N Engl J Med 1997; 337(6):396–407.

Sartipy P, Loskutoff DJ. Monocyte chemoattractant protein 1 in obesity and insulin resistance. Proc Natl Acad Sci USA 2003;100(12): 7265–7270.

Scherer P, Williams S, Fogliano M, et al. A novel serum protein similar to C1q, produced exclusively in adipocytes. J Biol Chem 1995;270: 26,746–26,749.

Schimmel RJ, Buhlinger CA, Serio R, et al. Activation of adenosine 3′,5′-monophosphate-dependent protein kinase and its relationship to cyclic AMP and lipolysis in hamster adipose tissue. J Lipid Res 1980;21(2):250–256.

Slavin BG, Ballard KW. Morphological studies on the adrenergic innervation of white adipose tissue. Anat Rec 1978;191(3):377–389.

Smith RE. Thermogenic activity of the hibernating gland in the cold-acclimated rat. Physiologist 1961;4:113.

Tontonoz P, Hu E, Graves RA, Budavari AI, Spiegelman BM. mPPARγ2: tissue-specific regulator of an adipocyte enhancer. Genes Dev 1994;8: 1224–1234.

van Liefde I, van Witzenberg A, Vauquelin G, et al. Multiple beta adrenergic receptor subclasses mediate the I-isoproteronol-induced lipolytic response in rat adipocytes. J Pharmacol Exp Ther 1992;262:552–558.

Weisberg SP, McCann D, Desai M, Rosenbaum M, Leibel RL, Ferrante AW, Jr. Obesity is associated with macrophage accumulation in adipose tissue. J Clin Invest 2003;112:1796–1808.

Wirsen C, Hamberger B. Catecholamines in brown fat. Nature 1967; 214(88):625–626.

Wolins NE, Skinner JR, Schoenfish MJ, et al. Adipocyte protein S3-12 coats nascent lipid droplets. J Biol Chem 2003;278(39):37,713–37,721.

Wu Z, Rosen ED, Brun R, et al. Cross-regulation of C/EBPα and PPARγ controls the transcriptional pathway of adipogenesis and insulin sensitivity. Mol Cell 1999;3:151–158.

Zhang Y, Proenca R, Maffei M, Barone M, Leopold L, Friedman JM. Positional cloning of the mouse obese gene and its human homologue. Nature 1994;372:425–432.

Zimmermann R, Strauss JG, Haemmerle G, et al. Fat mobilization in adipose tissue is promoted by adipose triglyceride lipase. Science 2004; 306:1383–1386.

GASTROENTEROLOGY

VI

SECTION EDITOR:
DAVID A. BRENNER

Abbreviations

VI. GASTROENTEROLOGY

3'NTR	3' noncoding region
5'NTR	noncoding 5' terminal region
5'UTR	5' untranslated region
5-ASA	5 aminosalicylic acid
ADV	adefovir
ALT	alanine transaminase
anti-HCV	antibody to HCV
AP-1	activator protein 1
apo	apolipoprotein
BCP	basal core promoter
bp	base pair
cag PAI	cag pathogenicity island
CARD15	C-terminal caspase recruitment domain
ccc	covalently closed circular
CF	cystic fibrosis
CFTR	cystic fibrosis transmembrane conductance regulator
CH-B	chronic hepatitis B
Csk	C-terminal SRC kinase
CTL	cytotoxic T-lymphocyte
DR	direct repeat
EIA	enzyme immunoassay
ER	endoplasmic reticulum
ERK	extracellular signal-regulated kinase
FDA	Food and Drug Administration
GP	glycoproteins
H.	*Helicobacter*
HBcAg	hepatitis B core antigen
HBeAg	hepatitis Be antigen
HBIg	hepatitis B immunoglobulin
HBsAg	hepatitis B surface antigen
HBV	hepatitis B virus
HCC	hepatocellular carcinoma
HCV	hepatitis C virus
HCW	health care worker
HFE	hemochromatosis gene
HH	hereditary hemochromatosis
HLA	human leukocyte antigen
HP	hereditary pancreatitis
HP-NAP	*H. pylori* neutrophil-activating protein
IBD	inflammatory bowel disease
IFN	interferon
IFN-α	interferon-α
IKK	inhibitor of κ kinase
IL	interleukin
IL-1	interleukin 1
J-HH	juvenile onset hereditary hemochromatosis
JNK	Jun n-terminal kinase
Le	Lewis
LHB	large-sized protein
LMV	lamivudine
LPS	lipopolysaccharide
MAP	mitogen activated protein
MHB	medium-sized protein
MHC	major histocompatibility complex
MHR	major hydrophilic region
MTP	microsomal triglyceride transport protein
NANBH	non-A non-B hepatitis
NAT	nucleic acid test
NS	nonstructural
nt	nucleotide
ORF	open reading frame
PAI	pathogenicity island
PAMP	pathogen-associated molecular receptor
pg	pregenomic
PKC	protein kinase C
PSTI	pancreatic secretory trypsin inhibitor
RIBA	recombinant immunoblot assay
ROI	reactive oxygen intermediate
RT	reverse transcriptase
SBDS	Shwachman-Bodian-Diamond Syndrome
SDS	Shwachman-Diamond Syndrome
SHB	small-sized protein
SIRS	systemic inflammatory response syndrome
SNP	single-nucleotide polymorphism
SOD	superoxide dismutase
SPINK1	serine protease inhibitor Kazal type 1
TCR	T-cell receptor
TFF1	trefoil factor 1
TfR1	transferrin receptor 1
TfR2	transferrin receptor 2
TGF	transforming growth factor
Th	T-helper
TLR	Toll-like receptor
TNF	tumor necrosis factor
Treg	regulatory T cells

52 Hepatitis C

JOHNSON YIU-NAM LAU, JANE WING-SANG FANG, MASASHI MIZOKAMI, ROBERT G. GISH, AND TERESA L. WRIGHT

"Reason, Observation, and Experience—the Holy Trinity of Science"

Robert G. Ingersoll (1825–1895)
In: Science—The Philosophy of Ingersoll.

SUMMARY

Hepatitis C virus (HCV) infection infects nearly four million people in the United States alone, is the most common cause of chronic liver disease, and also a common indication for liver transplantation in most of the larger transplant centers in this country. HCV infection is an immensely important public health problem. Rapid scientific advancements have been made in this area and our understanding of the virology, disease pathogenesis, diagnosis, diversity of clinical presentations, natural history, treatment, and prevention is evolving rapidly. This chapter will provide the reader with an update review of the various scientific and clinical aspects of HCV and the associated diseases.

Key Words: Assays; clinical; diagnostics; epidemiology; genotypes; hepatitis C; molecular; prevention; serology; treatment; viral hepatitis; virology.

HISTORY OF NON-A AND NON-B HEPATITIS/HEPATITIS C

Viral hepatitis has been a part of recorded history since the time of Hippocrates. Over the centuries, epidemics have devastated military and civilian communities throughout the world. The discovery of the Australia antigen by Blumberg and his colleagues in 1965 and its subsequent association with hepatitis B virus (serum hepatitis) heralded the onset of an accelerated era of hepatitis research. The discovery by Feinstone in 1973 of hepatitis A virus, the agent responsible for infectious hepatitis, failed to explain the large number of undefinable cases of posttransfusion hepatitis. Thus, the concept of non-A, non-B hepatitis (NANBH) developed in the early 1970s after the identification of hepatitis A and B made it obvious that many cases of hepatitis, particularly posttransfusion hepatitis, could not be accounted for, by either of these viruses.

In 1989, 14 yr after the initial proposal of the existence of such an infective agent, the virus responsible for virtually most, if not all, parenteral NANBH was identified by Choo et al. The breakthrough led to an explosion of research and discoveries about the virus, now designated as hepatitis C virus (HCV), and the disease,

From: *Principles of Molecular Medicine, Second Edition*
Edited by: M. S. Runge and C. Patterson © Humana Press, Inc., Totowa, NJ

NANBH now called hepatitis C. This chapter will highlight the role of molecular tools in the discovery of the virus, in the study of the virus and disease, in our understanding of the epidemiology and the virus–host interplay in clinical presentation, in the development of diagnostic tests, and perspectives in the treatment of hepatitis C.

DISCOVERY OF HCV

Advancements in the field of molecular biology provided the tools to search for the parenteral NANBH agent. In 1982, research workers from Chiron Corporation, in conjunction with the Center of Disease Control, initiated attempts to clone the NANBH virus genome from infectious chimpanzee liver homogenates and plasma using molecular techniques including subtractive hybridization methods. After screening more than 25×10^6 clones, it became apparent that the concentration of the putative NANBH virus nucleic acid in these samples was less than the limit of detection for such an approach. They proceeded to pool plasma samples from a chronically infected chimpanzee and titrated the infectivity of the pooled sample in other animals. A pool containing 10^6 chimpanzee infectious doses/mL was obtained for further studies.

Following extensive ultracentrifugation that was sufficient to pellet down the smallest of known infectious agents, total nucleic acid was extracted. Although an RNA virus was suspected from the results of physicochemical experiments, both extracted RNA and DNA were converted to cDNA and the fragments were cloned into a recombinant bacteriophage vector to form a cDNA library and expressed in the *Escherichia coli* bacteria. This library was screened with sera from patients with unequivocal NANBH in order to detect clones expressing NANBH viral peptides. More than one million clones were screened and five reactive clones were identified. One of these clones (5-1-1) coded for an antigen that bound circulating antibodies present in the serum of patients infected with NANBH. Importantly, chimpanzees infected experimentally with the NANBH agent, seroconverted to show reactivity to the 5-1-1 polypeptide following the onset of hepatitis, whereas those animals infected with either hepatitis A virus or hepatitis B virus did not seroconvert to this peptide. The other four clones obtained from the original screening were later shown not to have derived from the NANBH agent. Using the 5-1-1 clone as a probe, three other overlapping clones encoding at least a portion of the viral protein were identified. Another clone, c100-3, was constructed from these clones and expressed as a superoxide dismutase fusion protein in yeast for the

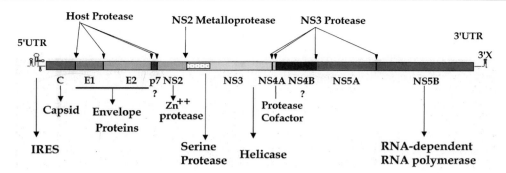

Figure 52-1 Genomic organization of HCV. The genome is around 9600 nucleotide long. The 5′ end consisted of an untranslated region (UTR) containing an internal ribosomal entry site (IRES), which is essential for viral initiation of polypeptide translation. The genome encodes a single open reading of around 3010 amino acids. The 5′ end of the genome consists of the structure genes, including capsid, two envelope proteins (E1 and E2) and p7. The junctions between the structural genes were cleaved by host proteases. Nonstructural (NS) gene 2 encodes a Zn^{2+} metalloprotease that cleaves the junction between NS2 and NS3. The viral protein NS3 consists of two enzymatic activities. The amino one-third is a serine protease, which cleaves the junction between the remaining NS part of the HCV polypeptide. The carboxy two-thirds encodes a helicase that is critical in the unwinding of the double-stranded RNA during viral replication. NS4A is a cofactor for NS3 protease. The functions of NS4B and NS5A are unknown but they are believed to be involved in the viral replication complex. The hydrophobic nature of NS4B suggests that NS4B might serves as a membrane anchor. NS5B encodes the viral RNA-dependent RNA polymerase. The terminal part of 3′ UTR consists of a highly conserved 98 nucleotide sequence which is believed to be critical for the binding of the replication complex and initiation of replication.

development of immunoassay for the detection of antiviral antibody. Both the 5-1-1 and c100-3 clones hybridized only with the RNA extracted from the infected liver, indicating that this agent was an RNA virus. The nucleotide sequence of the genomic RNA was determined by isolating overlapping cDNA clones using hybridization probes based on the sequence of previous clones. After 10 yr, the clinical description of parenteral NANBH, the agent was finally identified and named HCV.

In a parallel series of experiments at around the same time, research workers from Japan also cloned a portion of the viral genome from nucleic acids extracted from 100 L of pooled human sera derived from patients with clinical NANBH. A total of 29 clones were isolated, of which the sequences of 12 clones were later found to be similar to those cloned by the American team.

VIROLOGY OF HCV

STRUCTURE HCV is an enveloped virus of approx 50 nm in diameter visualized in electron microscopy. Immune electron microscopy has demonstrated both HCV core and envelope polypeptides in these particulate structures. HCV consists of a positive strand RNA encapsidated by the core (nucleocapsid peptides) in possibly icosahedral configuration, which is then covered by an envelope, made up of two viral glycoproteins (E1 and E2). The negative strand of HCV is produced as a replicative intermediate during replication, and is considered as a marker of ongoing viral replication.

GENOMIC ORGANIZATION HCV is a single-stranded positive sense RNA virus within the Flaviviridae family, which consists of positive strand RNA viruses encoding a single long polypeptide that is cleaved posttranslationally (Fig. 52-1). The genome of HCV is approx 9600 nucleotides and contains a single open reading frame encoding a large viral polypeptide precursor of around 3000 amino acids with regions at the 5′ and 3′ ends that are not translated. The cleavage of this protein by cellular and viral proteases results in a series of structural [nucleocapsid (C, p21) and the envelope 1 (E1, gp31) and envelope 2 (E2, gp70)], and nonstructural (NS) proteins (NS2, NS3, NS4A, NS4B, NS5A, and NS5B). The NS2 peptide is a metalloprotease essential for the

cleavage of the viral NS2/NS3 junction. The amino-terminus region of NS3 encodes a viral serine protease that is important in posttranslational cleavage of viral peptides from NS3 to NS5. The carboxyl two-third portion of NS3 functions as a helicase, which is essential for unwinding of viral RNA during replication. The NS5B protein functions as a viral RNA-dependent RNA polymerase. The function of the NS5A protein is unknown, but recent observations suggest that it has a role in the regulation of replication. The untranslated 5′ terminal region (5′UTR) and portions of the 3′ untranslated region (3′UTR) are the most conserved parts of the HCV genome and contain signals for replication and translation. The noncoding 5′ terminal region that consists of 349–352 bases has a highly complex secondary RNA structure with four stem root structures and contains an internal ribosomal entry site, the internal viral initiation for polypeptide synthesis. The 3′NTR of HCV consists of a hypervariable segment of approx 420 nucleotides, a poly-U element variable in size, and a recently discovered additional highly conserved region of 98 nucleotides, which is believed to be essential for replication.

The positive strand RNA of HCV has three potential functions: (1) as a template for synthesis of negative strand RNA during replication; (2) as a template for translation of viral proteins; (3) as genomic RNA to be packaged into new virions. As HCV replicates from RNA to RNA, there is no DNA intermediate and therefore, should have no potential for integration into the host cell genome.

REPLICATION Early events in viral binding to cell surface are still poorly understood. Knowledge of the mechanism of replication comes in part from studies in chimpanzees, and in part from extrapolation of the mechanisms adopted by other flaviviruses. HCV RNA is detectable within 3 d of infection in chimpanzees, and persists in serum during the peak of serum alanine transaminase (ALT) elevation. This is associated with the appearance of viral antigens in infected hepatocytes, the major site of HCV replication. The importance of extrahepatic reservoirs (such as peripheral blood mononuclear cells) of HCV replication is uncertain, and technical issues related to the specificity of methods cloud current studies. Through the low fidelity of viral polymerase and the host selection pressure, HCV mutates rapidly in adaptation to the changing virus–host interaction.

The cleavage of the viral polyprotein is achieved by host signal peptidase and two viral proteinases (NS2 and NS3). The function of the viral serine protease, which is located at the amino-terminus region of NS3, is enhanced by its cofactor NS4A. The viral replication machinery is established, when the nonstructural proteins are translated, cleaved cotranslationally, folded and assembled, which will then bind to the 3′NTR to initiate the replication. Mechanisms of viral packaging and release from the hepatocyte are poorly understood but host secretory mechanisms might be utilized by HCV for packaging and release of virions through budding from the Golgi apparatus.

GENOTYPES AND QUASISPECIES Like many other RNA viruses, HCV has an inherently high mutational rate through the poor fidelity of its viral polymerase that results in considerable heterogeneity throughout the genome; in addition, proofreading for mutations that is possible with double-stranded DNA does not occur on the RNA genome. However, constant virus–host interaction leads to clustering of molecular evolution, resulting in distinct distribution of the extent of sequence variations between isolates (Fig. 52-2). The first distinct diversion of the isolate is referred to as genotype. Each variation has different implications (e.g., silent or synonymous vs amino acid substitution or nonsynonymous) and the frequency of occurrence has also substantial impact to the virus fitness. When these are being considered using molecular evolutionary analysis, it appears that HCV isolates can be classified into different genotypes (clades). Current analysis showed that there are 6 major "types" (designated by Arabic numbers) with sequence similarities from 66 to 69% and more than 90 different "subtypes" (designated by a lower case letter) within these types, with sequence similarities from 77 to 80%. In this scheme, the first variant cloned by Choo et al. is designated type 1a.

Different HCV genotype infections have different geographic distribution, associated with different mode of acquisition and differences in responsiveness to antiviral therapy. The association between genotype and disease severity is not unclear. Nonetheless, all HCV genotypes have been found to be hepatotropic and pathogenic, and similar levels of viremia exist between patients infected with different genotypes. In the United States, genotype 1 is the most prevalent (approx 70% with an equal distribution of subtypes 1a and b). Genotypes 2 (10%) and 3 (6%) are less common.

Even within an individual patient, HCV exists as a collection of closely related, yet heterogeneous sequences, called quasispecies. The rate of nucleotide substitution varies significantly between various genomic regions, with an overall substitution rate of 10^{-2} mutations/nucleotide/yr. The highest proportion of mutations has been found in the E1 and E2 regions at both the nucleotide and the amino acid level, particularly in the hypervariable region (at the amino terminus end of E2. Even though this region only represents a minor part of E2/NS1 region, it accounts for about 50% of the nucleotide changes and 60% of the amino acid substitutions within the envelope region. The quasispecies nature of HCV might be one of the mechanisms by which the virus escapes immune responses. Other virus–host interaction

might also play a role in the viral quasispecies evolution. The clinical significance of genotypes and quasispecies continues to be an active area of investigation.

CHIMERAS, REPLICONS, AND INFECTIOUS CLONES Although an efficient cell culture system has not been developed, both replicons (capable of RNA amplification but not production of mature viruses) and chimeric viruses have been developed to enhance our understanding of HCV replication and gene expression. These experimental systems are helpful in the discovery and development of novel antiviral therapies. Infectious HCV clones demonstrated to infect chimpanzees have also been developed. These molecular tools will no doubt contribute to the understanding of the virus–host interactions, in both the mechanism of viral persistence and liver damage, and also to the development of improved antiviral therapies.

EPIDEMIOLOGY

The availability of molecular tools to detect antibody to HCV and viremia (i.e., HCV RNA) has allowed us to better define the epidemiology of HCV infection. In this section, the latest epidemiological findings are summarized. It has to be noted that different diagnostic tools are required for different settings and also other clinical factors, including coinfection with human immunodeficiency virus, might require other molecular tools in the overall evaluation of these patients.

INCIDENCE AND PREVALENCE OF INFECTION The worldwide seroprevalence of HCV infection, based on the detection of antibody to HCV (anti-HCV), is estimated to be 3%. However, marked geographical variation exists, ranging from around 1–2% in North America and 10–14% in North Africa. In the United States, the estimated seroprevalence of anti-HCV is approx 1.8% in the general population or 0.6% in volunteer blood donors. The incidence of acute hepatitis C is falling, from an estimated 180,000 cases per year in the mid-1980s (peak incidence) to approx 30,000 new cases per year in 1995, mainly attributed to risk reduction through blood donor screening, better education and the introduction of syringe-exchange programs. Currently less than 15,000 cases per year are identified attributable to harm reduction in high-risk communities.

TRANSMISSION The modes of transmission of HCV infection can be divided into percutaneous (blood transfusion and needlestick inoculation) and nonpercutaneous (sexual contact, perinatal exposure). The latter group might represent occult percutaneous exposure. Blood transfusion from unscreened donors and injection drug use are the two risk factors that were well documented. HCV was shown to be the etiological agent in more than 85% of cases of posttransfusion NANBH.

Percutaneous Transmission With the introduction of donor screening through anti-HCV testing, the risk of transfusion-related hepatitis has declined significantly, to approx 0.01–0.001% per unit of blood transfused, accounting for only 4% of all acute HCV infections.

The prevalence of HCV infection in injection drug users is 48–90%. Unlike transfusion-associated hepatitis, the prevalence of HCV associated with injection drug use has not declined and this population remains an important reservoir of HCV infection.

Figure 52-2 (opposite page) Phylogenetic tree for HCV isolates as constructed by (**A**) unweighed pair grouping method with arithmatic mean (UPGMA), (**B**) neighbor-joining method (NJ), and (**C**) maximal likelihood method (ML). Note that all HCV isolates clustered together into the same branch by all three methods. Based on this analysis, HCV can be classified into six major genotypes (given as 1–6; also called clades) and a series of subtypes (given as a, b, and so on).

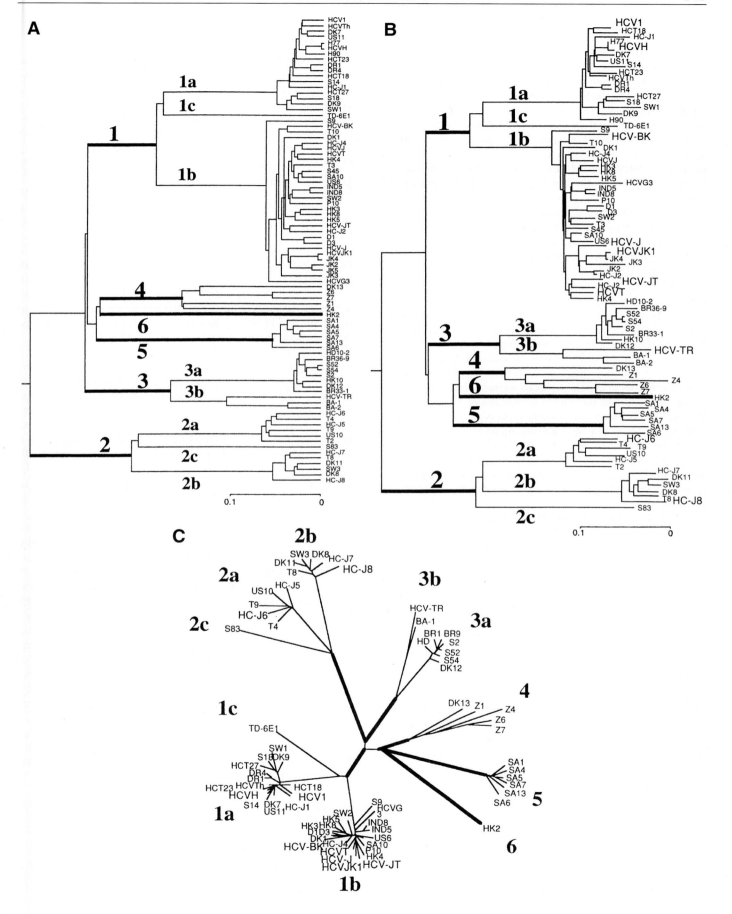

Chronic hemodialysis is associated with both endemic cases and, more rarely, sporadic outbreaks of HCV infection, with most studies showing a prevalence of 10–30%. Serological assays (testing for anti-HCV) might underestimate the prevalence of HCV infection in this relatively immunocompromised population and virological assays (for HCV RNA by polymerase chain reaction amplification [PCR] or transcription-mediated amplification [TMA]) might be necessary for more definitive diagnosis in dialysis patients.

Anti-HCV seroconversion rates have been 0–4% in longitudinal studies of health care workers with documented needle-stick exposures to anti-HCV-positive patients. If a sensitive, qualitative assay for HCV RNA is employed to detect infection, the risk of HCV acquisition after percutaneous exposure is up to 10%. Transmission might also occur from health care worker to patient. Because acute infection is often subclinical, nosocomial transmission might occur with greater frequency than has previously been recognized.

Nonpercutaneous Transmission   The nonpercutaneous modes of transmission include transmission between sexual partners and perinatal transmission. Nonpercutaneous transmission is inefficient; this is particularly true for sexual transmission of HCV, which although infrequent, clearly occurs. Sexual partners of low-risk index subjects without liver disease and without high-risk behavior (injection drug use or promiscuity) have anti-HCV prevalence ranging from 0 to 7%. Coinfection with human immunodeficiency virus and other high-risk behavior are associated with an increased risk with anti-HCV prevalence between 11 and 27%.

The efficiency of perinatal transmission of HCV infection is low, with a risk estimated to range between 0 and 10%. Because antibody to HCV can be passively transferred from mother to infant, detection of HCV viremia (i.e., HCV RNA) by a sensitive qualitative assay for HCV RNA in the infant should be the diagnostic tool of choice. Testing of the infant for anti-HCV before 18 mo is not recommended. The risk posed to the infant from breastfeeding is believed to be negligible.

SPORADIC HCV INFECTION   In earlier epidemiological reports, approx 40% of patients were reported to be without identifiable risk factors. More recent data suggest that the source of transmission is considered to be unknown for less than 10% of the newly identified patients. The high rate of unknown risk factors in previous reports might have been related to patients' denial of high-risk behavior. It is postulated that factors like alternative routes of illicit drug use (e.g., intranasal cocaine use), tattooing and body piercing, and other high-risk behavior involving body secretion/blood contact might be responsible for some of these cases.

PATHOGENESIS

VIRAL PERSISTENCE   HCV causes chronic infection in more than 45–80% of the infected patients. One determinant of viral persistence appears to be the quasispecies nature of the virus, which allows HCV to have the flexibility to evade the host defense and evolve consistently to adapt to the new environment. Other factors might include

1. Inadequate innate immune response.
2. Insufficient induction or maintenance of the immune response.
3. Viral evasion from efficient immune responses through mechanisms such as infection of immunologically privileged sites, viral interference with antigen processing or other immune responses, viral interference of the effectiveness of antiviral cytokines.

4. Amount of virus in inoculums.
5. Induction of immunological tolerance.

HEPATOCELLULAR DAMAGE   In general, viral infection can produce cellular injury by direct cytopathicity and indirect immune-mediated injury. Viral factors might play a role in the pathogenesis of disease. Viral proteins might directly impact cellular function. A correlation between serum HCV RNA levels and lobular inflammatory activity was reported but not all studies demonstrated such a correlation. A lack of correlation does not exclude the possibility of a direct cytopathic mechanism, as liver cell injury might require a certain critical level of intracellular HCV protein accumulation. Support for this comes from a report of severe liver dysfunction in an immunocompromised transplant recipient who, despite exhibiting subfulminant liver failure, had only moderate inflammation on biopsy yet very high levels of HCV viremia.

Immune-mediated mechanisms have also been implicated in HCV-induced hepatocellular damage. HCV infection elicits both innate and HCV-specific immune response, including antibody response and virus-specific CD8+ and CD4+ T-lymphocytes. Whereas, the cellular immune response is believed to play an important role in HCV pathogenesis, the importance of the antibody response in generating liver damage is less clear.

The HCV-specific CD8+ T-cell response is polyclonal, and directed against different epitopes of both structural and NS regions of the viral polyprotein, (core, envelope, NS3, NS4, and NS5) in the context of different major histocompatibility complex alleles. Recent studies using major histocompatibility complex tetramers estimated the frequency of HCV-specific CD8+ T-lymphocytes to range from 0.01 to 1.2% of total CD8+ T-lymphocytes. The CD4+ T-cell response against HCV is also multispecific and frequently found in patients with chronic hepatitis C. However, this CD4+ T-cell response is likely impaired as the proportion of chronic carriers able to mount an effective CD4+ T-cell response to HCV is very small.

Liver-infiltrating CD8+ and CD4+ lymphocytes are detected in portal, periportal, and lobular areas in patients with chronic HCV infection. CD8+ lymphocytes predominate, suggesting that cytotoxic T-lymphocytes (CTLs) are the main perpetrators of hepatocellular injury. Intrahepatic CD8+ lymphocytes recognizing multiple epitopes of the putative HCV core, E1, E2/NS1, and NS3 genomic regions have been cloned from chronically infected patients, and might represent a high proportion of the intrahepatic T-cell infiltrate. HCV-specific CD4+ T cells are rich in the liver, and the majority of these are intrahepatic CD4+ T cells secrete cytokines typical of Th1 cells, favoring HCV CD8+ T-cell activity in liver. Patients with detectable intrahepatic CTL activity show lower levels of viremia, higher ALT values, and more active liver disease than those without HCV-specific CTLs, suggesting a correlation between the CD8+ T-cell response and the degree of hepatocellular injury. Most of the intrahepatic HCV-specific CD8+ T-cells express the activation molecule CD69, which shows a very low expression in circulating virus-specific CD8+ T cells, suggesting that these cells become activated in the liver through their recognition of appropriate presentation of HCV-related epitopes.

CLINICAL FEATURES

HCV is an important public health problem because it is a major cause of chronic hepatitis, cirrhosis, hepatocellular carcinoma (HCC), and need for liver transplantation worldwide.

ACUTE AND CHRONIC INFECTION HCV accounts for about 20% of cases of acute hepatitis. Acute infection is rarely seen in clinical practice, as the vast majority of patients experience no clinical symptoms whereas others might present with nonspecific symptoms such as fatigue, nausea, and vomiting, indistinguishable from symptoms of other types of acute viral infections. HCV RNA appears in the blood within 2 wk of exposure and is followed by an increase in serum ALT levels (i.e., an indicator for hepatocellular damage) several weeks later. Serum ALT levels might exceed 1000 IU/L in 20% of the patients, and generally follow a fluctuating pattern during the first month. In those patients who develop jaundice, peak bilirubin levels are usually less than 12 mg/dL, and typically resolve in 1 mo. Fulminant hepatitis is very rare.

Approximately 45–80% of infected patients do not clear the virus by 6 mo and develop chronic hepatitis. Of these, the majority will have elevated or fluctuating ALT levels, whereas in one-third, persistently normal ALT values exist, despite continued liver injury and detectable viremia in the majority. The overwhelming complaint of patients with chronic infection is fatigue. The severity of this symptom is not necessarily related to the severity of the underlying liver disease. Other nonspecific symptoms include depression, nausea, anorexia, abdominal discomfort, and difficulty with concentration. Once patients develop liver cirrhosis, they are at risk for complications of portal hypertension (ascites, gastrointestinal bleeding, encephalopathy, and so on). Jaundice is rarely seen in chronic infection until significant hepatic decompensation has occurred. Liver transplantation should be considered when patients develop complications of portal hypertension or evidence of hepatic synthetic failure (reduction in serum albumin, rise in serum bilirubin, and/or prolongation of the prothrombin time as calculated as International Normalized Ratio [INR]).

EXTRAHEPATIC MANIFESTATIONS Approximately 1–2% of HCV-infected patients have extrahepatic manifestations. Reported extrahepatic manifestations include essential mixed cryoglobulinemia (that can result in membranoproliferative glomerulonephritis, leukocytoclastic vasculitis, peripheral neuropathy, and other organ injury), porphyria cutanea tarda, focal lymphocytic sialadenitis, Mooren's corneal ulcers, lichen planus, and diabetes mellitus. Some of these associations were clinical correlations and the exact causal relationship and the mechanism of the disease progress has not been established. In the case of essential mixed cryoglobulinemia and membranoproliferative glomerulonephritis, immune complexes induced by HCV (typically positive for rheumatoid factor) have been postulated to be the causal link. Anti-HCV antibodies are positive in 50–90% of patients with essential mixed cryoglobulinemia. In addition, cryoglobulins are found in about half of the patients infected with HCV and high concentration of HCV RNA has been found in the cryoprecipitate. Nonorgan specific autoantibodies are also frequently detected in patients with chronic HCV infection (antinuclear antibodies with a titer >1/40 in 21%, antismooth muscle antibody with a titer >1/40 in 21%, and antiliver kidney microsomal antigen in 5%).

DIAGNOSTICS

A number of immunological and molecular assays have been developed for the detection and assessment of hepatitis C status. The immunological or serological tests identify the presence of anti-HCV antibodies, which indicates previous exposure to the virus without differentiating between acute, chronic or resolved infection. In contrast, the molecular or virological assays detect specific viral nucleic acid sequences (HCV RNA), which indicate ongoing presence of the virus. Although serological assays are typically used for screening and first-line diagnosis, molecular/virological assays are needed in certain situations with the aim of confirming infection and/or monitoring therapy.

SEROLOGICAL TESTS There are two types of anti-HCV assays, the enzyme immunoassay (EIA) and the recombinant immunoblot assay (RIBA). Both detect antibodies against different HCV antigens from the core and nonstructural proteins and were developed using recombinant HCV antigens. Serological assays are typically used for screening and first-line diagnosis. Three generations of EIAs have been developed with increasing sensitivity. As first-generation EIAs lack sensitivity and specificity, confirmatory RIBAs were systematically used in samples positive in EIA. With the newer assays and the increased use of molecular assays, confirmatory RIBAs are seldom needed.

Screening Assays The latest EIA-3 assay uses recombinant antigens from the core, NS3/4A (c200) and NS5 (EIA-2 does not have this capture antigen) regions to provide better sensitivity for the detection of antibody to HCV. Even with these new assays, specificity might need to be confirmed in some populations, especially, those with low-risk. In this setting, confirmatory tests, typically molecular testing, are generally helpful.

Confirmatory Assays The RIBA tests use the same antigens as the corresponding EIA tests but in a strip or immunoblot assay format. Their sensitivity is generally lower than for EIA assays, but their specificity is better because the reactivity specific for the capture antigen can be visualized. The 4-antigen RIBA-2 (RIBA HCV 2.0 Strip Immunoassay, Chiron Corporation) was approved by the United States Food and Drug Administration in June 1993. This assay incorporated antigens 5-1-1, c100-3, c22-3, c33c and SOD (superoxide dismutase, as a control). With this assay, a specimen is considered positive if two bands or more are detectable, representing at least the presence of antibodies to two different HCV-derived capture antigens. If a specimen reacts with bands from only one region, such as 5-1-1 and c100-3 (both from the NS4 region), it is considered indeterminate. If a specimen reacts with the SOD band in addition to two or more HCV antigen bands, the result is also considered indeterminate. The third generation assay, RIBA-3 (RIBA HCV 3.0 Strip Immunoassay, Chiron Corporation) includes two recombinant antigens (c33c and NS5) and synthetic peptides from the nucleocapsid (c22) and the NS4 (c100-3) regions. It has been approved for use by blood banks as a supplemental test for EIA-3-positive samples. This new RIBA format is able to identify correctly HCV-negative and HCV-positive results in those samples that are RIBA-2 indeterminate.

VIROLOGICAL TESTS As HCV cell culture systems have not been established, detection of viral RNA in serum has been used as a direct marker of the virus. Qualitative HCV RNA assays are optimized to produce maximal signal regardless of the amount of input HCV RNA. In comparison, quantitative assays are developed to yield reproducible and accurate quantification values regardless of the input concentration of virus. Thus, these two types of assays are developed differently. Viral detection (i.e., qualitative result) is accomplished by target amplification methods such as the PCR-based AMPLICOR assay (Cobas Amplicor HVC Kit, Roche Diagnostics) or by the TMA-based VERSANT assay (Versant HCV RNA 3.0 Assay, Bayer Diagnostics). The qualitative PCR test for HCV might detect as few as 50 International Units (IU)/mL. The VERSANT assay employing TMA has a sensitivity of 10 IU/mL. To achieve these results, specific procedures directed to preserving the integrity of HCV RNA should be followed carefully, including separation of serum or plasma from whole blood within 4 h of venipuncture, and rapid storage of specimens at –70°C.

Qualitative assays for HCV RNA are used for confirmation of diagnosis and for assessment of viral clearance at the end of therapy and at follow-up to therapy (i.e., 6 mo after cessation of therapy). Ninety-five percent of viral loads at baseline are within the range of 33,500–3,700,000 IU/mL; therefore, the sensitivity of either of the qualitative assays should be sufficient to detect HCV RNA in a confirmatory application. In comparison, the TMA-based assay detected HCV RNA in (7–30% of) relapsers at the end of treatment when the PCR-based assay detected none. In this setting, very high sensitivity is important in detection of residual HCV RNA at the end of therapy.

The quantitative HCV RNA tests allow measurement of viral load and they are useful in monitoring the effectiveness of antiviral therapy and in evaluating the course of clinical disease. The branched DNA (bDNA) VERSANT assay (Bayer Diagnostics) uses capture and target probes directed to the conserved 5′ UTR and core regions in a microwell format. HCV RNA captured to the microwell supports the formation of very large hybridization complexes that include synthetic branched DNA oligonucleotides (signal amplification). These large hybrids contain many copies of probes that are labeled with alkaline phosphatase. Following addition of a chemiluminescent substrate, light is emitted in proportion to the number of HCV RNA molecules in the original specimen; the quantity of HCV RNA is determined by comparison of chemiluminescence from the specimen with a standard curve containing calibrators with known amount of target. The third generation assay, registered with the FDA, has been shown to measure down to 615 IU/mL with a dynamic range of over 4 logs (upper limit of detection 7.7×10^6 IU/mL).

The Amplicor HCV Monitor, v 2.0 quantitative assay provides a semiquantitative measurement of viral RNA. HCV RNA is reverse transcribed and amplified by end point PCR (i.e., with a specific number of amplification cycles) using primers from the most conserved region (in 5′ UTR) of the HCV genome. This reaction produces very large numbers of double-stranded DNA that has the same sequence as a portion of the HCV RNA in the specimen. The assumption is that the amount of amplicon produced is directly proportional to the amount of HCV RNA in the specimen. A quantitation standard (with a known number of HCV RNA targets) is added to each specimen and coamplified with the target. An internal control also is added to each specimen and is used to indicate if there are inhibitors of the RT-PCR steps in the reaction. A microwell plate detection system with chemiluminescent label is used for quantification of amplicons produced. The amount of viral RNA present in the amplified sample is calculated based on the signal from HCV RNA in the specimen and on the signal generated from the quantification standard. The lower limit of detection of the AMPLICOR assay is approx 600 IU/mL.

Recently, kinetic or real-time PCR methodologies have been applied to quantification of HCV RNA. Amplification by PCR is geometric and nucleotide and/or enzyme might become rate limiting during the reaction; the rate of accumulation of amplicons might decrease during the reaction and with higher input numbers of HCV RNA. Thus, end point PCR assays have a limited dynamic range of 2.5–3 $\log_{10}$ units. In comparison, real-time PCR assays

are carried out like end point assay except that signal from amplicons is detected during amplification. The fractional PCR cycle in which signal exceeds a critical threshold value (Ct), marks the start of the exponential phase of target amplification. A lower Ct indicates a higher input concentration of HCV RNA. The quantity of HCV RNA in a specimen is calculated based on the Ct for the specimen and the Ct for the Quantification Standard (with a known number of HCV target molecules). Alternatively, quantification might be based on the Ct for the specimen and the Ct's for a series of calibrators. Fluorescence energy transfer is used in many probe systems, including TaqMan, employed with the real time PCR technology. The assay is designed to avoid the problems associated with rate limitation resulting from enzyme and/or nucleotide depletion and, thus, is reported to be linear. Roche Molecular Systems and Abbott Diagnostics employ real time PCR in their Analyte Specific Reagents or kits. Bayer Diagnostics currently is developing assays that employ real time technologies.

Quantitative assays are employed in monitoring the efficacy of therapy often by showing changes in viral load between baseline (i.e., start of therapy) and during therapy. Linearity of assay response (i.e., degree to which the assay standard curve approximates a straight line) provides the clinician and patient accurate results regardless of the level of virus; changes in viral load reflect actual changes in the patient. The bDNA-based assay is linear (slopes of about 1) whereas the Amplicor HCV Monitor assay might exhibit nonlinear performance at viral loads greater than 500,000 IU/mL. Real-time PCR-based assays are linear.

An immunoassay that provides quantification values for HCV core antigen has been introduced as an indirect measure of viral load. This assay has a sensitivity of approx 20,000 IU/mL. Thus, the 2-$\log_{10}$ stopping rule at week 12 of therapy is employed in assessing nonresponse could be employed only in patients with viral loads of ≥2,000,000 IU/mL at baseline. To date, this assay has limited application because it is an indirect measure of virus and it is considerably less sensitivity than are the quantitative assays.

To permit universal standardization of HCV RNA quantitation units, a recent collaborative study established the World Health Organization (WHO) International Standard for HCV RNA quantitation. A lyophilized genotype 1 sample was accepted as the candidate standard and was assigned a titer of 10^5 IU/mL. This standard has been used to calibrate HCV RNA panels and by industrial manufacturers to express HCV RNA load in IU/mL in their assays (226). The goals of standardization are to allow for generalization of findings from clinical studies with one assay to patient management with all of the assays and to permit clinicians to use results from any of the assays in monitoring patients.

HCV GENOTYPING Differentiation of the HCV genotypes is accomplished by direct sequencing, differential PCR using type-specific primers, detection of PCR products with type-specific probes (available commercially, the Line Probe Assay), restriction fragment length polymorphism analysis, and serotyping with type-specific antibody. These techniques use targets in the 5′ UTR, NS4, NS5, and core regions. Of the many methods available for genotyping, direct sequencing coupled with phylogenetic tree analysis is regarded as the gold standard. However, sequencing methods are technically demanding and time-consuming. A study comparing sequencing, type-specific primers, serotyping, and restriction fragment length polymorphism analysis, demonstrated more than 90% concordance between methods.

SELECTION OF SEROLOGICAL AND VIROLOGICAL TESTS
Initial diagnostic testing of HCV infection is currently made by detecting specific antibody by EIA. For low-risk patients, a negative EIA test is sufficient to rule out infection. A positive EIA for low-risk patients should be confirmed by RIBA assay or molecular testing. For high-risk patients, individuals with recent exposure or immunocompromised patients (including HIV, chronic hemodialysis patients, transplant patients), a negative EIA should be confirmed and molecular test such as PCR or TMA-based qualitative test is the choice.

SCREENING IN BLOOD BANKS
With the latest EIA and RIBA assays, the number of false positive or indeterminate test results is very low. One major limitation of these assays however is the existence of a window period by which the patient might transmit the virus before antibodies are detectable. With recent assays, the average delay is approx 80 d. For this reason, many blood banks throughout the world have instituted testing all donors with qualitative PCR or TMA assays.

DIAGNOSIS IN IMMUNOCOMPROMISED PATIENTS
Antibody tests underestimate the prevalence of HCV infection in immunocompromised populations and detection of viral RNA is frequently required for diagnosis. Antibody assays also lack sensitivity in the transplant setting, as these patients are immunosuppressed. Molecular/virological assays for HCV RNA are the assays of choice.

LIVER HISTOLOGY
The range of histological findings in patients with chronic HCV infection is broad, from minimal periportal lymphocytic inflammation to active hepatitis with bridging fibrosis, hepatocyte necrosis, and frank cirrhosis. Steatosis, lymphoid aggregates, and bile duct damage are frequently found in the liver biopsies of patients with this infection, but there is considerable overlap with the histological findings in patients with chronic HBV infection and occasionally with autoimmune hepatitis. The role of a liver biopsy in the management of HCV-infected patients is still not settled although most physicians perform a liver biopsy before initiating treatment. This recommendation is waning somewhat for patients with genotypes 2 and 3, in which the viral response is much higher with a shorter course of therapy. The potential risks associated with a liver biopsy (1:3000 chance of bleeding, 1:12,000 chance of death) contrast with the importance of the information generated by this means. Recent consensus conferences have stated that a liver biopsy is recommended in patients with chronic hepatitis C and abnormal serum ALT levels so that correct staging and grading can be performed. This information is particularly relevant when considering antiviral therapy or when other causes of liver disease might be present. A posttreatment liver biopsy is not necessary as most trials have demonstrated that viral sustained response is generally associated with stable or improved histological findings. In patients with normal serum ALT levels, liver biopsy might also provide information about the stage of disease, particularly if antiviral therapy is being considered. Although fibrosis progression appears to be slow in these patients, only 20% have an absolutely normal liver, and a small percentage (<15%) have significant liver damage, and it is in these patients that treatment might be undertaken. In patients in whom the diagnosis of cirrhosis is established (ascites, splenomegaly, spider angioma, low platelet count, low prothrombin time, reduction of portal flow speed, nodularity of the liver), histological confirmation is usually not needed.

NATURAL HISTORY
An understanding of the natural history of infection is essential for guiding physicians when counseling patients about their prognosis and assessing the need for therapeutic intervention. Infection with HCV, once established, persists in the vast majority. Disease progression is largely silent with patients often identified only on routine biochemical screening or during the course of blood donation. The natural history of chronic HCV infection, as evaluated through different approaches (e.g., through referral centers, military recruits, pregnant women who received HCV contaminated immunoglobulins, and children with cardiac surgery who acquired HCV through transfusion), appears to show that HCV usually is a slowly progressive disease in 10–25% of the patients, and these patients might develop end-stage liver disease more than two to three decades. The remaining patients will have a benign evolution over decades.

For factors associated with disease progression, age (older than 40 yr), male gender, obesity (fatty liver), and increased alcohol intake (>50 g/d) have been documented as associated variables. Immunosuppression is clearly linked with more aggressive disease. Patients with humoral immunodeficiency (hypo γ-globulinemic patients) or cellular immune impairment (liver or kidney transplant recipients, HIV infected patients with low CD4 count) have shown rates of liver disease progression significantly faster than those observed in immunocompetent patients.

For patients with compensated HCV-related cirrhosis, the prognosis of patients in the short-term might be good. Actuarial survival is 91% at 5 yr and 79% after 10 yr in the absence of clinical decompensation. Survival drops to 50% at 5 yr among those who develop clinical decompensation. The cumulative probability of developing an episode of clinical decompensation is approx 5% at 1 yr, increasing to 30% at 10 yr from the diagnosis of cirrhosis. The risk of developing HCC is 1–4%/yr once cirrhosis is established.

For patients with persistently normal serum ALT levels (around one-third of the patients), most will have some degree of histologicaly proven chronic liver damage ranging from mild chronic hepatitis to cirrhosis. Disease progression appears to be slower in these patients than in those with abnormal serum ALT levels, and progression to cirrhosis is unlikely.

For renal transplant recipients, elevated serum ALT levels are more common in anti-HCV positive than in anti-HCV negative patients (median 48 and 14%, respectively). There are also reported differences in patient and graft survival between anti-HCV positive and anti-HCV negative kidney transplant recipients, the increased mortality being related to liver dysfunction.

HCV is evolving as an important issue in liver transplantation. Chronic HCV infection is the most common indication for liver transplantation in the United States. Recurrence of HCV following liver transplantation is universal. Viremia level increased by one log after liver transplantation. In a small proportion of patients (5%), an accelerated course of liver injury leading to rapid development of liver failure, reminiscent of that previously described in HBV-infected recipients with fibrosing cholestatic hepatitis has been observed. Disease progression is significantly faster than that observed in immunocompetent patients, and the time to develop cirrhosis is short in this population. Although histological evidence of liver injury will develop in approximately half of the patients within the first year posttransplantation, severe graft dysfunction in the short-term is infrequent. With longer follow-up (5–7 yr), a significant proportion of patients, ranging from 8 to

30%, develop HCV related graft-cirrhosis. The risk of decompensation once the transplant patient has developed clinically compensated cirrhosis is approx 40% at 1 yr.

For patients coinfected with HCV and human immunodeficiency virus undergoing active antiretroviral therapy, chronic hepatitis C is a growing cause of morbidity and mortality in this population. It was also observed that hepatic decompensation develop more rapidly in coinfected patients than in those with HCV infection alone but the mechanism responsible for this clinical observation was not known.

TREATMENT

The primary goal of therapy is to eradicate infection early in the course of the disease to prevent progression to end-stage liver disease and eventually to HCC. However, this is a long-term goal and cannot be measured in short-term clinical studies. In this context, normalization of serum ALT levels, loss of HCV RNA, and improvements in histological findings have been employed as the current standard therapeutic end points. Current data suggest that the achievement of these end points will translate into long-term benefit from therapy, as measured by reduction in the rate of disease progression, reduction in the need for liver transplantation, reduction in rate of development of HCC and improvement in survival. Indeed, several studies have shown that in patients with sustained biochemical and virological responses, the durability of the response is more than 95% for up to 10 yr. A lesser goal of therapy is to reduce the secondary spread of infection by eradicating the viremia.

Interferon-α based regimens constitute the cornerstone of our current antiviral therapies. There are several types of interferon-α available, including recombinant forms (interferon α-2a, α-2b, and consensus interferon) and naturally occurring forms (lymphoblastoid interferon). Interferons are naturaly occurring proteins, which exert a wide array of antiviral, antiproliferative, and immunomodulatory effects. For years, interferon-α given in monotherapy was the standard treatment in patients with chronic hepatitis C, with results considered modest at best. A modified version of interferon, pegylated interferon-α, which consists of interferon-α bound to a molecule of polyethylene glycol of varying length and with different order of branches has been developed. This process of pegylation increases the half-life of the molecule and reduces the volume of distribution. This altered pharmacokinetic profile provides more uniform and prolonged plasma levels, which in turn have led to weekly dosing of this product. Such a profile with better drug exposure is leading to better therapeutic efficacy compared to the unmodified interferon-α.

Ribavirin is a broad-spectrum antiviral agent with activity against both DNA and RNA viruses. In immunocompetent patients with chronic HCV infection, ribavirin resulted in improved serum ALT levels but the effect was transient and no significant direct antiviral activity was observed. Ribavirin is known to induce hemolysis, a side effect that is dose limiting. Because of this side effect, ribavirin is contraindicated in patients with a past history of myocardial infarction or cardiac arrhythmia. Ribavirin is also potentially teratogenic and patients and partners are required to avoid pregnancy during therapy and for 6 mo after cessation of treatment. Ribavirin has a long cumulative half-life. It is excreted by the kidney and cannot be removed by hemodialysis. Hence, ribavirin is contraindicated in patients with a serum creatinine of greater than 1.5 mg/dL.

Although neither interferon-α nor ribavirin monotherapy is very effective in the treatment of chronic HCV infection, the combination of these two drugs improves the treatment response rate by many folds and is currently the gold standard for the treatment of chronic HCV infection in individuals who have not received any previous treatment (i.e., treatment naive). The current recommendation for patients with HCV genotype 1 infection is pegylated interferon-α injection (dosing depends on the preparation: 180 μg weekly for pegylated interferon-α2a; and 1.5 μg/kg weekly for pegylated interferon-α2b) for 48 wk in combination with oral ribavirin (1000–1200 mg daily with pegylated interferon-α2a and 800 mg daily with pegylated interferon-α2b). Trials using pegylated interferon-α2a have compared safety and efficacy of 800 mg vs 1000–1200 mg of ribavirin daily, and for genotype 1 infection, results suggest superiority of the higher dose. Given these findings, it is likely that 1000–1200 mg of ribavirin is necessary for optimizing outcomes in these patients whether given in combination with pegylated interferon-α2b or -α2a. The recommendation for patients with HCV genotypes 2 and 3 infection is similar to patients with HCV genotype 1 infection except that 24 wk of therapy, and a dose of ribavirin at 800 mg appear adequate. Overall, the long-term sustained response (defined as normal serum ALT and with no detectable HCV RNA 6 mo after cessation of therapy) is around 55%. For patients with HCV genotype 1 infection, the long-term sustained response is around 40% and for patients with genotypes 2 and 3 infection, the long-term sustained response is around 80%. Adherence to full dose and duration of therapy can improve the sustained virological response rate by another 10%.

Factors associated with a better treatment outcome include low pretreatment serum HCV RNA levels, genotypes 2 and 3 infection, absence of cirrhosis, female gender and age less than 40 yr. African-Americans have generally been shown to respond less well to treatment than Caucasians, whether the treatment is interferon or pegylated interferon plus ribavirin. It should also be noted that with the current combination of pegylated interferon-α and ribavirin therapy, patients with HCV-related cirrhosis and patients with "transition to cirrhosis" have shown similar response rate as noncirrhotic patients, although there have been few studies focusing specifically on outcomes in patients with advanced liver disease. Thus, the presence of clinically compensated cirrhosis should not exclude patients from antiviral therapy.

Regarding indications, theoretically all patients with ongoing HCV infection with persistent elevation of serum ALT levels are potential candidates of antiviral therapy. However, given that (1) our therapies are still imperfect in terms of efficacy, and are associated with significant side effects; and (2) the natural history of hepatitis C is benign in the majority of patients, both physicians and patients need to evaluate the potential benefit, the costs, and the risks before initiating therapy. Ironically, patients with the lowest likelihood of progression are precisely the ones who are most likely to respond. In contrast, those with the least likelihood of responding or with the least tolerance of side effects of treatment are often the ones with the greatest need. In patients with a low chance of disease progression (immunocompetent, less than 40 yr of age, female gender, no alcohol consumption, minimal histological inflammation, and fibrosis), there are as many arguments to recommend starting treatment as there are to defer treatment until safer and more effective therapies are available.

There are certain situations in which the guidelines regarding treatment are not yet well developed, in part because studies in certain patient populations are still underway and complete results have not yet been published in the peer-reviewed literature. These include patients with active substance abuse (alcohol and injection drug use), those with clinically decompensated cirrhosis, those with very mild liver disease and those with coinfection with other viruses such as HIV and/or hepatitis B. As the need for treatment is high in many of these subpopulations, results from carefully conducted clinical trials are greatly needed. Clearance of virus in a larger percentage of patients might ultimately require the development of HCV therapies with different mechanisms of action to those that are currently available.

At present, combination therapy using the nonpegylated interferon in combination with oral ribavirin has been approved for the treatment of children with chronic HCV infection. Patients with HIV coinfection are frequently being treated in the context of randomized controlled trials. Preliminary data suggest that although sustained viral clearance is achievable, overall responses to peginterferon plus ribavirin are lower than those observed in HIV-negative patients. Interferon has produced short-term improvement in the signs and symptoms of cryoglobulinemia in those patients demonstrating a virological response, although recurrence of viremia and cryoglobulinemia is the rule when treatment is discontinued. Interferon has been used successfully in the treatment of HCV-associated membranoproliferative glomerulonephritis. There is a theoretical rationale for treating patients with acute HCV infection as the majority will develop persistent infection and chronic liver disease. The few studies that have been conducted in patients with acute HCV have used different dosage and duration of interferon therapy. Whereas, most are uncontrolled case series, high rates of remission have also been reported. The Manns study showed clearance of virus in 98% of a small number of treated patients; these patients were selected for the presence of icterus.

In patients who have relapsed after a course of interferon monotherapy, combination therapy is the treatment of choice. There are no FDA-approved treatments for nonresponders to previous treatment with interferon alone, or interferon-α/ribavirin combination therapy. If retreatment is undertaken with peginterferon plus ribavirin in those who have failed a previous course, viral clearance is achievable, particularly in patients with genotype non-1 infection, those who have failed previous interferon monotherapy rather than interferon plus ribavirin combination therapy and those who have demonstrated some degree of treatment sensitivity with a reduction in HCV RNA levels during the first course of therapy.

Monitoring before and during therapy is important in the overall management of patients with chronic HCV infection. Before starting therapy, blood tests should be conducted to establish baseline status, including liver biochemistry, complete blood count, viral load (with a quantitative HCV RNA test), and thyroid-stimulating hormone level. A pregnancy test is needed to rule out pregnancy before initiating ribavirin therapy in women. Strongly worded counseling needs to take place for partners who potentially could be involved in conception during ribavirin treatment to utilize a dual method of contraception to prevent pregnancy. HCV genotyping will help in selecting the best treatment strategy (i.e., dosage of ribavirin and duration of therapy). During the first month of therapy, a complete blood count should be done weekly as most side effects occur within this period of time, particularly hemolytic anemia related to ribavirin therapy. Approximately 9–23% of patients, depending on the ribavirin dose, will have a fall in hemo-

globin to less than 10 g/dL with a mean decrease of approx 3 g/dL. As dose reductions of ribavirin have the potential to compromise response to combination therapy, adjunctive treatments such as erythropoietin are being increasingly used to manage side effects in patients receiving HCV treatment. After the first month, liver biochemistry and a complete blood count should be performed monthly, and thyroid-stimulating hormone level every 3 mo. Modifications of doses should be done according to the severity of side effects. The recent NIH Guidelines recommend that viral load should be assessed at week 12 of therapy. Several studies of therapy with pegylated interferon plus ribavirin showed that patients in whom the viral load did not decrease by at least 2 $\log_{10}$ almost invariably (97–100% negative predictive value) were nonresponders with the full course of therapy. At the end of treatment and at 6 mo postdiscontinuation of treatment, serum HCV RNA testing with sensitive, qualitative assay should be carried out to assess treatment response. If sustained response is achieved, it is recommended that serum HCV RNA testing be performed annually for at least 2 yr after completion of therapy. A repeat liver biopsy following treatment is rarely necessary.

Newer therapies are being developed for anti-HCV infection. A number of the HCV viral peptides in the replication machinery are good targets for novel therapy development. Current efforts are focusing on targeting HCV internal ribosomal entry site, NS3 protease, NS3 helicase, and NS5B RNA-dependent RNA polymerase. Molecular approaches utilizing antisense, ribozyme, and small inhibitory RNA directed against the HCV genome are also being tested. A number of immunomodulators are also being tested for their ability to booster the host immune response. These include HCV-specific immune stimulation, i.e., therapeutic vaccine, as well as non-HCV specific immunomodulation using various cytokines. Efforts are also directed at developing a safer version of ribavirin, a prodrug of ribavirin that is predominately released by the deaminase enzyme system in the liver.

PREVENTION

GENERAL MEASURES   As there is no effective prophylactic vaccine and no effective postexposure prophylaxis, major efforts should be placed on counseling both HCV-infected patients and those at risk of infection on the general measures. Adequate sterilization of medical and surgical equipment is mandatory. Efforts should also be made to modify injection practices involved in folk medicine, rituals, and cosmetic procedures. Persons at high-risk of HCV infection such as recipients of blood/blood product transfusions before 1990, drug users, and sexual partners of persons infected with HCV should be tested for antiHCV. HCV-infected patients should be instructed to avoid sharing razors and toothbrushes and to cover any open wounds. Given the low rate of vertical transmission, pregnancy is not contraindicated in HCV-infected women. No recommendations have been issued regarding the mode of delivery. Breast-feeding is not contraindicated. It is recommended that HCV-infected patients be vaccinated against hepatitis A and B, given the increased risk of severe liver disease if superinfection with these viruses occurs.

PASSIVE IMMUNOPROPHYLAXIS   Immune serum globulin has not been studied clinically in the prevention of HCV infection. Nevertheless, there are several lines of evidence suggesting that such measures are unlikely to be effective. Studies from the 1970s of immune serum globulin as a measure of prophylaxis against posttransfusion NANBH failed to demonstrate any significant benefit. The neutralizing immune response to HCV infection even in healthy adults appears to be weak and hence it would seem unlikely that immune serum globulin would contain sufficient neutralizing antibody to be effective. Finally, HCV has an inherently high nucleotide substitution rate that would predictably facilitate rapid escape from humoral immune recognition. Despite this scientific rationale, polyclonal immunoglobulins containing anti-HCV are being tested to decrease the incidence of recurrent HCV viremia 1-yr post-transplantation, preliminary results have not been encouraging and long-term protection has not been reported. Whether such immune sera will be protective in the setting of exposure to virus remains to be determined.

ACTIVE IMMUNOPROPHYLAXIS Vaccine development for HCV appears to encounter the same difficulties encountered in the development of human immunodeficiency virus vaccine. The absence of natural protective immunity in chimpanzees that recovered from HCV infection to challenges with both heterologous and homologous strains of virus bodes poorly for vaccine development. Nevertheless, neutralizing antibodies to HCV can be elicited during natural infection and have been demonstrated to be effective at preventing viral transmission to experimental animals, when used to neutralize virus in vitro. Substantial efforts are currently directed to the development of prophylactic HCV vaccines.

"Science has radically changed the conditions of human life on earth. It has expanded our knowledge and our power but not our capacity to use them with wisdom"
J. William Fulbright (1905–1995)
In: Old Men and New Realities

ACKNOWLEDGMENTS

The authors thank all their colleagues who share their data, knowledge, and passion that drives the advancement of basic and clinical science with them. Many scientists and clinicians secured our knowledge on HCV. Neither space nor time has allowed us to be comprehensive. For those significant contributions that we failed to mention, we apologize.

SELECTED REFERENCES

Alberti A, Chemello L, Benvegnu L. Natural history of hepatitis C J Hepatol 1999;31:17–24.

Alter HJ, Seeff LB. Recovery, persistence, and sequelae in hepatitis C infection: a perspective on long-term outcome. Semin Liv Dis 2000; 20:17–35.

Alter MJ, Kniszon-Moran D, Nainan OV, et al. The prevalence of hepatitis C virus infection in the United States, 1999 through 1994. N Engl J Med 1999;341:556–562.

Bellentani S, Tiribelli C. The spectrum of liver disease in the general population: lesson from the Dionysos study. J Hepatol 2001;35:531–537.

Berenguer M, Prieto M, Rayon JM, et al. Natural history of clinicaly compensated HCV-related graft cirrhosis following liver transplantation. Hepatology 2000;32:852–858.

Berebguer M, Lopez-Labrador FX, Wright TL. Hepatitis C and liver transplantation. J Hepatol 2001;35:666–678.

Bouvier-Alias M, Patel K, Dahari H, et al. Clinical utility of total HCV core antigen quantification: a new indirect marker of HCV replication. Hepatology 2002;36:211–218.

Bukh J, Miller RH, Purcell RH. Genetic heterogeneity of hepatitis C virus: quasispecies and genotypes. Semin Liver Dis 1995;15:41–63.

Bukh J, Forns X, Emerson SU, Purcell RH. Studies of hepatitis C virus in chimpanzees and their importance for vaccine development. Intervirology 2001;44:132–142.

Centers for Disease Control and Prevention. Recommendations for prevention and control of hepatitis C virus (HCV) infection and HCV-related chronic disease. MMWR 1998;47(No. RR-19).

Comanor L, Hendricks DA. Hepatitis C virus RNA tests: performance attributes and their impact on clinical utility. Expert Rev Mol Diagn 2003;3:689–702.

Davis GL, Lau JYN. Choice of appropriate endpoints of response to interferon-α therapy in chronic hepatitis C virus infection. J Hepatol 1995;22(suppl 1):110–114.

Davis GL, Lau JYN. Factors predictive of response to interferon. Hepatol 1997;26:122S–127S.

Davis GL, Esteban-Mur R, Rustgi V, et al. Interferon alfa-2b alone or in combination with ribavirin for the treatment of relapse of chronic hepatitis C. N Engl J Med 1998;339: 1493–1499.

Di Bisceglie AM, McHutchinson J, Rice CM. New therapeutic strategies for hepatitis C. Hepatology 2002;35:224–231.

Elbeik T, Surtihadi J, Destree M, et al. Multicenter evaluation of the performance characteritics of the Bayer VERSANT HCV RNA 3.0 assay (bDNA). J Clin Micro 2004;42:563–569.

Fang JWS, Chow V, Lau JYN. Virology of hepatitis C virus. Semin in Liver Dis 1997;1:493–514.

Farci P, Alter HJ, Wong D, et al. A long-term study of hepatitis C virus replication in non-A, non-B hepatitis. N Engl J Med 1991;325: 98–104.

Gish RG. Standards of treatment in chronic hepatitis C. Semin Liver Dis 1999;19:35–47.

Gretch DR. Diagnostic tests for hepatitis C. Hepatology 1997;26:43S–47S.

Hadziyannis SJ, Sette H Jr, Morgan TR, et al. Pegasys International Study Group. Peginteron alpha2a and ribavirin combination therapy in chronic hepatitis C: a randomized study of treatment duration and ribavirin dose. Ann Intern Med 2004;1(140):346–355.

Hoofnagle JH. Therapy for acute hepatitis C. N Engl J Med 2001;345: 1495–1497.

Jonas MM. Hepatitis C in children. In: Hepatitis C, Liang TJ and Hoofnagle JH, eds. Biomed Res Rep. San Diego, CA: Academic Press, 2000, pp. 389–404.

Koziel MJ. Cytokines in viral hepatitis. Semin Liver Dis 1999;19:157–169.

Krajden M, Ziermann R, Khan A, et al. Qualitative detection of hepatitis C virus RNA: comparison of analytical sensitivity, clinical performance, and workflow of the COBAS Amplicor HCV test version 2.0 and the HCV RNA transcription-mediated amplification qualitative assay. J Clin Micro 2002;40:2903–2907.

Lau JYN, Mizokami M, Kolberg JA, et al. Application of six hepatitis C virus subtyping systems to sera of patients with chronic hepatitis C in the United States. J Infect Dis 1995;171:281–289.

Lau JYN, Davis GL, Prescott LE, et al. Distribution of hepatitis C virus genotypes in United States patients with chronic hepatitis C seen in tertiary referral centers. Ann Intern Med 1996;124:868–876.

Lau JYN, Standring DN. Development of novel therapies for hepatitis C. In: Hepatitis C, Liang TJ, Hoofnagle JH, eds. Biomed Res Rep 2000: San Diego, CA: Academic Press: pp. 453–467.

Lauer GM, Walker BD. Hepatitis C virus infection. N Engl J Med 2001;345:41–52.

Lee SG, Antony A, Lee N, et al. Improved version 2.0 qualitative and quantitative AMPLICOR reverse transcription-PCR tests for hepaitis C virus RNA: calibration to international units, enhanced genotype reactivity, and performance characteristics. J Clin Micro 2000;38: 4171–4179.

Lindenbach BD, Rice CM. Evasive maneuvers by hepatitis C virus. Hepatology 2003;38:3669–3679.

McHutchison JG, Gordon SC, Schiff ER, et al. Interferon alfa-2b alone or in combination with ribavirin as initial treatment for chronic hepatitis C. International Hepatitis Interventional Therapy Group. N Engl J Med 1998;339:1485–1492.

McHutshinson JG, Poynard T. Combination therapy with interferon plus ribavirin for the initial treatment of chronic hepatitis C. Semin Liver Dis 1999;19:57–65.

Mizokami M, Gobojori T, Lau JYN. Molecular evolutionary Virology - its application to the study of hepatitis C virus. Gastroenterology 1994;107:1181, 1182.

Morishima C, Chung M, Ng KW, et al. Stengths and limitations of commercial tests for hepatitis C virus RNA quantification. J Clin Micro 2004;42:421–425.

National Institutes of Health Consensus Develeopment Conference Statement: Management of Hepatitis C. Hepatology 2002;36(Suppl): S3–S20.

Nelson DR, Lau JYN. Host immune response to hepatitis C virus. Viral Hepatitis Reviews 1996;2:37–48.

Nelson DR, Marousis CG, Davis GL, et al. The role of hepatitis C virus-specific cytotoxic T-lymphocytes in chronic hepatitis C. J Immunol 1997;158:1473–1481.

Nelson DR, Lau JYN. Pathogenesis of chronic hepatitis C virus infection. Antiviral Therapy 1998;3:25–35.

Pawlotsky JM, Bouvier-Alias M, Hezode C, et al. Standardization of hepatitis C virus RNA quantitation. Hepatology 2000;32:654–659.

Pawlotsky JM. Use and interpretation of hepatitis C diagnostic assays. Clin Liver Dis 2003;7:127–137.

Poynard T, Bedossa P, Opolon P, for the OBSVIRC, METAVIR, CLINIVIR, and DOSVIRC groups. Natural history of liver fibrosis progression in patients with chronic hepatitis C. Lancet 1997;349: 825–832.

Poynard T, Marcellin P, Lee SS, et al. Randomized trial of interferon alpha 2b plus ribavirin for 48 weeks or for 24 weeks versus interferon alpha 2b plus placebo for 48 weeks for treatment of chronic infection with hepatitis C virus. International Hepatitis Interventional Therapy Group (IHIT) Lancet 1998;352:1426–1432.

Robert W, McMurray. Hepatitis C-Associated Autoimmune Disorders. Rheumatic Diseases Clinics of North America 1998;24:353–374.

Reed KE, Rice CM. Overview of hepatitis C virus genome structure, polyprotein processing, and protein properties. Curr Top Microbiol Immunol 2000;242:55–84.

Rossi SJ, Wright TL. New developments in the treatment of hepatitis C. Gut 2003;52:756, 757.

Robertson B, Myers G, Howard C, et al. Classification, nomenclature, and database development for hepatitis C virus (HCV) and related viruses: proposals for standardization. Arch Virol 1998;143: 2393–2403.

Sarrazin C, Hendricks DA, Sedarati F, Zeuzem S. Assessment, by transcription-mediated amplification, of virologic response in patients with chronic hepatitis C virus treated with peginterferon α-2a. J Clin Micro 2002;39:2850–2855.

Seeff LB, Buskell-Bales Z, Wright EC, et al. Long-term mortality after transfusion-associated non-A, non-B hepatitis. The National Heart, Lung, and Blood Institute Study Group. N Engl J Med 1992;327:1906–1911.

Seeff LB. Natural history of hepatitis C. Am J Med 1999;107:10S–15S.

Sherman KE, Rouster SD, Horn PS. Comparison of methodologies for quantification of hepatitis C virus (HCV) RNA in patients coinfected with HCV and human immunodeficiency virus. Clin Infect Dis 2002;35:482–487.

Simmonds P, Alberti A, Bonino F, et al. Nomenclature of genotypes for hepatitis C virus (correspondence). Hepatology 1994;19: 1321–1324.

Shiffman ML. Management of interferon therapy non-responders. Clin Liver Dis 2001;5:1025–1043.

Thomas DL, Astemborski J, Rai J, et al. The natural history of hepatitis C virus infection: host, viral, and environmental factors. JAMA 2000; 34:809–816.

Walker MP, Appleby TC, Zhong W, Lau JYN, Hong Z. Hepatitis C virus therapies: current treatments, targets and future perspectives. Antiviral Chem Chemother 2003;14:1–21.

Zignego A, Bréchot C. Extrahepatic Manifestations of HCV Infection: Facts and controversies. J Hepatol 1999;31:369–376.

53 Molecular Diagnostics in Hepatitis B

SCOTT BOWDEN AND STEPHEN LOCARNINI

SUMMARY

An estimated 400 million people are chronically infected with hepatitis B virus (HBV) and many will suffer serious liver disease as a consequence. HBV is an enveloped, partially double-stranded DNA virus, which replicates via reverse transcription of an RNA intermediate. The error rate of the reverse transcriptase generates a heterogeneous population of variants, endowing HBV with the ability to evade immune or antiviral selection pressure. Whereas HBV infection can be diagnosed by serological assays, the introduction of new antiviral agents to treat chronic infection requires monitoring by sensitive DNA amplification assays designed for quantification of HBV DNA in serum and liver tissue.

Key Words: Antiviral therapy; drug resistance; HBV ccc DNA; HBV genome organization; HBV genotypes; HBV viral load.

INTRODUCTION

More than 400 million people worldwide are chronically infected with the hepatitis B virus (HBV), making hepatitis B one of the most common infectious diseases. Of these chronic carriers, only 1–2% will annually spontaneously clear hepatitis B surface antigen (HBsAg). Ultimately, more than half of the HBsAg-positive patients will die of hepatocellular carcinoma (HCC) or liver failure. Host factors such as age, immunosuppression, and gender can contribute to patient outcome. Over the past decade there has been increasing interest in the role of virological factors such as load and specific mutations in particular regions of the viral genome on the clinical course and outcome of persistent infection.

HBV is an enveloped, partially double-stranded DNA virus, which is the prototype member of the family *Hepadnaviridae*. The virus replicates its DNA genome via an RNA intermediate, an unusual strategy that generates a heterogeneous population of genetic variants during the normal course of infection and provides enormous potential for adaptation to changing environments and response to particular selection pressures. This property endows the virus with the ability to evade host immunity and resist conventional antiviral strategies. However, the extreme genetic economy of the HBV genome, achieved by the use of overlapping reading frames, is a major constraint on HBV evolution and as such could be exploited to improve existing therapeutic approaches, in particular by the use of combination treatments targeting different parts of the virus life cycle. Studies on the pathogenesis of chronic hepatitis B

From: *Principles of Molecular Medicine, Second Edition*
Edited by: M. S. Runge and C. Patterson © Humana Press, Inc., Totowa, NJ

(CH-B) have revealed a complex interaction between the virus, the hepatocyte, and the host's immune response. This chapter describes the organization of the HBV genome, the role of the proteins it encodes, and the common variants produced by exogenous selection pressure. New antiviral therapies available for the treatment of CH-B are discussed with the molecular technologies necessary to assess their efficacy. Finally, promising techniques for investigating the intricacies of the HBV life cycle in the liver are highlighted.

THE VIRUS AND ITS GENOME

VIRION MORPHOLOGY Three types of virus-associated particles are found in serum of an HBV-infected individual. (1) HBV virions measuring 42 nm in diameter, comprising an outer envelope formed by the HBsAg. This envelope surrounds an inner nucleocapsid consists of the hepatitis B core antigen (HBcAg) that contains the packaged viral genome and an endogenous viral DNA polymerase; (2) abundant spherical particles of approx 22 nm in diameter that are in a 10^4–10^6-fold excess over the HBV virions; and (3) filamentous structures of approx 20–22 nm in diameter and of variable length. The latter two forms of subviral particles consist of virus-derived glycoproteins (GP) of HBsAg and do not contain the HBV genome and are thus not infectious. The purified 22 nm particles are highly immunogenic and when administered to normal individuals in the form of the hepatitis B vaccine, are able to induce a neutralizing anti-HBs antibody response.

HBV GENOME The HBV genome is a circular, partially double-stranded relaxed circular DNA molecule of approx 3200 nucleotides (nt) in length (Fig. 53-1). The two linear DNA strands are held in a circular configuration by a 226-bp cohesive overlap between the 5' ends of the two DNA strands that contain two 11-nt direct repeats called DR1 and DR2. All known complete HBV genomes are gapped, nicked, and circular, comprising 3181–3221 nt depending on the genotype (Table 53-1). Within the virion, the minus strand of the genomic DNA has a fixed length with defined 5' and 3' ends, and a terminal redundancy of 8–9 nt. The minus strand is not a closed circle and has a nick near the 5' end of the plus strand. The viral DNA polymerase is covalently bound to the 5' end of the minus strand. The 5' end of the plus strand contains an 18-base long oligoribonucleotide, which is capped in the same manner as mRNA. The 3' end of the plus strand is not at a fixed position so most viral genomes contain a single-stranded gap region of variable size from 20 to 80% of the genomic length, which may be filled in by the endogenous viral DNA polymerase.

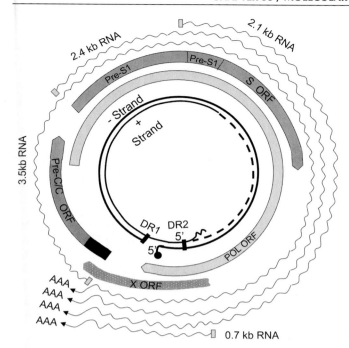

Figure 53-1 The organization of the hepatitis B virus genome. The inner circles represent the complete minus-sense strand of the genomic DNA with the viral polymerase attached to the 5′ end and the incomplete plus-sense strand with the capped RNA oligonucleotide at the 5′ end. The direct repeat sequences are designated DR1 and DR2. The four open reading frames (core [Pre-C/C], envelope [Pre-S/S], polymerase [POL], and X) are shown as the discrete thicker arrows around the genomic DNA. The outer thin circular lines depict the viral RNA transcripts, the core and pgRNA (3.5 kb), the Pre-S mRNA (2.4 kb), the S mRNA (2.1 kb) and the X mRNA (0.7 kb). Note that the transcripts all end at a common polyadenylation site (AAA).

The minus strand of HBV encodes four major open reading frames (ORFs) that carry all the protein-coding capacity of the virus: the envelope (pre-S1, pre-S2, and S), the core, the X protein and the polymerase. These overlap in a frame-shifted manner with one another, so that the minus strand is read 1.5 times. The longest ORF encodes the viral polymerase (Pol) whereas the ORF for the envelope (Pre-S/S) gene is completely located within the Pol ORF. The ORF for the core (Pre-Core/Core–Pre-C/C) and X genes partially overlap the Pol ORF. HBV is able to encode more than one protein from an ORF by using multiple internal AUG or start codons, creating additional start sites for protein biosynthesis. Thus, nested sets of proteins with different N-termini are synthesized. This gene overlap, although genetically economical, places constraints on the mutation and evolution rates.

Regulatory Elements Controlling Viral Replication Multiple regulatory elements involved in the regulation and expression of each individual HBV gene are located throughout the whole length of the viral genome. Because every region of the HBV genome is a protein-encoding sequence, all *cis*-acting regulatory elements reside within gene sequences. HBV genomic expression is regulated by two enhancers (*Enh*I and II), four promoters, a glucocorticoid response element, a negative regulatory element, and a CCAAT element. The four promoters, consists of the basal core promoter (BCP), the Pre-S1, Pre-S2/S, and X promoters, control the corresponding four major mRNA species of 3.5 kb (Pre-C/C and pregenomic [pg] RNA), 2.4 kb (Pre-S1 mRNA), 2.1 kb (Pre-S2/S

mRNA), and 0.7 kb (X mRNA) (*see* Fig. 53-1). HBV transcription is dependent to a large extent on liver-enriched transcription factors. All of these mRNA species are capped, unspliced, and share a common polyadenylation signal. Three other regulatory elements that also control HBV replication are located on the viral RNAs: the polyadenylation signal, posttranscriptional regulatory element, and the encapsidation signal (ε). The pgRNA serves as the template for reverse transcription.

Regulation of viral gene expression also occurs at the level of translation. The pgRNA serves as the mRNA not only for the viral core protein but also for the viral polymerase, which initiates from an AUG located in the distal portion of the core gene, although not in the same reading frame as core. Reading of the polymerase ORF appears to be inefficient compared to that of the core ORF. However, because core particles are assembled from 240 core subunits and only one or perhaps two polymerase proteins, pgRNA may serve as an mRNA for the translation, on average, of approx 200–300 core polypeptides before allowing the translation of a polymerase polypeptide. Because the polymerase preferentially binds to the 5′ end of its own mRNA to initiate reverse transcription and packaging, synthesis of the polymerase is probably sufficient to stop further translation of the pregenome.

Pre-S/S ORF HBsAg comprises the small (SHBs), medium (MHBs), and large (LHBs)-sized proteins (Fig. 53-2), all of which exist in two forms differing in their degree of glycosylation. N-linked glycosylation and glucosidase processing are necessary for virion, but not subviral particle secretion. The 22-nm spherical form contains approx 89% of SHBs, 10% of MHBs, and 1% of LHBs. The filamentous forms consist of the same ratio of proteins as the virion envelope, comprising approx 70% of SHBs, 10% of MHBs, and 20% of LHBs.

The 2.4-kb mRNA transcript encodes the LHBs whereas the 2.1-kb mRNA transcript encodes the MHBs and SHBs (*see* Fig. 53-2). The synthesis and assembly of the viral envelope, the small particles, and filaments occur in the endoplasmic reticulum (ER) membranes with the resultant assembled viral proteins budding into the ER lumen. The SHBs domain is 226 amino acids long and is the most abundant protein of the three HBV-associated particles. The SHBs are found in glycosylated (GP27) and nonglycosylated (P24) forms. They contain a high number of cysteine residues that are crosslinked with each other, forming a conformational loop that is the major antigenic determinant of the HBsAg (from amino acid residues 98–170), referred to as the major hydrophilic region. The most characterized mutation associated with vaccine escape, sG145R, is located within this region.

The MHBs containing the Pre-S2 domain are a minor component of the virion or subviral particles and consists of SHBs with a 55 amino acid N-terminal extension. The MHBs are either doubly or singly glycosylated (GP36 and GP33) and are required for virus secretion. However, this protein is not required for infectivity or virus assembly. The MHBs are considerably more immunogenic than SHBs, and Pre-S2-containing HBs particles generated from animal cell lines have been used in some countries as a prophylactic vaccine. The LHBs contain an additional 108 or 119 amino acids (depending on the subtype/genotype; *see* Table 53-1) in comparison to MHBs at its N terminus. The LHBs are mainly glycosylated (GP42) and myristylated, and are essential for viral infection, assembly, and release. A small amount of this protein is nonglycosylated (P39). A number of B- and T-cell epitopes have been mapped to LHBs, MHBs, and SHBs. The Pre-S1 region contains

Table 53-1
Overview of the Eight Major Genotypes of HBV

Genotype	Subtype	Genome length (nt)	HBV Proteins (no. of amino acids)			Frequency of mutation[a]		Global distribution
			PreS1[b]	Pol	Core	PC	BCP	
A	adw2, ayw1	3221	119	845	185	Uncommon (C1858)	Common	Western Europe, USA, Central Africa, India
B	adw2, ayw1	3215	119	843	183	Common (T1858)	Common	Japan, Taiwan, Indonesia, China, USA
Bj	adw2, aywl	3215	119	843	183	Common	Uncommon	Japan
Ba	adw2, aywl	3215	119	843	183	Low	Uncommon	China, Taiwan, Indonesia, Vietnam
C	adw2, adr, ayr	3215	119	843	183	Common T/C1858	Common	East Asia, Taiwan, Korea, China, USA, Japan, Polynesia
D	ayw	3182	108	832	183	Common T1858	Common	Mediterranean region, India, USA
E	ayw	3212	118	842	183	ND	ND	West Africa
F	adw, ayw	3215	119	843	183	Uncommon (C1858)	ND	Central and South America, Polynesia
G	adw	3248	108	842	195	Very common (insertion)	ND	USA, Europe
H	adw	3215	119	843	183	ND	ND	Central, South America

HBV, hepatitis B virus; ND, not described; Pol, polymerase.
[a]PC, Precore mutations such as G1896A; BCP, basic core promoter mutations such as A1762T, G1764A; common (up to 50% of isolates); uncommon (less than 10% of isolates); very common (most isolates).
[b]Pre-S2, 55aa; S, 226aa.

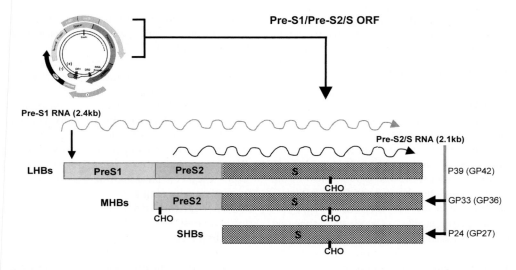

Figure 53-2 Pre-S1/Pre-S2/S open reading frames. The Pre-S/S open reading frame can be divided into Pre-S1, Pre-S2, and S domains by three in-frame start codons. The proteins encoded by the open reading frame are expressed from two mRNA transcripts. The larger 2.4-kb Pre-S1 mRNA leads to expression of the large-sized proteins, whereas the Pre-S2/S 2.1-kb mRNA encodes medium-sized proteins and small-sized proteins. MHBs are translated using the first start codon and SHBs from the internal start codon. LHBs can be detected as a nonglycosylated species (P39) but its major form is glycosylated (GP42). SHBs are found in both glycosylated (GP27) and nonglycosylated (P24) forms, whereas MHBs are glycosylated either at one (GP33) or two (GP36) sites.

two important epitopes. One at amino acid residues 58–100 is thought to be recognized by antibodies involved in viral clearance. The other, at residues 21–47 is thought to be the hepatocyte binding domain. The N terminus of Pre-S2 can bind to the fibronectin found in liver sinusoids, providing some degree of host tissue specificity. Interestingly, most of the Pre-S2 is not essential for viral replication or virion infectivity whereas only residues 109–113 are indispensable.

There are four different alleles within the *S* gene: r, d, y, and w. The determinants d/y and w/r are mutually exclusive, thus forming two allelic groups. The "a" determinant (amino acid residues 107–149) is part of all HBs subtypes and can be divided into two alleles that differ at amino acid 126 being either threonine or isoleucine. The main subtypes are designated ayw, ayr, adw, and adr. The clinically most important determinant of HBsAg is the "a" determinant (Fig. 53-3). During the natural course of infection,

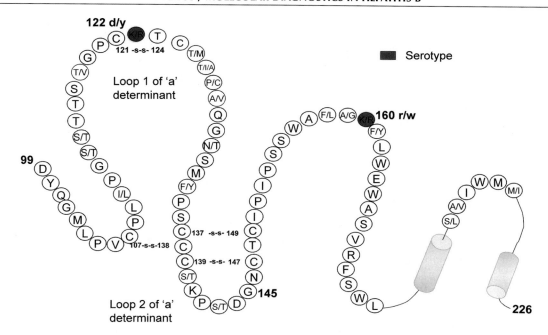

Figure 53-3 Schematic model of hepatitis B surface antigen. The two loops of the "a" determinant are stabilized by disulphide bridges (s–s) between cysteine residues. The C-terminal end of the protein has two alpha helices (shown as cylindrical structures). Serotype-specific epitopes are located in the "a" determinant. A point mutation that converts K122 to R122 (K122R) changes the *d* subtype to *y* and a similar mutation at K160R changes subtype *w* to *r*. These produce the four major subtypes of hepatitis B virus—*adw, adr, ayw,* and *ayr.* The location of the glycine residue that is modified to arginine (G145R) in virus associated with vaccine escape is shown. (Modified from Wallace et al., 1997.)

antibodies against all the determinants are produced, but only the antibodies against the "a" determinant are protective against a challenge with other HBV subtypes. The "antigenic" conformation of the "a" determinant is regarded as a two-loop structure stabilized by disulphide bridges between Cys-107 and Cys-138 (first loop) and Cys-139 and Cys-147 (second loop) whereas Cys-137 binding to Cys-149 stabilizes the interaction (*see* Fig. 53-3). If this conformation is altered, then anti-HBs produced previously against the native "a" determinant are no longer protective.

Pre-C/C ORF The Pre-C/C ORF encodes the core protein (P21), which is the major polypeptide of the nucleocapsid and is expressed as the HBcAg (Fig. 53-4). The HBc protein is 183, 185, or 195 amino acids long, depending on the genotype of the virus (*see* Table 53-1). ORF C is preceded by a short, upstream, in-phase ORF known as the precore region from which the soluble hepatitis Be antigen (HBeAg) is synthesized (*see* Fig. 53-4). Both the core (HBcAg) and precore (HBeAg) proteins are targets for immune-mediated viral clearance mechanisms.

Translation of the precore region from the 3.5-kb Pre-C/C mRNA results in a 25-kDa polypeptide. The first 19 amino acids of the precore protein represent a secretion signal that allows for the translocation of the precore protein into the lumen of the ER (*see* Fig. 53-4). The signal sequence is cleaved off by a host cell signal peptidase and the protein is secreted through the ER and Golgi apparatus. A further modification of the C terminus results in the secretion of a heterogeneous population of proteins (15–18 kDa), which is serologically defined as HBeAg. The precore protein is not essential to viral replication and thus can be regarded as an "accessory protein."

The HBc protein is translated in the cytosol from the 3.5-kb pg mRNA after which these proteins initially form dimers, followed by multimerization to form the nucleocapsid. The HBc protein has

been crystallized and the nucleocapsid protein has been mapped using cryoelectron microscopy. The multimerization of the HBc protein can occur independently of the encapsidation of the pgRNA–Pol complex. The core protein can be divided into two major domains, the N-terminal assembly domain (up to amino acid 144) and the C-terminal arginine-rich region involved in RNA–DNA binding interactions. The core protein can self-assemble into capsids, and two icosahedral shells of different sizes have been observed: particles with a $T = 3$ symmetry containing 90 homodimers of 32 nm, and particles with a $T = 4$ symmetry consisting of 120 homodimers of 36 nm.

Pol ORF The *Pol* gene is the longest ORF, spanning almost 80% of the genome, and overlaps the three remaining ORFs (*see* Fig. 53-1). Codons 834–845 in the Pol ORF have sequence homology to known reverse transcriptases (rts) and most parts of the ORF are essential for viral replication. The Pol protein is translated from the pgRNA (*see* Fig. 53-4). The 90-kDa product of the Pol ORF is a multifunctional protein that has at least four domains: (1) the N-terminal domain that encodes the terminal protein, which is covalently linked to the 5′ end of the minus strand of virion DNA. This part of the Pol ORF is necessary for priming minus-strand synthesis; (2) an intervening domain with no specific recognized function, referred to as the spacer or tether region; (3) the third domain that encodes the RNA- and DNA-dependent DNA polymerase activities, i.e., the rts; and (4) the C-terminal domain that encodes RNase H activity that cleaves the RNA in the RNA/DNA hybrids during the reverse transcription process.

The terminal protein's role in protein priming reverse transcription includes the provision of the substrate tyrosine at amino acid 63 of the HBV Pol for the formation of the covalent bond between the enzyme and the first nucleotide (G) of the minus-strand DNA. The DNA polymerase domain contains the amino-acid motif YMDD,

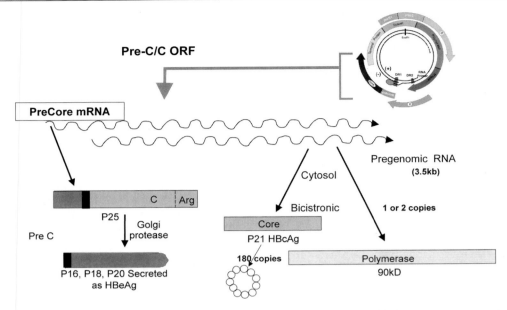

Figure 53-4   Core (Pre-C/C) open reading frame. The pregenomic RNA acts as a bicistronic mRNA. It codes for the polymerase protein and, by using an internal start codon, it also produces a translation product corresponding to the core protein (hepatitis B core antigen or P21). Multiple copies of the core protein can self-assemble into particles. Initiation of translation from the precore mRNA leads to production of a precore polypeptide (P25). The N terminus of this polypeptide has a signal sequence that targets it to the secretory pathway. The signal sequence is cleaved off by a host cell signal peptidase and the C terminus of the polypeptide is further cleaved by Golgi proteases to produce a heterogeneous population of proteins (P16, P18, and P20) known collectively as hepatitis Be antigen.

which is essential for rt activity. The RNase H domain, as well as being involved in degrading the RNA template, has other functions, including playing a role in viral RNA packaging, optimizing the priming of minus-strand DNA synthesis and in elongation of the minus-strand viral DNA.

Several cytotoxic T-lymphocyte (CTL) epitopes have been mapped to the polymerase protein. Six CTL epitopes within the rt or the RNase H domains of the viral polymerase have been described in patients with acute hepatitis. The epitope (GLSRYVARL) appears most relevant for interferon responsiveness and viral clearance. It has been suggested that Ser-457, Ala-461, or Arg-462 are contact sites for the T-cell receptor. If these critical amino acids are changed by mutation, then the T-cell receptor binding activity will be reduced and the CTL-mediated immune response attenuated and/or blunted.

The advent of nucleoside per nucleotide analog treatment has resulted in the outgrowth of otherwise minor quasispecies with mutations in the HBV *Pol* gene. Antiviral resistance to lamivudine (LMV) has been mapped to the YMDD locus in HBV Pol. Using the newly described nomenclature system, the major mutations within the rt gene that were selected during LMV therapy results in changes designated rtM204I/V (domain C, methionine at position 204 replaced by isoleucine or valine) with or without rtL180M (domain B). The domain B mutation rtL180M is also selected during famciclovir treatment. Recently, the development of adefovir (ADV)-resistant HBV with changes in the domain D (rtN236T) and domain B (rtA181T/V) of the viral polymerase has been described as has entecavir resistant virus with changes in domains B and C (rtS184G and rtS202I).

X ORF   The X ORF produces a 0.7-kb mRNA transcript encoding a polypeptide 154 amino acids in size (HBx) with a predicted molecular weight of 16–19 kDa (*see* Fig. 53-1). When first identified, the function of the X protein was unknown and thus, the X designation was assigned. HBx is the second accessory protein

of HBV and is dispensable for virus production in vitro, but is a critical component of the infectivity process in vivo. The C-terminal portion of the protein seems to be associated with the transactivating properties of X whereas the N terminus appears to act as a negative regulator of transactivation. HBx can act in the cytosol and in the nucleus. HBx behaves as a transcriptional transactivator for a number of viral and cellular gene promoters through direct interaction with transcription factors such as RPB5 subunit of RNA polymerase II, TATA-binding protein, and ATF/CREB (nuclear pathways). The cytoplasmic pathways are divided into protein kinase C (PKC)-dependent and -independent mechanisms. HBx interacts directly with inactive cytosolic PKC thereby activating it. In the PKC-independent cytosolic pathway, HBx is involved in the activation of signal transduction pathways, such as the Ras/Raf/MAP kinase cascade. The Ras pathway leads to the phosphorylation and activation of the transactivating domain of *c-jun*.

HBx is a multifunctional viral regulator that modulates transcription, cell responses to protein degradation, and signaling pathways. Such regulation of viral and cellular genes affects viral replication and viral proliferation, directly or indirectly. HBx has been implicated in the development of HCC and affects cell cycle checkpoints, cell death, and carcinogenesis. Although the precise mechanism remains uncertain, the HBx-associated transactivation activity may lead to alterations in cellular gene expression that contribute to cell transformation. HBx can bind to and inactivate the transcription factor and tumor suppressor, p53. In addition, the HBx can dampen the immune response by interfering with the ubiquitin-proteolysis pathway following binding with a 26S proteasome complex.

VIRAL GENOTYPES

There are eight recognized genotypes of HBV designated A to H, which vary by 8% at the nucleotide level over the entire genome.

These HBV genotypes have unique insertions or deletions. For example, HBV genotype A varies from the other genotypes by an insertion of 6 nt in the terminal protein region of the polymerase gene, whereas HBV genotype D has a 33-nt deletion in the spacer region of the polymerase gene, and HBV genotypes E and G have a 3-nt deletion in the same region (*see* Table 53-1). HBV genotype G also has a 36-nt insertion in the N terminus of the core gene. Genotype H has been defined and is most similar to genotype F. The HBV genotype designation is based on the entire genomic sequence. Thus, it is more reliable than the serological subtype nomenclature used previously, which was based on the immunore-activity of particular antibodies to a limited number of amino acids in the envelope protein. The relationship between the four major HBV subtypes (*adw, adr, ayw,* and *ayr)* and genotypes has been determined (*see* Table 53-1).

Important pathogenic and therapeutic differences do exist among HBV genotypes. For example, genotype C is associated with more severe liver disease than genotype B in Taiwan, whereas genotype D is associated with more severe liver disease than genotype A in India. Genotypes C and D are associated with a lower response rate to interferon therapy compared with genotypes B and A. Recombination between two HBV genotypes has been reported for genotypes B and C and genotypes A and D generating even more diversity. Furthermore, there is evidence for the widespread distribution of related hepatitis viruses in primates, implying that these viruses may have a common origin and that cross-species transmission of hepadnaviruses may have occurred among hominoids.

COMMON HBV MUTANTS

Viral and host factors, as well as exogenous selection pressures, typically define the predominate species in an infected individual. Exogenous pressures include nucleoside per nucleotide analog treatment, as well as immune-based intervention such as hepatitis B immunoglobulin, and vaccination. The presumably immune-based selection pressure that results in the reduction or loss in HBeAg and eventual elimination of HBsAg are probably responsible for the selection of particular mutants such as those associated with CH-B.

Viral rts lack proofreading function and are inherently error-prone, which ensures that HBV populations exist in the host as heterogeneous mixtures known as quasispecies. The HBV mutation frequency has been estimated to be approx $1.4–3.2 \times 10^{-5}$ nt substitutions/site/yr, approx 10-fold higher than other DNA viruses. The magnitude and rate of virus replication are also important in the process of mutation generation, with the total viral load in serum frequently approaching 10^{11} virions/mL. Most estimates place the mean half-life of the serum HBV pool at approx 1–2 d, so that the daily rate of *de novo* HBV production may be as great as 10^{11} virions. The high viral loads and turnover rates, coupled with poor replication fidelity, all influence mutation generation and the extent of the HBV quasispecies pool. However, these are less than for other retroviruses, mainly because of the constraints imposed by the overlapping reading frames.

MUTATIONS IN THE BCP REGION AND PRECORE GENE
Two major groups of mutations have been identified that result in reduced or blocked HBeAg expression. The first major group includes a translational stop codon mutation at nt 1896 (codon 28: TGG; tryptophan) of the precore gene. The single base substitution (G-to-A) at nt 1896 gives rise to a translational stop codon (TGG to TAG; TAG = stop codon) in the second last codon (codon 28) of the precore gene located in the ε structure. The ε structure is a highly

conserved stem loop structure critical in viral replication, with the nucleotide G1896 forming a bp with nt 1858 at the base of the stem loop. In HBV genotypes B, D, E, G, and some strains of genotype C, the 1858 is a thymidine (T) (*see* Table 53-1). Thus, the stop codon mutation created by G1896A stabilizes the ε structure (T–A). In contrast, the precore stop codon mutation is rarely detected in HBV genotype A, F, and some strains of HBV genotype C, as the nucleotide at position 1858 is a cytidine (C), maintaining the preferred Watson–Crick basepairing (G–C). Other less common mutations have been found such as precore codon 17 (G1862T), which can alter the processing of the precore proteins in the Golgi apparatus. Interestingly, the mutation at the precore codon 29 (G1899A) has been found in isolation or in association with the G1896A or G1862T, but its significance is unclear as it has no translational effect.

The second major group of mutations affects the BCP at nt1762 and nt1764 resulting in a transcriptional reduction of the Pre-C/C mRNA. Mutations in the BCP, such as A1762T plus G1764A, may be found in isolation or in conjunction with precore mutations, depending on the genotype. The double mutation of A1762T plus G1764A results in a decrease in HBeAg production, but not disappearance and interestingly, an increase in viral load. In general, this pattern of mutation is often found in genotype A-infected individuals. BCP mutants display reduced binding of liver-specific transcription factors resulting in less Pre-C/C mRNA transcripts and, thus, less precore protein. However, this mutation does not affect the transcription of pgRNA or the translation of the core or polymerase protein. By removing the inhibitory effect of the precore protein on HBV replication, the BCP mutations appear to enhance viral replication by suppressing Pre-C/C mRNA relative to pgRNA.

MUTATIONS IN THE CORE GENE
The core protein can be divided into two major domains, the N-terminal domain up to amino acid position 144, and the functionally important arginine-rich C-terminal domain. The C-terminal domain (up to amino acid 164) is required for encapsidation of the pgRNA and seems to stabilize the capsid by protein–nucleic acid interactions. The remaining C terminus (up to amino acid 173) appears important for the synthesis of plus-strand DNA and subsequent genomic replication.

The core protein contains a number of important B-cell and CTL epitopes. During the elimination phase of CH-B, escape mutations within those epitopes are readily selected. These "hot spots" have been linked to major CTL (aa 18–30) and T-helper (T_H) cell (aa 50–70) regions and to two B-cell (HBc/eI and HBc/e2) epitopes at residues 75–90 and 120–140, respectively. The HBcAg and HBeAg are highly cross-reactive at the T-cell level. The HBeAg probably presents immunogenic epitopes to the T cells, thus "protecting" the HBcAg-expressing hepatocytes against the immune system. After selection of the HBeAg-negative mutant(s), the epitopes of the HBcAg come under intense pressure from the immune system. Thus, the frequency of core gene mutations is typically associated with the presence of precore stop codon mutations, HBeAg-negativity, and active liver disease.

MUTATIONS IN THE X GENE
The X-ORF overlaps the C terminus of the *Pol* gene and the N terminus of the *C* gene (*see* Fig. 53-1). Depending on the extent of the mutation(s) within the X region, mutations can affect three genes at once. X-region deletions can create fusion proteins between the pol and the core proteins (PC-proteins) or between the pol and a 3′-truncated HBx (PX-proteins).

Typically, mutations in the X region involve the regulatory elements that control replication. Because the BCP encompasses nts

1742–1802 and overlaps with the X gene in the concomitant reading frame, the A1762T plus G1764A BCP mutations also cause changes in the X gene at xK130M and xV131I. Additionally, nearly all deletions/insertions in the BCP shift the X-gene reading frame and lead to the production of truncated X proteins. These shortened X proteins lack the domain in the C terminus (aa 130–140) that is required for the transactivation activity of HBxAg.

The two direct repeat sequences, DR-1 and DR-2, lie within the BCP sequence and are considered important in reverse transcription. Between DR-1 and DR-2 lies the cohesive end region of the HBV genome and this appears to be a preferred site for viral integration into host DNA. Interestingly, the cohesive end region near DR-1 contains a preferred cleavage site for topoisomerase I that can catalyze illegitimate recombinations between HBV and cellular DNA; following viral integration, deletions in this region have been found.

MUTATIONS IN THE ENVELOPE GENE The Pre-S sequences exhibit the highest heterogeneity of the HBV genome. Point mutations, deletions, and genetic recombinations within the *Pre-S* genes have been identified in HBV DNA sequences analyzed from the sera of chronic carriers. Deletions within the Pre-S region can affect the S promoter causing an imbalance in envelope assembly resulting in intracellular retention and accumulation of HBsAg. Viral genomes, which cannot synthesize Pre-S2 proteins, occur frequently, and can be the dominant virus populations in chronic carriers. The Pre-S2 region overlaps the spacer region of the Pol protein that is not essential for enzyme activity. It has been speculated that the loss of the highly immunogeneic Pre-S2 protein reflects an immunological escape mechanism.

All hepatitis B vaccines contain the major HBsAg, and an immune response to the major hydrophilic region located from residue 99–170 induces protective immunity. Mutations within this epitope have been selected during vaccination and also following treatment of liver transplant patients with hepatitis B immunoglobulin. Most isolates have a mutation from glycine to arginine at residue 145 of HBsAg (sG145R) or aspartate to alanine at residue 144 (sD144A). The sG145R mutation has been associated with vaccine failure. Mutations that abolish or alter the two-loop structure of the "a" determinant can affect anti-HBs binding. Such effects include changes in the hydrophobicity, the electrical charge, the acidity of the loops, addition of possible additional N-glycosylation sites (glycine-130 to Asn), or changing the stability of the disulphide bridge (Cys-147 to Gly). Finally, mutations near the "a" determinant, such as an insertion of eight amino acids between Thr-123 and Cys-124, two amino acids between Cys-121 and Lys-122 or of arginine between Pro-120 and Cys-121 can disturb the secondary structure of the "a" determinant.

POLYMERASE MUTATIONS: ANTIVIRAL DRUG RESISTANCE The advent of nucleoside per nucleotide analog treatment has resulted in the outgrowth of otherwise minor quasispecies with mutations in the HBV *Pol* gene. Antiviral resistance to LMV has been mapped to the YMDD locus, the catalytic site in the C domain of HBV polymerase, whereas resistance to ADV is associated with mutations in the D domain of the enzyme. Mutations within the rt gene that were selected during LMV therapy cause changes that are designated rtM204I/V/S (Domain C) +/–rtL180M (Domain B), whereas rtN236T (D-domain) and rtA181T are the major changes associated with ADV-resistant virus.

Lamivudine Resistance LMV resistance increases progressively during treatment at rates between 14 and 32% annually,

approaching 100% after 48 mo treatment. Factors that increase the risk of development of resistance include high pretherapy serum HBV DNA levels and ALT levels and incomplete suppression of viral replication. LMV resistance does not confer cross-resistance to ADV.

Mutations that confer LMV resistance decrease in vitro sensitivity to LMV from at least 20-fold to greater than 100-fold. The rtM204I substitution has been detected in isolation, but rtM204V and rtM204S are found only in association with other changes in the B or A domains. Numerous other secondary changes in the rt sequence also occur in conjunction with rtM204V/I/S, and some of these are probably compensatory.

Lamivudine resistance is mainly owing to steric hindrance resulting from the replacement of the methionine residue in the YMDD motif with either of the branched amino acids valine or isoleucine, which decrease the ability of the polymerase to bind the nucleoside analog in the deoxynucleotide triphosphate binding pocket relative to the natural substrate.

Adefovir Dipivoxil Resistance HBV resistance to ADV occurs less frequently (approx 2% after 2 yr, 5% after 3 yr, and 16% after 4 yr) than resistance to LMV. ADV resistance is conferred by substitution of threonine for asparagine at codon 236 (rtN236T), which is located in the D domain of the polymerase a change that does not significantly affect sensitivity to LMV, and/or the rtA181V/T change, which is located in the B domain of the enzyme. The mechanism of resistance by N236T has been determined to be indirect perturbation of the triphosphate binding site whereas indirect steric hindrance accounts for resistance owing to rtA181V/T. Both mutations, either together or separately, decrease sensitivity to the drug by less than 10-fold.

Entecavir Resistance Resistance to entecavir has been observed in two patients who had already failed to respond to LMV. The viral load increase was associated with clinical deterioration and rising levels of serum ALT. Sequencing of the HBV pol gene at the time of viral breakthrough confirmed LMV resistance and identified several unique mutations associated with entecavir resistance.

- Patient A: rtI169T (B-domain) and rtM250V (E-domain).
- Patient B: rtT184G (B-domain) and rtS202I (C-domain).

These changes have been confirmed to associated with entecavir resistance by using in vitro phenotypic assays.

Telbivudine Resistance Telbivudine is the β-L isomer of thymidine. After 24 wk of therapy, it results in a 4–6 log drop in HBV DNA levels. Resistance occurred at the rate of 5% per annum and resulted in the selection of the rtM204I mutation, indicating cross-resistance with LMV.

Pol-Env Link The envelope gene lies completely within the *Pol* gene but in a frame-shifted manner. Thus, mutations in one gene have the potential to affect the product(s) of the other gene. For example, some mutations in the *Pol* gene that confer drug-resistance affect the immunogenicity of the envelope gene products (Fig. 53-5). Conversely, immune selection can influence antiviral drug sensitivity. Cases of transmission of drug-resistant HBV have been reported. The clinical and public health importance of drug resistance is clear; improved treatment strategies are urgently required to ensure prevention of resistance.

Pathogenicity of Drug Resistant HBV: Role of Compensatory Mutations Compensatory mutations that partly or wholly restore the level of viral fitness have been documented during therapy for HIV infections and similar scenarios have been described for HBV.

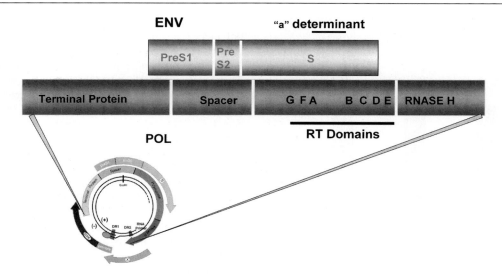

Figure 53-5 The Pol–Env link. The genomic organization of HBV is such that the Pre-S/S open reading frame (ENV) is completely overlapped by the polymerase (POL) open reading frame. Resistance to nucleoside/nucleotide analogs is caused by changes in the reverse transcriptase domain of the polymerase and this has the potential to select viruses with changes in the overlapping *S* gene, which may affect the *a* determinant. Similarly, changes to the *S* gene caused by immune selection may have the ability to modify drug sensitivity by altering the *Pol* gene and affecting the RT domain.

A high frequency of the co-occurrence of rtL80V/I (domain A) and rtL180M has been observed in conjunction with the M204V/I changes that confer LMV resistance in treated Japanese patients (genotype C). The presence of double and triple changes was associated with higher viral loads, increased LMV resistance, and disease exacerbation. Longitudinal studies showed that the mutations responsible for these sequence changes occurred almost simultaneously, just before viral breakthrough and also that the mutants were displaced by wild-type genotype C HBV after completion of therapy.

Similar observations have been recorded for liver transplant patients who developed life-threatening HBV recurrence. HBV isolates from these patients had compensatory mutations that enhanced their in vitro replication efficiency in the presence of LMV. Even greater enhancement and drug dependency occurred when mutations resulting in sG145R or sP120T, key changes in the envelope protein, were also present.

Mutations that abolish or decrease the expression of HBeAg affect replication efficiency. HBeAg-negative CH-B, which is common in the Mediterranean region, is usually characterized by lower serum HBV DNA levels than those found during HBeAg-positive CH-B. A group of HBeAg-negative CH-B patients have been studied who were infected with genotype D HBV that contained both BCP and precore stop codon mutations. Development of LMV resistance in these patients was associated with relatively rapid increases in viremia, frequently culminating in biochemical breakthrough, severe hepatic flares, and disease progression. In vitro studies confirmed that the presence of the typical precore mutation (G1896A) could compensate for the replication deficiency in LMV-resistant HBV quasispecies. Several case studies have confirmed that drug resistant HBV mutants are capable of causing severe, even fatal, disease, challenging the notion that drug resistant HBV mutants, and other minority quasispecies are benign.

These reports and the observed enhanced replication of HBV in the presence of LMV as well as the precore mutant have led to the conclusion that multiple mutations are continually selected during inadequate antiviral therapy and that these can act as compensatory mutations having the potential to restore replication competence.

MOLECULAR DIAGNOSTICS—SERUM COMPARTMENT

The natural history of CH-B can be divided into replicative and nonreplicative stages. As there is no practical measure of HBV infectivity, assays of serum HBV DNA by sensitive molecular methods have provided an indication of the level of viral replication. Also, the detection of particular viral proteins in an infected liver by immunohistochemical techniques can indicate the presence of active replication.

Development of potent chemotherapy to control CH-B, primarily using nucleoside per nucleotide analogs, has made it necessary to use more sophisticated methods for monitoring their effectiveness than traditional biochemistry and serology markers. Sensitive nucleic acid tests (NATs) are available to detect HBV DNA, employing signal or target amplification technologies, and each has advantages and disadvantages. Generally, the signal amplification assays have reduced sensitivity compared to the target amplification assays, which in turn suffer from a restricted upper range. Furthermore, the various assays may express the results in different units making comparisons difficult and highlighting the need for standardization.

New generation amplification assays have become commercially available that have been standardized to the World Health Organization international reference standard. These include an improved chemiluminescent signal amplification assay (Bayer VERSANT HBV 3.0 test) and assays exploiting the greater dynamic range intrinsic to kinetic or real-time PCR (Roche COBAS TaqMan HBV test and Artus RealArt HBV LC PCR reagents) (Fig. 53-6).

BAYER VERSANT HBV 3.0 TEST This amplification assay employs a series of sequential nucleic acid hybridization steps to produce a chemiluminescent signal that is proportional to the amount of HBV DNA in the original sample. The first step involves denaturation of the partially double-stranded HBV DNA so that

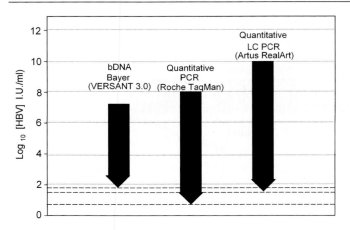

Figure 53-6 Dynamic range (expressed in IU/mL) of commercially available quantitative hepatitis B virus DNA assays. The Bayer VERSANT 3.0 bDNA assay relies on signal amplification whereas the Roche TaqMan and Artus RealArt assays rely on target amplification by real-time polymerase chain reaction.

target synthetic DNA oligonucleotides (probes) can bind to single-stranded portions of the HBV DNA. The target probes are a mix of two separate oligonucleotides and each oligonucleotide has two binding regions. Both have a region for specific hybridization to HBV DNA; one probe also has region to hybridize to a capture probe that is immobilized on the plastic surface of a microwell plate and the other probe has a portion complementary to a highly branched synthetic oligonucleotide (hence bDNA), which is subsequently added to the mix. The branches of the bDNA oligonucleotides are designed to have repeat sequences that allow multiple hybridization of another oligonucleotide (label probe) that is conjugated with alkaline phosphatase. On addition of a chemiluminescent substrate, a signal is generated and by comparison to a standard curve, a viral load can be determined. The assay has a wide dynamic range reporting in both copies/mL and International Units (IU)/mL. The lower limit of the assay is 357 IU/mL (2×10^3 copies/mL) and the upper limit is 17,587,100 IU/mL (10^8 copies/mL).

Signal amplification assays do offer some advantages over the target or nucleic acid amplification assays. There is no need for an extensive sample preparation to purify the DNA and because no amplicons (amplified subunits of DNA) are generated, there is no need for the stringent contamination control procedures employed for target amplification assays such as PCR.

ROCHE COBAS TAQMAN HBV TEST   This commercial assay supercedes the previous COBAS AMPLICOR HBV MONITOR assay, which relied on coamplification of a modified HBV DNA standard of known copy number to allow quantification. The MONITOR end point PCR assay suffered from a limited upper dynamic range mainly because of the saturation effects inherent in such technology. The development of real-time or kinetic PCR has overcome many of these deficiencies. In kinetic PCR, product is detected as it accumulates by the use of fluorescent-based detection chemistry. This allows a signal to be monitored following each thermal cycle without having to sample directly from each tube, which also reduces the contamination risks. The Roche COBAS TaqMan HBV test uses a dual fluorophore labeled probe that is designed to anneal to one strand of the HBV sequence generated from the PCR primers. The reporter fluorophore's emissions are extinguished by the nearby downstream quencher fluorophore,

resulting in no signal being produced. However, as the Taq DNA polymerase generates the complementary strand, the endonuclease activity of the enzyme cleaves the reporter off the probe and its emissions are no longer quenched, resulting in a measurable signal. The signal is proportional to the amount of amplicons generated, which is proportional to the amount of original target. Quantification is achieved using a linearized HBV plasmid Quantitation Standard DNA, which is incorporated with each sample and is carried through sample preparation, amplification and detection steps. The linear range of the assay is from approx 30 IU/mL to an upper limit of 1.1×10^8 IU/mL.

ARTUS REALART HBV LC PCR REAGENTS   This kit contains ready-for-use reagents for the quantification of HBV DNA by real-time PCR specifically using the Roche LightCycler™ instrument (Roche Diagnostics, Mannheim, Germany). The assay uses the fluorescence resonance energy transfer technology to monitor the fluorescence intensity. Dual probes are used where the 3′ end of one probe has a donor fluorophore and the 5′ end of the second probe has an acceptor fluorophore. The probes are designed to hybridize adjacent to one another on a strand of HBV DNA. If specific HBV DNA is present, on excitation the donor fluorophore transfers energy to the acceptor that emits a signal of defined wavelength for detection. The kit also provides an internal control, which is added to the lysed sample, to monitor DNA purification and to check for any inhibition of the PCR. Quantification is achieved by reference to a standard curve generated from supplied controls. The dynamic range of the assay is from 2×10^2 to an upper limit of 10^9 IU/mL.

VIRAL LOAD—CLINICAL SIGNIFICANCE   HBV DNA can be detected in acute infection before any serological marker and this may be of some use in the investigation of nosocomial outbreaks. In practice, acute infection can be diagnosed by serological detection of HBcIgM and usually HBsAg is also present. In chronic infection, the presence of HBeAg is a reliable indicator of active replication. Seroconversion from HBeAg positive to anti-HBe was presumed to be part of the immunoelimination phase of CH-B that preceded virus clearance and loss of HBsAg. Instead, it became evident that many patients without HBeAg had HBeAg-negative CH-B in which disease was ongoing, although characteristically it was associated with a lower viral load than the HBeAg-positive CH-B.

A number of workers have attempted to examine whether there is a threshold level of HBV DNA that can be used to discriminate between active and inactive disease, because markers such as HBeAg and serum transaminase levels have proved inadequate. It has been proposed some patients could be characterized as having inactive disease when they have detectable HBsAg, but without HBeAg and no transaminase elevations, and have HBV DNA levels below 10^5 copies/mL (approx 2×10^4 IU/mL). However, as previously demonstrated, many cases of HBeAg-negative CH-B have transaminase flares, meaning that there must be a greater reliance on HBV DNA levels. Evaluation of a large group of untreated patients with HBeAg-negative CH-B using regular testing of transaminase levels and histological examination when indicated, led to the conclusion that HBV DNA levels of 3×10^4 copies/mL (approx 6×10^3 IU/mL) represented a better cut off to classify a patient into the inactive carrier state.

The ability to measure HBV DNA levels has also allowed strategies to be designed to reduce the risk of virus transmission from HBV-infected healthcare workers (HCWs) to patients. Clearly, if all HCWs who were HBsAg positive were excluded from performing exposure prone procedures, there would be little opportunity for HBV transmission. However, it can be argued that the loss of expertise of highly qualified and experienced HCWs does affect the health care system, particularly in developing countries where replacement personnel may not be available. Thus, efforts have been made to establish guidelines for the management of HBV-infected HCWs based on HBV DNA levels. Many countries exclude HBeAg-positive HCWs from certain health care duties but HBV transmission has been documented to take place from HCWs negative for HBeAg. A European consensus panel agreed that each country could individually determine a HBV DNA level cut off for HCWs performing exposure prone procedures but proposed that a maximum level of 10^4 copies/mL (approx 2×10^3 IU/mL) would provide a balanced risk management strategy. This value would take into account that transmission rarely occurred with viral loads greater than 10^5 copies/mL (approx 2×10^4 IU/mL) and provided a 1 log safety margin to account for possible intermittent flares of activity, assay variation or early development of resistance while on anti-HBV therapy. Others consider this to be a conservative estimate and counter propose that a level of 10^5 copies/mL (approx 2×10^4 IU/mL) is associated with a minimal increase in risk.

VIRAL LOAD—USES IN ANTIVIRAL THERAPY Histological examination of liver tissue and determination of serum transaminase levels are both important measures to use in assessing a patient's eligibility for antiviral therapy. Importantly, detection and quantification of serum HBV DNA should also be one of the prerequisites for eligibility because it provides the clinician with a practical tool to monitor the effectiveness of treatment.

Kinetics of Viral Load Decay on Therapy One of the most promising areas in the evaluation of antiviral therapy is the examination of the kinetics of decline in viral load. Serial viral load measurements from patients prior to therapy show that viremia is maintained at an approximately constant level, even though that level can vary from patient to patient. This indicates that there is a dynamic equilibrium between virus production and clearance that maintains this steady-state relationship. The equilibrium is disturbed by the introduction of antiviral therapy and the analysis of the rate of decline in viral load allows predictions to be made about drug efficacy using mathematical models. In simplified models, there are at least two phases of viral load decay. The initial phase corresponds to clearance of circulating virus; the rate, and magnitude of the decline reflects the drug's efficacy. The second slower phase is thought to correspond to the eradication of infected cells. For HBV, this most likely represents immune elimination of infected cells, possibly aided by natural cell turnover. Unlike the viral dynamics of other blood-borne viruses, such as HIV or HCV, there appears to be greater variation in the phases with HBV infection and more complex mathematical models have been developed to explain these features. It is hoped that application of these models will provide predictive data on treatment outcome and allow the design of more effective treatment regimes.

Monitoring Effectiveness of Treatment Treatment of chronic HBV infection with either LMV or ADV produces a rapid decrease in viremia, corresponding to the first phase of viral decay. A small proportion of patients show loss of HBeAg and normalization of serum transaminase levels. However, during the second slower phase, drug-resistant virus can appear. The emergence of drug resistance may be signaled by clinical deterioration or increasing serum transaminases. A superior indicator of the development of resistance is a relapse of HBV DNA levels in the face of ongoing

therapy. Development of resistant virus can be confirmed by sequence analysis of the polymerase gene after PCR amplification in which characteristic mutations have been reported for many of the newer anti-HBV agents. A sensitive reverse hybridization line probe assay is also available but this detects only the common mutations that confer LMV resistance. Although empirically an increase in HBV DNA levels on therapy may be presumed to be resulting from the development of resistant virus, it is also important to verify that it is not because of noncompliance.

Defining End Points The development of nucleoside per nucleotide analogs as anti-HBV agents has prompted reappraisal of the traditional end points used to assess drug efficacy. For treatment with interferon, HBeAg loss or seroconversion 6 mo after therapy usually defines successful response. Treatment with the new anti-HBV agents produces a rapid decline in viremia, often to levels undetectable by even the new generation NATs. HBeAg seroconversion is uncommon and may be reversible when treatment ceases and is thus an unreliable marker. Histological examination of liver tissue can be useful but biopsies are invasive and cannot be performed on a frequent basis. Consideration has been given to using serum HBV DNA levels as an efficacy end point and although it has proven a useful tool, there is insufficient correlation with treatment responses to justify its use as a sole predictor.

OCCULT INFECTION Several case reports have described how some patients show clinical evidence of CH-B infection, despite remaining serologically HBsAg-negative. The use of sensitive NATs demonstrated that in many instances the presence of HBV DNA could be detected. Cases such as these were defined as having occult HBV infection. Several explanations have been proposed to account for the contradictory testing profile. One possibility was that mutations in the surface gene were sufficient to allow HBsAg to evade serological detection. However, studies employing sequence analysis have shown there are few instances of changes to the relevant epitopes of HBsAg. Furthermore, although mutations to regulatory elements in the HBV genome may have an indirect effect on HBsAg synthesis, these too appear to be rare.

The most significant finding in most studies of occult infection is that of a very low level of virus replication. This may be because of an incomplete immune response that allows a low level of virus replication or even an enduring cellular response that requires a low level of persistent virus replication. The clinical significance of occult hepatitis B has not been determined, although it appears that transmission of infection from patients with occult infection can occur.

QUASISPECIES Rt, an essential enzyme in the life cycle of HBV, lacks proofreading capacity and results in an estimated mutation rate of 10^{-3}–10^{-5} misincorporations per nucleotide copied. Mathematical analysis of viral load decay following antiviral therapy predicts greater than 10^{11} virus particles are produced per day. These features of HBV replication mean that heterogeneous genetic variants are generated, which are termed quasispecies. Quasispecies generation is a continuous process with competition and selection resulting in evolutionary flexibility. For HBV, the quasispecies diversity is constrained by overlapping reading frames, meaning that a mutation modifying a protein encoded by one reading frame can have a deleterious effect in the overlapping reading frame. Nevertheless, the high rates of virus production ensure that a large number of viable mutants are produced. Under selection pressure, such as from the host immune system or antiviral therapy, high quasispecies variability allows a rapid response resulting in a new dominant quasispecies that can be further refined by selection.

QUANTIFICATION OF HBsAg HBV infection leads to overexpression of HBsAg, which is found in vast excess over virions in the blood. Before development of automated assays, quantifying HBsAg was carried out by modifying radioimmunoassays or by Laurell electrophoresis. In acute hepatitis B, peak concentrations of HBsAg decrease within 16–20 d in resolving infection as the host immune system responds. In patients with acute hepatitis B who become carriers, no such decrease is seen. Automated assays have been adapted to the quantification of HBsAg, allowing greater throughput of samples. Using such assays, HBsAg levels were found to be higher in HBeAg-positive CH-B carriers than in HBeAg-negative CH-B carriers. Importantly, HBsAg levels in both sets of patients showed a good correlation with serum HBV DNA levels, potentially providing an inexpensive alternative to the HBV DNA NATs, worthy of further investigation.

MOLECULAR DIAGNOSTICS—LIVER COMPARTMENT

IMMUNOHISTOCHEMISTRY Components of HBV that reflect replication can be demonstrated in liver biopsy sections using specialized techniques. Various HBV DNA and RNA replicative intermediates can be demonstrated by PCR and/or *in situ* hybridization. Viral proteins such as HBsAg, HBcAg, HBeAg, HBx, and Pre-S proteins can all be demonstrated by immunohistochemistry. Immunodetection of HBsAg and HBcAg in hepatocytes can provide useful information about the replicative status of HBV and is usually performed as part of a histopathological diagnosis of patients with CH-B. The pattern of antigen distribution relates somewhat to the stage of infection. Patients in the nonreplicative phase have little or no demonstratable HBcAg in the liver. In the replicative phase, HBcAg is found in the hepatocyte nuclei, and when replication is very high, in the cytoplasm as well. Cytoplasmic HBcAg tends to correlate with the activity of the liver disease. HBsAg is found in the hepatocyte cytoplasm, but it tends to be inversely related to the amount of HBcAg and to the disease activity. Patients with abundant HBcAg generally have less HBsAg overall and less per cell than those with little or no HBcAg. Patients in the nonreplicative phase of infection, with integration of HBV DNA into the hepatocyte genome, often have hepatocytes with abundant cytoplasmic HBsAg. These cells have uniformly pale, eosinophilic cytoplasm with a "ground-glass" appearance on routine hematoxylin-eosin stains. In immunostains they appear dark and discrete, compared to the pale and diffuse staining pattern of the replicative phase. Both surface and core antigens typically have a patchy distribution within the liver, and more than one pattern may be found in the same biopsy.

The cellular localization of HBcAg and HBeAg generally coincide but there are important differences at a subcellular level. HBeAg is usually detected in the nucleus and/or cytoplasm and intense or strong cytoplasmic HBeAg-staining is associated with a high serum HBV DNA level and inactive liver disease. HBcAg can also be detected in the nucleus and/or cytoplasm, but strong cytoplasmic HBcAg expression is typically associated with active liver disease. The proportion of hepatocytes expressing HBsAg correlates inversely with viremia and HBsAg and HBcAg are usually expressed independently within the lobule. Thus, cytoplasmic HBcAg (and not HBeAg) is the target for immune system-mediated cytolysis of hepatocytes. Cytoplasmic HBeAg is not associated with liver damage, but instead with high levels of HBV replication. Finally, the degree of expression of HBcAg in the hepatocyte nucleus does reflect the level of viral replication in CH-B

INTRAHEPATIC HBV COVALENTLY CLOSED CIRCULAR DNA HBV infection is not directly cytopathic, so HBV DNA can persist in the hepatocyte as long as the cell survives. In an interesting study, a commercially available HBV PCR assay was modified to investigate the levels of HBV DNA in frozen liver tissue. Subgroups of patients with CH-B were examined, including those with active replication, as defined by detection of serum HBV DNA and liver HBcAg reactivity, and those with "suppressed" replication, which included patients on antiviral therapy and patients coinfected with hepatitis D virus. Although patients with active virus replication had the highest levels of intrahepatic viral DNA, patients with suppressed HBV activity maintained relatively high levels of intrahepatic HBV DNA. The mean difference in serum HBV DNA levels between the two groups was more than 300-fold, whereas the mean difference in intrahepatic DNA levels was only approx 3-fold.

It is likely that the major component of the intrahepatic HBV DNA in the suppressed patient groups is the covalently closed circular (ccc) replicative form found in the nucleus. This viral form is produced from the partially double-stranded genomic HBV DNA found in the viral nucleocapsid. On infection, the genomic DNA is transported to the hepatocyte nucleus in which it is converted by host cell enzymes into a fully double-stranded form. From this, a ccc DNA molecule is generated that associates with cellular histones and other nuclear proteins to form a viral minichromosome. This viral replicative form, the HBV ccc DNA, remains in the nucleus and serves as the transcriptional template for HBV RNA production. The hepatocyte RNA polymerase II transcribes all the viral mRNA from the HBV ccc DNA, including the terminally redundant primary transcript, the pgRNA. This RNA molecule is encapsidated in precursors of the virus core and is reverse transcribed by the viral polymerase to form the single-stranded minus-sense DNA. The RNA is degraded by the viral RNase H and the remaining minus-strand DNA becomes the template for the synthesis of a plus-strand DNA of variable length.

Assembled nucleocapsids containing the partially double-stranded HBV DNA can follow either of two pathways. They can become enveloped by the HBV surface proteins and be secreted from the cell or be recycled back to the nucleus in which the HBV DNA is converted into ccc DNA as part of an intracellular conversion pathway to maintain a ccc DNA pool. Once a pool of 5–50 copies has been established, nucleocapsids associate with envelope proteins, rather than being recycled, and leave the cell as virions. The determinant of which pathway the nucleocapsid follows appears to be the amount of pre-S protein. The greater the number of viral ccc DNA molecules, the greater the level of RNA transcripts, resulting in more pre-S protein available to associate with nucleocapsids.

The pool of viral ccc DNA molecules in the cell nucleus is the likely reason for the relapse of viremia after treatment with nucleoside and nucleotide analogs. HBV replication does not use a semiconservative mechanism, thus, antiviral therapy with such agents can only affect newly synthesized DNA and not the pre-existing HBV ccc DNA pool. Elimination of viral ccc DNA might be achieved if production of new virions could be completely blocked; ccc DNA would be eventually lost by either decay or death of the infected hepatocyte. Two major means of removal of viral ccc DNA have been proposed, a cytokine-induced noncytolytic clearance of virus from infected cells, and the killing of infected cells by virus-specific cytotoxic T cells.

The critical role played by intrahepatic viral ccc DNA has motivated researchers to develop assays for its detection and quantification. Assays for hepadnaviral ccc DNA have been developed for the woodchuck and duck hepatitis B models and applied to the investigation of the mechanism of clearance of infection. Studies using the woodchuck model showed that in transient infection a high proportion of infected hepatocytes were destroyed and replaced by uninfected cells, derived by cell division from the remaining infected hepatocytes. Some support that this mode of eradication of infection also occurs with antiviral therapy has been shown in chronically infected woodchucks treated with nucleoside analogs. The amount of viral ccc DNA decreased substantially whereas the amount of residual integrated viral DNA remained the same, suggesting a turnover of infected hepatocytes and compensatory accumulation of uninfected cells. Furthermore, in chronically infected ducks treated with a cytotoxic antiviral drug, the loss of infected hepatocytes was more rapid and showed in surviving animals that cell death and regeneration of uninfected cells play a role in recovery from infection.

For the assessment of HBV ccc DNA, a selective PCR assay was devised. Techniques that may have been applicable with animal models may not necessarily apply to patients in which the amount of sample available is limited, usually biopsy tissue, and the copy number of viral ccc DNA is low. Assays have been adapted to the real-time PCR format that provides for a greater dynamic range and more accurate quantification. In contrast to some of the studies in animal models, investigation of 48 wk treatment with the nucleotide analog ADV showed that there was a significant decrease in HBV ccc DNA levels, yet the number of immunostaining cells remained similar to that of pretreatment. This suggests a role for a noncytolytic mechanism of clearance rather than destruction of infected cells. Consistent with this is the finding of a more rapid elimination of HBV ccc DNA than that of HBsAg-positive hepatocytes in HBV infected chimpanzees. However, this phase of the elimination was followed by a second phase in which there was a peak of hepatocyte turnover and a surge of interferon-γ CD8+ T cells associated with loss of remaining viral ccc DNA. The study illustrates that the two mechanisms of eradication of infection, noncytopathic clearance of intracellular virus and immune-mediated destruction of hepatocytes, are not mutually exclusive.

PCR assays for HBV ccc DNA can have many uses. In patients being treated for CH-B, assessing the level of viral ccc DNA may indicate drug efficacy and help decide treatment duration. Insights into the mechanisms of elimination of HBV ccc DNA may identify potential targets for intervention. Assays require further standardization and validation before they can be considered part of a patient management strategy.

CONCLUSIONS

Hepatitis B is a vaccine preventable disease, yet it remains the commonest form of viral hepatitis and a worldwide public health problem. Acute infection can produce symptoms including fever, jaundice, and malaise that may spontaneously resolve within 6 mo. A number of people do not resolve the infection and become chronic carriers; this group is at risk of developing severe complications such as cirrhosis and HCC. Chronic carriers also represent a pool of infectious virus. Infection acquired early in life is likely to lead to chronic infection, so in countries hyperendemic for hepatitis B, transmission from chronically infected mothers to their babies helps perpetuate the carrier cycle.

Despite the availability of an efficacious vaccine that prevents HBV infection, help for those who already have CH-B relies on control of their disease by antiviral chemotherapy. The first effective antiviral agent used to treat CH-B was α-interferon. It is effective in eliminating HBV infection in a proportion of patients but is associated with considerable side effects. This has led to the search for other less toxic agents for the control of CH-B.

HBV replicates by reverse transcription of an RNA transcript. This provides the opportunity for inhibition of replication by nucleoside and nucleotide analogs, many of which have been previously evaluated for the treatment of HIV infection. Antiviral therapy with agents such as LMV and ADV result in a dramatic drop in serum HBV DNA levels, which has required the development of sensitive NATs to assess their efficacy. The replication strategy of HBV also means that a heterogeneous population of genetic variants, or quasispecies, is generated although this is constrained to some degree by the genomic organization of overlapping reading frames, which allows the virus to respond to the selection pressure placed on it by antiviral therapy. Here too technology can play a role in being able to detect clinically significant variants, particularly detection of the early development of resistance. Combination therapy with nucleoside per nucleotide analogs has been an effective approach to combat problems associated with resistance in the treatment of HIV infection and this has already been initiated against CH-B in preliminary clinical trials. Treatment with interferon has been revisited with the development of pegylated versions that reduce the frequency of injection and appear to show improved efficacy. The use of sensitive and standardized NATs will be important in determining optimal combination therapy and may play some role in defining therapeutic end points.

Assessment of liver damage can be determined by the histological examination of tissue from a liver biopsy. Immunohistochemical demonstration of viral proteins can also provide some indication of the stage of HBV replication. Molecular technology has been applied to the investigation of HBV replication in liver tissue. A number of assays have been developed to measure the replicative intermediate HBV ccc DNA. These assays need to be validated and standardized before their full potential can be realized. The ability to measure this important intermediate may provide information on treatment efficacy and an understanding of the mechanisms involved in the elimination of viral ccc DNA.

Further studies of HBV replication may shed light on the nature of other chronic viral infections. Analysis of the results from patients treated with combination therapy could provide a basis for improved combination therapy for treatment of HIV infection, rather than vice versa, as is the current situation. Likewise, an understanding of how HBV causes immune-mediated liver disease may aid in the prevention of complications such as cirrhosis and HCC caused by hepatitis C virus. Clearly, many questions remain to be answered with this fascinating pathogen.

SELECTED REFERENCES

Alberti A. Can serum HBV-DNA be used as a primary end point to assess efficacy of new treatments for chronic hepatitis B? Hepatology 2003;38:18–20.

Bartenschlager R, Schaller H. Hepadnaviral assembly is initiated by polymerase binding to the encapsidation signal in the viral RNA genome. EMBO J 1992;11:3413–3420.

Beasley R, Lin C, Hwang L, Chien C. Hepatocellular carcinoma and hepatitis B virus. Lancet 1981;2:1129–1133.

Birnbaum F, Nassal M. Hepatitis B virus nucleocapsid assembly: primary structure requirements in the core protein. J Virol 1990;64:3319–3330.

Brechot C, Thiers V, Kremsdorf D, Nalpas B, Pol S, Paterlini-Brechot P. Persistent hepatitis B virus infection in subjects without hepatitis B surface antigen: clinically significant or purely "occult"? Hepatology 2001;34:194–203.

Carman WF, Jacyna MR, Hadziyannis S, et al. Mutation preventing formation of hepatitis B e antigen in patients with chronic hepatitis B infection. Lancet 1989;2:588–591.

Carman WF, Zanetti AR, Karayiannis P, et al. Vaccine-induced escape mutant of hepatitis B virus. Lancet 1990;336:325–329.

Chang LJ, Pryciak P, Ganem D, Varmus HE. Biosynthesis of the reverse transcriptase of hepatitis B viruses involves *de novo* translational initiation not ribosomal frameshifting. Nature 1989;337:364–368.

Crowther R, Kiselev N, Bottcher B, et al. Three-dimensional structure of hepatitis B virus core particles determined by electron cryomicroscopy. Cell 1994;77:943–950.

Das K, Xiong X, Yang H, et al. Molecular modeling and biochemical characterization reveal the mechanism of hepatitis B virus polymerase resistance to lamivudine (3TC) and emtricitabine (FTC). J Virol 2001;75:4771–4779.

Fattovich G, Brollo L, Giustina G, et al. Natural history and prognostic factors for chronic hepatitis type B. Gut 1991;32:294–298.

Ganem D, Schneider R. Hepadnaviridae: The Viruses and Their Replication. In: Knipe DM, Howley PM, eds. Fields Virology, vol. 2, Philadelphia: Lippincott-Raven, 2001; pp. 2923–2970.

Gauthier J, Bourne EJ, Lutz MW, et al. Quantitation of hepatitis B viremia and emergence of YMDD variants in patients with chronic hepatitis B treated with lamivudine. J Infect Dis 1999;180:1757–1762.

Goodman Z. Histopathology of hepatitis B virus infection. In: Lai CLS, ed. Human Virus Guides, vol. 1, London: International Medical Press, 2002:131–143.

Guidotti LG, Rochford R, Chung J, Shapiro M, Purcell R, Chisari FV. Viral clearance without destruction of infected cells during acute HBV infection. Science 1999;284:825–829.

Gunther S, Fischer L, Pult I, Sterneck M, Will H. Naturally occurring variants of hepatitis B virus. Adv Virus Res 1999;52:25–137.

Hadziyannis SJ, Lieberman HM, Karvountzis GG, Shafritz DA. Analysis of liver disease, nuclear HBcAg, viral replication, and hepatitis B virus DNA in liver and serum of HBeAg vs. anti-HBe positive carriers of hepatitis B virus. Hepatology 1983;3:656–662.

Hino O, Ohtake K, Rogler CE. Features of two hepatitis B virus (HBV) DNA integrations suggest mechanisms of HBV integration. J Virol 1989;63:2638–2643.

Jung M, Pape G. Immunology of hepatitis B infection. Lancet Infect Dis 2002;2:43–50.

Kann M, Gerlich W. Hepadnaviridae: structure and molecular virology. In: Zuckerman A, Thomas H, eds. Viral Hepatitis. London: Churchill Livingstone, 1998:77–105.

Koike K, Tsutsumi T, Fujie H, Shintani Y, Kyoji M. Molecular mechanism of viral hepatocarcinogenesis. Oncology 2002;62(Suppl. 1):29–37.

Lok AS, Akarca U, Greene S. Mutations in the pre-core region of hepatitis B virus serve to enhance the stability of the secondary structure of the pre-genome encapsidation signal. Proc Natl Acad Sci USA 1994;91:4077–4081.

Lok AS, Heathcote EJ, Hoofnagle JH. Management of hepatitis B: 2000—summary of a workshop. Gastroenterology 2001;120:1828–1853.

Milich DR, McLachlan A, Stahl S, et al. Comparative immunogenicity of hepatitis B virus core and E antigens. J Immunol 1988;141:3617–3624.

Naoumov NV, Portmann BC, Tedder RS, et al. Detection of hepatitis B virus antigens in liver tissue. Gastroenterology 1990;99:1248–1253.

Newbold JE, Xin H, Tencza M, et al. The covalently closed duplex form of the hepadnavirus genome exists *in situ* as a heterogeneous population of viral minochromosomes. J Virol 1995;69:3350–3357.

Nowak MA, Bonhoeffer S, Hill AM, Boehme R, Thomas HC, McDade H. Viral dynamics in hepatitis B virus infection. Proc Natl Acad Sci USA 1996;93:4398–4402.

Richman DD. The impact of drug resistance on the effectiveness of chemotherapy for chronic hepatitis B. Hepatology 2000;32:866,867.

Rossner MT. Review: hepatitis B virus X-gene product: a promiscuous transcriptional activator. J Med Virol 1992;36:101–117.

Saldanha J, Gerlich W, Lelie N, Dawson P, Heermann K, Heath A. An international collaborative study to establish a World Health Organization international standard for hepatitis B virus DNA nucleic acid amplification techniques. Vox Sang 2001;80:63–71.

Schaller H, Fischer M. Transcriptional control of hepadnavirus gene expression. Curr Top Microbiol Immunol 1991;168:21–39.

Schlicht HJ, Bartenschlager R, Schaller H. Biosynthesis and enzymatic functions of the hepadnaviral reverse transcriptase. In: McLachlan A, ed. Molecular Biology of the Hepatitis B Viruses. Boca Raton, FL: CRC Press, 1991:171–180.

Seeger C, Mason WS. Hepatitis B virus biology. Microbiol Mol Biol Rev 2000;64:51–68.

Shaul Y. Regulation of hepadnavirus transcription. In: McLachlan A, ed. Molecular Biology of the Hepatitis B Virus. Boca Raton, FL: CRC Press, 1991:193–211.

Stuyver LJ, Locarnini SA, Lok A, et al. Nomenclature for antiviral-resistant human hepatitis B virus mutations in the polymerase region. Hepatology 2001;33:751–757.

Summers J, Mason WS. Replication of the genome of a hepatitis B-like virus by reverse transcription of an RNA intermediate. Cell 1982;29:403–415.

Summers J, Mason WS. Residual integrated viral DNA after hepadnavirus clearance by nucleoside analog therapy. Proc Natl Acad Sci USA 2004;101:638–640.

Summers J, Smith PM, Horwich AL. Hepadnavirus envelope proteins regulate covalently closed circular DNA amplification. J Virol 1990;64:2819–2824.

Summers J, Jilbert AR, Yang W, et al. Hepatocyte turnover during resolution of a transient hepadnaviral infection. Proc Natl Acad Sci USA 2003;100:11,652–11,659.

Tuttleman JS, Pourcel C, Summers J. Formation of the pool of covalently closed circular viral DNA in hepadnavirus-infected cells. Cell 1986;47:451–460.

Wallace WA, Carman WF. Surface variation of HBV: scientific and medical relevance. Viral Hepat Rev 1997;3:5–16.

Wang GH, Seeger C. Novel mechanism for reverse transcription in hepatitis B viruses. J Virol 1993;67:6507–6512.

Werle B, Bowden D, Locarnini S, et al. Persistence of viral cccDNA during the natural history of chronic hepatitis B and slow decline with adefovir dipivoxil therapy. Gastroenterology 2004;126:1750–1758.

Will H, Reiser W, Weimer T, et al. Replication strategy of human hepatitis B virus. J Virol 1987;61:904–911.

Wu TT, Coates L, Aldrich CE, Summers J, Mason WS. In hepatocytes infected with duck hepatitis B virus, the template for viral RNA synthesis is amplified by an intracellular pathway. Virology 1990;175:255–261.

Wynne SA, Crowther RA, Leslie AG. The crystal structure of the human hepatitis B virus capsid. Mol Cell 1999;3:771–780.

Zoulim F, Saputelli J, Seeger C. Woodchuck hepatitis virus X protein is required for viral infection in vivo. J Virol 1994;68:2026–2030.

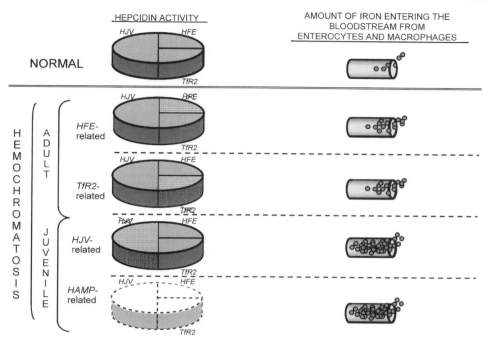

Figure 54-2   A unifying pathogenic model for all forms of hereditary hemochromatosis/hepcidin as common denominator. In this model HFE, transferrin receptor 2, and HJV are each independent but complementary modulators of hepcidin activity (pie chart); this activity is ultimately responsible for the rate of iron release from intestine and macrophages into the bloodstream. Relevant contribution of each gene to hepcidin synthesis/activity has been arbitrarily set in the figure. Owing to the severity of HJV-related hemochromatosis, hemojuvelin is likely the major regulator of hepcidin function. Loss of either HFE or TfR2 (e.g., *HFE-* or *TfR2*-related hereditary hemochromatosis) will result in appreciable increase or iron influx into the bloodstream, whereas residual hepcidin activity is sustained by normal HH genes. Owing to its dominant effect on hepcidin synthesis/activity, loss of hemojuvelin (e.g., *HJV*-related HH) will cause a much more dramatic effect on iron release from macrophages and enterocytes. Similarly, complete loss of hepcidin (e.g., *HAMP*-related HH), in spite of normal HFE, TfR2, and HJV, will inevitably lead to uncontrolled, massive release of iron into the circulation.

but complementary modulators of hepcidin activity. If so, the loss of one might be partially compensated by the presence of the other, and in the presence of normal *HAMP* some hepcidin upregulation could thus be achieved (*see* Fig. 54-2).

The scenario depicted above also allows intriguing speculation on more subtle phenotypic differences that could result from various combinations of HH-gene mutations.

CONCLUSION

For much of the 20th century, HH was regarded as a monogenic disorder characterized by excess tissue deposits of iron inevitably producing organ damage. This view has been shattered by the identification of similar phenotypes associated with mutations of at least four different iron-metabolism genes (*HFE, TfR2, HAMP, HJV*) and the increasing appreciation of the disease's multifactorial nature. HH is an autosomal-recessive disorder of iron metabolism, polygenic in nature, characterized by early progressive expansion of the plasma iron compartment, followed by progressive parenchymal iron deposits with the potential for severe organ damage, nonimpaired erythropoiesis, and optimal response to therapeutic phlebotomy. These features distinguish HH from all other known iron overload states in humans. Regardless of the underlying genetic variability, HH should be considered a unique clinicopathological syndromic entity and not divided into subtypes based exclusively on genetic criteria.

The precise molecular mechanisms responsible for the HH metabolic abnormality in the presence of nonfunctional HH genes

and the interplay of HFE, TfR2, hemojuvelin, and hepcidin in the control of iron trafficking, remains to be elucidated. Animal genetics and availability of murine models of HH will likely solve many of the unanswered questions in HH.

ACKNOWLEDGMENTS

This work was supported by grants from European Community n. QLK1-2001-00444, Ministero dell'Università e Ricerca Scientifica e Tecnologica, Rome, and Telethon.

SELECTED REFERENCES

Bridle KR, Frazer DM, Wilkins SJ, et al. Disrupted hepcidin regulation in HFE-associated haemochromatosis and the liver as a regulator of body iron homoeostasis. Lancet 2003;361:669–673.

Cairo G, Recalcati S, Montosi G, Castrusini E, Conte D, Pietrangelo A. Inappropriately high iron regulatory protein activity in monocytes of patients with genetic hemochromatosis. Blood 1997;89: 2546–2553.

Camaschella C, Roetto A, Cali A, et al. The gene TFR2 is mutated in a new type of haemochromatosis mapping to 7q22. Nat Genet 2000;25:14, 15.

Davies PS, Zhang AS, Anderson EL, et al. Evidence for the interaction of the hereditary haemochromatosis protein, HFE, with the transferrin receptor in endocytic compartments. Biochem J 2003;373:145–153.

Feder JN, Gnirke A, Thomas W, et al. A novel MHC class I-like gene is mutated in patients with hereditary haemochromatosis. Nat Genet 1996;13:399–408.

Gehrke SG, Kulaksiz H, Herrmann T, et al. Expression of hepcidin in hereditary hemochromatosis: evidence for a regulation in response to serum transferrin saturation and non-transferrin-bound iron. Blood 2003;102:371–376.

Hayashi A, Wada Y, Suzuki T, Shimizu A. Studies on familial hypotrans-ferrinemia—unique clinical course and molecular pathology. Am J Hum Genet 1993;53:201–213.

Kawabata H, Yang R, Hirama T, et al. Molecular cloning of transferrin receptor 2. A new member of the transferrin receptor-like family. J Biol Chem 1999;274:20,826–20,832.

Knisely AS, Mieli-Vergani G, Whitington PF. Neonatal hemochromatosis. Gastroenterol Clin North Am 2003;32:877–889.

Lebron JA, Bennett MJ, Vaughn DE, et al. Crystal structure of the hemochromatosis protein HFE and characterization of its interaction with transferrin receptor. Cell 1998;93:111–123.

Lynch SR, Skikne BS, Cook JD. Food iron absorption in idiopathic hemochromatosis. Blood 1989;74:2187–2193.

McLaren GD, Nathanson MH, Jacobs A, Trevett D, Thomson W. Regulation of intestinal iron absorption and mucosal iron kinetics in hereditary hemochromatosis. J Lab Clin Med 1991;117:390–401.

Merryweather-Clarke AT, Cadet E, Bomford A. et al. Digenic inheritance of mutations in HAMP and HFE results in different types of haemochromatosis. Hum Mol Genet 2003;12:2241–2247.

Merryweather-Clarke AT, Pointon JJ, Shearman JD, Robson KJH. Global prevalence of putative haemochromatosis mutations. J Med Genet 1997;34:275–278.

Montosi G, Donovan A, Totaro A, et al. Autosomal-dominant hemochromatosis is associated with a mutation in the ferroportin (SLC11A3) gene. J Clin Invest 2001;108:619–623.

Muckenthaler M, Roy CN, Custodio AO, et al. Regulatory defects in liver and intestine implicate abnormal hepcidin and Cybrd1 expression in mouse hemochromatosis. Nat Genet 2003;34:102–107.

Nicolas G, Viatte L, Lou DQ, et al. Constitutive hepcidin expression prevents iron overload in a mouse model of hemochromatosis. Nat Genet 2003;34:97–101.

Online Mendelian Inheritance in Man at http://www.ncbi.nlm.nih.gov/omim.

Papanikolaou G, Samuels ME, Ludwig EH, et al. Mutations in HFE2 cause iron overload in chromosome 1q-linked juvenile hemochromatosis. Nat Genet 2004;36:77–82.

Park CH, Valore EV, Waring AJ, Ganz T. Hepcidin, a urinary antimicrobial peptide synthesized in the liver. J Biol Chem 2001;276:7806–7810.

Parkkila S, Waheed A, Britton RS, et al. Immunohistochemistry of HLA-H, the protein defective in patients with hereditary hemochromatosis, reveals unique pattern of expression in gastrointestinal tract. Proc Natl Acad Sci USA 1997;94:2534–2539.

Pietrangelo A, Casalgrandi G, Quaglino D, et al. Duodenal ferritin synthesis in genetic hemochromatosis. Gastroenterology 1995;108:208–217.

Pietrangelo A. Hereditary hemochromatosis—a new look to an old disease. N Engl J Med 2004;350(23):2383–2397.

Pigeon C, Ilyin G, Courselaud B, et al. A new mouse liver-specific gene, encoding a protein homologous to human antimicrobial peptide hepcidin, is overexpressed during iron overload. J Biol Chem 2001;276:7811–7819.

Roetto A, Papanikolaou G, Politou M, et al. Mutant antimicrobial peptide hepcidin is associated with severe juvenile hemochromatosis. Nat Genet 2003;33:21, 22.

Sheldon J. Haemochromatosis. London: Oxford University Press, 1935.

Simon M, Le Mignon L, Fauchet R, et al. A study of 609 HLA haplotypes marking for the hemochromatosis gene: (1) Mapping of the gene near the HLA-A locus and characters required to define a heterozygous population and (2) hypothesis concerning the underlying cause of hemochromatosis-HLA association. Am J Hum Genet 1987;41:89–105.

von Recklinghausen FD. Uber Haemochromatose. Taggeblatt der (62) Versammlung deutscher Naturforscher and Aerzte in Heidelberg 1889:324, 325.

Yoshida K, Furihata K, Takeda S, et al. A mutation in the ceruloplasmin gene is associated with systemic hemosiderosis in humans. Nat Genet 1995;9:267–272.

Zhang AS, Davies PS, Carlson HL, Enns CA. Mechanisms of HFE-induced regulation of iron homeostasis: Insights from the W81A HFE mutation. Proc Natl Acad Sci USA 2003;100:9500–9505.

55 Pancreatic Exocrine Dysfunction

David C. Whitcomb and Jonathan A. Cohn

SUMMARY

Pancreatic exocrine dysfunction can present clinically either as an acute illness, a destructive process, or a condition such as pancreatic insufficiency or chronic abdominal pain. Acute pancreatitis is associated with injury to the pancreas through direct trauma, occasional viral infections, hyperlipidemia, cholelithiasis, alcohol abuse, hypercalcemia, or other factors that trigger intrapancreatic trypsinogen activation in susceptible individuals or that activate the immune system directly. Research is moving toward developing new methods to prevent idiopathic pancreatitis in highly susceptible individuals. Gene testing can already identify asymptomatic individuals in whom the risk of developing pancreatitis is increased by several 100-fold.

Key Words: Cystic fibrosis (CF); hereditary pancreatitis (HP); pancreatic exocrine dysfunction; Shwachman–Diamond Syndrome (SDS).

INTRODUCTION

The pancreas is a retroperitoneal gland with both endocrine and exocrine functions. Pancreatic endocrine secretions are released from the islets into the circulation where they are essential for regulating intermediary metabolism. Pancreatic exocrine secretions (pancreatic juice), produced by the concerted action of pancreatic acinar and ductal cells, are delivered into the duodenum via a ductal system where they are essential for normal digestion of complex nutrients. Different pancreatic enzymes promote the efficient digestion of carbohydrates, lipids, proteins, and other nutrients (Table 55-1). Many of these digestive enzymes have the potential to digest components of the pancreas itself. Such autodigestion is normally prevented by several mechanisms. For example, most digestive enzymes exist in an inactive (proenzyme, i.e., zymogens) form until they reach the duodenum. Other mechanisms either prevent activation of proenzymes inside the pancreas, inhibit enzymes such as trypsin directly, limit diffusion of prematurely activated digestive enzymes, or rapidly flush activated digestive enzymes out of the ductal system. If any of these protective mechanisms fails, this can increase susceptibility to recurrent acute pancreatitis and lead to chronic pancreatitis.

Pancreatic exocrine dysfunction can present clinically either as an acute illness (acute pancreatitis), a destructive process (chronic pancreatitis), or a condition (pancreatic insufficiency, chronic abdominal pain, and so on). Acute pancreatitis is associated with injury to the pancreas through direct trauma, occasional viral infections, hyperlipidemia, cholelithiasis, alcohol abuse, hypercalcemia, or other factors that trigger intrapancreatic trypsinogen activation in susceptible individuals or that activate the immune system directly (e.g., an infection). The clinical course of acute pancreatitis is variable, and is related to both the degree of pancreatic injury and intensity of the inflammatory response.

The primary risk factors for chronic pancreatic diseases are genetic, through classic Mendelian diseases or complex genetic traits that together predispose susceptible individuals to chronic inflammation, fibrosis, and pancreatic dysfunction. The major Mendelian genetic diseases include hereditary pancreatitis (HP), cystic fibrosis (CF), some forms of early onset chronic pancreatitis associated with homozygous *SPINK1* mutations, and Shwachman–Diamond syndrome (SDS). In these conditions, the responsible gene is known and information is rapidly emerging concerning the role of the gene's protein product in normal pancreatic physiology and mutation-associated dysfunction that leads to pancreatic pathology.

ACUTE PANCREATITIS

Acute pancreatitis is defined clinically as pancreatic inflammation characterized by the sudden onset of abdominal pain in association with elevation of pancreatic enzyme concentration in blood or urine. In approx 80% of the cases, acute pancreatitis is *mild* and recovery is expected. However, in the remaining cases, acute pancreatitis is *severe* and can produce potentially life-threatening complications. The keys to clinical management are early recognition of a severe episode of acute pancreatitis, anticipation of complications, and prevention of recurrence.

CLINICAL FEATURES Acute pancreatitis usually causes epigastric abdominal pain of acute onset. The pain tends to be constant and may radiate to the mid-back. Vomiting occurs in 80% of cases and provides little pain relief. Abdominal tenderness with guarding occurs in half of cases but tends to be less severe than anticipated based on either the severity of pain or the degree of pancreatic inflammation (by abdominal CT, MRI, or ultrasound) and this discrepancy between symptoms and signs on the physical examination results from the retroperitoneal location of the pancreas.

DIAGNOSIS In a patient presenting with typical abdominal pain, a serum amylase or lipase level more than 2.5 times the upper limit of normal strongly suggests the diagnosis of acute pancreatitis.

From: *Principles of Molecular Medicine, Second Edition*
Edited by: M. S. Runge and C. Patterson © Humana Press, Inc., Totowa, NJ

Table 55-1
Pancreatic Digestive Proteins

Proteinases
Trypsin(ogen)
Chymotrypsin(ogen)
(Pro)carboxypeptidases
(Pro)elastases
Kalikreinogen

Pancreatic α-amylase

Pancreatic lipase

Other enzymes
(Pro)colipase I, II
(Pro)phospholipase A_2
Ribonuclease
Deoxyribonuclease I

Table 55-2
Causes of Acute Pancreatitis

Mechanical
Gallstones
Biliary microlithiasis
Post-ERCP (multifactorial)
Pancreatic cancer
Anatomical predisposition
  Pancreas divisum
  Annular pancreas
  ? Sphincter of Oddi dysfunction

Toxins
Chronic alcohol abuse (multifactorial)
Scorpion bite
Medications
  Anticholinesterases
  L-Asparaginase
  Azathioprine
  Dideoxyinosine (DDI)
  Estrogen
  6-Mercaptopurine
  Salicylates
  Thiazide diuretics
  Valproic acid
  Vinca alkaloids
  Other (idiosyncratic reactions)

Hereditary
Trypsinogen gene mutations (others ?)

Metabolic
Hyperlipidemia (triglycerides >1000)
Hypercalcemia

Trauma
Blunt abdominal trauma
Penetrating ulcer
Postoperative/post-ERCP

Infections
Mycoplasma pneumoniae
Virus (mumps, coxsackie, CMV, HSV, HIV)
Bacteria
Mycobacterium avium-intracellulare

Vascular
Vasculitis (e.g., connective tissue diseases)
Hypotension (postoperative: e.g., CABG)
Infarction
Abdominal aortic aneurysm

Idiopathic
Unknown

CT with intravenous contrast is the most sensitive method of assessing the degree of pancreatic injury, pancreatic necrosis, and local extrapancreatic complications. Nonetheless, most experts recommend that the initial diagnosis is made on clinical and laboratory grounds rather than by CT because intravenous contrast worsens the severity of pancreatic injury early in the course of pancreatitis in animal models. In most cases, acute pancreatitis is associated with an identifiable cause, with gallstones and alcohol ingestion being the most common factors in adults (Table 55-2), and trauma, structural anomalies, viruses, medications, and systemic diseases being most common in children. Early identification of the cause of pancreatitis may prove beneficial in preventing ongoing pancreatic injury and also in preventing recurrence.

MOLECULAR PATHOPHYSIOLOGY   The first advance in understanding the nature of acute pancreatitis came in 1896 when Chiari proposed that pancreatic inflammation was triggered by digestive enzyme-mediated autodigestion of the pancreas rather than infection. This hypothesis has proven to be correct in most cases of acute pancreatitis, although viral and bacterial pancreatitis also occur. In the cases in which premature activation of digestive enzymes appears to play a central role, the problem may occur anywhere along the pathway between the site of digestive proenzyme (zymogen) synthesis within the acinar cell to the ampula of Vater where the zymogens normally enter the duodenum.

In pancreatic physiology, trypsin is the key molecule controlling zymogen activation. Many protective mechanisms focus on limiting the activation of trypsinogen (the proenzyme) to trypsin (the active enzyme) and on eliminating active trypsin from within the pancreas. Activation of trypsin normally occurs in the intestinal lumen where an intestinal brush border enzyme, *enterokinase,* cleaves a small trypsinogen activation peptide from trypsinogen to generate trypsin. Trypsin also activates trypsinogen, and trypsin efficiently activates all other pancreatic digestive enzymes. This process is desirable in the intestine but disastrous within the pancreas.

Trypsin activity is controlled within the pancreatic acinar cell by being synthesized in the inactive form as trypsinogen. Human trypsinogen can slowly autoactivate to trypsin, which can initiate the zymogen activation cascade. This is prevented by three mechanisms. The first is packaging of zymogens within dense granules in a semicrystallized form that is separated from some of the lysozomal enzymes that have the capacity to directly activate trypsinogen. The second is synthesis of pancreatic secretory trypsin inhibitor (PSTI), also know as serine protease inhibitor Kazal type 1 (SPINK1). This specific trypsin inhibitor is regulated as an acute phase protein and the ratio of SPINK1 to trypsin is therefore dependent on the status of the immune system and inflammation. The third mechanism is trypsin autolysis. The trypsin molecule has two globular domains connected by a peptide chain containing an arginine at codon 122. This arginine serves as target for a second trypsin and therefore serves as a self-destruct site when R122 is exposed. Cleavage at this site permanently inactivates trypsin (Fig. 55-1). Accessibility of R122 to cleavage appears to be regulated by calcium. Low calcium levels (e.g., inside the acinar cell) favor autolysis whereas high levels (e.g., inside the pancreatic duct

both may help to prevent precipitation of proteins as the pancreatic juice flows through the ducts. Beyond this, data from in vitro models suggests that alkalinization of the lumen of the pancreatic duct system may also be important for maintaining normal acinar cell function during exocytosis. Finally, ductal fluid secretion tends to flush zymogen proteins out of the pancreas.

In CFTR-related idiopathic chronic pancreatitis, inadequate ductal CFTR function also probably plays an early role in pathogenesis. Maintaining flow through the ducts may be especially important in individuals who have increased risk for intraductal trypsin activation (e.g., resulting from PSTI mutations). When these individuals also have reduced CFTR function (e.g., resulting from CFTR mutations), flow through the pancreatic duct is slow and this promotes injury by prolonging pancreatic exposure to any activated trypsin that occurs in the duct lumen. Thus, mutations of the *CFTR* and *PSTI* genes tend to have additive (independent) impact on pancreatitis risk. This agrees well with the distinct sites in the exocrine pancreas for the protein products of these genes: CFTR is ductal whereas PSTI is acinar.

In SDS, the primary site of pancreatic injury is the acinus rather than the duct. Acinar replacement is prominent; inflammation and gland destruction are atypical. Thus, the exocrine insufficiency of SDS mainly affects enzyme secretion rather than bicarbonate secretion, whereas the opposite pattern is seen in CF.

MANAGEMENT Pain control is often the predominant issue in treating chronic pancreatitis. Structural causes for pain include ductal obstruction resulting from strictures, tumor, pseudocysts, or stones, and a parenchymal compartment syndrome in which exocrine tissue is encased by fibrosis. Pain resulting from structural causes is typically intermittent and often occurs when serum cholecystokinin levels increase after a fat- or protein-rich meal. Medical therapy for this type of pain can include using gastric acid suppression, pancreatic enzyme supplements, and narcotics to reduce pancreatic secretion, whereas surgical options include procedures designed to relieve areas of ductal obstruction or fibrotic encasement. Chronic pancreatitis can also cause pain because of inflammation. This pain can be severe and unremitting, and surgical resection and celiac ganglion ablation are important management options.

Pancreatic insufficiency and diabetes mellitus are also common problems in chronic pancreatitis. Pancreatic enzyme replacement is the cornerstone of therapy for pancreatic insufficiency. Widely used enzyme preparations include a combination of lipase, amylase, and proteases. Because lipase is rapidly degraded at low pH, replacement enzymes are commonly administered either as enteric-coated microspheres or in combination with an H_2-receptor antagonist. Moderate enzyme doses are usually sufficient to achieve partial correction of steatorrhea with marked improvement in nutrition. Complete correction of steatorrhea is usually not possible even when very high enzyme doses are administered. High enzyme doses should be used with caution because they have been associated with colonic strictures. The management of diabetes is reviewed in Chapter 32.

The high prevalence of *CFTR* and *PSTI* mutations in idiopathic pancreatitis suggests that many patients with this condition could benefit from genetic testing. Potential benefits include helping patients understand their disease, promoting prompt detection of extrapancreatic CFTR-related conditions, identifying CF carriers for genetic counseling, and identifying occasional CF patients in whom pancreatitis occurs before the onset of lung disease. *CFTR* gene testing may also improve medical care in cases in which physicians might otherwise suspect undisclosed alcoholism as the cause of pancreatitis. *CFTR* mutation testing is more likely to be positive in younger CF patients who have extrapancreatic evidence of reduced CFTR function (e.g., borderline sweat testing). False-negative tests are more likely in non-Caucasians because the assays widely used for CF carrier screening are less sensitive in these populations. It is also unclear if the limited number of *CFTR* gene mutations that are included in CF screening panels is sufficient for determining risk of pancreatitis.

FUTURE DIRECTIONS Research is moving toward developing new methods to prevent idiopathic pancreatitis in highly susceptible individuals. Gene testing can already identify asymptomatic individuals in whom the risk of developing pancreatitis is increased by several 100-fold. As more is learned about the subsets of *CFTR* and *PSTI* genotypes associated with highest pancreatitis risk, the predictive power of gene testing will continue to improve, enabling identification of highly susceptible individuals prior to the onset of their first pancreatitis symptoms. Once identified, these individuals can be studied to learn about early events in the pathogenesis of this condition as a key step toward developing and evaluating preventive therapy. Specific questions being addressed by ongoing research include the following: Is the risk of pancreatitis increased in CF carriers who have one normal CFTR allele? Should CFTR-related idiopathic pancreatitis be classified as a form of CF? Can CFTR or PSTI gene testing be used to guide therapy in patients with pancreatitis? Do individuals with CFTR or PSTI mutations have increased susceptibility to alcoholic or drug-related pancreatitis?

SELECTED REFERENCES

Bachem MG, Schneider E, Gross H, et al. Identification, culture, and characterization of pancreatic stellate cells in rats and humans. Gastroenterology 1998;115:421–432.

Bhatia E, Choudhuri G, Sikora SS, et al. Tropical calcific pancreatitis: strong association with SPINK1 trypsin inhibitor mutations. Gastroenterology 2002;123:1020–1025.

Boocock GR, Morrison JA, Popovic M, et al. Mutations in BDS are associated with Shwachman–Diamond syndrome. Nat Genet 2003;33:97–101.

Cipolli M. Shwachman–Diamond syndrome: clinical phenotypes. Pancreatology 2001;1:543–548.

Cohn JA, Friedman KJ, Noone PG, Knowles MR, Silverman LM, Jowell PS. Relation between mutations of the cystic fibrosis gene and idiopathic pancreatitis. N Engl J Med 1998;339:653–658.

Durie PR. Inherited and congenital disorders of the exocrine pancreas. Gastroenterologist 1996;4:169–187.

Etemad B, Whitcomb DC. Chronic pancreatitis: diagnosis, classification, and new genetic developments. Gastroenterology 2001;120:682–707.

Frey CF. Current management of chronic pancreatitis. Adv Surg 1995; 28:337–370.

Gorry MC, Gabbaizedeh D, Furey W, et al. Mutations in the cationic trypsinogen gene are associated with recurrent acute and chronic pancreatitis. Gastroenterology 1997;113:1063–1068.

Kingsnorth A. Role of cytokines and their inhibitors in acute pancreatitis. Gut 1997;40:1–4.

Kloppel G, Maillet B. Pseudocysts in chronic pancreatitis: A morphological analysis of 57 resection specimens and 9 autopsy pancreata. Pancreas 1991;6:266–274.

Kusske AM, Rongione AJ, Reber HA. Cytokines and acute pancreatitis. Gastroenterology 1996;110:639–642.

Marino CR, Matovcik LM, Gorelick FS, Cohn JA. Localization of the cystic fibrosis transmembrane conductance regulator in pancreas. J Clin Invest 1991;88:712–716.

Mews P, Phillips P, Fahmy R, et al. Pancreatic stellate cells respond to inflammatory cytokines: Potential role in chronic pancreatitis. Gut 2002;50:535–541.

Noone PG, Zhou Z, Silverman LM, Jowell PS, Knowles MR, Cohn JA.
    Cystic fibrosis gene mutations and pancreatitis risk: Relation to epithe-
    lial ion transport and trypsin inhibitor gene mutations. Gastroenterology
    2001;121:1310–1319.
Papachristou GI, Whitcomb DC. Predictors of severity and necrosis in
    acute pancreatitis. Gastroenterol Clin North Am 2004;33:871–890.
Pfutzer RH, Barmada MM, Brunskill AP, et al. SPINK1/PSTI polymor-
    phisms act as disease modifiers in familial and idiopathic chronic pan-
    creatitis. Gastroenterology 2000;119:615–623.
Ranson JH, Rifkind KM, Roses DF, Fink SD, Eng K, Spencer FC.
    Prognostic signs and the role of operative management in acute pan-
    creatitis. Surg Gynecol Obstet 1974;139:69–81.
Rinderknecht H. Pancreatic secretory enzymes. In: Go VLW, Dimagno
    EP, eds. The Pancreas: Biology, Pathobiology, and Disease, 2nd ed.
    New York: Raven, 1993; pp. 219–251.
Sainio V, Kemppainen E, Puolakkainen P, et al. Early antibiotic treatment
    in acute necrotising pancreatitis. Lancet 1995;346:663–667.
Schneider A, Suman A, Rossi L, et al. SPINK1/PSTI mutations are asso-
    ciated with tropical pancreatitis and type II diabetes mellitus in
    Bangladesh. Gastroenterology 2002;123:1026–1030
Sharer N, Schwarz M, Malone G, et al. Mutations of the cystic fibrosis
    gene in patients with chronic pancreatitis. N Engl J Med 1998;339:
    645–652.
Slaff J, Jacobson D, Tillman CR, Curington C, Toskes P. Protease-specific
    suppression of pancreatic exocrine secretion. Gastroenterology
    1984;87:44–52.
Stern RC, Eisenberg JD, Wagener JS, et al. A comparison of the efficacy
    and tolerance of pancrelipase and placebo in the treatment of steator-
    rhea in cystic fibrosis patients with clinical exocrine pancreatic insuf-
    ficiency. Am J Gastroenterol 2000;95:1932–1938.
Sutton R, Criddle D, Raraty MG, Tepikin A, Neoptolemos JP, Petersen
    OH. Signal transduction, calcium and acute pancreatitis. Pancreatology
    2003;3:497–505.
Whitcomb DC, Ermentrout DB. A mathematical model of the pancreatic
    duct cell generating high bicarbonate concentrations in pancreatic
    juice. Pancreas 2004;29:e30–e40.
Whitcomb DC, Gorry MC, Preston RA, et al. Hereditary pancreatitis is
    caused by a mutation in the cationic trypsinogen gene. Nat Genet
    1996;14:141–145.
Whitcomb DC, Lowe M. Pancreatitis: acute and chronic. In: Walker WA,
    Durie PR, Hamilton JR, Walker-Smith JA, Watkins JB, eds. Pediatric
    Gastrointestinal Disease: Pathophysiology, Diagnosis, Management.
    Hamilton, BC: Decker, 2000; pp. 1584–1597.
Witt H, Luck W, Hennies HC, et al. Mutations in the gene encoding the
    serine protease inhibitor, Kazal type 1 are associated with chronic
    pancreatitis. Nat Genet 2000;25:213–216.

56 Small and Large Bowel Dysfunction

DEBORAH C. RUBIN

SUMMARY

The study of inflammatory bowel diseases (IBD) has advanced greatly, with the identification of the first disease susceptibility gene for Crohn's disease, the tentative identification of other susceptibility loci for IBD, the creation of new animal models of IBD using gene knock out and transgenic technology, and the application of cellular and molecular techniques to develop novel therapies for IBD. This chapter summarizes the important molecular and genetic developments relevant to the study of IBD, celiac sprue, lactase deficiency, glucose–galactose malabsorption, and abetalipoproteinemia as several prominent examples of how molecular technology can help advance the practice of gastrointestinal medicine.

Key Words: Abetalipoproteinemia; celiac sprue; Chrohn's disease; glucose–galactose malabsorption; inflammatory bowel diseases (IBD); lactase deficiency; ulcerative colitis.

INTRODUCTION

The application of molecular biological and genetic techniques to the study of the luminal gastrointestinal tract epithelium has led to exciting advances in several broad areas. The study of inflammatory bowel diseases (IBD) has advanced greatly, with the identification of the first disease susceptibility gene for Crohn's disease, the tentative identification of other susceptibility loci for IBD, the creation of new animal models of IBD using gene knockout and transgenic technology, and the application of cellular and molecular techniques to develop novel therapies for IBD. The molecular mechanisms underlying intestinal digestion and absorption of nutrients have been further clarified by the cloning and characterization of enterocytic genes that play critical roles in the digestion and absorption of luminal nutrients. Their chromosomal localization, structure, and regulation of expression have been at least partially characterized. These studies have provided the groundwork for understanding the pathophysiology of several rare but well-described genetic disorders of small intestinal transport, and have begun to clarify the mechanisms underlying more common gastrointestinal problems such as lactase deficiency. This chapter summarizes the important molecular and genetic developments relevant to the study of IBD, celiac sprue, lactase deficiency, glucose–galactose malabsorption, and abetalipoproteinemia as several prominent

From: *Principles of Molecular Medicine, Second Edition*
Edited by: M. S. Runge and C. Patterson © Humana Press, Inc., Totowa, NJ

examples of how molecular technology can help advance the practice of gastrointestinal medicine.

INFLAMMATORY BOWEL DISEASE

CLINICAL PRESENTATION   The IBDs include Crohn's disease and ulcerative colitis. These are chronic inflammatory disorders of the gastrointestinal tract that are manifested by symptoms of diarrhea and abdominal pain. Although the clinical presentation may be quite similar, important differences in their underlying pathophysiology result in unique complications and long-term sequelae. In ulcerative colitis, the colon is the primary affected organ, but Crohn's disease can occur in any part of the gastrointestinal tract from mouth to anus. Ulcerative colitis is characterized by a predominantly superficial mucosal inflammation. In Crohn's disease, the inflammatory process is transmural and granulomatous, affecting all layers of the gastrointestinal tract, from mucosa to serosa.

The etiology of these disorders is unknown. The identification of C-terminal caspase recruitment domain (CARD15/NOD2) as a Crohn's disease susceptibility factor has supported the roles of genetic factors and immune responses to luminal gut flora in its pathogenesis (*see* IBD Gene Discovery). A variety of disease-susceptibility chromosomal loci have been identified by linkage analysis of families with IBD. Several of these contain immune regulatory gene clusters. Studies of mice with targeted disruption of cytokine or T-cell receptor genes, or of chimeric transgenic mice in which there is disruption of the N cadherin gene or overexpression of tumor necrosis factor (TNF)-α, have provided promising new models of IBD. These novel systems may help clarify the etiology and pathogenesis of these disorders and aid in the design of new therapeutic agents.

EPIDEMIOLOGY   There are marked geographic differences in the incidence of IBD. The highest incidence rates are found in northern Europe and North America among Caucasians, ranging from 2 to 10/100,000. Prevalence of ulcerative colitis in these regions is 37–246 cases/100,000 person-years, and Crohn's disease is 26–199 cases/100,000. The incidence of IBD in southern Europe, Asia, and the developing world is low but has been rising. IBD appears to be more common in Jews of European or Ashkenazic origin, but not of Sephardic (African and Mediterranean) origin. The peak age of onset is from 15–25 yr, and a second peak between 55 and 65 yr of age has been suggested. There is a slight female predominance in the prevalence of both disorders. Although the disease is most common in Caucasians, the incidence in African Americans appears to be increasing, and in some pediatric studies reaches that of Caucasians.

Asian and Hispanic Americans continue to have a lower incidence of IBD. Environmental risk factors include cigarette smoking, which increases the risk of Crohn's disease but appears to be protective in ulcerative colitis. Other studies support the possible involvement of mycobacteria in Crohn's disease pathogenesis.

CROHN'S DISEASE

Location of Disease, Signs, and Symptoms   Crohn's disease can affect any part of the gastrointestinal tract. The most frequently involved sites are the ileocolon (40%), the small intestine alone (30%), or the colon alone (25%). Other regions of the gastrointestinal tract may also be involved, including the mouth, esophagus, and stomach. Anal involvement is common. Inflammation may involve the bowel in a segmental fashion, with "skip" areas of normal small and large intestine intermixed with patches of inflamed mucosa. Symptoms resulting from the inflammatory process include abdominal pain (especially in the right lower quadrant owing to terminal ileal involvement) and diarrhea. Other frequent symptoms include fever, weight loss, and malaise. A variety of extraintestinal manifestations including arthritis, uveitis/iritis, and skin diseases such as erythema nodosum and pyoderma gangrenosum are associated with IBD. Signs of active Crohn's disease include right lower quadrant abdominal fullness, mass or tenderness, and a chronically ill appearance.

There are multiple causes of diarrhea in Crohn's disease. Enhanced secretion occurs in the small bowel and colon because of inflammation. Patients with ileal disease or ileal resection may malabsorb bile salts, as specific receptors and transport proteins are expressed only in the ileum. Unabsorbed bile acids then enter the colon in which they produce a secretory diarrhea. Extensive terminal ileal involvement or resection of greater than 100 cm of ileum results in fatty acid diarrhea because of excessive loss of bile salts that cannot be replaced by enhanced hepatic production. Fat malabsorption may also result from bacterial overgrowth because of strictures of the small bowel leading to deconjugation of bile salts. Crohn's disease has also been associated with lactase deficiency, resulting in maldigestion of milk and milk products. Undigested lactose then produces an osmotic diarrhea.

Complications   The transmural inflammatory process characteristic of Crohn's disease leads to many complications. Inflammation may lead to ulceration through all layers of the bowel, resulting in the formation of fistulous tracts. Fistulas can form between the gut and any neighboring organ. Enteroenteric, enterocolonic, and enterocutaneous fistulas are frequently found in Crohn's disease. Less common are enterovesicular and enterovaginal fistulae. Strictures of the small or large bowel may result from chronic inflammation and can lead to intestinal obstruction. If severe and unremitting despite conservative management, strictures may require surgical resection to permit the continuation of normal enteral nutrition.

Perforation of the small bowel or colon may precipitate the onset of an acute abdomen requiring immediate surgical intervention. Alternatively, perforations and fistulas may produce intra-abdominal abscesses, another common complication of Crohn's disease. Abscesses may occur anywhere in the peritoneal cavity and must be drained to control sepsis.

Patients who have undergone surgical resection or who have extensive small bowel inflammation, fistulas, or strictures may suffer from short bowel syndrome with excessive diarrhea, volume loss, and malabsorption. These patients frequently require treatment with total parenteral nutrition to maintain a normal nutritional and fluid and electrolyte status. As indicated, loss of functional ileum may lead to fat malabsorption. Because of these complications, surgery is avoided whenever possible.

Kidney stones are most frequently made up of oxalate and are found in patients with ileal disease and fat malabsorption. Calcium, which normally binds to oxalate to produce insoluble calcium oxalate, is instead bound by fatty acids. This leads to the formation of sodium oxalate, which is readily absorbed through the colon, leading to hyperoxaluria and stone formation.

ULCERATIVE COLITIS

Location of Disease, Signs, and Symptoms   Ulcerative colitis is characterized by a continuous mucosal inflammatory process affecting the colon. Inflammation may be confined to the rectum alone (ulcerative proctitis), may extend from the rectum to the left colon, or may involve the entire colon. Unlike Crohn's disease, at least part of the rectum is always involved and the inflammatory process is continuous in affected areas (i.e., there are no "skip" regions). Abdominal pain, diarrhea, and gastrointestinal bleeding are common clinical presentations of this disorder. Anorexia and weight loss are occasionally present but are not common. Unlike Crohn's disease, which frequently follows a low-grade, chronic course, ulcerative colitis patients may present with fulminant colitis necessitating urgent colectomy. Physical findings include abdominal tenderness and grossly bloody stool on rectal examination. In fulminant cases, abdominal distention, massive hemorrhage, fever, and tachycardia may be present.

Complications   *Toxic megacolon* may occur in patients with acute fulminant colitis. The colon becomes atonic and dilated resulting from severe inflammation and can perforate if untreated. Toxic megacolon requires emergent surgical consultation and in many cases, removal of the colon. *Strictures* may result from chronic inflammation. *Colon cancer* is an important complication of long-standing ulcerative colitis. Although the precise risk of colon cancer is not clear, it is increased in patients with disease for greater than 8–10 yr, and is higher in patients with pancolitis compared with left-sided colitis alone. To prevent colon cancer either prophylactic colectomy or yearly colonoscopic screening for dysplasia/cancer is recommended depending on the patient's preference and disease activity. An important advance has been the development of the ileoanal anastomosis. Instead of an ileostomy, bowel continuity is maintained by creating an ileal reservoir in place of the rectum. This has led to greater acceptance for surgical options in the treatment of ulcerative colitis.

Extraintestinal Manifestations   There are multiple extraintestinal manifestations of IBD, including arthritis, skin and ocular diseases, liver involvement, kidney stones, and osteoporosis. The arthritic complaints include colitic arthritis, ankylosing spondylitis, and sacroiliitis. The large joints are generally involved in colitic arthritis. Arthritic complaints generally respond to adequate treatment of the bowel disease. Symptoms resulting from ankylosing spondylitis and sacroiliitis may be severe and more refractory to treatment. Skin manifestations of IBD include pyoderma gangrenosum and erythema nodosum. Ocular diseases are predominantly uveitis and episcleritis. Liver involvement may manifest as sclerosing cholangitis or pericholangitis. Cholesterol gallstones occur in Crohn's disease if there is ileal involvement or after resection, resulting in bile salt malabsorption. Finally, kidney stones may form in patients with small intestinal Crohn's disease and fat malabsorption, and are usually made up of calcium oxalate or urate. Osteoporosis may result from chronic fat malabsorption leading to calcium and vitamin D deficiency and from chronic corticosteroid therapy.

DIAGNOSIS

History and Physical Examinations A history of bloody diarrhea, abdominal pain, and fever should lead to a strong suspicion for ulcerative colitis. Symptoms in Crohn's disease are frequently more indolent and chronic, including intermittent diarrhea and fevers, abdominal pain, and weight loss. Physical findings in ulcerative colitis may include abdominal tenderness, and in fulminant disease, distention, decreased bowel sounds and an acute abdomen. In Crohn's disease, abdominal tenderness and an inflammatory abdominal mass may be present, particularly in the right lower quadrant. The perianal and perirectal regions should be examined for signs of fistulization and abscess. Signs of extraintestinal disease, including arthritis, ocular inflammation, and skin nodules or ulcers may be detected.

Laboratory and Pathological Examinations There is no specific laboratory test that is diagnostic of ulcerative colitis or Crohn's disease. An elevated white blood cell count can be seen in active disease or may be an indicator of sepsis because of perforation or abscess formation in Crohn's disease. Anemia may result from gastrointestinal bleeding or nutrient deficiencies (e.g., vitamin B12 owing to ileal Crohn's disease, decreased iron absorption in duodenal Crohn's disease). Erythrocyte sedimentation rate may be elevated in active disease. Nutritional parameters such as blood total protein and albumin levels may also be deranged in Crohn's disease.

Pathological specimens (endoscopic biopsies or surgical resection) may reveal evidence of active inflammation. Characteristic of colitis are crypt abscesses, in which neutrophils invade the crypts. Granulomas are more characteristic of Crohn's disease. Crypt atrophy and distortion are also seen, as is acute and chronic inflammation with lymphocytes and eosinophils, and mucin depletion. Ulceration of the mucosa occurs in ulcerative colitis, but the presence of transmural inflammation is most characteristic of Crohn's disease.

Radiological and Endoscopic Studies Evaluation of the mucosa for the presence of active disease can be achieved by endoscopic examination. In patients with symptoms of colitis, colonoscopy may aid in the initial diagnosis and is required to determine the extent of disease activity. The mucosal surface is observed for the presence of erythema, edema, granularity, friability, and ulceration. The extent of colonic involvement may help differentiate Crohn's disease from ulcerative colitis. The presence of "skip" areas, in which normal mucosa is intermixed with inflamed mucosa, is most characteristic of Crohn's disease, whereas in ulcerative colitis, inflammation is continuous. During colonoscopy, the terminal ileum may be entered and evaluated for involvement by Crohn's disease. Direct visualization of the upper gastrointestinal tract by routine upper endoscopy or small bowel enteroscopy may also help to establish the presence of Crohn's disease.

Radiological examination is an important part of the diagnostic evaluation of patients with IBD. Contrast studies are useful for detecting strictures and fistulae, as well as assessing disease activity in regions of the small intestine that are inaccessible to routine endoscopy. Patients with ulcerative colitis may demonstrate typical findings on barium enema, including straightening and shortening of the colon, loss of normal haustrations, and inflammatory polyps or malignancy. Mucosal detail is more difficult to assess with radiography, and endoscopic examination is generally preferred. In patients with very active colitis, radiographic examination is avoided because of the fear of inducing toxic megacolon owing to the introduction of air and barium. Similarly, colonoscopic testing is performed with caution and usually in a limited manner. Computerized axial tomographic scanning is an important diagnostic modality particularly for abscess detection in Crohn's disease. If accessible, CT-directed drainage of abscess collections may be performed.

GENETIC BASIS As confirmed by the discovery of the *CARD15/NOD2* gene mutation that confers susceptibility to Crohn's disease (*see* IBD Gene Discovery), genetic factors clearly play a role in the pathogenesis of IBD. Genetic predisposition to Crohn's disease was suggested by studies indicating an increased incidence in families, specific ethnic groups, and in twins. Of patients with IBD, approx 10–20% have a family history, and the risk for first degree relatives to develop IBD is 2–5%. Twin studies indicate that monozygotic twins have a higher concordance rate than dizygotic twins. The complex clinical manifestations of these diseases suggest a heterogeneous genetic basis.

MOLECULAR PATHOPHYSIOLOGY The etiology of the IBDs is unknown. One widely accepted hypothesis is that IBD results from an abnormal host immune response to normal gut components such as microflora, nutrients, or cellular constituents. Intestinal bacterial flora is postulated to be particularly important in activating the mucosal immune system in IBD. This may also be accompanied by a primary defect in gut permeability that allows antigens to nonspecifically "leak" through the mucosa and thereby stimulate an inflammatory response.

IBD GENE DISCOVERY: CARD15 AND IBD SUSCEPTIBILITY GENES A major advance in the study of Crohn's disease pathophysiology has been the identification of *CARD15/NOD2* as the first Crohn's susceptibility gene. *CARD15/NOD2*: encodes an intracellular protein that is involved in bacterial detection via peptidoglycan recognition. *CARD15/NOD2*: may play an important role in generating a protective response following exposure to bacteria. There are three genetic variants associated with Crohn's disease; 10–30% of patients with Crohn's disease are heterozygotes for one of these variants, and a smaller percentage of patients are homozygous or compound heterozygotes for these mutations. Yet, even homozygotes have only a 1 in 25 risk for developing disease, indicating the requirement for additional genetic and/or environmental factors. Interestingly, *CARD15/NOD2*: mutations are most consistently associated with the presence of ileal disease.

Other susceptibility loci for IBD have been identified by whole genome scanning techniques. There are presently seven loci, termed IBD1-7, that meet linkage criteria. These chromosomal regions include, for example, human leukocyte antigen (HLA) and cytokine gene clusters, which have been postulated to fit the role of disease susceptibility genes. However, the specific genes and mutations have not been identified.

Animal Models of IBD The specific role of a gene can be determined in the whole animal in "loss of function" experiments that utilize embryonic stem cell techniques. Mutations in specific target genes can be created in these cells to delete the gene or produce a sequence that encodes a nonfunctional protein. The mutated stem cells are injected into a mouse blastocyst and grown in a host mouse. Heterozygous mice are then backcrossed to create homozygous mutants.

In this manner, targeted deletion of various immune mediator genes has been performed. Interestingly, when interleukin (IL)-2, IL-10, major histocompatibility complex (MHC) class II or T-cell receptor α- or β-genes are deleted, gross inflammation of the bowel is produced in mice. IL-2 is produced by activated T cells and is an important regulator of immune responses. It increases T-cell

Table 56-1
Comparison of Crohn's Disease and Ulcerative Colitis

Clinical feature	Crohn's disease	Ulcerative colitis
Site of involvement	Entire gastrointestinal tract	Colon only
Pathology	Transmural inflammation, granulomas	Mucosal inflammation
Extraintestinal manifestations	Skin	Skin
	Eyes	Eyes
	Joints	Joints
Complications	Strictures, fistulae, abscesses	Strictures, colon cancer, toxic megacolon
Treatment	Surgical removal of diseased segments avoided because of disease recurrence	Surgical removal of diseased colon is curative

proliferation, leads to differentiation of B cells, and activates macrophages, natural killer cells, and lymphokine-activated killer cells. IL-10 is produced by T-helper cell subset 2, macrophages, keratinocytes, Ly-1 B cells, and thymocytes. It increases MHC class-II expression on B cells, and suppresses macrophage activation in vitro. IL-10 inhibits IL-1, IL-6, and TNF-α production by activated macrophages. Deletion of the IL-2 or IL-10 gene produces inflammation of the intestine, but with different clinical features. Deletion of IL-2 led to colonic disease, with diarrhea, rectal prolapse, and bleeding. Pathological examination of the colon showed crypt abscesses, ulceration, goblet cell depletion, and epithelial dysplasia. MHC class-II expression, normally limited to the small intestine, was seen in the colon. In contrast, deletion of IL-10 led to a chronic enterocolitis affecting the entire gastrointestinal tract with growth retardation and iron deficiency anemia. Mucosal inflammation with villus loss, mucosal gastrointestinal erosions, and crypt hyperplasia were found in small intestine and colon. MHC class-II expression was aberrantly enhanced in a small bowel and colonic epithelium. The onset of disease in the majority of mice was relatively rapid; by 3–4 wk, growth retardation was noted.

Interestingly, in both models, maintenance in a pathogen-free environment greatly diminished the intestinal inflammation. IL-10 mice had disease limited to the proximal colon only, and IL-2 mice were free of disease. A third model of IBD was generated in T-cell receptor α- or β-mutants, which lack αβ-T cells. These mice developed colonic inflammation but no diarrhea or bleeding. TNF has been implicated as a key pathogenic mediator in Crohn's disease and a model of TNF overexpression has been developed. These TNF$^{\Delta ARE}$ mice bear an endogenous deletion in the 3'AU rich region in the TNF gene resulting in high circulating TNF levels. These mice develop a specific Crohn's disease-like phenotype with chronic transmural ileitis.

Not only can immune cell defects produce intestinal inflammation, but disruption of the protective epithelial barrier may also lead to IBD. A dominant-negative N-cadherin mutant was linked to an intestine specific promoter and thus was selectively disrupted in the gut, in villus as well as crypt cells. This resulted in markedly decreased expression of E-cadherin with gross disruption of the epithelial barrier and severe mucosal inflammation. The small intestine was selectively affected with lymphoid hyperplasia, blunted villi, cryptitis and crypt abscesses, mucosal ulcerations, and eventually adenoma formation.

Although these models of IBD are diverse, they support several hypotheses regarding the etiology of these disorders. Disruption of the epithelial barrier can lead to intestinal inflammation even in the presence of a normal immune system. Selective immune defects that lead to the unopposed action of B cells can produce inflammation of the gut. Also the intestine is clearly vulnerable to inflammation because of constant external antigen exposure and the presence of luminal substances.

MANAGEMENT

Medical Therapy   Because the underlying cause of IBD is still unknown, therapy is presently directed toward controlling the intestinal inflammatory response (Table 56-1). One of the mainstays of treatment is oral and enema compounds containing 5-aminosalicylic acid (5-ASA), available in several different forms. These compounds are effective in the treatment of mild-to-moderate ulcerative or Crohn's colitis as single agents. They are used in conjunction with corticosteroids in the treatment of severe disease. Although their precise mechanism of action is unknown, they are thought to inhibit leukotriene synthesis via their inhibition of neutrophil lipoxygenase, particularly leukotriene B4. *Sulfasalazine* was the first of these agents and consists of 5-ASA bound to a sulfapyridine residue to prevent its premature absorption in the small intestine. Colonic bacteria are required to release the 5-ASA component. However, many side effects result predominantly from the sulfapyridine component, including dose-related effects, such as headache, nausea, vomiting, anorexia, fever, and rash. Idiosyncratic, hypersensitivity responses include rash, hemolytic and aplastic anemia, and agranulocytosis. Also, long-term usage in young men is frequently limited by its adverse effects on sperm count and morphology. Therefore, several compounds have been formulated containing 5-ASA alone, with various modifications to facilitate its delivery to the small intestine and colon, or preferentially to the ileum and colon, without excessive systemic absorption before reaching its preferred site. These include *Pentasa*, *Asacol*, and *Dipentum*. Pentasa and Asacol are released by pH-dependent mechanisms. Pentasa is an ethylcellulose-coated form of mesalamine (5-ASA) that is released throughout the small intestine and colon. Asacol is coated with an acrylic-based resin that dissolves at pH 7.0 or greater, facilitating its release only at the terminal ileum and colon. Dipentum consists of two 5-ASA molecules linked by an azo bond that is cleaved in the colon. These newer formulations clearly have fewer side effects than sulfasalazine and, thus, have led to an expanded pharmacological armamentarium. Mesalamine in enema form (Rowasa enemas) is a valuable treatment for ulcerative proctitis.

Corticosteroids are important in the therapy of moderate to severe IBD because of their broad anti-inflammatory actions. They are used in the treatment of active ulcerative colitis as well as Crohn's disease of the small and large bowel. Owing to the numerous side effects attendant with chronic glucocorticoid usage, long-term therapy for IBD is avoided. There is no data supporting its use in maintaining disease remission, unlike 5-aminosalicylate containing compounds in colitis.

Antibiotics are critical for the treatment of infectious complications of Crohn's disease, such as sepsis, abscess formation, and small bowel bacterial overgrowth. Metronidazole has been used successfully to treat perianal disease and colonic Crohn's disease. With the recognition of the importance of bacterial flora in Crohn's pathogenesis, antibiotics have increasingly been used as treatment for active disease.

Immunosuppressive agents such as azathioprine and its metabolite, 6-mercaptopurine, are used in Crohn's disease and to a lesser extent, in ulcerative colitis, for steroid-dependent and poorly controlled patients. Treatment is generally begun in patients who cannot be tapered from corticosteroids because of recurrent symptoms and who have major side effects, such as osteoporosis, hypertension, cataracts, glucose intolerance, and so on. Alternatively, immunosuppressive agents may be added to treat the patient with refractory disease inadequately treated with corticosteroid and 5-ASA compounds. Immunosuppressive agents are also used in patients with ulcerative colitis and refractory proctitis, but less commonly.

Other agents for active ulcerative colitis and Crohn's disease include methotrexate and cyclosporine. There are data that support the use of intravenous cyclosporine for severe colitis as a last-ditch medical effort to avoid surgical intervention. Methotrexate may be used as an alternative medication for steroid-dependent patients to induce and maintain a steroid-free remission.

The addition of infliximab, a chimeric monoclonal antibody to human TNF-α, has remarkably expanded the Crohn's disease treatment repertoire and is an excellent example of how understanding the molecular pathophysiology of disease leads to improved treatment regimens. As indicated, TNF is a major proinflammatory immune regulator with a prominent role in Crohn's disease. Infliximab infusion can induce remission in refractory Crohn's disease and can heal fistulous disease. Optimal treatment regimens, designed to maximize efficacy and minimize side effects, are being developed. This drug has been approved to maintain remission in Crohn's disease.

Surgical Treatment In fulminant ulcerative colitis that is refractory to medical therapy, total colectomy may be unavoidable. In addition, surgical resection may be required for corticosteroid-dependent patients with ulcerative colitis who have major steroid-induced side effects. Colectomy may also be performed in patients with colonic dysplasia or carcinoma, or prophylactically to prevent colon cancer in patients with >10 yr history of active ulcerative colitis. As an alternative to prophylactic colectomy, yearly colonoscopic screening for colon cancer may be performed after 8–10 yr of disease. The major problems with this approach are that cancers in ulcerative colitis arise from flat mucosa and, therefore, may be missed and accurate grading of dysplasia is difficult. Colectomy is curative in ulcerative colitis and ileoanal anastomotic procedures eliminate the need for an

ileostomy. This surgical procedure is not an option for patients with Crohn's disease, as there is a high incidence of recurrent disease in the ileal pouch leading to diarrhea, bleeding, pain, severe malfunction of the pouch, and eventually, the need for revision. In addition, surgery is *not* curative in Crohn's disease because it recurs commonly in all parts of the intestinal tract. Therefore, the approach to patients with Crohn's disease is very cautious and surgical intervention is avoided whenever possible. However, limited resection is often performed to relieve obstruction resulting from strictures to repair perforations or for abscess drainage.

FUTURE DIRECTIONS Significant research developments include the generation of animal models that recapitulate many of the features of human IBD, the identification of CARD15 mutations in CD, and the localization of new chromosomal susceptibility loci for IBD. The novel mouse models have proven useful for elucidating the pathogenesis of these disorders and for designing more effective therapies. The identification of the gene(s) that are responsible for the familial risk of IBD will undoubtedly continue to be a major research focus, as the key to developing new diagnostic and therapeutic approaches.

CELIAC SPRUE

Celiac sprue (also called celiac disease or gluten-sensitive enteropathy) is a chronic disease of the small intestinal mucosa resulting from exposure to dietary proteins contained in wheat, rye, and barley. The alcohol soluble component of wheat-derived gluten, or gliadin, and similar proteins derived from rye, barley, and oats, are toxic to the mucosa of susceptible individuals. In classic celiac sprue, the small bowel demonstrates complete villus atrophy and marked crypt hyperplasia, resulting in malabsorption and diarrhea. It is clear that specific host genetic factors are required in combination with exposure to gliadin to damage the epithelium. Linkage to histocompatibility antigen loci has been recognized for many years. The antigen recognized by the antiendomysial antibody has been identified as tissue transglutaminase. Data suggest that deamidation of gliadin proteins by tissue transglutaminase is required for the generation of epitopes that are recognized by CD4+ T cells. A specific 33 amino acid peptide has been identified that is derived from alpha gliadin by digestion with gastric and pancreatic enzymes, is not further proteolyzed into smaller fragments despite continued exposure to these enzymes, reacts with tissue transglutaminase and induces gut-derived T cells from patients with celiac sprue. These discoveries may have therapeutic implications to permit the development of a novel, antigen-specific immunotherapy.

CLINICAL PRESENTATION Patients with celiac sprue exhibit a broad spectrum of clinical presentations. In children, the disease tends to occur in the first 3 yr of life. In adults, the peak incidence is in the third decade, but may occur at any age. In the classic clinical presentation, extensive loss of normal villi throughout the small intestine leads to gross malabsorption and steatorrhea, severe weight loss, wasting, multiple vitamin deficiencies, and abdominal distention. The vitamin deficiencies may lead to anemia (B12, folate, iron), or a bleeding diathesis (vitamin K). Neurological symptoms such as peripheral neuropathy and paresthesias are also common. In other cases, patients may be asymptomatic or complain only of mild abdominal discomfort, malaise, bloating, and diarrhea. Those with more patchy proximal intestinal involvement may present simply with iron or folate deficiency, or osteomalacia. Relatives of patients with celiac sprue who are screened for the disease often have mild illness or may be completely asymptomatic.

Celiac sprue is frequently associated with other disorders. Dermatitis herpetiformis is characterized by severely pruritic papulovesicular lesions of the skin. The majority of afflicted patients show intestinal biopsy findings characteristic of celiac sprue. These patients are often only mildly affected by the gut lesion and may even be asymptomatic. Isolated nutrient deficiencies may be the only clinical manifestation. Both the intestinal and skin lesions resolve with gluten withdrawal.

Other diseases that are associated with celiac sprue include insulin-dependent diabetes mellitus (50-fold higher incidence of celiac disease in patients with diabetes), thyroid disease, and selective IgA deficiency, which share similar HLA haplotypes. Complications of celiac sprue include the development of T-cell lymphoma or other gastrointestinal malignancies. Ulcerative jejunoileitis is a serious complication resulting in ulceration and stricture of the small bowel with bleeding, perforation, and obstruction. Finally, patients may become refractory to removal of gluten from the diet and may require treatment with corticosteroids or immunosuppressive agents.

EPIDEMIOLOGY Celiac sprue is most prevalent in Caucasians, particularly in Northern Europe. The highest prevalence has been reported in Ireland at a frequency of 1/300 but the more typical incidence in Europe is 1–2/10,000 population. Asians from India and Pakistan are also frequently affected, but the disease is rare in Japanese, Chinese, and Africans. A study of Minnesota residents who were symptomatic and had celiac sprue documented by biopsy and response to a gluten-free diet revealed an incidence of celiac sprue of 1.2/100,000 person-years in the United States, with a prevalence of 21.8/100,000. Studies have indicated a decrease in the prevalence of childhood celiac sprue in several European countries, perhaps because of changes in feeding or other unidentified environmental factors.

DIAGNOSIS A valuable test for the diagnosis of celiac sprue is the small intestinal biopsy. Forceps biopsies of the duodenum or proximal jejunum can be obtained during routine upper endoscopy or peroral capsule biopsy techniques may be used. Biopsy should be performed before the initiation of gluten withdrawal and can also be repeated after removal of gluten from the diet to document an adequate response. Typical findings on biopsy are absence or atrophy of villi, crypt elongation and hyperplasia, and increased immune cell infiltrate. There is a marked increase in intraepithelial lymphocytes and infiltration of the lamina propria with lymphocytes, eosinophils, and macrophages. Because the biopsy findings in celiac sprue are not unique and can be seen in tropical sprue, lymphoma, viral or eosinophilic gastroenteritis, common variable immunodeficiency, or parasitic infection, the clinical response to removal of gluten in conjunction with biopsy is critical for definitively making the diagnosis. Rechallenge with gluten and rebiopsy is rarely recommended (except in equivocal cases).

Antibody tests are used in conjunction with small bowel biopsy to confirm the diagnosis. Serum antigliadin antibodies are positive in approx 90% of patients with untreated sprue but are also found in other disorders such as sarcoidosis and rheumatoid arthritis. Antiendomysial antibodies, which are recognized to be directed against the autoantigen tissue transglutaminase, are also elevated in patients with histological abnormalities on biopsy, detecting more than 95% of untreated patients. Tissue transglutaminase antibodies are virtually pathognomonic of celiac disease.

GENETIC BASIS Genetics plays an important role in celiac sprue, but in conjunction with environmental and other factors.

Approximately 8–12% of family members of patients with celiac sprue are also affected, as determined by intestinal biopsy. Interestingly, only 50% of all family members with abnormal biopsies manifest symptoms of the disease. In identical twins, there is 70% concordance for celiac sprue, indicating that factors other than genetics play a role in disease susceptibility.

The linkage of celiac sprue with specific MHC genes has been recognized for years. There is a strong association with HLA class-II haplotypes, particularly HLA DQ2 and HLADQ8. In Northern Europeans, the DR w17 and DQ w2 serological specificities are very common. HLA DQ2 is present in 90% of patients with celiac sprue. Molecular analysis indicates that a specific DQ α- and β-chain molecule encoded by DQA1*0501 and DQB1*0201 is found in 99% of Scandinavians with sprue. In southern European populations, the same HLA-DQ molecule is expressed on an HLA-DR7 and DR5 (or DR11/DR7, DR12/DR7) haplotype, as opposed to HLA DR3, DQ2 (or HLA-DR17) in northern Europeans. These molecules are necessary but not sufficient for developing the disease, because HLA identical siblings have only 40–50% concordance for this disease, and only a small percentage of the population that carries these alleles develops sprue. In addition, some populations do not demonstrate the same very high percentage of patients with HLA-DQ2, but instead are DR4 positive. Sequence analysis of the HLA DQ alleles from patients with celiac disease revealed no mutations when compared with normal individuals. This suggests that molecules encoded in regions outside of this HLA locus are required for generating the disease and there may be different genetic subgroups.

MOLECULAR PATHOPHYSIOLOGY The biochemistry of gluten and gliadin has been intensively studied to identify the protein moieties that are responsible for toxicity. The alcohol soluble component of gluten, gliadin, appears to be responsible for the disease. Several reports have shown that there are three peptides derived from alpha gliadin (located between amino acids 57 and 75, with the sequences PFPQPQLPY, PQPQLPYPQ, and PYPQPQLPY) that are deamidated by tissue transglutaminase and are recognized by CD4+ T cells from patients with celiac disease. Reports suggest that deamidation is required for T-cell stimulation, as it results in the production of negatively charged amino acids that are required for binding to the HLA-DQ2 molecule. A 33 amino acid peptide was identified that is derived from alpha gliadin by digestion with gastric and pancreatic enzymes, is not further proteolyzed into smaller fragments despite continued exposure to these enzymes, reacts with tissue transglutaminase and induces gut-derived T cells from patients with celiac sprue. However, it is likely that other peptides can also induce disease, as indicated by the diversity of antigenic responses in children.

Based on its sequence homology to A-gliadin, another environmental factor that may play a role in the pathogenesis of celiac sprue is a history of adenovirus 12 infection. There is a region of homology between the adenovirus serotype 12 E1b protein to A-gliadin that spans 12 amino acids, with eight identical residues. In addition, almost 90% of patients with untreated celiac sprue had serological evidence of prior adenovirus 12 infection, compared with only 17% of disease controls. These data suggest that mechanisms of molecular mimicry may be involved in the pathogenesis of this disorder, in which T cells recognize peptides in common to gliadin and viral proteins. However, adenovirus 12 DNA has not been detected in intestinal samples, and peptide challenge with an oligopeptide derived from the homologous region has not been shown to produce intestinal injury.

MANAGEMENT Removal of all gluten from the diet is the primary therapy for celiac sprue. Wheat, rye, oats, and barley-containing products must be eliminated from the diet because gluten and other related prolamins can produce injury. This restricted diet must be maintained lifelong. Patients may initially exhibit lactose intolerance because of villus atrophy and brush border enzyme deficiency, but this should resolve with treatment.

DISORDERS OF SMALL INTESTINAL ABSORPTION AND TRANSPORT

The brush border of the small intestinal enterocyte contains disaccharidases, peptidases, and transport proteins that are responsible for the absorption of ingested nutrients. Progress has been made in clarifying the molecular basis of several disorders characterized by selective malabsorption of carbohydrates or lipids. This section presents a summary of advances in understanding the pathophysiology underlying several of the more common of these defects.

LACTASE DEFICIENCY

Clinical Features and Epidemiology Lactase is one of the best-studied of the brush border enzymes. It is responsible for the hydrolysis of lactose into glucose and galactose. Several clinical categories of lactase deficiency have been described. Congenital lactase deficiency is a rare autosomal-recessive disorder, resulting in milk intolerance from birth. Much more common is the onset of diminished enzyme activity in childhood or adolescence and lasting into adulthood, also known as adult-onset hypolactasia. Loss of brush border lactase activity may also result from other small intestinal disorders, such as Crohn's disease, celiac sprue, viral illnesses, or other infections.

Loss of lactase activity beginning in childhood/adolescence occurs in the majority of humans throughout the world except for Caucasian populations. In particular, most white northern Europeans and their descendants in North America and Australia (populations that were traditionally cattle farmers and thus persistent milk drinkers) retain high lactase activity lifelong. The prevalence of lactase deficiency throughout the world supports the hypothesis that the decline in lactase activity with age is a normal event in response to weaning, common to all land mammals. Persistence of lactase activity has therefore been postulated to be the result of a genetic mutation that occurred in milk-drinking populations, leading to a survival advantage because milk-drinkers might be healthier.

Ingestion of milk and milk products in deficient individuals leads to abdominal pain, diarrhea, bloating, and excessive flatulence because of unabsorbed lactose in the lumen. This results in increased small bowel fluid. Fermentation of lactose in the colon produces hydrogen, methane, and carbon dioxide gas. Removal of lactose-containing products in the diet leads to resolution of these symptoms.

Diagnosis A *lactose tolerance test* may be performed, which consists of administering 50 g of lactose orally. If sufficient lactase activity is present, blood glucose levels will rise by more than 20 mg/dL during a 2-h period. Lactase deficiency is diagnosed by the lack of serum glucose elevation and frequently, the onset of symptoms of malabsorption, with gas, diarrhea, bloating, and abdominal pain. If the serum glucose increases yet symptoms also occur, one must consider occult diabetes mellitus. Alternatively, a

trial of dietary lactose avoidance may be attempted. After restriction of oral intake of milk and milk products, the patient is assessed for symptom resolution. Finally, small bowel biopsy allows for definitive diagnosis, but is unnecessary given the adequacy of the other two approaches.

Genetic Basis and Molecular Pathophysiology As determined by population and family studies, adult-onset hypolactasia is an autosomal-recessive trait, and persistence of lactase activity is autosomal-dominant. The molecular basis for lactase persistence/nonpersistence has been the subject of intensive investigation. In the majority of studies, lactase-specific activity and protein levels correlate very well with mRNA, indicating transcriptional regulation of lactase expression. A single-nucleotide polymorphism located at −14 Kb upstream from the start of lactase transcription, in the intron of another neighboring gene known as minichromosome maintenance (which plays a role in cell-cycle control), is highly associated with lactase persistence in Finnish populations. Individuals with low lactase activity were homozygous for a cytidine at this site, whereas lactase persistent individuals had either C/T or T/T. Another association was noted at a single-nucleotide polymorphism at −22018, with a G to A substitution. These substitutions were also associated with higher levels of lactase mRNA expression. Thus *cis*-acting elements appear to be responsible for the persistence/nonpersistence phenotype, based on differences in level of expression of lactase from one allele compared with the other. Studies have also focused on characterizing transacting factors that regulate lactase expression, because, for example, levels of NF-LPH-1, an intestine-specific transactivator that binds to a sequence close to the TATA box, are high in newborn pigs with high lactase activity and low in adult pigs with low lactase activity. Still other data suggest that there is a second phenotype of lactase deficiency, in which post-translational processing of lactase-phlorizin is altered. Thus, the precise molecular mechanisms underlying lactase persistence/nonpersistence are under investigation.

Management The treatment of symptomatic lactase deficiency consists of removal of lactose-containing nutrients from the diet (Table 56-2) and/or the use of oral enzyme replacement therapy. It is preferable to continue some milk and dairy food ingestion because of their rich calcium stores, especially in children and in women who are prone to osteoporosis. Lactase oral preparations are available in capsules or tablets and can be chewed. Replacement pills are taken with meals and titrated to diminish symptoms. Lactase may also be added directly to milk and ingested after an overnight incubation, or pretreated milk can be purchased.

Future Directions The ready availability of oral lactase capsules and the ease of treatment of symptoms by dietary avoidance or supplementation makes more sophisticated approaches to treatment, such as gene therapy, unnecessary. The major research interest still lies in determining how epidemiological observations are linked to genetics; i.e., what are the genetic alterations that lead to lactase persistence in the milk-drinking populations of the world, and are there differences among different ethnic or racial groups. These are questions of great interest to population and evolutionary geneticists.

GLUCOSE–GALACTOSE MALABSORPTION

Clinical Features Glucose–galactose malabsorption is a rare congenital disorder in which enterocytic transport of glucose and galactose is absent, because of mutation of the gene encoding the

Table 56-2
Medical Therapy for Inflammatory Bowel Disease

5-Aminosalicylic acid compounds
  Sulfasalazine (Azulfidine)
  Mesalamine
    Oral (Pentasa, Asacol, Dipentum)
    Enema (Rowasa)
    Suppository (Rowasa)

Glucocorticoids
  Oral
  Enema
  Suppository
  Intravenous

Antibiotics
  Metronidazole

Immunosuppressive agents
  Azathioprine
  6-Mercaptopurine
  Cyclosporine
    Oral
    Enema
    Intravenous
  Methotrexate
    Intramuscular
    Oral
    Infliximals

Na$^+$/glucose cotransporter sodium glucose transporter (SGLT)-1. This disease is characterized by the onset of profuse watery diarrhea in newborns that responds to the removal of dietary sources of glucose and galactose. Diarrhea usually develops within 4 d of birth. The diarrhea is so severe that dehydration is frequent. As in other diseases of carbohydrate absorption, the presence of unabsorbed sugars leads to an increase osmotic load in the small intestine with increased luminal fluid. Laboratory findings include an acidic stool pH because of colonic bacterial metabolism of unabsorbed sugar. In addition, sugar is found in the urine, consistent with the expression of SGLT-1 in the kidney. Oral monosaccharide tolerance tests reveal that absorption of glucose and galactose but not fructose is impaired.

Genetics and Molecular Pathophysiology Glucose–galactose malabsorption is an autosomal-recessive disease. The precise incidence of this disorder has not been determined but it is clearly rare, as indicated by the few case reports in the literature. Frequently, there is a history of consanguineous marriage.

Expression cloning of the cDNA that encodes SGLT-1, the Na$^+$/glucose cotransporter provided a major breakthrough in understanding pathophysiology of this disorder. Specific mutations in SGLT-1 lead to loss of transporter function in humans, resulting in glucose and galactose malabsorption. Analysis of cDNA reverse transcribed from RNA from intestinal biopsies of two affected sisters showed a single missense mutation, with a single base change from G to A at position 92, changing an aspartate to an asparagine. Their parents were heterozygous for this mutation. The autosomal-recessive inheritance of this disorder was confirmed. The mutant SGLT1 mRNA was expressed in *Xenopus laevis* oocytes and compared with the normal SGLT1 mRNA for ability to transport a glucose analog, α-methyl-D-glucopyranoside. As anticipated, the mutant SGLT1 demonstrated no detectable transport activity.

Subsequently, 30 other patients have been screened for mutations in SGLT1. The mutations included missense, nonsense, and frameshift mutations, and some occurred in splice sites at intron–exon boundaries. Two areas were identified as "hot spots" for missense mutations, between residues 289–304 and 369–405. Analysis of the mutant proteins indicated that loss of transporter activity was owing either to the production of truncated or nonfunctional protein, to defective trafficking of the transporter, or to defects in the transport cycle. The SGLT1 gene has been localized to chromosome 22 on the distal q arm.

Management The treatment of glucose–galactose malabsorption is the immediate removal of lactose, glucose, and galactose containing substances from the diet. Fructose is well tolerated, and a fructose-based formula is substituted with rapid resolution of symptoms. There are reports of increasing tolerance to glucose and galactose with age. Rechallenge with small amounts of these sugars may be possible.

Future Directions The cloning of the SGLT-1 cDNA and the identification of naturally occurring mutations has already led to notable advances in the knowledge of the basic mechanisms of sugar transport. The regulation of expression of this and other cotransporters, their mode of insertion in the membrane, and structure–function correlation are all possible to address in the research laboratory. With the identification of the SGLT1 gene, gene therapy may eventually be considered. However, in the near future, this is unlikely because of the relative ease of treatment by elimination diets as well as the rarity of this disorder.

ABETALIPOPROTEINEMIA

Clinical Features Abetalipoproteinemia is a rare disorder, characterized by the absence of apolipoprotein (apo) B containing lipoproteins in plasma. Patients present in infancy with diarrhea resulting from severe fat malabsorption, poor weight gain, and acanthocytosis. Atypical retinitis pigmentosa and spinocerebellar degeneration become apparent at older ages. Ocular symptoms include decreased night and color vision, and neurological signs of ataxia, spastic gait and dysmetria, loss of deep tendon reflexes, and decreased vibratory and proprioceptive sense appear in the second decade. Spontaneous hemorrhage characteristic of a bleeding diathesis may occur because of vitamin K deficiency.

Diagnosis The hallmark of this disorder is an abnormal plasma lipid profile in association with signs of spinocerebellar degeneration and a pigmented retinopathy. Total cholesterol and triglyceride plasma levels are extremely low and there is an absence of apo B containing plasma lipoproteins, including chylomicrons, very low-density lipoproteins, and low-density lipoproteins. Most patients are anemic because of enhanced hemolysis of abnormal red blood cells (acanthocytes). Fat malabsorption leads to deficiency of fat soluble vitamins. In particular, vitamins E, K, and A are affected as they are transported in chylomicrons. Vitamin E deficiency is most severe because its absorption from the intestine, transport to the liver, and circulation in the plasma are dependent on apo B containing lipoproteins. Vitamin E deficiency is clinically important because it is thought to be responsible for the development of neurological and retinal sequelae. Intestinal biopsy reveals lipid laden enterocytes but normal villi, and is useful for distinguishing this disorder from other intestinal illnesses associated with fat malabsorption.

Genetics and Molecular Pathophysiology Abetalipoproteinemia is a rare autosomal-recessive disorder. Consanguinity is common in these families. An absence of plasma lipoproteins containing apo B led to the hypothesis that this disorder is because of a defect in the *apo B* gene. However, linkage between apo B and abetalipoproteinemia in families has not been established by restriction fragment length polymorphism analysis and defects in the *apo B* gene have not been identified. Because assembly or secretion of apo B containing lipoproteins were most likely defective in this disorder, the microsomal triglyceride transport protein (MTP) was examined in affected individuals. This gene, located on chromosome 4q22-24, encodes a protein that catalyzes the transport of triglyceride, cholesteryl ester, and phospholipid between membranes. It is a heterodimer made up of a protein disulphide isomerase and a unique 97-kd subunit that appears to be responsible for the lipid transport activity. This larger subunit shares homology with lipovitellin 1, a member of the lipid-binding lipovitellin complex that serves as a source for lipid in the developing embryo. MTP activity and particularly the 97-kd subunit, normally present in microsomes from liver and intestine, are absent in intestinal biopsies from patients. Sequence analysis of cDNA and genomic DNA from patients with abetalipoproteinemia revealed homozygous frameshift and nonsense mutations in the gene encoding the 88-kd subunit, resulting in truncated proteins. Two missense mutations have also been identified. Analysis of additional patients indicated frameshift and splice site mutations, most of which lead to the formation of a truncated protein. Transfection of Cos-1 cells with mutant MTP cDNAs lacking part of the carboxy terminus shows decreased lipid transfer activity, supporting the hypothesis that alterations of this protein are the primary cause of abetalipoproteinemia.

Management A low-fat diet and supplementation with high doses of vitamin E as well as vitamins A and K are required. In particular, it is critical to avoid vitamin E deficiency as this appears to be the primary cause of the severe and irreversible neurological and ocular changes characteristic of this disease.

Future Directions The cloning of the cDNA encoding the MTP raises the possibility of gene therapy in the future. Although many of the devastating neurological and ocular sequelae may be avoided by high doses of vitamin E, there may be a role for gene replacement in refractory patients. Also, rapid, definitive diagnosis is crucial, so that prenatal screening of siblings may be useful. Finally, because patients with MTP deficiency have very low cholesterol and triglyceride levels, identification of selective inhibitors of its activity may prove a valuable addition to the treatment of hypercholesterolemia.

SELECTED REFERENCES

Ahmad T, Tamboli C, Jewell D, Colombel JF. Clinical relevance of advances in genetics and pharmacogenetics of IBD. Gastroenterology 2004;126(6):1533–1549.

Anderson RP, Dgano P, Godkin AJ, Jewell DP, Hill AVS. In vivo antigen challenge in celiac disease identifies a single transglutaminase-modified peptide as the dominant A-gliadin T-cell epitope. Nat Med 2000;6:337–342.

Berriot-Varoqueaux N, Aggerbeck LP, Samson-Bouma ME, Wetterau JR. The role of the microsomal triglyceride transport protein in abetalipoproteinemia. Annu Rev Nutr 2000;20:663–697.

Boll W, Wagner P, Mantei N. Structure of the chromosomal gene and cDNAs coding for lactase-phlorizin hydrolase in humans with adult-type hypolactasia or persistence of lactase. Am J Hum Genet 1991;48:889–902.

Cho JH, Nicolae Dl, Gold LH. Identification of novel susceptibility loci for inflammatory bowel disease on chromosomes 1p, 3q, and 4q: Evidence for epistasis between 1p and IBD1. Proc Natl Acad Sci USA 1998;95:7502–7507.

Enattah NS, Sahi T, Savilahti E, Terwilliger JD, Peltonen L, Jarvela I. Identification of a variant associated with adult-type hypolactasia. Nat Genet 2002;30:233–237.

Evans L, Grasset E, Heyman M, Dumontier AM, Beau JP, Desjexu JF. Congenital selective malabsorption of glucose and galactose. J Pediatr Gastroenterol Nutr 1985;4:878–886.

Grand RJ, Montgomery RK, Chitkara DK, Hirschhorn JN. Changing genes; losing lactase. Gut 2003;52:621, 622.

Green PHR, Jabri B. Coeliac disease. Lancet 2003;362:383–391.

Hediger MA, Coady MJ, Ikeda TS, Wright EM. Expression cloning and cDNA sequencing of the Na/glucose cotransporter. Nature 1987;330: 379–381.

Hugot JP. Genetic origin of IBD. Inflamm Bowel Dis 2004,10:S11–S15.

Hugot JP, Laurent-Puig P, Gower-Rousseau C, et al. Mapping of a susceptibility locus for Crohn's disease on chromosome 16. Nature 1996; 379(6568):821–823.

Kagnoff MF, Harwood JI, Bugawan TL, Erlich HA. Structural analysis of the HLA-DR, -DQ, and -DP alleles on the celiac disease-associated -DR3 (Drw17) haplotype. Proc Natl Acad Sci USA 1989;86:6274–6278.

Loftus EV. Clincial epidemiology of inflammatory bowel disease: incidence, prevalence and environmental influences. Gastroenterology 2004;126: 1504–1517.

Martin MG, Turk E, Lostao P, Kerner C, Wright EM. Defects in Na/glucose cotransporter (SGLT1) trafficking and function cause glucose-galactose malabsorption. Nat Genet 1996;12:216–220.

Mowat AM. Coeliac disease—a meeting point for genetics, immunology, and protein chemistry. Lancet 2003;361:1290–1292.

Pizarro TT, Arseneau KO, Bamias G, Cominelli F. Mouse models for the study of Crohn's disease. Trends Mol Med 2003;9:218–222.

Rader DJ, Brewer HB. Abetalipoproteinemia: new insights into lipoprotein assembly and vitamin E metabolism from a rare genetic disease. JAMA 1993;270:865–869.

Sadlack B, Merz H, Schorle H, Schimpl A, Feller AC, Horak I. Ulcerative colitis-like disease in mice with a disrupted interleukin-2 gene. Cell 1993;75:253–261.

Shamir R. Advances in celiac disease. Gastroenterol Clin North Am 2003;32:931–947.

Shan L, Molberg O, Parrot I, et al. Structural basis for gluten intolerance in celiac sprue. Science 2002;297:2275–2279.

Sharp D, Blinderman L, Combs KA, et al. Cloning and gene defects in microsomal triglyceride transfer protein associated with abetalipoproteinemia. Nature 1993;365:65–69.

Sollid LM. Coeliac disease: dissecting a complex inflammatory disorder. Nat Rev Immunol 2002;2:647–655.

Strober W, Ehrhardt RO. Chronic intestinal inflammation: an unexpected outcome in cytokine or T cell receptor mutant mice. Cell 1993;75:203–205.

Swallow DM. Genetics of lactase persistence and lactose intolerance. Annu Rev Genet 2003;37:197–219.

Troelsen JT, Olsen J, Noren O, Sjostrom H. A novel intestinal trans-factor (NF-LPH-1) interacts with the lactase-phlorizin hydrolase promoter and co-varies with the enzymatic activity. J Biol Chem 1992;267: 20,407–20,411.

Turk E, Zabel B, Mundlos S, Dyer J, Wright EM. Glucose/galactose malabsorption caused by a defect in the Na+/glucose cotransporter. Nature 1991;350:354–356.

Wetterau JR, Aggerbeck LP, Bouma M, et al. Absence of microsomal triglyceride transfer protein in individuals with abetalipoproteinemia. Science 1992;258:999–1001.

57 The Molecular Mechanisms of *Helicobacter pylori*-Associated Gastroduodenal Disease

PETER B. ERNST

SUMMARY

In 1984, Barry Marshall and Robin Warren proposed a role for *Helicobacter pylori* in gastroduodenal disease leading to an avalanche of research intended to prove or disprove their theory. The result has been a series of advances that have updated our understanding of these diseases and completely modernized the clinical approach to their management. In recognition of this impact, Marshall and Warren received the Nobel Prize for Physiology or Medicine in 2005. This chapter summarizes some important findings that have advanced our knowledge in this field with emphasis on the host response and the immunopathogenesis of gastroduodenal disease.

Key Words: Adaptive immunity; B cells; bacterial colonization; cytokines; epithelium; gastric; immunopathogenesis; innate immunity; persistence; T cells.

INTRODUCTION

In 1984, Marshall and Warren proposed a role for *Helicobacter pylori* in gastroduodenal disease. The result has been a series of advances that have updated the understanding of these diseases and completely changed the clinical approach to their management. Many aspects of the pathogenesis of these diseases have been dissected to the molecular level with key pathogenic mechanisms being validated by the association of some genes with the development of gastric cancer. There has been particular emphasis on understanding the molecular structures associated with the organism and their role in modifying the host responses. The gastric immune and inflammatory response have emerged as key elements in the pathogenesis of gastritis and epithelial cell damage that are accepted as being an integral component in the disease process. This chapter summarizes some of the important findings that have advanced the knowledge in this field, with special emphasis on the host response.

Gastric secretions have evolved to facilitate the acid and peptic degradation of luminal contents. This environment precludes the successful colonization by most micro-organisms but *H. pylori*

From: *Principles of Molecular Medicine, Second Edition*
Edited by: M. S. Runge and C. Patterson © Humana Press, Inc., Totowa, NJ

has evolved to survive in this niche. Although *H. pylori* colonizes the majority of humanity, the lack of colonization by a more diverse flora may have limited the selective pressures shaping the evolution of gastric immune and inflammatory responses. Therefore, most research has focused on the interaction between a single species of bacteria and the host response. This approach has forced investigators to compare their findings in the stomach to observations in other tissues infected with a range of organisms.

Epidemiological studies have provided convincing evidence that *H. pylori* is associated with, and indeed responsible for, several gastroduodenal diseases ranging from a generally benign, subclinical gastritis to peptic ulcers and several types of gastric cancer. Advances from experiments manipulating the organism and examining its interaction in cell lines or animal models have shown that infection activates multiple pathways leading to changes in epithelial cell morphology, tight junctions, cytokines, and epithelial cell turnover. Clearly, the molecular pathogenesis involves many factors and complementary interactions among the bacteria and various elements of the host response.

EPIDEMIOLOGY

The majority of new *H. pylori* infections occur in children; however, in the absence of specific clinical signs associated with infection, the details concerning the mode of transmission are less clear. Vomitus, saliva, and feces are the presumed sources of direct transmission particularly in crowded housing conditions. Generally, infection correlates inversely to socioeconomic conditions as lifetime infection rates in countries with a strong economy have dropped toward 10%, although rates in countries with emerging economies approach 80–90%. Once established, the infection persists for life unless antibiotic therapy is administered.

Most infected individuals experience subclinical gastritis although gastroduodenal ulceration may occur in 10–15% of the infected population. Gastric cancer is less frequent with approx 1% of infected individuals developing adenocarcinoma whereas even less experience gastric maltoma. In fact, *H. pylori* has been recognized as a type-I carcinogen by the World Health Organization. One study has even suggested that *H. pylori* is a necessary condition for noncardia gastric cancer. The geographic distribution of these

***Signaling Pathways Activated in Response to* H. Pylori**
H. pylori infection is linked to the activation of NF-κB and AP-1 in gastric epithelial cell lines by several signaling mechanisms. These include p21-activated kinase 1, which associates with and activates Nck-interacting kinase thereby activating the kinases inhibitor of kappa kinase α and inhibitor of kappa kinase β leading to phosphorylation and degradation of the inhibitory protein IκBα and the release of activated NF-κB. Mitogen-activated protein (MAP) kinase cascades regulate a range of cell functions including proliferation, inflammatory responses and cell survival. *Cag*-positive *H. pylori* activates the extracellular signal-regulated kinase (ERK), Jun n-terminal kinase and p38 MAP kinase pathways, and ERK and p38 regulate IL-8 production in gastric epithelial cells. The VacA toxin is sufficient to induce the phosphorylation of p38 and ERK1/2 although this signaling pathway seems to be independent of the vacuolization induced by this toxin. Kinases such as ERK and p38 can participate in the activation of the transcription factor AP-1 and the regulation of several genes that encode proteins that drive inflammation. FR167653, a p38α MAP kinase inhibitor, reduced both neutrophil infiltration and gastric mucosal injury in *H. pylori*-infected Mongolian gerbils. Thus, not only is p38 MAP kinase important in regulating the host inflammatory response to *H. pylori* infection, but this and other kinases can become therapeutic targets that attenuate inflammation and the ensuing tissue damage associated with infection.

Although infection with intact bacteria stimulates several signaling pathways, more attention is given to the role of specific virulence factors such as those associated with the *cag* PAI because *H. pylori* that carry the *cag* PAI are associated with increased IL-8 expression in gastric mucosal biopsy specimens. The only identified effector protein able to translocate via the *cag* PAI is the CagA protein. Following its translocation into the cytoplasm, CagA is tyrosine phosphorylated by host Src kinases and interacts with SHP-2—a phosphatase involved in cell signaling and regulating epithelial cell morphology—as well as Grb2 and C-terminal SRC kinase (Csk). Interaction with Grb2 results in the activation of the Ras/ERK pathway that contributes to an increase in proliferation whereas the activation of C-terminal SRC kinase may provide a negative feedback on CagA phosphorylation. Heterogeneity in the phosphorylation sites within CagA may vary by geographic distribution and results in an altered ability to interact with SHP-2 and modify intracellular signaling. It is intriguing to speculate that heterogeneity in the CagA protein may account for some of the geographic differences in disease. Researchers would suggest that interference with SHP-2 signaling favors gastric hyperplasia. Together, these studies point to fascinating molecular interactions to be investigated in the context of gastric cancer.

H. pylori can stimulate IL-8 directly via other bacterial factors. One such factor is designated outer inflammatory protein A (oipA), which induces epithelial cell IL-8 production, and does not appear to depend on the *H. pylori cag* PAI. Strains that express *oipA* were related to bacterial density, mucosal IL-8 levels, neutrophil infiltration, and clinical presentation. However, little activation of epithelial cell signaling via NF-κB occurs in the absence of the *cag* PAI. Subsequent studies have shown that specific bacterial products led to the activation of different transcription factors that collaborate to enhance IL-8 production. For example, the *cag* PAI and *oipA* are both required for the full activation of IL-8 but the former achieves this through both NF-κB and AP-1, whereas the latter was required to recruit activation by a STAT1-IRF1-ISRE response element.

Although the *cag* PAI facilitates the translocation of CagA, this bacterial protein *per se* has no effect on IL-8 and it is likely that other bacterial proteins translocate and contribute to the *cag* PAI-dependent signaling leading to IL-8 production. Together, these experiments illustrate the level of complexity that is emerging as individual bacterial factors are being aligned with overlapping or distinct signaling pathways that will define the epithelial cell phenotype during infection.

Beyond the Epithelium—Host Responses in the Lamina Propria   Although several epithelial receptors for *H. pylori* have been described, they do not appear to fully account for the magnitude of the inflammatory response to an organism that resides predominantly in the lumen. Some bacteria may infect epithelial cells whereas significant amounts of bacterial material may "leak" around epithelial cells and reach the lamina propria in which it can activate underlying phagocytes including neutrophils and macrophages. One candidate bacterial factor is the *H. pylori* neutrophil-activating protein (HP-NAP). This is a 150-kDa decamer protein that stimulates chemotaxis of monocytes and neutrophils. It also promotes neutrophil adhesion to endothelial cells and NADPH oxidase complex assembly at the plasma membrane, leading to subsequent production of reactive oxygen intermediates. In the context of the inflammatory environment during *H. pylori* gastritis, an additional observation made by investigators was that TNF-α and IFN-γ primed neutrophils and potentiated the effect of HP-NAP.

With the recruitment and activation of macrophages and neutrophils, other inflammatory mediators are released. As mentioned, reactive oxygen intermediates, NO, and some of its metabolites are important in the host defense against microbes. Increased expression of iNOS, the inducible isoform of NO synthase, is observed in the gastric mucosa during infection with *H. pylori*. NO and O_2^-, which may be produced by infiltrating neutrophils, react to form peroxynitrite, $ONOO^-$, a potent oxidant and reducing agent. Although these products have potent antimicrobial effects, uncontrolled or inappropriate production, however, could play a role in the gastric mucosal damage observed during *H. pylori* infection. For instance, the catabolism of urea by urease provides CO_2 that rapidly neutralizes the bactericidal activity of the peroxynitrate and forms $ONO-OCO_2$. Thus, urease may sustain bacterial colonization, however, this reaction enhances the nitration potential of $ONOO^-$ and may favor mutagenesis.

Cytokines from the epithelial cells complement those released in the lamina propria. For example, neutrophils are not only activated by IL-8 but also by other chemokines such as ENA-78 and Gro-α that can be produced by the epithelium, the adjacent myofibroblasts, or the macrophages within the lamina propria. Other cytokines are induced in macrophages, for example, urease induces TNF-α and IL-6 whereas heat shock protein 60 induces IL-6. Intact bacteria can induce the production of chemokines that recruit T cells as well as IL-12 and IL-18—two cytokines that favor the selection of T-helper (Th)1 cells. Thus, intact bacteria or bacterial factors trigger a broad cytokine response within the lamina propria as well.

Gastric T-Cell Responses   As adaptive responses develop, different Th cell subsets emerge as defined by characteristic patterns of cytokine secretion. At the risk of oversimplifying many complicated signaling events, Th1 cells promote cell-mediated immune responses mainly through the production of IFN-γ and TNF-α, whereas Th2 cells produce IL-4, IL-5, IL-10, and

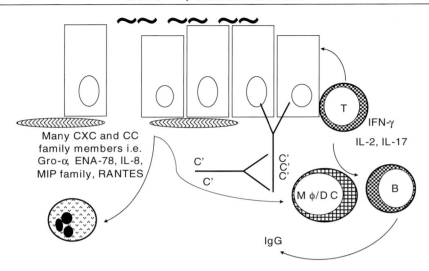

Figure 57-4   The immunopathogenesis of gastritis and epithelial cell damage. This figure shows the various means by which the gastric immune and inflammatory responses mediate epithelial cell damage. First, through direct effects, Th1 cells can induce epithelial cell death via Fas/Fas ligand interactions. T-cell-derived cytokines not only enhance the induction of apoptosis but also upregulate the expression of receptors such as class II major histocompatibility complex increase bacterial binding and favor the induction of apoptosis by *H. pylori*. In addition, Th1 cells complement the effects of *H. pylori* by stimulating epithelial cells to produce cytokines that recruit and activate neutrophils. In turn, activated neutrophils impart an oxidative stress that damages epithelial cells as well as cellular DNA. Finally, gastric T cells can modulate B-cell responses possibly leading to the production autoantibodies including those of the IgG class that can activate complement (C') and contribute to immune-complex-mediated inflammation. From this model, it is clear how genetic polymorphisms that increase the expression of cytokines that drive inflammation (i.e., IL-1β, tumor necrosis factor-α, IL-8) or decrease the expression of those that prevent inflammation (i.e., IL-10) contribute to an increase in gastritis. As gastritis is believed to favor the development of adenocarcinoma, it makes sense that these polymorphisms are associated with increased rates of gastric cancer. IFN, interferon; IL, interleukin; TNF, tumor necrosis factor.

transforming growth factor-β. The Th2 cells can promote mucosal IgA or IgE responses as well as diminish the inflammation caused by Th1 cytokines.

Th1 Cells Predominate in the Stomach   Studies suggest that the gastric mucosa is preconditioned to favor Th1 cell development because IL-12- and IFN-γ-producing cells are present at baseline and increase during infection. One hypothetical explanation is that infection selectively blocks Th2 development. In fact, *H. pylori* can interfere with Stat6 activation by IL-4, which could impair Th2 development. *H. pylori* infection is also associated with increased gastric IL-18 transcripts in the antral mucosa. This effect is independent of the *cag*-status of the infecting strain. Thus, IL-12 and IL-18 may contribute to the predominant Th1 response observed during *H. pylori* infection. Other cytokines that enhance Th1 responses, such as IL-23 and IL-27, remain to be studied in human tissue.

Interactions between bacteria, epithelial cells, and intercellular mediators play an important role in controlling the host response. This principle was demonstrated in a study characterizing the IL-17 response to infection. Biologically active IL-17, a cytokine produced by activated CD4+ T lymphocytes, is increased in the mucosa of *H. pylori*-infected patients. IL-17 is capable of activating NF-κB and MAP kinases that can initiate IL-8 expression by gastric epithelial cells thereby providing a positive feedback to epithelial cells and additional neutrophil recruitment. In addition, the activation of transcription factors by IL-17 may contribute to the increased levels of numerous other proinflammatory cytokines and enzymes observed during *H. pylori* infection, such as IL-1β, TNF-α, and cyclooxygenase-2. Similarly, Th1 cells produce IFN-γ and TNF-α that can increase the expression of many genes in the epithelium including

IL-8. Thus, the gastric T-cell response can complement the direct effects of the bacteria on the epithelium.

Pathogenic Effects of Th1 Cells   The inability of Th1 responses to clear infection suggests that T-cell activation may contribute to more severe gastroduodenal diseases (Fig. 57-4). This idea is supported by animal studies showing that protective immunity induced by vaccines for *Helicobacter* spp rely on Th cells other than Th1 cells possibly including Th2 cells. Other studies have implicated the Th1 cytokines IFN-γ and TNF-α in the activation of epithelial cell gene expression including IL-8 production. In addition, these cytokines enhance bacterial binding, apoptosis, as well as inflammation, atrophy and dysplasia in an animal model. Th1 cytokines, such as IFN-γ and TNF-α, also augment *H. pylori*-induced gastric epithelial death via apoptosis. Further, TNF-α, IFN-γ, and IL-1β upregulate gastric mucosal Fas antigen expression. Because Th1 cells express higher levels of FasL than Th2 cells, the relative increase in Th1 cells during *H. pylori* infection may induce epithelial cell death through Fas–FasL interactions.

Although B cells have been studied the most in the context of autoreactivity, proton-pump-specific Th1 cells in the gastric mucosa may act as effector cells in the targeted destruction of the H+,K+-ATPase in autoimmune gastritis. However, during *H. pylori* infection, in the absence of any organ-specific autoimmunity, T cells reactive to H+,K+-ATPase were not detected. This led to the conclusion that T-cell autoreactivity arises more selectively.

Potential Beneficial Effects of Other Th Subsets   In contrast to the pathogenic effects of Th1 cells, the anti-inflammatory effects of cytokines associated with Th2 cells, or possibly other regulatory subsets of Th cells can attenuate gastric inflammation. More direct evidence suggests that IL-4 can decrease gastritis and the effects of this cytokine may be mediated by the release of somatostatin. These interesting studies illustrate the important convergence of the flora, the host response, and other physiological mediators to modulate mucosal homeostasis. Additional studies will determine if the manipulation of T-cell responses can control the changes in epithelial cell atrophy and dysplasia in these animal models.

The fact that the gastric response can be modified by Th2 cells raises the question regarding the role of other T-cell subsets, such as regulatory T cells (Treg), in the pathogenesis of disease associated with *H. pylori* infection. Depletion of Treg in neonatal mice leads to autoimmune gastritis implying that Treg play an important role in the control of gastritis. The report that infection with *H. pylori* improves the autoimmune gastritis induced in neonatal mice suggests that infection may indeed stimulate a subset of anti-inflammatory T cells that impair excessive inflammation that could otherwise lead to the spontaneous clearance of the organism. There are several precedents for this in immunity and future studies may prove such a mechanism exists for prolonging *H. pylori* infection.

Gastric B-Cell Responses   Normally, antibodies in the gastrointestinal tract are of the IgA isotype, as IgA antibodies are highly adapted for mucosal protection. IgA has structural features that allow them to be transported selectively into the lumen with mucosal secretions, resist acid proteolysis and enzymatic degradation, and block bacterial attachment or neutralize toxins in the lumen. Moreover, they confer protective immunity without activating complement and stimulating deleterious amounts of inflammation. During infection with *H. pylori,* IgA producing cells are increased; however, IgG and IgM are also detected along with activated complement. Therefore, local immune complexes may be contributing to gastroduodenal inflammation and tissue damage during infection.

Direct evidence for autoantibody production in response to *H. pylori* requires the identification of the self-antigens that are recognized by these antibodies. Given the structural homology between Le antigens on *H. pylori* and host cells, an obvious hypothesis is that these antigens will contribute to the described autoreactive responses. Indeed in the mouse models, immunization with *H. pylori* induces antibody-producing cells that recognize Le$^{x/y}$ that are capable of inducing gastritis. Furthermore, an antibody response directed to gastric parietal cells during *H. pylori* infection correlates with increased corpus atrophy. In addition, ferrets naturally infected with *H. mustelae* generate antigastric antibodies that recognize parietal cells. The cellular target for these antibodies in mice appears to be the β-chain of the gastric H$^+$,K$^+$-ATPase localized in the parietal cell canaliculi in the corpus. Anti-Le antibodies have been described in humans and occur independently of the Le phenotype of the host. However, they do not appear to account for autoreactivity. Thus, it seems logical that autoantibodies induced in mice may recognize different targets within the gastric mucosa and may even cross-react with human gastric tissue. However, the autoantibodies induced in humans may have a completely different specificity.

Independent reports have shown that gastric antibodies can resemble rheumatoid factors because they recognize other antibodies. Thus, a complex of antibodies recognized by adjacent antibodies could trigger immune complex-mediated inflammation. Other investigators have shown that antibodies associated with *H. pylori* infection recognize gastric epithelial cells.

Moreover, monoclonal antibodies that recognize *H. pylori* cross-react to both human and murine gastric epithelial cells. Adoptive transfer of monoclonal antibodies to recipient mice induces gastritis as does the transfer of B-cells recognizing heat shock proteins from subjects with maltoma. Two groups have suggested that the level of autoantibodies in humans correlates with the severity of the gastritis. Thus, direct and indirect evidence supports the idea that autoantibodies can be induced during infection.

Is There an Immunological Basis for Persistence?   With few exceptions, infection with *H. pylori* persists for the life of the host unless there is some intervention with antibiotics. This has led investigators to ask if a form of immunological avoidance or tolerance exists that prevents immunity from developing. Although infection leads to the recruitment and activation of innate responses that could lead to potentially protective, adaptive responses, there is evidence that *H. pylori* disrupts the processes that could contribute to immunity. As discussed, several bacterial factors including catalase and urease antagonize innate host responses. Virulent strains of *H. pylori* also impair phagocytosis. The VacA toxin impairs antigen presentation by macrophages by inhibiting the Ii-dependent pathway mediated by newly synthesized class II MHC molecules. Moreover, *H. pylori* express antigenic molecules that mimic host molecules, such as Lewis antigens, and self-antigens normally stimulate T cells to release cytokines that protect from autoimmune reactions. However, the cytokine profile associated with *H. pylori* infection does not obviously resemble the expected version in a tolerant environment. For example, IL-4, IL-10, and transforming growth factor-β (which could mediate an anti-inflammatory effect) are not expressed to the same levels as the proinflammatory cytokines like IFN-γ and TNF-α. That is not to say that the expression of potentially anti-inflammatory cytokines that exists is not sufficient to impair immune responses and favor persistence but some additional data are required to support this model. Additionally, the infected gastric mucosa is characterized by chronic, active inflammation. Thus, tolerance, if it has occurred, may be relative.

Some evidence for a role in immune avoidance for the persistence of *H. pylori* can be found in animal models in which infection is cleared by immunization procedures that induce a substantial amount of gastritis. It remains to be determined if immunity is resulting from a higher degree of inflammation than what is observed in response to "natural" infection or whether protection results from a specific and selected response induced by the immunization.

Another perspective is that the T-cell responses may not be inappropriate but they may lack a level of coordination necessary to achieve immunity. Some groups have demonstrated that the bacteria are able to inhibit the growth of T cells and actually lead to the induction of apoptosis. This process has been demonstrated using cell lines and attributed to very specific patterns of gene expression including the induction of FasL and Fas on T cells that would enable apoptosis to proceed. Although studies suggest this can occur directly in a redox-sensitive manner, other reports suggest that peptides from *H. pylori* activate monocytes to produce oxygen radicals that impair the expression of CD3 zeta chain of the T-cell receptor complex as well as induce T-cell apoptosis. Support for the loss of T cells by apoptosis is given by the presence of apoptotic T cells in the gastric mucosa as well as the expression of Fas and FasL that was detected on biopsy specimens by immunohistochemistry.

VacA impairs T-cell growth and function independently of apoptosis in a T-cell line by inhibiting nuclear translocation of a transcription factor activation required for IL-2 production. Related studies illustrate the complexity of these events as the effects on cell lines differ from T cells isolated from human peripheral blood in that the toxin impairs IL-2-dependent expansion in freshly isolated T cells but not IL-2 production nor their survival. Others have shown that exposure of human T cells to *H. pylori* decreases their proliferative response by decreasing the expression of the CD3 zeta chain of the T-cell receptor complex.

These reports support the model that *H. pylori* interferes with normal T-cell activation in several ways; however, the answer may lie in the T cells within the gastric mucosa because cell lines and peripheral blood are a model that is often not replicated within the tissue. For example, some antigen-specific T-cell responses can be induced in the gastric mucosa. Nonetheless, it is still possible that the effect of the organism as well as the cytokine milieu disrupt the coordination that is required for the development of an effective, antigen-specific T-cell response.

CONCLUSION

The evidence presented above illustrates several changes associated with *H. pylori* infection that contribute to gastritis and alterations in epithelial cell biology. It is clear that these responses are induced by many different factors, which points to the importance of several pathways and the lack of an exclusive target that deserves preferential attention. There is the chance that a "final common pathway" may emerge as a key target that advances the understanding of the complex pathogenesis of gastroduodenal diseases. Insights at the molecular level will improve the understanding of the pathogenesis of these disorders and provide novel opportunities for diagnosis, treatment and modeling of gastrointestinal diseases consequential to chronic inflammation.

ACKNOWLEDGMENTS

The author and some of the work referred to are supported by the National Institutes of Health Grants DK50980, DK56703, and RR00175.

SELECTED REFERENCES

Aihara M, Tsuchimoto D, Takizawa H, et al. Mechanisms involved in *Helicobacter pylori*-induced interleukin-8 production by a gastric cancer cell line, MKN45. Infect Immun 1997;65:3218–3224.

Allen LA, Schlesinger LS, Kang B. Virulent strains of *Helicobacter pylori* demonstrate delayed phagocytosis and stimulate homotypic phagosome fusion in macrophages. J Exp Med 2000;191:115–128.

Amieva MR, Vogelmann R, Covacci A, Tompkins LS, Nelson WJ, Falkow S. Disruption of the epithelial apical-junctional complex by *Helicobacter pylori* CagA. Science 2003;300:1430–1434.

Andersen-Nissen E, Smith KD, Strobe KL, et al. Evasion of Toll-like receptor 5 by flagellated bacteria. Proc Natl Acad Sci USA 2005; 102:9247–9252.

Appelmelk BJ, Faller G, Claeys D, Kirchner T, Vandenbroucke-Grauls CM. Bugs on trial: the case of *Helicobacter pylori* and autoimmunity. Immunol Today 1998;19:296–299.

Appelmelk BJ, Simoons-Smit I, Negrini R, et al. Potential role of molecular mimicry between *Helicobacter pylori* lipopolysaccharide and host Lewis blood group antigens in autoimmunity. Infect Immun 1996; 64:2031–2040.

Argent RH, Kidd M, Owen RJ, Thomas RJ, Limb MC, Atherton JC. Determinants and consequences of different levels of CagA phosphorylation for clinical isolates of *Helicobacter pylori*. Gastroenterology 2004;127:514–523.

Atherton JC, Cao P, Peek RM, Tummuru MK, Blaser MJ, Cover TL. Mosaicism in vacuolating cytotoxin alleles of *Helicobacter pylori*. Association of specific *vac*A types with cytotoxin production and peptic ulceration. J Biol Chem 1995;270:17,771–17,777.

Bamford KB, Fan XJ, Crowe SE, et al. Lymphocytes in the human gastric mucosa during *Helicobacter pylori* have a T helper cell 1 phenotype. Gastroenterology 1998;114:482–492.

Basak C, Pathak SK, Bhattacharyya A, Pathak S, Basu J, Kundu M. The secreted peptidyl prolyl cis,trans-isomerase HP0175 of *Helicobacter pylori* induces apoptosis of gastric epithelial cells in a. J Immunol 2005;174:5672–5680.

Berstad AE, Brandtzaeg P, Stave R, Halstensen TS. Epithelium related deposition of activated complement in *Helicobacter pylori* associated gastritis. Gut 1997;40:196–203.

Beswick EJ, Das S, Pinchuk IV, et al. *Helicobacter pylori*-induced IL-8 production by gastric epithelial cells up-regulates CD74 expression. J Immunol 2005;175:171–176.

Betten A, Bylund J, Cristophe T, et al. A proinflammatory peptide from *Helicobacter pylori* activates monocytes to induce lymphocyte dysfunction and apoptosis. J Clin Invest 2001;108:1221–1228.

Blaser MJ. The biology of cag in the *Helicobacter pylori*-human interaction. Gastroenterology 2005;128:1512–1515.

Blaser MJ, Atherton JC. *Helicobacter pylori* persistence: biology and disease. J Clin Invest 2004;113:321–333.

Bliss CM Jr, Golenblock DT, Keates S, Linevsky JK, Kelly CP. *Helicobacter pylori* lipopolysaccharide binds to CD14 and stimulates release of interleukin-8, epithelial neutrophil-activating peptide 78, and monocyte chemotactic protein 1 by human monocytes. Infect Immun 1998;66:5357–5363.

Boncristiano M, Paccani SR, Barone S, et al. The *Helicobacter pylori* vacuolating toxin inhibits T cell activation by two independent mechanisms. J Exp Med 2003;198:1887–1897.

Boren T, Falk P, Roth KA, Larson G, Normark S. Attachment of *Helicobacter pylori* to human gastric epithelium mediated by blood group antigens. Science 1993;262:1892–1895.

Brandt S, Kwok T, Hartig R, Konig W, Backert S. NF-kappaB activation and potentiation of proinflammatory responses by the *Helicobacter pylori* CagA protein. Proc Natl Acad Sci USA 2005;102:9300–9305.

Brenner H, Arndt V, Stegmaier C, Ziegler H, Rothenbacher D. Is *Helicobacter pylori* infection a necessary condition for noncardia gastric cancer? Am J Epidemiol 2004;159:252–258.

Ceponis PJ, McKay DM, Menaker RJ, Galindo-Mata E, Jones NL. *Helicobacter pylori* infection interferes with epithelial Stat6-mediated interleukin-4 signal transduction independent of cagA, cagE, or VacA. J Immunol 2003;171:2035–2041.

Chiou CC, Chan CC, Sheu DL, Chen KT, Li YS, Chan EC. *Helicobacter pylori* infection induced alteration of gene expression in human gastric cells. Gut 2001;48:598–604.

Claeys D, Faller G, Appelmelk BJ, Negrini R, Kirchner T. The gastric H+, K+-ATPase is a major autoantigen in chronic *Helicobacter pylori* gastritis with body mucosa atrophy. Gastroenterology 1998;115:340–347.

Clyne M, Drumm B. Absence of effect of Lewis A and Lewis B expression on adherence of *Helicobacter pylori* to human gastric cells. Gastroenterology 1997;113:72–80.

Clyne M, Dillon P, Daly S, et al. *Helicobacter pylori* interacts with the human single-domain trefoil protein TFF1. Proc Natl Acad Sci USA 2004;101:7409–7414.

Correa P. Human gastric carcinogenesis: a multistep and multifactorial process—First American Cancer Society Award Lecture on Cancer Epidemiology and Prevention. Cancer Res 1992;52:6735–6740.

Correa P. Bacterial infections as a cause of cancer. J Natl Cancer Inst 2003;95:E3.

Covacci A, Telford JL, Del Giudice G, Parsonnet J, Rappuoli R. *Helicobacter pylori* virulence and genetic geography. Science 1999; 284:1328–1333.

Cover TL. The vacuolating cytotoxin of *Helicobacter pylori*. Molecular Microbiology 1996;20:241–246.

Cover TL, Krishna US, Israel DA, Peek RM Jr. Induction of gastric epithelial cell apoptosis by *Helicobacter pylori* vacuolating cytotoxin. Cancer Res 2003;63:951–957.

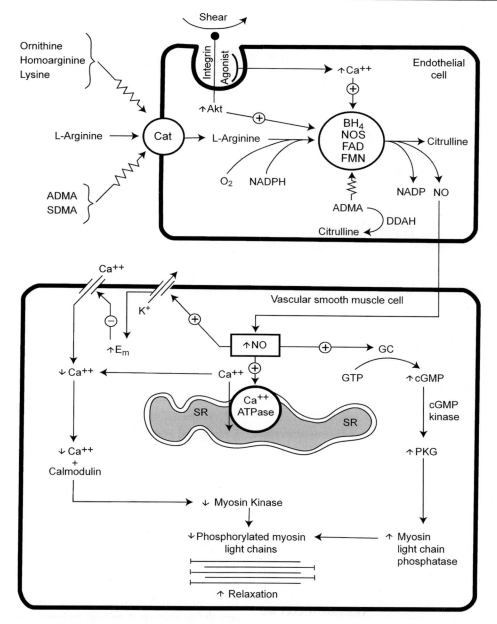

Figure 58-1 Cell diagram showing some pathways for NOS regulation in endothelial cells and for NO action in VSMCs. For details, *see* Molecular Targets for NO in Renal Blood Vessels.

activates cGMP kinase (G kinase) to stimulate protein kinase G (PKG) (Fig. 58-1). PKG activates myosin light chain phosphatase that dephosphorylates one of the light chains of each myosin head, which is also called the regulatory chain. This dephosphorylation dissociates the cross-bridges between the myosin head and the actin filaments, and prevents the attachment–detachment cycling of the myosin head with the actin filament. This leads to relaxation of the vascular smooth muscle cells (VSMCs) that is detected in pharmacological studies as an EDRF response. NO also reduces $IC_{Ca^{2+}}$ in VSMCs.

NO directly activates (1) a Ca^{2+} ATPase on the membrane of the sarcoplasmic reticulum, thereby sequestering cytoplasmic Ca^{2+} in the SR; (2) a Ca^{2+}-dependent K^+ channel in the cell membrane, thereby increasing the membrane potential (E_m); (3) inactivating L-type voltage-gated Ca^{2+}-channels; and (4) sodium–potassium ATPase. In addition, NO inhibits phospholipase C, causing decreased turnover of phosphoinositides.

NO can interact with many other heme-centered enzymes. For example, NO changes the affinity of hemoglobin for O_2. NO binds to thiol groups, forming *S*-nitrosothiols that modify the actions of the target protein and stabilize NO by protecting it from oxidative attack, thereby prolonging its biological action. The interaction of NO with O_2^- forms peroxynitrite ($ONOO^-$) which effectively terminates many of NO's actions. However, $ONOO^-$ is a potent oxidative and nitrosative agent that attacks tyrosine epitopes to form nitrotyrosine modification of proteins. These can be detected immunologically to provide insight into O_2^- and NO interactions in the kidney. Nitrotyrosine modification can also alter function. For example, prostacyclin synthase (PGI_2-S) is inactivated by $ONOO^-$ at a concentration of only 50 n*M*.

Molecular Targets for NO in the Tubular Cells NO interacts with heme-centered enzymes, such as GC, expressed in tubular and juxtaglomerular cells to generate cGMP. cGMP can inhibit

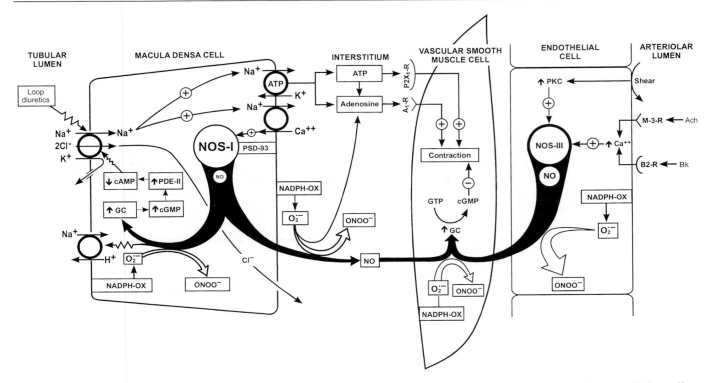

Figure 58-2   Cell diagram showing some pathways whereby NO generated by nNOS in the MD or eNOS in the vascular endothelium affects the tubuloglomerular feedback response or afferent arteriolar tone. For details, *see* Molecular Targets for NO in the Tubular Cells.

phosphodiesterase (PDE)-II in the cells of the thick ascending limb of the loop of Henle and the macula densa (MD). PDE-II metabolizes and inactivates cAMP (Fig. 58-2). The ensuing decrease in cAMP decreases the phosphorylation of the Na$^+$/K$^+$/2Cl$^-$ cotransporter in the luminal cell membrane, and thereby leads to its inactivation. NO also activates Ca^{2+}-activated K$^+$channels that increase E_m and thereby enhance Na$^+$ entry and reabsorption. Similar events in the juxtaglomerular cells of the afferent arteriole have complex effects on renin secretion. Renin secretion initially is decreased after NO by actions of cGMP to activate G-kinase and PKG. Later, renin secretion is stimulated via actions of cAMP to enhance protein kinase A. This occurs because NO inhibits PDE-III, thereby leading to a gradual increase in cAMP accumulation.

NO Measurement   NO released into the bloodstream reacts rapidly with hemoglobin to form nitrosohemoglobin which, on reduction, releases NO$_2^-$ which can be further oxidized to NO$_3^-$. Cellular release of NO$_2^-$ + NO$_3^-$ (NO$_x$) and renal excretion of NO$_x$ during consumption of a NO$_x$-deficient diet are methods to quantitate NO generation. NOS activity in the tissues can be studied directly from the release of labeled citrulline from labeled arginine, from the partial pressure of NO measured with a porphyrinic NO-sensitive electrode, by the use of fluorescent dyes, such as diaminofluorescein-2, which are trapped within cells and fluoresce on reaction with NO, by spectrophotometric changes that occur when NO interacts with test proteins such as hemoglobin, by generation of NO signaling molecules such as cGMP, and from functional responses to blockade of NOS with competitive antagonists such as L-nitroarginine methyl ester.

Distribution of NOS Isoforms in the Kidney   Type-I (neuronal) NOS is heavily expressed in MD cells. Other sites include the cortical and inner medullary collecting ducts and Bowman's

capsule of the glomerulus. There is a lower level of expression in the efferent arteriole. Type-III (endothelial) NOS is expressed primarily in the endothelial cells of the arterioles and capillaries of the kidney. eNOS is expressed also in the cells of the thick ascending limb, collecting ducts, and proximal tubules. Type-II (inducible) NOS can be widely expressed in the glomeruli, vessels, and tubules on challenge with lipopolysaccharide or cytokines. Basal expression is apparent in cells of the thick ascending limb, and the proximal and distal nephron.

Regulation of NO Generation and Action   NO generation is closely regulated. Cellular arginine uptake is mediated via cationic amino transporters (CATs) expressed on cell membranes (Figs. 58-1 and 58-2). There is competition for transport among the cationic amino acids, such as ornithine, lysine, and homoarginine, and with the dimethyl arginines, asymmetric dimethyl arginine (ADMA), and symmetric dimethyl arginine. All of these can inhibit arginine uptake and NO action (Fig. 58-1). Endothelial NOS in vascular endothelial cells is activated by a rise in IC$_{Ca^{2+}}$ by agonists, such as acetylcholine, acting on M-3 receptors or bradykinin (Bk) acting on B$_2$ receptors. Sheer stress is transduced by integrins expressed in caveolae, which activates Akt-1 which phosphorylates and activates eNOS. NOS activity in tubular or vascular cells can be inhibited by lack of availability of essential cofactors, notably BH$_4$, which, during oxidative stress, is converted to the inactive form, dihydrobiopterin.

ADMA is an endogenous inhibitor of NOS and CAT. ADMA (but not symmetric dimethyl arginine, which is ineffective as a NOS inhibitor) is metabolized to citrulline by dimethylarginine dimethylaminohydrolase (DDAH), which is widely expressed in the kidney at sites of NOS expression.

The tubuloglomerular feedback response is a unique renal mechanism, whereby delivery and reabsorption of Cl$^-$ at the MD segment leads to the elaboration of a mediator that vasoconstricts the adjacent afferent arteriole. Mediators include adenosine acting on type-1 receptors and adenosine triphosphate acting on purinergic type-2 receptors. The tubuloglomerular feedback response contributes to renal autoregulation and to adaptation of renal hemodynamics to changes in salt intake. Defects in tubuloglomerular feedback underlie salt-sensitive hypertension. Neuronal NOS also is activated in the MD during Cl^- reabsorption. The ensuing increase in NO generation blunts the tubuloglomerular feedback response both by inhibiting vasoconstriction of the adjacent afferent arteriole and by inhibiting the generation of the tubuloglomerular feedback signal by blocking the luminal Cl^- transporter (Fig. 58-2). An overactive tubuloglomerular feedback response in the spontaneously hypertensive rat (SHR) or the Dahl salt-sensitive rat can be ascribed to a blunted NO action in the juxtaglomerular apparatus because of enhanced inactivation of NO by O_2^-. This overactive tubuloglomerular feedback response likely contributes to renal vasoconstriction and hypertension.

Activation mechanisms for nNOS have been studied in the MD. Basal activity is negligible, but becomes substantial during delivery and reabsorption of NaCl at this segment. Reabsorption via the luminal $Na^+/K^+/2Cl^-$ cotransporter increases cell $[Na^+]$, which activates basolateral Na^+/Ca^{2+} countertransport, thereby increasing $IC_{Ca^{2+}}$ and activating NOS. nNOS is coexpressed with a protein having a postsynaptic density of 93 along the basolateral aspect of the MD cell. Its interaction with the PDZ domain on nNOS dimerizes and activates the enzyme (Fig. 58-2).

NO is inactivated rapidly in renal tubular epithelial cells by interaction with O_2^-. NADPH oxidase is responsible for much of the O_2^- generation in the renal cortex. As studied most fully in the leukocyte, this enzyme requires assembly of a complex of five protein subunits with a small guanidine triphosphatase activating protein rac-1. When activated, NADPH oxidase reduces O_2 to O_2^-. All the major protein components of NADPH oxidase are expressed in VSMCs and endothelial cells of the renal vessels and in the distal nephron, most prominently in the MD. Other prominent sites of NADPH oxidase expression include interstitial fibroblasts and mesangial cells (Fig. 58-2). Expression of NADPH oxidase along the luminal aspect of MD and thick ascending limb cells may protect the luminal cotransporters from phosphorylation and inactivation by NO, whereas expression in the interstitium, VSMC, and endothelial cells limits the access of NO generated in the MD or the endothelial cells to GC expressed in the VSMCs of the adjacent afferent arteriole (Fig. 58-2). Thus, the expression and activation of NADPH oxidase are important factors that limit the biological actions of NO in the juxtaglomerular apparatus.

Regulation of NOS Expression A low salt intake increases the expression of nNOS in the MD and renal cortex, but reduces its expression in the cortical collecting ducts. Despite its upregulation during salt restriction, the expression of nNOS in the MD is unresponsive to angiotensin (Ang) II infusion or to blockade of Ang II type-1 receptors (AT1-Rs). The upregulation of nNOS may be a response to reduced bioactive NO, because NO inhibits NOS activity and expression. The expression of nNOS in the MD is downregulated in the reduced renal mass model of chronic renal insufficiency, but is upregulated in several models of hypertension, including the poststenotic kidney of rats with Goldblatt hypertension and the SHR. However, oxidative stress that accompanies hypertension in these models enhances $ONOO^-$ deposition and prevents the action of NO to vasodilate the afferent arteriole.

In contrast, nNOS is upregulated in the MD in models of early insulinopenic diabetes mellitus, where it mediates glomerular hypertension and hyperfiltration via blunting of the vasoconstrictive tubuloglomerular feedback response.

Expression of eNOS in endothelial cells of the afferent arteriole also is upregulated by salt restriction but, unlike nNOS in the MD, this can be ascribed to Ang II action on AT1-R, because it is prevented by blockade of AT1-R with losartan. eNOS expression is upregulated in models of early insulinopenic diabetes mellitus and in some models of hypertension, such as the SHR.

Dietary salt restriction upregulates nNOS expression in the MD. However, its activity in the regulation of afferent arteriolar tone is absent, but can be restored by microperfusion of the NOS substrate, L-arginine, into the MD. The limitation of NOS activity in the MD during salt restriction by arginine availability can be ascribed to a reduced plasma arginine concentration and a reduced cellular uptake of L-arginine from the tubular lumen. Hepatic cells metabolize available arginine to ornithine and urea and thereby limit plasma levels of arginine. During dietary salt restriction there is an upregulation of the high-capacity CAT transporter for arginine expressed on hepatic cells. This may enhance hepatic arginine uptake from the portal system sufficiently to facilitate its metabolism and restrict its plasma level. The reduced plasma levels of arginine are accompanied by increases in ornithine and in urea appearance. Dietary salt restriction reduces the expression of CAT-2A in the thick ascending limb and MD cells of the loop of Henle. This restricts the uptake of arginine from the tubular fluid into these cells and contributes to the reduced activity of nNOS during salt restriction. These adaptations may be important because reduced NOS activity could contribute to the reduced renal blood flow and the enhanced renal NaCl reabsorption during salt deficiency.

Despite overexpression of nNOS in the MD, and of eNOS in the endothelium, the renal blood flow, and the tubuloglomerular feedback of the SHR are independent of NOS, as indicated by little or no response to blockade of NOS with drugs such as L-nitroarginine methyl ester. NOS activity in the juxtaglomerular apparatus of the SHR is not limited by the availability of arginine or BH_4 but can be restored in full by microperfusion into the juxtaglomerular apparatus of the antioxidant SOD mimetic, tempol.

The renal oxidative stress in the SHR and the Ang II infused rat or mouse has been attributed to an upregulation of NADPH-oxidase that is mediated by AT1-R. Ang II upregulates the $p22^{phox}$ and Nox-1 components of NADPH oxidase in the kidney, but downregulates Nox-4 and extracellular and mitochondrial-SOD. Ang II type-2 receptors have contrary effects and therefore are protective of the development of oxidative stress.

Renovascular Actions of NO The renal preglomerular (afferent) and postglomerular (efferent) arterioles are vasodilated tonically by NO, as indicated by a sharp increase in their resistances during blockade of NOS. An enhanced renal NO generation contributes to renal vasodilatation in normal pregnancy, during infusion of amino acids, and in early diabetes mellitus. Conversely, a reduced NO bioactivity contributes to renal vasoconstriction in many models of hypertension, such as prolonged Ang II infusion in the rat, the SHR, lead-induced hypertension, and the Dahl salt-sensitive rat and in models of chronic renal failure. There is a reduced total body NO generation in humans with essential hypertension and chronic renal failure. The NO that dilates the renal afferent arteriole may derive either from the adjacent vascular endothelial cell or the adjacent MD cell (Fig. 58-2). Despite these widespread effects of NO to regulate afferent arteriole tone, NO is not implicated in renal autoregulation.

Role of NO in Tubular Function   Most investigators have concluded that NO reduces tubular NaCl and fluid reabsorption. However, this is often complicated by secondary effects. For example, the increase in blood pressure (BP) that accompanies NOS inhibition systems reduces tubular NaCl reabsorption. Effects of NO on segmental NaCl tubular reabsorption are controversial. Both stimulation and inhibition have been reported in the proximal tubule and collecting ducts. Blockade of NOS in the proximal tubule can impair luminal Na^+/H^+ exchange leading to impaired reabsorption of Na^+ and HCO_3^- and development of a metabolic acidosis contrast. Stimulation of NO generation from eNOS in the adjacent peritubular capillary endothelium by Bk enhances basolateral HCO_3^- uptake. Higher concentrations of NO in the proximal tubule inhibit Na^+/K^+ ATPase. In the collecting ducts, NO, via cGMP, inhibits the luminal entry of Na^+ via the epithelial sodium channel, but also paradoxically can enhance Na^+ entry secondary to an increase in the basolateral potassium conductance that hyperpolarizes the cell. Studies in the thick ascending limb of the loop of Henle uniformly demonstrate inhibition owing to blockade by NO of the luminal $Na^+/K^+/2Cl^-$ cotransporter, Na^+/H^+ exchanger, and K^+ channel and the basolateral Na^+/K^+ ATPase. NO increases cGMP and cAMP, which promote phosphorylation and inactivation of the luminal transporters (Fig. 58-2). NO likely derived from nNOS within mitochondria in tubular epithelial cells competes with O_2 for cytochrome-c reductase and diminishes cellular O_2 usage. A reduction in NO in the kidney increases O_2 usage and reduces the efficiency with which the kidney uses O_2 for tubular Na^+ reabsorption. Consequently, there is a fall in the pO_2 of the kidney cortex.

Effects of NO on Renin Secretion   NO has site- and time-dependent effects on the secretion of renin from the afferent arteriole. NO can stimulate renin secretion from the juxtaglomerular cells via inhibition of PDE-III and elevation of cAMP, or may inhibit it via the cGMP/PKG pathway. Activation of nNOS in the MD by luminal perfusion of L-arginine enhances the secretion of renin. This may represent the effects of MD NO to activate COX-2 whose product, prostacyclin (PGI_2), stimulates renin secretion. In contrast, acute activation of eNOS in endothelial cells leads to cGMP-dependent inhibition of renin secretion. However, during prolonged stimulation of eNOS, the initial inhibition is followed by enhanced release.

Role of NO in Pathophysiology and Disease   A decrease in intrarenal NO activity in blood vessels, the MD and renal tubules accompanies many models of hypertension and contributes to renal vasoconstriction and enhanced tubular NaCl reabsorption. Inhibition of NOS in normal animals shifts the relationship between BP and salt so as to induce salt sensitive hypertension. In contrast, correction of oxidative stress in hypertensive models with an SOD mimetic that enhances NO bioactivity shifts the relationship back to the normal state, thereby correcting salt sensitivity and lowering BP. An increase in NO in the kidney contributes to hyperfiltration in models of early diabetes mellitus. In models of postischemic or endotoxic renal insufficiency, where oxidative stress is prominent, massive overproduction of NO in the kidney is implicated in the associated tubular damage that may be mediated by $ONOO^-$.

CYCLOOXYGENASE

COX is a fatty acid mono-oxygenase. It is widely distributed in the kidney and elsewhere. On cell activation by increased sheer stress, transmural pressure, peptides such as Ang II, Bk, or endothelin, cytokines or hypoxia, phospholipase A_2 hydrolyzes membrane phospholipids to free arachidonic acid that is metabolized by COX to prostaglandin (PG) endoperoxides. The initial COX product is prostaglandin G_2 but this is rapidly rearranged to the stable prostaglandin H_2 (PGH_2), which not only activates thromboxane-prostanoid receptors, but also is the substrate for three important classes of enzymes. Prostaglandin E_2 synthase generates prostaglandin E_2 (PGE_2), PGI_2-S generates PGI_2, and thromboxane A_2 synthase generates TxA_2.

COX ISOFORMS IN THE KIDNEY   Two COX isoforms are expressed in the kidney. COX-1 is widely expressed constitutively in body tissues. In most organs, COX-1 is responsible for basal PG synthesis. COX-2 is termed inducible because in most organs there is negligible basal COX-2 expression until stimulation with lipopolysaccharide or cytokines when COX-2 becomes the predominant source of PGs. However, as with NOS, the kidney is unusual in having high basal expression of the inducible isoform, which contributes importantly to basal renal PG productions.

COX-1 is located in the endoplasmic reticulum of the endothelial and VSMCs of the afferent and efferent arterioles and larger arteries, and in the glomerulus, the medullary collecting ducts, and medullary interstitial cells. Major sites of COX-2 expression include the MD cells, some adjacent thick ascending limb cells and medullary interstitial cells. COX-2 is expressed more widely in the embryonic kidney. Mice with targeted disruption of the gene for COX-2, but not COX-1, suffer nephron hypoplasia and renal atrophy, implying an important role for COX-2 products in renal development.

REGULATION OF COX ACTIVITY   COX activity is enhanced by peroxides, but high concentration of O_2^- leads to its irreversible inactivation. In low concentrations, NO stimulates COX activity and vascular PGI_2 generation. However, in high concentrations, as during iNOS induction, NO can inactivate COX. COX-1 activity is determined by the availability of arachidonate. The net effect of inhibition of COX-1-derived PGs in the blood vessels is usually vasoconstriction, likely owing primarily to inhibition of PGI_2 synthesis in resistance vessels. COX-1 activity in the collecting ducts is increased by arginine vasopressin (AVP). An ensuing increase in PGE_2 activates adenylate cyclase to generate cAMP which antagonizes the effects of AVP to enhance water permeability and terminates other effects of AVP. PGE_2 also inhibits the activity of the luminal Na^+ entry channel. Thus, blockade of COX-1 enhances tubular reabsorption of fluid and NaCl.

COX-2 activity is determined by enzyme expression, which is stimulated by serum, growth factors, lipopolysaccharide, tumor promoters, and peptides that include Ang II, Bk, and endothelin, whereas glucocorticoids inhibit expression. COX-2 expression in the MD is stimulated by dietary salt restriction. Remarkably, this effect is enhanced during blockade of AT1-R which indicates that Ang II has a negative feedback effect on COX-2 expression at this site. In contrast, Ang II stimulates expression of COX-2 in the thick ascending limb and blood vessels. A reduction in extracellular $[Cl^-]$ at the thick ascending limb stimulates COX-2 expression by increasing p38 mitogen-activated protein kinase activity. Negative feedback inhibition of COX-2 expression in the MD by Ang II is signaled via nuclear transcription factor-κB and is reinforced by Ang II-induced aldosterone secretion, which also inhibits COX-2 expression. Expression of COX-2 in the interstitial cells of the renal medulla is enhanced by dehydration or an increase in interstitial osmolality. The ensuing increase in PGE_2

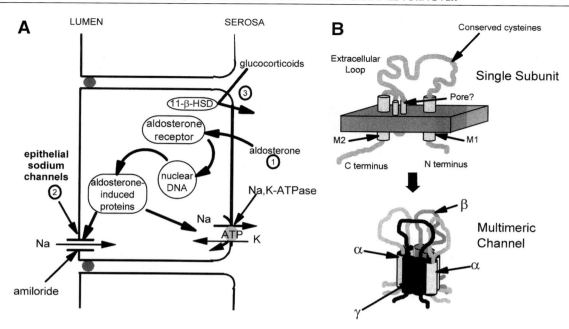

Figure 59-2   Mechanism of Aldosterone's Action and ENaC structure. (**A**) Aldosterone mechanism and pathology. Aldosterone enters principal cells (**A**) and interacts with cytosolic aldosterone receptors. The aldosterone-bound receptors interact with nuclear DNA to promote gene expression. The aldosterone-induced gene products activate sodium channels (**B**) and sodium pumps to increase sodium reabsorption. (**A**) Abnormalities of the adrenals and certain tumors can lead to primary hyper- or hypo-aldosteronism. (**B**) Loss of function mutations in sodium channels can lead to both pseudophypoaldosteronism; gain of function mutations produce pseudohyperaldosteronism (Liddle's syndrome). (**C**) Defects in 11-β-hydroxysteroid dehydrogenase (**C**) produces Apparent Mineralocorticoid Excess because glucocorticoids can then interact with aldosterone receptors to stimulate sodium channels. (**B**) Structure of ENaC. Each subunit has only two predicted membrane spanning domains, an unusual topology for an ion channel. Topologic analyses suggest that the amino and carboxy terminal regions of the ENaCs are cytoplasmic, and that each subunit has a large extracellular loop present among the membrane spanning regions. The α-, β-, and γ-ENaC have cysteine rich regions within putative extracellular loops, which are postulated to form intersubunit disulfide bonds that are important in oligomerization of Na channels. The three ENaCs also possess proline rich regions within their intracellular C-terminal domains that are important for interaction with accessory proteins that regulate the stability of functional channels in the apical membrane of renal cells. The three homologous ENaC subunit proteins form a heteromultimeric channel protein apparently made up of two α-, one β-, and one γ-subunit.

the physiological condition. In some cases, the reason for the excess blood volume is clear. For example, glomerular diseases often lead to inappropriate release of renin and an increase in angiotensin II and aldosterone levels with increases in collecting tubule sodium reabsorption, and ultimately, an increase in blood pressure. A tumor of the adrenal cortex can produce excess aldosterone causing an increase in blood pressure. A specific gain of function mutation in the sodium reabsorptive mechanism in the collecting duct also leads to excess sodium reabsorption and profound hypertension. Three examples illustrate types of defects that can complicate the control mechanism for maintaining total body sodium and mean blood pressure. First, excess renin production is a problem with the sensing mechanism for the system. Second, excess production of aldosterone is a defect in the signaling mechanism that lies between the sensor (pressure sensors in the large vessels and the kidney) and the effector (distal nephron sodium reabsorption); and the third example is a defect in the effector system (distal nephron sodium reabsorption). In each case, the defect is easily identified and correcting the underlying pathology usually corrects the hypertension. Table 59-1 provides a list of identifiable genetic defects in the regulation of sodium balance that lead to increases or decreases in blood pressure. Despite the relatively extensive list of known genetic defects, the etiology of hypertension is unclear. In most cases, renin angiotensin and aldosterone levels are normal or even reduced

and yet blood pressure is elevated as if the set-point of the control loop sensing blood pressure and varying sodium reabsorption is inexplicably high. The relatively normal levels of circulating renin, angiotensin II, and aldosterone imply that the defect in the regulation of sodium reabsorption lies beyond aldosterone interacting with the cells of the collecting tubule. Hypertension research has attempted to define the components controlling sodium reabsorption in response to aldosterone.

MOLECULAR BIOLOGY AND STRUCTURE OF EPITHELIAL NA CHANNELS

cDNAs for epithelial Na channels (ENaCs) were originally described by investigators who used expression cloning methods to isolate three separate cDNAs from rat distal colon. They designated the three cDNAs α-, β-, and γ-rat ENaC. Coinjection into *Xenopus* oocytes with cRNAs prepared from all three cDNAs induces expression of amiloride-sensitive Na channels that possess characteristics virtually identical to those observed in renal cortical collecting tubule principal cells. The three subunits show limited sequence homology to each other although, across species, the same subunit has significant (70–90%), amino acid sequence homology (some regions do have only limited homology). Each subunit has only two predicted membrane spanning domains, an unusual topology for an ion channel. Topologic analyses suggest that the amino and carboxy-terminal regions of the ENaCs are cytoplasmic,

Table 59-1
Genetic Bases for Changes in Blood Pressure

Genetic bases for hypertension		
Syndrome	*Defect*	*Characteristics*
Apparent mineralocorticoid excess	Loss of function mutation of 11-β-hydroxysteroid dehydrogenase	Aldosterone receptors in renal principal cells are not only activated by aldosterone, but can be activated by normal levels of circulating glucocorticoids promoting constitutive sodium reabsorption with profound early-onset hypertension and growth arrest. Responsive to mineralocorticoid (aldosterone) receptor antagonists, for example, spironolactone, eplerenone.
Liddle's	Gain of function mutation in the β- or γ-subunit of ENaC	Constitutive sodium reabsorption regardless of circulating aldosterone levels with profound early-onset hypertension Responsive to Midamor (amiloride HCl).
T594M β–ENaC	Single amino acid mutation in β-subunit of ENaC with moderate gain of function	Increased collecting duct sodium reabsorption with mild to moderate hypertension. Most prevalent in individuals of African descent. Responsive to Midamor (amiloride HCl).
Glucocorticoid-remediable aldosteronism	Elevated aldosterone owing to an abnormal activation of aldosterone synthase by ACTH	Early-onset hypertension that can be controlled by administration of glucocorticoids (to reduce ACTH production).
Aldosterone synthase polymorphisms	Gain of function leading to increased circulating aldosterone	Increased sodium reabsorption with mild hypertension. Most prevalent in men. More prevalent in individuals of Japanese descent. Responsive to mineralocorticoid (aldosterone) receptor antagonists, for example, spironolactone, eplerenone.
11-β-hydroxylase deficiency	Loss of function mutation leading to abnormal accumulation of 11-deoxycorticosterone that activates aldosterone receptors	Activation of aldosterone receptors leads to sodium retention and early-onset hypertension. Associated accumulation of androgens leads to masculinization of females *in utero* and both sexes postnatally. May be responsive to the aldosterone receptor antagonist, eplerenone, but spironolactone would exacerbate androgenic effects.
Pseudohypoaldosteronism Type II (Gordon's syndrome)	Loss of function mutation in With No K [lysine] kinases	Loss of With No K [lysine] kinase (WNK) function leads to activation of distal nephron thiazide-sensitive sodium chloride cotransporter causing sodium retention, hypertension, and hyperkalemia. Responsive to thiazides.
α-Adducin polymorphism	Structural protein that activates Na K-ATPase	Increased Na pump activity modestly increases sodium reabsorption to produce mild hypertension.
Hypertension exacerbated in pregnancy	Mutation in mineralocorticoid receptor that makes receptor more sensitive to aldosterone	Early-onset hypertension greatly exaggerated by pregnancy because progesterone also binds to the mutant receptor and promotes additional sodium reabsorption. The aldosterone receptor antagonist, spironolactone, acts as an agonist for the mutant receptor; effect of eplerenone has not been examined.
SGK	Two activating mutations	SGK inhibits ENaC degradation so activation causes accumulation of ENaC and an increase in renal sodium reabsorption with consequent hypertension. Possibly responsive to Midamor (amiloride HCl).
Various single nucleotide polymorphisms in the genes for renin, ACE, and angiotensin II receptor	Presumably slightly altered function of the genes controlling angiotensin production and sensitivity	Statistically significant increases in blood pressure. Some single nucleotide polymorphisms are more prevalent. in African Americans, others more prevalent in European Americans, and a few prevalent in both populations. Responsive to ACE inhibitors (e.g., captopril, and lotensin) and angiotensin II receptor inhibitors (e.g., losartan), and volume reduction with thiazide diuretics.

(Continued)

Table 59-1 *(Continued)*

	Genetic bases for hypotension	
Syndrome	*Defect*	*Characteristics*
Pseudohypoaldosteronism type I (dominant)	Loss of function mutation of the mineralocorticoid receptor	Salt wasting, hypotension, severe neonatal symptoms.
Pseudohypoaldosteronism type I (recessive)	Partial loss of function mutation of the α-subunit of ENaC	Salt wasting, hypotension, hyperkalemia, excess fluid secretion from airways, loss of salt taste, serious symptoms at all ages.
Aldosterone synthase	Loss of function leading to decreased circulating aldosterone	Decreased sodium reabsorption with severe hypotension and occasionally shock because of reduced intravascular volume.
Steroid 21-hydroxylase	Loss of function leading to decreased synthesis of aldosterone	Decreased sodium reabsorption with severe hypotension and other endocrine abnormalities.
Gitelman's syndrome	Loss of function of distal nephron thiazide-sensitive NaCl transporter	Salt wasting and mild hypotension in homozygotes.

ACTH, adrenocorticotropin hormone.

and indicate that each subunit has a large extracellular loop present between the two membrane spanning regions. The α-, β-, and γ-ENaC have cysteine rich regions within putative extracellular loops that are postulated to form intersubunit disulfide bonds necessary for oligomerization of Na channels. The three ENaCs also possess proline-rich regions within their intracellular C-terminal domains that are important for interactions between the subunits and accessory proteins that regulate the stability of functional channels in the apical membrane of kidney cells.

CELLULAR REGULATION OF ENaC

Sodium transport across the Na^+ reabsorbing, tight epithelia such as the distal nephron or colon is the major factor determining total body Na^+ content and thus, long-term blood pressure regulation. Sodium reabsorption in the distal nephron is a two step process (Fig. 59-2). First, sodium enters renal cells from the tubular lumen through ENaCs that are positioned in the apical membrane. Sodium is then actively transported out of the cell by Na K-ATPase on the basolateral membrane.

ENaC ACTIVITY IS IMPORTANT FOR CONTROLLING BLOOD SODIUM LEVELS AND MEAN BLOOD PRESSURE
ENaC is usually the rate-limiting step for Na^+ transport; and so represents the primary point for control of total body sodium balance and mean blood pressure. In fact, abnormalities in ENaC function can lead to disorders of total body Na^+ homeostasis, blood volume, blood pressure, and lung clearance (e.g., Liddle's syndrome and Pseudohypoaldosteronism Type I). An increase in ENaC activity or gain of function such as found in Liddle's syndrome leads to excessive salt reabsorption by the renal distal tubule, body fluid retention, and increased blood pressure. It has been suggested that in some African Americans with salt-sensitive hypertension, excessive sodium reabsorption is associated with ENaC hyperactivity. The clinical profile of these subjects includes low circulating levels of renin and angiotensin II and is consistent with this hypothesis. Also consistent is the observation that patients respond to treatment with diuretics like amiloride or triamterene whereas ACE inhibitors are ineffective. The control of ENaC activity, therefore, is important for understanding the pathophysiology of these disorders and hypertension in general.

REGULATION OF NA CHANNELS BY SMALL G PROTEINS
The small G proteins are single subunit proteins ranging in size from approx 20–30 kDa. There are several major categories of small G proteins that can participate in many aspects of cellular function including cell growth and differentiation. The first small G proteins described were the Ras proteins: there are three major categories of Ras proteins, H-, N-, and K-Ras proteins. All Ras proteins are post-translationally modified by the attachment of lipophilic groups (usually isoprenyl residues) to the C-terminal end plus subsequent methyl esterification of the C-terminus; these modifications are necessary for the biological function of the protein. After they are conjugated to methyl and isoprenyl groups, Ras proteins can be activated by GTP. Interestingly, methylation of isolated patches of membrane causes an increase in the activity of ENaC. This methylation-induced activation of ENaC is augmented simply by raising the cytosolic content of GTP. Thus, methylation of apical membranes excised as cell-free patches leads to an increase in ENaC activity. The response to methylation is augmented by GTP indicating that the small G protein regulates ENaC activity.

Evidence shows that one specific Ras protein, K-Ras2A, is a target for methylation in kidney cells and that Ras methylation is induced by aldosterone. K-Ras does contain the consensus amino acid sequence for methylation, a CAAX box (a methylated cysteine residue followed by two aliphatic residues, followed by any residue at the C-terminal end of a protein). The process requires both GTP and methylation before K-Ras activity rises. Inhibition of K-Ras2A expression in kidney cells reduces ENaC activity whereas augmenting K-Ras expression increases ENaC activity. These results indicate that the mechanism by which K-Ras is activated and identification of the signaling molecules that are activated by K-Ras are important steps in the understanding ENaC activity regulation.

Activation and Regulation of K-Ras   To be active, K-Ras must be methylated and changes in the rate of K-Ras methylation control the amount of membrane-associated K-Ras. Only the methylated, membrane-associated form binds GTP to increase its activity further. Thus, changes in the activity of the enzyme that methylates K-Ras, isoprenyl-cysteine-*O*-carboxy-methyl-transferase, alter K-Ras-induced ENaC activity. One way of regulating active, membrane-associated methyl transferases is to control the cytosolic concentrations of the end product of methylation, S-adenosyl-homocysteine (SAH). SAH is produced when the endogenous methyl donor, S-adenosyl-methionine, transfers its methyl group to a target protein. SAH is a potent inhibitor of all methyl transferases. The primary determinant of the SAH concentration in cells is generally not the rate of SAH production by methyl transferases, but rather, the rate of their degradation by another enzyme, S-adenosyl-L-homocysteine hydrolase or SAH hydrolase. For this reason, the extent of protein methylation can be controlled by changing the activity of SAH hydrolase rather than altering the intrinsic activity of the methyl transferase. Increased activity of the methyl transferase (measured as a rise in V_{max}) does occur when there is protein kinase C-mediated phosphorylation of the methyl transferase. In response to aldosterone, there is an increase in the activity of SAH hydrolase ensuring that the activity of the methyl transferase is not inhibited by the accumulation of its enzymatic product, SAH. How the SAH hydrolase is activated in response to aldosterone is unclear, though additional transcription and translation are not necessary.

The Mechanism for K-Ras Activation of ENaC Although K-Ras2A is necessary for ENaC activation, the mechanism by which K-Ras activates ENaC is not clear. The simplest mechanism would be a direct interaction of ENaC with K-Ras. It is likely, however, that other signaling elements lie between Ras and ENaC (any such element would have to be closely associated with ENaC in cell-free patches because it is possible to activate ENaC via Ras methylation in such patches). The traditional effector for Ras is Raf kinase and notably, Raf activation could activate the mitogen-activated protein kinase pathway, which in turn can activate other genes. Activation of the mitogen-activated protein kinase pathway, however, actually inhibits ENaC activity so K-Ras activation of Raf kinase does not appear to be responsible for K-Ras-mediated activation of ENaC. Another pathway leading to direct activation of ENaC is K-Ras2A-mediated activation of inositol lipid kinases that produce phosphatidylinositol bisphosphate (PIP$_2$) and phosphatidylinositol trisphosphate (PIP$_3$). For example, Ras proteins are known to activate several lipid kinases including phosphatidylinositol (PI)-3-kinase and PIP-5-kinase. Application of PIP$_2$ or PIP$_3$ to the cytosolic surface of excised cell patches strongly activates ENaC via an increase in the probability of an open channel.

Regulation of Na Channels by Inositol Lipids PIP$_2$ and PIP$_3$ are ubiquitous components of eukaryotic membrane phospholipids. The traditional view of phosphoinositide metabolism suggests that PI is sequentially phosphorylated by PI-4-kinase and PI-5-kinase to produce PI-4,5-bisphosphate or PIP$_2$. Once formed, PIP$_2$ can be phosphorylated to produce PI-3,4,5-triphosphate or PIP$_3$ via PI-3-kinase or it can be hydrolyzed by phospholipase C to produce 1,4,5-inositol trisphosphate (IP$_3$) and diacylglycerol. It was previously assumed that the sole purpose of PIP$_2$ production was to act as a precursor for IP$_3$ whhereas the remaining diacylglycerol would activate protein kinase C. It is clear that PIP$_2$ is a signaling molecule by itself and can directly activate other effector and signaling proteins. In particular, PIP$_2$ can bind to ion channels and modify their activity. The best-studied interactions in this case are between PIP$_2$ and K channels. PIP$_2$ binds the C-terminal domains of these K channels to increase channel activity; PIP$_2$ is absolutely required for the gating of these K$^+$ channels. The binding of the anionic PIP$_2$ to K$^+$ channels appears to involve, but is not limited to, electrostatic interactions. PIP$_2$ also modulates the activity of ENaC through similar interactions with hydrophobic and positively charged residues in the cytosolic tails of the β- and γ-subunits.

PHOSPHOINOSITIDE METABOLISM IS IMPORTANT FOR ENaC ACTIVITY 4,5-PIP$_2$ is just one of the inositol phospholipids that are produced by different inositol lipid kinases. PI-3-kinase is present in kidney cells. Inhibition of this enzyme with a specific PI-3-kinase inhibitor, LY-294002, blocks the basal rate and insulin-stimulated rate of Na$^+$ transport. The products of PI-3-kinase include PI-3-P (PIP), PI-3,4-P (PIP$_2$), and PI-3,4,5-P (PIP$_3$). These observations imply that phosphoinositides are involved in regulation of ENaC activity.

THE MOLECULAR BASIS FOR ENaC REGULATION BY ALDOSTERONE The mineralocorticoid, aldosterone, is the primary hormonal regulator of total body sodium balance. Increases in the circulating levels of the steroid specifically increase Na$^+$ reabsorption at the apical membrane by a two-phase reaction: an initial phase that increases transport four- to sixfold in the first 2–6 h followed by a late phase at 12–48 h, which increases transport another three to fourfold. The mechanisms for the early and late phases appear to be different. Aldosterone, like other steroid hormones, enters target cells (in the case of the kidney, the major targets are the principal cells of the collecting duct) and binds to cytosolic, mineralocorticoid receptor complexes. In mammalian principal cells, mineralocorticoid receptors are not activated by circulating glucocorticoids, because the enzyme, 11-β-hydroxysteroid dehydrogenase, changes the glucocorticoid structure to a form that does not bind aldosterone receptors. The enzyme does not change the aldosterone structure. After binding aldosterone, there is a conformational change in the aldosterone receptor. In its new conformation, it acts as a DNA binding protein and interacts with mineralocorticoid response elements. Binding to the mineralocorticoid response elements leads to changes in gene expression. For example, an increase in Na$^+$ transport can be measured within 1 h of exposure to aldosterone, by a mechanism that depends on gene transcription and translation. The induced gene products are referred to as aldosterone-induced proteins. Aldosterone and increased intracellular sodium also promote expression of the sodium pump during long-term exposure.

Many attempts have been made to identify the aldosterone-induced proteins. The relationship between the genes identified and the mechanism by which aldosterone increases Na$^+$ transport is often unclear. Originally, it was hypothesized that aldosterone induces ENaC synthesis and insertion into the cell membrane. Although the evidence from electrophysiological measurements remains somewhat controversial, the available biochemical evidence suggests that the number of sodium channel proteins in the apical membrane does not change after aldosterone treatment (at least in the first 2–4 h when the increase in sodium transport is most dramatic). The evidence suggests instead that the early effects of aldosterone are indirect and that the proteins that are synthesized are modulatory proteins that convert poorly transporting ENaC in the apical membrane into channels that readily transport sodium.

The three homologous ENaC subunit proteins form a heteromultimeric channel protein apparently made up of two α-, one β-, and one γ-subunit (although there is some disagreement about the exact stoichiometry). The most obvious link between aldosterone and increased ENaC activity would be a post-translational modification of the channels leading to an increase in the probability that the channels are open and hence, transporting sodium. A second hypothesis is that most or all of the ENaC channel subunits are present but dispersed in the apical membrane and aldosterone promotes the assembly of a channel complex, which transports sodium.

upstream of exon 1 and drives transcription of isoforms UT-A1, UT-A3, UT-A4, UT-A5, and UT-A6. and promoter II, which is located within intron 12 and drives transcription of isoform UT-A2. To date, no mutations in any of the UT-A isoforms have been reported in people. However, single nucleotide polymorphisms in UT-A2 are associated with variation in blood pressure in men, but not in women.

UT-A1 is the best studied and largest UT-A protein and is expressed in the apical membrane of the inner medullary collecting duct. UT-A1 is stimulated by cyclic AMP when expressed in *Xenopus* oocytes. UT-A3 is also expressed in the inner medullary collecting duct and stimulated by cAMP. A UT-A1/UT-A3 double knock-out mouse has a severe impairment in urine concentrating ability. Despite its name, UT-A2 was the first cloned urea transporter cDNA. UT-A2 is expressed in thin descending limbs and is not stimulated by cyclic AMP analogs. A UT-A2 knock-out mouse has a mild impairment in urine concentrating ability.

Lithium causes a marked reduction in AQP2 protein abundance. Lithium also causes a marked reduction in UT-A1 and UT-B protein abundances and interferes with vasopressin's ability to phosphorylate UT-A1. In inner medullary collecting ducts from normal rats, vasopressin rapidly increases UT-A1 phosphorylation and urea transport. However, in inner medullary collecting ducts from lithium-fed rats, vasopressin does not increase UT-A1 phosphorylation. Thus, lithium causes NDI by decreasing the abundance of several critical transport proteins involved in the urine concentrating mechanism, AQP2, UT-A1, and UT-B. The reduction in AQP2 decreases water reabsorption across the collecting duct apical membrane in response to vasopressin, thereby reducing transepithelial water reabsorption. The reduction in UT-A1 and phosphorylated UT-A1 decreases urea reabsorption across the inner medullary collecting duct in response to vasopressin, thereby reducing inner medullary interstitial urea accumulation, which reduces urine concentrating ability. The reduction in UT-B decreases urea recycling and the efficiency of countercurrent exchange, which reduces urine concentrating ability. Unfortunately, if lithium-induced NDI is not diagnosed quickly and lithium therapy stopped, the acquired NDI often becomes irreversible.

ACKNOWLEDGMENTS

This work was supported by National Institutes of Health Grants R01-DK41707, R01-DK63657, and P01-DK61521 (to JMS) and by the Canadian Institutes of Health Research Grant MT-8126 and the Kidney Foundation of Canada (to DGB). Address for correspondence: Dr. Jeff M. Sands, Emory University School of Medicine, Renal Division, WMRB Room 338, 1639 Pierce Drive, NE, Atlanta, GA 30322 USA. Phone: 404-727-2525; FAX: 404-727-3425; E-mail: jsands@emory.edu.

SELECTED REFERENCES

Aridor M, Balch WE. Integration of endoplasmic reticulum signaling in health and disease. Nat Med 1999;5:745–751.

Arthus M-F, Lonergan M, Crumley MJ, et al. Report of 33 novel *AVPR2* mutations and analysis of 117 families with X-linked nephrogenic diabetes insipidus. J Am Soc Nephrol 2000;11:1044–1054.

Bagnasco SM. Gene structure of urea transporters. Am J Physiol Renal Physiol 2003;284:F3–F10.

Bagnasco SM, Peng T, Janech MG, Karakashian A, Sands JM. Cloning and characterization of the human urea transporter UT-A1 and mapping of the human *Slc14a2* gene. Am J Physiol Renal Physiol 2001;281:F400–F406.

Bagnasco SM, Peng T, Nakayama Y, Sands JM. Differential expression of individual UT-A urea transporter isoforms in rat kidney. J Am Soc Nephrol 2000;11:1980–1986.

Bernier V, Lagace M, Lonergan M, Arthus MF, Bichet DG, Bouvier M. Functional rescue of the constitutively internalized V2 vasopressin receptor mutant R137H by the pharmacological chaperone action of SR49059. Mol Endocrinol 2004;18:2074–2084.

Bichet DG, Arthus M-F, Lonergan M, et al. X-linked nephrogenic diabetes insipidus mutations in North America and the Hopewell hypothesis. J Clin Invest 1993;92:1262–1268.

Bichet DG, Birnbaumer M, Lonergan M, et al. Nature and recurrence of AVPR2 mutations in X-linked nephrogenic diabetes insipidus. Am J Hum Genet 1994;55:278–286.

Bichet DG, Fujiwara TM. Nephrogenic diabetes insipidus. In: Scriver CR, Beaudet AL, Sly WS, Vallee D, Childs B, Kinzler KW et al., eds. The Metabolic and Molecular Bases of Inherited Disease. New York: McGraw-Hill, 2001; pp. 4181–4204.

Bode HH, Crawford JD. Nephrogenic diabetes insipidus in North America: the Hopewell hypothesis. N Engl J Med 1969; 280:750–754.

Brown D. The ins and outs of aquaporin-2 trafficking. Am J Physiol Renal Physiol 2003;284:F893–F901.

Crawford JD, Bode HH. Disorders of the posterior pituitary in children. In: Gardner LI, ed. Endocrine and Genetic Diseases of Childhood and Adolescence. Philadelphia: W.B. Saunders, 1975; pp. 126–158.

Deen PMT, Verdijk MAJ, Knoers NVAM, et al. Requirement of human renal water channel aquaporin-2 for vasopressin-dependent concentration of urine. Science 1994;264:92–95.

Deen PMT, Croes H, van Aubel RAMH, Ginsel LA, van Os CH. Water channels encoded by mutant aquaporin-2 genes in nephrogenic diabetes insipidus are impaired in their cellular routing. J Clin Invest 1995;95:2291–2296.

Fenton RA, Chou CL, Stewart GS, Smith CP, Knepper MA. Urinary concentrating defect in mice with selective deletion of phloretin-sensitive urea transporters in the renal collecting duct. Proc Natl Acad Sci USA 2004;101:7469–7474.

Fenton RA, Stewart GS, Carpenter B, et al. Characterization of the mouse urea transporters UT-A1 and UT-A2. Am J Physiol Renal Physiol 2002;283:F817–F825.

Fujiwara TM, Bichet DG. Molecular biology of hereditary diabetes insipidus. J Am Soc Nephrol 2005;16:2836–2846.

Galluci E, Micelli S, Lippe C. Non-electrolyte permeability across thin lipid membranes. Arch Int Physiol Biochim 1971;79:881–887.

Hoekstra JA, van Lieburg AF, Monnens LA, Hulstijn-Dirkmaat GM, Knoers VV. Cognitive and psychosocial functioning of patients with congenital nephrogenic diabetes insipidus. Am J Med Genet 1996;61:81–88.

Holtzman EJ, Kolakowski LF, O'Brien D, Crawford JD, Ausiello DA. A null mutation in the vasopressin V2 receptor gene (AVPR2) associated with nephrogenic diabetes insipidus in the Hopewell kindred. Hum Mol Genet 1993;2:1201–1204.

Ito M, Yu RN, Jameson JL. Mutant vasopressin precursors that cause autosomal dominant neurohypophyseal diabetes insipidus retain dimerization and impair the secretion of wild-type proteins. J Biol Chem 1999;274:9029–9037.

Kamsteeg EJ, Wormhoudt TA, Rijss JP, van Os CH, Deen PM. An impaired routing of wild-type aquaporin-2 after tetramerization with an aquaporin-2 mutant explains dominant nephrogenic diabetes insipidus. EMBO J 1999;18:2394–2400.

Karakashian A, Timmer RT, Klein JD, Gunn RB, Sands JM, Bagnasco SM. Cloning and characterization of two new mRNA isoforms of the rat renal urea transporter: UT-A3 and UT-A4. J Am Soc Nephrol 1999;10: 230–237.

Kim Y-H, Kim D-U, Han K-H, et al. Expression of urea transporters in the developing rat kidney. Am J Physiol Renal Physiol 2002;282:F530–F540.

Kimoto Y, Constantinou CE. Effects of [1-desamino-8-D-arginine]vasopressin and papaverine on rabbit renal pelvis. Eur J Pharmacol 1990;175:359–362.

Klein JD, Gunn RB, Roberts BR, Sands JM. Down-regulation of urea transporters in the renal inner medulla of lithium-fed rats. Kidney Int 2002;61:995–1002.

Klein JD, Sands JM, Qian L, Wang X, Yang B. Upregulation of urea transporter UT-A2 and water channels AQP2 and AQP3 in mice lacking urea transporter UT-B. J Am Soc Nephrol 2004;15:1161–1167.

Kokko JP, Rector FC. Countercurrent multiplication system without active transport in inner medulla. Kidney Int 1972;2:214–223.

Kuwahara M, Iwai K, Ooeda T, et al. Three families with autosomal dominant nephrogenic diabetes insipidus caused by aquaporin-2 mutations in the C-terminus. Am J Hum Genet 2001;69:738–748.

Kuznetsov G, Nigam SK. Folding of secretory and membrane proteins. N Engl J Med 1998;339:1688–1695.

Lucien N, Sidoux-Walter F, Olives B, et al. Characterization of the gene encoding the human Kidd blood group urea transporter protein: evidence for splice site mutations in Jk_null individuals. J Biol Chem 1998;273:12,973–12,980.

Lucien N, Sidoux-Walter F, Roudier N, et al. Antigenic and functional properties of the human red blood cell urea transporter hUT-B1. J Biol Chem 2002;277:34,101–34,108.

Marr N, Bichet DG, Lonergan M, et al. Heteroligomerization of an aquaporin-2 mutant with wild-type aquaporin-2 and their misrouting to late endosomes/lysosomes explains dominant nephrogenic diabetes insipidus. Hum Mol Genet 2002;11:779–789.

McIlraith CH. Notes on some cases of diabetes insipidus with marked family and hereditary tendencies. Lancet 1892;2:767, 768.

McKusick VA. Online Mendelian Inheritance in Man OMIM, (TM). McKusick-Nathans Institute for Genetic Medicine, Johns Hopkins University (Baltimore, MD) and National Center for Biotechnology Information, National Library of Medicine (Bethesda, MD), 2000. World Wide Web URL: http://www.ncbi.nlm.nih.gov/omim/.

Morello J-P, Bichet DG. Nephrogenic diabetes insipidus. Annu Rev Physiol 2001;63:607–630.

Mulders SB, Knoers NVAM, van Lieburg AF, et al. New mutations in the AQP2 gene in nephrogenic diabetes insipidus resulting in functional but misrouted water channels. J Am Soc Nephrol 1997;8:242–248.

Mulders SM, Bichet DG, Rijss JPL, et al. An aquaporin-2 water channel mutant which causes autosomal dominant nephrogenic diabetes insipidus is retained in the golgi complex. J Clin Invest 1998;102:57–66.

Nakayama Y, Naruse M, Karakashian A, Peng T, Sands JM, Bagnasco SM. Cloning of the rat Slc14a2 gene and genomic organization of the UT-A urea transporter. Biochem Biophys Acta 2001;1518:19–26.

Niaudet P, Dechaux M, Leroy D, Broyer M. Nephrogenic diabetes insipidus in children. In: Czernichow P, Robinson AG, eds. Frontiers of Hormone Research. Basel: Karger, 1985; pp. 224–231.

Nielsen S, Frokiaer J, Marples D, Kwon ED, Agre P, Knepper M. Aquaporins in the kidney: from molecules to medicine. Physiol Rev 2002;82:205–244.

Ohzeki T, Igarashi T, Okamoto A. Familial cases of congenital nephrogenic diabetes insipidus type II: remarkable increment of urinary adenosine 3',5'-monophosphate in response to antidiuretic hormone. J Pediatr 1984;104:593–595.

Okusa MD, Crystal LJT. Clinical manifestations and management of acute lithium intoxication. Am J Med 1994;97:383–389.

Olives B, Mattei M-G, Huet M, et al. Kidd blood group and urea transport function of human erythrocytes are carried by the same protein. J Biol Chem 1995;270:15,607–15,610.

Olives B, Neau P, Bailly P, et al. Cloning and functional expression of a urea transporter from human bone marrow cells. J Biol Chem 1994;269:31,649–31,652.

Pallone TL, Turner MR, Edwards A, Jamison RL. Countercurrent exchange in the renal medulla. Am J Physiol Regul Integr Comp Physiol 2003;284:R1153–R1175.

Ranade K, Wu KD, Hwu CM, et al. Genetic variation in the human urea transporter-2 is associated with variation in blood pressure. Hum Mol Genet 2001;10:2157–2164.

Reeves WB, Andreoli TE. Nephrogenic diabetes insipidus. In: Scriver CR, Beaudet AL, Sly WS, Valle D, eds. The Metabolic and Molecular Bases of Inherited Disease. New York: McGraw-Hill, 1995; pp. 3045–3071.

Rittig R, Robertson GL, Siggaard C, et al. Identification of 13 new mutations in the vasopressin-neurophysin II gene in 17 kindreds with familial autosomal dominant neurohypophyseal diabetes insipidus. Am J Hum Genet 1996;58:107–117.

Sands JM. Molecular approaches to urea transporters. J Am Soc Nephrol 2002;13:2795–2806.

Sands JM. Molecular mechanisms of urea transport. J Membr Biol 2003;191:149–163.

Sands JM. Urea transporters. Annu Rev Physiol 2003;65:543–566.

Sands JM. Renal urea transporters. Curr Opin Nephrol Hypertens 2004;13:525–532.

Sands JM, Gargus JJ, Fröhlich O, Gunn RB, Kokko JP. Urinary concentrating ability in patients with Jk(a-b-) blood type who lack carrier-mediated urea transport. J Am Soc Nephrol 1992;2:1689–1696.

Sands JM, Layton HE. Urine concentrating mechanism and its regulation. In: Seldin DW, Giebisch G, eds. The Kidney: Physiology and Pathophysiology. Philadelphia: Lippincott, Williams and Wilkins, 2000; pp. 1175–1216.

Sands JM, Nonoguchi H, Knepper MA. Vasopressin effects on urea and H2O transport in inner medullary collecting duct subsegments. Am J Physiol Renal Physiol 1987;253:F823–F832.

Sidoux-Walter F, Lucien N, Nissinen R, et al. Molecular heterogeneity of the Jk_null phenotype: expression analysis of the Jk(S291P) mutation found in Finns. Blood 2000;96:1566–1573.

Stephenson JL. Concentration of urine in a central core model of the renal counterflow system. Kidney Int 1972;2:85–94.

Tamarappoo BK, Verkman AS. Defective aquaporin-2 trafficking in nephrogenic diabetes insipidus and correction by chemical chaperones. J Clin Invest 1998;101:2257–2267.

Timmer RT, Klein JD, Bagnasco SM, et al. Localization of the urea transporter UT-B protein in human and rat erythrocytes and tissues. Am J Physiol Cell Physiol 2001;281:C1318–C1325.

Timmer RT, Sands JM. Lithium intoxication. J Am Soc Nephrol 1999;10:666–674.

Uchida S, Sohara E, Rai T, Ikawa M, Okabe M, Sasaki S. Impaired urea accumulation in the inner medulla of mice lacking the urea transporter UT-A2. Mol Cell Biol 2005;25:7357–7363.

van Lieburg AF, Knoers NVAM, Monnens LAH. Clinical presentation and follow-up of 30 patients with congenital nephrogenic diabetes insipidus. J Am Soc Nephrol 1999;10:1958–1964.

van Os CH, Deen PM. Aquaporin-2 water channel mutations causing nephrogenic diabetes insipidus. Proc Assoc Am Physicians 1998;110:395–400.

Waring AG, Kajdi L, Tappan V. Congenital defect of water metabolism. Am J Dis Child 1945;69:323–325.

Weil A. Ueber die hereditare form des diabetes insipidus. Arch Klin Med 1908;93:180–290.

Weil A. Ueber die hereditare form des diabetes insipidus. Virchows Arch Path Anat Physiol Klin Med 1884;95:70–95.

Wieth JO, Funder J, Gunn RB, Brahm J. Passive transport pathways for chloride and urea through the red cell membrane. In: Bolis K, Bloch K, Luria SE, Lynen F, eds. Comparative Biochemistry and Physiology of Transport. Amsterdam: Elsevier/North-Holland, 1974; pp. 317–337.

Williams RM, Henry C. Nephrogenic diabetes insipidus transmitted by females and appearing during infancy in males. Ann Intern Med 1947;27:84–95.

Yang B, Bankir L, Gillespie A, Epstein CJ, Verkman AS. Urea-selective concentrating defect in transgenic mice lacking urea transporter UT-B. J Biol Chem 2002;277:10,633–10,637.

You G, Smith CP, Kanai Y, Lee W-S, Stelzner M, Hediger MA. Cloning and characterization of the vasopressin-regulated urea transporter. Nature 1993;365:844–847.

Zhang C, Sands JM, Klein JD. Vasopressin rapidly increases the phosphorylation of the UT-A1 urea transporter activity in rat IMCDs through PKA. Am J Physiol Renal Physiol 2002;282:F85–F90.

61 Glomerulonephritis and Smad Signaling

HUI Y. LAN AND RICHARD J. JOHNSON

SUMMARY

Transforming growth factor-β and its signaling pathway, Smads, is the major mechanism mediating fibrosis. However, the involvement of other signaling pathways and the interplay among these pathways in fibrosis remain largely unclear. In this chapter, we focus on the current understanding of the molecular basis of transforming growth factor-β signaling and its crosstalk pathways in renal fibrosis, which may be also applicable to a wide arrange of other disease conditions involving fibrosis. In addition, results from current studies also suggest that Smad signaling may be a final common pathway of fibrosis and targeting the Smad pathway may provide a new therapeutic strategy for tissue and/or organ fibrosis.

Key Words: Diabetes; fibrosis; gene therapy; hypertension; kidney disease; TGF-β; signaling pathways; Smads.

INTRODUCTION

Fibrosis is the final common pathway leading to end-stage disease in a variety of tissues and organs including heart, liver, lung, skin, and kidney, regardless of the initial causes of damage. The common pathological feature of fibrosis is the accumulation of extracellular matrix (ECM) in tissues. ECM is made from collagen types I, III, and IV, fibronectin, and laminin and this response is mediated by multiple factors, involving several signaling pathways. Reports have identified transforming growth factor (TGF)-β and its signaling pathway, Smads, as one of the major mechanisms mediating fibrosis. The involvement of other signaling pathways and the interplay among different pathways to produce fibrosis remain largely unclear. This chapter focuses on the understanding of the molecular basis of TGF-β signaling and its crosstalk pathways in producing fibrosis in the kidney. These pathways may also be applicable to a wide range of other conditions including pulmonary fibrosis, hepatic fibrosis and cirrhosis, and cardiovascular sclerosis.

TGF-β AND RENAL FIBROSIS

TGF-β, a multifunctional cytokine with fibrogenic properties, has long been considered a key mediator in the pathogenesis of renal fibrosis. Increased TGF-β expression is a feature of many human and experimental renal diseases, including diabetic and hypertensive nephropathy. TGF-β stimulates ECM deposition by increasing the synthesis of ECM proteins and acting to inhibit their degradation. In addition, TGF-β mediates renal fibrosis through the transformation of tubular epithelial cells to ECM-producing myofibroblasts. The important role of TGF-β in producing renal fibrosis is demonstrated by the finding that fibrosis can be induced by the overexpression of TGF-β_1 within the normal rat kidney. This fibrosis can be prevented or ameliorated by blocking TGF-β activity with a neutralizing TGF-β antibody, decorin, or by antisense strategies. In a number of experimental kidney disease models TGF-β plays a central role in renal fibrosis.

TGF-β SIGNALING

The discovery that Smad proteins are the intracellular mediators and regulators of TGF-β signaling has provided important insights into the specific mechanisms by which TGF-β mediates the fibrogenic response. As shown in Fig. 61-1, TGF-β exerts its biological effects by signaling through the type-I and -II serine/threonine kinase receptors, TβRI and TβRII. TGF-β binds to receptor II, which then recruits and phosphorylates TβRI. The activated TβRI directly initiates signals to downstream intracellular substrates, receptor-regulated Smads (R-Smads) including Smad2 and -3. Activated R-Smads interact with the common partner, Smad4 (Co-Smad), to form a heteroligomer and these complexes are translocated into the nucleus to regulate target gene expression and initiate the fibrogenic process. Activation of the TGF-β signaling pathway can also lead to the expression of inhibitory Smads (I-Smads) including Smad6 and -7. In mammals, Smad2 and -3 are TGF-β/activin-specific R-Smads, whereas Smad1/5/8 are the bone morphogenetic protein (BMP)-specific R-Smads. Smad4 is the only one that functions as a Co-Smad. Smad6 (preferential inhibitor of the signaling processes initiated by BMP) and Smad7 (a potent inhibitor of signaling initiated by TGF-β or BMP) both act as inhibitory factors (I-Smads) and function as antagonists of R-Smads and Co-Smad signaling. It has been shown that Smad7 can act by specifically inhibiting Smad2 and -3 phosphorylation. The inhibition results from blocking their access to TβRI or by causing degradation of TβRI. Thus, overexpression of Smad7 may be a strategy that will terminate TGF-β signaling, thereby blocking TGF-β-mediated fibrosis.

The structure of the Smad family is highly conserved. Smad2 and -3 are the two R-Smads that are activated by TβRI. They are structurally very similar, with 91% of their amino acid sequences identical. Both contain an N-terminal "mad homology 1" domain,

From: *Principles of Molecular Medicine, Second Edition*
Edited by: M. S. Runge and C. Patterson © Humana Press, Inc., Totowa, NJ

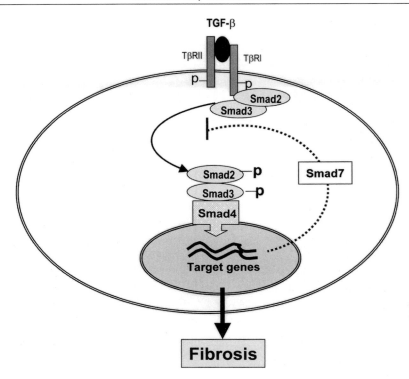

Figure 61-1   TGF-β signaling and fibrosis. Binding of TGF-β to receptor II causes phosphorylation of TβRI that results in phosphorylation of receptor-associated Smads (R-Smads), Smad2 and -3. Activated R-Smads form heteroligomers with the common partner Smad4 to translocate into the nucleus and regulate target gene expression including ECM genes and inhibitory Smad6 and -7. These I-Smads inhibit Smad2 and -3 phosphorylation by blocking their access to TβRI or by causing degradation of TβRI, thereby blocking TGF-β-mediated fibrosis.

which has DNA-binding activity, and a C-terminal mad homology 2 (MH2) domain that is responsible for translocation of the Smad complex into the nucleus in which it regulates transcription of target genes. TβRI-mediated phosphorylation of the C-terminal sequence of R-Smads, SSXS, leads to Smad2 and -3 activation. Smad4 lacks the SSXS sequence and therefore cannot be phosphorylated by the TβRI. The interaction between R-Smads (Smad2/3) and Co-Smad (Smad4) is primarily mediated by the mad homology 2 domain. Once within the nucleus, the Smads can function as transcriptional transactivators or coactivators, and may also directly bind to DNA, resulting in activation of the target genes that are the next step in producing fibrosis.

TGF-β SIGNALING IN RENAL FIBROSIS

It is clear that TGF-β mediates tissue fibrosis through Smad signaling pathway. Many ECM genes contain activator protein-1 binding sites in their regulatory regions; their induction by TGF-β has been shown to be Smad3 dependent. This conclusion is further supported by the finding that mice that are null for Smad3 are protected against radiation-induced fibrosis on the skin. In the context of fibrosis in the kidney, both Smad2 and -3 are strongly activated in human diabetic kidney (Fig. 61-2) or in the rat following obstruction of the kidney (Fig. 61-3). Activation of Smad2 and -3 within the kidney, therefore, can contribute to the development of glomerulosclerosis, tubulointerstitial fibrosis, and vascular sclerosis (Figs. 61-2 and 61-3), indicating that this TGF-β signaling system is a critical pathway leading to tissue fibrosis. In vitro, it has been shown that TGF-β-induced collagen matrix production by mesangial cells and tubular epithelial cells is mediated by Smad2 and -3. In addition, glucose-mediated collagen matrix production by mesangial

cells, tubular epithelial cells, endothelial cells, or vascular smooth muscle cells is also dependent on the activation of Smad2 and -3. Activation of Smads is required for TGF-β-induced, tubular epithelial cell–myofibroblast transition, an important process for tubulointerstitial fibrosis. The functional role of Smad2 and -3 in initiating fibrosis is delineated by results demonstrating that blockade of Smad2/3 activation by overexpression of Smad7 results in abrogation of bleomycin-induced lung fibrosis in mice and in fibrosis following obstructive kidney disease in rats. All of these reports provide strong evidence supporting a critical role for TGF-β/Smad signaling in the development of tissue scarring.

The precise role of individual Smads and the interplay among them in initiating the fibrotic process remains largely unknown. Although both Smad2 and -3 are structurally very similar, their modes of actions and the phenotypes of Smad2 and -3 are distinct. Smad3 regulates gene activity directly by binding to DNA, whereas Smad2 activates transcription by binding to other transcription factors that, in turn, can bind DNA and modulate gene activity. The distinct activities of Smad2 and -3 are highlighted by the finding that Smad2$^{-/-}$ mice are embryonic lethal, whereas Smad3$^{-/-}$ mice are viable but have impaired immunity. Similarly, different genes are regulated by different Smads or combinations of Smads in vitro. For example, in mouse embryo fibroblasts, the induction of matrix metalloproteinase-2 by TGF-β is selectively dependent on Smad2, whereas the induction of c-*fos* is dependent on Smad3, and both Smad2 and -3 are required for inducing the plasminogen activator inhibitor-1. Interestingly, the absence of Smad3 has no effect on TGF-β-induced inhibition of mammary epithelial cell proliferation, but without Smad3 there is decreased cell apoptosis but no compensatory changes in the expression or

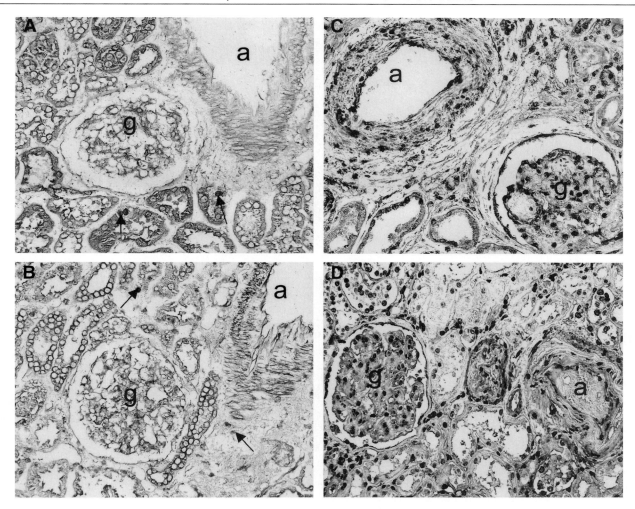

Figure 61-2 Smad2 and -3 activation in diabetic and hypertensive nephropathy. In the normal human kidney, activated Smad2 (**A**) and -3 (**B**) cells (black nuclear location) are rare (arrows). In contrast, in diabetic (**C**) and hypertensive (**D**) nephropathy, activation (black nuclear location) of Smad2 (**C**) and -3 (**D**) are prominent, contributing to glomerulosclerosis, tubulointerstitial fibrosis, and vascular sclerosis. (g, glomerulus; a, artery)

activation of Smad2. These findings suggest that epithelial cell Smad3 is not required for the influence of TGF-β on proliferation, but Smad3 contributes in a nonredundant manner to the induction of apoptosis. Interestingly, TGF-β-induced vascular endothelial growth factor expression by renal tubular epithelial cells depends on Smad3, but not Smad2, whereas TGF-β-induced thrombospondin-1 expression is stimulated by Smad2, but not Smad3. Although both Smad2 and -3 are required for TGF-β-induced tubular mesenchymal transition, Smad2 regulates a loss of an epithelial gene E-cadherin, but Smad3 contributes to *de novo* expression of a mesenchymal gene, α-SMA. Thus, Smad2 and -3 seem to work in a nonredundant manner, but both may be required in certain pathophysiological processes.

TGF-β-INDEPENDENT SMAD SIGNALING IN RENAL AND VASCULAR FIBROSIS

Smad2 and -3 can also be activated by a non-TGF-β-dependent pathway. Advanced glycation end products (AGEs), the molecules that are key mediators of diabetic complications, can also activate Smads directly and independently of TGF-β. For example, AGEs can induce a rapid activation of Smad2 and -3 in tubular epithelial cells, mesangial cells, or vascular smooth muscle cells; activation

is evident at 5 min and peaks by 30 min. This rapid activation of Smads occurs in the absence of TGF-β and a neutralizing TGF-β antibody will not block AGE-induced Smad activation. Importantly, the finding that AGEs, but not TGF-β, can activate Smads in both TβRI and TβRII mutant cells supports the presence of a TGF-β-independent Smad signaling pathway as a mediator of renal and vascular complications of diabetes. The mechanism by which AGEs activate Smad directly and independently of TGF-β has been uncovered; AGEs signal through the receptor for AGEs (RAGE) to induce Smad activation rapidly via the extracellular signal-regulated kinase (ERK)/p38 mitogen-activated protein (MAP)-Smad crosstalk pathway. For example, AGE-induced activation of Smad2/3 can be blocked by a neutralizing anti-RAGE antibody or by specific MAP kinase (MAPK) inhibitors of ERK1/2 (PD98059) and p38 (SB203580). AGEs are able to activate Smad2/3 after exposure for 24 h via the TGF-β-dependent mechanism. Thus, AGEs could mediate diabetic complications directly via the MAPK-Smad signaling pathway or indirectly through the classic TGF-β-Smad signaling pathway. Interestingly, substantial inhibition of AGE-induced Smad activation and collagen production by inhibitors of ERK/p38 MAPK or, to a lesser extent, by an anti-TGF-β antibody indicates that the MAPK-Smad

Normal   **Control vector**   **Smad7**

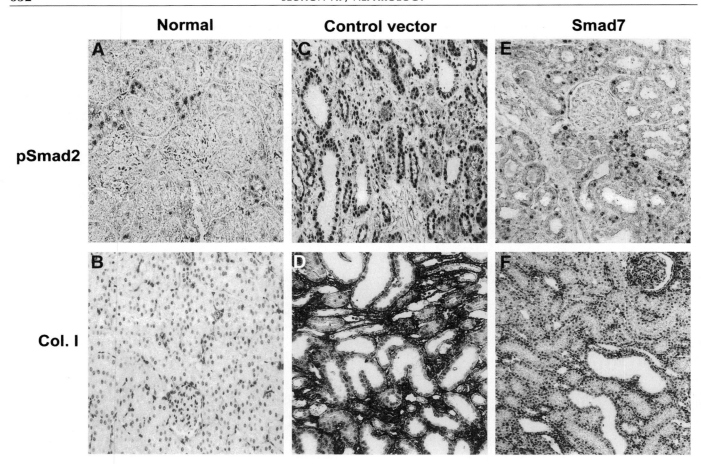

Figure 61-3   Overexpression of Smad7 inhibits Smad2 and -3 activation and renal fibrosis in a rat obstructive nephropathy. The left ureter was ligated and the left kidney was transfected with either Smad7 (treated animals) or empty vectors (control animals) in a mixture of Optison followed immediately by ultrasound as described. Smad7 transgene expression was induced by doxycycline in the drinking water for 7 d. In the normal rat kidney, phosphorylated Smad2 (pSmad2 nuclear location) are rare (**A**) with minor collagen I accumulation in tubulointerstitium (**B**). In contrast, marked activation of pSmad2 is found in tubulointerstitium (**C**), contributing to tubulointerstitial fibrosis (**D**). Significantly, kidney treated with Smad7 substantially prevents Smad2 activation (**E**) and tubulointerstitial fibrosis (**F**).

signaling crosstalk pathway is a key mechanism involved in the pathogenesis of AGE-mediated diabetic scarring. These findings also indicate that the Smad crosstalk pathway may play a critical role in development of the end-stage organ or in the tissue scarring characteristic of diabetes. Viewed in this fashion, anti-TGF-β therapy may not be sufficient to block diabetic complications.

The importance of MAPK-Smad signaling and crosstalk in initiating fibrosis has been demonstrated by finding a relationship between angiotensin (Ang)-II and Smads in the development of kidney and cardiovascular fibrosis. Preliminary studies demonstrate that, like AGEs, Ang-II-mediated collagen matrix production by both renal and vascular cells is Smad-dependent. Ang-II signals through its type 1 receptor to activate Smad2 and -3 within 5 min by a direct mechanism that is independent of TGF-β but dependent on ERK/p38 and MAPK. Ang-II is also able to activate Smad2 and -3 at 24 h, by a mechanism that is TGF-β dependent. Thus, activation of Smads via MAPK-Smad crosstalk pathways may be critical for developing diabetic- or hypertension-induced kidney and vascular sclerosis as shown in Fig. 61-2. In fact, increased Smad2 and -3 activation has been demonstrated in the scarred tissue that results following myocardial infarction;

this activation was attenuated by Ang-II signals through its type-1 receptor antagonists. In an obstructive kidney of rats, Ang-II has been shown to play a role in generating renal fibrosis and blockade of Smad2 and -3 activation by the overexpression of Smad7 substantially inhibits renal fibrosis. Direct evidence for a role of Smads in Ang-II-mediated fibrosis comes from the observation that mice null for Smad3 do not develop Ang-II-induced cardiovascular cell or kidney scarring. Together, these studies constitute strong evidence that there is crosstalk between Ang-II (or AGEs) and TGF-β signaling pathways that result in cardiovascular and renal scarring. These data also demonstrate the importance of a functional interaction between the MAPK and Smad signaling pathways in the process of fibrosis. Smad signaling may be a common pathway for the pathogenesis of tissue scarring, as shown in Fig. 61-4.

Mechanisms whereby Smads act as signal integrators to form the crosstalk pathways among fibrogenic molecules have been suggested from a number of studies. This is a complicated area however, because activation of Smads can be regulated by other signaling pathways, such as the MAPK pathway, the Janus-activated kinase/signal transducer and activator of transcription

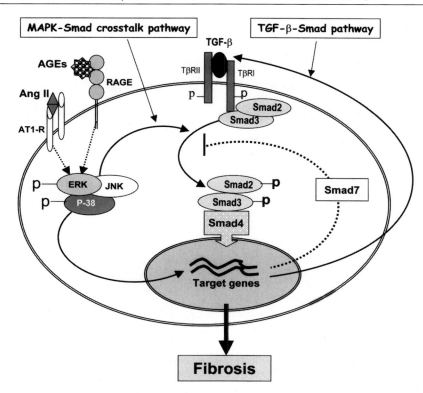

Figure 61-4 Smad signaling as a common pathway of fibrosis. Although TGF-β signals through TβRs to activate Smads to mediate fibrosis, both AGEs and Ang-II signal through their individual receptors to activate Smads via the MAP kinases (MAPK)-Smad signaling crosstalk pathway, in addition to the classic TGF-β-dependent Smad signaling pathway. Overexpression of the inhibitory Smad7 blocks Smad signaling and fibrosis generally.

pathway, and the nuclear factor-κB pathway. Of these pathways, the interaction between MAPK and Smad signaling pathways is the best delineated. It has been shown that signals derived from growth factor receptors with tyrosine kinase activities are capable of modulating Smad-dependent effects. Presently, the mechanism involves activation of a kinase downstream of mitogen-activated protein kinase (MEK)-1, the upstream activator of the ERK/MAPK pathway and results in the phosphorylation of Smad2. Phosphorylation of Smad1, -2, and -3 by Ras-activated ERK1/2 in its linker region will inhibit nuclear translocation of these transcription factors. In contrast, the intracellular kinase, mitogen-activated protein kinase kinase (MEKK)-1, can participate in Smad2-dependent transcriptional events. MEKK-1 is also capable of selectively activating Smad2-dependent transcriptional activity in cultured endothelial cells by a mechanism that is independent of TβRI-mediated responses. These responses do not require the presence of the C-terminal SSXS motif of Smad2, (the site of TβRI-mediated phosphorylation) and are positively regulated by the MEK1-ERK pathway. Activation of Smad2 by MEKK-1 results in enhanced Smad2–Smad4 interactions, nuclear localization of the Smad2–Smad4 complex, and the stimulation of Smad transcriptional coactivator interactions. Notably, overexpression of Smad7 can inhibit the MEKK-1-mediated stimulation of Smad2 transcriptional activity. For example, an inhibitor of the ERK1/2 pathway, U0126, or inhibitors of the p38 MAPK pathway, SB203580 and SKF86002, will block TGF-β-induced, aggrecan gene expression during chondrocyte differentiation. Other evidence for crosstalk between the ERK/MAPK pathway

and the Smad pathways is that both pathways are required for TGF-β$_1$-induced, furin gene transactivation.

A variety of other kinases have been implicated in TGF-β signaling; jun N-terminal kinase (JNK) is rapidly activated by TGF-β in a Smad-independent manner and JNK can phosphorylate Smad3 outside of the SSXS motif. Smad3 phosphorylation by JNK will facilitate, both Smad3 activation by the TGF-β receptor complex, and its nuclear accumulation. In fact, JNK cooperates with the Smad signaling to induce Smad7 transcription via the activator protein-1 element, and hence inhibits ERK activity. These results indicate that inhibitory Smad7 is negatively regulated by ERK, but positively regulated by JNK. Thus, there is an interdependent relationship between the MAPK and Smad pathways in TGF-β-mediated transcription. Overall, signaling by TGF-β-like factors is regulated in both positive and negative pathways, and is tightly controlled temporally and spatially through multiple mechanisms at the extracellular, membrane, cytoplasmic, and nuclear levels. Positive regulation might prove to be critical for amplification of signaling by TGF-β and involve activation of R-Smads 2/3, whereas negative regulation may play an important role in restriction and termination of TGF-β signaling via activation of I-Smad7.

SMADS AS A CENTRAL PATHWAY OF FIBROSIS AND AS A NOVEL THERAPEUTIC TARGET FOR TISSUE SCARRING

As shown in Fig. 61-4, Smad signaling may act as a central pathway that leads to fibrosis regardless of the initial pathogenic cause. Because Smad7 can act as a negative regulator of Smad signaling, overexpression of Smad7 might inhibit Smad2 and -3 activation to terminate Smad signaling and block Smad-mediated ECM production. In vitro, overexpression of Smad7 will block the fibrogenic effects of TGF-β in tubular epithelial or mesangial cells of the kidney. In vivo, overexpression of Smad7 using a gene transfer technique can inhibit Smad2 and -3 activation in bleomycin-induced TGF-β-dependent lung fibrosis or in a model of obstructive nephropathy in rats. A novel, effective, and inducible gene therapy that specifically blocks TGF-β/Smad signaling and fibrosis in obstructive nephropathy in rats, has been accomplished by transferring a doxycycline-regulated Smad7 using an ultrasound-microbubble-mediated system. This technique substantially increases the transfection rate and transgene expression by up to 1000-fold compared with the naked DNA transfer strategy. Using this technique, investigators transfected a doxycycline-regulated Smad7 gene into the kidney and induced the Smad7 transgene expression to a therapeutic level by controlling the doses of doxycycline in the drinking water. In the rat obstructive nephropathy model (Fig. 61-3), progressive renal fibrosis that is routinely induced by both TGF-β and Ang-II, is blocked by the expression of the doxycycline-induced Smad7 transgene. There also is complete inhibition of Smad2 and -3 activation plus complete inhibition of myofibroblast proliferation and collagen matrix production. In the rat diabetic nephropathy model, renal injury is mediated by multiple factors including AGEs, high glucose, TGF-β and/or Ang II. Overexpression of Smad7, however, results in complete inhibition of Smad2 and -3 activation and collagen matrix accumulation in both glomeruli and tubulointerstitium. Thus, Smad signaling could be a central pathway to organ fibrosis. Targeting Smad signaling could provide a therapeutic strategy to prevent or combat the scarring resulting in an end-stage organ.

Overexpression of Smad7 is also able to inhibit immune and inflammatory responses. Ultrasound-microbubble-mediated, doxycycline-induced Smad7 transgene expression results in substantial inhibition of inflammation in the kidney including suppression of inflammatory cytokines (IL-1, tumor necrosis factor-α), adhesion molecules (intercellular adhesion molecule-1and vascular cell adhesion molecule-1), chemotactic molecule (osteopontin), and macrophage and T-cell accumulation in the obstructed kidney model in rats. These changes are associated with inhibition of nuclear factor (NF)-κB activation and indicate that Smad7 may have a unique role in initiating antifibrosis and antiinflammatory and immunosuppressive effects. Inhibition of Smad2 and -3 by Smad7 may terminate fibrosis, but the ability of Smad7 to inhibit NF-κB activation may be a key mechanism by which Smad7 could act to resolve renal inflammation. It is possible that overexpression of Smad7 leads to an increase in IkBa, the endogenes inhibitor of NF-κB activity; the mechanism for Smad7 effects would involve inhibition of IkBa degradation resulting in inactivation of the survival factor, NF-κB. This response would result in cell apoptosis and suppression of NF-κB-driven inflammation.

It should be noted that extensive and uncontrollable overexpression of Smad7 could cause massive cell death through apoptosis, consistent with reports that Smad7 is an inducer of cell apoptosis. This response may be associated with inhibition of a survival factor NF-κB plus the activation of the JNK pathway. Consequently, it will be critical to control the degree of Smad7 transgene expression in order to maintain a physiological balance

among the TGF-β, NF-κB, and JNK signaling crosstalk pathways when using a strategy involving overexpression of Smad7. The degree of Smad7 transgene expression could be controlled by varying the concentrations of doxycycline in vitro or in vivo if the inducible gene is used. Both the in vitro and in vivo results imply that inducible Smad7 gene therapy using the ultrasound-microbubble technique might provide a novel, safe, and effective therapeutic strategy for controlling or preventing both inflammatory and fibrotic diseases.

CONCLUSION

The discovery of TGF-β signaling through Smads has markedly improved the understanding of the molecular mechanisms that lead to tissue scarring. Identifying the activity of individual Smads may lead to improved understanding of the specific role for each Smad in the pathophysiologic process of fibrosis, inflammation, and even cancer. Identification of specific Smad-signaling crosstalk pathways will enable recognition of the molecular mechanisms and the complicated processes in the pathogenesis of diseases. In organ fibrosis, Smad signaling probably represents a common pathway of tissue scarring. In this case, TGF-β binds directly to its receptor, resulting in activation of Smad2 and -3 to induce extracelllular matrix production, whereas AGEs, Ang-II, and other growth factors/molecules could bind to their individual receptors to activate Smads via the MAPK-Smad crosstalk pathway. These responses ultimately lead to tissue injury. In contrast, overexpression of Smad7 can terminate Smad signaling by blocking Smad2 and -3 activation. This response would inhibit the fibrotic effects of TGF-β, high glucose, AGEs, and Ang-II. These findings suggest that fibrosis is regulated positively by Smad2 and -3, but negatively by Smad7. The ability of Smad7 to block experimental models of renal and lung fibrosis indicates that targeting Smad signaling may provide a new therapeutic strategy for tissue and/or organ fibrosis.

SELECTED REFERENCES

Border WA, Noble NA. Evidence that TGF-beta should be a therapeutic target in diabetic nephropathy. Kidney Int 1998;54:1390, 1391.

Bottinger EP, Bitzer M. TGF-beta signaling in renal disease. J Am Soc Nephrol 2002;13:2600–2610.

Chen R, Huang C, Morinelli TA, Trojanowska M, Paul RV. Blockade of the Effects of TGF-beta1 on Mesangial Cells by overexpression of Smad7. J Am Soc Nephrol 2002;13:887–893.

Dixon IM, Hao J, Reid NL, Roth JC. Effect of chronic AT(1) receptor blockade on cardiac Smad overexpression in hereditary cardiomyopathic hamsters. Cardiovasc Res 2000;46:286–297.

Flanders KC, Sullivan CD, Fujii M, et al. Mice lacking Smad3 are protected against cutaneous injury induced by ionizing radiation. Am J Pathol 2002;160:1057–1068.

Funaba M, Zimmerman CM, Mathews LS. Modulation of Smad2-mediated signaling by extracellular signal-regulated kinase. J Biol Chem 2002;277:41,361–41,368.

Isono M, Chen S, Won Hong S, Iglesias-de la Cruz MC, Ziyadeh FN. Smad pathway is activated in the diabetic mouse kidney and Smad3 mediates TGF-beta-induced fibronectin in mesangial cells. Biochem Biophys Res Commun 2002;296:1356–1365.

Kavsak P, Rasmussen RK, Causing CG, et al. Smad7 binds to Smurf2 to form an E3 ubiquitin ligase that targets the TGF-beta receptor for degradation. Mol Cell 2000;6:1365–1375.

Kretzschmar M, Doody J, Timokhina I, Massagué J. A mechanism of repression of TGFβ/Smad signaling by ongenic ras. Genes Dev 1999;13:804–816.

63 The Pathophysiology of Acute Renal Failure

DIDIER PORTILLA, GUR P. KAUSHAL, ALEXEI G. BASNAKIAN,
AND SUDHIR V. SHAH

SUMMARY

Acute renal failure (ARF) is a syndrome that can be defined as an abrupt decrease in renal function sufficient to result in retention of nitrogenous waste in the body. ARF can result from a decrease of renal blood flow, intrinsic renal parenchymal diseases, or obstruction of urine flow. There has been little progress in preventing and treating ARF, but with a better understanding of cell injury mechanisms and by carefully defining populations at risk for developing ARF, treatment strategies could be developed.

Key Words: ARF; GFR; inflammatory cells; kidney; mitochondria; sublethal cell injury.

INTRODUCTION

Acute renal failure (ARF) is a syndrome that can be defined as an abrupt decrease in renal function sufficient to result in retention of nitrogenous waste (e.g., blood urea nitrogen and creatinine) in the body. ARF can result from a decrease of renal blood flow (prerenal azotemia), intrinsic renal parenchymal diseases (renal azotemia), or obstruction of urine flow (postrenal azotemia). The most common intrinsic renal disease that leads to ARF is referred to as acute tubular necrosis (used interchangeably with ARF in this chapter), a clinical syndrome in which there is an abrupt and sustained decline in glomerular filtration rate occurring within minutes to days following an acute ischemic or nephrotoxic insult. Its clinical recognition requires exclusion of prerenal and postrenal causes of azotemia, followed by exclusion of other causes of intrinsic ARF (e.g., glomerulonephritis, acute interstitial nephritis, or vasculitis). Ischemic ARF is associated with a mortality rate of about 50% in hospitalized patients and 70–80% in patients in intensive care units. This rate has essentially remained constant over the last 50 yr. Although the high mortality rate is due in part to the presence of comorbid conditions, there is evidence that ARF is responsible for the high mortality rate. The most common pathophysiological mechanism involved in the development of ARF is the presence of a complex interplay between altered renal hemodynamics, inflammation, and tubular dysfunction (Fig. 63-1). Advances have improved the understanding of the mechanisms involved in the development of ARF.

From: *Principles of Molecular Medicine, Second Edition*
Edited by: M. S. Runge and C. Patterson © Humana Press, Inc., Totowa, NJ

ROLE OF THE VASCULAR ENDOTHELIUM

Blood flow to the kidney accounts for 25% of the cardiac output, the majority going to the kidney cortex with very small amounts going into the medullary portion of the kidney. Measurement of PO_2 in the medulla of normal kidneys reveals a relatively hypoxic region (PO_2 values as low as 5–15 mmHg). The critically low PO_2 coupled with high energy demands of the medullary portion of the kidney results in increased susceptibility of the cortico-medullary portion of the kidney to injury.

Following an ischemic insult, total renal blood flow is reduced to 40–50% of normal value during reperfusion both in animal models and in human ischemic ARF. This "no-reflow" phenomenon has been observed after ischemia in other organs as well. Using intravital videomicroscopy of renal microcirculation during the immediate reperfusion period, investigators demonstrated profound and sustained deceleration of blood flow yielding a temporary loss of capillary patency and shifts in blood flow through postischemic capillaries from orthograde to the retrograde direction. These patterns of capillary blood flow in the postischemic kidney may explain the mechanisms of no-reflow phenomenon. Other evidence of abnormal "vascular reactivity" in the ischemic kidney includes a profound loss of acetylcholine-induced vasodilatation of the ischemic renal vasculature, inhibition of vasorelaxation in response to stimuli that generate endothelium-derived relaxing factor, and reduced production of nitric oxide in response to bradykinin.

The potential role of endothelial cells in producing ischemia/reperfusion injury was suggested by the finding that endothelial cells undergo swelling to narrow the lumen. Other support for the ischemia/reperfusion pathophysiologic cause of ARF includes the significant improvement in the peritubular capillary blood flow in the postischemic period in animals that had been transplanted with human umbilical vein endothelial cells and human embryonic kidney cells which stably expressed human endothelial or type-III NO synthase (eNOS). The observation that endothelial cells can rescue the function of an ischemic organ illustrates the principle of cell–cell interaction in which the dysfunction of one cell type affects the functions of other cells. Furthermore, implantation of cells expressing the functional eNOS (even though the cells are not endothelial cells *per se*) can ameliorate renal dysfunction following acute ischemia, also implicating eNOS in the pathophysiology of ARF.

Ischemia/Reperfusion

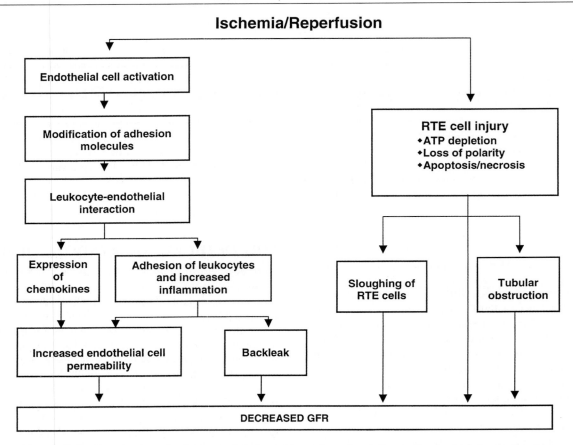

Figure 63-1 Complex interplay between altered renal hemodynamics, inflammation, and tubular dysfunction.

Study results provide further support for the role of microvascular endothelium in the pathophysiology of ischemic ARF. They demonstrated high circulating levels of von Willebrand factor (a marker for endothelial cell injury) plus increase in F-actin aggregates found in the basolateral aspects of renal microvascular endothelial cells within the first 24 h of ischemic injury. In addition, there were structural changes in vascular endothelial-cadherin at endothelial cell–cell junctions as early as 2 h, which were accompanied by a marked increase in microvascular permeability, resulting in interstitial edema. These observations implicate an important role of endothelial cells and could result in new therapeutic modalities for treatment of ARF.

PATHOLOGICAL ROLE OF INFLAMMATORY CELLS

Studies in experimental acute tubular necrosis previously suggested that inflammatory cells did not play an important role in renal tubular injury. Newer studies, however, support a role for inflammatory cells in ARF. Histological evaluation has shown that the accumulation of neutrophils occurs within the first 4 h and is maximal at 24–48 h of ischemia/reperfusion injury to the kidney. Most of the neutrophil accumulation occurs in the outer medulla and in the cortex. Leukocyte depletion achieved by antineutrophil serum protected the kidney, establishing a cause–effect relationship between neutrophil accumulation and tissue injury during ischemia/reperfusion. Studies using pharmacological agents support the idea that decreased neutrophil infiltration leads to prevention of ischemia/reperfusion injury. For example, administration of α-melanocyte-stimulating hormone has been associated with a

reduction of neutrophil infiltration and kidney injury after ischemic/reperfusion.

The adherence of leukocytes to the vascular endothelium is an early critical process resulting in the outer medullary congestion present in ischemic ARF. Leukocytes increase endothelial permeability leading to erythrocyte aggregation and edema as well as obstruction of the vasa recta. Neutrophils also release reactive oxygen species, proteases, elastases, myeloperoxidase, and other enzymes that damage tissue. In addition, increases in leukotriene B4 and platelet-activating factor produced by monocytes or platelets can increase vascular permeability and upregulate the expression of adhesion molecules to promote further inflammation.

The adhesion of neutrophils to endothelial cells occurs through a complex series of events involving the presence of several classes of adhesion molecules including selectins, mucin and other selectin ligands and integrins, plus members of the Ig superfamily. CD11/CD18 integrins and intracellular adhesion molecule (ICAM)-1 are also important molecules participating in the pathogenesis of ischemic renal injury. Protection from ischemic/reperfusion injury occurs in animals that are given antibodies to CD11a, CD11b, and ICAM-1 or antisense oligonucleotides to ICAM-1; ICAM-1-deficient mice are also protected. Activation of adenosine A2 receptors on endothelial cells reduces adherence factors and, ultimately, neutrophil accumulation. Hence neutrophil adherence to endothelial cells plays an important role in the pathogenesis of ischemic reperfusion injury.

Besides neutrophils, other inflammatory cells participate in ischemia/reperfusion injury. Biopsies of human kidneys with acute tubular necrosis reveal the presence of lymphocytes, but whether these cells directly participate in organ injury or whether macrophages and T cells appear only in the recovery phase of ARF is controversial. Indirect evidence for a role for T lymphocytes in ischemic ARF includes studies showing that lymphocyte-related cytokines are upregulated in the postischemic kidney. Moreover, CD4/CD8 knockout mice are protected from ischemia/reperfusion injury. In addition, administration of a selectin ligand resulted in attenuated postischemic renal dysfunction and decreased mortality. In contrast to these reports, mice that are deficient in the recombination-activating gene, RAG-1, have no T- or B-cells and do not produce immunoglobulins or T-cell proteins, but still experience tubular necrosis and neutrophil infiltration when subjected to ischemia-reperfusion.

Taken together, the studies in humans or rodent models of ARF support the idea that endothelial cell injury is accompanied by increased leukocyte and perhaps T-cell-endothelial cell interactions that compromise blood flow to the corticomedullary junction.

MECHANISMS OF TUBULAR CELL INJURY

SUBLETHAL CELL INJURY The apical brush border of the proximal tubule is a site of early morphological change, with patchy loss of apical microvilli that occurs within minutes of acute renal ischemia. Subsequently, there is complete loss of the apical microvilli that are shed into the tubular lumen. These same morphological alterations of the proximal tubule brush border occur in the postischemic renal allografts of patients.

Alterations in the actin cytoskeleton are dramatic. In in vivo as well as in vitro models, there is a disassociation of the heterodimeric capping protein from the actin cytoskeleton during renal ischemia. Dephosphorylation of ezrin and actin depolimerizing factor have been observed in hypoxic tubules and could account for the loss of the cytoskeletal support of the microvillar surface membrane with subsequent microvillar collapse following acute ischemic injury. In addition to the microvillar actin disruption, there is loss of the cortical actin cytoskeleton response to ischemia in vivo or ATP depletion in vitro. Investigators also found conversion of G-actin to F-actin and aggregation of F-actin molecules in the cytoplasm of the cell; redistribution of ankyrin and fodrin, two proteins that anchor NaK-ATPase; redistribution of NaK-ATPase to the apical domain; and inactivation of Rho-GTPase with disruption of the tight junction complex during ATP depletion in vitro. Following ATF depletion, plasma membrane protrusions or blebs containing cytosol and endoplasmic reticulum are formed, reflecting disruption of volume regulation mechanisms and cytoskeleton organization.

The multiple alterations in renal epithelial cell cytoskeletal structure and its surface membrane polarity may contribute to the decrease in the glomerular filtration rate of ARF. Increased paracellular permeability could be the result of changes in tight junctions whereas loss of the integrity of the epithelial cell layer from sloughing of viable cells may contribute to back-leak of the glomerular filtrate. Finally, the loss of cell polarity and the redistribution of β_1 integrin impairs cell adhesion, resulting in clumping of sloughed and nonsloughed cells within the tubular lumen, leading to tubular obstruction.

LETHAL INJURY: APOPTOTIC AND NECROTIC PATHWAYS In ARF induced by ischemia, endotoxemia, nephrotoxins, or other causes, renal tubular epithelial cells die during a catastrophic breakdown of regulated cellular homeostasis known as necrosis. In freshly isolated proximal tubules subjected to hypoxia/reoxygenation, investigators described the formation of pathological plasma membrane pores, or so-called "death channels," these pores can be blocked by glycine at physiological levels. Late in hypoxic stress, an irreversible state of proximal tubule cell injury develops, signified by lysosomal disruption, bleb coalescence and subsequent bleb rupture, followed by loss of membrane permeability. The abrupt failure of the plasma membrane permeability barrier releases cytosolic contents and a collapse of all of the plasmalemmal and electrical and ionic gradients. In this form of cell death, cells swell and there is loss of plasma membrane integrity and rupture of cells releasing a variety of inflammatory mediators.

The modern era of cell death began with the landmark publication by Kerr, Wyllie, and Currie in which they coined the term *apoptosis* and made a distinction between necrosis and apoptosis based on morphological criteria. In apoptosis, cells shrink, lose their microvilli and cell junctions, and explode into a series of membrane-bound, condensed apoptotic bodies. These bodies are phagocytosed by adjacent viable cells with minimal leakage of the contents of the dead cell, thereby invoking no inflammation. Because apoptosis does not evoke inflammation, it is an important mechanism in embryogenesis and normal tissue turnover.

One of the major advances in understanding cell death has been the recognition that the pathways traditionally associated with apoptosis can be critical in determining the type of cell injury associated with necrosis; the same insult may result in mild injury resulting in apoptosis or severe injury, producing necrosis. Thus, the pathway is determined by both the nature and severity of insults. It appears likely that the pathways that lead to apoptotic or necrotic cell death are activated almost simultaneously but there are some common pathways.

The important role that apoptosis plays in renal function during ischemic ARF was highlighted by an infusion of GTP before inducing ischemic reperfusion injury. There was substantial functional protection and amelioration of apoptosis but not necrosis. Administration of guanosine also prevented the expression of p53, whereas a p53 inhibitor, pifithrin, selectively modified apoptosis and ameliorated renal function if it was given within 14 h of the initial insult. These results suggest that amelioration of apoptosis rather than necrosis will account for the major mechanism that protects renal function during ischemic ARF.

DNA FRAGMENTATION AND ENDONUCLEASES IN RENAL TUBULAR EPITHELIAL CELL INJURY

Several reports have demonstrated chromatin condensation, the morphological hallmark of apoptosis, in models of ARF including ischemia/reperfusion injury. However, much of the evidence for the activation of apoptotic mechanisms in cell injury is based on the demonstration of endonuclease activation resulting in oligonucleosome-length DNA fragmentation (approx 200 bp) as one of the biochemical hallmarks of apoptosis. For example, DNA fragmentation in the kidney cortex, or the typical ladder pattern of DNA, has been detected within 12 h after beginning reperfusion.

Key questions are whether endonuclease activation is related to cell death and whether an attempt to halt this process would prevent cell death. The 200 bp ladder, commonly used because of its simplicity, actually measures very late events and only approx 40 double-strand DNA breaks per cell have been shown to be lethal. The role of endonucleases in kidney epithelial cell injury is linked to the biochemical and cellular mechanisms of oxidant injury. For example, hydrogen peroxide in the presence of iron contained in

DNA yields site-specific generation of hydroxyl radicals that damage DNA. In hydrogen peroxide-induced injury, endonuclease activation is an early event leading to DNA fragmentation, and endonuclease inhibitors can prevent hydrogen peroxide-induced DNA strand breaks, DNA fragmentation, and cell death. Endonuclease activation may be important in reactive oxygen mechanisms leading to tubular cell injury.

Subsequently, it was demonstrated that hypoxia/reoxygenation injury of freshly isolated rat proximal tubules results in DNA strand breaks and nuclear DNA fragmentation that precedes cell death. This injury increased DNA degrading activity and this new activity was found in molecules with an apparent molecular mass of 15 kDa. Endonuclease inhibitors protected against DNA damage induced by hypoxia/reoxygenation injury and provided significant protection against cell death. There also is a role of endonuclease in a model of chemical hypoxia. Taken together, endonuclease activation resulting in DNA damage and cell death is an integral part of hypoxia/reoxygenation injury. Despite unequivocal evidence of endonuclease activation, the morphologic features of apoptosis including chromatin condensation were not observed. This result is consistent with studies indicating that chromatin condensation and DNA fragmentation may be triggered through separate metabolic pathways. Cells with morphological features of either apoptosis or necrosis will have evidence of endonuclease activity.

ENDONUCLEASES IN THE KIDNEY Limited information is available regarding the identity of the endonuclease(s) responsible for DNA fragmentation in the kidney. Evidence for two major endonucleases exists in kidneys and kidney cells, a 15 kDa endonuclease just discussed and a 30–34 kDa DNase I-like endonuclease. The 30 kDa is mainly a cytoplasmic enzyme, whereas the 15 kDa endonuclease is located in the nuclei. Because the 30 kDa enzyme is similar to a DNase I by its biochemical characteristics, the role of DNase I in renal injury is being examined. The activity of 30 kDa endonuclease is increased during ischemia/reperfusion injury in the rat kidney and at least in vitro renal tubular epithelial cells that had been transfected with a phosphorothioated DNase I antisense construct were protected against DNA damage and cell death.

CASPASES IN RENAL TUBULAR EPITHELIAL CELL INJURY

A specific class of proteases, the "caspases" (cysteine aspartate-specific proteases), were found to be involved in apoptosis in genetic studies of the nematode *Caenorrhabditis elegans*. Caspases are a family of structurally related cysteine proteases that play a central role in the execution of apoptosis. When cells are subjected to a pro-apoptotic stimulus, the procaspases are proteolytically processed to the active forms; at least fourteen caspases encoded by distinct genes have been cloned and sequenced in mammals, caspase-2, -8, -9, and -10 have large prodomains and initiate the activation of downstream caspases. Caspase-3, -6, and -7 contain smaller domains that have been identified as effecter or executioner caspases. The executioner caspases are the major active caspases detected in apoptotic cells and are widely regarded as mediators of apoptosis by cleaving and inactivating intracellular proteins that are essential for cell survival and proliferation. The specificity of downstream executioner caspases to cleave cellular proteins is unique. For example, following activation, caspase-3 primarily recognizes DEVD or DMQD tetrapeptide sequences whereas caspase-6 recognizes and cleaves the VEID tetrapeptide sequence after the aspartate residue in the target proteins.

There is increasing evidence for a role for caspases in hypoxic renal tubular cell injury. Exposure of freshly isolated renal tubular epithelial cells to hypoxia results in caspase activation, cell membrane damage, and necrotic cell death. A pan-caspase inhibitor attenuates the hypoxia-induced increase in caspase activity in these cells and provides protection against hypoxia-induced cell membrane damage, as determined by release of lactic dehydrogenase from the cells. Chemical hypoxia induced by treatment with antimycin A increases caspase activity that precedes DNA damage and cell death. Caspase inhibitors prevent hypoxia-induced DNA fragmentation as measured either by agarose gel electrophoresis or by *in situ* labeling of cell nuclei. Partial ATP depletion results in marked increase in activation of caspase-8 and the caspase inhibitors provide marked protection against cell death. Activation of caspase-3 by hypoxia or ATP depletion was accompanied by the translocation of Bax, a member of the Bcl-2 family, from the cytosol to the mitochondria and the release of cytochrome-*c* from mitochondria to the cytosol.

There is differential regulation of caspase activities in kidneys subjected to ischemia/reperfusion injury. Caspase-3 activity was significantly increased in the rat and murine models of renal ischemia/reperfusion injury whereas administration of the pan-caspase inhibitor, Z-VAD-FMK, at the time of reperfusion significantly prevented caspase-1 and -3 activities and provided marked protection against ischemic ARF. A rat model of ischemia/reperfusion injury indicated that prolonged ischemia induces proapoptotic mechanisms, including increases in the Bax/Bcl-2 ratio, caspase-3 expression, poly(ADP-ribose) polymerase cleavage, DNA fragmentation, and apoptotic cell number in renal proximal and distal tubules. Besides caspase-3, the proinflammatory caspase-1 is involved; it participates in the proteolytic cleavage of the precursor forms of the proinflammatory cytokines, IL-I β and -18, resulting in the active forms of these cytokines. Because caspase-1 mediated formation of IL-1β and -18 is associated with inflammation in renal ischemia/reperfusion, caspase-1 may play an important role in this form of injury. Results from caspase-1$^{-/-}$ mice have been inconsistent.

MITOCHONDRIA: CENTRAL COORDINATORS OF CELL DEATH

Mitochondria can play a key role in the decision of cells to undergo apoptosis or necrosis by regulating the apoptotic process (Fig. 63-2). When mitochondrial ATP formation by oxidative phosphorylation ceases, anoxic and ischemic injury result. In the case of the proximal tubule, glycolytic capacity is limited and the lack of hexokinase further limits the cell's potential to generate ATP from sources other than fatty acids. Uncoupled respiration has been postulated as a potential mechanism contributing to cell death because it represents a more severe form of metabolic disruption to mitochondria than the inhibition of ATP production.

Uncoupling causes collapse of pH and electrical gradients across the mitochondrial inner membrane and activates the mitochondrial F1F0 ATPase. Indirect evidence for the presence of uncoupling during ischemic ARF includes the presence of an increased expression of uncoupling protein-2 detected in a microarray analysis of ischemic kidney cortex tissue. Profound inhibition of fatty acid oxidation and increased accumulation of long-chain fatty acids and long-chain acylcarnitines have been demonstrated in ischemic ARF in vivo and in freshly isolated tubules responding to hypoxic injury. Accumulation of long-chain fatty acid metabolites is likely to be toxic and contribute to mitochondrial dysfunction during ischemic ARF.

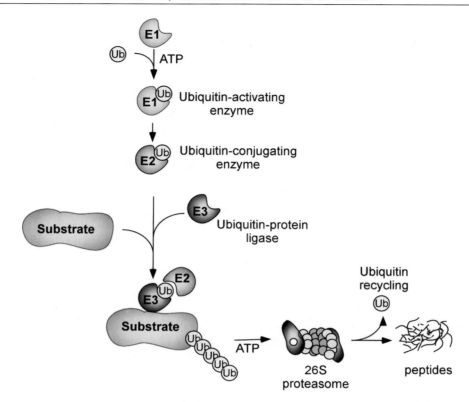

Figure 64-1 General scheme of protein degradation by the ubiquitin-proteasome system. Substrates that are degraded by the ubiquitin-proteasome system first undergo covalent addition of a polyubiquitin chain by a series of reactions that involve (1) ATP-dependent activation of ubiquitin by an E1 ubiquitin activating enzyme; (2) transfer of activated ubiquitin to the ε-NH$_2$ group of a lysine residue in the substrate and subsequent poly-ubiquitin chain formation by combinations of E2 ubiquitin conjugating enzymes and E3 ubiquitin protein ligase complexes (E3s can be monomeric or multimeric complexes). Substrate specificity is conferred by the various combinations of E2s and E3s; (3) recognition of the poly-ubiquitin chain by subunits of the 19S regulatory complex, which attaches to the end of a 20S core proteasome to form the 26S proteasome; and (4) unfolding, insertion and degradation of the substrate by the 26S proteasome (a process that requires ATP) to yield small peptides that are further degraded by peptidases. Ubiquitin chains are released from the protein and recycled.

Evidence that the ubiquitin-proteasome system is activated to break down muscle protein in kidney failure and other catabolic conditions comes from studies involving measurements of rates of protein degradation in isolated muscles incubated with inhibitors of the different proteolytic pathways. For example, muscles isolated from rats with chronic renal failure were incubated with inhibitors of calcium-dependent and lysosomal proteases and the rate of protein degradation was measured. With these inhibitors, there was a small and parallel decrease in the rates of protein degradation in muscles of both the chronically uremic rats and the sham-operated, pair-fed rats. However, these inhibitors did not block the accelerated rate of proteolysis stimulated by kidney failure. In contrast, when an inhibitor of the proteasome (i.e., MG132) was added or when ATP generation was blocked, the accelerated rate of protein degradation was eliminated and this occurred even in the presence of inhibitors of the calcium-activated and lysosomal proteases. Notably, the rate of protein degradation in muscles of the control rats was also suppressed to a low rate, indicating that the ubiquitin-proteasome system is responsible for the degradation of the bulk of protein in muscle. Additional evidence that the ubiquitin-proteasome system is activated in muscle of rats with various wasting conditions includes:

1. Increased conjugation of ubiquitin to muscle proteins.
2. Increased levels of the proteins that are components of the system.

3. Increased levels of mRNAs that encode ubiquitin and other component proteins of the system.
4. Return of these responses to control levels or lower when the condition causing accelerated muscle proteolysis is attenuated.

Two genes encoding ubiquitin protein ligases (i.e., E3s) have been identified in experiments based on microarray or differential display analyses of muscles undergoing atrophy. One of these proteins, muscle ring finger 1 (MuRF1 or atrogin-1), is a ring finger protein that interacts with titin, a large myofibrillar protein that has several functions. The other newly identified protein, atrogin-1 (also called muscle atrophy F-box [MAFbx]), belongs to the F-box (SCF) family of proteins that includes components of the multi-subunit skp-cullin-F box E3 ligases. Consistent with the role of the ubiquitin-proteasome system as the principal mechanism degrading muscle protein, the mRNA for atrogin-1 is specifically expressed in skeletal and cardiac muscle and its expression is increased >10-fold in muscles undergoing atrophy. Moreover, overexpression of atrogin-1 in C2C12 muscle cells resulted in thinner myotubes, reminiscent of muscle atrophy whereas muscles of mice with null alleles for either MuRF1/atrogin-1 do undergo atrophy in response to muscle denervation, but the degree of muscle wasting was attenuated in comparison with that in wild-type mice. Given the complexity of the pool of muscle proteins, it is likely that multiple ubiquitin conjugation systems are involved when the proteolytic process is accelerated.

The mechanisms leading to activation of the ubiquitin-proteasome system in conditions leading to muscle atrophy are poorly understood. For example, the "rate-limiting" step in muscle proteolysis has not been identified. Potentially important steps include:

1. Availability of muscle protein substrates because actomyosin and myofibrils are not degraded by the system, so the substrates actin and myosin must be liberated before they are degraded by the ubiquitin-proteasome system.
2. Recognition and polyubiquitination of substrate proteins by combinations of E2 and E3 enzymes acting in concert.
3. The proteolytic capacity of the cell related to changes in the levels of the many components of the system.

There are clues or insights into how catabolic signals activate this proteolytic system.

One potential clue is the frequent observation that mRNAs encoding various components of the system (e.g., ubiquitin, ubiquitin-conjugating enzymes, subunits of the 26S proteasome) are increased in each model of different conditions causing accelerated loss of muscle protein. This finding has been extended to patients with catabolic conditions (e.g., head trauma and sepsis) and includes patients with chronic renal failure. These subjects not only have evidence of muscle protein losses but also have higher levels of pathway mRNAs in muscle. At least in chronic kidney failure, removal of the catabolic stimulus, metabolic acidosis, was associated with a coordinated decrease in mRNA level for ubiquitin and muscle proteolysis suggesting the two responses are linked. Specifically, patients with end-stage renal disease receiving chronic ambulatory peritoneal dialysis were treated to remove the metabolic acidosis associated with kidney failure over 1 mo. This treatment yielded an increase in body weight and a simultaneous reduction in the level of ubiquitin mRNA in their muscle.

Several extracellular signals could accelerate proteolysis through the ubiquitin-proteasome system in muscle. In kidney failure, metabolic acidosis, and diabetes (or possibly insulin resistance), cytokines are potential signals acting directly or indirectly to stimulate muscle proteolysis and increase pathway mRNAs. Besides these mechanisms, glucocorticoids play a role because they can regulate the ubiquitin-proteasome system in muscle but their role varies depending on their level in animals. For example, when glucocorticoids are present in the high physiologic range, they are necessary for the activation of proteolysis plus the increase in pathway mRNAs in muscle, but their role is permissive because glucocorticoids require the presence of an additional catabolic signal (e.g., acidosis, cytokines, or a low level of insulin). In contrast, if rats are given pharmacologic doses of glucocorticoids, muscle atrophy does occur and levels of mRNAs encoding components of the ubiquitin-proteasome system in muscle are higher, at least transiently. The clinical relevance of glucocorticoids derives from reports that catabolic conditions upregulate the glucocorticoid signaling system in muscle; the number of glucocorticoid receptors is increased in muscle of rats with experimental sepsis following cecal ligation and puncture. Moreover, the proteolytic response in muscles was blocked by giving septic rats the glucocorticoid receptor antagonist, RU486, suggesting that a positive feedback system is activated in the muscle.

In addition to glucocorticoids, factors that stimulate expression of the components of the ubiquitin-proteasome pathway and enhance muscle protein degradation could include a decrease in muscle cell pH (or some other ion change linked to a fall in extracellular pH) or

impairment of insulin signaling. There is evidence in kidney cells that acidification can activate gene transcription via specific signaling pathways. The impact of intracellular acidification in stimulating the ubiquitin-proteasome pathway was investigated by examining chronically uremic rats with the same characteristics as rats expressing accelerated muscle proteolysis and higher levels of mRNAs for the components of the ubiquitin-proteasome system in muscle. Using nuclear magnetic resonance (NMR), pH measurements were taken in the intact muscle of these rats and the pair-fed, sham-operated control rats. It was neither subnormal nor was there a delay in recovery of cell pH when the muscle was stimulated to tetany in order to drop muscle cell pH acutely. Although there could be a change in pH in some compartment of muscle that was not measured, these results do not support a direct role for changes in pH causing stimulation of the ubiquitin-proteasome pathway or transcription of genes.

It has been shown that both acidosis and kidney failure can impair insulin signaling. The latter is important because an acute decrease in insulin markedly stimulates protein degradation and the expression of mRNAs encoding components of the ubiquitin-proteasome pathway in muscle. Furthermore, studying the signals that activate muscle protein loss in acute diabetes shows that stimulation of the ubiquitin-proteasome pathway, including the increase in muscle levels of mRNAs for components of the system, was not blocked when the development of metabolic acidosis was prevented by feeding acutely diabetic rats $NaHCO_3$. The stimulation of the ubiquitin-proteasome system in acutely diabetic rats, like those with metabolic acidosis, required glucocorticoids to activate the system.

CATABOLIC SIGNALS INITIATE A PROGRAM OF TRANSCRIPTIONAL RESPONSES IN MUSCLE

Whether greater amounts of ubiquitin-proteasome pathway mRNAs arise from increased message stabilization or transcriptional activation was revealed from evaluation of nuclear run-off assays using nuclei isolated from the hindquarter muscle of rats with acute diabetes or chronic renal failure. In both cases, there was increased transcription of the ubiquitin and the proteasome C3 subunit genes in comparison with rates measured in muscles of pair-fed control rats. In L6 muscle cells, dexamethasone, a potent glucocorticoid, was found to increase the transcription of the ubiquitin (*UbC*) and proteasome C3 subunit genes, leading to increased levels of these proteins. It has also been reported that there is no difference in the rate of disappearance of ubiquitin mRNA when extensor digitorum longus muscles from septic and sham-operated control rats are incubated in the presence of actinomycin to inhibit transcription. This finding indicates that the increase in mRNA is not attributable to message stabilization or post-transcriptional events. Thus, muscle atrophying conditions activate a program of specific transcriptional responses in muscle.

Genes encoding several components of the ubiquitin-proteasome system in rodents and humans have been characterized (e.g., proteasome C3 and C5 subunits, *UbC*). Surveys of their promoter regions reveal cis-acting elements with the potential for responding to inflammatory or stress-related signals. It has also been reported that CCAAT enhancer binding proteins, (C/EBP)-β and -δ, and activator protein-1, are activated in muscle of rats with sepsis; these are the same transcription factors that mediate inflammatory responses. The role of glucocorticoids in the activation of these factors was examined by giving septic rats an oral dose of RU486, a glucocorticoid receptor antagonist. RU486 blocked the

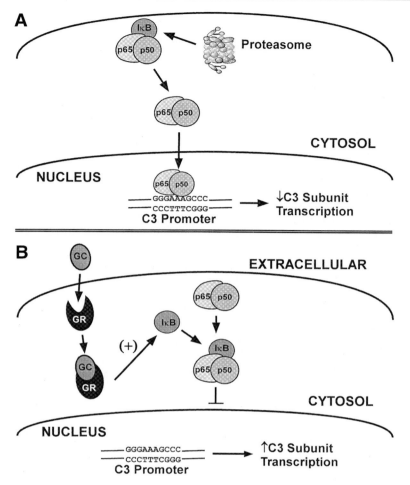

Figure 64-2 Mechanism of proteasome C3 subunit transactivation by glucocorticoids. (**A**) In muscle, NF-κB is activated by proteasome-mediated degradation of IκB, a cytosolic inhibitor protein. NF-κB then translocates to the nucleus in which it binds to sites in the C3 subunit promoter and suppresses transcription. (**B**) Glucocorticoids prevent the proteasome-mediated degradation of IκB, thus inhibiting NF-κB nuclear translocation. Sequestration of NF-κB in the cytosol results in stimulation of proteasome C3 subunit expression.

activation of C/EBP-β and -δ but did not block the activation of activator protein-1. These findings suggest that stress-related mediators play a part in activating the program of transcriptional responses in muscle occurring in response to cachectic signals.

NF-κB IS A NEGATIVE REGULATOR OF THE PROTEASOME C3 SUBUNIT EXPRESSION Glucocorticoids are potent regulators of gene expression and can influence transcription by multiple mechanisms. Investigations of the role of glucocorticoids in the transcriptional responses of the ubiquitin-proteasome system in muscle included studying the influence of glucocorticoids on the regulation of the proteasome C3 subunit in L6 muscle cells. Inspection of the human C3 proteasome subunit promoter region did not identify a classic glucocorticoid response element despite the fact that glucocorticoids-induced expression of this subunit in L6 muscle cells. However, there was a region of the C3 subunit promoter between –400 and –256 bp (+1 = transcription start site) that was essential for stimulation by dexamethasone. This region contains several nuclear factor (NF)-κB-like binding sites, notable because glucocorticoid receptors and NF-κB can exert mutually antagonistic effects to repress or activate gene transcription. Further examination of a binding site at –322/–313 using mobility shift assays revealed that incubating cells to dexamethasone for

only 20 min decreased the formation of a DNA–NF-κB complex. This antagonism of NF-κB binding to the promoter region persisted for at least 24 h. Because glucocorticoids act to stimulate the transcription of the proteasome C3 subunit, these findings indicate that NF-κB must act as a repressor of C3 subunit transcription (Fig. 64-2A). Thus, glucocorticoids act to stimulate transcription by antagonizing the transrepression by NF-κB of the C3 subunit of the proteasome. This mechanism was confirmed by demonstrating that overexpressing NF-κB subunits or activating cellular production of NF-κB with cytokines reduced transcription of the C3 proteasome subunit. In contrast, blocking NF-κB activity stimulated transcription of this gene.

How do glucocorticoids antagonize NF-κB transactivation? No evidence exists for a direct interaction between the glucocorticoid receptor and NF-κB subunits nor did dexamethasone increase the transcription of inhibitor of κB (IκB). However, glucocorticoids increased the amount of IκB protein in the cytosol with a concurrent increase in the amount of cytosolic NF-κB p65 subunit, leading to the conclusion that glucocorticoids enhance proteasome C3 subunit transcription by causing a sequestration of inactive NF-κB in the cytosol (Fig. 64-2B). Subsequent studies of muscle from septic and control rats recapitulated the findings with L6 muscle cells and confirmed that NF-κB serves as a suppressor of proteasome C3 subunit transcription in muscle of intact animals.

GLUCOCORTICOIDS INCREASE UBC TRANSCRIPTION BY A SP1-DEPENDENT MECHANISM　Three independent genes (i.e., *UbA*, *UbB*, and *UbC*) encode protein products that are processed to yield "free" ubiquitin protein. Among these genes, *UbC* mRNA has typically increased the most in response to conditions causing muscle atrophy. The human *UbC* promoter region has been characterized, including a number of potential binding sites for factors that could regulate transcription. By cloning the rat *UbC* promoter, conservation of a number of the potential response elements was found, including multiple sites for NF-κB, other inflammatory class transcription factors, and specificity factor 1 (Sp1). As in the case of the proteasome C3 subunit, however, there was a conspicuous absence of consensus glucocorticoid response elements in the rat or human *UbC* promoter even though dexamethasone stimulated transcription of the *UbC* gene in L6 muscle cells. These findings prompted investigation of the cis-acting elements that confers glucocorticoid responsiveness. Initially, in vivo genomic footprinting assays were performed in L6 muscle cells to identify regions of the *UbC* promoter that undergo structural changes in response to dexamethasone. Surprisingly, these bases were located in a potential Sp1 binding site. This location suggested that dexamethasone induces a change in the binding of Sp1 and results of promoter deletion and mutational analysis coupled with mobility shift assays did show that dexamethasone increases the in vitro binding of Sp1 to a *UbC*-specific DNA probe. The importance of Sp1 in mediating the transactivation of the *UbC* promoter was confirmed when an inhibitor of Sp1 binding, mithramycin, was shown to prevent the dexamethasone-induced increase in *UbC* gene activity. Mithramycin also decreased the levels of free ubiquitin protein and ubiquitin conjugated to endogenous muscle cell proteins. Thus, it is clear that a mechanism for increased *UbC* expression by dexamethasone involves Sp1.

Sp1 has traditionally been considered a ubiquitous transcription factor involved in the basal transcription of many genes. To determine how glucocorticoids increase Sp1 binding to the *UbC* promoter, the total cellular content of Sp1 was measured and the distribution of Sp1 between the cytosol and nucleus was examined. Dexamethasone did not change the amount or distribution of Sp1 in L6 cells, suggesting that glucocorticoids do not simply augment the level of Sp1 in the nucleus. There are reports that Sp1 binding activity is modulated by phosphorylation. Moreover, activation of the p42/44 mitogen-activated protein (MAP) kinase (i.e., extracellular signal regulated kinase [ERK] 1/2) signaling pathway has been linked to increased Sp1-mediated transcription and glucocorticoids can stimulate ERK activity. Examination of the role of MAP kinase/ERK kinase (MEK)1/2, the kinases upstream of ERK, using a MEK1/2 inhibitor, U0126 revealed that treating L6 muscle cells with U0126 blocked the induction of *UbC*-driven luciferase activity by dexamethasone. In contrast, transfecting L6 cells to express constitutively active MEK1 mimicked dexamethasone by inducing *UbC* transcription. These findings demonstrate that glucocorticoids stimulate *UbC* transcription by a mechanism involving both Sp1 and MEK1. A potential signaling scheme for this response is shown in Fig. 64-3.

CONCLUSIONS

Studies involving a variety of models of pathological states consistently indicate that catabolic conditions causing loss of muscle

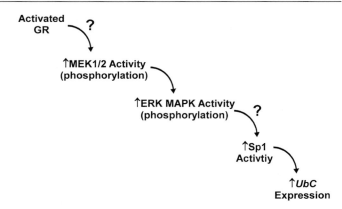

Figure 64-3　Potential mechanism of Ubiquitin C (*UbC*) transactivation by glucocorticoids. Glucocorticoids increase Sp1 binding to the *UbC* promoter. MEK1/2 is involved in the transactivation process but the mechanism is unknown. In the potential scheme shown, glucocorticoids bind to their receptor, which indirectly stimulates MEK1/2, which activates ERK1/2, resulting in the phosphorylation of Sp1. Phosphorylation of Sp1 increases its ability to bind to the *UbC* promoter, thus enhancing its transcription.

protein induce a concomitant program of transcriptional responses that result in higher levels of the mRNAs that encode components of the ubiquitin-proteasome system. The transactivation mechanisms for many of these conditions have not been defined and are likely to be complex. The mechanism by which glucocorticoids induce the *UbC* and proteasome C3 subunit genes differ substantially. In the case of the proteasome C3 subunit, glucocorticoids act by antagonizing NF-κB, a suppressor of subunit transcription. Conversely, glucocorticoids induce *UbC* by increasing the binding of Sp1 and the mechanism requires components of a MAP kinase pathway linked to cell growth and survival. Although the importance of the increase in mRNAs encoding components of the ubiquitin-proteasome system in terms of proteolysis is debated, the majority of evidence indicates that catabolic signals that accelerate protein degradation via the ubiquitin-proteasome pathway initiate a program of selective transcriptional responses in muscle. The impressive concordance between studies performed with cultured muscle cells and studies involving experimental animals and patients suggests that there is strong evolutionary pressure to maintain these "stress"-related responses. Understanding the mechanisms leading to activation of transcription could lead to improved methods of preventing the loss of muscle protein.

ACKNOWLEDGMENT

This work was supported by the National Institutes of Health through grants DK50740, DK63658, and DK37175.

SELECTED REFERENCES

Alvestrand A. Carbohydrate and insulin metabolism in renal failure. Kidney Int Suppl 1997;62:S48–S52.

Bailey JL, England BK, Long RC Jr, Weissman J, Mitch WE. Experimental acidemia and muscle cell pH in chronic acidosis and renal failure. Am J Physiol 1995;269:C706–C712.

Bailey JL, Wang X, England BK, Price SR, Ding X, Mitch WE. The acidosis of chronic renal failure activates muscle proteolysis in rats by augmenting transcription of genes encoding proteins of the ATP-dependent, ubiquitin-proteasome pathway. J Clin Invest 1996;97:1447–1453.

Bodine SC, Latres E, Baumhueter S, et al. Identification of ubiquitin ligases required for skeletal muscle atrophy. Science 2001;294:1704–1708.

Cecchin F, Ittoop O, Sinha MK, Caro JF. Insulin resistance in uremia: insulin receptor kinase activity in liver and muscle from chronic uremic rats. Am J Physiol 1988;254:E394–E401.

DeFronzo RA, Alvestrand A, Smith D, Hendler R. Insulin resistance in uremia. J Clin Invest 1981;67:563–568.

Du J, Mitch WE, Wang X, Price SR. Glucocorticoids induce proteasome C3 subunit expression in L6 muscle cells by opposing the suppression of its transcription by NF-κB. J Biol Chem 2000;275:19,661–19,666.

Glickman MH, Ciechanover A. The ubiquitin-proteasome proteolytic pathway: destruction for the sake of construction. Physiol Rev 2002;82(2): 373–428.

Gomes MD, Lecker SH, Jagoe RT, Navon A, Goldberg AL. Atrogin-1, a muscle-specific F-box protein highly expressed during muscle atrophy. Proc Natl Acad Sci USA 2001;98(25):14,440–14,445.

Hasselgren PO. Glucocorticoids and muscle catabolism. Curr Opin Clin Nutr Metab Care 1999;2:201–205.

Jagoe RT, Goldberg AL. What do we really know about the ubiquitin-proteasome pathway in muscle atrophy? Curr Opin Clin Nutr Metab Care 2001;4(3):183–190.

Jagoe RT, Lecker SH, Gomes M, Goldberg AL. Patterns of gene expression in atrophying skeletal muscles: response to food deprivation. FASEB J 2002;16(13):1697–1712.

Karin M, Chang L. AP-1-glucocorticoid receptor crosstalk taken to a higher level. J Endocrinol 2001;169(3):447–451.

Marinovic AC, Zheng B, Mitch WE, Price SR. Ubiquitin (UbC) expression in muscle cells is increased by glucocorticoids through a mechanism involving Sp1 and MEK1. J Biol Chem 2002;277(19):16,673–16,681.

May RC, Kelly RA, Mitch WE. Metabolic acidosis stimulates protein degradation in rat muscle by a glucocorticoid-dependent mechanism. J Clin Invest 1986;77:614–621.

McKay LI, Cidlowski JA. Cross-talk between nuclear factor-κB and steroid hormone receptors: mechanisms of mutual antagonism. Mol Endocrinol 1998;12(1):45–56.

Mehrotra R, Kopple JD. Nutritional management of maintenance dialysis patients: why aren't we doing better? Annu Rev Nutr 2001;21:343–379.

Mitch WE, Bailey JL, Wang X, Jurkovitz C, Newby D, Price SR. Evaluation of signals activating ubiquitin-proteasome proteolysis in a model of muscle wasting. Am J Physiol 1999;276:C1132–C1138.

Mitch WE, Goldberg AL. Mechanisms of muscle wasting: The role of the ubiquitin-proteasome pathway. N Engl J Med 1996; 335(25):1897–1905.

Mitch WE, Price SR. Mechanisms activated by kidney disease and the loss of muscle mass. Am J Kidney Dis 2001;38(6):1337–1342.

Nenoi M, Mita K, Ichimura S, et al. Hetergeneous structure of the polyubiquitin gene UbC of Hela S3 cells. Gene 1996;175:179–185.

Penner CG, Gang G, Wray C, Fischer JE, Hasselgren PO. The transcription factors NF-kappaB and AP-1 are differentially regulated in skeletal muscle during sepsis. Biochem Biophys Res Commun 2001;281(5): 1331–1336.

Pickering WP, Price SR, Bircher G, Marinovic AC, Mitch WE, Walls J. Nutrition in CAPD: serum bicarbonate and the ubiquitin-proteasome system in muscle. Kidney Int 2002;61(4):1286–1292.

Price SR, Bailey JL, Wang X, et al. Muscle wasting in insulinopenic rats results from activation of the ATP-dependent, ubiquitin proteasome proteolytic pathway by a mechanism including gene transcription. J Clin Invest 1996;98:1703–1708.

Samson SL, Wong NC. Role of Sp1 in insulin regulation of gene expression. J Mol Endocrinol 2002;29(3):265–279.

Solomon V, Goldberg AL. Importance of the ATP-ubiquitin-proteasome pathway in the degradation of soluble and myofibrillar proteins in rabbit muscle extracts. J Biol Chem 1996;271(43):26,690–26,697.

Varshavsky A. The N-end rule and regulation of apoptosis. Nat Cell Biol 2003;5(5):373–376.

Wiborg O, Pedersen MS, Wind A, Berglund LE, Marcker KA, Vuust J. The human ubiquitin multigene family: some genes contain multiple directly repeated ubiquitin coding sequences. EMBO J 1985;4: 755–759.

65 Mechanisms of Renal Allograft Rejection

Daniel R. Goldstein, Anirban Bose, and Fadi G. Lakkis

SUMMARY

The immune response to donor antigens leads to the rejection of transplanted organs. The earliest event in this response is the activation of the innate immune system. Innate activation culminates in the migration of antigen presenting cells to the recipient's secondary lymphoid tissues where they trigger the adaptive immune response. The principal events of this response are the activation of T and B lymphocytes, which generate effector cells that inflict immediate damage. Adaptive immunity also produces long-lived memory lymphocytes that cause either acute or chronic rejection. Here, we will summarize the cellular and molecular mechanisms of the innate and adaptive responses that lead to graft rejection.

Key Words: Adaptive immunity; antigen presenting cells; B cells; cytokines; innate immunity; lymphocytes; memory; natural killer cells; rejection; T cells; transplantation.

INTRODUCTION

Transplanting an organ from one member of a species into a nonidentical member of the same species results in a donor-specific immune response referred to as alloimmunity. If left untreated, alloimmune responses lead to the rejection of the transplanted organ (the allograft). The central mediator of the alloimmune response is the T lymphocyte. On activation by donor antigens (alloantigens) presented on antigen-presenting cells (APCs), allospecific T lymphocytes proliferate and differentiate into effector cells or provide help to other cells that inflict damage on the allograft. This chapter provides an overview of the cellular and molecular mechanisms underlying the immune response that leads to allograft rejection.

OVERVIEW OF THE ALLOIMMUNE RESPONSE

The alloimmune response, like any other immune response to a foreign antigen, occurs in two broad phases: the innate and adaptive phases (Fig. 65-1). In the innate phase, inflammation in the transplanted organ activates APCs and induces their maturation and migration to secondary lymphoid organs (the spleen and lymph nodes). The adaptive immune response is initiated when APCs activate antigen-specific T cells within secondary lymphoid organs leading to effector cell generation and their migration to the allograft where they mediate rejection. The majority of effector T cells eventually undergoes apoptosis and the few that survive

From: *Principles of Molecular Medicine, Second Edition*
Edited by: M. S. Runge and C. Patterson © Humana Press, Inc., Totowa, NJ

become long-lived memory T cells that endanger the survival of a subsequent organ transplant.

Before describing the molecular and cellular mechanisms of the innate and adaptive immune responses to a transplanted organ, it is important to define "alloantigen." The principal non-self-antigens responsible for initiating alloimmune responses are the major histocompatibility complex (MHC) proteins, known as human leukocyte antigens (HLAs) in man. MHC proteins are encoded by a family of highly polymorphic genes and are divided into two classes. MHC class-I antigens are expressed on the vast majority of nucleated cells whereas MHC class-II antigens are expressed primarily on APCs such as dendritic cells (DCs), macrophages, and B-lymphocytes. MHC class-II expression is also induced on activated T cells and, in humans, on endothelial cells. The physiologic function of MHC molecules is to bind antigenic peptides and present them to T lymphocytes. In fact, the T-cell receptor for antigen (TCR) does not interact with whole antigens but instead recognizes small antigenic peptides bound to the grooves of MHC molecules present on APCs. In general, exogenous antigens (e.g., circulating foreign proteins) are taken up by APCs, degraded within endocytic vesicles, and presented by class-II molecules, whereas endogenous antigens (e.g., viral proteins produced within the cell cytosol) are presented by class-I molecules. The highly polymorphic MHC ensures that humans mount immune responses against a wide array of pathogens. Unfortunately, the same polymorphism forms the basis of tissue incompatibility between members of the same species. T cells of one individual recognize the non-self-MHC present on another individual's tissues as foreign, leading to the phenomenon of transplant rejection. In addition to MHC, non-MHC polymorphic molecules, known as minor histocompatibility antigens, also initiate alloimmune responses. Single or multiple minor histocompatibility differences between the donor and the recipient lead to the rejection of MHC-matched organs. A classic example of minor histocompatibility antigens is the HY antigen expressed on male but not female cells.

THE INNATE IMMUNE RESPONSE TO A TRANSPLANTED ORGAN

CELLULAR AND MOLECULAR COMPONENTS OF INNATE IMMUNITY The innate immune system acts as "the first line of defense" against foreign antigens, whether an allograft or an invading microbial pathogen. The cellular components of this phase of the immune system consist of APCs such as DCs and macrophages, natural killer (NK) cells, and neutrophils. These cells reside in

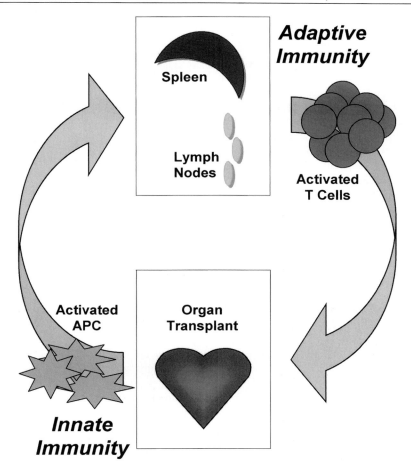

Figure 65-1 Innate and adaptive immune mechanisms lead to allograft rejection. Ischemia-reperfusion injury and inflammation in a newly transplanted organ activates APC, which then migrate to secondary lymphoid organs (the spleen and lymph nodes). In the secondary lymphoid organs, APC activate antigen-specific T cells, which then differentiate into effector cells that migrate to the allograft and cause its rejection.

tissues and are activated, in an antigen-nonspecific manner, by local inflammation that is induced by infections and other noxious stimuli. A set of innate immune receptors, toll-like receptors (TLRs), plays a central role in innate immunity. These receptors are germline-encoded, transmembrane, and intracellular receptors that are critical for the detection of microbial pathogen products, often referred to as pathogen-associated molecular patterns (PAMPS). PAMPS include bacterial lipopolysaccharide, lipoproteins, peptidoglycans, flagellin, and unmethylated cytosine-guanine (cPG) nucleic acids. TLRs are a form of pathogen recognition receptors that are expressed by APCs. To date, at least 10 TLRs have been identified with individual specificity for different microbial products. Once ligated by PAMPS, TLRs initiate a signaling pathway via the universal signal adaptor protein, MyD88, which induces the translocation of nuclear factor-κB and the expression of proinflammatory cytokines (tumor necrosis factor-α, IL-1, 6, 8, and 12). These cytokines induce DCs to mature, migrate to the draining secondary lymphoid tissues, and express surface proteins essential for T-cell costimulation (such as CD40, CD80, and CD86). In secondary lymphoid organs, DCs activate naïve T cells, thus initiating the adaptive phase of the immune response.

INNATE IMMUNITY IN TRANSPLANTATION Evidence supports the concept that TLRs can be activated by pathogen-unrelated, endogenous signals such as heat-shock proteins, heparan sulfate, surfactant, and the contents of necrotic cells.

Therefore, it is possible that TLRs may play a role in initiating the immune response to a transplanted organ. Consistent with this hypothesis, investigators have demonstrated that rejection of minor mismatched (HY antigen-mismatched) skin allografts is critically dependent on signaling via MyD88, the adaptor protein required for TLR signaling. Specifically, they demonstrated that female mice that had no MyD88 were not able to reject male allografts from MyD88-deficient donors. Furthermore, the inability to reject these allografts was owing to reduced accumulation of mature DCs in draining lymph nodes and impaired expansion of antigraft-reactive T cells. Thus, the initiation of the alloimmune response to minor mismatched transplant antigens is dependent on innate immune mechanisms that trigger the maturation and migration of APCs. It is not clear whether the rejection of fully MHC-mismatched allografts also depends on TLR signaling via Myd88. In addition, the nature of the ligands that stimulates TLRs in the transplant setting is not known.

The role of other cellular components of the innate immune response (monocyte/macrophages, neutrophils and NK cells) has also been investigated in murine transplantation models. None of these cellular components has been found to be indispensable for the rejection of either allografts or xenografts. However, studies have shown that graft infiltration with these cell types precedes T-cell infiltration, consistent with the idea that they may orchestrate effector T-cell migration and function. For example, NK cells activated by non-self-antigens secrete interferon (IFN)-γ, which stimulates local production of chemokines that recruit APCs and effector T cells to the site of inflammation.

Soluble components of innate immunity have also been investigated in the rejection of vascularized allografts. The complement system, a set of plasma proteins used to attack extracellular pathogens, has been shown to be critical for the rejection of renal allografts in mice. Specifically, donor allografts that were deficient in C3, a critical protein for complement activation, underwent significantly delayed allograft rejection compared to wild-type donor allografts. If the recipients were C3-deficient, wild-type allografts were rejected in a normal tempo demonstrating that local expression of complement within the graft is important for the rejection process. However, it is not clear whether complement activation plays a role in initiating the immune response (e.g., by activating and mobilizing APCs) or in the effector phase of rejection (e.g., by enhancing the recruitment of effector T cells). The complement cascade is also critical in hyperacute rejection of vascularized allografts and xenografts. In this case, recipients have preformed antibodies against donor transplant antigens. A classic example is the hyperacute rejection of ABO-incompatible allografts, whereby preformed antibodies deposit on the donor endothelium and initiate the complement cascade leading to platelet activation, thrombin deposition, and hemorrhagic infarction of the organ.

THE ADAPTIVE IMMUNE RESPONSE TO A TRANSPLANTED ORGAN

The first stage in the adaptive phase of the alloimmune response is the activation of alloreactive T cells by APCs. This process occurs within the organized structures of secondary lymphoid organs (the spleen, lymph nodes, and mucosal lymphoid tissues). On activation, antigen-specific T cells begin to expand in a logarithmic fashion (the expansion phase) and acquire effector functions that allow them, with the help of B-lymphocytes and other mononuclear cells, to eliminate the foreign antigen (the effector phase). T-cell expansion, however, does not continue indefinitely but quickly halts as autoregulatory mechanisms to ensure that most effector T cells generated during the immune response are eliminated by apoptosis (the regulatory phase). The few T cells that survive the death phase become long-lived memory T cells that confer life-long protection against the foreign antigen (the memory phase). There are cellular and molecular mechanisms underlying the stages of the adaptive immune response to a transplanted organ.

THE EXPANSION PHASE OF THE ALLOIMMUNE RESPONSE

Allorecognition Foreign transplant antigens (alloantigens) are recognized by and activate recipient T lymphocytes via two pathways (Fig. 65-2). In the direct pathway, the recipient's T lymphocytes are triggered by alloantigens expressed on *donor* APCs, commonly referred to as passenger leukocytes, which migrate out of the transplanted organ to the host's secondary lymphoid tissues. These alloantigens are intact allo-MHC molecules complexed to endogenous peptides derived from either histocompatibility antigens or from conserved proteins common to all members of the same species (self-peptides). It is the polymporphic MHC in the latter case that confers "foreignness" to the MHC-peptide complex and leads to the activation of alloreactive T cells. In the indirect pathway, alloantigens are shed by donor cells, taken up and processed by *recipient* APCs, and presented to recipient T lymphocytes in the groove of self-MHC molecules. Although the direct

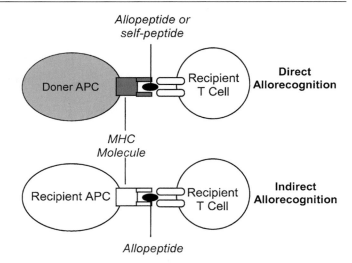

Figure 65-2 The direct and indirect pathways of allorecognition. Both pathways contribute to the initiation of the alloimmune response. However, the direct pathway leads to a more robust immune response by activating a larger number of T cells.

pathway appears to mount a more vigorous immune response, either pathway of allorecognition is sufficient for graft rejection.

The prevailing view had been that T-cell activation occurs within the transplanted organ and does not require the presence of secondary lymphoid organs. However, studies have challenged this point. Investigators found that mice that lacked all secondary lymphoid organs (splenectomized alymphoplastic mice) did not reject fully vascularized heart allografts but ignored them as if they were self. Using different mutant strains of mice (splenectomized, lymphotoxin-α (LTα$^{-/-}$), and lymphotoxin-β receptor (LTβR$^{-/-}$)-deficient mice), other investigators found that allograft rejection was severely delayed in the absence of secondary lymphoid organs although it did eventually occur. The discrepancy between these two studies may be owing to the differences in the mutations present in the recipient mice. Both the LTα$^{-/-}$ and the LTβR$^{-/-}$ mice have accumulations of CD4 T cells that may be already activated and thus not require the presence of secondary lymphoid organs to initiate allograft rejection. Nonetheless, both studies demonstrate that secondary lymphoid organs are important for initiating the adapting alloimmune response. Homing of activated APCs to the spleen and draining lymph nodes following transplantation is guided by the chemokine receptor CCR7 and its ligand, secondary lymphoid chemokine. SLC is expressed on the endothelium of the afferent lymphatic system, including high endothelial venules in lymph nodes, where it directs the entry of both activated APCs and naïve T cells. APC–T cell interaction within the T cells' zones of secondary lymphoid organs then initiates the alloimmune response.

T Lymphocyte Activation The first event in APC–T cell interaction that leads to T-cell activation is the binding of the TCR to the MHC–peptide complex on the APC (Fig. 65-3). The ability of the TCR to trigger intracellular signaling in T lymphocytes is dependent on the TCR 2 (TCRz) chain and on noncovalent interactions with the membrane molecule CD3 (Fig. 65-3). The intracellular signaling pathways initiated by the TCRz chain and CD3 include protein kinases, phospholipases, and calcineurin, which is a calcium-dependent protein phosphatase. The clinically important immunosuppressive agents, cyclosporine and tacrolimus, exert their immunosuppressive effects by inhibiting calcineurin

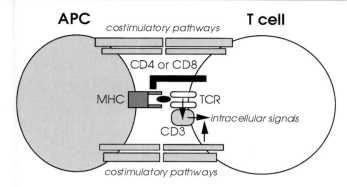

Figure 65-3 T cell activation. Recognition of the foreign MHC–peptide complex by the TCR is the first step in T-cell activation, often referred to as signal 1. The TCR is dependent on the accessory molecule CD3 to deliver intracellular signals that are necessary but not sufficient for triggering T cell proliferation. Additional stimulation, often referred to as signal 2, is required for T-cell proliferation and is delivered by costimulatory molecules present on T cells. Costimulatory molecules are engaged by counter-receptors expressed on activated APCs.

action. The CD4 and CD8 molecules, expressed on the surface of distinct T cell types, often referred to as CD4 helper (Th) and CD8 cytotoxic T lymphocytes (CTL), bind to nonpolymorphic regions of MHC class-II and -I molecules, respectively, and enhance signaling via the TCR-CD3 complex (Fig. 65-3).

TCR-CD3 interaction with the foreign MHC-peptide complex, however, is not sufficient for T-cell proliferation and differentiation into helper or cytotoxic cells. Additional help has to be provided by costimulatory molecules expressed on T lymphocytes (Fig. 65-3). The ligands for costimulatory molecules are present on professional APCs. These costimulatory pathways contribute to the formation of a tight "immunological synapse" between APCs and T lymphocytes. The synapse guarantees that TCR engagement by the MHC-peptide complex is sustained long enough to induce T-cell proliferation. Others have argued that costimulatory molecules provide intracellular signals that are distinct from those delivered by the TCR.

Although many costimulatory molecules have been identified, the ones that are well studied and proven to be critical for the induction of alloimmunity are CD28 and the CD40 ligand (CD40L or CD154). During APC-T cell interaction, B7-1 (CD80) and B7-2 (CD86) on APCs bind to CD28 on the surface of resting T lymphocytes. CD28 crosslinking facilitates T-cell activation by recruiting membrane and intracellular kinase-rich raft microdomains to the site of TCR engagement, resulting in enhanced and sustained TCR-CD3 signaling followed by increased IL-2 production and T-cell proliferation. Proof that the CD28-B7 costimulatory pathway is critical for allograft rejection derives from studies showing markedly prolonged allograft survival in experimental animals treated with CTLA4Ig, a recombinant fusion protein that binds B7-1 and B7-2 with high affinity and prevents their interaction with CD28. Unlike CD28, the costimulatory molecule CD40L is expressed only on activated T lymphocytes. Its counter-receptor, CD40, is a glycoprotein present on the surface of professional APCs and endothelial cells. Studies indicate that the crosslinking of CD40 by CD40L mediates the immunologic functions of this costimulatory pathway. First, CD40 engagement on DCs upregulates B7-1 and B7-2 expression and induces IL-12 production. These activation steps enhance the ability of DCs to induce the proliferation of CD4+ T cells and the differentiation of CD8+ T cells

into CTL. Second, CD40 ligation on B-lymphocytes by T cells is essential for the generation of adaptive humoral immune responses characterized by immunoglobulin isotype switching from IgM to IgG. Third, CD40 ligation on monocytes or macrophages by T cells augments their pro-inflammatory activities, and CD40 engagement on endothelial cells by T cells upregulates cell adhesion molecules, which are essential for the migration of leukocytes into sites of inflammation. That the CD40L–CD40 costimulatory pathway plays a crucial role in allograft rejection is demonstrated by studies showing that monoclonal antibodies, which block CD40L–CD40 interaction, significantly prolong allograft survival in rodents and nonhuman primates. CD28 and CD40L are not the only costimulatory molecules present on T lymphocytes. Other membrane proteins such as 4-1BB, ICOS, OX40L, and CD70L provide costimulation for T cells, and murine studies indicate that allograft survival can be prolonged by blocking the binding of these molecules to their ligands on APCs.

Cytokines Cytokines produced by APCs and activated alloreactive T lymphocytes act in an autocrine or paracrine fashion to enhance APC functions, T-cell proliferation, and T-cell differentiation into effector cells. The role of cytokines in allograft rejection has been largely inferred from their in vitro functions and from in vivo experiments in which cytokine expression is correlated with acute rejection. These studies however have led to contradictory results owing to the complexity of cytokine cascades triggered after transplantation. In vivo experiments using cytokine gene-knockout mice and cytokine-neutralizing antibodies point to two main conclusions: (1) cytokine actions are highly redundant; and (2) a single cytokine may have multiple actions and thus, influence the activation, effector, and regulatory phases of the alloimmune response. The redundancy phenomenon is supported by data showing that cytokine gene-knockout mice that lack IL-2, IL-4, or IFN-γ reject allografts vigorously, despite the fact these cytokines have indispensable immunostimulatory functions in vitro. One important exception to cytokine redundancy is that IFN-γ is necessary for the acute rejection of MHC class-II-incompatible allografts. This unique requirement for IFN-γ in the rejection process can be attributed to its essential role in inducing or upregulating MHC class-II expression on APCs and endothelial cells. The observation that a single cytokine could have multiple and sometimes opposing actions derives from experiments showing that immunostimulatory cytokines such as IFN-γ and IL-2 also have essential immunoregulatory roles in vivo. For example, IL-2 is a T-cell mitogen that also programs T lymphocytes for apoptosis. The absence of IL-2 in vivo does not lead to immunodeficiency but, instead, results in the accumulation of activated T lymphocytes, autoimmunity, and failure to accept allografts longterm.

THE EFFECTOR PHASE OF THE ALLOIMMUNE RESPONSE
The effector pathways that lead to allograft rejection involve a multiplicity of mechanisms, classified here according to the principal cell type that is responsible for tissue destruction.

Cytotoxic T Cells CD8+ CTL recognize their targets in a MHC-restricted, antigen-specific manner. The end-result of the interaction between a CTL and an allograft is the apoptosis of target cells. Two pathways of apoptosis have been described. In the first, activated CD8+ T cells synthesize perforin and granzymes that are then stored in intracellular granules. This transformation is assisted by IFN-γ and IL-2 secreted by CD4+ Th cells. On contact with alloantigen presented in the context of MHC class-I molecules, the granules release their contents, and perforin forms pores in the target cell membrane. In addition to their ability to cause osmotic lysis of target cells, perforin-induced pores allow granzymes, a family of proteases released simultaneously with perforin from CTL granules, to enter the cytoplasm where they cause the release of cytochrome c from the mitochondria and trigger target cell apoptosis. In the second pathway, CTL induce target cell apoptosis via the FasL-Fas pathway. Fas, a member of the tumor necrosis factor (TNF) family of death receptors, is constitutively expressed on most cells whereas FasL is expressed on T cells following their activation. The binding of FasL on the CTL to Fas on the target cell leads to apoptosis via caspase-dependent pathways.

Although perforin, granzymes, and FasL appear to be necessary components of the killing machinery in vitro, their role in acute allograft rejection in vivo is not obligatory. Mice that lack either perforin or FasL reject allografts at the same rate as their wildtype counterparts. The nonobligatory roles of these cytotoxic molecules point to the redundancy of the system. This may occur because of the presence of other cytotoxic molecules, for example TNF-related apoptosis inducing ligand (TRAIL), or because other cell types mediate allograft rejection in the absence of CTL-mediated cytotoxicity.

Monocytes and Macrophages Monocytes that infiltrate an organ transplant differentiate into macrophages that participate in graft rejection. They form an integral part of the infiltrate that characterizes delayed type hypersensitivity (DTH) responses. DTH responses are orchestrated by CD4+ T cells. Activated CD4+ T lymphocytes stimulate macrophages via the CD40L-CD40 pathway and by secreting IFN-γ and lymphotoxin. Macrophages then release a host of mediators that include cytokines (TNF, IL-1, 6, 10, 12, and 15), chemokines, reactive oxygen species, nitric oxide, proteolytic enzymes, and extracellular matrix proteins that lead to fibrosis. Nitric oxide can be cytotoxic by itself at sufficiently high local concentrations. TNF induces expression of adhesion molecules on endothelial cells, enhances intravascular thrombosis, and activates neutrophils, eosinophils, and macrophages. Like TNF, IL-1 mediates local tissue inflammation. IL-6 stimulates the growth of activated B-cells at a late stage in their differentiation into plasma cells. IL-12 induces IFN-γ production by NK and T cells and enhances the generation of CTLs. IL-15 serves as a mitogen to NK and T cells, particularly CD8+ memory T cells.

Natural Killer Cells NK cells are a lymphocyte subset, which expresses neither T- nor B-lymphocyte markers. They are activated by IL-2, IL-15 and type-1 IFNs. They release IFNγ on stimulation by IL-12. IFN-γ in turn induces chemokine secretion by cells of the graft, particularly endothelial cells, leading to the recruitment of more activated T cells. Inflammatory chemokines shown to play a significant role in allograft rejection include CXCR3 ligands (IP-10, MIG, and I-TAC) and to some extent CCR5 ligands (the MIP-1 family of chemokines). Like CTLs, NK cells kill target cells by releasing perforins and granzymes. In addition, they secrete TNF, which induces apoptosis of cells expressing the TNF receptor. NK cells recognize their target cells in two different ways. First, by expressing low affinity receptor for the constant (Fc) portion of IgG, they bind to and kill antibody-coated target cells (antibody-dependent cell-mediated cytotoxicity or ADCC). Second, NK cells also express receptors that recognize MHC class-I molecules complexed to self peptides. Many of these receptors, however, are inhibitory such that NK cells are shut down when they engage self MHC proteins. This implies that NK cells react to non-self by recognizing the absence of self-peptides in the grooves of MHC class-I molecules. Although NK cell depletion does not significantly alter acute rejection, they may play a subtle role in chronic rejection.

B Cells and Alloantibodies Antibodies directed against donor HLA molecules (alloantibodies) pose the greatest threat to a transplanted organ. Alloantibody generation is generally the consequence of sensitization. Sensitization occurs in patients who have been previously exposed to human HLA proteins in the form of transfusions, pregnancy or prior organ transplants. B cells that recognize specific HLA molecules via their B-cell receptor for antigen (membrane-bound immunoglobulins), internalize the HLA-antibody complex, cleave it into allopeptides, and present it in the context of MHC class-II molecules to CD4+ T cells. The production of IL-2, IL-4, and IL-5 by activated CD4+ T cells and T–B interactions via CD40–CD40L leads to B-cell maturation, proliferation, isotype switching, and the production of harmful alloantibodies. The most dramatic example of antibody-mediated allograft damage is hyperacute rejection, initiated by preformed donor-specific antibodies present in the recipient at the time of transplantation. Preformed antibodies that cause hyperacute rejection include anti-ABO and anti-HLA IgG antibodies, particularly those targeted against class-I HLA. Complement and coagulation cascades are activated leading to widespread endothelial damage, intravascular thrombosis, and graft necrosis. Alloantibodies cause tissue damage by activating the complement cascade or by mediating ADCC. In nonsensitized recipients, humoral rejection has been described as a cause of both acute and chronic rejection, but their relative importance is not known. B-cell-deficient mice, for example, are capable of vigorous acute allograft rejection. Chronic transplant arteriosclerosis, on the other hand, does not develop in B-cell-deficient mice, suggesting that alloantibodies play an important role in chronic rejection. In humans, humoral renal allograft rejection is diagnosed by staining for the complement component C4d in biopsy specimens.

Eosinophils Eosinophils are recruited into the allograft by the cytokines IL-4, 5, and 13, which are produced by Th2-type CD4+ T cells. Th2-mediated cellular rejection can occur in experimental models in the absence of CD8+ or CD4+ Th1 cells and is characterized by an eosinophilic infiltrate. The clinical significance of this finding is not known, but hypereosinophilia has been reported to precede acute rejection, and activated eosinophils and IL-5 expression have been observed in acutely rejecting allografts.

THE REGULATORY PHASE OF THE ALLOIMMUNE RESPONSE Expansion of antigen-specific lymphocytes and their differentiation into effectors in response to foreign antigen is followed by rapid clonal contraction. Deletion of the majority of activated/effector lymphocytes ensures that collateral damage to the host does not occur during immune responses. Elimination of the antigen that initially triggered lymphocyte stimulation is the ultimate means by which primary immune responses are terminated. Several down-regulatory mechanisms, however, participate in cases of large or persistent antigen loads such as a transplanted organ. These mechanisms include cell surface molecules and cytokines, which regulate proliferation and survival of activated T lymphocytes. There is also evidence that regulatory T cells that suppress immune responses may exist.

Activation-Induced Cell Death Apoptosis of activated and effector T cells is perhaps the most conspicuous means by which immune responses are regulated. Repeated stimulation of T lymphocytes by antigen results in the apoptosis of activated T cells instead of their continued proliferation. This phenomenon is known as antigen- or activation-induced cell death (AICD). AICD is in large part mediated by interaction between the cell surface molecule Fas (CD95), a "death" receptor, and its ligand (FasL). Antigenic stimulation upregulates Fas expression and induces *de novo* FasL expression on T lymphocytes. FasL-Fas binding then leads to apoptosis of activated T lymphocytes. Other membrane molecules that trigger T cell apoptosis include members of the TNF receptor (TNFR) family such as CD30, TNF receptor-related apopotosis-mediating protein, and the TRAIL receptor (DR4).

Among cytokines that act on T cells, IL-2 is essential for AICD, a function not shared by other T cell mitogenic cytokines such as IL-4, 7, 9, and 15, which also engage the common cytokine receptor γ-chain (γc). Although IL-2 is a potent mitogen to resting CD4+ and CD8+ T lymphocytes, it programs these cells to undergo apoptosis when restimulated with antigen. It does so by upregulating death-transducing receptors such as Fas and TNFR and by down-regulating death-inhibiting molecules such as FLIP and γc. IL-2-deficient mice are not capable of long-term allograft acceptance because of impaired alloantigen-induced apoptosis of activated T cells. Similarly, allograft acceptance cannot be achieved in IFN-γ-deficient mice because of exaggerated T-cell expansion in response to alloantigen. It is still debated whether IFN-γ regulates immune responses by promoting alloantigen-induced apoptosis of activated T cells, by limiting their proliferation, or both. The cyto-toxic molecule perforin also contributes to the apoptosis of acti-vated T cells by effecting the suicide or fratricide of both CD8+ and CD4+ T cells. Perforin gene-knockout mice have dysregulated immune responses and are unable to accept allografts even with potent immunosuppression.

Inhibition of T-Cell Proliferation and Differentiation

Another mechanism by which immune responses are regulated is the inhibition of T-cell proliferation. The T-cell surface molecule CTL antigen-4 (CTLA4 or CD152) has emerged as an important inhibitor of activated T-cell proliferation. CTLA4 is homologous to CD28 and shares the same ligands, B7-1 and B7-2. Unlike CD28, CTLA4 is expressed on the plasma membrane only on activated T cells, has a much higher affinity to B7 proteins, and delivers a negative signal that turns off the proliferation of activated T cells. Thus, early in the immune response B7-1 and B7-2 interact with CD28 receptors on naïve T cells to effect costimulation, whereas later the high-affinity interaction between B7 proteins and CTLA4 on activated T cells leads to inhibition of cell cycling. The CTLA4-B7-negative feedback pathway is essential for the optimal induc-tion of peripheral tolerance to protein antigens and to transplanted organs. A regulatory cytokine of paramount importance, TGFβ, is a potent inhibitor of activated T-cell differentiation into effector cells. TGFβ has been shown to downregulate alloimmune responses in several murine transplantation models.

Suppressor T Cells   There has been an explosive resurgence of the concept that regulatory/suppressor T cells that modulate immune responses exist. The most commonly described suppressor phenotype is the CD4+ T cell constitutively expressing CD25+ on its surface, often referred to as Treg. Other regulatory populations have also been described, including Tr1 cells that seem to suppress immune responses by secreting TGF-β and IL-10. In addition, CD8+ regulatory/suppressor T cells may exist. CD4+CD25+ Treg cells appear to mediate their suppressive effects by direct cell–cell interaction but the exact mechanism by which they inhibit the pro-liferation of other T cells is not known. An increasing body of evi-dence suggests that Treg have a role in maintaining self-tolerance, neonatal tolerance, and long-term allograft acceptance. A transcrip-tional regulator, Foxp3, which is uniquely associated with Treg has been identified. Genetic deletion of Foxp3 leads to absence of Treg

Table 65-1
Advantages of Memory T Cells Over Naïve T Cells

Characteristic	Naïve T cell	Memory T cell
Survival	Months to years	Years to lifetime
	Dependent on TCR interaction with MHC/antigen	Not dependent on TCR interaction with MHC/antigen
Migration	Secondary lymphoid tissues	Both lymphoid and nonlymphoid tissues
Response and effector function	Requires stimulation with antigen	Requires restimulation with antigen but is faster and larger in magnitude than naïve T cells
In vivo protection against foreign antigen	Long-lived but relatively inefficient	Long-lived and efficient

AICD, activation-induced cell death; MHC, major histocompatibil-ity complex; TCR, T-cell receptor for antigen.

and massive expansion of autoreactive, pathogenic T cells. The generation of suppressor T-cell clones may be the result of interac-tion of naïve T cells with immature DCs or the elusive plasmacy-toid DC, DC2.

THE MEMORY PHASE OF THE ALLOIMMUNE RESPONSE

A cardinal feature of the adaptive immune response is the genera-tion of memory lymphocytes. Although the vast majority of effec-tor T cells undergoes apoptosis as the primary immune response dissipates, few lymphocytes survive to become long-lived mem-ory T cells. Memory T cells that recognize microbial antigens pro-vide the organism with long-lasting protection against potentially fatal infections. Conversely, memory T cells that recognize donor alloantigens jeopardize the survival of life-saving organ trans-plants by mediating both acute and chronic rejection.

Memory T cells have several inherent advantages over their naïve counterparts that endow them with the ability to clear a for-eign antigen, whether a microbial pathogen or an allograft, in a vig-orous fashion (Table 65-1). The first advantage is that their response to a foreign antigen (recall response) is greater in magnitude and faster than the naïve T-cell response. Memory T cells generate a considerable number of effector T cells, capable of cytokine secre-tion cytolytic activity, or both, within hours of antigenic restimula-tion, whereas naïve T cells generate a smaller number of effectors at a much slower pace (days). Second, memory T cells have a survival advantage over their naïve counterparts. Antigen-specific memory T-cell populations persist for years to lifetime in humans and their survival appears to be antigen- and MHC-independent. Mature naïve T-cell populations also persist for a relatively long period of time (months to few years in humans) but their survival is depend-ent on constant, low-grade stimulation with MHC–self-peptide complexes. Third, the circulation of naïve T cells is restricted to sec-ondary lymphoid tissues, the site where they are activated by for-eign antigens presented by APC; memory T cells circulate through both secondary lymphoid tissues and peripheral nonlymphoid tis-sues. Unlike naïve T cells, memory T cells can directly encounter foreign antigen and mount a productive immune response within nonlymphoid tissues. The migratory advantage of memory T cells, therefore, allows them to detect and eliminate a foreign intruder substantially before it reaches secondary lymphoid tissues. The acti-vation, survival, and migration advantages of memory T cells confer the organism with enhanced protection against foreign antigens long after the primary immune response has dissipated.

The same advantages of memory T cells that make them efficient at eliminating microbial pathogens enable them to rapidly reject foreign tissues. Unlike inbred mice, outbred animals including humans, harbor a significant number of memory T cells that are alloreactive. These memory T cells generally arise if an individual is exposed to alloantigens via pregnancy, blood transfusion, or a previous organ transplant. However, alloreactive memory T cells also exist in individuals who have never been exposed to foreign tissues. It is proposed that such alloreactivity in the T-cell memory pool is caused largely by cross-reactivity; repeated exposure to viral and bacterial antigens over time leads to the development of memory T cells that also recognize alloantigens. This phenomenon, commonly referred to as heterologous immunity, has been demonstrated in murine infection models, and is supported by experimental findings in humans. Alloreactive memory T cells, whether generated by previous exposure to alloantigens or microbial infection, can cause acute and chronic rejection and interfere with the induction of immunologic tolerance (donor-specific unresponsiveness).

CONCLUSIONS

Despite advances in understanding the cellular and molecular mechanisms of allograft acceptance, long-term survival of transplanted organs remains an important clinical challenge. Moreover, transplantation tolerance and allograft acceptance in the absence of continuous immunosuppression have been elusive clinical goals. The reason for these seemingly insurmountable challenges stems from the properties of the alloimmune response. These properties include the large number of alloreactive T cells present in a given individual, the limitations of immunoregulatory mechanisms responsible for turning off the alloimmune responses, and

the fact that immune responses to foreign antigens, by virtue of evolutionary design, are destined to generate immunologic memory. The latter property is perhaps the most formidable obstacle to long-term allograft acceptance and transplantation tolerance. Therefore, an important but unmet challenge in clinical transplantation is whether selective deletion or suppression of alloreactive memory T cells can be accomplished without globally compromising the host's immune system.

SELECTED REFERENCES

Adams A, Williams A, Jones T, et al. Heterologous immunity provides a potent barrier to transplantation tolerance. J Clin Invest 2003;111: 1887–1895.

Chalasani G, Lakkis FG. Immunologic ignorance of organ allografts. Curr Opin Organ Transplant 2001;6:83–88.

Dai Z, Lakkis FG. The role of cytokines, CTLA-4, and costimulation in transplant tolerance and rejection. Curr Opin Immunol 1999;11:504–508.

Goldstein D, Tesar B, Akira S, Lakkis F. Critical role of the Toll-like receptor signal adaptor protein Myd88 in acute allograft rejection. J Clin Invest 2003;111:1571–1578.

Kaech SM, Wherry EJ, Ahmed R. Effector and memory T cell differentiation: Implications for vaccine development. Nat Rev Immunol 2002; 2:251–262.

Lakkis F. Where is the alloimmune response initiated? Am J Transplant 2003;3:241–242.

Lakkis FG. Role of cytokines in transplantation tolerance: lessons learned from gene-knockout mice. J Am Soc Nephrol 1998;9:2361–2367.

Lakkis FG, Arakelov A, Konieczny BT, Inoue Y. Immunologic 'ignorance' of vascularized organ transplants in the absence of secondary lymphoid tissue. Nat Med 2000;6:686–688.

Salama A, Remuzzi G, Harmon W, Sayegh M. Challenges to achieving clinical transplantation tolerance. J Clin Invest 2001;108:943–948.

Sayegh MH, Turka LA. The role of T-cell costimulatory activation pathways in transplant rejection. N Engl J Med 1998;338:1813–1821.

Womer KL, Velle JP, Sayegh MH. Chronic allograft dysfunction: mechanisms and new approaches to therapy. Semin Nephrol 2000;20:126–147.

MUSCULOSKELETAL | VIII

SECTION EDITOR:
DANIEL J. GARRY

Abbreviations

VIII. MUSCULOSKELETAL

ANC-1	Nuclear-anchoring protein in C. elegans
bHLH	basic helix–loop–helix
CaM	calmodulin
CaMK	Ca^{2+}/CaM-dependent protein kinase
CDK	cyclin-dependent protein kinase
CKI	cyclin-dependent protein kinase inhibitor
CPK	creatine phosphokinase
CsA	cyclosporin
DGC	dystrophin glycoprotein complex
ECM	extracellular matrix
ES	embryonic stem
FGF	fibroblast growth factor
FKHR	fork head homolog rhabdomyosarcoma
FKRP	fukutin-related protein
FSHD	facioscapulohumeral muscular dystrophy
GSK-3β	glycogen synthase kinase-3β
HDAC5	histone deacetylase 5
HGF/SF	hepatocyte growth factor/scatter factor
HLH	helix–loop–helix
Id	inhibitor of differentiation
IGF1	insulin growth factor 1
IGF2	insulin growth factor 2
IGF-2	insulin-like growth factor II
IGFs	insulin-like growth factors
IRS	intergroup Rhabdomyosarcoma Study
LGMD	limb-girdle muscular dystrophy
LOH	loss of heterozygosity
MEF2	muscle-enriched factor 2
MEF2	myocyte enhancer binding factor-2
MGF	mechano growth factor
mTOR	mammalian target of rapamycin
NFAT	nuclear factor of activated T cells
NMJ	neuromuscular junction
nNOS	neuronal nitric oxide synthase
NRF-1	nuclear respiratory factor
PABP2	poly(A) binding protein 2
PCR	polymerase chain reaction
PGC-1	peroxisome proliferator-activated receptor γ coactivator-1
PI-3K	phosphoinositide 3-kinase
PKC	protein kinase C
POMGnT1	O-mannose β-1,2-N-acetylglucosaminyltransferase
POMT1	O-mannosyltransferase
PPAR-γ	peroxisome proliferator-activated receptor γ
Rb	retinoblastoma protein
SEPN1	selenoprotein N
SERCA	sarcoplasmic reticulum calcium ATPase pump
Shh	sonic hedgehog
SP	side population
SR	sarcoplasmic reticulum
T	transverse
TGF-β	transforming growth factor-β

function in mammalian cells and specifically whether they have a similar role in the syncytial mammalian muscle fiber.

The connective tissue that surrounds each myofiber is contiguous with the myotendinous junction and ultimately the tendons themselves. Proteins important for attachment to the intracellular matrix are highly concentrated in the myotendinous junction. Integrins are heterodimeric proteins expressed in nearly all cell types. Integrins bind to two major types of proteins in the extracellular matrix, fibronectin, and laminin. In muscle, the most highly expressed integrin isoforms are the laminin receptor $\alpha_7\beta_1$ and fibronectin receptor $\alpha_5\beta_1$. Integrin $\alpha_7\beta_1$ is the major integrin expressed in mature muscle and is highly concentrated at the myotendinous junction in addition to being found at the plasma membrane of muscle. Muscle contraction produces the shortening of individual myofibers, and the connective tissue that surrounds each myofiber is important for force transmission. The register of thin and thick filaments is foreshortened and, thus, redundancy is present in sarcolemma surrounding each myofiber. Because not every myofiber extends the entire length of the muscle, the sheaths that surround each fiber necessarily must function in force transmission. Moreover, the myotendinous junctions transmit force of the entire muscle directly on the tendons and underlying bone.

THE SARCOMERE, THE UNIT OF CONTRACTION H&E staining of longitudinal myofibers shows cross striations that are perpendicular to the long axis of the myofiber (Fig. 67-1). Alternating light and dark bands comprise the cross-striations. The darker bands, or A bands, are so named for their anisotropic properties in that they are birefringent in polarized light. The light bands, called I bands or isotropic, do not polarize light. The Z band, (or Z disk, Z line), is a thin dark band that bisects each I band. Thin filaments are found in the I band, and the Z band is made up of actin binding proteins. Overlying the Z bands at the sarcolemma are specialized structures called costameres. Costameric patterning on the surface of myofibers reflects the underlying Z band structures and provides attachments from the Z band to the surface plasma membrane. In the center of the A band is a lighter area, the H band, which represents thick filaments without any overlapping thin filaments (Fig. 67-1).

Myosin and actin, the components of thick and thin filaments were among the first proteins to be purified and help contribute to the "domain" theory of protein function. Myosin is a hexamer with two heavy chains (220 kDa each) and four light chains (20–25 kDa each). The amino terminus of myosin is globular in nature and the two pairs of light chains bind at the junction between the globular head and the carboxy-terminal rod region. Within the head domain are the sequences required for ATP hydrolysis and actin binding. Proteolysis was used to separate the head region of myosin from the rod region and, using this approach, it was found that the rod region self-assembles with the periodicity of the intact myosin hexamer (143 Å). That is, the 850 amino acids that consist of the head region represent the enzymatically active region of the molecule, whereas the carboxy-terminal 1200 amino acids have an α-helical coiled nature responsible for macromolecular assembly. Thick filaments assemble bidirectionally, so that heads from myosin orient in opposite directions. A typical native thick filament assembles to a length not greater than 1–1.5 μm. Myosin binding protein C, a thick filament binding protein, may help regulate thick filament assembly or may help stabilize thick filaments once they are formed. The role of myosin binding protein C is especially important in the cardiomyocyte in

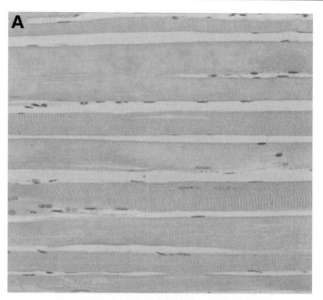

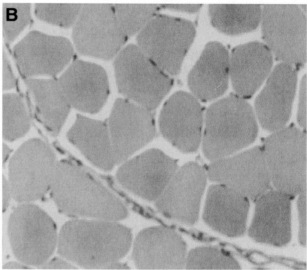

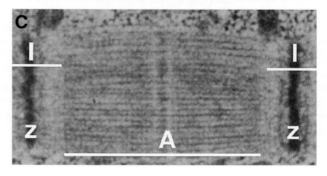

Figure 67-1 Shown are longitudinal (**A**) and transverse (**B**) cross-sections of human skeletal muscle. In the longitudinal section, the cross striations are visible. Each myofiber is a single cell that contains many nuclei located at the periphery of each myofiber. In transverse cross-sections each fiber is uniform in size, and fibers are tightly packed and encased in connective tissue (seen running from the upper left to the lower right of the section). Note the peripheral position of myonuclei. (**C**) shows an electron micrograph of a sarcomere, the unit of contraction. The Z band anchors the thin filaments. The thin filaments interdigitate with the myosin containing thick filaments. The A band represents overlapping thin and thick filaments. The I band is made up of only thin filaments that contain actin, tropomyosin, and the troponins.

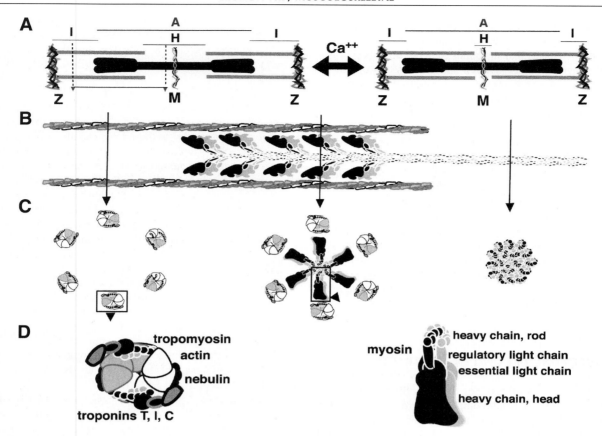

Figure 67-2 (**A**) Shows relaxation (left diagram) and contraction (right diagram) of the sarcomere. In the presence of calcium, a conformation change occurs in the thin filament that allows actin and myosin to interact. Through the myosin power stroke, the overlap between thick and thin filaments increases, and the sarcomere and muscle shorten. (**B**) Shows the myosin heads (gray and black) interacting with actin containing thin filaments. (**C**) Shows a cross-section of thin filaments, further highlighted in **D**. Thin filament regulatory proteins, tropomyosin and the troponins, regulate the actomyosin interface. Large proteins such as nebulin and titin anchor thick filaments. The middle panel of **C** shows a cross-section through a myosin thick filament surrounded by thin filaments. The right panel in **C** shows a cross-section through a myosin thick filament demonstrating the tight packing of myosin rod regions. Myosin is made up of two heavy chains and two each of regulatory and essential light chains. Hexamers of myosin tightly pack to form the thick filament.

which mutations in the cardiac form of myosin binding protein C lead to hypertrophic cardiomyopathy.

Thin filaments are made up of several different proteins, but filamentous actin is the major constituent. Monomeric, or G actin, is 43 kDa. Modulated by ionic strength and actin binding proteins, actin assembles to form a right-handed double helical filament (F actin). The pitch of the actin filament is 36 nm with seven actin monomers per strand. Along the grooves of the actin double helix are the thin filament regulatory proteins, troponins T, C, and I and tropomyosin. Tropomyosin is a rod-like molecule, and troponin T directly interacts with tropomyosin. Troponin C directly binds calcium providing calcium sensitivity to the actomyosin interaction.

From these biochemical observations and the structural observations of muscle, the sliding filament theory was proposed. In this model, the heads of myosin protrude from the thick filaments (Fig. 67-2). Protruding myosin heads directly interact with actin thin filaments to increase the overlap of thick and thin filaments, reducing the I band and effectively shortening the sarcomere and the muscle fiber as a whole. Force is transmitted parallel to the long axis of muscle. As the Z band anchors thin filaments, force is also to some degree transmitted perpendicular to the long axis of myofibers. The Z band also attaches to the plasma membrane at specialized structures called costameres. Further support for the sliding filament

model was found by examining the appearance of isolated thick filaments where protruding myosin heads could be seen. In the sliding filament model, the "rowing" movement of myosin protruding heads must occur within the myosin head or neck to be effective in moving the thick filaments along thin filaments. Although electron microscopy of muscle provided anatomic support for the sliding filament theory, demonstrating movement within the myosin head or neck region has been difficult.

A revolution in understanding myosin and actin function occurred with the development of in vitro motility assays that required only purified actin and myosin to visualize the movement of fluorescently labeled actin filaments along myosin fixed to a surface. These assays have provided data on the domains of myosin required for ATP hydrolysis and actin binding, and have allowed the identification of domains required for movement and force production. The crystal structure of the myosin head and structures of myosin heads with actin have been used to identify varying conformational states of the actomyosin interface and have provided support for the sliding filament theory.

One central question in myosin biology is to determine the length of the step that a myosin head can make along the length of actin filament for a hydrolysis of ATP (Fig. 67-3). This calculation, referred to as myosin step size, has been estimated from several

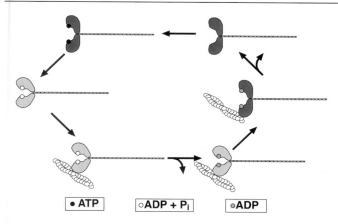

Figure 67-3 Shown is the ATPase cycle of the actomyosin interaction. After hydrolyzing ATP to ADP plus P_i, myosin undergoes a conformational change. The interaction of the myosin head with actin occurs. After release of P_i, myosin is thought to undergo an additional conformational change that moves actin along the actin thin filament. The distance that myosin can move along the actin thin filament per cycle of ATP hydrolysis is referred to as the myosin step size.

approaches. The estimates range from 5 to 15 nm, and this is in the context of a myosin that is approx 20 nm in length itself. There are at least 16 types of myosin molecules defined using electronic database searching and biochemical characterization. Myosins fall into two broad classes. The first, myosin I, are specialized motors for intracellular transport. These myosins have a head region similar to the myosin found in muscle, but have modified tail regions specialized for the cargo and vesicle attachment. The neck regions of myosin are also specialized in that this region may bind light chains or calmodulin to regulate the function of myosin. Muscle myosin, referred to as myosin II, represents the second class. These myosins have the specialized rod region that can form thick filaments. Thus, type-II myosins function as many motors together on a rod whereas type-I myosins may function as single heads or as single molecules with two heads. For example, myosin V has two heads and can take an enormous step of 36 nm. This large step can be accomplished while the second myosin head remains attached. The processivity of this myosin appears to differ from muscle myosin, and this is further supported by kinetic studies that show a slow release of adenosine 5′-diphosphate (ADP) to aid the processive nature of myosin V. Muscle myosin appears to have smaller step size, and a much faster release of ADP. Some estimates calculated the step size of muscle myosin to be as small as 5 nm. Other estimates, which argue that the arrangement of actin filaments influences measurements of myosin head step size, have calculated step sizes as large as 15–30 nm. These investigators reason that to achieve this larger step size, myosin actually takes "substeps" in its interactions with actin. Kinetic studies have not necessarily supported the presence of multiple small "substeps" although further experimentation is required to fully understand the interaction of myosin with actin and the molecular basis of biological movement.

Current structural studies focus on the neck region of myosin, as this appears to have regions capable of serving the lever function for movement. Comparisons of evolutionarily and functionally diverse myosins have revealed myosin VI as a molecule that contains a distinct lever region. In vitro studies of this myosin showed surprisingly that it moves in an opposite orientation relative to all other characterized myosins. Generally myosins move

toward the barbed end of actin filaments. In contrast, myosin VI moves toward the pointed end, supporting the idea that not all myosin molecules have the identical unidirectional movement. To date, myosin VI is the only myosin described capable of reverse movement.

ANCHORING THE SARCOMERE, PASSIVE FORCE, ELASTIC RECOIL, AND FORCE TRANSMISSION Titin is giant protein that spans the length of the sarcomere providing attachment from the sarcomere to the Z band and also to the membrane. Titin is alternatively spliced to produce a variety of protein forms that are several megadaltons in size. As an elongated structure, titin can span nearly 1 μm, close to the length of a sarcomere. Titin has a highly repetitive structure thought to impart elastic recoil properties of muscle. Actin-containing thin filaments are anchored to the Z band. A number of Z band-associated proteins have been identified that are important for skeletal muscle and cardiac muscle function. Titin has attachments along the Z band and can interact with proteins such as telethonin (T cap) and subunits of the calcium-activated protease, calpain. Mutations in titin, telethonin, and calpain 3 can lead to muscular dystrophy. Myotilin is a smaller protein that contains several immunoglobulin domains. Genetic mutations in myotilin also are associated with muscular dystrophy. The precise mechanism of how genetic defects in these proteins lead to muscle degeneration is not known, but their convergence on the Z band of muscle implies the importance of this muscular structure.

ANCHORING Z BANDS TO THE PLASMA MEMBRANE Z bands anchor the sarcomere to the plasma membrane. Concentrated over the Z band at the plasma membrane is the dystrophin glycoprotein complex (DGC). The specialized connections of the Z bands to the plasma membrane are referred to as costameres and can be visualized on longitudinal sections of muscle. Dystrophin, the protein product of the Duchenne muscular dystrophy locus, is a 427 kDa protein with an actin-binding domain found at its amino terminus. Within its elongated rod region are 24 spectrin repeats that are interrupted by hinge sites. Hinge sites are defined by breaks in the typical spectrin repeats and are thought to provide flexibility. Spectrin repeats are independently folding domains of roughly 100 amino acids that have a triple-helical bundled structure. Each spectrin repeat has a limited degree of flexibility. Spectrin repeats are named for the prototypical protein spectrin, a protein component of the erythrocyte membrane. Genetic defects in spectrin lead to instability of the erythrocyte membrane and to hemolytic anemia. Similarly, absence or reduction in the dystrophin component of the plasma membrane leads to instability of the muscle membrane producing muscle degeneration and muscular dystrophy. In skeletal muscle, regeneration can occur, but typically in Duchenne muscular dystrophy, regeneration is insufficient to match the ongoing degeneration and therefore, muscle wasting and weakness ensue.

The Dystrophin Glycoprotein Complex and its Role in Membrane Stability The DGC is a macromolecular structure that can be purified from the membrane fraction of muscle (Fig. 67-4). The DGC has cytoplasmic and transmembrane components. A major transmembrane component is the laminin receptor dystroglycan. Dystroglycan is made up of an α- and β-subunit produced by proteolytic cleavage of a single polypeptide. Dystroglycan is broadly expressed, is found in most tissue types and has an essential role in development where it organizes laminin in the extracellular matrix. In addition, in nonmuscle cells dystroglycan serves as a receptor for a number of pathogenic

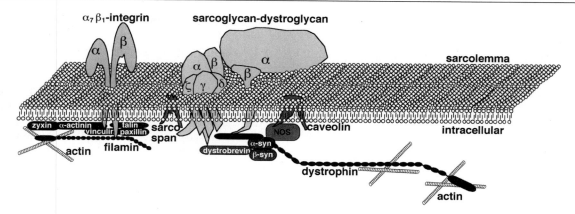

Figure 67-4   Shown is a schematic representation of the dystrophin glycoprotein complex and the integrin complex, two membrane-associated complexes in muscle that serve to connect the extracellular matrix to the membrane and the underlying cytoskeleton. Dystrophin attaches to dystroglycan. The sarcoglycan complex may stabilize the interaction of α and β dystroglycan. The integrin complex is concentrated at Z bands and at the myotendinous junction.

agents. In its intracellular portion, dystroglycan can directly bind to dystrophin. Dystroglycan can also bind Grb2, a protein implicated in Ras. In the central and peripheral nervous systems, α-dystroglycan is 120 kDa, whereas in skeletal muscle, the larger subunit of dystroglycan is 156 kDa, and this difference relates to differential glycosylation.

The sarcoglycan complex is a muscle specific subcomplex within the DGC, and mutations in the genes encoding α-, β-, γ- and δ-sarcoglycan lead to autosomal-recessive limb girdle muscular dystrophy. The precise role of the sarcoglycan complex is not fully understood, but like the entire DGC, the sarcoglycan complex likely has both mechanical and signaling roles for the maintenance and normal function of skeletal muscle membranes. Sarcospan is a four membrane-spanning tetraspanin protein. Other tetraspanin proteins have been demonstrated to interact with integrins. Mice engineered with a null mutation of sarcospan do not develop muscular dystrophy. A number of other tetraspanin proteins are expressed in muscle and compensatory upregulation of other tetraspanins may limit the expression of a phenotype from the loss of sarcospan. Mice have been engineered with null mutations in the sarcoglycan proteins and these mice recapitulate the human phenotypes. The *mdx* mouse is a spontaneously arising mutant that has a nonsense mutation 23 of the dystrophin gene, and, thus, makes no full-length dystrophin. These mice display an identical histopathology to what is seen in Duchenne muscular dystrophy, but do not develop overt muscle weakness, are fertile and have a nearly normal lifespan. Mouse models of dystrophin and sarcoglycan deficiency have proved useful for determining a DGC function in maintaining membrane stability in muscle.

The cytoplasmic face of the DGC includes a number of intracellular proteins including neuronal nitric oxide synthase (NOS or nNOS1), dystrobrevins, and the syntrophins. The syntrophins are PDZ domain containing proteins that can bind directly to nNOS. The dystrobrevins have homology to the carboxy-terminal region of dystrophin and bind directly to dystrophin and each other. The syntrophins bind directly to dystrophin and to dystrobrevin, thus forming a complex that anchors nNOS. Consistent with this, mutations in dystrophin displace nNOS from the plasma membrane. nNOS can also bind to caveolin, a small membrane-bound protein important for the formation of caveolae structures.

Dystrophin, dystroglycan, and laminin are thought to form a mechanical link that stabilizes the plasma membrane through its interaction with the extracellular matrix through the considerable deformation and stress faced through repeated muscle contraction. Mutations that reduce dystrophin result in destabilization of the remainder of the DGC including dystroglycan and sarcoglycan. The loss of the DGC is thought to render the membrane susceptible to contraction-induced damage. Supporting this, muscle lacking dystrophin displays a significant increase in membrane disruption and damage when subjected to eccentric contraction, resulting in a reduction in maximal force production. A common molecular feature between sarcoglycan mutant muscle and dystrophin mutant muscle is the loss of the sarcoglycan complex. Interestingly, in γ-sarcoglycan mutant muscle the sarcoglycan complex is largely destabilized but dystrophin, dystroglycan, and laminin are present. In similar eccentric contraction protocols, γ-sarcoglycan muscle does not demonstrate contraction-induced damage supporting a nonmechanical role for the sarcoglycan complex.

On the cytoplasmic face, muscle lacking for nNOS or the syntrophins does not develop muscular dystrophy. This may relate to compensatory upregulation of related proteins or may indicate that these subunits participate in alternative intracellular functions. Mice engineered to lack α-dystrobrevin develop a mild muscular dystrophy phenotype although the properties of membrane instability may be different than what is seen with sarcoglycan or dystrophin mutations.

At its amino terminus, dystrophin has a classic actin-binding site similar to that seen in α-actinin and other actin-binding proteins. Given the localization of dystrophin at the plasma membrane and especially its concentration overlying Z bands, dystrophin is thought to preferentially interact with γ-actin that forms part of the cytoskeletal network that is under the sarcolemma. Supporting this, when the plasma membrane is mechanically peeled from the underlying myofibrils, the under surface of the plasma membrane has a costameric arrangement of γ-actin (Fig. 67-5). Moreover, when dystrophin is mutant, the pattern of γ-actin is disrupted and is no longer associated with the plasma membrane, remaining instead affiliated with the myofibrillar structure including Z bands. Therefore, dystrophin participates in a mechanically strong linkage that includes γ-actin.

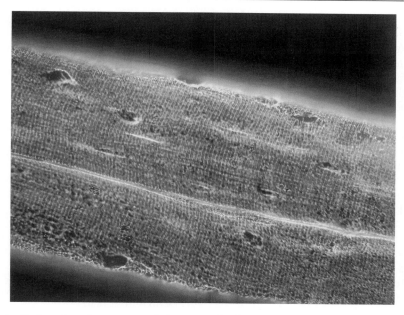

Figure 67-5 Shown is a longitudinal section of mouse muscle immunostained with an antibody for δ-sarcoglycan. The pattern of staining that runs perpendicular to the long axis of the myofiber represents the costameric pattern overlying Z bands. The dystrophin glycoprotein complex is concentrated more highly at costameres.

Dystrophin associates with actin not only through the amino-terminal actin-binding domain, but also through a side-to-side interaction with actin filaments along its rod. Utrophin is a chromosome-6 encoded homolog of dystrophin that is highly expressed in developing muscle and expressed at lower levels in mature muscle. The overall structural similarity between utrophin and dystrophin is substantiated as utrophin can substitute for dystrophin in the *mdx* mouse, a mouse model of muscular dystrophy. Utrophin is also concentrated at neuromuscular junctions (NMJs). The NMJ is a specialization for the organized delivery of neural input to muscle. Utrophin mutant mice have a reduction in the number of folds normally found in the NMJ and concomitant decrease in NMJ function. Moreover, mice doubly mutant for dystrophin and utrophin have a more severe phenotype indicating overlapping roles of dystrophin and utrophin.

NEURONAL CONTROL

Skeletal muscle requires neuronal input from motor neurons and from muscle spindles, receptors required for spatiotemporal proprioception. This input contributes directly to the development and relaxation of muscle groups for coordinated movement. Neural input also provides feedback on a longer time-scale to regulate gene expression and modify fiber typing for the requirements of repeated use. Hypertrophy and fiber recruitment occur in response to training. Muscle fibers fall into two major categories. Type-I fibers are slow twitch muscle with aerobic metabolism. In contrast, type-II fibers are modified for fast twitch function and thereby depend on anaerobic metabolism utilizing glycogenolytic pathways. The program of gene expression varies considerably between these two types of fibers and most human skeletal muscles contain a mixture of fiber types. Some fibers have intermediate properties and certain fiber types may be more susceptible to certain disease processes.

Slow and fast motorneurons provide input to type-I and type-II fibers, respectively. Denervation of muscle leads to atrophy. Gene expression profiling has identified genes and proteins that are uniquely upregulated in atrophic states. Regulation of muscle mass occurs during development and also is constantly regulated in adult states. Myostatin, a member of the type-β transforming growth factor family of proteins, is a negative regulator of muscle mass. Mice engineered that completely lack myostatin have muscle mass nearly 200% of normal. Adult mice treated with inhibitors of myostatin function can increase by muscle mass 20–30%. The ability to inhibit the negative regulation of muscle mass may prove useful in disease states. Myostatin is thought to act directly on muscle itself through paracrine mechanisms although further study is required to fully understand its scope of action.

The NMJ is a highly redundant structure to allow rapid transmission of neuronal input to the muscle. Acetylcholine receptors are the major receptor of this input. Molecules such as agrin participate in acetylcholine receptor clustering and regulation of receptor function. The intracellular surface kinases, such as MuSK, regulate acetylcholine function. The acetylcholine receptor is important in disease states such as myasthenia gravis where defects in receptor function can be induced through immune mediated or inherited mechanisms.

Neural input leads to membrane depolarization that, in turn, must lead to coordinated muscle membrane depolarization and intracellular calcium release. Depolarization of the membrane is directly propagated through membrane invaginations known as transverse (T) tubules. As T tubules contact the sarcoplasmic reticulum (SR) directly, this allows conformational changes in the calcium release channels of the SR.

REGULATION OF MUSCLE CONTRACTION BY CALCIUM

For coordinated activation of actomyosin interaction, intracellular calcium is tightly regulated. Such excitation contraction coupling occurs at regions where the intracellular sarcoplasmic reticulum, an extension of the endoplasmic reticulum, forms junctions with the sarcolemma. Tubular invaginations of the sarcolemma, T tubules, form a junction with two terminal cisternae regions of the SR forming a triad junction. Within the SR and the T tubule system, there are a number of proteins that regulate calcium sequestration and calcium release. Among these are the intracellular ryanodine receptor, a large >500 kDa protein that forms a tetramer and the dihydropyridine receptor, a voltage gated L-type calcium channel. Together, these proteins are important for the regulation of depolarization-induced calcium release as well as calcium-induced calcium release. Thus, these proteins are essential for coupling excitation and contraction through the release of calcium. Uptake after contraction is equally essential to maintaining tight control on the actomyosin interaction. For this role, the sarcoplasmic reticulum calcium ATPase pump (SERCA) is required. Triadin, junctin, mitsugumin, and junctophilin are proteins that participate in the formation of the triad junction facilitating the interaction of the T-tubular dihydropyridine receptor and the ryanodine receptor. Calsequestrin is a luminal protein that directly binds calcium. Together these proteins each participate in the regulation of the triad junction and play a role in excitation contraction coupling in skeletal muscle.

Highlighting the importance of calcium regulation to disease, mutations in the genes encoding both the ryanodine receptor and SERCA lead to muscle dysfunction and disease. Mutations in the ryanodine receptor lead to malignant hyperthermia in which a sudden increase in intracellular calcium can occur leading to hypercontraction. In Brody's disease, mutations in SERCA lead to abnormal relaxation characterized by painless muscle cramping and exercise-induced impairment of muscle relaxation. Brody patients frequently show an inability to relax skeletal muscle following contracture.

MYOCYTE NUCLEI

As in other eukaryotic cells, the nuclear membrane is made up of two distinct lipid bilayers, the inner and outer nuclear membranes. Facing the nucleus and associated with the inner nuclear membrane is a network of proteins that scaffolds nuclear contents. Lamins A and C are produced from a single gene and form higher order filamentous structures. As in most other terminally differentiated cells, lamins A and C are intermediate filament proteins that provide support to the mature myofiber inner nuclear membrane. Mutations in the gene encoding lamin A/C are a common cause of muscular dystrophy. Recent studies suggest that lamin A/C is important for the mechanical properties of myofiber nuclei. In addition, mutations in the gene encoding the nuclear membrane protein emerin cause an X-linked form of muscular dystrophy. Like lamin A/C, emerin is broadly expressed, yet mutations in this gene lead to a tissue specific phenotype. The identification of lamin A/C and emerin, and their role in muscle degeneration highlights the importance of nucleoskeleton.

CONCLUSIONS

The structure of skeletal muscle is unique and provides the machinery necessary for controlled movement. The cell biological aspects of skeletal muscle have emphasized both structural and nonstructural roles for a variety of proteins in the sarcomere, the Z band, the plasma membrane, and the nuclear membrane. The importance of these proteins to normal skeletal muscle function has been highlighted with the identification of a large number of genetic mutations that lead to skeletal muscle dysfunction and

disease. In general, many of these genetic defects have not targeted muscle development, as such mutations may prove too lethal for the organism's survival. However, muscle developmental paradigms are increasingly important with the characterization of pluripotent stem cells in muscle and the role of satellite cells for muscle regeneration. These topics are covered in Chapters 66 and 68.

SELECTED REFERENCES

Ahn AH, Kunkel LM. The structural and functional diversity of dystrophin. Nat Genet 1993;3:283–291.

Barral JM, Epstein HF. Protein machines and self assembly in muscle organization. Bioessays 1999;21:813–823.

Bodine SC, Latres E, Baumhueter S, et al. Identification of ubiquitin ligases required for skeletal muscle atrophy. Science 2001;294: 1704–1708.

Bonne G, Carrier L, Richard P, Hainque B, Schwartz K. Familial hypertrophic cardiomyopathy: from mutations to functional defects. Circ Res 1998;83:580–593.

Clark KA, McElhinny AS, Beckerle MC, Gregorio CC. Striated muscle cytoarchitecture: an intricate web of form and function. Annu Rev Cell Dev Biol 2002;18:637–706.

Durbeej M, Campbell KP. Muscular dystrophies involving the dystrophin-glycoprotein complex: an overview of current mouse models. Curr Opin Genet Dev 2002;12:349–361.

Emery AE. Emery-Dreifuss muscular dystrophy—a 40 year retrospective. Neuromuscul Disord 2000;10:228–232.

Ervasti JM. Costameres: The Achilles' heel of herculean muscle. J Biol Chem 2003;278:13,591–13,594.

Faulkner G, Lanfranchi G, Valle G. Telethonin and other new proteins of the Z-disc of skeletal muscle. IUBMB Life 2001;51:275–282.

Franzini-Armstrong C, Protasi F. Ryanodine receptors of striated muscles: A complex channel capable of multiple interactions. Physiol Rev 1997;77:699–729.

Gomes MD, Lecker SH, Jagoe RT, Navon A, Goldberg AL. Atrogin-1, a muscle-specific F-box protein highly expressed during muscle atrophy. Proc Natl Acad Sci USA 2001;98:14,440–14,445.

Gregorio CC, Antin PB. To the heart of myofibril assembly. Trends Cell Biol 2000;10:355–362.

Hack AA, Cordier L, Shoturma DI, Lam MY, Sweeney HL, McNally EM. Muscle degeneration without mechanical injury in sarcoglycan deficiency. Proc Natl Acad Sci USA 1999;96:10,723–10,728.

Hack AA, Groh ME, McNally EM. Sarcoglycans in muscular dystrophy. Microsc Res Tech 2000;48:167–180.

Henry MD, Campbell KP. Dystroglycan inside and out. Curr Opin Cell Biol 1999;11:602–607.

Houdusse A, Sweeney HL. Myosin motors: missing structures and hidden springs. Curr Opin Struct Biol 2001;11:182–194.

Huxley AF. Cross-bridge action: present views, prospects, and unknowns. J Biomech 2000;33:1189–1195.

Kron SJ, Spudich JA. Fluorescent actin filaments move on myosin fixed to a glass surface. Proc Natl Acad Sci USA 1986;83:6272–6276.

Lee SJ, McPherron AC. Myostatin and the control of skeletal muscle mass. Curr Opin Genet Dev 1999;9:604–607.

Leong P, MacLennan DH. Complex interactions between skeletal muscle ryanodine receptor and dihydropyridine receptor proteins. Biochem Cell Biol 1998;76:681–694.

Ma J, Pan Z. Junctional membrane structure and store operated calcium entry in muscle cells. Front Biosci 2003;8:D242–D255.

MacLennan DH, Abu-Abed M, Kang C. Structure-function relationships in Ca(2+) cycling proteins. J Mol Cell Cardiol 2002;34:897–918.

Mayer U. Integrins: redundant or important players in skeletal muscle? J Biol Chem 2003;278:14,587–14,590.

Muller FU, Kirchhefer U, Begrow F, Reinke U, Neumann J, Schmitz W. Junctional sarcoplasmic reticulum transmembrane proteins in the heart. Basic Res Cardiol 2002;97:I52–I55.

Pardo JV, Siliciano JD, Craig SW. A vinculin-containing cortical lattice in skeletal muscle: transverse lattice elements ("costameres") mark sites of attachment between myofibrils and sarcolemma. Proc Natl Acad Sci USA 1983;80:1008–1012.

Petrof BJ, Shrager JB, Stedman HH, Kelly AM, Sweeney HL. Dystrophin protects the sarcolemma from stresses developed during muscle contraction. Proc Natl Acad Sci USA 1993;90:3710–3714.

Rafael JA, Brown SC. Dystrophin and utrophin: genetic analyses of their role in skeletal muscle. Microsc Res Tech 2000;48:155–166.

Rando TA. The dystrophin-glycoprotein complex, cellular signaling, and the regulation of cell survival in the muscular dystrophies. Muscle Nerve 2001;24:1575–1594.

Rock RS, Rice SE, Wells AL, Purcell TJ, Spudich JA, Sweeney HL. Myosin VI is a processive motor with a large step size. Proc Natl Acad Sci USA 2001;98:13,655–13,659.

Rybakova IN, Patel JR, Ervasti JM. The dystrophin complex forms a mechanically strong link between the sarcolemma and costameric actin. J Cell Biol 2000;150:1209–1214.

Spudich JA. The myosin swinging cross-bridge model. Nat Rev Mol Cell Biol 2001;2:387–392.

Starr DA, Han M. ANChors away: an actin based mechanism of nuclear positioning. J Cell Sci 2003;116:211–216.

Starr DA, Han M. Role of ANC-1 in tethering nuclei to the actin cytoskeleton. Science 2002;298:406–409.

Trinick J, Tskhovrebova L. Titin: a molecular control freak. Trends Cell Biol 1999;9:377–380.

Walker ML, Burgess SA, Sellers JR, et al. Two-headed binding of a processive myosin to F-actin. Nature 2000;405:804–807.

Wells AL, Lin AW, Chen LQ, et al. Myosin VI is an actin-based motor that moves backwards. Nature 1999;401:505–508.

Whittemore LA, Song K, Li X, et al. Inhibition of myostatin in adult mice increases skeletal muscle mass and strength. Biochem Biophys Res Commun 2003;300:965–971.

Worman HJ, Courvalin JC. How do mutations in lamins A and C cause disease? J Clin Invest 2004;113:349–351.

Yanagida T, Kitamura K, Tanaka H, Hikikoshi Iwane A, Esaki S. Single molecule analysis of the actomyosin motor. Curr Opin Cell Biol 2000;12:20–25.

68 Stem Cells and Muscle Regeneration

CINDY M. MARTIN, THOMAS J. HAWKE, AND DANIEL J. GARRY

SUMMARY

Somatic (adult) stem cell populations are resident in postnatal tissues such as skeletal muscle and function in the maintenance and regeneration of the respective tissues. Use of transgenic and emerging technologies will enhance understanding of the regulation of the somatic stem cell populations and regenerative mechanisms in normal, aging and myopathic states. Furthermore, these studies may promote the use of adult stem cells for cell replacement therapies or for use as vehicles for gene replacement therapy.

Key Words: Aging; embryonic stem (ES); skeletal muscle; somatic; stem cell; regeneration.

INTRODUCTION

The ancient Greeks recognized the potential of tissue regeneration in the legend of Prometheus. As punishment for attempting to steal the secret of fire from the Gods, Prometheus was chained to the side of Mount Caucasus and sentenced to a life of eternal torture as vultures would feed on his liver during the daytime and at night his liver would undergo repair and regeneration. This ability for tissue regeneration remains an area of intense interest and research. Titans or champions of regeneration include the hydra, zebrafish, and the newt, which have the capability of regenerating entire limbs, heart, jaw, retina, and tail. Although a number of common pathways and networks are shared between urodeles (i.e., newts) and mammals, the regenerative capacity of humans and rodents is more limited and dependent on resident stem cell populations, a permissive niche or milieu and molecular networks to promote repair and regeneration of adult tissues such as skeletal muscle.

EMBRYONIC STEM CELLS: PROTOTYPIC STEM CELL POPULATION

Perhaps the most intensely studied stem cell population is the embryonic stem (ES) cell. ES cells are derived from the embryonic blastocyst and are pluripotent. The ES cells have a distinct molecular signature as they express Esg1, Utf1, Oct3/4, Nanog, Rex3, Tex20, and a number of additional factors that promote their unlimited proliferative capacity and multipotentiation. In addition, the ES cells are routinely cultured in the presence of feeder cells (growth arrested or mitotically inactive fibroblasts) to provide growth factors and chemokines, such as leukemia inhibitory factor, which maintain

From: *Principles of Molecular Medicine, Second Edition*
Edited by: M. S. Runge and C. Patterson © Humana Press, Inc., Totowa, NJ

the ES cell population in an undifferentiated and proliferative state. The extensive analyses of murine ES cells ultimately resulted in the isolation of human ES cells. A number of studies have been undertaken to further characterize the culture conditions, proliferative capacity, and the potential of human ES cells to contribute to alternative lineages using in vitro conditions. For example, although human ES cells grow more slowly (double every 36 h) than mouse ES cells (double every 12 h), the human and mouse ES cells are similar in their expression of high levels of telomerase, and their capability of self-renewal and multilineage differentiation in vitro (e.g., muscle, blood, fat, and so on) (Fig. 68-1). In contrast to the ES population, the somatic (adult) stem cell populations are more limited in their proliferative capacity and plasticity.

SOMATIC STEM CELLS FOR THE MAINTENANCE AND REPAIR OF ADULT TISSUES

Tissue-specific adult (somatic) stem cells are important in the growth, maintenance, and regeneration of postnatal and adult tissues. Nearly all adult tissues contain a resident stem cell population including the hematopoietic stem cells and stromal cells (bone marrow), neural stem cells (subventricular zone and hippocampus of the brain), epithelial stem cells (intestinal crypts), oval stem cells (liver), and satellite cells (skeletal muscle) (Fig. 68-1).

Myogenic progenitor cells (satellite cells) are resident in skeletal muscle as small mononuclear cells that occupy a peripheral location with respect to the adjacent multinucleated myotube (Fig. 68-2). The satellite cells can be identified using electron microscopy as they occupy a sublaminar (beneath the basal lamina) position with respect to the adjacent myofiber (Fig. 68-2). In neonatal skeletal muscle, approx 30% of the nuclei are satellite cells that fuse to the growing myofibers and contribute to postnatal growth of skeletal muscle. The satellite cells in adult skeletal muscle are reduced in number, representing approx 2–5% of the nuclei. The quiescent satellite cells are arrested at an early stage of the myogenic program such that they do not express any of the myogenic basic helix-loop-helix (bHLH) regulatory factors of the MyoD family (Myf5, MyoD, Myogenin, and Mrf4). Limited molecular markers for this cell population include Foxk1, m-cadherin, c-met, syndecan-4, Pax7, and CD34. Foxk1 and Pax7 are transcription factors that have important functional roles in the regulation of satellite cells. Using a gene disruption strategy (i.e., gene knockout), mice lacking the *forkhead/ winged helix transcription factor, Foxk1, have a severe growth deficit and impaired muscle regeneration. The impairment in muscle regeneration results from decreased numbers of satellite cells

MITOCHONDRIAL BIOGENESIS AND SLOW MUSCLE GENE EXPRESSION

Findings in peroxisome proliferator-activated receptor (PPAR)-γ coactivator-1α (PGC-1α) gene regulation and function have led to the consideration of PGC-1α as a key regulator of important features of skeletal muscle adaptation. PGC-1α is a transcriptional coactivator cloned originally by a yeast two-hybrid screen from a differentiated brown fat cell line using PPAR-γ as bait. PGC-1α mRNA and protein are highly expressed in slow, oxidative fibers compared to the fast, glycolytic fibers, consistent with the function of a gene involved in fiber-type specialization. Several different models have suggested the functional importance of PGC-1α in striated muscles. A possible association between polymorphism of the PGC-1α gene and type-II diabetes has also been suggested. PGC-1α protein interacts with many nuclear regulatory proteins, such as thyroid hormone receptor, estrogen receptor α, PPAR-γ, nuclear respiratory factor-1 (NRF-1) and CREB-binding protein. PGC-1α also stimulates the expression of multiple effector genes during various biological processes. The most striking property of PGC-1α function in skeletal muscle is that its overexpression in cultured myoblasts induces mitochondrial biogenesis, and overexpression in transgenic mice causes a remarkable fast-to-slow fiber-type switching and enhanced mitochondrial biogenesis. These findings suggest the possibility that increased expression of PGC-1α in skeletal muscle plays a key role in endurance exercise-induced skeletal muscle adaptation by promoting mitochondrial biogenesis and other genetic and biochemical events. The profound effect of PGC-1α overexpression probably results from the enhancement of the transactivation activities of regulatory proteins, such as NRF-1 and MEF-2, as well as the induction of the genes in encoding these transcription factors.

The importance of PGC-1α function in promoting the acquisition of slow-twitch muscle contractile and metabolic properties also is suggested by the observation that endurance exercise induces PGC-1α mRNA expression in the recruited skeletal muscle through transcriptional control. PGC-1α protein expression along with that of NRF-1 and NRF-2 are also increased in exercised skeletal muscle. Endurance exercise is likely to induce PGC-1α gene expression through a combination of transcriptional activation of the PGC-1α gene and increased protein stability. Studies to elucidate the signal transduction pathways and the molecular mechanism for exercise-induced PGC-1α gene expression in skeletal muscle will yield critically important information.

THE CA²⁺/CAM-DEPENDENT PROTEIN KINASE PATHWAY

Ca^{2+}/CaM, acting through calcineurin and Ca^{2+}/CaM-dependent protein kinase (CaMK) pathways, stimulates MEF-2 transactivation activity and downstream target genes, such PGC-1α (Fig. 69-3). Relatively little is known about the exact CaMK pathway(s) in exercise-induced skeletal muscle adaptation. A molecular mechanism for CaMK-induced activation of MEF-2 activity has been elucidated in cardiac myocytes. Phosphorylation of histone deacetylase 5 results in its binding with the intracellular chaperone protein 14-3-3 and promotes its nuclear export leading to derepression of MEF-2 activity. This mechanism plays a role in maintenance of mitochondrial biogenesis in the heart. However, the endogenous kinase that is responsible for transducing the signal and catalyzing the dephosphorylation of HDAC remains unknown. Furthermore, it is not known whether the same regulatory mechanism accounts for the adaptation in skeletal muscle in response to exercise training.

The effects of activated CaMKIV in skeletal muscle in inducing PGC-1α gene expression, enhancing mitochondrial biogenesis, and promoting myosin isoform switching in a transgenic mouse model have been described. In this model, a constitutively active form of CaMKIV was expressed in fast-twitch myofibers under the control of the muscle creatine kinase promoter. A significant increase in percentage of slow-twitch fibers in normally fast-twitch muscles and a marked increase in subsarcolemmal mitochondrial density were confirmed along with increases in various genetic and biochemical markers for a slow oxidative muscle phenotype, including a profound induction of PGC-1α mRNA. Another study reported that energy deprivation-induced mitochondrial biogenesis is dependent on an activation of the AMP-activated protein kinase pathway, which was associated with increased CaMKIV protein and PGC-1α mRNA expression. These data suggest a role for CaMK signaling in the acquisition of a slow-twitch muscle phenotype in adults, but do not identify the specific isoforms of CaMK that are relevant to this response.

CONCLUSIONS

Cell size and specialized characteristics of myofibers in adult skeletal muscles are controlled by multiple signaling pathways. Ca^{2+}-dependent activation of calcineurin-NFAT signaling and exercise-induced induction of PGC-1α are both involved in the activity-dependent induction and maintenance of fiber-type-specific gene expression. Satellite cell activity and intracellular signaling activities involving the PI-3K/Akt/mammalian target of rapamycin and PI-3K/Akt/GSK-3 pathways in mature myofibers appear to mediate skeletal muscle hypertrophy in response to hypertrophic stimuli, such as resistance exercise. The future challenge is to define relationships between these and other signaling pathways that are responsible for neuromuscular activity-mediated adaptations. Such knowledge may foster the development of novel therapeutics and preventive technologies to improve human fitness and health.

SELECTED REFERENCES

Adams GR, McCue SA. Localized infusion of IGF-I results in skeletal muscle hypertrophy in rats. J Appl Physiol 1998;84:1716–1722.

Baar K, Wende AR, Jones TE, et al. Adaptations of skeletal muscle to exercise: rapid increase in the transcriptional coactivator PGC-1. FASEB J 2002;16:1879–1886.

Barton ER, Morris L, Musaro A, Rosenthal N, Sweeney HL. Muscle-specific expression of insulin-like growth factor I counters muscle decline in mdx mice. J Cell Biol 2002;157:137–148.

Beals CR, Sheridan CM, Turck CW, Gardner P, Crabtree GR. Nuclear export of NF-ATc enhanced by glycogen synthase kinase-3. Science 1997;275:1930–1934.

Bodine SC, Stitt TN, Gonzalez M, et al. Akt/mTOR pathway is a crucial regulator of skeletal muscle hypertrophy and can prevent muscle atrophy in vivo. Nat Cell Biol 2001;3:1014–1019.

Chakravarthy MV, Abraha TW, Schwartz RJ, Fiorotto ML, Booth FW. Insulin-like growth factor-I extends in vitro replicative life span of skeletal muscle satellite cells by enhancing G1/S cell cycle progression via the activation of phosphatidylinositol 3′-kinase/Akt signaling pathway. J Biol Chem 2000;275:35,942–35,952.

Chin ER, Olson EN, Richardson JA, et al. A calcineurin-dependent transcriptional pathway controls skeletal muscle fiber type. Genes Dev 1998;12:2499–2509.

Coleman ME, DeMayo F, Yin KC, et al. Myogenic vector expression of insulin-like growth factor I stimulates muscle cell differentiation and myofiber hypertrophy in transgenic mice. J Biol Chem 1995;270: 12,109–12,116.

Czubryt MP, McAnally J, Fishman GI, Olson EN. Regulation of peroxisome proliferator-activated receptor gamma coactivator 1 alpha (PGC-1 alpha) and mitochondrial function by MEF2 and HDAC5. Proc Natl Acad Sci USA 2003;100:1711–1716.

Delling U, Tureckova J, Lim HW, De Windt LJ, Rotwein P, Molkentin JD. A calcineurin-NFATc3-dependent pathway regulates skeletal muscle differentiation and slow myosin heavy-chain expression. Mol Cell Biol 2000;20:6600–6611.

DeVol DL, Rotwein P, Sadow JL, Novakofski J, Bechtel PJ. Activation of insulin-like growth factor gene expression during work-induced skeletal muscle growth. Am J Physiol 1990;259:E89–E95.

Dunn SE, Chin ER, Michel RN. Matching of calcineurin activity to upstream effectors is critical for skeletal muscle fiber growth. J Cell Biol 2000;151:663–672.

Lin J, Wu H, Tarr PT, et al. Transcriptional co-activator PGC-1 alpha drives the formation of slow-twitch muscle fibres. Nature 2002;418:797–801.

Liu Y, Cseresnyes Z, Randall WR, Schneider MF. Activity-dependent nuclear translocation and intranuclear distribution of NFATc in adult skeletal muscle fibers. J Cell Biol 2001;155:27–39.

Lu J, McKinsey TA, Nicol RL, Olson EN. Signal-dependent activation of the MEF2 transcription factor by dissociation from histone deacetylases. Proc Natl Acad Sci USA 2000;97:4070–4075.

Markuns JF, Wojtaszewski JF, Goodyear LJ. Insulin and exercise decrease glycogen synthase kinase-3 activity by different mechanisms in rat skeletal muscle. J Biol Chem 1999;274:24,896–24,900.

McKinsey TA, Zhang CL, Lu J, Olson EN. Signal-dependent nuclear export of a histone deacetylase regulates muscle differentiation. Nature 2000;408:106–111.

Michael LF, Wu Z, Cheatham RB, et al. Restoration of insulin-sensitive glucose transporter (GLUT4) gene expression in muscle cells by the transcriptional coactivator PGC-1. Proc Natl Acad Sci USA 2001;98:3820–3825.

Molkentin JD, Lu JR, Antos CL, et al. A calcineurin-dependent transcriptional pathway for cardiac hypertrophy. Cell 1998;93:215–228.

Musaro A, McCullagh KJ, Naya FJ, Olson EN, Rosenthal N. IGF-1 induces skeletal myocyte hypertrophy through calcineurin in association with GATA-2 and NF-ATc1. Nature 1999;400:581–585.

Naya FJ, Mercer B, Shelton J, Richardson JA, Williams RS, Olson EN. Stimulation of slow skeletal muscle fiber gene expression by calcineurin in vivo. J Biol Chem 2000;275:4545–4548.

Pallafacchina G, Calabria E, Serrano AL, Kalhovde JM, Schiaffino S. A protein kinase B-dependent and rapamycin-sensitive pathway controls skeletal muscle growth but not fiber type specification. Proc Natl Acad Sci USA 2002;99:9213–9218.

Pilegaard H, Saltin B, Neufer PD. Exercise induces transient transcriptional activation of the PGC-1alpha gene in human skeletal muscle. J Physiol 2003;546:851–858.

Puigserver P, Rhee J, Lin J, et al. Cytokine stimulation of energy expenditure through p38 MAP kinase activation of PPARgamma coactivator-1. Mol Cell 2001;8:971–982.

Puigserver P, Wu Z, Park CW, Graves R, Wright M, Spiegelman BM. A cold-inducible coactivator of nuclear receptors linked to adaptive thermogenesis. Cell 1998;92:829–839.

Rommel C, Bodine SC, Clarke BA, et al. Mediation of IGF-1-induced skeletal myotube hypertrophy by PI(3)K/Akt/mTOR and PI(3)K/Akt/GSK3 pathways. Nat Cell Biol 2001;3:1009–1013.

Rosenthal SM, Cheng ZQ. Opposing early and late effects of insulin-like growth factor I on differentiation and the cell cycle regulatory retinoblastoma protein in skeletal myoblasts. Proc Natl Acad Sci USA 1995;92:10,307–10,311.

Rothermel B, Vega RB, Yang J, Wu H, Bassel-Duby R, Williams RS. A protein encoded within the down syndrome critical region is enriched in striated muscles and inhibits calcineurin signaling. J Biol Chem 2000;275:8719–8725.

Schiaffino S, Reggiani C. Molecular diversity of myofibrillar proteins: Gene regulation and functional significance. Physiol Rev 1996;76:371–423.

Semsarian C, Wu MJ, Ju YK, et al. Skeletal muscle hypertrophy is mediated by a Ca2+-dependent calcineurin signalling pathway. Nature 1999;400:576–581.

Serrano AL, Murgia M, Pallafacchina G, et al. Calcineurin controls nerve activity-dependent specification of slow skeletal muscle fibers but not muscle growth. Proc Natl Acad Sci USA 2001;98:13,108–13,113.

Shioi T, McMullen JR, Kang PM, et al. Akt/protein kinase B promotes organ growth in transgenic mice. Mol Cell Biol 2002;22:2799–2809.

Swoap SJ, Hunter RB, Stevenson EJ, et al. The calcineurin-NFAT pathway and muscle fiber-type gene expression. Am J Physiol Cell Physiol 2000;279:C915–C924.

Taigen T, De Windt LJ, Lim HW, Molkentin JD. Targeted inhibition of calcineurin prevents agonist-induced cardiomyocyte hypertrophy. Proc Natl Acad Sci USA 2000;97:1196–1201.

Tatsumi R, Anderson JE, Nevoret CJ, Halevy O, Allen RE. HGF/SF is present in normal adult skeletal muscle and is capable of activating satellite cells. Dev Biol 1998;194:114–128.

Tatsumi R, Hattori A, Ikeuchi Y, Anderson JE, Allen RE. Release of hepatocyte growth factor from mechanically stretched skeletal muscle satellite cells and role of pH and nitric oxide. Mol Biol Cell 2002;13:2909–2918.

Wu H, Kanatous SB, Thurmond FA, et al. Regulation of mitochondrial biogenesis in skeletal muscle by CaMK. Science 2002;296:349–352.

Wu H, Rothermel B, Kanatous S, et al. Activation of MEF2 by muscle activity is mediated through a calcineurin-dependent pathway. EMBO J 2001;20:6414–6423.

Wu Z, Puigserver P, Andersson U, et al. Mechanisms controlling mitochondrial biogenesis and respiration through the thermogenic coactivator PGC-1. Cell 1999;98:115–124.

Yang S, Alnaqeeb M, Simpson H, Goldspink G. Cloning and characterization of an IGF-1 isoform expressed in skeletal muscle subjected to stretch. J Muscle Res Cell Motil 1996;17:487–495.

Zong H, Ren JM, Young LH, et al. AMP kinase is required for mitochondrial biogenesis in skeletal muscle in response to chronic energy deprivation. Proc Natl Acad Sci USA 2002;99:15,983–15,987.

70 Muscular Dystrophies

Mechanisms

PETER B. KANG AND LOUIS M. KUNKEL

SUMMARY

Since the cloning of the gene responsible for Duchenne and Becker muscular dystrophy two decades ago, a number of other genes have been associated with various forms of muscular dystrophy. The protein products of these genes display a diversity of cellular localizations and functions, suggesting a complex pathophysiology within this class of disorders. Two recently identified functions of selected proteins include membrane repair and glycosylation, providing important insights into the disease process. A definitive cure remains elusive, but supportive therapies have become increasingly sophisticated, improving the quality of life and lengthening the life expectancy for many affected individuals.

Key Words: Becker; calpain; congenital muscular dystrophy; duchenne; dysferlin; dystroglycan; dystrophin; facioscapulo-humeral muscular dystrophy; limb-girdle; merosin; muscular dystrophy; sarcoglycan.

INTRODUCTION

The muscular dystrophies are a group of inherited primary diseases of muscle that are characterized clinically by progressive, chronic weakness, and pathologically by degeneration of muscle fibers with necrosis and connective tissue infiltration. This definition distinguishes muscular dystrophies from other primary diseases of muscle, including the congenital myopathies and inflammatory myopathies, although there are some areas of overlap.

The clinical course of muscular dystrophy varies widely between specific diseases from the rapidly fatal Walker–Warburg disease to the milder Becker muscular dystrophy. There are four major categories of muscular dystrophy: dystrophinopathies, limb-girdle muscular dystrophies (LGMD), congenital muscular dystrophies, and the syndromic muscular dystrophies (Table 70-1). These categories are largely based on the clinical characteristics of the diseases and do not reflect the differences in molecular and biochemical origins. An international collaborative effort in the mid-1980s led to positional cloning of dystrophin, the gene on the X-chromosome responsible for Duchenne muscular dystrophy. Since then, the genes that cause more than a dozen other types of muscular dystrophy have been described (summarized at http://www.dmd.nl/). These proteins, with other associated muscle

From: *Principles of Molecular Medicine, Second Edition*
Edited by: M. S. Runge and C. Patterson © Humana Press, Inc., Totowa, NJ

proteins that have not been shown to play a primary role in human disease, have been extensively studied (Fig. 70-1). The majority of the proteins produced by these genes appear primarily to be structural in function and are linked to each other in the vicinity of the sarcolemma. Some of these proteins may also play a role in cellular signaling and repair. Very few are enzymes.

DYSTROPHINOPATHIES

Duchenne muscular dystrophy is caused by mutations in the *DMD* gene on the X-chromosome. It is the most common muscular dystrophy, occurring in 1 in 3300 live male births. The high incidence is because of the large size of the gene, which has 79 exons and produces a 427-kDa protein called dystrophin. The majority of mutations are deletions that cluster in exons 2–20 and 44–53, areas in which the intronic sequences are unusually long, approaching 200 bp. Polymerase chain reaction amplification techniques concentrating on these exons identify about two-thirds of affected patients. The remainders have point mutations, deletions in other regions, and duplications.

Becker muscular dystrophy, a milder variant, is also associated with mutations in *DMD*. Shifting or preservation of the reading frame is more important than the size of the deletion in determining whether an affected child will have the Duchenne vs Becker phenotype; most children with Duchenne muscular dystrophy have a frameshift mutation, whereas those with Becker muscular dystrophy typically have a preserved translational reading frame.

The dystrophin protein is expressed in a number of organs besides muscle. Brain, Purkinje cells, and muscle produce the full-length 427 kDa protein. Retina, Schwann cells, glial cells, and kidney produce shorter isoforms. In skeletal muscle, dystrophin is located in the subsarcolemmal region and has four major domains: amino terminus, rod domain, cysteine-rich domain, and carboxy terminus. The amino terminus binds to actin, whereas the carboxy terminus binds to a protein complex that extends into the extracellular matrix. Dystrophin's main role appears to be structural, although there is evidence that it, with its associated proteins, may be involved in more dynamic functions such as regulating the perfusion and repair of muscle.

Clinically, Duchenne muscular dystrophy typically presents with gait abnormalities between the ages of 3–5 yr, although in retrospect parents may recall symptoms as early as 1 yr of age. The gait abnormalities may include toe walking, frequent falling

Table 70-1
Muscular Dystrophies

Disorder	Gene	Protein location	Function
Dystrophinopathies			
Duchenne MD	DMD	Subsarcolemma	Structural
Becker MD	DMD	Subsarcolemma	Structural
Dominant limb-girdle muscular dystrophies			
1A	TTID	Sarcomere	Structural
1B	LMNA	Nucleus	Structural
1C	CAV3	Sarcolemma	Structural
1D	? (6q23)	Unknown	Unknown
1E	? (7q)	Unknown	Unknown
1F	? (5q31)	Unknown	Unknown
Recessive limb-girdle muscular dystrophies			
2A	CAPN3	Cytoplasm	Protease
2B	DYSF	Sarcolemma	Unknown
2C	SGCG	Sarcolemma	Structural
2D	SGCA	Sarcolemma	Structural
2E	SGCB	Sarcolemma	Structural
2F	SGCD	Sarcolemma	Structural
2G	TCAP	Sarcomere	Structural
2H	TRIM32	Unknown	Ligase?
2I	FKRP	ER	Glycosylation
2J	TTN	Sarcomere	Structural
2K	POMT1	Golgi complex	Glycosylation
Congenital muscular dystrophies			
Ullrich disease	COL6A1, A2, A3	Extracellular	Structural
Rigid spine	SEPN1	ER	Unknown
Merosin-negative	LAMA2	Extracellular	Structural
MDC1C	FKRP	ER	Glycosylation
MDC1D	LARGE	Golgi complex	Glycosyltransferase
Fukuyama	FCMD	Golgi complex	Glycosylation
Muscle-eye brain	POMGnT1	Golgi complex	Glycosylation
Walker-Warburg	POMT1	Golgi complex	Glycosylation
	FCMD	Golgi complex	Glycosylation
	FKRP	ER	Glycosylation
Syndromic muscular dystrophies			
Emery-Dreifuss MD	EMD	Nucleus	Unknown
	LMNA	Nucleus	Structural
Facioscapulohumeral	? (4q35)	Unknown	Unknown
Oculopharyngeal MD	PABP2	Nucleus	Unknown

ER, endoplasmic reticulum; ?, gene not identified.

and tripping, waddling gait, and delayed walking. Examination is notable for weakness of the proximal muscles, most marked in the hip girdle in the early stages and more widespread with disease progression. Reflexes are initially normal or reduced and become absent in the later stages. Becker muscular dystrophy has a similar but milder presentation with a typical onset in later childhood or adolescence and a slower progression of weakness.

In suspected cases of Duchenne or Becker muscular dystrophy, initial laboratory evaluation should include measurement of muscle enzymes in the serum: creatine phosphokinase (CPK), aldolase, alanine aminotransferase, aspartate transaminase, and lactate dehydrogenase. The first two are most specific for muscle; the others are also produced in the liver. These enzymes are elevated in both diseases, but more markedly in Duchenne muscular dystrophy. The diagnosis may then be confirmed in about two-thirds of cases by polymerase chain reaction amplification of

the most commonly deleted exons on blood leukocytes. When this test is negative, a muscle biopsy with antibody staining for dystrophin confirms or excludes the diagnosis. Routine histochemical staining of muscle tissue reveals muscle necrosis and inflammation with replacement of muscle fibers by connective tissue. On antibody staining, dystrophin is virtually absent in Duchenne muscular dystrophy and present in abnormal size or amount in Becker muscular dystrophy. The need for about one-third of boys with Duchenne muscular dystrophy to undergo muscle biopsy, an invasive procedure that requires general anesthesia in children, is not ideal. Robust DNA sequencing of all 79 exons in children suspected of having Duchenne muscular dystrophy should enable more cases to be confirmed without muscle biopsy.

The course is progressive with Duchenne muscular dystrophy patients often surviving into early adulthood and Becker muscular dystrophy patients surviving well into adulthood. The most common causes of death are respiratory and cardiac complications.

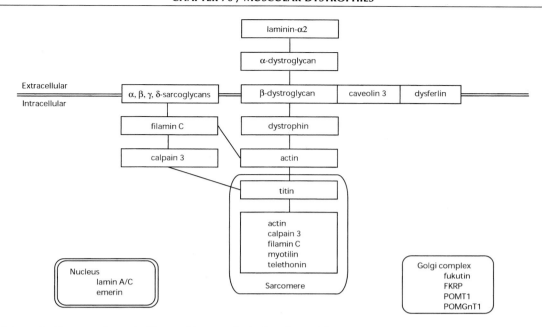

Figure 70-1 Schematic diagram of muscle fiber architecture, including dystrophin-associated protein complex and other proteins involved in the muscular dystrophies. Rounded rectangles indicate discrete cellular regions or compartments, single lines indicate physical associations between proteins, double lines indicate phospholipid membranes. FKRP, fukutin-related protein; POMT1, O-mannosyltransferase 1; POMGnT1, O-mannose β-1,2-N-acetylglucosaminyltransferase.

LIMB-GIRDLE MUSCULAR DYSTROPHIES

Clinically and histologically, the LGMDs are similar to the dystrophinopathies, with a progressive course of predominantly proximal weakness and signs of inflammation, necrosis, and connective tissue replacement on biopsy. The severity ranges widely from a mild course similar to Becker muscular dystrophy to a more rapidly progressive one that resembles Duchenne muscular dystrophy. Cardiac complications appear to be common in types 1B, 1D, 2G, and 2I, but the overall frequency is unclear because of the small number of patients reported for a number of subtypes. Intelligence is usually normal. The dystrophinopathies may be regarded as an X-linked recessive category of LGMD, but for historical reasons are usually classified separately. The genes that cause certain LGMDs (1B, 1C, 2B, and 2I) have also been shown to cause other diseases. Certain individual mutations in caveolin and dysferlin are associated with multiple phenotypes, suggesting the involvement of modifying factors.

AUTOSOMAL-DOMINANT LGMD (TYPE 1) Biochemically, the protein products of the identified autosomal-dominant LGMDs do not appear to have much in common. The common thread that runs through these disorders is the inheritance pattern and the generally mild course of disease compared with the autosomal-recessive LGMDs. Type 1 is much rarer than type 2, comprising less than 10% of cases.

LGMD type 1A is caused by mutations in the myotilin gene, whose protein product localizes to the Z-disk of the sarcomere. Myotilin's exact function is unknown, but the protein appears to play a structural role in the Z-disk. Mutations lead to abnormalities in the Z-disk, which may appear under light microscopy as rod-shaped structures similar to the rods found in nemaline myopathy.

Patients with LGMD type 1A have, in addition to muscle weakness, a distinctive dysarthric pattern of speech. The age of onset is usually in early adulthood. In the initial stages, the weakness is mostly proximal, but slowly spreads to involve distal muscles as the disease progresses. CPK levels are significantly elevated.

Mutations in the lamin A/C gene cause LGMD 1B, Emery–Dreifuss muscular dystrophy, cardiomyopathy, and lipodystrophy. A missense mutation in the lamin A portion of the gene has been identified as a cause of Hutchinson–Gilford progeria. The two protein products, lamins A and C, are produced by alternative splicing and localize to the nuclear lamina. The mechanism of disease is unclear, but may be related to impaired interactions with other nuclear proteins or dysfunctional filament assembly.

Cardiac complication rates are high in both LGMD 1B and Emery–Dreifuss muscular dystrophy. The two diseases are distinguished clinically by the absence of early contractures and a proximal pattern of weakness in LGMD 1B.

Mutations in the gene encoding caveolin 3 cause LGMD 1C, rippling muscle disease, distal myopathy, and hyper-CKemia. The same mutation in the caveolin gene has been shown to cause rippling muscle disease with distal myopathy in some individuals, and rippling muscle disease with LGMD in others. Caveolins are the proteins found in caveolae, which are 50–100 nm invaginations of the plasma membrane found in most cell types, including muscle. Caveolae are involved in membrane trafficking, sorting, transport, and signal transduction. Caveolin 3, a muscle-specific caveolin protein, forms a hairpin loop within the sarcolemma, enabling both the amino- and carboxy-terminal ends to face the cytoplasm. The protein coprecipitates with dystrophin, indicating a link to the dystrophin-associated protein complex. This connection is further supported by the development of dystrophin deficiency in mice when caveolin 3 is overexpressed. In mouse models, a deficiency of caveolin 3 leads to a deficiency of caveolae and abnormalities in the T-tubule system.

Onset of proximal muscle weakness in LGMD 1C is typically at 5 yr, with calf hypertrophy, Gowers' sign, and occasional reports of exercise intolerance. CPK levels are significantly elevated.

In LGMD 1D–1F, the genetic loci have been mapped, but the exact genes have not been identified. Genetic linkage has identified the locus responsible for LGMD 1D to a 3-cM region of 6q23. Two nearby laminins have been excluded as causes, but their proximity suggests that a previously unknown laminin may be the gene responsible. The most prominent symptoms are cardiac with dilated cardiomyopathy and cardiac conduction defects the most common manifestations. Sudden death may occur. Onset is typically in early adulthood, sometimes in late adolescence. Mild proximal muscle weakness frequently occurs, and may precede or follow the initial cardiac symptoms. Serum CPK levels are mildly elevated. The phenotype resembles that of LGMD 1B.

The genetic region of interest in LGMD 1E appears to be a 9-cM interval on 7q, although the odds ratio for this region is not ideal. Additional kindreds must be analyzed to confirm this finding and pinpoint the responsible gene. Clinical features in affected individuals include the classic pattern of proximal muscle weakness.

Vocal cord and pharyngeal weakness with autosomal-dominant distal myopathy has been localized to a 12-cM interval on 5q31. Although it is a distal myopathy with little evidence of inflammation on muscle biopsy, it is classified as LGMD 1F. The onset of symptoms is typically in middle adulthood. Clinical manifestations include voice change, finger extensor weakness, peroneal weakness, shoulder girdle weakness, and dysphagia. Serum CPK levels may be mildly elevated.

AUTOSOMAL-RECESSIVE LGMD (TYPE 2)   The autosomal-recessive LGMDs (type 2) are more common than the dominant forms, and generally have a more severe clinical course.

The gene encoding calpain 3 is mutated in LGMD 2A. Calpain 3 is a muscle-specific calcium-activated proteolytic enzyme, the first nonstructural protein demonstrated to cause LGMD. Calpain 3 has been shown to cleave filamin 2, but the exact pathogenesis of disease remains obscure; the enzyme is quickly degraded, and is, thus, difficult to study. In human muscle biopsy tissue and mouse models, calpain-3 deficiency is associated with myonuclear apoptosis and abnormal expression of the transcriptional factor nuclear factor-κB and its inhibitor (IκBα). Injection of Evans blue dye, which cannot cross intact membranes, into the mouse model revealed disruption of the sarcolemma, a phenomenon seen commonly in other muscular dystrophies. It is not clear whether the apoptotic cascade or membrane disruption is the more primary event.

LGMD 2A (calpainopathy), thought to be the most common form of LGMD, is characterized by progressive, predominantly proximal weakness, without cardiac or facial involvement. The severity varies widely and does not correlate consistently with the level of expression of calpain 3 in muscle.

Mutations in the gene encoding dysferlin cause LGMD 2B, Miyoshi myopathy, and distal myopathy with anterior tibial onset. Deletion of 1 bp causes both Miyoshi myopathy and distal myopathy with tibial onset in different kindreds, whereas missense mutations cause Miyoshi myopathy and LGMD 2B in different individuals within the same family. The gene is large, consisting of 55 exons and a 6243 bp open reading frame, and is expressed mainly in skeletal and cardiac muscles. The dysferlin protein plays an important role in the calcium-mediated process of membrane resealing, which is crucial for the stability of the muscle membrane.

LGMD 2B has a proximal pattern of weakness; Miyoshi myopathy tends to involve more distal muscles, particularly gastrocnemius. Difficulty standing on the toes is a common initial complaint of patients with Miyoshi myopathy. Onset is typically in childhood or

early adulthood. CPK levels are markedly elevated in all the phenotypes. The course is milder than in the other recessive LGMDs; only about 10% of patients lose the ability to ambulate.

The four sarcoglycanopathies are LGMDs 2C–2F and are linked to mutations in the genes encoding γ-, α-, β-, and δ-sarcoglycans, respectively. A fifth sarcoglycan (ε) has been identified. Mutations in ε-sarcoglycan cause a dystonia rather than a muscular dystrophy. The sarcoglycans form a complex that spans the sarcolemma. Because they are physically linked, a mutation in the gene encoding one sarcoglycan often causes a secondary deficiency in one or more of the others, especially when primary mutations in β- and δ-sarcoglycan are present. This frequently makes it difficult to diagnose a sarcoglycanopathy based entirely on antibody staining of muscle tissue, even though antibodies to all four disease-causing sarcoglycans are available. Of the four sarcoglycanopathies, α-sarcoglycanopathy frequently has a mild phenotype; all reported cases of δ-sarcoglycanopathy have been severe.

The telethonin protein localizes to the Z-disk of the sarcomere and is expressed in skeletal and cardiac muscles. Mutations in its gene cause LGMD 2G. Its specific function is unknown, but it interacts with titin, mutations of which cause LGMD 2J. Patients with LGMD 2G typically present in late childhood or adolescence with proximal weakness, sometimes accompanied by distal weakness that may resemble the phenotype of Miyoshi myopathy. A significant minority of patients lose the ability to ambulate independently in the third or fourth decade. Cardiac complications are common.

LGMD 2H is caused by mutations in the gene encoding *TRIM 32*, an E3 ubiquitin ligase expressed in skeletal and cardiac muscle. A deficiency of the enzyme could presumably cause the accumulation of its target protein, but histological examination has not revealed any unusual deposits in muscle fibers. The clinical disease is mild and slowly progressive. Mutations in the gene encoding fukutin-related protein (*FKRP*) cause both LGMD 2I and congenital muscular dystrophy 1C. In contrast to the genotype–phenotype correlations with dysferlin, different mutations in *FKRP* correspond to the two different phenotypes, suggesting that the mutations themselves are the primary determinants of the disease manifestations. Patients with LGMD 2I frequently have a C826A (Leu276Ileu) mutation. In more severely affected patients, the patterns of protein expression may resemble that of the more severe forms of congenital muscular dystrophy, with secondary deficiencies of laminin-α2 and α-dystroglycan observed on muscle tissue immunohistochemistry, Western blots, or both.

In the more severe form of LGMD 2I, children develop hypotonia, motor delays, and muscle hypertrophy (which sometimes causes macroglossia), usually in the first 2 yr of life. Clinically, they resemble patients with Duchenne muscular dystrophy, with cardiac complications and loss of ambulation in early adolescence. The milder form of LGMD 2I has been described in a Tunisian family, having a later onset and a slower progression, with preservation of ambulation in nearly all cases. CPK levels are markedly elevated in both forms.

A sarcomeric protein named titin has been demonstrated to be mutated in LGMD 2J. These patients have proximal weakness with elevated CPK levels. Immunohistochemistry of muscle tissue reveals a secondary deficiency of calpain 3.

A novel form of LGMD, LGMD2K, has recently been described in a small number of Turkish patients. Affected individuals tend to have mild proximal muscle weakness, mild muscle hypertrophy, and marked elevations in serum CK levels. Onset is between 1 and 3 yr, although this range may be expanded as further patients are identified. Patients remain ambulatory at least until late adolescence. Unusual features include microcephaly and mental retardation. However, brain imaging so far has not revealed any structural abnormalities. Histologically, there is a reduction of α-dystroglycan staining in muscle tissue. A mutation in *O*-mannosyltransferase-1 (*POMT1*) has been identified in this cohort (A200P).

The genetic causes of LGMD have most likely not been fully described. Other genes responsible for this syndrome may yet be identified.

CONGENITAL MUSCULAR DYSTROPHIES

Congenital muscular dystrophies generally share with the other muscular dystrophies the characteristic findings on routine muscle histology. As the name implies, patients typically present at birth with hypotonia and weakness. There are three broad categories of congenital muscular dystrophies, which may be distinguished by the immunohistochemical staining pattern of laminin-α2 on muscle biopsy and by the clinical course. The mild laminin-α2 (merosin)-positive congenital muscular dystrophies are associated with normal MRI findings and normal cognitive development. Patients with the moderately severe congenital muscular dystrophies typically have white matter changes on MRI and normal or slightly impaired cognitive development. This category includes the most common single variant, laminin-α2 (merosin)-negative congenital muscular dystrophy. The severe congenital muscular dystrophies are accompanied by significant structural brain lesions and mental retardation, and often have a rapidly progressive course. Immunohistochemical staining typically demonstrates reduced but not absent laminin-α2.

MILD CONGENITAL MUSCULAR DYSTROPHIES The laminin-α2 (merosin)-positive congenital muscular dystrophies are characterized by normal immunohistochemical staining of laminin-α2 on muscle biopsy. It is rare to have structural brain lesions, and intelligence is normal. Many cases of laminin-α2-positive congenital muscular dystrophy are not further classified, but the genetic origins of two distinct congenital muscular dystrophy syndromes, Ullrich disease, and rigid spine syndrome, have been identified.

Mutations in the collagen-VI α 1, 2, and 3 genes cause some cases of Ullrich disease. These findings correspond to the deficiencies of collagen VI demonstrated on immunohistochemistry of muscle tissue from affected patients. Collagen VI is widely expressed in all connective tissues and anchors collagen I/III fibrils to basement membranes. In contrast, collagen IV expression is upregulated, perhaps as a compensatory mechanism.

Patients with Ullrich disease present in infancy with marked hypotonia, motor delays, and muscle atrophy. The distinguishing clinical features of the disease include distal joint hyperextensibility and proximal joint contractures. Some are able to walk for several years, but all patients eventually are unable to walk. Intelligence is usually normal.

Rigid spine syndrome is caused by a mutation in the gene encoding selenoprotein N (*SEPN1*), which incorporates selenium in the form of selenocysteine. The function of this protein remains obscure, but selenium deficiency is known to cause cardiomyopathy in humans and muscular dystrophy in livestock. Patients affected with rigid spine syndrome generally have a mild degree of weakness, retaining the ability to walk and having little or no elevation in

the level of CPK. However, they tend to develop respiratory insufficiency requiring ventilation, perhaps related to selective involvement of the diaphragm. Multiminicore disease has also been linked to mutations in *SEPN1*.

Most children with laminin-α2 (merosin)-positive congenital muscular dystrophy have a mild course and do not have the phenotype of either Ullrich disease or rigid spine syndrome. These patients bear further study; other genetic loci may be identified in the future.

MODERATE CONGENITAL MUSCULAR DYSTROPHIES Primary mutations in the laminin-α2 (merosin) gene cause laminin-α2-negative congenital muscular dystrophy. Laminin-α2 is an extracellular matrix protein that is associated with α-dystroglycan. A deficiency of laminin-α2 on immunohistochemistry of muscle tissue does not necessarily imply a primary laminin-α2-negative congenital muscular dystrophy—this finding only indicates a protein deficiency, which may be caused by either a mutation in laminin-α2 or may be secondary to a mutation in an associated protein, as occurs in the severe forms of congenital muscular dystrophy and LGMD 2I. Many of the published cases of laminin-α2-negative congenital muscular dystrophy do not include mutation analysis. Thus, laminin-α2-negative congenital muscular dystrophy as a disease entity is in flux.

In the classic, severe form of primary laminin-α2-negative congenital muscular dystrophy, affected children present in the first 6 mo of life with hypotonia, muscle weakness, and contractures. The course is moderately severe; most patients never ambulate independently. Serum CPK levels are mildly to moderately elevated. Although these patients have diffuse white matter lesions evident on MRI, gray matter is generally preserved, and intelligence is typically normal, although mental retardation has been reported in some cases. Other less commonly encountered features include seizures, cardiac complications, and neuronal migration defects.

MDC1C with mutations in *FKRP* also spare cognitive function, although the muscular defect is severe and survival past the first decade may only be possible with assisted ventilation.

SEVERE CONGENITAL MUSCULAR DYSTROPHIES The three classic severe congenital muscular dystrophies, Fukuyama congenital muscular dystrophy, muscle-eye-brain disease, and Walker–Warburg syndrome, share in common a more severe course than the other congenital muscular dystrophies, brain abnormalities in both white and gray matter, and mental retardation. The genetic origins of all three have been described, and the protein products all localize to the Golgi apparatus, which is consistent with their putative role in protein glycosylation. Protein glycosylation appears to play a role in cell adhesion, growth, and differentiation. Muscle tissue from affected patients has secondary deficiencies in laminin-α2 and α-dystroglycan on immunohistochemistry.

Mutations in *FCMD*, the gene encoding fukutin on 9q31, cause Fukuyama congenital muscular dystrophy, and have also been associated with the Walker–Warburg phenotype. The most common molecular defect is a 3-kb retrotransposal insertion in the 3′ untranslated region of the gene. Some patients also have point mutations in the coding region. Both defects lead to an absence of protein expression in affected patients. The exact function of fukutin is unknown, although a deficiency of highly glycosylated α-dystroglycan has been noted in the muscle tissue of these patients, suggesting that fukutin may play a role in glycosylation.

Patients with Fukuyama congenital muscular dystrophy have severe hypotonia and weakness, and almost never walk independently. Cortical and cerebellar dysgenesis (especially micropolygyria), hydrocephalus, and white matter abnormalities are typical. Mental retardation and seizures are common. Patients may survive to early adulthood.

Mutations in the gene encoding O-mannose β-1,2-N-acetylglucosaminyltransferase (POMGnT1) have been demonstrated in patients with muscle-eye-brain disease. This enzyme, a Golgi glycosyltransferase, catalyzes the transfer of N-acetylglucosamine from UDP-GlcNAc to O-mannosyl glycoproteins, which is the second step in the biosynthesis of O-mannosylglycan, a component of α-dystroglycan.

Children with muscle-eye-brain disease have severe hypotonia and weakness, and most are, thus, unable to walk. The eye manifestations include myopia, glaucoma, optic disk pallor, and retinal hypoplasia. MRI commonly reveals lissencephaly, flattened brainstem, cerebellar hypoplasia, and white matter abnormalities. Mental retardation is universal and epilepsy is common. Patients usually survive into early adulthood.

The gene encoding POMT1 has been demonstrated to be mutated in individuals with Walker–Warburg syndrome from at least six different families. A handful of patients with mutations in FCMD and FKRP also fit the traditional clinical picture of Walker–Warburg syndrome. POMT1, like fukutin and POMGnT1, plays a role in glycosylation, as indicated by the absence of glycosylation of α-dystroglycan in the muscle tissue of affected patients. The amount of α-dystroglycan is also reduced in these muscles. POMT1 is ubiquitously expressed, but peak levels are found in fetal brain, skeletal and cardiac muscle, and adult testis, corresponding to several of the organs most affected.

Walker–Warburg syndrome is the most severe of all muscular dystrophies, with patients rarely surviving infancy. The mothers of affected patients often have a history of miscarriages. These children are born with severe hypotonia and weakness. Brain malformations include cobblestone lissencephaly, agenesis of the corpus callosum, cerebellar hypoplasia, hydrocephalus, and extensive white matter abnormalities. Buphthalmos, glaucoma, and other eye abnormalities are present, as are testicular defects. Serum CPK levels are moderately elevated.

SYNDROMIC MUSCULAR DYSTROPHIES

The syndromic muscular dystrophies do not share genetic or clinical features beyond those common to all the muscular dystrophies. Each one, however, has a distinct clinical presentation, which has traditionally enabled physicians to make the diagnosis before the genetic etiologies were identified.

EMERY–DREIFUSS MUSCULAR DYSTROPHY Defects in two distinct genes have been found to cause Emery–Dreifuss muscular dystrophy: EMD, located on Xq28, and LMNA. Mutations in LMNA are inherited in an autosomal-dominant pattern, and also cause LGMD 1B. EMD is ubiquitously expressed, but is most prevalent in skeletal muscle, heart, colon, testis, ovary, and pancreas.

The clinical presentation of Emery–Dreifuss muscular dystrophy is striking. The three characteristic findings are muscle weakness and atrophy in a humeroperoneal distribution, heart block, and contractures involving the posterior neck, elbows, and heel cords. The contractures are an early finding. Intelligence is preserved.

FACIOSCAPULOHUMERAL MUSCULAR DYSTROPHY The genetics and pathogenesis of facioscapulohumeral muscular dystrophy (FSHD) remain largely a mystery. In patients with FSHD, deletions in a D4Z4 tandem repeat sequence on 4q35 have

been identified. Each D4Z4 sequence is 3.3-kb long and contains two homeobox domains. Affected individuals have fewer than 11 D4Z4 repeats. The length of the deletion correlates with the severity of disease, and is stably inherited. However, this sequence does not contain a known coding region. The most likely mechanism appears to be position effect variegation, in which a number of genes upstream of the D4Z4 region on 4q35 are upregulated in the disease state. In normal individuals, a multiprotein complex consisting of Yin Yang1, high-mobility box 2, and nucleolin binds to an element within D4Z4 and mediates transcriptional repression of those other genes, including adenine nucleotide transporter 1 and FSHD region genes 1 and 2. When too few copies of D4Z4 exist, the baseline repression of these genes is disrupted, leading to their overexpression and potentially explaining the molecular basis of FSHD.

Patients with FSHD have a distinct pattern of muscle wasting and weakness. As the disease name suggests, the muscles most affected are in the face, shoulder girdle, and humerus. Pelvic girdle, forearm, and peroneal muscles are also affected later in the course. Intelligence is preserved. Sensorineural hearing loss and retinal telangiectasias may occur, requiring periodic hearing tests and ophthalmological evaluations. The majority of patients remain ambulatory. Variants of FSHD that have been linked to the same genetic locus are scapuloperoneal and scapulohumeral dystrophies.

OCULOPHARYGEAL MUSCULAR DYSTROPHY Oculopharyngeal muscular dystrophy is the only muscular dystrophy caused by a triplet repeat expansion. Although myotonic dystrophy is also caused by a triplet repeat expansion and involves muscle wasting and weakness, most muscle samples from these patients do not appear dystrophic on muscle biopsy and it is usually classified as a myotonic disorder. The gene linked to oculopharyngeal muscular dystrophy is poly(A)-binding protein 2, which in control subjects contains a $(GCG)_6$ repeat but in affected patients contains a $(GCG)_{8-13}$ expansion. The expansions are stably inherited and have low copy numbers, in contrast to other triplet repeat expansion diseases. The typical pattern of inheritance is autosomal-dominant, but the $(GCG)_7$ expansion on one allele may modify (worsen) the phenotype typically caused by a higher copy number on the other allele. The $(GCG)_7$ expansion, when present on both alleles, may behave as an autosomal-recessive disease trait.

Patients with oculopharyngeal muscular dystrophy typically present in late adulthood with dysphagia, ptosis, and proximal muscle weakness. The characteristic pathological findings are nuclear filament inclusions in muscle fibers.

CONCLUSION

Since the cloning of the gene encoding dystrophin, 20 other genes causing various forms of muscular dystrophy have been discovered, elucidating the genetic origins of many muscle diseases. Although these genes are in some ways heterogeneous, some interesting patterns emerge. Many are physically connected, either directly or indirectly, to dystrophin, including a large sarcolemmal and subsarcolemmal dystrophin-associated protein complex that appears to stabilize the sarcolemmal membrane and connect the internal cytoskeleton with the extracellular matrix. Many of the dystrophinopathies and LGMDs are linked to components of this complex, and ones that are not may have indirect connections yet to be described. Dysferlin is the first of what may be a number of proteins involved in the process of membrane resealing, which is critical for maintaining the integrity of the muscle membrane. The congenital muscular dystrophies are more severe and generally related to primary or secondary defects in the extracellular matrix, specifically laminin-α2 (merosin) and the glycosylation of α-dystroglycan.

The genotype–phenotype correlations raise interesting questions for further investigation. Several genes, *LMNA*, *DYSF*, and *FKRP*, cause markedly different phenotypes in different patients, raising the possibility that modifier genes may help determine the actual clinical presentation. The molecular basis of FSHD may be an extreme example of this. Conversely, Emery–Dreifuss muscular dystrophy may be caused by mutations on either of two genes, which are on entirely different chromosomes. Further study of the pathogenesis of these diseases may yield insights into the mechanisms of transcription regulation, as well as potential therapeutic approaches.

SELECTED REFERENCES

Balci B, Uyanik G, Dincer P, et al. An autosomal recessive limb girdle muscular dystrophy (LGMD2) with mild mental retardation is allelic to Walker-Warburg syndrome (WWS) caused by a mutation in the *POMT1* gene. Neuromuscul Disord 2005;15:172–275.

Bansal D, Miyake K, Vogel SS, et al. Defective membrane repair in dysferlin-deficient muscular dystrophy. Nature 2003;423:168–172.

Bashir R, Britton S, Strachan T, et al. A gene related to Caenorhabditis elegans spermatogenesis factor fer-1 is mutated in limb-girdle muscular dystrophy type 2B. Nat Genet 1998;20:37–42.

Beltrán-Valero de Bernabé D, Currier S, Steinbrecher A, et al. Mutations in the O-mannosyltransferase gene POMT1 give rise to the severe neuronal migration disorder Walker-Warburg syndrome. Am J Hum Genet 2002;71:1033–1043.

Bione S, Maestrini E, Rivella S, et al. Identification of a novel X-linked gene responsible for Emery-Dreifuss muscular dystrophy. Nat Genet 1994;8:323–327.

Bonne G, Di Barletta MR, Varnous S, et al. Mutations in the gene encoding lamin A/C cause autosomal dominant Emery-Dreifuss muscular dystrophy. Nat Genet 1999;21:285–288.

Brais B, Bouchard JP, Xie YG, et al. Short GCG expansions in the PABP2 gene cause oculopharyngeal muscular dystrophy. Nat Genet 1998;18:164–167.

Brockington M, Yuva Y, Prandini P, et al. Mutations in the fukutin-related protein gene (FKRP) identify limb girdle muscular dystrophy 2I as a milder allelic variant of congenital muscular dystrophy MDC1C. Hum Mol Genet 2001;10:2851–2859.

Burghes AH, Logan C, Hu X, Belfall B, Worton RG, Ray PN. A cDNA clone from the Duchenne/Becker muscular dystrophy gene. Nature 1987;328:434–437.

Bushby KMD, Beckmann JS. The 105th ENMC sponsored workshop: Pathogenesis in the non-sarcoglycan limb-girdle muscular dystrophies, Naarden, 12–14 April 2002. Neuromuscul Disord 2003;13:80–90.

Darras BT, Menache CC, Kunkel LM. Dystrophinopathies. In: Jones HR Jr, De Vivo DC, Darras BT, eds. Neuromuscular Disorders of Infancy, Childhood, and Adolescence: A Clinician's Approach. Boston: Butterworth-Heinemann, 2003; pp. 649–699.

De Sandre-Giovannoli A, Bernard R, Cau P, et al. Lamin A truncation in Hutchinson-Gilford progeria. Science 2003;300:2055–2058.

Demir E, Sabatelli P, Allamand V, et al. Mutations in COL6A3 cause severe and mild phenotypes of Ullrich congenital muscular dystrophy. Am J Hum Genet 2002;70:1446–1458.

Eriksson M, Brown WT, Gordon LB, et al. Recurrent *de novo* point mutations in lamin A cause Hutchinson-Gilford progeria syndrome. Nature 2003;423:293–298.

Feit H, Silbergleit A, Schneider LB, et al. Vocal cord and pharyngeal weakness with autosomal dominant distal myopathy: clinical description and gene localization to 5q31. Am J Hum Genet 1998;63:1732–1742.

Fisher J, Upadhyaya M. Molecular genetics of facioscapulohumeral muscular dystrophy (FSHD). Neuromuscul Disord 1997;7:55–62.

Frosk P, Weiler T, Nylen E, et al. Limb-girdle muscular dystrophy type 2H associated with mutation in TRIM32, a putative E3-ubiquitin-ligase gene. Am J Hum Genet 2002;70:663–672.

Gabellini D, Green MR, Tupler R. Inappropriate gene activation in FSHD: a repressor complex binds a chromosomal repeat deleted in dystrophic muscle. Cell 2002;110:339–348.

Hauser MA, Horrigan SK, Salmikangas P, et al. Myotilin is mutated in limb girdle muscular dystrophy 1A. Hum Mol Genet 2000;9:2141–2147.

Helbling-Leclerc A, Zhang X, Topaloglu H, et al. Mutations in the laminin α2-chain gene (LAMA2) cause merosin-deficient congenital muscular dystrophy. Nat Genet 1995;11:216–218.

Higuchi I, Shiraishi T, Hashiguchi T, et al. Frameshift mutation in the collagen VI gene causes Ullrich's disease. Ann Neurol 2001;50:261–265.

Jones KJ, Morgan G, Johnston H, et al. The expanding phenotype of laminin-α2 chain (merosin) abnormalities: case series and review. J Med Genet 2001;38:649–657.

Kobayashi K, Nakahori Y, Miyake M, et al. An ancient retrotransposal insertion causes Fukuyama-type congenital muscular dystrophy. Nature 1998;394:388–392.

Lim LE, Campbell KP. The sarcoglycan complex in limb-girdle muscular dystrophy. Curr Opin Neurol 1998;11:443–452.

Liu J, Aoki M, Illa I, et al. Dysferlin, a novel skeletal muscle gene, is mutated in Miyoshi myopathy and limb girdle muscular dystrophy. Nat Genet 1998;20:31–36.

Messina DN, Speer MC, Percak-Vance MA, McNally EM. Linkage of familial dilated cardiomyopathy with conduction defect and muscular dystrophy to chromosome 6q23. Am J Hum Genet 1997;61:909–917.

Minetti C, Sotgia F, Bruno C, et al. Mutations in the caveolin-3 gene cause autosomal dominant limb-girdle muscular dystrophy. Nat Genet 1998;18:365–368.

Moghadaszadeh B, Petit N, Jaillaird C, et al. Mutations in SEPN1 cause congenital muscular dystrophy with spinal rigidity and restrictive respiratory syndrome. Nat Genet 2001;29:17, 18.

Monaco AP, Neve RL, Colletti-Feener C, Bertelson CJ, Kurnit DM, Kunkel LM. Isolation of candidate cDNAs for portions of the Duchenne muscular dystrophy gene. Nature 1986;323:646–650.

Moreira ES, Wiltshire TJ, Faulkner G, et al. Limb-girdle muscular dystrophy type 2G is caused by mutations in the gene encoding the sarcomeric protein telethonin. Nat Genet 2000;24:163–166.

Muntoni F, Guicheney P. 85th ENMC international workshop on congenital muscular dystrophy: 6th international CMD workshop: 1st workshop of the myo-cluster project 'GENRE': 27–28 October 2000, Naarden, the Netherlands. Neuromuscul Disord 2002;12:69–78.

Lennon NJ, Kho A, Backsai BJ, et al. Dysferlin interacts with annexins A1 and A2 and mediates sarcolemmal wound-healing. J Biol Chem 2003;278:50,466–50,473.

Richard I, Broux O, Allamand V, et al. Mutations in the proteolytic enzyme calpain 3 cause limb-girdle muscular dystrophy type 2A. Cell 1995;81:27–40.

Speer MC, Vance JM, Grubber JM, et al. Identification of a new autosomal dominant limb-girdle muscular dystrophy on chromosome 7. Am J Hum Genet 1999;64:556–562.

Yoshida A, Kobayashi K, Manya H, et al. Muscular dystrophy and neuronal migration disorder caused by mutations in a glycosyltransferase, POMGnT1. Dev Cell 2001;1:717–724.

Zatz M, Vainzof M, Passos-Bueno MR. Limb-girdle muscular dystrophy: One gene with different phenotypes, one phenotype with different genes. Curr Opin Neurol 2000;13:511–517.

71 Rhabdomyosarcomas

STEPHEN J. TAPSCOTT

SUMMARY

Significant progress has been made in understanding the molecular biology of rhabdomyosarcomas and in improving therapeutic regimens for the treatment of these cancers. Alveolar rhabdomyosarcomas are associated with translocations that create a novel fusion protein of either PAX3 or PAX7 with the FKHR transcription factors, whereas, embryonoal rhabdomayosarcomas are associated with a loss of heterozygosity at 11p15.5. In addition, animal models suggest that the combination of factors that induce myogenesis with an abrogation of tumor suppressors such as p53 and Rb can lead to the formation of rhabdomyosarcomas. Historically, treatment stratification has been based on histological criteria, however, the increasing knowledge of distinct molecular phenotypes of rhabdomyosarcomas will likely inform treatment strategies in the future.

Key Words: Alveolar; embryonal; FKHR; muscle differentiation; PAX3; PAX7; rhabdomyosarcoma; tumor suppressors.

INTRODUCTION

Rhabdomyosarcomas are the most common soft tissue sarcomas in childhood, yet they are still a relatively rare tumor, with an incidence in the United States of 1.3–4.5/million children/yr. The histological classification of rhabdomyosarcoma has historically relied on the expression of genes associated with skeletal muscle in some of the tumor cells, giving a subset of cells the appearance of skeletal muscle cells or myoblasts. Several histological subcategories of rhabdomyosarcomas have also been recognized. Embryonal rhabdomyosarcomas occur most frequently during the first 3 yr after birth and account for about 50–60% of rhabdomyosarcomas. Additional distinctions can be made within the group of embryonal rhabdomyosarcomas, for example, there are the botyroid and spindle cell variants. Alveolar rhabdomyosarcomas are distinguished from embryonal rhabdomyosarcomas histologically by characteristic open spaces in pathology sections, reminiscent of alveoli in the lungs. Alveolar rhabdomyosarcomas account for approx 20% of rhabdomyosarcomas and have a bimodal incidence distribution with peaks at approx ages 3 and 15 yr. A third group of pleomorphic or primitive rhabdomyosarcomas is not easily distinguished from other small round cell tumors of childhood, such as neuroblastoma, Ewing's sarcoma, primitive neuroectodermal tumors, and non-Hodgkin's lymphoma based on

From: *Principles of Molecular Medicine, Second Edition*
Edited by: M. S. Runge and C. Patterson © Humana Press, Inc., Totowa, NJ

standard histology. For these primitive tumors, classification as rhabdomyosarcomas can be confirmed using antibodies or other molecular probes to genes characteristically expressed in skeletal muscle, such as desmin, or muscle creatine kinase.

MOLECULAR GENETICS OF ALVEOLAR RHABDOMYOSARCOMAS

Cytogenetic studies identified multiple abnormalities in cells from rhabdomyosarcomas; however, alveolar rhabdomyosarcomas had a characteristic translocation between chromosome 2 and 13, t(2;13)(q35;q14). Fine mapping of the breakpoint identified *PAX3* as a candidate gene on chromosome 2, leading to the demonstration that the rearrangement occurred within the PAX3 gene. Ultimately a novel chimeric transcript was identified, encoding the amino-terminal portion of the PAX3 protein from chromosome 2 and the carboxy-terminal portion of a gene on chromosome 13, with homology to the fork head family of genes.

PAX3 is a transcription factor that is expressed in the neural tube, neural crest derivatives, and in the muscle precursor cells that migrate from the somites into the limb bud. Dominant or semidominant mutations of *PAX3* in mice, the splotch mutant, and humans, the Waartenberg syndrome, are noted for defects in neural crest and neural tube development. Embryos homozygous for some alleles of splotch have deficient limb muscle formation that can be attributed to the inadequate generation or migration of limb muscle precursor cells. This may partly be the basis for limb deformities in human variations of the Waartenberg syndrome that are homozygous for *PAX3* mutations.

The t(2;13) in alveolar rhabdomyosarcomas creates a novel gene with the transcription start site and 5′ coding region of the PAX3 gene and the 3′ region of the fork head homolog rhabdomyosarcoma (*FKHR*) gene, a member of the fork head family of transcription factors, so-called because the prototype gene of the family was described as a mutation in *Drosophila melanogaster* that produced two spiked head structures (*see* Chapter 3). Additional vertebrate members of the fork head family include the hapatocyte nuclear factors (*HNF-3α*, *HNF-3β*, *HNF-3γ*) and brain factor-1. The fusion protein includes two DNA-binding domains in the carboxy-terminal half of the PAX3 protein, a paired box DNA-binding domain and a homeodomain, but disrupts the DNA-binding region of the FKHR protein. The carboxy-terminal portion of FKHR maintained in the fusion protein is rich in prolines and acidic amino acids, attributes consistent with an acidic activation domain, and transfection experiments demonstrate that the fusion protein is more potent than PAX3 as a transcriptional activator of reporter constructs driven by PAX3 binding sites. Further, DNA-binding studies show that the fusion protein binds to PAX3 binding sites, but that it has a mildly altered DNA-binding affinity compared to PAX3. Therefore, the PAX3-FKHR fusion protein may have oncogenic activity based on enhanced activation of genes regulated by PAX3 or through altered binding affinity to specific DNA sequences.

Although PAX3 is apparently expressed in the early migrating muscle progenitor cells, its role in development is not fully understood. Genetic experiments in mice indicate that PAX3 plays a critical role in specifying cells to become myoblasts, in part by regulating the expression of the myogenic basic helix–loop–helix (bHLH) protein MyoD. Although PAX3 plays a positive role in specifying myoblast fate, PAX3 expression inhibits myogenesis in cultured muscle cell lines and inhibits the ability of MyoD to activate the myogenic program in fibroblasts. The PAX3-FKHR fusion protein is a more potent inhibitor of myogenesis and MyoD activity in this system. Based on these observations and the developmental expression of PAX3 in the migrating muscle precursor cells, but not in skeletal muscle, it is possible that the normal function of PAX3 is to initiate and maintain an early phase of myogenesis and the fusion protein either enhances this activity or loses an element necessary to suppress this activity, resulting in an arrested state of development.

Although much less frequent than t(2;13), a t(1;13)(p36;q14) translocation has been described in some alveolar rhabdomyosarcomas. This translocation creates a fusion protein between PAX7 on chromosome 1 and FKHR that is structurally similar to the PAX3-FKHR fusion protein. PAX7 is also expressed in muscle precursor cells and is capable of binding to PAX3 sites either as a homodimer or as a heterodimer with PAX3. Genetic studies in mice revealed that PAX7 is necessary for the formation of muscle satellite cells, the cell population that regenerates skeletal muscle in the adult. Therefore, it appears that PAX3 and PAX7 both have central roles in specifying cells to become skeletal muscle. It is likely that each of the fusion proteins associated with alveolar rhabdomyosarcomas, PAX3-FKHR, and PAX7-FKHR, maintains some ability to initiate the skeletal muscle program but cannot sustain normal differentiation. The role of the FKHR protein is largely unknown, but it promotes myoblast fusion during terminal differentiation and dominant negative mutants of FKHR can prevent fusion. Therefore, the truncated FKHR fusion protein might block specific aspects of the program of terminal differentiation.

MOLECULAR GENETICS OF EMBRYONAL RHABDOMYOSARCOMAS

Most rhabdomyosarcomas are sporadic; however, the appearance of rhabdomyosarcomas in families with the Li-Fraumeni syndrome or the Beckwith-Wiedemann syndrome has provided valuable insights into the genetics of this tumor (see Chapter 7). Beckwith-Wiedemann syndrome (see Chapter 116) is associated with growth excess and a high incidence of tumors, including Wilms' tumor, hepatoblastoma, adrenal carcinoma, and rhabdomyosarcoma. Because of the association of Wilms' tumor with a locus on chromosome 11p13, this region was analyzed for loss of heterozygosity (LOH) in both rhabdomyosarcomas and in the Beckwith-Wiedemann syndrome. LOH of chromosome 11 was detected in a large portion of rhabdomyosarcomas, but the common region of LOH mapped to 11p15.5 similar to the mapping of the region of LOH for the Beckwith-Wiedemann syndrome. A preferential

retention of the paternal allele in both embryonal rhabdomyosarcomas and in the Beckwith-Wiedemann syndrome has led to the suggestion that LOH alters the level of gene expression maintained by an imprinted allele, either decreasing expression of a tumor suppressor gene by loss of the nonimprinted allele or increasing expression of a growth-promoting gene by duplication of the nonimprinted allele.

The presence of a tumor growth suppressor gene at 11p15 has been supported by transfer of subchromosomal fragments to rhabdomyosarcoma cells. Fragments of chromosome 11 that contain 11p15 suppress growth and xenograft tumor formation in embryonal rhabdomyosarcomas, although similar experiments have not been performed in alveolar rhabdomyosarcomas, nor has parental origin of the suppressing allele been analyzed.

The gene relevant to rhabdomyosarcoma formation at 11p15 has not been clearly identified, although some candidates have been studied. Insulin-like growth factor II (IGF-2) is a maternally imprinted gene that maps to 11p15, transcriptionally silent on the maternal allele and expressed from the paternal allele. Elevated levels of IGF-2 resulting from paternal disomy associated with LOH may give a growth advantage to cells and have been postulated as the cause of the somatic hypertrophy in the Beckwith-Wiedemann syndrome. IGF-2 has been shown to act as an autocrine growth factor in some rhabdomyosarcomas and loss of imprinting, i.e., expression of IGF-2 from both alleles has been demonstrated in alveolar rhabdomyosarcomas and embryonal rhabdomyosarcomas that do not have LOH at 11p15. The growth-promoting activity of increased IGF-2 levels may play a critical role in the generation of rhabdomyosarcomas; however, this model would not explain the somatic cell genetic experiments that implicate a tumor suppressor gene at 11p15.

A second candidate gene that maps to 11p15, H19, is unusual because the H19 transcript does not contain a conserved open reading frame and may function as a regulatory polyadenylated RNA. H19 is imprinted in the opposite manner to IGF-2, expressed from the maternal allele and silent on the paternal allele; therefore, loss of the maternal allele decreases H19 expression. Transfection of H19 into rhabdomyosarcoma cell lines suppresses both growth and tumorigenesis, making it a candidate for the 11p15 tumor suppressor.

Implicating imprinting as a critical factor in the LOH at 11p15 means that the transcription of numerous genes in the region might contribute to the transformed phenotype, and both H19 and IGF-2 may contribute to the generation of rhabdomyosarcomas. Many additional genes have been mapped to the 11p15.5 region, including the cyclin-dependent kinase inhibitor p57^{KIP2}, the nucleosome assembly protein hNAP2, and the retinoblastoma-associated protein RbAp48. Mutations of the p57 gene have been reported in Beckwith-Wiedemann syndrome and cause developmental abnormalities in mice that are similar to Beckwith-Wiedemann syndrome, indicating that p57 has a critical role in this syndrome. It remains to be determined whether altered expression of p57 or other genes in this region contributes to the generation of rhabdomyosarcomas.

RHABDOMYOSARCOMAS EXPRESS MYOD OR RELATED MYOGENIC FACTORS

Expression of the myogenic regulatory protein, MyoD, or one of the related members of this group of myogenic bHLH proteins, which consists of MyoD, Myf5, Myogenin, and MRF4, can be used to categorize less differentiated tumors as rhabdomyosarcomas, because almost all rhabdomyosarcomas express one or more of this group of proteins. The myogenic bHLH proteins are transcription factors that orchestrate the expression of genes that characterize skeletal muscle. Gene knockout experiments demonstrate that these genes are necessary for skeletal myogenesis, and the ability to convert nonmyogenic cells to skeletal muscle by expressing one of the myogenic bHLH proteins indicates that in many cell types, they are sufficient to mediate differentiation. In addition to activating expression of muscle structural genes, MyoD has been shown to mediate withdrawal from the cell cycle and induction of p21 expression. The role of these proteins in normal development is discussed in Chapter 92.

Given the ability of the myogenic proteins to activate transcription of skeletal muscle genes, the expression of MyoD in rhabdomyosarcomas can account for the low level of muscle differentiation seen in the tumor. In the tumors that have been analyzed, however, most of the cells in the tumor express MyoD, but do not terminally differentiate into postmitotic muscle cells, indicating that the program of muscle differentiation mediated by the MyoD family of transcription factors has been partially blocked. Analysis of the myogenic bHLH proteins in several tumors has demonstrated that they are not mutant, yet they are inefficient activators of muscle gene expression. Several molecular mechanisms have been identified that can prevent MyoD and related myogenic bHLH transcription factors from functioning. Relevant to the mutations that can cause rhabdomyosarcomas, normal Rb and p53 are necessary for muscle gene expression by MyoD, and amplified MDM2 can prevent MyoD transcriptional activity.

RB, P53, AND ONCOGENES   Just as the association of rhabdomyosarcomas with the Beckwith-Wiedemann syndrome focused attention on 11p15, the appearance of rhabdomyosarcomas in families with Li-Fraumeni syndrome suggested that p53 inactivation may be important for tumor formation. Analysis of p53 abnormalities, without respect to alveolar or embryonal histological types, indicated that approximately half of the tumors had abrogated normal p53 function. When histological subtype is considered, it appears that the frequency of p53 mutations is higher in the embryonal rhabdomyosarcomas. Differences between embryonal and alveolar rhabdomyosarcomas are further suggested by a higher frequency of N-myc amplification in alveolar rhabdomyosarcomas, whereas mutation in N-ras and K-ras appear to be more frequent in embryonal rhabdomyosarcomas.

Mouse models have indicated several different regulatory pathways that can contribute to the formation of rhabdomyosarcomas. Mice with a mutation that inactivates the p16INK4a and the p14ARF transcripts, two different transcripts from the same locus that, respectively, regulate pRB and p53 function, mainly develop lymphomas and fibrosarcomas. However, when combined with a transgene that expresses hepatocyte growth factor/scatter factor, the ligand for the c-MET receptor expressed on satellite cells and myoblasts, the INK4a/ARF mutation induces a high rate of rhabdomyosarcomas in mice. In this model, blocking both p53 and pRb activity in the presence of a constitutive myogenic growth factor was sufficient to generate rhabdomyosarcomas. This is similar to the finding that amplified MDM2 can contribute to rhabdomysarcomas by inhibiting the activity of both p53 and Rb when expressed in myoblasts. There are likely many different molecular pathways that can contribute to rhabdomyosarcoma

formation, as evidenced by the formation of rhabdomysarcomas in mice deficient in the Patched receptor that inhibits signaling by Sonic Hedgehog. Sonic Hedgehog is necessary to specify skeletal muscle cells in the developing embryo and acts, at least in part, by regulating the expression of the myogenic bHLH transcription factor Myf5, similar to the role of PAX3 in regulating the expression of the related myogenic transcription factor MyoD. One theme that emerges from these different models of rhabdomyosarcomas is the constitutive or aberrant activity of factors that induce myogenesis coupled with conditions that prevent normal terminal differentiation.

CONCLUSIONS

Therapy of rhabdomyosarcomas combines chemotherapy, radiation therapy, and surgery. The Intergroup Rhabdomyosarcoma Studies (IRS) utilized a risk-based design that increased therapeutic intensity in groups with marginally poorer prognosis. In addition to tumor staging based on invasiveness, involvement of lymph nodes, metastasis, and degree of surgical excision, tumor histology is a significant variable in predicting response to treatment. In IRS-II, the 5-yr survival rate was 95% for the favorable category of botyroid, 67% for embryonal, and approx 50% for alveolar and undifferentiated. IRS-III includes therapy intensification of the groups with the less favorable prognosis and has achieved survival rates for alveolar tumors comparable to embryonal ones.

One challenge remaining is to determine if survival can be improved and therapy-related complications minimized by using the available molecular markers to further refine risk-based therapy. An analysis of patients with metastatic alveolar rhabdomyosarcoma enrolled in the IRS-IV study revealed a more favorable outcome for those with a PAX7-FKHR translocation than those with a PAX3-FKHR translocation, whereas the type of translocation did not appear related to outcome in nonmetastatic disease. The availability of molecular methods to accurately identify fusion transcripts, gene amplifications, and gene mutations might permit the identification of other factors associated with response to therapy and survival.

Ideally further understanding of the molecular biology of rhabdomyosarcomas eventually will lead to rationally designed therapies. Perhaps the development of drugs that inhibit PAX3 expression or agents that degrade the PAX3-FKHR fusion transcript would be useful adjuvants to therapy.

SELECTED REFERENCES

Barr FG, Galili N, Holick J, Biegel JA, Rovera G, Emanuel BS. Rearrangement of the PAX3 paired box gene in paediatric solid tumor alveolar rhabdomyosarcoma. Nat Genet 1993;3:113–117.

Best LG, Hoekstra RE. Wiedemann-Beckwith syndrome: autosomal dominant inheritance in a family. Am J Med Genet 1981;9:291–299.

Bober E, Franz T, Arnold HH, Gruss P, Tremblay P. Pax-3 is required for the development of limb muscles: a possible role for the migration of dermomyotomal muscle progenitor cells. Development 1994;120: 603–612.

Clark J, Rocques PJ, Braun T, et al. Expression of members of the myf gene family in human rhabdomyosarcomas. Br J Cancer 1991;64: 1039–1042.

Crist W, Gehan EA, Ragab AH, et al. The third intergroup rhabdomyosarcoma study. J Clin Oncol 1995;13:610–630.

Davis RJ, D'Cruz CM, Lovell MA, Biegel JA, Barr FG. Fusion of PAX7 to FKHR by the variant t(1;13)(p36;q14) translocation in alveolar rhabdomyosarcoma. Cancer Res 1994;54:2869–2872.

Douglas EC, Valentine M, Etcubanas E, et al. A specific chromosomal abnormality in rhabdomyosarcomas. Cytogenet Cell Genet 1987;45: 148–155.

Epstein JA, Lam P, Jepeal L, Maas RL, Shapiro DN. Pax3 inhibits myogenic differentiation of cultured myoblast cells. J Biol Chem 1995; 270:11,719–11,722.

Felix CA, Kappel CC, Mitsudomi T, et al. Frequency and diversity of p53 mutations in childhood rhabdomyosarcoma. Cancer Res 1992;52: 2243–2247.

Fredericks WJ, Galili N, Mukhopadhyay S, et al. The PAX3-FKHR fusion protein created by the t(2;13) translocation in alveolar rhabdomyosarcomas is a more potent transcriptional activator that PAX3. Mol Cell Biol 1995;15:1522–1535.

Galili N, Davis RJ, Fredericks WJ, et al. Fusion of a fork head domain gene to PAX3 in the solid tumor alveolar rhabdomyosarcoma. Nat Genet 1993;5:230–235.

Hao Y, Crenshaw T, Moulton T, Newcomb E, Tycko B. Tumour-suppressor activity of H19 RNA. Nature 1993;365:764–767.

Koi M, Johnson LA, Kalikin LM, Little PF, Nagamura Y, Feinberg AP. Tumor cell growth arrest caused by subchromosomal transferable DNA fragments from chromosome 11. Science 1993;260:361–364.

Koufos A, Hansen MF, Copeland NG, Jenkins NA, Lampkin BC, Cavenee WK. Loss of heterozygosity in three embryonal tumours suggests a common pathogenetic mechanism. Nature 1985;316: 330–334.

Loh WE, Scrable HJ, Livanos E, et al. Human chromosome 11 contains two different growth suppressor genes for embryonal rhabdomyosarcoma. Proc Natl Acad Sci USA 1992;89:1755–1759.

Mulligan LM, Matlashewski GJ, Scrable HJ, Cavenee WK. Mechanisms of p53 loss in human sarcomas. Proc Natl Acad Sci USA 1990;87:5863–5867.

Scrable H, CaveneeW, Ghavimi F, Lovell M, Morgan K, Sapienza C. A model for embryonal rhabdomyosarcoma tumorigenesis that involves genome imprinting. Proc Natl Acad Sci USA 1989;86:7480–7484.

Scrable H, Witte D, Shimada H, et al. Molecular differential pathology of rhabdomyosarcoma. Genes Chromosomes Cancer 1989;1:23–35.

Seale P, Sabourin LA, Girgis-Gabardo A, Mansouri A, Gruss P, Rudnicki MA. Pax7 is required for the specification of myogenic satellite cells. Cell 2000;102:777–786.

Sharp R, Recia JA, Jhappan C, et al. Synergism between INK4a/ARF inactivation and aberrant HGF/SF signaling in rhabdomyosarcomagenesis. Nat Med 2002;8:1276–1280.

Sorensen PHB, Lynch JC, Qualman SJ, et al. PAX3-FKHR and PAX7-FKHR gene fusions are prognostic indicators in alveolar rhabdomyosarcoma: a report from the Children's Oncology Group. J Clin Oncol 2002;20:2672–2679.

Stratton MR, Fisher C, Gusterson BA, Cooper CS. Detection of point mutations in N-ras and K-ras genes of human embryonal rhabdomyosarcomas using oligonucleotide proges and the polymerase chain reaction. Cancer Res 1989;49:6324–6327.

Tapscott SJ, Thayer MJ, Weintraub H. Deficiency in rhabdomyosarcomas of a factor required for MyoD activity and myogenesis. Science 1993;259:1450–1453.

Zhan S, Shapiro DN, Helman LJ. Activation of an imprinted allele of the insulin-like growth factor II gene implicated in rhabdomyosarcoma. J Clin Invest 1994;94:445–448.

IX

ONCOLOGY

SECTION EDITOR:
W. STRATFORD MAY, JR.

Abbreviations

IX. ONCOLOGY

17-AAG	17-Allyamino-17-demethoxygeldanamycin
2-5A	2′-5′-oligoadenylate
ABL	Abelson
ADH	atypical ductal hyperplasia
ALCL	anaplastic large-cell lymphoma
ALK	anaplastic lymphoma kinase
ALL	acute lymphoblastic leukemia
AMACR	alpha-methylacyl coenzyme A racemase
AML	acute myeloid leukemia
α-MSH	α-melanocyte stimulating hormone
AO	anaplastic oligodendroglioma
AOA	mixed anaplastic oligoastrocytoma
AP-2	activator protein-2
APaf-1	apoptosis protease activating factor
APC	adenomatous polyposis coli
APL	acute promyelocytic leukemia
APO-3	apoptosis antigen 3
AR	androgen receptor
ARF	alternative reading frame
ART	antiretroviral therapy
AT	adenine-thymine
ATM	ataxia-telangectasia mutated
ATRA	all-*trans*-retinoic acid
BCL-2	B-cell leukemia/lymphoma gene
BCR	breakpoint cluster region
bFGF	basic fibroblast growth factor
BH	Bcl2 homology
bHLH	basic helix loop helix
BID	BH3 interacting domain death agonist
BIR	baculovirus inhibitor of apoptosis repeat
BL	Burkitt's lymphoma/leukemia
BM	bone marrow
BMSC	bone marrow stromal cell
BPH	benign prostatic hyperplasia
CAD	caspase-activated DNase
C-ALCL	cutaneous anaplastic large-cell lymphoma
CAMs	cell adhesion molecules
CBF	core binding factor
CCND1	cyclin D-1
CD	cluster designation
CDK	cyclin-dependent kinase
c-FLIP	c-FLICE-like inhibitory protein
CIITA	class II transactivator
CI	chromosomal instability
CIMP	CpG island methylator phenotype
CIN	cervical intraepithelial neoplasia

CIS	carcinoma *in situ*
CKI	CDK-inhibitor
CKI	cyclin-dependent kinase inhibitor
CLL	chronic lymphocytic leukemia
CML	chronic myelogenous leukemia
CMP	common myeloid progenitor
CTL	cytolytic T-cell
Cyt c	cytochrome *c*
DAPK	death-associated protein kinase
DCIS	ductal carcinoma *in situ*
Dex	dexamethasone
DISC	death-induced signaling complex
DLCL	diffuse large-cell lymphoma
DNMT	DNA methyltransferases
DR	death receptor
EB	end-binding protein
EBNA	Epstein-Barr virus nuclear antigen
EBV	Epstein-Barr virus
ECM	extracellular matrix
EGF	epidermal growth factor
EGFR	epidermal growth factor receptor
ER	estrogen receptor
ERE	estrogen response element
ERK	extracellular signal-regulated kinase
ET	endothelin
FAB	French–American–British
FAK	focal adhesion kinase
FAP	familial adenomatous polyposis
FAS.L	Fas ligand
FGF	fibroblast growth factor
FGF-2	fibroblast growth factor-2
FHIT	fragile histidine triad
FISH	fluorescence *in situ* hybridization
FLD	flexible loop domain
FN	fibronectin
FPD/AML	familial platelet defect with propensity to develop AML
FTI	farnesyl transferase inhibitor
G_0	non-proliferative state
G2	Gap2
GBM	glioblastoma multiforme
GC	germinal center
GM-CSF	granulocyte-macrophage colony-stimulating factor
GMP	granulocyte-monocyte progenitor
GPCR	G protein-coupled receptor
GRO	growth-regulated protein
GRP	gastrin-releasing peptide
GSK3β	glycogen synthase-3β kinase

GST	glutathione *S*-transferase	MMP	matrix metalloproteinase
H	*helicobacter*	MMR	mismatch repair
HAT	histone acetyl transferase	MOA	mixed oligoastrocytoma
HCV	hepatitis C virus	MRD	minimal residual disease
HDAC	histone deacetylase	MSI	microsatellite instability
HGF	hepatocyte growth factor	MSR1	macrophage scavenger receptor 1 gene
HHV-8	human herpesvirus 8	MTC	maternal-to-child
HIF	hypoxia-inducible factor-1	NE	neuroendocrine
HIV-1	HIV type 1	NF	nuclear factor
HNPCC	hereditary nonpolyposis colorectal cancers	NFAT	nuclear factor of activated T-cells
HPC	hereditary prostate cancer	NFκB	nuclear factor κB
HPC1	hereditary prostate cancer 1	NHL	non-Hodgkin's lymphoma
HPV	human papilloma virus	NK	natural killer
HSC	hematopoietic stem cell	NNB	non neoplastic brain
Hsp90	heat shock protein 90	NNK	4-(methylnitrosanino)-1-(3-pyridyl)-1-butanone
HTLV	human T-cell leukemia viruses	NPC	nasopharyngeal carcinoma
IAP	inhibitors of apoptosis	NPM	nucleophosmin
ICC	invasive cervical carcinoma	NS5A	nonstructural protein 5A
ICE	interleukin-Iβ-converting enzyme	NSCLC	non-small cell lung cancer
IFN	interferon	OMM	outer mitochondrial membrane
IGF	insulin-like growth factor	OPG	osteoprotegerin
IGF-1	insulin-like growth factor-1	PAH	polycyclic aromatic hydrocarbon
IGH	immunoglobulin H	PAI-1	type 1 plasminogen inhibitor
IgH	immunoglobulin heavy chain	PAR-1	protease-activated receptor 1
IgL	immunoglobulin light chain	PCD	programmed cell death
IKK	IκB kinase	PCL	plasma cell leukemia
IL	interleukin	PDGF	platelet-derived growth factor
ITAM	immunoreceptor-tyrosine-based activation motif	PDK	phosphoinsitol-dependent protein kinase
ITD	internal tandem duplications	Ph	Philadelphia chromosome
Jak	Janus tyrosine kinase	PI3K	phosphoinositide 3-kinase
JMML	juvenile myelomonocytic leukemia	PIA	proliferative inflammatory atrophy
JPS	juvenile polyposis syndrome	PIN	prostatic intraepithelial neoplasia
k-NN	nearest neighbor prediction model	PJS	Peutz-Jeghers syndrome
KS	Kaposi's sarcoma	PKB	protein kinase B
LC	light chain	PKC	protein kinase C
LCIS	lobular carcinoma *in situ*	PLC-γ	phospholipase C-γ
LDH-A	lactate dehydrogenase A	PML	promyelocytic leukemia
Lef	lymphoid enhancer factor	PR	progesterone receptor
LMO	cysteine-rich LIM-domain only	pRB	retinoblastoma gene product
LMP	latent membrane protein	PSA	prostate-specific antigen
LOH	loss of heterozygosity	PTEN	phosphatase and tensin homolog deleted on chromosome 10
LTR	long terminal repeat		
M	mitosis (when used in cell cycle discussions)	PTHrP	parathyroid hormone-related protein
MALT	mucosa-associated lymphoid tissue	PTK	protein tyrosine kinases
MAPK	mitogen-activated protein kinase	PTP	protein tyrosine phosphatase
MC1-R	melacortin-1 receptor	RANKL	receptor activator of nuclear factor-κB ligand
MCHR	melanocyte-stimulating hormone receptor	RAR	retinoic acid receptor
MCL	mantle cell lymphoma	RARα	retinoic acid receptor α
MCR	mutation cluster region	Rb	retinoblastoma protein or susceptibility gene
MDR	multidrug resistance		
MDS	myelodysplastic syndrome	RGP	radial growth phase
MGSA	melanocyte growth stimulatory activity	RNASEL	RNase L gene
MGUS	monoclonal gammopathy of unknown significance	ROS	reactive oxygen species
MHC II	major histocompatibility class II	RT	reverse transcriptase
Min	multiple intestinal neoplasia	RTK	receptor tyrosine kinase
MIP	macrophage inflammatory protein	S	synthesis (when used in cell-cycle discussions)
MIP-1α	macrophage inflammatory protein-1 α	SCC	squamous cell carcinoma
Mitf	microphthalmia-associated transcription factor	SCF	stem cell factor
MLL	mixed lineage leukemia	SCL	stem cell leukemic protein
MM	multiple myeloma	SCLC	small-cell lung cancer

SERM	selective ER modulator	TIMP-1	tissue inhibitor of metallproteinases
SH2	src-homology domain 2	T-LBL	T-lymphoblastic lymphoma
sIg	surface immunoglobulins	TM	transmembrane
siRNA	small-interfering RNA	TNF	tumor necrosis factor
SL-IC	SCID leukemia-initiating cells	TNFR	tumor necrosis factor receptor
SLL	small lymphocytic lymphoma	TRAIL	TNF-related apoptosis-inducing ligand
SRC	w/e	TRRAP	transactivating/transformation
Stat	signal transducer and activators of transcription		domain-associated protein
T-ALL	T-cell acute lymphoblastic leukemia	TSG	tumor suppressor gene
Tcf	T-cell factor	uPA	urokinase-type 1 plasminogen activator
TCR	T-cell receptors	uPAR	urokinase-type plasminogen activator receptor
TDLU	terminal duct lobular unit	UPR	unfolded protein response
TDT	terminal deoxynucleotidyl-transferase	UV	ultraviolet
TGFα	transforming growth factor α	VE	vascular endothelial
TGFβ	transforming growth factor-β	VEGF	vascular endothelial growth factor
TGFβRII	transforming growth factor-β receptor II	VGP	vertical growth phase
TIF2	transcriptional intermediary factor 2	WHO	World Health Organization

SOLID TUMORS

72 Apoptosis

W. STRATFORD MAY, JR. AND XINGMING DENG

SUMMARY

Cell growth represents the net effect of cell proliferation balanced by attrition from terminal differentiation and/or apoptotic cell death. Apoptosis is a genetically and biochemically regulated process known as programmed cell death. Successful execution of apoptosis is required for normal embryonic development, regulation of the immune response, control of cell numbers, the process of aging and senescence and the cell's ability to compensate for otherwise damaging stresses. This chapter focuses on mechanisms responsible for regulating apoptosis in the context of cancer and other pathology.

Key Words: Anoikis; apoptosis; autophagy; BCL-2; caspase; cell growth; cytolytic T-cells; natural killer; necrosis.

INTRODUCTION

Cell growth represents the net effect of cell proliferation balanced by attrition from terminal differentiation and/or apoptotic cell death. Apoptosis is a genetically and biochemically regulated process known as programmed cell death. Successful execution of apoptosis is required for normal embryonic development, regulation of the immune response, control of cell numbers (e.g., in rapidly turning over cells in the GI tract, bone marrow, skin, and uterus), the process of aging and senescence and the cell's ability to compensate for otherwise damaging stresses (e.g., nutrient deprivation, or toxicant drug exposure and DNA damage). Indeed, dysregulation of apoptosis (i.e., too little or too much) can lead to disease pathology including developmental defects, chronic degenerative, and autoimmune diseases and malignancy. Specifically with respect to malignancy, disabling apoptosis affords the cancer cell not only a selective growth advantage but also resistance to chemoradiation treatment. This feature not only helps to ensure survival when the cancer cell finds itself in an otherwise inhospitable microenvironment, for example following metastases, but also when evading attack by the body's immune system. This chapter focuses on mechanisms responsible for regulating apoptosis in the context of cancer and other pathology.

CELL DEATH

NECROSIS AND APOPTOSIS
Cell death can result by two distinct processes, necrosis and apoptosis (Table 72-1). Necrosis is a functionally passive process, which occurs when cells are exposed to extreme physical and chemical environmental imbalances (e.g., hyperthermia, hypoxia) or as a result of forceful physical trauma (e.g., blunt trauma) that directly damages membranes and tissues. Such damage leads to an osmotic-type shock that results in the rapid influx of water and extracellular ions through damaged membranes including those of the organelles, which produces cell swelling and rupture with extrusion of cytoplasmic contents, including lysosomal enzymes, into the microenvironment. This triggers a secondary, local inflammatory response that may lead to the destruction of undamaged bystander cells. By contrast, apoptosis is an energy-dependent, active process that is highly regulated and not easily triggered. However, when activated its biochemical consequences lead to the cell's proteolytic destruction from within, primarily through the action of a specific set of proteases, the caspases. This type of cell suicide results from the destruction of key regulatory and structural proteins necessary for the maintenance of cell integrity and viability. The classic morphological features of apoptosis, which contrast with those of necrosis, include cell shrinkage, membrane blebbing, partitioning of nuclear and cytoplasm components into membrane bound apoptotic bodies (containing nuclear-ribosomal or organellar remnants), and specific internucleosomal degradation of cellular DNA, which is the classic molecular "hallmark" of this process. Because the apoptotic cell undergoes volume loss associated with nuclear and cytoplasmic condensation, this process has also been called "shrinkage necrosis." Ultimately the process leads to classic DNA degradation that yields a regular "ladder pattern" of fragmented genetic material that can be diagnostically recognized following gel electrophoresis of DNA as regularly separated, 180-bp fragments. Such DNA "laddering" is caused by the action of a specific class of endonucleases, the caspase-activated DNases (CADs), which are primarily activated by caspases but can also apparently be activated in a caspase-independent manner consistent with a caspase-independent form of apoptosis. Caspase-independent apoptosis is also initiated by leakage of mitochondrial proteins, including endonuclease G and apoptosis-inducing factor. However, rather than activate caspases these apoptogenic factors are translocated to the nucleus in which they can act to mediate characteristic DNA degradation. Therefore, unlike necrosis, apoptosis is a quiet process with respect to a lack of inflammation and damage to surrounding cells. Instead, the neighbor cells are actively recruited into this morbid process by specific "eat me" phospholipid signals displayed on the surface of the dying cell. Neighbor cells respond by engulfing and phagocytosing the corpse, resulting in its elimination without inflammatory fanfare or collateral injury.

From: *Principles of Molecular Medicine, Second Edition*
Edited by: M. S. Runge and C. Patterson © Humana Press, Inc., Totowa, NJ

Table 72-1
Types of Cell Death

Necrosis
   "Explosive" but passive process
   Cell swelling and lysis
   DNA intact
   Inflammation
Anoikis
   Apoptosis following loss of cell–cell contact
Autophagy
   Golgi, mitochondrial, endoplasmic reticulum membrane
      degradation
   Autophagic vacuoles formed
   May "blend" with apoptosis
Apoptosis
   Cell directed "suicide"
   Volume loss
   Membrane blebbing
   Chromatin condensation
   DNA fragmentation
   Apoptotic bodies
   Noninflammatory process
   Neighborhood cell engulfment

Table 72-2
Physiological Relevance of Apoptosis

Embryonic development
Regulation of immune system
   Immune cell development
   Cytolytic T-cell killing (e.g., immune surveillance,
      viral infections)
   Terminating active immune response
   Tight regulation/renewal of cell numbers (e.g., bone marrow,
      gastrointestinal, uterus, skin)
Compensatory response to cell stress
   Intrinsic pathway (e.g., Growth factor removal, external
      radiation therapy, chemotherapy)
   Extrinsic pathway (e.g., FAS.Ag, TNF-R activation)
Senescence/aging

Table 72-3
Apoptosis and Pathology

Insufficient (too little)
   Cancer
   Developmental defects
Excessive (too much)
   Neurodegenerative
   Autoimmune
   Cardiovascular
   Developmental defects
   AIDS (T4 cells)

ANOIKIS AND AUTOPHAGY Two other types of apoptotic-like cell death occur. Anoikis occurs in adherent cells (e.g., fibroblasts and some epithelial cells) that have lost their cell–cell or cell–matrix contact necessary for providing survival signals via integrin binding and "inside-out" survival signaling. Following loss of contact with its environmental substratum, the detached cell undergoes apoptosis. By contrast, autophagy was initially described in yeast and later found to operate in mammalian cells. Autophagy is a process whereby yeast cells are forced to engulf their own organelles in response to amino acid/nutrient starvation. Such recycling occurs in a unique "double-membrane" vesicle, the autophagosome, which surrounds and degrades organellar proteins in an attempt to replenish the depleted intracellular pool of amino acids/nutrients. This provides the affected cell with a means to survive, at least short term, until a more hospitable microenvironment becomes available. However, if uncompensated, by improved nutritional conditions, ongoing autophagy apparently will evolve into cell death indistinguishable from apoptosis.

CYTOLYTIC T CELLS AND NATURAL KILLER CELLS INDUCE APOPTOSIS Cytolytic T-cells (CTLs) and natural killer (NK) lymphocytes utilize a granule-mediated exocytosis pathway to destroy their target, including virally-infected and malignant cells, by inducing apoptosis. For example, after targeting a cell for immune destruction, CTLs and NK cells release their cytotoxic granules that contain perforin and serine proteases known as granzymes. Perforin, a pore forming protein, permeates the membrane of target cell to facilitate the entrance of the injected granzymes. Once inside the cell, granzyme B, for example, can cleave and activate procaspase-3, BH3 interacting domain (BID) death agonist and inhibitor of the CAD nuclease to initiate apoptosis. Other granzymes (i.e., granzymes A and C) can apparently induce a caspase-independent type of cell death.

PHYSIOLOGICAL RELEVANCE

Apoptosis is essential for the regulation of normal embryonic development as well as the maintenance of cellular and tissue homoeostasis in the adult organism (Table 72-2). Unbalancing

apoptosis by either inappropriate activation or a failure to activate apoptosis pathways can lead to either a shortening or lengthening, respectively, of cell survival. This can result in various pathological consequences, including developmental defects, chronic degenerative and autoimmune disorders, and tumor development (Table 72-3). For example, accelerated or excessive apoptosis has been causally linked to autoimmune disorders including rheumatoid arthritis, systemic lupus erythematosus, as well as the chronic neurodegenerative disorders including Alzheimer's, Parkinson's, and Huntington's disease (*see* BCL-2 Family Members Regulate Apoptosis Pathway). In addition, primary or secondary immunodeficiency diseases (e.g., HIV), infertility, as well as congenital developmental defects (e.g., limb bud malformation) may result. Furthermore, failure to execute apoptosis following appropriate cues, including developmental or injurious stress, is a characteristic feature of cancer cells that facilitates their prolonged survival and drug-resistant phenotype.

APOPTOSIS PATHWAYS

Accounting for its ancient importance, apoptosis is conserved in metazoans from worms to man. Apoptosis is triggered in response to developmental cues or environmental stresses (e.g., viral infections, toxicant treatment, and so on) that activate a compensatory elimination response. In addition, the mitochondrion has emerged as the principle organelle that assumes the functional role of master "sensor" organ that responds to cell stress. Indeed, it is the mitochondria that act as a clearinghouse for stress injuries that trigger the intrinsic pathway. As such, this organelle pulls "double duty" for the cell by functioning as the cell's major source of energy production and its potential death arsenal. Although the mitochondrion functions during normal, unperturbed cell growth to generate life-sustaining chemical energy in the form of ATP that results from

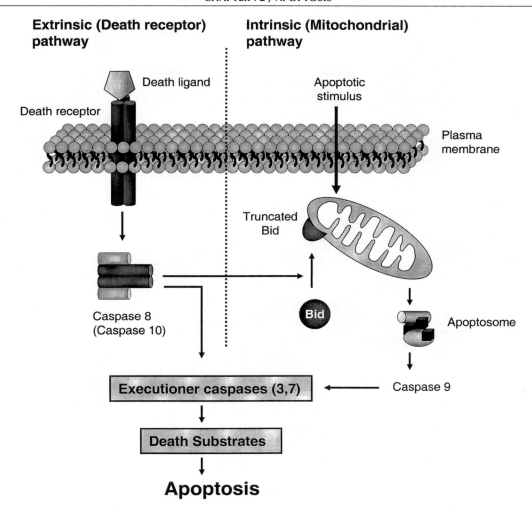

Figure 72-1 Apoptotic pathways. The extrinsic pathway is activated by binding of a death ligand (e.g., TNF-α, FAS.L, TRAIL) to its receptor, which sequentially triggers activation of the initiator caspase 8 followed by an executioner/effector caspase. The intrinsic pathway is activated following a death stimulus resulting from chemotherapy, irradiation or growth factor withdrawal that induces mitochondrial dysfunction characterized by leakage of apoptogenic factors, including cytochrome C, that lead to activation of initiator caspase 9 and effector caspase. Executioner caspases degrade specific substrates to bring about cell death. Cross talk between the extrinsic and intrinsic pathways can occur when caspase 8 cleaves cytosolic BID to truncated BID that is able to translocate to the mitochondria and trigger the intrinsic pathway. This serves to amplify the extrinsic pathway.

electron transfer and oxidative phosphorylation, it also sequesters and can release on cell injury factors that act as potent proapoptotic regulators. Perhaps surprisingly, such apoptogenic factors include the electron carrier cytochrome-C that not only serves as a major transducer of cellular energy but also as the key activator of procaspases when released into the cytosol. It is, therefore, critical to maintain mitochondrial integrity in order to protect cell survival. Apoptotic cell death proceeds through the highly regulated and coordinated signaling of two main pathways, the extrinsic and intrinsic pathways (Fig. 72-1). Although the net result of activation of either pathway will lead to cellular suicide via caspase activation, the regulatory components involved in the two pathways and their mechanism(s) of regulation are both varied and overlapping.

EXTRINSIC APOPTOTIC PATHWAY The extrinsic pathway is triggered by the binding of either soluble cytokines (tumor necrosis factor [TNF]-α, TNF-related apoptosis-inducing ligand [TRAIL]) or cell-bound death ligands (FAS.L) to their cognate surface receptors on target cells (*see* Fig. 72-1). TNF-α, and the FAS.L represent immune mediators produced by inflammatory

cells that are necessary for an appropriate immune response because they work with the effector immune cells that facilitate the removal of infected, neoplastic, aged or otherwise unwanted cells. Interestingly, the same cytokines also work to limit the immune attack by inducing the CTL to undergo apoptosis once its target is destroyed.

INTRINSIC APOPTOTIC PATHWAY By contrast, the intrinsic pathway is activated following either damage to an intracellular organelle (e.g., endoplasmic reticulum), DNA or the cytoskeleton following toxicant treatment or from the loss of growth factor–mediated survival signals. Mechanistically, the mitochondrion is able to "sense" cellular stress induced by damage to DNA, intracellular organelles (e.g., endoplasmic reticulum, Golgi, liposomes) or the cytoskeleton. This damage/stress results in the generation of an activated B-cell lymphoma (BCL)-2 homology (BH)-3-only proapoptotic member, (e.g., BID, BIM, and BAD), that translocates to the mitochondria to facilitate a BAX (or BAK) conformational change with oligomerization to form the "death pore" in the outer mitochondrial membrane (OMM). This

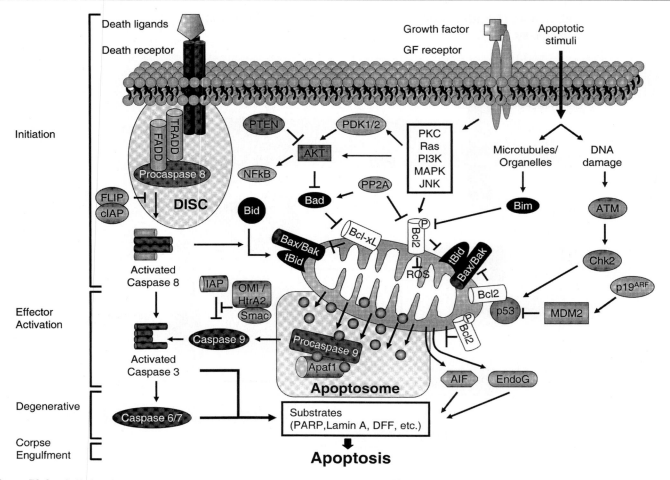

Figure 72-2 Cell signaling and apoptosis pathways are integrated. A schematic demonstrating interactions between growth and apoptotic signaling. Arrows (→) indicate stimulation and crosses (⊥) indicate inhibitory effects. The DISC and apoptosome platforms that enable activation of initiator caspases in extrinsic and intrinsic pathways, respectively, are indicated by light shading. Refer to text and other figures for details. Bcl2, B-cell lymphoma gene 2; GF, growth factor.

leads to leakage of intramembranous contents including cytochrome C and other apoptogenic factors that mediate activation of caspases. In this manner, the intrinsic pathway functions as the cell's compensatory response to overwhelming, nonrepairable damage and/or the prolonged depletion or loss of survival signals. The result is inducing its own death while sparing the undamaged neighbor cells the same fate.

To regulate mitochondrial integrity, the BCL-2 gene family has evolved as the principle guardians of the mitochondrion (Fig. 72-2). Interestingly, some of the members of this large gene family are antiapoptotic and function to maintain mitochondrial integrity by inhibiting the proapoptotic members that function to facilitate the release of apoptogenic mitochondrial intramembranous contents. Formation of a mitochondrial "death pore" with leakage of apoptogenic factors requires one of two proapoptotic members, BAX or BAK (*see* Caspase Proteases Mediate Apoptosis). Thus, although either BAX or BAK null mice are more resistant to toxicant treatment than wild type mice, BAX and BAK double knockout mice are highly resistant. The antiapoptotic BCL-2 family members of which BCL-2 is the prototype function to block mitochondrial dysfunction by binding to and inhibiting pore formation by BH3-only proapoptotic proteins interacting with BAX or BAK. In addition, BCL-2 can also function to block Ca²⁺ release from the endoplasmic reticulum that

can trigger apoptosis but the mechanism is not clear. Thus, the direct addition of proapoptotic BAX and BAK to isolated mitochondria induces cytochrome-C leakage in vitro, whereas overexpression of BCL-2 (or Bcl$_{XL}$, Mcl1, and so on) can block BAX or BAK induced cytochrome C release.

CASPASE PROTEASES MEDIATE APOPTOSIS

The intrinsic and extrinsic proteolytic doom that is created by apoptosis is mediated by a unique class of substrate-specific cysteine proteases known as caspases (i.e., c-terminal aspartate site cleaving proteases; *see* Fig. 72-1). Caspases are synthesized as inactive proenzymes that reside in the cytosol and can be activated by autoproteolysis. The identification and characterization of the caspases began with studies of one of the *C. elegans* death genes, Ced-3. Subsequent studies in mammalian cells led to the identification of the first human caspase, IL-Iβ-converting enzyme, now called Caspase 1. Iβ-converting enzyme is activated by autoproteolysis of its C terminus at a specific aspartate residue and the resulting heterodimer then specifically cleaves pro-IL-1β into the active, proinflammatory cytokine, IL-1β. More than 16 caspases have been identified, which cleave their substrates, which are either critical regulatory or structural proteins necessary for cell integrity. For example, cleavage of the nuclear lamins, PARP and DFF will lead to disruption of the

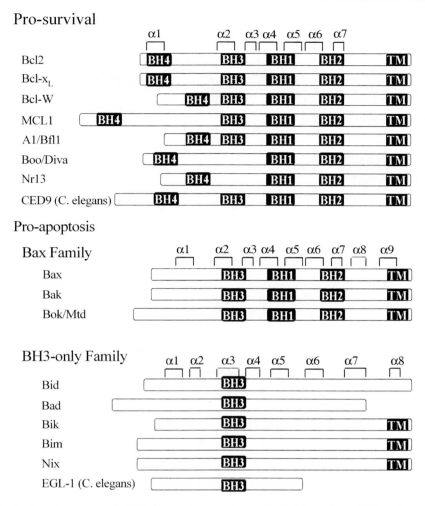

Figure 72-3 BCL-2 family. Anti- and proapoptotic BCL-2 members are shown. BCL-2 homology (BH) regions transmembrane domain and alpha helical structures are indicated.

nuclear envelope with classic DNA "ladder" degradation, whereas cleavage of α-Fodrin, MEKK, or FAK will affect growth signals that regulate and maintain cell shape. By degrading such substrates, caspases mediate intracellular liquefaction.

TWO CLASSES OF CASPASES Caspases are divided into initiators (e.g., caspases 8 and 10) and effectors (e.g., caspases 3, 6, and 7) based on their role in either initiating or executing apoptosis. In addition, different caspases have preferred aspartate cleavage sites, represented by a minimal putative tetrapeptide sequence (e.g., IETD for caspase 3; VETD for caspase 8), which is found in specific substrates. Activated caspases cleave their substrates on the C-terminal side of such aspartate residues. Once activated, the effector caspases target and degrade/inactivate key regulatory and structural polypeptides necessary for the maintenance of cell integrity. In addition to proteolysis of selected substrates and to ensure inactivation of the dying cell's genetic capabilities, effector caspase activation also results in activation of specific endonucleases, the CADs, which degrade cellular DNA to produce the "hallmark" molecular signature of apoptosis, DNA laddering.

CASPASE ACTIVATION Caspases are synthesized and remain in their inactive, proenzyme state during unstressed cell growth. However, developmental cues or noxious, toxicant stresses can trigger their activation. Procaspases are made up of an N-terminal

prodomain (long in length in case of initiator caspases and short for effector caspases) that is cleaved to yield a p20 and a p10 kDa domain molecule that heterodimerize. Autocleavage of the procaspases occurs at a specific internal aspartate site to yield the p20/p10 dimer that then forms a tetramer, which represents the mature form of the activated protease (Fig. 72-3). Initially, an initiator procaspase becomes activated, which cleaves and activates a downstream effector caspase. This serial activation is referred to as the "caspase cascade." Initiator caspase activation occurs on one of two different bioplatforms, the death-inducing signaling complex (DISC) in the extrinsic and the apoptosome in the intrinsic apoptotic pathway.

Death-mediating ligands including TNF-α, FAS ligand or TRAIL bind to their cognate surface receptors and induce aggregation of receptor-associated molecules. This creates an intracellular "platform," called the DISC, for the assembly of specific adapter and regulatory molecules (i.e., TRADD or FADD) necessary to achieve activation of procaspase 8 (Fig. 72-4). The DISC functions like a sponge to increase the local concentration of procaspase 8 or 10 and regulatory molecules and facilitate autocleavage and activation of the initiator caspases (i.e., induced proximity model). Once an initiator caspase is activated, it targets and cleaves cytosolic procaspase 3. Activated effector

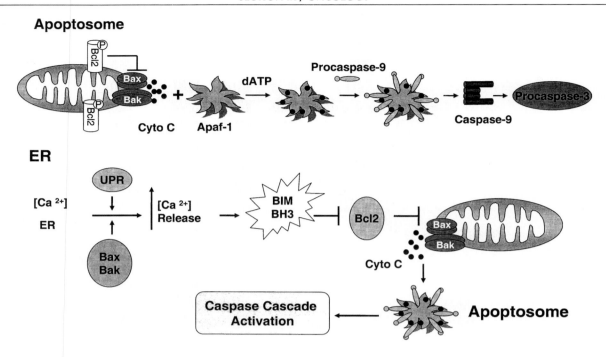

Figure 72-4 Apoptosome and endoplasmic reticulum. Dysregulation of the mitochondria or endoplasmic reticulum can lead to activation of the intrinsic apoptotic pathway. Bcl2, B-cell lymphoma gene 2; BH3, BCL-2 homology 3.

caspase 3 then proceeds to wreak intracellular proteolytic doom. Receptor-mediated activation of apoptosis occurs independently of the mitochondria in some cells called type-I cells (e.g., Thymocytes). Alternately, caspase 8 activation may lead to "recruitment" of the intrinsic/mitochondrial pathway in cells referred to as type-II cells (e.g., hepatocytes). This "recruitment" serves to amplify the extrinsic pathway and results from caspase 8 being able to directly activate caspase 3 and also being able to target and cleave the cytosolic BH-3 only proapoptotic molecule, BID, into its truncated, activated form, tBID. Activated tBID then is able to translocate from the cytosol to the mitochondrion where it binds and disrupts the interaction between BCL-2 (or other antiapoptotic members like Bcl$_{XL}$) and directly activates BAX (or BAK) (*see* Fig. 72-2). As a result, BAX (or BAK) becomes "functionally" released from inhibition and undergoes a structural conformational change that apparently facilitates its integral insertion into the OMM via its transmembrane domain. Insertion and oligomerization create the "death pore" through which the intramembranous contents are leaked into the cytosol to trigger activation of initiator procaspase 9.

For the intrinsic pathway, initiator and effector caspases are activated following a nonreceptor mediated stress event (e.g., toxicant treatment or withdrawal of growth factor survival signals) that results in mitochondrial dysfunction with release of cytochrome C and other apoptogenic factors. Release induces formation of the apoptosome complex that consists of apoptosis protease activating factor (APaf-1), cytochrome C, dATP, and procaspase 9. Following release from mitochondria, cytochrome-C, and Apaf-1 bind, allowing procaspase 9 to also bind Apaf-1 via its caspase activation and recruitment domain, a feature of all caspases. The "mature" apoptosome then facilitates the efficient autocleavage of procaspase 9, which in turn activates cytosolic procaspase 3 in a postmitochondrial mechanism.

INHIBITION OF CASPASES   As a safeguard against chance activation of caspases, normal cellular (and some viral) proteins known as inhibitors of apoptosis (IAP; e.g., including cFLIP, cIAP, and survivin) or the baculovirus p35 protein can inhibit caspases. Interestingly, IAP activity was initially recognized in a baculovirus gene product, p35, which inhibits the proteolytic activity of caspases following viral infection of insect cells. Caspase inhibition allows the virus to maximally replicate by overcoming this host-antiviral mechanism. Later, mammalian cells were also found to express a related activity, cIAP. The IAP contain common tandem repeats known as baculovirus inhibitory repeats that enable their binding to and inactivation of caspases (*see* Fig. 72-2). Cellular IAP may function by either directly inhibiting caspases or by targeting the caspase for ubiquitination and degradation by the proteosome. However, to ensure success of activated caspases, IAP activity can also be inhibited by mitochondrial factors also released along with apoptogenic factors, including SMAC/DIABLO and OMI/HtrA2. These inhibitors function to either directly block cIAP from binding to the activation site of a caspase or by competing with the cIAP once bound to an activated caspase. Because SMAC/DIABLO and OMI/HtrA2 are also sequestered in the mitochondria and released along with cytochrome-C (and other caspase activators), they help to ensure a feedforward functioning of the death pathway once activated.

DEATH RECEPTORS MAY ALSO BE ASSOCIATED WITH SURVIVAL SIGNALING   In addition to TNF-α and FAS.L, death ligand-induced apoptosis may also be triggered by TRAIL and apoptosis antigen 3 binding to their receptors, DR 4/5 or DR3. TRAIL or apoptosis antigen 3 binding also sequentially induces caspases 8 and 3 activation and can activate BID to "recruit" the intrinsic death pathway. Because some cancer cells are reported to maintain sensitivity to TRAIL-induced killing, exploitation of this vulnerability as a potential cancer treatment is being studied.

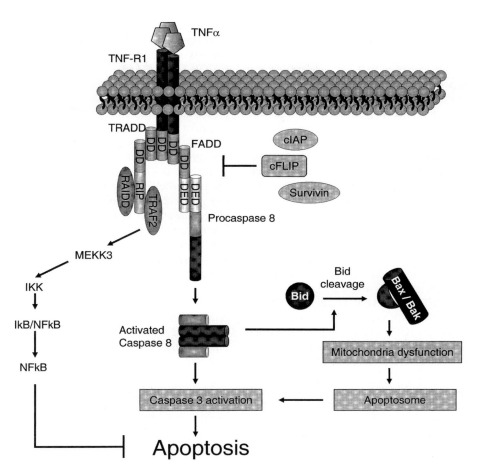

Figure 72-5 Apoptosis signaling through extrinsic death receptors. Binding of the death ligand TNF-α (or FAS.L or TRAIL) to the TNF receptor leads to the formation of the DISC. Made up of adapter molecules, TRADD or FADD bind to the death domain of the receptor and bind to procaspase 8 via its death effector domain (DED-DED). This leads to activation of initiator caspase 8 and triggering of the extrinsic pathway. In some cells, TNF-α binding to its receptor, TNF-R1, and TRADD may recruit RIP, RAIDD and TRAF2, which can result in NF-κβ activation and cell survival signaling that results in upregulation of NF-κβ genes including IAP and cFLIP that inhibit caspases.

However, although FAS.L and TRAIL or APO3L signaling induce apoptosis, TNF-α binding does not always induce cell death. Under certain circumstances, TNF-α can promote cell growth. The mechanism(s) by which TNF-α decides on death or growth appears to result from a cell-type specific type of differential signaling. Thus, while binding of the TRADD and FADD adapter protein to the intracytoplasmic portion of the TNF receptor will induce caspase 8 activation, TRADD binding to RIP and RAIDD may affect other regulators including TRAF2, that can stimulate nuclear factor (NF)-κβ and inhibitor of NF-κβ (Iκβ) kinase. Thus when activated, Iκβ kinase phosphorylates and releases Iκβ, inhibitor of NF-κβ, resulting in its transcriptional activation. This induces NF-κβ-responsive genes, including cFLIP and other IAP, whose activities help prevent procaspase 8 from being activated and results in blocking the TNF-α death signal (Fig. 72-5). However, when the NF-κβ signal falters or becomes weak, the preassembled TRADD-procaspase 8 complex can now activate caspase 8 to engage the extrinsic pathway. Such differential signaling by TNF-α indicates the delicate balance between life and death in certain cells. It also suggests a novel antitumor strategy whereby blocking TNF-α-mediated NF-κβ survival signaling in certain tumors could trip the activation of the extrinsic death pathway. When combined with the effects of chemo- or radiation therapy, this could potentially enhance their cytotoxicity.

BCL-2 FAMILY MEMBERS REGULATE APOPTOSIS PATHWAY

BCL-2 is the prototype and founding member of this large family of regulators of apoptosis (*see* Fig. 72-3). BCL-2 was discovered as the product of translocation of chromosome 14 and 18, t (14; 18) that characteristically occurs in up to 85% of human follicular BCLs. The resulting chromosomal fusion conjoins BCL-2 and the proximal immunoglobulin promoter, which functionally results in overexpression of BCL-2 in B cells. However, unlike other oncogenes, BCL-2 does not promote cell proliferation, rather it cooperates with oncogenes by enhancing cell survival. This unique property was discovered when it was demonstrated that forced expression of BCL-2 in IL-3 factor-dependent cells significantly delayed cell death following growth factor deprivation or on treatment with cytotoxic agents or irradiation. Because BCL-2 is primarily localized to mitochondria, with some expression in the endoplasmic reticulum and nuclear envelope, this highlighted mitochondria in the cell death process. The discovery of BCL-2 also sparked a new field of biomedical research in the mid 1980s and has led to the identification of a large family of structurally related BCL-2 proteins with both antiapoptotic and proapoptotic functions. For example, BCL-2, Bcl_{XL}, Mcl, and Al contain all four BH domains and are antiapoptotic and suppress cell death. Other members, including BAX, BAK, BAD, BID, and BIM that contain BH 1-3 or BH-3 only domains are proapoptotic and can induce cell death (*see* Figs. 72-2 and 72-3). Consistent with its oncogenic role in tumorigenesis, mice whose B cells overexpress the BCL-2 transgene develop a polyclonal follicular hyperplasia, and some even develop a monoclonal BCL that recapitulates the human lymphoproliferative disease. By contrast, BCL-2 null mice display early and massive apoptosis of their lymphocytes as well as other developmental defects including renal insufficiency and a deficiency in pigmentation of the melanocyte. Interestingly and of particular relevance to tumor biology, in addition to follicular lymphomas, many or even most human cancers including breast, lung, colon, prostate, melanoma, and leukemia also express high levels of BCL-2 (or other antiapoptotic members such as Bcl_{XL} or Mcll) albeit not as the result of a t(14;18) chromosomal translocation. Interestingly, in addition to functioning to suppress apoptosis, BCL-2 has two other properties: it can retard cell-cycle entry from G1 and has an antioxidant function such that its expression in cells is associated with decreased reactive oxygen species (ROS) levels.

ANTI- AND PROAPOPTOTIC FUNCTION OF BCL-2 MEMBERS   BCL-2 family members are classified based on their sharing of conserved BH domains, BH1-4 (*see* Fig. 72-3). Although antiapoptotic members contain all four BH domains, proapoptotic members contain either BH1-3 or a BH-3-only domain. The BH-3 domain is necessary for the proapoptotic function. Indeed, removing BCL-2's BH4 domain and leaving its BH3 domain unopposed, can convert BCL-2 into a proapoptotic BH1-3 containing molecule (like BAX or BAK). Solution and crystal structure of Bcl_{XL} and BCL-2 have revealed that the BH1, 2, and 3 domains fold to create a hydrophobic pocket that will accommodate the BH-3 domain of another proapoptotic family member such as BAX (or BAK), which results in the effective neutralization of its killing potential. Furthermore, it is the BH3-domain that apparently must be so shielded because synthetic BH-3-only containing peptides, or small organic molecules that can block BCL-2 (or Bcl_{XL}) and BAX (or BAK) heterodimerization, can also bring about apoptosis. This appears to result in the exposure of the α-helical BH-3 domain of BAX (or BAK) with subsequent integral insertion into the OMM to form the "death pore." Although BAX (or BAK) is required for mitochondrial disruption and apoptosis, simply overexpressing BAX or BAK in most cells is not sufficient to trigger apoptosis without a concurrent stress signal. This indicates that some type of post-transcriptional regulation is generally required for their activation.

BH-3 only proapoptotic members include BID, BAD, BIM, NOXA, and PUMA. When activated following stress, these proapoptotic members act as messengers to convey the death signal generated by a damaged organelle or DNA to the mitochondria. Functionally, when BAX (or BAK) becomes "activated" as a result of a conformational change in its structure triggered either by stress or binding to a BH-3-only containing molecule like tBID, BAX (or BAK) undergoes insertion and oligomerization within the OMM to create a "death" pore-like gateway through which mitochondrial contents, including cytochrome C and other apoptogenic factors, may leak to trigger caspase activation. Mechanistically, an accepted model holds that in viable, unstressed cells, BAX exists primarily in the cytosol or is only peripherally associated in monomeric form but not yet integrated into the OMM. Following a death stimulus, BAX undergoes a conformational change leading to exposure of its transmembrane domain that facilitates insertion into the OMM in which it

also may bind a BH3-only member like tBID to facilitate the oligomerization that produces pore formation. Because of the similarity between the α-helical structures of bacterial pore-forming toxic proteins and BAX, one general model holds that oligomerized BAX/BAK may form death pores large enough to release cytochrome C. This is considered a viable hypothesis because BAX forms pores in artificial lipid membranes that are capable of releasing cytochrome C. Another model implicates the well described mitochondrial permeability transition pore that forms between the inner and OMMs as a result of complexing between the voltage dependent anion channel, the adenine nucleotide transporter and cyclophilin D. This channel will leak ions and dissipate ion gradients and result in the collapse of the mitochondrial membrane potential ($\Delta\Psi_m$) that leads to mitochondrial swelling and rupture, with release of cytochrome-C along and apoptogenic activators. However, because cytochrome-C release precedes both permeability transition pore formation and loss of $\Delta\Psi_m$ that occurs during apoptosis, this is a less attractive mechanism to explain how cytochrome C is released and caspases are activated in apoptosis.

REGULATION OF BCL-2 MEMBERS BY PHOSPHORYLATION   Antiapoptotic BCL-2 (and MCL-1 and Bcl_{XL}) as well as proapoptotic BAD are regulated by phosphorylation (Fig. 72-6). For BCL-2, serum and growth factors such as IL-3 mediate its phosphorylation on serine 70, a site located within the flexible loop domain (FLD) that positively regulates its antiapoptotic function. The "regulatory" FLD domain lies between BH4 and BH3 regions in BCL-2 (*see* Fig. 72-4). Phosphorylation can be mediated by several growth factor-activated protein kinases, including the MAP kinases, ERK 1 and 2 and JNK1 and 2, as well as PKC and the CDC2 kinase. Multisite phosphorylation of BCL-2 in the FLD at serine 70, threonine 69 and serine 87 can also occur when cells are treated with microtubule disrupting agents such as paclitaxel and vincristine. As revealed by phosphomimetic or nonphosphorylatable BCL-2 mutants, phosphorylation at any of these sites can significantly enhance its antiapoptotic function. Mechanistically, phosphorylation appears to stabilize the BCL-2/BAX interaction as well as protect BCL-2 from degradation that can occur during apoptosis.

The majority of BCL-2 expressed in the cell is localized in the mitochondria with some in the endoplasmic reticulum and nuclear envelope. Interestingly, the majority of cellular ROS are generated (at least in nonphagocytic cells) in the mitochondria. In addition, although the mechanism is not clear, BCL-2 phosphorylation also regulates its antioxidant and cell cycle entry functions. That is, expression of wt and phosphomimetic but not nonphosphorylatable BCL-2 mutants in cells results in a significantly reduced level of cellular ROS and slower cell growth. Furthermore, slower growth results from BCL-2's ability to retard cell cycle entry from G1 and is closely associated with upregulation of the cyclin inhibitor p27 and downregulation of CdK2 activity. Increasing ROS levels in such slowly cycling cells by adding low concentrations of hydrogen peroxide directly to them can reverse the effect, suggesting that BCL-2's antioxidant function may play a role in regulating cell-cycle entry. This apparent functional linkage between BCL-2's antiapoptotic, cell-cycle retardation and antioxidant properties seem to underscore BCL-2's central role in managing cell stress and apoptosis. That is, cells can generally withstand the effects of an apoptotic-inducing stress better when they are not cycling and ROS levels are lower, as compared to cells undergoing DNA replication and/or cell mitotic division when ROS levels are elevated.

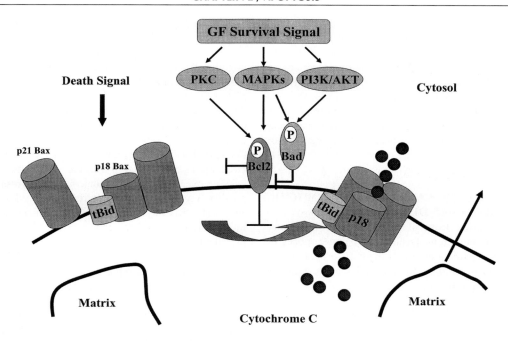

Figure 72-6 Regulation of BCL-2 and BAD by phosphorylation. Growth factors such as IL-3 can activate protein kinases to directly phosphorylate BCL-2 and BAD. BCL-2 phosphorylation blocks BAX oligomerization and "death pore" formation mediated by tBID that leads to cytochrome C release. BCL-2 also can block cleavage of full length p21 BAX to p18 BAX by a cathepsin-like protease. Phosphorylated BAD is inactive and sequestered in the cytosol. Following a death signal, BAD becomes dephosphorylated and can translocate to the mitochondria and bind and inhibit BCL-2's antiapoptotic function. BCL-2, B-cell lymphoma gene 2.

Whether other antiapoptotic BCL-2 members also may regulate the cell cycle and possess antioxidant effects is not clear.

BAX is the first proapoptotic member of the BCL-2 family to be identified as the heterodimeric binding partner of BCL-2. One popular model holds that BCL-2 binds and neutralizes BAX's proapoptotic activity. The ratio of anti- to proapoptotic activity blocking binding of BH3-only proapoptotic molecules (i.e., BCL-2/BAX) is thought to act like a survival "biorheostat" and set the threshold of cell susceptibility to activation of the intrinsic pathway. Growth factors cannot only provide survival signals to activate antiapoptotic and suppress proapoptotic members but also can transcriptionally increase expression of Bcl_{XL} (and BCL-2 and Mcl1) to facilitate survival. By contrast, stress-induced activation of p53 can induce upregulation of p53 responsive genes including the proapoptotic molecules BAX/PUMA and NOXA that can induce cell death. This outcome alters the BCL-2/BAX ratio such that increased BCL-2 (or Bcl_{XL}) or reduced BAX or (BAK) levels favor survival whereas reduced BCL-2 (or Bcl_{XL}) or increased BAX or (BAK) expression favor increased sensitivity to cytotoxic treatments. In the former case, tumor cells would potentially gain both a survival advantage and a drug-resistance phenotype advantage that could provide a selective growth advantage.

As mentioned, regulating the function of BH-3-only proapoptotic members can occur by several mechanisms including phosphorylation and sequestration away from the mitochondria or proteolytic activation with translocation to the mitochondria. For example, IL-3 addition to factor dependent cells induces multisite phosphorylation of BAD, which then bind to protein 14-3-3 in the cytosol away from the mitochondria. However, following growth factor withdrawal, a BAD PP2A-like phosphatase is activated that mediates dephosphorylation, which interrupts its binding to 14-3-3. That leads to BAD's translocation to mitochondria in which it can directly bind BCL-2

(or Bcl_{XL}) to disrupt the BCL-2:BAX interaction and lead to BAX activation. This causes "death pore" formation and mitochondrial dysfunction with activation of the intrinsic pathway as discussed.

Another BH-3-only molecule, BIM, can also be sequestered from the mitochondria by localizing to the myotubule-associated dynin light chain (LC8) that is part of the motor complex. Following drug treatment, the BIM-LC8 complex is released and BIM is translocated to the mitochondria in which it can now bind and inhibit BCL-2 (or Bcl_{XL}) interaction with to gain access to BAX (or BAK). Thus, activation and translocation of BH3-only proapoptotic molecules to mitochondria represents a common regulatory theme for BH-3 only proapoptotic molecules. Although antiapoptotic BCL-2 and Bcl_{XL} members potentially function to bind and neutralize BAX (or BAK), their activity can be overcome by a barrage of such activated BH-3-only molecules. This has prompted investigators to design novel agents that might target and block the BCL-2/ BAX interaction. Various strategies including antisense technology (e.g., BCL-2 antisense) and design and synthesis of cell permeable small molecule inhibitors of BCL-2 (or Bcl_{XL}) that bind to the BH-3 domain are being developed as potential cancer treatments. Additionally, stabilizing the BCL-2/ BAX interaction or inhibiting caspase activation may potentially preserve the vulnerable tissues in degenerative diseases where the intrinsic pathway is overactive.

p53 AND APOPTOSIS   Independent of its transcriptional role in mediating cell-cycle arrest and apoptosis, p53 apparently can also stimulate apoptosis when localized in the cytosol. This can occur by directly binding to BCL-2 (or $BCL-2_{XL}$) to promote the disassociation of BCL-2/BAX, which results in enhanced BAX proapoptotic activity (*see* Fig. 72-2). p53 not only resides in the nucleus where it functions as a transactivator but also surprisingly may accumulate in the cytosol. Even when deficient in transactivation function, p53 can directly bind BCL-2 (or BCL-2$_{XL}$) and lead to BAX activation and engagement of the intrinsic apoptotic program. Although the mechanism is not clear, p53 may facilitate binding of a BH-3 only proapoptotic molecule to Bcl$_{XL}$ (or BCL-2). Thus, the p53 tumor suppressor may pull "double duty" in regulating cellular responses to stress: first, by functioning in the nucleus as a transcriptioned regulator of genes involved in cell-cycle arrest, and DNA repair and apoptosis, second by working also in the cytosol as a proapoptotic regulator of the intrinsic death pathway.

APOPTOSIS AND DISEASE

GROWTH FACTOR SIGNALING AND APOPTOTIC PATHWAYS IN MALIGNANT DISEASE   Tumorigenesis is a multistep process resulting from a spontaneous or hereditary mutation or epigenetic alteration of cellular protoonocogenes or tumor suppressor genes. Mutations confer the transformed phenotype of the cancer cell that results from the cell having acquired at least two of the following properties:

1. Replicate in the absence of growth signals.
2. Overcome growth-inhibitory signals.
3. Avoid the host immune surveillance.
4. Maintain an adequate oxygen and nutrient supply necessary for invasion and metastases to unfamiliar microenvironments.
5. Avoid apoptotic cell death.

However, without thwarting apoptosis, the tumor cell would be unable to survive to exhibit its abnormal growth. Furthermore, because malignant cells can both multiply and survive under the most inhospitable of metabolic and microenvironmental conditions (e.g., hypoxia, nutrient depletion) and must be able to successfully defend themselves against or avoid the host antitumor immune response, it is not surprising that mutational or epigenetic alterations of these same genes may affect both proliferation and cell survival. In addition, because chemotherapy and irradiation mediate toxicity by triggering the intrinsic apoptotic pathway, blocking or inhibiting apoptosis in cancer cells may not only cooperate in oncogenicity but also confer a drug resistant phenotype. This linkage seems teleological because it results in conservation of energy and functional simplicity. However, with such interdependence comes the potential risk that mutation of a common component may substantially affect both processes.

Indeed, as discussed, either inactivating mutations or downregulation of proapoptotic genes, including BAX, have been identified in some cancers, which would result in a weakening of the cell's ability to efficiently undergo apoptosis following chemoradiation therapy. In addition, increased expression or an activating mutation of an antiapoptotic gene product like BCL-2 or Mcl-1 may potentially facilitate the development of the malignant phenotype by enhancing cell survival. Interestingly, in addition to lymphomas, BCL-2 is reported to be over/highly expressed in many other cancers, indicating that altered expression of BCL-2 or other antiapoptotic BCL-2 members is a common target in malignancies. Other antiapoptotic regulators may be involved in tumor cells. For example, the cIAP, including c-FLIP, are overexposed in some cancers and implicated in the resistance of tumor cells to chemotherapy-induced activation of caspases. Already well described mutations in critical oncogenes such as RAS, AKT, Myc, PI3K, NF-κβ, and MDM2, clearly lead to enhanced mitogenesis and to enhanced survival as a result of the downregulation of the intrinsic death pathway.

Furthermore, inactivating mutations of tumor suppressor genes including p53, p19^{ARF}, ATM, ChK2, and Rb also prevent cell-cycle inhibition and promote survival of cancer cells. Of particular note, p53 apparently can play a dual role in regulating apoptosis. Although an inactivating mutation of p53 not only inhibits its transcriptional activity and upregulation of proapoptotic genes like BAX, NOXA, PUMA, it may also block its newly described function to directly bind and prevent Bcl$_{XL}$ (or BCL-2) from neutralizing BAX's proapoptotic activity.

Moreover, mutations in transcriptional silencing of some of the positive regulators of the extrinsic (e.g., FAS Antigen/CD95, TRAIL-R1/R2, or proCaspase 8) or intrinsic (e.g., Apaf-1) apoptotic pathways have been reported in various cancers. Therefore, therapeutic targeting with the intent of inhibiting these proapoptotic regulators has the potential for enhancing cell death in cancer cells. This concept represents an active field of research among oncologists and has the potential to add a therapeutic approach to the anticancer armamentarium.

Finally, patients with a heterozygous mutation in the FAS antigen or those with initiator caspase-10 deficiency may develop an autoimmune lymphoproliferative syndrome characterized by ineffective lymphocyte apoptosis. In addition, mutation of caspase-8, another initiator caspase, can result in autoimmunity characterized by a developmental immunodeficiency resulting from defects in T-, B-, and NK-cell activation.

APOPTOSIS IN NONMALIGNANT DISEASES   Neurodegenerative disorders, including Alzheimer's, Parkinson's, Huntington's, and the prion disease, scrapie, represent diseases in which inappropriately enhanced apoptosis has been observed and may be causative. For example, in Alzheimer's and Huntington's disease, failure of proper folding of proteins within the endoplasmic reticulum that results from defects in chaperone protein partner binding, appears to lead to a misfolded or "unfolded" protein. This constitutes a form of organelle stress and stimulates the unfolded protein response, which is a normal, compensatory response leading to degradation of the misfolded products in an attempt to restore proper "protein homeostasis." However, when overwhelmed by too many "misfolded" proteins, the normal unfolded protein response may itself lead to cell damage of the endoplasmic reticulum and trigger endoplasmic reticulum-initiated apoptosis. For example, in Alzheimer's disease, neurotoxicity is associated with an abnormal accumulation of amyloid-β-peptides owing to a failure of appropriate cleavage of the normal amyloid precursor protein. This buildup results in local endoplasmic reticulum-lipid peroxidation, leads to increased Ca^{2+} release from the endoplasmic reticulum, and triggers activation of caspase-12, leading to mitochondrial dysregulation and neuronal cell death by activation of the intrinsic pathway. In Huntington's disease, a mutant Huntingtin protein fails to function normally in the formation of a clathrin complex involved in normal vesicular transport during neurotransmitter release from neurons. Malfunction of this protein appears to result in the activation of both the initiator caspase-8 and effector caspase-3 and is linked to the neurotoxic properties of mutant Huntingtin protein cleavage products. Finally, for at least one form of Parkinson's disease, the autosomal-recessive juvenile Parkinson's disease, protein homeostasis in the endoplasmic reticulum may be disrupted in a different way by utilizing the process of endoplasmic reticulum-associated protein degradation of ubiquitinated proteins by the proteosome pathway.

Activation of this pathway may result in the death of dopaminergic neurons characteristic of Parkinson's disease.

Neuronal cell death may also play a role in another neurodegenerative disorder, the prion disease scrapie. Although cellular prion protein, PrP^c, is ubiquitously expressed on the cell membrane as a glycosylphosphotidyl-inositol-linked glycoprotein, when misassembled into an abnormal conformer, PrP^{sc}, it is associated with prion-mediated apoptosis. Thus, although apoptosis appears to play a critical role in neurodegenerative diseases, whether it is causative or merely an effect of the disease is not clear. Nonetheless, blocking activation of caspases and apoptosis in such diseased tissues is an active strategy that, if successful, may at least slow the degenerative process.

ACKNOWLEDGMENT

We would like to thank Janice Taylor for her excellent administrative support in the preparation of this manuscript.

SELECTED REFERENCES

Alnemri ES, Livingston DJ, Nicholson DW, et al. Human ICE/CED-3 protease nomenclature. Cell 1996;87:171.

Ashkenazi A, Dixit VM. Death receptors signaling and modulation. Science 1998;281:1305–1308.

Bakhshi A, Jensen JP, Goldman P, et al. Cloning the chromosomal breakpoint of t(14:18) human lymphomas: clustering around JH on chromosome 14 and hear a transcriptional unit on 18. Cell 1985;41:899–906.

Boise LH, Gonzalez-Garcia M, Postema CE, et al. Bcl-x, a bcl-2-related gene that functions as a dominant regulator of apoptotic cell death. Cell 1993;74:597–608.

Bratton SB, Cohen GM. Apoptotic death sensor: an organelle's alter ego. Trends Pharmacol Sci 2001;22:306–315.

Cory S, Adams JM. The Bcl2 family: regulators of the cellular life-or-death switch. Nat Rev Cancer 2002;2:647–656.

Cory S, Huang DCS, Adama JM. The Bcl2 family: roles in cell survival and oncogenesis. Oncogene 2003;22:8590–8607.

Deng X, Gao F, Flagg T, May WS. Mono- and multi-site phosphorylation enhance Bcl2's anti-apoptotic and inhibition of cell cycle entry functions. Proc Natl Acad Sci USA 2004;101:153–158.

Du C, Fang M, Li Y, Li L, Wang X. Smac, a mitochondrial protein that promotes cytochrome c-dependent caspase activation by eliminating IAP inhibition. Cell 2000;102:33–42.

Enari M, Sakahira H, Yokoyama H, Okawa K, Iwamatsu A, Nagata S. A caspase-activated DNase that degrades DNA during apoptosis, and its inhibitor ICAD. Nature 1998;391:43–50.

Ferri KF, Kroemer G. Organelle-specific initiation of cell death pathways. Nat Cell Biol 2001;3:255–263.

Goldstein JC, Waterhouse NJ, Juin P, Evan GI, Green DR. The coordinate release of cytochrome c during apoptosis is rapid, complete and kinetically invariant. Nat Cell Biol 2000;2:156–162.

Hengartner MO. Programmed cell death in the nematode *C. elegans*. Recent Prog Horm Res 1999;54:213–222.

Heusel JW, Wesselschmidt RL, Shresta S, Russel JH, Ley TJ. Cytotoxic lymphocytes require granzyme B for the rapid induction of DNA fragmentation and apoptosis in allogeneic target cells. Cell 1994;76: 977–987.

Hockenbery D, Nunez G, Milliman C, Schreiber RD, Korsmeyer SJ. Bcl-2 is an inner mitochondrial membrane protein that blocks programmed cell death. Nature 1990;348:334–336.

Hsu H, Xiong J, Goeddel DV. The TNF receptor 1-associated protein TRADD signals cell death and NF-kappa B activation. Cell 1995;81: 495–504.

Huang DC, Strasser A. BH3-only proteins-essential initiators of apoptotic cell death. Cell 2000;103:839–842.

Kerr JF, Wyllie AH, Currie AR. Apoptosis: a basic biological phenomenon with wide-ranging implications in tissue kinetics. Br J Cancer 1972; 26:239–257.

Kornblau SM, Vu HT, Ruvolo P, et al. Bax and PKCα modulate the prognostic impact of Bcl2 expression in acute myelogenous leukemia. Clin Cancer Res 2000;6:1401–1409.

Levine AJ. P53, the cellular gatekeeper for growth and division. Cell 1997;88:323–331.

Levine B, Klionsky DJ. Development by self-digestion: molecular mechanisms and biological functions of autophagy. Dev Cell 2004;6: 463–477.

Meier P, Finch A, Evan G. Apoptosis in development. Nature 2000;407: 796–801.

Miyashita T, Reed JC. Tumor suppressor p53 is a direct transcriptional activator of the human bax gene. Cell 1995;80:293–299.

Nicholson DW. Caspase structure, proteolytic substrates and function during apoptotic cell death. Cell Death Differ 1999;6:1028–1042.

Salvesen GS, Dixit VM. Caspases: intracellular signaling by proteolysis. Cell 1997;91:443–446.

Takeshige K, Baba M, Tsuboi S, Noda T, Ohsumi Y. Autophagy in yeast demonstrated with proteinase-deficient mutants and conditions for its induction. J Cell Biol 1992;119:301–311.

Thornberry NA, Lazebnik Y. Caspases: enemies within. Science 1998; 281:1312–1316.

Vaux DL, Cory S, Adams JM. Bcl-2 gene promotes haemopoietic cell survival and cooperates with c-myc to immortalize pre-B cells. Nature 1988;335:440–442.

Vogelstein B, Lane D, Levine AJ. Surfing the p53 network. Nature 2000; 408:307–310.

Wang CY, Mayo MW, Baldwin AS. TNF- and cancer therapy-induced apoptosis: potentiation by inhibition of NF-κB. Science 1996;274: 777–784.

Wei MC, Zong WX, Cheng EH, et al. Proapoptotic BAX and BAK: a requisite gateway to mitochondrial dysfunction and death. Science 2001;292:727–730.

Zha J, Harada HK, Yang E, Jokel J, Korsemeyer SJ. Serine phosphorylation of death agonist BAD in response to survival factor results in binding to 14-3-3 not Bcl$_{XL}$. Cell 1996;87:619–628.

Zhang H, Huang Q, Ke N, et al. Drosophilia proapoptotic Bcl2/BAX homologue reveals evolutionary conservation of cell death mechanisms. J Biol Chem 2000;275:27,303–27,306.

73 Colorectal Cancer

SATYA NARAYAN

SUMMARY

Colorectal cancer is the third most common death-causing disease in the developed countries. It arises after a series of mutations in various tumor suppressor and proto-oncogenes, each of which are accompanied by specific alterations and pathological conditions. Recent advances have contributed a great deal of understanding of the molecular basis of events that lead to colorectal tumorigenesis. Mutation in the *adenomatous polyposis coli (APC)* gene is considered to be one of the earliest events in the development of colon cancer. The familial adenomatous polyposis and hereditary nonpolyposis colorectal cancer (HNPCC) are the most commonly inherited colorectal cancers. Familial adenomatous polyposis and HNPCC develop owing to mutations in *APC* and DNA mismatch repair (MMR) genes, respectively. The main functions of APC are known to regulate β-catenin protein levels through Wnt-signaling pathway, involved in cell migration and cell–cell adhesion, and chromosomal stability. Mutations in the *APC* gene disrupt the normal functioning of these pathways and thus are involved in the development of colon cancer. Colorectal cancer also develops owing to alterations in the transforming growth factor-β-signaling pathway. Mutations in the pro-apoptotic gene *Bax* is found in many colon tumors from HNPCC patients. A summary of the molecular genetics of the development of colorectal cancer is briefly discussed here.

Key Words: *Adenomatous polyposis coli*; chromosomal instability; colorectal cancer; familial adenomatous polyposis; hereditary nonpolyposis colorectal cancers; heterozygosity; microsatellite instability; mismatch repair; mutation cluster region; transforming growth factor-β.

INTRODUCTION

Prognosis of colorectal cancer depends on the tumor stage at the time of diagnosis with surgery being the most effective treatment. Colorectal cancers develop through a series of histologically distinct stages from "adenoma to carcinoma." The temporal order in which mutations occur in different genes relates to the progression through the histological stages of cancer from adenoma to carcinoma. Genes that are mutated at different stages of colorectal cancer development include tumor suppressor genes, proto-oncogenes, DNA repair genes, growth factors and their receptor genes, cell-cycle checkpoint genes, and apoptosis-related genes (Fig. 73-1). It is thought

From: *Principles of Molecular Medicine, Second Edition*
Edited by: M. S. Runge and C. Patterson © Humana Press, Inc., Totowa, NJ

that mutations in one of these genes set the stage for initiation and transformation of the normal colonic epithelial cells. Further accumulation of mutations in other genes then contributes to the progression of cancer through the adenoma-carcinoma-metastasis stages. During accumulation of genetic changes, a complex signaling network is established among inactivated and activated cellular pathways. Many cells bearing defective signaling pathways may go through programmed cell death or apoptosis and be removed from the normal population of cells; however, one of the target cells can go through the selection process and survive among other cells by overruling cell-cycle checkpoints and abrogating apoptosis pathways. After clonal expansion, the genetically modified single cell becomes a full-grown tumor.

Many colon cancer syndromes have been characterized based on their phenotypic, histological, and genetic changes. Among them, the most common and highly studied colon cancer syndromes are familial adenomatous polyposis (FAP) and hereditary nonpolyposis colorectal cancers (HNPCC), which are caused by mutations in the *adenomatous polyposis coli (APC)* and mismatch repair (MMR) genes, respectively. Other colon cancer syndromes include Peutz-Jeghers syndrome, juvenile polyposis syndrome, hereditary mixed polyposis syndrome, and Cowden's syndrome. These syndromes contain hamartomatous polyps and are inherited in an autosomal-dominant fashion. Mutations in serine-threonine kinase II, *STKII*, gene, Sma and Mad-related protein 4/deleted in pancreatic carcinoma 4, *Smad4/DPC4*, gene, and phosphatase and tensin homolog deleted on chromosome 10 *(pten)* gene, and *pten* gene are linked with Peutz-Jeghers syndrome, juvenile polyposis syndrome, and Cowden's syndromes, respectively. The inherited syndromes account for only 3–5% of all colon cancers, and the rest are the somatic colon cancers in which both alleles of the tumor suppressor genes are inactivated somatically. This chapter mainly discusses the functions of *apc* and *mmr* genes.

APC GENE MUTATIONS

Mutations in the *APC* gene on chromosome 5q21 locus are considered one of the earliest events in the initiation and progression of colorectal cancer. In FAP patients, allelic mutation of the *APC* gene followed by a loss of heterozygosity is a common feature. Notably, mutations in the *APC* gene also are found in 60–80% of sporadic colorectal cancers and adenomas. Patients with *APC* mutations are prone to hundreds to thousands of colorectal adenomas and early onset carcinoma. FAP patients also are prone to small intestinal adenomas (and carcinomas), intra-abdominal

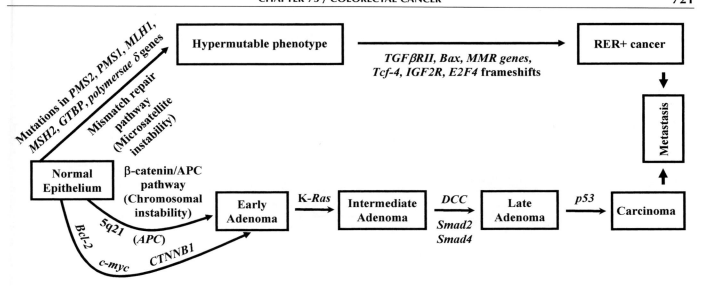

Figure 73-1   Model for genetic alterations in the development of colorectal cancer. Based on genetic analysis, at least two pathways are char-acterized in detail, which lead to colon cancer development. One pathway initiates with mutations in the adenomatous polyposis coli gene and CI followed by mutations in K-*ras*, deleted in colorectal cancer and *p53* genes. The second pathway is initiated by the mutations in the MMR genes and MSI followed by mutations in *TGFβIIR, Bax, Tcf-4, insulin-like growth factor 2 receptor,* and *E2F4* genes. Other pathways are less character-ized but a high degree of overlap is expected among them. At least seven gene mutations are needed to develop a normal epithelial cell into carci-noma. However, a cluster of gene mutations is observed in carcinoma and metastatic tumors. Bcl-2, B-cell leukemia/lymphoma 2; CTNNB1, β-catenin; GTBP, G/T mismatch-binding protein; MLH1, mutL homolog1; MSH2, mutS homolog2; PMS, postmeiotic segregation increased; RER, replication error (+).

desmoids and osteomas (Gardner's syndrome), congenital hyper-trophy of retinal pigment epithelium, fundic gland polyps in the stomach, pancreas and thyroid, dental abnormalities, and epidermal cysts.

APC is expressed constitutively within the normal colonic epithelium. The *APC* gene product is a 310-kDa-homodimeric protein localized in both the cytoplasm and the nucleus. The *APC* gene is inducible, which is transcriptionally upregulated by p53 in response to DNA damage. p53 is a negative regulator of normal cell growth and division. Although mutation in the *p53* gene is also widely present in colorectal cancers, its consequence on the expression of the wild-type or mutant *APC* gene is not clear. In the *Apc$^{Min/+}$* (Min, multiple intestinal neoplasia) mice model, an increased multiplicity and invasiveness of intestinal adenomas is often associated with deficiency for *p53*. Also, the occurrence of desmoid fibromas in these mice was strongly enhanced by *p53* deficiency. The structure of the APC protein with different protein interaction domains is given in Fig. 73-2. At the N-terminal site, the APC protein contains oligomerization and armadillo repeat-binding domains; at the C-terminal site there are EB1 and tumor suppressor protein DLG-binding domains. APC protein also contains three 15-amino acids and seven 20-amino acids repeat regions in which the latter is involved in the negative regulation of β-catenin protein levels in cells. APC functions as a nuclear-cytoplasmic shuttling protein and as a β-catenin chaperone. There are three APC nuclear export signals located in the 20-amino acid repeat region of 3, 4, and 7. The first 20-amino acid repeat in the *APC* gene is located at the 5'-end of the mutation cluster region (MCR) and often produces truncated proteins. An association exists between severe polyposis phenotype and germline muta-tions in the MCR. Selective pressure for an MCR mutant has been proposed based on the germline mutation in FAP. These findings suggest that a truncation mutation in MCR is necessary for APC

to lose β-catenin-binding and nuclear localization signals. These mutations produce loss of function and tumor progression.

APC REGULATION OF β-CATENIN LEVELS THROUGH Wnt-SIGNALING   APC acts as a negative regulator of β-catenin signaling in the transformation of colonic epithelial cells and in melanoma progression. The role of the Wingless/Wnt signaling pathway has been described in *Drosophila, Xenopus,* and in verte-brates. This pathway is important in organ development, cellular proliferation, morphology, motility, and the fate of embryonic cells. In a simple model shown in Fig. 73-3, Wingless/Wnt signaling reg-ulates the assembly of a complex consisting of axin (and its homologs Axinl and conductin), APC, β-catenin, and glycogen synthase-3β kinase (GSK3β). Axin (Axil/conductin) binds to form a complex with APC, β-catenin, and GSK3β to promote β-catenin phosphorylation and subsequent binding with slim (β-TrCP), which mediates its ubiquitination and degradation in the proteasome. GSK3β regulates this process by phosphorylating β-catenin, APC, and Axin (Axil/conductin) complex. Activation of the Wingless/Wnt signaling pathway inhibits GSK3β and stabilizes β-catenin. Mutations of β-catenin or truncation of APC, which occur both in colon cancer and melanoma cells, increases the stability and tran-scriptional activity of β-catenin. The stabilized pool of β-catenin associates with members of the T-cell factor (Tcf)–lymphoid enhancer factor (Lef) family of transcription factors. There are four known members of the Tcf and Lef family in mammals, one of which, the human *Tcf4* gene, is expressed specifically in colon cancer cells. The β-catenin/Tcf4 complex regulates the proto-oncogene and cell-cycle regulator *c-myc*, the G_1/S-regulating *cyclin D1*, the gene encoding the matrix-degrading metalloproteinase, *matrysin*, the AP-1 transcription factors *c-jun* and *fra-1*; and the urokinase-type plasminogen activator (uPA) receptor gene. From this discussion, it is clear that the inactivation of APC causes activation of β-catenin, which results in the constitutive activation of Tcf/Lef response genes.

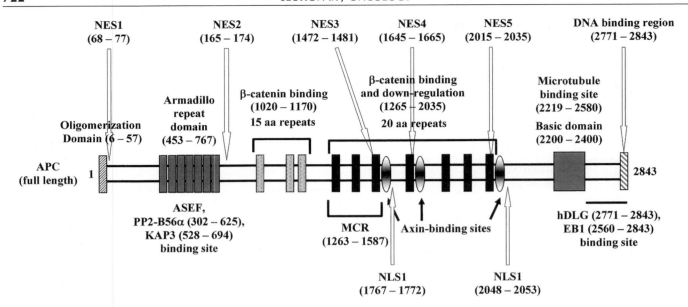

Figure 73-2   Structural features of the adenomatous polyposis coli protein. Most of the mutations in APC occur in the mutator cluster region and create truncated proteins. The truncated proteins contain APC-stimulated guanine nucleotide exchange factor and β-catenin-binding sites in the armadillo repeat domain but lose the β-catenin regulatory activity that is located in the 20-amino acids repeat domain. Somatic mutations are selected more frequently in FAP patients with germline mutations outside of the MCR. aa, amino acid; EB1, end-binding protein 1; hDLG, human disks large; KAP, kinesin superfamily associated protein; NES, nuclear export signal; NLS, nuclear localization signal; PP2-B56α, protein phosphatase 2 B56α-subunit.

In many cases colon tumors carrying mutations in the *APC* gene also carried increased levels of c-Myc, a known factor for cellular proliferation. A direct link has been established between *APC* gene mutation, β-catenin activation, and *c-myc* gene upregulation in colon cancer development. The increased expression of c-Myc through Wnt-signaling pathway upregulates the expression of *Cdk4* gene, whose product is responsible for cell-cycle regulation in G_1 phase. The *c-myc* gene encodes a transcription factor of helix-loop-helix leucine zipper family that binds as a heterodimer with Max to E boxes (CACGTG) on target promoters, for example *Cdk4* gene, and activates its expression. Max can also interact with Mad and Mxi1 and downregulate c-Myc target gene expression. It has been suggested that the increased levels of Cdk4 protein can phosphorylate pRB. The E2F/DP transcription factor then dissociates from the hyperphosphorylated pRB, which actively transcribes genes involved in cell-cycle progression through G_1 phase. It is also suggested that the increased levels of Cdk4 may sequester cell-cycle kinase inhibitor p21, p27, and p16. This sequestration may account for the ability of c-Myc overexpression to substitute for p16 deficiency as noted in mouse fibroblast transformation. Thus there is a link among *APC* gene mutation, β-catenin stabilization, *c-myc* gene activation, and Cdk4/cyclin D1/pRB/p16 pathway in colorectal cancer development.

APC INVOLVEMENT IN ACTIN CYTOSKELETAL INTEGRITY, CELL–CELL ADHESION, AND CELL MIGRATION   Actin cytoskeletal integrity is necessary to maintain the shape and adherence junctions of cells. The imbalance in actin cytoskeletal integrity can cause disturbance in cell–cell adhesion and cell migration. The role of APC in actin cytoskeletal maintenance is predicted through its interaction with β-catenin. β-catenin establishes a link between APC and actin by providing a bridge to β-catenin. In *Drosophila*, mutations in E-APC affect the organization of adherence junctions. Another link of APC with actin is shown through its interaction

with PDZ domain of DLG protein. Because APC colocalizes with DLG at the lateral cytoplasm in rat colon epithelial cells, the APC–DLG complex may participate in regulation of cell-cycle progression. Mutant APC lacking the S/TXV motif for DLG-binding exhibits weaker cell-cycle blocking activity at G_0/G_1 phase than the intact APC.

Interaction of APC with β-catenin and the members of the cadherin family of proteins have been implicated in cell–cell adhesion. The C-terminal domain of E-cadherin interacts with β- and γ-catenin, which associate with α-catenin and form an E-cadherin complex with actin cytoskeleton. This complex maintains the stable cell–cell adhesion. APC becomes a part of the cell–cell adhesion complex linked with E-cadherin, because it directly binds with β-catenin, γ-catenin, and actin filament. The tyrosine phosphorylation of β-catenin by epidermal growth factor, hepatocyte growth factor, and c-Met receptors is important in modulating cadherin-catenin complexes from membrane bound form to free cytosolic form. The phosphorylation of β-catenin at tyrosine residue, which is blocked by tyrosine phosphatase Pez, is involved in epithelial cell migration. If the Wnt-pathway and the epidermal growth factor receptor or c-Met receptors pathway are activated at the same time, then the degradation of β-catenin can be inhibited and it may translocate to the nucleus, bind to the Lef–Tcf transcription factor, and downregulate the transcription of E-cadherin gene, *CDH1*, expression. These complex interactions may finally result in the reduction in E-cadherin-mediated cell–cell adhesion and proliferation of cells.

Another important role for APC is in cell migration. Colonic epithelial cells, derived from a committed stem cell, divide in the lower two-thirds of the crypts and migrate rapidly to the surface to form a single layer. During migration, they differentiate into absorptive, secretory, Paneth, and endocrine cells. The function of a wild-type APC is necessary in maintaining the direction of

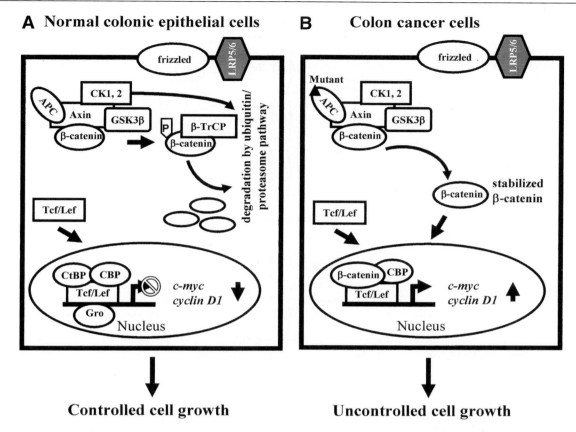

A Normal colonic epithelial cells

B Colon cancer cells

Controlled cell growth

Uncontrolled cell growth

Figure 73-3 A model for the Wnt-signaling pathway. (**A**) downregulation of β-catenin transactivation activity in normal colonic epithelial cells. β-Catenin remains in a complex of Axin/Axil/conductin, adenomatous polyposis coli, GSK3β and casein kinase 1 or 2 (CK1 or 2). In the absence of Wnt-signaling, GSK3β and CK1 or 2 kinases become active and phosphorylate β-catenin at serine and threonine residues in the N-terminal domain. Axin and APC promote phosphorylation of β-catenin by acting as a scaffold protein and bringing together enzyme(s) and substrate(s). The phosphorylated β-catenin then binds with F-box protein β-transducin repeat-containing protein of the Skp1-Cullin-F-box complex of ubiquitin ligases and undergoes proteasomal degradation. Even though Tcf–Lef transcription factor without β-catenin may bind to DNA in the absence of β-catenin, the repressors and corepressors such as carboxy-terminal-binding protein, CREB-binding protein, Groucho, and LDL receptor-related protein bind with Tcf–Lef and repress *c-myc* or *cyclin D1* gene expression to control cell-cycle progression. Some other known genes that are regulated by β-catenin/Tcf–Lef pathway include *Cyclin D1, CDH1, Tcf-1, c-jun, Fra-1, PPARd, Gastrin, uPAR, MMP7, Conductin, CD44, Id2, Siamois, Xbra, Twin,* and *Ubx.* (**B**) The role of mutations in the APC or β-catenin protein in the regulation of β-catenin level and its transactivation property in colon cancer cells. The mutant β-catenin escapes its degradation through the Wnt-pathway and becomes stabilized in the cytoplasm. The stabilized level of β-catenin then heterodimerizes with Tcf–Lef transcription factor and moves into the nucleus, where it actively transcribes cell-cycle-related genes causing cellular proliferation. The binding of β-catenin with Tcf–Lef inhibits the binding of carboxy-terminal-binding protein, CREB-binding protein, Groucho or LDL receptor-related protein and potentiates its transcriptional activity.

upward movement of these cells along the crypt-villus axis. Loss of wild-type APC functions resulting from loss of expression or mutations affects cell migration. Instead of migrating upward toward the gut lumen, these cells migrate aberrantly or less efficiently toward the crypt base in which they accumulate and form polyps. In time, they become aneuploid because of defects in chromosome segregation as well as acquire β-catenin stabilization and activation of genes for cell proliferation. The mechanisms by which APC might be involved in cell migration can be understood by its association with the kinesin superfamily associated protein KAP3 that has been established in cell–cell adhesion and migration. APC, mediated by KAP3, interacts with kinesin motor proteins that transport it as well as β-catenin along the microtubules to the growing ends of the cytoskeleton protruding into motile cell membranes. At the tip of microtubule, APC interacts with the end-binding protein, EB1, and protein tyrosine phosphatase (PTP)-BL. PTP-BL modulates the steady state levels of tyrosine phosphorylations of APC-associated proteins such as β-catenin and GSK3β.

In fact, GSK3β kinase activity has been implicated in microtubule dynamics. The mechanism by which mutated APC might play a role in the migration of colorectal tumor cells is predicted through its interaction with Rac-specific guanine nucleotide exchange factor ASEF. APC binds with ASEF and controls its activity. ASEF is activated in colorectal cancer cells containing truncated APC. Active ASEF decreases E-cadherin-mediated cell–cell adhesion and promotes cell migration. Thus, the dynamic association of APC, EB1, ASEF, catenins, EGFR or c-Met receptor, PTP-BL, and E-cadherin proteins at cell–cell adherence junctions and microtubule ends play an important role in cell–cell communication, cell migration, and carcinogenesis.

GENETIC INSTABILITY IN COLON CANCER PROGRESSION

Both sporadic and hereditary colorectal cancers exhibit a defined set of biological and genetic cell heterogeneity through a series of molecular events. Two specific pathologically distinct

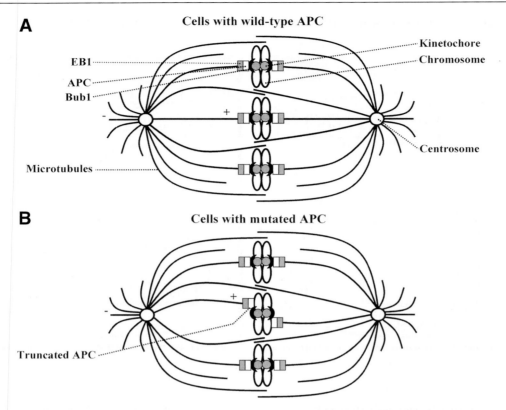

Figure 73-4   CI in cells carrying mutations in adenomatous polyposis coli gene. **(A)** A model for the interaction of APC with plus-end of micro-tubule through end-binding protein and with kinetochore of chromosome through budding uninhibited by benzimidazole 1 in normal colonic epithelial cells. APC can also bind microtubules directly via the C-terminal basic domain. **(B)** A disruption in the interaction between spindle microtubules and kinetochores because of expression of truncated form of APC in colon cancer cells.

genetic pathways for colorectal cancer have been identified—the chromosomal instability (CI) pathway and the microsatellite insta-bility (MSI) pathway. The CI and MSI are associated with two major inherited syndromes, FAP and HNPCC, respectively. The MSI leads to a 1000-fold increase in the rate of subtle DNA changes, whereas CI enhances the rate at which gross chromosomal changes occur during cell division such as chromosome breaks, duplica-tion, rearrangements, and deletions. Findings describing these two pathways are discussed below.

APC **GENE MUTATION ASSOCIATED WITH CI** Aneuploidy, the abnormal number of chromosomes both quanti-tatively and qualitatively, is a common characteristic of colon cancer cells. It is thought that the aneuploidy in colon cancer cells arises during mitosis through a defective cell division leading to CI. CI is a common feature of approx 85% colorectal cancers, and it has been detected in the smallest adenoma, suggesting that CI may occur at very early stages of colorectal cancer development. The mechanism(s) by which CI is generated in colon cancer cells is largely unclear. Because the main feature of CI is aneuploidy, it has been suggested that it may arise because of structural changes to the chromosomes and abnormal mitosis. In this scenario, the wild-type APC is involved in maintaining the proper connection of microtubules with chromosomes. APC performs a bridging func-tion between microtubules and chromosomes. APC binds at the plus end of the microtubule through EB1, stretches it to the chro-mosomes, and inserts them into kinetochores after binding with benzimidazole 1 (Bub1). APC colocalizes to kinetochores and forms complexes with Bub1 and Bub3, the two mitotic checkpoint

proteins. The successful complex formation facilitates proper growth of spindle formation and helps in maintaining euploidy (Fig. 73-4A). Once the *APC* gene is mutated, the truncated APC protein loses its ability to bind with Bub1 and it is unable to prop-erly maintain the attachment of microtubules at kinetochores, resulting in defect in segregation of chromosomes (Fig. 73-4B).

Another observation noted with CI was that after blocking apop-tosis in either $Apc^{Min/+}$ or $Apc1638T$ ES cells, the number of aber-rant chromosomes were much greater than in control ES cells that were unable to undergo apoptosis. From these findings, a multiple-hit hypothesis of colorectal cancer development has been suggested. The chromosome segregation defect in colon cancer cells with mutated *APC* gene could lie dormant until an additional genetic-hit suppresses the mitotic checkpoint or the apoptosis of defective cells. In this regard, the proper functioning of the hSecurin, a protein necessary for the completion of the anaphase portion of mitosis, is critical to maintain euploidy, because the loss of hSecurin is often associated with the loss of chromosomes at a high frequency. Furthermore, telomere dysfunction promotes CI that triggered early carcinogenesis in the $Apc^{Min/+}$ $Terc^{-/-}$ mouse models, whereas telo-merase activation restored genomic stability to a level permissive for tumor progression, suggesting that early and transient telomere dysfunction is a major mechanism underlying CI of human cancers. Thus, multiple factors may influence colorectal cancer development from normal epithelial cells to adenoma to carcinoma stages.

MMR GENE MUTATIONS ASSOCIATED WITH MSI   MSI is characterized by the size variation of microsatellites in tumor DNA as compared to matching normal DNA because of defects in

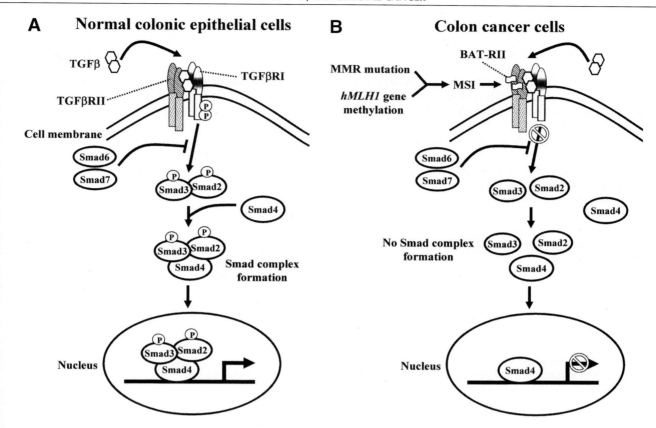

Figure 73-5 TGF-β signaling in normal colonic epithelium and cancer cells. **(A)** The functional pathway of TGF-β signaling in normal colonic epithelial cells. TGF-β ligand-binding with TGF-β receptor II recruits TGFβRI into a tetrameric receptor complex resulting in transphosphorylation and activation of TGFβRI. After phosphorylation, the TGFβRI becomes an active kinase that phosphorylates Smad2 and Smad3. Smad anchor for receptor activation (SARA), a scaffolding protein, facilitates interaction between Smad2, Smad3, and TGFβRI. Phosphorylated Smad2 and Smad3 allow the formation of homo- and heterodimerization complex, including Smad4. The Smad complex then translocates into nucleus, binds with DNA, and stimulates the expression of target genes including *p15* (inhibitor of cell-cycle kinase that controls cell cycle into G_1 phase) and *PAI-1* (inhibitor of protease 1 that degrades extracellular matrix proteins during metastasis). **(B)** The abnormal pathway of TGF-β signaling in colon cancer cells. Many colon cancer cells with MSI because of defective MMR activity induce mutations in *TGFβRII* gene. Often these are frameshift mutations that insert or delete one or two adenine bases located within a 10 bp polyadenine repeat region (base pairs 709–718, codons 125–128; referred to as BAT-RII) of *TGFβRII* gene. These mutations encode TGFβRII proteins that are truncated between 129 and 161 amino acids of the cytoplasmic domain, which causes functional inactivation of these proteins. Thus, the loss of TGF-β signaling may abolish cell-cycle control and induce metastasis of colon cancer cells by inhibiting *p15* and *PAI-1* gene expression, respectively. hMLH1, human mutL homolog1.

the MMR system. MMR system is critical for the maintenance of genomic stability. MMR increases the fidelity of DNA replication by identifying and excising single-base mismatches and insertion–deletion loops that may arise during DNA replication. Thus, the MMR system serves a DNA damage surveillance function by preventing incorrect base pairing or avoiding insertion–deletion loops by slippage of DNA polymerase. Once cells compromise with these functions, it may lead to accumulation of mutations resulting in the initiation of cancer. The MMR genes are involved in one of the most prevalent cancer syndromes in humans known as HNPCC or Lynch syndrome. HNPCC is characterized as an autosomal-dominant inherited disease with 85–90% gene penetrance for early onset of colorectal carcinoma. HNPCC accounts for approx 5–7% of cases of colorectal carcinoma. The molecular diagnosis of HNPCC is based on determining MMR genes for germline mutations. There are at least six different proteins required for the complete MMR system: hMSH2, hMLH1, hPMS1, hPMS2, hMSH3, and hMSH6 (GTBP). hMSH2 forms a heterodimer with either hMSH6 or hMSH3 (depending on the type of lesion to be repaired) and binds to the mismatch site. The

complex of hMSH2 with hMSH6 is called hMutSα, and it is required for the correction of single-base mispairs. The complex of hMSH2 with hMSH3 is called hMutSβ, and it is required for the correction of insertion–deletion loops. Subsequently, a heterodimer of hMLH1 and hPMS2 proteins are recruited by hMutSα or hMutSβ proteins to the mismatch recognition complex, which with other proteins are involved in excision, resynthesis, and ligation of DNA. Mutations in the hMLH1 and hPMS2 have been found in approx 90% of HNPCC cases. Mutations in other MMR genes have been less frequent in HNPCC patients. In many sporadic colon cancers, hypermethylation of the *hMLH1* gene promoter resulting in its transcriptional silencing has been observed more than mutations. Both mutations and methylation of *hMLH1* gene have been linked with MSI playing a causal role in the initiation of colorectal cancer. The CpG island methylator phenotype pathway has been suggested as a novel mutator pathway that predisposes to colonic tumorigenesis. In many cases of the sporadic colon cancers, the MSI can be induced by CpG island methylator phenotype, followed by *hMLH1* gene's promoter methylation, loss of *hMLH1* gene expression, and resultant MMR deficiency.

Mutation rate in cells with MMR deficiency are 100- to 1000-fold greater than in normal cells. There are many targets of MMR gene inactivation; however, the precise stage of tumorigenesis in which mutation of the wild-type MMR gene occurs is not clear. There are four well-studied gene targets of MMR, whose mutations in the microsatellite region have been found in colorectal cancers carrying a mutated *hMLH1* gene. These gene targets are the transforming growth factor-β receptor-II (*TGF-IIβ*), insulin-like growth factor II receptor, antiapoptotic gene *Bax*, *Tcf-4*, and the cell-cycle regulator *E2F4*.

Altered TGF-β Signaling in MSI Cells   In colon cancers, TGF-β signaling potently inhibits the growth of normal epithelial cells; because the tumor cells are frequently resistant to TGF-β, they cause preneoplastic lesions, increase motility and spread cancer. The structural basis for TGF-β resistance in colon cancers is defined resulting from somatic mutations that inactivate TGF-β receptor II (TGFβRII). In human colon cancer cell lines with high rates of MSI, mutations in the *TGFβRII* gene were found. These are primarily frameshift mutations that add or delete one or two adenine bases within or from a 10 bp polyadenine repeat in the cysteine-rich coding region (codons 125–128) of the *TGFβRII* gene. These mutations produce truncated proteins that lack the cytoplasmic domain. As much as 90% of the colorectal cancers with MSI have a mutated *TGFβRII* gene. TGFβIIR responses are connected with Smads, tumor suppressor gene products, which help to initiate TGFβ-mediated gene transcription (Fig. 73-5). The transcriptional regulation of type-1 plasminogen inhibitor (*PAI-1*) and cyclin-dependent kinase inhibitor *p15* genes are controlled by TGFβ signaling. PAI-1 is the primary inhibitor of tissue-type plasminogen activator and uPA. TGFβ inhibits cell proliferation by inducing a G_1-phase cell-cycle arrest acting through increased expression of *p15*. Thus, the loss of TGFβIIR or Smad4 can abolish TGFβ-signaling and advocate cell proliferation and development of colorectal cancer.

Mutations in Proapoptotic Gene BAX in MSI Cells   Of tumors with MSI, approx 50% are found with mutations in the *Bax* gene. These mutations produce frameshift mutations within a coding region of eight nucleotide stretch of guanine residues, G_8. Bax heterodimerizes with antiapoptotic protein Bcl2 and induces apoptosis. In the presence of apoptotic signals, BH3 domain proteins tBid are activated and bound with Bax. The interaction of tBid with Bax brings conformational changes in Bax, and this promotes its translocation to the mitochondria. Bax oligomerizes and inserts into the outer mitochondrial membrane in which it forms channels to release cytochrome *c* (Cyt c) into the cytoplasm. The released Cyt c forms a complex called apoptosome with Apaf-1, dATP, and procaspase 9. The apoptosome recruits and processes procaspase 9 to form a holoenzyme complex, which in turn recruits and activates the effector caspases leading to apoptosis. Thus, the expression of mutated Bax protein may fail to release Cyt c and increase the Bax-Bcl2 ratio resulting in the escape from apoptosis and inducing initiation of colorectal carcinogenesis.

CONCLUSIONS

Development of colorectal cancer is a complex, multistep process in which several gene defects coordinate in genotypic and phenotypic outcome. Mutations in many tumor suppressor and protooncogenes in the development of sporadic and hereditary colorectal cancers are well established; however, their precise role in this process is unclear. For example, it is established that mutations

in *APC* gene may be necessary for the early onset of FAP. Mutations in the *APC* gene perhaps set a stage for mutations in other genes such as K-*ras*, deleted in colorectal cancer, and *p53*. However, the mechanism(s) by which *APC* gene mutations may contribute to the accumulation of mutations in the genes associated with the colon cancer progression remain unclear. Mutations in the MMR genes can be linked to an increased rate of mutations; however, MMR negative cells develop resistance to apoptosis rather than accumulation of mutations. Thus, MMR gene mutations and their role in MSI and apoptosis need further investigation in context with apoptosis and cell-cycle-related genes. These studies will provide a better understanding of colorectal cancer development and its intervention by genetic or chemotherapeutic means.

SELECTED REFERENCES

Ben-Ze'ev A, Geiger B. Differential molecular interactions of beta-catenin and plakoglobin in adhesion, signaling and cancer. Curr Opin Cell Biol 1998;10:629–639.

Bright-Thomas RM, Hargest R. APC, β-catenin and hTcf-4; an unholy trinity in the genesis of colorectal cancer. Eur J Surg Oncol 2003;29:107–117.

Buermeyer AB, Deschenes SM, Baker SM, Liskay RM. Mammalian DNA mismatch repair. Annu Rev Genet 1999;33:533–564.

Cain K, Bratton SB, Cohen GM. The Apaf-1 apoptosome: a large caspase-activating complex. Biochimie 2002;84(2–3):203–214.

Dikovskaya D, Zumbrunn J, Penman GA, Nathke IS. The adenomatous polyposis coli protein: in the limelight out at the edge. Trends Cell Biol 2001;11:378–384.

Erdmann KS, Kuhlmann J, Lessmann V, et al. The adenomatous polyposis coli-protein (APC) interacts with the protein tyrosine phosphatase PTP-BL via an alternatively spliced PDZ domain. Oncogene 2000;19: 3894–3901.

Fearon ER, Vogelstein B. A genetic model for colorectal tumorigenesis. Cell 1990;61:759–767.

Fodde R, Kuipers J, Rosenberg C, et al. Mutations in the APC tumour suppressor gene cause chromosomal instability. Nat Cell Biol 2001;3: 433–438.

Hannon GJ, Beach D. p15INK4B is a potential effector of TGF-beta-induced cell cycle arrest. Nature 1994;371:257–261.

Henderson BR. Nuclear-cytoplasmic shuttling of APC regulates β-catenin subcellular localization and turnover. Nat Cell Biol 2000;2:653–660.

Hermeking H, Rago C, Schuhmacher M, et al. Identification of CDK4 as a target of c-MYC. Proc Natl Acad Sci USA 2000;97:2229–2234.

Huber O, Bierkanp C, Kemler R. Cadherins and catenins in development. Curr Opin Cell Biol 1998;8:685–691.

Ilyas M, Straub J, Tomlinson IP, Bodmer WF. Genetic pathways in colorectal and other cancers. Eur J Cancer 1999;35:1986–2002.

Jaiswal AS, Narayan S. p53-dependent transcriptional regulation of the APC promoter in colon cancer cells treated with DNA-alkylating agents. J Biol Chem 2001;276:18,193–18,199.

Jallepalli PV, Waizenegger IC, Bunz F, et al. Securin is required for chromosomal stability in human cells. Securin is required for chromosomal stability in human cells. Cell 2001;105:445–457.

Kawasaki Y, Sato R, Akiyama T. Mutated APC and ASEF are involved in the migration of colorectal tumour cells. Nat Cell Biol 2003;5:211–215.

Kawasaki Y, Senda T, Ishidate T, et al. ASEF, a link between the tumor suppressor APC and G-protein signaling. Science 2000;289:1194–1197.

Korinek V, Barker N, Morin PJ, et al. Constitutive transcriptional activation by a β-catenin-Tcf complex in APC$^{-/-}$ colon carcinoma. Science 1997;275:1784–1787.

Lamlum H, Ilyas M, Rowan A, et al. The type of somatic mutation at APC in familial adenomatous polyposis is determined by the site of the germline mutation: a new facet to Knudson's 'two-hit' hypothesis. Nat Med 1999;5:1071–1075.

Lynch HT, de la Chapelle A. Genetic susceptibility to non-polyposis colorectal cancer. J Med Genet 1999;36:801–818.

Markowitz S, Wang J, Myeroff L, et al. Inactivation of the type II TGF-beta receptor in colon cancer cells with microsatellite instability. Science 1995;268:1336–1338.

Morin PJ, Sparks AB, Korinek V, et al. Activation of β- catenin-Tcf signaling in colon cancer by mutations in β-catenin or APC. Science 1997;275:1787–1790.

Moss SF, Liu TC, Petrotos A, Hsu TM, Gold LI, Holt PR. Inward growth of colonic adenomatous polyps. Gastroenterology 1996;111:1425–1432.

Narayan S, Jaiswal AS. Activation of adenomatous polyposis coli (*APC*) gene expression by the DNA-alkylating agent *N*-methyl-*N'*-nitro-*N*-nitrosoguanidine requires p53. J Biol Chem 1997;272:30,619–30,622.

Narayan S, Roy D. Role of *APC* and DNA mismatch repair genes in the development of colorectal cancers. Mol Cancer 2003;2:42–56.

Kaplan KB, Burds AA, Swedlow JR, Bekir SS, Sorger PK, Nathke IS. A role for the adenomatous polyposis coli protein in chromosome segregation. Nat Cell Biol 2001;3:429–432.

Neufeld KL, White RL. Nuclear localizations of the adenomatous polyposis coli protein. Proc Natl Acad Sci USA 1997;94:3034–3039.

Palombo F, Iaccarino I, Nakajima E, Ikejima M, Shimada T, Jiricny J. hMutSbeta, a heterodimer of hMSH2 and hMSH3, binds to insertion/deletion loops in DNA. Curr Biol 1996;6:1181–1184.

Polakis P. Wnt signaling and cancer. Genes Dev 2000;14:1837–1851.

Rampino N, Yamamoto H, Ionov Y, et al. Somatic frameshift mutations in the BAX gene in colon cancers of the microsatellite mutator phenotype. Science 1997;275:967–969.

Rosin-Arbesfeld R, Townsley F, Bienz M. The APC tumour suppressor has a nuclear export function. Nature 2000;406:1009–1012.

Souza RF, Appel R, Yin J, et al. Microsatellite instability in the insulin-like growth factor II receptor gene in gastrointestinal tumours. Nat Genet 1996;14:255–257.

Souza RF, Yin J, Smolinski KN, et al. Frequent mutation of the E2F-4 cell cycle gene in primary human gastrointestinal tumors. Cancer Res 1997;57:2350–1353.

Veigl ML, Kasturi L, Olechnowicz J, et al. Biallelic inactivation of hMLH1 by epigenetic gene silencing, a novel mechanism causing human MSI cancers. Proc Natl Acad Sci USA 1998;95:8698–8702.

Wadham C, Gamble JR, Vadas MA, Khew-Goodall Y. The protein tyrosine phosphatase Pez is a major phosphatase of adherens junctions and dephosphorylates beta-catenin. Mol Biol Cell 2003;14:2520–2529.

Wijnhoven BP, Dinjens WN, Pignatelli M. E-cadherin-catenin cell–cell adhesion complex and human cancer. Br J Surg 2000;87:992–1005.

Zhang F, White RL, Neufeld KL. Phosphorylation near nuclear localization signal regulates nuclear import of adenomatous polyposis coli protein. Proc Natl Acad Sci USA 2000;97:12,577–12,582.

Zhang L, Yu J, Park BH, Kinzler KW, Vogelstein B. Role of BAX in the apoptotic response to anticancer agents. Science 2000;290:989–992.

74 Breast Cancer

Yi Huang and Nancy E. Davidson

SUMMARY

Breast cancer is the most common malignancy among Western women. Like other human cancers, breast cancer results from the accumulation of a series of genetic and/or epigenetic changes to genes with diverse functions, ultimately evolving to a malignant state. Recent scientific advances have offered many new approaches to identify and target a growing number of these genetic and epigenetic alterations in breast cancer. It is expected that this improved understanding of breast cancer biology will enhance risk assessment, prevention, diagnosis, and treatment of this disease.

Key Words: Breast cancer; breast cancer susceptibility genes; ductal carcinoma *in situ* (DCIS); endocrine therapies; epigenetic alterations; growth factor receptors; hormone regulation; hormone resistance; invasive breast cancer; oncogenes; steroid hormone receptors; tumor suppressor genes.

INTRODUCTION

Breast cancer is the most common malignancy and a leading cause of mortality in women in the Western world. More than 200,000 American women were diagnosed with breast cancer in 2004. The incidence of breast cancer varies with multiple factors including gender, age, ethnicity, family history, reproductive factors, socioeconomic class, exogenous and endogenous hormones, radiation exposure, genetic susceptibility, and so on. Like other human cancers, breast cancer is recognized as a genetic disease in that it is thought to result from a progressive accumulation of genetic changes. Initiation of breast cancer results from uncontrolled cell proliferation and/or aberrant programmed cell death as a consequence of cumulative alterations of tumor suppressor gene and/or protooncogene expression. Epigenetic changes such as DNA methylation or chromatin modeling can also contribute to modified gene expression. These changes can modulate expression of a variety of critical genes with diverse functions. Previously, the only biological factor of clinical import in breast cancer was steroid receptor expression because it has been an important predictive factor of response to endocrine therapy. But over the last two decades, enormous advances have been made in the understanding of breast cancer at the molecular level. This understanding has revealed a large number of new targets that may play a role as risk, prognostic, or predictive factors and/or aid in the development of new effective therapies of breast cancer.

From: *Principles of Molecular Medicine, Second Edition*
Edited by: M. S. Runge and C. Patterson © Humana Press, Inc., Totowa, NJ

BREAST CANCER PATHOLOGY AND DEVELOPMENT

The natural history of breast cancer involves a sequential progression of epithelial changes. Epithelial hyperplasia may be one of the first steps in breast carcinoma development. Hyperplasia without atypia (also termed usual or typical hyperplasia) is characterized by myoepithelial and epithelial growth, resulting in increased cellularity of the terminal duct lobular unit. Atypical ductal hyperplasia is associated with an increased risk of breast cancer progression and could represent the next step toward breast carcinoma. Ductal carcinoma *in situ* (DCIS) is a malignant proliferation of a subgroup of epithelial cells without invasion through basement membrane into stroma. DCIS is thought to be a precursor of invasive ductal carcinoma in some cases. Different histological patterns of DCIS have been described and differences in biological behavior have been ascribed to these patterns. For example, comedo DCIS is generally a high-grade lesion characterized by clusters of large epithelial cells with central necrosis, reflecting cell death because of the deprivation of essential metabolites, and is thought to be associated with poorer outcome. The noncomedo DCIS, like cribriform and micropapillary DCIS, are usually low grade with a relatively low mitotic rate. Histological grade is judged to be a more important determinant of outcome than the particular pattern of DCIS. In some cases, extended growth of DCIS into a breast lobule makes it difficult to distinguish DCIS from lobular carcinoma *in situ* (LCIS), a neoplastic proliferation of epithelial cells in the terminal duct lobular unit. In contrast to DCIS, cells of LCIS are usually regular with small, rounded nuclei and defined border. LCIS is felt to be a marker for the propensity to develop invasive breast cancer in the future.

Accumulated genetic changes combined with other factors may lead to the development of invasive carcinoma. Infiltrating duct carcinomas are the most common type of invasive breast cancer, accounting for 60–80% of all breast cancers. The second most common type of invasive breast cancer (approx 10% of breast cancers) is invasive lobular carcinoma. Classic lobular carcinoma cells are small with rounded nuclei and dense chromatin. Generally, lobular carcinoma has slightly better overall survival rate than ductal tumors. Medullary carcinoma, comprising 5–7% of breast malignancies, is a circumscribed entity with extensive infiltration of lymphocytes and plasma cells. Other types of uncommon invasive breast carcinomas include tubular, adenoid cystic, mucinous, papillary, and metaplastic carcinomas. A hallmark of all invasive breast carcinomas is disruption of the basement membrane, which suggests that cancer cells

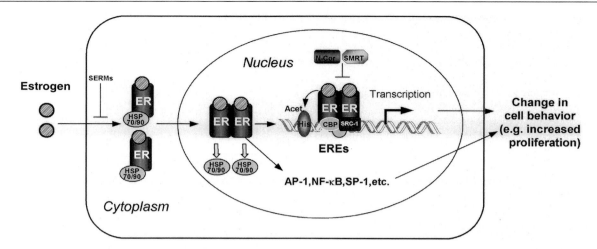

Figure 74-1 Mechanisms of ligand-dependent activation of ERs. Binding of agonist to ER complex can induce ER-conformational change, which results in the disassociation of chaperones (hsp90 or hsp70) and ER dimerization. Coactivators of ER such as steroid receptor coactivator-1 and CREB-binding protein can form a complex with receptor dimers, which in turn binds to EREs of target genes. The coactivator complex activates gene transcription via interaction with basal transcription factors and stimulation of histone (His) acetylation (Acet.). ER corepressors N-Cor and silencing mediator of retinoid and thyroid receptors can suppress transcription of ER target genes by interacting with ER dimers and forming a complex with histone deacetylase. Ligand-bound ER may also activate genes without EREs ("nonclassic" activation) via the interaction of ER with other transcription factors such as activating protein-1 (AP-1) NF-κB, or SP1, which subsequently activates target genes that do not contain EREs but encompass specific binding sites for AP-1, NF-κB, or SP1. ER-mediated gene expression usually promotes the breast cell proliferation that may ultimately lead to breast tumorigenesis. Selective ER modulators can selectively inhibit the ligand–receptor interaction, thereby preventing estrogen molecules from binding to these receptors. CBP, CREB-binding protein; HSP, heat shock protein; N-CoR, nuclear receptor corepressor.

may have acquired the ability to metastasize to distant sites. Metastatic tumors can become fatal when they disrupt the function of vital organs.

HORMONE REGULATION

ESTROGEN RECEPTOR Estrogen receptors (ER) are members of the steroid receptor superfamily. Two isoforms of ER (ERα and ERβ) have been identified. Although ERα and ERβ have only 30% overall sequence similarity, their DNA-binding and ligand-binding domains are highly homologous, suggesting that the two receptors likely share similar ligands and DNA-binding activity. Most of the knowledge about ER activity and function in breast cancer has been obtained from studies on ERα; much less is known about ERβ.

The ER is a nuclear transcription factor that regulates the expression of a number of genes involved in regulation of cell proliferation and differentiation. Binding of a ligand to ER results in a ligand–ER complex that subsequently induces an ER-conformational change, disassociation of chaperones such as hsp90 or hsp70, and receptor dimerization (Fig. 74-1). Activated ER dimers can bind to the estrogen response elements (EREs) of target genes and regulate their transcription. Some nuclear proteins interact with ER and function as coactivators or corepressors of ER. Identified coactivators include SRC-1, SRC-2, SRC-3 (AIB-1), CREB-binding protein/p300, TRIP-1, TIF-2, and others. N-Cor and silencing mediator of retinoid and thyroid receptors are corepressors that can interact with ER and inhibit ER-activated transcription. Coactivators may either directly acetylate histones or recruit other molecules containing such activity, whereas corepressors have the opposite function by forming complexes with histone deacetylases (HDACs). Ligand-bound ER may also activate genes without EREs in their promoter region ("nonclassic" activation). In that situation, ligand binding to ER leads to its interaction with other transcription factors such as AP-1, nuclear factor (NF)-κB, or SP1, which subsequently activate

target genes that do not contain EREs but rather encompass specific binding sites for AP-1, NF-κB, or SP1. Finally, some signaling in the estrogen pathway may take place through the membrane.

Because of the pivotal role that ER plays in breast cancer progression, development of specific agents targeting ER or its ligands has become an important strategy for breast cancer treatment. Applied endocrine therapies include depletion of the ligand, estrogen, (by oophorectomy or luteinizing hormone releasing hormone analogs in premenopausal women or aromatase inhibitors in postmenopausal women), steroidal antiestrogens that destroy ER such as fulvestrant (also known as ICI 182,780), and selective ER modulators (SERMs) like tamoxifen. SERMs selectively stimulate or inhibit the ER in different target tissues. A SERM may interfere with ER activity in breast cells but activate the ER in other target tissues like uterus, bone, and liver. The most widely used SERM is tamoxifen, which can selectively inhibit the ligand–ER interaction in breast, thereby preventing estrogen molecules from binding to these receptors. But unlike estrogen, the binding of tamoxifen to ER does not cause the ER to acquire the altered conformation that allows it to bind properly to coactivators. As a result, ER target genes that stimulate cell proliferation cannot be activated. Most studies show that early-stage breast cancer patients with ER-expressing tumors benefit from tamoxifen treatment with longer disease-free and overall survival. However, tamoxifen has no obvious impact on the outcome of ER-poor tumors. Thus assessment of ER status in breast cancer patients has been of major utility to predict the potential response to hormonal therapy.

Unfortunately *de novo* or acquired hormone resistance is a feature of some breast cancers. Approximately 30% of breast cancers lack ER-gene expression (ER-negative). Tumors lacking ER protein are usually associated with higher growth rate, poorer differentiation, and worse clinical outcome. Thus, ER expression has been a possible prognostic factor for early breast cancer patients. Genetic changes that could account for the loss of ER in breast cancer include deletions, insertions, point mutations, or rearrangements of ER gene. However, these alterations do not occur frequently enough to explain the loss of ER expression in a substantial fraction of breast cancers. As discussed later, inactivation of ER-gene expression may result from hypermethylation of the ER-CpG island in promoter region or other epigenetic mechanisms. Support for this possibility comes from in vitro studies showing re-expression of the ER gene in ER-negative human breast cancer cell lines by using inhibitors of DNA methyltransferase or HDAC. In addition, studies using sensitive PCR-based assays have shown that CpG island methylation is a common feature of primary breast cancers that lack ER-protein expression by immunohistochemistry and ligand-binding assays. A number of mechanisms may account for hormone resistance in the presence of ER: a shift to dependence on other growth regulatory pathways, inappropriate balance of coactivators and corepressors, or other defects in the ER-transcriptional pathway.

PROGESTERONE RECEPTOR The progesterone receptor (PR) gene also belongs to the nuclear receptor superfamily. Two isoforms of PR, PRA, and PRB, arise from two different transcription initiation sites within the same gene. Like ER, PR can also bind to ligand and target DNA to function as a transcription factor. About half of ER-positive tumors are reported to express both ER and PR genes (ER-positive/PR-positive) and these tumors are more differentiated and more responsive to hormonal therapy. About 25–30% of primary breast tumors are negative for both ER and PR. These tumors are generally associated with poorer differentiation and worse clinical outcome than ER-positive/PR-positive tumors (Table 74-1). Clinical trials have confirmed the value of PR gene expression in predicting the response of breast tumors to hormonal therapy. Elevated PR levels significantly correlate with increased response to tamoxifen in patients with ER-positive metastatic breast cancer. In ER-negative/PR-positive tumors, response to hormonal therapy is commonly observed, although responses are not as frequent as with tumors expressing both ER and PR (Table 74-1). As the ER gene is a critical regulator of PR expression, loss of ER or abrogation of the ER pathway is one mechanism for loss of PR expression. As with ER, the inactivation of PR gene in some breast tumors may also be a consequence of genetic changes or epigenetic modifications like CpG island methylation in the PR promoter region. The mechanism of methylation is of potential interest in accounting for the differential loss of PR in ER-positive/PR-negative phenotype.

ONCOGENES AND GROWTH FACTOR RECEPTORS

The identification of alterations to a number of protooncogenes and growth factor receptors in breast carcinoma has highlighted a number of signal transduction cascades that have important roles in normal mammary growth and mammary tumorigenesis.

THE HER FAMILY The members of the *erb*-B/epidermal growth factor receptor (EGFR)/class I family of receptor tyrosine kinases include HER1 (EGFR/*c-erb*-B1), HER2 (*c-erb*-B2/neu), HER3 (*c-erb*-B3), and HER4 (*c-erb*-B4) and share significant sequence homology to each other. HER2/*neu* has emerged as one of the most important oncogenes in breast cancer. The molecular mechanisms by which overexpression of HER2/*neu* induces cell transformation are not completely understood but may involve the formation of heterodimers of HER2/*neu* with other members of HER family and subsequent activation of several signaling pathways leading to cell proliferation. Although various ligands with selectivity for one of the HER receptors have been recognized, no

Table 74-1
Frequency of ER and PR Expression in Breast Cancer and Response to Hormonal Therapy

Tumor phenotype	Frequency of phenotype	Response rate to hormonal therapy
ER+/PR+	40%	75–80%
ER+/PR–	30%	20–30%
ER–/PR+	Less than 5%	40–50%
ER–/PR–	25–30%	Less than 10%

Adapted from Lapidus RG, Nass SJ, Davidson NE, 1998 with permission.

ligand has been identified that directly binds to HER2/*neu*. The major HER2/*neu* activated signaling pathways are summarized in Fig. 74-2. Several downstream substrates such as the adaptor molecules, Grb2, and/or Shc, can complex with activated HER dimer via src homology-2 domains. Interaction between the guanine-nucleotide exchange factor, son of sevenless, and Shc/grb2 catalyzes the activation of the ras-GTP complex that subsequently activates the serine-threonine kinase *Raf-1* and mitogen-activated protein kinase (MAPK) pathways. HER2/HER3 heterodimer can phosphorylate and activate the p85 unit of phosphoinositide 3-kinase (PI3K), an important enzyme for generation of an intracellular second message. MAPK and PI3K activation by HER2/*neu* leads to enhanced cell proliferation through the activation of a number of nuclear targets, including c-fos, c-jun, c-*myc*, cyclin D1, and so on. The direct activation of phospholipase C-γ (PLC-γ) by HER2/*neu* also appears to mediate the transforming potential of HER2/*neu* although the exact role of PLC-γ is not clear. The induced activity of these pathways may reflect the most important cellular effects of HER2/*neu* receptor activation in breast cancer cells.

Amplification of the HER2/*neu* gene occurs in approx 20–30% breast carcinomas. Since the first report in 1987 of the correlation of HER2/*neu* gene amplification with poorer clinical outcome in a multivariate analysis in node-positive breast cancer patients, a number of prognostic studies have given mixed results on this finding. Others have addressed the possibility that HER2 overexpression correlates with absence of ER expression or tamoxifen resistance in an ER-expressing tumor. A possible mechanism for the latter is that HER2/*neu* overexpression can upregulate MAPK. MAPK then phosphorylates ER, leading to ligand-independent activation of ER and loss of the inhibitory effect of tamoxifen on ER-mediated transcription. These findings imply a role for HER2/*neu* overexpression as a potential predictive marker for hormone therapy and suggest that the possible utility of combinations of anti-HER2/*neu* and endocrine therapy in clinical practice.

Increasing attention has been given to the HER2/*neu* receptor as a direct therapeutic target in breast cancer overexpressing HER2/*neu*. One such approach, use of the anti-HER2 monoclonal antibody, trastuzamab, is effective in the treatment of HER2-positive metastatic breast cancer. Trastuzamab can inhibit both PI3K and MAPK activation induced by HER2/*neu* and arrest cells at G_1 phase. Preclinical and clinical studies suggest that the combination of trastuzamab with certain chemotherapeutic agents such as paclitaxel may significantly improve the therapeutic efficacy over chemotherapy alone.

Other studies have focused on the role of the EGFR/HER1 gene in breast cancer. HER1 overexpression is associated with loss of ER expression and, like HER2/*neu*, HER1 expression may

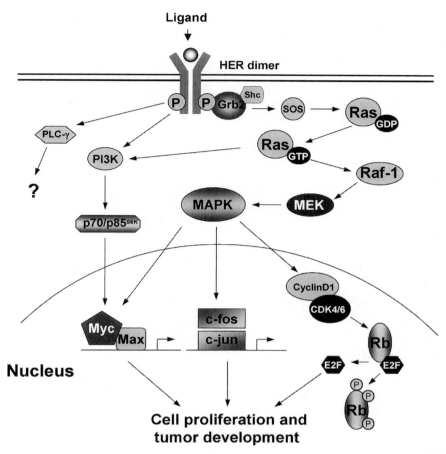

Figure 74-2 The major signal transduction pathways activated by HER2/*neu* heterodimers. Ligand induction of HER2/*neu*-containing dimerization induces phosphorylation on specific tyrosine residues in the C-terminus of the dimer. Downstream signaling substrates grb2 and/or Shc can complex with activated receptor tyrosine kinases via src homology-2 domains. Interaction between SOS and Shc/grb2 catalyzes the activation of ras-GTP complex. Subsequent activation of *Raf-1* and MAP kinase pathways by ras leads to cell proliferation and breast tumor progression through activation of a number of nuclear targets, including *c-fos*, *c-jun*, *myc*, cyclin D1, E2F, and so on. Another pathway is the PI3K, whose activation results in increased pro-survival signals. In addition, PLC-γ mediates the transforming potential of HER2 via uncertain pathways. CDK, cyclin-dependent kinase; HER, Hercgulin; MEK, MAPK/ERK kinase; Rb, retinoblastoma protein; P, phosphate; PI3K, phosphoinositide 3-kinase; SOS, son of sevenless.

also be associated with endocrine resistance. Attempts to target HER1 by the small molecule tyrosine kinase inhibitor, gefitinib, have shown modest effects in heavily pretreated advanced breast cancer patients. Combined approaches with trastuzamab, endocrine therapy, or cytotoxics are under evaluation.

C-MYC The proto-oncogene c-*myc* belongs to the *myc* gene family that also includes B-*myc*, L-*myc*, N-*myc*, and S-*myc*. c-*myc* is a nuclear transcription factor that, when dimerized with Max, binds to a specific DNA sequence in the promoter region of target genes that are involved in regulating cell proliferation and apoptosis. Cell transformation may occur when c-*myc* is aberrantly expressed or genetically altered.

c-*myc* amplification has been found in approx 20% of primary human breast cancers and occurs more frequently in tumors that lack ER and/or PR expression. The transformation of normal cells by c-*myc* generally requires the coactivation and/or amplification of other important oncogenes like HER2/*neu*, cyclin D1 gene (*ccnd1*), and *ras*, and so on. The tumor suppressor *BRCA1* can also physically interact with c-*myc* and repress c-*myc*-mediated transcription. However, loss of p53 in breast cells seems to have negligible effect on c-*myc*-induced mammary carcinogenesis. Although

several studies have indicated a relationship between c-*myc* gene amplification and poor prognosis, other studies did not find such a correlation. This may reflect complex and differential effects of c-*myc* on different proteins and signaling pathways that may ultimately have divergent, even opposite functions.

RAS The *Ras* proto-oncogene family, including the N-, H- and K-*Ras* genes, encodes small GTP binding proteins that regulate many cellular processes, including proliferation, differentiation, cytoskeleton organization, and membrane trafficking. The *Ras* protein interacts with a variety of factors, including *Raf*, PI3-kinase, and Ral-GDS and can activate several important proproliferation pathways like MEK/Erk, Akt/PKB, and so on. The role of *Ras* genes in human breast carcinogenesis is not completely clear. Although alteration of *Ras* gene expression has been reported to be associated with aggressive features of breast carcinoma, the incidence of significant *Ras* oncogenic mutations in human breast cancer is rare. Increased *Ras* activity in breast cancer cells has also been reported to occur through HER2/*neu* signaling mediation. Expression of activated *Ras* in ER-positive breast cancer cells results in increased estrogen-independent growth of cells in vitro. This might be caused by *Ras*-induced Erk activity and the activation of Erk-regulated ER coactivator, AIB1. *Ras* signaling is a potential target in breast cancer treatment as *Ras* protein processing farnesyltransferase inhibitors inhibit growth of breast tumor cells in vitro and are under evaluation in advanced breast cancer clinical trials.

CYCLIN D1   Cyclin D1 protein is encoded by *CCND1* gene and was first implicated in tumorigenesis following localization to chromosome 11q13, a region that is commonly amplified in human breast cancer. Cyclin D1, complexed with either cyclin-dependent kinase (CDK)4 or CDK6, controls cell cycle progression in the G1 phase by enabling the enzymes to phosphorylate retinoblastoma protein (Rb), a pivotal factor in cell-cycle regulation (*see* Fig. 74-2). Knockout studies have shown the important role of cyclin D1 in normal mammary gland physiology. Overexpression of *CCND1* gene has been found in approx 50% of human mammary carcinomas. Preliminary studies on primary breast cancers indicate that lobular carcinomas universally overexpress *CCND1*, whereas overexpression in ductal carcinomas is confined to ER-positive cases.

TUMOR SUPPRESSOR GENES AND BREAST CANCER SUSCEPTIBILITY GENES

Although activation of oncogenes is accepted as one essential mechanism to transform normal breast cells, it is clear that inactivation or alteration of tumor suppressor genes may also play an important role in breast cancer progression. Dozens of tumor suppressor genes have been identified and the investigation into the function of tumor suppressor genes in breast cancer has provided invaluable information.

p53   The most commonly mutated tumor suppressor gene in human tumors is p53. Wild-type p53 functions to maintain the genomic stability and has been called "guardian of the genome." When DNA damage occurs, p53 acts as a cell-cycle checkpoint to arrest the cells in the G_1 phase for damage repair or to eliminate the damaged cells by triggering apoptotic pathways. Several independent pathways activate p53 under certain circumstances, including an ataxia-telangectasia mutated/human homolog of the Rad53 (Chk2)-dependent pathway activated by DNA double-strand breaks, an INK4 and p14^{ARF} dependent pathway, and a pathway activated by ultraviolet light or cytotoxic antitumor agents. Increased protein levels and DNA binding affinity of p53 may be caused by reduced mouse double minute 2-dependent proteolytic degradation.

Involvement of p53 in breast cancer development was first reported when germline mutations in this gene were revealed to be responsible for Li–Fraumeni syndrome, a hereditary cancer syndrome that includes elevated risk of breast cancer. This clinical finding implies an important role for p53 in mammary carcinogenesis. However, comprehensive meta-analysis showed that only approx 20% of primary breast cancers express mutant p53 protein. Although loss of heterozygosity (LOH) in the p53 gene is a common phenomenon in primary breast cancer, the majority of cases with LOH retain one wild-type p53 allele. Several studies indicate that p53 mutations are rare in low-grade DCIS, but more frequent in high-grade DCIS. An increased rate of p53 mutations has been observed in cancers with germline *BRCA1/BRCA2* mutations, suggesting that the distribution and type of p53 changes may be affected by *BRCA1/BRCA2* status in breast cancer. Moreover, certain types of breast carcinoma like typical medullary carcinoma are associated with higher frequencies of p53 mutation.

Many studies support the prognostic significance of p53 mutations in breast cancer. There is evidence that tumors with missense p53 mutations affecting amino acids critical for DNA binding are associated with very aggressive phenotype and a short survival, whereas null mutations or other kinds of missense mutation display an intermediate clinical phenotype. Preclinical studies also suggest that analysis of p53 mutation status can provide valuable information to predict the response to DNA damaging chemotherapeutic drugs in breast cancer patients. It is hoped that molecular analysis of specific components in p53 signaling pathway may ultimately provide greater impact on the diagnosis, prognostication, and selection of optimal treatment for breast cancer patients.

RETINOBLASTOMA GENE   The Rb gene, the classic example of a tumor suppressor gene, is located on chromosomal band 13q14 and encodes for a 105 kDa protein. Hyperphosphorylation of Rb by cyclin-dependent kinases allows cells to progress from G_1 to S-phase. Unphosphorylated Rb restricts cell-cycle progression in G_1 by interacting with various proteins including the growth-stimulatory protein, E2F. Loss of Rb activity has been implicated in breast cancer progression. Structural abnormalities of the Rb gene including chromosomal loss and mutations have been reported in approx 20–30% of breast cancers. Other mechanisms like methylation of the Rb promoter may also result in down-regulation of Rb gene expression. Estrogen may not only lead to the phosphorylation of Rb but also increase Rb mRNA and protein levels in estrogen-dependent breast cancer cells, suggesting that regulation of Rb by estrogen may contribute to breast tumorigenesis.

BRCA1/BRCA2   It has been estimated that 5–10% of all breast cancers are linked to hereditary genetic predisposition. In the early 1990s, two breast cancer susceptibility genes, *BRCA1* and *BRCA2*, were identified. Germline mutation of either of these two genes followed by somatic inactivation of the remaining wild type allele may lead to the cancer phenotype that accounts for some inherited breast cancer cases. Although *BRCA* mutations are rare, women who carry these mutations have a very high lifetime risk of developing breast cancer. Clinical features that imply a genetic alteration of *BRCA1* and *BRCA2* include bilateral breast cancer, breast cancer development at an unusually young age, and ovarian cancer. It is not clear why germline mutations of *BRCA1* and *BRCA2* genes, which are transmitted in an autosomal-dominant fashion, predispose particularly to breast or ovarian cancer. It is possible that other factors or exposures like reproductive factors and hormonal influences play a role.

The *BRCA1* and *BRCA2* genes are located on chromosome 17q21 and 13q12-q13, respectively. *BRCA1/2* proteins are thought to function as tumor suppressors and are involved in repair of DNA damage and maintenance of chromosome integrity. The understanding of the role of *BRCA1* and *BRCA2* in DNA repair is summarized in Fig. 74-3. When DNA damage occurs, *BRCA1* is phosphorylated by ataxia-telangiectasia (ATM) mutated protein kinase. Phosphorylated *BRCA1* in turn activates DNA repair machinery through formation of a complex with *BRCA2*, *BRCA1*-associated RING domain, *Rad51* and/or *Rad50*, which are key proteins for mitotic recombination and DNA break repair. Loss of *BRCA1* or *BRCA2* function in breast cells leads to chromosomal instability and triggers checkpoint activation. If the checkpoint function is intact, critical checkpoint genes like p53 and p21 may be activated and induce cell-cycle arrest. However, mutation of *BRCA* genes frequently results in an accelerated accumulation of secondary genetic changes. When such secondary genetic changes occur to critical checkpoint genes like p53, the checkpoint cannot be activated and

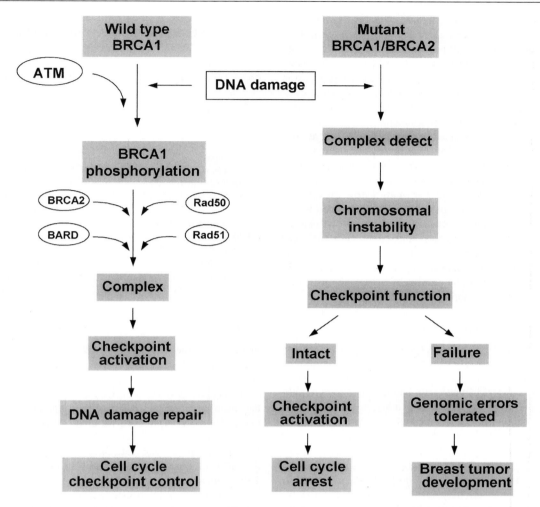

Figure 74-3 Function of breast cancer susceptibility genes *BRCA1* and *BRCA2* in DNA repair. In response to DNA damage, *BRCA1* is phosphorylated by ataxia-telangectasia mutated protein kinase. Phosphorylated *BRCA1* activates DNA damage repair by recombination with *BRCA2*, BRCA1-associated RING domain, Rad50 and/or Rad51. The complex might be involved in DNA-damage cell-cycle checkpoint. Mutations in *BRCA1* and/or *BRCA2* may cause a complex recombination defect in response to DNA damage and would lead to chromosomal instability. If the checkpoint function is intact, important checkpoint genes such as p53 and p21 can be activated and induce cell-cycle arrest. When such a checkpoint has already been disabled (e.g., p53 mutation), the chromosomal errors may be tolerated and lead to uncontrolled neoplastic progression.

uncontrolled cell growth may result. In support of this, an increased frequency and accelerated onset of breast tumors accompanying p53 inactivation has been observed in *BRCA1* knockout mice.

The identification of *BRCA1* and *BRCA2* makes predictive genetic testing possible for individuals in families where a disease-associated mutation is identified. However, *BRCA1* and *BRCA2* mutations are found in a limited proportion (<50%) of inherited breast cancer families, suggesting that *BRCA1/2* mutations are unlikely to be the only genetic change in inherited breast cancer. In addition, somatic mutations of *BRCA1* and *BRCA2* are absent in sporadic breast cancer. To better understand the genetics of inherited breast cancer as well as the development of sporadic breast cancer, it is important to identify other potential breast cancer susceptibility genes or nongenetic factors, whose activities may contribute to the greater burden of breast cancer.

GENETIC CHANGES IN BREAST CANCER ADHESION, INVASION, AND METASTASIS

Normal breast epithelial cells are arrayed in a very orderly manner and are cemented in position by a number of cell adhesion and basement proteins; the development of invasive breast cancer requires loss of adhesive properties and the acquisition of a motile and invasive phenotype. Mutations in the cognate genes may lead to the malfunction of adhesion proteins. Two types of cell adhesion proteins related to breast cancer invasion are the cadherins and integrins. E-cadherin (E-Cad) is a member of the cadherin superfamily and plays a critical role in initiating and maintaining cell–cell contacts and suppressing invasion. The E-Cad gene is located on chromosome 16q22.1, a region frequently associated with LOH in sporadic breast cancer. Loss of E-Cad resulting from inactivating mutations has been detected in early breast carcinomas. CpG hypermethylation of the E-Cad gene correlates with loss of E-Cad expression in breast cancers that lack E-Cad mutations. Re-expression of E-Cad in E-Cad-negative breast cancer cells in laboratory models decreases motility and invasiveness, suggesting a metastasis suppressor role of this protein in breast cancer development. Another important class of cell adhesion molecules is integrin receptors that are actively involved in regulation of cell–cell and cell–stromal interactions. Integrins form heterodimers that provide a transmembrane link between cytoskeleton and specific extracellular matrix proteins. Among these dimers, $\alpha_2\beta_1$ and α_6 integrins (especially $\alpha_6\beta_1$ and $\alpha_6\beta_4$) have been most clearly implicated in breast cancer progression. The cross-talk between integrins and receptors for some important growth factors, hormones, and cytokines may contribute to breast cancer invasion and metastasis. In particular, findings show that the integrins activate the PI3-K/Akt/PKB signaling pathway, which plays a pivotal role in invasive breast carcinoma development.

Enzymatic proteolysis degrades extracellular matrix, permitting cells to traverse the basement membrane, a critical step in breast cancer invasion and metastasis. Three major groups of proteolytic enzymes implicated in breast invasion and metastasis include cathepsins, serine proteinases, and matrix metalloproteinases. In addition, several factors may affect tumor cell motility, including autocrine mobility factor, hepatocyte growth factor, chemoattractants and their receptors, and so on. Research has demonstrated that protein kinase C is also activated in metastatic breast carcinomas. Further understanding of the molecular mechanisms underlying the metastatic process of invasive breast carcinoma will be important for therapy development.

EPIGENETIC ALTERATIONS

Although much work has focused on genetic alterations as previously outlined, more attention has been focused on the contribution of epigenetic modifications to breast tumorigenesis. Indeed epigenetic changes such as DNA hypermethylation and histone modifications may modify gene expression with a higher frequency than genetic changes. Although both genetic and epigenetic changes are heritable, a critical difference between genetic and epigenetic changes is that epigenetic changes are potentially reversible. The role of DNA hypermethylation as an epigenetic regulator of gene expression is the most studied. In the promoter region of many genes, CpG dinucleotides are frequently found to cluster into CpG islands, which extend about 500–3000 bp. Cytosines in these CpG islands may be methylated through the actions of three active DNA methyltransferases (DNMT). DNMT1 is highly conserved in human cells and is mainly responsible for maintenance of DNA methylation. DNMT 3a and 3b are active in *de novo* DNA methylation rather than methylation maintenance. CpG methylation is frequently associated with transcription repression through several possible mechanisms. First, methylation may directly interfere with the transcription initiation at the promoter area of a gene by reducing the binding affinity of sequence-specific transcription factors such as AP-1, NF-κB, and E2F. Also CpG methylation recruits transcriptional corepressors like mSin3A, DMAP1, TSG101, and Mi2. In addition, sequence-independent changes in chromatin structure and histone acetylation and methylation have emerged as an important mechanism to mediate silencing of gene expression. Several methyl-CpG-binding proteins including MeCP2 and MBD1/2a/2b/3 have been identified to function as transcriptional repressors through association with members of HDACs family.

As shown in Table 74-2, studies of DNA hypermethylation alterations in human breast cancer specimens have identified many key breast tumorigenesis-related genes as targets for epigenetic downregulation. Altered cell proliferation is fundamental to breast cancer cell growth and expression of some growth control genes may be epigenetically regulated. For example, loss of tumor suppressor gene p16 expression resulting from methylation of its promoter has been observed in approx 20–30% of primary breast cancers. Progressive methylation of p16 gene may cause human

Table 74-2
Some Epigenetically Regulated Breast Tumor Genes

Gene	Function
Breast cancer type 1 (BRCA1)	DNA damage repair, cell-cycle checkpoint control
p53	Regulation of cell-cycle and apoptosis
p16	Regulation of cell-cycle and senescence, tumor suppressor
Homeo box A5	Regulation of apoptosis
Cyclin D2 (CCND2)	Cell-cycle regulation
Stratifin (14-3-3σ)	Cell-cycle regulation
Estrogen receptor-α and -β	Cell-growth regulation, hormonal therapy predictor
Progesterone receptor	Cell-growth regulation
RARβ	Apoptosis, growth inhibition
Transforming growth factor β receptor II	Regulation of proliferation and cell cycle
E-cadherin	Epithelial cell–cell adhesion
Tissue inhibitor of metalloproteinase-3	Inhibits tumor growth, angiogenesis, and invasion
Glutathione S-transferase PI	Carcinogen detoxification

mammary epithelial cells to escape from block of transient growth plateau (M0), leading ultimately to breast tumorigenesis. *Cyclin D2* is involved in regulation of transition from G1 to S during cell cycle. Hypermethylation of the CpG island in *cyclin D2* promoter has been detected in DCIS, suggesting that loss of *cyclin D2* expression is an early event in breast tumorigenesis. In sporadic breast cancer, DNA methylation has been proposed as an alternative mechanism to inactivate the *BRCA1* gene. One study showed that *BRCA1* promoter hypermethylation was present in approx 13% of unselected primary breast carcinomas.

As noted, steroid hormone receptors may also be epigenetically regulated. Both the ER and PR can be methylated in breast cancer specimens and methylation appears to correlate with gene expression. Use of methyltransferase inhibitors (5-aza-cytidine or 5-aza-2′-deoxycytidine) and HDAC inhibitors may lead to reexpression of ER mRNA in ER-negative breast cancer cells, suggesting that both DNA methylation and histone acetylation are actively involved in regulation of ER-gene transcription. The methylation of the PR has been demonstrated in approx 40% of PR-negative breast cancers. Also expression of retinoic acid receptor (RAR)-β is frequently reduced in breast cancer cells, and RAR-β promoter methylation is thought to be one of the major mechanisms leading to RAR downregulation and loss of response to retinoids.

A number of other critical genes related to breast tumorigenesis are also methylation targets. These include 14-3-3σ, p53, homeo box A5, E-Cad, Tissue inhibitor of metalloproteinase-3, transforming growth factor β receptor II, glutathione S-transferase PI, and so on. (Table 74-2). Knowledge of these methylated markers may provide a useful tool for risk assessment or breast cancer detection as aberrant methylation is felt to be a hallmark of malignancy and CpG island hypermethylation might be detected with higher specificity, sensitivity, and frequency. Also, because epigenetic changes are potentially reversible, strategies to reverse these changes in breast cancer could be a novel approach to treatment.

CONCLUSIONS

As with all cancers, the molecular mechanisms underlying the development of breast cancer are extremely complex. Breast cancer development is a sequential process whereby normal cells accumulate a series of genetic and/or epigenetic changes to genes with diverse functions, ultimately evolving to a malignant state. Damage to proto-oncogenes or tumor suppressor genes such as p53, *BRCA1/2*, *Myc*, and so on, may significantly increase the risk of developing breast carcinoma. Development of invasive and metastatic breast carcinoma may stem from altered expression of genes that regulate cell growth, death, adhesion, motility, and invasion. The management of breast cancer in the clinic is already dependent on the understanding of breast cancer biology. For example, detection of germline mutations in *BRCA1, BRCA2*, or p53 permits identification of high risk individuals who may wish to undertake surveillance or prevention strategies. Knowledge of the expression of the ER, PR, and HER2/*neu* proteins is a prerequisite for effective counseling about the use of targeted endocrine therapies or trastuzamab for breast cancer treatment. It is hoped that enhanced understanding of breast cancer biology will enhance risk assessment, prevention, diagnosis, and treatment. Finally, it is likely that new techniques such as cDNA microarray and proteomic analysis will permit refocusing from the assessment of a handful of genes and proteins to simultaneous consideration of multiple targets, deepening the understanding of breast cancer biology and its clinical implications.

SELECTED REFERENCES

Ali S, Coombes RC. Endocrine-responsive breast cancer and strategies for combating resistance. Nat Rev Cancer 2002;2:101–112.

Barnes DM, Gillett CE. Cyclin D1 in breast cancer. Breast Cancer Res Treat 1998;52:1–15.

Berx G, Van Roy F. The E-cadherin/catenin complex: an important gatekeeper in breast cancer tumorigenesis and malignant progression. Breast Cancer Res 2001;3:289–293.

Dang CV. c-Myc target genes involved in cell growth, apoptosis, and metabolism. Mol Cell Biol 1999;19:1–11.

Debies MT, Welch DR. Genetic basis of human breast cancer metastasis. J Mammary Gland Biol Neoplasia 2001;6:441–451.

Elledge RM, Fuqua SA. Estrogen and progesterone receptors. In: Harris JR, ed. Diseases of the Breast, Philadelphia, PA: Lippincott Williams and Wilkins, 2000; vol. 2. pp. 471–488.

Ellisen LW, Haber DA. Hereditary breast cancer. Annu Rev Med 1998;49: 425–436.

Jones PA, Baylin SB. The fundamental role of epigenetic events in cancer. Nat Rev Genet 2002;3:415–428.

Keen JC, Davidson NE. The biology of breast carcinoma. Cancer 2003;97: 825–833.

Lapidus RG, Nass SJ, Davidson NE. The loss of estrogen and progesterone receptor gene expression in human breast cancer. J Mammary Gland Biol Neoplasia 1998;3:85–94.

Liao DJ, Dickson RB. c-Myc in breast cancer. Endocr Relat Cancer 2000; 7:143–164.

Mallon E, Osin P, Nasiri N, Blain I, Howard B, Gusterson B. The basic pathology of human breast cancer. J Mammary Gland Biol Neoplasia 2000;5:139–163.

Margolese RG, Fisher B, Hortobayi GN, Bloomer WD. Neoplasms of the breast. In: Bast RC, Kufe DW, Pollock RE, Weichselbaum RR, Holland JF, Frei E, eds. Cancer Medicine. Canada: BC Decker Inc., 2000; pp. 1735–1822.

Mihara K, Cao XR, Yen A, et al. Cell cycle-dependent regulation of phosphorylation of the human retinoblastoma gene product. Science 1989;246:1300–1303.

Miki Y, Swensen J, Shattuck-Eidens D, et al. A strong candidate for the breast and ovarian cancer susceptibility gene BRCA1. Science 1994; 266:66–71.

Osborne CK. Steroid hormone receptors in breast cancer management. Breast Cancer Res Treat 1998;51:227–238.

Pharoah PD, Day NE, Caldas C. Somatic mutations in the p53 gene and prognosis in breast cancer: a meta-analysis. Br J Cancer 1999;80:1968–1973.

Reese DM, Slamon DJ. HER-2/neu signal transduction in human breast and ovarian cancer. Stem Cells 1997;15:1–8.

Slamon DJ, Clark GM, Wong SG, Levin WJ, Ullrich A, McGuire WL. Human breast cancer: correlation of relapse and survival with amplification of the HER-2/neu oncogene. Science 1987;235:177–182.

Sommer S, Fuqua SA. Estrogen receptor and breast cancer. Semin Cancer Biol 2001;11:339–352.

Vogelstein B, Lane D, Levine AJ. Surfing the p53 network. Nature 2000;408:307–310.

Welcsh PL, Owens KN, King MC. Insights into the functions of BRCA1 and BRCA2. Trends Genet 2000;16:69–74.

Widschwendter M, Jones PA. DNA methylation and breast carcinogenesis. Oncogene 2002;21:5462–5482.

Yang X, Yan L, Davidson NE. DNA methylation in breast cancer. Endocr Relat Cancer 2001;8:115–127.

75 Lung Cancer

Lei Xiao

SUMMARY

Lung cancer is the leading cause of cancer-related deaths worldwide today. An increasing understanding of the pathogenesis of lung cancer at the cellular and molecular levels has revealed that lung cancer arises as the result of the accumulation of multiple genetic and epigenetic alterations. These include chromosomal abnormalities, aberrant DNA methylation, the activation of proto-oncogenes, the inactivation of tumor suppressor genes, and changes in signal transduction pathways. This chapter provides a brief summary of the recent advances in understanding the molecular biology of human lung cancer with emphasis on tumor-acquired deregulation of cell proliferation and survival.

Key Words: Apoptosis; chromosomal abnormality; epigenetic alternation; lung cancer; oncogene; proliferation; signal transduction; telomerase; tumor suppressor gene; tumorigenesis.

INTRODUCTION

Lung cancer is the leading cause of cancer-related deaths worldwide today, with an estimated 169,500 new cases and 157,400 deaths predicted for 2001 in the United States. Human lung cancer is a disease of heterogeneous histology that can be divided into two major categories: small-cell lung cancer (SCLC) and non-small-cell lung cancer (NSCLC). SCLC represents approx 25% of all lung cancer worldwide. The remaining 75% of lung cancers fall into one of three major subtypes of NSCLC carcinomas: squamous cell carcinoma (SCC), adenocarcinoma, and large cell carcinoma. Tobacco smoking is the most important cause of lung cancer with 80–90% of the disease arising in cigarette smokers. Early epidemiological studies of the smoking-caused lung cancer indicated that SCC was the most frequently diagnosed type of lung cancer, followed by small cell carcinoma. Adenocarcinoma of the lung is the most common histological type of lung cancer in the world, and is the most frequent type of lung cancer in women, nonsmokers, and in young people.

SCLC is distinct from NSCLC in biology, response to therapy, and prognosis. SCLCs are neuroendocrine (NE) tumors that are strongly smoking associated and characterized by early metastasis and initial marked responsiveness to chemotherapy and radiation. However, nearly all patients with SCLC relapse develop resistance to cytotoxic therapies. The overall 5-yr survival rate is only 3–4%. NSCLCs, at large, lack NE features. They respond poorly to chemotherapy as compared with SCLCs. The treatment strategies of NSCLCs are based on the stage of diseases at the time of diagnosis, which include surgery, chemotherapy, radiotherapy, or combined therapy. Although great efforts have been made to improve patient survival, the overall treatment results have not changed significantly in the past 30 yr. The 5-yr lung cancer survival rate remains between 8 and 14%.

In the past decade an increasing understanding of the pathogenesis of lung cancer at the cellular and molecular levels has provided insight into the molecular process underlying lung tumorigenesis and progression. Lung cancer arises as the result of multiple genetic lesions because of exposure to cigarette smoke or other environmental carcinogens as well as inherited predisposition(s). It is becoming clear that genetic changes acquired by lung cancer are multiple, complex, and heterogeneous. These genetic abnormalities include chromosomal deletion and/or amplification, epigenetic changes in DNA methylation, the activation of proto-oncogenes and other growth promoting genes, and the inactivation of tumor suppressor genes (TSGs). NSCLC and SCLC exhibit distinct but overlapping patterns of genetic alterations. This chapter briefly reviews advances in the understanding of the molecular biology of human lung cancer with emphasis on tumor-acquired deregulation in cell growth and apoptosis.

ONCOGENES AND TSGS

Oncogenes are derived from the activation of proto-oncogenes through a variety of mechanisms, including DNA rearrangement, chromosomal translocation, point mutation, gene amplification, and overexpression, whereas TSGs are inactivated through biallelic alterations that are combinations of point mutation, deletion, epigenetic changes, and loss of heterozygosity (LOH). Activation of proto-oncogenes usually results in a dominant phenotype, leading to cellular transformation. In contrast, loss of function of TSGs leads to abrogation of the normal growth control. Alterations of either type of genes could result in dysregulated growth, which eventually can lead to malignancy along with other genetic changes.

ONCOGENES

The Ras Family   The Ras family of genes (N-*ras*, K-*ras*, and H-*ras*) encodes three GTP-binding proteins, which function as molecular switches that cycle between an active GTP-bound and an inactive GDP-bound form, and play a pivotal role in signal transduction. The critical difference between the oncogene and the proto-oncogene is a point mutation resulting in a single amino

From: *Principles of Molecular Medicine, Second Edition*
Edited by: M. S. Runge and C. Patterson © Humana Press, Inc., Totowa, NJ

acid substitution in codon 12, 13, or 61 of the Ras protein. Compared with normal Ras, mutant (oncogenic) Ras has impaired intrinsic guanosine triphosphatase activity, which catalyzes the hydrolysis of the bound GTP. Consequently, a higher proportion of oncogenic Ras exists in the cell as the active GTP-bound form, whereas normal Ras is usually in the inactive GDP-bound form. Thus, oncogenic Ras acts as a signal transducer that causes persistent activation of multiple effector-mediated signaling pathways, leading to cell proliferation, transformation, and other abnormal biological effects in the cell.

Activating mutations of the Ras gene family (major K-*ras*2) have been detected in >30% of NSCLCs, particularly adenocarcinomas. In contrast, *ras* mutations have never been detected in SCLC. The presence of a K-*ras* mutation seems to be an unfavorable prognostic factor and may be associated with tumor progression of NSCLC. This is probably, at least in part, because cells harboring Ras oncogenes become more resistant to radiotherapy and chemotherapy, suggesting that an abnormal Ras signaling may lead to certain cellular changes that are required for developing a resistance to treatment.

Given the relevance of *ras* oncogenes in lung cancer, the activated Ras proteins and/or their downstream signaling components have become attractive targets for therapeutic intervention. The major downstream targets activated by oncogenic Ras include the Raf-1/MEK (ERK-activating kinase)/ERK (extracellular signal-regulated kinase) pathway and the Raf-independent pathways such as the JNK/stress-activated protein kinase pathway. Activation of the Raf-1/MEK/ERK pathway is frequently associated with transformation of primary cells by Ras. However, the Raf-independent pathways seem particularly important for transformation of epithelial cells. This is important because all carcinomas including lung cancer are derived from their epithelial origin. Studies have pinpointed the importance of the JNK pathway in the growth control of lung cancer cells. The JNK/c-Jun/AP-1 pathway plays an essential role in mediating oncogenic Ras transforming function in lung cancer cells, and a significant growth-promoting role of JNK has also been demonstrated in human lung cancer cells. A major target of the JNK pathway is the AP-1 transcriptional activator, which is made up of homo- or heterodimers of the Jun and Fos family proteins. AP-1 activity is abundantly present in NSCLC cells but not in SCLC cells. The induction of AP-1 activity is associated with a transition from SCLC to NSCLC phenotype in an in vitro SCLC progression model. These data suggest that AP-1 is an important mediator of oncogenic Ras signaling and plays a role during lung cancer progression. It is hoped that a detailed understanding of the Raf-independent signal transduction pathways will serve to identify novel targets for therapeutic intervention.

The Myc Family Members of the *myc* gene family, c-*myc*, N-*myc*, and L-*myc*, are sequence-specific DNA-binding transcription factors that play important roles in cell cycle regulation, apoptosis, and differentiation. Myc proteins heterodimerize with other cellular proteins such as Max. The Myc–Max heterodimers bind to specific DNA sequences, leading to transcriptional activation of the targeted genes. The general mechanism of *myc* oncogene activation is gene amplification or genetic alterations that lead to increased transcription, which results in protein overexpression. Amplification of *myc* family genes is more frequently observed in SCLC than NSCLC, and has been associated with an adverse effect in survival of SCLC. High levels of c-*myc* mRNA have been detected in 58% of primary NSCLCs in comparison to nontumor lung epithelium, suggesting that *myc* gene expression may significantly affect the development of NSCLCs. Moreover, studies have suggested that L-*myc* polymorphism may play a role in the progression of NSCLC and in determining the different susceptibility to lung cancer in smokers.

Bcl-2 The Bcl-2 family of proteins are key regulators in programmed cell death, or apoptosis. The Bcl-2 family consists of proapoptotic and antiapoptotic subfamilies. The interactions between the pro- and antiapoptotic Bcl-2 members help determine cell fate during apoptosis. Bcl-2 is an antiapoptotic member that forms heterodimers with several proapoptotic Bcl-2 members such as Bax and Bak. The mechanisms by which Bcl-2 prevents apoptosis are not fully understood, but stabilizing the mitochondrial membrane and preventing the release of the proapoptotic proteins are possibilities.

Bcl-2 is expressed in the early stage of bronchial preneoplasia and is related to smoke exposure. Bcl-2 expression is more common in SCLCs (75%) than NSCLCs, whereas SCCs show a higher level of Bcl-2 expression than adenocarcinomas. There is no clear conclusion regarding the Bcl-2 status and a survival benefit for patients. However, an inverse correlation between Bcl-2 and Bax expression in low grade (high in Bax) and high grade (high in Bcl-2) of NE lung tumors suggests that Bcl-2 may be linked to the disease progression.

TUMOR SUPPRESSOR GENES

p53 and p14/ARF The p53 gene, located at chromosome 17p13.1, encodes a transcription factor that plays important roles in cell cycle control, DNA damage response, genome stability, and apoptosis. In response to DNA damage, p53 is phosphorylated and functions as a sequence-specific DNA-binding transcription factor that regulates the expression of several downstream genes including p21/Cip1/WAF1, MDM2, GADD45, Bax, and cyclin G, thereby leading to cell cycle arrest or apoptosis. Most p53 mutations identified in human cancers including lung cancer are missense and occur frequently in the DNA-binding domain. Many of these mutations completely abrogate the DNA binding and transactivation function of p53. Thus, transactivation of gene expression by p53 is thought to significantly influence its tumor suppressing activity.

Inactivation of p53 in lung cancer mainly occurs through point mutations or by small chromosomal deletions of the region containing the p53 gene. p53 mutations are present in approx 50% of NSCLCs and more than 90% of SCLCs. A significantly higher frequency of p53 mutations was observed in smokers compared with nonsmokers. Loss of p53 function is viewed as an early event in lung tumorigenesis. This is supported by the presence of p53 mutations and/or the accumulation of the p53 protein in preneoplastic lesions, such as bronchial epithelial dysplasia.

p14/ARF, encoded by the p16/INK4A locus via an alternative reading frame, is one of the major upstream regulators in the p53 growth-control pathway. As an inhibitor of HDM2 (Mdm2 in mice) that reduces p53 levels through proteasome-dependent degradation, p14/ARF prevents p53 degradation by binding to HDM2 and sequestering it in nucleoli, resulting in p53 activation/stabilization. Thus, dysregulation of p14/ARF in cancer provides an additional means of disrupting the p53 growth-control pathway. p14/ARF mutations were found in 19–37% of NSCLCs; the absence of p14/ARF protein was observed in 65% of SCLCs. However, mutations in the p53 gene and loss of p14/ARF expression are not always mutually exclusive suggesting the tumor suppressing function of p14/ARF may be p53 independent.

p16/INK4A and Rb   p16/INK4A and retinoblastoma (Rb) are key components of the cell cycle pathway of p16/INK4A-cyclin D1-CDK4-Rb, which plays an essential role in controlling G1 to S phase transition of the cell cycle. p16/INK4A is a member of a family of cyclin-dependent kinase (CDK) inhibitory proteins and functions by inhibiting the kinase activity of the CDK4/cyclin D1 complex. The cyclin D1-associated CDK4 and CDK6 can phosphorylate Rb, which inactivates Rb's ability to bind to a number of cellular proteins, including the E2F family of transcription factors, thereby releasing cells from the growth inhibitory stage (G0/G1) and promoting G1/S transition.

Inactivation of p16/INK4A has been observed in 30–70% of NSCLCs, whereas Rb inactivation is much more common in SCLCs (approx 90%) than in NSCLCs (15–30%). These findings suggest that the p16/INK4A-cyclin D1-CDK4-Rb pathway is inactivated predominantly through p16/ARF4A inactivation in NSCLC, whereas Rb inactivation appears to be the preferred mechanism in SCLC. Homozygous deletion and epigenetic alterations of promoter hypermethylation are the most common mechanisms for p16/INK4A inactivation. Deletion, nonsense mutations, and splicing abnormalities that lead to truncated (mutant) Rb proteins are responsible for alterations of the Rb gene. A reciprocal relationship between Rb inactivation and p16/INK4A expression has been observed in primary lung cancers, suggesting the inactivation of p16/INK4A and Rb are mutually exclusive.

Tumor Suppressor Genes at Chromosome 3p   Homozygous deletions in specific chromosomal regions may imply the presence of putative TSGs. Chromosome 3p contains several distinct deletion regions including 3p25-26, 3p21-22, and 3p14, which are frequently deleted in lung cancer. Homozygous deletions at 3p14.2 in lung cancer led to the discovery of the fragile histidine triad (FHIT) gene that encodes the protein diadenosine $5',5'$-P^1, P^3-triphosphate (Ap_3A) hydrolase. When introduced into cancer cells with a FHIT gene alteration, FHIT inhibits tumor growth through the induction of apoptosis and/or cell cycle arrest. This links the tumor-suppressor activity of FHIT to its proapoptotic function. Abnormal transcripts of FHIT were found in 40% of NSCLCs and 80% of SCLCs. In addition, approx 50% of primary lung tumors fail to express the FHIT protein, mainly owing to tumor-acquired promoter methylation. LOH of the FHIT gene is more common in smokers (80%) than in nonsmokers (approx 22%), indicating that the FHIT gene is a target for tobacco carcinogens and may occur early in lung tumorigenesis.

The RASSF1 (the Ras association domain family 1) gene, located at the lung tumor suppressor locus 3p21.3, consists of two major alternative transcripts, RASSF1A and RASSF1C. RASSF1A is epigenetically inactivated in >90% of SCLCs and 40% of NSCLCs. Reexpression of RASSF1A reduced the growth of human lung cancer cells in vitro and in vivo, supporting a role for RASSF1A as a TSG. RASSF1A binds Ras in a GTP-dependent manner and may serve as a novel Ras effector that mediates the apoptotic effects of oncogenic Ras. RASSF1A inactivation and K-ras activation are mutually exclusive events in the development of certain carcinomas. This observation further pinpoints the function of RASSF1A as a negative effector of Ras. Importantly, a significant correlation between RASSF1A promoter methylation and impaired lung cancer patient survival was reported, and RASSF1A silencing was correlated with several parameters of poor prognosis

and advanced tumor stage (e.g., poor differentiation, aggressiveness, and invasion). Thus, RASSF1A may serve as a useful marker for the prognosis of lung cancer patients.

In addition to RASSF1A, several candidate TSGs including FUS1, SEMA3B, 101F6, and NPRL2 are all located within 100 kb of RASSF1A in the 3p21.3 region. Data indicate that LOH at 3p, in particular the 3p21.3 region, is one of the earliest changes occurring in smoking-damaged, but histologically normal lung epithelium, suggesting that alterations in the expression of these putative TSGs are a critical early step in the development of lung cancer.

CHROMOSOME ABNORMALITIES

Numerous chromosomal abnormalities including common regions of chromosomal loss and LOH have been found in lung cancer. The chromosomal arms with the most frequent LOH are 1p, 3p, 4p, 4q, 5q, 8p, 9p (p16/INK4A), 9q, 10p, 10q, 13q (Rb), 15q, 17p (p53), 18q, 19p, Xp, and Xq. SCLC and NSCLC show distinct regions of frequent LOH, suggesting that SCLC and NSCLC frequently undergo different genetic alterations. Additionally, a much higher frequency of widespread chromosomal abnormalities has been found in lung adenocarcinoma from smokers than such tumors arising in nonsmokers. This observation supports the idea that lung cancers in nonsmokers arise through genetic alterations distinct from the common events in tumors from smokers.

The most consistent chromosomal abnormality in lung cancer has been the allele loss of chromosome 3p (3p12-26), found in more than 90% of SCLCs and more than 80% of NSCLCs. Several distinct regions on 3p show frequent allele loss or independent homozygous deletions in lung cancer, which represent strong evidence for the presence of potential TSGs. A number of putative TSGs including RASSF1A and FHIT have been cloned from these 3p deletion regions. It should be noted that 3p allele loss also occurs in the normal epithelium of smokers without lung cancer as well as preneoplastic lesions of the lung. A progressive increase in the frequency and the size of 3p allele loss was correlated with the increasing severity of histopathological preneoplastic/preinvasive changes. These observations suggest that 3p allele loss is an early event involved in the pathogenesis of lung cancer.

EPIGENETIC CHANGES (ABERRANT PROMOTER METHYLATION)

Epigenetic alterations in general and gene silencing events in particular are viewed as fundamental aspects of tumorigenesis. Tumor cells generally exhibit a global DNA hypomethylation and regional promoter hypermethylation that is associated with gene silencing. Aberrant methylation of CpG islands in promoter regions is one of the major mechanisms for silencing of TSGs in cancer cells. Methylation serves as an alternative to the genetic loss of a TSG function by deletion or mutation. TSGs that are frequently methylated in primary lung tumors include adenomatous polyposis coli, retinoic acid receptor beta, CDH13 (H-cadherin), FHIT, RASSF1A, p16/INK4A, death-associated protein kinase (DAPK), and others. The profile of methylated genes in NE tumors (SCLC and carcinoids) was very different from that of NSCLC, and significant differences in the methylation patterns also exist between the two major types of NSCLC (adenocarcinoma and SCC), indicating that distinct epigenetic alterations may contribute to the development of different subtypes of lung cancer.

A significantly reduced overall, and/or disease-free survival has been linked to the promoter hypermethylation of *DAPK* and *RASSF1A*. Methylated DNA sequences can be detected in primary tumors, circulating in serum DNA from lung cancer patients, in sputum samples before the onset of invasive lung cancer, in pre-neoplastic lesions of lung carcinomas, as well as in the smoking-damaged bronchial epithelium from cancer-free heavy smokers. Thus, an assessment of promoter hypermethylation of certain TSGs may be useful biomarkers for early diagnosis and risk assessment of lung cancer.

TELOMERASE

Telomerase is a specialized ribonucleoprotein polymerase that adds TTAGGG repeats at the ends of vertebrate chromosomal DNA called telomeres. Telomeres are important in maintaining stability of the chromosome, which undergo progressive shortening with cell division through replication-dependent sequence loss at DNA termini. Telomerase is thought to compensate for the loss of telomeric repeats and is associated with the acquisition of the immortal phenotype. Telomerase activity is detected in many types of human cancers. Almost all SCLCs and approx 80% of NSCLCs are telomerase positive. Telomerase activity has been directly correlated with malignant and metastatic phenotypes of human lung cancer. Telomerase RNA expression was present in 20% of hyperplasia, 53% of dysplasia, and 100% of microinvasion and carcinoma *in situ*. Lower levels of telomerase activity were detected in preneoplastic lung cancer lesions compared with invasive cancer. These findings indicate that dysregulation of telomerase expression increases along with lung tumor progression.

GROWTH FACTORS/RECEPTORS

Many growth factors or neuropeptides and their receptors are expressed and/or mutated in human lung cancer cells or in the adjacent stroma. This results in multiple autocrine and/or paracrine circuits that activate the positive growth signaling pathways and promote tumor cell growth. Neuropeptides and their specific G protein-coupled receptors (GPCR) play a key role in the regulation of SCLC growth, whereas peptide growth factors and receptor tyrosine kinases (RTKs) are more important for stimulating NSCLC growth. In the context of the multistage evolution of cancer, these autocrine and/or paracrine mitogens may play a role as tumor promoters in the early stages of lung tumorigenesis and/or later as growth stimulators in the unrestrained growth of the fully developed lung tumor.

NEUROPEPTIDE GROWTH FACTORS Neuropeptide growth factors include gastrin-releasing peptide (GRP) and bombesin-like peptides that have been extensively studied as neuropeptide mitogens in SCLC. Expression of GRP was demonstrated in 20–60% of SCLCs but less frequently in NSCLCs by immunohistochemical analysis. Neutralizing antibodies against GRP/bombesin and bombesin antagonists inhibit both in vitro and in vivo growth of SCLC cells. In addition, a high frequency (>50%) of coexpression of gastrin and its receptor CCK-B in SCLCs suggests that the neuropeptide autocrine signaling is a prominent driving force for SCLC proliferation.

GRP and bombesin-like peptides function as autocrine growth factors, which signal through the GPCRs. GRP and bombesin-like peptides bind to at least three GPCRs, including the GRP receptor, the bombesin receptor, and the neuromedin B receptor, which lead to the activation of multiple intracellular protein kinase pathways that ultimately converge on the regulation of some important cell cycle proteins. In particular, activation of protein kinase C (PKC) and the mitogen-activated protein kinase cascade play important roles in regulating neuropeptide autocrine growth signaling in SCLC cells.

RECEPTOR TYROSINE KINASES RTKs are key components of signaling pathways that regulate cell growth, differentiation, and survival. RTKs consist of an extracellular-, transmembrane-, and intracytoplasmic-domain and are activated through appropriate ligand binding. Ligand binding of the receptor results in dimerization and activation of tyrosine kinase activity through autophosphorylation of the intracellular tyrosine kinase domain of the receptor itself. The phosphotyrosine residues of activated RTKs play a crucial role in transducing extracellular signals to intracellular signaling molecules. Oncogenic activation of RTKs occurs through deletion, point mutations, as well as overexpression, which lead to persistent activation of the receptor-mediated signaling pathways independent of ligand binding, resulting in uncontrolled cell growth. A number of RTKs are overexpressed or mutated in human lung cancer cells. These RTKs are attractive targets for therapeutic intervention against lung cancer.

Epidermal Growth Factor Receptor Epidermal growth factor receptor (EGFR, also called *erBB1*) and heregulin receptor (*HER2/neu*) belong to the type-I EGFR family that regulates epithelial proliferation and differentiation. The EGFR is activated by binding the extracellular domain to one of several ligands, including EGF (betacellulin), transforming growth factor-α (epiregulin), and HB-EGF (amphiregulin). NSCLC tumors have been demonstrated to synthesize transforming growth factor-α and HB-EGF, and these growth factors seem to form an autocrine feedback loop with EGFR and, as a result, play an important role in the tumorigenesis.

The EGFR expression varies according to histological subtypes. Overexpression of EGFR was found frequently in 60–80% of NSCLCs but rarely in SCLCs. Overexpression of EGFR is one of the earliest and most consistent abnormalities in bronchial epithelium of high-risk smokers. It is present at the stage of basal cell hyperplasia and persists through squamous metaplasia, dysplasia, and carcinoma *in situ*. The prognostic significance of EGFR overexpression in NSCLC is unclear. However, patients with strong EGFR-expressing tumors tended to have shorter survival than the patients with slight- or nonexpressing tumors.

HER2/neu is highly expressed in approx 30% of NSCLC, particularly adenocarcinomas. High levels of HER2/neu expression are associated with a shortened survival time and with an intrinsic chemoresistance to three commonly used chemotherapeutic drugs (doxorubicin, etoposide, and cisplatin) in NSCLC. Coexpression of EGFR and HER2/neu also occurs in NSCLC tumors. HER2/neu and EGFR coexpression appears to have an additive effect on survival. High HER2/neu expression and high EGFR/HER2 coexpression gave unfavorable prognosis, indicating that HER2/neu and EGFR play a critical role in the biological behavior of NSCLCs.

Proto-Oncogene c-Kit c-Kit RTK is a class III receptor similar to platelet-derived growth factor receptor. c-Kit and its natural ligand, stem cell factor, form an autocrine loop that is implicated in the development of SCLC. Coexpression of c-Kit and stem cell factor was reported in up to 70% of SCLC tumor specimens and cell lines. Inhibition of c-Kit activation by several tyrosine kinase inhibitors led to growth suppression and cell death in SCLC cell lines.

Several additional growth factor/RTK autocrine loops that have been implicated in the growth regulation of lung cancer include insulin-like growth factors and their receptor IGF-R$_s$ as well as hepatocyte growth factor and its receptor c-Met.

DYSREGULATION OF APOPTOSIS

Apoptosis, or programmed cell death, is a highly specific and regulated process that plays an important role in the development and homeostasis of multicellular organisms as well as tumorigenesis. There is an increasing evidence that the control of apoptosis is disrupted in many tumor cells. The dysregulated apoptosis is thought to contribute to enhanced tumor progression and metastasis. Furthermore, it has become evident that resistance to apoptosis is one potential mechanism whereby tumor cells escape from chemotherapy-induced cytotoxicity, leading to cell survival. Development of drug resistance (intrinsic or *de novo*) in cancer cells may be because of their selective alterations in the expression and/or function of genes important to the apoptotic response. These changes may provide a selective advantage for tumor cells, thereby rendering them resistant to chemotherapy.

CASPASES-8   Apoptotic cell death is controlled by the activation of caspases, a family of aspartate-specific cysteine proteases. Caspases are normally expressed as latent zymogens and are activated by proteolytic cleavage at the onset of apoptosis. There are two well-characterized caspase-activating cascades that regulate apoptosis: one is mediated by cell surface death receptors and the other is regulated by the mitochondria. Chemotherapeutic drug-induced apoptosis is, in general, regulated via the mitochondrial pathway.

Caspase-8 is a so-called initiator caspase and plays an essential role in the death receptor-mediated apoptosis. However, studies indicate that activation of caspase-8 is also involved in drug-induced apoptosis. Caspase-8 mRNA expression is absent in most (79%) of SCLC cell lines, but retained in all NSCLC cell lines tested. Loss of caspase-8 gene expression is correlated with the absence of the protein. In addition, the absence of caspase-8 expression was also found in a subset of SCLC tumors but in none of NSCLC tumors. These observations suggest that inhibition of caspase-8 activity represents one potential mechanism by which lung tumor cells, especially SCLC cells, develop resistance to drug-induced apoptosis.

SERINE/THREONINE KINASES

Akt/PKB   The serine/threonine kinase Akt (or protein kinase B) is the cellular homolog of a retroviral oncogene product, v-Akt. Akt is commonly activated in response to growth factor stimulation and plays a key role in cancer progression by stimulating cell proliferation and inhibiting apoptosis. Constitutively activated Akt can contribute to tumorigenesis in vivo in a variety of tissues. The antiapoptotic function of Akt is mediated by phosphorylating various proteins involved in apoptosis, including proapoptotic Bcl-2 family member Bad, the forkhead transcription factor, and glycogen synthase kinase 3. Akt activation might inhibit apoptosis by promoting the increased expression of survival molecules or the degradation of proapoptotic molecules.

Constitutive Akt activity was found in premalignant and malignant human bronchial epithelial cells, but not in nonmalignant human bronchial epithelial cells. Furthermore, Akt is activated in primary human lung epithelial cells in vitro and in vivo by exposure to nicotine and to a tobacco-specific carcinogen, 4-(methylnitrosamino)-1-(3-pyridyl)-1-butanone. Nicotine activation of Akt also promotes the survival of human lung epithelial cells by suppressing apoptosis. The fact that phosphorylated Akt (an activated form) was detectable in 4-(methylnitrosamino)-1-(3-pyridyl)-1-butanone-induced murine lung tumors and in human lung cancers derived from smokers suggests that nicotine activation of Akt plays a role in lung tumorigenesis, and sustained Akt activation might be necessary for tumor maintenance. Thus, Akt and the PI3K/Akt pathway might be important molecular targets for lung cancer prevention and treatment.

Protein Kinase C   PKC is a family of at least 11 structurally related serine/threonine protein kinases that play crucial roles in transducing signals that regulate diversified biological functions, including proliferation, differentiation, and apoptosis. PKC is known to play a role in the regulation of two survival pathways, the PI3K/Akt and MEK/ERK pathways, and has been implicated in regulating drug resistance in cancer cells. Alterations in expression and/or activity of PKCs have been linked to the drug resistant phenotype in lung cancer cell lines and primary lung tumors. Studies suggest that the antiapoptotic effect of specific PKC isoforms, in particular the novel PKC isoforms (PKC-ε and PKC-δ), may contribute to chemoresistance in lung cancer cells. Forced expression of PKC-ε in SCLC cells conferred chemoresistance by effectively blocking drug-induced apoptosis, which was accompanied by the inhibition of cytochrome-*c* release from mitochondria and caspase activation, indicating that dysregulation of the mitochondrial pathway may be involved in PKC-ε-mediated survival. In contrast, inhibition of PKC-δ function with rottlerin, a PKC-δ specific inhibitor, or by a dominant negative mutant, increased apoptosis and dramatically sensitized NSCLC cells to chemotherapeutic drugs. These findings suggest that specific PKC isoforms may be targeted for the novel therapeutic intervention in order to overcome drug resistance in lung cancer.

Death-Associated Protein Kinase   The DAPK is a family of calmodulin-regulated serine/threonine protein kinases that functions as a positive mediator of programmed cell death and is ubiquitously expressed in various tissues. A unique autoinhibiting mechanism is thought to keep these death-promoting kinases silent in healthy cells and ensures their activation only in response to apoptotic signals. DAPK is involved in both death receptor and mitochondrial pathways of apoptosis. *DAPK* is located on chromosome 9q34.1, a region of frequent allelic loss in 50–64% of lung cancer, and is inactivated in a large fraction of lung cancer via aberrant promoter methylation. Promoter methylation of the DAPK gene in NSCLCs is associated with poor prognosis and an advanced pathological stage, but not with exposure to tobacco or asbestos, suggesting that DAPK may be important in the progression of NSCLC from early to late stage disease.

CONCLUSION

It is becoming clear that the development of lung cancer and its progression is the result of accumulations of multiple and complex genetic defects. Modern molecular and genetic techniques have identified numerous genes and proteins whose expression is altered in lung cancer and/or preneoplastic lesions. These molecular abnormalities have provided novel possibilities for translational research into the diagnosis, prognosis, and the treatment of the disease. Certainly, knowledge of the fundamental cellular and molecular biology of lung cancer will significantly advance with the information from the human genome project and the use of genome-wide techniques such as microarrays and proteomics. One major challenge is to successfully translate knowledge into clinical practice.

SELECTED REFERENCES

Alberg AJ, Samet JM. Epidemiology of lung cancer. Chest 2003;123: 21S–49S.

Bost F, McKay R, Dean N, Mercola D. The JUN kinase/stress-activated protein kinase pathway is required for epidermal growth factor stimulation of growth of human A549 lung carcinoma cells. J Biol Chem 1997;272:33,422–33,429.

Bost F, McKay R, Potapova O, et al. The Jun kinase 2 isoform is preferentially required for epidermal growth factor-induced transformation of human A549 lung carcinoma cells. Mol Cell Biol 1999;19:1938–1949.

Brambilla E, Gazzeri S, Lantuejoul S, et al. p53 mutant immunophenotype and deregulation of p53 transcription pathway (Bcl2, Bax, and Waf1) in precursor bronchial lesions of lung cancer. Clin Cancer Res 1998;4:1609–1618.

Brambilla E, Negoescu A, Gazzeri S, et al. Apoptosis-related factors p53, Bcl2, and Bax in neuroendocrine lung tumors. Am J Pathol 1996;149: 1941–1952.

Broers JL, Viallet J, Jensen SM, et al. Expression of c-myc in progenitor cells of the bronchopulmonary epithelium and in a large number of non-small cell lung cancers. Am J Respir Cell Mol Biol 1993;9:33–43.

Budihardjo I, Oliver H, Lutter M, et al. Biochemical pathways of caspase activation during apoptosis. Annu Rev Cell Dev Biol 1999;15: 269–290.

Chan DC, Gera L, Stewart JM, et al. Bradykinin antagonist dimer, CU201, inhibits the growth of human lung cancer cell lines in vitro and in vivo and produces synergistic growth inhibition in combination with other antitumor agents. Clin Cancer Res 2002;8:1280–1287.

Cho JY, Kim JH, Lee YH, et al. Correlation between K-ras gene mutation and prognosis of patients with nonsmall cell lung carcinoma. Cancer 1997;79:462–467.

Chun KH, Kosmeder JW II, Sun S, et al. Effects of deguelin on the phosphatidylinositol 3-kinase/Akt pathway and apoptosis in premalignant human bronchial epithelial cells. J Natl Cancer Inst 2003;95: 291–302.

Clark AS, West KA, Blumberg PM, Dennis PA. Altered protein kinase C (PKC) isoforms in non-small cell lung cancer cells: PKCδ promotes cellular survival and chemotherapeutic resistance. Cancer Res 2003;63:780–786.

Colgin LM, Reddel RR. Telomere maintenance mechanisms and cellular immortalization. Curr Opin Genet Dev 1999;9:97–103.

Cory S, Adams JM. The bcl2 family: regulators of the cellular life-or-death switch. Nat Rev Cancer 2002;2:647–656.

Crowell JA, Steele VE. AKT and the phosphatidylinositol 3-kinase/AKT pathway: important molecular targets for lung cancer prevention and treatment. J Natl Cancer Inst 2003;95:252, 253.

Dammann R, Li C, Yoon JH, et al. Epigenetic inactivation of a RAS association domain family protein from the lung tumour suppressor locus 3p21.3. Nat Genet 2000;25:315–319.

Dammann R, Schagdarsurengin U, Strunnikova M, et al. Epigenetic inactivation of the Ras-association domain family 1 (RASSF1A) gene and its function in human carcinogenesis. Histol Histopathol 2003;18:665–677.

Dempsey EC, Newton AC, Mochly-Rosen D, et al. Protein kinase C isozymes and the regulation of diverse cell responses. Am J Physiol Lung Cell Mol Physiol 2000;279:L429–L438.

Ding L, Wang H, Lang W, Xiao L. Protein kinase C-epsilon promotes survival of lung cancer cells by suppressing apoptosis through dysregulation of the mitochondrial caspase pathway. J Biol Chem 2002; 277:35,305–35,313.

Dong X, Mao L. Molecular biology of human lung cancer. In: Weitberg AB, ed. Cancer of the Lung, Totowa: Humana Press, 2002; pp. 103–127.

Evan GI, Vousden KH. Proliferation, cell cycle and apoptosis in cancer. Nature 2001;411:342–348.

Facchini FM, Spiro SG. Chemotherapy in small-cell lung cancer. In: Brambilla C, Brambilla E, eds. Lung Biology in Health and Disease: Lung Tumors, vol. 124. New York: Marcel Dekker, 1999; pp. 611–630.

Ferreira CG, Span SW, Peters GJ, et al. Chemotherapy triggers apoptosis in a caspase-8-dependent and mitochondria-controlled manner in the non-small cell lung cancer cell line NCI-H460. Cancer Res 2000;60:7133–7141.

Fontanini G, De Laurentiis M, Vignati S, et al. Evaluation of epidermal growth factor-related growth factors and receptors and of neoangiogenesis in completely resected stage I–IIIA non-small cell lung cancer: amphiregulin and microvessel count are independent prognostic indicators of survival. Clin Cancer Res 1998;4:241–249.

Franklin WA, Veve R, Hirsch FR, et al. Epidermal growth factor receptor family in lung cancer and premalignancy. Semin Oncol 2002;29 (Suppl 4):3–14.

Gazzeri S, Della Valle V, Chaussade L, et al. The human p19ARF protein encoded by the beta transcript of the p16INK4a gene is frequently lost in small cell lung cancer. Cancer Res 1998;58:3926–3931.

Girard L, Zochbauer-Muller S, Virmani AK, et al. Genome-wide allelotyping of lung cancer identifies new regions of allelic loss, differences between small cell lung cancer and non-small cell lung cancer, and loci clustering. Cancer Res 2000;60:4894–4906.

Grandori C, Eisenman RN. Myc target genes. Trends Biochem Sci 1997;22:177–181.

Greenlee RT, Hill-Harmon MB, Murray T, Thun M. Cancer statistics, 2001. CA Cancer J Clin 2001;51:15–36.

Grossi F, Loprevite M, Chiaramondia M, et al. Prognostic significance of K-ras, p53, bcl-2, PCNA, CD34 in radically resected non-small cell lung cancers. Eur J Cancer 2003;39:1242–1250.

Hanaoka T, Nakayama J, Mukai J, et al. Association of smoking with apoptosis-regulated proteins (Bcl-2, bax and p53) in resected non-small-cell lung cancers. Int J Cancer 2001;91:267–269.

Hecht SS. Tobacco smoke carcinogens and lung cancer. J Natl Cancer Inst 1999;91:1194–1210.

Hibi K, Takahashi T, Yamakawa K, et al. Three distinct regions involved in 3p deletion in human lung cancer. Oncogene 1992;7:445–449.

Hirsch FR, Scagliotti GV, Langer CJ, et al. Epidermal growth factor family of receptors in preneoplasia and lung cancer: perspectives for targeted therapies. Lung Cancer 2003;41(Suppl 1):S29–S42.

Hofmann J. Modulation of protein kinase C in antitumor treatment. Rev Physiol Biochem Pharmacol 2001;142:1–96.

Hung J, Kishimoto Y, Sugio K, et al. Allele-specific chromosome 3p deletions occur at an early stage in the pathogenesis of lung carcinoma. JAMA 1995;273:558–563.

Husgafvel-Pursiainen K, Boffetta P, Kannio A, et al. p53 mutations and exposure to environmental tobacco smoke in a multicenter study on lung cancer. Cancer Res 2000;60:2906–2911.

Jacobson DR. ras mutations in lung cancer. In: Brambilla C, Brambilla, E, eds. Lung Tumors. New York: Marcel Dekker, 1999; pp. 139–156.

Ji L, Nishizaki M, Gao B, et al. Expression of several genes in the human chromosome 3p21.3 homozygous deletion region by an adenovirus vector results in tumor suppressor activities in vitro and in vivo. Cancer Res 2002;62:2715–2720.

Jones PA, Baylin SB. The fundamental role of epigenetic events in cancer. Nat Rev Genet 2002;3:415–428.

Kalomenidis I, Orphanidou D, Papamichalis G, et al. Combined expression of p53, Bcl-2, and p21WAF-1 proteins in lung cancer and premalignant lesions: association with clinical characteristics. Lung 2001; 179:265–278.

Kashiwabara K, Oyama T, Sano T, et al. Correlation between methylation status of the p16/CDKN2 gene and the expression of p16 and Rb proteins in primary non-small cell lung cancers. Int J Cancer 1998;79: 215–220.

Kelley MJ, Johnson BE. Molecular genetics of lung cancer. In: Carney DN, ed. Lung Cancer. Boston: Arnold, 1995; pp. 245–266.

Khosravi-Far R, Campbell S, Rossman K, Der CJ. Increasing complexity of Ras signal transduction: involvement of Rho family proteins. Adv Cancer Res 1998;72:57–107.

Kim DH, Nelson HH, Wiencke JK, et al. Promoter methylation of DAP-kinase: Association with advanced stage in non-small cell lung cancer. Oncogene 2001;20:1765–1770.

Krystal GW, Hines SJ, Organ CP. Autocrine growth of small cell lung cancer mediated by coexpression of c-kit and stem cell factor. Cancer Res 1996;56:370–376.

Kumimoto H, Hamajima N, Nishimoto Y, et al. L-myc genotype is associated with different susceptibility to lung cancer in smokers. Jpn J Cancer Res 2002;93:1–5.

Levine AJ. p53, the cellular gatekeeper for growth and cell division. Cell 1997;88:323–331.

Lowy DR, Willumsen BM. Function and regulation of *ras*. Annu Rev Biochem 1993;62:851–891.

Mabry M, Nakagawa T, Nelkin B, et al. v-Ha-ras oncogene insertion: a model for tumor progression of human small cell lung cancer. Proc Natl Acad Sci U S A 1988;85:6523–6527.

Mao L, Hruban RH, Boyle JO, et al. Detection of oncogene mutations in sputum precedes diagnosis of lung cancer. Cancer Res 1994;54:1634–1637.

Mills NE, Fishman C, Rom WN, et al. Increased prevalence of K-ras oncogene mutations in lung adenocarcinoma. Cancer Res 1995;55:1444–1447.

Milner AE, Palmer DH, Hodgkin EA, et al. Induction of apoptosis by chemotherapeutic drugs: the role of FADD in activation of caspase-8 and synergy with death receptor ligands in ovarian carcinoma cells. Cell Death Differ 2002;9:287–300.

Minna JD, Roth JA, Gazdar AF. Focus on lung cancer. Cancer Cell 2002;1:49–52.

Mitsudomi T, Viallet J, Mulshine J, et al. Mutations of ras genes distinguish a subset of non-small-cell lung cancer cell lines from small-cell lung cancer cell lines. Oncogene 1991;6:1353–1362.

Nicholson SA, Okby NT, Khan MA, et al. Alterations of p14ARF, p53, and p73 genes involved in the E2F-1-mediated apoptotic pathways in non-small cell lung carcinoma. Cancer Res 2001;61:5636–5643.

Rathi A, Kazuo Y, Onuki N, et al. Telomerase and lung cancer. In: Brambilla C, Brambilla E, eds. Lung Biology in Health and Disease: Lung Tumors, vol. 124. New York: Marcel Dekker, 1999; pp. 269–277.

Risse-Hackl G, Adamkiewicz J, Wimmel A, Schuermann M. Transition from SCLC to NSCLC phenotype is accompanied by an increased TRE-binding activity and recruitment of specific AP-1 proteins. Oncogene 1998;16:3057–3068.

Robles AI, Linke SP, Harris CC. The p53 network in lung carcinogenesis. Oncogene 2002;21:6898–6907.

Roz L, Gramegna M, Ishii H, et al. Restoration of fragile histidine triad (FHIT) expression induces apoptosis and suppresses tumorigenicity in lung and cervical cancer cell lines. Proc Natl Acad Sci U S A 2002;99:3615–3620.

Rozengurt E. Autocrine loops, signal transduction, and cell cycle abnormalities in the molecular biology of lung cancer. Curr Opin Oncol 1999;11:116–122.

Rusch V, Klimstra D, Venkatraman E, et al. Overexpression of the epidermal growth factor receptor and its ligand transforming growth factor α is frequent in resectable non-small cell lung cancer but does not predict tumor progression. Clin Cancer Res 1997;3:515–522.

Sanchez-Cespedes M, Ahrendt SA, Piantadosi S, et al. Chromosomal alterations in lung adenocarcinoma from smokers and nonsmokers. Cancer Res 2001;61:1309–1313.

Sattler M, Ralgia R. Molecular and cellular biology of small cell lung cancer. Semin Oncol 2003;30:57–71.

Scheid MP, Woodgett JR. Pkb/akt: functional insights from genetic models. Nat Rev Mol Cell Biol 2001;2:760–768.

Sethi T, Langdon S, Smyth J, Rozengurt E. Growth of small cell lung cancer cells: Stimulation by multiple neuropeptides and inhibition by broad spectrum antagonists in vitro and in vivo. Cancer Res 1992;52(Suppl):2737s–2742s.

Seufferlein T, Rozengurt E. Galanin, neurotensin, and phorbol esters rapidly stimulate activation of mitogen-activated protein kinase in small cell lung cancer cells. Cancer Res 1996;56:5758–5764.

Sherr CJ. Cancer cell cycles. Science 1996;274:1672–1677.

Shih CM, Kuo YY, Wang YC, et al. Association of L-myc polymorphism with lung cancer susceptibility and prognosis in relation to age-selected controls and stratified cases. Lung Cancer 2002;36:125–132.

Shivapurkar N, Reddy J, Chaudhary PM, Gazdar AF. Apoptosis and lung cancer: a review. J Cell Biochem 2003;88:885–898.

Shivapurkar N, Toyooka S, Eby MT, et al. Differential inactivation of caspase-8 in lung cancers. Cancer Biol Ther 2002;1:65–69.

Shohat G, Shani G, Eisenstein M, Kimchi A. The DAP-kinase family of proteins: study of a novel group of calcium-regulated death-promoting kinases. Biochim Biophys Acta 2002;1600:45–50.

Sidransky D, Hollstein M. Clinical implications of the p53 gene. Annu Rev Med 1996;47:285–301.

Sklar M. Increased resistance to *cis*-diamminedichloroplatinum(II) in NIH 3T3 cells transformed by ras oncogenes. Cancer Res 1988;48:793–797.

Sklar M. The ras oncogenes increase the intrinsic resistance of NIH 3T3 cells to ionizing radiation. Science 1988;239:645–647.

Smit E, Postmus P. Chemotherapy of small cell lung cancer. In: Carney D, ed. Lung Cancer. Boston: Arnold, 1995; pp. 156–172.

Sozzi G, Sard L, De Gregorio L, et al. Association between cigarette smoking and FHIT gene alterations in lung cancer. Cancer Res 1997;57:2121–2123.

Tang X, Khuri FR, Lee JJ, et al. Hypermethylation of the death-associated protein (DAP) kinase promoter and aggressiveness in stage I non-small-cell lung cancer. J Natl Cancer Inst 2000;92:1511–1516.

Toyooka S, Toyooka KO, Maruyama R, et al. DNA methylation profiles of lung tumors. Mol Cancer Ther 2001;1:61–67.

Tsai CM, Chang KT, Wu LH, et al. Correlations between intrinsic chemoresistance and HER-2/neu gene expression, p53 gene mutations, and cell proliferation characteristics in non-small cell lung cancer cell lines. Cancer Res 1996;56:206–209.

Vaux DL, Korsmeyer SJ. Cell death in development. Cell 1999;96:245–254.

Vos MD, Ellis CA, Bell A, et al. Ras uses the novel tumor suppressor RASSF1 as an effector to mediate apoptosis. J Biol Chem 2000;275:35,669–35,672.

Weber JD, Jeffers JR, Rehg JE, et al. p53-independent functions of the p19(ARF) tumor suppressor. Genes Dev 2000;14:2358–2365.

West KA, Brognard J, Clark AS, et al. Rapid Akt activation by nicotine and a tobacco carcinogen modulates the phenotype of normal human airway epithelial cells. J Clin Invest 2003;111:81–90.

Wingo PA, Ries LA, Giovino GA, et al. Annual report to the nation on the status of cancer, 1973–1996, with a special section on lung cancer and tobacco smoking. J Natl Cancer Inst 1999;91:675–690.

Wistuba II, Behrens C, Virmani AK, et al. High resolution chromosome 3p allelotyping of human lung cancer and preneoplastic/preinvasive bronchial epithelium reveals multiple, discontinuous sites of 3p allele loss and three regions of frequent breakpoints. Cancer Res 2000;60:1949–1960.

Xiao L, Lang W. A dominant role for the c-JunNH2-terminal kinase in oncogenic Ras-induced morphologic transformation of human lung carcinoma cells. Cancer Res 2000;60:400–408.

Zochbauer-Muller S, Fong KM, Maitra A. 5' CpG island methylation of the FHIT gene is correlated with loss of gene expression in lung and breast cancer. Cancer Res 2001;61:3581–3585.

Zochbauer-Muller S, Gazdar AF, Minna JD. Molecular pathogenesis of lung cancer. Annu Rev Physiol 2002;64:681–708.

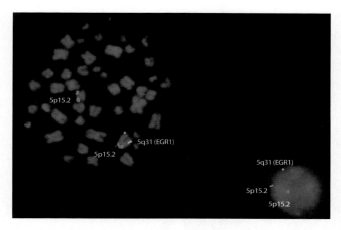

Figure 4-2 (*See* full caption on p. 28 and discussion on p. 28. in Ch. 4) FISH of a pediatric leukemia sample demonstrating that one chromosome 5 contains a deleted segment that includes the *EGR1* gene.

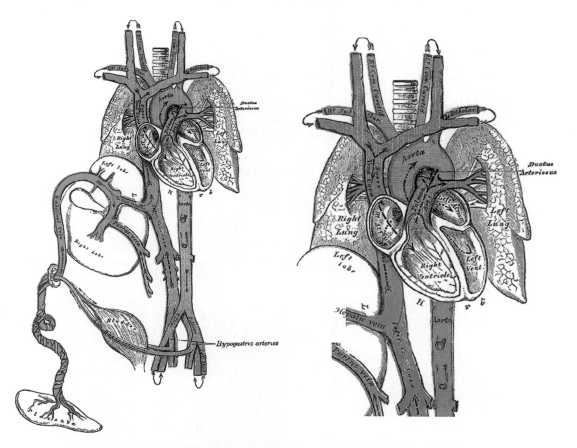

Figure 10-1 (*See* full caption on p. 91 and discussion on p. 90. in Ch. 10) (Left) Fetal circulation in the human. Oxygenated blood travels from the placenta to the fetus through the umbilical vein and then the ductus venosus.

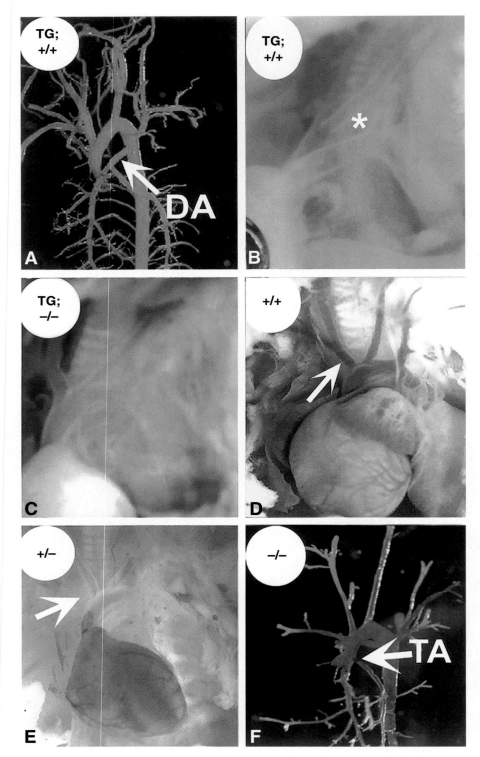

Figure 10-2 (*See* full caption on p. 94 and discussion on p. 93. in Ch. 10) Dosage sensitive role of *Tbx1* in the etiology of cardiovascular defects in mice.

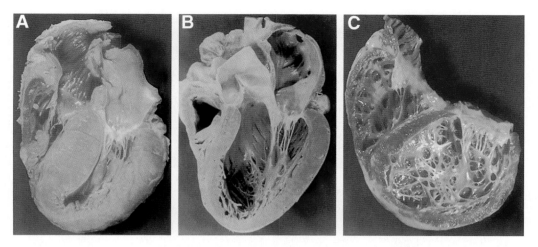

Figure 11-1 (*See* full caption on p. 99 and discussion on p. 98. in Ch. 11) Gross pathological specimens of a heart with (**A**) hypertrophic cardiomyopathy (HCM) and (**C**) dilated cardiomyopathy (DCM).

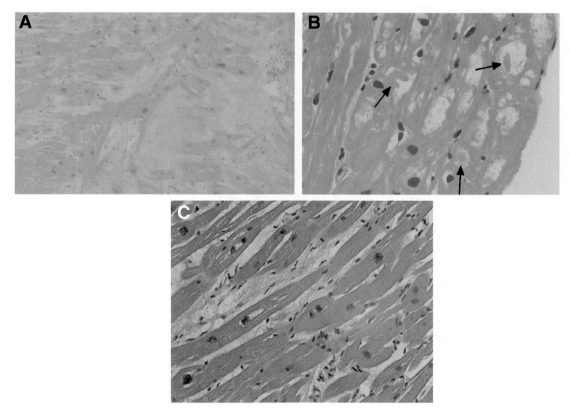

Figure 11-2 (*See* full caption on p. 99 and discussion on p. 98. in Ch. 11) Histopathology of distinct human cardiomyopathies revealed by hematoxylin and eosin staining.

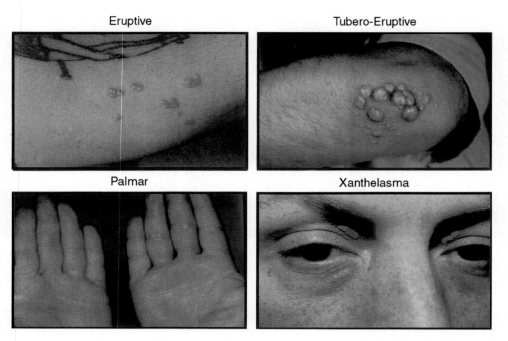

Figure 15-3 (*See* full caption on p. 132 and discussion on p. 131. in Ch. 15) Xanthomas. Several different types of xanthomas are shown.

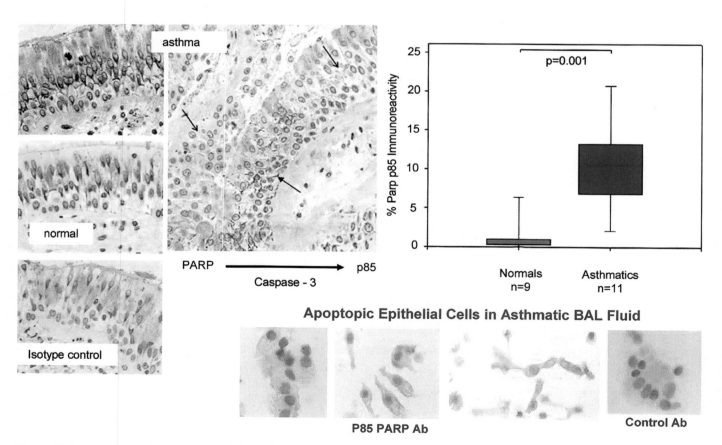

Figure 22-5 (*See* full caption on p. 207 and discussion on p. 207. in Ch. 22) Increased immunostaining for the caspase-3 p85 cleavage product of poly ADP-ribose polymerase in asthmatic mucosal biopsies and BAL epithelial cells.

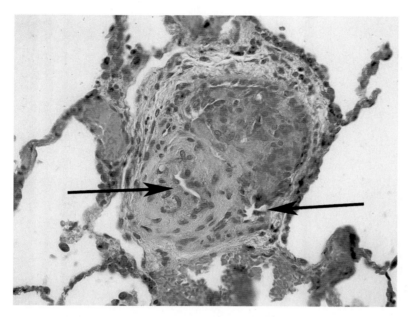

Figure 24-4 (*See* full caption on p. 227 and discussion on p. 226. in Ch. 24). Plexiform lesion. The end-stage of pulmonary hypertension is associated with the formation of occlusive intimal lesions.

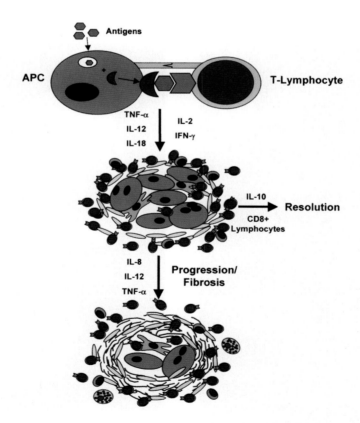

Figure 29-1 (*See* full caption on p. 270 and discussion on p. 269. in Ch. 29) Development of granulomatous inflammation.

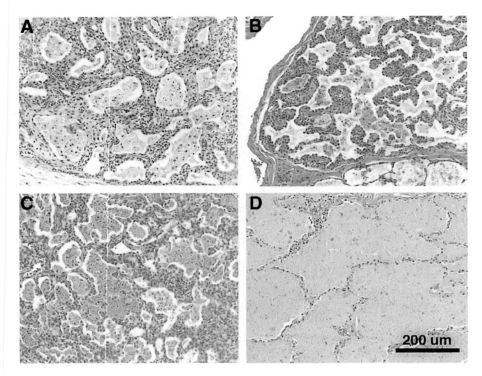

Figure 30-2 (*See* full caption on p. 280 and discussion on p. 278. in Ch. 30) Histopathology of surfactant abnormalities found in the lungs of human patients with **(A)** mutations in the *SFTPB* gene, **(B)** mutations in the *SFTPC* gene, **(C)** mutations in the *ABCA3* gene, **(D)** and antibodies to granulocyte macrophage-colony stimulating factor.

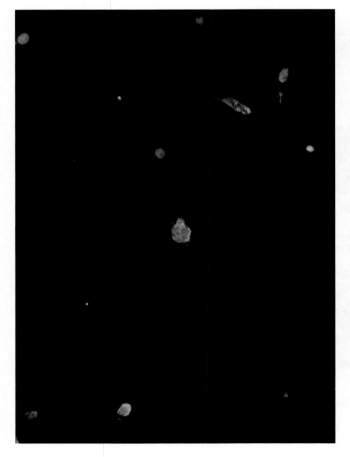

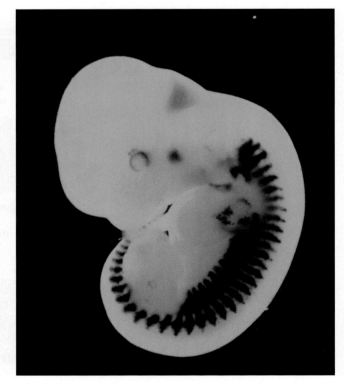

Figure 66-7 (*See* full caption on p. 670 and discussion on p. 669. in Ch. 66) Expression pattern of a myogenin-lacZ transgene in an 11.5-d mouse embryo.

Figure 66-1 (*See* full caption on p. 666 and discussion on p. 665. in Ch. 66) Activation of MHC expression in fibroblasts expressing exogenous MyoD.

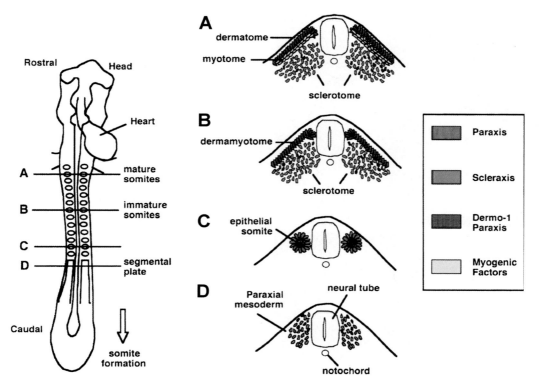

Figure 66-6 (*See* full caption on p. 669 and discussion on p. 668. in Ch. 66) Diagrammatic representation of somite maturation.

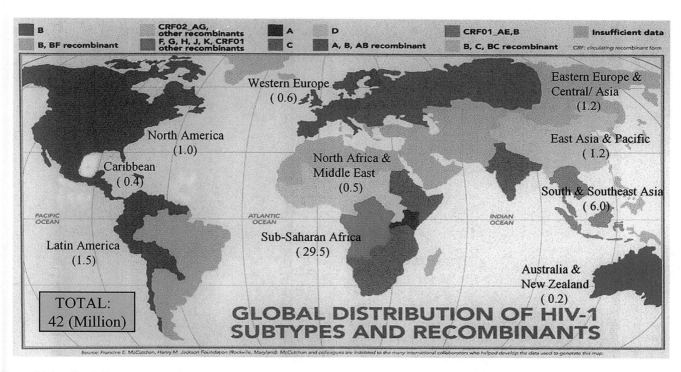

Figure 84-1 (*See* full caption on p. 819 and discussion on p. 818. in Ch. 84) Global epidemiology of HIV type 1 subtypes and estimated number of infected individuals (in millions) at the end of 2002 according to the International AIDS Vaccine Initiative and the Joint United Nations Programme on HIV/AIDS.

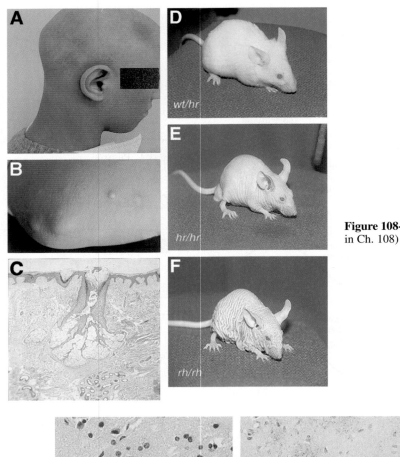

Figure 108-1 (*See* full caption on p. 1054 and discussion on p. 1053. in Ch. 108) Features of the hairless phenotype in humans and mice.

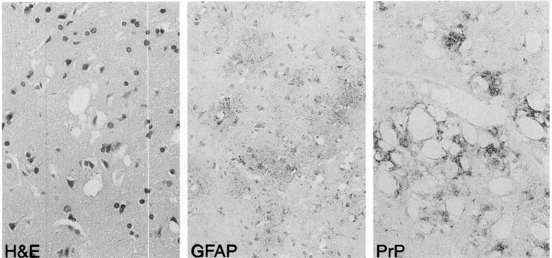

Figure 119-1 (*See* full caption on p. 1143 and discussion on p. 1142. in Ch. 119) Characteristic neuropathologic features of transmissible spongiform encephalopathies.

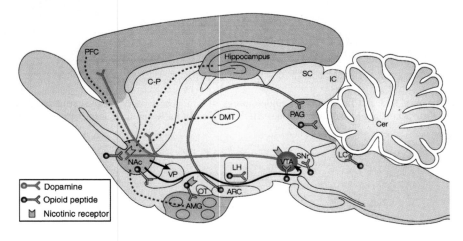

Figure 129-1 (*See* full caption on p. 1222 and discussion on p. 1220. in Ch. 129) Key neural circuits of addiction. *Dotted lines* indicate limbic afferents to the NAc.

76 Discoveries and Frontiers in Prostate Cancer Translational Sciences

Jonathan W. Simons

SUMMARY

With the application of molecular biology and biotechnologies to human prostate cancer research, new targets in the lethal phenotypes of prostate cancer have been rapidly ascertained. How many are pharmacologically amenable and can be blocked with clinical relevance remains to be discovered. For all the emergent genetic and protein target insights, perhaps the greatest challenges will be the participation of more men with prostate cancer in translational research clinical trials that evaluate the new science of therapeutics designed specifically for prostate cancer.

Key Words: Androgen receptor; benign prostatic hyperplasia; glutathione *S*-transferase; hereditary prostate cancer; polycyclic aromatic hydrocarbons; proliferative inflammatory atrophy; prostate cancer; prostatic intraepithelial neoplasia.

OVERVIEW

Prostate cancer is among the most common human neoplasias. In 1990, prostate cancer overtook lung cancer as the most common noncutaneous cancer diagnosed in US men. More than 30,000 US men were projected to die from prostate cancer in 2004; this is an estimated annual loss of 300,000 yr of life. Prostate cancer is truly a medical burden created from successful increases in *Homo sapiens'* life expectancy in the 20th century; less than 1% of cases are diagnosed under the age of 40. Specific genetic alterations in pathogenesis are reviewed later, but a key factor in human prostate cancer biology is time. Time is required to acquire the specific genetic alterations in the prostate epithelium to confer an invasive metastatic phenotype for human prostate cancer. Despite the decades it takes to emerge, prostate carcinogenesis begins early. Undiagnosed, microscopic foci of prostate cancer have been identified in autopsy series in men younger than 30 yr. The latency of most prostate cancer suggests very important gene–environment interactions may influence later steps in the development of the lethal phenotypes of prostate cancer. Prostate cancer initiation—manifested by a histologically identifiable lesion—is frequent, being detected at autopsy series in nearly one-third of men over age 45. The majority of these microscopic adenocarcinomas do not progress to clinically detectable tumors within the lifetime of these men. A critical question is: why not? Epigenetic and genetic factors that create clinically aggressive cancers from incidentally diagnosed ones are at the heart of investigation. The long latency period of prostate cancer affords a new opportunity for chemoprevention, and potentially dietary interventions as described later.

Despite its incidence and mortality in the developed world, prostate cancer has historically lagged behind others in molecular understanding of pathogenesis. With a significant push from the activism of national nonprofit organizations of prostate cancer survivors in the United States, federal funding has increased over 500% from its 1993 baseline to 2000. By 2003, a concomitant increase in new research models and basic understanding has affected the field and defined treatment targets for the future. Described later are discoveries that have generated new opportunities for translational research to reduce the morbidity and mortality of prostate cancer. A special emphasis is placed on implications for therapy in chemoprevention and the development of systemic therapies for advanced disease.

NEW CONCEPTS IN CARCINOGENESIS AND CHEMOPREVENTION

Prostate neoplasia develops in two different regions of the gland, with most lesions (approx 80%) found in the periphery that can be palpated, and most of the remaining cancers found in a periurethral region transition zone. Benign prostatic hyperplasia (BPH) originates in the transition zone of the prostate. Based primarily on this tissue difference in the incidence of benign growth and adenocarcioma formation, and the finding that stromal cell proliferation is typically a major component of BPH. BPH is not the precursor of prostate cancer. Rather, prostatic intraepithelial neoplasia (PIN) containing foci of dysplastic ductal and acinar cells is thought to be the precursor lesion of prostate cancer. PIN lesions have become critical for application of molecular probes to define the earliest changes in malignant transformation at the level of DNA and RNA alterations and protein expression.

The incidence of prostate cancer shows clear age, racial, and geographic dependencies. Prostate cancer is relatively uncommon in Asian populations and prevalent in Scandinavian countries, and the highest incidence (and mortality) rates known are in African Americans, being nearly twice higher than in white Americans.

From: *Principles of Molecular Medicine, Second Edition*
Edited by: M. S. Runge and C. Patterson © Humana Press, Inc., Totowa, NJ

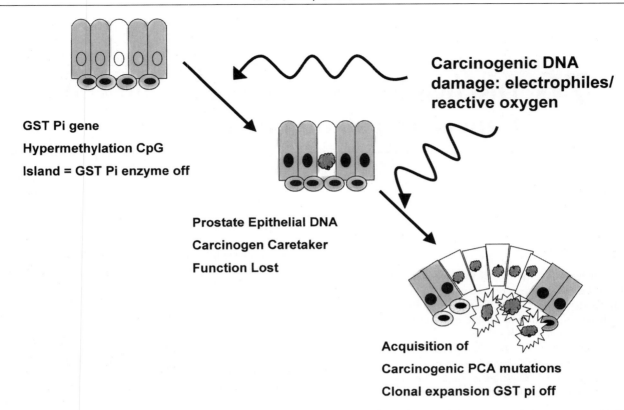

Figure 76-1   GST-π inactivation is the earliest known and essential step in prostate cancer carcinogenesis. Loss of "caretaker" function permits electrophilic attack and mutations to be introduced into prostate epithelial cell DNA. Chemoprevention strategies are oriented to restoring this protective function of GST-π.

Mortality rates vary significantly by country, ranging from the highest reported rates in Trinidad, to 23/100,000 in the United States, to less than one-fifth US rates in Japan.

Significant focus has been placed on interactions of diet and lifestyle and genes critical to prostate cancer tumorigenesis in the developed world. There is also species specificity to human prostate cancer risk. Despite the presence of a prostate in all male mammals, there is no reported high risk for prostate cancer in any other aging mammal in veterinary medicine except for the *Canis familiaris* (dog). Human lineage departed from other higher primates eight million years ago. *Homo sapiens* emerged only about 200,000 yr ago, and only in the past 15,000 yr have humans and dogs experienced dietary changes that might affect prostate cancer carcinogenesis. With civilization and departure from agrarian to urban dietary habits, cooked, smoked, processed, and stored meats became predominant dietary components during this time for man and, via leftovers, for dog. Polycyclic aromatic hydrocarbons and other components of burned red meat in particular are implicated as potential prostate cancer carcinogens; these are created in charbroiling fish and meat. As Asians cultures do not char meats in cooking, the reduced incidence of prostate cancer in Asian men has been speculated to be because of lesser lifetime exposure to intraprostatic polycyclic aromatic hydrocarbons. This would also help account for the increasing rates of prostate cancer in Asian Americans who immigrated to the United States and Western diets one generation ago.

Genetic alterations in prostate cancer tumorigenesis suggest a specific pattern for carcinogenesis in the prostate epithelium (Fig. 76-1). The most common genomic alteration in prostate cancer—and the first identified molecular event in prostate cancer—is the inactivation of the glutathione *S*-transferase (GST)-π gene. GSTs are enzymes that catalyze conjugation reactions between glutathione and various reactive chemical species. GSTs detoxify carcinogens, acting as "caretaker" genes to prevent carcinogen-induced DNA mutations and cancer development. The π-family of GSTs are ubiquitous, and have a critical role in genomic DNA damage defense. For example, GST-π knockout mice carrying disrupted genes exhibit increased skin cancers on cutaneous treatment with 7,12-dimethylbenzanthracene. Somatic inactivation of GST-π by transcriptional silencing associated with *de novo* CpG island hypermethylation occurs in more than 90% of prostate cancers. The loss of GSTP1 in PIN and prostate cancer exposes the cell to genomic damage inflicted by heterocyclic amine carcinogens, such as those present in "well-done" meats, and perhaps more importantly by reactive oxygen species produced by inflammatory cells in prostatitis (discussed later). Thus a unique feature of the prostate epithelium compared with other human cancers is how early in malignant transformation it loses a defined enzyme in detoxifying carcinogens.

Some high-grade PINs and early adenocarcinomas appear to arise from areas of proliferative inflammatory atrophy (PIA). PIA has been recognized as the lesion creating genetically damaged clones that form PIN. PIA has become a focus for carcinogenesis research in prostate cancer. Inflammation and other environmental factors may (1) lead to the destruction of prostate epithelial cells, (2) increase epithelial turnover, and (3) drive the increased prostate epithelial proliferation that occurs in PIA. Decreased G1/S checkpoint control protein p27(Kip1) has been found in PIA lesions. Increased oxidant and electrophile stress in the setting of increased proliferation rates in PIA lesions may be the presumed source for expanding clones that have accumulated new DNA mutations. Epithelial cells in PIA lesions characteristically exhibit several molecular signs of stress, including induced expression of GSTP1, GSTA1, and COX-2. Loss of GSTP1 expression via *de novo* GSTP1 CpG island hypermethylation seems to demarcate the switch from PIA to clonal, GSTP1-inactivated neoplasia in PIN or prostate adenocarcinoma. A major effort in ultimate chemoprevention of prostate cancer will be to block the epigenetic processes that drive PIA into PIN foci.

TRANSLATIONAL RESEARCH IMPLICATIONS: CHEMOPREVENTION

Significant implications for chemoprevention of prostate cancer have arisen from the finding that human prostate cancer is characterized by an early and near-universal loss of expression of the phase 2 enzyme GST-π. First, on prostate biopsies that are negative for adenocarcinoma, diagnostic loss of GST-π expression in high frequency of normal appearing cells may indicate epithelium at lifetime higher risk for developing prostate cancer. Second, investigators are pursuing a mechanism-based prostate cancer preventive strategy that involves induction of phase 2 enzymes within the prostate to compensate for the loss of GSTP1 expression via dietary supplementation. NAD[P]H: (quinone-acceptor) oxidoreductase/quinone reductase enzymatic activity can be measured after treating the human prostate cancer cell lines with known phase 2 enzyme-inducing agents from distinct chemical classes. The search for antioxidant micronutrients in tomatoes and cruciferous vegetables in high throughput screening is ongoing.

Given the interest in Cox-2 in chemoprevention of bowel and other tumors, the role of prostate cancer cell lines do not express basal levels of Cox-2 protein. Analysis of multiple primary human prostate cancer specimens by immunohistochemistry indicates there is no consistent overexpression of COX-2 in established prostate cancer or high-grade PIN, as compared with adjacent normal prostate tissue. Positive staining is observed only in scattered cells (<1%) in both tumor and normal tissue regions but was much more consistently observed in areas of PIA, lesions that have been implicated in prostatic carcinogenesis. Staining was also seen at times in macrophages. Western blotting and quantitative reverse transcriptase PCR analyses confirmed these patterns of expression. The chemoprevention effects—if any—of COX-2 inhibitors are likely to be mediated by modulating COX-2 activity in non-prostate cancer cells (either inflammatory cells or atrophic epithelial cells) or by affecting now recognized COX-2-independent pathways of NSAID action.

MOLECULAR GENETICS OF PROSTATE CANCER: RNASEL, MSR1

Inherited genes are estimated to account for perhaps 10% or more of the risk of prostate cancer. Its heterogeneous nature suggests that the predisposition to prostate cancer may involve multiple genes and variable phenotypic expression. Mendelian inheritance of prostate cancer has allowed genome wide searches for hereditary prostate cancer (HPC) genes. The high prevalence of sporadic cases of prostate cancer has made it very difficult to identify tumor suppressor genes that are involved in familial prostate cancer. Previously, there has been limited success in identifying high-risk susceptibility genes in prostate cancer analogous to BRCA1 or

BRCA2 for breast and ovarian cancer. Linkage studies have identified at least two genes in familial clusters of HPC. The discovery of these genes within the human genome could have broad implications for understanding sporadic prostate cancers. Germline mutations in the gene encoding 2′-5′-oligoadenylate (2-5A)-dependent RNase L gene (RNASEL) segregate in prostate cancer families with autosomal-recessive HPC1 (hereditary prostate cancer 1) region at 1q24-25. The RNASEL gene maps to the HPC-predisposition locus at 1q24-q25 (HPC1). RNASEL has inactivating truncation mutations in two families with linkage to HPC1. Inactive RNASEL alleles are present at a low frequency in the general population. Microdissected tumors with a germline mutation of RNASEL had loss of RNase L protein, and RNASEL activity was reduced in lymphoblasts from heterozygotes.

In addition to the 1q24-25 locus, deletions on human chromosome 8p22-23 in prostate cancer cells and linkage studies in families affected with HPC suggested this region is involved in prostate tumorigenesis. The macrophage scavenger receptor 1 gene (MSR1) is located at 8p22, and in families affected with HPC, six rare missense mutations and one nonsense mutation in MSR1 have been identified. Furthermore, in whites of European descent, MSR1 mutations were identified in 4% of individuals affected with non-HPC compared with 0.8% of unaffected men. Among African American men, these values were 12.5% and 1.8%, respectively. MSR1 genotype may confer major risk for prostate cancer in men from both African American and European descent. Pilot genetic testing with biotechnologies for allelotyping MSR1 and RNASEL are under development.

TRANSLATIONAL RESEARCH IMPLICATIONS OF GENETICS MOLECULAR EPIDEMIOLOGY OF HEREDITY AND PROSTATITIS

Both RNASEL and MSR1 created fascinating new hypotheses for prostate cancer carcinogenesis. Both were discovered by genome-wide searches and both genes unexpectedly are normally involved in host inflammatory responses to infections. The RNASEL gene encodes a single-stranded specific endoribonuclease involved in the antiviral actions of interferons. RNASEL is activated enzymatically after binding to unusual 5′-phosphorylated, 2-5As in viral infections. Virally mediated induction of cell apoptosis is defective in mouse cells lacking RNASEL. RNASEL mutations and some variants may allow genetically RNASEL –/– prostate epithelial cells to escape a potent apoptotic pathway created by a viral prostatitis. If they have become genetically altered, and are RNASEL defective in a normal apoptotic pathway, this might allow premalignant clones to survive in the context of prostatitis.

The finding of MSR1 germline mutations in HPC risk also suggests an impairment in macrophage function could be involved in pathogenesis of prostate cancer. In addition, normal macrophage functions have some protective effect. MSR1 is also involved in macrophage growth and maintenance, adhesion to the substratum, cell–cell interactions, phagocytosis, and pathogen clearance. Taken together, RNASEL and MSR1 have generated the hypothesis that inflammation from prostatitis could contribute to the DNA damage and survival of genetically altered prostate epithelial cells. In this hypothesis, the early loss of GST-π would confer susceptibility to DNA damage from reactive oxygen created by inflammatory intermediates in prostatitis. The testable implications are: (1) RNASEL –/– genotype carriers would have prostate cells that had lost an apoptotic signal in the milieu of interferon caused by

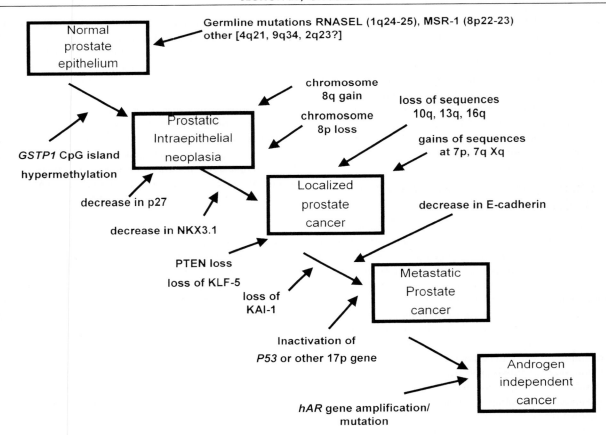

Figure 76-2   Multiple genetic alterations occur in prostate cancer progression. Many of these genomic alterations are not identified. GST, glutathione *S*-transferase.

prostatitis, and could survive with RNASE –/– mutations following prostatitis; and (2) MSR1 –/– genotype carriers might have persistent prostatitis from defects in macrophage clearance of infection in the prostate allowing far longer exposure to inflammatory oxygen free radicals. Although these predictions must be tested by genetic epidemiologists, the concept of genetic risk from prostatitis as a carcinogen for prostate cancer did not exist in the field in 2000. Of note, 9% of men 40–79 yr of age report suffering with symptomatic prostatitis. The key pathogens involved in the prostatitis—geographic differences in prostatic infection rates, population frequencies of the key alleles, and natural history of asymptomatic prostatitis and increased lifetime risk of prostate cancer—are not known. Also, though many cases of symptomatic prostatitis may be triggered by infections, pathogens are not always identified. Intensive molecular epidemiological studies have been launched on prostatitis as causative process in prostate cancer carcinogenesis, with a superimposed risk conferred by inheritance of RNASEL and MSR1 mutations or polymorphisms. *Helicobacter pylori* is a class I carcinogen for gastric cancer risk as a result of reactive oxygen damage from the bacterial infection on the gastric mucosal cells' DNA, not from insertion of oncogenes from the bacterium. The same concept of carcinogenesis from infection may apply to reactive oxygen intermediates' damage to the prostate epithelium from prostatitis. The epidemiological hunt for *H. pylori*—like bacterial and viral pathogens that could infect the prostate epithelium has begun.

In other genome-wide scans, genes on chromosomes 4q21, 9q34, and 2q23 also show evidence for some prostate cancer linkage in some families. Given the prevalence and extensive heterogeneity

in the genetic aspects of prostate cancer disease, global data sets from large numbers of prostate cancer families will be needed to effectively dissect inheritance of genes conferring increased risk. Many more genes in the human genome may modify prostate cancer lifetime risk than originally anticipated.

THERAPEUTIC TARGETS

PROGRESSION: NKX3.1, PTEN, KLF5: MOLECULAR RECLASSIFICATION AND THERAPEUTIC TARGETS   Despite the clinical use of Gleason Grade in prostate cancer pathology, its prognostic powers are limited. The majority of prostate biopsies are Gleason Grade 7, which cannot distinguish those tumors with metastatic potential from those without it. A molecular and mechanism-informing picture of prostate cancer is emerging that is likely to create a "Molecular Profiling with Gleason Grade" for prostate cancer. Figure 76-2 depicts this emerging molecular profile in prostate cancer progression. Tumor suppressor genes have been identified for prostate cancer progression including NKX3.1 from 8p21, PTEN from 10q23, p27/Kip1 from 12p13, and KLF5 from 13q21. In addition to their location in regions with frequent allelic losses, all have functional and/or genetic evidence supporting their contribution to prostate cancer progression. For example, Nkx3.1 homeobox gene plays an important role in normal differentiation of the prostatic epithelium; loss of function in differentiation may be an initiating event in prostate carcinogenesis. Nkx3.1 homeobox gene undergoes epigenetic inactivation through loss of protein expression. In transgeneic systems, loss of function of Nkx3.1 co-operates with loss of function of the Pten tumor suppressor gene in cancer progression in the activation of Akt (protein kinase).

Inactivation of the tumor suppressor gene PTEN is particularly of consequence in prostate cancer. Gene dose may have prognostic significance and create opportunities for the use of PTEN specific signal transduction inhibitors in prostate cancer. PTEN appears to be the most frequently mutated gene in advanced prostate cancer. Many clinical prostate cancers are –/+ for PTEN status. Experimentally, the gene dosage of PTEN mutations affects key downstream targets such as Akt, p27(Kip1), mTOR, FOXO3, and hypoxia-inducible factor (HIF)-1 involved in cell division, metabolic survival, angiogenesis and motility. The loss of the PTEN tumor suppressor phosphatase activity for phosphatidylinositol-3,4,5-trisphosphate allows AKT-1 signaling downstream and has become a major pathway for signal transduction inhibitor drug discovery for prostate cancer. Although the loss of a single allele of PTEN is haploinsufficient to suppress tumors experimentally, PTEN –/– prostate cancer tumors may have even more aggressive behavior than PTEN –/+ tumors. PTEN loss has dual consequences for the lethal phenotype of prostate cancer. PTEN also negatively controls the G1/S cell cycle transition as it regulates the levels of p27(KIP1), a cyclin-dependent kinase inhibitor. A ubiquitin ligase, the SKP-2 complex that mediates p27 ubiquitin-dependent proteolysis, is negatively regulated by PTEN phosphatase. Loss of PTEN affects SKP2 function and permits p27(KIP1) degradation and cell proliferation as well as increases AKT-1 downstream signaling. PTEN mutant, SKP-2 expressing, mTOR activated prostate cancer has become a major focus for development of signal transduction inhibitors. Researchers have discovered that mTOR inhibitors like CCI 779 are in vitro particularly effective against PTEN mutant prostate cancer cell lines in which mTOR is being activated by AKT-1. mTOR inhibitors like rapamycin and CCI 779 have entered phase I/II studies in advanced prostate cancer.

RNA ALTERATIONS IN PROSTATE CANCER: DIAGNOSTIC MARKERS AND THERAPEUTIC TARGETS

With transcriptome profiling using arrayed cDNA biotechnologies, multiple candidate biomarkers, and regulatory genes have been identified by comparing prostate cancer and normal prostate epithelium. The expression and clinical utility of one of the most highly overexpressed—α-methylacyl coenzyme A racemase (AMACR)—has already entered prospective testing. Overexpressed in prostate cancer by global profiling strategies, AMACR upregulation in prostate cancer was confirmed by both reverse transcriptase PCR and immunoblot analysis. These studies were enabled by large tumor banks created by the National Cancer Institutes' SPORES program in the 1990s. Immunohistochemical analysis demonstrated an increased expression of AMACR in malignant prostate epithelia relative to benign cells. Tissue microarrays to assess AMACR expression in specimens consisting of benign prostate, atrophic prostate, PIN, localized prostate cancer, and metastatic prostate cancer demonstrated differences in staining intensity between clinically localized prostate cancer compared with benign prostate tissue. AMACR protein expression in prostate needle biopsy specimens demonstrated 97% sensitivity and 100% specificity for detecting prostate cancer. In less than 4 yr from original discovery to reduction to clinical research in pathology, AMACR is appearing useful in the interpretation of prostate needle biopsy specimens that are diagnostically challenging.

AMACR also may be a new therapeutic target given its differential overexpression in prostate cancer. α-methylacyl-CoA racemase is an enzyme involved in β-oxidation of branched-chain fatty acids. Overexpressed AMACR from both clinical tissues and prostate cancer cell lines is wild type by DNA sequence analysis and enzymatically active. Small-interfering RNA (siRNA) against AMACR, but not control siRNAs, reduces the expression of AMACR and significantly impaired proliferation in androgen-responsive prostate cancer cell lines. Simultaneous inhibition of both the AMACR pathway by siRNA and androgen signaling by means of androgen withdrawal or antiandrogen suppressed the growth of prostate cancer cells in vitro to a greater extent than either treatment alone. AMACR and β-oxidation of fatty acids is important in the optimal growth of prostate cancer cells, and inhibition of this enzyme has the potential to be a complementary target with androgen ablation in prostate cancer treatment.

ANDROGEN RECEPTOR AND ANTIANDROGENS: DISSECTION OF RESISTANCE TO THERAPY AND NEW THERPEUTIC TARGETS

The mainstay of therapy for advanced prostate cancer is medical or surgical castration. Prostate cancer are hormone-dependent malignancies that respond to drugs that reduce circulating testosterone levels or prevent binding of this ligand to the androgen receptor (AR). Whereas effective, these approaches are not curative and, in almost all cases, clinical progression to an androgen refractory prostate cancer is eventually observed. Antiandrogens or androgen withdrawal causes apoptotic death of untreated prostate cancer cells. Growth of normal and neoplastic prostate is mediated by the AR, a ligand-dependent transcription factor activated by high affinity androgen binding. The AR is highly expressed in recurrent prostate cancer cells that proliferate despite reduced circulating androgen. Unlike breast cancer in which a significant percentage of tumors present with loss of estrogen receptors and progesterone receptors, AR expression is selected for in prostate cancer and retained in clinical progression.

Mechanisms of bypass of antiandrogen resistance whereas prostate cancer cells retain the nuclear expression of AR in patients treated with antiandrogens are being identified. The AR can drive prostate cancer progression through three mechanisms: AR overexpression via amplifications, point mutations in the AR gene, and ligand-independent activation of AR. AR gene amplification and mutations creating amino acid substitutions in the AR have been detected at some frequency in metastatic prostate cancers. These changes confer growth advantage to the tumor cells because of either hypersensitivity of AR to low, castrate-level androgens, or a realignment of the receptor conformation, leading to altered ligand specificity that enables adrenal androgens, nonandrogen steroids, or even nonsteroidal antiandrogens to act agonistically to increase AR activity. Persistence of signaling by the wild-type AR in therapy-resistant tumors may also be caused by receptor activity caused by cross talk of AR with multiple intracellular signaling cascades including the IL-6–IL-6 receptor intracellular signaling, phosphoinositide 3 kinase/Akt activation, and the receptor tyrosine kinase growth factors—activated mitogen-activated protein kinase (MAPK) pathways. These complex cross talk circuits in the absence of androgens may be essential pathways for prostate cancer progression in the absence of androgen. For example, epidermal growth factor (EGF) increases androgen dependent AR transactivation in the recurrent prostate cancer cell line CWR-R1 through a mechanism that involves a posttranscriptional increase in the p160 coactivator transcriptional intermediary factor (TIF) 2 /glucocorticoid receptor interacting protein (GRP) 1. Site-specific mutagenesis and selective MAPK inhibitors confirm EGF-induced increase in AR transactivation to phosphorylation of TIF2/GRIP1. EGF signaling increases the coimmunoprecipitation of TIF2 and AR, and AR stimulation by EGF can be

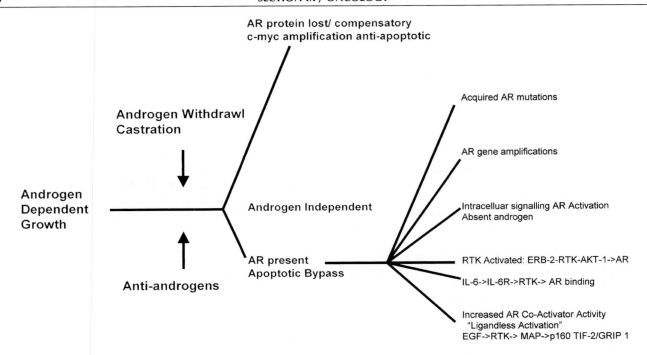

Figure 76-3   Androgen receptor expression is not, but antiandrogen resistance is a hallmark of the lethal phenotype of hormone refractory prostate cancer. In malignant progression, antiapoptotic effects of the androgen receptor are disconnected from the absence of circulating testosterone. Multiple mechanisms now permit a molecular profiling of the different phenotypes of hormone refractory prostate cancer for therapeutic development. IL, interleukin; MAPK, mitogen-activated protein kinase.

blocked by siRNA inhibition of TIF2/GRIP1 expression. EGF signaling through MAPK increases TIF2/GRIP1 coactivation of AR transactivation in recurrent prostate cancer. A molecular profile of different pathways of antiandrogen resistance has begun to emerge (Fig. 76-3).

Because a common element of these resistance mechanisms is restoration of antiapoptotic AR signaling, agents that target AR expression represent one of the most rational options for "final common pathway" targeting in disease progression following castration. Prior to ligand binding, AR exists in a complex with heat shock protein (Hsp) 90 and other cochaperones. The AR–Hsp90 interaction maintains AR in a high-affinity ligand-binding conformation that permits efficient response to dihydrotestosterone. Geldanamycin and 17-Allyamino-17-demethoxygeldanamycin (17-AAG) are inhibitors of the Hsp90 chaperone protein, a new class of antineoplastics. Pharmacological blockade of Hsp90 function causes the proteasomal degradation of proteins that require this chaperone for maturation or stability. Hsp90 chaperone "clients" include key proteins involved in tumor progression, including wild-type and mutated AR, Akt, and HIF-1. In murine models of prostate cancer, 17-AAG causes the degradation of these client proteins at nontoxic doses and inhibits the growth of hormone-naive and castration-resistant prostate cancer. In cancer cells Hsp90 exists in multi-chaperone complexes, but in normal, "unstressed" cells Hsp90 is in a latent, uncomplexed state. In vitro reconstitution of chaperone complexes with Hsp90 resulted in increased binding affinity to 17-AAG. These results suggest that prostate cancer cells contain Hsp90 complexes in an activated, high-affinity conformation that facilitates malignant progression, and that may represent a differentially expressed target that is essential for AR processing on which prostate cancer cell survival depends. 17-AAG has entered early clinical trials in hormone-

refractory prostate cancer with molecular surrogate end points including the degradation of AR. Other approaches to the blockade of AR signaling effects on antiapoptosis pathways are also under investigation.

NEW TARGETS IN HORMONE-REFRACTORY PROSTATE CANCER: INHIBITORS OF ANTIMICROTUBULIN DYNAMICS

Of prostate cancer patients with metastatic disease, more than 90% develop osseous bone metastases in the absence of significant visceral organ metastases. Historically, the median survival of patients with hormone-refractory osseous prostate cancer is 12–18 mo. Two major developments have changed the picture of slow progress in medical oncology drug development in hormone-refractory prostate cancer.

With more than 30 yr of National Cancer Institute-sponsored combination cytotoxic chemotherapy clinical trials failing to demonstrate phase III trial increase in overall survival, one class of agents shows reproducible clinical benefits. Antimicrotubule targeting drugs appear to favorably affect clinical course in osseous, hormone-refractory prostate cancer. Four independent phase II studies seem to confirm this observation. Docetaxel, which acts primarily by inhibiting microtubular depolymerization, alone or in combination with other antimicrotubule inhibitors like estramustine, consistently demonstrated a palliative response, a decrease in serum prostate-specific antigen (PSA) levels by 50% or greater in more than 60% of patients, a decrease in measurable disease and single institution observations of improved survival. Two large randomized phase III clinical trials are evaluating phase II data that overall survival is improved with the use of docetaxel. Regarding toxicity, few World Health Organization grade 3 or 4 hematological and gastrointestinal side effects and few thromboembolic events have been observed in a population that includes a high percentage of men over 70-yr old receiving treatment.

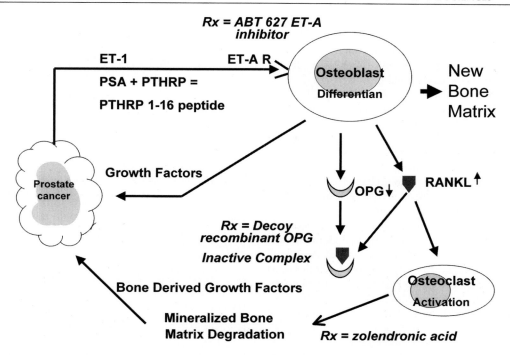

Figure 76-4 Osseous prostate cancer is the dominant form of metastatic disease. Disruption of activation of osteoclast and osteoblast interactions with the prostate cancer cells is a new strategy in cotargeting stroma and tumor interactions. PSA, prostate-specific antigen; Rx, treatment.

As hormone-refractory prostate cancer contains defects in apoptotic pathways—but does not have a high proliferative index (S fraction)—the question developed as to why microtubule-dynamics inhibitors would have activity in a tumor type that has a low fraction of cells in G2/M and moreover, why the clinical "signature" of activity would be reduction in PSA and pain in patients? A major emphasis is being placed on the mechanistic answer to this clinical question. For example, a novel class of microtubule inhibitors, 2 methoxyestradiol—which is a nonestrogenic metabolite—inhibits tumor growth and angiogenesis at concentrations that efficiently disrupt tumor microtubules in vivo. 2ME2, like paclitaxel and docetaxel, downregulates the transcription factor HIF in prostate cancer at the post-transcriptional level and inhibits HIF-1-induced transcriptional activation of vascular endothelial growth factor expression. Inhibition of HIF-1 protein levels occurs downstream of the 2ME2/tubulin interaction, as disruption of interphase micro-tubule s is required for HIF-α downregulation. 2ME2 is a small molecule inhibitor of a critical transcription factor in angiogenesis, and provides a new mechanistic link between the disruption of the microtubule cytoskeleton and inhibition of prostate cancer angio-genesis. 2ME2 has entered phase I trials for hormone-refractory prostate cancer. Effects of microtubule inhibitors in prostate cancer like docetaxel and 2ME2 may be at the level of disrupting inter-phase microtubules involved in HIF protein expression and the secretion of angiogenesis and HIF-1 regulated extracelluar growth factors—that cause prostate cancer pain and progression—as opposed to acting principally as cytotoxic drugs at mitosis. This has emerged as a new focus for drug discovery in prostate cancer. Chronic and lower dose treatment targeting microtubule disruption in hormone-refractory prostate cancer is a new avenue for clinical pharmacological investigation.

TARGETING BONE METASTASIS: COTARGETING STROMA AND TUMOR Despite 100 yr of description of the unique features of prostate cancer bone metastases with its predominant osteoblastic response around metastatic deposits of tumor and hallmark radio-opaque osteoblastic and sclerotic lesions on X-rays of bone, only recently molecular biology has been applied to understanding and revealing disruption of key pathways that may be unique to hormone-refractory prostate cancer survival in bone. The pathophysiological circuitry of the prostate cancer bone metastasis is beginning to be dissected (*see* Fig. 76-3). Studies show prostate cancer survival in the bone requires bidirec-tional signaling from stromal–epithelial interactions. These inter-actions appear to be critical for prostate cancer cells to survive and proliferate in the prostate and bone. Attacking both epithelial and stromal elements simultaneously is a unique approach to metastatic prostate cancer therapy, and proof of concept has been developed. Cotargeting both tumor cells and stroma requires identifying new tumor and stromal targets.

Castrate levels of testosterone increase the activity of bone-destroying cells, osteoclasts, and subsequent bone loss. The hypothesis is being tested that androgen deprivation therapy, by derepressing osteoclastic bone resorption and the release of growth factors, may increase the metastatic progression of prostate cancer to bone. In addition, osteoclastogenesis creates bone resorption and as the bone matrix is a storehouse of prostate cancer candidate and confirmed growth factors, bone metastatic progression may be promoted (Fig. 76-4). Targeting the inhibition of activated osteoclasts in prostate cancer bone metastases has shown clinical benefit. Zoledronic acid as a bisphosphonate decreases the risk of skeletal-related events, including spinal cord compressions and pathological fractures in men with bone metastases and disease progression after first-line hormonal therapy. These studies have been conducted in advanced hormone-refractory prostate cancer; whether osteoclast inhibition can improve survival with early treatment is under phase III testing.

Efforts are underway to further block the osteoclastic activation using recombinant proteins as new therapeutics for cotargeting.

For example, osteoprotegerin (OPG) is a decoy receptor that is a member of the tumor necrosis factor receptor family. OPG, an osteoblast-secreted decoy receptor, specifically binds to osteoclast differentiation factor and inhibits osteoclast maturation that is required for bone resorption around a metastasis. OPG prevents the binding of the receptor activator of nuclear factor-κB ligand (RANKL) to the RANK receptor on osteoclasts. Recombinant OPG decoy receptors given intravenously may disrupt the RANKL activation pathway created by prostate cancer and this approach is entering clinical trials in hormone-refractory prostate cancer.

Within the bone metastasis, prostate cancer cells secrete PSA and parathyroid hormone-related protein (PTHrP). PTHrP is a critical peptide factor for osteoclastic activation and osteolytic bone destruction. PSA however is a serine protease, which cleaves PTHrP into peptide fragments. One of these peptides, amino acids 1–16, has amino acid homology to endothelin, and binds to the endothelin receptor on osteoblasts and acts as an osteoblast mitogen. A unique difference between osseous breast metastases and prostate cancer is that PSA and the prostate-specific related exocrine serine protease hK2 converts PTHrP from an osteolytic to an osteoblastic signal in prostate cancer bone metastases.

A new picture for therapeutics is emerging for the treatment of prostate cancer bone metastases by cotargeting prostate cancer secreted agonists acting on the osteoblast. Transforming growth factor β, released from the metastasis degraded bone matrix, induces prostate cancer production of factors that promote the unique histological features of prostate cancer bone metastases, including osteoblastic responses and dysregulated new bone matrix formation. Three factors involved in prostate cancer bone metastases secreted by the tumor include endothelin-1, adrenomedullin, and insulin-like growth factor binding protein 3. The osteoblast receptors for all three ligands are being evaluated as potential targets for cotargeting blockade of prostate cancer bone metastases.

Of these three, disrupting the endothelin (ET)-1 axis using selective ET-1 A receptor antagonist ABT 627 (atrasentan) has entered phase III studies in hormone-refractory prostate cancer.

CONCLUSIONS

In some respects, prostate cancer offers unique challenges in oncology. The interactions of Western cooking, genes involved in infection and inflammation in the prostate, and human longevity are all new frontiers for understanding epigenetic influences on inherited risk and earlier detection. The discovery of the virtually universal inactivation of the GST-π gene at prostate cancer initiation has created the opportunity for new and mechanistic prostate epithelium-specific strategies of chemoprevention drug discovery. Intracellular signaling pathways in hormone-refractory prostate cancer are being dissected. Cotargeting stromal–tumor interactions in prostate cancer osseous metastases have emerged as a new paradigm in the medical oncology of prostate cancer. With the application of molecular biology and biotechnologies to human prostate cancer research, new targets in the lethal phenotypes of prostate cancer have been rapidly ascertained. How many are pharmacologically amenable and can be blocked with clinical relevance remains to be discovered. For all the emergent genetic and protein target insights, perhaps the greatest challenges will be the participation of more men with prostate cancer in translational research clinical trials that evaluate the new science of therapeutics designed specifically for prostate cancer.

SELECTED REFERENCES

Brooks JD, Goldberg MF, Nelson LA, Wu D, Nelson WG. Identification of potential prostate cancer preventive agents through induction of quinone reductase in vitro. Cancer Epidemiol Biomarkers Prev 2002;11(9):868–875.

Carducci MA, Padley RJ, Breul J, et al. Effect of endothelin-A receptor blockade with atrasentan on tumor progression in men with hormone-refractory prostate cancer: a randomized, phase II, placebo-controlled trial. J Clin Oncol 2003;21(4):679–689.

Carpten J, Nupponen N, Isaacs S, et al. Germline mutations in the ribonuclease L gene in families showing linkage with HPC1. Nat Genet 2002;30(2):181–184.

Chung LW, Hsieh CL, Law A, et al. New targets for therapy in prostate cancer: modulation of stromal-epithelial interactions. Urology 2003; 62(5 Suppl 1):44–54.

Coffey DS. Similarities of prostate and breast cancer: evolution, diet, and estrogens. Urology 2001;57(4 Suppl 1):31–38.

Culig Z. Role of the androgen receptor axis in prostate cancer. Urology 2003;62(5 Suppl 1):21–26.

DeMarzo AM, Nelson WG, Isaacs WB, Epstein JI. Pathological and molecular aspects of prostate cancer. Lancet 2003;361(9361): 955–964.

Dong JT. Chromosomal deletions and tumor suppressor genes in prostate cancer. Cancer Metastasis Rev 2001;20(3–4):173–193.

Gregory CW, Fei X, Ponguta LA, et al. Epidermal growth factor increases coactivation of the androgen receptor in recurrent prostate cancer. J Biol Chem 2004;279(8):7119–7130.

Guise TA, Chirgwin JM. Role of bisphosphonates in prostate cancer bone metastases. Semin Oncol 2003;30(5):717–723.

Hsieh CL, Gardner TA, Miao L, Balian G, Chung LW. Cotargeting tumor and stroma in a novel chimeric tumor model involving the growth of both human prostate cancer and bone stromal cells. Cancer Gene Ther 2004;11(2):148–155.

Iwamura M, Hellman J, Cockett AT, Lilja H, Gershagen S. Alteration of the hormonal bioactivity of parathyroid hormone-related protein (PTHrP) as a result of limited proteolysis by prostate-specific antigen. Urology 1996;48(2):317–325.

Kamal A, Thao L, Sensintaffar J, et al. A high-affinity conformation of Hsp90 confers tumour selectivity on Hsp90 inhibitors. Nature 2003; 425(6956):407–410.

Khan MA, Carducci MA, Partin AW. The evolving role of docetaxel in the management of androgen independent prostate cancer. J Urol 2003; 170(5):1709–1716.

Kim WS, Ordija CM, Freeman MW. Activation of signaling pathways by putative scavenger receptor class A (SR-A) ligands requires CD14 but not SR-A. Biochem Biophys Res Commun 2003;310(2):542–549.

Mabjeesh NJ, Escuin D, LaVallee TM, et al. 2ME2 inhibits tumor growth and angiogenesis by disrupting microtubules and dysregulating HIF. Cancer Cell 2003;3(4):363–375.

Mabjeesh NJ, Post DE, Willard MT, et al. Geldanamycin induces degradation of hypoxia-inducible factor 1alpha protein via the proteosome pathway in prostate cancer cells. Cancer Res 2002;62(9): 2478–2482.

Mamillapalli R, Gavrilova N, Mihaylova VT, et al. PTEN regulates the ubiquitin-dependent degradation of the CDK inhibitor p27(KIP1) through the ubiquitin E3 ligase SCF(SKP2). Curr Biol 2001;11(4): 263–267.

Nelson WG, DeWeese TL, DeMarzo AM. The diet, prostate inflammation, and the development of prostate cancer. Cancer Metastasis Rev 2002;21(1):3–16.

Nelson WG, De Marzo AM, Isaacs WB. Prostate cancer. N Engl J Med 2003;349(4):366–381.

Nelson JB, Hedican SP, George DJ, et al. Identification of endothelin-1 in the pathophysiology of metastatic adenocarcinoma of the prostate. Nat Med 1995;1(9):944–949.

Neshat MS, Mellinghoff IK, Tran C, et al. Enhanced sensitivity of PTEN-deficient tumors to inhibition of FRAP/mTOR. Proc Natl Acad Sci USA 2001;98(18):10314–10319.

Rubin MA, Zhou M, Dhanasekaran SM, et al. alpha-Methylacyl coenzyme A racemase as a tissue biomarker for prostate cancer. JAMA 2002;287(13):1662–1670.

Schluter KD, Katzer C, Piper HM. A N-terminal PTHrP peptide fragment void of a PTH/PTHrP-receptor binding domain activates cardiac ET(A) receptors. Br J Pharmacol 2001;132(2):427–432.

Smith MR, McGovern FJ, Zietman AL, et al. Pamidronate to prevent bone loss during androgen-deprivation therapy for prostate cancer. N Engl J Med 2001;345(13):948–955.

Solit DB, Zheng FF, Drobnjak M, et al. 17-Allylamino-17-demethoxygeldanamycin induces the degradation of androgen receptor and HER-2/neu and inhibits the growth of prostate cancer xenografts. Clin Cancer Res 2002;8(5):986–993.

Trotman LC, Niki M, Dotan ZA, et al. Pten dose dictates cancer progression in the prostate. PLoS Biol 2003;1(3):E59.

Visakorpi T. The molecular genetics of prostate cancer. Urology 2003; 62(5 Suppl 1):3–10.

Walsh PC. Germline mutations and sequence variants of the macrophage scavenger receptor 1 gene are associated with prostate cancer risk. J Urol 2003;169(4):158–190.

Xiang Y, Wang Z, Murakami J, et al. Effects of RNase L mutations associated with prostate cancer on apoptosis induced by 2′-5′-oligoadenylates. Cancer Res 2003;63(20):6795–6801.

Xu J, Gillanders EM, Isaacs SD, et al. Genome-wide scan for prostate cancer susceptibility genes in the Johns Hopkins hereditary prostate cancer families. Prostate 2003;57(4):320–325.

Xu J, Zheng SL, Komiya A, et al. Common sequence variants of the macrophage scavenger receptor 1 gene are associated with prostate cancer risk. Am J Hum Genet 2003;72(1):208–212.

Yin JJ, Mohammad KS, Kakonen SM, et al. A causal role for endothelin-1 in the pathogenesis of osteoblastic bone metastases. Proc Natl Acad Sci USA 2003;100(19):10954–10959.

Zha S, Ferdinandusse S, Denis S, et al. Alpha-methylacyl-CoA racemase as an androgen-independent growth modifier in prostate cancer. Cancer Res 2003;63(21):7365–7376.

Zha S, Gage WR, Sauvageot J, et al. Cyclooxygenase-2 is upregulated in proliferative inflammatory atrophy of the prostate, but not in prostate carcinoma. Cancer Res 2001;61(24): 8617–8623.

http://www.prostatecancerfoundation.org

77 Cutaneous Melanoma

MOIRA R. JACKSON AND STEPHEN P. SUGRUE

SUMMARY

The incidence of cutaneous melanoma is increasing significantly and responds poorly to current therapies. At the root of this problem is the transformation of melanocytes, which normally synthesize melanin to protect the skin against ultra violet (UV) damage, into highly invasive cells which can colonize many different regions of the body, reminiscent of their neural crest origin. Paradoxically, UV radiation increases the incidence of melanoma and the penetrance of melanoma susceptibility genes such as CDKN2A. Abnormal expression of cadherins, integrins, and other cell adhesion and matrix proteins are key in melanoma cell transformation and in transendothelial migration, a key step in metastasis.

Key Words: Melanocyte; epidermis; radial growth phase; E-cadherin; CDKN2A; melanoma; UV radiation; vertical growth phase; N-cadherin; vasculogenic mimicry.

INTRODUCTION

The alarming increase in the incidence of melanoma presents a significant healthcare and research challenge. Over the last five decades melanoma rates have steadily risen in the United States and Western countries. Melanomas represent the fifth most common cancer in men and the sixth most common in women, with lifetime risks of 1.72 and 1.22, respectively. The incidence rates have risen more rapidly than mortality rates most likely owing to surgical resection in the earliest stages. Melanoma affects a relatively young population, it demonstrates a propensity to metastasize, and it exhibits a poor response to therapies. Once melanoma has successfully metastasized the survival rate is small. Research has revealed numerous genetic and molecular details defining the precise mechanisms of melanoma progression and importantly has revealed potential targets for specific new therapies. These include genetic deletions initially detected after studying familial melanoma, epigenetic alterations, and differences in levels of a variety of proteins involved in signaling pathways, oncogenes, cytokines, adhesion complex proteins, matrix molecules, and factors determining the formation of vascular supply to the tumors.

Cutaneous melanomas arise from the malignant transformation of the pigment producing melanocytes, which are located and evenly distributed in the basal epidermal layer of human skin, accounting for 1–2% of the epidermis. Melanocytes express adhesion proteins, which enable them to form connections with

From: *Principles of Molecular Medicine, Second Edition*
Edited by: M. S. Runge and C. Patterson © Humana Press, Inc., Totowa, NJ

neighboring keratinocytes. The result of these melanocyte-keratinocyte connections is to control the rate of melanocyte division and migration and to maintain epidermal homeostasis. Cutaneous melanoma occurs when melanocyte division escapes normal control mechanisms, melanocytes proliferate unchecked, invade the underlying connective tissue compartment, and metastasize to numerous distant locations throughout the body.

All melanocytes are derived from the neural crest of the embryo. The neural crests are a multipotent population of cells that through extensive cell expansion and migration seed many distinct locations throughout organism. Progressive restrictions in the developmental potencies of neural crest cells are regulated by the action of external cytokines on the target progenitor cells. The selection and expansion of migratory melanogenic precursors to the skin depends on the local action of the cytokine endothelin-3 and the restriction to melanogenic lineage is reversible. Much like their ancestral neural crest cells, metastatic melanoma can colonize numerous visceral (lung, liver, small intestine) and nonvisceral sites (skin, lymph nodes, bones, and brain).

The study of melanoma initiation and progression has been defined to five steps in melanoma development. First, melanoma begins at a common, acquired or congenital, nevus with structurally normal melanocytes. Second, there is the change to a dysplastic nevus with structural and architectural atypia. Interestingly, a strong correlation exists of density (number/area) of dysplastic nevi and risk of melanoma development. The third step is referred to as the radial growth phase (RGP). By histological criteria, the RGP melanoma is considered to be at the early stage of primary melanoma development. RGP melanoma cells are primarily confined to the epidermis and are metastatically incompetent. The fourth step is called the vertical growth phase (VGP). By histological criteria, VGP melanoma is the advanced stage of primary melanoma. VGP melanoma is an important transition from RGP to a more aggressive condition, which is characterized by tumor cell invasion into the underlying dermis and subcutaneous tissue (Fig. 77-1). The fifth and final step in melanoma development is formation of metastatic melanoma, when the melanoma cells successfully migrate to additional distant locations.

There are significant molecular and biological differences between RGP and VGP melanoma cells and these differences have profound prognostic and therapeutic implications. In RGP neoplastic cells spread in the epidermis or demonstrate limited invasion of the dermis as single cells or small clusters of cells. In VGP, cancer cells expand in the dermis and generate significant tumor nodules.

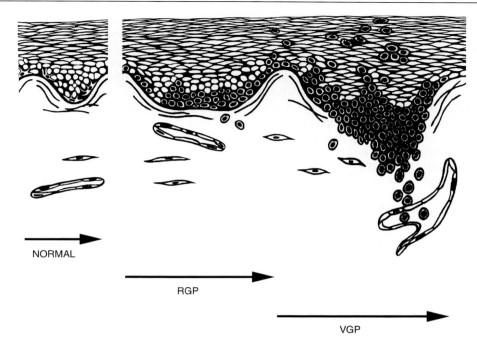

Figure 77-1 Progression of cutaneous melanoma. In normal skin, melanocytes are interspersed between keratinocytes along the dermal–epidermal border. Their dendritic processes transport melanosomes to more apical keratinocytes. During the RGP melanocytes lose their dendritic processes and proliferate in a horizontal direction predominantly within the epidermis. They have not yet acquired metastatic potential. As tumors progress to the more aggressive VGP, melanoma cells invade the underlying dermis and become metastatically competent.

Unlike the aggressive VGP melanoma cells, the RGP melanoma cells are difficult to maintain in tissue culture, have low colony forming ability, are nontumorigenic in nude mice, and do not have competence to metastasize. In the case of RGP tumors the disease can be cured by proper surgical excision. VGP cells acquire metastatic capability and may be resistant to common methods of therapy. Not surprisingly, the molecular details that may account for the transition from RGP to VGP have received much attention.

ETIOLOGY OF MELANOMA

The total risk of melanoma is determined through the interplay between genetic factors and exposure to sunlight. Ultra violet (UV) irradiation can cause DNA damage and the specific genetic background can predispose to susceptibility to UV irradiation. Differences in the relative exposure to UV radiation by latitude may contribute to the wide geographic variation in melanoma incidence rates. For example, the incidence of melanoma in Queensland Australia is notably high (lifetime incidence 1/15 or 1/20). The latitude of the residence and fair skin of the majority of the population have therefore combined to significantly increase the lifetime risk of developing melanoma for a person living in Queensland.

UV RADIATION One of the most crucial factors predisposing to melanoma development is the degree and timing of exposure to UV radiation, with childhood and/or intermittent exposures being key factors. Both UVA and UVB wavelengths can be harmful and cause DNA damage and/or immunosuppression. UVA, although having the ability to penetrate deeper into the tissue and cause immediate and persistent pigment darkening, does not seem to cause direct damage. UVA may, however, cause damage through the creation of reactive oxygen species. UVB (280–320 nm) is considered to represent the most carcinogenic waveband, inducing erythema, or sunburn, historically associated with skin cancer risk.

UVB exposure is commonly associated with direct DNA damage. Nucleic acids and proteins absorb light within the UVB range, peaking at 260 and 280 nm, respectively (figures familiar to the molecular biologist). UVB causes two types of DNA lesions via creation of photoproducts between adjacent pyrimidine residues and pyrimidine dimers. Both lesions can lead to genetic mutations such as $C > T$ or $CC > TT$ transitions, the latter representing the hallmark of UV-induced mutagenesis.

Melanin affords protection from UV radiation. In dark-colored skin, melanocytes accomplish a highly organized presentation of melanosomes throughout the epidermis producing an effective protective screen from damaging UV. Melanin, because it effectively absorbs both UV photons and free radicals induced by UV irradiation, protects the skin from sun damage. There are two types of melanin, eumelanin found in dark skin and hair and pheomelanin found in red hair and freckled individuals. Eumelanin synthesis is upregulated by α-melanocyte-stimulating hormone (MSH) binding to the G protein-coupled melacortin-1 receptor (MC1-R). Loss-of-function mutations of MC1-R prevent eumelanin production and are associated with most red-hair phenotypes. Nonfunctional MC1-R has been linked to enhanced cytotoxic effects of UV, as well as an increased incidence of melanoma.

So why are melanocytes themselves sensitive to UV? Melanocytes may in fact respond to UV light differently than other cell types. Melanocytes produce the antiapoptotic protein B-cell leukemia/lymphoma gene (BCL-2) at high levels, which might explain the melanocytes' relatively high resistance to apoptosis subsequent to extensive UV-induced DNA damage. Both BCL-2 and its regulator microphthalmia-associated transcription factor (MITF) have been demonstrated to be critical to melanocyte survival; deficiency of either gene in mice leads to a depletion of melanocytes. The cellular decision to undergo apoptosis or cell cycle arrest and DNA repair in melanocytes may also differ from other cell types. In fibroblasts the decision seems to be via dose dependent p53-dependent induction of p21 at low UVB doses, but Bax, not p21, is induced at higher UVB doses leading to apoptosis. The elevated levels of BCL-2 in melanocytes may allow mutant melanocytes the opportunity to survive a high dose of UVB. The survival of melanocytes may serve to maintain the integrity of the skin's sole source of melanin, ensuring uninterrupted protection from subsequent UV irradiation, but risking propagating severely damaged melanocytes and melanoma development.

MELANOMA SUSCEPTIBILITY GENES   It is estimated that 10% of melanoma cases report a first or second degree relative with melanoma. Two genes that confer susceptibility to melanoma have been identified within the high-risk families, CDKN2A and CDK4. Of these melanoma families the CDKN2A locus, one of the earliest and most frequently encountered defects at chromosome 9p21, accounts for susceptibility in 25–40%, whereas mutations in the CDK4 gene have been documented in far fewer kindreds. Transgenic animals deficient in the CDKN2A (NK4a/ARF locus) develop cutaneous melanoma within a quarter of the time taken for wild-type mice to develop similar tumors. The CDKN2A gene is unique in that alternative splicing of exon 1B can result in two different proteins being transcribed in two different reading frames. The protein encoded by mRNA lacking exon 1B is the cyclin-dependent kinase inhibitor 2A, called p16/INK4a, which is involved in the retinoblastoma pathway. The protein encoded by inclusion of exon 1B of CDNK2A is called p14/ARF (**a**lternative **r**eading **f**rame) and is involved in the p53 pathway.

The p16/INK4a protein functions as a negative regulator of CDK4 activation by competing with cyclin D1 for CDK4 binding. Inhibition of CDK4 activity prevents phosphorylation of the retinoblastoma gene product (pRB). Phosphorylation of pRB results in the dissociation of pRB and E2F transcription factors and thus enables transcription of E2F target genes and progression of cells from G1 to S phase. Thus, p16/INK4a is considered as a tumor suppressor because it controls cell-cycle progression via this critical pathway. Loss of p16/INK4a results in hyperphosphorylation of pRB and, in turn, the uncontrolled activation of E2F-mediated transcription, resulting in excessive cellular growth. p16/INK4a may also play a role at the G2/M transition point in the cell cycle and loss of this protein may result in a lack of DNA repair following UV exposure as cells continue through successive divisions.

The p14/ARF protein appears to sequester Mdm2 in the nucleus so that it is not available to bind p53, an essential step in the nuclear export and proteosomal degradation of p53. Thus, a loss of p14/ARF would accelerate p53 degradation and reduce p53-mediated apoptosis. There is evidence that p14/ARF may be an independent melanoma predisposition gene. There is one report of a germline mutation that exhibited melanoma without other tumors. In addition, there is an unequivocal report of a germline deletion of p16/INK4a in the absence of concomitant loss of either CDKN2A or CDKN2B in a case of melanoma with neurilemmoma in the thoracic wall. p14/ARF may also influence the penetrance of CDKN2A mutation in mice. p14/ARF haploinsufficiency in a p16/INK4a null background suggests cooperation between p16/INK4a and p14/ARF.

Mutation in the gene encoding CDK4 itself, mapping to 12q14, has also been detected in three families predisposed toward melanoma development. Interestingly, the CDK4 mutations documented in the three families all occur at codon 24, which change

arginine to either cysteine or histidine. Arginine at that position seems critical for interaction with p16/INK4a. Thus these mutations abrogate the capacity of p16/INK4a to associate with CDK4, reinforcing that loss of this inhibitory interaction as integral to melanoma susceptibility.

As mentioned, UV radiation increases the incidence of melanoma. It also increases the penetrance of known melanoma susceptibility genes such as CDKN2A. These increases may simply reflect an increase in mutational burden that would lead to a higher probability of accumulating sufficient additional mutations required for cancer to develop or a more direct mechanism may exist. For example, UV radiation induces p16/INK4A expression in human skin where it is involved in UV-induced G2 phase cell-cycle arrest. Mutations in the MSH receptor may also predispose toward melanoma development. Interaction of α-MSH with MSH receptor results in signaling responses that potentiate the UV-induced increase in p16 expression. In vitro experiments also indicate increased binding of p21 with cyclin E/cdk2 and cyclin A/cdk2 as well as p27 with cyclin E/cdk2 in transformed melanoma cells following exposure to UVB. Thus, the activities of cyclin-dependent kinases and transition through the cell cycle are key processes influenced by UV radiation in melanoma.

TUMOR INITIATION AND PROGRESSION   Advances in genomic technologies have afforded the identification of many melanoma associated gene expression changes. The ability of transcription factors to control gene expression through gene activation or repression can enhance tumor formation and progression, and act to promote proliferation, migration, or to inhibit apoptosis.

Oncogenes are derived from genes with a role in cellular homeostasis that have undergone point mutations, amplifications, or promoter translocations that result in constitutive activation or inactivation of key regulatory pathways. The most commonly activated oncogenes in melanoma are those related to the RAS/mitogen-activated protein kinase (MAPK) signaling pathway, which conducts cellular signaling from growth factor receptors. Oncogenic events in melanoma typically include activating mutations in N-RAS. These mutations maintain the proteins in the GTP-bound state, thus constitutively active. In the mouse model, melanocyte-specific expression of mutated Ha-RAS was carried out in an INK4a null environment resulting in mice that develop high frequency of spontaneous cutaneous melanoma. The accumulating data derived from both human and murine models suggest that RAS activation contributes not only to growth advantage but also to tumor maintenance.

B-RAF is mutationally activated by point mutations in up to 60% of examined primary melanoma cell lines. B-RAF acts downstream of Ras in the MAPK pathway transducing signals from Ras through MAPK/ERK kinase to MAPK. Constitutive active B-RAF results in activation of downstream effectors that contribute to cell proliferation and inhibition of apoptosis. However, high frequency B-RAF mutation has been demonstrated in nevi, which are benign melanocytic proliferations. These data suggest that active B-RAF alone may not be sufficient to drive the transformation, but mutation in B-RAF may represent an early, perhaps prerequisite, step in the initiation of melanoma. In contrast however, B-RAF mutations were reported in only 10% of the earliest RGP melanomas, suggesting that B-RAF mutations may correlate with tumor progression and not initiation.

Downstream of the RAS/MAPK is Cyclin D1, an important regulator of the G1/S transition. Acral melanomas (those occurring in the hands and feet), unlike cutaneous melanomas, are characterized by gene amplifications, frequently exhibiting amplifications of Cyclin D1. As mentioned, Cyclin D1 complexes with CDK4 to mediate the phosphorylation of pRB. Intriguingly, interfering with Cyclin D1 expression in a murine xenograft model of melanoma led to apoptosis and tumor regression, highlighting the role of this pathway in tumor maintenance.

Gain or loss of transcription factor gene function plays a major role in melanoma progression. Abnormal expression of transcription factors can in turn modulate several genes involved in tumor growth and metastasis. Alterations in activity/expression of transcription-related genes including activator protein (AP)-2, calcium/cAMP response element binding (CREB) protein, ATF-1, ATF-2 SNAI, MITF, and nuclear factor (NF)-κB have all been implicated to be involved in melanoma progression.

The role of AP-2 in progression of melanoma has received much attention and it is now accepted that AP-2 is a major transcriptional regulator of genes involved in melanoma progression. Highly metastatic melanoma cells do not express AP-2 and transfection of AP-2 into highly metastatic melanoma cells inhibits their growth and metastatic potential in nude mice. The transition of melanomas from radial to VGP is associated with the loss of c-KIT and the overexpression of melanoma cell adhesion molecule MCAM/MUC18. Interestingly, there appears to be a direct association between cKIT and AP-2 and an inverse correlation between AP-2 and MCAM/MUC18 and both these genes have AP-2 binding sites. AP-2 also regulates other genes involved in the progression of human melanoma such as E-cadherin, p21WAF, IGFR-1, matrix metalloproteinase (MMP)-2, and vascular endothelial growth factor (VEGF).

CREB expression correlates directly with metastatic potential of murine melanoma cells, and ATF is not detected in normal melanocytes but is easily found in metastatic melanoma cells. CREB/ATF-1 can act either as positive or negative regulators of transcription. CREB factors are thought to contribute to the acquisition of the metastatic phenotype in human melanoma by upregulating MMP-2 and MCAM/MUC18 expression, both of which have CRE regions in their promoters. CREB/ATF-1 may also act as survival factors for human melanoma cells.

A variety of additional transcription factors may also affect melanoma progression. Overexpression of SNAIL suppresses expression of E-cadherin, thus, significantly increasing the metastatic potential of melanoma cells. MITF plays an important role in the differentiation of melanocytes and other neural crest-derived cells by regulating tyrosinase, tyrosinase-related proteins, and dopachrome tautomerase, all involved in melanin synthesis. NF-κB regulates IL-8 and VEGF in melanoma cells and so plays a significant role in the progression of human melanoma.

Hence, loss of AP-2 and overexpression or hyperactivity of CREB/ATF-1, AFT-2, SNAIL, MITF, and NF-κB in metastatic melanoma cells may work in concert to regulate several genes contributing to the development of the malignant phenotype.

AUTOCRINE AND PARACRINE REGULATION BY CYTOKINES AND GROWTH FACTORS IN MELANOMA

Malignant melanoma cells express different growth factors and cytokines and their receptors at different stages of tumor progression, which by autocrine and paracrine effects enable them to grow autonomously and confer competence to metastasis. Autocrine growth factors (fibroblast growth factor [bFGF], melanocyte growth stimulatory activity/growth regulated protein [MGSA/GRO], IL8 and sometimes IL-6, platelet-derived growth factor [PDGF]-A, IL-10) produced by melanoma cells stimulate proliferation of the producing cell itself whereas paracrine growth factors (e.g., PDGF, EGF, transforming growth factor [TGF]-β, IL-1, granulocyte-macrophage colony-stimulating factor [GM-CSF], IGF-1, NGF, VEGF) modulate the microenvironment to benefit tumor growth and invasion. Paracrine effects include angiogenesis, stroma formation, activation of proteolytic enzymes, adhesion or motility and metastasis formation. Some growth factors have inhibitory effects on melanocytes and early lesions (IL-1, IL-6, TGF-β, oncostatin-M [OSM] tumor necrosis factor, and interferon) but not on advanced stage melanomas and in some cases they switch to an autocrine stimulator (IL-6, TGF-β). Understanding the involvement of different growth factors and cytokines in the molecular mechanism of melanoma progression may provide insight into new therapeutic approaches.

Autonomous overexpression of growth factors and their receptors are key events in melanocytic transformation. FGF-2 is a prime example of this process, whereby a normally repressed gene is activated and signals via its receptor in an autocrine manner, stimulating tumor growth. Overexpression of TGF-α, TGF-β, IGF-1, IGF-2, EGF, PDGF, and MGSA/GRO and their receptors have also been found in melanoma analyses.

A survey of expression patterns from melanoma tumors revealed that increased expression of WNT5A levels correlated with increased motility and invasiveness of the melanoma cells. In a series follow-up experiments, the levels of WNT5A were demonstrated to affect the motility characteristics of cells. The WNT5A effect may also be mediated through protein kinase C (PKC), which is thought to be associated with the cell's cytoskeletal organization, and that the PKC pathway also appeared to be downstream of the Frizzled5 (WNT5A receptor). These data may have uncovered an unexplored pathway in melanoma progression.

MELANOMA CELL ADHESION AND CELL MIGRATION

Progression of cutaneous melanoma is associated with alterations in the expression profiles of many types of cell adhesion molecules. Cadherins traverse the cell membrane and form calcium-dependent homotypic or heterotypic connections with identical proteins on neighboring cells and are connected to the actin cytoskeleton via α- and β- or γ-catenins. E-cadherin is the predominant cadherin expressed on keratinocytes and nontransformed melanocytes. During the transformation of a melanocyte to a melanoma cell, expression of E-cadherin falls and is replaced by N-cadherin. The switch from E-cadherin expression to mostly N-cadherin seems to be an important step in melanoma cell transformation. Indeed, the level of N-cadherin expression seems to correlate with stage of transformation of melanoma cells and with their migratory capability. Aggressive melanoma cell lines revert back to more quiescent cells following transfection with wild-type E-cadherin. Studies using melanoma cell lines have demonstrated an upregulation of the E-cadherin transcriptional repressor SNAIL is associated with reduced E-cadherin protein levels. Melanoma cells also express hepatocyte growth factor and its receptor c-Met, which act in an autocrine manner via PI3K and MAPK signaling to downregulate both E-cadherin and desmoglein, thus, dissociating keratinocytes from melanoma cells. Furthermore, the E2A gene product can also repress E-cadherin expression during the transition from an epithelioid to a mesenchymal phenotype observed in melanoma.

Not only are cadherin protein levels and localization important but their degree and nature of glycosylation may also be salient to melanoma progression. N-cadherin is heavily glycosylated and different types of glycosylation have been observed in melanoma cell lines from different stages of melanoma or different sites of metastasis. In vitro experiments have also shown that altering E-cadherin glycosylation can contribute to the suppression of metastasis in a murine melanoma cell line.

Normally vascular endothelial (VE)-cadherin is expressed only on endothelial cells and on placental trophoblast, both of which are exposed to circulating blood. VE-cadherin is expressed on the surfaces of melanoma cells, and cells expressing it appear to line channels within the tumor resembling blood. VE-cadherin expression and the ability to form channels has been correlated with aggressive melanoma metastasis. Clearly, strategies targeting restoration of E-cadherin expression or abrogation of N-cadherin or VE-cadherin function could have great therapeutic value.

Cadherins are linked to the actin cytoskeleton via catenins. β- and γ-catenins also act as modulators of transcription via the TCF/LEF-1 transcription complex. Thus, β-catenin is an essential component of the Wnt signaling pathway and its levels within the cytoplasm are tightly controlled. Phosphorylation of β-catenin by glycogen synthase kinase an essential step in its interaction with adenomatous polyposis coli and axin and subsequent degradation by ubiquitination and the 26s proteosome pathway. Mutations in β-catenin or adenomatous polyposis coli may result in increased cytoplasmic levels of β-catenin, which can then interact with TCF/LEF-1 in the nucleus and influence target genes that facilitate tumor survival and progression. Although mutations in the CTNNB1 gene that encodes β-catenin are rare in melanoma, increase in nuclear β-catenin is frequently observed during melanoma progression. It is thought that the increases in nuclear β-catenin are likely attributable to post-translational modifications. Interestingly, the presence of serine phosphorylation of β-catenin in malignant melanoma is an indication of a poor prognosis. LEF-1 transcripts are also increased in actively migrating melanoma cells perhaps because of increased levels of nuclear β-catenin. β-catenin-LEF-1-mediated regulation of MITF may also be pertinent to melanoma cell growth. Furthermore, transcripts of ICAT, a specific inhibitor of β-catenin-TCF signaling, in malignant melanoma are low or even absent. Interestingly, the ICAT gene is located at 1p36.2, one of the loci initially identified in loss of heterozygosity studies of familial melanoma.

One of the hallmarks of the progression of melanoma tumors from the nonmetastatic RGP to the potentially metastatic VGP is the downregulation of $\alpha_6\beta_1$ and $\alpha_v\beta_1$ integrins and increased expression of β_3-integrins. Several groups have observed a correlation between β_3-integrin levels and melanoma progression. Expression of the $\alpha_{IIb}\beta3$-integrin appears to enhance melanoma tumor cell survival, promoting increased adherence and migration. In addition, levels of the vitronectin receptor $\alpha_v\beta_3$ correlate directly with both tumor thickness and progression in melanoma and are indicative of a poor prognosis. $\alpha_v\beta_3$-integrin is detected in all metastatic lesions and may prove an effective target for therapeutic intervention. Activation of $\alpha_v\beta_3$-initiates signals that promote metastasis through the phosphorylation of focal adhesion kinase and activation of SRC. Integrin-linked kinase is associated with β_1- and β_3-integrins and its activation results in increased expression of LEF-1 and its downstream transcriptional targets, which include the E-cadherin repressor SNAIL.

Melanoma cells also express several other adhesion molecules including MUC18/MCAM, ALCAM, and L1. Upregulation of MUC18/MCAM expression correlates with E-cadherin loss and metastasis from melanoma cell tumors in nude mice. Signaling via MUC18/MCAM can lead to focal adhesion kinase activation and downstream signaling. ALCAM has been shown to be expressed in metastasizing but not in nonmetastasizing melanoma cell tumors in nude mice by differential display.

Migration of melanoma cells involves, and may require, the degradation and remodeling of the extracellular matrix. MMPs and their inhibitors and components of the plasminogen activation system play leading roles in this process. Melanoma cells increase their ability to bind active MMPs that can degrade matrices in their path. Increased levels of active MMP-2 correlate with melanoma progression. Moreover, expression of MT1-MMP associated with MMP-2 activation increases tumor growth and vascularization in melanoma cells. Poorly aggressive melanoma cells do not appear to synthesize MMP-9 but do produce its inhibitor, tissue inhibitor of metalloproteinases-1. As melanoma progresses, this balance is reversed and cells derived from primary tumors increase MMP-9 synthesis whereas their production of tissue inhibitor of metalloproteinases decreases. Alendronate, a bisphosphonate, inhibits several MMPs and can reduce invasion of a melanoma cell line in vitro.

Components of the plasminogen activation system can also regulate cellular migration. Immunocytochemical studies indicate that both activators and inhibitors and urokinase-type plasminogen activator receptor are upregulated in primary cutaneous melanoma. Increased uPA and urokinase-type plasminogen activator receptor immunostaining may correlate with increased invasive potential, whereas the inhibitor PAI1 tends to be enriched at the periphery of the lesion in which keratinocytes may still have some level of communication and control over neighboring melanocytes. Levels of PAI1 in particular correlate with different stages of melanoma progression and may be used prognostically. Elevated levels of protease-activated receptor (PAR)-1, the thrombin receptor, are also detected in metastatic human melanoma cells lines. Cleavage of PAR-1 by thrombin activates signaling cascades that affect levels of growth factors, integrins and MMPs and promote invasion. AP-2, a repressor acting on the PAR-1 promoter in nonmetastatic melanoma cells, is downregulated in highly metastatic melanoma cells. Malignant melanoma cells also express tissue factor, which can activate thrombin, which may act as a growth factor in human melanoma cells.

METASTASIS   Transendothelial migration is an essential step in the metastasis of melanoma. It involves adhesion to and then migration (diapedesis) across the endothelial monolayer. Many factors that are upregulated in melanoma tumors play a role in melanocyte chemotaxis and adhesion to endothelium or communication between melanomal and endothelial cells in vitro. Endothelial cells secrete chemokines that induce melanoma cell chemotaxis. One of the most crucial of these is IL-8, which acts through the CXCR1 receptor on melanoma cells. There is also evidence that interactions between melanoma cells and polymorphonuclear cells play a role in the adhesion of both cell types to the endothelium before transendothelial migration. As melanoma cells adhere to the endothelium, levels of VE-cadherin and PECAM between adjacent endothelial cells are diminished allowing melanoma cells to send membrane protrusions between endothelial cells. Melanoma cells appear to adhere to endothelium via N-cadherin, $\alpha_v\beta_3$-integrin, cell adhesion molecule L1, and MCAM/ MUC18. Furthermore, several members of the tetraspanin superfamily (CD9, CD81, and CD151) localize to these heterotypic points of contact in two- and three-dimensional cocultures of melanoma cells and endothelial cells, and antibodies against CD9 inhibit melanoma cell transmigration.

TUMOR PERFUSION

Tumor growth requires adequate perfusion of blood and an ever-increasing network of vessels to convey that blood. Microvascular density within tumors is prognostically significant in the staging and diagnosis of melanoma. In general, histological examinations of highly aggressive melanoma samples show a greater density of microvessels than nonaggressive tumors. Doppler studies also indicate that greater blood flow is associated with poorer outcome. Thus, angiogenesis is considered one of the key targets for therapeutic intervention.

ANGIOGENESIS Melanoma cells synthesize a multitude of proteins, which are themselves angiogenic or cleave other proteins to produce factors that can influence angiogenesis. Levels of two well-characterized angiogenic cytokines, VEGF and FGF-2, are constitutively higher in transformed melanocytes than in normal melanocytes, and elevated serum levels of VEGF and FGF-2 are strongly correlated with poor overall prognosis of melanoma. Invasive melanomas also display higher levels of immunostaining for VEGF when compared with noninvasive tumors. Although VEGF is primarily angiogenic, FGF-2 also has an autocrine role in melanoma cell survival and proliferation; both factors are, therefore, required to maintain tumor growth. The three isoforms of MGSA/GRO are also known to stimulate angiogenesis, whereas experiments in mouse models have demonstrated significant roles for endothelial cell-selective adhesion molecule and IL-1β, IL-1α and the IL-1 receptor in the angiogenic response in melanoma cell-derived tumors. Neovascularization in melanoma is also achieved by reducing key antiangiogenic molecules. Indeed, invasion of both melanoma cells and endothelial cells is abrogated by angiostatin treatment.

VASCULOGENIC MIMICRY "Vasculogenic mimicry" is the phrase coined to describe the apparent formation of a network of channels within metastatic cutaneous lesions, which resemble the vasculogenic networks formed by differentiating endothelial cells in the embryo. This is a fascinating example of the plasticity of aggressive melanoma cells and constitutes an angiogenesis-independent pathway of facilitating tumor perfusion and preventing necrosis. Evidence of vasculogenic mimicry in tumors has a most unfavorable prognosis.

These channels are not lined by endothelial cells, yet erythrocytes and plasma can be detected within them raising the possibility that some anastomoses may occur between both endothelia-lined and nonendothelia-lined "vessels." They are formed by aggressive melanoma cells expressing VE-cadherin. Downregulation of VE-cadherin abrogates the ability of melanoma cells to form them. Introduction of aggressive melanoma cells into an ischemic environment (the hindlimb of a nude mouse) results in the expression of VE-cadherin and other endothelial associated genes and cell fate determination molecules reminiscent of embryonic vasculogenesis. Melanoma cells capable of engaging in vasculogenic mimicry express several endothelial-associated growth factors and their receptors including EphA2 and CD34. Notch 4 is also highly expressed by malignant melanoma cells undergoing neovascularization, and

inhibiting tumor vasculogenic mimicry is relatively unaffected by endostatin and, thus, any therapy targeting tumor perfusion must also consider the characteristics of these nonendothelial lined channels. MMP-2 and MT1-MMP-dependent cleavage of the laminin-5γ2 chain produced fragments that could induce vasculogenic mimicry in poorly aggressive tumor cells in vitro if grown on an aggressive tumor cell conditioned matrix. Interestingly, the application of chemically modified tetracyclins, which inhibit MMP activity, also inhibits generation of fragments of laminin-5γ2 chain and the induction of vasculogenic mimicry-associated genes in less aggressive cell lines. Clearly, the microenvironment plays a significant role in neovascularization and targeting factors in the environment of aggressive melanomas may be a useful therapeutic adjunct.

SELECTED REFERENCES

Baldi A, Santini D, Battista T, et al. Expression of AP-2 transcription factor and of its downstream target genes c-kit, E-cadherin and p21 in human cutaneous melanoma. J Cell Biochem 2001;83(3):364–372.

Bar-Eli M. Gene regulation in melanoma progression by the AP-2 transcription factor. Pigment Cell Res 2001;14(2):78–85.

Bastian BC. Understanding the progression of melanocytic neoplasia using genomic analysis: from fields to cancer. Oncogene 2003;22(20):3081–3086.

Bennett DC. Human melanocyte senescence and melanoma susceptibility genes. Oncogene 2003;22(20):3063–3069.

Bishop DT, Demenais F, Goldstein AM, et al. Geographical variation in the penetrance of CDKN2A mutations for melanoma. J Natl Cancer Inst 2002;94(12):894–903.

Bittner M, Meltzer P, Chen Y, et al. Molecular classification of cutaneous malignant melanoma by gene expression profiling. Nature 2000;406 (6795):536–540.

Chin L, Pomerantz J, Polsky D, et al. Cooperative effects of INK4a and ras in melanoma susceptibility in vivo. Genes Dev 1997;11(21):2822–2834.

Ciolczyk-Wierzbicka D, Gil D, Hoja-Lukowicz D, Litynska A, Laidler P. Carbohydrate moieties of N-cadherin from human melanoma cell lines. Acta Biochim Pol 2002;49(4):991–998.

Davies H, Bignell GR, Cox C, et al. Mutations of the BRAF gene in human cancer. Nature 2002;417(6892):949–954.

Degen WG, van Kempen LC, Gijzen EG, et al. MEMD, a new cell adhesion molecule in metastasizing human melanoma cell lines, is identical to ALCAM (activated leukocyte cell adhesion molecule). Am J Pathol 1998;152(3):805–813.

Demunter A, Libbrecht L, Degreef H, De Wolf-Peeters C, van den Oord JJ. Loss of membranous expression of beta-catenin is associated with tumor progression in cutaneous melanoma and rarely caused by exon 3 mutations. Mod Pathol 2002;15(4):454–461.

Dong J, Phelps RG, Qiao R, et al. BRAF oncogenic mutations correlate with progression rather than initiation of human melanoma. Cancer Res 2003;63(14):3883–3885.

Dupin E, Le Douarin NM. Development of melanocyte precursors from the vertebrate neural crest. Oncogene 2003;22(20):3016–3023.

Dupin E, Real C, Glavieux-Pardanaud C, Vaigot P, Le Douarin NM. Reversal of developmental restrictions in neural crest lineages: Transition from Schwann cells to glial-melanocytic precursors in vitro. Proc Natl Acad Sci USA 2003;100(9):5229–5233.

Ferrier CM, van Muijen GN, Ruiter DJ. Proteases in cutaneous melanoma. Ann Med 1998;30(5):431–442.

Folberg R, Hendrix MJ, Maniotis AJ. Vasculogenic mimicry and tumor angiogenesis. Am J Pathol 2000;156(2):361–381.

Gruss C, Herlyn M. Role of cadherins and matrixins in melanoma. Curr Opin Oncol 2001;13(2):117–123.

Halaban R. The regulation of normal melanocyte proliferation. Pigment Cell Res 2000;13(1):4–14.

Hayward NK. Genetics of melanoma predisposition. Oncogene 2003; 22(20):3053–3062.

Heikkila P, Teronen O, Moilanen M. Bisphosphonates inhibit stromelysin-1 (MMP-3), matrix metalloelastase (MMP-12), collagenase-3 (MMP-

13) and enamelysin (MMP-20), but not urokinase-type plasminogen activator, and diminish invasion and migration of human malignant and endothelial cell lines. Anticancer Drugs 2002;13(3):245–254.

Hendrix MJ, Seftor EA, Hess AR, Seftor RE. Molecular plasticity of human melanoma cells. Oncogene 2003;22(20):3070–3075.

Hendrix MJ, Seftor EA, Hess AR, Seftor RE. Vasculogenic mimicry and tumour-cell plasticity: lessons from melanoma. Nat Rev Cancer 2003; 3(6):411–421.

Hendrix MJ, Seftor EA, Meltzer PS, et al. Expression and functional significance of VE-cadherin in aggressive human melanoma cells: role in vasculogenic mimicry. Proc Natl Acad Sci USA 2001;98(14): 8018–8023.

Herlyn M, Berking C, Li G, Satyamoorthy K. Lessons from melanocyte development for understanding the biological events in naevus and melanoma formation. Melanoma Res 2000;10(4):303–312.

Hersey P, Zhang XD. How melanoma cells evade trail-induced apoptosis. Nat Rev Cancer 2001;1(2):142–150.

Hess AR, Seftor EA, Gardner LM, et al. Molecular regulation of tumor cell vasculogenic mimicry by tyrosine phosphorylation: role of epithelial cell kinase (Eck/EphA2). Cancer Res 2001;61(8):3250–3255.

Hsu MY, Meier F, Herlyn M. Melanoma development and progression: a conspiracy between tumor and host. Differentiation 2002;70(9–10): 522–536.

Hsu MY, Meier FE, Nesbit M, et al. E-cadherin expression in melanoma cells restores keratinocyte-mediated growth control and down-regulates expression of invasion-related adhesion receptors. Am J Pathol 2000; 156(5):1515–1525.

Ichihashi M, Ueda M, Budiyanto A, et al. UV-induced skin damage. Toxicology 2003;189(1–2):21–39.

Jean D, Gershenwald JE, Huang S, et al. Loss of AP-2 results in up-regulation of MCAM/MUC18 and an increase in tumor growth and metastasis of human melanoma cells. J Biol Chem 1998;273(26):16,501–16,508.

Jhappan C, Noonan FP, Merlino G. Ultraviolet radiation and cutaneous malignant melanoma. Oncogene 2003;22(20):3099–3112.

Johnson JP. Cell adhesion molecules in the development and progression of malignant melanoma. Cancer Metastasis Rev 1999;18(3):345–357.

Kamada S, Shimono A, Shinto Y, et al. BCL-2 deficiency in mice leads to pleiotropic abnormalities: accelerated lymphoid cell death in thymus and spleen, polycystic kidney, hair hypopigmentation, and distorted small intestine. Cancer Res 1995;55(2):354–359.

Kannan K, Sharpless NE, Xu J, O'Hagan RC, Bosenberg M, Chin L. Components of the Rb pathway are critical targets of UV mutagenesis in a murine melanoma model. Proc Natl Acad Sci USA 2003;100(3): 1221–1225.

Krimpenfort P, Quon KC, Mooi WJ, Loonstra A, Berns A. Loss of p16Ink4a confers susceptibility to metastatic melanoma in mice. Nature 2001; 413(6851):83–86.

Kurschat P, Mauch C. Mechanisms of metastasis. Clin Exp Dermatol 2000;25(6):482–489.

Li G, Ho VC. p53-dependent DNA repair and apoptosis respond differently to high- and low-dose ultraviolet radiation. Br J Dermatol 1998;139(1):3–10.

Li G, Satyamoorthy K, Herlyn M. N-cadherin-mediated intercellular interactions promote survival and migration of melanoma cells. Cancer Res 2001;61(9):3819–3825.

Li G, Satyamoorthy K, Meier F, Berking C, Bogenrieder T, Herlyn M. Function and regulation of melanoma-stromal fibroblast interactions: when seeds meet soil. Oncogene 2003;22(20):3162–3171.

Li G, Schaider H, Satyamoorthy K, Hanakawa Y, Hashimoto K, Herlyn M. Downregulation of E-cadherin and Desmoglein 1 by autocrine hepatocyte growth factor during melanoma development. Oncogene 2001;20(56):8125–8135.

Longo N, Yanez-Mo M, Mittelbrunn M, et al. Regulatory role of tetraspanin CD9 in tumor-endothelial cell interaction during transendothelial invasion of melanoma cells. Blood 2001;98(13):3717–3726.

Luca MR, Bar-Eli M. Molecular changes in human melanoma metastasis. Histol Histopathol 1998;13(4):1225–1231.

MacDougall JR, Bani MR, Lin Y, Muschel RJ, Kerbel RS. 'Proteolytic switching': opposite patterns of regulation of gelatinase B and its inhibitor TIMP-1 during human melanoma progression and consequences of gelatinase B overexpression. Br J Cancer 1999;80(3–4): 504–512.

Maniotis AJ, Folberg R, Hess A, et al. Vascular channel formation by human melanoma cells in vivo and in vitro: vasculogenic mimicry. Am J Pathol 1999;155(3):739–752.

McGary EC, Lev DC, Bar-Eli M. Cellular adhesion pathways and metastatic potential of human melanoma. Cancer Biol Ther 2002;1(5):459–465.

McGill GG, Horstmann M, Widlund HR, et al. BCL-2 regulation by the melanocyte master regulator MITF modulates lineage survival and melanoma cell viability. Cell 2002;109(6):707–718.

Meier F, Satyamoorthy K, Nesbit M, et al. Molecular events in melanoma development and progression. Front Biosci 1998;3:D1005–D1010.

Mollaaghababa R, Pavan WJ. The importance of having your SOX on: role of SOX10 in the development of neural crest-derived melanocytes and glia. Oncogene 2003;22(20):3024–3034.

Nakayama K, Negishi I, Negishi I, Kuida K, Sawa H, Loh DY. Targeted disruption of BCL-2 alpha beta in mice: Occurrence of gray hair, polycystic kidney disease, and lymphocytopenia. Proc Natl Acad Sci USA 1994;91(9):3700–3704.

Nierodzik ML, Chen K, Takeshita K, et al. Protease-activated receptor 1 (PAR-1) is required and rate-limiting for thrombin-enhanced experimental pulmonary metastasis. Blood 1998;92(10):3694–3700.

Nyormoi O, Bar-Eli M. Transcriptional regulation of metastasis-related genes in human melanoma. Clin Exp Metastasis 2003;20(3):251–263.

Pavey S, Gabrielli B. Alpha-melanocyte stimulating hormone potentiates p16/CDKN2A expression in human skin after ultraviolet irradiation. Cancer Res 2002;62(3):875–880.

Pavey S, Russell T, Gabrielli B. G2 phase cell cycle arrest in human skin following UV irradiation. Oncogene 2001;20(43):6103–6110.

Perez-Moreno MA, Locascio A, Rodrigo I, et al. A new role for E12/E47 in the repression of E-cadherin expression and epithelial-mesenchymal transitions. J Biol Chem 2001;276(29):27,424–27,431.

Pollock PM, Harper UL, Hansen KS, et al. High frequency of BRAF mutations in nevi. Nat Genet 2003;33(1):19–20.

Pollock PM, Hayward N. Mutations in exon 3 of the beta-catenin gene are rare in melanoma cell lines. Melanoma Res 2002;12(2):183–186.

Polsky D, Cordon-Cardo C. Oncogenes in melanoma. Oncogene 2003;22(20):3087–3091.

Poser I, Dominguez D, de Herreros AG, Varnai A, Buettner R, Bosserhoff AK. Loss of E-cadherin expression in melanoma cells involves up-regulation of the transcriptional repressor Snail. J Biol Chem 2001;276(27):24, 661–24,666.

Ramjeesingh R, Leung R, Siu CH. Interleukin-8 secreted by endothelial cells induces chemotaxis of melanoma cells through the chemokine receptor CXCR1. FASEB J 2003;17(10):1292–1294.

Randerson-Moor JA, Harland M, Williams S, et al. A germline deletion of p14(ARF) but not CDKN2A in a melanoma-neural system tumour syndrome family. Hum Mol Genet 2001;10(1):55–62.

Reifenberger J, Knobbe CB, Wolter M, et al. Molecular genetic analysis of malignant melanomas for aberrations of the WNT signaling pathway genes CTNNB1, APC, ICAT and BTRC. Int J Cancer 2002;100(5):549–556.

Reinke V, Lozano G. Differential activation of p53 targets in cells treated with ultraviolet radiation that undergo both apoptosis and growth arrest. Radiat Res 1997;148(2):115–122.

Rizos H, Puig S, Badenas C, et al. A melanoma-associated germline mutation in exon 1beta inactivates p14ARF. Oncogene 2001;20(39): 5543–5547.

Sanders DS, Blessing K, Hassan GA, Bruton R, Marsden JR, Jankowski J. Alterations in cadherin and catenin expression during the biological progression of melanocytic tumours. Mol Pathol 1999;52(3):151–157.

Sandig M, Voura EB, Kalnins VI, Siu CH. Role of cadherins in the transendothelial migration of melanoma cells in culture. Cell Motil Cytoskeleton 1997;38(4):351–364.

Sauter ER, Yeo UC, von Stemm A, et al. Cyclin D1 is a candidate oncogene in cutaneous melanoma. Cancer Res 2002;62(11):3200–3206.

Seftor EA, Meltzer PS, Schatteman GC, et al. Expression of multiple molecular phenotypes by aggressive melanoma tumor cells: role in vasculogenic mimicry. Crit Rev Oncol Hematol 2002;44(1):17–27.

Seftor RE, Seftor EA, Hendrix MJ. Molecular role(s) for integrins in human melanoma invasion. Cancer Metastasis Rev 1999;18(3):359–375.

mature epithelial cells. It is thus plausible that high levels of expression of CDX2 as a consequence of the t(12;13) chromosomal translocation dysregulates *HOX* expression in hematopoietic progenitors and results in leukemia. Evidence to support this includes the ability CDX2 to induce leukemia in murine retroviral transduction models. Although CDX2 is not normally expressed in hematopoietic cells, its family member CDX4 has been cloned, and appears to play a similar role in hematopoietic development as CDX2 does in the gut. Of note, CDX4 appears to either be downstream or epistatic with MLL in regulation of *HOX* gene expression in hematopoietic cells.

C/(EBP)α Mutations in AML   C/EBPα is a hematopoietic transcription factor required for normal myeloid lineage development. Loss of function results in severe neutropenia owing to lack of maturation of the myeloid lineage. Point mutations in *C/EBPα* have been identified in a fraction of M2 AML cases that confer dominant negative properties, and would be predicted to impair differentiation of myeloid lineage cells. Data indicate that *C/EBPα* mutations confer a favorable prognosis.

GATA-1 Mutations in AML *GATA-1* mutations are associated with a subset of acute megakaryoblastic leukemias (FAB M7), in particular leukemias arising in patients with Down syndrome (constitutional trisomy 21). These mutations appear to result in loss of function or dysregulation of GATA-1, and are thought to contribute to leukemogenesis. The mechanism through which hypomorphic alleles of *GATA-1* contribute to leukemogenesis in the context of +21 is not known. *GATA-1* mutations have only been associated with Down syndrome, and have not been observed in other infant acute megakaryoblastic leukemias.

TRANSCRIPTIONAL REGULATORY PROTEINS IN CHROMOSOMAL TRANSLOCATIONS   The observation of mutations and gene rearrangements affecting the function of transcription factors important for normal hematopoietic development suggests that the target genes for these transcription factors, and their mutated counterparts, are important in disease pathogenesis. However, an interesting class of mutations has been observed in AML involving components of the transcriptional apparatus with no apparent DNA binding specificity. These include fusion genes involving transcriptional coactivators such as CMP, p300, MOZ, and TIF2, and transcriptional modulators such as MLL.

MLL Gene Rearrangements   11q23 translocations involving the *MLL* locus have been observed in several AML FAB subtypes, but occur most commonly in the M4 myelomonocytic and M5 monoblastic leukemias. In addition, t(4;11)(q21;q23) is the single most common cytogenetic abnormality in infants with acute leukemia, occurring in approx 70–80% of these cases. 11q23 translocations are also observed frequently in therapy-related leukemias in patients who have previously been treated with chemotherapy drugs that inhibit topoisomerase II, especially the epipodophyllotoxins.

MLL is a large protein (molecular weight approx 430 kDa), and contains several functional motifs that suggest that MLL has properties of a transcriptional regulatory protein. These include N-terminal adenine–thymine (AT)-hook motifs that bind to AT-rich sequences in the minor groove of DNA; a region of homology with DNA methyltransferases; two regions of homology to the *Drosophila trithorax* gene referred to as PHD or LAP domains; and a C-terminal SET domain. There are also transcriptional activation and repression domains. Targeted disruption of *Mll* in mice results in embryonic lethality at day E10.5, and *Mll*

heterozygous mice have growth retardation, bidirectional homeotic transformations of the axial skeleton, and sternal malformations. In the *Mll* homozygous deficient mice, expression of *Hoxa7* and *Hoxc9* is abolished, whereas in *Mll* heterozygous mice, there is posterior shift of the anterior boundaries of expression of these genes. These findings indicate that MLL is a positive regulator of *HOX* gene expression during development, and provide evidence that MLL-related fusions might aberrantly regulate *HOX* genes in leukemogenesis.

MLL is involved in more than 40 different chromosomal translocations, with a diverse spectrum of partners. In addition, there is partial tandem duplication of *MLL* sequences in a subset of AML patients with trisomy 11 or a normal karyotype that duplicates the amino terminal AT hooks, the methyltransferase and repression domains of MLL. These findings suggest that the critical transforming event may be related to rearrangement of MLL itself, as opposed to contributions from the diverse fusion partners.

In support of this hypothesis, the MLL gene product is a propeptide that is cleaved by a novel protease, taspase 1. There appears to be aberrant regulation of *HOX* gene expression by noncleaved MLL, and it has been suggested that the *MLL* fusion genes and the *MLL* partial tandem duplications are surrogates for the noncleaved MLL protein. This hypothesis would explain in part the similarity in phenotype of most of the MLL fusions in AML, and also indicates that a critical transforming event in leukemia is dysregulation of *HOX* gene expression. The fusion partners might then contribute to lineage specificity or other phenotypic aspects of transformation related to *MLL* gene rearrangements.

As noted, most infant leukemias harbor the t(4;11)(q21;q23) that results in expression of the *MLL-AF4* fusion gene. Analysis of global patterns of gene expression indicates that these leukemias represent a distinct subclass of leukemia that can be readily delineated from AML or acute lymphoblastic leukemia by gene expression profiles. These data, and information on the target genes that are overexpressed in infant leukemia with the MLL-AF4 fusion such as FLT3, suggest novel approaches to therapy of this subtype of leukemia.

Important data on mechanisms of transformation by *MLL* fusion genes have been generated in retroviral transduction models of leukemia. Transduction of *MLL-ENL* fusion into primary murine bone marrow cells results in immortalization as assessed by serial replating assays, whereas constructs containing either N-terminal *MLL, ENL* alone, or vector controls could not maintain proliferative capacity beyond three passages. Furthermore, transplantation of *MLL-ENL*-transduced bone marrow into syngeneic recipient mice resulted in AML. These experiments were extended to analyze the importance of *HOX* family members in leukemogenesis by transduction of murine backgrounds genetically deficient in *HoxA9* or *HoxA7*. Transduction of *MLL* fusion genes into these backgrounds results in a marked attenuation of the leukemia phenotype, and demonstrates a critical requirement for certain *Hox* family members for leukemia transformation mediated by at least a subset of *MLL* fusion genes. These studies have been further extended to characterize the target cell for transformation. Retroviral transduction with *MLL-ENL* of purified committed progenitors that have no inherent capacity for self-renewal, such as common myeloid progenitors (CMP) or granulocyte-monocyte progenitors (GMP) confers properties of self-renewal. These data indicate that certain leukemia oncogenes can reprogram committed hematopoietic progenitors to acquire properties of leukemic stem cells.

The leukemogenic potential of *MLL* fusions has also been demonstrated in *Mll-AF9* knockin mouse model, in which chimeric animals developed AML within 6–9 mo.

GENE REARRANGEMENTS INVOLVING TRANSCRIPTIONAL COACTIVATORS IN AML The recruitment of transcriptional coactivators and corepressors by transcription factors involved in leukemia suggests a critical role for these proteins in leukemogenesis. In keeping with the recurring theme that the diverse and numerous chromosomal translocations in leukemia may share targets and functional activity, there are chromosomal translocations involving proteins that directly modulate and facilitate regulated gene expression.

Fusion genes associated with AML that directly involve coactivators include *MLL-CBP, MLL-p300, MOZ-CBP,* and *MOZ-TIF2*. Each of these involves a transcriptional coactivator with intrinsic histone acetyl transferase activity, and in the case of MOZ-TIF2, CBP or p300 can be recruited through interaction with the LXXLL motif in TIF2. The transforming properties of these fusion proteins are not well understood. Loss of function of CBP is responsible for the Rubenstein-Taybi syndrome that predisposes to the development of colon cancer, suggesting that CBP has properties of a tumor suppressor. This observation might suggest that the fusion genes involving coactivators act as dominant negative proteins. However, data also supports the hypothesis that MOZ-TIF2 may represent a gain of function for CBP based on mutational analysis in cell culture and murine models of leukemia. It has been demonstrated that MOZ nucleosome binding activity and TIF2 interactions with CBP are required for leukemogenesis, whereas MOZ histone acetyl transferase activity is not. These data suggest that the leukemogenicity of the fusion is based on recruitment of CBP to MOZ nucleosome binding sites. In addition, transduction of MOZ-TIF2 into committed hematopoietic progenitors, but not nonleukemogenic point mutants of MOZ-TIF2, confers properties of leukemic stem cells to this population that lacks the capacity for self-renewal. This observation extends the paradigm first reported for MLL-ENL, and may provide a platform for further characterization of self-renewal programs in normal and leukemic stem cells.

GAIN OR LOSS OF GENETIC MATERIAL IN AML The molecular basis of leukemogenesis in patients with numerical chromosomal abnormalities, such as monosomy 7, trisomy 8, or trisomy 21 is poorly understood, but may be related to changes in gene dosage of one or more genes, or duplication or loss of mutant genes. Identification of the gene(s) responsible for AML or MDS associated with recurrent chromosomal deletions, including 5q-, 7q-, and 20q-, is extraordinarily difficult. Efforts have focused on identification of classical tumor suppressor genes at these loci, in which there is loss of function of one allele owing to deletion, and of the other owing to mutation. The lack of success in identifying a *bona fide* tumor suppressor thus far, and observations that haploid gene dosage can contribute to hematopoietic phenotypes such as the FPD/AML syndrome, suggests that haploinsufficiency of one or more genes in the deleted regions may contribute to the leukemic phenotype.

COOPERATING MUTATIONS IN AML

Mutations in signal transduction intermediates associated with AML are not sufficient to cause AML. Rather, expression of these alleles alone, such as the FLT3-ITD, oncogenic Ras, or mutant PTPN11 results in a myeloproliferative phenotype. The phenotypes are similar, and include neutrophilia with normal maturation and differentiation, extramedullary hematopoiesis, and lack of self-renewal capacity as assessed by serial replating or serial transplantation assays. These mutations form a functional and epidemiological complementation group, in that only rarely do two of these mutations occur in the same patient.

In contrast, a second complementation group of mutant genes associated with AML has been identified that primarily involves hematopoietic transcription factors or transcriptional coactivators. These proteins, exemplified by RUNX1-ETO, PML-RARα, MLL-ENL, or MOZ-TIF2, are not sufficient to cause AML in cell culture or murine models of disease, but do appear to contribute to impaired hematopoietic differentiation and self-renewal potential of AML cells.

However, mutations from each of these complementation groups are often identified in the same AML patient, suggesting that mutant genes from each of these classes cooperates to engender the AML phenotype. From murine models of AML based on human genotypes, there is evidence for cooperation between these complementation groups. BCR-ABL cooperates with NUP98-HOXA9 to cause AML in a murine model of chronic myelogenous leukemia in myeloid blast crisis, as does TEL-PDGFβR and RUNX1-ETO. FLT3 mutations associated with t(15;17) and PML-RARα expression are common in human APL, and retroviral transduction of FLT3-ITD into a Cathepsin G PML-RARα transgenic mouse background results in APL with shortened latency and complete penetrance, consistent with cooperative effects. These data suggest cooperation between these two complementation groups in AML, and that molecular therapies targeted against each of the classes of mutation may be additive or synergistic in treatment of AML. For example, it may be feasible to treat APL patients with FLT3 mutations with a combination of small molecule inhibitors of FLT3 and ATRA.

THE LEUKEMIA STEM CELL Normal hematopoiesis is a hierarchy that has at its root the self-renewing hematopoietic stem cell (HSC) from which all other hematopoietic elements are derived. These cells are rare and often quiescent in normal adult bone marrow. Emerging evidence indicates that in AML, as in normal hematopoietic development, a hierarchy is governed by the so-called leukemic stem cell. Furthermore, the existence of cancer stem cells has also been demonstrated in several other contexts, including breast cancer and central nervous system tumors. There are important clinical implications of these observations. First, these data suggest that the bulk of any given tumor is made up of clonogenic progenitors that do not have the capacity to self-renew. Although cancer therapy is usually assessed by the efficiency of reduction of disease burden, the reduction and elimination of the cancer stem cell population will likely be the most important goal toward preventing disease relapse. Thus, it is important to understand the relationship of the normal stem cell and the respective cancer stem cell, to understand mechanisms of self-renewal in these populations, and to develop therapeutic strategies that specifically target this critical population of cells.

Leukemic stem cells exist among a primitive population of hematopoietic progenitors in human AML. Using murine models in which human AML cells are transplanted into immunodeficient recipient (NOD-SCID) mice, SCID leukemia-initiating cells (SL-IC) can be identified that occur at a frequency of about 1 in 10^5 AML cells. These cells are phenotypically identical to those of the AML patient from which they were derived, and can reconstitute the AML phenotype in recipient animals. SL-ICs reside in a primitive compartment of hematopoietic progenitors identifiable by flow cytometric analysis as CD34$^+$/CD38$^-$ cells. Several lines of evidence have suggested that the target cell for transformation is the HSC itself. For example, the SL-IC is immunophenotypically similar to a normal HSC, and CD34$^+$ progenitors derived from AML patients often contain the diagnostic cytogenetic abnormality. In addition, there is theoretical support for the stem cell as a target for transformation, in that this population already has properties of self-renewal, and is long lived, which would allow for acquisition of the multiple mutations that are required for leukemic transformation.

However, other data provide a counterpoint to the HSC as a target for transforming events in AML. Expression of certain leukemia oncogenes in committed hematopoietic progenitors that are destined to apoptotic cell death can confer properties of self-renewal to these cells. As discussed previously, the *MLL-ENL* fusion gene can confer properties of leukemic stem cells in CMP or GMP that are irrevocably committed to terminal differentiation and apoptotic cell death, as demonstrated by the ability to serially replate in methylcellulose cultures, and to cause AML that can be serially transplanted into secondary recipient mice. The leukemias are immunophenotypically identical, regardless of the starting cell population (purified HSC, CMP, or GMP populations isolated by high speed multiparameter flow cytometry) that is transduced. These data suggest that the certain leukemia oncogenes like the *MLL-ENL* fusion can commandeer programs of self-renewal in committed progenitors, and enforce phenotypic expression of markers associated with the HSC. These findings provide a platform for identification of the transcriptional programs that control self-renewal. These in turn may allow for development of therapies that selectively target the leukemic stem cell, and may also provide insight into strategies to confer properties of self-renewal to adult somatic cells for therapeutic benefit, such as tissue regeneration.

SUMMARY AND FUTURE DIRECTIONS

A virtual explosion has been seen in the identification and characterization of disease alleles in AML in cell culture and murine models of leukemia. These insights have provided a platform for development of molecularly targeted therapies of AML that may improve clinical outcome. ATRA in the treatment of APL is one proof-of-principle example for this approach, and will hopefully be a harbinger for the development of additional efficacious treatments, such as FLT3 inhibitors and others. The data indicating that at least two mutations cooperate to cause the AML phenotype suggest strategies for independently targeting multiple pathways that contribute to AML, using animal models as a platform for testing combination therapies. Finally, the seminal observation that AML contains a small, but well-defined, population of cells with stem cell-like properties may allow for development of therapies that target this critical population.

SELECTED REFERENCES

Aasland R, Gibson TJ, Stewart AF. The PHD finger: implications for chromatin-mediated transcriptional regulation. Trends Biochem Sci 1995;20:56–59.

Abe A, Emi N, Tanimoto M, Terasaki H, Marunouchi T, Saito H. Fusion of the platelet-derived growth factor receptor beta to a novel gene CEV14 in acute myelogenous leukemia after clonal evolution. Blood 1997;90(11):4271–4277.

Abu-Duhier F, Goodeve A, Wilson G, et al. FLT3 internal tandem duplication mutations in adult acute myeloid leukaemia define a high-risk group. Br J Haematol 2000;111:190–195.

Ahuja HG, Hong J, Aplan PD, Tcheurekdjian L, Forman SJ, Slovak ML. t(9;11)(p22;p15) in acute myeloid leukemia results in a fusion between NUP98 and the gene encoding transcriptional coactivators p52 and p75-lens epithelium-derived growth factor (LEDGF). Cancer Res 2000;60:6227–6229.

Amann JM, Nip J, Strom DK, et al. ETO, a target of t(8;21) in acute leukemia, makes distinct contacts with multiple histone deacetylases and binds mSin3A through its oligomerization domain. Mol Cell Biol 2001;21:6470–6483.

Araki T, Mohi MG, Ismat FA, et al. Mouse model of Noonan syndrome reveals cell type- and gene dosage-dependent effects of Ptpn11 mutation. Nat Med 2004;10:849–857.

Armstrong SA, Staunton JE, Silverman LB, et al. MLL translocations specify a distinct gene expression profile that distinguishes a unique leukemia. Nat Genet 2002;30:41–47.

Ayton PM, Cleary ML. Transformation of myeloid progenitors by MLL oncoproteins is dependent on Hoxa7 and Hoxa9. Genes Dev 2003;17:2298–2307.

Beaupre DM, Kurzrock R. RAS and leukemia: from basic mechanisms to gene-directed therapy. J Clin Oncol 1999;17:1071–1079.

Beghini A, Peterlongo P, Ripamonti CB, et al. C-kit mutations in core binding factor leukemias. Blood 2000;95:726, 727.

Bhatia M, Wang JC, Kapp U, Bonnet D, Dick JE. Purification of primitive human hematopoietic cells capable of repopulating immune-deficient mice. Proc Natl Acad Sci USA 1997;94:5320–5325.

Bonnet D, Dick JE. Human acute myeloid leukemia is organized as a hierarchy that originates from a primitive hematopoietic cell. Nat Med 1997;3:730–737.

Borrow J, Shearman AM, Stanton VP Jr, et al. The t(7;11)(p15;p15) translocation in acute myeloid leukaemia fuses the genes for nucleoporin NUP98 and class I homeoprotein HOXA9. Nat Genet 1996;12:159–167.

Braun BS, Tuveson DA, Kong N, et al. Somatic activation of oncogenic Kras in hematopoietic cells initiates a rapidly fatal myeloproliferative disorder. Proc Natl Acad Sci USA 2004;101:597–602.

Brown D, Kogan S, Lagasse E, et al. A PMLRARalpha transgene initiates murine acute promyelocytic leukemia. Proc Natl Acad Sci USA 1997;18:2551–2556.

Caligiuri MA, Strout MP, Schichman SA, et al. Partial tandem duplication of ALL1 as a recurrent molecular defect in acute myeloid leukemia with trisomy 11. Cancer Res 1996;56:1418–1425.

Carapeti M, Aguiar RCT, Goldman JM, Cross NCP. A novel fusion between MOZ and the nuclear receptor coactivator TIF2 in acute myeloid leukemia. Blood 1998;91:3127–3133.

Castilla LH, Garrett L, Adya N, et al. The fusion gene Cbfβ blocks myeloid differentiation and predisposes mice to acute myelomonocytic leukemia. Nat Genet 1999;23:144–146.

Castilla LH, Wijmenga C, Wang Q, et al. Failure of embryonic hematopoiesis and lethal hemorrhages in mouse embryos heterozygous for a knocked-in leukemia gene CBFB-MYH11. Cell 1996;87: 687–696.

Chan IT, Kutok JL, Williams IR, et al. Conditional expression of oncogenic K-ras from its endogenous promoter induces a myeloproliferative disease. J Clin Invest 2004;113:528–538.

Chase A, Reiter A, Burci L, et al. Fusion of ETV6 to the caudal-related homeobox gene CDX2 in acute myeloid leukemia with the t(12;13)(p13;q12). Blood 1999;93:1025–1031.

Cobaleda C, Gutierrez-Cianca N, Perez-Losada J, et al. A primitive hematopoietic cell is the target for the leukemic transformation in human Philadelphia-positive acute lymphoblastic leukemia. Blood 2000;95:1007–1013.

Corral J, Lavenir I, Impey H, et al. An Mll-AF9 fusion gene made by homologous recombination causes acute leukemia in chimeric mice: a method to create fusion oncogenes. Cell 1996;85:853–861.

Cozzio A, Passegue E, Ayton PM, Karsunky H, Cleary ML, Weissman IL. Similar MLL-associated leukemias arising from self-renewing stem cells and short-lived myeloid progenitors. Genes Dev 2003;17:3029–3035.

Dash A, Gilliland DG. Molecular genetics of acute myeloid leukaemia. Best Pract Res Clin Haematol 2001;14:49–64.

Dash AB, Williams IR, Kutok JL, et al. A murine model of CML blast crisis induced by cooperation between BCR/ABL and NUP98/HOXA9. Proc Natl Acad Sci USA 2002;99:7622–7627.

Davidson AJ, Ernst P, Wang Y, et al. cdx4 mutants fail to specify blood progenitors and can be rescued by multiple hox genes. Nature 2003;425:300–306.

de The H, Lavau C, Marcio A, Chomienne C, Degos L, Dejean A. The PML-RAR-alpha fusion mRNA generated by the t(15;17) translocation in acute promyelocytic leukaemia encodes a functionally altered RAR. Cell 1991;66:675–684.

Deguchi K, Ayton PM, Carapeti M, et al. MOZ-TIF2-induced acute myeloid leukemia requires the MOZ nucleosome binding motif and TIF2-mediated recruitment of CBP. Cancer Cell 2003;3:259–271.

Dyck JA, Maul GG, Miller WH, Jr, Chen JD, Kakizuka A, Evans RM. A novel macromolecular structure is a target of the promyelocyte-retinoic acid receptor oncoprotein. Cell 1994;76:333–343.

Geary CG, Harrison CJ, Philpott NJ, Hows JM, Gordon-Smith EC, Marsh JC. Abnormal cytogenetic clones in patients with aplastic anaemia: Response to immunosuppressive therapy. Br J Haematol 1999;104:271–274.

Giles RH, Dauwerse JG, Higgins C, et al. Detection of CBP rearrangements in acute myelogenous leukemia with t(8;16). Leukemia 1997;11:2087–2096.

Gilliland DG. Proteolytic processing in development and leukemogenesis. Cell 2003;115:248–250.

Gilliland DG, Griffin JD. The roles of FLT3 in hematopoiesis and leukemia. Blood 2002;100:1532–1542.

Griffin JD. Point mutations in the FLT3 gene in AML. Blood 2001;97:2193A–2193A.

Griffith J, Black J, Faerman C, et al. The structural basis for autoinhibition of FLT3 by the juxtamembrane domain. Mol Cell 2004;13:169–178.

Grignani F, De Matteis S, Nervi C, et al. Fusion proteins of the retinoic acid receptor-alpha recruit histone deacetylase in promyelocytic leukaemia. Nature 1998;391:815–818.

Grisolano JL, O'Neal J, Cain J, Tomasson MH. An activated receptor tyrosine kinase, TEL/PDGFbetaR, cooperates with AML1/ETO to induce acute myeloid leukemia in mice. Proc Natl Acad Sci USA 2003;100:9506–9511.

Grisolano JL, Wesselschmidt RL, Pelicci PG, Ley TJ. Altered myeloid development and acute leukemia in transgenic mice expressing PML-RAR alpha under control of cathepsin G regulatory sequences. Blood 1997;89:376–387.

Hanson RD, Hess JL, Yu BD, et al. Mammalian Trithorax and polycomb-group homologues are antagonistic regulators of homeotic development. Proc Natl Acad Sci USA 1999;96:14,372–14,377.

He LZ, Guidez F, Tribioli C, et al. Distinct interactions of PML-RARalpha and PLZF-RARalpha with co-repressors determine differential responses to RA in APL. Nat Genet 1998;18:126–135.

He LZ, Tolentino T, Grayson P, et al. Histone deacetylase inhibitors induce remission in transgenic models of therapy-resistant acute promyelocytic leukemia. J Clin Invest 2001;108:1321–1330.

He LZ, Tribioli C, Rivi R, et al. Acute leukemia with promyelocytic features in PML/RARalpha transgenic mice. Proc Natl Acad Sci USA 1997;94:5302–5307.

Hiebert SW, Reed-Inderbitzin EF, Amann J, Irvin B, Durst K, Linggi B. The t(8;21) fusion protein contacts co-repressors and histone deacetylases to repress the transcription of the p14ARF tumor suppressor. Blood Cells Mol Dis 2003;30:177–183.

Higuchi M, O'Brien D, Kumaravelu P, Lenny N, Yeoh E-J, Downing JR. Expression of a conditional AML1-ETO oncogene bypasses embryonic lethality and establishes a murine model of human t(8;21) acute myeloid leukemia. Cancer Cell 2002;1:63–74.

Hsieh JJ, Ernst P, Erdjument-Bromage H, Tempst P, Korsmeyer SJ. Proteolytic cleavage of MLL generates a complex of N- and C-terminal fragments that confers protein stability and subnuclear localization. Mol Cell Biol 2003;23:186–194.

Karp JE. Farnesyl protein transferase inhibitors as targeted therapies for hematologic malignancies. Semin Hematol 2001;38:16–23.

Kasper LH, Brindle PK, Schnabel CA, Pritchard CE, Cleary ML, van Deursen JM. CREB binding protein interacts with nucleoporin-specific FG repeats that activate transcription and mediate NUP98-HOXA9 oncogenicity. Mol Cell Biol 1999;19:764–776.

Kelly LM, Yu JC, Boulton CL, et al. CT53518, a novel selective FLT3 antagonist for the treatment of acute myelogenous leukemia (AML). Cancer Cell 2002;1:421–432.

Kiyoi H, Naoe T, Nakano Y, et al. Prognostic implication of FLT3 and N-RAS gene mutations in acute myeloid leukemia. Blood 1999;93:3074–3080.

Kottaridis PD, Gale RE, Frew ME, et al. The presence of a FLT3 internal tandem duplication in patients with acute myeloid leukemia (AML) adds important prognostic information to cytogenetic risk group and response to the first cycle of chemotherapy: analysis of 854 patients from the United Kingdom Medical Research Council AML 10 and 12 trials. Blood 2001;98:1752–1759.

Lapidot T, Sirard C, Vormoor J, et al. A cell initiating human acute myeloid leukaemia after transplantation into SCID mice. Nature 1994;367:645–648.

Lavau C, Szilvassy SJ, Slany R, Cleary ML. Immortalization and leukemic transformation of a myelomonocytic precursor by retrovirally transduced HRX-ENL. EMBO J 1997;16:4226–4237.

Levis M, Allebach J, Tse KF, et al. A FLT3-targeted tyrosine kinase inhibitor is cytotoxic to leukemia cells in vitro and in vivo. Blood 2002;99:3885–3891.

Liang J, Prouty L, Williams BJ, Dayton MA, Blanchard KL. Acute mixed lineage leukemia with an inv(8)(p11q13) resulting in fusion of the genes for MOZ and TIF2. Blood 1998;92:2118–2122.

Lin RJ, Nagy L, Inoue S, Shao W, Miller WH, Evans RM. Role of the histone deacetylase complex in acute promyelocytic leukaemia. Nature 1998;391:811–814.

Liu P, Tarle SA, Hajra A, et al. Fusion between transcription factor CBFB/PEBP2B and a myosin heavy chain in acute myeloid leukemia. Science 1993;261:1041–1044.

Loh ML, Vattikuti S, Schubbert S, et al. Mutations in PTPN11 implicate the SHP-2 phosphatase in leukemogenesis. Blood 2004;103:2325–2331.

Mazo AM, Huang DH, Mozer BA, Dawid IB. The trithorax gene, a trans-acting regulator of the bithorax complex in Drosophila, encodes a protein with zinc-binding domains. Proc Natl Acad Sci USA 1990;87:2112–2116.

Melnick A, Carlile GW, McConnell MJ, Polinger A, Hiebert SW, Licht JD. AML-1/ETO fusion protein is a dominant negative inhibitor of transcriptional repression by the promyelocytic leukemia zinc finger protein. Blood 2000;96:3939–3947.

Meshinchi S, Woods WG, Stirewalt DL, et al. Prevalence and prognostic significance of Flt3 internal tandem duplication in pediatric acute myeloid leukemia. Blood 2001;97:89–94.

Meyers S, Lenny N, Hiebert SW. The t(8;21) fusion protein interferes with AML-1B-dependent transcriptional activation. Mol Cell Biol 1995;15:1974–1982.

Michaud J, Wu F, Osato M, et al. In vitro analyses of known and novel RUNX1/AML1 mutations in dominant familial platelet disorder with predisposition to acute myelogenous leukemia: Implications for mechanisms of pathogenesis. Blood 2002;99:1364–1372.

Mrozek K, Heinonen K, Bloomfield CD. Clinical importance of cytogenetics in acute myeloid leukaemia. Best Pract Res Clin Haematol 2001;14:19–47.

Nakamura T, Largaespada DA, Lee MP, et al. Fusion of the nucleoporin gene NUP98 to HOXA9 by the chromosome translocation t(7;11)(p15;p15) in human myeloid leukaemia. Nat Genet 1996;12:154–158.

Neubauer A, Dodge RK, George SL, et al. Prognostic importance of mutations in the ras proto-oncogenes in de novo acute myeloid leukemia. Blood 1994;83:1603–1611.

Neubauer A, Greenberg P, Negrin R, Ginzton N, Liu E. Mutations in the ras proto-oncogenes in patients with myelodysplastic syndromes. Leukemia 1994;8:638–641.

Nucifora G, Dickstein JI, Torbenson V, Roulston D, Rowley JD, Vardiman JW. Correlation between cell morphology and expression of the AML1/ETO chimeric transcript in patients with acute myeloid leukemia without the t(8;21). Leukemia 1994;8:1533–1538.

O'Farrell A, Abrams T, Yuen H, et al. SUGEN compounds SU5416 and SU11248 inhibit Flt3 activity: therapeutic application in AML. Blood 2001;89:118a.

Okuda T, Cai Z, Yang S, et al. Expression of a knocked-in AML1-ETO leukemia gene inhibits the establishment of normal definitive hematopoiesis and directly generates dysplastic hematopoietic progenitors. Blood 1998;91:3134–3143.

Okuda T, van Deursen J, Hiebert SW, Grosveld G, Downing JR. AML1, the target of multiple chromosomal translocations in human leukemia, is essential for normal fetal liver hematopoiesis. Cell 1996;84: 321–330.

Osato M, Asou N, Abdalla E, et al. Biallelic and heterozygous point mutations in the runt domain of the AML1/PEBP2alphaB gene associated with myeloblastic leukemias. Blood 1999;93:1817–1824.

Pabst T, Mueller BU, Zhang P, et al. Dominant-negative mutations of C/EBPalpha, encoding CCAAT/enhancer binding protein-alpha, in acute myeloid leukemia. Nat Genet 2001;27(3):263–270.

Pandolfi PP. Histone deacetylases and transcriptional therapy with their inhibitors. Cancer Chemother Pharmacol 2001;48:S17–S19.

Pandolfi PP. Transcription therapy for cancer. Oncogene 2001;20: 3116–3127.

Preudhomme C, Sagot C, Boissel N, et al. Favorable prognostic significance of CEBPA mutations in patients with de novo acute myeloid leukemia: A study from the Acute Leukemia French Association (ALFA). Blood 2002;100:2717–2723.

Rawat VP, Cusan M, Deshpande A, et al. Ectopic expression of the homeobox gene Cdx2 is the transforming event in a mouse model of t(12;13)(p13;q12) acute myeloid leukemia. Proc Natl Acad Sci USA 2004;101:817–822.

Rowley JD, Reshmi S, Sobulo O, et al. All patients with the t(11;16) (q23;p13.3) that involves MLL and CBP have treatment-related hematologic disorders. Blood 1997;90:535–539.

Saha V, Chaplin T, Gregorini A, Ayton P, Young BD. The leukemia-associated-protein (LAP) domain, a cysteine-rich motif, is present in a wide range of proteins, including MLL, AF10, and MLLT6 proteins. Proc Natl Acad Sci USA 1995;92:9737–9741.

Salomoni P, Pandolfi PP. The role of PML in tumor suppression. Cell 2002;108:165–170.

Schichman SA, Canaani E, Croce CM. Self-fusion of the ALL1 gene. A new genetic mechanism for acute leukemia. JAMA 1995;273: 571–576.

Sebti SM, Hamilton AD. Farnesyltransferase and geranylgeranyltransferase I inhibitors in cancer therapy: important mechanistic and bench to bedside issues. Expert Opin Investig Drugs 2000;9:2767–2782.

Song WJ, Sullivan MG, Legare RD, et al. Haploinsufficiency of CBFA2 causes familial thrombocytopenia with propensity to develop acute myelogenous leukaemia. Nat Genet 1999;23:166–175.

Speck NA, Gilliland DG. Core-binding factors in haematopoiesis and leukaemia. Nat Rev Cancer 2002;2:502–513.

Stirewalt DL, Radich JP. The role of FLT3 in haematopoietic malignancies. Nat Rev Cancer 2003;3:650–665.

Taki T, Sako M, Tsuchida M, Hayashi Y. The t(11;16)(q23;p13.3) translocation in myelodysplastic syndrome fuses the MLL gene to the CBP gene. Blood 1997;89:3945–3949.

Tallman MS, Nabhan C, Feusner JH, Rowe JM. Acute promyelocytic leukemia: Evolving therapeutic strategies. Blood 2002;99:759–767.

Tartaglia M, Niemeyer CM, Fragale A, et al. Somatic mutations in PTPN11 in juvenile myelomonocytic leukemia, myelodysplastic syndromes and acute myeloid leukemia. Nat Genet 2003;34: 148–150.

Thirman MJ, Gill HJ, Burnett RC, et al. Rearrangement of the MLL gene in acute lymphoblastic and acute myeloid leukemias with 11q23 chromosomal translocations. N Engl J Med 1993;329:909–914.

Thorsteinsdottir U, Sauvageau G, Humphries RK. Hox homeobox genes as regulators of normal and leukemic hematopoiesis. Hematol Oncol Clin North Am 1997;11:1221–1237.

Tschiersch B, Hofmann A, Krauss V, Dorn R, Korge G, Reuter G. The protein encoded by the Drosophila position-effect variegation suppressor gene Su(var)3-9 combines domains of antagonistic regulators of homeotic gene complexes. EMBO J 1994;13:3822–3831.

Wang Q, Stacy T, Binder M, Marin-Padilla M, Sharpe AH, Speck NA. Disruption of the Cbfa2 gene causes necrosis and hemorrhaging in the central nervous system and blocks definitive hematopoiesis. Proc Natl Acad Sci USA 1996;93:3444–3449.

Wechsler J, Greene M, McDevitt MA, et al. Acquired mutations in GATA1 in the megakaryoblastic leukemia of Down syndrome. Nat Genet 2002;32:148–152.

Weis K, Rambaud S, Lavau C, et al. Retinoic acid regulates aberrant nuclear localization of PML-RAR alpha in acute promyelocytic leukemia cells. Cell 1994;76:345–356.

Weisberg E, Boulton C, Kelly LM, et al. Inhibition of mutant FLT3 receptors in leukemia cells by the small molecule tyrosine kinase inhibitor PKC412. Cancer Cell 2002;1:433–443.

Yamamoto Y, Kiyoi H, Nakano Y, et al. Activating mutation of D835 within the activation loop of FLT3 in human hematologic malignancies. Blood 2001;97:2434–2439..

Yergeau DA, Hetherington CJ, Wang Q, et al. Embryonic lethality and impairment of haematopoiesis in mice heterozygous for an AML1-ETO fusion gene. Nat Genet 1997;15:303–306.

Yu BD, Hess JL, Horning SE, Brown GA, Korsmeyer SJ. Altered Hox expression and segmental identity in Mll-mutant mice. Nature 1995;378:505–508.

Zelent A, Guidez F, Melnick A, Waxman S, Licht JD. Translocations of the RARalpha gene in acute promyelocytic leukemia. Oncogene 2001;20:7186–7203.

Zhu J, Koken MH, Quignon F, et al. Arsenic-induced PML targeting onto nuclear bodies: Implications for the treatment of acute promyelocytic leukemia. Proc Natl Acad Sci USA 1997;94:3978–3983.

Zimonjic DB, Pollock JL, Westervelt P, Popescu NC, Ley TJ. Acquired, nonrandom chromosomal abnormalities associated with the development of acute promyelocytic leukemia in transgenic mice. Proc Natl Acad Sci USA 2000;97(24):13,306–13,311.

80 Acute Lymphoblastic Leukemia

ALEXANDER E. PERL AND DONALD SMALL

SUMMARY

Advances in the understanding of childhood acute lymphoblastic leukemia (ALL) have transformed the disease from a rapidly progressive and usually lethal disorder to a disease with an 80% cure rate. These improved outcomes are owing to the development of multiagent, dose-intensive chemotherapy regimens, central nervous system prophylaxis, and improved supportive care. In parallel to the improved understanding of therapeutic approaches to ALL, knowledge of the pathogenesis of ALL has increased dramatically. But uncovering the molecular mechanisms behind this disease has not yet produced targeted therapies that specifically act on these elements, as has been the case, for example, with tyrosine kinase inhibition for chronic myelogenous leukemia. Such novel treatment approaches are needed in particular in adult ALL, which although morphologically indistinguishable from pediatric disease, has a considerably poorer response to chemotherapy and remains incurable in >50% of the cases. These differences are in part resulting from differing molecular pathogenesis, which results in a higher proportion of tumors with de novo pan-drug resistance

Key Words: Acute lymphoblastic leukemia; chemotherapy; chronic myelogenous leukemia; *E2A-PBX1*; *Tel-AML1*; tumor suppressor.

INTRODUCTION

Acute lymphoblastic leukemia (ALL) is the most common malignancy among children and represents 80 and 10–20%, respectively, of childhood and adult acute leukemias. Advances in the understanding of childhood ALL have transformed the disease from a rapidly progressive and usually lethal disorder to a disease with an 80% cure rate. These improved outcomes are resulting from the development of multiagent, dose-intensive chemotherapy regimens, central nervous system (CNS) prophylaxis and improved supportive care. In parallel to the improved understanding of therapeutic approaches to ALL, knowledge of the pathogenesis of ALL has increased dramatically. But uncovering the molecular mechanisms behind this disease has not yet produced targeted therapies that specifically act on these elements, as has been the case, for example, with tyrosine kinase inhibition for chronic myelogenous leukemia (CML). Such novel treatment approaches are needed in particular in adult ALL, which although morphologically indistinguishable from pediatric disease, has a considerably poorer response to chemotherapy and

From: *Principles of Molecular Medicine, Second Edition*
Edited by: M. S. Runge and C. Patterson © Humana Press, Inc., Totowa, NJ

remains incurable in >50% of the cases. These differences in part result from differing molecular pathogenesis, which results in a higher proportion of tumors with *de novo* pan-drug resistance.

ALL is characterized by the accumulation of malignant precursors of either B or T lymphocytes in bone marrow and/or peripheral blood. Although some maturation might occur in the periphery, the proliferating cells generally are arrested in early developmental stages within the marrow. The primitive cells crowd out the normal marrow elements, causing pancytopenia. Tumor infiltration frequently causes splenomegaly, hepatomegaly, and diffuse lymphadenopathy. Patients usually present with a few weeks of nonspecific symptoms such as fatigue, often resulting from anemia, or may have a flu-like syndrome. Fever, petechial rash, bleeding, or easy bruising owing to cytopenias may also prompt medical evaluation. Bone pain might also be present, especially in children. Leukostasis or leptomeningeal spread causing focal neurological deficits can occur at diagnosis, but is uncommon.

Complete blood counts usually point to the diagnosis, showing pancytopenia of mature cells and often circulating blasts. However, the WBC is variable, and might be decreased, normal, or elevated. Marked elevation of leukocyte count with >100,000 cells/mm^3 is not unusual. Lactate dehydrogenase is typically elevated and there may be evidence of disseminated intravascular coagulation or spontaneous tumor lysis with hyperuricemia, hyperkalemia, and hyperphosphatemia. A bone marrow aspirate and biopsy with immunophenotyping and cytogenetic analysis is used to confirm diagnosis. Lumbar puncture is mandatory to assess the presence of leukemic cells in the CNS, which, with the testes, can serve as a sanctuary site.

Untreated ALL is rapidly fatal, with death usually occurring in weeks to a few months. Therapy consists of several dose-intense cycles of multiagent, noncross-resistant chemotherapy. Many classes of chemotherapeutic agents share activity in ALL including anthracyclines, steroids, alkylating agents, vinca alkaloids, topoisomerase II inhibitors, asparaginase, antimetabolites, and purine analogs. With current treatment strategies, approx 80% of children with ALL are cured. In adults, the rate is closer to 30%, virtually all of them who are younger than 60 yr. The goal of therapy is to induce complete remission as defined by the elimination of leukemic blasts by diagnostic surveillance techniques and restoration of normal peripheral blood counts. Because of advances in laboratory detection of minimal populations of leukemic cells, it is somewhat difficult to compare the success rates of remission induction therapies to those in the past, when morphological data was primarily used. This is because the flow cytometric and molecular probing techniques in use are considerably more sensitive to minimal populations of tumor cells. Indeed, current assays are capable of detecting as few as one leukemic cell among 1 million normal cells. Regardless, historic data show excellent responses to induction chemotherapy, with approx 98% of children and 80% of adults entering a complete remission, as defined by <5% blasts in the marrow and recovery of normal peripheral blood counts.

Induction chemotherapy is followed by several cycles of consolidation therapy, as well as prophylaxis of the CNS with intrathecal chemotherapy, high-dose systemic agents with CNS penetration, or radiation therapy. Treatment is typically given with minimal breaks between cycles for approx 6 mo, and is followed by maintenance therapy with low-dose oral chemotherapy for as long as 3 yr.

Once in remission, selected patients with high-risk profiles benefit from myeloablative chemotherapy and allogeneic stem cell transplantation. Relapsed disease may be treated again with dose-intense combination chemotherapy. However, except in unusual circumstances such as relapses following durable remissions, isolated CNS relapses, or relapses greater than 1 yr from the end of therapy, patients with relapsed disease generally cannot be cured unless an allogeneic stem cell transplant successfully follows the patient's second remission.

EPIDEMIOLOGY

According to the National Cancer Institute's Surveillance Epidemiology and End Results program, approx 3600 cases of ALL are diagnosed annually, with approx two-thirds of cases occurring in children. The annual disease incidence in children is measured at 28 cases per million, making it the most common pediatric malignancy. For unclear reasons, this incidence has increased by approx 50% over the last three decades. The disease is slightly more common in males (ratio of 1.3/1), and whites (regardless of Hispanic origin) are affected about twice as often as blacks. The peak incidence is in children ages 2–3. In adults, the disease is rare, and accounts for about 10–20% of the 11,000 cases of acute leukemia diagnosed yearly. Of adult ALL diagnoses, more than two-thirds occur before age 45. The incidence reaches a nadir by middle age and increases slightly thereafter.

There are no clearly implicated risk factors for ALL other than ionizing radiation, chemotherapy (especially topoisomerase II inhibitors), and benzene exposure. These identified risk factors, however, make up a small fraction of all cases. Certain karyotypic abnormalities, such as trisomy 21 (Down syndrome) carry an increased risk of acute leukemia, which may be myeloid or lymphoid. Patients with congenital DNA repair abnormalities (e.g., Bloom syndrome or ataxia telangiectasia) are also at increased risk for ALL, among other malignancies.

DIAGNOSIS AND MOLECULAR MARKERS OF DISEASE

A diagnosis of ALL requires the presence of more than 20% lymphoid blasts in a bone marrow aspirate. In most cases of ALL, the diagnosis is not difficult because of the predominance of these blasts. The French–American–British (FAB) morphological criteria (L1-3) were developed to categorize the disease based on morphological appearance. With the exception of the L3 morphology (mature B cell, or Burkitt leukemia), these descriptions are unfortunately neither predictive of clinical behavior nor useful to guide therapy. The FAB classifications largely have been supplanted by immunopheno-

typic diagnosis and cytogenetic analysis to risk stratify patients. Indeed, the World Health Organization classification of ALL focuses primarily on immunophenotype and karyotype (Fig. 80-1).

Unlike the myeloblasts of acute myeloid leukemia (AML), which may have Auer rods and cytoplasmic granulation, there are no morphological features that unmistakably identify malignant lymphoid blasts from their normal counterparts. The absence of staining for either myeloperoxidase or monocyte-associated esterases as well as the presence of terminal deoxynucleotidyl-transferase staining is useful in identifying ALL cells. The major morphological differential diagnosis is undifferentiated AML (M0), which may not stain for any myeloid markers but should be terminal deoxynucleotidyl-transferase negative. Immunophenotyping is critical for accurate diagnosis and has decreased the number of patients mistakenly assigned an inappropriate treatment regimen. The presence of lymphoid surface markers and immunoglobulin or T-cell receptor gene rearrangements are the most sensitive and specific findings used to confirm diagnosis of ALL.

No surface markers are truly lineage specific, however, and therefore the overall pattern of surface expression of multiple cluster designation (CD) antigens is used to determine the leukemia phenotype. It is not uncommon for both lymphoid and myeloid antigens to be aberrantly coexpressed, but the predominant lineage markers are used to identify the pedigree of the leukemic cells. Such distinctions are important, as therapeutic approaches to AML and the different subtypes of ALL differ radically, with significant differences in treatment outcome. In general, the strong expression of one of the common lymphoid markers (CD10, also known as the common ALL antigen, or CALLA) can be used as a sensitive screen for ALL, although patients with progenitor-B cell, precursor-T, or mature B-ALL may lack this marker. The presence of early B or T-cell antigens (e.g., CD19 or CD7, respectively) helps assign a lineage, although more specific antigen expression (surface immunoglobulin, cytoplasmic CD79a, Cμ, or CD5) helps to define the stage of maturational arrest. ALL that shows mixed lineage expression of both myeloid and lymphoid antigens is being increasingly noted and may represent a distinct diagnostic entity. When such expression is associated with mixed lineage leukemia (MLL) gene rearrangements at chromosome 11q23 (e.g., t[4;11]), a particularly poor risk group is defined, as is covered in greater detail later in this chapter.

RISK STRATIFICATION OF PEDIATRIC DISEASE

The therapeutic approach to treat children with ALL depends on a detailed relapse risk assessment. Because pediatric ALL therapies are frequently curative, yet have narrow therapeutic toxic ratios, selection of appropriate therapeutic intensity is especially important in these patients. A low-risk subset, when identified, can hopefully receive less intensive therapy without an unacceptable increase in relapse rate. The consequence of overtreating ALL in low-risk patients includes cognitive impairment, growth retardation, infection, as well as the gamut of transplant-related complications for those who may inappropriately receive this therapy. The greatest risk of undertreating high risk patients is, of course, relapse and the development of drug resistance, which lowers cure rates.

Cytogenetic and molecular profiling has generated a more accurate predictive model for risk stratification for ALL than FAB morphology or immunophenotyping. The most common

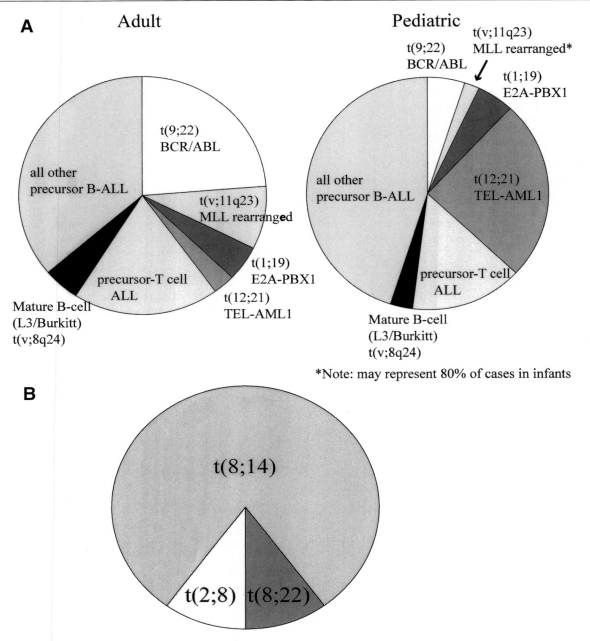

Figure 80-1 **(A)** Realtive incidence of adult and pediatric ALL subtypes. **(B)** Realtive incidence of c-*myc* translocations (chromosome band 8q24) in mature B-cell (Burkitt) ALL.

identifying molecular markers are specific, recurring translocations. Certain translocations confer favorable risk, such as t(12;21) (TEL-AML1). Others, such as t(9;22) (BCR-ABL) and t(v;11q23) (MLL rearranged), identify poor risk biology that necessitates more aggressive treatment approaches. The role of these particular translocations in leukemogenesis is expanded later.

Another prognostic marker is the overall number of chromosomes or ploidy. Hyperdiploid leukemia (i.e., those containing at least 50 chromosomes) has a particularly good prognosis, hypodiploid (<45 chromosomes) indicates poor prognosis, those between these extremes being intermediate. The presence of specific trisomies (e.g., chromosome 4,10) might account for the good prognostic significance of the hyperdiploid patients.

Previously, mature-B (L3 or Burkitt) and T lineage ALL were considered poor risk groups. Lineage-directed therapy has improved the cure rates for these diseases substantially. Both have an excellent cure rate and are considered standard risk leukemia at most centers. This finding validates the in-house directed therapeutic approach.

As in AML, WBC count at diagnosis is prognostically important in ALL. Elevated WBC indicates high tumor burden and is likely a continuous variable, with higher cell counts indicating higher risk. In adult disease, WBC counts above 30,000/mm^3 have been identified as a negative risk factor. Pediatric studies have indicated WBC elevation more than 20–25,000/mm^3 likely confers increased risk. The independence of leukocytosis as a risk factor is not entirely certain, as it usually correlates with particular genetic abnormalities that portend unfavorable prognosis. Examples of these include translocations or partial tandem duplications of the MLL gene and the BCR/ABL fusion.

Age also appears to be an important prognostic factor. Adults and children younger than 1 yr typically develop high-risk disease. The cure rates for infant ALL (<20%) stand in stark contrast to that of older children (>80%). A probable explanation is the frequency of unfavorable cytogenetics. In the case of infant leukemias, this is generally results from MLL rearrangements. Similarly, children younger than 2 or older than 9 yr, adolescents, and adults are also less likely to have favorable karyotypes or ploidy, though the particular abnormalities are more heterogeneous than is the case for infants. Unfavorable disease biology and the inability to tolerate dose intensive therapy may largely explain the poorer prognosis associated with adult patients.

As mentioned, cytogenetics are invaluable in risk-stratifying ALL. It should be noted; however, that cytogenetic analysis is challenging in this disease owing to the relative difficulty of growing cells before analysis and the overall poor quality of metaphases in cells that are informative. For this reason, fluorescence *in situ* hybridization (FISH) has become a particularly powerful tool. The major translocations are easily identified by FISH probes and this allows rapid and accurate assignment of a risk profile to an individual case.

Last, perhaps the most important risk assessment tool is the response to chemotherapy. The speed of marrow response is a potent prognostic marker and can be informative as early as 1 wk following initiation of therapy. Minimal residual disease (MRD), assessed through flow cytometry or quantitative molecular studies, has proven highly prognostic in a number of studies. Slow marrow response to chemotherapy generally indicates the presence of drug resistance and is a poor prognostic marker, regardless of other prognostic indices. Overall, a period of more than 4 wk to achieve remission indicates a very high risk for relapse.

LEUKEMOGENESIS

Although the topic of stem cell origin of solid tumors is a relatively new concept, leukemia provides the most solid evidence of the existence of malignant stem cells. Among this evidence is the morphological and immunophenotypic similarity of blasts to normal hematopoietic stem cells as well as the capacity of malignant cells to differentiate in vitro to multiple hematopoietic lineages with the addition of growth factors. Such differentiation capacity may be seen in vivo and serves as the therapeutic rationale in some forms of AML (e.g., all-trans retinoic acid for acute promyelocytic leukemia). However, there has been no established therapeutic differentiating agent for ALL.

What remains controversial is the cell of origin of more mature leukemias. A long-held belief is that the malignant cell in acute leukemia is a normally differentiating cell that encounters genetic damage during its development and is arrested in its progression to terminal differentiation at the stage in which the critical genetic "hit" occurs. Underlying this logic, the stage at which differentiation block occurs determines the maturity of the proliferating cells.

In contrast, an emerging theory holds that even acute leukemias involving more mature cells arise from primitive stem cells whose progeny, owing to the genetic aberrations in the stem cell, possess limited differentiation ability. Although the accumulating cells may show some capacity for differentiation, a small number of genetically disordered parental cells remain at a very primitive stage of

development. It is these leukemic stem cells that have unlimited self renewal capacity and supply the tumor with an unending supply of daughter cells. These progeny make up the majority of the cells seen clinically. Evidence to support this latter position includes demonstration of identical clonal karyotypic abnormalities in both patients' leukemic cells and their leukemic progenitors in the CD34$^+$/CD38$^-$ compartment. Indeed, it is only these immature CD34$^+$/38$^-$ cells that are able to propagate leukemia in NOD/SCID murine transplantation models.

Another concept with increasing acceptance in leukemia is that of multistep transformation. CML in lymphoid blast crisis provides one example of leukemogenesis that occurs at the stem-cell level, yet ultimately acquires genetic abnormalities that produce a disease molecularly similar to, if not indistinguishable from, a subtype of ALL.

Regardless of which theory of leukemogenesis is correct, one generally accepted concept is that leukemia, like all other cancers, arises from multiple genetic abnormalities. The work of Vogelstein in the 1980s suggested that the progression from normal colonic epithelial cell to adenoma, carcinoma *in situ*, and finally to invasive and metastatic tumor occurs through predictable, stepwise mutational events. This hypothesis can be generalized to acute leukemia, although the particular combinations of mutations appear to be more heterogeneous than in colon cancer. This finding reflects the diversity of tumor biologies encompassed within leukemia. The ability to perform karyotypic analysis on blood cells has added significantly to the understanding of these mutational "hits" in leukemogenesis. Such analyses show recurring karyotypic signatures that, although not entirely specific to a particular tumor type, predict within a particular diagnosis the phenotype and therapeutic response.

The most common karyotypic abnormalities in leukemia are translocations and deletions. When deletions cause tumor suppressor loss, inappropriate progression through the cell cycle and dysregulated growth occur. This is a common finding in both solid tumors and leukemia. By contrast, translocations are unusual in solid tumors, but relatively common in leukemia. Translocations produce chromosomal fusions that generally fall into two categories. The first type occurs when genes are removed from their normal transcriptional control and rearranged to loci in which new promoters inappropriately activate their transcription. This causes abnormal gene expression levels. The inappropriate activation of *myc* by its fusion with the immunoglobulin heavy chain gene through the t(8;14) translocation commonly found in Burkitt lymphoma/leukemia is one such example. The second type of translocation involves fusion of one part of each gene to encode a novel protein product that alters normal cellular survival, proliferation, and differentiation. The *PML-RARα* fusion in M3 AML that blocks differentiation is an example of the latter mechanism.

Studies involving cell lines consistently show malignant transformation following transfection with many fusion proteins commonly seen in ALL. It can be argued, however, that cell lines are already immortalized and represent partially transformed cells. Therefore it is difficult to determine if any of the transfected gene products truly transformed the cells. When fusion genes are used alone to transform primary murine bone marrow cells, few, if any, accurately generates a model of human leukemia. This is true for the most common translocation-generated fusion genes seen in ALL, including *BCR-ABL*, *TEL-AML1*, and *E2A-PBX1*. Often leukemia develops, but only after a long latency. This emphasizes the need for multiple cooperative mutations to produce a full-fledged leukemia.

In leukemia, the types of cooperative mutations primarily fall into two categories, those affecting growth and/or survival pathways and those impairing differentiation. It is hypothesized that both types of mutations must be present to induce leukemia, although several mutations of each type may occur in a particular tumor cell.

TRANSLOCATIONS AND ASSOCIATED FUSION PROTEINS

A common finding in leukemias is the presence of distinct, recurrent chromosomal translocations. A consequence of these translocations is the formation of either novel oncoproteins or a change in the expression level of normal proteins by inappropriate transcriptional regulation. As might be expected, the genes most often involved in these alterations are those associated with cellular growth, differentiation, apoptosis, or cell-cycle regulation. In the next section, the most common and well-understood translocations and gene rearrangements are discussed.

TEL-AML1 (Also Known As ETV6/CBFA2) *Tel-AML1* is a gene fusion product that occurs from an often cryptic t(12;21) (p13;q22) translocation. Although difficult to detect by classic cytogenetics, molecular probes demonstrate the gene product in approx 25% of pediatric pre-B-cell ALL and less than 5% of adult disease. Tel-AML1 is a member of the core binding factor (CBF) leukemias. This group of diseases is characterized by translocations that encode chimeric proteins that serve as repressors of CBF activity. Inactivation of CBF both impairs differentiation and inhibits p53 function, which in turn inhibits apoptosis and may contribute to cell-cycle checkpoint dysregulation. Other CBF leukemias include AML with inv(16) (FAB M4Eo/*CBFβ-SMMHC*), t(8;21) (*AML1-ETO*), and t(3;21) (*AML1-EVI1*). When seen in isolation, these all represent favorable karyotypes with above average responses and disease free survivals in response to standard chemotherapy, with the lone exception of t(3;21). The *TEL* gene is a member of the *ETS* family of transcription factors. *TEL* is widely expressed in both hematological and nonhematological tissues and serves a critical step in yolk sac angiogenesis during fetal development. Its function is dependent on an N-terminal helix-loop-helix domain known as the pointed domain. In the postembryonic period, *TEL* serves a critical role in establishing bone marrow hematopoiesis. *AML1* is a transcription factor with significant structural homology in its DNA binding domain to the *Drosophila* runt domain. *AML1* heterodimerizes with *CBFβ* to increase its affinity and binds the enhancer core sequence *TGT/CGGT*. Through DNA binding, AML1/CBFβ helps activate and coordinate lineage-specific transcription, including such genes as IL-3, neutrophil elastase, myeloperoxidase, CSF-1 receptor, and the subunits of the T-cell antigen receptor.

In the t(12;21) translocation, *TEL* fuses in-frame with nearly the entire *AML1* gene. By unclear mechanisms, fusion with *TEL* reverses *AML1's* activity, and the chimeric protein acts as a transcriptional repressor of AML1 targets. The TEL pointed domain is critical for this change in activity. The pointed domain can also cause heterodimerization between nontranslocated *TEL* and *TEL-AML1*. Although it seems that this would lead to loss of function of the nontranslocated *TEL*, *TEL* deletions are commonly seen in the nontranslocated allele, suggesting a possible role for TEL as a tumor suppressor. On closer examination, however, this does not seem to hold true by Knudson's classic definition of the term. In this model, mutational inactivation of the remaining allele would

be predicted in cases of ALL that featured *TEL* loss of heterozygosity but did not contain *TEL-AML1*. A loss of heterozygosity analysis; however, did not find such mutations among 33 cases examined.

E2A-PBX1 Of both adult and pediatric ALL, approx 5% contain the translocation t(1;19)(q23;p13.3), which encodes the fusion protein E2A-PBX1. This was previously thought to represent a poor prognostic marker, but intensification of therapy in pediatric patients has overcome its effects on outcome. The results of high dose chemotherapy with stem cell rescue in adults may also have this effect, but because the incidence of this cytogenetic marker is relatively low, it is difficult to draw a firm conclusion. The mechanism by which this translocation contributes to leukemogenesis involves both gain of function via upregulating transcription of a *HOX* gene cofactor as well as the loss of one copy of intact *E2A*, a candidate tumor suppressor gene.

E2A encodes two transcription factors, E12 and E47, through alternative splicing. Each protein is a member of the class I basic helix-loop-helix family and has two activation domains. Targeted disruption of this gene in mice causes early B-lineage maturational arrest with an inability to develop either immunoglobulin DJ rearrangements or CD19 expression, demonstrating its importance in early B-cell differentiation. E2A also has important functions in later B cells, including immunoglobulin class switching and plays a role in early T-cell development and maturation. Finally, *E2A* null mice almost invariably develop thymomas and aggressive T-cell lymphomas by 3 mo. Restoration of E2A functionality in cell lines derived from *E2A* null mice leads to rapid induction of apoptosis, confirming the tumor suppressor function of this gene. E2A's ability to activate expression of inhibitors of cyclin-dependant kinases (CDKs) such as Kip family genes (e.g., p27, p21) may provide a mechanism for how it serves as a tumor suppressor.

PBX1 is not normally expressed in lymphoid cells, though its function can be inferred from the role played by similar proteins in these cells (PBX2 and 3) and through its *Drosophila* homolog, *EXD*. *EXD* serves as a required cofactor for activation of several *HOX* homeodomain genes. Its sequence is highly conserved in the human gene *PBX1*. Numerous *HOX* genes, such as *HOXA9* and A10, are oncogenic when overexpressed.

In the formation of *E2A-PBX1* by translocation, a novel fusion protein is generated in which the expression of a putative oncogene cofactor falls under control of a heavily transcriptionally active gene. This activity seems to be increased further by an inability of cells to regulate the shuttling of *E2A-PBX1* between the nucleus and cytosol. Normally, *PBX1's* location is tightly regulated. However, the fusion product loses such controls and remains permanently located in the nucleus. There, opportunities for interactions with *HOX* genes would be favored and the activity of the chimeric gene is further augmented. In addition to these gain-of-function changes in the fusion protein, the loss of one allele of *E2A* might have a significant effect on cell-cycle regulation owing to its status as a tumor suppressor. The *E2A-PBX1* fusion may sequester *E2A* cofactors, such as *P300*, and, thus, further impair the ability of the remaining *E2A* to regulate transcription (Fig. 80-2).

Interestingly, murine transgenic and retroviral transduction models of *E2A-PBX1* fail to reliably generate B-cell neoplasms. As in the *E2A* null mice, T-cell lymphomas are most commonly generated. Further, there is a long latency period before the onset of malignancy, favoring the idea that the fusion protein requires

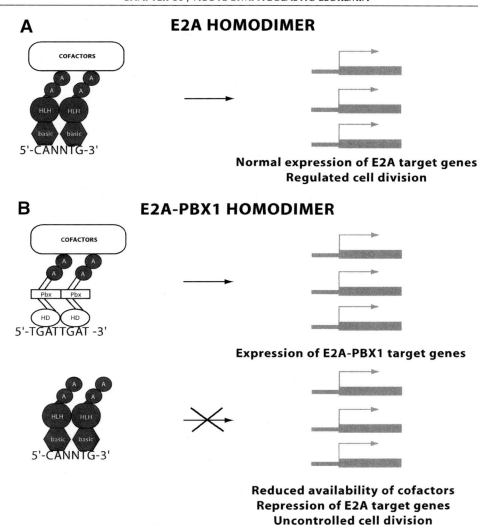

A   **E2A HOMODIMER**

COFACTORS

5'-CANNTG-3'

**Normal expression of E2A target genes
Regulated cell division**

B   **E2A-PBX1 HOMODIMER**

COFACTORS

Pbx   Pbx

HD   HD

5'-TGATTGAT -3'

Expression of E2A-PBX1 target genes

HLH   HLH

basic   basic

5'-CANNTG-3'

**Reduced availability of cofactors
Repression of E2A target genes
Uncontrolled cell division**

Figure 80-2   t(1;19) E2A/PBX1 and leukemogenesis. In normal hematopoiesis (upper figure), E2A binds DNA avidly, activating target genes that include cyclin-dependent kinase inhibitors to slow progress through the cell cycle. The t(1;19) fusion of E2A/PBX1 (lower figure) may contribute to leukemogenesis by several mechanisms. These include transactivation of Hox target genes via association with PBX1 as well as impaired wild-type E2A DNA binding, causing transcriptional repression of E2A targets (e.g., p21) and inappropriate progression through cell cycle. Sequestration of E2A cofactors by the fusion protein may contribute to the latter effect. (Reproduced with permission from Aspland SE, Bendall HH, Murre C. The role of E2A-PBX1 in leukemogenesis. Oncogene 2001;20:5708–5717. Copyright 2001 Macmillan Publishers.)

further mutational events to complete malignant transformation in vivo. The inability to demonstrate leukemogenesis of this fusion protein casts some doubt regarding gain-of-function activity of the fusion protein and may instead favor the hypothesis that loss of *E2A* underlies the malignant phenotype. Further support of this mechanism is seen in T-cell acute lymphoblastic leukemia (T-ALL) that contains rearrangements of the stem cell leukemic protein (*SCL*) gene, a transcription factor that also dimerizes with, and likely inactivates, E2A. This topic is covered in more detail in later sections.

MLL   Translocations and partial tandem duplications of the *MLL* gene at chromosome 11q23 are seen in both AML and ALL and immunophenotypically often results in aberrant coexpression of both myeloid and lymphoid antigens. For this reason the malignancy may be called an mixed lineage leukemia (MLL). Sequencing of the *MLL* gene shows marked structural homology to the drosophila gene trithorax, which positively regulates several *HOX* genes. In murine models, overexpression of a number of

HOX genes has been implicated in leukemogenesis. Although *MLL* is purported to serve as an analog of trithorax in humans, its function and mechanism of action have not been completely defined. A *MLL* (–/–) knockout mouse embryo has been developed that is characterized by defective yolk sac hematopoiesis with a differentiation block at the stage of early hematopoietic progenitor cells. This suggests an important role for *MLL* in the establishment of normal hematopoiesis. In leukemia, translocations of *MLL* generally fuse an intact promoter and amino terminus up to the breakpoint cluster region (BCR) between exons 5 and 11 with a partner gene's carboxy terminus. A variety of genes combine with *MLL*, and greater than 30 different translocation partners have been described. Although the multiple fusion partners may suggest that the contribution of specific translocations to leukemogenesis is to disrupt or destabilize *MLL* function, it should be noted that heterozygous *MLL* knockout mice do not develop leukemia or other cancers.

MLL rearrangement leukemias in some cases arise following DNA topoisomerase II inhibitor therapy, usually with a short latency from exposure (in comparison to alkylating agent, benzene, or radiation-induced leukemia) that would suggest that few if any additional mutations are necessary for transformation. This and other lines of evidence favor a gain-of-function from translocation partners as the contribution of *MLL* toward leukemic transformation.

The most common *MLL* fusion partner in ALL is *AF4* on chromosome 4q21, which is a member of a transcriptional transactivating gene family. The presence of t(4;11)(q21;q23) is an ominous prognostic marker in ALL, as it is associated with hyperleukocytosis, extramedullary disease, early relapse following induction chemotherapy, and poor overall survival. This risk seems to be age-dependent, because infants and children over age 10 who harbor t(4;11) have a particularly poor prognosis, but patients with this karyotype between the ages of 1 and 10 fare no worse than standard risk ALL.

Gene expression profiling of infant leukemias harboring MLL gene rearrangements identified a distinct expression pattern that discriminates the disease from either AML or ALL. Interestingly, one of the most differentially expressed genes is *FLT3*, a receptor tyrosine kinase that is commonly mutated in AML, causing constitutive kinase activation, cellular proliferation, apoptotic inhibition, and impaired differentiation. Internal tandem duplications mutations of FLT3 strongly predict elevated WBC count in AML and are a negative prognostic marker in all FAB categories, with the possible exception of M3. In the case of infant MLL, *FLT3*-internal tandem duplications were not seen but other kinase activating mutations do occur. Highly overexpressed wild-type FLT3 may also be, in part, responsible for this phenotype. Data suggests that coexpression of *FLT3* ligand by leukemic cells may create an autocrine loop that creates constitutive kinase activation in the absence of receptor mutation. *FLT3*-selective tyrosine kinase inhibitors are cytotoxic to infant MLL cells both in vitro and in a murine model, and these inhibitors will undergo human clinical trials in infant leukemia.

The t(4:11)(q21;q23) is also the most common translocation that occurs in therapy-related ALL following topoisomerase II treatment. Indeed, 80% of leukemias that follow topo II exposure demonstrate *MLL* gene rearrangements. Within the BCR of the *MLL* gene lie 11 sequences that resemble topoisomerase II consensus binding sites and one complete consensus site. Treating leukemia cell lines with topo II inhibitors causes double-stranded breaks most commonly at these sites. Sequencing of the MLL gene in treatment-related leukemias shows this to be the region most often rearranged. As with infant leukemias, topo II-induced leukemias commonly relapse following standard chemotherapy and are usually treated with allogeneic bone marrow transplantation once a patient achieves a complete remission.

BCR-ABL and the Philadelphia Chromosome   Nowell and Hungerford first noted the truncation of chromosome 22 in patients with CML in 1960, and this was the first recurrent cytogenetic abnormality described in cancer. This morphological change is known as the Philadelphia chromosome and was later found to be due to a recurrent translocation. The Philadelphia chromosome is seen in 95% of CML cases. t(9;22)(q34;q11) is also the most common and prognostically important translocation in adult ALL. Though uncommon in pediatric ALL, it is present in approx 35% of adults with B-lineage ALL. The translocation portends a poor prognosis because of pan-drug resistance that leads to early relapse. When feasible, allogeneic stem cell transplantation

is recommended as therapy for ALL patients with this karyotype, regardless of the age at presentation.

The two genes involved in this fusion are the *BCR*, which is a gene of unknown function, and *ABL*, a cytoplasmic tyrosine kinase with structural homology to *src* kinases. Several different translocations of these genes are seen, with some predilection for particular malignancies. In CML, the most common gene product is p210BCR-ABL, a 210-kDa protein. The most common ALL fusion protein is known as p190*BCR-ABL*, which is a 190-kDa protein. The difference in molecular weights of the fusions results from differences in the portion of the *BCR* gene incorporated into the gene product. Sequencing of the various fusion products has enabled the development of FISH and reverse transcriptase PCR probes for these fusions. This allows for greater diagnostic accuracy, because there can be false negative results from cytogenetic analysis, allowing increased sensitivity for detection of MRD and early relapse. Because the presence or absence of BCR-ABL affects therapeutic recommendations, such probes have allowed for more effective risk-stratification of ALL patients, and consequently better cure rates with more appropriate therapy.

Both p210 and p190 fusion oncoproteins, and indeed all *BCR-ABL* fusion proteins that have been studied, constitutively activate the *ABL* tyrosine kinase, leading to several pathways of downstream signaling. These downstream targets include *PI3K/AKT*, *Ras/Raf/MAPK*, *myc*, *BCL2*, and *STAT5*, among others. As differentiation blockade is not a feature of CML, BCR-ABL signaling is not thought to significantly impair differentiation. Instead, antiapoptotic and proliferative signals are primarily induced by the constitutively activated kinase.

In vitro transformation by BCR-ABL has been well described. Structural analysis of the ABL kinase demonstrates SH2 and SH3 domains, an SH1 tyrosine kinase domain, and an F-actin binding region. The SH2 and SH3 domains are responsible for protein–protein interactions, and likely regulate the activity of the kinase as well as the specificity of binding with several effector molecules. As noted, the tyrosine kinase bears structural similarity to *src* kinases and is involved in activation of signaling of several growth and apoptosis regulatory pathways. BCR-ABL kinase activity is upregulated as much as sevenfold above that of the wild type kinase. The F-actin binding domain likely serves as a nuclear export signal region and is responsible for *ABL* kinase normally shuttling between cytosol and nucleus. With nuclear localization, the protein interacts with cell-cycle regulatory proteins. In contrast, the fusion oncoprotein does not localize to the nucleus. This restricted cytoplasmic localization may either prevent it from inhibiting cell-cycle progression or may prevent access to negative kinase regulators within the nucleus.

Although the normal function of *BCR* is unknown, its structure contains elements that are likely critical for malignant transformation. Among these features are a coiled-coil oligomerization motif that is responsible for dimerization of BCR, a phosphoserine, and phosphothreonine-rich SH2 domain, and a tyrosine residue at position 177. This tyrosine residue is a potential phosphorylation site that interacts strongly with the adaptor protein GRB2 to link BCR-ABL with the RAS-MAP kinase pathway.

The development of imatinib (Gleevec, or STI-571) has been a major breakthrough in the understanding as well as the therapy for CML. The drug will ultimately play a role in the treatment of Ph (+) ALL. Imatinib is a small molecule that competitively inhibits adenosine triphosphate binding to the active site of BCR-ABL, thus abrogating the constitutive activation of the kinase. Imatinib induces apoptosis in vitro in *BCR-ABL*-containing cell lines and patient samples, and reverses the myeloproliferative state induced by forced *BCR-ABL* expression in a murine model. Human trials of the drug demonstrate normalization of hematological parameters in patients in 95% of patients with chronic phase and 50–80% of patients in accelerated phase CML.

In blast crisis CML, imatinib may induce short-lived hematological responses in patients. Following such disease stabilization, some patients may safely undergo allogeneic transplantation. These responses in blast phase occur with greater frequency than with other agents, including chemotherapy, interferon-α or the combination of these agents, and many hematological remissions are associated with major or complete cytogenetic responses. As a new drug, long-term follow-up is needed to see if these changes are associated with improved survival and/or cure. It should be noted that although the cytogenetic responses are better than any therapy agent short of allogeneic transplantation, the percentage of patients treated with imatinib in chronic phase who revert to undetectable levels of *BCR-ABL* transcripts by reverse transcriptase PCR is low.

As imatinib is active against both p210 and p190, trials of the drug in ALL are ongoing. Phase II data show activity of the agent in Ph (+) ALL, although resistance to the drug is acquired rapidly. Analysis of CML patients treated with imatinib demonstrates at least five mechanisms for resistance to the drug, with mutations in the adenosine triphosphate binding site of *BCR-ABL* that render the kinase inaccessible to the inhibitor being the most common. Other mechanisms include *BCR-ABL* amplification, mutations of additional genes causing *BCR-ABL*-independent growth, increased expression of α-1 acid glycoprotein, which binds imatinib, and increased expression of MDR-1/p-glycoprotein, which pumps the drug out of cells.

SCL Rearrangement in T-ALL   In contrast to the frequent chromosomal rearrangements in B-lineage ALL, less than one-thirds of T-ALL cases show evidence of recurrent translocations. In addition, no association between karyotype and prognosis has been seen and therefore no treatment strategy exists that discriminates the various T-ALL patients into high, standard, and low risk. Although gene expression profiling analysis of T-ALL has shown distinct expression patterns within this group, suggesting that different mechanisms of leukemogenesis occur, the significance of these differences is clinically unknown. The most common translocations in T-ALL involve the T-cell receptor gene on chromosome 14q11. A number of transcription factors, including *LMO2*, *LYL-1*, and *SCL* (also known as *Tal-1*) each translocate to this locus, resulting in inappropriate expression and/or creation of a fusion product with altered characteristics.

SCL rearrangements are perhaps the best characterized among the putative oncogenes in T-ALL. The *SCL* gene encodes a class B, basic helix-loop-helix transcription factor that is normally lineage-restricted to fetal hematopoietic and vascular progenitor cells as well as the CNS. It serves a crucial role in establishing fetal hematopoiesis and is expressed in adult erythroid, mast cell, and megakaryocytic lines. Of note, it is not normally expressed in thymocytes. Forced expression and antisense in vitro experiments show that *SCL* plays a role in hematopoietic proliferation, differentiation, and apoptosis. SCL forms heterodimers with class B basic helix-loop-helix proteins, such as the products of the *E2A* gene, E47, and E12. The heterodimers bind DNA at E box motifs

to transactivate target genes. In addition to binding DNA, the heterodimers of SCL-E2A bind several other proteins, including the lim domain proteins LDB-1 and LMO-2. This binding forms a large protein complex that bridges between the SCL/E2A heterodimer and the zinc finger transcription factor GATA-1. *SCL*, *LMO-2*, and *GATA-1* are expressed in nearly identical tissues and deficiency of each is embryonically lethal owing to failed hematopoiesis. This suggests a common role in early hematopoietic regulation.

Aberrant expression of SCL is a common occurrence in T-ALL and may occur owing to translocation within the T-cell receptor delta locus [t(1;14)(p33;q11)]. Another common mechanism involves a cryptic 90 kB deletion. This removes both the 5′ regulatory elements of *SCL* and the entire coding region of the ubiquitously expressed *SIL* gene, which lies immediately upstream. The karyotypically silent fusion product, *SIL-SCL*, falls under transcriptional control of the *SIL* promoter, leading to aberrant *SCL* expression. As is the case with B-precursor ALL featuring the fusion gene *E2A-PBX1*, there is controversy concerning whether the oncogenicity of aberrantly expressed SCL owes inappropriate activation of *E2A* target genes by the DNA-binding protein complex formation. As noted, *E2A* also serves a role similar to a tumor suppressor gene. Therefore, the formation of heterodimers with SCL may cause sequestration of E2A proteins and impair their ability to regulate the cell cycle.

Interestingly, transgenic models with forced *SCL* expression do not generate tumors. In addition, tumors are not seen when the *SIL* promoter is used to express *SCL* in murine T cells. Coexpression of SCL and similar basic helix-loop-helix transcription factors such as *LDB-1* and *LMO-2* do however greatly facilitate tumor formation. These other genes normally are silent in T cells but their coexpression can sometimes be seen in T-ALL. This finding further supports cooperative, multistep oncogenesis in T-ALL. The finding of T-ALL in two patients with severe combined immunodeficiency syndrome (SCIDS) treated by gene therapy further supports the cooperative role of LMO-2. In both patients the retrovirus used to replace their adenosine deaminase (ADA) deficiency resulted in insertional mutagenises in the *LMO-2* locus with resulting upregulation through the retroviral promoter.

c-*myc*/Immunoglobulin Translocations in L3 ALL   Burkitt's lymphoma and FAB L3 (Burkitt-type) ALL share molecular mechanisms to the extent that they can be considered phenotypic variants of a single disease, Burkitt's lymphoma/leukemia. The characteristic cytogenetic finding in BL is a balanced translocation between c-*myc* and one of the immunoglobulin loci, leading to markedly increased c-*myc* expression. The c-*myc* gene codes for a 64-kDa basic helix-loop-helix transcription factor that normally resides at chromosome 8q24. Of patients with BL, 80% show the classic translocation between c-*myc* and *IGH* [t(8;14)(q24,q32)] and approx 20% of patients show evidence of a variant translocation (Fig. 80-1B). These variants are divided evenly among translocations that pair *myc* with either the *IGK* [t(2;8)(p12;q24)] or *IGL* [t(8;22)(q24;q11)] loci. Through translocation, c-*myc* falls downstream of immunoglobulin enhancer sequences that are particularly active in mature B cells. This places c-*myc* under new transcriptional regulation, ultimately causing its overexpression, increased activation of *myc* targets, and cellular proliferation.

Enhanced c-*myc* function in BL occurs not only by translocation, but also by mutational stabilization that impairs *myc* turnover. Normally, *myc* turnover is regulated by phosphorylation at threonine-58. This event targets *myc* for ubiquitination and proteosomal degradation. Thr-58 is a mutational hot spot in BL. Such point mutations are thought to impair phosphorylation, leading to escape from proteolysis and prolonged *myc* half-life. An additional method for increased *myc* activity is deletion of its negative regulatory elements. This is most clearly seen in BL that features t(8;14). The c-*myc* breakpoint in this translocation frequently lies downstream of a negative regulatory exon 1 and intron 1 sequence. Because the truncated gene that translocates lacks the negative regulatory element, it escapes this control. In other cases, the negative regulatory elements may be present but are mutated and thus inactivated.

Once overexpressed, c-*myc* not only interacts with components of the RNA polymerase transcriptional complex, but perhaps more importantly dimerizes with a small, basic helix-loop-helix leucine zipper known as MAX. Through this interaction, c-*myc* acquires DNA binding capacity. *myc*/MAX heterodimers bind the E-box DNA motif CACGTG to activate transcription. Additionally, the N-terminal domain of c-*myc* interacts with transactivating/transformation domain-associated protein, which plays a crucial role in *myc* oncogenesis. Transactivating/transformation domain-associated protein, in turn, recruits the GCN5 histone acetyltransferase to cause chromatin remodeling by increased histone acetylation in promoter regions, and transactivation of c-*myc* targets.

Upregulated *myc* activity is associated with enhanced cell proliferation and survival, increased metabolism, and arrested differentiation. In contrast to aberrant expression in cancer cells, c-*myc* expression is tightly regulated in normal cells in cell cycle and repressed in those undergoing terminal differentiation. Microarray analysis of cells engineered to conditionally express *myc* has identified multiple targets involved in cell-cycle control. Among these is cyclin D2, which is induced, and the cyclin-dependent kinase inhibitor p21, which is repressed. Using targeted homologous recombination, a c-*myc* (–/–) cell line was created that shows a threefold reduction in growth rate that was associated with significant lengthening of G_1 and G_2 and profound reductions in the activity of cyclin-dependent kinases during the G_0-S transition. By contrast, cell lines that overexpress c-*myc* show hyperphosphorylation of the retinoblastoma susceptibility gene, a shortened G_1 phase, and rapid progression through the cell cycle.

It should be noted that cell lines engineered with conditional *myc* knockouts do not experience cell-cycle arrest on loss of c-*myc*. Instead the speed of progression through the cell cycle is slowed. The speed of cell-cycle progression (and in particular G_1 phase) in tumors that overexpress c-*myc* may have profound implications for genomic instability. Studies using forced, transient c-*myc* overexpression in embryonic fibroblasts showed that the cells were readily transformed. Surprisingly, this effect persisted in the fibroblasts for over 30 d after removal of c-*myc* expression. This finding was associated with acquired karyotypic abnormalities such as polycentric chromosomes and hypersensitivity to DNA damaging agents. These data suggest that abbreviation of G_1 owing to *myc* overexpression may directly cause mutations. Alternatively, c-*myc* overexpression may contribute to oncogenesis by allowing tumor cells to speed past cell-cycle checkpoints, thereby predisposing to the propagation of "second-hit" mutations to daughter cells. Such mutations may be lesions responsible for the transformation seen in vitro long after the effect of overexpressed c-*myc* was removed. The extent to which this finding is true in human BL is unclear as most of these malignancies are not aneuploid.

TUMOR SUPPRESSOR LOSS AND CELL-CYCLE REGULATION Central to oncogenesis in many tumor types is the loss of tumor suppressor gene function. These genes regulate appropriate entry into and progression through the cell cycle, thus, keeping growth in check and ensuring that cells with damaged DNA do not replicate until repaired. Loss of proper cell-cycle checks and balances is a common finding in cancer, including ALL. As could be predicted, cell-cycle control is extensively regulated, so there are many genes whose function is crucial for inhibiting inappropriate progression. Mutational inactivation, deletion, or transcriptional silencing by promoter hypermethylation all contribute to tumor suppressor loss and leukemogenesis in ALL. The particular perturbations of cell-cycle regulation, however, appear to be tumor type-specific, as some of the most common aberrations in solid tumors are only rarely seen in hematological malignancies and vice versa.

The retinoblastoma susceptibility gene, plays a crucial role in cell-cycle regulation. RB functions to prevent $G_1 \rightarrow S$ progression in the cell cycle. This action depends on the RB protein remaining in an unphosphorylated state. Several kinases phosphorylate and inactivate RB, thus promoting entry to the cell cycle. Principal among these are CDK 4 and 6, whose action, in turn, is facilitated by cyclin D1 (also known as BCL-1). CDK 4/6 inhibitors provide a check to this activity and maintain RB in its active, unphosphorylated state. Among the inhibitors of CDK 4/6 are a group of genes known as the *INK4* family and the *KIP* family genes, which are downstream targets of *p53*. *p53*, in concert with genes such as *MDM-2*, *ATM*, *Chk1*, *Chk2*, and *p14ARF* acts to halt cell-cycle progression in response to DNA damage. *P14ARF* arises from alternative splicing of the *INK4* gene *p16*, showing a connection between these two regulatory pathways and demonstrating the potential for significant dysregulation of growth control owing to homozygous deletion of this locus.

About half of ALL cases feature decreased levels of *Rb* expression and many show abnormalities of cell-cycle regulatory genes that affect Rb phosporylation. The mechanism for decreased *Rb* expression in ALL is unclear as mutations and deletions of the gene are rare in this disease. Loss of Rb function, however, is well documented and the mechanisms have been elucidated in many cases. These include overexpression of CDKs, loss-of-function of CDK inhibitors such as INK4 or KIP family genes or those upstream of these targets (*see* Fig. 80-2). Among the *INK4* family, *p15* and *p16* appear to be the genes most frequently altered in ALL. In particular, p15 promoter hypermethylation and homozygous deletion of either *p15* or *p16* appear to be the principal ways through which loss of *INK4* family-controlled CDK inhibition occurs. *P15* hypermethylation occurs in approx 40% of B-cell precursor ALL and T-cell ALL, and deletion of either *p15* or *p16* occurs in up to 50% of T-ALL. In contrast, homozygous deletion of *p15* or *p16* occurs less frequently in mature B-cell neoplasms (<25%) and is generally not seen in AML, myelodysplastic syndrome, or CML outside of lymphoid blast crisis. Hypermethylation of *p16* is generally rare in hematological malignancies, regardless of histology.

p53 is known as the "guardian of the genome." Its role serves to halt the cell cycle in the face of DNA damage until repair is completed. This function is crucial to protect against the propagation of mutations to daughter cells. Mutational inactivation of *p53* is the most common genetic abnormality in cancer. It is somewhat surprising, therefore, that *p53* mutations are rarely seen in hematological malignancies and indeed are found in less than 5% of

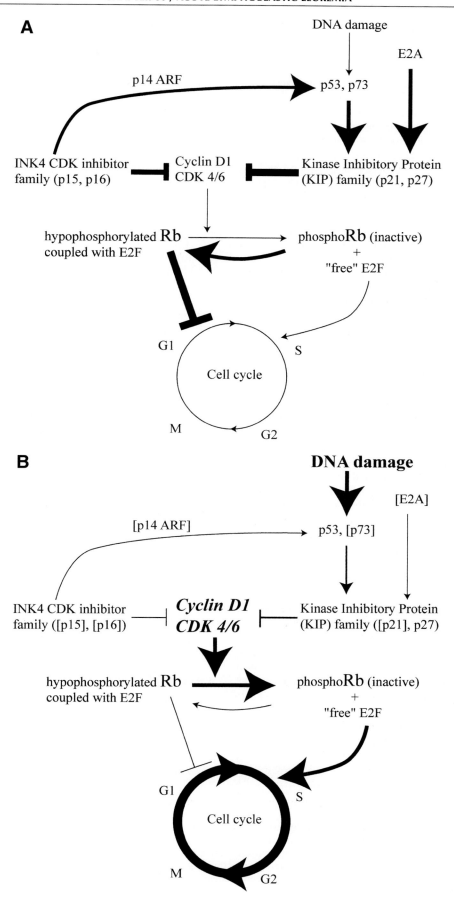

ALL samples. Although *p53* mutations are rarely seen in ALL, loss of p53 effect through mutation, deletion, or methylation of regulators of its pathway, is commonly encountered.

p73 is a tumor suppressor gene that shares much structural homology with p53, including its DNA-binding, oligomerization, and transactivating domains. It also shares several downstream targets, including *KIP* family genes such as *p21*. Hypermethylation of CPG islands in the *p73* promoter region causes transcriptional silencing and is found in as many as 62% of T-cell ALL. Independent of *p73*, loss of *p21* function might also occur through methylation in up to 41% of patients with ALL. Methylation-induced p21 silencing was found to be an independent risk factor for ALL relapse, regardless of therapy type. Finally, *p14ARF* deletion occurs concomitant to *p16* deletion as noted. This gene serves as an upstream regulator whose inactivation results in *p53* inhibition (Fig. 80-3).

GENE EXPRESSION PROFILING AND OTHER NEW DIRECTIONS IN ALL
An exciting new area in the understanding of leukemia biology is gene expression profiling. ALL, and indeed all cancers, represents a heterogeneous collection of biological mechanisms that are grouped together because of a common histological appearance. However, the similar morphological appearance and clinical presentation masks the diversity of biological mechanisms responsible for this presentation. This diversity is true even among tumor types that share common immunophenotypes or translocations. Although two leukemias may share a particular gene rearrangement, the additional mutational events required to fully transform the cells to leukemia are frequently divergent.

RNA expression profiling has allowed for precise determination of an expression "fingerprint" for a particular tumor and the ability to see similarities between, and differences among, multiple patient samples. This approach has been useful not only in terms of confirming and validating other diagnostic modalities, but also in terms of risk-stratifying patients within subgroups. The traditional karyotypic classifications can be recapitulated through gene expression profiling. Interestingly, some data appears to define additional subcategories among patients, in particular karyotypic groups that predicted later relapse or transformation to therapy-related AML. In addition, novel groupings outside of the known chromosomal rearrangements are seen. Although the underlying mechanisms of these tumors is not yet known, several putative oncogenes have been identified by this approach that otherwise would have escaped detection. Although the ramifications of these findings herald a new era in leukemia diagnostics, the predictive ability of this technology needs to be validated prospectively. Furthermore, the reproducibility of these techniques can be operator dependent. Therefore their applicability to clinical practice remains to be established.

Expression profiling is likely to be eventually integrated into diagnostics and may eventually play a role in prognostication. Real-time quantitative PCR allows the ongoing surveillance of pediatric and adult ALL patients with defined translocations who are in morphological remission. MRD sensitivities with this technique can be as low as detecting one cancer cell among 10^5–10^6 normal cells.

This is a 10- to 100-fold improvement in sensitivity over flow cytometric analysis. Using PCR, MRD positivity following induction chemotherapy correlates strongly with future relapse. Low or negative MRD in the same patient population is associated with extended disease free survival. A similar increased risk for relapse after allogeneic transplant is seen in patients who have demonstrable MRD at the time of transplantation. These results might argue for additional pretransplant therapy or alternative treatment. Gene expression profiling from samples taken at diagnosis may also ultimately lead to the ability to prognosticate among patients who are MRD positive. With this approach, those who have residual disease but are still likely to be cured are spared excessive treatment and those who are likely to relapse despite therapy may be given more appropriate treatment.

CONCLUSION

Advances in the understanding of leukemia biology have steadily advanced the care of childhood ALL, transforming the disease from a universally fatal condition into among the most curable of cancers in a period of two decades. Improvements in the therapy for poor risk ALL patients, particularly infants and adults, is still desperately needed. ALL remains a collection of many disease processes with a deceptively common histopathological appearance. Through improved understanding of the molecular mechanisms through which leukemogenesis occurs, novel therapeutic approaches will be developed and cure rates will likely continue to rise. Ultimately, the field may strive for a goal of matching targeted therapies to molecular subcategories. By this approach, it is hoped the treatment of even good risk leukemic patients will become less toxic although sustaining a high level of efficacy.

SELECTED REFERENCES

Andersen MK, Christiansen DH, Jensen BA, Ernst P, Hauge G, Pedersen-Bjergaard J. Therapy-related acute lymphoblastic leukaemia with MLL rearrangements following DNA topoisomerase II inhibitors, an increasing problem: report on two new cases and review of the literature since 1992. Br J Haematol 2001;114:539–543.

Andreasson P, Schwaller J, Anastasiadou E, Aster J, Gilliland DG. The expression of ETV6/CBFA2 (TEL/AML1) is not sufficient for the transformation of hematopoietic cell lines in vitro or the induction of hematologic disease in vivo. Cancer Genet Cytogenet 2001;130: 93–104.

Armstrong SA, Kung AL, Mabon ME, et al. Inhibition of FLT3 in MLL. Validation of a therapeutic target identified by gene expression based classification. Cancer Cell 2003;3:173–183.

Armstrong SA, Staunton JE, Silverman LB, et al. MLL translocations specify a distinct gene expression profile that distinguishes a unique leukemia. Nat Genet 2002;30:41–47.

Aspland SE, Bendall HH, Murre C. The role of E2A-PBX1 in leukemogenesis. Oncogene 2001;20:5708–5717.

Bain G, Engel I, Robanus Maandag EC, et al. E2A deficiency leads to abnormalities in alphabeta T-cell development and to rapid development of T-cell lymphomas. Mol Cell Biol 1997;17:4782–4791.

Bain G, Maandag EC, Izon DJ, et al. E2A proteins are required for proper B cell development and initiation of immunoglobulin gene rearrangements. Cell 1994;79:885–892.

Figure 80-3 **(A)** Simplified model of cell cycle regulation in normal cells. In normal hematopoiesis, DNA damage induces cell cycle arrest at the G1 → S checkpoint. Rb and p53 play a central role in the mechanism that halts cell cycle to allow time for DNA repair. Bars indicate inhibition and arrows stimulation. **(B)** Simplified model of disrupted cell cycle regulation in ALL. In contrast to the normal regulatory signals outlined in Fig. 80-3A, G1 → S checkpoint control is disordered in ALL owing to Rb phosphorylation. Mechanisms that promote this phosphorylation include overexpression (shown in italics) of cyclin-dependent kinases (CDK). In addition, reduced expression levels (shown in brackets) of CDK inhibitors and other tumor suppressors through either promoter hypermethylation or deletion contribute to Rb phosphorylation and loss of its negative regulatory function. Hyperphosphorylated Rb promotes inappropriate progression through cell cycle and dysregulated cellular proliferation. Bars indicate inhibition and arrows stimulation.

Ballerini P, Blaise A, Busson-Le Coniat M, et al. HOX11L2 expression defines a clinical subtype of pediatric T-ALL associated with poor prognosis. Blood 2002;100:991–997.

Barton LM, Gottgens B, Green AR. The stem cell leukaemia (SCL) gene: a critical regulator of haemopoietic and vascular development. Int J Biochem Cell Biol 1999;31:1193–1207.

Basecke J, Griesinger F, Trumper L, Brittinger G. Leukemia- and lymphoma-associated genetic aberrations in healthy individuals. Ann Hematol 2002;81:64–75.

Begley CG, Green AR. The SCL gene: from case report to critical hematopoietic regulator. Blood 1999;93:2760–2770.

Boxer LM, Dang CV. Translocations involving c-myc and c-myc function. Oncogene 2001;20:5595–5610.

Brisco MJ, Condon J, Hughes E, et al. Outcome prediction in childhood acute lymphoblastic leukaemia by molecular quantification of residual disease at the end of induction. Lancet 1994;343:196–200.

Cave H, van der Werff ten Bosch J, Suciu S, et al. Clinical significance of minimal residual disease in childhood acute lymphoblastic leukemia. European Organization for Research and Treatment of Cancer—Childhood Leukemia Cooperative Group. N Engl J Med 1998;339:591–598.

Cobaleda C, Gutierrez-Cianca N, Perez-Losada J, et al. A primitive hematopoietic cell is the target for the leukemic transformation in human philadelphia-positive acute lymphoblastic leukemia. Blood 2000;95:1007–1013.

Coller HA, Grandori C, Tamayo P, et al. Expression analysis with oligonucleotide microarrays reveals that myc regulates genes involved in growth, cell cycle, signaling, and adhesion. Proc Natl Acad Sci USA 2000;97:3260–3265.

Corn PG, Kuerbitz SJ, van Noesel MM, et al. Transcriptional silencing of the p73 gene in acute lymphoblastic leukemia and Burkitt's lymphoma is associated with 5′ CpG island methylation. Cancer Res 1999;59:3352–3356.

Dimartino JF, Cleary ML. MLL rearrangements in haematological malignancies: lessons from clinical and biological studies. Br J Haematol 1999;106:614–626.

Drexler HG. Review of alterations of the cyclin-dependent kinase inhibitor INK4 family genes p15, p16, p18 and p19 in human leukemia-lymphoma cells. Leukemia 1998;12:845–859.

Engel I, Murre C. Ectopic expression of E47 or E12 promotes the death of E2A-deficient lymphomas. Proc Natl Acad Sci USA 1999;96:996–1001.

Ernst P, Wang J, Korsmeyer SJ. The role of MLL in hematopoiesis and leukemia. Curr Opin Hematol 2002;9:282–287.

Faderl S, Kantarjian HM, Manshouri T, et al. The prognostic significance of p16INK4a/p14ARF and p15INK4b deletions in adult acute lymphoblastic leukemia. Clin Cancer Res 1999;5:1855–1861.

Falini B, Mason DY. Proteins encoded by genes involved in chromosomal alterations in lymphoma and leukemia: clinical value of their detection by immunocytochemistry. Blood 2002;99:409–426.

Fearon ER, Burke PJ, Schiffer CA, Zehnbauer BA, Vogelstein B. Differentiation of leukemia cells to polymorphonuclear leukocytes in patients with acute nonlymphocytic leukemia. N Engl J Med 1986;315:15–24.

Felix CA, Lange BJ. Leukemia in infants. Oncologist 1999;4:225–240.

Felsher DW, Bishop JM. Transient excess of myc activity can elicit genomic instability and tumorigenesis. Proc Natl Acad Sci USA 1999;96:3940–3944.

Ferrando AA, Neuberg DS, Staunton J, et al. Gene expression signatures define novel oncogenic pathways in T cell acute lymphoblastic leukemia. Cancer Cell 2002;1:75–87.

Foa R, Vitale A, Mancini M, et al. E2A-PBX1 fusion in adult acute lymphoblastic leukaemia: biological and clinical features. Br J Haematol 2003;120:484–487.

Friedman AD. Leukemogenesis by CBF oncoproteins. Leukemia 1999;13:1932–1942.

Gambacorti-Passerini CB, Gunby RH, Piazza R, Galietta A, Rostagno R, Scapozza L. Molecular mechanisms of resistance to imatinib in Philadelphia-chromosome-positive leukaemias. Lancet Oncol 2003;4:75–85.

Gilliland DG, Griffin JD. The roles of FLT3 in hematopoiesis and leukemia. Blood 2002;100:1532–1542.

Gregory MA, Hann SR. c-Myc proteolysis by the ubiquitin-proteasome pathway: stabilization of c-Myc in Burkitt's lymphoma cells. Mol Cell Biol 2000;20:2423–2435.

Haase D, Feuring-Buske M, Konemann S, et al. Evidence for malignant transformation in acute myeloid leukemia at the level of early hematopoietic stem cells by cytogenetic analysis of CD34+ subpopulations. Blood 1995;86:2906–2912.

Hahn WC, Weinberg RA. Rules for making human tumor cells. N Engl J Med 2002;347:1593–1603.

Hann I, Vora A, Harrison G, et al. Determinants of outcome after intensified therapy of childhood lymphoblastic leukaemia: results from Medical Research Council United Kingdom acute lymphoblastic leukaemia XI protocol. Br J Haematol 2001;113:103–114.

Harrison CJ. The detection and significance of chromosomal abnormalities in childhood acute lymphoblastic leukaemia. Blood Rev 2001;15:49–59.

Hecht JL, Aster JC. Molecular biology of Burkitt's lymphoma. J Clin Oncol 2000;18:3707–3721.

Hochhaus A, Kreil S, Corbin AS, et al. Molecular and chromosomal mechanisms of resistance to imatinib (STI571) therapy. Leukemia 2002;16:2190–2196.

Hoelzer D, Thiel E, Loffler H, et al. Prognostic factors in a multicenter study for treatment of acute lymphoblastic leukemia in adults. Blood 1988;71:123–131.

Kantarjian HM, Cortes J, O'Brien S, et al. Imatinib mesylate (STI571) therapy for Philadelphia chromosome-positive chronic myelogenous leukemia in blast phase. Blood 2002;99:3547–3553.

Karn J, Watson JV, Lowe AD, Green SM, Vedeckis W. Regulation of cell cycle duration by c-myc levels. Oncogene 1989;4:773–787.

Knechtli CJ, Goulden NJ, Hancock JP, et al. Minimal residual disease status before allogeneic bone marrow transplantation is an important determinant of successful outcome for children and adolescents with acute lymphoblastic leukemia. Blood 1998;92:4072–4079.

Krug U, Ganser A, Koeffler HP. Tumor suppressor genes in normal and malignant hematopoiesis. Oncogene 2002;21:3475–3495.

Lang SE, McMahon SB, Cole MD, Hearing P. E2F transcriptional activation requires TRRAP and GCN5 cofactors. J Biol Chem 2001;276:32,627–32,634.

Larson RC, Lavenir I, Larson TA, et al. Protein dimerization between Lmo2 (Rbtn2) and Tal1 alters thymocyte development and potentiates T cell tumorigenesis in transgenic mice. EMBO J 1996;15:1021–1027.

Levis M, Small D. FLT3: ITDoes matter in leukemia. Leukemia 2003;17:1738–1752.

Loh ML, Rubnitz JE. TEL/AML1-positive pediatric leukemia: prognostic significance and therapeutic approaches. Curr Opin Hematol 2002;9:345–352.

Maloney KW, McGavran L, Odom LF, Hunger SP. Different patterns of homozygous p16INK4A and p15INK4B deletions in childhood acute lymphoblastic leukemias containing distinct E2A translocations. Leukemia 1998;12:1417–1421.

Mateyak MK, Obaya AJ, Sedivy JM. c-Myc regulates cyclin D-Cdk4 and -Cdk6 activity but affects cell cycle progression at multiple independent points. Mol Cell Biol 1999;19:4672–4683.

McHale CM, Wiemels JL, Zhang L, et al. Prenatal origin of TEL-AML 1-positive acute lymphoblastic leukemia in children born in California. Genes Chromosomes Cancer 2003;37:36–43.

McNeil DE, Cote TR, Clegg L, Mauer A. SEER update of incidence and trends in pediatric malignancies: acute lymphoblastic leukemia. Med Pediatr Oncol 2002;39:554–557; discussion 552–553.

Mercola M, Wang XF, Olsen J, Calame K. Transcriptional enhancer elements in the mouse immunoglobulin heavy chain locus. Science 1983;221:663–665.

Michaud J, Scott HS, Escher R. AML1 interconnected pathways of leukemogenesis. Cancer Invest 2003;21:105–136.

Moos PJ, Raetz EA, Carlson MA, et al. Identification of gene expression profiles that segregate patients with childhood leukemia. Clin Cancer Res 2002;8:3118–3130.

Mori H, Colman SM, Xiao Z, et al. Chromosome translocations and covert leukemic clones are generated during normal fetal development. Proc Natl Acad Sci USA 2002;99:8242–8247.

Nimmanapalli R, Bhalla K. Novel targeted therapies for Bcr-Abl positive acute leukemias: beyond STI571. Oncogene 2002;21: 8584–8590.

Nowell PH, Hungerford DA. Chromosome studies on normal and leukemic human leukocytes. J Natl Cancer Inst 1960;25:85–109.

O'Brien S, Druker B. Current status of trials of imatinib mesylate (STI571, Gleevec) alone and in combination. In: Broudy V, ed. Hematology 2002: American Society of Hematology Education Program Book. Washington, DC: American Society of Hematology, 2002, pp. 111–119.

O'Brien SG, Guilhot F, Larson RA, et al. Imatinib compared with interferon and low-dose cytarabine for newly diagnosed chronic-phase chronic myeloid leukemia. N Engl J Med 2003;348:994–1004.

Ottmann OG, Druker BJ, Sawyers CL, et al. A phase 2 study of imatinib in patients with relapsed or refractory Philadelphia chromosome-positive acute lymphoid leukemias. Blood 2002;100:1965–1971.

Pane F, Intrieri M, Quintarelli C, Izzo B, Muccioli GC, Salvatore F. BCR/ABL genes and leukemic phenotype: from molecular mechanisms to clinical correlations. Oncogene 2002;21:8652–8667.

Pui CH, Chessells JM, Camitta B, et al. Clinical heterogeneity in childhood acute lymphoblastic leukemia with 11q23 rearrangements. Leukemia 2003;17:700–706.

Pui CH, Evans WE. Acute lymphoblastic leukemia. N Engl J Med 1998; 339:605–615.

Pui CH, Frankel LS, Carroll AJ, et al. Clinical characteristics and treatment outcome of childhood acute lymphoblastic leukemia with the t(4;11)(q21;q23): a collaborative study of 40 cases. Blood 1991; 77:440–447.

Ren R. The molecular mechanism of chronic myelogenous leukemia and its therapeutic implications: studies in a murine model. Oncogene 2002;21:8629–8642.

Roman-Gomez J, Castillejo JA, Jimenez A, et al. 5′ CpG island hypermethylation is associated with transcriptional silencing of the p21(CIP1/WAF1/SDI1) gene and confers poor prognosis in acute lymphoblastic leukemia. Blood 2002;99:2291–2296.

Roumier C, Fenaux P, Lafage M, Imbert M, Eclache V, Preudhomme C. New mechanisms of AML1 gene alteration in hematological malignancies. Leukemia 2003;17:9–16.

Rubnitz JE, Pui CH, Downing JR. The role of TEL fusion genes in pediatric leukemias. Leukemia 1999;13:6–13.

Salesse S, Verfaillie CM. BCR/ABL: from molecular mechanisms of leukemia induction to treatment of chronic myelogenous leukemia. Oncogene 2002;21:8547–8559.

Sanchez-Beato M, Sanchez-Aguilera A, Piris MA. Cell cycle deregulation in B-cell lymphomas. Blood 2003;101:1220–1235.

Schiffer CA, Hehlmann R, Larson R. Perspectives on the treatment of chronic phase and advanced phase CML and Philadelphia chromosome positive ALL(1). Leukemia 2003;17:691–699.

Stegmaier K, Takeuchi S, Golub TR, Bohlander SK, Bartram CR, Koeffler HP. Mutational analysis of the candidate tumor suppressor genes TEL and KIP1 in childhood acute lymphoblastic leukemia. Cancer Res 1996;56:1413–1417.

Tissing WJ, Meijerink JP, den Boer ML, Pieters R. Molecular determinants of glucocorticoid sensitivity and resistance in acute lymphoblastic leukemia. Leukemia 2003;17:17–25.

Van Etten RA. Studying the pathogenesis of BCR-ABL+ leukemia in mice. Oncogene 2002;21:8643–8651.

Vogelstein B, Fearon ER, Hamilton SR, et al. Genetic alterations during colorectal-tumor development. N Engl J Med 1988;319:525–532.

Whitman SP, Strout MP, Marcucci G, et al. The partial nontandem duplication of the MLL (ALL1) gene is a novel rearrangement that generates three distinct fusion transcripts in B-cell acute lymphoblastic leukemia. Cancer Res 2001;61:59–63.

Wiemels JL, Cazzaniga G, Daniotti M, et al. Prenatal origin of acute lymphoblastic leukaemia in children. Lancet 1999;354:1499–1503.

Wiemels JL, Greaves M. Structure and possible mechanisms of TEL-AML1 gene fusions in childhood acute lymphoblastic leukemia. Cancer Res 1999;59:4075–4082.

Xie Y, Davies SM, Xiang Y, Robison LL, Ross JA. Trends in leukemia incidence and survival in the United States (1973–1998). Cancer 2003;97:2229–2235.

Yeoh EJ, Ross ME, Shurtleff SA, et al. Classification, subtype discovery, and prediction of outcome in pediatric acute lymphoblastic leukemia by gene expression profiling. Cancer Cell 2002;1:133–143.

Zajac-Kaye M, Gelmann EP, Levens D. A point mutation in the c-myc locus of a Burkitt lymphoma abolishes binding of a nuclear protein. Science 1988;240:1776–1780.

Zheng R, Levis M, Piloto O, et al. FLT3 ligand causes autocrine signaling in acute myeloid leukemia cells. Blood 2004;103:267–274.

81 Chronic Myelogenous Leukemia

Brian J. Druker

SUMMARY

Chronic myelogenous leukemia is a clonal hematopoietic stem disorder characterized by excess numbers of myeloid cells that over time, lose the capacity for terminal differentiation. A series of discoveries led to the identification of the BCR-ABL tyrosine kinase as the cause of the disease and this provided the impetus for the development of specific agents that target this abnormality. This has also led to improved methods for diagnosis and molecular monitoring of patients with the disease.

Key Words: Allogeneic stem cell transplant; BCR-ABL; chronic myelogenous leukemia; imatinib; molecular monitoring; Philadelphia chromosome; RT-PCR; tyrosine kinase; tyrosine kinase inhibitors.

INTRODUCTION

Chronic myelogenous leukemia (CML) was the first malignancy to be associated with a specific chromosome abnormality. This abnormality, known as the Philadelphia (Ph) chromosome, results from a reciprocal translocation between chromosomes 9 and 22. This finding led to the identification of *BCR–ABL* as the causative molecular event of this disease and ultimately to the development of a therapy that targets this pathogenetic event. These developments are reviewed along with the understanding of the signal transduction pathways impacted by the BCR–ABL fusion protein.

CLINICAL FEATURES OF CML

CML is a malignant, clonal hematopoietic stem cell disorder. It accounts for 15–20% of all cases of leukemia, with an annual incidence of 1–1.5 cases/100,000. Although CML affects all age groups, the median age at diagnosis for patients not selected by referral is close to 60 yr of age. Clinically, the course of CML is divided into three phases. Most patients present in the chronic or stable phase of the disease, which after a variable length of time progresses through an accelerated phase to an invariably fatal acute leukemia, also known as blast crisis.

During the chronic phase, leukemic cells retain the capacity to differentiate normally with the peripheral blood smear showing a full spectrum of myeloid cells from blasts to neutrophils with blasts comprising less than 5% of the white blood cell differential. Basophilia is invariably present and eosinophilia is common. After

From: *Principles of Molecular Medicine, Second Edition*
Edited by: M. S. Runge and C. Patterson © Humana Press, Inc., Totowa, NJ

a median of 4–5 yr in untreated patients, there is a transition from chronic phase CML to an accelerated or blastic phase. The accelerated phase is a transitional period that is poorly defined. The transition of CML to blastic phase is accompanied by the loss of the capacity of the malignant clone for terminal differentiation. Approximately 65% of patients evolve to blastic crisis with myeloid blasts, 30% have lymphoid blast crisis, and 5% of cases have biphenotypic, undifferentiated or T-cell blasts. Blastic phase CML responds poorly to cytotoxic chemotherapy. Median survival of patients in blastic phase is 3–6 mo, although patients with lymphoid blast crisis have a somewhat better outcome.

MOLECULAR PATHOGENESIS OF CML

MOLECULAR ANATOMY OF BCR–ABL TRANSLOCATIONS

In 1960, Nowell and Hungerford described a consistent chromosomal abnormality in CML patients, an acrocentric chromosome that was thought to be a chromosomal deletion. This was the first example of a chromosomal abnormality linked to a specific malignancy. As chromosomal banding techniques improved, it became apparent that the abnormality was a shortened chromosome 22. Rowley later clarified that the shortened chromosome, the so-called Ph chromosome, was the product of a reciprocal translocation between the long arms of chromosomes 9 and 22, t(9:22) (q34;q11) (Fig. 81-1). The molecular consequence of this translocation is the fusion of the *abl* gene from chromosome 9 to sequences on chromosome 22, *bcr*, giving rise to a chimeric *bcr–abl* gene.

The breakpoints within the *ABL* gene at 9q34 can occur anywhere over a large (>300 kb) area at its 5′ end, either upstream of the first alternative exon Ib, downstream of the second alternative exon Ia, or, more frequently, between the two (Fig. 81-2). Regardless of the exact location of the breakpoint, splicing of the primary hybrid transcript yields an mRNA molecule in which *BCR* sequences are fused to the second exon of *ABL*, exon a2. In the majority of patients with CML and in approximately one-third of patients with Ph chromosome positive acute lymphoblastic leukemia (ALL), the break occurs within a 5.8-kb area spanning *BCR* exons 13 and 14, originally referred to as exons b2 and b3, and also known as the major BCR (M-*BCR*). Depending on the site of the translocation, fusion transcripts with either *BCR* exon b2 or b3 fused to *ABL* exon a2 can be formed. Each of these fusion mRNAs are transcribed into a 210-kd chimeric protein (p210$^{\text{BCR–ABL}}$). In the remaining patients with ALL and rarely in patients with CML, characterized clinically by prominent monocytosis, the breakpoints are further upstream in the 54.4-kb region

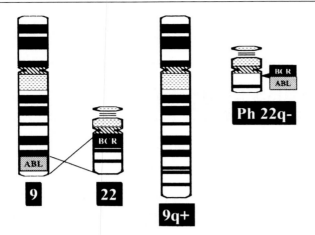

Figure 81-1 Schematic diagram of the translocation that creates the Ph chromosome. BCR, breakpoint cluster region. (Reproduced with permission from Deininger MW, Druker BJ. Specific targeted therapy of chronic myelogenous leukemia with imatinib. Pharmacol Rev 2003; 55:401–423.)

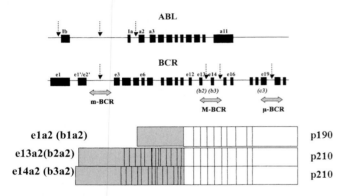

Figure 81-2 Structure of the *BCR* and *ABL* genes showing locations of the breakpoints and various mRNAs created. (Reproduced with permission from Deininger MW, Goldman JM, Melo JV. The molecular biology of chronic myeloid leukemia. Blood 2000;96:3343–3356. Copyright American Society of Hematology.)

between *BCR* exons 1 and 2, also known as the minor BCR (m-*BCR*). The resultant e1a2 mRNA is translated into a 190-kd protein (p190$^{BCR–ABL}$). A third BCR (μ-*BCR*) has been identified downstream of exon 19, giving rise to a 230-kd fusion protein (p230$^{BCR–ABL}$) associated with some, but not all cases of the rare Ph chromosome-positive chronic neutrophilic leukemia.

ANIMAL MODELS OF CML Several experimental approaches have demonstrated the ability of *BCR–ABL* to cause leukemia. In one set of experiments, transgenic mice that express *BCR–ABL* developed a rapidly fatal acute leukemia. Using a different approach, a *BCR–ABL*-expressing retrovirus was used to infect murine bone marrow. These *BCR–ABL*-expressing marrow cells were used to repopulate irradiated mice. The transplanted mice developed a variety of myeloproliferative disorders, including a CML-like syndrome. Although these approaches demonstrate the leukemogenic potential of *BCR–ABL*, it is possible that secondary changes are required for leukemia to develop. Researchers have placed *BCR–ABL* under the control of a tetracycline repressible promoter. Mice expressing this transgene develop a reversible leukemia dependent on the presence or absence of tetracycline, thus demonstrating the leukemic potential of *BCR–ABL* as a sole oncogenic abnormality.

BCR–ABL SIGNALING AND CML PATHOGENESIS

BCR–ABL functions as a constitutively activated tyrosine kinase and significant advances have been made in determining the signaling pathways that are activated by BCR–ABL kinase activity (Fig. 81-3). Numerous substrates and binding partners have been identified and efforts are being directed at linking these pathways to the specific pathological defects that characterize CML. The pathological defects identified in CML cells include increased proliferation or decreased apoptosis of a hematopoietic stem or progenitor cell leading to a massive increase in myeloid cell numbers. Because patients have circulating immature myeloid progenitors, it has been postulated that there is a defect in adherence of myeloid progenitors to marrow stroma. An example of a cellular pathway that links to an increased proliferative rate is activation of the RAS pathway. STAT-5 (signal transducer and activator of transcription) mediated upregulation of the antiapoptotic molecule BCL$_{XL}$ and phosphorylation of and inactivation of the proapoptotic molecule BAD promoter by AKT are postulated to lead to a protection from programmed cell death. CML cells also exhibit reduced adhesion to fibronectin, possibly as a downstream effect of CRKL phosphorylation. Despite the seemingly endless expansion of the list of pathways activated by BCR–ABL and the increasing complexity that is being revealed in these pathways, all of the transforming functions of BCR–ABL are dependent on its tyrosine kinase actvity.

MOLECULAR BIOLOGY OF DISEASE PROGRESSION Clonal cytogenetic abnormalities besides a single Ph chromosome may be acquired in patients with CML as their disease progresses; up to 80% of patients with overt blastic transformation have additional cytogenetic abnormalities. The molecular basis of disease progression is poorly defined in the majority of patients. Up to 25% of patients with myeloid blastic transformation of CML have point mutations or deletions in the *p53* tumor suppressor gene. As many as 50% of patients with lymphoid transformation show homozygous deletion in the *p16* tumor suppressor gene. Alteration of the retinoblastoma, *Rb*, tumor suppressor gene is associated with the rare megakaryoblastic transformation. Amplification of the *MYC* proto-oncogene appears to be rare. However, none of these lesions explains the loss of differentiation that is the most striking feature of transformation to blast crisis.

TREATMENT OPTIONS FOR CML

The treatment of CML has rapidly evolved. Standard treatment options for patients in the chronic phase are allogeneic stem cell transplantation, imatinib, chemotherapy such as hydroxyurea and busulfan, or interferon-α-based regimens. Allogeneic stem cell transplantation remains the only proven, curative therapy for CML. The overall survival for patients transplanted using a matched donor, whether sibling or unrelated is about 60–70% at 5 yr. The major risk factors for early mortality are increasing age and a higher degree of mismatch between the donor and recipient. Patients transplanted in the blast phase of disease have a 5-yr survival of less than 10% owing to a high percentage of relapses. Thus, transplant is most commonly recommended for younger patients with suitably matched donors in the chronic phase of the disease and ideally, within 1 yr of diagnosis. As the average age of onset of CML is greater than 50 yr of age, this factor, plus the inability to identify a suitably matched donor limits this option to a minority of patients. Thus, approximately one-third of patients with CML are transplanted and less than 20% of CML patients are cured with current treatment options.

Hydroxyurea is an efficacious, well-tolerated cytoreductive agent that can control blood counts in the majority of patients but does

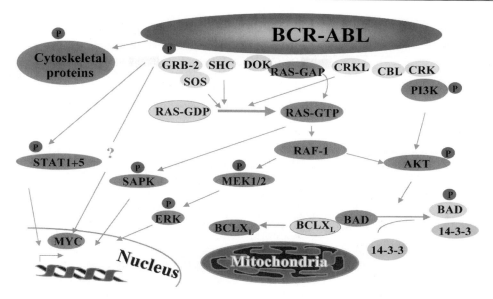

Figure 81-3 Signaling pathways affected by BCR–ABL expression. (Reproduced with permission from Deininger MW, Goldman JM, Melo JV. The molecular biology of chronic myeloid leukemia. Blood 2000;96:3343–3356. Copyright American Society of Hematology.)

little to alter the natural history of the disease. Interferon-α-based regimens induce complete hematological responses in 70–80% of patients and prolong survival by up to 20 mo as compared with hydroxyurea therapy. Patients achieving a major cytogenetic response (a reduction in the percentage of Ph chromosome positive bone marrow metaphases to <35%) may obtain the greatest survival benefit; however, major cytogenetic responses occur in only 20–30% of interferon-treated patients. Interferon therapy is associated with a well-described set of side effects, which are intolerable in up to 20% of interferon-treated patients.

IMATINIB: MOLECULAR BIOLOGY TO THERAPY From the above discussion, it should be clear the BCR–ABL possesses many characteristics of an ideal therapeutic target. It is expressed in the majority of patients with CML and it has been shown to cause CML. BCR–ABL functions as a constitutively activated tyrosine kinase and mutagenic analysis has shown that this activity is essential for the transforming function of the protein. Thus, an inhibitor of the BCR–ABL kinase would be predicted to be an effective and selective therapeutic agent for CML (Fig. 81-4).

Imatinib mesylate (Gleevec, Glivec, formerly STI571) is a relatively specific inhibitor of the BCR–ABL tyrosine kinase. Other tyrosine kinases inhibited by imatinib include the platelet-derived growth factor receptor, KIT, and ARG (*ABL*-related gene). Preclinical data showed significant specific activity against *BCR–ABL*-expressing cells lines in vitro and in vivo. In addition, imatinib could select for the growth of *BCR–ABL*-negative hemato-poietic cells from CML patient samples in colony forming assays and long-term marrow cultures.

Based on the favorable preclinical data, imatinib was tested in phase-I and -II clinical trials in CML patients. These studies showed that imatinib has significant activity in all phases of CML. The results of the phase-II trials are summarized in Table 81-1. These data demonstrate that virtually all patients in the chronic phase of the disease achieve a complete hematological response with the majority obtaining a major or complete cytogenetic response, and these responses have been durable. In patients with more advanced disease, the majority of patients respond to imatinib, but

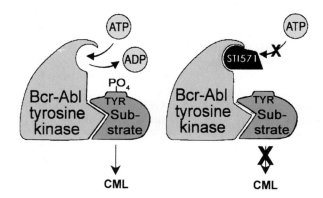

Figure 81-4 Schematic representation of the mechanism of action of the BCR–ABL tyrosine kinase and its inhibition by imatinib. TYR, tyrosine.

Table 81-1
Phase-II Results With Imatinib

	Chronic phase (IFN failure) (%)	Accelerated phase (%)	Blast crisis (%)
CHR	96	40	9
MCR	64	28	16
CCR	48	20	7
Disease progression	13	50	90

IFN, interferon; CHR, complete hematological response; MCR, major cytogenetic response (Philadelphia chromosome positive metaphases ≤35%); CCR, complete cytogenetic response.

Results reported are with a median follow-up of 36 mo.

in patients with blast phase disease, the majority relapse while on therapy with imatinib.

A phase-III randomized study, comparing imatinib at 400 mg/d with interferon-α plus cytarabine (Ara-C) in newly diagnosed patients with chronic phase CML, enrolled 1106 patients from June 2000 to January 2001. Five hundred and fifty-three patients were randomized to each treatment. With a median follow-up of

Table 81-2
Phase III Results of Imatinib Vs Interferon-α Plus Cytarabine (Ara-C) for Newly Diagnosed Chronic Phase CML Patients

	Imatinib 400 mg (%)	Interferon + Ara-C (%)
CHR	97	69
MCR	87	35
CCR	76	14
Intolerance	3	31
Progressive disease	3	8.5

CHR, complete hematological response; MCR, major cytogenetic response (Philadelphia chromosome positive metaphases <35%); CCR, complete cytogenetic response. Intolerance leading to discontinuation of first-line therapy. Progressive disease to accelerated phase or blast crisis. (All of these differences are highly statistically significant with $p < 0.001$). Results reported are with a median follow-up of 19 mo.

19 mo, patients randomized to imatinib had statistically significant better results than patients treated with interferon-α plus Ara-C in all parameters measured (Table 81-2) including rates of complete hematological response, major and complete cytogenetic responses, tolerance of therapy, and freedom from disease progression. Despite the fact that 76% of patients randomized to imatinib achieved a complete cytogenetic response, the majority of these patients had detectable leukemia as analyzed by reverse transcriptase (RT)-PCR for *BCR–ABL* transcripts. When analyzed by log reduction in *BCR–ABL* transcript levels, 55% of patients achieved at least a three-log reduction in *BCR–ABL* levels, but only 5% have undetectable *BCR–ABL* transcript levels.

RESISTANCE TO IMATINIB THERAPY In evaluating relapse mechanisms, patients can be separated into two categories, those with persistent inhibition of the BCR–ABL kinase (BCR–ABL independent) and those with reactivation of the BCR–ABL kinase (BCR–ABL dependent) at relapse. In the largest studies of resistance or relapse, several consistent themes emerge. In patients with primary resistance, that is, patients who do not respond to imatinib therapy, BCR–ABL-independent mechanisms are most common. In contrast, the majority of patients who relapse on therapy with imatinib reactivate the BCR–ABL kinase. In these studies, greater than 50% and perhaps as many as 90% of patients with hematological relapse have *BCR–ABL* point mutations in at least 25 different amino acids scattered throughout the *ABL* kinase domain. Other patients have amplification of *BCR–ABL* at the genomic or transcript level.

In patients who relapse as a consequence of reactivation of the BCR–ABL kinase, the BCR–ABL kinase remains a good target. Alternate ABL kinase inhibitors have already been synthesized and two have advanced to clinical trials. One of these compounds, AMN107, was synthesized based on the knowledge of the crystal structure of the ABL kinase in complex with imatinib. This information was used to synthesize an ABL inhibitor that is approx 30-fold more potent than imatinib. An alternate approach was to profile existing compounds for activity against the ABL kinase. This led to the recognition that many SRC inhibitors are also inhibitors of the ABL kinase. One of these dual SRC/ABL inhibitors, dasatinib (BMS-354825), is over 100-fold more potent against ABL than imatinib. Both AMN107 and dasatinib inhibit most of the common imatinib-resistant BCR–ABL kinase domain mutations except T315I and have shown significant activity in imatinib-resistant patients in early clinical trials. Additional clinical trials are

examining the combination of imatinib with agents that target downstream signaling pathways activated by BCR–ABL.

It should be noted that the studies described above represent a minority of CML patients. Most of the patients described in the studies of resistance had advanced phase disease. In contrast, the majority of patients diagnosed with CML will be in the chronic phase, most will obtain a complete cytogenetic response with imatinib, and very few have relapsed. However, only a minority attain a molecular remission. Hypotheses for the mechanism of molecular persistence can also be divided into BCR–ABL-dependent and -independent mechanisms. For example, stem cell quiescence has been postulated as a potential BCR–ABL-independent mechanism of resistance to imatinib. BCR–ABL-dependent mechanisms of molecular persistence include the possibility that low levels of BCR–ABL kinase activity prevent cells from proliferating, but are sufficient to protect cells from apoptosis. This could be because of imatinib's inability to completely inhibit the BCR–ABL kinase or to the fact that stem cells express high levels of P-glycoprotein that result in efflux of imatinib. Each of these scenarios suggests specific therapeutic interventions to overcome molecular persistence.

MOLECULAR DIAGNOSIS AND MONITORING OF CML

The traditional method of diagnosing CML and monitoring disease status is the cytogenetic analysis of bone marrow-derived metaphases for the presence of the Ph chromosome. However, cytogenetics are negative in approx 10% of patients at diagnosis and at least half of these patients will have a *BCR–ABL* fusion detectable by either fluorescence *in situ* hybridization (FISH) or RT-PCR.

FISH analyses relies on the colocalization of large genomic probes specific to the *BCR* and *ABL* genes. FISH has several advantages over conventional cytogenetics. It can be performed on peripheral blood and on metaphase or interphase cells. Comparison of marrow and blood samples by FISH analysis shows high concordance. One potential problem with FISH is the random colocalization of the signals from the *BCR* and *ABL* probes such that 8–10% of normal cells appear positive. This has been circumvented, in part, with D-FISH, which uses probes that span the breakpoint region. However, at diagnosis, in which the majority of cells are *BCR–ABL* positive, FISH is a highly accurate diagnostic test, as false negative results are rare and false positives are not a concern when greater than 90% of cells are positive.

RT-PCR can be used to amplify the region around the splice junction between *BCR* and *ABL*. The high sensitivity of this technique makes it the ideal for the detection of minimal residual disease. RT-PCR and quantitative RT-PCR have been used to detect residual CML cells following allogeneic stem cell transplantation. Whether persistence of *BCR–ABL* transcripts beyond 6 mo is predictive of relapse has not been resolved, but a rising level of *BCR–ABL* transcripts by quantitative RT-PCR after transplant is highly predictive of relapse. Similar to FISH, peripheral blood and marrow RT-PCR values show a high level of concordance. As the majority of patients treated with imatinib will be cytogenetically and FISH negative, PCR is frequently the only means to monitor patients on imatinib therapy. Further, *BCR–ABL* transcript levels correlate with progression-free survival; thus, quantitative PCR monitoring is currently recommended for the majority of patients with CML on imatinib therapy. Current efforts are being directed at increasing the availability of standardized PCR testing.

CONCLUSIONS

From the discovery of the Ph chromosome to molecularly targeted therapy of CML with imatinib, there is perhaps no other disease that has been so well characterized at the molecular level and in which the knowledge of the molecular biology has been exploited in the diagnosis, monitoring, and therapy of the disease. The current task for patients and their treating physicians is to make increasingly difficult decisions between treatment options. For the future, the goals will be to continue to improve and apply the knowledge of the molecular and immunological features of this disease to further improve treatment outcomes.

SELECTED REFERENCES

Ben-Neriah Y, Daley GQ, Mes-Masson A-M, Witte ON, Baltimore D. The chronic myelogenous leukemia-specific P210 protein is the product of the bcr/abl hybrid gene. Science 1986;233:212–214.

Chronic Myeloid Leukemia Trialists' Collaborative Group. Interferon alfa versus chemotherapy for chronic myeloid leukemia: a meta-analysis of seven randomized trials. J Natl Cancer Inst 1997;89:1616–1620.

Daley GQ, Van Etten RA, Baltimore D. Induction of chronic myelogenous leukemia in mice by the P210bcr/abl gene of the Philadelphia chromosome. Science 1990;247:824–830.

de Klein A, van Kessel AG, Grosveld G, et al. A cellular oncogene is translocated to the Philadelphia chromosome in chronic myelocytic leukemia. Nature 1982;300:765–767.

Deininger MW, Druker BJ. Specific targeted therapy of chronic myelogenous leukemia with imatinib. Pharmacol Rev 2003;55:401–423.

Deininger MW, Goldman JM, Melo JV. The molecular biology of chronic myeloid leukemia. Blood 2000;96:3343–3356.

Dewald GW, Wyatt WA, Juneau AL, et al. Highly sensitive fluorescence *in situ* hybridization method to detect double BCR/ABL fusion and monitor response to therapy in chronic myeloid leukemia. Blood 1998;91: 3357–3365.

Druker BJ, Lydon NB. Lessons learned from the development of an abl tyrosine kinase inhibitor for chronic myelogenous leukemia. J Clin Invest 2000;105:3–7.

Druker BJ, Sawyers CL, Kantarjian H, et al. Activity of a specific inhibitor of the Bcr–Abl tyrosine kinase in the blast crisis of chronic myeloid leukemia and acute lymphoblastic leukemia with the Philadelphia chromosome. N Engl J Med 2001;344:1038–1042.

Druker BJ, Talpaz M, Resta D, et al. Efficacy and safety of a specific inhibitor of the Bcr–Abl tyrosine kinase in chronic myeloid leukemia. N Engl J Med 2001;344:1031–1037.

Hansen JA, Gooley TA, Martin PJ, et al. Bone marrow transplants from unrelated donors for patients with chronic myeloid leukemia. N Engl J Med 1998;338:962–968.

Heisterkamp N, Jenster G, ten Hoeve J, Zovich D, Pattengale PK, Groffen J. Acute leukaemia in bcr/abl transgenic mice. Nature 1990;344:251–253.

Hochhaus A, Kreil S, Corbin AS, et al. Molecular and chromosomal mechanisms of resistance to imatinib (STI571) therapy. Leukemia 2002;16: 2190–2196.

Horowitz MM, Rowlings PA, Passweg JR. Allogeneic bone marrow transplantation for CML: a report from the International Bone Marrow Transplant Registry. Bone Marrow Transplant 1996;17(Suppl 3): S5, S6.

Huettner CS, Zhang P, Van Etten RA, Tenen DG. Reversibility of acute B-cell leukaemia induced by BCR–ABL1. Nat Genet 2000;24: 57–60.

Kantarjian H, Sawyers C, Hochhaus A, et al. Hematologic and cytogenetic responses to imatinib mesylate in chronic myelogenous leukemia. New Engl J Med 2002;346:645–652.

Kelliher MA, McLaughlin J, Witte ON, Rosenberg N. Induction of a chronic myelogenous leukemia-like syndrome in mice with v-abl and BCR/ABL. Proc Natl Acad Sci USA 1990;87:6649–6653.

Nowell PC, Hungerford DA. A minute chromosome in human chronic granulocytic leukemia. Science 1960;132:1497–1501.

O'Brien SG, Guilhot F, Larson RA, et al. Imatinib compared with interferon and low-dose cytarabine for newly diagnosed chronic-phase chronic myeloid leukemia. New Engl J Med 2003;348:994–1004.

O'Hare T, Walters DK, Stoffregen EP, et al. In vitro activity of Bcr–Abl inhibitors AMN107 and BMS-354825 against clinically relevant imatinib-resistant Abl kinase domain mutants. Cancer Res 2005;65: 4500–4505.

Rowley JD. A new consistent abnormality in chronic myelogenous leukaemia identified by quinacrine fluorescence and giemsa staining. Nature 1973;243:290–293.

Sawyers CL, Hochhaus A, Feldman E, et al. Imatinib induces hematologic and cytogenetic responses in patients with chronic myeloid leukemia in myeloid blast crisis: results of a phase II study. Blood 2002;99: 3530–3539.

Schoch C, Schnittger S, Bursch S, et al. Comparison of chromosome banding analysis, interphase- and hypermetaphase-FISH, qualitative and quantitative PCR for diagnosis and for follow-up in chronic myeloid leukemia: a study on 350 cases. Leukemia 2002;16:53–59.

Shah NP, Nicoll JM, Nagar B, et al. Multiple BCR–ABL kinase domain mutations confer polyclonal resistance to the tyrosine kinase inhibitor imatinib (STI571) in chronic phase and blast crisis chronic myeloid leukemia. Cancer Cell 2002;2:117–125.

Shtivelman E, Lifshitz B, Gale RP, Canaani E. Fused transcript of abl and bcr genes in chronic myelogenous leukaemia. Nature 1985;315:550–554.

Silver RT, Woolf SH, Hehlmann R, et al. An evidence-based analysis of the effect of busulfan, hydroxyurea, interferon, and allogeneic bone marrow transplantation in treating the chronic phase of chronic myeloid leukemia: developed for the American Society of Hematology. Blood 1999;94:1517–1536.

Talpaz M, Silver RT, Druker BJ, et al. Imatinib induces durable hematologic and cytogenetic responses in patients with accelerated phase chronic myeloid leukemia: results of a phase 2 study. Blood 2002;99: 1928–1937.

van Rhee F, Szydlo RM, Hermans J, et al. Long-term results after allogeneic bone marrow transplantation for chronic myelogenous leukemia in chronic phase: a report from the Chronic Leukemia Working Party of the European Group for Blood and Marrow Transplantation. Bone Marrow Transplant 1997;20:553–560.

82 Non-Hodgkin's Lymphoma and Chronic Lymphocytic Leukemia

Ayad M. Al-Katib and Anwar N. Mohamed

SUMMARY

This chapter describes non-Hodgkin's lymphoma (NHL) and chronic lymphocytic leukemia (CLL). NHL is a complex and heterogeneous group of disorders characterized by clonal proliferation of lymphocytes at different stages of maturation. There are approx 30 types of NHL with varying clinical, pathological, and genetic features. Understanding some of its biological features has provided insights into the clinical behavior of NHL. CLL is a neoplasm of monomorphic small, round lymphocytes of B cell origin in 98% of the cases. It is the most frequent type of leukemia in the United States and Europe where the majority of patients are older than 50; it has a male:female ratio of 2:1. CLL remains an incurable, chronic disease with a variable survival depending on clinical stage at presentation.

Key Words: Anaplastic large-cell lymphoma; B-cell; Burkitt; chronic lymphocytic leukemia; diffuse large-cell lymphoma; mantle-cell lymphoma; non-Hodgkin's lymphoma; T-cell.

NON-HODGKIN'S LYMPHOMA

Non-Hodgkin's lymphoma (NHL) is a complex and heterogeneous group of disorders characterized by clonal proliferation of lymphocytes at different stages of maturation. There are approx 30 types of NHL with varying clinical, pathological, and genetic features. Understanding some of its biological features has provided insights into the clinical behavior of NHL. For example, lymphomas with high proliferative indices (like Burkitt's and lymphoblastic lymphomas) present with rapidly growing tumor masses, referred to clinically as high-grade lymphomas, and are rapidly fatal if not successfully treated. Histologically, these lymphomas have diffuse architecture, intermediate or large-cell morphology with large numbers of visible mitotic figures. In contrast, lymphomas with low proliferative indices (follicular and small lymphocytic lymphomas [SLLs]) have indolent clinical courses measured in years, affect older patients, and have small, mature-looking cell morphology. Ironically, the "aggressive," rapidly growing lymphomas are curable whereas the indolent ones remain incurable with available therapeutic strategies.

Classification of NHL has been constantly changing. Each classification system becomes quickly outdated as new insights into the biological and genetic features of these disorders change the understanding of them and lead to recognition of new entities. The most recent classification is that of the World Health Organization (WHO) incorporating the latest advances in the understanding of the pathogenesis of NHL. Lymphomas are now viewed as distinct clinico-pathological genetic entities, each with distinct morphological, immunophenotypic and genetic features. Unique biological and genetic features of each lymphoma are aides to a more precise diagnosis and subtyping of NHL. It has also helped explain key biological behaviors of certain lymphomas. For example, rearrangement of *C-MYC* oncogene resulting from t(8;14) translocation may explain the high proliferative index and the high-grade nature of Burkitt's lymphoma. Understanding the molecular and genetic pathways of NHL may be more useful than improving diagnostic precision and delineation of new entities. Exploiting genetic abnormalities, which are at the root of lymphomagenesis, for therapy is already a reality. Clinicians, therefore, may not be able to dismiss knowledge of specific chromosomal translocations and oncogene rearrangements as important only for the experimentalists. It is possible that physicians will eventually treat NHL based on its genetic and immunophenotypic profile with a combination of antigene and monoclonal antibody reagents instead of a combination of cytotoxic agents. Anti-CD20 monoclonal antibody is now a standard therapy for certain B-cell lymphomas and bcl_2 antisense oligonucleotides are in clinical trials, ushering in a new era for NHL treatment.

This chapter addresses established molecular and genetic pathways of NHL. It should be noted, however, that genetic aberrations are final common pathways leading to the expansion of malignant clones. There are a variety of upstream events that are important etiological factors. Environmental factors, like exposure to pesticides, immune suppression, and the role of immune surveillance and bacterial infections like *Helicobacter pylori* are but few examples. The role of such factors, however, is not the focus of this chapter.

MOLECULAR PATHOGENESIS OF B-CELL NHL Acquired chromosomal translocation in lymphoma is a well-recognized mechanism that leads to activation of protooncogene. Similar to

From: *Principles of Molecular Medicine, Second Edition*
Edited by: M. S. Runge and C. Patterson © Humana Press, Inc., Totowa, NJ

Table 82-1
Chromosomal Translocations and Genes Rearranged in Association
With Histological Subtypes of B-Cell Non-Hodgkin's Lymphoma

Chromosomal translocations	Genes involved	Histology
T(3;14)(q27;q32)	BCL6;IGH	Diffuse large B cell
T(3;22)(q27;q11)	BCL6;IGL	Diffuse large B cell
t(2;3)(p12;q37)	IGK;BCL6	Diffuse large B cell
t(3;4)(q27;p13)	BCL2;RHOH	Diffuse large B cell
t(3;6)(q27;p22)	BCL6;H1F1	Diffuse large B cell
t(3;6)(q27;p21.2)	BCL6;PIM-1	Diffuse large B cell
t(14;18)(q32;q21)	IGH;BCL2	Follicular B cell
t(18;22)(q21;q11)	BCL2;IGL	Follicular B cell
t(2;18)(p12;q21)	IGK;BCL2	Follicular B cell
t(11;14)(q13;q32)	BCL1;IGH	Small lymphocytic, mantle
t(8;14)(q24;q32)	CMYC;IGH	Burkitt, small noncleaved
t(2;8)(p12;q24)	IGK;CMYC	Burkitt, small noncleaved
t(8;22)(q24;q11)	CMYC;IGL	Burkitt, small noncleaved
t(14;19)(q32;q3)	IGH;BCL3	CLL, small noncleaved NHL
t(9;14)(p13;q32)	PAX5;IGH	Lymphoplasmacytic
t(2;14)(p13;q32)	BCL11A;IGH	Mixed small/large cell/CLL
t(11;18)(q21;q21)	API2;MALT	MALT lymphoma
t(1;14)(p22;q32)	BCL10;IGH	MALT lymphoma
t(10;14)(q24;q32)	LYT10;IGH	Variable, B-cell lymphoma

acute myeloid leukemia, the translocations in NHL are usually balanced, reciprocal recombination between two chromosomal sites; in rare cases the translocations are complex affecting more than two chromosomes. The chromosomal translocations in lymphoma are usually nonrandom and associated with a specific clinicopathological category of NHL. The most commonly affected chromosome is 14, found in more than 50% of NHLs. In most instances, the translocations relocate transcriptional control genes to the vicinity of highly active promoter/enhancer elements of the immunoglobulin genes. The common consequence of the translocation is the dysregulated expression of the protooncogene sequences by two mechanisms: by changing the level of protooncogene expressed in normal cells or by activation of protooncogene that is physiologically not expressed in normal cells. A wide variety of translocation partner chromosomes recombined with 14q32 have been described in NHL; common to the majority of these cases is a B-lineage immunophenotype reflecting the rearrangement of the immunoglobulin H (IGH) locus at 14q32. Several protooncogenes were cloned and identified from the partner sites of the translocations. As already established, t(8;14) (q24;q32), commonly associated with Burkitt lymphoma/ leukemia, juxtaposes the *C-MYC* oncogene on 8q24 to the IGH locus in 14q32 resulting in the overexpression of the transcription factor c-myc protein. Subsequently, the chromosomal translocation t(11;14)(q13;q32), causing rearrangement of the *BCL1* gene locus and overexpression of cyclin D-1 (CCND1)/ PRAD1 protein, was shown to be highly characteristic of mantle-cell lymphoma (MCL). The most frequent chromosomal translocation in NHL is the t(14;18)(q32;q21), detected in up to 85% of follicular lymphoma and in 30% of diffuse large-cell lymphoma (DLCL). Molecular analysis of the t(14;18) breakpoints identified *BCL2* gene on chromosome 18q21 that is overexpressed because of its relocation next to the transcriptionally active IGH locus on chromosome 14q32. Later, functional studies revealed that increased production of bcl2 protein in B cells carrying this translocation prolongs their survival by blocking the programmed cell death.

Other significant translocations in lymphoma are t(3;14) and its variant, which are mainly seen in DLCL. The translocations involve rearrangement of *BCL6* protooncogene with various immunoglobulin loci. Several less common translocations have been also identified in lymphoma, for example, t(14;19), t(12;14), t(9;14) (Table 82-1). In all these recombination, the oncogene activation operates through a similar mechanism by bringing the oncogene under the control of constitutive regulatory sequences of immunoglobulin loci. The exception to the deregulation model of B-NHL translocations is the t(11;18) of mucosa-associated lymphoid tissue (MALT) lymphoma, which causes gene fusion resulting in a chimeric protein with oncogenic properties. Some of the well-characterized chromosomal translocations in B-NHL are described below.

t(8;14), C-MYC and Burkitt's Lymphoma The t(8;14) (q24;q32) is a highly consistent and specific translocation in Burkitt's lymphoma which plays a key role in the genesis of both the endemic (African) and the nonendemic (sporadic) forms, and obviously is not Epstein-Barr virus-dependent. The t(8;14) repositions the *C-MYC* protooncogene from its normal site on chromosome 8q24 to the vicinity of a highly active immunoglobulin enhancer on chromosome 14q32. In 75–85% of Burkitt's cases, the t(8;14) is responsible for *C-MYC* activation; however, two variant translocations t(2;8) and t(8;22) can produce the same effect in the remaining 15–25% of cases. However, t(2;8) and t(8;22) variant translocations move the *immunoglobulin-κ and immunoglobulin-λ* light chain genes respectively to the *C-MYC* locus on chromosome 8q24. *C-MYC* oncogene belongs to a small gene family with closely related members. The human *C-MYC* oncogene has three exons and two promoters, P1 and P2, controlling the transcription of the gene. The choice of the promoter depends on the myc protein level. P2 promoter is the most active and generates a 2.25-kb transcript, whereas P1 promoter produces a 2.4-kb transcript. The position of the molecular breakpoints in relation to the *C-MYC* gene on chromosome 8 and the *IGH* gene on 14q differ with the geographic origin of the disease. In endemic

Burkitt's lymphoma, the breakpoints occur some distance 5' to C-MYC exon 1, whereas the breakpoints on chromosome 14 usually occur in the IGH joining regions (J_H). In sporadic and AIDS-related Burkitt's lymphoma, the t(8;14) breakpoints occur between exon 1 and 2 of C-MYC gene on chromosome 8 and within the IGH switch μ switch region on chromosome 14. In the two variant translocations, the breakpoints on 8q are located at variable distance 3' of the C-MYC locus. The breakpoints on chromosomes 2 and 22 occur at 5' of the immunoglobulin-κ and immunoglobulin-λ gene constant region segments, respectively. Therefore, C-MYC gene is translocated to der(14) in t(8;14), whereas in variant translocation, C-MYC remains on der(8). Because the immunoglobulin enhancers are constitutively active in mature B cells, their relocation close to C-MYC oncogene in Burkitt's lymphoma results in high levels of c-myc RNA and protein expression. In addition, C-MYC may be dysregulated by point mutations in the sequences of the gene by other mechanisms, further contributing to increased C-MYC activity.

The c-myc protein is a transcription factor of the helix-loop-helix/leucine zipper family that activates transcription through its heterodimerization with a partner protein, MAX. C-MYC dysregulation influences multiple cellular processes, including cell proliferation, apoptosis, and cellular metabolism. Furthermore, data have revealed that C-MYC regulates genes involved in cell growth, division, death, and adhesion, all of which contribute to cellular transformations. The role of c-myc protein in cell cycle regulation is complex but its expression is strongly associated with increased cellular proliferation. C-MYC overactivity promotes cell cycle progression, and therefore, it inhibits cellular differentiation. Another indirect mechanism that inhibits differentiation may be the repression of genes that have direct control on cellular differentiation such as C/EBPα. C-MYC also regulates a variety of metabolic pathways. The most relevant one in Burkitt's lymphoma is lactate dehydrogenase A, an enzyme highly expressed in Burkitt's lymphoma. The high level of lactate dehydrogenase A seems to help the cells to survive hypoxic conditions. C-MYC may also regulate genes that are involved in nucleotide and protein synthesis and iron metabolism, some of which are required for cellular transformation. Another hallmark of C-MYC overexpression is the induction of a high-level cellular apoptosis. This may be reflected by the starry-sky appearance characteristic of Burkitt's lymphoma which results from a high rate of apoptotic cell death. In addition, increased expression C-MYC leads to maintenance of telomerase expression, an enzyme that contributes to the immortalization of cells by protecting the end of the chromosomes.

As in the case of other specific neoplasia-associated translocations, additional chromosomal alterations superimposing the t(8;14) translocation are seen in most cases and become more numerous during disease progression. The most frequent secondary aberrations seen in >30% of cases are structural rearrangements of chromosome 1, often leading to partial gain in the long arm (q) of chromosome 1. Other recurrent abnormalities seen in association with t(8;14) are trisomy 7, 8, 12, and 18. Chromosome 6q abnormalities, particularly deletions, are frequent in Burkitt's lymphoma, suggesting the presence of suppressor genes in this lesion. Another area of secondary involvement seen in approx 30% Burkitt's lymphoma cases is alterations of the short arm (p) of chromosome 17, the site of the p53 gene, which correlate with the frequency of p53 mutations in Burkitt's tumors. BCL-6 gene on chromosome 3q27 is mutated in 30–50% of Burkitt's tumors causing dysregulation of BCL-6 expression.

These secondary genetic changes seem not to be specific for Burkitt's lymphoma, however, they are nonrandom and their appearance predicts clonal evolution associated with disease progression and clinical deterioration.

t(11;14) Translocation and the BCL1 Gene   The t(11;14) (q13;q34) involves a breakpoint on chromosome 14 within the IgH gene and the Bcl_1 region on chromosome 11. The breakpoints of the t(11;14) were initially shown to juxtapose the joining region of IgH to a region of 11q13 designated as BCL1 (B-cell lymphoma/leukemia). Most of the rearrangements occur in the major translocation cluster region on 11q13. To identify a putative oncogene associated with the translocation, studies on a chromosome 11 inversion, inv(11) (p15;q13) in parathyroid adenomatosis, led to the characterization of PRAD-1. Analysis of the PRAD-1 sequence showed high homology with D-type cyclins and therefore the gene was renamed CCND1 but is sometimes still referred to as CCND1/ PRAD-1. The coding region of CCND1 is not altered by the t(11;14) translocation but CCND1 expression is abnormally induced by the translocation presumably reflecting the influence of the B-cell specific IgH gene enhancer from chromosome 14. The gene encodes a 295 amino acid, 36-kDa protein. CCND1 is not normally expressed in lymphocytes or myeloid cells but is expressed in high levels in MCL with t(11;14) (q13;q34) translocation attesting to the critical role of this translocation in the pathogenesis of MCL. Although some MCL cases express aberrant transcripts, most express two major CCND1 mRNA transcripts of 4.5 and 1.5 kb. Both transcripts contain the whole coding region of the gene but differ in the 3' length of untranslated region.

CCND1 is involved in cell-cycle control. Specifically, it participates in accelerating G1 progression and G1-S transition by forming complexes with cyclin-dependent kinases 4 and 6 (CDK 4/6). These complexes (a regulatory subunit, the cyclin, and a catalytic subunit, CDK) promote phosphorylation of the retinoblastoma protein (Rb). Phosphorylation of the tumor suppressor Rb leads to its deactivation and release of its inhibitory effect on E2F. Uninhibited by Rb, the transcription factor E2F activates DNA synthesis, thus permitting the cell cycle to progress into S phase (Fig. 82-1). There are two families of negative cell-cycle regulatory proteins that inhibit the CCND1/CDK4/6 activity (cyclin-dependent kinase inhibitors, CKIs). One of these families is the INK 4 (inhibitor of CDK4), which consists of four proteins: p15INK4b, p16INK4a, p18INK4c, and p19INK4d. Generally, these proteins compete with D-type cyclins for binding to the CDK subunit; p8INK4c and p19INK4d are clearly related and preferentially bind CDK6. The other family is Cip/Kip (for CDK interacting protein/kinase inhibitory protein) consisting of three proteins: p21Cip1, p27Kip1, and p57Kip2; p21Cip1 was the first CKI identified. It is also known as Waf1 (wild-type p53-activated fragment) to indicate its involvement in p53-dependent DNA damage-induced G1 arrest. The amount of p21Cip1 increases following exposure to DNA damaging agents in wild-type but not in mutant p53-containing cells. As such, p21Cip1 is an effector molecule of p53 at the G1 checkpoint. Regulation of the p27Kip1, however, is complex, including transcriptional, translational, proteolytic, and localization mechanisms. The targeted disruption of p57Kip2 in mice showed a role for this CKI in the control of the commitment/withdrawal decision as well as differentiation and apoptosis in particular tissues.

The t(11;14)(q13;q34) translocation and the resultant overexpression of CCND1 is characteristically seen in MCL. This is a

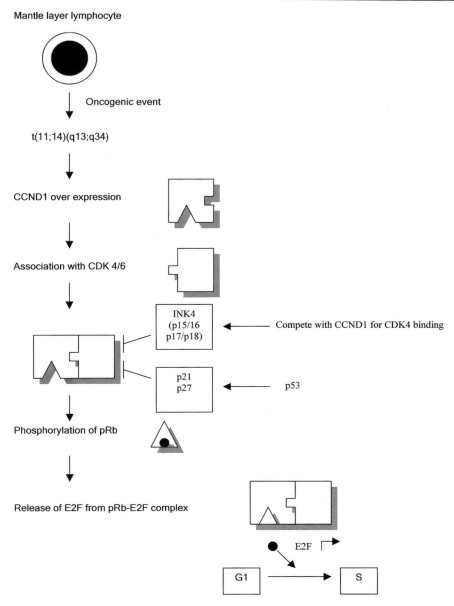

Figure 82-1 Genetic and molecular pathogenesis of MCL. The normal counterpart of MCL is thought to be the mantle layer of lymphocytes that surrounds the germinal center of lymphoid follicles. An "oncogenic" event yet unidentified leads to t(11;14) translocation and overexpression of cyclin D1 gene (CCND1). CCND1 associates with cyclin-dependent kinases 4 and 6 (CDK 4/6) resulting in binding and phosphorylation of the retinoblastoma tumor suppressor gene (pRb). Phosphorylation (inactivation) of pRb releases its inhibitory effect on the transcription factor E2F, which then permits the progression of cells from G1 to S phase. The CCND1/CDK4/6 complex is inhibited by two families of proteins, the inhibitors of CDK4 (INK4), which compete with CCND1 for CDK4/6 binding; and p21/p27. p21 is under the control of p53. INK4, inhibitor of CDK4.

B-cell neoplasm that arises from the mantle cell layer surrounding the germinal center of secondary lymphoid follicles. MCL includes 3–10% of NHL and occurs in middle-aged to older individuals. The most common sites of involvement are lymph nodes, spleen, bone marrow (with or without blood involvement), and gastrointestinal tract. The neoplastic cells are monoclonal B cells with rearranged Ig heavy and light chain genes and unmutated variable region genes indicating a pregerminal center B cell in the majority of cases. MCL is usually CD5+, FMC7+, CD10–, CD23–, Bcl2+, bcl6–. The coexpression of bcl$_1$ and bcl$_2$ makes this lymphoma one of the most difficult to treat. It has the worst features of both low-grade (incurability) and high-grade (aggressive growth) lymphomas. These biological characteristics can be explained by the coexpression of both bcl1 (which enhances proliferation) and bcl2 (which prevents programmed cell death and imparts resistance to chemotherapy). MCL has a median survival of 3–5 yr. The most consistently reported adverse histopathological prognostic parameter is a high mitotic rate (>10–37.5/15 hpf), blastoid variant and peripheral blood involvement (leukemic phase) at diagnosis. Secondary chromosomal abnormalities are identified including 13q 14 deletion, 17p deletion and total or partial plus 12; the latter being associated with shorter survival. At the molecular level, there is some evidence that deregulation of some regulatory elements involved in CCND1-driven G1-S transition are of prognostic importance in MCL. Examples include p53 mutations, loss of p21 waf1 and p16INK4a expression and deletion of p16INK4a gene.

Although t(11;14) (q13;q34) is characteristic for MCL, it is not exclusive. This translocation has been reported, albeit with much less frequency, in other lymphoproliferative disorders including splenic marginal zone lymphoma, occasional cases of chronic lymphocytic leukemia (CLL), prolymphocytic leukemia, DLCL, and multiple myeloma. However, CCND1 overexpression in these disorders is rare. Detection of CCND1, therefore, is a useful marker in the differential diagnosis of MCL from other B-cell leukemias and lymphomas. This test can be performed on small biopsy samples with limited material using immunohistochemical staining techniques.

t(14;18)(q32;q21) and the BCL2 Gene in Lymphoma   The BCL2 protooncogene was identified through the molecular analysis of breakpoints involved in the t(14;18) chromosomal translocation, which is found in the majority of follicular lymphomas. Two other translocations, t(2;18) and t(18;22), are rare variants and all share the same clinical significance. This genomic aberration juxtaposes the BCL2, normally located on chromosome 18q21, under the control of the IGH gene enhancer on 14q32, leading to upregulation of the BCL2 gene in lymphoid cells. The breakpoints on chromosome 14 are all 5′ of one of the J segments in IGH gene. As a result, the IGH constant region with an intact enhancer remains on the der(14)t(14;18). The BCL2 gene consists of three exons and most of the breakpoints are clustered in the 3′ untranslated region of the gene (70% of cases) or more distal in 3′ of exon 3 (in 30% of cases). The t(14;18) does not affect the coding sequences of the BCL2 gene but relocates BCL2 to the der(14) next to immunoglobulin enhancer, which stimulates the expression of BCL2. The role of bcl2 protein in lymphomagenesis remained unclear for several years after the discovery of the gene. Several studies have since demonstrated that overexpression of bcl2 protein does not alter the proliferation activity of the bearing cells but acts to prolong their survival. Subsequently, BCL-2 was confirmed to be an apoptosis inhibitor causing cell accumulation rather than transformation. The bcl-2 protein is the founding member of a large family of highly conserved proteins, several members of which appear to play important positive and negative roles in the control of cell death. The striking discovery of BCL2 function has defined a new class of oncogenes, antiapoptotic genes, that protects against cell death. The dysregulation of the antiapoptotic genes has expanded the research field of genetic alterations that contribute to cancer development.

The BCL2 gene encodes a membrane-associated protein found in the endoplasmic reticulum and mitochondrial membranes. The effects of BCL2 overexpression on mitochondrial control of cell death are multifunctional and may act directly on mitochondrial membrane permeability, a process often associated with the release of cytochrome-c and subsequent cell death. Furthermore, BCL2 may have some role in the regulation of basal mitochondrial energy metabolism as previous studies suggested that bcl2 protein might regulate proton transport across the inner mitochondrial membrane. BCL2 is also capable of inhibiting cytochrome-c release pathways independent of mitochondrial permeability transition, such as Bid- and Bax-mediated cytochrome-c release. In addition, bcl2 protein cooperates with other oncoproteins such as c-myc to immortalize pre-B cell. Bcl2 protects cultured cells from c-myc-induced apoptosis, an activity that may explain that concomitant overexpression of both c-myc and bcl2 in lymphocytes of transgenic mice results in synergistic tumorigenesis, generating lymphoid tumors much more aggressively than either transgene alone.

Experimental studies have revealed that transgenic mice carrying BCL2/IGH gene fusion develop a polyclonal follicular lymphoproliferation, however, over time the hyperplasia transformed into monoclonal B-cell lymphoma. This suggests that BCL2 activation is not sufficient for follicular lymphoma development but an initiating factor leading to cell immortalization through prolonged cell survival. This may be supported by observations that the majority of follicular lymphoma displayed additional genetic changes at initial diagnosis. The number and the type of secondary chromosomal alterations seen in association with t(14;18) are variable among cases but have nonrandom patterns, and are seen in different combinations. The most frequent secondary abnormalities are gains of chromosomes 7, X, followed by chromosomes 18/der(18)t(14;18), 5, 12, and 21. The majority of structural aberrations seen in t(14;18) lymphoma are unbalanced rearrangements mostly affecting 1p and/or 1q, deletions of 6q, 9p, 10q, and 13q.

Moreover, the type and frequency of the secondary abnormalities as well as the complexity and the ploidy of the karyotype are correlated with the morphological evolution of the t(14;18) follicular lymphoma. For example, gain of chromosome 7 in t(14;18) lymphoma is the most frequent abnormality seen in later disease and strongly associates with transformation to diffuse pattern. Gains of chromosomes 5 and 12, 13q- and 17p- are markers associated with expression of a higher-grade histology. Obviously most of the secondary abnormalities associated with t(14;18) are unbalanced, leading to gain or loss of genetic material. The molecular mechanisms associated with gains may include simple gene dose effects or duplication of active mutated oncogenes causing proliferation of selective cell populations leading to histological transformation. However, loss of active suppressor genes seems the likely underlying mechanism associated with deletions. The 17p abnormalities may reflect alterations of the p53 gene, which has been associated with follicular center cell lymphoma transformation. Rearrangements of 9p21 region harboring the p15 and p16 tumor-suppressor gene loci, leading to deletions, mutations, and hypermethylation of these genes with loss of the protein expression are important secondary genetic events in the progression of t(14;18) follicular lymphoma. Deletions of 6q are frequent in t(14;18) lymphoma as well as in other lymphoid neoplasms. Three distinct regions of minimal common deletions are identified, suggesting three separate tumor suppressor genes of importance in follicular lymphoma progression. Another less frequent but valuable genetic marker seen in t(14;18) lymphoma is the Burkitt's-type translocation t(8;14) or its variants. The later translocation is considered as clonal genetic evolution causing activation of C-MYC oncogene that is implicated in histological progression to blastic/blastoid transformation of follicular lymphoma.

t(11;18), API2-Malt Genes and MALT Lymphoma   The t(11;18)(q21;q21) is the most common translocation found in marginal zone lymphoma of MALT. The t(11;18) occurs in 30–40% of gastric lymphomas, and is also found in MALT lymphoma of other mucosal sites but rarely in nodal B-cell lymphoma. The t(11;18) is one of the determinant factors in the treatment and outcome of gastric MALT because the lymphomas carrying t(11;18) are resistant to H. pylori eradication therapy. A remarkable finding is that the t(11;18) is the sole chromosomal alteration in most cases suggesting the importance of the translocation in the pathogenesis of MALT lymphoma. The breakpoints of t(11;18) translocation were found to involve API2 gene at 11q21, and a previously unknown gene, MALT, at 18q21. Unlike other lymphoma-associated translocations, the t(11;18)

a subset of what was initially called malignant histiocytosis led to the recognition of a clinically distinctive category of T-cell lymphoma, known as ALCL.

The chromosomal alterations can be detected by conventional cytogenetics, Southern blot, PCR, and/or by FISH. FISH has revolutionized the field of genetics. Conventional cytogenetics requires fresh tumor tissues, and is limited in some cases by the inability of malignant cells to divide in culture, like in CLL and/or poor chromosome morphology. The diagnostic ability of FISH is increasingly used in clinical cytogenetics for the detection of chromosomal aberrations on metaphase and interphase cells and also can be performed on fresh or aged specimens, frozen or paraffin-embedded tissues. FISH is target-specific and has the ability to detect a cryptic rearrangement that would not be possible by classic banded chromosomes. For example, MCL has an aggressive clinical course and is refractory to standard chemotherapy; therefore, it is important to distinguish this disease from other B-cell neoplasms. Several studies have shown the superiority of FISH over PCR and conventional cytogenetic techniques in detecting t(11;14) */IGH-CCND1* fusion, a genetic marker associated with MCL.

The genetic abnormalities can also be used as markers in staging and in detection of minimal residual disease. PCR to detect t(14;18)/*BCL2* rearrangement is being used to monitor patients undergoing bone marrow transplants for follicular lymphoma. In addition, the genetic abnormalities may affect the clinical outcome of disease and can identify high-risk patients. The presence of 13q- in CLL and multiple myeloma is an independent adverse prognostic factor. The t(11;18) in gastric lymphoma is associated with a low frequency of transformation to large-cell lymphoma but at the same time this translocation predicts failure of antibiotic therapy in eradicating this type of *H. pylori* infection-associated lymphoma. The t(2;5) in ALCL is associated with good prognosis. The use of microarray gene chip technology has also entered the clinical arena where biopsy of lymphoma tissue from patients can be screened for thousands of genes utilizing automated technology. Although still available only on a research basis, this technology allows for gene profiling of lymphoid malignancies and grouping of gene families according to function. By analyzing hundreds of cases and comparing results with normal lymphocytes, important data is emerging to enable grouping of lymphomas according to genetic profiles. The advantage of such technology lies in its large-scale screening ability and its automation. Finally, the future goal is to exploit knowledge of genetic defects clinically by designing new therapies targeting genetic mechanisms unique to each lymphoid disorder. Research efforts in this direction include the introduction of antisense oligonucleotides to bcl2 as therapeutic agents in clinical trials. Such strategy is aimed at downregulating bcl2, which can also be used to inhibit other oncogenes. There are also efforts to neutralize key gene products pharmacologically with small synthetic molecules that bind to key gene products and neutralize their function.

SELECTED REFERENCES

Aalto Y, El-Rifa W, Vilpo L, et al. Distinct gene expression profiling in chronic lymphocytic leukemia with 11q23 deletion. Leukemia 2001; 15:1721–1728.

Athanasiou E, Kotoula V, Hytiroglou p, Kouidou S, Kaloutsi V, Papadimitriou CS. *In situ* hybridization and reverse transcription-polymerase chain reaction for cycline D1 mRNA in the diagnosis of mantle cell lymphoma in paraffin-embedded tissues. Mod Pathol 2001; 14:62–70.

Barrans SL, O'Connor SJ, Evans PA, et al. Rearrangement of the BCL6 locus at 3q27 is an independent poor prognostic factor in nodal diffuse large B-cell lymphoma. Br J Haematol 2002;117:322–332.

Crossen PE. Genes and chromosomes in chronic B-cell leukemia. Cancer Genet Cytogenet 1997;94:44–51.

Du M-Q, Isaccson PG. Gastric MALT lymphoma: from aetiology to treatment. Lancet Oncol 2002;3:97–104.

Hecht JL, Aster JC. Molecular Biology of Burkitt's lymphoma. J Clin Oncol 2000;18:3707–3721.

Horsman DE, Connors JM, Pantzar T, Gascoyne RD. Analysis of secondary chromosomal alterations in 165 cases of follicular lymphoma with t(14;18). Genes Chromosomes Cancer 2001;30:375–382.

Husson H, Carideo EG, Neuberg D, et al. Gene expression profiling of follicular lymphoma and normal germinal center B cells using cDNA arrays. Blood 2002;99:282–289.

Jaffe ES, Harris NL, Stein H, Vardiman JW (eds). World Health Organization Classification of Tumours: Pathology and Genetics of Tumours of Haematopoietic and Lymphoid Tissues. Lyon: IARC Press, 2001.

Kowaltowski AJ, Cosso RG, Campos CB, Fiskum G. Effect of Bcl-2 overexpression on mitochondrial structure and function. J Biol Chem 2002;277:42,802–42,807.

Kramer MH, Hermans J, Wijburg E, et al. Clinical relevance of BCL2, BCL6 and MYC rearrangements in diffuse large B-cell lymphoma. Blood 1998;92:3152–3162.

Kuppers R, Klein U, Hansmann ML, Rajewsky K. Cellular origin of human B-cell lymphomas. N Engl J Med 1999;341:1520–1529.

Kutok JL, Aster JC. Molecular biology of anaplastic lymphoma kinase-positive anaplastic large cell lymphoma. J Clin Oncol 2002;20:3691–3702.

Ladanyi M. The *NPM/ALK* gene fusion in the pathogenesis of anaplastic large cell lymphoma. Cancer Surv 1997;30:59–75.

Mohamed AN, Palutke M, Eisenberg L, Al-Katib A. Chromosomal analysis of 52 follicular lymphoma with t(14;18), including blastic/blastoid variant. Cancer Genet Cytogenet 2001;126:45–51.

Sanchez-Beato M, Sanchez-aguilera A, Piris MA. Cell cycle deregulation in B-cell lymphomas. Blood 2003;101:1220–1235.

Stein H, Foss HD, Durkop H, et al. CD30(+) anaplastic large cell lymphoma: a review of its histopathologic, genetic, and clinical features. Blood 2000;96:3681–3695.

Tsujimoto Y, Croce CM. Molecular genetics of human B-cell neoplasia. Curr Top Microbiol Immunol 1986;132:183–192.

Tsujimoto Y, Yunis J, Onorato-Showe L, Erikson J, Nowell PC, Croce CM. Molecular cloning of the chromosomal breakpoint of B-cell lymphomas and leukemias with the t(11;14) chromosome translocation. Science 1984;224:1403–1406.

Vidal A, Koff A. Cell-cycle inhibitors: three families united by a common cause. Gene 2000;247:1–15.

Wessendorf S, Schwaenen C, Kohlhammer H, et al. Hidden gene amplifications in aggressive B-cell non-Hodgkin lymphomas detected by microarray-based comparative genomic hybridizatin. Oncogene 2003; 22:1425–1429.

83 Multiple Myeloma

A Story of Genes and the Environment

KENNETH H. SHAIN AND WILLIAM S. DALTON

SUMMARY

Multiple myeloma (MM) is characterized by the clonal expansion of mature B cells within bone marrow. This malignancy is believed to arise from mutations involving nonrandom translocations between specific oncogenes and immunoglobulin coding regions of B cells. Further mutations parallel a relatively well-described progression from benign MGUS to MM and secondary plasma cell leukemia. Current literature suggests that in addition to genetic adaptations, specific effectors of the bone marrow microenvironment might contribute significantly to both MM pathogenesis as well as to treatment failure. Within this chapter we discuss the molecular and biochemical factors that contribute to malignant potential of MM.

Key Words: Adhesion; apoptosis; cell cycle; cyclin D; c-maf; FGFR; IL (interleukin)-6; MGUS (monoclonalgammopathy of unknown significance); myeloma; multidrug resistance; MMSET; microenvironment; oncogenes; Ras; STAT.

INTRODUCTION

Multiple myeloma (MM) is a hematopoietic malignancy characterized by the clonal expansion of mature B cells, a low proliferative index, clonal secretion of Ig, osteolytic bone destruction, and ultimate development of drug resistance. MM cells are thought to arise from postgerminal center (GC) plasma cells that have undergone immunoglobulin class switching and somatic hypermutation. Importantly, it is through these normal DNA recombinatorial processes of B-cell differentiation (Ig class switching and somatic hypermutation) that the initial transforming events in MM have been proposed to originate. Evidence for this hypothesis has been demonstrated through the identification of numerous immunoglobulin heavy chain (IgH) and light chain (IgL) translocations in MM and the premalignant monoclonal gammopathy of unknown significance (MGUS). Like their normal plasma cell counter parts, MM cells home to the bone marrow (BM) remaining closely associated with their physical extracellular environment. MM cells become BM independent only in the most terminal phases and only after the acquisition of secondary or tertiary transforming mutations. These later DNA alterations are frequently somatic mutations and secondary Ig-translocations leading to the

From: *Principles of Molecular Medicine, Second Edition*
Edited by: M. S. Runge and C. Patterson © Humana Press, Inc., Totowa, NJ

constitutive activity of oncogenes. Further, the unique BM dissemination has been proposed to be integral in MM disease progression. The BM is rich in cytokines, growth factors, and other soluble factors, as well as in adhesive matrices including fibronectin (FN), hyaluronan and bone marrow stromal cells (BMSCs) that can support MM expansion. Therefore, the roles of both genetic and environmental effectors in MM pathogenesis are the focus of intense research. Research continues on the potential interplay between the genetically altered MM cell and its environment, leading to the identification of specific molecular and biochemical determinants that might serve as potential therapeutic targets. This chapter reviews some of the best-understood individual genetic and environmental aspects of MM. A working model is proposed of how these individual aspects form a potential network of pro-cancer effects promoting progression of this complex and terminal malignancy.

MM is a BM resident malignancy of plasma cells, diagnosed at a rate of approx 14,000 new cases per year, making it the second most prevalent hematopoietic malignancy, accounting for 15% of all hematopoietic cancers. This plasma cell dyscrasis occurs at higher rates in blacks than whites and is unbiased by gender. It is a disease primarily of older individuals with a median age of diagnosis of 68 yr for men and 70 yr for women, and is characterized by a number of clinical factors: focused skeletal destruction, hypercalcemia, clonal immunoglobulin production (M-component), urinary Bence-Jones protein, renal insufficiency, anemia, hypoγ-globulinemia, and recurrent infections. These clinical findings result from the unfettered expansion of a mutant Ig-secreting (99% of MM) plasma cell population within the BM. MM cells overgrow the BM compartment and in turn alter production of hematopoietic cells (anemia and hypoγ-globulinemia) leading to weakness and recurrent infection. Further, the primary presenting symptom of MM patients is bone pain as a result of localized osteolytic destruction in load-bearing structures such as the femur, pelvis, or vertebrae. Osteolytic lesions result from alterations in cytokine/chemokine signaling in the BM; as a result the osteoblast/osteoclast ratio is reduced favoring bone destruction. The subsequent osteoporosis manifests in bone weakness and pain, and clinically in hypercalcemia, a major factor in renal insufficiency. A number of the clinical signs can be successfully treated. Unfortunately, the most unavoidable characteristic of MM is its finality. Despite tremendous effort by clinicians and researchers, MM patient therapy is plagued by the ultimate development of

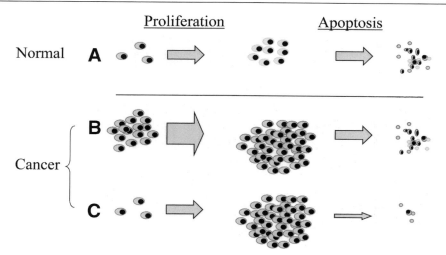

Figure 83-1 Cancer results from the imbalance in cellular fate. Tissue homeostasis is maintained through a balance between the number of cells produced and the number of cells eliminated. Under normal conditions the number of proliferating cells is equal to the number of cells undergoing apoptosis (**A**). To this end, the total population of cells does not increase. In contrast, in cancer tissue, homeostasis is subverted resulting in the uncontrolled expansion of a population of cells. This expansion occurs as a result of a dysregulation of the processes governing progression through the cell cycle (**B**) or of the processes promoting cell death (**C**). In scenarios **B** and **C**, the net effect of increasing the number of dividing cells or decreasing the number of dying cells is an increase in the overall population.

progressive disease, making MM one of the most challenging cancers to treat. The resiliency of MM to therapy has fostered a great deal of research into delineating the mechanisms by which MM cells evade and eventually become resistant to multiple regimens of chemotherapy. Improvements in the treatment of myeloma largely have been based on data collected from research investigating of the molecular and cellular determinants of MM, with new novel therapies under clinical investigation. MM disease progression and the phenomenon of multidrug resistance (MDR) have both genetic and environmental components.

As a cancer, MM adheres to a basic principle: MM cells have escaped the normal restraints governing proliferation and death. In the typical "life" of a normal cell, it proliferates, differentiates for a given task, and then is eliminated through a process termed apoptosis or programmed cell death (PCD). Under normal conditions the number of cells dividing equals the number of cells dying thereby maintaining tissue homeostasis. To this end, the expansion of a malignant population of cells results from the deregulation in progression through the cell cycle (uncontrolled proliferation) or in the mechanisms that promote cell death (decreased number of cells being eliminated) (Fig. 83-1). Cancers require alterations in both of these homeostatic controls. MM is no exception; its progression requires (1) the acquisition/utilization of mechanisms that drive MM cells through the cell cycle arrest afforded terminally differentiated B cells during normal maturation and (2) the acquisition/utilization of mechanisms that protect MM cells from both physiological and therapeutic effectors of PCD. In MM it has been proposed that these initial requirements are fulfilled by the translocation of a gene(s) that normally functions as determinants of cell proliferation or cell survival to regions juxtaposed to active Ig-enhancer elements, thereby facilitating the superfluous expression and subsequent function of that gene product (*an oncogene*). These translocations most frequently involve IgH (14q32) and to a lesser extent IgL (22q11 [λ], 2p11 [λ]) enhancer elements and a limited number of oncogenes including cyclin D_1 (11q13), cyclin D_3 (6q21), FGFR3/MMSET (4p16.3), c-maf (16q23), and others. IgH

translocations connected with these oncogenes account for approx 75% of MM disease. Additional mutations are acquired throughout the course of the disease including chromosome 13 deletion, activating somatic mutations, and secondary Ig-translocations demonstrating a step-wise model for MM pathogenesis (Fig. 83-2). Importantly, although MM is a genetic disease by definition, it is apparent that both DNA mutations and the BM microenvironment contribute to the deregulation of life and death of MM cells. The MM BM microenvironment provides a myriad of soluble and physical growth and survival factors. Soluble factors such as interleukin (IL)-6, IL-10, granulocyte-macrophage colony stimulating factor, insulin-like growth factor (IGF)-1, vascular endothelial growth factor, fibroblast growth factor (FGF), and macrophage inflammatory protein-1α, are associated with MM expansion. Interactions between MM cells and specific extracellular matrix components and BMSCs have been demonstrated to protect cells from both physiological and chemotherapeutic mediators of apoptosis. Taken together, these data suggest that the MM microenvironment plays a significant role in the disease pathogenesis by providing a "sanctuary" for BM resident MM cells. Therefore, delineation of the specific molecular pathways utilized by the environmental effectors might provide an avenue to better attack the advance of MM. This chapter discusses the understanding of how genetic and environmental determinants influence MM progression through their influence on rates of cell proliferation and cell turnover.

CELL CYCLE PROGRESSION AND APOPTOSIS

Cancer is a disease that requires the inappropriate cell replication and sensitivity to apoptosis. Each process has specific constituents governing the transmission of signals within the cell. To better understand the mechanisms utilized by MM cells to overcome replication and PCD, a brief introduction to some of the molecular determinants of theses processes is presented. These determinants can be divided into two general categories: those that drive cell cycle progression or apoptosis-"the gas pedals" so to speak and those that stop cell cycle progression or apoptosis-"the

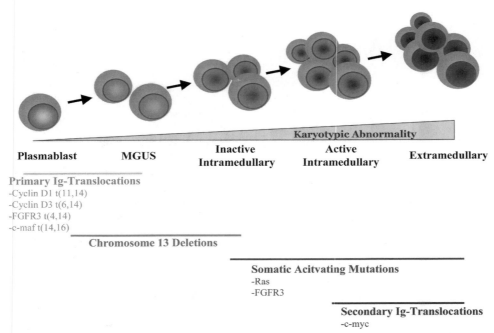

Figure 83-2 A multi-step progression of multiple myeloma (MM). MM can be staged from the pre-malignant MGUS, to smoldering/indolent MM, to an inactive intramedullary then active intramedullary stage, and finally to extramedullary disease (secondary plasma cell leukemia). Importantly, progression through this model parallels an accumulation of karyotypic abnormalities. Identification of a number of these karyotypic alterations has revealed a multi-step pathogenesis of MM. Examination of patient DNA has demonstrated a progression from primary Ig-translocations (cyclin D1 t[11q13], cyclin D3 [6p21], FGFR3 [4p16.3], and c-maf [16q23]), chromosome 13 deletions, activating somatic mutations (Ras and FGFR mutations), and secondary Ig-translocations or insertions (c-myc). Importantly, these are the most prevalent mutations observed. It is not proposed that these are the only causative DNA alterations associated with MM progression. FGFR, fibroblast growth factor receptor; MGUS, monoclonal gammopathy of unknown significance.

brakes." In the context of cell regulatory factors the "gas pedals" are termed oncogenes because they promote oncogenesis. In contrast, the "brakes" are denoted tumor suppressors as they oppose the actions cellular proliferation and survival thereby suppressing oncogenesis. To this end, overexpression (increased activity) of oncogenes and deletion (decreased activity) of tumor suppressors are requirements of cancer progression. For regulators of PCD the nomenclature would be reversed.

CELL CYCLE (G_1) Cellular replication entails succession through the four phases of the cell cycle, G_1, synthesis (S), Gap2 (G_2), and mitosis (M) and in some cases progression from a quiescent or nonproliferative state (termed G_0). Entry into and exit from the phases of the cell cycle involves a network of transient and sequential biochemical events modulating progression through two-phase transitions ($G_{1/0}$-S and G_2-M). Under normal conditions this process is stimulated by extracellular stimuli, frequently extracellular mitogens (cytokines and growth factors) that bind and activate transmembrane receptors. Ligand binding facilitates activation of signaling cascades that promote the expression of transiently expressed proteins termed cyclins. Interactions between cyclins and their constitutively expressed cyclin-dependent kinase (CDK) partners mediate progression through the cell cycle. Progression from G_1 to S requires expression of one or more of the D-type cyclins (cyclin D1, D2, D3), cyclin binding to the appropriate CDK (CDK4 or CDK6), and subsequent kinase activity mediated by the formation of cyclin D/CDK4/6 heterodimers (Fig. 83-3). Cyclin D/CDK heterodimers phosphorylate the tumor suppressor retinoblastoma protein (Rb). Rb is a molecular guardian blocking progression through the cell cycle. In its hypophosphorylated state, Rb inhibits

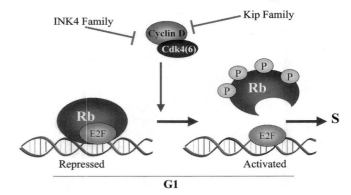

Figure 83-3 Cyclin D/cyclin-dependent kinase-4(6) regulation of G1-S progression. Progression from G_1 to S requires expression of the D-type cyclins (cyclin D1, D2, or D3). The transiently expressed cyclins bind to specific cyclin-dependent kinase inhibitors (CDKs [CDK4 or CDK6]), and subsequent kinase activity is mediated by the formation of cyclin D/CDK4/6 heterodimers. Cyclin D/CDK phosphorylates the retinoblastoma protein (Rb). Hypophosphorylated Rb inhibits cell cycle progression by repressing transcription of genes necessary for subsequent phases by sequestering E2F transcription factors. Phosphorylated Rb releases E2F facilitating transcription of genes required for DNA synthesis and succession through G_2 and mitosis.

cell cycle progression by repressing transcription of genes necessary for subsequent phases by sequestering E2F transcription factors. On phosphorylation by cyclin D/CDK4(6), Rb releases E2F facilitating transcription of genes required for DNA synthesis and succession through G_2 and mitosis, including thymidine kinase, dihydrofolate reductase, c-Myc, c-Myb, c-Fos, cyclin A, and the G_2/M transition gate keepers, cyclin B and p34[cdc2] (cdc2). Therefore, expression of D-type cyclins is an initiating event in cell division, as such overexpression of one of the D-type cyclins would increase the proliferative potential of a cell.

CYCLIN-DEPENDENT KINASE INHIBITORS   Just as cyclins and CDKs drive cell cycle progression, the cell governs transit through the cycle. As mentioned, Rb attenuates cell cycle progression as a transcriptional repressor. Cell cycle progression is also regulated by CDK-inhibitors (CKIs), a super family of proteins including the INK family (p15[INK4B] [CDKN2B], p16[INK4A] [CDKN2A], p18[INK4C] [CDKN2C], and p19[INK] [CDKN2D]), the Kip family (p27[Kip1] and p57[Kip2]), and p21[waf]. CKIs attenuate cell cycle progression by inhibiting the interactions between cyclins and CDKs. Hence CKIs block cell cycle progression, acting as brakes to allow for "checks" on energy supplies, metabolites, and DNA integrity before copying DNA. Because of their function in arresting cellular proliferation, CKIs are tumor suppressor genes. Oncogenesis often correlates with decreased expression of CKIs promoting uncontrolled progression through the cell cycle. Tumor suppressor dysfunction frequently involves homozygous deletion or loss of heterozygocity of the gene. Interestingly, p15[INK4B], p16[INK4A], and 18[INK4C] deletions are rarely observed in MM. However, the expression of the INK-family is silenced in up to 75% of MM and MM cell lines. The decreased expression of these factors results from hypermethylation of their promoters. Promoter methylation alters the chromatin structure surrounding the promoter selectively inhibiting access to the DNA. A study examining MGUS patient samples demonstrated p16[INK4A] methylation in 19%, p15[INK4B] methylation in 36%, and both promoters were methylated in 6.5% of patients examined, suggesting that loss of this family of tumor suppressors might be important in early progression of MM.

APOPTOTIC SIGNALING   Uncontrolled proliferation is only one regulatory system dysregulated in cancer (MM). MM expansion also depends on alterations in the mechanisms executing PCD. Dysregulation of apoptotic signaling affords MM cells' resistance to antitumor immune responses mediated by cytotoxic lymphocytes and to chemotherapeutic drugs. Physiological and chemotherapeutic mediators of apoptosis share a well-characterized sequence of biochemical events culminating in cell destruction. Under physiological conditions the antitumor immune response mediated by cytotoxic T cells and natural killer cells can implement apoptosis through the crosslinking of death receptors with transmembrane death ligands or soluble versions of death ligands. Death receptors constitute the tumor necrosis factor receptor/nerve growth factor receptor family including tumor necrosis factor receptor 1, tumor necrosis factor receptor 2, CD95/Fas/Apo-1, death receptor (DR) 4 (TRAIL-R1), and DR5 (TRAIL-R2). Crosslinking of death receptors by their cognate ligands (TNF-α, CD95L/FasL/Apo1L, or TRAIL/Apo2L, respectively) induces aggregation of specific molecular determinates and initiation of a proteolytic cascade of events involving a family of cysteine-aspartate specific proteases or caspases (Fig. 83-4). Ligation of death receptors induces receptor multimerization and recruitment of the adapter protein Fas-associated death domain containing protein (FADD) and procaspase-8, the initial proteolytic enzyme in the apoptotic cascade. DR localization of procaspase-8 mediates a proximity-induced cleavage of procaspase-8 and initiation of a zymogen cascade. Activation of procaspase-8 propagates cell death through proteolytic cleavage of downstream effector caspases, most notably procaspase-3. Activation of procaspase-3 by caspase-8 can occur directly (type I) or indirectly (type II) through a mitochondrial-dependent mechanism depending on the cell type and the DR stimulated. Mitochondria are important components of the apoptotic cascade as they are targeted by cytotoxic agents used in the clinic. Indeed, mitochondria are the major point of convergence between DR and chemotherapeutic drug-mediated apoptosis. Additionally, studies have demonstrated that therapeutic agents can also stimulate DR and death ligand expression facilitating DR crosslinking. Targeting of the mitochondria by either DRs or therapeutic drugs primarily entails cleavage and/or activation of proapoptotic members of the Bcl-2 family. Caspase-8 targets Bim; drugs have been demonstrated to activate Bax, Bak, Bim, and other small death-inducing Bcl-2 family proteins. Doxorubicin stimulates conformational changes of Bak and Bax facilitating mitochondrial targeting. These proteins induce mitochondrial permeability transition, mediating release of cytochrome-c and other proapoptotic effectors from mitochondria. Cytosolic cytochrome-c precipitates the formation of a large (approx 700 kDa) complex containing multiple apoptotic protease activating factor-1 and caspase-9 molecules, termed the apoptosome. Apoptosome aggregation results in a dATP-dependent cleavage and activation of caspase-9, which in turn targets effector caspases, procaspases-7 and -3. Active caspase-3 (-7) targets cytosolic, cytoskeletal, and nuclear factors facilitating cell death.

ANTI-APOPTOTIC EFFECTORS   Uncontrolled activation of the earlier-mentioned apoptotic cascade would rapidly destroy a cell. Therefore, this cell death pathway must be tightly regulated to protect from spontaneous activation. To this end, the apoptotic effectors ("gas pedals") that drive this cascade are modulated by numerous proteins ("brakes") acting at specific stages of the cell death cascade to regulate the inappropriate activation of PCD. Regulation apoptosis can be divided into two categories; those that are specific to DR-mediated apoptosis (death-induced signaling complex formation and caspase-8 activation) and those that are common to both DR and chemotherapeutic drug-mediated PCD (mitochondrial and postmitochondrial events) phases of the cell death cascade.

Regulation of CD95-Mediated Apoptotic Signaling   DR-induced PCD can be regulated at several levels (Fig. 83-5). Ligand crosslinking is inhibited by soluble CD95, soluble CD95L, as well as CD95-specific decoy receptor-3s (DcR-3). Regulation of DR expression also correlates with cellular sensitivity to ligand crosslinking. In MM, heterologous CD95 expression within a given MM cell population affords low CD95 expressing cells a survival advantage to DR ligation as compared to higher expressing cells. Further, specific mutations in the death domain of CD95 have been identified in MM patient samples that might negatively affect receptor signaling. Other potential mechanisms to CD95 resistance have also been identified in other model systems. Posttranslational modification of CD95 by the ubiquitin-like protein Sentrin/SUMO has been suggested to repress apoptotic signaling from CD95 by blocking recruitment and activation of apoptotic effectors. c-FLIP (c-FLICE-like inhibitory protein), an anti-apoptotic protein that shares significant similarity with procaspases -8 and -10, is proposed to inhibit CD95-mediated apoptosis by competing with procaspase-8 for FADD, thereby preventing or reducing the participation of procaspase-8 in the death-induced signaling complex and blocking activation of the proteolytic cascade. Expression of c-FLIP also directly contributes to expansion of hematopoietic tumors in vivo by protecting cells from CD95-mediated antitumor

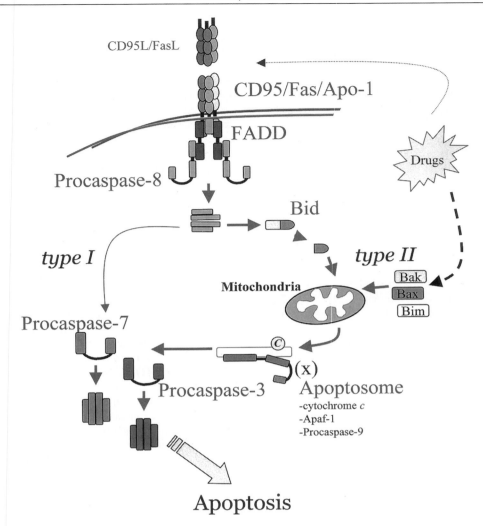

Figure 83-4 Apoptosis (extrinsic and intrinsic pathways). Cell death mediated by death ligands (extrinsic pathway of apoptosis) proceeds following ligand binding to specific death receptors. Receptor binding facilitates death-induced signaling complex formation initiating caspase-8 cleavage. Active caspase-8 propagates the cell death cascade by activating the downstream effector caspase-3, either directly or indirectly through mitochondria. Mitochondrial induced apoptosis (intrinsic pathway) represents a shared portion apoptotic pathway between death receptors and chemotherapeutic agents. Prevailing dogma indicates that most drugs activate the intrinsic pathway of programmed cell death by "directly" targeting the mitochondria facilitating the release of cytochrome-*c*, apoptosome formation, catalytic activation of procaspases-3 and -7, and subsequent cellular destruction. Other apoptotic-signaling components might also play a role in drug-mediated apoptosis. Apoptotic signaling from the CD95/Fas/Apo-1 death receptor has been demonstrated to mediate the cytotoxicity of certain drugs.

immune responses, demonstrating a direct correlation between cellular sensitivity to DR-mediated apoptosis and tumorigenesis.

Mitochondrial and Postmitochondrial Regulation
Regulatory factors that act downstream of the death-induced signaling complex might also contribute to resistance to CD95- and chemotherapeutic-mediated apoptosis (*see* Fig. 83-5). As discussed, mitochondria are one of the pivotal components of the apoptotic cascade. A growing number of reports suggest that regulation of mitochondrial events might be of the utmost importance in dictating cellular fate in response to both DR and drug-induced apoptosis. The Bcl-2 family of proteins regulates mitochondrial membrane integrity. This family of proteins contains proteins that both promote (Bax, Bak, Bik, Bid, and Bad-apoptotic family members) and inhibit (Bcl-2, Bcl-X$_L$, Mcl-1, and A1/bfl-1-anti-apoptotic family members) mitochondrial membrane permeability transition and apoptosis. Mitochondrial function and mitochondrial cytochrome-*c*

are maintained by a balance between or equilibrium between proapoptotic and antiapoptotic Bcl-2 family members. In response to apoptotic stimuli such as DR ligation or chemotherapeutic agents, cytosolic proapoptotic Bcl-2 family members target the mitochondria pushing the balance in favor of cell death thereby mediating mitochondrial membrane permeability transition and the release of apoptotic effectors including cytochrome-*c*. As such, an imbalance in this equilibrium would either stimulate cell death (increased proapoptotic activity) or conversely inappropriate cell survival through increased expression of antiapoptotic family members. Therefore, cellular fate is dependent on the expression and/or activity of the Bcl-2 family.

Postmitochondrially, the inhibitors of apoptosis (IAP) family of proteins has been demonstrated to block the activity of the caspases-9, -3, and -7. The IAP are considered a subset of anti-apoptotic members within the BIR-containing protein family, a

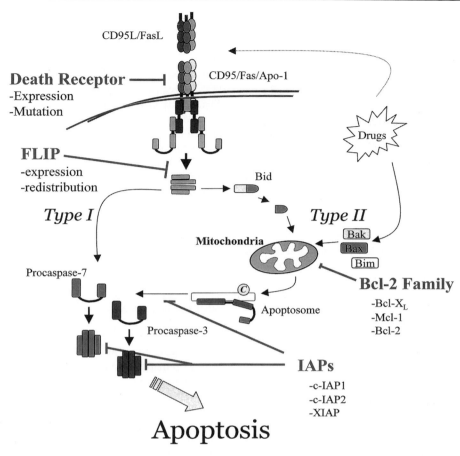

Figure 83-5 Regulators of the apoptotic cascade. Cellular control of CD95 and chemotherapeutic drug-mediated apoptosis has been demonstrated at both the initiation of the extrinsic cascade (DISC formation and caspase-8 activation), initiation of the intrinsic cascade (mitochondrial events), and in the execution phases (postmitochondrial) of the apoptotic cascade.

group of polypeptides characterized by the existence of one or more baculovirus inhibitor of apoptosis repeat domains. Baculovirus inhibitor of apoptosis repeat domains are protein–protein interaction domains important for at least some of the anti-apoptotic properties of IAP. A second important molecular structure of IAP is the carboxy-terminal RING domain. The RING domain promotes polyubiquitination of associated substrates; a covalent marker for 26S proteosome targeting and proteolytic degradation. IAP (XIAP, c-IAP1, and c-IAP2) are a unique group of antiapoptotic effectors in that they have multiple mechanisms through which they attenuate apoptosis dependent on the target molecule. The baculovirus inhibitor of apoptosis repeat 3 domain of XIAP associates with the small subunit of caspase-9 (exposed after proteolytic processing of caspase-9 in the apoptosome) and inhibits caspase-9 activity. Further, a sequence adjacent to the baculovirus inhibitor of apoptosis repeat 2 domain of XIAP (and c-IAP1 and c-IAP2) interacts with the substrate binding site of caspases-3 and -7 thereby inhibiting their apoptotic activity. Additionally, the RING domain of these antiapoptotic determinants also mediates poly-ubiquitinization of caspases-3 and -7 facilitating their degradation (inactivation). From this body of information it is apparent that IAP influence cellular sensitivity to apoptosis through multiple avenues (note: IAP have other antiapototic, proapoptotic, and apoptosis-independent functions not discussed here). Apoptotic regulatory factors, including those affecting initiating events of both the extrinsic (FLIP) and intrinsic apoptotic cascades (Bcl-2, Bcl-X$_L$, and Mcl-1), as well as

the execution phase of apoptosis (IAP), provide important checkpoints for cellular commitment to death. Whether through genetic alterations in genes or through communication with the tumor microenvironment, tumor progression (immune evasion and drug resistance) frequently involves the deregulation of these endogenous checks on PCD.

GENETIC CONTRIBUTION

MM is a cancer of plasma cells initiated by genetic "mistakes." These mistakes, in turn, disconnect the homeostatic controls governing cell growth and death. MM, as well as other B-cell neoplasms, has been proposed to occur as a result of mutations incurred during the normal processes of B-cell differentiation. Maturation of a B cell from a naive B cell to a long-lived memory B cell involves three independent DNA recombination events: VDJ recombination, GC-associated somatic hypermutation, and GC-associated isotype switch recombination resulting in the expression of an immunoglobulin with unique antigen-binding specificity (i.e., VDJ recombination and somatic hypermutation, and antibody activity [isotype class switching]). Analysis of MM chromosomal structure demonstrates that the primary mutations occur through reciprocal nonrandom IgH-translocations (and to a lesser extent IgL) with oncogenes at DNA breakpoints that correspond to sequences of DNA specific for somatic hypermutation (JH-regions) and switch recombination (switch regions). These data suggest that MM originates from B cells that have entered GCs having undergone VDJ recombination and that the transforming mutations result from mistakes incurred primarily during somatic hypermutation and somewhat less frequently during switch recombination. Interestingly, the oncogenes involved in these Ig-translocations predominantly involve proteins that drive proliferation (cyclin D1, cyclin D3, c-maf, and FGFR3/MMSET), suggesting that escape from the quiescence of normal long lived memory B cells is an important early event in MM pathogenesis.

MM staging has been based on a number classification systems: Durie and Salmon, Kyle and Greipp, and British Columbia Cancer Agency, and on criteria set by the International Myeloma Group based primarily on degree of plasmacytosis, concentration of Ig (M-protein), the presence or absence of bone lesions, and end organ tissue impairment. From these criteria MM can be staged from the premalignant MGUS, to smoldering/indolent MM, to an inactive intramedullary then active intramedullary stage, and finally to extramedullary disease (secondary plasma cell leukemia). Importantly, progression through this model parallels an accumulation of karyotypic abnormalities (*see* Fig. 83-2). Furthermore, acquisition of specific genetic alterations is associated with the multi-step pathogenesis of MM involving primary Ig-translocations, chromosome 13 deletions, activating somatic mutations, and secondary Ig-translocations or insertions. Therefore, clinical staging of MM correlates with biochemical and molecular changes within the MM cell population that afford cells a more malignant phenotype (progression to the next stage of disease).

MONOCLONAL GAMMOPATHY OF UNKNOWN SIGNIFICANCE

MGUS represents the putative premalignant precursor to MM. MGUS progresses to frank MM at a rate of approx 1%/yr and nearly one-third of patients with MGUS progress to MM, although not all MM has a premalignant history. Therefore, MGUS might not be a prerequisite for MM. However, examination of MGUS provides novel insight into the genetic requirements of plasma cell transformation and the early requirements for MM. Karyotyping of MGUS patient specimens demonstrated the existence of primary Ig-translocations involving specific oncogenes. These reciprocal Ig-translocations put the expression of oncogenes under constitutively active IgH or IgL enhancer elements, thereby ensuring the overexpression of the participating oncogene. Karyotypic analysis demonstrated IgH translocations with cyclin D1 t(11q13) in 20% of MM tumors, cyclin D3 (6p21) in 5%, FGFR3 (4p16.3) in 15%, and c-maf (16q23) in 13% of MM tumors. Ig-translocations are absent in 25% of tumors indicating that unidentified genetic alterations can participate in transformation of plasma cells (or limitations in genetic analysis of MM cells). The remaining MM tumor translocation associated gene loci are with MUM1/IRF-4 (6p25), IRTA1 and IRTA2 (1q21-24), mafB (20q12), and others; however, the significance of these translocations is not well understood. The major oncogenes (cyclin D1, cyclin D3, FGFR3, and c-maf) accounting for 75% of observed Ig-translocations are all molecules with roles in controlling cell proliferation. As discussed, expression of D-type cyclins is an initial event marking entry into and progression through the cell cycle. To this end, overexpression of cyclins D1 or D3 would overcome endogenous regulatory mechanisms and drive inappropriate cell division. FGFR3, one of four bFGF (basic FGF) binding cell surface tyrosine kinase receptors, is not usually expressed of MM cells. FGFR3 signaling through signal transducer and activators of transcription (Stat) and the

Ras/Raf/ERK1/2 pathways support growth of both human fibroblasts and hematopoietic cells. Constitutive FGFR3 signaling substitutes for IL-6, a major MM growth and apoptotic factor, in MM cell lines. Importantly, in MM cells with translocations involving FGFR3 (4p16), levels of cyclin D2 are elevated, demonstrating a link between initial Ig-translocations and cell cycle progression. The role of MMSET has not been clearly defined, however, evidence has demonstrated MMSET gene translocations independent of FGFR3, suggesting MMSET translocation is important in the transforming potential of t(4,14) translocations. c-Maf is a transcription factor that associates with jun and fos, components of AP-1, an important mitogenic transcription factor. c-Maf is the cellular homolog to the transforming avian maf retrovirus product, v-maf. Similarly to FGFR3/MMSET/Ig-translocations, elevated levels of cyclin D2 are observed in MM cells with c-maf/Ig-translocations. Examination of t(11,14), t(6,14), t(4,14), and t(14,16) Ig-translocations demonstrates that these primary transforming events directly or indirectly regulate progression through the cell cycle through the inappropriate regulation of D-type cyclin expression. Of note, this does not exclude FGF3R/MMSET and c-maf translocations from other potential transforming actions.

INTRAMEDULLARY MM

Intramedullary MM represents the next step in MM pathogenesis with identifiable genetic alterations (increase in karyotypic abnormality). Intramedullary MM is divided into two stages, an inactive and active phase defined by their proliferating cell-labeling index. Genetic analysis of metaphase MM cells of inactive intramedullary MM initially demonstrated increased rates of chromosome 13 deletions as compared to MGUS. However, a report examining 72 MGUS and smoldering MM patients with metaphase fluorescent *in situ* hybridization analysis showed that approx 50% had chromosome 13 deletion numbers equivalent to those observed in MM. These data suggest that although chromosome deletions might be subsequent to Ig-translocations, they might occur earlier than previously proposed. Although the specific requirements of chromosome 13 deletion are not completely elucidated, the tumor suppressor Rb locus is located on chromosome 13. Further, examination of MM patients demonstrated that Rb (13q14) deletion correlated with a more severe prognosis when coupled with cyclin D1 amplification.

Progression from inactive to active intramedullary MM is associated with the accumulation of somatic mutations (often point mutations) most frequently resulting in the constitutive activation of the GTPase Ras (N-Ras, K-Ras) and less frequently FGFR3. Interestingly, examination of human MM cell lines demonstrated that mutations in either Ras or FGFR3, but not both, are present, suggesting that they serve overlapping functions. In one study, Ras mutations (N12-Ras and K61-Ras) were observed in 54.5% of MM at diagnosis. This was compared to only 12.5% of MGUS and smoldering MM examined. Further, examination following relapse demonstrated 81% of MM with Ras mutations. FGFR3 Ig-translocations represent one of the primary genetic events in MM pathogenesis (plasma cell to MGUS); somatic mutations later in MM might lead to ligand independence and constitutive signaling from this oncogenic receptor. Two of three identified FGFR3 mutations were demonstrated to confer constitutive kinase activation in MM cell lines when overexpressed and all three mutations were capable of supporting fibroblast growth in colony-forming assays. Because of the proliferative activity of Ras and FGFR3 mutations, acquisition of these genetic changes has been proposed to afford the increased proliferation of active intramedullary MM cells.

EXTRAMEDULLARY MM

Extramedullary growth has primarily been associated with secondary Ig-translocations. Unlike primary translocation these DNA malformations are infrequently reciprocal and are often complex involving multiple chromosomes. Therefore, these translocations are unlikely to manifest from the DNA recombinatorial events that mediate primary Ig-translocations. Secondary translocation of the oncogene *c-myc* (8q24.1) is most commonly observed and therefore has served as a paradigm for progression from intramedullary disease to extramedullary disease (secondary plasma cell leukemia), and on to human myeloma cell lines. c-Myc is not expressed in normal memory B cells, however, genetic alterations in *c-myc* are found in as many as 45% of advanced MM and in 86% of human myeloma cell lines. Importantly, the observation of *c-myc* translocation late in MM pathogenesis and the coordinate BM independent growth suggest that the constitutive expression of *c-myc* might provide the necessary growth and survival stimuli previously supplied by the BM microenvironment.

BONE MARROW MICROENVIRONMENT

Cancer requires alterations in the homeostatic mechanism controlling cell growth and cell death. The previous section discussed elegant work elucidating the genetic aspects of MM pathogenesis. The oncogenes associated with the proposed initiating events of MM are primarily involved in regulation of cellular proliferation (cyclin D1, cyclin D3, FGFR3, and c-maf). However, MM is a disease associated with a decreased propensity for cell death. Taken together these observations indicate that nongenetic (environmental) factors within the BM might influence the response of MM cells to apoptotic stimuli. Additionally, MM cells only escape the confines of the BM in terminal stages associated with highly proliferative c-myc mutations. This pattern of growth suggests that factors within the BM might also contribute significantly to MM disease pathogenesis through progrowth effects. This section reviews some of the major soluble factors and adhesive matrices that promote proliferation and prevent PCD.

SOLUBLE FACTORS IN MM   The BM microenvironment of MM supplies a myriad of soluble factors that contribute to MM proliferation and survival. IL-6, a B-cell differentiation factor, is the primary growth and survival factor in MM. Other soluble factors including IGF-1, bFGF, granulocyte-macrophage colony stimulating factor and hepatocyte growth factor fulfill a similar role in MM growth and survival. The prominent role of IL-6 in MM disease has increased interest in the delineation of the signal cascades elicited following IL-6 receptor crosslinking. Signaling by IL-6 signaling requires the formation of a protein complex consisting of two IL-6, two IL-6R alpha (IL-6Rα/gp80) and two gp130 molecules (IL-6β) (Fig. 83-6). Intracellular signaling by IL-6 is mediated entirely through the gp130-subunit. Gp130 is a transmembrane signaling subunit required for signaling by IL-6R family members (leukemia inhibitory factor, ciliary neurotrophic factor, Oncostatin M, IL-11, and cardiotrophin-1). Gp80 and gp130 interactions stimulate phosphorylation of specific gp130 tyrosine residues by members of the Janus tyrosine kinase (Jak) family of nonreceptor tyrosine kinases (Jak1, Jak2, and Tyk2) that are constitutively associated with gp130. Phosphorylated tyrosine residues of gp130 function as docking sites for a number

of cytosolic proteins, including Stat proteins, SHC (adaptor protein), phosphoinositide 3-kinase (PI3K), and src-homology domain 2-containing protein tyrosine phosphatase 2. Biochemical signaling events initiated by these gp130-associated proteins can independently regulate cell survival and proliferation. Recruitment of SHP2 to gp130 has also been implicated in the activation of both the Ras/MAPK and PI3K/Akt (protein kinase B) signaling cascades. However, both might also occur independently of SHP2. Therefore, IL-6 mediated gp130 signaling primarily activates three cascades, each established growth and survival signaling pathways (Jak/Stat3, PI3K/Akt, and Ras/MAPK [ERK1/2]).

Signal Transducer and Activators of Transcription   Stats are family of src-homology domain 2-containing cytoplasmic proteins activated through phosphorylation of specific tyrosine residues by receptor associated tyrosine kinases (Jaks), growth factor tyrosine kinases (epidermal growth factor receptor, platelet-derived growth factor receptor), or nonreceptor tyrosine kinases (Src and Abl). The Stat family consists of seven members characterized by four highly homologous domains, a cooperative domain, a central DNA-binding domain, a dimerization domain (src-homology domain 2 domain containing region), and a trans-activation domain. Stat phosphorylation induces homo- or heterodimerization (IL-6 signaling primarily involves Stat3 and to a lesser extent Stat1), nuclear translocation, DNA binding, and expression of genes involved in cell proliferation, survival, differentiation, development, and specific components of the immune response. The ability of Stats to promote neoplastic growth involves the expression of factors that control both cell survival and proliferation. Stat activity correlates with resistance to apoptosis mediated by CD95 ligation, interferon-γ, ultraviolet irradiation, as well as chemotherapeutic drugs. The primary prosurvival targets of IL-6 induced Stat3 activity in MM are Mcl-1 and Bcl-X$_L$, two antiapoptotic members of the Bcl-2 family. The role of Bcl-X$_L$ in MM survival was demonstrated in studies examining Jak/Stat3 signaling in U266 IL-6 dependent MM cell line. Inhibition of Jak kinase activity or Stat3 DNA binding with Jak2 kinase inhibitor AG490 or Stat3 dominant negative (Stat3β), respectively, resulted in specific down-regulation of Bcl-X$_L$ expression and increased sensitivity to CD95-mediated apoptosis, demonstrating a novel role for IL-6/Jak2/Stat3-signaling in CD95 resistance in MM. Further, as Bcl-X$_L$ has been demonstrated to block apoptosis mediated by certain cytotoxic agents, it is likely that Stat3-mediated Bcl-X$_L$ expression similarly correlates with endogenous resistance to chemotherapy. Mcl-1 is also an important downstream target of IL-6/Jak/Stat3 signaling in MM.

Jak/Stat-signaling also plays an important role in proliferation mediated by IL-6 in MM. Stimulation of Stat3 activity by nonreceptor protein tyrosine kinases mediates the expression of two key cell cycle regulatory proteins, cyclin D1 and c-myc. Stat3-dependent regulation of the D-type cyclins has been demonstrated in several cell models. In MM, IL-6 regulated Jak/Stat3 signaling specifically regulates cyclin D1 expression that, in turn, promotes cell proliferation. Treatment of IL-6-dependent MM cells with the Jak2 inhibitor AG490 inhibited Jak kinase activity and Stat3 signaling. The reduction in Stat3 signaling correlated with the downregulation of cyclin D1 and accumulation of cells in G1-phase of the cell cycle. To this end, Stat3-induced cyclin D1 expression might be an important effector of IL-6-mediated cellular proliferation in MM. c-myc is another potent oncogene involved in the regulation of the cell cycle targeted by Stat3 transactivation. c-myc controls a number of

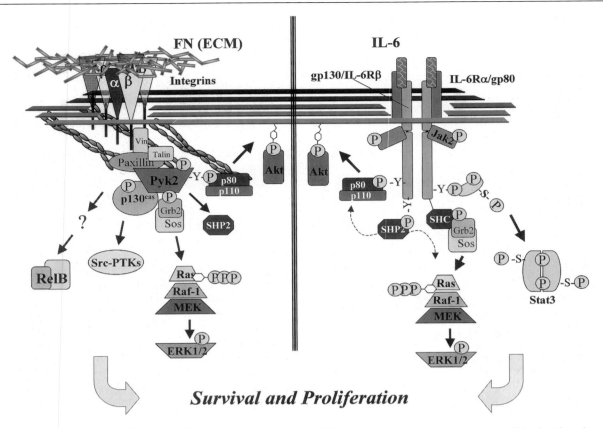

Survival and Proliferation

Figure 83-6   IL-6 and integrin-mediated signaling cascades. IL-6, a B-cell differentiation factor, has long been established as the primary growth and survival factor in MM. IL-6 signaling requires the formation of a protein complex consisting of two IL-6, two IL-6Rα (IL-6Rα/gp80) and two gp130 molecules (IL-6β). IL-6 signaling is mediated entirely through the gp130-subunit. IL-6Rα and gp130 interactions stimulates phosphorylation of specific gp130 tyrosine residues by members of the Janus tyrosine kinase (Jak) family of nonreceptor tyrosine kinases (Jak1, Jak2, and Tyk2) constitutively associated with gp130. Phosphorylated tyrosine residues of gp130 function as docking sites for a number of cytosolic proteins, including Stat3, SHC, PI3K, and SHP2. These three signaling cascades independently regulate cell survival and proliferation. Importantly these cascades are utilized by a number of other proMM survival factors. Ligand bound FNα and β-integrin heteromultimers facilitate the aggregation of a host of signaling and cytoskeletal proteins. Integrins lack intrinsic kinase activity, therefore, focal adhesions utilize associated nonreceptor protein tyrosine kinases (PTK) and receptor tyrosine kinases for intracellular signaling. Integrin signaling in MM involves Pyk2/RAFTK. Pyk2/RAFTK and associated with p130^Cas are recruited to focal adhesions with the docking/cytoskeletal protein paxillin following integrin ligand crosslinking in MM cells. β₁-integrin occupancy stimulates Pyk2/RAFTK tyrosine phosphorylation and the recruitment of the Src PTKs p53/56^Lyn and p59^Fyn to Pyk2/p130^Cas complexes. SHP2 also aggregates at focal adhesions in MM. Further, in other cell models, integrin stimulation has been shown to mediate a Pyk2/RAFTK-dependent activation of PI3K and ERK1/2 phosphorylation through the recruitment of Grb2/SOS and activation of Ras. Stat, signal transducer and activators of transcription.

aspects of G1 (cell cycle) progression, including increased activity of cyclin D/CDK4 complexes. As c-myc secondary Ig-translocations are observed in a large percentage of extramedullary MM and HMCLs, it is speculated that IL-6 and other BM effectors might modulate the expression of c-myc or c-myc-like activities thereby supporting MM expansion.

Phosphotidylinositol-3 Kinase   PI3K is an inositol phospholipid phosphotransferase demonstrated to participate in MM survival and proliferation following IL-6 crosslinking primarily through the activation of Akt/protein kinase B and its downstream effectors. PI3K is a heterodimeric protein consisting of an adapter subunit (p85) and a kinase domain containing subunit (p110). On IL-6R stimulation the p85-subunit of PI3kinase associates with gp130 recruiting the p110-subunit. The PI3K heterodimer phosphorylates the 3′ OH ring of inositol phospholipids forming phosphotidylinositol (3,4,5) 3-phosphate and phosphotidyinositol (3,4) 2-phosphate on the inner leaflet of the plasma membrane. The cytosolic serine/threonine kinase Akt is recruited to the plasma membrane through

interactions between the pleckstrin homology, PH, domain of Akt and the 3′-phosphorylated inositol phospholipids. Plasma membrane localized Akt is a substrate for phosphoinsitol-dependent protein kinase (PDK) 1 or PDK2. Phosphorylated (active) Akt subsequently phosphorylates a number of key determinants involved in MM proliferation and survival. Several Akt substrates have been associated with survival. Direct phosphorylation of the proapoptotic Bcl-2 family member Bad attenuates its apoptotic activity through cellular redistribution. Phosphorylation of procaspase-9 suppresses its apoptotic properties. Akt phosphorylation of FKHRL-1, a member of the Forkhead family of transcription factors, inhibits its transcriptional activity by targeting it for nuclear export. DNA associated unphosphorylated FKHRL-1 (nuclear) promotes expression of the DR ligand FasL, the proapoptotic Bcl-2 family member Bim, and the CKI p27^KIP1. So, Akt phosphorylation and nuclear export of FKHRL-1 would negatively regulate the expression of FasL, Bim, and p27^KIP1 potentially promoting survival and growth of IL-6 stimulated cells. Interruption of this cascade by molecular or pharmacological inhibitors of PI3K/Akt signaling induces cell cycle arrest and apoptosis demonstrating a prominent role of this IL-6 induced pathway in MM expansion. Interestingly, the expression of the tumor suppressor PTEN, a dual specificity phosphatase (phosphotyrosine and phospholipids) shown to negatively regulate Akt signaling through the dephosphorylation of phosphoinositol phospholipids, was decreased in a number of MM cell lines. Further, the decreased levels of PTEN correlated with increased Akt signaling, suggesting that MM cells with decreased PTEN expression/activity might be more sensitive to PI3K/Akt activating stimuli.

Ras/ERK1/2   Activating Ras mutations are observed in greater than 50% of MM patients. These mutations maintain Ras in an active GTP-bound state. In this constitutively active state Ras promotes succession to a more pathogenic stage of intramedullary disease. Proliferative and anti-apoptotic signaling from IL-6 has also been shown to involve activation of one of the Ras isoforms (N-Ras, K-Ras, and H-Ras). Ras is a GTPase that is active when GTP is bound and inactive on GTP hydrolysis (GDP-bound). The ability of Ras to modulate signaling is dependent on plasma membrane localization facilitated by lipid modification. The lipid modification involves recognition of four conserved carboxy-terminal amino acids, proteolytic removal of the three terminal amino acids, and the linkage of farnesyl or geranylgeranyl lipid moieties to the terminal cysteine of Ras by farnesyl transferases or genranylgeranyl transferases, respectively. IL-6-mediated Ras activation requires the gp130 association and phosphorylation of SHC. SHC and the constitutively associated Grb2 protein recruit the guanine nucleotide exchange factor Sos to IL-6R complexes. Sos facilitates the exchange of GDP for GTP for membrane bound Ras. GTP-bound Ras (active) initiates a serine/threonine kinase cascade resulting in activation of ERK1/2 (MAPK). Interruption of this kinase cascade blocks IL-6 mediated MM cell proliferation. Further, constitutive activation of ERK1/2 signaling by the overexpression of activated Ras in IL-6 MM cell lines can compensate for the proliferative and antiapoptotic functions of IL-6. IL-6 and the signaling cascades elicited following receptor binding serve as a paradigm for cytokine and growth factor signaling in MM. Other soluble factors have been implicated in MM disease progression, all of which primarily elicit cellular response through the activation of these signaling effectors or similar signaling cascades.

ADHESION AND MM SURVIVAL   Cell adhesion molecules (CAMs) consisting of the immunoglobulin family, cadherins, selectins, hyaluronate receptors, receptor tyrosine phosphatases, and integrins mediate interactions between cells and their physical environment. CAMs coordinate homing, lodging, differentiation, and survival of MM in the BM through specific homotypic and heterotypic interactions with environmental ligands. Integrins are the most well characterized members of this superfamily of surface glycoproteins. Integrins are heterodimeric (α and β) membrane receptors communicating the physical extracellular environment to intracellular events, including cytoskeletal rearrangements and signal cascades that control cell migration, cell growth, and survival. Twenty-two potential integrin receptors have been identified, comprised of specific dimers derived from 18 α-subunits and 8 β-subunits. Integrin binding requires transition from a low to high affinity ligand-binding state, allowing cell adhesion to extracellular matrix components such as FN, vitronectin, laminin, and collagens, or other CAMs. Stimulation of high affinity ligand binding involves a process termed "inside-out signaling." The cytoplasmic tails of integrins are indirectly targeted by the small

prenylated GTPases Ha-ras, R-ras, and Rap, mediating conformational changes in the extracellular ligand-binding domain and thereby modulating adhesion (negatively or positively). Ligand-associated α and β integrin heteromultimers facilitate the aggregation of a host of signaling and cytoskeletal proteins. As integrins lack intrinsic kinase activity these unique molecular aggregates, termed focal adhesions, utilize associated nonreceptor protein tyrosine kinases and receptor tyrosine kinases for intracellular signaling. Signals originating from focal adhesions in anchorage-dependent cells primarily involve focal adhesion kinase, a nonreceptor PTK recruited to focal adhesions in association with cytoskeletal proteins talin, paxillin, and vinculin. Focal adhesion kinase is a docking protein involved in recruitment of integrin-signaling associated factors such as p130^{cas} (Crk-associated substrate), Ras through Grb2/Sos, Src, and PI3K. However, in MM as opposed to focal adhesion kinase, the related nonreceptor PTK Pyk2/RAFTK (proline rich tyrosine kinase 2/RAFTK/CAKβ) modulates integrin multimerization. Pyk2/RAFTK is constitutively associated with p130^{Cas} and recruited to focal adhesions with paxillin following integrin ligand crosslinking in MM cells. β_1 integrin occupancy stimulates Pyk2/RAFTK tyrosine phosphorylation and the recruitment of the Src protein tyrosine kinases p53/56^{Lyn} and p59^{Fyn} to Pyk2/p130^{Cas} complexes. It has also been shown that integrin stimulation of MM cells facilitates the recruitment of the tyrosine phosphatase SHP2. In other cell models, integrin stimulation mediates a Pyk2/RAFTK-dependent activation of PI3kinase and ERK1/2 phosphorylation through the recruitment of Grb2/SOS and activation of Ras. However, the downstream effectors of integrin-mediated Pyk2RAFTK activation and the consequences of this activation on the cytoprotective effects of integrin adhesion have yet to be directly linked. β_1-integrin-mediated adhesion to FN of MM cells was demonstrated to stimulate nuclear localization and transcriptional activity of RelB, a member of the NF-κB family of transcription factors. The FN-mediated increases in RelB transcriptional activity correlated with elevated expression of the NF-κB regulated anti-apoptotic effector c-IAP, the CAMs syndecan-4 and CD83, as well as the cytokines IL-8 and IL-6. NF-κB activation has also been associated with adhesion of MM cells to BMSC, facilitating secretion of IL-6 by the BMSCs. From these studies it is apparent that integrin-mediated (or BMSCs') interactions with the physical environment can elicit a number of signaling cascades that might directly or indirectly confer a growth or survival advantage to adherent MM cells.

Most data indicates that MM integrin adhesion is associated with cell survival in response to both physiological and chemotherapeutic mediators of apoptosis. One important characteristic of a tumor is the ability to evade tumor-specific immune responses. MM cell adhesion to the extracellular matrix component FN confers resistance to CD95-mediated apoptosis. CD95-mediated caspase activation and apoptosis was reduced following β_1-integrin-mediated adhesion of hematopoietic cancer cell lines to FN. This resistance was associated with the intracellular trafficking of c-FLIP$_L$ from a membrane-associated subcellular location to a cytosolic location where c-FLIP$_L$ could be recruited to the death-induced signaling complex and inhibits apoptosis. FLIP expression is also regulated by adhesion and IGF-1 stimulation at the levels of RNA synthesis, suggesting that c-FLIP expression might be regulated at multiple levels by multiple BM effectors.

MULTIDRUG RESISTANCE

The failure of MM chemotherapy is defined by the phenomenon of MDR. Treatment of MM is characterized by initial response to chemotherapy, eventual relapse, and expansion of a therapy-resistant population of cells. MM cells become refractory to therapy through the acquisition of genetic changes that alter cellular susceptibility to cytotoxic therapy in the face of cytotoxic insult. This selective process results in acquisition of mechanisms that mediate resistance to multiple classes of therapeutic agents, or acquired MDR. The mechanisms of acquired MDR have been primarily elucidated using in vitro systems that have identified molecular changes within individual cells selected under prolonged exposure to cytotoxic insult. The mechanisms of acquired MDR in MM can be divided into three subcategories: reduced drug accumulation at target, alterations in drug target, and inhibition of apoptotic signaling pathways (Table 83-1). It is important to understand that although these mechanisms of acquired MDR have been categorized, within a given cell drug resistance frequently (if not always) results from multiple mechanisms.

In contrast to selected mechanisms of MDR or perhaps more appropriately in concert with acquired MDR, the environment has been demonstrated to modulate MM cell sensitivity to therapeutic drugs. As discussed, the BM environment produces cytokines, growth factors, chemokines, and adhesive matrices with the potential to confer a selective advantage to BM resident MM cells. An increasing number of these extrinsic effectors have been demonstrated to mediate drug resistance in MM (*see* Table 83-1). IL-6 and its associated signaling cascades modulate MM cell sensitivity to a number of drugs including dexamethasone (Dex). IGF-1, FGF, and hepatocyte growth factor also confer resistance to Dex through the activation of specific signaling cascades. Adhesion to specific BM extracellular matrixs attenuates the cytotoxic effects of the multitude of therapeutic agents, a phenomenon termed CAM drug resistance. These data indicated that the BM microenvironment might be a powerful mediator of a *de novo* MDR. Importantly, this de novo drug resistance might provide an initial resistance to MM cell in the face of therapeutic insult. In so doing the BM microenvironment might confer a selective advantage to resident MM cells allowing acquisition of more stable and durable mechanisms of MDR (acquired mechanisms). By targeting these effectors or the subsequent signaling cascades disruption of the survival network afforded MM cells by the BM might result, and in turn provide more successful treatment.

CONCLUSION

MM is a complex disease as demonstrated by the number of tumorigenic mechanisms presented in this chapter. Physicians and researchers using the reductionist theory have been examining MM, breaking down the disease and its manifestations to their most basic parts. Using this ideology MM research has revealed many molecular and biochemical factors involved. A handful of these molecular determinants and the mechanism by which they might individually contribute to MM pathogenesis have been presented. Importantly, synthesis of this enormous volume of data has given insight into the disease complexity. Progression from a maturing GC localized B cell to extremeduallry MM does not occur through a single event; a step-wise succession of genetic alterations occurs. Primary Ig-translocations involving a nonrandom set of oncogenes facilitates the earliest transforming steps in MM. These events are frequently

Table 83-1
Multidrug Resistance (MDR) in MM

Mechanisms of acquired MDR[a]

Reduced drug accumulation at target
  P-glycoprotein
  Multidrug resistance protein 1 (MRP1)
  Breast cancer resistance protein (BCRP)
  Lung resistance protein (LRP)/major vault protein (MVP)
  Drug detoxification
  CD98 expression
Alterations in drug target
  Reduced topoisomerase II expression
  Decreased glucocorticoid receptor (GR) expression
  Deleted GR ligand binding domain
Anti-apoptotic proteins
  Increased Bcl-2 family members
  Decreased CD95 expression[b]

Mechanisms of de novo MDR[a]

Soluble factors
  Interleukin-6
    PI3K/Akt
    Ras/ERK1/2
    Jak/Stat3: Bcl-X_L and Mcl-1
    SHP2: RAFTK
  Insulin-like growth factor (IGF)[b]
    Insulin receptor substrate
    Ras/ERK1/2
  Interferon α (IFN α)
    Jak/Stat3: Mcl-1
  Granulocyte-macrophage colony-stimulating factor[b]
  Hepatocyte growth factor[b]
    PI3K/Akt
  Fibroblast growth factor
  Macrophage inflammatory protein 1-α[b]
    PI3K/Akt
    Ras/ERK1/2
Direct cell contact
  Integrin-mediated adhesion
    Increased p27^{Kip1}
    Intracellular redistribution of topo IIβ
    Intracellular redistribution of c-FLIP$_L$[b]
  Hyaleronon (a glucosaminoglycan)
    Increased IL-6 stability/concentration at receptor
  Bone marrow stromal cells (BMSC)
    Production of IL-6

[a]Represents only mechanisms identified in MM.
[b]Antiapoptotic, however, no direct link to drug resistance has been established.

paired with deletion or silencing of tumor suppressor genes. The acquisition of activating somatic mutations that might promote mitogen-independent growth are observed in more advanced stages of cancer. Finally, complex secondary Ig-translocations promoting the expression of c-myc (frequently) are observed in the most advanced stages of MM correlating with BM-independent growth. Importantly, these B cells (and MM cells) do not undergo genetic changes without other processes also occurring. Until the most terminal phases of MM, cells remain primarily in the BM. MM is not simply a mutated cell, it is a genetically altered cell residing in an environment rich in cytokines, growth factors, other soluble factors, as well as physical matrices. Therefore, it is likely that these environmental factors support MM growth and survival throughout the

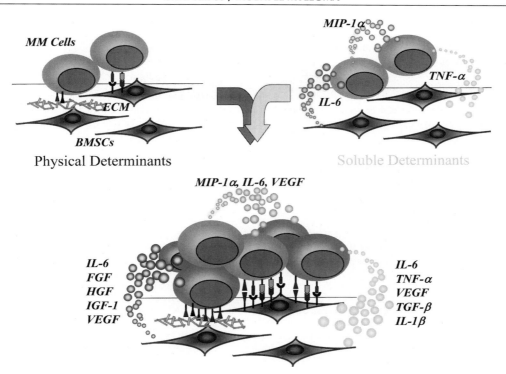

Figure 83-7 Myeloma bone marrow (BM) microenvironment: a network of promultiple myeloma (MM) survival determinants. The MM microenvironment plays a significant role in the disease pathogenesis by providing a "sanctuary" for BM resident MM cells. The environmental effectors have been proposed to constitute a network of paracrine and autocrine signaling, as well as regulatory events mediated by adhesion of MM cells to bone marrow stromal cells (BMSCs) or to adjacent MM cells that control MM cell growth and survival. FGF, fibroblast growth factor; ECM, extracellular matrix; HGF, hepatocyte growth factor; IGF-1, insulin-like growth factor-1; IL, Interleukin; MIP-1α, macrophage inhibitory protein-1α; TNF-α, tumor necrosis factor-α; VEGF, vascular endothelial growth factor.

course of intramedullary disease facilitating the acquisition of subsequent transforming genetic alterations.

Adding to the complexity, MM is not a single cell reacting to a single environmental cue. MM cells are constantly in contact with their physical environment and bathed with a multitude of soluble determinants. These environmental effectors have been proposed to constitute a network controlling MM proliferation and survival (Fig. 83-7). This network involves paracrine and autocrine signaling, as well as regulatory events mediated by adhesion of MM cells to BMSC (or to adjacent MM cells). Interestingly, cell adhesion is an important catalyst in the proposed survival network. Interactions between MM cells and BMSC induce production of the pro-expansion factor IL-6 by BMSCs. IL-6 signaling increases the adherent potential of MM cell lines to FN through an increase in macrophage inflammatory protein-1α secretion. Importantly, IL-6 mediated macrophage inflammatory protein-1α production was dependent on adhesion to FN, suggesting that FN-adhesion altered the manner in which the cell "interpreted" IL-6 stimulation. A number of soluble/adhesive networks have been elucidated. As with IL-6, MM cell adhesion to BMSCs modulates vascular endothelial growth factor secretion. Further, MM cell proliferation paralleled increased vascular endothelial growth factor levels. Vascular endothelial growth factor produced by MM cells also participates in paracrine signaling to adjacent BMSC, stimulating production of IL-6 by BMSCs. The cytokines IL-1β, TGF-β, and TNF-α produced by MM also facilitate BMSC secretion of IL-6. Moreover, TNF-α regulates increased adhesion of MM cells to BMSC through the expression of specific CAMs on both MM cells

and BMSCs. The glucosaminoglycan hyaluronan was shown to contribute to MM cell resistance to Dex through the stabilization of IL-6 demonstrating a coordinated antiapoptotic effect involving both soluble and physical BM determinants in drug resistance. Together these studies suggest that MM progression might be mediated through a complex network. Further evidence for this hypothesis was demonstrated in experiments examining the antiapoptotic nature of specific coculturing conditions between MM cell lines and BMSCs. In these studies the degree of MM cell resistance to mitoxantrone was dependent on the coculture condition examined. MM cells were cultured alone, cocultured with BMSCs in transwells chambers (inhibiting adhesion), and directly cocultured with BMSCs (facilitating adhesion). MM cells cocultured in the absence or in the presence of intercellular contact with BMSCs were protected from mitoxantrone. MM cells cultured alone were unprotected. However, MM cells adhered to BMSCs were significantly more resistant to chemotherapeutic drugs than cells maintained in transwell chambers (not adhered). These data suggest that soluble factors and physical determinants might function in concert, potentiating the proliferative and/or protective effects of the individual constituents. MM must not be considered simply a genetic disease or a disease with one effector. MM is a complex disorder that requires an understanding of how genetic and environmental determinants contribute to tumorigenesis. Moreover, the significant role of the BM microenvironment in MM suggests that therapies designed to disrupt specific signaling cascades, ligand-receptor binding, or interactions between cells and the physical environment might be important targets in MM therapy.

SELECTED REFERENCES

Anderson KC, Lust JA. Role of cytokines in multiple myeloma. Semin Hematol 1999;36(1 Suppl 3):14–20.

Anwar AR, Moqbel R, Walsh GM, Kay AB, Wardlaw AJ. Adhesion to fibronectin prolongs eosinophil survival. J Exp Med 1993;177(3): 839–843.

Aoudjit F, Vuori K. Matrix attachment regulates Fas-induced apoptosis in endothelial cells. A role for c-flip and implications for anoikis. J Cell Biol 2001;152(3):633–644.

Astier A, Avraham H, Manie SN, et al. The related adhesion focal tyrosine kinase is tyrosine-phosphorylated after beta1-integrin stimulation in B cells and binds to p130cas. J Biol Chem 1997;272(1):228–232.

Astier A, Manie SN, Law SF, et al. Association of the Cas-like molecule HEF1 with CrkL following integrin and antigen receptor signaling in human B-cells: potential relevance to neoplastic lymphohematopoietic cells. Leuk Lymphoma 1997;28(1,2):65–72.

Avraham H, Park SY, Schinkmann K, Avraham S. RAFTK/Pyk2-mediated cellular signalling. Cell Signal 2000;12(3):123–133.

Bergsagel PL, Kuehl WM. Chromosome translocations in multiple myeloma. Oncogene 2001;20(40):5611–5622.

Billadeau D, Jelinick DF, Shah N, LaBien TW, Van Ness B. Introduction of an activated N-ras oncogene alters the growth characteristics of the IL-6-dependent myeloma cell line ANBL-6. Cancer Res 1995; 55(16):3640–3646.

Bloem AC, Lamme T, de Smet M, et al. Long-term bone marrow cultured stromal cells regulate myeloma tumour growth in vitro: studies with primary tumour cells and LTBMC-dependent cell lines. Br J Haematol 1998;100(1):166–175.

Catlett-Falcone R, Landowski TH, Oshiro MM, et al. Constitutive activation of Stat3 signaling confers resistance to apoptosis in human U266 myeloma cells. Immunity 1999;10(1):105–115.

Chauhan D, Anderson KC. Mechanisms of cell death and survival in multiple myeloma (MM): therapeutic implications. Apoptosis 2003;8(4): 337–343.

Chauhan D, Uchiyama H, Urashima M, Yamamoto K, Anderson KC. Regulation of interleukin 6 in multiple myeloma and bone marrow stromal cells. Stem Cells 1995;13(Suppl 2):35–39.

Clark EA, King WG, Brugge JS, Symons M, Hynes RO. Integrin-mediated signals regulated by members of the rho family of GTPases. J Cell Biol 1998;142(2):573–586.

Dalton WS. The tumor microenvironment: focus on myeloma. Cancer Treat Rev 2003;29(Suppl 1):11–19.

Dalton WS, Bergsagel PL, Kuehl WM, Anderson KC, Harousseau JL. Multiple myeloma. Hematology (Am Soc Hematol Educ Program) 2001;157–177.

Dalton WS, Jove R. Drug resistance in multiple myeloma: approaches to circumvention. Semin Oncol 1999;26(5 Suppl 13):23–27.

Damiano JS, Cress AE, Hazlehurst LA, Shtil AA, Dalton WS. Cell adhesion mediated drug resistance (CAM-DR): role of integrins and resistance to apoptosis in human myeloma cell lines. Blood 1999;93(5): 1658–1667.

Damiano JS, Dalton WS. Integrin-mediated drug resistance in multiple myeloma. Leuk Lymphoma 2000;38(1,2):71–81.

Dankbar B, Padro T, Leo R, et al. Vascular endothelial growth factor and interleukin-6 in paracrine tumor-stromal cell interactions in multiple myeloma. Blood 2000;95(8):2630–2636.

de la Fuente MT, Casanova B, Garcia-Gila M, Silva A, Garcia-Pardo A. Fibronectin interaction with alpha4beta1 integrin prevents apoptosis in B cell chronic lymphocytic leukemia: correlation with Bcl-2 and Bax. Leukemia 1999;13(2):266–274.

Derksen PW, de Gorter DJ, Meijer HP, et al. The hepatocyte growth factor/Met pathway controls proliferation and apoptosis in multiple myeloma. Leukemia 2003;17(4):764–774.

Ferlin M, Noraz N, Hertogh C, Brochier J, Taylor N, Klein B. Insulin-like growth factor induces the survival and proliferation of myeloma cells through an interleukin-6-independent transduction pathway. Br J Haematol 2000;111(2):626–634.

Ganju RK, Hatch WC, Avraham H, et al. RAFTK, a novel member of the focal adhesion kinase family, is phosphorylated and associates with

signaling molecules upon activation of mature T lymphocytes. J Exp Med 1997;185(6):1055–1063.

Gonzalez M, Mateos MV, Garcia-Sanz R, et al. De novo methylation of tumor suppressor gene p16/INK4A is frequent finding in multiple myeloma patients at diagnosis. Leukemia 2000;14(1):183–187.

Guillerm G, Gyan E, Wlolwiec D, et al. p16/INK4A and p15/INK4B gene methylations in plasma cells from monoclonal gammopathy of undetermined significance. Blood 2001;98(1):244–246.

Gupta D, Treon SP, Shima Y, et al. Adherence of multiple myeloma cells to bone marrow stromal cells upregulates vascular endothelial growth factor secretion: therapeutic applications. Leukemia 2001;15(12): 1950–1961.

Hallek M, Bergsagel PL, Anderson KC. Multiple myeloma: increasing evidence for a multistep transformation process. Blood 1998;91(1):3–21.

Hatch WC, Ganju RK, Hiregowdara D, Avraham S, Groopman JE. The related adhesion focal tyrosine kinase (RAFTK) is tyrosine phosphorylated and participates in colony-stimulating factor-1/macrophage colony-stimulating factor signaling in monocyte-macrophages. Blood 1998;91(10):3967–3973.

Hazlehurst LA, Damiano JS, Buyuksal I, Pledger WJ, Dalton WS. Adhesion to fibronectin via beta1 integrins regulates p27kip1 levels and contributes to cell adhesion mediated drug resistance (CAM-DR). Oncogene 2000;19(38):4319–4327.

Hazlehurst LA, Valkov N, Wisner L, et al. Reduction in drug-induced DNA double-strand breaks associated with beta1 integrin-mediated adhesion correlates with drug resistance in U937 cells. Blood 2001; 98(6):1897–1903.

Hideshima T, Chauhan D, Schlossman R, Richardson P, Anderson KC. The role of tumor necrosis factor alpha in the pathophysiology of human multiple myeloma: therapeutic applications. Oncogene 2001;20(33): 4519–4527.

Hughes PE, O'Toole TE, Ylanne J, Shattil SJ, Ginsberg MH. The conserved membrane-proximal region of an integrin cytoplasmic domain specifies ligand binding affinity. J Biol Chem 1995 270(21):12,411–12,417.

Hughes PE, Renshaw MW, Pfaff M, et al. Suppression of integrin activation: a novel function of a Ras/Raf-initiated MAP kinase pathway. Cell 1997;88(4):521–530.

International Myeloma Working Group. Criteria for the classification of monoclonal gammopathies, multiple myeloma, and related disorders: a report of the International Myeloma Working Group. Br J Haematol 2003;121(5):749–757.

Jourdan M, Veyrune JL, Vos JD, Redal N, Couderc G, Klein B. A major role for Mcl-1 in the IL-6-induced survival of human myeloma cells. Oncogene 2003;22(19):2950–2959.

Katagiri K, Hattori M, Minato N, Irie S, Takatsu K, Kinashi T. Rap1 is a potent activation signal for leukocyte function-associated antigen 1 distinct from protein kinase C and phosphatidylinositol-3-OH kinase. Mol Cell Biol 2000;20(6):1956–1969.

Kaufmann SH, Earnshaw WC. Induction of apoptosis by cancer chemotherapy. Exp Cell Res 2000;256(1):42–49.

Keely PJ, Rusyn EV, Cox AD, Parise LV. R-Ras signals through specific integrin alpha cytoplasmic domains to promote migration and invasion of breast epithelial cells. J Cell Biol 1999;145(5):1077–1088.

Kinashi T, Katagiri K, Watanabe S, Vanhaesebroeck B, Downward J, Takatsu K. Distinct mechanisms of alpha 5beta 1 integrin activation by Ha-Ras and R-Ras. J Biol Chem 2000;275(29):22,590–22,596.

Klingbeil CK, Hauck CR, Hsia DA, Jones KC, Reider SR, Schlaepfer DD. Targeting Pyk2 to beta 1-integrin-containing focal contacts rescues fibronectin-stimulated signaling and haptotactic motility defects of focal adhesion kinase-null cells. J Cell Biol 2001;152(1):97–110.

Kramer A, Schultheis B, Bergmann J, et al. Alterations of the cyclin D/Rb/p16INK4A pathway in multiple myeloma. Leukemia 2002; 16(9):1844–1851.

Kulkarni MS, Daggett JL, Bender TP, Kuehl WM, Bergsagel PL, Williams ME. Frequent inactivation of the cdk-inhibitor p18 by homozygous deletion in multiple myeloma cell lines: ectopic p18 expression inhibits growth and induces apoptosis. Leukemia 2002;16(1): 127–134.

Landowski TH, Olashaw NE, Agrawal D, Dalton WS. Cell adhesion-mediated drug resistance (CAM-DR) is associated with activation of NF-kB (RelB/p50) in myeloma cells. Oncogene 2003;22(16): 2417–2421.

Lauta VM. A review of the cytokine network in multiple myeloma: diagnostic, prognostic, and therapeutic implications. Cancer. 2003;97(10): 2440–2452.

Lemoli RM, Fortuna A. C-kit ligand (SCF) in human multiple myeloma cells. Leuk Lymphoma 1996;20(5,6):457–464.

Li J, Avraham H, Rogers RA, Raja S, Avraham S. Characterization of RAFTK, a novel focal adhesion kinase, and its integrin-dependent phosphorylation and activation in megakaryocytes. Blood 1996;88(2): 417–428.

Liu L, Moesner P, Kovach NL, et al. Integrin-dependent leukocyte adhesion involves geranylgeranylated protein(s). J Biol Chem 1999;274(47): 33,334–33,340.

Lu ZY, Zhang XG, Rodriguez C, et al. Interleukin-10 is a proliferation factor but not a differentiation factor for human myeloma cells. Blood 1995;85(9):2521–2527.

Manie SN, Astier A, Haghayeghi N, et al. Regulation of integrin-mediated p130(Cas) tyrosine phosphorylation in human B cells. A role for p59(Fyn) and SHP2. J Biol Chem 1997;272(25):15,636–15,641.

Manie SN, Beck AR, Astier A, et al. Involvement of p130(Cas) and p105(HEF1), a novel Cas-like docking protein, in a cytoskeleton-dependent signaling pathway initiated by ligation of integrin or antigen receptor on human B cells. J Biol Chem 1997;272(7):4230–4236.

Mateos MV, Garcia-Sanz R, Lopez-Perez R, et al. P16/IN4A gene inactivation by hypermethylation is associated with aggressive variants of monoclonal gammopathies. Hematol J 2001;2(3):146–149.

Mitsiades C, Mitsiades N, Poulaki V, et al. Activation of NF-κB and upregulation of intracellular anti-apoptotic proteins via the IGF-1/Akt signaling in human multiple myeloma cells: therapeutic implications. Oncogene 2002;21(37):5673–5683.

Nefedova Y, Landowski TH, Dalton WS. Bone marrow-derived soluble factors and direct cell contract contribute to de novo drug resistance in myeloma cells by distinct mechanisms. Leukemia;17(6):1175–1182.

Ogata A, Chauhan D, Teoh G, et al. IL-6 triggers cell growth via the Ras-dependent mitogen-activated protein kinase cascade. J Immunol 1997;159(5):2212–2221.

Oshiro MM, Landowski TH, Catlett-Falcone R, et al. Inhibition of JAK kinase activity enhances Fas-mediated apoptosis but reduces cytotoxic activity of topoisomerase II inhibitors in U266 myeloma cells. Clin Cancer Res 2001;7(12):4262–4271.

Panaretakis T, Pokrovskajo K, Shoshan MC, Grander D. Activation of Bak, Bax, and BH3-only proteins in the apoptotic response to doxoxrubicin. J Biol Chem 2002;277(46):44,317–44,326.

Panka DJ, Mano T, Suhara T, Walsh K, Mier JW. Phosphatidylinositol-3 Kinase/Akt activity regulates c-FLIP expression in tumor cells. J Biol Chem 2001;276(10):6893–6896.

Pollett JB, Trudel S, Stern D, Li ZH, Stewart AK. Overexpression of the myeloma-associated oncogene fibroblast growth factor receptor 3 confers dexamethasone resistance. Blood 2002;100(10):3819–3821.

Ronchetti D, Greco A, Compasso S, et al. Deregulated FGFR3 mutants in multiple myeloma cell lines with t(4;14): comparative analysis of Y373C, K650E, and the novel G384D mutations. Oncogene 2001; 20(27):3553–3562.

Salgia R, Avraham S, Pisick E, et al. The related adhesion focal tyrosine kinase forms a complex with paxillin in hematopoietic cells. J Biol Chem 1996;271(49):31,222–31,226.

Santra M, Zahn F, Tian E, Barlogie B, Shaughnessy J. A subset of multiple myeloma harboring the t(4:14)(p16:q32) translocation lackes FGFR3 expression but maintains as IGH.MMSET fusion transcript. Blood 2003;101(6):2374–2376.

Salvesen GS, Duckett CS. IAP proteins: blocking the road to death's door. Nat Rev Mol Cell Biol 2002;3(6):401–410.

Schlapbach R, Spanaus KS, Malipiero U, et al. TGF-beta induces the expression of the FLICE-inhibitory protein and inhibits Fas-mediated apoptosis of microglia. Eur J Immunol 2000;30(12):3680–3688.

Sieg DJ, Ilic D, Jones KC, Damsky CH, Hunter T, Schlaepfer DD. Pyk2 and Src-family protein-tyrosine kinases compensate for the loss of FAK in fibronectin-stimulated signaling events but Pyk2 does not fully function to enhance FAK- cell migration. EMBO J 1998;17(20):5933–5947.

Shain KH, Dalton WS. Cell adhesion is a key determinant in de novo multidrug resistance (MDR): new tagets for the prevention of aquired MDR. Mol Cancer Ther 2001;1(1):69–78.

Shain KH, Landowski TH, Dalton WS. Adhesion-mediated intracellular redistribution of c-FLIP-long confers resistance to CD95-induced apoptosis in hematopoietic cancer cell lines. J Immunol 2002;168(5): 2544–2553.

Shou Y, Martelli ML, Gabrea A, et al. Diverse karyotypic abnormalities of the c-myc locus associated with c-myc dysregulation and tumor progression in multiple myeloma. Proc Natl Acad Sci USA 2000;97(1): 228–233.

Sonneveld P. Drug resistance in multiple myeloma. Pathol Biol (Paris) 1999;47(2):182–187.

Uchida T, Kinoshita T, Ohno T, Ohashi H, Nagai H, Saito H. Hypermethylation of p16/INK4A gene promoter during the progression of plasma cell dycrasia. Leukemia 2001;15(1):157–165.

Urashima M, Ogata A, Chauhan D, et al. Transforming growth factor-beta1: differential effects on multiple myeloma versus normal B cells. Blood 1996;87(5):1928–1938.

Vaux DL, Silke J. Mammalian mitochondrial IAP binding proteins. Biochem Biophys Res Commun 2003;304(3):499–504.

Vincent T, Molina L, Espert L, Mechti N. Hyaluron, a major non-protein glycosaminoglycan component of the extracellular matrix in human bone marrow, mediates dexamethasone resistance in multiple myeloma. Br J Haematol 2003;121(2):259–269.

Xu F, Gardner A, Tu Y, Michl P, Prager D, Lichtenstein A. Multiple myeloma cells are protected against dexamethasone-induced apoptosis by insulin-like growth factors. Br J Haematol 1997;97(2):429–440.

Yeh JH, Hsu SC, Han SH, Lai MZ. Mitogen-activated protein kinase kinase antagonized fas-associated death domain protein-mediated apoptosis by induced FLICE-inhibitory protein expression. J Exp Med 1998;188(10):1795–1802.

Zhang Z, Vuori K, Wang H, Reed JC, Ruoslahti E. Integrin activation by R-ras. Cell 1996;85(1):61–69.

84 HIV-1, AIDS, and Related Malignancies

MAUREEN M. GOODENOW AND JAMES J. KOHLER

SUMMARY

HIV type 1 (HIV-1) is a lentivirus that causes the global acquired immunodeficiency disease pandemic. HIV-1 infection of CD4$^+$ lymphocytes and macrophages modulates signal transduction pathways and immune response. Although rarely oncogenic itself, HIV-1 exacerbates clinical disease course in individuals dually infected by HIV-1 and hepatitis C virus, human papilloma virus, Epstein-Barr virus, or human herpesvirus-8. No vaccines or treatments to prevent or cure HIV-1 infection are available. Combinations of antiretroviral drugs reduce perinatal infection and HIV-1 associated morbidity and mortality. Increased survival among HIV-1 infected adults and children could lead to an increase in malignancies owing to chronic immune suppression, coinfection by oncogenic viruses, and/or persistent HIV-1 infection.

Key Words: Antiviral therapy; HIV-1; macrophages; signal transduction; virus–host cell interactions; quasispecies.

HIV-1 EPIDEMIOLOGY

HIV type 1 (HIV-1) is the etiological agent that causes AIDS. HIV-1 infection is a global pandemic afflicting more than 50 million adults, adolescents, and children. HIV-1 is spread primarily by sexual transmission, although maternal-to-child (MTC) transmission, needle sharing, and contaminated blood products also contribute to significant levels of infection. After 20 yr of the epidemic, there is no vaccine to prevent new infections and no cure for individuals once infected by the virus. Effective antiretroviral drugs that reduce significantly perinatal MTC transmission (but not pediatric infection by breast feeding) and control disease progression have been developed. Nonetheless, even prolonged suppression of HIV-1 replication fails to eliminate long-lived infected cells that can persist for years and serve as reservoirs for virus in children and adults. Continued viral replication results in evolution of genetic variants or quasispecies of HIV-1 that can evade drug therapies and immune response.

Although the HIV-1 epidemic extends worldwide, prevalence of infection is highest among populations in subSaharan Africa and other developing countries in Asia, South America, and the Indian subcontinent (Fig. 84-1). Seroprevalence varies dramatically but can reach levels as high as 9% in some countries in subSaharan Africa. A variety of subtypes of HIV-1, designated by

letters A through K, are defined by molecular characteristics of the virus in contrast to traditional classification of viruses based on serotypes. Subtypes of HIV-1 tended initially to be localized in specific countries or regions, but mobility of individuals and recombination between viral subtypes that produces circulating recombinant forms of HIV-1 are contributing to global drifts in virus populations. HIV-2 is genetically related to HIV-1, has a more limited geographic distribution that colocalizes with HIV-1 infection in Western Africa, and causes less aggressive immune suppression.

MOLECULAR VIROLOGY OF HIV-1

HIV-1 is a lentivirus that is similar to, but genetically more complex than, the family of animal and human oncogenic retroviruses. HIV-1 virions contain two copies of a single-stranded RNA genome, which encodes a number of functions that are vital for the virus life cycle (Fig. 84-2A). The *gag*, *pol*, and *env* regions encode a variety of proteins including matrix, capsid, and nucleocapsid required for virion structure; protease, reverse transcriptase (RT), and integrase enzymes that function in virion maturation, synthesis of the DNA form of the virus, and integration of viral DNA into the host cell genome, respectively; and glycoproteins gp120 and gp41, the surface and transmembrane components of the viral envelope (Env) proteins, which mediate infection of target cells that express CD4 and an appropriate coreceptor (Fig. 84-2B). The HIV-1 genome encodes no less than six additional proteins that provide regulatory (Tat and Rev) or accessory (Nef, Vpr, Vif, Vpu) functions. Long terminal repeat (LTR) elements flanking the viral genome regulate reverse transcription and integration. In addition, *cis*-acting transcriptional elements localized in the LTRs regulate expression of the viral genome by host cell mechanisms. Antiretroviral drugs approved for treatment of HIV-1 infection target multiple key steps in the virus life cycle (Fig. 84-3). Entry can be blocked by inhibitors of Env interactions with coreceptors or fusion between virus and host cell. Early steps in virus replication are targeted by a variety of RT inhibitors, whereas late steps in virion maturation that are essential for infectious virus are blocked by PR inhibitors.

HIV-1 IMMUNE DEFICIENCY AND AIDS

HIV-1 affects multiple lineages of hematopoietic cells by direct infection of T lymphocytes, thymocytes, and monocyte/macrophages that coexpress CD4 and CCR5 or CXCR4, chemokine receptors that function as coreceptors for HIV-1. Over time, HIV-1 infection produces significant declines in CD4 T lymphocytes that, in combination

From: *Principles of Molecular Medicine, Second Edition*
Edited by: M. S. Runge and C. Patterson © Humana Press, Inc., Totowa, NJ

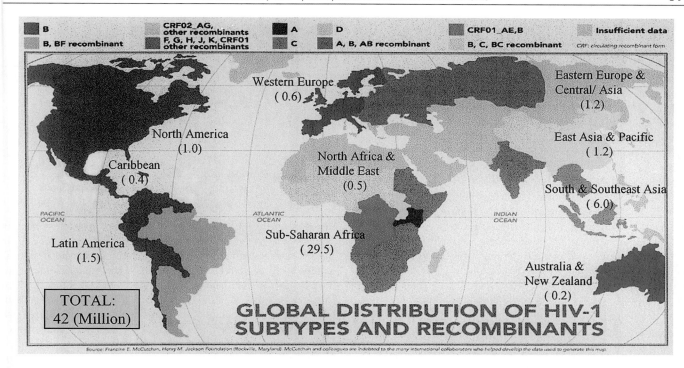

Figure 84-1 Global epidemiology of HIV type 1 subtypes and estimated number of infected individuals (in millions) at the end of 2002 according to the International AIDS Vaccine Initiative and the Joint United Nations Programme on HIV/AIDS. (Please *see* color insert.)

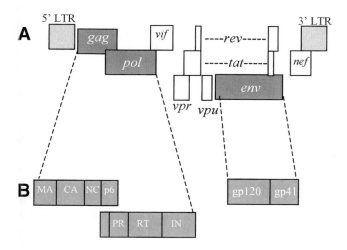

Figure 84-2 **(A)** HIV type-1 genome encodes three structural genes (*gag, pol, env*), in addition to accessory genes (*vif, rev, tat, nef, vpr, vpu*). Long terminal repeat elements flank the genome. **(B)** Gag proteins include matrix, capsid, and nuclear capsid. Pol proteins are protease, RT, and integrase. Envelope glycoproteins include surface gp120 and transmembrane gp41.

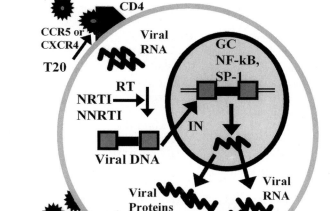

Figure 84-3 HIV type-1 viral life cycle. Virus infection is mediated at the cell surface by interactions between gp120 and receptor complex (CD4 plus CCR5 or CXCR4) on the surface of the host cell. DNA form of virus is a product of RT; integration into host genome is mediated by integrase. Regulation of HIV-1 gene expression involves host cell transcription factors such as glucocorticoid receptor (GC), or NF-κB and SP-1. Immature virions bud from the cell membrane. Processing by protease leads to mature, infectious virions. Inhibitors approved for clinical use include T20 (entry inhibitor, nucleotide and non-nucleoside RT inhibitors (NRTI or NNRTI), and protease inhibitors.

with indirect effects independent of infection of CD8 T cells, B lymphocytes, natural killer cells, and dendritic cells, contribute to global immune disregulation, profound immune dysfunction, and AIDS.

The Centers for Disease Control define AIDS in adults and adolescents by a spectrum of opportunistic infections and a heterogeneous group of malignancies, in particular Kaposi's sarcoma (KS), non-Hodgkin's lymphoma (NHL) including Burkitt's, immunoblastic, and primary brain lymphomas, and invasive cervical carcinoma (ICC). HIV-1 infection increases significantly the risk of developing KS, NHL, or ICC, and can exacerbate hepatocarcinoma and leukemia. Estimates place the occurrence of some type of malignancy in as many as 40% of persons with HIV/AIDS.

Pediatric HIV-1 disease is also accompanied by a significant increase in malignancies. Between 1981 and 1996, approx 2% of children with AIDS in the United States developed cancer. In contrast to adults, HIV-1 infected children present a somewhat different spectrum of malignancies. For example, NHL was the predominant malignancy among children with HIV-1 infection in a large multi-center case-control study. KS is the AIDS defining tumor in only a small number of children in the United States, but is highly associated with pediatric HIV infection among African children.

Non-AIDS-defining malignancies, including lung, skin, head and neck, conjunctival, testicular, hepatic, and breast cancers, as well as multiple myeloma, leukemia, and leiomyosarcomas, also increase morbidity and mortality among HIV-1 infected individuals with AIDS. Leiomyosarcomas (smooth muscle tumors) and lymphoproliferative disorders, which could progress to malignancy, appear more frequently in children than adults.

Epidemiology of AIDS and non-AIDS related malignancies differs significantly between developed and developing countries. A variety of environmental and economic factors could contribute to geographical differences. In addition, any association that might occur between different HIV-1 subtypes or circulating recombinant forms of HIV-1 and malignancies is unknown.

ETIOLOGY OF MALIGNANCIES ASSOCIATED WITH AIDS

HIV-1 can with low frequency contribute directly by insertional mutagenesis into a region of c-*fes* proto-oncogene to development of malignancy in some T-cell lymphomas and in macrophages in non-T-cell lymphomas. For the most part, herpesviruses are major etiological agents of human AIDS-defining malignancies (Table 84-1). Human herpesvirus-8 (HHV-8) infection contributes to increased risk for KS; Epstein-Barr virus (EBV) infection increases risk for NHL, including primary brain lymphomas and leiomyosarcomas in children; and cervical infection by high-risk human papilloma viruses (HPVs) increases risk for ICC among HIV-1 or HIV-2 infected women worldwide. A subset of human malignancies associated with HIV-1 infection involves coinfection by other viruses. For example, hepatitis C virus (HCV) infection increases the risk for hepatic carcinoma, whereas two types of human T-cell leukemia viruses (HTLV-1 and HTLV-2) contribute to leukemia/lymphomas. Coinfection by oncogenic viruses and HIV-1 is facilitated by the high prevalence of the viruses in similar geographic locations, by similar modes of transmission of the viruses, and the impact of HIV-1 related immune dysfunction on susceptibility to infection and disease progression by at least some of the oncogenic viruses.

ANTIRETROVIRAL THERAPY AND HIV-ASSOCIATED MALIGNANCY

Immune deficiency caused by chronic HIV-1 infection is a significant variable for risk of malignancy. Effective antiretroviral therapy (ART) for control of HIV-1 infection involves inhibitors that target RT, either alone or in combination with PR. No evidence implicates RT or PR inhibitors directly with increased risk for malignancy, as many of the studies of HIV-associated cancer risk were performed prior to widespread use of ART. Exposure

Table 84-1
Viral-Induced Malignancies Associated With HIV

Virus	AIDS-defining malignancies
EBV	NHL
	Hodgkin's disease
	Leiomyosarcoma
	CNS/Brain lymphomas
HHV-8	KS
HPV	Squamous cell neoplasia
	AIDS-associated malignancies
HCV	Hepatocellular carcinoma
Human T-cell leukemia virus	HTLV-1 associated myelopathy
	Tropical spastic paraparesis

in utero to zidovudine, one of the RT inhibitors that reduce significantly MTC transmission, provides no discernible risk factor for development of malignancies in children. Indeed, reduction and sustained control of HIV-1 viral burden by ART can result in reversal of immune suppression and a concomitant decline in risk for HIV/AIDS-related malignancies. For example, incidence of KS is exquisitely sensitive to immune deficiency and decreased significantly by ART. Incidence of NHL, including CNS or primary brain lymphoma, also decreases but requires longer periods of ART, implicating immune suppression as a risk factor. NHL is actually a heterogeneous group of malignancies, which could account for some reports that NHL is not markedly decreased by ART or that some HIV-1 infected individuals develop NHL despite suppressed viral replication and high CD4 T-cell counts. ART has no impact on high-risk HPV infection or development of cervical cancer, implying that factors unrelated to immune suppression or associated with processes independent of ART may contribute to some AIDS-related malignancies.

HIV INFECTION AND IMPACT ON SIGNALING CASCADES

HIV has direct and indirect impact on CD4+ cells of the lymphocytic and monocyte/macrophage lineages (Table 84-2). Infection of macrophages by HIV-1 is correlated with progressive functional impairments, which include defects in chemotaxis, cytokine production, expression of surface proteins, and antigen processing and presentation. HIV-1 blocks the transcription of major histocompatibility class II determinants, which has a significant immunosuppressive effect on macrophages. HIV-1 Tat protein can compete with class II transactivator binding and subsequently block the expression of major histocompatibility class II genes. Specifically, cyclin T1 together with CDK9 forms the positive transcription elongation factor b complex, which binds to class II transactivator and can also bind to the activation domain of Tat.

HIV alters a variety of signal transduction pathways at multiple stages in infection. Beginning with entry, binding of gp120 to CD4 plus the chemokine receptors CCR5 or CXCR4 results in activation of intracellular protein tyrosine kinases. Presumably, binding of Env glycoproteins to the receptor complex can mimic binding of ligands, and result in activation of heterotrimeric G proteins, calcium fluxes, and tyrsosine phosphorylation of Pyk2, phosphatidylinositol-3-kinase, and the Ras-independent Lck/Raf-1 signaling pathway that leads to the MEK/ERK pathway. Microarray studies demonstrate global activation with overexpression of c-jun, JNK, MEK,

Table 84-2
Viral Proteins and Their Cellular Targets

Virus	Viral protein	Target cell	Cellular targets
HIV-1	Env gp120	CD4+ lymphocytes	Protein tyrosine kinases, calcium fluxes
		Macrophages	Pyk2 phosphorylation; PI3; MEK/ERK pathway; STAT1, STAT3, STAT5; caspase-3 activation
	Nef	CD4+ lymphocytes	Calcium signaling; activate NFAT, c-*fos*, Jun-D
		Macrophages	TGF-β, IL-4, MIP-1α, MIP-1β
	Vpr	CD4+ lymphocytes	cAMP response element, G_2 arrest
	Tat	Monocytes	TNF-α, bFGF signaling pathways, type-IV collagenase
HHV-8	Homologs of IL-8 (vGPCR), bcl-2, IL-1, NCAMs	Endothelial-type cells	Cell proliferation, activation cascades, antiapoptosis signals, NF-AT
EBV	LMP1	B-lymphoid epithelial	Adhesion molecules, transferring receptor, TGF-β sensitivity, bcl-2 oncogene, CD40-CD40L signaling, NF-κB activation
	LMP2α/B	B cells	Inhibit lyn and syk kinases
	Unknown	Monocytes	Proapoptotic signaling
	Unknown	Dendritic cells	Inhibit DC development
HPV	E6	Keratinocytes, epithelial cells	P53 tumor suppressor activates TERT gene, IL-8 repression
	E7	Epithelial cells	p-RB, pCAF acetyltransferase, IL-8 repression
HCV	HCV core	Hepatocytes	Suppress immune response
		Macrophages	Reduce IFN-γ, IL-2
		Lymphocytes	Fas-mediated apoptosis
	NS5A	Lymphocytes	Inhibit PKR; phosphorylation of eIF-2α; CDK inhibitor p21/waf1; STAT2 activation; NF-κB, IFN-γ responsive genes
HTLV	Tax	T lymphocytes	Cytokine independent growth; transactivates NF-κB, CREB, cyclin D2, CDK2, p21; blocks G_1/S and G_2/M checkpoints; Jak1, Jak3, STAT3, STAT5, MIP-1α, C-C chemokine 3, IFN-γ, GM-CSF

DC, dendritic cell; FGF, fibroblast growth factor; GM-CSF, granulocyte-macrophage colony-stimulating factor; IFN, interferon; IL, interleukin; MIP, macrophage inflammatory protein; NCAM, neural cell adhesion molecules; NF, nuclear factor; TGF, transforming growth factor; TNF, tumor necrosis factor.

p38 MAPK, STAT, and JAK induced in HIV infected cells. Thus, HIV-1 entry into target cells modulates cellular signaling that may be necessary for replication or occur as a consequence of infection.

Gp120 induces not one, but at least three different STATs (STAT1, STAT3, and STAT5), with significant implications. First, each activated STAT represents a highly specific pathway that results in regulation of expression of a set of genes. Secondly, constitutive activation of STAT1, STAT3, and STAT5 is associated with malignant transformation induced by various oncoproteins. Cellular activation that is induced by HIV-1 precludes apoptosis. For example, envelope-mediated induction of infectious virus from purified resting CD4+ T cells occurs without the induction of classic markers of T-cell activation or progression through the cell cycle. Impairment of cell-cycle progression may occur in part through HIV-induced activation of caspase-3 and cleavage of focal adhesion kinase. Intracellular signals resulting from HIV-1 envelope may have immunopathogenic consequences including anergy, syncytium formation, apoptosis, and inappropriate cell trafficking. Activation of STAT regulated genes provides a model for interactions by HIV-1 and oncogenic viruses coinfection in development of malignancies.

In addition to the influences of Env, Nef, Vpr, and Tat proteins can also affect host cell signaling pathways. Specifically, Nef stimulates calcium signaling to activate transcription factors such as nuclear factor of activated T (NFAT) cells, nuclear factor-κB (NF-κB), IRF-1, IRF-2, c-Fos, and Jun-D, which positively regulate the viral LTR regulatory domain. In addition, several cytokines,

including transforming growth factor (TGF)-β and IL-4, together with the chemokines macrophage inflammatory protein (MIP)-1α and MIP-1β are upregulated by Nef in macrophages. Vpr can cooperate with Nef in NFAT-directed gene expression and upregulation of cAMP response element-directed transcription that may act by stabilizing interactions with CREB. Vpr also induces G2 arrest of lymphocytes through specific changes in gene expression patterns that differ from simple activation of stress response or cytokine response pathways. HIV Tat protein is secreted by infected cells, can act on other cells, independent of infection, and induces tumor necrosis factor (TNF)-α in human monocytes through protein kinase C and calcium pathways. HIV-1 Tat can enhance the endothelial cell growth and type-IV collagenase expression in response to basic fibroblast growth factor to induce KS-like lesions in transgenic mice.

Although HIV-1 infection alone is rarely oncogenic, the profound effects on host immunity, signal cascades, and gene expression could contribute to increased prevalence of malignancies because of coinfection with oncogenic viruses.

VIRUSES INVOLVED IN AIDS-DEFINING MALIGNANCIES

HUMAN HERPESVIRUS-8 The etiological agent of KS is HHV-8, also known as KS herpesvirus. HHV-8 is a double-stranded DNA virus that is a member of the γ-herpesvirus family, which also includes EBV. HHV-8 seroprevalence exceeds 40% among some populations in the regions surrounding the Mediterranean and in sub-Saharan Africa where KS is endemic. In North America, northern Europe, Southeast Asia, and the Caribbean, where incidence of KS is low, seroprevalence ranges from less than 1% to approx 20%. HHV-8 infection can be detected in neonates and seroprevalence among children tends to be somewhat lower than in adults, but increases with age prior to puberty. Pediatric infection would indicate that HHV-8 can be transmitted not only by sexual activity and blood, but also by maternal transmission and close family contacts among siblings.

Seroprevalence among individuals with HHV-8 associated disease, including KS, primary effusion lymphoma (a rare B-cell lymphoma), and multicentric Castleman's disease, can be as high as 100%. HHV-8 malignancies are highly sensitive to host immune suppression, particularly related to HIV-1 infection or transplantation, but not to HIV-2 infection. Seroprevalence of HHV-8 increases in HIV-1 infected individuals with KS, whereas HHV-8 viremia and HIV-1 infection are significant risk factors for developing KS.

HHV-8 has a genome of approx 165 kb and encodes a remarkable number of proteins with functional homology to host cell genes that regulate cell proliferation, activation, and survival (*see* Table 84-2). For example, the HHV-8 genome includes homologies to human cyclin D, an IL-8-like G protein coupled receptor (vGPCR), bcl-2, no less than three chemokines, a variety of cytokines related to IL-1 and interferon (IFN) regulatory factors, as well as complement-binding proteins and neural cell adhesion molecule-like adhesion molecules. KS is a complex malignancy included spindle-formed cells expressing endothelial cell markers, newly formed blood vessels, and infiltrates of cells with characteristics of smooth muscle cells, macrophages, or dendritic cells. Only a minor subset of cells in a KS lesion express viral genes leading to a paracrine model of tumorigenesis in which expression of viral gene products by some cells affects regulation of surrounding cells. A paracrine mechanism could also provide a model for synergy between HIV-1 and HHV-8 infection in view of the different host cells targeted by each virus. Consistent with this model, HIV-1 Tat protein is secreted by infected cells, activates KS cell growth, and can collaborate with HHV-8 vGPCR protein to activate NFAT, a transcription factor expressed by a variety of cell types that is involved in regulation of expression of cytokine and adhesion molecule genes.

EPSTEIN-BARR VIRUS EBV is an ubiquitous human γ-herpesvirus that infects more than 90% of the world's population. Although infection is generally subclinical, EBV causes infectious mononucleosis and lymphoproliferative disorders in immunologically compromised individuals. EBV is etiologically linked to human malignancies involving lymphoid and epithelial cell origin, including Burkitt's lymphoma, T-cell lymphoma, nasopharyngeal carcinoma, post-transplant lymphoma, AIDS-associated lymphomas, parotid gland carcinoma, and gastric carcinoma. EBV strains are classified as type 1 or type 2, based on major sequence differences in the EBV nuclear antigen 2 (EBNA-2) and EBNA-3C genes. Type-1 EBV shows more potent transforming efficiency in vitro than type 2 and appears to predominate in the general Caucasian and Asian populations. Type-2 infection is more prevalent in immunocompromised patients; and both types are relatively common in equatorial Africa and New Guinea.

Several lines of evidence implicate a close association between HIV-induced immune suppression and EBV-associated lymphomas. Compared to healthy individuals, HIV-1 infected subjects usually have a higher EBV viral load and/or number of EBV-infected cells both in the peripheral blood compartment and lymphoid tissues. Expansion of EBV-positive B cells is probably because of chronic B-cell stimulation driven by HIV-1 antigens (especially in ART-treated individuals that results in increased CD4+ immune cells but the continuance of a high viral load) and an impaired immunosurveillance against EBV. Individuals newly diagnosed with Hodgkin's lymphoma demonstrate stronger EBV association together with poorer survival and more aggressive clinical characteristics. EBV is responsible for lymphoproliferative disorders including cases of Burkitt's lymphoma in Africa, and is associated with higher frequencies of T-cell activation and IL-4-producing cells in the periphery, and higher susceptibility to activation-induced apoptosis. High viral burden with EBV is associated with the development of malignancy in HIV-infected children. In addition, EBV has a causal role in the oncogenesis of smooth muscle tumors (leiomyosarcomas), which represent the second most prevalent malignancy of children with AIDS. An association between some EBV tumors and immune suppression stresses the importance of immune responses in keeping a balance between the oncogenic virus and the infected host.

EBV binding to monocytes influences the differentiation stage of monocytes and inhibits development of dendritic cells from monocyte precursors by a unique interference that is independent of *de novo* synthesis of viral proteins or mRNAs. More specifically, exposure to EBV induces proapoptotic signaling in monocytes, which correlates with an aberrant response to both granulocyte-macrophage colony-stimulating factor and IL-4.

Genetic analyses define the genes of EBV that are essential for B-lymphocyte transformation and their potential functions and biochemical properties (*see* Table 84-2). The EBV genome encodes a unique set of latent genes designated as latent membrane proteins (LMP)-1, 2A and 2B that confer oncogenic potential and the ability to induce immortalization of B-lymphocytes in vitro. Globally, LMP1 has oncogenic properties that alter the phenotype of B-cell activation antigens, adhesion molecules, transferrin receptor and sensitivity to TGF-β, whereas inhibiting apoptosis through the induction of expression of *bcl*-2 oncogene. In addition, LMP1 mimics the signaling pathways that are activated by CD40-CD40L interaction, resulting in the activation of NF-κB. In fact, an increased ability of LMP1 variants to activate NF-κB is correlated with advanced nasopharyngeal carcinoma cases. Host cell factors, such as STAT genes, could influence the switch to latent, transforming gene expression of LMP1 and cellular proliferation.

LMP2 proteins exist in two forms, LMP2A and 2B, as a result of alternatively spliced mRNAs that contain exons located at both ends of the linear EBV genome. LMP2A has a 119 amino acid N-terminal cytoplasmic domain that contains an immunoreceptor-tyrosine-based activation motif. In B and T cells, cellular immunoreceptor-tyrosine-based activation motif s functionally bind Lyn and Syk kinases leading to activation of multiple signal transduction cascades. However, LMP2A can competitively sequester and degrade Lyn and Syk kinases, thereby inhibiting lymphoctye activation.

HUMAN PAPILLOMA VIRUSES HPV is a group of DNA tumor virus related to simian virus 40 and other polyomaviruses. HPVs are sexually transmitted and certain types of HCV are the etiological agent of cervical intraepithelial neoplasia (CIN), the precursor of cervical cancer, as well as ICC. Greater than 90% of CIN and ICC in women worldwide contain HPV DNA. Infection by HIV-1 leads to a higher prevalence and prolonged persistence of cervical HPV infection, increased levels of HPV, and increased incidence of high grade CIN. Although HIV-1 infection and immune suppression are associated with overall prevalence of HPV, effective ART for HIV-1 fails to diminish the prevalence or pathogenesis of HPV.

HPV is classified into more than 90 different types, which present low- or high-risk for development of neoplasia. High-risk types are predominantly HPV 16, 18, 31, and 45, although HPV 16 is by far the most prevalent in premalignant CIN and occurs in about half of ICC. In addition, risk analysis indicates that HPV 26, 53, and 66, previously typed as low risk, should be classified as high-risk types. Prevalent and incident detection of HPV 16, unlike other types of HPV, displays only a weak association with immune status among HIV-1 seropositive women, raising the possibility that HPV 16 avoids host immunity, which would contribute to the significant relationship between this HPV 16 and malignancy.

High-risk HPV genomes encode two early proteins, E6 and E7 that are expressed concurrently, effect growth control of infected cells, and contribute to immortalization and transformation of a variety of cells, including keratinocytes and epithelial cells, by a variety of mechanisms (see Table 84-2). The HPV 16 E6 oncoprotein is 151 amino acids, contains two zinc-finger motifs, and binds to p53 tumor suppressor protein that activates p53 degradation by a ubiquitin-dependent pathway. E6 also activates expression of the TERT gene that encodes the catalytic subunit of the telomerase enzyme, which maintains chromosomal telomere length and inhibits senescence. HPV E7 is a multifunctional, 98-amino acid phosphoprotein. E7 binding to pRB, a tumor suppressor protein, releases transcription factors that promote progression of cells through the G1/S boundary into S-phase of the cell cycle. E7 also interacts with p300/CBP-associated factor acetyltransferase, a coactivator for a variety of transcription factors, including p53. In addition to functions as oncoproteins, HPV 16 E6 and E7 cooperatively repress IL-8 transcription. IL-8 is an inflammatory chemokine involved in initiation of local immune responses. Repression of IL-8 gene expression could contribute to HPV escape from immune surveillance.

The host cell range for HIV-1 and HPV differ, making direct effects by HIV-1 an unlikely explanation for increased HPV pathogenesis. More likely, the overall impact by HIV-1 on cytokines and factors modulates the cellular milieu to favor HPV replication and/or progression of HPV-mediated initiation of premalignant lesions.

VIRUSES INVOLVED IN AIDS-ASSOCIATED MALIGNANCIES

HEPATITIS C VIRUS HCV is a significant public health concern, affecting more than 170 million people worldwide and approx 4 million Americans. HCV causes chronic hepatitis, which can progress to cirrhosis and hepatocellular carcinoma, the fifth most common cancer in the world. Coinfection with HCV in HIV-infected persons occurs frequently as these viruses share routes of transmission and target cells. In the United States alone, 20–25% of HIV-1 infected people are estimated to be coinfected with HCV, whereas worldwide, 6.5–13 million individuals are estimated to be coinfected with HCV and HIV. The prevalence of chronic HCV infection is more than 50% among HIV-infected intravenous drug users. Effective ART and prolonged chronic HIV disease state increases HCV-related morbidity and mortality. Although HIV and HCV can be transmitted by percutaneous exposure to blood,

through sexual intercourse, and from mother to child, relative efficiency of transmission by these routes varies. HCV, for example, is reportedly 10 times more infectious than HIV through percutaneous blood exposures.

HCV has little known effect on HIV disease, but infection with HIV adversely affects the outcome of hepatitis C infection, resulting in higher HCV RNA viral load and accelerated hepatopathology. HIV-associated decline in CD4$^+$ T helper lymphocytes and defective CD4$^+$ proliferation and apoptosis constitute critical factors of immunosuppression that correlate with ineffective host immune response to HCV and progression to end-stage liver disease. Interestingly, HCV/HIV coinfection results in decreased response to IFN therapy, although IFN therapy has protective effects against HCV-related cirrhosis independent of the patient's HIV status.

ART-associated hepatotoxicity can diminish effectiveness of HIV therapy and cause significant morbidity and mortality. Drug-induced hepatotoxicity may be more common among persons with HIV–HCV coinfection who are receiving PR inhibitors. Enhanced drug-induced hepatotoxicity among individuals coinfected with HIV and HCV may result from decreased drug metabolism, or increased susceptibility to mitochondrial dysfunction.

In addition to hepatocytes, various immune cells including macrophages, B cells, and T cells support HCV replication. HCV core protein is the first protein expressed during the early phase of infection (see Table 84-2). Through Fas-binding, HCV augments signaling mediated through caspase-3 activity, which increases susceptibility to Fas-mediated apoptosis. Therefore, HCV core protein has a demonstrated effect on immune responsiveness.

A late stage, nonstructural protein 5A (NS5A) is a serine phosphoprotein that binds and inhibits the homodimerization and kinase activity of the double-stranded RNA-dependent protein kinase, a major intracellular enzyme that mediates the antiviral action of IFN, phosphorylation of eIF-2α, and the attenuation of cellular protein synthesis. Furthermore, NS5A protein downregulates transcription of cell-cycle regulatory genes (i.e., the cyclin-dependent kinase inhibitor p21/waf1 gene) and mediates activation of transcription factors including STAT-3 and NF-κB. Arguably, NF-κB and/or STAT-3 may regulate gene expression of survival factors to further promote an antiapoptotic environment in the cells and favor oncogenesis.

HUMAN T-CELL LEUKEMIA VIRUS HTLV type 1 (HTLV-1) is a retrovirus that serves as the etiological agent for adult T-cell leukemia and the neurological disorder HTLV-1 associated myelopathy/tropical spastic paraparesis. HTLV-1 mediates transformation or transition from a cytokine-dependent to an independent phase of growth through its virally encoded 40 kDa regulatory phosphoprotein, Tax (see Table 84-2). Tax transactivates cellular genes driven by transcription factors such as CREB, NF-κB, and serum response factor. In addition, Tax alters expression of cell-cycle regulatory proteins, upregulating cyclin D2, cyclin E, CDK2, CDK4, CDK6, and p21$^{Waf1/Cip1/Sdi1}$, and downregulating cyclin D3 and p18. Thus, Tax blocks the G$_1$/S and G$_2$/M cell-cycle check points, linking Tax expression to chromosomal abnormalities and abnormal cell division. Upregulation of p21 results in at least two independent mechanisms of regulation: the enhancement of NF-κB activation and/or CREB signaling, and the excitation of antiapoptotic machinery. Further evidence suggests that HTLV-1-transformed T cells become functionally redundant for proliferation through the Jak3-STAT5 pathway, as AG-490 treatment has no effect on Jak3/STAT5 activation. In fact, Jak1, Jak3, and STATs

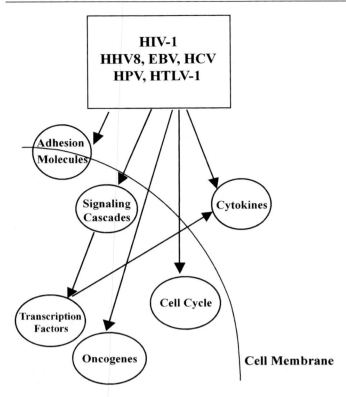

Figure 84-4 Cellular pathways induced by HIV type 1 and associated oncogenic viruses. HHV-8, human herpesvirus-8; EBV, Epstein-Barr virus; HCV, hepatitis C virus; HPV, human papilloma virus; HTLV-1, human T-cell leukemia viruses.

3 and 5 are constitutively activated in HTLV-1-transformed cells, rendering infected peripheral blood T cells IL-2 independent.

HTLV type 2 (HTLV-2) is endemic in some native American Indian and African tribes and has a high prevalence among HIV-1 infected individuals. HTLV-2 infection can potentially interfere with the replicative capacity of HIV-1 by upregulating the secretion of HIV-1 suppressive chemokines, in particular, C-C chemokine ligand 3/macrophage-inflammatory protein-1α (MIП-1α). HTLV-2 induces the secretion of IFN-g and granulocyte-macrophage colony stimulating factor, which in turn results in the activation of STAT1 or STAT5, respectively.

CONCLUSIONS

HIV-1 infection leads to immune dysfunction by multiple mechanisms that extend beyond attrition of CD4 T lymphocytes. Interactions by viral proteins with signal transducing and gene expression pathways may be necessary for HIV-1 replication or a consequence of infection. Nevertheless, the outcomes of HIV infection can modulate the cellular environment to promote malignancy by coinfecting oncogenic viruses (Fig. 84-4).

Increased survival by HIV-1 infected adults and children could lead to an increase in malignancies, because of chronic immune suppression, coinfection with oncogenic viruses, and/or persistent HIV-1 infection. Chemotherapy treatments of malignancies in HIV-1 infected children and adults are complicated by potential interactions with antiretroviral drugs, novel toxicities, metabolic abnormalities associated with ART, and immune suppression caused by HIV-1, as well as limited direct data for many drugs

about dose and indications for use in pediatric patients. Even mild immunosuppression is associated with decreased ability to control HPV, which could have implications for treatment of women by ART that prolongs life, but increases by years mild immunosuppression and risk of HPV-associated neoplasia and ICC. Certainly management of individuals with HIV infection and malignancies needs to be examined. Continued surveillance of HIV-1 infected individuals throughout the world is imperative to identify any changes in prevalence of malignancies.

ACKNOWLEDGMENTS

Authors acknowledge funding from PHS R01 awards HD032259, AI065265, AI047723; T32 CA09126; American Foundation for AIDS Research; University of Florida Center for Research for Pediatric Immune Deficiency; Stephany W. Holloway University Chair for AIDS Research.

SELECTED REFERENCES

Castro K, Ward J, Slutsker L, et al. 1993 revised classification system for HIV infection and expanded surveillance case definition for AIDS among adolescents and adults. MMWR 1992;41:1–19.

Ablashi DV, Chatlynne LG, Whitman JE Jr, Cesarman E. Spectrum of Kaposi's sarcoma-associated herpesvirus, or human herpesvirus 8, diseases. Clin Microbiol Rev 2002;15:439–464.

Aquaro S, Calio R, Balzarini J, Bellocchi MC, Garaci E, Perno CF. Macrophages and HIV infection: therapeutical approaches toward this strategic virus reservoir. Antiviral Res 2002;55:209–225.

Arendt CW, Littman DR. HIV: master of the host cell. Genome Biol 2001;2:1030.1–1030.4.

Ariyoshi K, Schim vdL, Cook P, et al. Kaposi's sarcoma in the Gambia, West Africa is less frequent in human immunodeficiency virus type 2 than in human immunodeficiency virus type 1 infection despite a high prevalence of human herpesvirus 8. J Hum Virol 1998;1:193–199.

Barillari G, Sgadari C, Palladino C, et al. Inflammatory cytokines synergize with the HIV-1 Tat protein to promote angiogenesis and Kaposi's sarcoma via induction of basic fibroblast growth factor and the alpha v beta 3 integrin. J Immunol 1999;163:1929–1935.

Benekli M, Baer MR, Baumnan H, Wetzler M. Signal transducer and activator of transcription proteins in leukemias. Blood 2003;101:2940–2954.

Benhamou Y, Bochet M, Di Martino V, et al. Liver fibrosis progression in human immunodeficiency virus and hepatitis C virus coinfected patients. Hepatology 1999;30:1054–1058.

Bennasser Y, Badou A, Tkaczuk J, Bahraoui E. Signaling pathways triggered by HIV-1 Tat in human monocytes to induce TNF-a. Virology 2002;303:174–180.

Berretta M, Cinelli R, Martellotta F, Spina M, Vaccher E, Tirelli U. Therapeutic approaches to AIDS-related malignancies. Oncogene 2003; 22:6646–6659.

Biggar RJ, Frisch M. Estimating the risk of cancer in children with AIDS. JAMA 2000;284:2593–2594.

Blankson JN, Persaud D, Siliciano RF. The challenge of viral reservoirs in HIV-1 infection. Annu Rev Med 2002;53:557–593.

Blattner WA. Human retroviruses: their role in cancer. Proc Assoc Am Physicians 1999;111:563–572.

Boshoff C, Chang Y. Kaposi's sarcoma-associated herpesvirus: a new DNA tumor virus. Annu Rev Med 2001;52:453–470.

Bovolenta C, Camorali L, Lorini A, et al. Constitutive activation of STATs upon in vivo human immunodeficiency virus infection. Blood 1999; 94:4202–4209.

Bovolenta C, Pilotti E, Mauri M, et al. Retroviral interference on STAT activation in individuals coinfected with human T cell leukemia virus type 2 and HIV-1. J Immunol 2002;169:4443–4449.

Bowman T, Garcia R, Turkson J, Jove R. STATs in oncogenesis. Oncogene 2000;19:2474–2488.

Brayfield BP, Phiri S, Kankasa C, et al. Postnatal human herpesvirus 8 and human immunodeficiency virus type 1 infection in mothers and infants from Zambia. J Infect Dis 2003;187:559–568.

Casoli C, Vicenzi E, Cimarelli A, et al. HTLV-II down-regulates HIV-1 replication in IL-2-stimulated primary PBMC of coinfected individuals through expression of MIP-1alpha. Blood 2000;95:2760–2769.

Centers for Disease Control and Prevention. Revised classification system for human immunodeficiency virus infection in children less than 13 years of age. MMWR Morb Mortal Wkly Rep 1994;43:1–12.

Centers for Disease Control and Prevention. Updated U.S. public health service guidelines for the management of occupational exposures to HBV, HCV, and HIV and recommendations for post-exposure prophylaxis. MMWR Morb Mortal Wkly Rep 2001;50:1–52.

Cesarman E, Mesri EA, Gershengorn MC. Viral G protein-coupled receptor and Kaposi's sarcoma: a model of paracrine neoplasia? J Exp Med 2000;191:417–422.

Chan SW, Blackburn EH. New ways not to make ends meet: telomerase, DNA damage proteins and heterochromatin. Oncogene 2002;21:553–563.

Chen S, Tuttle DL, Oshier JT, et al. Transforming growth factor-β1 increases CXCR4 expression, stromal-derived factor-1α-stimulated signaling and human immunodeficiency virus-1 entry in human monocyte-derived macrophages. Immunol 2005;114:565–574.

Chiao EY, Krown SE. Update on non-acquired immunodeficiency syndrome-defining malignancies. Curr Opin Oncol 2003;15:389–397.

Cicala C, Arthos J, Ruiz M, et al. Induction of phosphorylation and intracellular association of CC chemokine receptor 5 and focal adhesion kinase in primary human CD4+ T cells by macrophage-tropic HIV envelope. J Immunol 1999;163:420–426.

Cicala C, Arthos J, Selig SM, et al. HIV envelope induces a cascade of cell signals in non-proliferating target cells that favor virus replication. Proc Natl Acad Sci USA 2002;99:9380–9385.

Coberley CR, Kohler JJ, Brown JN, et al. Impact on genetic networks in human macrophages by a CCR5 strain of human immunodeficiency virus type 1. J Virol 2004;78:11477–11486.

Connor EM, Sperling RS, Gelber R, et al. Reduction of maternal-infant transmission of human immunodeficiency virus type 1 with zidovudine treatment. Pediatric AIDS Clinical Trials Group Protocol 076 Study Group. N Engl J Med 1994;331:1173–1180.

Critchlow CW, Hawes SE, Kuypers JM, et al. Effect of HIV infection on the natural history of anal human papillomavirus infection. AIDS 1998;12:1177–1184.

Davis CB, Dikic I, Unutmaz D, et al. Signal transduction due to HIV-1 envelope interactions with chemokine receptors CXCR4 or CCR5. J Exp Med 1997;186:1793–1798.

Dean M, Jacobson LP, McFarlane G, et al. Reduced risk of AIDS lymphoma in individuals heterozygous for the CCR5-delta32 mutation. Cancer Res 1999;59:3561–3564.

Di M, Rufat P, Boyer N, et al. The influence of human immunodeficiency virus coinfection on chronic hepatitis C in injection drug users: A long-term retrospective cohort study. Hepatology 2001;34: 1193–1199.

Dukers NH, Rezza G. Human herpesvirus 8 epidemiology: what we do and do not know. AIDS 2003;17:1717–1730.

Dyson N, Guida P, Munger K, Harlow E. Homologous sequences in adenovirus E1A and human papillomavirus E7 proteins mediate interaction with the same set of cellular proteins. J Virol 1992;66:6893–6902.

Engels EA, Biggar RJ, Marshall VA, et al. Detection and quantification of Kaposi's sarcoma-associated herpesvirus to predict AIDS-associated Kaposi's sarcoma. AIDS 2003;17:1847–1851.

Ensoli B, Buonaguro L, Barillari G, et al. Release, uptake, and effects of extracellular human immunodeficiency virus type 1 Tat protein on cell growth and viral transactivation. J Virol 1993;67:277–287.

Ensoli B, Gendelman R, Markham P, et al. Synergy between basic fibroblast growth factor and HIV-1 Tat protein in induction of Kaposi's sarcoma. Nature 1994;371:674–680.

Fassone L, Cingolani A, Martini M, et al. Characterization of Epstein-Barr virus genotype in AIDS-related non-Hodgkin's lymphoma. AIDS Res Hum Retroviruses 2002;18:19–26.

Fowler MG. Prevention of perinatal HIV infection. What do we know? Where should future research go? Ann N Y Acad Sci 2000;918:45–52.

Franceschi S, Dal Maso L, Arniani S, et al. Risk of cancer other than Kaposi's sarcoma and non-Hodgkin's lymphoma in persons with AIDS in Italy. Cancer and AIDS Registry Linkage Study. Br J Cancer 1998;78:966–970.

Frankel AD, Pabo CO. Cellular uptake of the tat protein from human immunodeficiency virus. Cell 1988;55:1189–1193.

Freeman RB Jr. Diagnosing hepatocellular carcinoma: a virtual reality. Liver Transpl 2002;8:762–764.

Frisch M, Biggar RJ, Goedert JJ. Human papillomavirus-associated cancers in patients with human immunodeficiency virus infection and acquired immunodeficiency syndrome. J Natl Cancer Inst 2000; 92: 1500–1510.

Gale M Jr, Blakely CM, Kwieciszewski B, et al. Control of PKR protein kinase by hepatitis C virus nonstructural 5A protein: molecular mechanisms of kinase regulation. Mol Cell Biol 1998;18:5208–5218.

Garcia R, Jove R. Activation of STAT transcription factors in oncogenic tyrosine kinase signaling. J Biomed Sci 1998;5:79–85.

Ghosh AK, Steele R, Meyer K, Ray R, Ray RB. Human hepatitis C virus NS5A protein modulates cell cycle regulatory genes and promotes cell growth. J Gen Virol 1999;80:1179–1183.

Gichangi PB, Bwayo J, Estambale B, et al. Impact of HIV infection on invasive cervical cancer in Kenyan women. AIDS 2003;17:1963–1968.

Gires O, Zimber-Strobl U, Gonnella R, et al. Latent membrane protein 1 of Epstein-Barr virus mimics a constitutively active receptor molecule. EMBO J 1997;16:6131–6140.

Glaser SL, Clarke CA, Gulley ML, et al. Population-based patterns of human immunodeficiency virus-related Hodgkin lymphoma in the Greater San Francisco Bay Area, 1988–1998. Cancer 2003;98: 300–309.

Gong G, Waris G, Tanveer R, Siddiqui A. Human hepatitis C virus NS5A protein alters intracellular calcium levels, induces oxidative stress, and activates STAT-3 and NF-kB. Proc Natl Acad Sci USA 2001;98: 9599–9604.

Gonzalez CE, Adde M, Taylor P, Wood LV, Magrath I. Impact of chemotherapy for AIDS-related malignancies in pediatric HIV disease. Ann N Y Acad Sci 2000;918:362–366.

Goodenow MM, Rose SL, Tuttle DL, Sleasman JW. HIV-1 fitness and macrophages. J Leukoc Biol 2003;74:657–666.

Gottlieb GS, Sow PS, Hawes SE, et al. Molecular epidemiology of dual HIV-1/HIV-2 seropositive adults from Senegal, West Africa. AIDS Res Hum Retroviruses 2003;19:575–584.

Graham CS, Baden LR, Yu E, et al. Influence of human immunodeficiency virus infection on the course of hepatitis C virus infection: a meta-analysis. Clin Infect Dis 2001;33:562–569.

Granovsky MO, Mueller BU, Nicholson HS, Rosenberg PS, Rabkin CS. Cancer in human immunodeficiency virus-infected children: a case series from the Children's Cancer Group and the National Cancer Institute. J Clin Oncol 1998;16:1729–1735.

Hahn CS, Cho YG, Kang BS, Lester IM, Hahn YS. The HCV core protein acts as a positive regulator of Fas-mediated apoptosis in a human lymphoblastoid T cell line. Virology 2000;276:127–137.

Hammer SM, Yeni P. Antiretroviral therapy: where are we? AIDS 1998; 12(Suppl. A):S181–S188.

Hanson IC, Antonelli TA, Sperling RS, et al. Lack of tumors in infants with perinatal HIV-1 exposure and fetal/neonatal exposure to zidovudine. J Acquir Immune Defic Syndr Hum Retrovirol 1999;20:463–467.

Hawes SE, Critchlow CW, Faye Niang MA, et al. Increased risk of high-grade cervical squamous intraepithelial lesions and invasive cervical cancer among African women with human immunodeficiency virus type 1 and 2 infections. J Infect Dis 2003;188:555–563.

He J, Choe S, Walker R, Di Marzio P, Morgan DO, Landau NR. Human immunodeficiency virus type 1 viral protein R (Vpr) arrests cells in the G2 phase of the cell cycle by inhibiting p34cdc2 activity. J Virol 1995;69:6705–6711.

Henderson S, Rowe M, Gregory C, et al. Induction of bcl-2 expression by Epstein-Barr virus latent membrane protein 1 protects infected B cells from porgrammed cell death. Cell 1991;65:1107–1115.

Sparano JA (ed.) HIV and HTLV-1 Associated Malignancies. Norwell: Kluwer Academic Publishers, 2001.

Huang SM, McCance DJ. Down regulation of the interleukin-8 promoter by human papillomavirus type 16 E6 and E7 through effects on CREB binding protein/p300 and P/CAF. J Virol 2002;76:8710–8721.

Jenson HB, Leach CT, McClain KL, et al. Benign and malignant smooth muscle tumors containing Epstein-Barr virus in children with AIDS. Leuk Lymphoma 1997;27:303–314.

Johnson RJ, Stack M, Hazlewood SA, et al. The 30-base-pair deletion in Chinese variants of the Epstein-Barr virus LMP1 gene is not the major effector of functional differences between variant LMP1 genes in human lymphocytes. J Virol 1998;72:4038–4048.

Jowett JB, Planelles V, Poon B, Shah NP, Chen ML, Chen IS. The human immunodeficiency virus type 1 vpr gene arrests infected T cells in the G2 + M phase of the cell cycle. J Virol 1995;69:6304–6313.

Kanazawa S, Peterlin BM. Repression of MHC determinants in HIV infection. Microbes Infect 2001;3:467–473.

Kanazawa S, Okamoto T, Peterlin BM. Tat competes with CIITA for the binding to P-TEFb and blocks the expression of MHC class II genes in HIV infection. Immunity 2000;12:61–70.

Kapasi AA, Patel G, Franki N, Singhal PC. HIV-1 gp120-induced tubular epithelial cell apoptosis is mediated through p38-MAPK phosphorylation. Mol Med 2002;8:676–685.

Kawata S, Ariumi Y, Shimotohno K. p21Waf1/Cip11/Sdi1 prevents apoptosis as well as stimulates growth in cells transformed or immortalized by human T-cell leukemia virus type 1-encoded Tax. J Virol 2003;77:7291–7299.

Kemp K, Akanmori BD, Hviid L. West African donors have high percentages of activated cytokine producing T cells that are prone to apoptosis. Clin Exp Immunol 2001;126:69–75.

Kieff E, Rickinson AB. Epstein-Barr virus and its replication. In: Knipe DM, Howley PM, eds. Field's Virology. Philadelphia, PA: Lippincott/ Williams and Wilkins, 2001; pp. 2511–2573.

Kinter AL, Umscheid CA, Arthos J, et al. HIV envelope induces virus expression from resting CD4+ T cells isolated from HIV-infected individuals in the absence of markers of cellular activation or apoptosis. J Immunol 2003;170:2449–2455.

Kirk O, Pedersen C, Cozzi-Lepri A, et al. Non-Hodgkin lymphoma in HIV-infected patients in the era of highly active antiretroviral therapy. Blood 2001;98:3406–3412.

Kirken RA, Erwin RA, Wang L, Wang Y, Rui H, Farrar WL. Functional uncoupling of the Janus kinase 3-Stat5 pathway in malignant growth of human T cell leukemia virus type 1-transformed human T cells. J Immunol 2000;165:5097–5104.

Kohler JJ, Tuttle DL, Coberley CR, Sleasman JW, Goodenow MM. Human immunodeficiency virus type 1 (HIV-1) induces activation of multiple STATs in CD4+ cells of lymphocyte or monocyte/ macrophage lineages. J Leukoc Biol 2003;73:407–416.

Lahti AL, Manninen A, Saksela K. Regulation of T cell activation by HIV-1 accessory proteins: Vpr acts via distinct mechanisms to cooperate with Nef in NFAT-directed gene expression and to promote transactivation by CREB. Virology 2003;310:190–196.

Lahti AL, Mannimen A, Saksela K. Regulation of T cell activation by HIV-1 accessory proteins: Vpr acts via distinct mechanisms to cooperate with Nef in NFAT-directed gene expression and to promote transactivation by CREB. Virology 2003;310:190–196.

Laux G, Perricaudet M, Farrell PJ. A spliced Epstein-Barr virus gene expressed in immortalized lymphoctyes is created by circularization of the linear viral genome. EMBO J 1988;7:769–774.

Levitsky V, Masucci MG. Manipulation of immune responses by Epstein-Barr virus. Virus Res 2002;88:71–86.

Levy JA. HIV infection and development of cancer. HIV and the Pathogenesis of AIDS. Washington: American Society for Microbiology, 1998; pp. 285–310.

Lewis MJ, Gautier VW, Wang XP, Kaplan MH, Hall WW. Spontaneous production of C-C chemokines by individuals infected with human T lymphotropic virus type II (HTLV-II) alone and HTLV-II/HIV-1 coinfected individuals. J Immunol 2000;165:4127–4132.

Li LQ, Liu D, Hutt-Fletcher L, Morgan A, Masucci MG, Levitsky V. Epstein-Barr virus inhibits the development of dendritic cells by promoting apoptosis of their monocyte precursors in the presence of GM-CSF and IL-4. Blood 2002;99:3725–3734.

Lin TS, Mahajan S, Frank DA. STAT signaling in the pathogenesis and treatment of leukemias. Oncogene 2000;19:2496–2504.

Littman DR. Chemokine receptors: keys to AIDS pathogenesis? Cell 1998;93:677–680.

Macsween KF, Crawford DH. Epstein-Barr virus-recent advances. Lancet Infect Dis 2003;3:131–140.

Mann DA, Frankel AD. Endocytosis and targeting of exogenous HIV-1 Tat protein. EMBO J 1991;10:1733–1739.

Mbulaiteye SM, Parkin DM, Rabkin CS. Epidemiology of AIDS-related malignancies: An international perspective. In: Krown SE, Von Roenn JH, eds. Hematology/Oncology Clinics of North America. Philadelphia: WB Saunders Company, 2003; pp. 673–696.

McClain KL. Epstein-Barr virus and HIV-AIDS-associated diseases. Biomed Pharmacother 2001;55:348–352.

McClain KL, Leach CT, Jenson HB, et al. Association of Epstein-Barr virus with leiomyosarcomas in children with AIDS. N Engl J Med 1995;332:12–18.

McMurray HR, McCance DJ. Human papillomavirus type 16 E6 activates TERT gene transcription through induction of c-Myc and release of USF-mediated repression. J Virol 2003;77:9852–9861.

Migone TS, Lin JX, Cereseto A, et al. Constitutively activated Jak-STAT pathway in T cells transformed with HTLV-I. Science 1995;269:79–81.

Miller ED, Smith JA, Lichtinger M, Wang L, Su L. Activation of the signal transducer and activator of transcription 1 signaling pathway in thymocytes from HIV-1-infected human thymus. AIDS 2003;17:1269–1277.

Miller WE, Cheshire JL, Baldwin AS Jr, Raab-Traub N. The NPC derived C15 LMP1 protein confers enhanced activation of NF-kB and induction of the EGFR in epithelial cells. Oncogene 1998;16:1869–1877.

Mofenson LM. Technical report: perinatal human immunodeficiency virus testing and prevention of transmission. Committee on Pediatric Aids. Pediatrics 2000;106:E88.

Monga HK, Rodriguez-Barradas MC, Breaux K, et al. Hepatitis C virus infection-related morbidity and mortality among patients with human immunodeficiency virus infection. Clin Infect Dis 2001;33:240–247.

Mueller BU. Cancers in children infected with the human immunodeficiency virus. Oncologist 1999;4:309–317.

Munoz N, Bosch FX, de Sanjose S, et al. Epidemiologic classification of human papillomavirus types associated with cervical cancer. N Engl J Med 2003;348:518–527.

Ng VL, McGrath MS. The immunology of AIDS-associated lymphomas. Immunol Rev 1998;162:293–298.

Ockenga J, Tillmann HL, Trautwein C, Stoll M, Manns MP, Schmidt RE. Hepatitis B and C in HIV-infected patients. Pre-valence and prognostic value. J Hepatol 1997;27:18–24.

Okano M. Overview and problematic standpoints of severe chronic active Epstein-Barr virus infection syndrome. Crit Rev Oncol Hematol 2002;44:273–282.

Orenstein JM. The macrophage in HIV infection. Immunobiology 2001;204:598–602.

Palefsky JM. Cervical human papillomavirus infection and cervical intraepithelial neoplasia in women positive for human immunodeficiency virus in the era of highly active antiretroviral therapy. Curr Opin Oncol 2003;15:382–388.

Pati S, Foulke JS Jr, Barabitskaya O, et al. Human herpesvirus 8-encoded vGPCR activates nuclear factor of activated T cells and collaborates with human immunodeficiency virus type 1 Tat. J Virol 2003;77: 5759–5773.

Patrick DR, Oliff A, Heimbrook DC. Identification of a novel retinoblastoma gene product binding site on human papillomavirus type 16 E7 protein. J Biol Chem 1994;269:6842–6850.

Persaud D, Zhou Y, Siliciano JM, Siliciano RF. Latency in human immunodeficiency virus type 1 infection: no easy answers. J Virol 2003;77:1659–1665.

Petit AJ, Tersmette M, Terpstra FG, de Goede RE, van Lier RA, Miedema F. Decreased accessory cell function by human monocytic cells after infection with HIV. J Immunol 1988;140:1485–1489.

Pollock BH, Jenson HB, Leach CT, et al. Risk factors for pediatric human immunodeficiency virus-related malignancy. JAMA 2003;289:2393–2399.

Polyak S, Chen H, Hirsch D, George I, Hershberg R, Sperber K. Impaired class II expression and antigen uptake in monocytic cells after HIV-1 infection. J Immunol 1997;159:2177–2188.

Popik W, Pitha PM. Exploitation of cellular signaling by HIV-1: Unwelcome guests with master keys that signal their entry. Virology 2000;276:1–6.

Table 86-1
Landmarks in the History of PNH

Year	Scientist	Issue
1678	Schmidt	First clinical report
1882	Strübing	First detailed description
1911	Marchiafava	Recognition as disease entity
1937	Ham; Dacie	Specific diagnostic test
1956	De Sandre	PNH erythrocytes are AchE deficient
1965	Lewis and Dacie	PNH granulocytes are NAP-deficient
1966	Rosse and Dacie	Two types of PNH erythrocytes
1967	Lewis and Dacie	Relation with aplastic anemia
1970	Oni and Luzzatto	Evidence of clonal origin
1983	Nicholson-Weller	PNH cells are DAF-deficient
1984	Rotoli and Luzzatto	In vitro evidence of clonal origin
1986	Medof	Relation to GPI-anchoring system
1989	Rotoli and Luzzatto	The survival advantage hypothesis
1990	Van der Schoot	Cytometry of GPI-deficient cells
1992, 1993	Ueda; Hillmen	PNH lymphoblastoid cell lines
1993	Kinoshita	Cloning of the *PIG-A* gene
1994	Bessler and Luzzatto	*PIG-A* gene organization and mutations
1999	Araten	PNH cells in normal individuals
2001	Bessler	Mouse models
2001, 2002	Karadimitris; Risitano	Clonal T-cell expansion in PNH patients

AchE, acetylcholinesterase; DAF, decay accelerating factor (CD55); GPI, glycosyl-phosphatidylinositol; NAP, neutrophil alkaline phosphatase; PIG-A, phosphatidylinositol glycan class A; PNH, paroxysmal nocturnal hemoglobinuria.

have only one allele and females have only one functional allele (as result of X-chromosome inactivation). Although females have two *PIG-A* alleles, only half of the mutation will occur in the functional X; thus, the risk of having the disease is the same in both genders. Because a defect causing a metabolic block is generally recessive, it is unlikely (although not impossible) that a double mutation targeting both alleles of an autosomal gene in the same cell may occur in vivo.

PIG-A MUTATIONS IN PNH Practically all types of mutations have been found in the *PIG-A* gene of PNH cells: small deletions or insertions producing frameshift, nucleotide substitutions resulting in stop codon, missense mutations causing amino acids substitutions or new sites for alternative splicing, large deletions. Most of the mutations occur in exon 2, probably because it is the largest; however, no particular clustering of mutations has emerged, and almost all mutations are unique to each patient (private mutations) (*see* Fig. 86-1).

Comparing the type of mutations found in PNH with those found in glucose-6-phosphate dehydrogenase deficiency, another (this time inherited) X-linked disorder of a housekeeping gene, shows a clear discrepancy. In PNH, a vast majority of mutations have extremely severe functional consequences, (i.e., production of truncated proteins), whereas missense mutations are rare; in glucose-6-phosphate dehydrogenase deficiency almost all mutations are missense, leading to single amino acid substitutions with conserved (although possibly altered) function. Two considerations may be relevant to this discrepancy: (1) In hereditary disorders, a complete absence of the product of a housekeeping gene is probably lethal; thus, only mutations with residual activity are seen. By contrast, if a mutation is somatically acquired, it will not affect organ development and, once occurred, it will affect the genetic make-up of only a small fraction of somatic cells, which may survive although with some functional abnormality. (2) If missense mutations in PNH are rare, this means that for a clonal

expansion to take place, the gene must be seriously damaged. Indeed, the rare missense mutations found in PNH patients are associated with a marked reduction of GPI-linked proteins, indicating that they affected mRNA stability or protein function, or both.

MOLECULAR PATHOPHYSIOLOGY

The *PIG-A* mutation responsible for PNH arises in a multipotent hematopoietic stem cell, which is capable of differentiating along several lineages; maturation along erythroid, myeloid, and megakaryocytic lineages is almost always preserved, whereas lymphoid differentiation (along B- and/or T lineages) is observed in a minority of patients. As a consequence of the damage of the GPI-anchor synthesis pathway, all the affected cells in any state of maturation are deficient in all the GPI-linked molecules, and deficiency is often complete. More than 20 different proteins sharing the GPI-anchoring system have been described on the surface of human blood cells (Fig. 86-3). The understanding of their functional significance is limited; in many cases, the study of PNH patients or cells was an important source of information.

HEMOLYSIS IN PNH PATIENTS Intravascular hemolysis is the most characteristic clinical feature of PNH; it is because of increased susceptibility of PNH erythrocytes to complement-mediated lysis. This abnormality is caused by the absence on red cell membrane of two complement-regulatory proteins, CD59/MIRL (membrane inhibitor of reactive lysis) and CD55/DAF (decay accelerating factor), which are both GPI-linked. This membrane abnormality renders PNH erythrocytes extremely sensitive to complement activation, which translates in vivo into a hemolytic state and in vitro into red cell destruction in acified serum (Ham test). A low level of complement activation is probably a constant physiologic phenomenon, which is greatly amplified during inflammatory or infectious diseases; thus, PNH erythrocytes are chronically lysed with paroxystic exacerbations. It is unclear why exacerba-

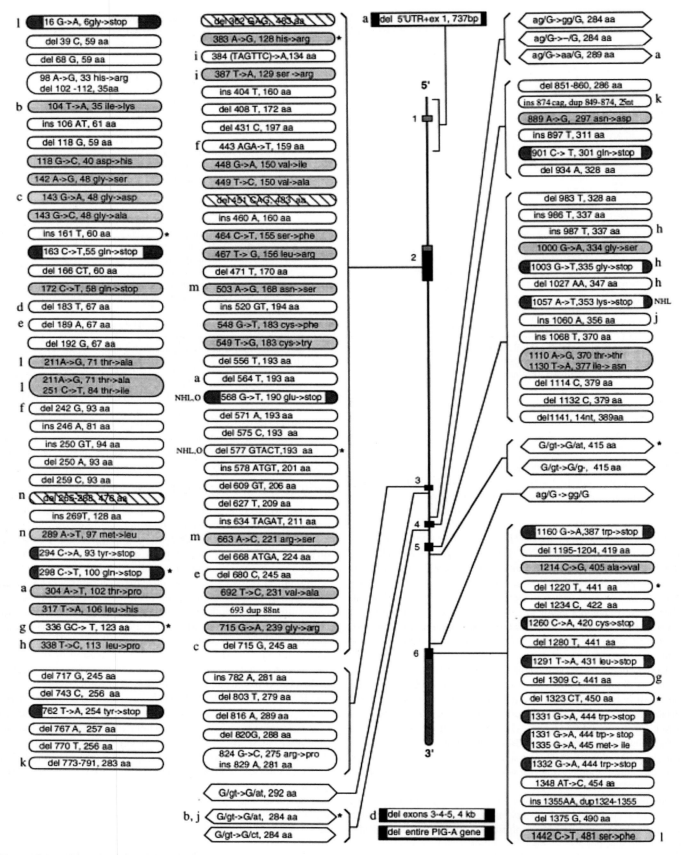

Figure 86-1 Phosphatidylinositol glycan class A gene structure and mutations. The genomic gene spans approx 17 kb. Exons (thick blocks, numbered) and introns (thin lines) are represented in the central bar; untranslated exon regions are in gray. Three mRNA transcripts arising from alternative splicing were found by Bessler et al., (1994) who also described an unproductive pseudogene mapped to 12q21. Mutations found to

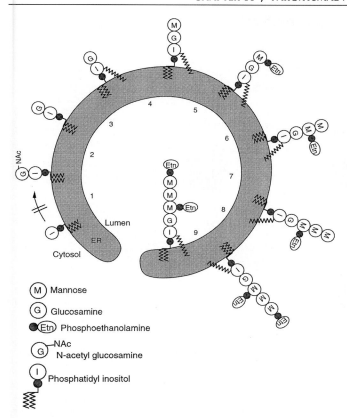

M Mannose

G Glucosamine

Etn Phosphoethanolamine

G NAc
    N-acetyl glucosamine

I Phosphatidyl inositol

Figure 86-2 Glycosyl-phosphatidylinositol-anchor biosynthesis. The anchor synthesis is a multistep (1–9) process that occurs in the endoplasmic reticulum (ER), starting on the cytoplasmic side, then flipping into the luminal side. The anchor is transferred *en bloc* on the C-terminal of the protein, which is cleaved of a short sequence of 20–30 amino acids led by a signal sequence called ω. Although GPI-deficient cell lines obtained by experimental mutagenesis have shown defects in any step of the synthesis, all paroxysmal nocturnal hemoglobinuria patients studied so far are defective in the first step (⫫→).

tions occur mainly during the night. In a functional hierarchy, CD59 plays a major role, as discovered by studying rare inherited conditions in which a single molecule is lacking. A CD59-deficient patient had a PNH-like picture, whereas subjects deficient of CD55 on red cell membrane (those carrying the rare Inab blood group phenotype) show no hyperhemolysis. Although CD59 and CD55 are deficient also on leukocytes, there is no evidence of reduced leukocyte life-span in PNH patients, probably because nucleated cells have an additional transmembrane (i.e., non-GPI-linked) molecule (CD46) that protects them from complement activation. Sensitivity to complement is the best known, but not the only defect, of PNH cells. Table 86-2 lists other molecules that are deficient and their specific function, when known.

HEMATOPOIESIS IN PNH PATIENTS   A wide spectrum of clinical picture emerges when several PNH patients are compared with each other, ranging from almost asymptomatic individuals to severely ill subjects. Several mechanisms are responsible for such phenotypic heterogeneity:

1. The coexistence of a variable percentage of normal cells, which are progeny of residual GPI+ stem cells.
2. A selective destruction of particles succumbing to the activated complement attack (this is particularly true for PNH red cells after a paroxysm of hemolysis).
3. The type of molecular lesion in the *PIG-A* gene, leading to PNH cells with a variable sensitivity to complement-mediated lysis (PNH II and PNH III populations).
4. The degree of commitment of the stem cell having the *PIG-A* mutation; if the mutation occurs in a totipotent stem cell, even lymphocytes will carry the PNH defect, whereas a mutation in a multipotent myeloid cell will not produce PNH lymphocytes.

In theory, a mutation in a more committed progenitor could generate a monolineage PNH; however, patients with a purely myeloid *PIG-A*-deficient clone, giving rise to only granulocytes and/or platelets may remain undetected, as the sparing of the erythroid lineage implies lack of the typical symptoms suggesting PNH.

PNH hematopoiesis is certainly clonal, but clonal does not necessarily mean monoclonal. Initial observations that more than one abnormal cell population may be present in a single PNH patient were first inferred by functional studies based on different sensitivity to complement-mediated lysis and then by flow cytometry in the early 1990s. The final confirmation of such an unusual pattern came from DNA analysis, which documented the simultaneous presence of two or even more different *PIG-A* mutations in several PNH patients, each originating a distinct multilineage PNH clone. A mechanism that may explain the expansion of more clones carrying the same functional defect but arising from different mutations is selection. A theory based on this mechanism was developed for PNH in 1989 and termed the "relative advantage," later the "escape" hypothesis; it is supported by several pieces of circumstantial evidence, but still requires a direct confirmation. According to this theory, a mutation in the *PIG-A* gene might be a fairly common phenomenon, which has no biological consequences, because the mutated cell has no chance of expanding in the presence of a vast majority of normal cells. However, if normal hematopoiesis is inhibited by a primary cause (as in idiopathic aplastic anemia [AA]), and if the killing mechanism is directly or indirectly mediated by one or more proteins that are GPI-linked on the surface of progenitor cells, *PIG-A* mutated cells survive, undergoing clonal expansion. Because only cells severely GPI-deficient are able to survive, in PNH serious molecular lesions (i.e., frameshift, stop codon, and deletion) prevail over single amino acid substitutions. Several observations indirectly support this theory; in patients with a B-cell lymphoproliferative disorder treated by Campath-1H (a monoclonal antibody that kills lymphocytes targeting the GPI-linked protein CD52), severely GPI-deficient T cells emerged; they were cloned and showed mutations in the *PIG-A* gene. When a banked blood specimen that had been drawn before monoclonal antibody treatment was searched for the *PIG-A* deficient clone, a few cells carrying the same molecular defect were detected. On Campath-1H discontinuation, the GPI-deficient T cells gradually disappeared. Thus, this model elucidates most features of the PNH pathogenesis: the preexistence of *PIG-A*

Figure 86-1 (*Continued*)   date are displayed. ⊂⊃: small deletion or insertion and resulting in frameshift and truncated protein; ◼⊃: nonsense mutation; ⟨⊃: mutation causing altered splicing; ◼◼: vast deletion; ▨▨: deletion, in frame; ▰▰: missense mutation. *Mutations found in more than one patient. A small letter outside the box identifies multiple mutations found in a single patient. Only one polymorphism has been described (55C→T, 19 arg→trp).

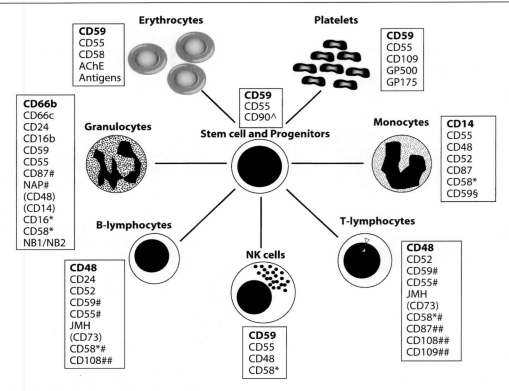

Figure 86-3   GPI-linked molecules on blood cell surface. For each cell type, the molecules are listed in order of sensitivity for detecting deficient cells (in bold, highest sensitivity; molecules in parenthesis, weak expression; *, also transmembrane; #, increased on cell activation; ##, expressed only on cell activation. ^, approx 25% of early hematopoietic progenitors express CD90, which is the analog of murine Thy-1. §, in our hands, CD59 was often present on PNH monocytes. A few molecules have been omitted that need better knowledge of their lineage-restricted expression (ULBPs, PRV-1, PrP^c, TRAIL-R3).

mutated cells, their expansion under a selective pressure negatively acting on normal cells by a mechanism to which the mutated cells are resistant (for the absence of CD52), and the gradual disappearance of the mutated clone once the selective mechanism has been removed. The existence of a few (10–50 cells per million) PNH cells in peripheral blood of healthy individuals has been documented by analyzing cytometrically a large number of granulocytes. A nested PCR technique confirmed the clonality of these cells by identifying the specific *PIG-A* mutation. The absence of an intrinsic genomic instability in PNH patients has been shown by comparison with another bone marrow failure disorder, Fanconi anemia (FA). The measurement of *PIG-A* spontaneous mutation rate in B-lymphoblastoid cell lines derived from PNH or FA patients showed a normal rate of mutation in PNH patients, contrasting with a markedly elevated rate in FA patients. Thus, the development of PNH cannot be attributed to increased risk of *PIG-A* mutations, but only to the expansion of pre-existing rare mutant clones. The finding that FA patients, although having both more *PIG-A* mutated stem cells and reduced marrow cellularity, do not develop PNH, strongly supports the escape theory: because bone marrow failure in FA is owing to a mechanism that does not involve GPI-linked molecules, there is no growth advantage for the mutated cells.

Murine Models of PNH   To explore experimentally the growth of PNH hematopoietic stem cells, murine models have been generated. A complete knockout animal could not be produced, demonstrating that *pig-a* is necessary for embryogenesis. When the mouse *pig-a* gene was inactivated in embryonic stem (ES) cells with the conventional knockout gene targeting technique, in vitro studies

demonstrated that *pig-a* deficient ES cells were able to differentiate into mature cells of various hematopoietic lineages, showing that *pig-a* is not necessary for differentiation and maturation of hematopoietic progenitors. When tested in vivo, with chimeras obtained by inserting *pig-a* knocked out ES cells during early embryonic development, in the few surviving chimeras the proportion of GPI-deficient blood cells was low at birth and decreased with aging, proving that there is no absolute growth advantage for PNH cells as compared with normal cells coexisting in the same organism. Mice showing in vivo expansion of *pig-a* mutated hematopoiesis, thus better mimicking the human PNH disease, have been obtained with a more sophisticated approach. A conditional inactivation of the murine *pig-a* gene was implemented using the Cre recombinase and its specific recombination sites, loxP. When the Cre/loxP system was targeted to the hematopoietic stem cells or the erythroid/megakaryocytic lineage using tissue-specific c-FES and GATA-1 regulatory sequences, respectively, the generation of mice having almost 100% of red cells with the PNH phenotype was obtained. Such mice are under investigation to answer open questions in PNH pathophysiology.

In Vitro Decreased Susceptibility of PNH Cells to Immune Effector Mechanisms   Several contradictory data have been produced on a putative differential sensitivity of normal and PNH hematopoiesis to inhibitory stimuli. Susceptibility to apoptosis has been reported increased, normal, or decreased in different models; it has been shown that human cell lines carrying the PIG-A mutation are less susceptible to NK-mediated killing compared with their normal counterpart, a phenomenon that was reverted by transfection with a *PIG-A* cDNA. In a more sophisticated model, GPI-deficient

IRP2 levels rise when cellular iron stores are depleted. Binding of either of these proteins to the ferritin IREs prevents assembly of the translational initiation complex on the ferritin mRNA.

Interestingly, these same IRPs are involved in a very different translational regulatory mechanism when they bind to IREs located in the 3′ UTR of TFR mRNA. Under conditions of cellular iron depletion, IRP binding stabilizes TFR mRNA by preventing endonucleolytic degradation. This results in increased TFR translation and placement of more TFR molecules on the cell surface to mediate iron uptake. Thus, the same protein regulators act to modulate ferritin and TFR gene expression coordinately as appropriate for iron status. There are also IREs in the 3′ UTR of some isoforms of DMT1 mRNA and in the 5′ UTR of ferroportin mRNA, which are thought to regulate translation in a manner similar to TFR and ferritins, respectively.

SYSTEMIC IRON HOMEOSTASIS Iron balance must also be regulated at the level of the entire organism. Systemic iron homeostasis requires complex signals between remote tissues including the intestine, bone marrow, and liver. Because humans have no mechanism for deliberate iron excretion, regulation of iron availability requires coordinate control of intestinal absorption, and mobilization of iron from stores (particularly macrophages, hepatocytes). Four conditions are known to modulate absorption and release: deviation of the levels of stores from normal, increased need for iron for erythropoiesis, inflammation, and hypoxia. Following on nomenclature of Finch, these will be referred to as *stores, erythroid, inflammatory,* and *hypoxia regulators,* respectively. These can coexist, e.g., in the setting of iron deficiency anemia, when both the *stores* and *erythroid regulators* should act to increase iron availability. There appears to be a hierarchy of activity; the *stores regulator* can modulate iron absorption and availability modestly, over a range of no more than threefold, whereas the *erythroid regulator* is much more potent, capable of increasing iron absorption as much as 10-fold or more. When increased iron stores and iron-restricted erythropoiesis occur simultaneously, as in the rare disorder atransferrinemia (severe deficiency of serum transferrin), the more powerful *erythroid regulator* predominates, and intestinal iron absorption is markedly increased in spite of tissue iron overload.

Previously, these regulators were observed as clinical phenomena, but not understood on a molecular level. In 2001, a new iron-regulatory hormone was discovered, designated hepcidin because it is produced in the liver and bears similarity to antimicrobial peptides. The primary activity of hepcidin appears to be to inhibit intestinal iron absorption and cellular iron release. Levels of hepcidin are modulated by each of the four known regulators. Expression of hepcidin is increased in iron overload (*stores regulator*) and inflammation (*inflammatory regulator*), presumably to compensate for excess iron and to keep iron away from invading pathogens, respectively. Activation of the *inflammatory regulator* and consequent elevation of hepcidin levels likely explains some, if not all, of the features of the anemia of inflammation (also called the anemia of chronic disease). Expression of hepcidin is decreased in response to iron-restricted erythropoiesis (*erythroid regulator*) and hypoxia (*hypoxia regulator*), likely as a measure to boost production of oxygen-carrying red blood cells. These activities are summarized in Fig. 87-2.

Although hepcidin is undoubtedly important, there are clearly other components of systemic iron-regulatory networks. These have been ascertained through study of genetic iron overload disorders, a heterogeneous collection of diseases triggered by single gene mutations (Table 87-2). Most of these disorders are characterized by

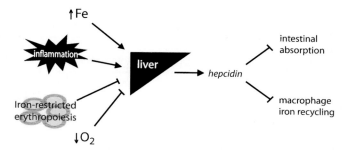

Figure 87-2 Regulation and activity of hepcidin. Hepcidin is produced in the liver. Its production is induced by iron overload (↑Fe) and inflammation and diminished in response to iron-restricted erythropoiesis and hypoxia (↓O$_2$). Hepcidin acts to interrupt both intestinal iron absorption and macrophage recycling.

increased intestinal iron absorption leading to deposition of excess iron in parenchymal cells of the liver, heart, and endocrine glands. Iron toxicity, presumably associated with increased production of oxygen free radicals, causes hepatic fibrosis and cirrhosis, hepatocellular carcinoma, cardiomyopathy, diabetes mellitus, and, rarely, hypogonadotropic hypogonadism. Treatment is aimed at decreasing the body iron burden through serial phlebotomies, removing approx 200 mg of iron as hemoglobin in every 500 mL of blood drawn.

The prototype iron overload disorder is hereditary hemochromatosis resulting from mutations in the hemochromatosis disease gene (HFE). HFE encodes an atypical major histocompatibility class I-like molecule that complexes with β-2 microglobulin but has no known role in immunoregulation. Approximately one in eight individuals of Northern European descent carry a missense mutation that results in a cysteine to tyrosine substitution in amino acid 282 of the HFE protein (C282Y). Patients who are homozygous for the C282Y mutation are at significant risk for the development of clinical hemochromatosis, though estimates of disease penetrance vary markedly, from <1% to almost 50%. This wide range is owing, in part, to different definitions of clinical hemochromatosis. Severely affected individuals are unusual.

The normal role of HFE in iron homeostasis is not well understood, but there are several important clues. First, studies in mouse models have shown that the C282Y mutation results in a loss of HFE activity. Second, the HFE molecule forms a protein—protein complex with TFR. However, the function of the HFE/TFR complex is controversial. Data from several groups suggest that HFE precludes transferrin binding and, therefore, decreases iron uptake through the transferrin cycle, whereas data from another group suggest that HFE serves to make the transferrin cycle more efficient. This issue has not been resolved. Finally, studies indicate that patients and mice with HFE hemochromatosis have inappropriately low levels of hepcidin. Accordingly, forced expression of hepcidin in HFE mutant mice prevents hemochromatosis. Taken together, these observations suggest that HFE is normally involved in the regulation of hepcidin expression, and that loss of normal regulation leads to a failure to limit iron absorption and cellular iron release in HFE hemochromatosis. However, much remains to be learned about how this occurs.

A similar iron overload disorder is observed in patients who are homozygous for any of a number of different mutations in the gene encoding transferrin receptor 2 (TFR2). TFR2 is a close relative of TFR that shares some of its properties. TFR2 can mediate cellular

Table 87-2
Genes Mutated in Patients With Iron Overload

Gene (Online Mendelian inheritance in man database designation)	Inheritance	Chromosomal location	Role in iron homeostasis	Clinical test
HFE (HFE1)	Autosomal-recessive	6p21	Regulates levels of hepcidin	Genetic study for C282Y mutation and for H63D polymorphism
Hemojuvelin (HFE2)	Autosomal-recessive	1q21	Not known - regulates levels of hepcidin?	N/A
Hepcidin (HFE2B)	Autosomal-recessive	19q13	Hormone that controls iron absorption, release of iron from macrophage stores	N/A
Transferrin Receptor 2 (HFE3)	Autosomal-recessive	7q22	Resembles the transferrin receptor involved in cellular iron uptake; role not clear	N/A
Ferroportin (HFE4)	Autosomal-dominant (distinct pathology)	2q32	Iron transporter	N/A

N/A, test not yet available.

iron uptake from transferrin less efficiently than TFR, but its role in vivo is uncertain. It is primarily expressed in the liver and in hematopoietic precursor cells. Both TFR and TFR2 normally exist in cells as protein dimers, and heterodimers made up of one molecule of TFR and one molecule of TFR2 form at low levels. However, unlike TFR, TFR2 cannot form a protein–protein complex with HFE. The relationship between TFR2 and hepcidin, if any, has not been elucidated.

Aggressive, early-onset, "juvenile hemochromatosis" is rare in comparison to other iron overload disorders. Juvenile hemochromatosis is pathologically similar to HFE and TFR2 hemochromatosis, but iron loading is accelerated and severe complications typically present in the second decade of life. Patients are more likely to have cardiac and endocrine complications, and somewhat less likely to develop cirrhosis. Juvenile hemochromatosis is caused by homozygosity for loss-of-function mutations in either of two genes. Perhaps not surprisingly, one of these is hepcidin itself. As predicted from mice lacking hepcidin, absence of hepcidin in human patients leads to severe iron overload.

The gene mutated in other families with juvenile hemochromatosis encodes a novel protein, termed hemojuvelin. Curiously, the only known protein related to hemojuvelin is a chicken protein (called RGM, for repulsive guidance molecule) involved in axonal patterning in the developing nervous system. The expression pattern of hemojuvelin gives little additional information about its function in iron homeostasis; it is expressed at highest levels in skeletal muscle, heart, and liver. Patients homozygous for hemojuvelin mutations also have inappropriately low levels of hepcidin suggesting that hemojuvelin, like HFE, may participate in the regulation of hepcidin expression. However, hemojuvelin remains enigmatic.

A fifth genetic iron overload disorder differs from the first four in several regards. Inheritance follows an autosomal-dominant, rather than recessive pattern. Iron loading occurs first in tissue macrophages and only later affects parenchymal cells. This disorder is usually less aggressive, perhaps owing to the distinct pathology. It results from missense mutations in ferroportin. No truncation or nonsense mutations have been identified, suggesting that the disease results from alteration of protein function, rather than from a complete loss of one ferroportin allele. The most likely explanation is that the missense mutations preferentially

inactivate ferroportin in macrophages, but have little if any effect on the activity of ferroportin in intestinal iron absorption. A unique ferroportin mutation, Q248H, has been detected in African and African-American patients with iron overload. This mutation may explain a previously described disorder, originally termed "Bantu siderosis," which is prevalent in individuals in sub-Saharan Africa and exacerbated by ingestion of an alcoholic beverage brewed in nongalvanized steel drums.

Although genetic iron overload disorders are relatively common as a group, genetic iron deficiency disorders are rare. There are several case reports of patients with inherited iron deficiency, but genetic analysis has failed to reveal mutations in any of the known genes of iron metabolism. It seems likely that elucidation of the molecular etiology of genetic iron deficiency will also contribute to the overall understanding of the intricate networks governing iron homeostasis.

SELECTED REFERENCES

Abboud S, Haile DJ. A novel mammalian iron-regulated protein involved in intracellular iron metabolism. J Biol Chem 2000;275:19,906–19,912.

Bahram S, Gilfillan S, Kuhn LC, et al. Experimental hemochromatosis due to MHC class I HFE deficiency: immune status and iron metabolism. Proc Natl Acad Sci USA 1999;96:13,312–13,317.

Bennett MJ, Lebron JA, Bjorkman PJ. Crystal structure of the hereditary haemochromatosis protein HFE complexed with transferrin receptor. Nature 2000;403:46–53.

Beutler E, Barton JC, Felitti VJ, et al. Ferroportin 1 (SCL40A1) variant associated with iron overload in African-Americans. Blood Cells Mol Dis 2003;31:305–309.

Bridle KR, Frazer DM, Wilkins SJ, et al. Disrupted hepcidin regulation in HFE-associated haemochromatosis and the liver as a regulator of body iron homeostasis. Lancet 2003;361:669–673.

Camaschella C, Roetto A, Cali A, et al. The gene TFR2 is mutated in a new type of haemochromatosis mapping to 7q22. Nat Genet 2000; 25:14, 15.

Canonne-Hergaux F, Gruenheid S, Ponka P, Gros P. Cellular and subcellular localization of the Nramp2 iron transporter in the intestinal brush border and regulation by dietary iron. Blood 1999;93:4406–4417.

Cazzola M, Invernizzi R, Bergamaschi G, et al. Mitochondrial ferritin expression in erythroid cells from patients with sideroblastic anemia. Blood 2003;101:1996–2000.

Donovan A, Brownlie A, Zhou Y, et al. Positional cloning of zebrafish ferroportin1 identifies a conserved vertebrate iron exporter. Nature 2000;403:776–781.

Finch C. Regulators of iron balance in humans. Blood 1994;84: 1697–1702.

Fleming MD, Romano MA, Su MA, Garrick LM, Garrick MD, Andrews NC. Nramp2 is mutated in the anemic Belgrade (b) rat: Evidence of a role for Nramp2 in endosomal iron transport. Proc Natl Acad Sci USA 1998;95:1148–1153.

Fleming MD, Trenor CC, Su MA, et al. Microcytic anemia mice have a mutation in Nramp2, a candidate iron transporter gene. Nat Genet 1997;16:383–386.

Giannetti AM, Snow PM, Zak O, Bjorkman PJ. Mechanism for multiple ligand recognition by the human transferrin receptor. PLoS Biol 2003;1:E51.

Gordeuk V, Mukiibi J, Hasstedt SJ, et al. Iron overload in Africa. Interaction between a gene and dietary iron content. N Engl J Med 1992;326: 95–100.

Gordeuk VR, Caleffi A, Corradini E, et al. Iron overload in Africans and African-Americans and a common mutation in the SCL40A1 (ferroportin 1) gene. Blood Cells Mol Dis 2003;31:299–304.

Gunshin H, Mackenzie B, Berger UV, et al. Cloning and characterization of a mammalian proton-coupled metal-ion transporter. Nature 1997; 388:482–488.

Haile DJ. Regulation of genes of iron metabolism by the iron-response proteins. Am J Med Sci 1999;318:230–240.

Harris ZL, Durley AP, Man TK, Gitlin JD. Targeted gene disruption reveals an essential role for ceruloplasmin in cellular iron efflux. Proc Natl Acad Sci USA 1999;96:10,812–10,817.

Harris ZL, Takahashi Y, Miyajima H, Serizawa M, MacGillivray RT, Gitlin JD. Aceruloplasminemia: molecular characterization of this disorder of iron metabolism. Proc Natl Acad Sci USA 1995;92:2539–2543.

Kaplan J. Mechanisms of cellular iron acquisition: another iron in the fire. Cell 2002;111:603–606.

Kawabata H, Yang R, Hirama T, et al. Molecular cloning of transferrin receptor 2. A new member of the transferrin receptor-like family. J Biol Chem 1999;274:20,826–20,832.

Levi S, Corsi B, Bosisio M, et al. A human mitochondrial ferritin encoded by an intronless gene. J Biol Chem 2001;276:24,437–24,440.

Levy JE, Jin O, Fujiwara Y, Kuo F, Andrews NC. Transferrin receptor is necessary for development of erythrocytes and the nervous system. Nat Genet 1999;21:396–399.

Levy JE, Montross LK, Cohen DE, Fleming MD, Andrews NC. The C282Y mutation causing hereditary hemochromatosis does not produce a null allele. Blood 1999;94:9–11.

McKie AT, Barrow D, Latunde-Dada GO, et al. An iron-regulated ferric reductase associated with the absorption of dietary iron. Science 2001; 291:1755–1759.

McKie AT, Marciani P, Rolfs A, et al. A novel duodenal iron-regulated transporter, IREG1, implicated in the basolateral transfer of iron to the circulation. Mol Cell 2000;5:299–309.

Montosi G, Donovan A, Totaro A, et al. Autosomal-dominant hemochromatosis is associated with a mutation in the ferroportin (SLC11A3) gene. J Clin Invest 2001;108:619–623.

Muckenthaler M, Gray NK, Hentze MW. IRP-1 binding to ferritin mRNA prevents the recruitment of the small ribosomal subunit by the cap-binding complex eIF4F. Mol Cell 1998;2:383–388.

Muckenthaler M, Roy CN, Custodio AO, et al. Regulatory defects in liver and intestine implicate abnormal hepcidin and Cybrd1 expression in mouse hemochromatosis. Nat Genet 2003;34:102–107.

Ned RM, Swat W, Andrews NC. Transferrin receptor 1 is differentially required in lymphocyte development. Blood 2003;102(10): 3711–3718.

Nicolas G, Bennoun M, Devaux I, et al. Lack of hepcidin gene expression and severe tissue iron overload in upstream stimulatory factor 2 (USF2) knockout mice. Proc Natl Acad Sci USA 2001;98: 8780–8785.

Nicolas G, Chauvet C, Viatte L, et al. The gene encoding the iron regulatory peptide hepcidin is regulated by anemia, hypoxia, and inflammation. J Clin Invest 2002;110:1037–1044.

Nicolas G, Viatte L, Bennoun M, Beaumont C, Kahn A, Vaulont S. Hepcidin, a new iron regulatory peptide. Blood Cells Mol Dis 2002;29: 327–335.

Nicolas G, Viatte L, Lou DQ, et al. Constitutive hepcidin expression prevents iron overload in a mouse model of hemochromatosis. Nat Genet 2003;34:97–101.

Njajou OT, Vaessen N, Joosse M, et al. A mutation in SLC11A3 is associated with autosomal dominant hemochromatosis. Nat Genet 2001; 28:213–214.

Papanikolaou G, Samuels ME, Ludwig EH, et al. Mutations in HFE2 cause iron overload in chromosome 1q-linked juvenile hemochromatosis. Nat Genet 2004;36:77–82.

Pearson HA, Lukens JN. Ferrokinetics in the syndrome of familial hypoferremic microcytic anemia with iron malabsorption. J Pediatr Hematol Oncol 1999;21:412–417.

Pigeon C, Ilyin G, Courselaud B, et al. A new mouse liver-specific gene, encoding a protein homologous to human antimicrobial peptide hepcidin, is overexpressed during iron overload. J Biol Chem 2001;276: 7811–7819.

Roetto A, Papanikolaou G, Politou M, et al. Mutant antimicrobial peptide hepcidin is associated with severe juvenile hemochromatosis. Nat Genet 2003;33(1):21, 22.

Roy CN, Weinstein DA, Andrews NC. 2002 E. Mead Johnson Award for Research in Pediatrics Lecture: the molecular biology of the anemia of chronic disease: a hypothesis. Pediatr Res 2003;53:507–512.

Theil EC. Ferritin: at the crossroads of iron and oxygen metabolism. J Nutr 2003;133:1549S–1553S.

Vogt TM, Blackwell AD, Giannetti AM, Bjorkman PJ, Enns CA. Heterotypic interactions between transferrin receptor and transferrin receptor 2. Blood 2003;101:2008–2014.

Vulpe CD, Kuo YM, Murphy TL, et al. Hephaestin, a ceruloplasmin homologue implicated in intestinal iron transport, is defective in the sla mouse. Nat Genet 1999;21:195–199.

West AP Jr, Bennett MJ, Sellers VM, Andrews NC, Enns CA, Bjorkman PJ. Comparison of the interactions of transferrin receptor and transferrin receptor 2 with transferrin and the hereditary hemochromatosis protein HFE. J Biol Chem 2000;275:38,135–38,138.

Zhou XY, Tomatsu S, Fleming RE, et al. HFE gene knockout produces mouse model of hereditary hemochromatosis. Proc Natl Acad Sci USA 1998;95:2492–2497.

88 Correction of Genetic Blood Defects by Gene Transfer

MARINA CAVAZZANA-CALVO, SALIMA HACEIN-BEY-ABINA,
ADRIAN J. THRASHER, PHILIPPE LEBOULCH, AND ALAIN FISCHER

SUMMARY

Gene therapy has been proposed as an appealing tool for introducing a normal gene into affected hematopoietic stem cells to correct their inherited defect. Theoretically, in the absence of a related human leukocyte antigen identical donor, gene therapy could be an alternative given the accessibility and the information available on the hematopoietic stem cell biology. This chapter describes the progress and limits of the gene therapy approach applied to some genetic blood defects that appear to be good targets for this strategy.

Key Words: ADA; Fanconi anemia; gene therapy; hematopoietic stem cells; SCD; SCID.

RATIONALE FOR THE GENE THERAPY OF GENETIC BLOOD DISEASE

Gene therapy has been proposed as an appealing tool for introducing a normal gene into affected hematopoietic stem cells (HSC) to correct their inherited defect.

In addition to some particular forms of T-cell primary immunodeficiencies, the blood genetic defects potentially curable by this strategy include Fanconi anemia (FA), hemoglobinopathies, and phagocyte disorders. The treatment of choice for all these nonmalignant hematological disorders consists in allogeneic stem cell transplantation from a related or unrelated human leukocyte antigen (HLA)-matched donor. In the presence of a related HLA-genoidentical donor, this treatment leads to a high rate of disease cure with most patients being long-term survivors. Theoretically, in the absence of a related HLA-identical donor, gene therapy could be an alternative given the accessibility and the information available on the HSC biology. In practice, this option is only partially available taking the following issues into account: need to provide a selective growth advantage to transduced cells, uncertain identification of the human stem cells, poor knowledge on HSC self-renewal, limited transduction efficiency of HSC by the available oncoretrovirus type C derived vector, and need to carefully assess the risk/benefit balance in relationship with the severe adverse events (SAE) that occurred in the X-linked severe

combined immunodeficiency (SCID)-X1 clinical trial. This chapter describes the progress and limits of the gene therapy approach applied to some genetic blood defects that appear to be good targets for this strategy.

SEVERE COMBINED IMMUNODEFICIENCY DISEASE

SCID is a heterogenous group consisting at least nine different forms united by one common characteristic: the complete block in T-cell development that is always associated with a direct or indirect impairment of B-cell immunity (Fig. 88-1 and Table 88-1). Consequently these patients are highly susceptible to infection with many micro-organisms, causing early mortality, usually within the first year of life, unless treated by HSC transplantation. HSC transplantation from related HLA-genoidentical donor, for instance, is highly successful as reported in the European survey. Otherwise, the transplantation-related mortality can vary from 5–70% depending on age at treatment, newborn patients having the best outcome; presence of active viral infections; lung impairment; disease type (B+ vs B– SCID forms); and degree of HLA disparity. Overall 5-yr survival from haploidentical hematopoeitic stem cell transplant is approx 70–75%. Moreover, SCID patients treated by a haploidentical transplant present a long-term decline of the immunological reconstitution and an infrequent correction of the B-cell immunity because of several contributing factors such as the likely absence of stem cells engraftment in the absence of fully myeloablative conditioning regimen, and the potential allogeneic damage to the thymic epithelium. Therefore, several groups have developed active preclinical research to try to establish alternative treatments based on the "ex vivo retrovirus transduction" of autologous HSC. SCID indeed appeared as good candidates for this approach for several reasons: they are monogeneic diseases, the involved genes have been mostly identified and these disease are lethal, HSC are accessible for manipulation, although an immune response against the transgene is not expected and more importantly, the presence of a growth selective advantage for transduced cells has been well demonstrated by clinical and preclinical studies.

ADENOSINE DEAMINASE DEFICIENCY Adenosine deaminase (ADA) deficiency was the first disease to be treated

From: *Principles of Molecular Medicine, Second Edition*
Edited by: M. S. Runge and C. Patterson © Humana Press, Inc., Totowa, NJ

SCID Diseases and Mechanisms

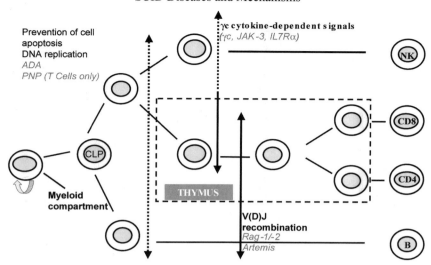

Figure 88-1   X-linked SCID and mechanisms.

Table 88-1
Characteristics of the Different SCID Conditions

	Disease	*Gene*	*Inheritance*
T(−),B(+)			
NK(−)	SCID-X1	γc	XL
NK(−)	SCID	Jak3	AR
NK(+)	SCID	IL7Rα	AR
NK(+)	SCID	?	AR
T(−),B(−)			
Myeloid(−), NK(−)	Reticular dysgenesis	?	AR
NK (variable)	ADA	Adenosine deaminase	AR
NK(+)	Alymphocytosis	RAG-1 or RAG-2	AR
NK(+)	Alymphocytosis	Artemis	AR
NK(+)	SCID	CD45	AR

ADA, adenosine deaminase; AR, autosomal-recessive; IL, interleukin; NK, natural killer; SCID, severe combined immunodeficiency; SCID-X1, X-linked severe combined immunodeficiency; XL, X-chromosome linked.

using gene therapy, following identification of the disease gene. This enzyme is responsible for detoxification of metabolites in the murine salvage pathway and its deficiency is responsible for the selective accumulation of deoxy ATP, which inhibits cell division and induces cell death by apoptosis. In this disease, there is a premature death of early lymphoid precursor cells caused by the accumulation of toxic metabolites. Other tissues and organs can be damaged in ADA deficiency such as the thymic epithelium, the lung, and the liver. This widespread toxicity can explain in part the rather poor prognosis of allogeneic bone marrow transplantation and thus justify the search for other therapeutic strategies including enzymatic substitution with polyethylene glycol-conjugated bovine-ADA (PEG–ADA) and gene therapy. Five gene therapy clinical trials have been conducted since 1990. The first two consisted of repeated infusions of peripheral T cells transduced ex vivo with an ADA–cDNA retroviral vector.

Two patients have been enrolled in the M. Blaese's trial and each of them received a total of approx 10^{11} cells over a period of approx 2 yr. During and after treatment they continued to receive PEG–ADA, therefore, conclusions on the clinical benefit are difficult to establish. In one patient, levels of transduced positive cells ranged from 20 to 40% of his circulating lymphocytes whereas the second one had <1% of transduced cells. Nevertheless, important information, up to 12 yr postgene therapy for the gene therapy field, has been provided by this pioneer trial. No adverse event occurred despite the injection of huge numbers of autologous modified T cells transduced with a first generation retroviral vector. The life span of human T cells can be prolonged, up to 12 yr following in vitro induction of their division. The Moloney retroviral promoter can drive transgene expression for long periods of time without silencing the gene. Immunodeficient patients with oligoclonal repertoire can mount efficient immune responses both against the retroviral envelope and the fetal calf serum used in the transduction procedure, confounding the interpretation of the clinical results and requiring changes in retroviral vector design and culture conditions to try to circumvent these problems.

In the second protocol performed by Bordignon's group, six patients received multiple infusions of autologous transduced peripheral blood lymphocytes as well as HSC. Among them, in one patient, who received 3.3×10^9 transduced peripheral blood lymphocytes, PEG–ADA treatment could be discontinued. The discontinuation led to a selective growth advantage of gene-transduced T lymphocytes although absolute CD34+ T-cell counts comparable to age-matched control were not reached. Some improvements of the immunological tests were also noted. Both protocols showed the limits of this strategy and opened the way to the HSC gene therapy of ADA patients. Three protocols attempted to target autologous HSC; however, the PEG–ADA substitutive treatment administered simultaneously is likely to have exerted a deleterious effect by decreasing or abrogating the presumed advantage conferred to the transduced cells. Other factors that could have contributed to the loss of benefit are the nonoptimal ex vivo transduction protocol and the retroviral vector used that could have been silenced in vivo. Candotti et al. enrolled four ADA patients in an optimized protocol. Higher levels of transduction have been achieved by using the vector called MND-ADA, which contains five mutations in the long terminal repeat. Frequency of circulating transduced cells is in the 1×10^{-5} order of magnitude. Despite these technical improvements, patients were maintained under PEG–ADA treatment and showed no clear changes in their immunological status after 1 yr of follow-up; it will be interesting to follow the consequences of PEG–ADA discontinuation.

All these limiting factors have been circumvented by Aiuti et al. who showed that gene therapy in the absence of concomitant PEG–ADA treatment, with a mild myeloablation can successfully treat ADA deficiency. Four patients have been treated and longer follow-up in two showed a significant correction of the immune deficiency. Whether this success is owing to PEG–ADA omission and/or to the addition of a mild myeloablation is unknown. Expression of ADA by T cells alone may not be sufficient to correct the overall metabolic ADA deficiency; therefore, myeloablation, by increasing the level of hematopoietic correction, is likely to be a contributing factor.

X-LINKED SEVERE COMBINED IMMUNODEFICIENCY

SCID-X1 is the most frequent form of SCID accounting for 50% of cases. Absence of mature T and natural killer (NK) lymphocytes associated with a normal B-cell differentiation are the main characteristics of this disease, which results from mutations of the gene encoding the γ-common (γc-chain) subunit of the hematopoietic cytokine receptors family. The γc-chain is shared by several receptors of this family including the interleukin (IL)-2, IL-4, -7, -9, -15, and -21. The defective IL-7 and -15 induced growth and proliferation signaling are responsible for the early block observed in T and NK differentiation pathway, respectively.

The role of the γc-chain in the survival, proliferation, and differentiation of the lymphoid precursors led to the expectation that its expression could confer a major selective growth to the transduced cells over nontransduced counterparts. This expectation was fulfilled in a well-documented case of reversion of a point mutation that naturally occurred in a boy with an attenuated form of SCID-X1. In this case, the mutation reversion occurred in a single T-cell progenitor, after the branching point of the NK, as the patient presented low circulating numbers of oligoclonal T cells expressing the normal γc molecule, although NK cells were absent and γc expression on B lymphocytes and monocytes, which all carried the original mutation, was not detectable. This clonal reversion allowed limited but sustained immunological functions up to 6 yr of age after which the patient has been successfully transplanted.

In addition to this observation, a number of preclinical studies provided clear data in favor of this approach. All confirmed that the ex vivo transduction of γc-deficient HSC restored the differentiation of NK and T cells without any detectable adverse effect. The first clinical trial was initiated in March 1999. Ten children under the age of 1 yr were enrolled by May 2002. Detailed analysis of the gene therapy results of the first five treated patients has been reported. A second clinical trial was established in the United Kingdom and enrolled four patients affected by the classic form of SCID-X1. These two trials were proposed for SCID-X1 patients lacking an HLA-identical donor. The protocol consisted of marrow harvesting; CD34-cell positive selection; preactivation in the presence of early acting cytokines as stem cell factor, FLT3-L, megakaryocyte growth and developmental factor, IL-3 or IL-6; and three cycles of infection with the supernatant containing the

defective amphotrophe or GALV retroviral vector in sterile bags coated with CH-296 fibronectin fragment. After ex vivo transduction, cells were infused to the patients who did not receive any myeloablative therapy.

In 13 out of the 14 treated patients, transduced T cells appeared 60–90 d after treatment and their counts reached the normal or close to normal range within 4–6 mo following gene transfer, remaining stable thereafter. The different T-cell subsets, including T-cell receptor (TCR) αβ and γδ+ cells were detected in normal proportions and were found functional as evidenced by proliferation in the presence of mitogens and of immunization antigens. Despite a very low (approx 1%) transduction rate of B lymphocytes, the treated children developed B-cell antibody responses, enabling a majority of patients to discontinue intravenous immunoglobulin therapy. Conversely, the NK-cell restoration appeared limited over time; following a rapid normalization of the NK-cell counts after gene therapy (i.e., approx d 45–60), the NK-cell compartment declined. Two explanations that are not mutually exclusive can account for this result, i.e., a limited expansion capacity of the NK-precursor cell and the potential lack of a γc-dependent hematopoietic cell able to sustain NK-cell development or survival.

As a consequence of the development of T- and B-cell immune responses, a favorable clinical outcome ensued allowing the patients to resume normal growth and to enjoy a normal life despite cessation of all treatment. Although these findings indicate that immunological correction of SCID-X1 condition by gene therapy is achievable, two SAE occurred 3 yr after gene therapy, which forced reassessment of the delicate balance between risk/benefit of this powerful therapeutic approach. Two children developed a clonal T-cell lymphoproliferation owing, at least in part, to the consequences of insertional mutagenesis. The two patients who developed this clonal lymphoproliferation have been treated by conventional chemotherapy and are in complete remission. The retrovirus vector integrated close to the LMO_2 (LIM domain only) transcription factor and induced its aberrant expression on immature T cells. This transcription factor is a master gene in embryonic and adult hematopoiesis and is involved in acute T-lymphoblastic leukemia both in mice and in humans. Additional factors must have contributed to these SAE justifying the transitional hold of this clinical trial and close monitoring of the other treated patients whereas the search continues for other contributive factors, such as age, disease, and genetic susceptibility μo_2. Altogether these studies should lead to a precise evaluation of the risk as well as a modification of the vectors to decrease or prevent the occurrence of these adverse events.

JAK 3 DEFICIENCY

This form of SCID is characterized by an immunological phenotype identical to that of SCID-X1 described earlier. The Jak-3 protein tyrosine kinase is indeed associated to γc and mediates cytokine-induced signaling. The results obtained after transferring the JAK3 gene in vitro and in vivo argue in favor of using this therapeutic approach. In support of this, it was found that the retroviral transduction of the cDNA into Epstein-Barr Virus Jak-3(–) lineages restored the expression and phosphorylation of this protein and caused these cells to proliferate in response to IL-2 and IL-4. The transduction of bone marrow cells in Jak3 (–) mice induced T- and B-lymphocyte differentiation and restored their functions. This result clearly demonstrates the existence of a selective advantage for ex vivo corrected hematopoietic cells and represented the first animal model demonstration of the concept. One study performed by the same groups in a larger number of animals has excluded the possibility of any toxic effect. One 3-yr-old child has been enrolled in a clinical trial. No correction has been observed possibly because of the relative old age of the patient.

SCID WITH T AND B ALYMPHOCYTOSIS Of patients suffering from SCID, approx 20% have complete absence of mature T- and B-lymphocytes, whereas NK cells are present in normal numbers and are functional. Inheritance is autosomal-recessive and the thymus in these patients is hypoplastic. The phenotype is reminiscent of that of natural mutant SCID mice, characterized by a lack of T and B differentiation. This form may be subdivided into two groups on the basis of cell sensitivity to ionizing radiation, distinguishing SCID with normal sensitivity to ionizing radiation and SCID with increased sensitivity. The ionizing radiation causes double-strand breaks in the DNA and their repair involves proteins that are also necessary for *rearranging the genes* involved in the formation of TCR and B-cell receptor encoding genes.

The molecular basis of the genetic defect presented by subjects who are suffering from SCID with increased sensitivity to ionizing radiation has been identified; radiosensitive SCID is caused by mutation of the Artemis gene. Patients suffering from T(–) B(–) SCID, but not showing any abnormal sensitivity to ionizing radiation, present mutations in the genes coding for the RAG1 and RAG2 proteins responsible for initiating the V(D)J recombination process. These SCID conditions are good candidates for gene therapy because a selective advantage should be also confered to transduced cells, and unregulated expression of this protein should not be toxic because the V(D)J recombination is obtained solely through the combined action of the RAG1 and RAG2 proteins and Artemis ubiquitously expressed. Mice transgenic for one of these two proteins do not show any lymphohematopoietic abnormalities. The preliminary data obtained after Rag2 gene transfer into the hematopoeitic cells of RAG2-deficient mice showed that normal cell and humoral immunity was restored and remained stable for more than 1 yr without any detectable toxicity.

WISKOTT–ALDRICH SYNDROME

Wiskott–Aldrich syndrome (WAS) is a rare inherited disease characterized by immune dysregulation and microthrombocytopenia. In its less severe form, known as X-linked thrombocytopenia, mutations in the same gene produce the characteristic platelet abnormality but minimal immunological disturbance. Clinical manifestations of the immune disorder in WAS include susceptibility to pyogenic, viral, and opportunistic infection, eczema, autoimmune phenomena, and increased incidence of B-cell lymphoproliferative disease. The most invariable abnormality is thrombocytopenia (platelet count usually <70,000/mm^3 in the absence of splenectomy) with small platelet volume (mean platelet volume usually <5 fL), that is present from birth. As a consequence, the majority of patients present with related complications, which vary from minor bruising to life-threatening gastrointestinal or intracranial hemorrhage. In general, a platelet count of <10,000/mm^3 is predictive of severe bleeding complications, although higher counts are not necessarily protective. A progressive decrease in T-cell number (in peripheral blood and lymphoid tissue) and function during childhood is associated with restricted defects in proliferative responses of WAS T cells (particularly CD3-mediated proliferation, but also depressed responses

to mitogens), deficient antibody responses to polysaccharide and protein antigens, and low or absent levels of isohemagglutinins. Quantitative abnormalities of immunoglobulin levels evolve in many patients, manifesting typically as low levels of IgM and increased levels of IgA, IgD, and IgE. Immune dysregulation may also manifest as food allergy, or as autoimmune disease, including hemolytic anemia, vasculitis, inflammatory polyarthritis, and inflammatory bowel disease. The median survival for WAS patients is approx 15–25 yr, and the usual causes of death (unrelated to transplantation procedures) are infection, bleeding, and malignancy, with a considerable variability in disease severity.

The WAS gene encodes a proline-rich intracellular protein, WASp, which belongs to a defined family of more widely expressed proteins involved in transduction of signals from receptors on the cell surface to the actin cytoskeleton. WASp itself is expressed exclusively in hematopoietic cells, including stem and progenitor cells.

The molecular control of actin filament assembly and disassembly is of necessity highly regulated and coordinated, as reflected in the complex modular domain structure of WASp that supports its role as a platform for integration of signals from diverse input pathways. The activity of WASp is modulated by multiple signals, including binding of the Rho GTPase Cdc42 in the GTP-bound state, phosphatidylinositol-4,5-bisphosphate, SH-2 domain containing proteins, and tyrosine and serine phosphorylation. In the activated configuration, WASp triggers actin polymerization through binding to the actin related protein, Arp2/3 complex. This initiates actin nucleation, which is the rate-limiting step in polymerization of monomeric G-actin. The biological mechanisms responsible for the pathophysiology of WAS are therefore linked to deficient actin polymerization in hematopoietic cells. As a result, WASp-deficient cells exhibit profound cytoskeletal defects leading to abnormalities of chemotaxis, migration, phagocytosis, receptor-mediated (including TCR) signaling, and platelet function.

CONVENTIONAL TREATMENT Conventional therapy includes the use of prophylactic antibiotics and immunoglobulin for infections, and platelet transfusion in circumstances of life-threatening hemorrhage (e.g., intracranial) or prior to surgical procedures. Splenectomy is usually effective in increasing platelet numbers and reducing bleeding complications, but also increases the risk of infection. The only curative therapy for WAS is allogeneic stem cell transplantation. Survival rates following transplantation from HLA-identical sibling donors and matched HLA-unrelated donors in WAS approach 90%. However, transplantation with HLA-nonidentical grafts, and transplantation in older patients results in an exceptionally high incidence of graft rejection, graft-vs-host disease (GVHD) and Epstein-Barr virus-related lymphoproliferative disease (39% of HLA-nonidentical transplants, European Group for Bone Marrow Transplant Registry).

GENE THERAPY For those patients without an HLA-matched donor source, stem cell gene therapy is a highly attractive proposition. Emerging preclinical data suggest that this will be feasible. Interestingly, several reports suggest that "corrected" T cells from classic WASp-null patients have significant growth and survival advantages over mutant cells. For example, in one member of a classic WAS kindred, in vivo reversion of a 6-bp deletion led to the reconstitution of WASp expression in the majority of circulating T cells (presumably derived from a single precursor), but not in myeloid cells, B lymphocytes, or NK cells. In a second example, a second site mutation in a precursor resulted in deletion of the disease causing primary mutation, and reconstitution of functional WASp. A small fraction of the total T-cell population expressed WASp, but this was enriched in the CD45RO fraction indicating an advantage for acquisition of immunological memory. Correction of cells by gene transfer (stem cells or lineage restricted T-cell populations) would, therefore, be expected to provide similar survival pressures. It has previously been suggested that selective pressures may also exist for homing of stem cell populations, which may, therefore, positively influence the engraftment potential for corrected cells. This is supported by serial murine transplantation and competitive reconstitution experiments demonstrating that WASp-null bone marrow cells, including HSCs, have decreased homing and engraftment capacities.

Reconstitution of cytoskeletal defects by gene transfer has been reported for lymphoblastoid cell lines, and reconstitution of anti-CD3 mediated proliferation in WAS T cells and T-cell lines derived from patients. Partial correction of a murine model in terms of antigen receptor-mediated proliferation of WAS T cells has been demonstrated following gene transfer to HSCs. All these studies have used conventional γ-retroviral vectors, and although adverse effects have not been reported, some concerns remain related to transgene toxicity. Certainly, in cell lines, overexpression of WASp leads to polymerization of actin in highly abnormal structures. A mutation in WASp that results in its constitutive activation has been shown to predispose to myelodysplasia and genetic instability. The identification of natural regulatory sequences or promoters that mimic physiological gene expression is, therefore, an important goal for optimization of safety, and will be facilitated by the development of sophisticated lentivirus-based vector systems. In preliminary studies, such systems have been used to demonstrate correction of cytoskeletal defects in WASp-null T-cell lines, macrophages, and osteoclasts, and are being tested in murine models in preparation for clinical studies.

HEMOGLOBINOPATHIES

Thalassemias and sickle cell disease (SCD) were the earliest monogenic disorders considered for gene therapy. These hemoglobinopathies are associated with high morbidity and mortality throughout the world. β-Thalassemia is caused by various mutations or deletions within the adult β-globin gene or its controling elements that result in decreased expression levels and the accumulation of toxic, unbound α-globin chains. This in turn causes ineffective erythropoiesis and hemolytic anemia requiring lifelong red cell transfusions. Premature death occurs from complications of iron loading in spite of iron chelation therapy. Although patients' survival has improved, β-thalassemia remains a serious public health problem.

SCD was the first genetic disorder to be understood at the protein and subsequently DNA levels: the substitution of valine for glutamic acid in human β-globin codon 6. In homozygotes, the abnormal hemoglobin (Hb) HbS ($\alpha_2 \beta_2^s$) polymerizes in long fibers on deoxygenation within red blood cells, which become deformed (sickled), rigid, and adhesive, thereby triggering microcirculation occlusion, anemia, infarction, and organ damage. SCD is one of the most prevalent autosomal-recessive disorders worldwide. In certain regions of tropical Africa, the frequency of heterozygotes reaches 40%, as heterozygosity confers a protective advantage against malaria. In the United States, approx 1 out of 13 African Americans carries the mutated gene, which is also common among individuals of Mediterranean, Middle-Eastern, or Indian descent. SCD patients still suffer from high morbidity and increased mortality despite progress in symptomatic disease management and partial pharmacological inhibition of sickle cell formation with hydroxyurea and butyrate derivatives. For both β-thalassemia and SCD, the only hope of cure remains allogenic bone marrow transplantation from a related, HLA-matched donor. However, only a small subset of patients have a compatible donor and those who do still face the risk of severe and often lethal consequences of GVHD.

The idea of a gene therapy for the β-hemoglobinopathies was in principle straightforward: integrating in the HSC chromosomes a normal β-globin gene or an antisickling gene, for β-thalassemia and SCD, respectively, with sufficiently high expression in the red blood cell lineage. Retroviral vectors were the vector of choice, because they were the only effective means to integrate genes into the HSC genome. Regarding the choice of the antisickling gene, various globin chains are known to inhibit HbS polymerization. Human γ-globin is a much stronger inhibitor of HbS polymerization than human β-globin, because it is excluded from the polymer and it interferes with its formation through intermolecular contacts. Previously, β-globin gene transfer into HSC in mice has been too low to warrant instigation of a clinical trial. The most important technical challenge has been to design stable vectors containing the functional globin gene and the necessary regulatory elements, such as the β-locus control region (LCR), to achieve high-level and stable globin gene expression in developing erythroblasts. The first (β-globin/LCR) retroviral vectors tested were notoriously unstable with low titers and multiple rearrangements of the integrated proviral structure. Unwanted splicing of the retroviral RNA prior to packaging into virions was found to be the main mechanism of instability of (β-globin/LCR) retroviral vectors. Also, mutagenesis of the main cryptic splice sites can prevent this instability. A similar result was achieved by sequence permutation of LCR elements.

Even with these stable LCR retroviral vectors, initial reports have indicated that despite the inclusion of elements from the LCR into the retroviral vectors, the level of β-globin expression was suboptimal, decreased over time and was suffering from position effect variegation, which is a reflection of the effects of flanking chromatin in differentiated cells and of chromatin remodeling at the site of integration in the progeny of pluripotential cells. To avoid in vivo HSC β-globin gene silencing, ex vivo preselection of retrovirally-transduced stem cells using GFP expression (green fluorescent protein gene marker) juxtaposed to the β-globin/LCR segment was investigated. All mice engrafted with preselected cells showed sustained expression of human β-globin and GFP in red cells.

To allow larger LCR elements to be successfully transferred in an effort to surmount the limitations observed in long-term β-globin gene expression, the use of RNA export elements such as the Rev protein of HIV together with its Rev-responsive element has been proposed. Extending previous evidence on the utility of lentiviral vectors for gene transfer to HSCs, HIV-based lentiviral vectors carrying a Rev-responsive element allowed successful transfer of large LCR fragments with dramatic amelioration of β-thalassemia in transplanted mouse β-thalassemia models of various severity. When a high-titer (β-globin/LCR) lentiviral vector was used to achieve multiple provirus copy integration (approx 2–3/HSC), balanced expression opposing variegation was achieved with high,

liver, kidneys, dental, and immune systems. SDS is the second most common cause of exocrine pancreatic insufficiency in children next to cystic fibrosis, occurring at an estimated incidence of 1/100,000–200,000. It is an autosomal-recessive disorder with the SDS locus mapped to chromosome 7.

Clinical Features Hematological abnormalities are varied regarding cytopenia and cell lines affected, many of which are detected in the neonatal period. Neutropenia is also a required diagnostic feature and approx 25% of patients develop marrow failure and aplastic anemia. There is also an increased risk of MDS and AML as with other congenital aplastic anemia syndromes.

Diagnosis Peripheral blood smears display varying degrees of cytopenias with neutropenia being the most common abnormality, occurring in 88–100% of cases. Anemia is usually normocytic, but macrocytosis is also found. Thrombocytopenia is seen in 25–90% of patients. Pancytopenia, seen in up to 65% of patients, is a poor prognostic sign and carries a higher chance of developing severe aplastic anemia if present. Hypoplasia and fatty infiltration are typically seen in varying degrees, and severity of cytopenia does not necessarily correlate with bone marrow findings. Many findings suggest that SDS is actually an MDS from its onset because it is a stem-cell disorder with peripheral cytopenia, ineffective hematopoiesis, scattered foci of dysplastic changes in the marrow, varying degrees of marrow cellularity, and a risk of transformation into acute leukemia. If dysplasia is a prominent feature, it signifies malignant myeloid transformation, which for SDS means more advanced stages of MDS.

Genetics Several different cytogenetic abnormalities have been reported in patients with SDS. Of these patients, 24% had isochromosome 7q[i(7q)], a finding uncommon in AML, acute lymphocytic leukemia, or MDS without SDS. It is likely a specific clonal marker for SDS given its high occurrence rate and is probably related to the SDS gene locus being at 7q11. Other chromosome 7 abnormalities have been described including monosomy 7, combined i(7q) and monosomy 7, and deletions or translocations involving the long arm of chromosome 7. This population of patients with chromosome 7 abnormalities has a high likelihood of developing subsequent MDS or AML. The exact mechanism of malignant myeloid transformation is not known, but it is possible the SDS gene product is required for the development and maintenance of stem cells or progenitor cells of other tissues. The SDS gene locus has been mapped to the centromeric region of chromosome 7 (7p10-7q11). Several mutations in the gene responsible for SDS, called *SBDS*, have been reported. The gene contains five exons and encodes a 250 amino acid protein of uncharacterized function. It is speculated that the *SBDS* gene product is involved in RNA metabolism. There is also a pseudogene, *SBDSP,* located in a duplicated genomic segment of 305 kb that shares 97% nucleotide identity with *SBDS*. Originally, SDS was thought to be a result of gene mutations involving a region within exon 2 of the *SBDS* gene. These mutations resulted from gene conversions owing to recombination with the *SBDSP* pseudogene. Although these data were from patients of European ancestry, other data from Japanese patients have identified two recurrent mutations (96-97insA, 258 + 2T→C) and three novel mutations (292-295delAAAG, 183-184TA→CT + 201A→G, and 141C→T + 183-184TA→CT + 201A→G). These mutations occurred in various locations between intron 1 and exon 3, not just within exon 2 as previously described. Additional studies are needed to help elucidate the exact mechanism by which these genetic mutations lead to the SDS phenotype.

Management Frequent monitoring of cytopenias and supportive care are mainstays of therapy for the hematological problems in patients with SDS. For severe neutropenia, growth factor support is often used and intravenous antibiotics are given if infection occurs. Occasional responses to immunosuppression have been reported but are rare. PBSCT is the only curative option for the hematological complications of SDS. PBSCT has been used more commonly during the MDS phase of the syndrome. Of seven patients transplanted during an MDS phase, one had a matched-related donor and was alive at 2 yr follow-up. Of the six receiving unrelated transplants, two were alive at 12 and 41 mo, whereas the other four died. Treatment for patients progressing to acute leukemia is standard induction therapy with an effort toward PBSCT as soon as possible.

MYELODYSPLASTIC SYNDROMES

MDSs are a group of hematological conditions characterized by one or more peripheral blood cytopenias with accompanying bone marrow dysfunction. They can occur *de novo* or secondary to treatment with chemotherapy or radiation therapy for other diseases. The secondary form of MDS usually has a poorer prognosis than *de novo* forms. Approximately one-third of cases of MDS progress to acute myeloid leukemia. The annual incidence is approx 4.1/100,000 with most series showing a male predominance. This compares to approx 2.1/100,000 for acute leukemia.

CLINICAL FEATURES MDS occurs predominantly in patients older than 60 yr. Common findings include anemia, fatigue, dizziness, exercise intolerance, and easy bruising (*see* Fig. 89-1). All are sequelae of peripheral cytopenias and not disease specific. Often patients are asymptomatic and diagnosed from routine blood work. Neutropenia is responsible for a high incidence of infections in patients with MDS. Autoimmune phenomena including arthritis, pericarditis, iritis, myositis, and peripheral neuropathy. Cutaneous vasculitis can occur although hepatosplenomegaly is an uncommon finding on physical exam.

DIAGNOSIS Normocytic or macrocytic anemia with a low reticulocyte count is almost uniformly present. About 50% of cases are present with neutropenia. Granulocytes often display decreased segmentation with reduced or absent granulation, a finding known as the pseudo-Pelger-Huet anomaly. Some degree of thrombocytopenia is present in approx 25% of cases. The bone marrow is usually hypercellular with single or multilineage dysplasia. The diagnosis of MDS should be considered in any patient with cytopenias of unclear etiology with a diagnostic work up including a peripheral blood smear and bone marrow biopsy with cytogenetics.

GENETICS Chromosomal abnormalities occur in up to 70% of MDS cases. The most common abnormalities are del(5q) and monosomy or del(7q). Trisomy 8, del(17p), and del(20q) are also frequently seen. Trisomy 8, del(5q), and del(7q) are seen in both MDS and AML; however, balanced translocations are distinct for AML and almost never seen in MDS. With the exception of the 5q-syndrome (deletion of the long arm of chromosome 5), cytogenetic changes do not typically correlate with any specific morphological subtype of MDS. In the 5q-syndrome, 80% of patients have refractory anemia and only approx 15% of these patients transform to acute leukemia. Although the majority of cases have an interstitial del(5)(q13q33), other deletions including del(5)(q15q33) and del(5)(q22q33) have been described. The mutations necessary for leukemic transformation in MDS are not known. Changes in the N-ras oncogene, p53 and *IRF-1* tumor suppressor genes, *Bcl-2*

Table 89-2
International Prognosis Scoring System
in Myelodysplastic Syndrome

Variable	0	0.5	1.0	1.5	2.0
Marrow blasts (%)	<5	5–10	–	11–20	21–30
Karyotype	Good	Intermediate	Poor	–	–
Cytopenias	0–1	2–3	–	–	–

Risk group	IPSS score	Median survival (yr)
Low	0	5.7
Intermediate-1	0.5–1.0	3.5
Intermediate-2	1.5–2.0	1.2
High	>2.5	0.4

Karyotypes: Good = normal, –Y, del(5q), del(20q); poor = complex (>3 abnormalities) or abnormal chromosome 7; intermediate = all others.

Cytopenias: neutrophils <1800/uL, platelets <100,000/uL, hemoglobin <10 g/dL.

apoptotic gene, and transcription factor genes such as *EVI1* and *MLL* have all been implicated.

PROGNOSIS Patients without cytogenetic abnormalities have a low likelihood of developing AML although complex cytogenetic abnormalities increase the chance of transformation to AML and are associated with refractory disease and subsequently shortened survival times. Overall, progression to AML occurs in 20–35% of patients. Prognosis is best for del(5q) and del(20q) abnormalities, intermediate for other single cytogenetic abnormalities, and poor if complex abnormalities are present. Single cytogenetic defects of chromosome 7, especially involving 7q32 also yield poor outcomes. There is an international prognostic scoring system (IPSS) for MDS based on percent marrow blasts, number of cytopenias, and types of cytogenetic abnormalities present (Table 89-2). Median survival times for good, intermediate, and poor outcome groups are 3.8, 2.4, and 0.8 yr, respectively, and correlate most strongly with the frequency of marrow blasts.

MANAGEMENT The four goals of treatment for MDS are to control symptoms resulting from cytopenias, improve quality of life with low toxicity, improve overall survival, and slow progression to AML. Treatment assessment should be based on age, performance status, and IPSS-defined risk category. Furthermore, treatments are categorized into high intensity (intensive chemotherapy regimens and stem cell transplant) vs low intensity (growth factor support and low intensity chemotherapy). In general, patients younger than 60 yr of age with a good performance status who have an IPSS intermediate to high-risk profile should be offered high intensity therapy. Those with low-risk IPSS profiles generally receive low intensity therapy. Those older than age 60 most often get low intensity therapy, although each patient must be evaluated individually. Supportive care with growth factors, antibiotics as needed for infections, and transfusional support are given to poor performance status patients. Treatments such as 5-azacytidine appear to delay the time to development of AML and reduce the frequency of transfusions by promoting cell differentiation through methylation of DNA.

AGNOGENIC MYELOID METAPLASIA/ MYELOFIBROSIS

There are both malignant and nonmalignant causes of collagen deposition within the bone marrow leading to myelofibrosis. The idiopathic form of myelofibrosis, also known as agnogenic myeloid metaplasia (AMM), is discussed here. This is a malignant disorder of the hematopoietic stem cell that leads to a nonclonal fibrosis of the marrow characterized by anemia, splenomegaly, and extramedullary hematopoiesis. First described in the late 1800s, it is classified with other myeloproliferative disorders including essential thrombocythemia, polycythemia vera, and chronic myelogenous leukemia. Essential thrombocythemia and polycythemia vera can develop into AMM. All of the myeloproliferative disorders are at risk for transformation into acute leukemia as well. The annual incidence of AMM is approx 0.5/100,000 with a median age at diagnosis of 60 yr. Noted risk factors include exposure to radiation, benzene, and thorium dioxide (used as a radioactive contrast agent). Viral origins for AMM and the other myeloproliferative disorders remain speculative.

CLINICAL FEATURES Symptoms of fatigue, weakness, palpitations, and dyspnea are not uncommon and may be disproportionate to the degree of anemia (*see* Fig. 89-1). Splenomegaly is typically present and may be massive in nature leading to early satiety and weight loss. Despite the multitude of symptoms that can be involved in AMM, at least 25% of patients are asymptomatic at presentation and the diagnosis is made by routine lab screening. Exam findings include pallor, jaundice, hepatosplenomegaly, petechiae, and easy bruising. Thrombosis of the portal or hepatic veins as well as increased portal blood flow from an enlarged spleen resulting from extramedullary hematopoiesis secondary to marrow fibrosis may occur and cause portal hypertension.

DIAGNOSIS The characteristic peripheral blood smear in AMM shows teardrop-shaped red blood cells with poikilocytosis. Immature myeloid cells and large platelets are also seen. The bone marrow often produces a "dry tap" secondary to fibrosis. The core biopsy shows patchy cellularity with clusters of dysplastic megakaryocytes. Reticulin stains are positive for varying degrees of fibrosis.

GENETICS No consistent cytogenetic abnormalities have been noted with AMM, although trisomy 8, 9, and 21 have been described. Other abnormalities including del(13q) and del(20q) have been reported. Although the hematopoiesis in AMM has a clonal nature, the fibrosis in AMM is thought to be a chronic reactive stromal process. Collagen deposition is increased within the marrow stroma with greater amounts of collagen types I, III, IV, and V present. This increased collagen deposition at sites of clustered megakaryocytes in AMM led to the search for possible cytokines that could explain the pathogenesis of fibrosis in this disorder. Platelet-derived growth factor, transforming growth factor (TGF)-β, and fibroblast growth factor-acidic are all cytokines contained within platelet granules. These cytokines can induce marrow fibroblast proliferation leading to AMM. Specifically, TGF decreases the synthesis of enzymes that degrade collagen and increases expression of certain genes responsible for creating various form of collagen. Other actions of TGF include stimulating increases in platelet-derived growth factor from endothelial cells within the marrow. This may allow for augmentation of fibroblast proliferation and increased collagen deposition as well. TGF-β may also cause a TPO-induced myelofibrosis as seen in mouse models. The bone marrow stem cells from wild-type and TGF-β null mice were infected with a retrovirus encoding TPO protein and engrafted into lethally irradiated hosts. Over time, myelofibrosis was seen in the spleen and marrow of all mice engrafted with wild-type cells vs no fibrosis in mice engrafted with TGF-β null cells. AMM is associated with changes in megakaryocytopoiesis with accumulation of megakaryocytes within the marrow. This adds to the thought that activation of stromal cells by cytokines released by megakaryocytes may be the etiology of AMM. GATA-1 is a transcription factor with differentiating effects on erythroid and megakaryocytic cell lines. Mice with the GATA-1^{low} mutation develop a myelofibrosis-like disease suggesting that alterations in GATA-1 expression may also contribute to AMM pathogenesis. An exact gene locus responsible for AMM has not been elucidated, although candidate genes being studied include retinoblastoma, p53, p16, and RAS.

MANAGEMENT Treatment is instituted once a patient develops symptoms from severe anemia or thrombocytopenia, symptomatic splenomegaly, or from symptomatic extramedullary hematopoiesis, which can be in various tissues of the body. For suitable candidates, allogeneic stem cell transplant represents the only curative option. This is typically attempted in young patients with a matched sibling. Agents such as hydroxyurea and IFN have been used to reduce symptomatic splenomegaly and improve peripheral cell counts. Growth factor support has also been used with limited success in those who are not candidates for stem cell transplant. Certain subsets of patients with severe thrombocytopenia, refractory associated hemolytic anemia, portal hypertension with gastrointestinal bleeding, and symptomatic, massive splenomegaly should be considered for splenectomy. Symptoms of more than 50% of patients improve despite the transient decrease in blood counts frequently following such a procedure. If a patient is inoperable, splenic irradiation may be a reasonable alternative. Median survival for AMM is approx 5 yr. The presence of circulating early precursors cells, severe anemia, and cytogenetic abnormalities decreases survival by as much as 50%.

OTHER CAUSES OF BONE MARROW FAILURE/PERIPHERAL CYTOPENIAS

DIAMOND–BLACKFAN ANEMIA Diamond–Blackfan anemia (DBA), a rare congenital hypoplastic anemia, presents in infancy at an incidence of 4–5/million live births. Dominant and recessive inheritance is found in approximately one-fourth of cases. Patients have a moderate-to-severe macrocytic anemia, occasional neutropenia and thrombocytosis with erythroid hypoplasia in a normocellular bone marrow. Head and upper extremity anomalies are present in one-fourth of individuals. Linkage studies including families with dominant and recessive inheritance patterns have localized the DBA gene to chromosome 19q13. In 25% of dominantly inherited DBA, mutations in a critical 1 Mb region coding for ribosomal protein S19 are found with up to 60 mutations across the entire gene having been described. The protein is ubiquitously expressed in hematological and nonhematological tissues, but it remains unclear how defects in this gene cause problems with erythropoiesis.

KOSTMANN SYNDROME Kostmann syndrome (KS) is an autosomal-recessive disorder notable for severe neutropenia resulting in frequent bacterial infections and early death. Bone marrow shows normal erythroid and platelet precursors with absent or markedly reduced myeloid cells. Increased risks of MDS and/or AML exist for these patients. Some evidence of a defect in the GCSF receptor exists although the data are inconclusive and contradictory. Expression of Bcl-2 is decreased in myeloid progenitor cells of patients with KS although mitochondrial release of cytochrome *c* and apoptosis are increased compared with controls. Additionally,

treatment with GCSF improved both Bcl-2 expression and progenitor cell survival although partially reversing cytochrome *c* release from mitochondria. This points to a possible role for mitochondria-dependent apoptosis in the pathogenesis of KS and lends support to the use of hematopoietic growth factors in treating the syndrome. Although the exact genetic mechanism of KS remains unclear, treatment with recombinant GCSF can have a positive impact on the lives of patients with this disorder, and stem cell transplant is used only in rare circumstances in which treatment with GCSF is unsuccessful.

CONGENITAL AMEGAKARYOCYTIC THROMBOCYTOPENIA Congenital amegakaryocytic thrombocytopenia (CAMT) is a rare disorder that presents in infancy with isolated thrombocytopenia and progresses into pancytopenia later in childhood. TPO is important for megakaryopoiesis as well as early hematopoiesis with high levels of TPO found in the sera of patients with CAMT. Assays for reactivity to TPO in platelets and early progenitor cells in patients with CAMT were negative. Further flow analysis found an absence of the TPO surface receptor c-mpl in patients with this disorder. Several point mutations in the c-mpl gene lead to complete loss of receptor function. It is postulated that this is the cause of the thrombocytopenia and progressive pancytopenia seen in CAMT. For example, one point mutation leads to an exchange of arginine 102 to proline, which may alter protein folding and subsequent binding of TPO to its receptor.

NUTRITIONAL CAUSES OF PANCYTOPENIA Severe nutritional deficiencies can result in single or multilineage cytopenias. Three prominent deficiencies include vitamin B12, folate, and iron. With B12 and folate deficiencies, patients typically present with a megaloblastic anemia that results from impaired DNA synthesis. Hereditary forms of B12 deficiency exist, such as Imerslund–Grasbeck's disease (megaloblastic anemia 1) that is inherited in an autosomal-recessive pattern and caused by malabsorption of intrinsic factor-B12 complex. A disease specific mutation called P1297L (FM1) in the IF-B12 receptor, cubilin, results in loss of affinity of the mutant receptor for the IF-B12 complex and thus decreased absorption of B12. Hematological findings of B12/folate deficiency include a macrocytic anemia, elevated lactate dehydrogenase and bilirubin from ineffective erythropoiesis, normal to low reticulocyte count, and normal to low leukocytes and platelets. Neutrophils are typically hypersegmented (>5% of neutrophils with five or more lobes or 1% with six or more lobes). Bone marrow biopsy shows a hypercellular marrow with megaloblastic erythroid hyperplasia. Iron deficiency results from many causes with blood loss being the most common etiology. Malabsorption of iron is uncommon but does occur with such disease entities as celiac sprue. The anemia is microcytic/hypochromic in nature. Symptoms such as fatigue, dyspnea, and poor exercise tolerance ensue as the anemia progresses. With severe anemia from any nutritional deficiency, pancytopenia may occur and disorders such as MDS, AML, and aplastic anemia must be excluded.

SELECTED REFERENCES

Ballmaier M, Germeshausen M, Schulze H, et al. *c-mpl* mutations are the cause of congenital amegakaryocytic thrombocytopenia. Blood 2001; 97(1):139–146.

Carlsson G, Aprikyan AA, Tehranchi R, et al. Kostmann syndrome: severe congenital neutropenia associated with defective expression of Bcl-2, constitutive mitochondrial release of cytochrome c, and excessive apoptosis of myeloid progenitor cells. Blood 2004;103(9):3355–3361.

Deeg HJ, Seidel K, Casper J, et al. Marrow transplantation from unrelated donors for patients with severe aplastic anemia who have failed immunosuppressive therapy. Biol Blood Marrow Transplant 1999; 5(4):243–252.

Dokal I. Dyskeratosis congenita in all its forms. Br J Haematol 2000; 110(4):768–769.

Dror Y, Freedman MH. Shwachman-Diamond Syndrome. Br J Haematol 2002;118(3):701–713.

Fogarty PF, Yamaguchi H, Wiestner A, et al. Late presentation of dyskeratosis congenita as apparently acquired aplastic anemia due to mutations in telomerase RNA. Lancet 2003;362(9396):1628–1630.

Greenberg P, Cox C, LeBeau MM, et al. International scoring system for evaluating prognosis in myelodysplastic syndromes. Blood 1997; 89(6): 2079–2088.

Heaney ML, Golde DW. Myelodysplasia. N Engl J Med 1999;340(21): 1649–1660.

Kristiansen M, Aminoff M, Jacobsen C, et al. Cubilin P1297L mutation associated with hereditary megaloblastic anemia 1 causes impaired recognition of intrinsic factor-vitamin B12 by cubilin. Blood 2000; 96(2):405–409.

Li Y, Youssoufian H. MxA overexpression reveals a common genetic link in four Fanconi anemia complementation groups. J Clin Invest 1997; 100(11):2873–2880.

Nakashima E, Mabuchi A, Makita Y, et al. Novel *SBDS* mutations caused by gene conversion in Japanese patients with Shwachman-Diamond syndrome. Hum Genet 2004;114(4):345–348.

Saunthararajah Y, Nakamura R, Nam JM, et al. HLA-DR15 (DR2) is over-represented in myelodysplastic syndrome and aplastic anemia and predicts a response to immunosuppression in myelodysplastic syndrome. Blood 2002;100(5):1570–1574.

Sieff CA, Nisbet-Brown E, Nathan DG. Congenital bone marrow failure syndromes. Br J Haematol 2000;111(1):30–42.

Storb R, Etzioni R, Anasetti C, et al. Cyclophosphamide combined with antithymocyte globulin in preparation for allogeneic marrow transplants in patients with aplastic anemia. Blood 1994;84(3):941–949.

Tefferi A. Myelofibrosis with myeloid metaplasia. N Engl J Med 2000; 342(17):1255–1265.

Vannucchi A, Bianchi L, Cellai C, et al. Development of myelofibrosis in mice genetically impaired for GATA-1 expression (GATA-1^{low} mice). Blood 2002;100(4):1123–1132.

Vulliamy T, Marrone A, Goldman F, et al. The RNA component of telomerase is mutated in autosomal dominant dyskeratosis congenita. Nature 2001;413(6854):432–435.

Young NS. Acquired aplastic anemia. Ann Intern Med 2002;136(7): 534–546.

91 Advances in Transfusion Safety

Lorna M. Williamson and Jean-Pierre Allain

SUMMARY

Although transfusion is now extremely safe, the tools of molecular biology are continually being harnessed to improve diagnosis and therapy. Viral genome testing has been introduced in the developed world for HIV and HCV, to detect donors in the infectious "window period" before sero-conversion. Pathogen inactivated fresh frozen plasma and platelets are already available, but alloimmunization has halted trials of pathogen-inactivated red cells. Development of synthetic oxygen carriers has included perflurocarbons, and crosslinked, polymerized or mutated human or bovine hemoglobin, either free or encapsulated. No perfect replacement for the human red cell is yet on the horizon.

Key Words: Bacterial transmission; blood substitutes; perflurocarbons; hemoglobin solutions; nucleic acid viral testing; pathogen inactivation; transfusion safety; transfusion-transmitted parasites; transfusion-transmitted viruses.

INTRODUCTION

For many years, there were few changes to the way blood for transfusion was processed and tested. Whole blood donations were separated into red cells, platelets, and plasma, while virus testing usually consisted of serological assays for either viral antigens or antibodies in the donor. The viral safety of blood, already high in the more affluent parts of the world, potentially took a quantum leap with the development of rapid, automatable genome amplification assays on the one hand, and pathogen inactivation techniques on the other. Meantime, there was a search to find a way of avoiding human blood transfusion altogether, by developing alternative ways of transporting oxygen from the lungs to the tissues. This chapter outlines the rapid change in these fields in the last two decades, and attempts to set these into the context of policy making for national blood supplies.

RED CELL SUBSTITUTES

WHAT IS NEEDED AND WHY "Artificial blood," meaning a synthetic oxygen carrier, has been the holy grail of transfusion research for decades. Innovation in this area was originally driven by military requirements for a long shelf life battlefield solution that would need neither refrigeration nor matching with the recipient. The publicity surrounding transfusion-transmitted infections since the 1980s (HIV, hepatitis B and C, West Nile virus [WNV], and

From: *Principles of Molecular Medicine, Second Edition*
Edited by: M. S. Runge and C. Patterson © Humana Press, Inc., Totowa, NJ

now prions) provided a new impetus to these developments. Now many countries face chronic blood shortages. In developed countries, this is primarily because of an imbalance between the blood requirements of an aging population and a diminishing donor base, whereas in the developing world, lack of infrastructure to collect, test, and store blood safely is a major issue. So the need for alternatives to human blood remains.

However, the task facing developers of oxygen carriers is daunting. The human red cell is a miracle of evolution; its shape, the gas exchange properties of its membrane, and the complex interactions between oxygen, CO_2, 2,3 diphosphoglycerate (2,3 DPG), the vessel wall, and hemoglobin itself make the creation of a substitute a challenging task. Moreover, it has become increasingly clear that a "one size fits all" solution will not work, and that the specification of a product for transfusion dependent patients could differ from what is needed for acute hemorrhage. Virtually all development in this area has focused on acute replacement, and the term "bridge oxygenator" has appeared to describe solutions designed to maintain tissue oxygenation until the patient can receive conventional red cell transfusion.

Two classes of compounds have been extensively studied as potential oxygen carriers: perfluorocarbons and hemoglobin solutions. Each type has its merits and problems (Table 91-1). A number of promising first generation compounds of both types failed clinical trials, forcing a return to basic research on the events in the microvasculature that determine outcome in acute severe blood loss. Much more is now understood concerning the optimal characteristics of synthetic oxygen carriers, and although none is yet licensed in either Europe or North America, second generation products may perhaps fulfill early hopes.

PHYSIOLOGICAL RESPONSE TO HEMORRHAGE In acute hemorrhage, physiological responses designed to preserve the blood supply to vital organs at the expense of peripheral perfusion are automatic. Peripheral vasoconstriction is mediated by autonomic reflexes. At less than 50% blood loss, fluid shifts into circulation to maintain blood volume, so hematocrit and viscosity fall. This reduces the shear forces exerted on the endothelium, resulting in a reduction of production and release of natural vasodilators such as nitric oxide (NO) and prostacyclin. Peripheral resistance therefore rises further, and tissue blood flow slows even more, until a point is reached when oxygen supply is insufficient for tissue demands. Then anaerobic respiration takes over, leading to buildup of CO_2 and lactic acid. Once established, this state of metabolic acidosis is difficult to treat.

Table 91-1
Advantages and Disadvantages of Hemoglobin Solutions and Perfluorocarbons

Advantages	Disadvantages
Hemoglobin solutions	
High capacity for O_2 and CO_2	Short plasma half-life
Functions at physiological pH	Potential renal toxicity
Oncotic activity	Vasoactivity
Absent red blood cell antigens	Auto-oxidation
Prolonged shelf life	
Virus inactivation possible	
Perfluorocarbons	
Large-scale production	Need to be emulsified
Low production costs	Particles not uniform size
Prolonged shelf life	High FiO_2 required
Minimal infection risk	Low O_2 capacity at physiological O_2
Minimal antigenicity	Rapid plasma clearance

FIRST GENERATION HEMOGLOBIN SOLUTIONS   Some hemoglobin solutions were initially developed by military or academic institutions, but all are now licensed to commercial companies for development (Table 91-2). They have most commonly used outdated human blood donations as the source of hemoglobin, although one company (Biopure) uses bovine blood, whereas another (Somatogen) used recombinant technology. The biological challenges to the development of a hemoglobin solution include the following.

1. Free hemoglobin dissociates into α/β dimers that oxidize rapidly and are cleared by the kidney, resulting in a short half-life and in renal toxicity if their concentration reaches critical levels. Various mechanisms have therefore been used to crosslink the α/β-subunits through either the α- or β-chains, using chemicals or recombinant technology.

2. In the absence of 2,3 DPG, the oxygen dissociation curve of free hemoglobin is left shifted when compared to hemoglobin in red cells. Early investigators considered this as a potentially useful characteristic, but this increase in oxygen affinity means that oxygen does not readily off-load from the carrier to the tissues. Strategies taken to reverse this shift include pyridoxylation, site-directed mutagenesis, polymerization, and internal crosslinking, all discussed later. A completely different approach is to use bovine hemoglobin, which, although having 90% sequence homology with human hemoglobin, responds allosterically to chloride ion rather than to 2,3 DPG. Therefore, at physiological chloride concentrations, its oxyhemoglobin dissociation curve resembles that of human hemoglobin within red cells.

3. Free hemoglobin exerts considerable oncotic pressure, drawing fluid from the tissues into the circulation.

A variety of modifications were therefore introduced into the molecule by different companies to counteract the problems previously outlined (Fig. 91-1).

Chemical Crosslinking of α- or β-Chains   This not only prevents dimerization in vivo but in theory could stabilize the molecule sufficiently to permit viral inactivation. The HemAssist product developed by Baxter used 3,5 *bis* (dibromosalicyl) fumarate to crosslink the α-chains. The dimensions of the crosslinker meant that it reacted only with Lysα$_1$ 99 and Lysα$_2$ 99 in the internal cavity of

the molecule, binding the two halves together. This also had the useful effect of raising the P_{50} (Fig. 91-2), but the product had significant vasoactivity in animal studies of shock. Phase III clinical trials in stroke and trauma gave disappointing results, and development of the product was discontinued in 1998.

The Hemolink product developed by Haemosol in Canada uses open ring (oxidized) raffinose to crosslink specific amino acids in the β-chains in the 2,3 DPG pocket, which also has the effect of raising the P_{50}. The *O*-raffinose is also used to polymerize the molecule.

Polymerization   Polymerization can be achieved through the use of crosslinkers that target surface amino groups. Polymers of various lengths can be produced using gluteraldehyde, as the reaction can be quenched using lysine. This strategy has been employed by Northfield Laboratories to polymerize human hemoglobin (PolyHeme). This product is also pyridoxylated, which raises the P_{50}, resulting in a product similar to human blood in terms of oxygen affinity and colloid oncotic pressure. Gluteraldehyde polymerization is also used by Biopure for production of their bovine hemoglobin product (Hemopure). This product can transport oxygen to the tissues effectively, and even in low doses can raise arterial pressure and lower cardiac index. It was reported to be life saving in a case of severe autoimmune hemolytic anemia, and has been licensed in South Africa for orthopedic surgery. Currently, a trial is proposed in which Hemopure is used in cardiac surgery to improve tissue oxygenation by diffusion through an atheromatous obstruction in coronary arteries. Finally, as mentioned, the HemoLink product is polymerized using *O*-raffinose.

Recombinant Technology   Building on ideas generated at the UK's Medical Research Council laboratories in Cambridge, Somatogen (and later Baxter Healthcare) developed a human hemoglobin solution produced in *Escherichia coli*, using synthetic genes encoding the human α- and β-globin polypeptides and expressed from a single operon. The purified recombinant hemoglobin had the correct stoichiometry of the α- and β-globin polypeptides, which associated into soluble tetramers, and incorporated heme. Each globin chain also contained an additional methionine as an extension to the amino terminus. The recombinant hemoglobin had an high-performance liquid chromatography profile essentially identical to that of human hemoglobin A and comigrated with hemoglobin A on polysaccharide gel electrophoresis. The visible spectrum and oxygen affinity were similar to that of native human hemoglobin A, but the recombinant protein showed a reduction in Bohr and phosphate effects, possibly because of the presence of the methionine at the amino termini of the α- and β-chains.

Because the oxygen affinity of this free hemoglobin in the absence of 2,3 DPG was too high to allow adequate oxygen offloading in the tissues, a variant was created using an expression vector containing one gene encoding the naturally occurring Asn-108β to Lys mutation (hemoglobin Presbyterian), which reduces the oxygen affinity and enhances the Bohr effect slightly. In addition, to prevent α β-dimerization and renal toxicity, and to increase the half-life, the product was made using one duplicated, tandemly fused α-globin gene, resulting in end-to-end fusion of the two α-globin-subunits. The short distance (2–6 Å) between the N-terminal residue of one α-chain and the C-terminal residue of the other allowed the insertion of a glycine residue as a bridge. Despite these elegant modifications, this product led to gastrointestinal side effects, and Baxter discontinued its development at the same time as studies on HemAssist were stopped.

Table 91-2
Red Cell Substitutes and Their Current Status

Company	Product	Source	Modification	Development status
Perfluorocarbons				
Alliance Pharmaceutical Corporation	Oxygent	–	Emulsified perflubron	Phase III cardiac surgery, hemodilution, hemorrhage
Hemogen	Oxyfluor	–	–	Discontinued
Hemoglobin solutions				
Apex Bioscience (now Curacyte)	PHP	Human	Pyridoxylated; conjugated to polyoxyethylene, binds NO	Phase IIc, shock
Baxter Healthcare	HemAssist	Human	α-α crosslinked with "diaspirin"	Discontinued 1998 at phase III stage
Biopure	Hemopure	Cow	Gluteraldehyde-polymerized; purified to remove tetramers	Phase III with hemodilution, +compassionate use; Licensed for surgery in South Africa; FDA license submitted; Trial planned in cardiac surgery
Biopure	Oxyglobin	Cow	Gluteraldehyde-polymerized	Licensed for use in dogs
Enzon	PEG-hemoglobin	Cow	PEG; tetramer	Not in active development
Hemosol	Hemolink	Human	*O*-raffinose to crosslink β-chains and to polymerize; tetramers remain	Phase III cardiac surgery, studies with erythropoietin in renal failure and surgery
Northfield Laboratories	PolyHeme	Human	Pyridoxylated; gluteraldehyde polymerized; purified to remove tetramers	Phase III trauma
Sangart	Hemospan (MP4)	Human	PEG; polymer; virus treated with riboflavin	Phase II, orthopedics, Sweden, and now USA
	Hemospan PS	Human	Hemospan + pentastarch	
Somatogen/Baxter	Optro-r hemoglobin-1.1	Recombinant	Tetramer; α-chains fused end to end; β-chain mutation	Discontinued 1998
Synzyme	Hemozyme	Human	Polymerized	Preclinical

FDA, Food and Drug Administration; PEG, polyethylene glycol; PHP, pyridoxal hemoglobin polyoxyethylene.

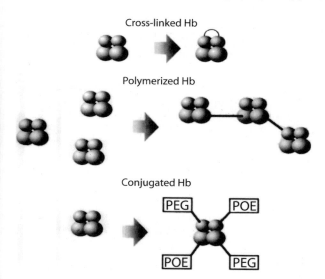

Figure 91-1 Internally crosslinked, polymerized, and surface-modified hemoglobins. (Reprinted with permission from Blackwell Publishing from Stowell CP, Levin J, Spiess BD, Winslow RM. Progress in the use of blood substitutes. Transfusion 2001;41[2]:287–299.)

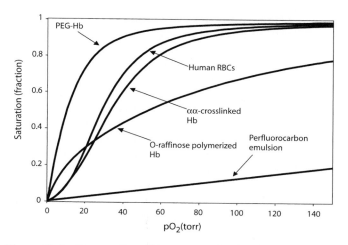

Figure 91-2 Oxygen dissociation curves of various hemoglobins and perfluorocarbon. Note that all hemoglobins give sigmoid curves, whereas perflurocarbon gives a linear relationship. (Reprinted with permission from Blackwell Publishing from Stowell CP, Levin J, Spiess BD, Winslow RM. Progress in the use of blood substitutes. Transfusion 2001;41[2]:287–299.)

Surface Modification The 42 lysine amino groups on the surface of hemoglobin are targets for attachment of small molecules such as polyethylene glycol (PEG) and polyoxyethylene (POE), which stabilize the tetramer and increase the molecular weight. The resulting increase in oncotic pressure and viscosity was considered therapeutically useful in expanding the plasma volume. It was also thought that this type of modification would render the molecule less visible to the reticulo-endothelial system, minimizing its antigenicity. Products in this category include bovine hemoglobin modified by PEG, which was manufactured by Enzon, but this may no longer be in active development. However, a human hemoglobin solution designated pyridoxal hemoglobin polyoxyethylene developed by Apex Bioscience is in phase IIc trial in shock.

Encapsulation To prevent the renal toxicity and short half-life associated with free hemoglobin, attempts have been made to enclose hemoglobin in liposomes consisting of synthetic lipids in various combinations. Phosphotidylcholine has been used to produce bilamellar spheres loaded with a hemoglobin solution, whereas the addition of cholesterol increases elasticity and half-life. In theory, the oxygen affinity could be modulated by the inclusion of 2,3 DPG, whereas methemoglobin reductase could be added to prevent oxidation. However, there are technical difficulties in controlling the size of the liposomes, and it is not yet clear what effects the clearance of large amounts of phosphotidylcholine would have on the reticuloendothelial system. These products remain at the preclinical stage of development.

PROBLEMS WITH FIRST GENERATION OF SUBSTITUTES AND NEW APPROACH TO HEMOGLOBIN SUBSTITUTES

Many first generation compounds failed clinical trial because of unacceptable hypertension, bradycardia, chest and abdominal pain and nausea/vomiting. At first these effects were thought to be owing to contaminants, but are now considered to be the result of reflex vasoconstriction. Discoveries regarding the functioning of the microvasculature, facilitated by new techniques for viewing small vessels, have changed the thinking behind the ideal properties of a hemoglobin substitute.

1. Identification of NO as the endothelium-derived relaxing factor. The heme group binds NO with high affinity, and this is especially true of free hemoglobin. This property of free hemoglobin contributes to the hypertensive properties of some solutions.

2. The realization that diffusion of cell-free oxygenated hemoglobin can be harmful, as it leads to constriction of precapillary arterioles and thus reduces tissue perfusion. Significant amounts of oxygen leave the circulation at the precapillary arteriolar stage. These vessels are rich in nerve endings, and appear to be extremely sensitive to oxygen. The so-called facilitated diffusion of oxygen that is bound to the free hemoglobin can be limited by increasing both the diameter of the hemoglobin molecule itself and the viscosity of the solution. Modified hemoglobin molecules of different radii have varying vasoactive properties, even though their interaction with NO is the same. Widespread prearteriolar vasoconstriction in the presence of a normal blood volume leads to hypertension; conversely vasoconstriction with an inadequate blood volume results in shock, volume depletion and ultimately collapse of the nonmuscular capillary walls, which rely on vascular pressure to keep them open. To overcome this undesirable side effect, oxygen availability from the hemoglobin substitute should be less than that from natural red cells. Oxygen availability to the precapillary arterioles can be limited by increasing the oxygen affinity of the molecule and decreasing its concentration in the solution.

3. Production of vasodilators stimulated by shear forces on the endothelium can be maintained by having a solution of fairly high viscosity. At rest, therefore (though not during exercise), the maintenance of microvascular blood flow, vascular volume and acid–base balance are more important than

Table 91-3
Past and Current Concepts in the Design of a Blood Substitute

Parameter	Considered optimal for first generation oxygen carriers	Considered optimal for second generation oxygen carriers
Oxygen binding	Like blood: P50 28 mmHg	P50 5–10 mmHg
Viscosity	Like water: 1 cP	Like blood: 4 cP
Oncotic pressure	Like blood: 15 mmHg	Increased
Hemoglobin concentration	Like blood: 15 g/dL	As low as possible

Modified from Winslow RM. Current status of blood substitute research: toward a new paradigm. J Intern Med 2003;253(5):508–517.

oxygen carrying capacity. These observations change the theoretical requirements of an oxygen carrier (Table 91-3). This logic has determined the design of the modified hemoglobin solution Hemospan (MP4, Sangart, see Table 91-2).

Made from outdated red cells, this compound has the lysine residues thiolated then further surface modified by the addition of PEG. It is subjected to pathogen reduction using the riboflavin technique. This solution has a P_{50} of only 4 mmHg, which is predicted to limit early oxygen off-loading at the arteriolar stage. The large increase in radius as a result of the PEG also limits the undesirable oxygen diffusion, maintains plasma viscosity, and hence shear forces on the endothelium, and confers a half-life of 43 h. The compound resulted in 100% survival and absence of hypertension in a hemorrhagic rat model (Fig. 91-3), and in primate studies, no vasoconstriction or hypertension was seen. The compound is now in phase II clinical trial in orthopedic surgery in Sweden, and a trial in the United States is planned.

PERFLUOROCARBONS The perfluorocarbon class of compounds is characterized by a linear or cyclic carbon backbone that is highly fluorinated, with other halogens sometimes also present.

They can dissolve large amounts of oxygen and CO_2 whereas being chemically and biologically inert. Their properties were famously displayed in images of a mouse living and breathing "underwater" in a beakerful of oxygenated fluorocarbon. At a pO_2 of 100 torr, dissolved oxygen can reach 10 mL/dL, compared with 0.5 mL/dL for plasma and 20 mL/dL in blood with a hemoglobin concentration of 15 g/dL. Unlike hemoglobin, the oxygen dissociation curve is linear (see Fig. 91-2), so if the patient can breathe very high levels of inspired oxygen, greater amounts of oxygen can be carried. However, because fluorocarbons are immiscible with plasma, they have to be emulsified by mixing with a surfactant (usually a phospholipid) to produce particles of submicron size, although precise size is difficult to control. The surfactant can comprise a high percentage of the solution by weight, and may not be totally biologically inert.

The original compound, Fluosol-DA, was licensed by the US Food and Drug Administration in 1990 for use in percutaneous transluminal coronary angioplasty, but became obsolete and was withdrawn for this purpose in 1994. Clinical trials in acute hemorrhage demonstrated no improvement in clinical outcome. Later compounds have smaller particle size, which should reduce flu-like symptoms attributable to cytokine and complement activation, and greater solubility for oxygen. Oxygent (Alliance Pharmaceuticals) is an emulsion of perflubron (perfluoro-octyl bromide) and egg yolk phospoholipid. It is in a phase II/III clinical trial to assess

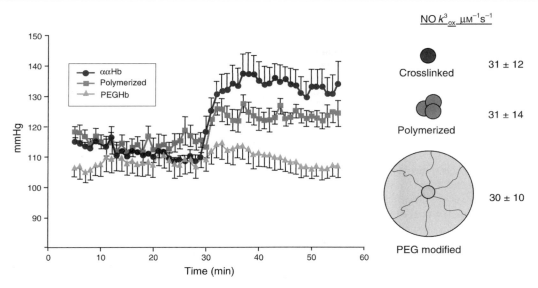

Figure 91-3 Mean arterial pressure response in the rat to infusion of three modified hemoglobins. The sizes of the molecules are drawn to scale relative to each other, and the association rate constants for NO are given at the right. (Reprinted with permission from Blackwell Publishing from Winslow RM. Current status of blood substitute research: toward a new paradigm. J Intern Med 2003;253[5]:508–517.)

whether its use can increase the permitted degree of acute normovolemic hemodilution, thus improving the extent of blood saving. A further trial is designed to examine its effect in acute hemorrhage. Another fluorocarbon (Oxyfluor) was designed to absorb the microbubbles that form on cardiopulmonary bypass circuits and are thought to be responsible for neurovascular complications. This is no longer in development.

ONGOING ISSUES IN THE DEVELOPMENT OF A BLOOD SUBSTITUTE

How to Evaluate the Product Regulatory authorities increasingly expect clinical end points from studies of new products. One of the difficulties is that the red cells used as controls have not themselves been subjected to studies of similar rigor, and there are no established criteria for assessing their efficacy. Mortality and transfusion avoidance have been used in some trials, but other end points may evolve as different clinical scenarios are studied.

Short Half-Life Short half-life is still a major problem. Even the best substitutes (encapsulated/surface modified) have circulatory half-lives of only 2–3 d, with most being only 12–24 h. This still restricts the usage to acute hemorrhage, with no sign of a product to treat chronic anemias.

A Safe and Reliable Source of Start Material Although not an issue for perfluorocarbons, of which there is limitless supply, sourcing adequate amounts of human hemoglobin is a challenge. With optimal stock management, outdates are low (<2% in England), and for safety reasons, the donor exclusion criteria cannot be relaxed to increase supply. Yields of free hemoglobin from outdated red cells are rarely more than 50%, so targeted blood collections would have to be organized to provide start material.

The use of bovine blood seems questionable at this point, as possible prion transmission is a key concern of blood suppliers. Accredited bovine spongiform encephalopathy-free herds could be developed, but the possibility of unknown bovine agents exists. Recombinant technology remains a possibility once the optimal formulation is established, but it is uncertain whether any process could be adequately scaled up to meet demand.

The Safety/Cost Balance In the two decades of development of blood substitutes, blood itself has become increasingly safe from the virus point of view. The residual risk of HIV, HBV, and HCV is now 1 in 10^{5-6}/U in many parts of the world. Even when a new agent emerged (WNV in the United States and Canada in 2002), genome testing was in place within 12 mo. Developed countries are questioning the spiraling costs of blood components, and the high costs of steps providing only small incremental increases in safety. In the United States, virus inactivated pooled solvent detergent fresh frozen plasma (FFP) did not become an established product, and is now withdrawn. In Europe, in which one pathogen inactivation system is now licensed for platelets, uptake is limited, and cost-effectiveness is one factor in this. Ironically, the parts of the world that might gain most benefit from a blood substitute are unlikely to be able to afford it. Another related issue is the safety of the products themselves. As blood safety increases, the acceptance of possible serious side effects of a blood substitute will fall.

Further Advances in Knowledge of the Red Cell Intriguingly, a recent study suggested that red cells themselves may be able to respond to hypoxia by releasing NO generated from the reduction of nitrite by deoxyhemoglobin. It remains to be seen whether this newly discovered property of red blood cells will present another obstacle in the search for an artificial oxygen carrier.

SUMMARY Although it might be considered disappointing to not have a single licensed blood substitute, a great deal has been learned about the physiology of oxygen delivery to tissues and the sequence of events when it goes wrong. The next decade may see one or more products reach the clinic. Issues of cost-effectiveness, safety, and availability will ultimately determine whether these products become true blood substitutes or niche products for a limited number of patients.

GENOMIC DETECTION OF VIRAL AGENTS

METHODS Methods enabling the detection of the genome of infectious agents have been developed, initially in research, then for diagnostics, and finally for blood screening. Methods such as direct hybridization and its more sensitive version called "branched

Table 91-4
Impact of HCV and HIV NAT on Blood Safety

| Country | Author | Number screened (millions) | Estimated risk/million transfusions | | | |
| | | | HCV | | HIV | |
			Pre NAT	Post NAT	Pre NAT	Post NAT
United States	Stramer	35.7	4.3	0.61	0.75	0.52
France	Pillonel	4.9	1.0	0.15	0.71	0.4

HCV, hepatitis C virus; NAT, nucleic acid testing.

DNA" are not adapted to the mass screening approach required for testing in the transfusion context. Methods including amplification such as PCR, ligase chain reaction, transcription mediated amplification, or nucleic acid sequence-based amplification have been developed and used in transfusion, in which requirements of high sensitivity, high specificity, and high throughput need to be met. Quantitative PCR based on the use of Taqman probes has been introduced and seems to be well adapted to the demand of the transfusion market.

Nucleic acid testing (NAT) was first introduced in 2000 for the detection of the hepatitis C virus (HCV) genome. Soon after other NAT targets such as HIV, hepatitis B virus (HBV), and WNV were added, creating a momentum for the development of multiplex NAT, enabling simultaneous detection of genomes of two (duplex) or three (triplex) different viruses in a single reaction tube.

Automation is critical in blood screening for transfusion. No system is available to integrate all three basic steps of NAT: nucleic acid extraction, amplification, and detection, in a unique automated instrument. A fair amount of manual operation remains that will be eliminated when the prototype automated instruments become commercially available.

SAMPLES The considerable cost of NAT on a large scale led to the development of the concept of plasma pool testing by which mixtures of individual plasma samples from blood or plasma donations are mixed and tested in a pool. The pool size ranges from 8 to 512 depending on the target genome and the method used. Pooling has a clear impact on test sensitivity. This inherent lack of sensitivity was overcome in different ways: one was extreme sensitivity of assays with the attached toll on specificity, the other was concentration of targets by various methods, the most popular being ultracentrifugation. When NAT targeted viruses such as HCV or HIV that replicate very rapidly to viral load above 10^5 copies/mL, pooling did not substantially affect screening efficacy, although most national blood transfusion organizations progressively reduced the number of samples per pool from 96 to 48, 24, and 16. The lower viral load observed with HBV and WNV during the infectious window period led blood services to reduce further pool size to 8 or 10 samples. Ultimately, individual donation NAT already implemented by some blood organizations will likely become the rule, particularly with the relative decrease in costs introduced by multiplexing.

IMPLEMENTATION OF NAT IN TRANSFUSION NAT was first introduced in the late 1990s by the plasma derivative industry following the transmission of HCV by intravenous IgG that was not virally inactivated. NAT of various sensitivities was applied to large pools of plasmas prepared for fractionation. Later, despite the initial reticence of both regulators and the blood bank community, NAT applied to HCV RNA was mandated by the EU and US regulatory bodies but the pool size was not specified, only a clinical sensitivity of 5000 IU/mL was to be achieved by the methods used. In 2004, all EU countries have implemented HCV NAT. HIV NAT

was simultaneously implemented in France, Germany, and the United States, soon followed by other countries such as Australia, Japan, and more European countries.

The WNV epidemics in the United States that spread between 1999 and 2003 raised a new level of concern regarding transmissibility of emerging viruses by transfusion, and in a 6-mo period, commercial NATs under investigational new drug regulation were implemented in July 2003 in the United States and Canada. The epidemiology of WNV in other areas such as Western Europe does not warrant a similar approach.

Discussions are ongoing to determine the usefulness of NAT for other transfusion transmissible viruses with known residual risk such as HBV and human erythroviruses that include parvovirus B19. HBV DNA screening is already implemented in Japan, Germany, Austria, and Luxemburg. The successive implementation of several NATs in addition to the serological screening assays is adding not only to the financial burden, but also to the complication of operations, therefore increasing the risk of errors. Following implementation of HCV, HIV, and HBV NAT, the rate of errors has become a major factor in calculating residual risk of viral transmission by transfusion. Complete automation is expected to reduce that risk. However, as the number of NATs is likely to continuously increase, alternative strategies such as pathogen inactivation need to be considered, both from a safety and a financial point of view.

IMPACT OF NAT ON BLOOD SAFETY The impact of NAT on the safety of the blood supply has been estimated in several countries. Owing to the rarity of transmission cases, no direct assessment can be done and only calculated estimates can be provided. Table 91-4 indicates preliminary results from France and the United States.

In the present circumstances of a widespread epidemic, epidemiological review of the WNV NAT implemented in North America revealed that several hundred viremic donations had tested positive, and it is estimated that approx 1000 cases per year of transmission would be avoided. This result contrasts with the 5 and 55 cases avoided per year with the HIV and HCV NAT, respectively.

Emerging viral infections originating either from new viruses (mostly animal) breaking into humans or from previously unknown viruses recently discovered are candidate for additional NAT. However, before implementation, several criteria need to be met. The emerging virus should be pathogenic, transmissible by transfusion, in relatively low prevalence, and infectious/persistent for a long enough period of time. The recent severe acute respiratory system, SARS, infection epidemic falls into the first category; although no evidence of transfusion transmission has been provided. The second category includes GB virus-C, TT virus, and SEN virus. The first virus is of low prevalence but no evidence of pathogenicity has been found, whereas the other two, which are in the same family of human circoviridae, are ubiquitous and with no identified pathogenicity.

MOLECULAR DETECTION OF BACTERIALLY INFECTED BLOOD Bacterial infection of blood components is relatively frequent in platelet concentrates because this product is stored at 20°C under constant agitation, which is highly favorable to growth of aerobic bacteria. Among the many methods developed to detect bacterial contamination, the most effective practiced method is culture, with detection either by accumulation of CO_2 or consumption of O_2. These methods are very sensitive, but require a period of natural bacterial growth to amplify the number of bacteria to a detectable level. This procedure takes time (at least 24 h), a major handicap for a product whose shelf life is only 5 d. Molecular methods including an amplification step can overcome this drawback but the diversity of bacterial genome makes it difficult to cover a large spectrum of organisms. Methods targeting the 16S ribosomal (r)RNA have been proposed, whereas others use a universal bacterial rRNA probe. To date, despite a sensitivity of 6–500 organisms/100 μL, these methods do not cover a sufficiently large spectrum of bacteria and are considered expensive and labor intensive. Considerable development is needed before molecular methods can be considered as suitable replacement for methods involving culture.

MOLECULAR DETECTION OF PARASITES IN TRANSFUSION MEDICINE Parasites are transmissible by transfusion but are mostly limited to circumscribed geographic areas. However, immigration from endemic areas and intensive travel have resulted in a real risk of malarial transmission from African and Asian tropical areas in the Northern hemisphere and of *Trypanosoma cruzi* transmission from Central and South America to the Northern part of the American continent. Rules of donor exclusion according to place of origin or traveling have been implemented, but the yield is poor and the number of undeserved donor deferrals high. Various methods have been proposed to distinguish between donors presenting with and without a real risk of transmission. In the case of malaria, antibody detection identifies individuals who have been infected in the past but are not necessarily infectious, whereas antigen detection or thick blood smear are not sufficiently sensitive and, for the latter, discouragingly labor intensive. Genomic amplification methods have therefore been developed using nested PCR or quantitative PCR to detect one parasite per 100 μL of whole blood. The cost-effectiveness of such methods has been evaluated but their clinical efficacy remains to be assessed.

T. cruzi infection is highly immunogenic, with infection occurring mostly in young children. The presence of antibodies in a blood donation is considered synonymous with infectious risk, and high-performance assays are systematically used in endemic areas. Molecular methods have not been considered to help in the deferral of at risk blood donors.

A similar situation is found with tick-transmitted parasites such as Babesia that is endemic in the Northern hemisphere.

PATHOGEN REDUCTION OF BLOOD COMPONENTS Although they have resulted in extensive reductions in risk, donor selection and testing have not eliminated pathogen transmission by transfusion. With the continual discovery of new pathogens, it is clear that the addition of a new test for each adds complexity and loss of donations and donors with false positive reactions. Pathogen inactivation is an adjunct and in some cases a possible alternative to developing individual tests and donor exclusion criteria to address each pathogen individually.

Since the early 1990s, a long series of compounds have been evaluated for their ability to inactivate viruses or other infectious agents without unacceptable loss of cellular function. The last and

Table 91-5
Pathogen Inactivation Methods for Blood Components

Component	Compound	Phase of development
Platelet	Amotosalen (S59)	Clinical practice EU
RBC	FRALE (S303)	Interrupted
RBC	Inactive (PEN 110)	Interrupted
FFP	Amotosalen (S59)	Phase 3 completed; submitted for EU license
FFP	Solvent detergent	Clinical practice EU, discontinued in United States
FFP	Methylene blue	Clinical practice EU

EU, European Union; FFP, fresh frozen plasma; RBC, red blood cell.

most promising generation of such compounds targets nucleic acids directly, which are altered and made unable to replicate. In addition to having the potential to inactivate viral and bacterial nucleic acids, compounds such as Psoralens (S59), Inactine, and Riboflavin can inactivate parasites and leucocytes, particularly lymphocytes responsible for transfusion-associated graft-vs-host disease, a universally fatal complication. These follow other chemicals such as methylene blue or solvent detergent-based methods already in use. Because solvent/detergent is effective by disrupting viral (and possibly bacterial) membranes, the spectrum of activity is limited to enveloped viruses.

Among the compounds listed in Table 91-5, Solvent detergent and methylene blue can only be used in fresh frozen plasma as it disrupts cell membranes. Clinical use of Amotosalen has been started in some European countries, following CE marking. Published randomized trial results indicate efficacy of the system, and although there is a systematic reduction of platelet yield compared to standard products, this difference did not seem to affect clinical efficacy in preventing bleeding. In vitro and in animals, no evidence of oncogenic or other toxicities have been found in short- and long-term studies. However, clinical trials of two different pathogen reduction systems for red cells (S303 and Inactine) have both been suspended following development of red cell alloantibodies. The long-term future of pathogen reduction of red cells and platelets remains to be seen.

SELECTED REFERENCES

Allain-JP. Genomic screening for blood-borne viruses in transfusion settings. Clin Lab Haematol 2000;22(1):1–10.

Allain JP, Seghatchian J. Current strategies on pathogen removal/inactivation: an overview. Transfus Apheresis Sci 2001;25(3):195–197.

Allain JP, Thomas I, Sauleda S. Nucleic acid testing for emerging viral infections. Transfus Med 2002;12(4):275–283.

Blajchman MA. Incidence and significance of the bacterial contamination of blood components. Dev Biol (Basel) 2002;108:59–67.

Centers for Disease Control and Prevention (CDC). Detection of West Nile virus in blood donations- United States, 2003. MMWR 2003;52(38): 769–773.

Looker D, Abbott-Brown D, Cozart P, et al. A human recombinant hemoglobin designed for use as a blood substitute. Nature 1992;356:258–260.

McCullough J, Vesole DH, Benjamin RJ, et al. Therapeutic efficacy and safety of platelets treated with photochemical process for pathogen inactivation: the SPRINT trial. Blood 2004;104(5):1534–1541.

Mullon J, Giacoppe G, Clagett C, MacCune D, Dillard T. Transfusions of polymerised bovine hemoglobin in a patient with severe autoimmune hemolytic anaemia. N Engl J Med 2000;342(22):1638–1643.

Nagababu E, Ramasamy S, Abernethy DR, Rifkind JM. Active nitric oxide produced in the red cell under hypoxic conditions by deoxyhemoglobin-mediated nitrite reduction. J Biol Chem 2003;278(47):46,349–46,356.

Pillonel J, Laperche S. Groupe "Agents Transmissibles par Transfusion" de la Societe francaise de transfusion sanguine; etablissement francais du sang; Centre de transfusion sanguine des armees. [Trends in residual risk of transfusion-transmitted viral infections (HIV, HCV, HBV) in France between 1992 and 2002 and impact of viral genome screening (Nucleic Acid Testing)]. Transfus Clin Biol 2004;11(2):81–86.

Stramer SL. NAT update: where are we today? Dev Biol (Basel) 2002; 108:41–56.

Vandegriff KD, Malavalli A, Wooldridge J, Lohman J, Winslow RM. MP4, a new nonvasoactive PEG-Hb conjugate. Transfusion 2003;43(4): 509–516.

van Rhenen D, Gulliksson H, Cazenave JP, et al. Transfusion of pooled buffy coat platelet components prepared with photochemical pathogen inactivation treatment: The EuroSPRITE trial. Blood 2003;101(6):2426–2433.

Winslow RM. Blood substitutes: refocusing an elusive goal. Br J Haematol 2000;111:387–396.

Table 92-2
Examples of Autoimmune Diseases

	Antigen/autoimmune mechanism	Immunomodulatory therapy
Multisystem diseases		
Systemic lupus erythematosus	Auto-antibodies against DNA, histones, ribosomes result in arthritis, renal disease, and vasculitis.	Corticosteroids, azathioprine, cyclophosphamide, rituximab
Rheumatoid arthritis	Unknown antigen in joint synovium. The immune response results in destructive arthritis.	Corticosteroids, azathioprine, cyclosporine, methotrexate, etanercept, infliximab, leflunomide, anti-IL-1 (anakinra)
Polyarteritis nodosa	Hepatitis B virus surface antigen. Vasculitis of medium and small-sized vessels results in systemic disease.	Corticosteroids, cyclophosphamide
Organ-specific autoimmune diseases		
Diabetes mellitus type I	Antigen in β cells in the pancreas. Immune response by TH1 cells, CTL, and antibodies results in destruction of insulin-producing cells.	Vaccination with different peptides is being attempted to try to prevent total destruction of the β cells.
Multiple sclerosis	Myelin basic protein; T-cell-mediated immune response results in repeated episodes of CNS demyelination.	Corticosteroids, IFN, daclizumab, natalizumab
Guillain-Barre syndrome	Antibodies directed against components of peripheral or cranial nerve myelin.	Plasma exchange and administration of intravenous Ig are beneficial; corticosteroids are not.
Anti-GBM antibody disease (Goodpasture's syndrome)	Protein in the basement membrane collagen type IV. Antibody and complement-mediated inflammation of glomeruli and lung alveoli results in glomerulonephritis and pulmonary hemorrhage.	Plasmapheresis to eliminate the antibody present, combined with cyclophosphamide and corticosteroids
Idiopathic thrombocytopenic purpura	Platelet membrane proteins (gpIIb/IIIa integrin). Antibodies cause opsonization and phagocytosis of platelets.	Corticosteroids, intravenous Ig
Graves disease	TSH receptor. Antibodies bind to TSH receptors and cause thyroid hormone secretion.	None for the hyperthyroidism; corticosteroids for the ophthalmopathy

These derivatives of the glucocorticoid hormones are the mainstay of treatment of autoimmune diseases. They may be used at very small doses (e.g., prednisone 5–10 mg daily) as anti-inflammatory agents, at intermediate doses (e.g., prednisone 0.5–1 mg/kg daily) as immunosuppressive agents and at very high doses (e.g., methyl-prednisolone 500–1000 mg daily) as lymphocyte-depleting agents. Glucocorticoids enter the cell and bind with the steroid receptor, which resides in the cytoplasm, forming a complex with the heat-shock protein, Hsp90. After binding, the glucocorticoid-steroid receptor complex translocates to the nucleus, in which it binds to specific DNA sequences in the promoter regions of steroid-responsive genes, resulting in the activation of the transcription of multiple genes and the suppression of many more. The overall result is a decrease in the synthesis of proinflammatory cytokines, including IL-1, tumor necrosis factor (TNF)-α, IL3, GM-CSF, and chemokines. At very high doses, steroids may induce lympho-cyte apoptosis, and this mechanism may play a role in the effect of the very high doses ("pulses") of methylprednisolone used for the treatment of acute attacks of multiple sclerosis or lupus glomerulonephritis.

Agents That Interfere With Antigen Processing and Presentation Most agents in this category are experimental. The interaction between APCs and lymphocytes can be targeted at

several points, including preventing the interaction between CD40 on B cells and CD40 ligand (CD154) on activated T cells using an anti-CD154 antibody (ineffective in a randomized controlled trial in lupus); and preventing effective costimulation by blocking CD80 and CD86 (B7.1, B7.2) on APCs by the use of CTLA4-Ig (promising in rheumatoid arthritis and psoriasis).

Agents That Interfere With T-Cell Activation Probably the most important drugs in medical transplantation are the calcineurin inhibitors, cyclosporine A and tacrolimus. Cyclosporine A and tacrolimus (FK506) act by reducing the expression of cytokine genes that are normally expressed during T-cell activation, includ-ing IL-2, the most important T-cell growth factor. These drugs are most effective to prevent immune activation, and accordingly are much more important in transplantation (to prevent rejection) than in autoimmunity (in which the immune response is already in progress). Cyclosporine and tacrolimus bind to different target pro-teins called immunophilins (cyclosporine to cyclophilin, tacrolimus to the FK-binding protein), but both result in the binding and inhi-bition of calcineurin, a phosphatase that becomes activated in T cells after T-cell receptor binding. Calcineurin activates a number of tran-scription factors, and its inhibition prevents effective T-cell activa-tion and clonal expansion. Tacrolimus and cyclosporine act on the same step of T-cell activation, and they have similar efficacy. The

Table 92-3
Selected Immunomodulators

	Description/mechanism of action	Uses
Interference with antigen processing and presentation		
CTLA4-Ig	Fusion molecule that binds CD80 and CD86 on the surface of APCs blocking the interaction with CD28 that would deliver a costimulatory signal to the T cell	Phase II studies in rheumatoid arthritis, psoriasis and transplantation
Anti-CD40 ligand	Blocks the interaction between CD40 on macrophages and B cells and CD40 ligand (CD154), which is expressed on activated T cells	Animal models, including xenotransplantation
Efalizumab (anti-LFA-1)	Binds to LFA-1, preventing LFA-1-ICAM interaction, resulting in blocking T-cell adhesion, trafficking and activation	Phase III trials in psoriasis, I/II in transplantation and rheumatoid arthritis
Natalizumab (anti α-4 integrin)	Humanized monoclonal antibody prevents the interaction between α-4 integrin on the surface of inflammatory cells and VCAM-1 on vascular endothelial cells, preventing leukocyte migration across the blood–brain barrier in multiple sclerosis.	Approved for use in remitting-relapsing multiple sclerosis; was withdrawn from the market owing to serious side effects
Interference with T-cell activation		
Cyclosporine A	Binds to cyclophilin. The complex cyclosporine-cyclophilin binds and inhibits calcineurin, preventing the activation of the transcription factor nuclear factor of activated T cells (NFAT). This blocks the activation of T cells and the production of IL-2.	Prevention of solid organ rejection and of GVHD. Approved for rheumatoid arthritis and psoriasis; often used in several other autoimmune diseases
Tacrolimus (FK506)	Tacrolimus binds the protein FKBP, and this complex binds and inhibits calcineurin. Same effect as cyclosporine	Prevention of solid organ rejection and of GVHD. Approved (topical) for atopic dermatitis. Often used in several other autoimmune diseases
Inhibition of T-cell proliferation		
Rapamycin (Sirolimus)	Rapamycin binds the intracellular protein FKBP. The complex rapamycin-FKBP binds MTOR, arresting cell cycle between G1 and S	Prevention of rejection in solid organ transplant; prophylaxis of GVHD, treatment of steroid-refractory GVHD
Leflunomide	Inhibits the *de novo* pathway of pyrimidine synthesis, suppressing T-cell proliferation	Effective in rheumatoid arthritis. Experimental use in solid organ transplant
Azathioprine	Antimetabolite through purine synthesis inhibition	Prevention of rejection in solid organ transplant
Mycophenolate mofetil (MMF)	Antimetabolite through purine synthesis inhibition, selective for lymphocytes	Prevention of rejection in solid organ transplant; prevention of GVHD
Methotrexate	Antifolate antimetabolite.	Induction and maintenance in solid organ transplantation; prevention of GVHD, treatment of rheumatoid arthritis and vasculitis
Dacluzimab	Humanized monoclonal antibody directed against CD25 (part of the IL-2 high-affinity receptor)	In solid organ transplant it has been used as part of the induction regimen; in allo-HSCT, it has been used as treatment of steroid-refractory GVHD.
Basiliximab	Monoclonal antibody directed against CD25 (part of the IL-2 high-affinity receptor)	In solid organ transplant it has been used as part of the induction regimen.
Lymphocyte depletion		
Antithymocyte immunoglobulin	Polyclonal immunoglobulin obtained from horse or rabbit	Treatment of aplastic anemia. Treatment of acute rejection in renal transplantation
Muronomab-CD3	Anti-CD3 monoclonal antibody	Treatment of acute rejection in solid organ transplantation. Treatment of GVHD in allo-HSCT

(Continued)

Table 92-3 *(Continued)*

	Description/mechanism of action	*Uses*
Alemtuzumab (Campath-1H)	Humanized monoclonal antibody directed against CD52	FDA-approved only as antineoplastic in chronic lymphocytic leukemia; it has been used to treat some autoimmune diseases, including autoimmune cytopenias, refractory rheumatoid arthritis and vasculitis. In allo-HSCT it has been used to prevent GVHD.
Other agents		
Corticosteroids	Multiple mechanisms of action. Steroid complexes with cytosolic receptors and translocates to the nucleus, binding to glucocorticoid response elements in the promoter regions of cytokine genes. The result is prevention of T-cell recruitment and activation.	The basic drugs used to prevent and treat solid organ recjection, prevent GVHD and treat a wide variety of autoimmune diseases
Etanercept	Recombinant form of the extracellular domain of human p75 tumor necrosis factor receptor fused to the Fc fragment of human immunoglobulin G1. Blocks TNF-α action	Used in rheumatoid arthritis, psoriasis and ankylosing spondylitis. Experimental in other autoimmune diseases
Infliximab	Chimeric antibody against human TNF-α. Blocks TNF-α action	Used in Crohn's disease (an autoimmune colitis) and ankylosing spondylitis. In allo-HSCT it has been used to treat steroid-refractory GVHD.

FKBP, FK-binding protein.

combination of both drugs would not be expected to be more active that either of them at optimal dose, and is typically not used.

Agents That Interfere With T-Cell Proliferation One of the consequences of T-cell activation is proliferation. T-cell proliferation may be inhibited in different ways. IL-2, the T-cell growth factor, which is released in the course of T-cell activation, may be blocked by the monoclonal antibodies daclizumab or basiliximab, directed against CD25 (the α chain of the IL-2 receptor). Blockade of the interaction between IL-2 and its high-affinity receptor (which is expressed only on activated T cells) inhibits the proliferation of activated T cells. These antibodies are used to prevent rejection in solid organ transplant, and they may act in a synergistic way with the calcineurin inhibitors.

Sirolimus (rapamycin) binds (like tacrolimus) to FK-binding protein, but the rapamycin–FK-binding protein complex does not interfere with calcineurin. Instead, it binds another intracellular protein, MTOR, (the mammalian target of rapamycin), which regulates the cell cycle. The final effect is arrest of cells in the G1 phase of the cell cycle. As it acts at a different step than cyclosporine and tacrolimus, the combination of rapamycin with either of these agents would be expected to result in more potent T-cell inhibition.

Leflunomide interferes with the *de novo* pathway of pyrimidine synthesis, limiting T-cell clonal expansion on activation. As rapamycin, it results in G1 phase arrest. This drug has been used successfully in rheumatoid arthritis, but its use in transplantation has been more limited because of safety concerns.

Azathioprine and mycophenolate mofetil (MMF) are antimetabolites that act by inhibiting purine synthesis. Azathioprine effectively blocks the *de novo* synthesis of adenine and guanine nucleotides, and it has effects on all replicating cells (commonly resulting in the undesirable side effects of leucopenia and thrombocytopenia). MMF is metabolized to mycophenolic acid, which blocks a lymphocyte-specific isoform of inosine monophosphate dehydrogenase, inhibiting the synthesis of guanine nucleotides in lymphocytes only. Given its similar mechanism of action and efficacy with reduced toxicity, MMF has replaced azathioprine in transplantation.

Cyclophosphamide is a cytotoxic drug from the nitrogen mustard family of compounds. It kills lymphocytes and many other dividing cells. Its toxicity has contributed to decreasing use, but it is still the treatment of choice for some severe autoimmune diseases (lupus nephritis and Wegener's granulomatosis).

Other Immunomodulatory Agents TNF-α blockade has emerged as an extremely useful form of therapy in some autoimmune diseases, namely rheumatoid arthritis, psoriatic arthritis, ankylosing spondylitis, and inflammatory bowel disease. Blockade of TNF may be attained pharmacologically by one of two agents, infliximab and etanercept. Infliximab is a humanized monoclonal antibody that binds to TNF-α and prevents it from acting. It showed efficacy in the treatment of enteric fistulas in Crohn's disease, a type of inflammatory bowel disease. Etanercept is a recombinant fusion protein that combines the extracellular domain of the TNF receptor (TNFR p75) with an immunoglobulin IgG1 Fc fragment. It also acts by binding free TNF. It has shown great benefit in rheumatoid arthritis, ankylosing spondylitis, and psoriatic arthritis, but not in Crohn's disease.

Anakinra is a recombinant IL-1 receptor antagonist (IL-1Ra). It competes with IL-1 for binding to the IL-1 receptor, and in this way it can block the effects of IL-1. It is effective in rheumatoid arthritis.

Lymphocyte depletion may be attempted with antilymphocyte immunoglobulin (ATG), a polyclonal immunoglobulin obtained by immunizing horses or rabbits with human thymic extract, or with monoclonal antibodies directed against CD3, CD4, CD52, or CD20. Antilymphocyte globulin is profoundly immunosuppressive, and its indications are limited to organ transplantation and aplastic anemia.

Anti-CD3 monoclonal antibody has also been used in organ transplantation. Anti-CD4 monoclonal antibodies were used unsuccessfully in multiple sclerosis and rheumatoid arthritis, in which they resulted in long-term CD4 depletion without clinical benefit, but newer humanized versions of anti-CD4 are being tested in psoriasis. The anti-CD52 rat monoclonal alemtuzumab (Campath-1h) causes significant, long-lasting lymphocyte depletion and has been used in refractory rheumatoid arthritis and transplantation.

SOLID ORGAN AND STEM CELL TRANSPLANTATION In transplantation, as in autoimmunity, there is a harmful immune response that needs to be suppressed. However, there are two very important practical differences. First, in the case of solid organ rejection (and its equivalent in hematopoietic cell transplantation, GVHD) the timing and intensity of the immune response are predictable, so prevention is an option. In fact, prevention is the best alternative, as it has been proven that controlling immune responses is much more difficult than avoiding them. Second, animal models of transplantation are more similar to the human conditions than animal models of autoimmunity. This has allowed for a smooth transition between experiments and clinical practice in transplantation immunology that is not present in autoimmune diseases.

Solid Organ Transplantation Transplantation is the treatment of choice for end-organ damage in many clinical conditions. Kidney, liver, heart, and lung transplantation have become standard medical–surgical procedures. Pancreatic islet cell and intestine transplantation are experimental procedures that are becoming closer to standard of care. Other than donor availability, rejection is the main obstacle to successful transplantation. An immune response to the transplanted organ may take place by one of two mechanisms, called direct and indirect. The direct pathway involves the recognition of donor HLA antigens on donor APCs by the recipient's T cells. This direct recognition of nonself MHC molecules on the transplanted organ is thought to be the most important pathway for rejection, as a significant fraction of the T-cell repertoire is directed against allo-MHC molecules. The indirect pathway involves the activity of the recipient's professional APCs that process and present a variety of donor antigens from the graft.

Organ rejection after transplantation may take one of three forms: hyperacute, acute, and chronic. The immunopathogenesis of the three differs. Hyperacute rejection (typically occurring within hours after the procedure) is caused by pre-existing antibodies directed against donor endothelial antigens. The binding of the antibodies to the endothelium in the blood vessels of the transplanted organ causes complement activation, endothelial damage, inflammation, thrombosis, and vascular occlusion that result in irreversible ischemic damage. This form of rejection is not amenable to immunomodulation, and it must be prevented by screening transplant recipients for the presence of antibodies. Acute rejection begins after a few days, and is caused by T cells (both CD4 and CD8) that are activated mainly by the direct or recognition pathway of alloantigens as previously outlined. This is the predictable response that can be prevented by immunomodulation. Episodes of acute rejection may occur for years after transplant, and continued immunosuppression is required for prevention. When an episode of acute rejection ensues despite prophylaxis, more intensive immunosuppression is required. Chronic rejection represents an immunological phenomenon only partially, is not responsive to therapy and requires retransplant or removal of the damaged organ.

Prevention of Acute Rejection The standard regimen includes triple therapy with corticosteroids, calcineurin inhibitor (cyclosporine/tacrolimus) and an antilymphoproliferative agent (MMF, azathioprine, or rapamycin [Sirolimus]). Some groups add "induction with antibody," using ATG, anti-CD3 or anti-CD25 monoclonal antibodies to minimize the risk of acute rejection. It is not known if any one of these antibody therapies results in a better long-term outcome. The possibility of corticosteroid-free immunosuppression for organ transplantation has been explored for islet cell transplantation for diabetes according to the so-called Edmonton protocol, which combines sirolimus, tacrolimus, and daclizumab. Steroid elimination is a desirable goal in all transplants, and more studies are being done using this approach for transplants other than islet cell.

Treatment of Acute Rejection Once acute rejection begins, the treatment has to be directed against already activated T cells, although keeping the possible blockages on proliferation and activation, to prevent the expansion of the immune response. High-dose intravenous glucocorticoids are the treatment of choice for acute rejection, although the exact regimen of choice is unclear (relatively few comparative studies have been done). The mechanism of action of such high dose of steroids is not known, although there is evidence that they cause lymphocyte apoptosis and elimination of dendritic cells from the peripheral blood.

Allogeneic Bone Marrow (Hematopoietic Stem Cell) Transplantation Allo-HSCT has become the treatment of choice for a variety of hematological malignancies. It can also cure several nonmalignant hematological conditions and immunodeficiencies. In this procedure, precursor hematopoietic cells are administered to the patient. If the transplant is successful, the stem cells engraft and develop into myeloid blood cells and lymphocytes. A new immune system, derived from the stem cells of the donor, develops over time. This immune system is able to contribute significantly to the effective control of the leukemia, lymphoma, or solid tumors present in the recipient (GVL effect). However the donor's immune system may also recognize the recipient as "foreign," and unleash a multi-organ attack called GVHD, which has emerged as the main obstacle for the wide use of this therapeutic modality.

The MHC proteins are the most important initiators of the GVHD response, and consequently stem cell transplants are performed ideally using donors that are HLA identical to the recipient. The presence of mismatched "minor histocompatibility antigens" explains why GVHD still occurs in up to one-third of transplants, even when the donor and the recipient are "HLA identical." Minor histocompatibility agents are also the explanation for the fact that GVHD is much more common when unrelated (i.e., not family) donors are used, even if they are a "perfect" HLA match. Siblings that share HLA antigens are likely to share also a significant fraction of minor antigens; the same is not true for unrelated individuals. GVHD is the mirror image of solid organ rejection. Strong evidence from animal models suggests that the host's APCs are the ones that activate the donor's T lymphocytes (note this is equivalent to the "indirect" pathway described in solid organ transplantation). Compared with solid organ rejection, however, GVHD has one critical complicating factor. Whereas a rejected organ can be removed or replaced, thus eliminating the rejection episode, when the new immune system engrafted with the stem cells is directed against the recipient, the only possible option is to control the untoward immune response.

Most individuals who need an HSCT do not have an HLA-identical sibling. This requires the use of some other source of stem cells: an unrelated donor, a family member with some common HLA, or stem cells obtained from newborns' cord blood. With unrelated donors, whether they are HLA-matched (matched-unrelated donor transplant) or partially mismatched, the frequency of GVHD, as expected, increases significantly. Lastly, when used as treatment of cancer or leukemia, part of the beneficial effect of allo-HSCT is mediated by an immunologically mediated GVL effect. Lower incidence of GVHD has been associated with a higher incidence of leukemia relapse after transplantation. Hence, allo-HSCT presents a unique challenge in that the immune response cannot be completely abrogated without a significant loss in effectiveness. In a way, and at the population level (as opposed to individual cases), GVHD is the price one has to pay to develop a significant GVL.

Prevention of Acute GVHD The attempts to prevent GVHD start by selecting a donor that is as closely HLA matched to the recipient as possible, there are several possible ways of preventing GVHD. Acute GVHD is caused by T cells already present in the administered stem cell (or bone marrow) infusion. It follows that lymphocyte depletion of the graft is a possible approach to prevent GVHD. Indeed, when lymphocyte depletion results in a dose of CD3+ cells of 3×10^4 cells/kg, it is possible to completely prevent GVHD, even in the presence of one HLA mismatch. In fact, in stem cell transplant from an unrelated donor, T-lymphocyte depletion is a commonly used strategy, which unfortunately generates its own set of problems (graft dysfunction, usually caused by rejection, delayed immune reconstitution, with its attendant risks of infection, and post-transplant EBV-related lymphoproliferative disorder, and leukemia relapse).

In the case of transplant from an HLA-identical sibling, a pharmacological approach to the prevention of GVHD is most often used. The standard of care is dual therapy with either cyclosporine or tacrolimus combined with methotrexate. In the standard approach, cyclosporine is initiated before the infusion of stem cells with the aim of preventing T-cell activation, and methotrexate is then added. Methotrexate, by inhibiting purine biosynthesis, is supposed to prevent the proliferation of any T-cell that might have encountered antigen and undergone activation. The combination indeed is more effective than cyclosporine alone to prevent GVHD and the addition of methylprednisolone to cyclosporine and methotrexate may result in still lower rates of acute GVHD, confirming the potential for synergistic activity of immunosuppressive agents with different targets.

Treatment of Acute GVHD Despite the use of prophylaxis, GVHD still develops in 25–50% of HLA-matched sibling transplants. In 20–40%, it is severe enough to require systemic treatment. Corticosteroids are the treatment of choice, at a dose equivalent to 2 mg of methylprednisolone/kg/d. Patients who do not respond to steroids ("steroid-refractory" GVHD) have a particularly poor prognosis, and no treatment has established efficacy in this setting, even if many different immunosuppressive agents have been used. The agents used include many of the immunomodulator agents mentioned earlier (rapamycin, infliximab, daclizumab, alemtuzumab, ATG, and anti-CD3) as well as other experimental monoclonal antibodies including anti-CD3, anti-CD147, denileukin diftitox (human IL-2 fused to diphtheria toxin), and others.

Chronic Graft-vs-Host Disease Chronic GVHD may appear after acute GVHD or *de novo* a few months after transplantation. It typically involves the skin (with scleroderma-like features), the eyes, and mouth (with sicca syndrome similar to Sjoegren's) and the liver (with chronic cholestasis or hepatitis). The lungs may also be involved with a pattern of progressive obliteration of small airways. The cause of chronic GVHD is less well

understood, and it has many features of autoimmune diseases. Treatment involves intense immunosuppression, usually using corticosteroids, combined with some other immunosuppressive agents in resistant cases. Photopheresis is another immunomodulatory technique often beneficial in chronic GVHD. In this procedure the patient's peripheral blood mononuclear cells are extracted by pheresis, exposed to the photoreactive agent methoxsalen and ultraviolet A (UVA) radiation, and then reinfused. It is unknown how photopheresis results in immunomodulation, but in chronic GVHD it seems to allow decreasing the dose of steroids. Methoxsalen, after being exposed to UVA radiation at the proper wavelength, irreversibly cross-links DNA thymine bases and arrests cell proliferation. Some findings suggest that the reinfusion of peripheral blood mononuclear cells after exposure to UVA-activated methoxsalen results in an immune response against proliferating T-cell clones. According to this theory, activated clones of T cells undergo apoptosis during the procedure, are phagocytized by monocytes and dendritic cells and presented to other T cells to induce an immune response against the activated T-cell clones. Extracorporeal photopheresis is licensed for the treatment of cutaneous T-cell lymphoma, in which it is supposed to act in a similar way, except in this case it would target a malignant, instead of activated, T-cell clone.

SELECTED REFERENCES

A controlled trial of interferon gamma to prevent infection in chronic granulomatous disease. The International Chronic Granulomatous Disease Cooperative Study Group. N Engl J Med 1991;324(8):509–516.

Autran B, Carcelain G, Combadiere B, Debre P. Therapeutic vaccines for chronic infections. Science 2004;305(5681):205–208.

Aversa F, Tabilio A, Velardi A, et al. Treatment of high-risk acute leukemia with T-cell-depleted stem cells from related donors with one fully mismatched HLA haplotype. N Engl J Med 1998;339(17):1186–1193.

Bacigalupo A, Van Lint MT, Frassoni F, Marniont A. Graft-versus-leukemia effect following allogeneic bone marrow transplantation. Br J Haematol 1985;61(4):749–751.

Baron F, Storb R, Little MT. Hematopoietic cell transplantation: five decades of progress. Arch Med Res 2003;34(6):528–544.

Barquet N, Domingo P. Smallpox: the triumph over the most terrible of the ministers of death. Ann Intern Med 1997;127(8 Pt 1):635–642.

Blattman JN, Greenberg PD. Cancer immunotherapy: a treatment for the masses. Science 2004;305(5681):200–205.

Brock MV, Borja MC, Ferber L, et al. Induction therapy in lung transplantation: A prospective, controlled clinical trial comparing OKT3, antithymocyte globulin, and daclizumab. J Heart Lung Transplant 2001; 20(12):1282–1290.

Buckley RH. Primary cellular immunodeficiencies. J Allergy Clin Immunol 2002;109(5):747–757.

Cascinelli N, Belli F, MacKie RM, Santinami M, Bufalino R, Morabito A. Effect of long-term adjuvant therapy with interferon alpha-2a in patients with regional node metastases from cutaneous melanoma: a randomised trial. Lancet 2001;358(9285):866–869.

Childs RW, Barrett J. Nonmyeloablative allogeneic immunotherapy for solid tumors. Annu Rev Med 2004;55:459–475.

Childs R, Chernoff A, Contentin N, et al. Regression of metastatic renal-cell carcinoma after nonmyeloablative allogeneic peripheral-blood stem-cell transplantation. N Engl J Med 2000;343(11): 750–758.

Coiffier B, Lepage E, Briere J, et al. CHOP chemotherapy plus rituximab compared with CHOP alone in elderly patients with diffuse large-B-cell lymphoma. N Engl J Med 2002;346(4):235–242.

Coyle TS, Nam TK, Camouse MM, Stevens SR, Baron ED. Steroid-sparing effect of extracorporeal photopheresis in the treatment of graft-vs-host disease. Arch Dermatol 2004;140(6):763, 764.

Cunningham D, Humblet Y, Sienna S, et al. Cetuximab monotherapy and cetuximab plus irinotecan in irinotecan-refractory metastatic colorectal cancer. N Engl J Med 2004;351(4):337–345.

Davidson A, Diamond B. Autoimmune diseases. N Engl J Med 2001; 345(5):340–350.

Dudley ME, Wunderlich JR, Robbins PF, et al. Cancer regression and autoimmunity in patients after clonal repopulation with antitumor lymphocytes. Science 2002;298(5594):850–854.

Francis RJ, Sharma SK, Springer C, et al. A phase I trial of antibody directed enzyme prodrug therapy (ADEPT) in patients with advanced colorectal carcinoma or other CEA producing tumours. Br J Cancer 2002;87(6):600–607.

Gordon LI, Molina A, Witzig T, et al. Durable responses after ibritumomab tiuxetan radioimmunotherapy for CD20+ B-cell lymphoma: long-term follow-up of a phase 1/2 study. Blood 2004;103(12):4429–4431.

Hiraoka A, Ohashi Y, Okamoto S, et al. Phase III study comparing tacrolimus (FK506) with cyclosporine for graft-versus-host disease prophylaxis after allogeneic bone marrow transplantation. Bone Marrow Transplant 2001;28(2):181–185.

Ho VT, Soiffer RJ. The history and future of T-cell depletion as graft-versus-host disease prophylaxis for allogeneic hematopoietic stem cell transplantation. Blood 2001;98(12):3192–3204.

Holland SM. Update on phagocytic defects. Pediatr Infect Dis J 2003; 22(1):87, 88.

Kalden JR, Schattenkirchner M, Sorensen H, et al. The efficacy and safety of leflunomide in patients with active rheumatoid arthritis: a five-year followup study. Arthritis Rheum 2003;48(6):1513–1520.

Kreitman RJ, Wilson WH, Bergeron K, et al. Efficacy of the anti-CD22 recombinant immunotoxin BL22 in chemotherapy-resistant hairy-cell leukemia. N Engl J Med 2001;345(4):241–247.

Letvin NL, Walker BD. Immunopathogenesis and immunotherapy in AIDS virus infections. Nat Med 2003;9(7):861–866.

Leussink VI, Jung S, Merschdorf U, Toyka KV, Gold R. High-dose methylprednisolone therapy in multiple sclerosis induces apoptosis in peripheral blood leukocytes. Arch Neurol 2001;58(1):91–97.

Locatelli F, Bruno B, Zecca M, et al. Cyclosporin A and short-term methotrexate versus cyclosporin A as graft versus host disease prophylaxis in patients with severe aplastic anemia given allogeneic bone marrow transplantation from an HLA-identical sibling: results of a GITMO/EBMT randomized trial. Blood 2000;96(5): 1690–1697.

Mikuls TR, Moreland LW. TNF blockade in the treatment of rheumatoid arthritis: Infliximab versus etanercept. Expert Opin Pharmacother 2001;2(1):75–84.

Mosmann TR, Coffman RL. TH1 and TH2 cells: different patterns of lymphokine secretion lead to different functional properties. Annu Rev Immunol 1989;7:145–173.

Nash RA, Antin JH, Karanes C, et al. Phase 3 study comparing methotrexate and tacrolimus with methotrexate and cyclosporine for prophylaxis of acute graft-versus-host disease after marrow transplantation from unrelated donors. Blood 2000;96(6):2062–2068.

Phan GQ, Yang JC, Sherry RM, et al. Cancer regression and autoimmunity induced by cytotoxic T lymphocyte-associated antigen 4 blockade in patients with metastatic melanoma. Proc Natl Acad Sci USA 2003; 100(14):8372–8377.

Present DH, Rutgeerts P, Targan S, et al. Infliximab for the treatment of fistulas in patients with Crohn's disease. N Engl J Med 1999; 340(18): 1398–1405.

Ratanatharathorn V, Nash RA, Przepiorka D, et al. Phase III study comparing methotrexate and tacrolimus (prograf, FK506) with methotrexate and cyclosporine for graft-versus-host disease prophylaxis after HLA-identical sibling bone marrow transplantation. Blood 1998;92(7):2303–2314.

Rosenberg SA, Lotze MT, Muul LM, et al. A progress report on the treatment of 157 patients with advanced cancer using lymphokine-activated killer cells and interleukin-2 or high-dose interleukin-2 alone. N Engl J Med 1987;316(15):889–897.

Rosenberg SA, Lotze MT, Yang JC, et al. Prospective randomized trial of high-dose interleukin-2 alone or in conjunction with lymphokine-activated killer cells for the treatment of patients with advanced cancer. J Natl Cancer Inst 1993;85(8):622–632.

Ruutu T, Volin L, Parkkali T, Juvonen E, Elonen E. Cyclosporine, methotrexate, and methylprednisolone compared with cyclosporine and methotrexate for the prevention of graft-versus-host disease in bone marrow transplantation from HLA-identical sibling donor: a prospective randomized study. Blood 2000;96(7):2391–2398.

Shapiro AM, Lakey JR, Ryan EA, et al. Islet transplantation in seven patients with type 1 diabetes mellitus using a glucocorticoid-free immunosuppressive regimen. N Engl J Med 2000;343(4): 230–238.

Shlomchik WD, Couzens MS, Tang CB, et al. Prevention of graft versus host disease by inactivation of host antigen-presenting cells. Science 1999;285(5426):412–415.

Storb R, Deeg HJ, Whitehead J, et al. Methotrexate and cyclosporine compared with cyclosporine alone for prophylaxis of acute graft versus host disease after marrow transplantation for leukemia. N Engl J Med 1986;314(12):729–735.

Suda T, Chida K, Matsuda H, et al. High-dose intravenous glucocorticoid therapy abrogates circulating dendritic cells. J Allergy Clin Immunol 2003;112(6):1237–1239.

Van Lint MT, Uderzo C, Locasciulli A, et al. Early treatment of acute graft-versus-host disease with high- or low-dose 6-methylprednisolone: a multicenter randomized trial from the Italian Group for Bone Marrow Transplantation. Blood 1998;92(7):2288–2293.

Volpin R, Angeli P, Galioto A, et al. Comparison between two high-dose methylprednisolone schedules in the treatment of acute hepatic cellular rejection in liver transplant recipients: a controlled clinical trial. Liver Transpl 2002;8(6):527–534.

Washburn K, Speeg KV, Esterl R, et al. Steroid elimination 24 hours after liver transplantation using daclizumab, tacrolimus, and mycophenolate mofetil. Transplantation 2001;72(10):1675–1679.

Weinblatt ME, Kremer JM, Bankhurst AD, et al. A trial of etanercept, a recombinant tumor necrosis factor receptor:Fc fusion protein, in patients with rheumatoid arthritis receiving methotrexate. N Engl J Med 1999;340(4):253–259.

Weisdorf DJ, Nesbit ME, Ramsay NK, et al. Allogeneic bone marrow transplantation for acute lymphoblastic leukemia in remission: prolonged survival associated with acute graft-versus-host disease. J Clin Oncol 1987;5(9):1348–1355.

93 HIV Molecular Biology, Treatment, and Resistance

Frank Maldarelli

SUMMARY

HIV has infected more than 40 million individuals on six continents since emerging in 1981, with an estimated 15,000 new infections transmitted daily. The rapid spread and lethal nature of the HIV-1 pandemic has made the development of useful and widely available therapy a compelling imperative. As such, many of the molecular mechanisms of HIV replication have been investigated as potential therapeutic targets. This chapter summarizes key molecular events in HIV replication, their use as therapeutic targets, and the inevitable emergence of resistance to therapy.

Key Words: Drug resistance; HIV; integrase; non-nucleoside reverse transcriptase inhibitor (NNRTI); nucleoside reverse transcriptase inhibitors (NRTI); *vif*.

INTRODUCTION

HIV has infected more than 40 million individuals on six continents since emerging in 1981, with an estimated 15,000 new infections transmitted daily. Untreated, HIV infection results in a progressive, inexorable immunodeficiency culminating in death from opportunistic infections or neoplastic diseases. Over half of all infected individuals have already died and, without intervention, the remainder are expected to succumb in the next 10–15 yr. The rapid spread and lethal nature of the HIV-1 pandemic has made the development of useful and widely available therapy a compelling imperative. As such, many of the molecular mechanisms of HIV replication have been investigated as potential therapeutic targets. This chapter summarizes key molecular events in HIV replication, their use as therapeutic targets, and the inevitable emergence of resistance to therapy.

HIV is a lentivirus member of the retroviruses, a family of RNA viruses that replicate via a DNA intermediate using a viral encoded reverse transcriptase (RT). Infection with two distinct HIV variants, HIV-1 and HIV-2, have been described in humans; HIV-1 is a pandemic strain found worldwide, and accounts for the majority of infections. Sequence homology studies have subdivided HIV-1 into three principal groups: M (main), O (other), and N (non-M, non-O); Group M has been further subdivided into 10 distinct subtypes. HIV-2 represents a related, but clearly distinct virus of with two principal subtypes (A and B), which have a limited geographic

circulation, principally in West Africa. The precise origin(s) of HIV remain uncertain; simian immunodeficiency viruses similar to HIV-1 and HIV-2 are present in many primate species, and convincing evidence supports the theory that independent zoonotic transmission events from primates to humans are responsible for HIV-1 and HIV-2 epidemics, and perhaps for HIV-1 M, N, and O groups as well. Interestingly, the simian immunodeficiency viruses presumed precursors of HIV infect and replicate to high titer in their natural primate hosts without inducing severe immunodeficiency. As such, there is no single viral component or replication event that is intrinsically or universally pathogenic. Instead, in the cross-species transmission, the combination of new host and viral factors resulted in a highly virulent outcome.

HIV-1 transmission occurs when virus or virus-infected cells directly contacts susceptible host cells, either as exposed mucosa during sexual transmission, or lymphoid elements during blood-borne transmission. Within days, HIV-1 replication expands from local sites of infection principally to lymphoid tissue (lymph nodes, gut associated lymphoid tissue, thymus, spleen) and to central nervous system elements. Wide dissemination of HIV-1 results in relatively high viral and humoral response, viremia declines to a surprisingly stable "set point" characteristic of the individual. Over time, the consequence of persistent HIV-1 infection is a progressive immune deficiency. HIV-induced immunodeficiency is difficult to quantitate, but CD4 cell concentrations represent a useful and reasonable measure of immunity. In general, morbidity and mortality from HIV infection are secondary to opportunistic infections and neoplastic diseases, although HIV replication alone may be responsible for central nervous system disorders including dementia. The relative risk of opportunistic infection or characteristic neoplasm increases with degree of CD4 lymphopenia; AIDS is a specific diagnosis requiring the presence of specific infections (e.g., *Pneumocystis* pneumonia), neoplasms (e.g., Kaposi sarcoma), or decline in CD4 cell counts to <200 cells/µL.

The precise mechanism of CD4 lymphopenia during HIV infection remains uncertain. Although viral cytopathic effects are likely to contribute to cell death in vivo, the fraction of CD4 cells that are HIV infected (typically 1:1000–1:10,000) is relatively small, suggesting direct cell killing does not account for the significant CD4 lymphopenia. Alternative possibilities for the progressive loss of CD4 cells include: (1) bystander effects, with killing of uninfected cells proximal to, or in contact with, infected cells and (2) induction

From: *Principles of Molecular Medicine, Second Edition*
Edited by: M. S. Runge and C. Patterson © Humana Press, Inc., Totowa, NJ

HIV Replication Cycle

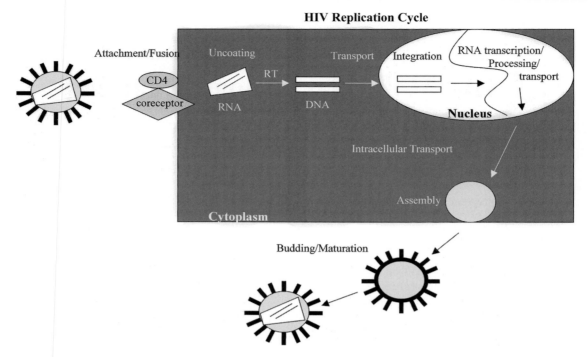

Figure 93-1   Replication cycle of HIV showing binding at cell surface membranes, entry via fusion, reverse transcription, transpost and integration, HIV expression, translation of HIV proteins, and assembly and maturation. The HIV replication cycle may be completed in as little as 1 d. RT, reverse transcriptase.

of apoptosis occurring in immune cells that have become nonspecifically activated but that have not encountered antigen.

As morbidity and mortality from HIV infection is closely related to CD4 cell numbers, strategies to counteract the CD4 lymphopenia directly through the use of growth factors, notably IL-2, have been explored as potential therapy to directly counteract HIV-induced immunodeficiency. IL-2 therapy results in sustained increases in peripheral CD4 cell numbers and expansion in the pool of CD4 naïve and central memory cells. Large multinational studies are underway to determine whether the numerical increases in CD4 cell concentrations induced by IL-2 correspond to improvement in morbidity and mortality from HIV infection.

MOLECULAR EVENTS OF HIV REPLICATION

HIV-1 replication may be divided into a series of molecular events, including attachment and fusion, uncoating, reverse transcription, integration, RNA expression and transport, virion assembly, virion budding, and virion release (Fig. 93-1). Many of these steps have been investigated as potential therapeutic targets for HIV infection.

HIV-1 replication is initiated by virions or infected cells interacting with specific host cell receptors. HIV-1 entry is mediated by multimeric complexes of gp120–gp41 glycoprotein on the virion surface and has been dissected into two stages: attachment and membrane fusion.

ENTRY OF HIV   During the attachment phase of entry, gp120 engages two surface proteins expressed on host cells, a primary receptor, CD4, and a coreceptor. HIV-1 coreceptors are cytokine receptors and are principally divided into two broad types: X4, (CXCR4), and R5 (CCR5). Essentially all HIV bind to CD4 (rare CD4-independent variants have been identified), and coreceptor specificity defines the range of cell type infection (Fig. 93-2)

and cytopathicity in vitro. HIV with R5 specificity infects both macrophage and lymphocytes, whereas R4 viruses infect lymphocytes. R5 viruses are critically involved at the time of infection; large genetic surveys have demonstrated that individuals homozygous for a mutation in CCR5 that prevents HIV binding have a very low risk of infection, suggesting R5 viruses act as the initial inoculum in an infection. During chronic HIV infection, both R5 and X4 viruses circulate in an infected individual. In general, R5 viruses have been associated with slower disease progression, and a switch from R5 to X4 has been associated with accelerated CD4 cell decline and disease progression. Dual tropic viruses capable of using either CCR5 or CXCR4 have been reported with marked cytopathicity. Additionally, several alternative molecules have been identified that may be used infrequently as coreceptors. The residues involved in coreceptor specificity have been identified, and can be assigned either phenotypically or predicted by bioinformatics techniques.

Inhibition of attachment and entry has been investigated as an important therapeutic target. Direct inhibition of gp120-CD4 binding in vitro has been achieved in vitro typically using specific antibody, but in vivo studies have not been widely successful. In contrast, small molecule inhibitors of gp120-coreceptor binding have been identified for both X4 and R5 coreceptors; competitive inhibitors of R5 binding are in phase I trials. Fortunately, some R5 inhibitors appear to be quite specific and do not have detectable R5 agonist activity, so they bind to CCR5 without interfering with normal host CCR5 signaling activity. One concern in the development of all coreceptor inhibitors, however, is that use of one coreceptor inhibitor may shift viral populations to use the alternative coreceptor; for example, use of a CCR5 inhibitor could result in a change in circulating HIV so that it exclusively uses CXCR4; the consequences of such a drug-induced coreceptor switch are unknown.

SUMMARY AND FUTURE DIRECTIONS

HIV infection carries out a relatively complex replication program using unique viral-encoded functions and exploiting host machinery. Several steps in HIV replication have been targeted for therapy, and several more are under investigation. Antiretroviral therapy has matured over the last 15 yr from transiently effective monotherapy to sustained suppression with combinations of antiretroviral agents. Therapy remains, however, severely limited. Despite suppressive therapy, HIV infection remains incurable, and available therapies are at risk of failure from the emergence of resistance. New strategies to effectively deal with resistance are clearly necessary, and novel approaches to HIV infection will be essential to eradicate infection.

SELECTED REFERENCES

Bishop KN, Holmes RK, Sheehy AM, Davidson NO, Cho SJ, Malim MH. Cytidine deamination of retroviral DNA by diverse APOBEC proteins. Curr Biol 2004;14(15):1392–1396.

Coffin JM, Hughes SH, Varmus HE, eds. Retroviruses, New York: Cold Spring Harbor Press, 1997.

De Clercq E. Antiviral drugs in current clinical use. J Clin Virol 2004; 30(2):115–133.

Gallant JE, Gerondelis PZ, Wainberg MA, et al. Nucleoside and nucleotide analogue reverse transcriptase inhibitors: A clinical review of antiretroviral resistance. Antivir Ther 2003;8(6):489–506.

Kao S, Khan MA, Miyagi E, Plishka R, Buckler-White A, Strebel K. The human immunodeficiency virus type 1 Vif protein reduces intracellular expression and inhibits packaging of APOBEC3G (CEM15), a cellular inhibitor of virus infectivity. J Virol 2003;77(21):11,398–11,407.

KewalRamani VN, Coffin JM. Virology. Weapons of mutational destruction. Science 2003;301(5635):923–925.

Maldarelli F. HIV drug resistance. In: Zeichner S, Read J, eds. Handbook of Pediatric HIV Care, London: Cambridge University Press, 2004; pp. 334–354.

Schrofelbauer B, Yu Q, Landau NR. New insights into the role of Vif in HIV-1 replication. AIDS Rev 2004;6(1):34–39.

Sharp PM, Bailes E, Chaudhuri RR, Rodenburg CM, Santiago MO, Hahn BH. The origins of acquired immune deficiency syndrome viruses: where and when? Philos Trans R Soc Lond B Biol Sci 2001; 356(1410):867–876.

Shulman N, Winters M. A review of HIV-1 resistance to the nucleoside and nucleotide inhibitors. Curr Drug Targets Infect Disord 2003; 3(4):273–281.

94 Cellular and Molecular Aspects of Pneumonia

MARCUS J. SCHULTZ AND TOM VAN DER POLL

SUMMARY

Immunotherapy aimed at modulation of immune responses may serve as an important adjuvant to antibiotic therapy in the treatment of pneumonia. Alveolar macrophages and polymorphonuclear cells play a prominent role in innate immunity in the lungs. These cells need to communicate in mounting an effective host defense against invading pathogens. Cytokines, chemokines, and colony-stimulating factors play a critical role in this process. Side-products of the coagulation cascade also enhance local inflammation. Activation of the complement system results in the formation of several proinflammatory mediators that can attract and activate polymorphonuclear cells, and formation of molecules with antimicrobial activity.

Key Words: Chemokines; coagulation; complement; cytokines; factor VII; fibrinolysis; granulocyte colony-stimulating factor; IL-10; plasminogen activator inhibitor-1; pneumonia; tissue factor; tumor necrosis factor-α.

INTRODUCTION

The airways are continuously exposed to respiratory pathogens, either by inhalation or by (micro)aspiration. Infectious agents that have passed structural defenses enter the terminal airways, in which they may cause pneumonia, one of the most common infectious diseases.

The growing number of immunocompromised patients susceptible to pneumonia, and a rise of antibiotic resistance among microorganisms have made the treatment of pneumonia more difficult. Hence, there is a need for novel therapeutic approaches for lower respiratory tract infections. Immunotherapy aimed at modulation of the immune response may serve as an important adjuvant to antibiotic therapy in the treatment of pneumonia. However, new therapeutics for patients with pneumonia must be approached with caution because underlying cellular and molecular mechanisms of pneumonia are not fully understood.

Pulmonary host defense includes both innate and specific immune responses. Innate immune responses are primarily responsible for the elimination of bacterial pathogens from the alveolar spaces; specific immune responses are involved in eradication of encapsulated pathogens, and pathogens that survive after phagocytosis. This chapter focuses on innate immune responses (Table 94-1). Innate defenses consist of structural defenses, antimicrobial molecules, and phagocytosis by resident alveolar macrophages (AMs) and recruited polymorphonuclear cells (PMNs). AMs and PMNs play a prominent role in innate immunity in the lungs. These cells can phagocytose and kill microorganisms, and PMNs can release the microbicidal contents of their granules. AMs and PMNs need to communicate in mounting an effective host defense against invading pathogens. Proinflammatory and anti-inflammatory cytokines, chemokines (cytokines with chemotactic activities), and colony-stimulating factors play a critical role in this process. Side-products of the coagulation cascade also enhance local inflammation. Finally, activation of the complement system results in the formation of several proinflammatory mediators that can attract and activate PMNs, and formation of molecules with antimicrobial activity (e.g., the membrane attack complex). Furthermore, several complement components can induce the production of cytokines, chemokines, and other proinflammatory cytokines by several cell types.

Potential immunomodulating strategies that may hold promise for patients with pneumonia are aimed at targeting AMs, the cytokine network, the coagulation cascade, and the complement system. This chapter discusses such strategies during experimental respiratory infections. Most of this knowledge has been obtained from animal studies; only a limited number of human studies have been performed in the last decade.

TARGETING AMs IN PNEUMONIA

Respiratory pathogens that have entered the terminal airways are first encountered by AMs. AMs play a central role in pulmonary host defense. The recruitment of large numbers of PMNs in the alveolar space from the marginated pool of leukocytes in the pulmonary circulation is initiated when the microbial challenge is too large or too virulent to be contained by the AMs alone. These recruited PMNs provide auxiliary phagocytic capacities, critical for the effective eradication of pathogens. AMs can bind, phagocytose, and kill pathogens, and, thus, can directly influence the bacterial load. Furthermore, AMs can also secrete a large range of inflammatory mediators. Some of these mediators act directly on respiratory pathogens, whereas others exert their effects indirectly by recruiting PMNs. Finally, AMs can phagocytose apoptotic PMNs. From this it can be concluded that AMs (or AM-derived

From: *Principles of Molecular Medicine, Second Edition*
Edited by: M. S. Runge and C. Patterson © Humana Press, Inc., Totowa, NJ

Table 94-1
Components of the Innate Host Defense in the Lungs

Structural defenses
- Antimicrobial molecules (e.g., surfactant-associated proteins, defensins)
- Mucociliary clearance
- Sneezing/coughing

Soluble components
- Proinflammatory cytokines, including colony-stimulating factors[a]
- Anti-inflammatory cytokines[a]
- Chemokines[a]
- Leukotrienes
- Nitric oxide
- Complement[a]
- Coagulation factors[a]

Cellular components
- AMs[a]
- PMNs
- Epithelial cells

[a]Discussed in this chapter.

substances) play a regulating role in the pathogenesis of pneumonia, both in the initiation of the inflammatory response, and in its resolution.

AMs CONTRIBUTE TO THE RECRUITMENT OF PMNS DURING PNEUMONIA Compared with control rats, PMN numbers were decreased in bronchoalveolar lavage fluids (BALF) of AM-depleted rats after instillation of a sublethal dose of *Pseudomonas aeruginosa* into the airways, concordant with significantly decreased levels of tumor necrosis factor (TNF)-α and macrophage inflammatory protein (MIP)-2 mRNA expression in one study. In another study, in which AMs from lipopolysaccharide (LPS)-exposed mice were transferred to the lungs of naive recipient mice, nearly a threefold increase in the number of PMNs in BALF was found compared with instillation of AMs from unexposed mice.

AMs AND BACTERIAL CLEARANCE/SURVIVAL IN EXPERIMENTAL PNEUMONIA MODELS Evidence exists for the importance of AMs in host defense against different respiratory pathogens. In particular studies in which rodents were treated with a mixture of clodronate and liposomes via the airways, resulting in a selective depletion of AMs by induction of programmed cell death (apoptosis), have provided valuable information. Impaired survival was found in mice depleted of AMs in a murine *Streptococcus pneumoniae* pneumonia model. In this model, PMN-recruitment was largely increased in AM-depleted mice, but no difference in bacterial outgrowth could be observed. By contrast, in a murine *Mycoplasma* pneumonia model, AM-depletion resulted in elevated outgrowth of *Mycoplasma* from the lungs. AM-depletion exacerbated the *Mycoplasma* infection in *Mycoplasma*-resistant mice by reducing killing of the pathogen to a level comparable to that in *Mycoplasma*-susceptible mice without AM-depletion, suggesting that defective AM-function is the likely explanation for the difference between susceptible and resistant mice. Interestingly, higher numbers of PMNs in lavage fluids were recovered from the AM-depleted mice, indicating that the differences in killing of the invading pathogen could not be explained by an effect on the recruitment of PMNs. In a murine *Klebsiella pneumoniae* pneumonia model, AM depletion influenced mortality dramatically, with 100% lethality after 3 d in AM-depleted mice compared with 100% long-term survival in nondepleted mice. This was

accompanied by an increased outgrowth of *K. pneumoniae* from lungs and blood in AM-depleted mice, and similar to the former study, an increase in PMN-influx into the pulmonary compartment. Similar data were reported on a murine pneumonia model with *P. aeruginosa*, in which AM depletion resulted in a delayed bacterial clearance compared with control mice. However, it was also demonstrated that early after the initiation of pneumonia, compared with control mice, AM-depleted mice had lower concentrations of chemokines and fewer PMNs in BALF, and a significant improvement in lung edema. Importantly, although AM depletion improved early-phase inflammation, (late) survival was not altered. These data illustrate both the beneficial and deleterious effects of AMs during the orchestration of inflammation during pneumonia. Depletion of AMs in the early phase of *Pseudomonas* pneumonia may initially improve lung injury, but may worsen the eventual outcome, as seen in the models of pneumonia with this pathogen, and other pathogens like *K. pneumoniae*, *S. pneumoniae*, and *M. pneumoniae*.

AMs AND RESOLUTION OF INFLAMMATION Whereas initially AMs readily phagocytose and (thereby) eliminate certain inhaled pathogens, they later represent important effector cells in the resolution process. The (previously mentioned) observation of overzealous and persistent PMN-infiltration in the absence of AMs may be related to the equally important function of AMs during resolution of inflammation. To reinstitute tissue homeostasis, all processes involved in the initiation of inflammation must be reversed and one important prerequisite for resolution to occur is the removal of extravasated PMNs. Several lines of evidence support the hypothesis that PMNs undergo apoptosis followed by rapid clearance by AMs. Apoptosis thereby provides an injury-limiting mechanism because the membrane of PMN remains intact, preventing potentially injurious granule contents from being released. The role of AMs as regulator of inflammation has further been illustrated by studies demonstrating that AMs engulf apoptotic PMNs and release anti-inflammatory mediators. These data indicate that the role of AMs in host defense is not limited to the generation of the initial inflammatory response, but extends to regulation of inflammation, including elimination of phagocytosed pathogens.

No human studies on targeting AMs or AM-functions during pneumonia have been performed.

TARGETING THE CYTOKINE NETWORK IN PNEUMONIA

Cytokines are small proteins produced by many different cell types (including AMs and PMNs), having effects on a large variety of (immune) cells. Cytokines are considered to be involved in the early response after the recognition of a pathogen (e.g., TNF and interleukin [IL]-1β), in the recruitment of immune cells to the site of infection (the so-called chemokines, such as IL-8), or in the activation of AMs and recruited PMNs (e.g., TNF, IL-1β, interferon [IFN]-γ, IL-12, IL-17, IL-18, IL-6, and IL-10). Cytokines are considered to have proinflammatory or anti-inflammatory properties, or both. Colony-stimulating factors are a cytokine family required for the proliferation and differentiation of hematopoietic progenitor cells. This family includes granulocyte macrophage colony-stimulating factor, granulocyte colony-stimulating factor (G-CSF), and IL-3. G-CSF plays an important role in maintaining the normal PMN-count in blood and enhancing the functional properties of PMNs.

ACTIVATION OF THE CYTOKINE NETWORK DURING PNEUMONIA

The early response cytokines TNF and IL-1β, both typical proinflammatory cytokines, have been studied extensively in the context of pulmonary host defense. Increased expression of TNF and IL-1β has been observed in bacterial pneumonia, both in animals and in humans. TNF and IL-1β play important roles during host defense because these cytokines can activate AMs and PMNs, leading to augmented phagocytosis, oxidative burst, protein release, and bacterial killing; contribute to the recruitment of PMNs by stimulating the expression of adhesion molecules; and induce the production of chemokines.

Chemokines are low molecular weight cytokines involved in the recruitment of immune cells to the site of infection. Certain chemokines (e.g., IL-8, epithelial neutrophil activating protein-78 in humans; MIP-2 and KC in mice) exhibit chemotactic and activating effects on PMNs. Elevated chemokine levels have been detected in lungs of mice with experimental pneumonia; elevated levels of IL-8 have also been found in BALF of patients with pneumonia, and IL-8 levels correlated with PMN-counts in, as well as PMN-chemotactic activity of pleural fluid.

IFN-γ is a cytokine mainly produced by antigen-activated T and natural killer cells. The secretion of IFN-γ is induced by TNF and IL-12. IFN-γ exerts several immune regulatory activities, including activation of phagocytes, stimulation of antigen-presentation by increasing the expression of major histocompatibility complex molecules class I and II on antigen-presenting cells, orchestration of leukocyte–endothelium interactions and stimulation of the respiratory burst. Macrophages are stimulated by IFN-γ to secrete TNF and IL-12, setting up a paracrine positive-feedback cycle. Like the production of TNF, IL-1β, and chemokines, the production of the proinflammatory cytokine IFN-γ is enhanced during murine pneumonia. Similarly, the expression of another proinflammatory cytokine, IL-12, is enhanced in bacterial pneumonia. IL-17 is a cytokine that induces granulopoiesis via G-CSF production and stimulates the production of chemokines. The release of IL-17 in the lungs in pneumonia has been demonstrated before. IL-18 is another proinflammatory cytokine, with many similarities to IL-1. IL-18 is expressed constitutively in lungs and IL-18 concentrations increase marginally during experimental pneumonia. Nonetheless, findings suggest that either constitutively expressed IL-18 influences the innate immune response during respiratory tract infection or that the modest rise in IL-18 levels is biologically significant in the context of murine pneumonia. IL-6 is both a proinflammatory and an anti-inflammatory cytokine. The production of IL-6 is under the influence of TNF and IL-1β. Many cell types, including macrophages, T and B cells, and parenchymal cells produce IL-6. Like the other cytokines, IL-6 is produced in the lung during pneumonia.

IL-10 is a typical anti-inflammatory cytokine. IL-10 attenuates the production of TNF, IL-1β, chemokines, IFN-γ, and IL-12, and has potent inhibitory effects on PMNs resulting in reduced phagocytosis and bacterial killing. IL-10 is produced in the pulmonary compartment in mice with pneumonia.

AMs from patients with pneumonia produce G-CSF spontaneously, whereas AMs from healthy individuals only produce G-CSF on stimulation with LPS. It has been hypothesized that production of TNF and IL-1, which subsequently stimulates AMs to produce G-CSF, is one of the major roles of local macrophages: in this hypothesis, G-CSF acts locally during pneumonia to recruit PMNs to the infected lung and subsequently activate the recruited PMNs.

ROLE OF PROINFLAMMATORY CYTOKINES DURING PNEUMONIA

Proinflammatory cytokines appear to play a protective role in pulmonary host defense. Indeed, systemic neutralization of TNF-attenuated host defense in pulmonary bacterial infections with *S. pneumoniae* and *K. pneumoniae* resulting in decreased survival, although administration of low doses of exogenous TNF, or augmentation of local expression of TNF in the lungs through gene therapy significantly diminished mortality and enhanced bacterial clearance from the pulmonary compartment during severe pneumonia with these pathogens. Similarly, IL-1 receptor type I deficient mice demonstrated an impaired clearance of *S. pneumoniae* and a reduced capacity to form inflammatory infiltrates. Treatment with a neutralizing anti-TNF antibody made IL-1 receptor-deficient mice extremely susceptible to pneumococcal pneumonia, more so than IL-1 receptor knockout mice treated with a control antibody and wild-type mice treated with anti-TNF, indicating that the concurrent action of TNF and IL-1 is required for an adequate host defense against pneumococcal pneumonia.

Comparable data are present for IL-12, IFN-γ, IL-17, IL-18, and IL-6. Neutralization of IL-12 attenuated bacterial clearance and increased mortality of mice with *K. pneumoniae* pneumonia, whereas overexpression of IL-12 reduced mortality. In accordance, IL-12 knockout mice had a normal host defense against *S. pneumonia*; bacterial outgrowth from lung tissue and survival was similar to wild-type mice in a pneumonia model with this pathogen. The role of IFN-γ in the setting of bacterial pneumonia is less clear. Although in one study IFN-γ knockout mice demonstrated higher mortality compared to wild-type mice, and in other studies local overexpression of IFN-γ in rats resulted in increased bacterial clearance from the pulmonary compartment, other data suggest that endogenous IFN-γ may impair an effective pulmonary defense in pneumonia. Indeed, pulmonary clearance of *S. pneumoniae* was attenuated in IFN-γ-R knockout mice, as well as in IFN-γ knockout mice compared to wild-type mice. IL-17 receptor-deficient mice were exquisitely sensitive to intranasally administered *K. pneumoniae* with 100% lethality after 48 h compared with 40% mortality in control mice. The IL-17 receptor-deficient mice displayed a significant delay in PMN recruitment into the lungs, associated with significant reduction in local G-CSF and MIP-2 levels. From these data it can be concluded that IL-17 receptor signaling is critical for host defense against *K. pneumoniae*. IL-18 deficient mice demonstrated a reduced clearance of *S. pneumoniae* and were more susceptible to progression to systemic infection at 24 and 48 h after an intranasal challenge with this pathogen. Although survival was not different between knockout mice and wild-type mice, these data suggest that IL-18 plays a protective role in the early host response during pneumococcal pneumonia. Evidence for the importance of IL-6 in host defense during pneumonia was obtained from a study on *S. pneumoniae* pneumonia in IL-6 knockout mice. IL-6 knockout mice had more bacteria in their lungs after an intranasal challenge with this pathogen, and died significantly earlier than normal mice.

ROLE OF CHEMOKINES DURING PNEUMONIA

Several studies suggest a regulating role for chemokines in pneumonia: administration of chemokine neutralizing antibodies resulted in a reduction in PMN influx, which was associated with an attenuation of bacterial clearance from the lung, and an increased incidence of bacteremia in several murine pneumonia models. Local chemokine overexpression in the lung of transgenic mice led to an increase in PMN influx after intratracheal administration of bacteria, which was associated with a striking improvement in survival, increased bacterial clearance from the lungs, and reduced incidence of bacteremia.

ROLE OF ANTI-INFLAMMATORY CYTOKINES IN PNEUMONIA   Evidence exists that the anti-inflammatory cytokine IL-10 plays a detrimental role in the clearance of bacteria during pulmonary infections; administration of exogenous IL-10 reduced survival and increased outgrowth of bacteria in lungs of mice with *S. pneumoniae* pneumonia. Conversely, neutralization of endogenous IL-10 led to enhanced clearance of bacteria and improved survival in mice with pulmonary infection with *K. pneumoniae* or *S. pneumoniae*. Thus, although the proinflammatory cytokines and chemokines appear to play a protective role in pulmonary host defense by initiating a protective inflammatory reaction, the anti-inflammatory cytokines demonstrate a detrimental role in the innate immunity against respiratory pathogens by resolving the immune responses.

From the point of view that after the initiation and, if necessary, reinforcement of the inflammatory reaction, there is a need for innate immune responses to be stopped when the invading pathogens have been erased from the pulmonary compartment, it is logical that both proinflammatory and anti-inflammatory cytokines are produced locally in an inflammatory reaction. This fine-tuning of inflammation is necessary to protect the host from an overzealous reaction.

IS THE ROLE OF CYTOKINES COMPARABLE WITH ALL TYPES OF PNEUMONIA?   The majority of the aforementioned models on the role of different cytokines involved infection with *S. pneumoniae* or *K. pneumoniae*. Importantly, the role of these cytokines may be different during pneumonia with other pathogens. Indeed, although endogenous TNF was important for clearance of *S. pneumoniae* and *K. pneumoniae* from mouse lungs, TNF impaired host defense mechanisms during pneumonia with *P. aeruginosa*. Similarly, although IL-1 receptor I-deficient mice demonstrated an impaired bacterial clearance and a reduced capacity to form inflammatory infiltrates during infection with *S. pneumoniae*, during infection with *P. aeruginosa* IL-1 receptor I-deficient mice demonstrated an enhanced bacterial clearance. Results from two studies demonstrate opposite roles for IL-18 during pneumococcal pneumonia and during pneumonia caused by *P. aeruginosa*, comparable to the results previously mentioned. Whereas in pneumococcal pneumonia the absence of endogenous IL-18 resulted in a reduced clearance of *S. pneumoniae*, in IL-18 deficient mice challenged with *P. aeruginosa* enhanced bacterial clearance was found. Furthermore, although endogenous IL-10 hampered bacterial clearance in mouse models of *S. pneumoniae* and *K. pneumoniae*, IL-10 improved host defense in a model of pneumonia caused by *P. aeruginosa*.

These data suggest that in more gradually developing pneumonias, such as that caused by *S. pneumoniae* and *K. pneumoniae*, a certain proinflammatory cytokine response within the pulmonary compartment is required to combat the invading microorganism, whereas in a more acute form of pneumonia, such as caused by *P. aeruginosa*, an excessive inflammatory response contributes to an adverse outcome. However, it must be emphasized that the murine *Pseudomonas* pneumonia model has some potential flaws, because a rather large amount of bacteria must be installed into the airways to induce pneumonia in mice, using lower inocula, bacteria are cleared from the airways and no pneumonia will develop;

and because compared with the other experimental pneumonia models in which pneumonia develops in some days, in this model an acute pneumonia develops within 6–24 h; and *Pseudomonas* almost invariably causes pneumonia in the immunocompromised host, whereas the vast majority of mouse models used previously healthy immunocompetent animals. Hence, experimental models of *Pseudomonas* pneumonia described in the literature may not adequately mimic the clinical situation.

GCS-F: RESULTS FROM PRECLINICAL AND CLINICAL STUDIES   In animal models of pneumonia, G-CSF is important for survival of pneumonia. Indeed, in a *S. pneumoniae* pneumonia model, administration of G-CSF before challenge improved survival in splenectomized mice. Furthermore, during infection with *K. pneumoniae*, IL-17 receptor-deficient mice were more likely to die compared with control mice, which was associated with significant reduction in local G-CSF levels.

Based on favorable effects of G-CSF in preclinical studies, several clinical studies with G-CSF in patients with pneumonia have been performed, unfortunately all with disappointing results. One was a randomized, placebo-controlled, multicenter trial of G-CSF up to 10 d as an adjunct to antibiotics in patients with pneumonia. Although G-CSF accelerated radiological improvement and appeared to reduce serious complications, such as empyema, adult respiratory distress syndrome (ARDS), and disseminated intravascular coagulation, mortality and length of hospitalization were not affected. In a second study G-CSF was compared with standard therapy in hospitalized adult patients with multilobar community-acquired pneumonia. In this study only a trend toward reduction of mortality in patients with pneumococcal bacteremia was seen in the study group. In another study, use of G-CSF did not reduce mortality and frequency of nosocomial infections in neutropenic patients requiring intensive care medicine. Finally, in two double-blind, randomized studies in patients with pneumonia and sepsis, there was no reduction of mortality or complications in the study group as compared with controls.

Thus only animal studies have shown beneficial effects of certain strategies aiming at modulation of the cytokine network. Unfortunately, results from these additive therapies are dependent on the causative pathogen, or may even be detrimental (Table 94-2). G-CSF has failed to improve mortality or any other important outcome measure in patients suffering from pneumonia.

TARGETING THE COAGULATION SYSTEM IN PNEUMONIA

Local changes in coagulation and fibrinolysis during pneumonia are remarkably similar to systemic changes in coagulation and fibrinolysis during sepsis and changes found in BALF of patients with ARDS. Interestingly, pathways responsible for local activation of coagulation and inhibition of fibrinolysis during pneumonia, both responsible for enhanced fibrin formation in the airways, are thought to be similar to those in the systemic compartment during sepsis (Fig. 94-1).

ACTIVATION OF COAGULATION AND INHIBITION OF FIBRINOLYSIS IN PNEUMONIA   In humans with pneumonia, increased local thrombin generation has been observed. Next to activation of coagulation, inhibition of fibrinolysis has been demonstrated. Like in the systemic procoagulant state during sepsis, during pneumonia expression of tissue factor is suggested to play a key role in thrombin generation in the bronchoalveolar compartment. In one study of mechanically ventilated patients

Table 94-2
Cytokines Influence Host Defense During Respiratory Tract Infections, Although Their Role May Vary Depending on the Pathogen

Cytokine	*Streptococcus pneumoniae*	*Klebsiella pneumoniae*	*Pseudomonas aeruginosa*
TNF	+	+	+/−
IL-1β	+	?	−
Chemokines	?	+	+
IL-10	−	−	+/−
IL-6	+	?	?
IL-12	0	+	?
IL-17	?	+	?
IL-18	+	?	−
IFN-γ	+/−	?	+/−

+, indicates a beneficial role in case of respiratory infection with the specified pathogen; −, indicates a detrimental role in case of respiratory infection with the specified pathogen; +/−, indicates conflicting data; ?, indicates that there are no data on the effect of this cytokine; 0, indicates no effect.

IFN, interferon; IL, interleukin; TNF, tumor necrosis factor.

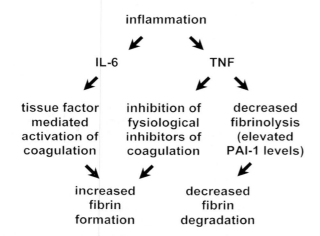

Figure 94-1 Schematic presentation of pathways involved in enhanced fibrin formation in sepsis and pneumonia. Coagulation activation is stimulated by IL-6, although inhibition of fibrinolysis is under control of TNF-α. It is uncertain if inhibition of natural inhibitors of coagulation is a feature of local inflammation in the lung. PAI, plasminogen activator inhibitor.

who developed pneumonia, tissue factor expression preceded the clinical manifestation of pneumonia, suggesting that this response indeed is important in the pathogenesis of pneumonia. Disturbed local fibrin turnover is also substantially resulting from depression of fibrinolysis. In the lung, the most important plasminogen activator appears to be urokinase-type plasminogen activator (u-PA). Although plasminogen activator inhibitor (PAI) type-1 is in almost all tissues the principal inhibitor of fibrinolysis, in the bronchoalveolar compartment PAI-2 seems to play an important role as well. Both PAI-1 and PAI-2 are increased in ARDS and pneumonia, and are probably derived from AMs and lung epithelial cells, fibroblasts, and endothelial cells, respectively. Markedly enhanced levels of PAI-1 and PAI-2 were noted in BALF from mechanically ventilated patients with pneumonia, compared with healthy controls. Also noted is that the depression of bronchoalveolar fibrinolysis

precedes the clinical occurrence of pneumonia. In this study, PAI-1 levels decreased before the clinical diagnosis of pneumonia was made.

DOES DISTURBED FIBRIN TURNOVER IN PNEUMONIA INFLUENCE HOST DEFENSE? Although fibrin formation accompanies pneumonia, the importance of local coagulopathy in host defense during pneumonia is not known. Accumulation of fibrin may upregulate local inflammation during respiratory tract infections. In this way fibrin formation may play a positive role in pulmonary host defense.

As yet, studies on the role of activation of coagulation in the pathogenesis of pneumonia are lacking and studies on the role of inhibition of fibrinolysis in the pathogenesis of pneumonia are sparse. However, u-PA and the u-PA receptor play an essential role in experimental murine pneumococcal pneumonia. U-PA receptor deficiency was associated with reduced PMN-recruitment, enhanced bacterial outgrowth, extensive dissemination of infection, and reduced survival. In contrast, u-PA deficient mice showed enhanced host defense in this model, associated with more PMN-influx and less outgrowth of bacteria. These results suggest that the function of u-PA receptor in the response to infection is particularly pronounced when this receptor is unoccupied by u-PA. That these mechanisms are independent of fibrinolytic activity is illustrated by similar experiments in plasminogen or PAI-1 deficient mice that showed no effect on the immune response to infection.

The relationship between inflammation and coagulation is a two-way interaction: activation of coagulation (and inhibition of fibrinolysis) is, at least in part, under the control of TNF and IL-6. However, activation of coagulation can also importantly modulate inflammatory activation. In this context, therapy aimed at normalization of local abnormalities in coagulation and fibrinolysis may have a detrimental influence on pulmonary host defense.

Future studies are necessary to draw firm conclusions on whether modulation of the local fibrin formation during respiratory tract infections has beneficial effects on morbidity and mortality.

TARGETING THE COMPLEMENT CASCADE IN PNEUMONIA

The complement cascade is another important part of the immune system; it plays a significant role in the elimination of invading pathogens. Patients and animals deficient in complement system components are more susceptible to bacterial infections, and have increased morbidity and mortality on bacterial challenge. Three separate pathways can activate complement: (1) the "classic" pathway, in which activation occurs when antibody/antigen complexes interact with the first complement component (C1), (2) the "alternative" pathway, an antibody-independent, self-amplifying pathway that can be activated by a variety of mechanisms (e.g., biomaterials, yeast cell walls, tissue type-PA), and (3) the "lectin" pathway, also an antibody-independent pathway, which is activated by binding of mannose-binding lectin to carbohydrate structures on the surface of bacteria, yeast, protozoa, and viruses (Fig. 94-2). The three previously described pathways merge at C3, which is cleaved into C3a and C3b. C3b stimulates cleavage of C5 into C5a and C5b, and the addition of C6, C7, C8, and multiple C9 units results in the formation of C5b-9, also known as the "membrane-attack complex." Apart from the formation of this important membrane-attack complex, important for killing invasive pathogens, several side-products are produced on complement activation (e.g., C3a, C5a), all with proinflammatory properties.

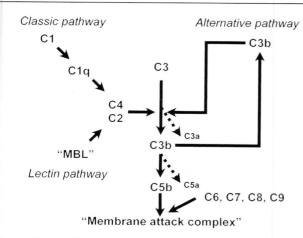

Classic pathway   *Alternative pathway*

Lectin pathway

"Membrane attack complex"

Figure 94-2 Schematic presentation of complement pathways. Three pathways of complement activation ("classic," "alternative," and "lectin") merge at complement component C3, eventually leading to the formation of the important "membrane-attack complex." Important side-products are C3a and C3b. Mannose-binding lectin, MBL. (Adapted and modified with permission from ref. Bhole D, Stahl GL. Therapeutic potential of targeting the complement cascade in critical care medicine. Crit Care Med 2003;31:S97–S104.)

C3a and C5a primarily act on white blood cells; although C3a mostly interacts with eosinophils, C5a interacts with PMNs. C5a attracts PMNs, increases PMN adherence to the endothelium, and stimulates the production/release of reactive oxygen species, granule content, and leukotrienes. Furthermore, C5a induces the production of cytokines and chemokines.

ACTIVATION OF THE COMPLEMENT SYSTEM DURING SEPSIS AND PNEUMONIA   Activation of complement, mainly via the classic pathway, is clearly involved in the pathogenesis of sepsis. Indeed, increased plasma levels of activated complement components have been found after injection of LPS in animals and in septic patients. It is speculated that overzealous activation of the complement system is responsible for morbidity and mortality during sepsis, and several animal studies support this hypothesis. Activation of the complement system has also been described in patients with acute lung injury or pneumonia; in a study on trauma patients, in patients developing ARDS significantly higher C3 concentrations and a higher C3a/C3 ratio were found in the first few hours after multiple trauma. Follow-up BALF demonstrated strongly increased C3a levels during the first 24 h, mainly in ARDS patients and, to a lesser degree, in non-ARDS patients. In a study of neutropenic febrile patients, activated complement components were measured in BALF, revealing higher C3a and C5a levels in patients who developed pneumonia. Similar results have been shown in mechanically ventilated patients developing pneumonia. In this study, in patients with pneumonia, BALF levels of C3a were higher as compared with patients not developing pneumonia. Moreover, local levels of C3a rose toward the diagnosis of pneumonia.

TARGETING THE COMPLEMENT SYSTEM   There is evidence that therapeutic targeting of the complement cascade may be of value in the treatment of patients with pulmonary diseases. In an aspiration model in rats, complement inhibition by recombinant human soluble complement receptor type 1 or complement depletion by *cobra venom* factor, significantly reduced lung edema, protein accumulation in BALF, and improved tissue oxygenation.

Similar results were found in mice. In addition, in a study on septic primates, anti-C5a antibody treatment not only attenuated some of the systemic manifestations of sepsis but also ARDS.

C5a receptor deficient mice, in comparison to control mice, were unable to clear intrapulmonary-instilled *P. aeruginosa*, despite a marked increase in neutrophil influx, and died because of pneumonia. These C5a-receptor-deficient mice challenged with sublethal inocula of *Pseudomonas* become super-infected with secondary bacterial strains. Targeting the complement cascade is an interesting approach that needs attention in the near future.

CONCLUSION

Immunotherapy, aimed at modulating the immune response, may serve as an important adjuvant to antibiotic therapy in the treatment of infectious diseases. Immunomodulating therapy for patients with pneumonia must be approached with caution because underlying cellular and molecular mechanisms of pneumonia are not fully understood. This chapter discussed several components of pulmonary host defense. Thus far, only G-CSF has reached the status of immunomodulating agent in clinical studies, and results were negative. Future studies are needed to show whether immunomodulation can be safely and successfully used in patients with pneumonia.

SELECTED REFERENCES

Alper CA, Abramson N, Johnston RB Jr, Jandl JH, Rosen FS. Increased susceptibility to infection associated with abnormalities of complement-mediated functions and of the third component of complement (C3). N Engl J Med 1970;282:350–354.

Amura CR, Fontan PA, Sanjuan N, et al. Tumor necrosis factor alpha plus interleukin 1 beta treatment protects granulocytopenic mice from *Pseudomonas aeruginosa* lung infection: role of an unusual inflammatory response. APMIS 1995;103:447–459.

Amura CR, Fontan PA, Sanjuan N, Sordelli DO. The effect of treatment with interleukin-1 and tumor necrosis factor on *Pseudomonas aeruginosa* lung infection in a granulocytopenic mouse model. Clin Immunol Immunopathol 1994;73:261–266.

Bengtson A, Lannsjo W, Heideman M. Complement and anaphylatoxin responses to cross-clamping of the aorta. Studies during general anaesthesia with or without extradural blockade. Br J Anaesth 1987;59:1093–1097.

Beutler B. TNF, immunity and inflammatory disease: lessons of the past decade. J Investig Med 1995;43:227–235.

Bhole D, Stahl GL. Therapeutic potential of targeting the complement cascade in critical care medicine. Crit Care Med 2003;31:S97–S104.

Boehm U, Klamp T, Groot M, Howard JC. Cellular responses to interferon-gamma. Annu Rev Immunol 1997;15:749–795.

Boutten A, Dehoux MS, Seta N, et al. Compartmentalized IL-8 and elastase release within the human lung in unilateral pneumonia. Am J Respir Crit Care Med 1996;153:336–342.

Brieland JK, Remick DG, Freeman PT, et al. In vivo regulation of replicative *Legionella pneumophila* lung infection by endogenous tumor necrosis factor alpha and nitric oxide. Infect Immun 1995;63:3253–3258.

Broaddus VC, Hebert CA, Vitangcol RV, et al. Interleukin-8 is a major neutrophil chemotactic factor in pleural liquid of patients with empyema. Am Rev Respir Dis 1992;146:825–830.

Broug-Holub E, Kraal G. In vivo study on the immunomodulating effects of OM-85 BV on survival, inflammatory cell recruitment and bacterial clearance in Klebsiella pneumonia. Int J Immunopharmacol 1997;19:559–564.

Chapman HA Jr, Bertozzi P, Reilly JJ Jr. Role of enzymes mediating thrombosis and thrombolysis in lung disease. Chest 1988;93:1256–1263.

Chapman HA Jr, Stone OL. A fibrinolytic inhibitor of human alveolar macrophages. Induction with endotoxin. Am Rev Respir Dis 1985;132:569–575.

Cox G, Crossley J, Xing Z. Macrophage engulfment of apoptotic neutrophils contributes to the resolution of acute pulmonary inflammation in vivo. Am J Respir Cell Mol Biol 1995;12:232–237.

Cox G. IL-10 enhances resolution of pulmonary inflammation in vivo by promoting apoptosis of neutrophils. Am J Physiol 1996;271:L566–L571.

Czermak BJ, Sarma V, Pierson CL, et al. Protective effects of C5a blockade in sepsis. Nat Med 1999;5:788–792.

Dale DC, Liles WC, Summer WR, Nelson S. Review: granulocyte colony-stimulating factor—role and relationships in infectious diseases. J Infect Dis 1995;172:1061–1075.

Dehoux MS, Boutten A, Ostinelli J, et al. Compartmentalized cytokine production within the human lung in unilateral pneumonia. Am J Respir Crit Care Med 1994;150:710–716.

Gosselin D, DeSanctis J, Boule M, et al. Role of tumor necrosis factor alpha in innate resistance to mouse pulmonary infection with Pseudomonas aeruginosa. Infect Immun 1995;63:3272–3278.

Greenberger MJ, Kunkel SL, Strieter RM, et al. IL-12 gene therapy protects mice in lethal Klebsiella pneumonia. J Immunol 1996;157:3006–3012.

Greenberger MJ, Strieter RM, Kunkel SL, et al. Neutralization of IL-10 increases survival in a murine model of Klebsiella pneumonia. J Immunol 1995;155:722–729.

Greenberger MJ, Strieter RM, Kunkel SL, et al. Neutralization of macrophage inflammatory protein-2 attenuates neutrophil recruitment and bacterial clearance in murine Klebsiella pneumonia. J Infect Dis 1996;173:159–165.

Gruson D, Hilbert G, Vargas F, et al. Impact of colony-stimulating factor therapy on clinical outcome and frequency rate of nosocomial infections in intensive care unit neutropenic patients. Crit Care Med 2000;28:3155–3160.

Gunther A, Mosavi P, Heinemann S, et al. Alveolar fibrin formation caused by enhanced procoagulant and depressed fibrinolytic capacities in severe pneumonia. Comparison with the acute respiratory distress syndrome. Am J Respir Crit Care Med 2000;161:454–462.

Harmsen AG. Role of alveolar macrophages in lipopolysaccharide-induced neutrophil accumulation. Infect Immun. 1988;56:1858–1863.

Hashimoto S, Pittet JF, Hong K, et al. Depletion of alveolar macrophages decreases neutrophil chemotaxis to Pseudomonas airspace infections. Am J Physiol 1996;270:L819–L828.

Haslett C. Granulocyte apoptosis and its role in the resolution and control of lung inflammation. Am J Respir Crit Care Med 1999;160:S5–S11.

Hebert JC, O'Reilly M, Gamelli RL. Protective effect of recombinant human granulocyte colony-stimulating factor against pneumococcal infections in splenectomized mice. Arch Surg 1990;125:1075–1078.

Heideman M, Norder-Hansson B, Bengtson A, Mollnes TE. Terminal complement complexes and anaphylatoxins in septic and ischemic patients. Arch Surg 1988;123:188–192.

Hickman-Davis JM, Michalek SM, Gibbs-Erwin J, Lindsey JR. Depletion of alveolar macrophages exacerbates respiratory mycoplasmosis in mycoplasma-resistant C57BL mice but not mycoplasma-susceptible C3H mice. Infect Immun 1997;65:2278–2282.

Hopken UE, Lu B, Gerard NP, Gerard C. The C5a chemoattractant receptor mediates mucosal defence to infection. Nature 1996;383:86–89.

Huber-Lang M, Sarma VJ, Lu KT, et al. Role of C5a in multiorgan failure during sepsis. J Immunol 2001;166:1193–1199.

Huber-Lang MS, Sarma JV, McGuire SR, et al. Protective effects of anti-C5a peptide antibodies in experimental sepsis. FASEB J 2001;15:568–570.

Huffnagle GB, Toews GB, Burdick MD, et al. Afferent phase production of TNF-alpha is required for the development of protective T cell immunity to Cryptococcus neoformans. J Immunol 1996;157:4529–4536.

Hussain N, Wu F, Zhu L, Thrall RS, Kresch MJ. Neutrophil apoptosis during the development and resolution of oleic acid-induced acute lung injury in the rat. Am J Respir Cell Mol Biol 1998;19:867–874.

Idell S. Endothelium and disordered fibrin turnover in the injured lung: Newly recognized pathways. Crit Care Med 2002;30:S274–S280.

Kiehl MG, Ostermann H, Thomas M, Birkfellner T, Kienast J. Inflammatory mediators in BAL fluid as markers of evolving pneumonia in leukocytopenic patients. Chest 1997;112:1214–1220.

Kilgore KS, Park JL, Tanhehco EJ, et al. Attenuation of interleukin-8 expression in C6-deficient rabbits after myocardial ischemia/reperfusion. J Mol Cell Cardiol 1998;30:75–85.

Knapp S, Leemans JC, Florquin S, et al. Alveolar macrophages have a protective antiinflammatory role during murine pneumococcal pneumonia. Am J Respir Crit Care Med 2003;167:171–179.

Kolls JK, Lei D, Nelson S, et al. Adenovirus-mediated blockade of tumor necrosis factor in mice protects against endotoxic shock yet impairs pulmonary host defense. J Infect Dis 1995;171:570–575.

Kolls JK, Lei D, Nelson S, Summer WR, Shellito JE. Pulmonary cytokine gene therapy. Adenoviral-mediated murine interferon gene transfer compartmentally activates alveolar macrophages and enhances bacterial clearance. Chest 1997;111:104S.

Kolls JK, Lei D, Stoltz D, et al. Adenoviral-mediated interferon-gamma gene therapy augments pulmonary host defense of ethanol-treated rats. Alcohol Clin Exp Res 1998;22:157–162.

Kooguchi K, Hashimoto S, Kobayashi A, et al. Role of alveolar macrophages in initiation and regulation of inflammation in Pseudomonas aeruginosa pneumonia. Infect Immun 1998;66:3164–3169.

Kyriakides C, Wang Y, Austen WG Jr, et al. Sialyl Lewis(x) hybridized complement receptor type 1 moderates acid aspiration injury. Am J Physiol Lung Cell Mol Physiol 2001;281:L1494–L1499.

Laichalk LL, Danforth JM, Standiford TJ. Interleukin-10 inhibits neutrophil phagocytic and bactericidal activity. FEMS Immunol Med Microbiol 1996;15:181–187.

Laichalk LL, Kunkel SL, Strieter RM, et al. Tumor necrosis factor mediates lung antibacterial host defense in murine Klebsiella pneumonia. Infect Immun 1996;64:5211–5218.

Lauw F, Branger J, Florquin S, et al. IL-18 improves the early antimicrobial host response to pneumococcal pneumonia. J Immunol 2002;168:372–378.

Le J, Vilcek J. Tumor necrosis factor and interleukin 1: cytokines with multiple overlapping biological activities. Lab Invest 1987;56:234–248.

Levi M, Schultz MJ, Rijneveld AW, van der Poll T. Bronchoalveolar coagulation and fibrinolysis in endotoxemia and pneumonia. Crit Care Med 2003;31:S238–S242.

Levi M, van der Poll T, ten Cate H, et al. Differential effects of anticytokine treatment on bronchoalveolar hemostasis in endotoxemic chimpanzees. Am J Respir Crit Care Med 1998;158:92–98.

Marshall BC, Sageser DS, Rao NV, Emi M, Hoidal JR. Alveolar epithelial cell plasminogen activator. Characterization and regulation. J Biol Chem 1990;265:8198–8204.

Mohr M, Hopken U, Oppermann M, et al. Effects of anti-C5a monoclonal antibodies on oxygen use in a porcine model of severe sepsis. Eur J Clin Invest 1998;28:227–234.

Moore TA, Newstead MW, Strieter RM, et al. Bacterial clearance and survival are dependent on CXC chemokine receptor-2 ligands in a murine model of pulmonary Nocardia asteroides infection. J Immunol 2000;164:908–915.

Murray HW. Interferon-gamma, the activated macrophage, and host defense against microbial challenge. Ann Intern Med 1988;595–608.

Nelson S, Belknap SM, Carlson RW, et al. A randomized controlled trial of filgrastim as an adjunct to antibiotics for treatment of hospitalized patients with community-acquired pneumonia. CAP Study Group. J Infect Dis 1998;178:1075–1080.

Nelson S, Heyder AM, Stone J, et al. A randomized controlled trial of filgrastim for the treatment of hospitalized patients with multilobar pneumonia. J Infect Dis 2000;182:970–973.

Nelson S. Novel nonantibiotic therapies for pneumonia: Cytokines and host defense. Chest 2001;119:419S–425S.

Obertacke U, Joka T, Zilow G, Kirschfink M, Schmit-Neuerburg KP. The role of C3a in pulmonary alveoli following trauma. Prog Clin Biol Res 1989;308:43–49.

Oswald IP, Wynn TA, Sher A, James SL. Interleukin 10 inhibits macrophage microbicidal activity by blocking the endogenous production of tumor necrosis factor alpha required as a costimulatory factor for interferon gamma-induced activation. Proc Natl Acad Sci USA 1992;89:8676–8680.

Rabinovici R, Neville LF, Abdullah F, et al. Aspiration-induced lung injury: Role of complement. Crit Care Med 1995;23:1405–1411.

Ralph P, Nakoinz I, Sampson-Johannes A, et al. IL-10, T lymphocyte inhibitor of human blood cell production of IL-1 and tumor necrosis factor. J Immunol 1992;148:808–814.

Ren Y, Savill J. Proinflammatory cytokines potentiate thrombospondin-mediated phagocytosis of neutrophils undergoing apoptosis. J Immunol 1995;154:2366–2374.

Rijneveld AW, Florquin S, Branger J, et al. TNF-alpha compensates for the impaired host defense of IL-1 type I receptor-deficient mice during pneumococcal pneumonia. J Immunol 2001;167:5240–5246.

Rijneveld AW, Florquin S, Bresser P, et al. Plasminogen activator inhibitor type-1 deficiency does not influence the outcome of murine pneumococcal pneumonia. Blood 2003;102(3):934–939.

Rijneveld AW, Lauw FN, Schultz MJ, et al. The role of interferon-gamma in murine pneumococcal pneumonia. J Infect Dis 2002;185:91–97.

Rijneveld AW, Levi M, Florquin S, et al. Urokinase receptor is necessary for adequate host defense against pneumococcal pneumonia. J Immunol 2002;168:3507–3511.

Rodriguez JL, Miller CG, DeForge LE, et al. Local production of interleukin-8 is associated with nosocomial pneumonia. J Trauma 1992;33:74–81.

Root RK, Lodato RF, Patrick W, et al. Multicenter, double-blind, placebo-controlled study of the use of filgrastim in patients hospitalized with pneumonia and severe sepsis. Crit Care Med 2003;31:367–373.

Rubins JB, Pomeroy C. Role of gamma interferon in the pathogenesis of bacteremic pneumococcal pneumonia. Infect Immun 1997;65:2975–2977.

Saadi S, Holzknecht RA, Patte CP, Platt JL. Endothelial cell activation by pore-forming structures: pivotal role for interleukin-1alpha. Circulation 2000;101:1867–1873.

Sacks T, Moldow CF, Craddock PR, Bowers TK, Jacob HS. Oxygen radicals mediate endothelial cell damage by complement-stimulated granulocytes. An in vitro model of immune vascular damage. J Clin Invest 1978;61:1161–1167.

Sawa T, Corry DB, Gropper MA, et al. IL-10 improves lung injury and survival in Pseudomonas aeruginosa pneumonia. J Immunol 1997;159:2858–2866.

Schultz MJ, Levi M, van der Poll T. Anticoagulant therapy for acute lung injury or pneumonia. Curr Drug Targets 2003;4:315–321.

Schultz MJ, Rijneveld AW, Speelman P, Deventer SJ, van der Poll T. Endogenous interferon-gamma impairs bacterial clearance from lungs during Pseudomonas aeruginosa pneumonia. Eur Cytokine Netw 2001;12:39–44.

Schultz MJ, Wijnholds J, Peppelenbosch MP, et al. Mice lacking the multidrug resistance protein 1 are resistant to Streptococcus pneumoniae-induced pneumonia. J Immunol 2001;166:4059–4064.

Schultz M, Millo J, Levi M, et al. Local activation of coagulation and inhibition of fibrinolysis in the lung during ventilator-associated pneumonia. San Diego: Interscience Conference on Antimicrobial Agents and Chemotherapy, 2002.

Schultz MJ, Rijneveld AW, Florquin S, et al. Role of interleukin-1 in the pulmonary immune response during Pseudomonas aeruginosa pneumonia. Am J Physiol Lung Cell Mol Physiol 2002;282:L285–L290.

Schultz MJ, Knapp S, Florquin S, et al. Interleukin-18 impairs the pulmonary host response to Pseudomonas aeruginosa. Infect Immun 2003;71:1630–1634.

Skerrett SJ, Martin TR, Chi EY, et al. Role of the type 1 TNF receptor in lung inflammation after inhalation of endotoxin or Pseudomonas aeruginosa. Am J Physiol 1999;276:L715–L727.

Smedegard G, Cui LX, Hugli TE. Endotoxin-induced shock in the rat. A role for C5a. Am J Pathol 1989;135:489–497.

Standiford TJ, Wilkowski JM, Sisson TH, et al. Intrapulmonary tumor necrosis factor gene therapy increases bacterial clearance and survival in murine gram-negative pneumonia. Hum Gene Ther 1999;10:899–909.

Stevens JH, O'Hanley P, Shapiro JM, et al. Effects of anti-C5a antibodies on the adult respiratory distress syndrome in septic primates. J Clin Invest. 1986;77:1812–1816.

Takashima K, Tateda K, Matsumoto T, et al. Role of tumor necrosis factor alpha in pathogenesis of pneumococcal pneumonia in mice. Infect Immun. 1997;65:257–260.

Tan AM, Ferrante A, Goh DH, Roberton DM, Cripps AW. Activation of the neutrophil bactericidal activity for nontypable Haemophilus influenzae by tumor necrosis factor and lymphotoxin. Pediatr Res 1995;37:155–159.

Tazi A, Nioche S, Chastre J, Smiejan JM, Hance AJ. Spontaneous release of granulocyte colony-stimulating factor (G-CSF) by alveolar macrophages in the course of bacterial pneumonia and sarcoidosis: endotoxin-dependent and endotoxin-independent G-CSF release by cells recovered by bronchoalveolar lavage. Am J Respir Cell Mol Biol 1991;4:140–147.

Tonnesen MG, Anderson DC, Springer TA, et al. Adherence of neutrophils to cultured human microvascular endothelial cells. Stimulation by chemotactic peptides and lipid mediators and dependence upon the Mac-1, LFA-1, p150,95 glycoprotein family. J Clin Invest 1989;83:637–646.

Tsai WC, Strieter RM, Mehrad B, et al. CXC chemokine receptor CXCR2 is essential for protective innate host response in murine Pseudomonas aeruginosa pneumonia. Infect Immun 2000;68:4289–4296.

Tsai WC, Strieter RM, Wilkowski JM, et al. Lung-specific transgenic expression of KC enhances resistance to Klebsiella pneumoniae in mice. J Immunol 1998;161:2435–2440.

Tsai WC, Strieter RM, Zisman DA, et al. Nitric oxide is required for effective innate immunity against Klebsiella pneumoniae. Infect Immun 1997;65:1870–1875.

van der Poll T, Keogh CV, Buurman WA, Lowry SF. Passive immunization against tumor necrosis factor-alpha impairs host defense during pneumococcal pneumonia in mice. Am J Respir Crit Care Med 1997;155:603–608.

van der Poll T, Marchant A, Keogh CV, Goldman M, Lowry SF. Interleukin-10 impairs host defense in murine pneumococcal pneumonia. J Infect Dis 1996;174:994–1000.

van der Poll T, Keogh CV, Guirao X, et al. Interleukin-6 gene-deficient mice show impaired defense against pneumococcal pneumonia. J Infect Dis 1997;176:439–444.

Wessels MR, Butko P, Ma M, et al. Studies of group B streptococcal infection in mice deficient in complement component C3 or C4 demonstrate an essential role for complement in both innate and acquired immunity. Proc Natl Acad Sci USA 1995;92:11,490–11,494.

Wunderink R, Leeper K Jr, Schein R, et al. Filgrastim in patients with pneumonia and severe sepsis or septic shock. Chest 2001;119:523–529.

Ye P, Rodriguez FH, Kanaly S, et al. Requirement of interleukin 17 receptor signaling for lung CXC chemokine and granulocyte colony-stimulating factor expression, neutrophil recruitment, and host defense. J Exp Med 2001;194:519–527.

Zilow G, Joka T, Obertacke U, Rother U, Kirschfink M. Generation of anaphylatoxin C3a in plasma and bronchoalveolar lavage fluid in trauma patients at risk for the adult respiratory distress syndrome. Crit Care Med 1992;20:468–473.

Zisman DA, Strieter RM, Kunkel SL, et al. Ethanol feeding impairs innate immunity and alters the expression of Th1- and Th2-phenotype cytokines in murine Klebsiella pneumonia. Alcohol Clin Exp Res 1998;22:621–627.

95 Molecular Pathogenesis of Fungal Infections

Brahm H. Segal

SUMMARY

Opportunistic fungal infections are a major cause of morbidity and mortality in the immunocompromised. Fungi have evolved complex and coordinated mechanisms to survive in the environment and the mammalian host. These include the ability to adhere to and colonize a variety of sites (e.g., skin, gastrointestinal mucosa, and intravenous catheters), invade tissue, establish localized disease, and disseminate. Fungi must adapt to "stressors" in the host, including nutrient acquisition, pH, and reactive oxygen and nitrogen intermediates. Knowledge of the immunopathogenesis of fungal infections has paved the way to promising preclinical studies and clinical trials of immunotherapy. The availability of genomic databases for key fungal pathogens will shed light on fungal pathogenesis and response to stressors both from host defense pathways and antifungal drugs, and will identify promising targets for drug development.

Key Words: Antifungal agents; *Aspergillus*; *Candida*; *Cryptococcus*; dimorphic fungi; drug development; genomics; vaccine; virulence factors.

FUNGAL INFECTIONS

Opportunistic fungal infections are a major cause of morbidity and mortality in immunocompromised patients. McNeil et al. evaluated trends in mortality because of invasive mycosis in the United States between 1980 and 1997 based on an analysis of death certificates. During the study period the annual number of deaths associated with an invasive mycosis increased from 1557 to 6534. In patients with AIDS, *Pneumocystis jiroveci* (formerly *P. carinii,* more appropriately classified as a fungus than a protozoan based on genetic similarity) and *Cryptococcus neoformans* accounted for the majority of opportunistic mycoses associated with mortality. Even before the availability of protease inhibitors targeted against HIV, there was a decrease in mortality from opportunistic mycoses associated with HIV infection; this may be related to the availability of early antiretroviral regimens with modest efficacy and antimicrobial prophylaxis. Among those without HIV infection, there has been a dramatic increase in mortality due invasive aspergillosis and "other mycoses," presumably related to the increase in patients receiving potent immunosuppressive therapy for malignancy and transplantation.

From: *Principles of Molecular Medicine, Second Edition*
Edited by: M. S. Runge and C. Patterson © Humana Press, Inc., Totowa, NJ

Opportunistic yeasts produce a spectrum of clinical disease that ranges from superficial and mucosal infections to disseminated disease. Oral mucosal candidiasis usually reflects severe T-cell depression commonly associated with AIDS or high-dose systemic corticosteroids. *Candida* spp. are endogenous flora that may gain access to the bloodstream through breaches in anatomical barriers. The bowel is the principal portal of entry in patients with acute leukemia receiving mucotoxic regimens.

Host defense against *C. neoformans* is also principally dependent on T-cell immunity. Immunoglobulins directed against capsular epitopes and complement facilitate phagocytosis of the organism, and play a role in host defense. The principal portal of entry for *C. neoformans* is by inhalation, with subsequent spread to the blood and central nervous system.

Endemic dimorphic fungi are so named because of their characteristic geographic distribution. These organisms include *Histoplasma capsulatum, Coccidioides immitis, Blastomyces dermatitidis, Paracoccidioides brasiliensis,* and *Penicillium marneffei.* Dimorphic refers to their existence in nature in the fruiting mycelial stage and conversion to the yeast stage at body temperature. Because some of these pathogens may be quiescent during the initial infection and only manifest clinically during depression of cell-mediated immunity, a detailed travel history is essential.

Filamentous fungi (molds) are ubiquitous soil inhabitants whose conidia (spores) we inhale on a regular basis. The sinopulmonary tract is the most common portal of entry. The respiratory mucosa and alveolar macrophages constitute the first line of host defense against conidia. At the hyphal stage, circulating neutrophils are most important in controlling infection. *Aspergillus* infection and other filamentous fungi are a major cause of morbidity and mortality in highly immunocompromised patients. Patients at risk include those with prolonged neutropenia, hematopoietic stem cell transplant (HSCT) recipients (mostly allogeneic), solid organ transplant recipients (particularly lung), advanced AIDS, and chronic granulomatous disease (CGD).

Most filamentous fungal infections are caused by *Aspergillus* spp. Prolonged and persistent neutropenia is a critical risk factor for aspergillosis. Invasive aspergillosis has become the leading cause of infection-related mortality in allogeneic HSCT recipients, with most cases occurring in the postengraftment rather than the neutropenic period, with immunosuppressive therapy for GVHD being a principal risk factor.

Zygomycosis is also being observed with increased frequency in patients with hematological malignancies and allogeneic HSCT at some centers in association with use of voriconazole, an agent with a broad spectrum of antifungal activity but poor activity against zygomycetes. Infections by less common pathogenic fungi including dark-walled moulds, *Scedosporium* species, and *Fusarium* species have increased over the past 20 yr among patients with hematological malignancies and allogeneic HSCT recipients.

This chapter will focus on the major mechanisms of virulence in pathogenic fungi. Because of the key importance of host defense against opportunistic fungi, host–pathogen interactions will be discussed and related to novel strategies aimed at immune augmentation, including vaccine development. Recent developments in the antifungal armamentarium and new opportunities for drug discovery created by a greater understanding of the molecular pathogenesis of fungal infections and genomics will be discussed.

FUNGAL VIRULENCE FACTORS IN RELATION TO HOST DEFENSE

Both the pathogen and the host contribute to microbial pathogenesis. Nowhere else is this more true than in mycology. Thus, a "virulence factor" or a "virulence gene" occurs in the context of the specific host. All of the major opportunistic fungal pathogens are associated with a broad range of virulence factors, which enable the pathogen to adhere to the host cell or foreign body surfaces (such as *Candida* biofilms adhering to intravenous catheters), invade, damage tissue, and disseminate. Virulence factors enable the pathogen to survive within a hostile host environment and specific host conditions including body temperature (37°C), pH within the tissue, nutrient deficiency, reactive oxidants, and numerous nonoxidant-dependent host defense pathways (e.g., defensins, cathepsins, elastases, and other neutrophil granule constituent proteins). Fungal genes that mediate resistance to antifungal agents are also legitimately classified as "virulence factors" in the specific context of exposure to the relevant drug.

Falkow proposed the following criteria for Koch's molecular postulates:

1. The phenotype or property under investigation should be associated with pathogenic members of a genus or species.
2. Specific inactivation of the gene or genes associated with the suspected virulence trait should lead to a measurable loss in pathogenicity or virulence.
3. Reversion or allelic replacement of the mutated gene should lead to restoration of pathogenicity.

The second and third criteria are routinely evaluated by generating "knockout" and "knockin" strains in which the relevant gene is inactivated or restored, respectively.

Most opportunistic fungi grow in the environment independent of an animal host. Casadevall et al. used the term, "dual use" virulence factors to describe certain virulence factors that confer a survival advantage both in the environment and in animals. In *C. neoformans*, virulence in animals may have originated from factors that enabled persistence in amoeboid and nematode predators. For example, following ingestion by *Acanthamoeba castellani*, *C. neoformans* replicates and forms polysaccharide-containing vesicles in the cytoplasm, a process mirrored by the interaction between macrophages and ingested cryptococci.

Virulence genes require a context. For example, a wild-type strain of *Aspergillus fumigatus* and a strain with a deleted gene of interest will likely both be nonvirulent in normal mice challenged via the intratracheal route. However, if mice are first rendered neutropenic,

we may discover that the deletant strain is less virulent than the wild-type strain. Genes that permit *Candida* spp. to adhere to epithelial surfaces are a prerequisite for infection. In an immunocompetent person, this virulence factor may permit asymptomatic colonization of mucosal surfaces without clinical relevance. In healthy women, this virulence factor may be a requisite for vaginitis. In advanced AIDS, this virulence factor may be a requisite for disabling oral mucosal and esophageal candidiasis. In a patient receiving cytotoxic chemotherapy, this virulence factor may facilitate candidemia and disseminated candidiasis arising from defects in the gastrointestinal mucosa.

Host damage can result from microbial factors, host response, or both. Casadevall and Pirofski elegantly illustrated the limitations of the "microorganism-centered" and "host-centered" paradigms. They proposed the "damage-response" framework of microbial pathogenesis in which the host relevant outcome of the host–microorganism interaction is determined by the amount of damage to the host.

ADHESION

Adhesion is a prerequisite to colonization and invasion. Inhaled pathogens (e.g., filamentous fungi, dimorphic fungi, *C. neoformans*) generally establish infection by adhering to respiratory epithelium. *Candida* spp. colonize the gastrointestinal and vaginal tracts, the skin, and foreign bodies (e.g., catheters). Understanding the molecular biology of adherence is of key importance in development of drugs and immunotherapy aimed at inhibiting adhesion.

There is strong evidence for the importance of adherence in *Candida* virulence. There is a correlation between the degree of endothelial cell adherence and virulence of different *Candida* spp. Several adhesins of *C. albicans* have been characterized. Mutants deficient in genes encoding these adhesins showed decreased adherence to host cell substrates in vitro and decreased virulence in animal models. *Hwp1p* mediates adherence to buccal epithelial cells by acting as a substrate for transglutaminase. *EAP1* mediates adherence to polystyrene and renal epithelial cells. *CaMnt1p* mediates O-linked mannosylation of proteins and plays a role in *C. albicans* cells adhering to each other and to host epithelial cells. *CaMnt1p* null mutants had reduced virulence in systemic infection in mouse and guinea pigs. Reduced virulence of null mutants in guinea pigs was associated with decreased ability to reach and/or adhere to internal organs. *Csf4* is a putative glycosidase that plays a role in adherence and filamentation; a null mutant had attenuated virulence in disseminated candidiasis in mice.

The *C. albicans ALS* gene family consists of at least eight members that encode cell surface proteins characterized by three domains. The N-terminus contains a putative signal peptide, the central region consists of a variable number of tandem repeats, and the C-terminus is serine-threonine rich and contains a glycosylphosphatidylinositol anchor. The Als proteins have diverse substrate specificities for adherence that is conferred by the N-terminal domain. Sheppard et al. suggested an analogy between Als proteins and antibodies. The Als proteins contain hypervariable regions (similar conceptually to the hypervariable region of antibodies) that mediate substrate specificity. The genetic variability in the Als family enables binding to multiple proteins, which may in turn enable adherence to a broader range of anatomic surfaces during infection.

Als proteins may therefore be attractive targets for drug development and vaccine development aimed at inducing antibody responses that target key Als epitopes and inhibit adherence to host tissue. A vaccine made up of the recombinant N-terminus of *Als1p* reduced fungal burden and improved survival in experimental candidiasis in both immunocompetent and immunocompromised mice. The vaccine-mediated protection by enhancing cell mediated, but not humoral, immunity.

Candidemia is a major cause of nosocomial infection related morbidity and mortality. The two major portals of entry are breaches in the gastrointestinal tract (such as occurs following mucotoxic antineoplastic chemotherapy) and intravenous catheter-associated infections. *Candida* biofilms are *bona fide* virulence factors in the context of catheter-associated candidal infections. *Candida* biofilm production occurs through specific maturation phases and requires the generation of a polysaccharide extracellular matrix. Mature *Candida* biofilms have a heterogeneous architecture in terms of the relationship between fungal cells and matrix. Similar in concept to other biofilm-producing pathogens such as staphylococci, *Candida* biofilms facilitate pathogen adherence to foreign bodies such as catheters, leading to a persistent nidus of infection that may be refractory to antimicrobials. Biofilm formation is also important in the development of denture stomatitis.

Mukherjee et al. showed that *C. albicans* biofilms mediate resistance to fluconazole in vitro, and that resistance involves a complex interaction between azole efflux pumps and the maturity of the biofilm. At early time-points of biofilm production, wild-type *C. albicans* was resistant to fluconazole, but strains deficient in drug efflux pumps were resistant. At later time-points, all strains were resistant indicating that drug resistance was independent of the efflux pumps. Lipid formulations of amphotericin B and echinocandins retain antifungal activity even in the presence of mature biofilms; the clinical importance of this finding merits further study.

Blastomyces dermatiditis is an extracellular dimorphic fungus that can cause progressive pulmonary, soft tissue, and disseminated infection. BAD1 (formerly WI-1), a 120-kDa protein, is a major adhesin and immune modulator in *B. dermatiditis*. It contains tandem repeat sequences homologous to invasin, an adhesin of *Yesernia* species . BAD1 is released extracellularly before association with the yeast surface and mediates attachment to CD18 and CD14 receptors on human macrophages. Genetically engineered BAD1-deficient strains of *B. dermatitidis* bind poorly to the lung ex vivo and to macrophages in vitro, and have greatly diminished virulence following experimental infection in mice. BAD1 also modulates host immunity. Early in the course of infection, BAD1suppressed host tumor necrosis factor (TNF)-α production through transforming growth factor (TGF)-β-dependent and independent mechanisms. Deletion of the C-terminal epidermal growth factor (EGF)-like domain of BAD1 prevented localization of BAD1 to the yeast surface and impaired yeast adherence to macrophages. However, the deletant strain and the purified deletant protein suppressed TNF-α production in phagocytes and in the lung as effectively as BAD-1-reconstituted wild-type strains and retained virulence in experimental infection in mice. Thus, the requirements for adhesion and immune modulation by BAD1 occur in discreet domains.

MORPHOLOGICAL ADAPTATION

Morphogenesis and phenotypic switching allow opportunistic fungi to adapt to different environments and survive in the infected host. These changes in structure are under complex genetic control. The ability of *C. albicans* to transform from the yeast to the filamentous phenotype confers the ability to penetrate host tissue and escape phagocytosis by macrophages. Filamentation occurs in response to several stimuli, including elevated temperature, growth in serum, pH changes, and the presence of an extracellular matrix. Mutants in the hyphal-regulating transcriptional factors, *Efg1P* and *Cph1P*, are unable to grow in the filamentous form in serum and other media at 37°C, but can filament in matrix at lower temperatures. These mutants have attenuated virulence in systemic infection in mice.

Hyphal growth in *C. albicans* is influenced by the local topography, and may be important for mucosal invasion and growth along indwelling catheters. In artificial membranes, reorientation of the hyphal tip occurs in response to scratches and pores, referred to as "thigmotrophism." Thigmotrophism may require activation of stretch-sensitive calcium channels. *CZF1p*, a zinc finger protein, is important in mediating hyphal development when *C. albicans* is grown within matrix. During growth within matrix, *Efg1p* may inhibit filamentation, and *CZF1p* reverses this inhibition.

The dimorphic fungi exist in the yeast form at body temperature and in the filamentous form at lower temperatures. *C. immitis* is endemic in the Southwestern United States. The tissue form is the spherule. Arthroconidia are inhaled from the environment in which they convert into spherules. Spherules enlarge (20–100 μm) and segment internally into hundreds of endospores. Mature endospores rupture through the spherule in which they can extend the local infection or disseminate. The spherule prevents access of neutrophils to maturing endospores, and following rupture, endospores are themselves covered by a matrix from the inner spherule wall which may also aid in evading phagoctyosis. The potential for *C. immitis* to widely disseminate has prompted the search for extracellular fungal proteinases that may be targets for inhibitors or vaccines.

A randomized placebo-controlled study involving 2867 subjects from endemic regions showed no benefit of the formalin-killed spherule vaccine in preventing coccidioidomycosis. Additional candidate vaccines for coccidioidomycosis are being developed, with efforts focused on identifying immunodominant Coccidioides antigens to be used in subunit vaccines (Cox, Magee, 2004). Studies in multiple laboratories have shown that antigen 2/proline-rich antigen (Ag2/PRA) as both protein and DNA vaccines provide significant protection in experimental coccidioidomycosis. The completed and genomic sequence of *C. immitis* may facilitate identifying new candidate antigens for vaccine development.

C. neoformans is unique among the pathogenic fungi in having a polysaccharide capsule that is a major virulence factor that allows the pathogen to evade phagocytosis. Acapsular variants of *C. neoformans* have attenuated virulence. The *C. neoformans* capsule also interferes with dendritic cell (DC) activation and maturation, a mechanism by which the fungus may suppress an effective T-cell response. The capsule is made up of primarily of glucuronoxylomannan (GXM). GXM has an α-1,3 linked mannose backbone that is O-acetylated and substituted with single-side chains of xylose and glucouronic acid. The degree of acetylation and xylose substitution can vary, producing four serotypes. Serial isolates of *C. neoformans* from chronically infected patients show changes in virulence, karyotype, and capsular polysaccharide structure, suggesting that structural changes occur during chronic infection. "Phenotypic switching" (high frequency reversible changes in colony morphology) has been described in several strains of *C. neoformans*. For example, phenotypic switching in *C. neoformans* SB4 is associated with changes in colony morphology that

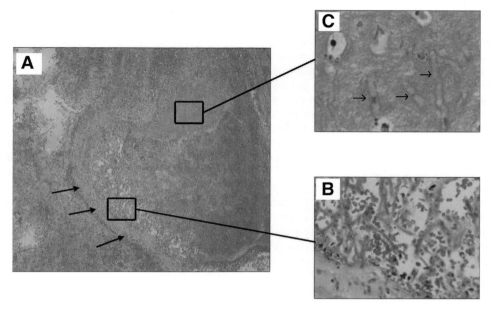

Figure 95-1   Invasive pulmonary aspergillosis in an allogeneic hematopoietic stem cell transplant recipient at autopsy. **(A)** Lower power view shows arterial thrombosis (Hematoxylin & Eosin, 40×). Arrows, vessel wall. **(B)** Higher power magnification shows hyphae invading the arterial wall (×200) and **(C)** invasive hyphae (arrows) within the thrombus (×400). (Reproduced with permission from Segal BH, Walsh TJ. Current approches to diagnosis and treatment of invasive aspergillosis. Am J Respir Crit Care Med. 2006; in press.)

included: (1) smooth, (2) wrinkled, and (3) serrated. The wrinkled phenotype was the most virulent in experimental infection. Infection of rats with serrated *C. neoformans* produced the most intense inflammatory responses characterized by granuloma formation and necrosis. Wrinkled *C. neoformans* produced a minimal inflammatory response. Thus, phenotypic switching affects *C. neoformans* virulence and the host inflammatory response, which may confer an advantage in establishing chronic infection and evading host defense. Antibodies directed against capsular epitopes confer protection in murine cryptococcal infection. Murine IgG1 (Mab 18B7) was well-tolerated in a Phase I dose-escalating trial in patients with cryptococcal meningitis.

ANGIOINVASION

Filamentous fungi have a propensity to angioinvasion in the highly immunocompromised host, leading to thrombosis, infarction, and coagulative necrosis (Fig. 95-1). Conidia are inhaled, germinate, and transform into the hyphal stage. In the susceptible host (e.g., severe neutropenia), hyphae (but not conidia) are capable of invading surrounding tissue and blood vessels. The molecular mechanisms underlying angioinvasion are poorly understood. Lopes Bezerra and Filler, showed that both *A. fumigatus* conidia and hyphae induced endothelial cell microfilament changes and subsequent endocytosis in vitro. Endocytosed conidia and hyphae caused endothelial cell injury, but only hyphae (either live or killed) activated endothelial cell tissue factor, a key mediator of thrombosis.

C. albicans stimulates multiple endothelial responses, including expression of leukocyte adhesion molecules and production of prostaglandins and proinflammatory cytokines. *C. albicans* hyphae are endocytosed by endothelial cells in vitro. Als1 mediates adherence to endothelial and epithelial cells. Sanchez et al. noted a relationship between *C. albicans* virulence in hematogenous infection in animals and endothelial damage in vitro. *C. albicans* did not stimulate endothelial cell tissue factor activity. The ability to

induce endothelial cell tissue factor activity may be why vascular thrombosis is characteristic of invasive aspergillosis but not invasive candidiasis. Interestingly, tissue invasive aspergillosis in CGD is not angioinvasive in contradistinction to neutropenia and other immunocompromised conditions in which angioinvasion occurs. Further studies aimed at defining pathogen/endothelial cell interactions at the molecular level will be important in designing therapeutic modalities aimed at preventing angioinvasion.

DAMAGE

PHOSPHOLIPASES   Most pathogenic fungi are saprophytes, living on decayed animal or plant material for nutrition. Extracellular degradative enzymes such as proteinases and phospholipases cause host cell damage. These enzymes break down epithelial mucosa and extracellular matrix, a requirement to establish infection, and likely increase the availability of host-derived nutrients. Because the vast majority of pathogenic fungi exist in the environment and are not dependent on an animal host for their life cycle, these degradative enzymes likely have a dual use purpose in the saprophytic setting.

Extracellular phospholipases are virulence factors in pathogenic fungi and have been implicated as virulence factors in pathogens including clostridia, *Pseudomonas aeruginosa*, *Rickettsia rickettsii* (agent of Rocky Mountain spotted fever), *Rickettsia prowazekii, Toxoplasma gondii, Entamoeba histolytica*, and *Listeria monocytogenes*. Fungal phospholipases enhance virulence through damage of host cell membranes. Other potential mechanisms of virulence include phospholipase-mediated signal transduction and augmentation of the host inflammatory response. There is precedent for these effects in bacteria and *E. histolytica*.

Birch et al. suggested that *A. fumigatus* produces extracellular phospholipases A, B, C, and D based on phospholipid degradation products. Phospholipase C (PLC) activity (assessed using p-nitrophenylphosphorylcholine as a substrate) was initially observed at

30 h after growth and increased during stationary phase. PLC activity was greater at 37°C than at lower temperatures. The authors noted the pathological similarities of necrotizing fasciitis and clostridial gangrene, ecthyma gangrenosum caused by *P. aeruginosa* and invasive aspergillosis regarding angioinvasion, infarction, and tissue necrosis. Because each of these pathogens produces extracellular PLC, the authors speculated that PLC may account for some of the pathological characteristics of invasive aspergillosis. Extracellular PLC activity was higher in clinical strains of *A. fumigatus* whereas phospholipid acyl hydrolase activity was higher in environmental strains, suggesting that specific phospholipases may influence host trophism.

Ibrahim et al. showed that *C. albicans* strains exhibiting increased phospholipase B (PLB) activity had greater virulence in experimental disseminated candidiasis in mice. Genetically engineered mutants of *PLB1* had diminished virulence in mice, and reintroduction of a functional *PLB1* gene into the null mutant restored virulence. PLB expression during *Candida* invasion of the gastrointestinal tract of infant mice was localized to the growing hyphal tips. PLB production is under complex regulatory control and is influenced by nutritional supplementation, pH, and growth phase.

PLB is also a pathogenic factor in *C. neoformans*, promoting survival and replication in macrophages in vitro. It likely contributes to cryptococcal virulence through lysis of host defense cells, and may help evade macrophage host defenses by increasing fungal eicosanoid production, leading to down-modulation of macrophage function. Using a *PLB1* null mutant and a *PLB1* reconstituted *C. neoformans* strain, Santangelo et al. showed that PLB was required for spread to draining lymph nodes and hematogenous dissemination following endotracheal challenge in mice. Secreted PLB in *C. neoformans* has three phospholipase activities in the one protein: PLB, lysophospholipase, and lysophospholipase transacylase. Only inhibitors of PLB had antifungal activity in vitro.

Phospholipases are promising therapeutic targets. Approaches include identification of inhibitors by chemical screening or by inhibitor design based on the tertiary structure of the protein. Hanel et al. identified phospholipase inhibitors with antifungal activity from the β-blocker category of drugs. These agents when combined with fluconazole were more effective than fluconazole alone in murine disseminated candidiasis. Vaccine development may exploit fungal antigens distinct from mammalian phospholipases. Because phospholipases are released during infection, their detection may facilitate early diagnosis of invasive fungal infection.

PROTEASES Many pathogenic fungi secrete proteases during infection, though the function of specific proteases in vivo is often difficult to determine. Secreted endoproteases (which cleave internal peptides within a polypeptide) consist of aspartic proteases of the pepsin family, serine proteases, and metalloproteases. Pathogenic fungi also secrete aminopeptidases, carboxypeptidases, and dipeptidylpeptidases. Secreted proteases play an important role in the pathogenicity of dermatophytes, which grow exclusively on keratinized tissue such as skin, nails, and hair. Proteases from dermato phytes are similar to those from other fungi such as *Aspergillus* species, but with different substrate specificities.

In *C. albicans*, secreted aspartyl proteinases (SAPs) are encoded by at least 10 genes and contribute to virulence. The *C. albicans* SAPs. Two distinct groups are clustered within the family. SAP1-SAP3 have 67% similarity and SAP4-SAP6 are 89% identical. Different SAP proteins mediate adherence and tissue damage and are differentially regulated under a variety of in vitro growth conditions. SAP4-SAP6 are upregulated after phagocytosis by murine macrophages and their respective null mutants are killed more efficiently following ingestion. Ripeau et al. showed that *C. albicans* SAPs were differentially expressed during oral infection in wild type and transgenic mice expressing HIV-1. Schofield et al. also detected differences in *SAP* and *PLB* gene expression in experimental oroesophageal vs gastric *C. albicans* infection.

Naglik et al. evaluated the in vivo expression of genes encoding the SAPs and PLB in 137 human subjects with oral or vaginal candidiasis or carriage. They demonstrated differential expression of these genes in active disease and by anatomic location. Because *Candida* spp. can infect multiple tissues (skin, endothelial cells, and visceral organs in hematogenous infection), a spectrum of proteolytic enzymes under differential regulation may facilitate entry into a greater repertoire of niches. The genome of *C. albicans* is sequenced and DNA microarrays have been generated. These will further increase our understanding of gene regulation in host cell interactions.

Protease inhibitors used to treat HIV infection also inhibit *Candida* SAPs. In addition to their salutary role in controlling HIV replication and enabling reconstitution of cellular immunity, protease inhibitors may also reduce the frequency of oral mucosal candidiasis through inhibition of SAPs. De Bernardis et al. longitudinally evaluated *Candida* isolates from the oral cavity of HIV-infected patients receiving antiretroviral therapy with and without protease inhibitors. Protease inhibitors reduced SAP expression in vivo, but did not eliminate *Candida* carriage or affect susceptibility to antifungal agents. More potent inhibitors of the *Candida* SAP enzymes may be more effective antifungals. SAPs may also be promising targets for vaccine development. Vilanova et al. showed that immunization of mice with SAP2 elicited immunoglobulin responses that correlated with protection following experimental systemic *C. albicans* infection.

A. fumigatus conidia are internalized in vitro by lung epithelial cells. Uptake into those nonprofessional phagocytes may facilitate evasion of host defense in the lung. *A. fumigatus* secretes a variety of proteases, including an alkaline serine protease, a metalloproteinase, an aspartic protease, and elastases. Their likely roles in mammalian infection are to degrade the extracellular matrix layer in the respiratory mucosa. Kogan et al. showed that *A. fumigatus* secretes proteases that perturb the organization of the actin cytoskeleton in A549 pneumocytes, leading to formation of actin aggregates, cell blebbing, and disruption of focal adhesion sites. These changes were blocked by antipain, a serine and cysteine protease inhibitor. Antipain also reduced *Aspergillus*-induced A549 cell death and detachment from matrix, suggesting an important role for *A. fumigatus* proteases in causing lung epithelial cell damage and breaching the epithelia barrier.

SURVIVAL UNDER STRESS

IRON ACQUISITION The ability of microbes to compete with their hosts to acquire iron is a major requirement for pathogenicity. Siderophores (low molecular weight ferric iron chelating agents) involved in iron acquisition under iron-limited conditions are virulence factors in a wide variety of plant and animal pathogens.

Ramanan and Wang identified two genes, *CaFTR1* and *CAFTR2*, that encode high affinity iron permeases in *C. albicans*. *CaFTR1* is induced under iron-limited conditions and repressed when iron supplies are adequate, whereas *CaFTR2* is regulated in the reverse.

CaFTR1, but not *CaFTR2*, is required for growth in iron-deficient medium. *CaFTR1* null mutants are unable to establish systemic infection in mice. Like many bacteria, *C. albicans* is able to use hemin and hemoglobin as iron sources. *RBT5* encodes a mannosylated protein induced under iron starvation that is necessary in using hemin and hemoglobin as iron stores. Iron-starvation inducible heme-binding proteins are conserved in other *Candida* spp. and in *S. cerevisiae*.

Addition of hemoglobin to *C. albicans* cultures increases adhesion to several host proteins. This activity is mediated by a cell surface hemoglobin receptor and is independent of iron acquisition. Hemoglobin induces the expression of several genes, including a heme oxygenase that facilitates acquisition of iron from heme and hemoglobin. Iron is also required for endothelial injury by *C. albicans* in vitro. The siderophore iron transporter of *C. albicans* (SIT1) mediates uptake of ferrichrome-type siderophores and is required for epithelial cell invasion in vitro, but was not required for systemic infection in mice. This suggests that different iron acquisition mechanisms exist during mucosal infection compared with hematogenous infection in which other sources of iron, such as heme, are available.

Iron acquisition pathways in filamentous fungi are less well defined at the molecular level than those in *Candida*. *A. fumigatus* survival in human serum requires siderophores that extract iron from transferrin. Five siderophores were purified from *A. fumigatus* culture medium, the two major ones were triacetylfusarinine and ferricrocin. Of the filamentous fungi, zygomycosis (also termed, "mucormycosis") is most frequently associated with iron overload states and deferoxamine (an iron chelator) therapy. Boelaert et al. showed that *Rhizopus* (a member of the zygomycetes) uses deferoxamine as a siderophore. The iron-deferoxamine complex abolishes the fungistatic effect of serum on *Rhizopus* and accelerates in vitro growth. The effect of the iron chelate complex on iron uptake and growth in vitro were far more impressive for *Rhizopus* than *A. fumigatus,* and close to nil in *C. albicans*. Deferoxamine also aggravated experimental *Rhizopus* infection in guinea pigs. Renal failure reduces clearance of the iron chelate, which may account for the increased frequency of zygomycosis in dialysis patients receiving deferoxamine.

MELANIN Melanins have attracted considerable interest as virulence factors in pathogenic fungi. They are widely produced by several pathogenic fungi, including *C. neoformans, Aspergillus* species, *Sporothrix schenckii*, and the dark-walled moulds. The majority of melanins produced by fungi are derived from the 1,8-dihydroxynaphthalene pathway. In *C. neoformans*, melanin is produced when laccase (laccases are copper containing proteins that require oxygen to oxidize phenols and other substrates) catalyzes the oxidation of certain aromatic compounds, including L-DOPA (a brain catecholamine), to quinones that then polymerize to melanin.

C. neoformans has provided an excellent model to understand the role of melanin in pathogenicity. Melanization has been associated with protection of *C. neoformans* against environmental stressors, including ultraviolet radiation, temperature extremes, oxygen and nitrogen free radicals, silver nitrate (a toxic heavy metal in the environment), and enzymatic degradation by predator microbes in the environment. The diverse protective effects of melanin likely have dual roles in facilitating survival of *C. neoformans* in the environment and in animals. Laccase, an essential enzyme for melanin synthesis in *C. neoformans*, is

tightly associated with the cell wall and accessible for interaction with host cells. Salas et al. showed that the laccase gene *CNLAC1* was an essential virulence factor in cryptococcal infection in mice.

Melanin may also have an anti-inflammatory role facilitating evasion of host defense. Synthetic melanin reduced the production of several proinflammatory cytokines (TNF-α, IL-1B, and IL-6) following stimulation of monocytes with endotoxin. By conferring protection against reactive oxidant and nitrogen species, it may enhance the ability of *C. neoformans* to survive within host phagocytes. Melanins may also reduce susceptibility of fungi to antifungal agents. Van Duin et al. showed that nonmelanized *C. neoformans* and *H. capsulatum* had increased susceptibility to amphotericin B and caspofungin. Fungal melanins bind to amphotericin B and caspofungin in vitro, which may attenuate their antifungal activity.

REACTIVE OXYGEN AND NITROGEN INTERMEDIATES
Host phagocytes produce reactive oxygen and nitrogen intermediates in response to infection. To survive in this milieu, mechanisms that scavenge or detoxify reactive intermediates are essential. Superoxide dismutases (enzymes that catalyze the conversion of superoxide to hydrogen peroxide) and catalases (enzymes that detoxify hydrogen peroxide) are produced by most bacteria and fungi. *C. albicans* possesses an inducible nitric oxide defense mechanism involving flavohemoglobin genes. Melanin may also scavenge reactive oxygen and nitrogen intermediates in *C. neoformans*.

Narasipura et al. showed that a strain of *C. neoformans* deficient in the Cu, Zn superoxide dismutase gene *(SOD1)* was more susceptible to neutrophil killing in vitro and had attenuated virulence in a mouse model. The *SOD1* null mutant was also deficient in laccase, urease, and phospholipase, raising the possibility that *SOD1* has a signaling role related to the expression of other virulence genes.

The essential role of reactive oxygen intermediates in host defense is illustrated in CGD, an inherited disorder of the NADPH oxidase characterized by recurrent life-threatening bacterial and fungal infections, almost all of which produce catalase. The importance of catalase in the CGD pathogens was posited to relate to the ability of catalase to scavenge the pathogen-produced hydrogen peroxide within the CGD phagolyosome. Activation of the NADPH oxidase in neutrophils leads to the release of cationic granule proteins into the phagolysozome, among which are elastase and cathepsin G that are bound to the anionic proteoglycan matrix in the inactivated state. Mice deficient in the cationic granule proteins (but with an intact NADPH oxidase) recapitulate the CGD phenotype in terms of susceptibility to bacterial and fungal infections. Activation of preformed granule proteases is likely to be one of the principal mechanisms of NADPH oxidase-mediated host defense. Catalase-deficient *Aspergillus nidulans* were just as virulent as the wild-type strain in experimental pulmonary infection in the p47$^{phox-/-}$ mouse model of CGD. This finding raises the possibility of redundant pathogen-derived reactive oxygen scavengers that may compensate for the lack of catalase.

Gliotoxin, a toxin produced by *A. fumigatus* and other fungi, has immunosuppressive properties that may facilitate evasion of host defense, including inhibition of the NADPH oxidase. It inhibits p47^{phox} phosphorylation and its subsequent translocation to the membrane-bound flavocytochrome, a key step in NADPH oxidase assembly and activation. Gliotoxin also inhibits ingestion of *A. fumigatus* by macrophages, inhibits cytotoxic T-lymphocyte cytotoxicity, induces apoptosis of thymocytes, splenocytes, and mesenteric lymph node cells, and can selectively deplete bone marrow of mature lymphocytes in mice. Gliotoxin inhibits activation of NF-κB (a transcriptional factor that is a key mediator of cytokine and inflammatory responses) in T and B cells. Stanzani et al. showed that *A. fumigatus* extract suppressed human cellular immune responses via gliotoxin-mediated apoptosis of antigen presenting cells; they suggest that in addition to evading host defense during infection, gliotoxin may cause a more global immunosuppression predisposing to other opportunistic infections.

ADAPTATION TO pH   For organisms that grow over a wide range of pH, mechanisms are required to sense and respond appropriately. Pathogenic fungi usually encounter a wide range of pH in the environment and in animal hosts. *C. albicans* causes infection in diverse anatomic sites with different pH, including the oral cavity, gastrointestinal tract, and vaginal tract. Pathogenic fungi with a host intracellular stage may be exposed to the acidic environment within the phagolysozome. For example, *A. fumigatus* conidia can survive and germinate in the acidic phagosomes of respiratory epithelial cells in vitro.

The ability to respond to alkaline environments is governed by signal transduction pathways. The pacC pathway has been extensively studied as a model of pH regulation in *A. nidulans*. The *pal* gene family consists of six members encoding proteins that signal under alkaline conditions to activate by proteolytic cleavage the zinc finger transcriptional factor PacC. This in turn upregulates "alkali-expressed genes" and prevents the expression of "acid-expressed genes." Mutations inactivating *pacC* or the pal signaling pathway lead to absence of expression of alkaline genes and derepression of acid genes, resulting in "acidity mimicry." Constituitively expressed *pacC* mutations, which bypass control of the pal pathway, lead to constant activation of alkaline genes, "alkaline mimicry." *pacC* has homology to other transcription factors, including the inflammatory regulator NF-κB and the sterol regulatory element binding protein that mediates lipid metabolism.

Homologues of the pal/pacC system are present in a variety of filamentous fungi, *S. cerevesia*, and *Candida* spp. Ramon et al. showed that *CaRIM101*, the *pacC* homologue in *C. albicans*, is activated under alkaline conditions. Null mutants were unable to regulate gene expression in response to pH and were defective in filamentous growth, a key virulence factor. CaRIM101 null mutants had attenuated virulence in mice and were less damaging to endothelial cells than wild-type strains. The CaRIM101 pathway also mediates pH-independent responses, including resistance to high concentrations of lithium and to the drug, hygromycin B.

CALMODULIN AND CALCINEURIN   Calcium signaling via calmodulin and calcineurin is critical for regulation of stress responses in fungi. Calmodulin is a 17-kDa Ca^{2+} binding protein that is highly conserved throughout evolution that regulates transcription factors, protein kinases, phosphatases, and cytoskeletal components. Calcineurin is a serine–threonine phosphatase that is also highly conserved, is activated following binding with Ca^{2+}/calmodulin, and has important cell signaling functions.

Studies in *C. albicans* and *C. neoformans* show that calcineurin is important for virulence, but acts through distinct mechanisms in each fungus. In *C. albicans*, Ca^{2+}/calmodulin signaling is important for transition from the yeast to the filamentous form. *C. albicans* calcineurin mutants had significantly reduced virulence in systemic infection in mice. Calcineurin was not required for survival at 37°C, filamentation, host-cell adhesion and invasion, or germ

tube formation, but was required to colonize and grow in kidneys of infected animals and to grow in serum in vitro. In contrast, in *C. neoformans* calcineurin is required for growth at 37°C and for maintenance of cell-wall integrity. Strains lacking calcineurin are avirulent in animal models.

Calcineurin inhibitors (cyclosporin A and tacrolimus) are used widely as immunosuppressive agents to prevent rejection of transplanted organs and GVHD. These agents have antifungal activity in vitro against *C. albicans*, *C. neoformans*, *S. cerevesiae*, and *A. fumigatus*, and can act synergistically with existing antifungal agents. Development of fungal-specific calcineurin inhibitors merits further study, but may be limited by the significant homology of eukaryotic calcineurins.

Heat shock proteins (HSP) are molecular chaperones that are often upregulated during physiologic stress and regulate folding, transport, and degradation of a diverse set of client proteins, many of which function in cell signaling. Cowen and Lindquist showed that fungal Hsp90, in combination with its client protein, calcineurin, exerts distinct effects on drug resistance in evolutionarily distant fungal pathogens. It potentiated the emergence of resistance to fluconazole (a cell membrane acting agent) in *S. cerevisiae* and *C. albicans* by enabling mutations in the ergosterol biosynthetic pathway to have immediate phenotypic effects. Hsp90 was also required for resistance to an echinocandin (a cell wall acting agent) in *Aspergillus terreus*. Hsp90 likely confers resistance by enabling adaptive changes in protein structure in response to drugs that alter the fungal cell membrane and cell wall. That Hsp90-mediated drug resistance is exerted through calcineurin raises the prospect of novel drug combinations that pair inhibitors of these "stress" pathways with "conventional" antifungal agents that target fungal biosynthetic pathways.

PATHOGEN RECOGNITION AND POTENTIAL FOR IMMUNE AUGMENTATION

Toll-like receptors (TLR) are a conserved family of receptors that recognize common protein and DNA pattern motifs present in microbes, and initiate signaling for cytokine production and T-cell and DC maturation. During phagocytosis, TLRs recognize pathogen specific motifs within the vacuole, distinguish between pathogens, and trigger an appropriate inflammatory response. TLRs have homology to IL-1R1 and share a similar signaling cascade leading to activation of NF-κB and mitogen activated protein kinases, a process that mediates gene expression and regulation of inflammatory responses.

TLR-dependent antifungal pathways are highly conserved in nature as demonstrated by their presence in Drosophila. TLRs recognize motifs on *Candida* and *Cryptococcus* species and regulate inflammatory responses. TLR4-defective mice are more susceptible to *C. albicans* infection, and this is associated with impaired chemokine expression and neutrophil recruitment.

Aspergillus conidia, but not hyphae, stimulate macrophages to produce proinflammatory cytokines TNF-α and IL-1 in a TLR4-dependent fashion. In contrast, *Aspergillus* hyphae, but not conidia, stimulated production of the anti-inflammatory cytokine IL-10 through TLR2-dependent mechanisms. The authors consider that this switch from a proinflammatory to an anti-inflammatory state during germination may help *Aspergillus* evade host defense. Wang et al. reported that both CD14 and TLR4, but not TLR2, mediate activation of human monocytes by *A. fumigatus* hyphae. Other investigators found that both TLR2 and TLR4 recognize *Aspergillus* hyphae, stimulate proinflammatory cytokines in effector cells, and stimulate neutrophil recruitment.

Gomez BL, Nosanchuk JD. Melanin and fungi. Curr Opin Infect Dis 2003;16:91–96.

Green CB, Cheng G, Chandra J, Mukherjee P, Ghannoum MA, Hoyer LL. RT-PCR detection of Candida albicans ALS gene expression in the reconstituted human epithelium (RHE) model of oral candidiasis and in model biofilms. Microbiology 2004;150:267–275.

Grow WB, Moreb JS, Roque D, et al. Late onset of invasive aspergillus infection in bone marrow transplant patients at a university hospital. Bone Marrow Transplant 2002;29:15–19.

Hanel H, Kirsch R, Schmidts HL, Kottmann H. New systematically active antimycotics from the beta-blocker category. Mycoses 1995;38:251–264.

Herbrecht R, Denning DW, Patterson TF, et al. Voriconazole versus amphotericin B for primary therapy of invasive aspergillosis. N Engl J Med 2002;347:408–415.

Heymann P, Gerads M, Schaller M, Dromer F, Winkelmann G, Ernst JF. The siderophore iron transporter of Candida albicans (Sit1p/Arn1p) mediates uptake of ferrichrome-type siderophores and is required for epithelial invasion. Infect Immun 2002;70:5246–5255.

Hissen AH, Chow JM, Pinto LJ, Moore MM. Survival of Aspergillus fumigatus in serum involves removal of iron from transferrin: the role of siderophores. Infect Immun 2004;72:1402–1408.

Hogan LH, Josvai S, Klein BS. Genomic cloning, characterization, and functional analysis of the major surface adhesin WI-1 on Blastomyces dermatitidis yeasts. J Biol Chem 1995;270:30,725–30,732.

Hoyer LL. The ALS gene family of Candida albicans. Trends Microbiol 2001;9:176–180.

Ibrahim AS, Spellberg BJ, Avenissian V, Fu Y, Filler SG, Edwards JE Jr. Vaccination with recombinant N-terminal domain of Als1p improves survival during murine disseminated candidiasis by enhancing cell-mediated, not humoral, immunity. Infect Immun 2005;73:999–1005.

Ibrahim AS, Mirbod F, Filler SG, et al. Evidence implicating phospholipase as a virulence factor of Candida albicans. Infect Immun 1995;63:1993–1998.

Imhof A, Balajee SA, Fredricks DN, Englund JA, Marr KA. Breakthrough fungal infections in stem cell transplant recipients receiving voriconazole. Clin Infect Dis 2004;39:743–746. Epub 2004 Aug 13.

Jantunen E, Ruutu P, Niskanen L, et al. Incidence and risk factors for invasive fungal infections in allogeneic BMT recipients. Bone Marrow Transplant 1997;19:801–808.

Jiang B, Bussey H, Roemer T. Novel strategies in antifungal lead discovery. Curr Opin Microbiol 2002;5:466–471.

Jiang C, Magee DM, Ivey FD, Cox RA. Role of signal sequence in vaccine-induced protection against experimental coccidioidomycosis. Infect Immun 2002;70:3539–3545.

Johnson SM, Kerekes KM, Zimmermann CR, Williams RH, Pappagianis D. Identification and cloning of an aspartyl proteinase from Coccidioides immitis. Gene 2000;241:213–222.

Jones T, Federspiel NA, Chibana H, et al. The diploid genome sequence of Candida albicans. Proc Natl Acad Sci USA 2004;101:7329–7334. Epub 2004 May 3.

Kogan TV, Jadoun J, Mittelman L, Hirschberg K, Osherov N. Involvement of secreted Aspergillus fumigatus proteases in disruption of the actin fiber cytoskeleton and loss of focal adhesion sites in infected A549 lung pneumocytes. J Infect Dis 2004;189:1965–1973. Epub 2004 May 11.

Kontoyiannis DP, Lionakis MS, Lewis RE, et al. Zygomycosis in a tertiary care cancer center in the era of Aspergillus-active antifungal therapy: A case control observational study of 27 recent cases. J Infect Dis 2005;191:1350–1360.

Kraus PR, Heitman J. Coping with stress: calmodulin and calcineurin in model and pathogenic fungi. Biochem Biophys Res Commun 2003;311:1151–1157.

Kuhn DM, Ghannoum MA. Candida biofilms: antifungal resistance and emerging therapeutic options. Curr Opin Investig Drugs 2004;5:186–197.

Kuhn DM, George T, Chandra J, Mukherjee PK, Ghannoum MA. Antifungal susceptibility of Candida biofilms: unique efficacy of amphotericin B lipid formulations and echinocandins. Antimicrob Agents Chemother 2002;46:1773–1780.

Kunert J, Kopecek P. Multiple forms of the serine protease Alp of Aspergillus fumigatus. Mycoses 2000;43:339–347.

Larsen RA, Pappas PG, Perfect J, et al. Phase I evaluation of the safety and pharmacokinetics of murine-derived anticryptococcal antibody 18B7 in subjects with treated cryptococcal meningitis. Antimicrob Agents Chemother 2005;49:952–958.

Leidich SD, Ibrahim AS, Fu Y, et al. Cloning and disruption of caPLB1, a phospholipase B gene involved in the pathogenicity of Candida albicans. J Biol Chem 1998;273:26,078–26,086.

Lemaitre B, Nicolas E, Michaut L, Reichhart JM, Hoffmann JA. The dorsoventral regulatory gene cassette spatzle/Toll/cactus controls the potent antifungal response in Drosophila adults. Cell 1996;86:973–983.

Li F, Palecek SP. EAP1, a Candida albicans gene involved in binding human epithelial cells. Eukaryot Cell 2003;2:1266, 1267.

Li M, Martin SJ, Bruno VM, Mitchell AP, Davis DA. Candida albicans Rim13p, a protease required for Rim101p processing at acidic and alkaline pHs. Eukaryot Cell 2004;3:741–751.

Lo HJ, Kohler JR, DiDomenico B, Loebenberg D, Cacciapuoti A, Fink GR. Nonfilamentous C. albicans mutants are avirulent. Cell 1997;90:939–949.

Lopes Bezerra LM, Filler SG. Interactions of Aspergillus fumigatus with endothelial cells: Internalization, injury, and stimulation of tissue factor activity. Blood 2004;103:2143–2149. Epub 2003 Nov 20.

Maertens J, Raad I, Petrikkos G, et al. Efficacy and safety of caspofungin for treatment of invasive aspergillosis in patients refractory to or intolerant of conventional antifungal therapy. Clin Infect Dis 2004;39:1563–1571. Epub 2004 Nov 9.

Mambula SS, Sau K, Henneke P, Golenbock DT, Levitz SM. Toll-like receptor (TLR) signaling in response to Aspergillus fumigatus. J Biol Chem 2002;277:39,320–39,326.

Marr KA, Boeckh M, Carter RA, Kim HW, Corey L. Combination antifungal therapy for invasive aspergillosis. Clin Infect Dis 2004;39:797–802. Epub 2004 Aug 27.

Marr KA, Carter RA, Boeckh M, Martin P, Corey L. Invasive aspergillosis in allogeneic stem cell transplant recipients: changes in epidemiology and risk factors. Blood 2002;100:4358–4366.

Marty FM, Cosimi LA, Baden LR. Breakthrough zygomycosis after voriconazole treatment in recipients of hematopoietic stem-cell transplants. N Engl J Med 2004;350:950–952.

McNeil MM, Nash SL, Hajjeh RA, et al. Trends in mortality due to invasive mycotic diseases in the United States, 1980–1997. Clin Infect Dis 2001;33:641–647. Epub 2001 Jul 30.

McWhinney PH, Kibbler CC, Hamon MD, et al. Progress in the diagnosis and management of aspergillosis in bone marrow transplantation: 13 years' experience. Clin Infect Dis 1993;17:397–404.

Meier A, Kirschning CJ, Nikolaus T, Wagner H, Heesemann J, Ebel F. Toll-like receptor (TLR) 2 and TLR4 are essential for Aspergillus-induced activation of murine macrophages. Cell Microbiol 2003;5:561–570.

Mohagheghpour N, Waleh N, Garger SJ, Dousman L, Grill LK, Tuse D. Synthetic melanin suppresses production of proinflammatory cytokines. Cell Immunol 2000;199:25–36.

Monod M, Togni G, Hube B, Sanglard D. Multiplicity of genes encoding secreted aspartic proteinases in Candida species. Mol Microbiol 1994;13:357–368.

Monod M, Capoccia S, Lechenne B, Zaugg C, Holdom M, Jousson O. Secreted proteases from pathogenic fungi. Int J Med Microbiol 2002;292:405–419.

Monod M, Paris S, Sanglard D, Jaton-Ogay K, Bille J, Latge JP. Isolation and characterization of a secreted metalloprotease of Aspergillus fumigatus. Infect Immun 1993;61:4099–4104.

Monod M, Paris S, Sarfati J, Jaton-Ogay K, Ave P, Latge JP. Virulence of alkaline protease-deficient mutants of Aspergillus fumigatus. FEMS Microbiol Lett 1993;106:39–46.

Mora-Duarte J, Betts R, Rotstein C, et al. Comparison of caspofungin and amphotericin B for invasive candidiasis. N Engl J Med 2002;347:2020–2029.

Mukherjee J, Scharff MD, Casadevall A. Protective murine monoclonal antibodies to Cryptococcus neoformans. Infect Immun 1992;60:4534–4541.

Mukherjee PK, Chandra J, Kuhn DM, Ghannoum MA. Differential expression of Candida albicans phospholipase B (PLB1) under various environmental and physiological conditions. Microbiology 2003a;149: 261–267.

Mukherjee PK, Chandra J, Kuhn DM, Ghannoum MA. Mechanism of fluconazole resistance in Candida albicans biofilms: phase-specific role of efflux pumps and membrane sterols. Infect Immun 2003b;71: 4333–4340.

Mukherjee PK, Seshan KR, Leidich SD, Chandra J, Cole GT, Ghannoum MA. Reintroduction of the PLB1 gene into Candida albicans restores virulence in vivo. Microbiology 2001;147:2585–2597.

Mullbacher A, Eichner RD. Immunosuppression in vitro by a metabolite of a human pathogenic fungus. Proc Natl Acad Sci USA 1984;81:3835–3837.

Mylonakis E, Barlam TF, Flanigan T, Rich JD. Pulmonary aspergillosis and invasive disease in AIDS: Review of 342 cases. Chest 1998;114: 251–262.

Naglik JR, Rodgers CA, Shirlaw PJ, et al. Differential expression of Candida albicans secreted aspartyl proteinase and phospholipase B genes in humans correlates with active oral and vaginal infections. J Infect Dis 2003;188:469–479. Epub 2003 Jul 14.

Narasipura SD, Ault JG, Behr MJ, Chaturvedi V, Chaturvedi S. Characterization of Cu,Zn superoxide dismutase (SOD1) gene knockout mutant of Cryptococcus neoformans var. gattii: role in biology and virulence. Mol Microbiol 2003;47:1681–1694.

Netea MG, Van Der Graaf CA, Vonk AG, Verschueren I, Van Der Meer JW, Kullberg BJ. The role of toll-like receptor (TLR) 2 and TLR4 in the host defense against disseminated candidiasis. J Infect Dis 2002;185:1483–1489.

Netea MG, Warris A, Van der Meer JW, et al. Aspergillus fumigatus evades immune recognition during germination through loss of toll-like receptor-4-mediated signal transduction. J Infect Dis 2003;188: 320–326.

Newman SL, Chaturvedi S, Klein BS. The WI-1 antigen of Blastomyces dermatitidis yeasts mediates binding to human macrophage CD11b/CD18 (CR3) and CD14. J Immunol 1995;154:753–761.

Noverr MC, Cox GM, Perfect JR, Huffnagle GB. Role of PLB1 in pulmonary inflammation and cryptococcal eicosanoid production. Infect Immun 2003;71:1538–1547.

Nucci M, Marr KA, Queiroz-Telles F, et al. Fusarium infection in hematopoietic stem cell transplant recipients. Clin Infect Dis 2004;38:1237–1242. Epub 2004 Apr 15.

Odds FC, Van Gerven F, Espinel-Ingroff A, et al. Evaluation of possible correlations between antifungal susceptibilities of filamentous fungi in vitro and antifungal treatment outcomes in animal infection models. Antimicrob Agents Chemother 1998;42:282–288.

Odom A, Muir S, Lim E, Toffaletti DL, Perfect J, Heitman J. Calcineurin is required for virulence of Cryptococcus neoformans. Embo J 1997;16:2576–2589.

Okumura Y, Ogawa K, Nikai T. Elastase and elastase inhibitor from Aspergillus fumigatus, Aspergillus flavus and Aspergillus niger. J Med Microbiol 2004;53:351–354.

Ostrosky-Zeichner L, Marr KA, Rex JH, Cohen SH. Amphotericin B: Time for a new "gold standard". Clin Infect Dis 2003;37:415–425. Epub 2003 Jul 22.

Ozinsky A, Underhill DM, Fontenot JD, et al. The repertoire for pattern recognition of pathogens by the innate immune system is defined by cooperation between toll-like receptors. Proc Natl Acad Sci USA 2000;97:13,766–13,771.

Pahl HL, Krauss B, Schulze-Osthoff K, et al. The immunosuppressive fungal metabolite gliotoxin specifically inhibits transcription factor NF-kappaB. J Exp Med 1996;183:1829–1840.

Pappagianis D. Evaluation of the protective efficacy of the killed Coccidiodes immitis spherule vaccine in humans. The Valley Fever Vaccine Study Group. Am Rev Respir Dis 1993;148:656–660.

Patterson TF, Kirkpatrick WR, White M, et al. Invasive aspergillosis. Disease spectrum, treatment practices, and outcomes. I3 Aspergillus Study Group. Medicine (Baltimore) 2000;79:250–260.

Patterson JE, Peters J, Calhoon JH, et al. Investigation and control of aspergillosis and other filamentous fungal infections in solid organ transplant recipients. Transpl Infect Dis 2000;2:22–28.

Penalva MA, Arst HN Jr. Regulation of gene expression by ambient pH in filamentous fungi and yeasts. Microbiol Mol Biol Rev 2002;66: 426–446.

Pendrak ML, Yan SS, Roberts DD. Sensing the host environment: recognition of hemoglobin by the pathogenic yeast Candida albicans. Arch Biochem Biophys 2004;426:148–156.

Peng T, Shubitz L, Simons J, Perrill R, Orsborn KI, Galgiani JN. Localization within a proline-rich antigen (Ag2/PRA) of protective antigenicity against infection with Coccidioides immitis in mice. Infect Immun 2002;70:3330–3335.

Perfect JR. Treatment of non-Aspergillus moulds in immunocompromised patients, with amphotericin B lipid complex. Clin Infect Dis 2005; 40(Suppl 6):S401–S408.

Popolo L, Gilardelli D, Bonfante P, Vai M. Increase in chitin as an essential response to defects in assembly of cell wall polymers in the ggp1delta mutant of Saccharomyces cerevisiae. J Bacteriol 1997;179:463–469.

Ramanan N, Wang Y. A high-affinity iron permease essential for Candida albicans virulence. Science 2000;288:1062–1064.

Ramon AM, Porta A, Fonzi WA. Effect of environmental pH on morphological development of Candida albicans is mediated via the PacC-related transcription factor encoded by PRR2. J Bacteriol 1999;181: 7524–7530.

Reeves EP, Lu H, Jacobs HL, et al. Killing activity of neutrophils is mediated through activation of proteases by K+ flux. Nature 2002;416: 291–297.

Rhodes JC, Oliver BG, Askew DS, Amlung TW. Identification of genes of Aspergillus fumigatus up-regulated during growth on endothelial cells. Med Mycol 2001;39:253–260.

Riggle PJ, Andrutis KA, Chen X, Tzipori SR, Kumamoto CA. Invasive lesions containing filamentous forms produced by a Candida albicans mutant that is defective in filamentous growth in culture. Infect Immun 1999;67:3649–3652.

Ringden O. Ten years' experience with liposomal amphotericin B in transplant recipients at Huddinge University Hospital. J Antimicrob Chemother 2002;49(Suppl 1):51–55.

Ripeau JS, Fiorillo M, Aumont F, Belhumeur P, de Repentigny L. Evidence for differential expression of candida albicans virulence genes during oral infection in intact and human immunodeficiency virus type 1-transgenic mice. J Infect Dis 2002;185:1094–1102. Epub 2002 Mar 21.

Rogers PD, Barker KS. Evaluation of differential gene expression in fluconazole-susceptible and -resistant isolates of Candida albicans by cDNA microarray analysis. Antimicrob Agents Chemother 2002;46: 3412–3417.

Romani L. Immunity to fungal infections. Nat Rev Immunol 2004;4:1–23.

Romani L, Bistoni F, Gaziano R, et al. Thymosin alpha 1 activates dendritic cells for antifungal Th1 resistance through toll-like receptor signaling. Blood 2004;103:4232–4239. Epub 2004 Feb 24.

Rosas AL, Casadevall A. Melanization affects susceptibility of Cryptococcus neoformans to heat and cold. FEMS Microbiol Lett 1997;153:265–272.

Salas SD, Bennett JE, Kwon-Chung KJ, Perfect JR, Williamson PR. Effect of the laccase gene CNLAC1, on virulence of Cryptococcus neoformans. J Exp Med 1996;184:377–386.

San-Blas G, Travassos LR, Fries BC, et al. Fungal morphogenesis and virulence. Med Mycol 2000;38:79–86.

Sanchez AA, Johnston DA, Myers C, Edwards JE Jr., Mitchell AP, Filler SG. Relationship between Candida albicans virulence during experimental hematogenously disseminated infection and endothelial cell damage in vitro. Infect Immun 2004;72:598–601.

Sanford JE, Lupan DM, Schlageter AM, Kozel TR. Passive immunization against Cryptococcus neoformans with an isotype-switch family of monoclonal antibodies reactive with cryptococcal polysaccharide. Infect Immun 1990;58:1919–1923.

Santangelo R, Zoellner H, Sorrell T, et al. Role of extracellular phospholipases and mononuclear phagocytes in dissemination of cryptococcosis in a murine model. Infect Immun 2004;72:2229–2239.

Schofield DA, Westwater C, Warner T, Nicholas PJ, Paulling EE, Balish E. Hydrolytic gene expression during oroesophageal and gastric candidiasis in immunocompetent and immunodeficient gnotobiotic mice. J Infect Dis 2003;188:591–599. Epub 2003 Jul 24.

Segal BH, Holland SM. Invasive aspergillosis in chronic granulomatous disease. The Aspergillus website. http://www.aspergillus.man.ac.uk Jan. 26, 2006.

Segal BH, Leto TL, Gallin JI, Malech HL, Holland SM. Genetic, biochemical, and clinical features of chronic granulomatous disease. Medicine (Baltimore) 2000;79:170–200.

Segal BH, Barnhart LA, Anderson VL, Walsh TJ, Malech HL, Holland SM. Posaconazole as salvage therapy in patients with chronic granulomatous disease with invasive filamentous fungal infection. Clin Infect Dis 2005;40:1684–1688.

Shaukat A, Bakri F, Young P, et al. Invasive filamentous fungal infections in allogeneic hematopoietic stem cell transplant recipients after recovery from neutropenia: clinical, radiologic, and pathologic characteristics. Mycopathologia 2005;159:181–188.

Sheppard DC, Yeaman MR, Welch WH, et al. Functional and structural diversity in the Als protein family of Candida albicans. J Biol Chem 2004;279:30,480–30,489. Epub 2004 May 5.

Shoham S, Huang C, Chen JM, Golenbock DT, Levitz SM. Toll-like receptor 4 mediates intracellular signaling without TNF-alpha release in response to Cryptococcus neoformans polysaccharide capsule. J Immunol 2001;166:4620–4626.

Silva AJ, Benitez JA. Th1-type immune response to a Coccidioides immitis antigen delivered by an attenuated strain of the non-invasive enteropathogen Vibrio cholerae. FEMS Immunol Med Microbiol 2005;43:393–398.

Silva AJ, Mohan A, Benitez JA. Cholera vaccine candidate 638: intranasal immunogenicity and expression of a foreign antigen from the pulmonary pathogen Coccidioides immitis. Vaccine 2003;21:4715–4721.

Spellberg BJ, Ibrahim AS, Avenissian V, et al. The anti-Candida albicans vaccine composed of the recombinant N terminus of Als1p reduces fungal burden and improves survival in both immunocompetent and immunocompromised mice. Infect Immun 2005;73:6191–6193.

Staab JF, Bradway SD, Fidel PL, Sundstrom P. Adhesive and mammalian transglutaminase substrate properties of Candida albicans Hwp1. Science 1999;283:1535–1538.

Stanzani M, Orciuolo E, Lewis R, et al. Aspergillus fumigatus suppresses the human cellular immune response via gliotoxin-mediated apoptosis of monocytes. Blood 2005;105:2258–2265. Epub 2004 Nov 16.

Steenbergen JN, Shuman HA, Casadevall A. Cryptococcus neoformans interactions with amoebae suggest an explanation for its virulence and intracellular pathogenic strategy in macrophages. Proc Natl Acad Sci USA 2001;98:15,245–15,250. Epub 2001 Dec 11.

Steinbach WJ, Schell WA, Blankenship JR, Onyewu C, Heitman J, Perfect JR. In vitro interactions between antifungals and immunosuppressants against Aspergillus fumigatus. Antimicrob Agents Chemother 2004;48:1664–1669.

Stevens DA. Vaccinate against aspergillosis! A call to arms of the immune system. Clin Infect Dis 2004;38:1131–1136. Epub 2004 Apr 5.

Tauszig-Delamasure S, Bilak H, Capovilla M, Hoffmann JA, Imler JL. Drosophila MyD88 is required for the response to fungal and Gram-positive bacterial infections. Nat Immunol 2002;3:91–97.

Tkalcevic J, Novelli M, Phylactides M, Iredale JP, Segal AW, Roes J. Impaired immunity and enhanced resistance to endotoxin in the absence of neutrophil elastase and cathepsin G. Immunity 2000;12: 201–210.

Tsunawaki S, Yoshida LS, Nishida S, Kobayashi T, Shimoyama T. Fungal metabolite gliotoxin inhibits assembly of the human respiratory burst NADPH oxidase. Infect Immun 2004;72:3373–3382.

Ullmann BD, Myers H, Chiranand W, et al. Inducible defense mechanism against nitric oxide in Candida albicans. Eukaryot Cell 2004;3: 715–723.

Underhill DM, Ozinsky A, Hajjar AM, et al. The Toll-like receptor 2 is recruited to macrophage phagosomes and discriminates between pathogens. Nature 1999;401:811–815.

van Duin D, Casadevall A, Nosanchuk JD. Melanization of Cryptococcus neoformans and Histoplasma capsulatum reduces their susceptibilities to amphotericin B and caspofungin. Antimicrob Agents Chemother 2002;46:3394–3400.

Vecchiarelli A, Pietrella D, Lupo P, Bistoni F, McFadden DC, Casadevall A. The polysaccharide capsule of Cryptococcus neoformans interferes with human dendritic cell maturation and activation. J Leukoc Biol 2003;74:370–378.

Wald A, Leisenring W, van Burik JA, Bowden RA. Epidemiology of Aspergillus infections in a large cohort of patients undergoing bone marrow transplantation (see comments). J Infect Dis 1997;175: 1459–1466.

Walsh TJ, Groll A, Hiemenz J, Fleming R, Roilides E, Anaissie E. Infections due to emerging and uncommon medically important fungal pathogens. Clin Microbiol Infect 2004;10(Suppl 1):48–66.

Walsh TJ, Goodman JL, Pappas P, et al. Safety, tolerance, and pharmacokinetics of high-dose liposomal amphotericin B (AmBisome) in patients infected with Aspergillus species and other filamentous fungi: maximum tolerated dose study. Antimicrob Agents Chemother 2001;45: 3487–3496.

Wang Y, Casadevall A. Decreased susceptibility of melanized Cryptococcus neoformans to UV light. Appl Environ Microbiol 1994a;60:3864–3866.

Wang Y, Casadevall A. Susceptibility of melanized and nonmelanized Cryptococcus neoformans to nitrogen- and oxygen-derived oxidants. Infect Immun 1994b;62:3004–3007.

Wang JE, Warris A, Ellingsen EA, et al. Involvement of CD14 and toll-like receptors in activation of human monocytes by Aspergillus fumigatus hyphae. Infect Immun 2001;69:2402–2406.

Wasylnka JA, Moore MM. Uptake of Aspergillus fumigatus Conidia by phagocytic and nonphagocytic cells in vitro: quantitation using strains expressing green fluorescent protein. Infect Immun 2002;70: 3156–3163.

Wasylnka JA, Moore MM. Aspergillus fumigatus conidia survive and germinate in acidic organelles of A549 epithelial cells. J Cell Sci 2003; 116:1579–1587.

Weissman Z, Kornitzer D. A family of Candida cell surface haem-binding proteins involved in haemin and haemoglobin-iron utilization. Mol Microbiol 2004;53:1209–1220.

Winkelstein JA, Marino MC, Johnston RB Jr, et al. Chronic granulomatous disease: report on a national registry of 368 patients. Medicine (Baltimore) 2000;79:155–169.

Wuthrich M, Filutowicz HI, Warner T, Deepe GS Jr, Klein BS. Vaccine immunity to pathogenic fungi overcomes the requirement for CD4 help in exogenous antigen presentation to CD8+ T cells: implications for vaccine development in immune-deficient hosts. J Exp Med 2003;197:1405–1416.

Yamada A, Kataoka T, Nagai K. The fungal metabolite gliotoxin: Immunosuppressive activity on CTL-mediated cytotoxicity. Immunol Lett 2000;71:27–32.

Yoshida LS, Abe S, Tsunawaki S. Fungal gliotoxin targets the onset of superoxide-generating NADPH oxidase of human neutrophils. Biochem Biophys Res Commun 2000;268:716–723.

Yuen KY, Woo PC, Ip MS, et al. Stage-specific manifestation of mold infections in bone marrow transplant recipients: risk factors and clinical significance of positive concentrated smears. Clin Infect Dis 1997;25:37–42.

Zhu X, Gibbons J, Garcia-Rivera J, Casadevall A, Williamson PR. Laccase of Cryptococcus neoformans is a cell wall-associated virulence factor. Infect Immun 2001;69:5589–5596.

DERMATOLOGY | XII

SECTION EDITORS:
LUIS A. DIAZ AND LOWELL A. GOLDSMITH

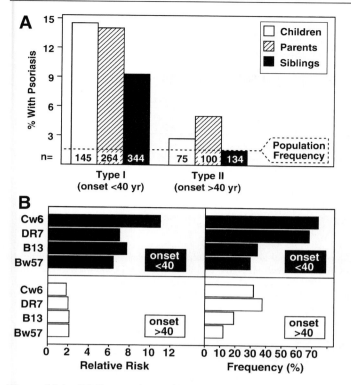

Figure 96-4 (**A**) Increased prevalence of affected relatives in early-onset (Type I) compared with late-onset (type II) psoriasis. (**B**) Increased relative risk and frequency of human leukocyte antigen-Cw6, DR7, B13, and B57 in juvenile onset psoriasis. (Reproduced with permission from Elder et al., Arch Dermatol 1994;130:216–224. Copyright © 1994, American Medical Assocation.)

Several lines of evidence argue for ongoing T-cell activation by antigen in the lesion itself. Psoriatic lesions contain increased numbers of activated dendritic antigen-presenting cells (APCs) and memory (antigen-activated) T cells. These memory T cells have been observed to proliferate in direct contact with APCs (Fig. 96-7). Also, expansion of T cells in psoriatic lesions is oligoclonal, as judged by the presence of specific rearrangements of the variable region of the β-chain of the T-cell receptor. These clones persist over time and in different lesions of the same patient, and are clearly expanded in skin lesions compared to the peripheral blood. This is the strongest evidence for ongoing T-cell activation by antigens (as opposed to cytokines alone) in psoriatic lesions. These observations fit with the genetic evidence implicating HLA-Cw6 in psoriasis, as HLA Class I molecules are involved in antigen presentation, and CD8+ T cells, which recognize antigen in the context of HLA Class I, predominate in psoriatic epidermis. However, APCs usually take up antigens and present them in the context of MHC Class II, whereas MHC Class I is involved in the presentation of intracellular peptides such as those derived from viruses. An alternative pathology of "cross-presentation" has been implicated in tumor immunity. It is possible that this pathway is also involved in psoriasis.

Major abnormalities of APCs are also present in psoriatic lesions. APC numbers and activity are markedly increased in lesional psoriatic skin, and both are rapidly reduced by cyclosporine treatment. TNF-α stimulates maturation of immature Langerhans cells by promoting migration to the nodes and by inducing the key accessory molecules B7-1 (CD80) and B7-2 (CD86) on the surface of

APC. These important molecules provide a "second signal" for T-cell activation (Fig. 96-8). TNF-α is also involved in recruiting a second class of APCs from the peripheral blood into the dermis once an infection is underway, and this class of APC appears to be markedly increased in psoriatic lesions. Once activated, T cells produce IFN-γ, which in turn stimulates APCs and monocyte/macrophages to produce TNF-α. TNF-α can also be directly produced by a subset of CD8+ T cells. Thus, once activated, T cells appear to perpetuate a "vicious circle" of increased antigen presentation in psoriasis (*see* Fig. 96-7).

Shortly after activation by antigen, T cells differentiate along one of two pathways, termed T1 and T2. The T1 pathway evolved to activate macrophages to eliminate intracellular pathogens, whereas the T2 pathway evolved to promote antibody-mediated protection against extracellular parasites. Cytokines play a crucial role in determining not only which pathway a differentiating T cell will utilize, but also how that cell will regulate effector responses and how the balance between T1 and T2 differentiation will be maintained. IFN-γ and IL-12 can be considered key cytokines of the T1 pathway, whereas IL-4, -10, and -11 can be considered key cytokines of the T2 pathway. Expression of IFN-γ and IL-12 strongly predominate over IL-4, -10, and -11 in psoriatic lesions, indicative of a T1 pattern. Although the precise reason for T1 dominance is not clear, psoriasis can be triggered by streptococcal and viral infections of the upper respiratory tract, and APCs activated by viruses and certain bacteria produce large amounts of IL-12. In turn, IL-12 stimulates the production of IFN-γ by NK cells. Because NK cells are regulated by HLA-C and HLA-B, it is possible that the genetic defect at PSORS1 relates to inappropriate stimulation of NK cells, resulting in excessive production of IFN-γ and maintenance of the T1 state. Recently, IL-23 has also been implicated in psoriasis. IL-23 shares its p40 subunit with IL-12.

There appear to be three interrelated defects leading to the vicious circle of T-cell activation in psoriasis: (1) maintenance of antigen presentation at an inappropriately high level because of (2) a T1 state of T-cell differentiation dictated and maintained by the actions of IFN-γ and TNF-α. This chronic state of increased antigen presentation facilitates (3) breakdown of immunological tolerance, allowing self-peptides that resemble those of an initiating pathogen to cross-react with memory T cells activated by the initial, possibly infectious, stimulus.

As discussed, keratinocyte hyperproliferation is a prominent feature of psoriasis. Three theories have been advanced to explain how T-cell activation could trigger keratinocyte hyperproliferation in psoriasis. First, soluble factors from psoriatic T cells could stimulate keratinocyte proliferation. Second, keratinocytes might be injured by T cells as they invade the epidermis. Third, macrophages might perforate the basement membrane, leading to leakage of fibronectin into the epidermal compartment. Either of these latter events could activate the keratinocyte wound healing program, resulting in hyperproliferation. Activation of this program is accompanied by increased autocrine signaling through the epidermal growth factor receptor, leading to increased proliferation and upregulation of vascular endothelial growth factor. This, in turn, increases permeability and elongation of the dermal capillaries. Finally, cytokines such as IFN-γ and TNF-α stimulate keratinocytes to produce chemokines such as IL-8, which promote chemotaxis of polymorphonuclear leukocytes into the upper epidermis, and Mig and IP-10, which promote chemotaxis of T cells and macrophages into the dermis and epidermis. Thus, it appears that a persistent

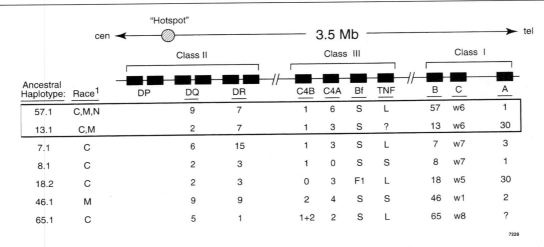

Figure 96-5 Map of the MHC, showing ancestral haplotypes. Depiction of MHC loci are incomplete and distances between them are not to scale. "Hotspot" indicates a region of high recombination resulting in loss of LD between HLA-DP and the remainder of the MHC. (Data from Degli-Epsoti et al., Immunogenetics 1992;36:345–356, Human Immunology 1992;34:242–252, and Wu et al., Hum Immunol 1992;33:89–97.) cen, centromere; tel, telomere; Mb, megabases; C, Caucasoid, M, Mongoloid; MHC, major histocompatibility complex; N, Negroid; TNF, tumor necrosis factor.

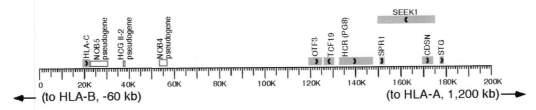

Figure 96-6 Gene map of the PSORS1 region. Note the existence of a cluster of genes extending from 100 to 160 kb telomeric to human leukocyte antigen-C. Open boxes indicate pseudogenes; shaded boxes indicate genes. Arrowheads indicate direction of gene transcription.

state of type 1 T-cell activation, centrally involving IFN-γ and TNF-α, can explain essentially all features of the chronic psoriatic plaque: T-cell activation, keratinocyte hyperproliferation, and vascular changes (*see* Fig. 96-7).

MANAGEMENT

In view of its genetic basis, lifelong duration, and low mortality, avoidance of toxicity is a cornerstone of psoriasis therapy. Treatment of moderate to severe psoriasis can entail substantial toxicity and demands thoughtful choices. Standard and novel psoriasis therapies are reviewed below in light of the immunological paradigm of psoriasis presented.

EMOLLIENTS Emollients have long played an important role in psoriasis therapy, presumably by improving barrier function. Loss of epidermal barrier function is a trigger for keratinocyte production of various proinflammatory cytokines including IL-8 and TNF-α.

CORTICOSTEROIDS/RETINOIDS/VITAMIN D Corticosteroids inhibit lymphocyte activation and the maturation of dendritic APCs. Systemic steroids were initially popular but are now little used because of their well-known systemic complications, as well as "rebound" flaring of disease on their withdrawal. In their stead, many different topical corticosteroid preparations of varying potency have been developed. Irrespective of their cellular site(s) of action, it is now clear that steroids, retinoids, and vitamin D derivatives exert their beneficial effects through binding to specific nuclear receptors, which serve as ligand-dependent transcription factors. The synthetic retinoid etretinate has been used to treat psoriasis

systemically since the 1970s. Topical vitamin D3 derivatives and topical retinoids emerged as useful treatments for psoriasis in the 1990s. Steroids, retinoids, and vitamin D derivatives all have profound effects on keratinocyte growth and differentiation as well as on inflammation and immunity.

ULTRAVIOLET LIGHT Ultraviolet (UV) light treatment continues to be a mainstay of therapy for moderate-to-severe psoriasis. Therapy combining UVB light (290–320 nm) with crude coal tar was introduced in 1925, and the combination of psoralens with lower-energy UVA light (320–400 nm) followed in 1974. Initially, both psoralen UVA and B were thought to act directly on keratinocyte proliferation. However, both therapies induce immunosuppression, either by promoting apoptosis of activated T cells or by deviating the T-cell response from T1 to T2 through decreased production of IL-12 and increased production of IL-4.

METHOTREXATE Methotrexate is a highly effective oral antipsoriatic drug whose main dose-limiting toxicity is hepatic fibrosis. Methotrexate was initially thought to exert its effects through inhibition of keratinocyte proliferation. However, it is effective under doses and schedules of administration that fail to inhibit keratinocyte proliferation in vitro. It appears that this drug exerts profound anti-inflammatory effects by promoting the extracellular accumulation of adenosine.

CYCLOSPORINE/FK506 As discussed, CsA exerts potent antipsoriatic effects, with nearly immediate clearing of psoriasis when used in high doses. The drug is effective at doses as low as 2.5 mg/kg/d; however, renal toxicity is a problem even at low

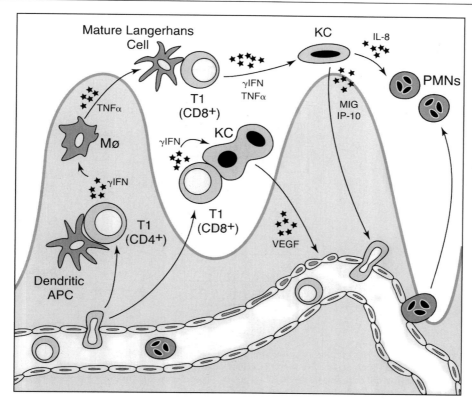

Figure 96-7 Immunopathogenesis of psoriasis. T cells are activated by mature Langerhans cells in the epidermis and by dermal dendritic cells in the dermis. T cells entering the lesion have a memory phenotype and are differentiated along the T1 pathway because of the influence of IL-12 produced by macrophages and dendritic cells, and interferon (IFN)-γ produced by T cells (and/or NK cells). Activated CD8⁺ epidermal T cells can produce tumor necrosis factor (TNF)-α directly, whereas dermal CD4⁺ T cells produce IFN-γ, thereby stimulating TNF-α production by macrophages (Mφ) and dendritic APCs. IFN-γ might also promote keratinocyte proliferation, although epidermal injury produced by migrating epidermal T cells might also play an important role. Activated keratinocytes synthesize vascular endothelial growth factor, which might function to support the hyperactive dermal capillaries. The actions of IFN-γ and TNF on suprabasal keratinocytes cause them to secrete chemoattractants such as IL-8, Mig and IP-10. *See* text for additional details. (Adapted with permission from Krueger JG. The immunologic basis for the treatment of psoriasis with new biologic agents. J Am Acad Dermatol 2002;46:1–23.) KC, Kupffer cell; PMNs, polymorphonuclear leukocytes; APC, antigen-presenting cell; VEGF, vascular endothelial growth factor.

doses with long-term use. CsA binds to cyclophilin, which is particularly abundant in T cells. The resulting complex inhibits the calmodulin-dependent protein phosphatase regulatory subunit calcineurin B, leading to the inability to translocate a component of the transcription factor NF-AT from the cytoplasm to the nucleus. This blockade of T-cell signaling greatly reduces the output of IL-2, which interacts with its receptor to expand the responding clone by stimulating T-cell proliferation. CsA also reduces expression of B7-1 and B7-2 and inhibits the production of IL-12 by dendritic APCs at clinically relevant doses. The former effect would reduce the overall levels of T-cell activation, whereas the latter would shift the T-cell maturation response from T1 to T2. FK506 is another calcineurin blocker, i.e., 5–10 times more potent than cyclosporine, but its therapeutic ratio is no better than that of CsA.

BIOLOGICALS Recombinant DNA and protein expression technologies have made it possible to manufacture large quantities of exact replicas of human proteins or fragments thereof, known as "biologicals," thereby avoiding the problem of hypersensitivity to foreign proteins. The principal biologicals in use are "humanized" monoclonal antibodies and fusion proteins. One type of fusion protein combines a human protein with a toxin, whereas the other fuses human receptors for proteins to the Fc portion of human immunoglobulin. A variety of immunosuppressive and anti-inflammatory

proteins are being developed, and three have entered clinical use for the treatment of psoriasis and/or psoriatic arthritis, based on the immunopathological model of psoriasis previously presented. Because they are proteins, biologicals cannot be delivered orally or topically. Nevertheless, their target specificity allows them to be effective with only limited systemic toxicity, which is generally related to decreased immunological surveillance.

ANTI-TNF AGENTS Two anti-TNF-α biologicals have demonstrated substantial antipsoriatic efficacy in clinical trials: infliximab, a chimeric anti-TNF-α monoclonal antibody, and etanercept, a TNF-α receptor-immunoglobulin fusion protein. Etanercept has received FDA approval for use in psoriatic arthritis. With either agent, half to three-fourths of patients obtain a 75% reduction in involved total body surface area within 12 wk of treatment. This is approximately the same response obtained with cyclosporine, presumably because of interference with the antigen- and cytokine-driven vicious circle of T-cell activation depicted in Fig. 96-7.

Another biological approved for the treatment of psoriasis is alefacept, a fusion protein combining the extracellular domain of LFA-3 and the Fc portion of IgG. LFA-3 normally binds CD2 to provide T-cell costimulation (*see* Fig. 96-8). Alefacept might function by interfering with the CD2-LFA-3 interaction, or by causing NK cells to lyse CD2⁺ memory T cells. Consistent with loss of

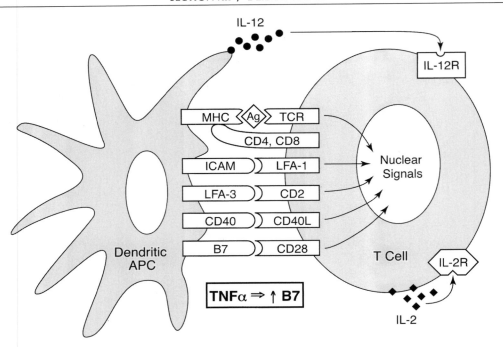

Figure 96-8 T-cell activation by APCs. The complex of antigenic peptide and major histocompatibility complex (MHC) binds to the T-cell receptor in the context of coreceptors CD4 (helper T-cells) or CD8 (suppressor/cytotoxic T-cells). The interaction of intercellular adhesion molecules and LFA-1 is critical for increasing the duration of the MHC-Ag-T-cell receptor recognition event, and is therefore depicted as part of the first signal. Interactions of CD2 with LFA-3, CD40 ligand (CD40L) with CD40, and CD28 with B7 send additional signals to the nucleus through different signal transduction pathways and are therefore called "Signal 2." When Signals 1 and 2 are received simultaneously, the T cell is activated, producing cytokines such as IL-2 and, in the case of psoriasis, IFN-γ, and TNF-α. IL-2 interacts with its own high-affinity receptor to promote T-cell proliferation, whereas IFN-γ and TNF-α support antigen presentation, keratinocyte proliferation, and the production of cytokines by keratinocytes (*see* text and Fig. 96-7). APC, antigen-presenting cell; TCR, T-cell receptor.

immunological memory, alefacept induces relatively long-term remissions in individuals who are helped by the drug.

Numerous additional biologicals are under development for psoriasis and other inflammatory disorders. These agents target various molecules responsible for T-cell activation and/or survival, control of the Th1/Th2 balance, or elaboration of the inflammatory response. Targets for blockade not already discussed earlier include LFA-1 and B7-1 (T-cell costimulation), CD3, CD4, IL-2 and IL-2 receptor (T-cell proliferation), IFN-γ, IL-12/IL-23, IL-12 (T-cell differentiation), and IL-8 (chemotaxis). In addition, IL-10 and -11 have yielded promising results in early therapeutic trials, as they should promote T2 differentiation.

FUTURE DIRECTIONS

The actions of nearly all antipsoriatic drugs can be understood in terms of immunosuppressive and/or anti-inflammatory effects, with T-cell activation as a likely primary target through the ternary complex of APC, antigen, and T-cell receptor in the context of appropriate accessory signals. Thus it is not surprising that various novel molecular approaches to blocking this activation event are in clinical trials. In addition to the biological agents described, studies suggest that picrolemus, an orally administered congener of FK506 that functions similarly to CsA, might be more specifically targeted to the skin than FK506. This agent might prove effective against psoriasis with fewer side effects than CsA.

As a genodermatosis, the question remains whether psoriasis will prove to be amenable to gene therapy. Direct correction of genetic defects might prove difficult if (as appears to be the case for PSORS1) the etiological allele is a common variant with important

immunological functions. However, it might be feasible to introduce the various biologics discussed into the skin at the level of the gene, rather than the cognate protein. Under this scenario, gene therapy for psoriasis deserves serious consideration.

SELECTED REFERENCES

Baadsgaard O, Gupta AK, Taylor RS, Ellis CN, Voorhees JJ, Cooper KD. Psoriatic epidermal cells demonstrate increased numbers and function of non-Langerhans antigen-presenting cells. J Invest Dermatol 1989;92:190–195.

Capon F, Munro M, Barker J, Trembath R. Searching for the major histocompatibility complex psoriasis susceptibility gene. J Invest Dermatol 2002;118:745–751.

Christophers E, Mrowietz U. Psoriasis. In: Freedberg IM, Eisen AZ, Wolff K, et al., eds. Dermatology in General Medicine. 6th ed., New York: McGraw-Hill, 2003, pp.407–427.

Cookson WO, Ubhi B, Lawrence R, et al. Genetic linkage of childhood atopic dermatitis to psoriasis susceptibility loci. Nat Genet 2001;27: 372, 373.

Elder JT, Nair RP, Henseler T, et al. The genetics of psoriasis 2001: the odyssey continues. Arch Dermatol 2001;137:1447–1434.

Krueger JG. The immunologic basis for the treatment of psoriasis with new biologic agents. J Am Acad Dermatol 2002;46:1–23.

Morganroth GS, Chan LS, Weinstein GD, Voorhees JJ, Cooper KD. Proliferating cells in psoriatic dermis are comprised primarily of T cells, endothelial cells, and factor XIIIa⁺ perivascular dendritic cells. J Invest Dermatol 1991;96:333–340.

Nickoloff BJ, Naidu Y. Perturbation of epidermal barrier function correlates with initiation of cytokine cascade in human skin. J Am Acad Dermatol 1994;30:535–546.

Nickoloff BJ, Wrone-Smith T. Injection of pre-psoriatic skin with CD4⁺ T cells induces psoriasis. Am J Pathol 1999;155:145–158.

Piepkorn M, Pittelkow MR, Cook PW. Autocrine regulation of keratinocytes: the emerging role of heparin-binding, epidermal growth factor-related growth factors. J Invest Dermatol 1998;111: 715–721.

Prinz JC. Psoriasis vulgaris—a sterile antibacterial skin reaction mediated by cross-reactive T cells? An immunological view of the pathophysiology of psoriasis. Clin Exp Dermatol 2001;26: 326–332.

Speckman RA, Wright Daw JA, Helms C, et al. Novel immunoglobulin superfamily gene cluster, mapping to a region of human chromosome 17q25, linked to psoriasis susceptibility. Hum Genet 2003;112: 34–41.

Tajima K, Amakawa R, Ito T, Miyaji M, Takebayashi M, Fukuhara S. Immunomodulatory effects of cyclosporin A on human peripheral blood dendritic cell subsets. Immunology 2003;108:321–328.

Walters IB, Ozawa M, Cardinale I, et al. Narrowband (312-nm) UV-B suppresses interferon gamma and interleukin (IL) 12 and increases IL-4 transcripts: differential regulation of cytokines at the single-cell level. Arch Dermatol 2003;139:155–161.

Winchester R. Psoriatic arthritis. In: Freedberg IM, Eisen AZ, Wolff K, et al., eds. Dermatology in General Medicine, 6th ed., New York: McGraw-Hill, 2003, pp. 427–436.

97 Atopic Dermatitis

KEFEI KANG, DONALD Y. M. LEUNG, AND KEVIN D. COOPER

SUMMARY

Atopic dermatitis, also known as atopic eczema, is a chronic inflammatory skin disease frequently seen in patients with a personal or family history of asthma and allergic rhinitis. There have been extraordinary strides made in the understanding of the immunopathogenesis of allergic diseases. In particular, this constellation of inherited illnesses is associated with activation of a specific group of cytokine genes encompassing IL-3, IL-4, IL-5, IL-13, and granulocyte-macrophage colony-stimulating factor. The molecular basis for selective activation of this cytokine gene cluster and their immunological consequences are being investigated. However, it is clear that allergic diseases result from a polygenic inheritance pattern that involves cytokine-gene activation and other less-well-defined gene products as well. In addition, the clinical expression of allergic diseases is highly dependent on a complex interaction between the host and its environment, for example, allergen exposure. This chapter reviews some of these developments and their clinical implications.

Key Words: Atopic dermatitis; eczema; eosinophil; keratinocytes; langerhans' cells; lymphocyte; mast cells; monocytes; pruritus; xerosis.

INTRODUCTION

Atopic dermatitis, also known as atopic eczema, is a chronic inflammatory skin disease frequently seen in patients with a personal or family history of asthma and allergic rhinitis. The term atopic dermatitis was first introduced in 1933 by Hill and Sulzberger in recognition of this close association between atopic dermatitis and respiratory allergy. Eczema (to boil out) is commonly used to refer to atopic dermatitis, but includes spongiotic dermatitis other than atopic dermatitis, so the term atopic eczema is used to specify that the type of eczema is the atopic dermatitis form, while retaining the commonly used parlance. There have been extraordinary strides made in the understanding of the immunopathogenesis of allergic diseases. In particular, this constellation of inherited illnesses is associated with activation of a specific group of cytokine genes encompassing IL-3, IL-4, IL-5, IL-13, and granulocyte-macrophage colony-stimulating factor (GM-CSF). The molecular basis for selective activation of this cytokine gene cluster and their immunological consequences are being investigated. However, it is clear that allergic diseases result from a polygenic inheritance pattern that involves cytokine-gene activation and other less-well-defined gene products as well. In addition, the clinical expression of allergic diseases is highly dependent on a complex interaction between the host and its environment, for example, allergen exposure. This chapter reviews some of these developments and their clinical implications.

DIAGNOSIS

Because of the lack of distinguishable clinical and laboratory parameters, the diagnosis of atopic dermatitis is largely based on the constellation of the major and minor clinical features. Although there are suggested features that are essential and important for the diagnosis, fully agreeable criteria need to be established. Progressive approaches to the diagnosis have been suggested by various study groups organizations, beginning with the widely used criteria of Hanifin and Rajika (Table 97-1). The Williams guidelines are useful for epidemiological studies (Table 97-2) and a simplification was used by Hanifin for United States-based epidemiology. A hierarchy of features for the diagnosis of pediatric atopic dermatitis has been suggested (Table 97-3).

Approximately 50% of patients develop atopic dermatitis by the first year of life, and an additional 30% between ages 1–5 yr. Nearly 80% of patients with atopic dermatitis eventually develop allergic rhinitis or asthma later in childhood. Many of these patients outgrow their skin disease as they are developing respiratory allergy. This observation is consistent with the concept that the clinical expression of allergic disease is determined in part from local tissue allergen sensitization and compartmentalization of the immune response in the skin vs the respiratory mucosa.

CLINICAL FEATURES

CLINICAL REACTION PATTERNS Several types of inflammatory skin lesions are commonly seen in atopic dermatitis. Acute lesions are intensely pruritic and characterized by erythematous papules over erythematous skin. These are associated with extensive excoriations, erosions, and serous exudate. Subacute dermatitis is characterized by erythematous, excoriated, scaling papules. Chronic dermatitis is characterized by thickened skin, accentuated skin markings (lichenification), and fibrotic papules. Acute episodes may occur during the chronic stage. At all stages of atopic dermatitis, patients usually have dry skin. Dyspigmentation is common. Skin distribution and reaction patterns vary according to the patient's age and disease chronicity. During infancy, the atopic dermatitis is generally more acute and primarily involves

From: *Principles of Molecular Medicine, Second Edition*
Edited by: M. S. Runge and C. Patterson © Humana Press, Inc., Totowa, NJ

Table 97-1
Diagnostic Features of Atopic Dermatitis (Hanifin and Rajika)

Major features (3 of 4 present)
Pruritus
Typical morphology and distribution of skin lesions
Chronic or chronically relapsing dermatitis
Personal or family history of atopy

Minor features (3 of 23 present)
Xerosis
Ichthyosis/palmar hyperlinearity/keratosis pilaris
Immediate (type I) skin test reactivity
Elevated serum IgE
Early age of onset
Tendency toward cutaneous infections/impaired cell-mediated
   immunity
Tendency toward nonspecific hand or foot dermatitis
Nipple eczema
Cheilitis
Recurrent conjunctivitis
Dennie-Morgan infraorbital fold
Keratoconus
Anterior subcapsular cataract
Orbital darkening
Facial pallor/erythema
Pityriasis alba
Anterior neck folds
Ichthyosis when sweating
Intolerance to wool and lipid solvents
Perifollicular accentuation
Food intolerance
Course influence by environmental/emotional factors
White dermagraphism/delayed blanch

From ref. Hanifin JM, Rajka G. Diagnostic features of atopic dermatitis. Acta Derm Venereol 1980;92:44–47 with permission.

Table 97-2
Diagnostic Guidelines of Atopic Dermatitis

Must have
An itchy skin condition (or parental report of scratching or rubbing
   in a child)
Plus 3 or more of the following
History of involvement of the skin creases such as folds of elbows,
   behind the knees, fronts of ankles, or around the neck (including
   cheeks in children under 10 yr)
A personal history of asthma or hay fever (or history of atopic
   disease in a first-degree relative in children under 4 yr)
A history of general dry skin in the last year
Visible flexural eczema (or eczema involving the cheek/forehead and
   outer limbs on children under 4 yr)
Onset under the age of 2 yr (not used if child is under 4 yr)

From Williams HC, Burney PGJ, Pembroke AC, et al. The UK Working Party's diagnostic criteria for atopic dermatitis III. Independent hospital validation. Br J Dermatol 1994;131:406–416 with permission.

the face, scalp, and the extensor surfaces of the extremities. In older patients who have had long-standing skin disease, the rash is characterized by the chronic form of dermatitis with lichenification and localization to the flexural areas of the extremities. Facial and hand dermatitis can remain problematic.

PRURITUS Intense itching is the hallmark of atopic dermatitis. Patients with atopic dermatitis have a reduced threshold for

Table 97-3
Hierarchy of Clinical Features for Diagnosis of Pediatric Atopic Dermatitis (American Academy of Dermatology Consensus Conference on Pediatric Atopic Dermatitis)

Essential features, must be present, and if complete, are sufficient
for diagnosis
   Pruritus
   Eczematous changes
Typical and age-specific patterns (facial, neck, and exterior
involvement in infants and children; current or prior flexural
lesions in adult/any age; sparing of groin and axillary regions)
Chronic or relapsing course

Important features, seen in most cases for support of the diagnosis
   Early age of onset
   Atopy (IgE reactivity)
   Xerosis

Associated features, help in suggesting the diagnosis
   Keratosis pilaris/ichthyosis/palmar hyperlinearity
   Atypical vascular responses
   Perifollicular accentuation/lichenification/prurigo
   Ocular/periorbital changes
   Perioral/ periaucular lesions

On the exclusion of other skin conditions such as contact dermatitis, seborrhoeic dermatitis, cutaneous lymphoma, and so on, the diagnosis is proposed to be established based on the above features presented at International Atopic Dermatitis Symposium, Portland, Oregon, USA, 2001.

pruritus. It is often worse in the evening and may be exacerbated by allergens, reduced humidity, excessive sweating, and irritants, for example, wool, acrylic, soaps, and detergents. The rubbing and scratching shown as superficial erosions or hemorrhagic crusts may initiate or exacerbate pathogenic events leading to the rash of atopic dermatitis. The mechanisms of pruritus remain unclear. Neuropeptides (NPs) are small amino acid compounds functioning as neurotransmitters and neuromodulators. They are also widely distributed in skin peripheral nerves. Vasoactive intestinal peptide (VIP), calcitonin gene-related peptide, and substance P (SP) are the most abundant NPs in human skin. VIP and calcitonin gene-related peptide are mainly around skin blood vessels, and eccrine sweat glands. Various inflammatory cells such as mononuclear leukocytes, mast cells, and eosinophils, important in mediating allergic disease, are also able to synthesize NP precursors in the skin and finally release smaller biologically active peptides. In atopic dermatitis, VIP levels are significantly higher in lesional skin and SP positive nerve fibers are present in most cases of atopic dermatitis. Close appositions of nerve fibers and mast cells were observed in atopic dermatitis skin. Further, α-melanocyte stimulating hormone, another NP produced in the skin, stimulates a dose-dependent release of histamine from isolated human skin mast cells. Taken together, higher availability of NPs in atopic dermatitis and an abnormal sensitivity of mast cells and blood vessels to these peptides may be involved in the mechanisms of pruritus. In addition to these molecules, anti-inflammatory drugs such as corticosteroids and calcineurin inhibitors are much more effective than antihistamines in controlling pruritus. Thus inflammation itself may lead to the release of a number of molecules involved in pruritus.

XEROSIS The xerosis in atopic dermatitis is different from icthyosis and from the dry skin in older individuals. It refers to persistent and generalized fine scaliness without visible clinical inflammation (but histologically shows spongiosis) associated with an impaired barrier function of the stratum corneum. This is present in about 70% of atopic dermatitis patients. This barrier-disrupted skin shows markedly higher transepidermal water loss and lower skin surface hydration levels. Sphingomyelin (SM) deacylase activities are significantly increased in atopic dermatitis epidermis. This SM deacylase triggers metabolism of SM resulting in a ceramide deficiency that is closely associated with skin dryness in atopic dermatitis patients. The barrier-disrupted skin may cause atopic dermatitis skin to be highly susceptible to environmental offenders such as irritants, allergens, and microbes. Interestingly, percutaneous sensitization and elicitation with different allergens through barrier-disrupted skin vs normal intact skin differentially regulates the balance of T-helper type I (Th1) and Th2 cytokine expression. For example, picryl chloride induces a decrease of the expression of IL-2 and interferon (IFN)-γ but not for IL-4; house dust mite induces an increase of IL-4 but not IL-2 or IFN-γ. These data suggest that barrier-disrupted skin in atopic dermatitis not only causes dryness of the skin but also is actively involved in induction of Th2 dominant immune responses through the entry of environmental allergens.

ROLE OF ALLERGENS

Serum IgE levels are elevated in 80–85% of patients with atopic dermatitis; about 85% of patients have positive immediate skin tests or radioallergosorbent test® (RAST) for specific IgE to a variety of food and inhalant allergens. However, positive immediate skin tests to specific allergens do not always indicate clinical sensitivity and patients who outgrow atopic dermatitis frequently continue to have positive skin tests. Indeed, there is a distinction between symptomatic and asymptomatic hypersensitivity based on the observation that atopic dermatitis patients with positive food skin tests do not always have positive challenges to the foods implicated by IgE responses. These clinical observations suggest that the relationship between IgE and clinical disease is not exclusively dependent on IgE-mediated mast-cell degranulation.

Well-controlled, double-blind, placebo-controlled food challenge studies have, however, demonstrated that food allergens can exacerbate skin rashes in at least a subset of patients, particularly young children with atopic dermatitis. Importantly, elimination of putative food allergens in such patients results in significant improvement of their skin disease. As patients grow older, they outgrow their food allergy, but a majority of them become sensitized to inhalant allergens. Although sensitization to inhalant allergens in most cases reflects the development of coexisting respiratory allergy for example, asthma or allergic rhinitis, clinical studies suggest that inhalation or contact with aeroallergen may play a role in the exacerbation of atopic dermatitis.

CUTANEOUS INFECTIONS

Patients with atopic dermatitis have an increased tendency to develop viral, fungal, and bacterial skin infections. These infections are generally localized to the skin. Deep-seated infections suggest the possibility of hyperimmunoglobulinemia E syndrome or another immunodeficiency syndrome. Superficial fungal infections also appear to occur more frequently in atopic individuals. The potential importance of these dermatophyte infections is suggested by the reported reduction of atopic dermatitis skin severity following treatment with antifungal agents such as ketoconazole.

Viral infections include herpes simplex, vaccinia, warts, molluscum contagiosum, and papilloma virus. A potentially serious viral infection is herpes simplex, which can cause eczema herpeticum. Eczema vaccinatum is another severe and potentially fatal virus complication of atopic dermatitis with a mortality rate of 10–30% if untreated. Because of a potential risk of bioterrorist attack with smallpox, immunization of live vaccinia virus is being recommended for wide scale use. Atopic dermatitis patients should avoid contact with recent vaccinees and are advised not to receive vaccinia unless there is immediate risk of exposure to smallpox.

Considerable attention has focused on the contribution of *Staphylococcus aureus* colonization and infection to the severity of atopic dermatitis. *S. aureus* is found in more than 90% of atopic dermatitis skin lesions. Honey-colored crusting, extensive serous weeping, folliculitis, and pyoderma indicate bacterial infection usually secondary to *S. aureus* in patients with atopic dermatitis. The importance of *S. aureus* in atopic dermatitis is supported by the observation that not only patients with impetiginized atopic dermatitis, but also atopic dermatitis patients without superinfection, show clinical response to combined treatment with anti-staphylococcal antibiotics and topical corticosteroids.

Furthermore, *S. aureus* also secretes a group of toxins (staphylococcal enterotoxins: SEA, SEB) and toxic shock syndrome toxin-1 known to act as superantigens that stimulate marked activation of T cells and macrophages. Nearly half of atopic dermatitis patients produce IgE directed to these staphylococcal toxins. These findings suggest that local production of staphylococcal enterotoxins at the skin surface could cause IgE-mediated histamine release and thereby trigger the itch-scratch cycle that can exacerbate atopic dermatitis.

The mechanism of atopic dermatitis susceptibility to microbes has been studied regarding endogenous antimicrobial peptides known as cathelicidins and β-defensin. These peptides have significant antimicrobial activity against *S. aureus*. Antimicrobial peptide expression was significantly decreased in acute and chronic lesions from atopic dermatitis patients, but increased in psoriasis. This deficiency in the expression of antimicrobial peptides may account for the susceptibility of atopic dermatitis patients to skin infection with *S. aureus*.

IMMUNOHISTOLOGY

IMMUNOHISTOLOGICAL FINDINGS The histological features of atopic dermatitis depend on the acuity and therefore the duration of the skin lesion. Uninvolved or clinically normal skin of atopic dermatitis patients is histologically abnormal and demonstrates mild hyperkeratosis, epidermal hyperplasia, and a sparse dermal cellular infiltrate consisting primarily of T lymphocytes. Acute lesions are characterized by marked intercellular edema (spongiosis) of the epidermis, and intracellular edema noted as ballooning of the keratinocytes. A sparse epidermal infiltrate consisting primarily of T lymphocytes is frequently observed. In the dermis, there is a marked perivenular inflammatory-cell infiltrate consisting predominantly of lymphocytes, and occasional monocyte-macrophages. Eosinophils, basophils, and neutrophils are rarely present in the acute lesion. In chronic lichenified lesions, the epidermis is hyperplastic with elongation of the rete ridges, prominent hyperkeratosis, and minimal spongiosis. Increased numbers of Langerhans cells (LCs) are present in the epidermis, and macrophages dominate the dermal mononuclear cell infiltrate. Mast cells are increased in number but are generally fully granulated. Endothelial cells of the superficial venular plexus and deep venules are hypertrophied with enlarged nuclei and prominent nucleoli.

PATTERNS OF CYTOKINE EXPRESSION IN ATOPIC DERMATITIS SKIN LESIONS

In humans and mice, two types of CD4+ T-cell clones have been described, based on their pattern of cytokine secretion. Th1 cells secrete IL-2 and IFN-γ, but not IL-4, and IL-5. In contrast, Th2 cells produce IL-4, IL-5, and IL-13, but not IFN-γ. The patterns of cytokines expressed locally play a critical role in modulating the nature of tissue inflammation. Therefore, an analysis of cytokine expression at different clinical stages of atopic dermatitis is important for elucidation of its immunopathogenesis. The *in situ* hybridization technique has been used to investigate the expression of IL-4, IL-5, and IFN-γ mRNA in skin biopsies from clinically normal (uninvolved), acute (erythematous atopic dermatitis lesions of <3-d duration), and chronic (>2-wk duration) skin lesions of patients with atopic dermatitis. As compared with normal control skin, uninvolved skin of patients with atopic dermatitis had a significant increase in number of cells expressing IL-4 and IL-13, but not IL-5 or IFN-γ, mRNA. Acute and chronic skin lesions, when compared to normal skin or uninvolved skin of atopic dermatitis patients, in addition to having significantly greater numbers of cells that were positive for mRNA for IL-4 and IL-13, also had increased IL-5 producing cells. However, neither acute atopic dermatitis nor uninvolved atopic dermatitis skin contained significant numbers of IFN-γ mRNA-expressing cells. As compared with acute atopic dermatitis, chronic atopic dermatitis skin lesions had significantly fewer IL-4 and IL-13 mRNA-expressing cells, but significantly greater IL-5 and IFN-γ mRNA-expressing cells. These data indicate that although cells in acute and chronic atopic dermatitis lesions are associated with increased activation of IL-4, IL-5, and IL-13 genes, acute skin inflammation in atopic dermatitis is associated with a predominance of IL-4 and IL-13 expression, while maintenance of chronic inflammation is predominantly associated with increased IL-5 and IFN-γ producing cells accompanied by the infiltration of eosinophils and macrophages. Studies on the expression of cytokine receptor mRNA have shown that a high expression of IL-4 receptor is associated with acute atopic dermatitis while IL-5 and GM-CSF receptors are increased in chronic atopic dermatitis.

Studies have demonstrated overexpression of IL-16 in acute skin lesions, which may promote CD4+ T-cell recruitment into the lesions. The overexpression of IL-12 and GM-CSF in chronic lesions is likely to enhance cell survival of eosinophils and macrophages in skin lesions, and may promote alteration in dendritic cells.

Confirming the findings in clinically acute vs chronic dermatitis, the biphasic pattern of T-cell activation has also been demonstrated in studies of atopic patch test reaction sites (Table 97-4). At early time points, 24 h after allergen application, increased expression of IL-4 mRNA and protein, which is derived from Th2 cell clones, is observed. In contrast, IFN-γ mRNA is strongly overexpressed at greater than 48 h but not at early time-points, suggesting early emergence of a mixed Th1 plus Th2 cytokine profile.

Interestingly, the increased expression of IFN-γ mRNA in atopic patch test lesions is preceded by a peak of IL-12 expression coinciding with the infiltration of macrophages and eosinophils, and both cell types are known to express IL-12. These observations give rise to the proposition that initiation of atopic dermatitis is driven by allergen-induced activation of Th2 type cells, and that the chronic type-I inflammatory response is driven by the infiltration of IL-12 expressing eosinophils and macrophages accompanying the initial Th2 response (Fig. 97-1).

Table 97-4
Cells and Cytokines in Atopic Dermatitis Skin Lesions

Cell type	Uninvolved	Acute	Chronic
	Nature of skin lesion		
T cells	+	+++	++
Eosinophils	−	+	+++
Macrophages	−	++	+++
	Cytokine gene expression		
IL-4/IL-13	+	++++	+++
IL-5	−	++	+++
IFN-γ	−	−	++
IL-12	−	−	++
IL-16	+	+++	++
GM-CSF	−	+	++

MOLECULAR BASIS OF IMMUNO-REGULATION

Based on observations from the previously mentioned immunohistological studies, T cells and T cell-derived cytokines play a central role in immune responses in atopic dermatitis. These responses intimately orchestrate the role of other immune competent cells such as antigen-presenting cells (APCs), eosinophils, mast cells, keratinocytes, and endothelial cells.

As with CD4+ T cells, increasing evidence suggests that CD8+ T cells can secrete either a Th1-like cytokine pattern or a Th2-like pattern. It has been recommended that T cells be referred to as type I (IFN-γ, IL-2 predominant) and type II (IL-4, IL-5, IL-10, IL-13 predominant), respectively, rather than referring to Th1, Tc1$_{(cytotoxic)}$ and Th2, Tc2$_{(suppressor)}$. In addition to the studies on cytokine production by Th1 and Th2 cells, the factors responsible for the polarization of the specific immune response into a predominant type-I or type-II profile have been extensively studied. Atopic dermatitis is a distinct model of type-I/II profile alterations in skin disease. The following focuses on underlying immunoregulatory abnormalities of cytokines and chemokines released from activation of T cells and other populations of immune competent cells in the different stages of atopic dermatitis (*see* Fig. 97-1).

LANGERHANS' CELLS LC are the predominant dendritic APC residing in the epidermis. In normal skin, there is a compartmentalization of LC phenotypes with epidermal LC: CD1a^{high}, CD1b−, CD36−, whereas dermal LCs are CD1a^{low}, CD1b+, and CD36−. In atopic dermatitis lesional skin, however, in addition to LC expressing CD1a^{high}, in both epidermis and dermis, a group of cells is frequently present at a distinct stage of maturation. APC in atopic dermatitis lesions with this type of phenotype have been termed inflammatory dendritic epidermal cells (IDECs) expressing both CD1a and CD1b as well as CD36, CD32, and high FcεR1. The difference between LC and IDEC has been studied by the activity of protein-tyrosine kinases (PTK). Atopic FcεR1^{high} LC, after FcεR1 ligation, uniquely restrict PTK activity to target phospholipase C-γ (PTK substrate) for phosphorylation. Interestingly, IDEC only showed moderate PTK levels when compared with LC from normal skin. Furthermore, low to moderate PTK levels were observed in monocyte-derived DC, suggesting that IDEC may derive from circulating monocytes and may be different from LC. This implies that a functional FcεR1 signaling pathway in LC may only be active in atopic dermatitis. As a consequence, FcεR1 ligation leads to calcium mobilization and subsequent NF-kB activation in these cells. Thus, LC in atopic dermatitis may

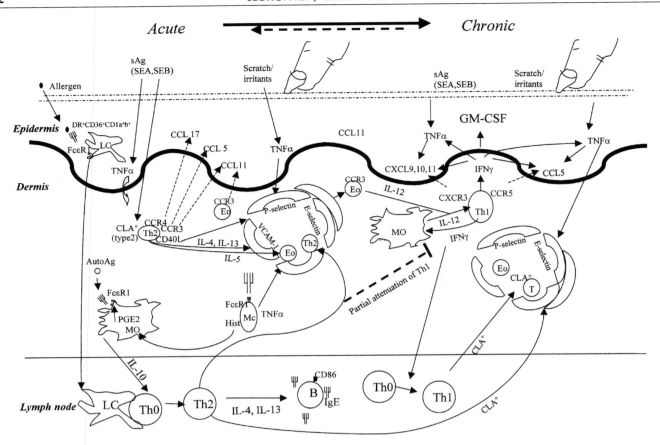

Figure 97-1   Molecular basis of immunopathogenesis in acute and chronic atopic dermatitis. In acute stage of atopic dermatitis, LC in the epidermis enable capture of allergens and autoantigens, which are then internalized, processed and packaged in major histocompatibility complex molecules on LC surface and induce activation of T cells in the draining lymph nodes. Increased monocyte PGE2 and IL-10 secretion directs T cell differentiation initially toward Th2 (CCR3+, CCR4+) with IL-4, IL-5, and IL-13 over-expression. Th2 cells (with cutaneous lymphocyte antigen molecule, CLA+) are recruited to the skin preferentially with the help of chemokines produced by various cells in the skin, such as CCL17 (thymus and activation regulated chemokine), CCL-11 (eotaxin-1), and CCL5 (RANTES). B cells are associated with the production of IgE with the help of IL-4, and IL-13 secreted from Th2 cells. CD86 upregulation on B cells is associated with IgE synthesis. Activated keratinocytes also can be stimulated by nonspecific irritants, such as scratch and superantigens, and produce TNF-α, GM-CSF, and chemokines critical for type-II T cells (early) and type-I T cells (late). Moreover, activated mast cells (e.g., crosslinking with FcεR1 on the cell surface) highly release TNF-α, IL-4, and IL-13, and together with CD40L on activated T cells enhance the expression of P-selectin, E-selectin, and VCAM-1 on endothelial cells. These molecules further promote recruitment of cells from the blood. Atopic dermatitis has a tendency toward chronicity with frequently relapsing course. In chronic stages, GM-CSF is overproduced in the thickened epidermis and can function to sustain APCs as well as eosinophils and other leukocytes. Eosinophils are elevated in atopic dermatitis blood and migrate into the dermis along with monocytic cells and T cells. Eosinophils are a source of IL-12, allowing a transition to induction of Th1 differentiation with IFN-γ production. In turn, IFN-γ promotes monocytic/macrophagic cell IL-12, further promoting Th1 differentiation. Activated keratinocytes and mast cells produce TNF-α, upregulating the expression of P-selectin, and E-selectin, on endothelial cells, thus recruiting more leukocytes from the blood. Moreover, TNF-α, particularly in combination with IFN-γ promotes production of chemokines such as CXCL9 (Mig), 10 (IP-10), 11 (I-TAC), ligands for CXCR3, and CCL5, a ligand for CCR5 on Th1 cells, resulting in further recruitment of cells capable of type-I immune responses. However, this type-I immune response may differ from conventional DTH because of partial attenuation by predominant Th2 responses in atopic dermatitis.

act in two ways to influence inflammatory reactions by IgE-mediated antigen focusing, which allows for T-cell activation at much reduced antigen concentrations, and by production of proinflammatory cytokines and chemokines.

Further, LC bearing FcεR1 are also an important bridge for IgE to mediate delayed-type hypersensitivity (DTH) to allergens. T cells reacting to major histocompatibility complex-bound peptides from allergenic proteins may be expressed in eczematous skin lesions after application of aeroallergens to clinically uninvolved skin of atopic patients. Of course, the heightened state of activity of LC in atopic dermatitis lesional skin would also facilitate activation of T-cells reactive to foreign microbial antigens presented in classic fashion (bacteria, fungi), as well as T-cells reactive to

superantigens and self-peptides, such that a complex, multiantigenic polyclonal T-cell response is generated.

MONOCYTES/MACROPHAGES   In addition to LC, monocytes also have increased expression of high affinity IgE receptors in atopic dermatitis. Interestingly, this FcεRI aggregation prevents generation of monocyte-derived dendritic cells implying that this receptor is modulating the differentiation of monocytes. Furthermore, monocytes are the source of increased prostaglandin E (PGE) 2 secretion in atopic dermatitis; PGE2 secretion is correlated with abnormally increased cAMP-phosphodiesterase (PDE) activity in mononuclear leukocytes, particularly in monocytes of atopic dermatitis patients. In addition, histamine subsequently induces elevation of cAMP via stimulation of H_2 receptors on monocytes. The increased cAMP-PDE activity and PGE2 secretion and cross-linking of FcεRI on monocytes results in increased atopic monocyte secretion of IL-10; IL-10 in turn inhibits Th1 response development and accentuates IL-4 secretion by Th2 cells and is likely active in initiating and flaring lesions and in the poor responses to fungal and viral infections in atopic dermatitis. In chronic lesions, however, monocytes are stimulated with IFN-γ from Th1 T lymphocytes, and may act in concert with eosinophils to produce IL-12 to further convert to Th1 phenotype during the chronic stage of the disease.

LYMPHOCYTES As mentioned, the predominant cell infiltrating atopic dermatitis skin is the T lymphocyte. Circulating T lymphocytes of atopic dermatitis patients are in a relatively more activated state, compared with those from normal control subjects. This heightened T-cell activation state is revealed by their elevated levels of secretory IL-2R, L-selectin, and the cell surface expression of HLA-DR, CD40L, and CLA, a phenotype of the homing antigen/allergen-reactive memory cells. This implies that a population of activated circulating T lymphocytes could represent skin-associated T-cell subset expansion with a low threshold for activation within the skin in patients with atopic dermatitis. Evidence for the relationship between CLA and cutaneous T-cell responses in atopic dermatitis comes from analysis of the CLA phenotype of circulating memory T cells in atopic dermatitis vs asthmatic patients who were sensitized with the house dust mite. When peripheral blood CLA$^+$CD3$^+$CD45RO$^+$ T cells were separated from CLA$^-$CD3$^+$CD45RO$^+$ T cells, the mite-specific T-cell proliferation response in patients with atopic dermatitis sensitized to dust mite was localized to CLA$^+$ T cells. In contrast, mite-sensitive asthmatics had strong mite-dependent proliferation responses in their CLA$^-$ T-cell subset. The link between CLA expression and skin disease-associated T-cell effector function in atopic dermatitis was demonstrated by the observation that freshly isolated circulating CLA$^+$ T cells in atopic dermatitis patients, but not normal controls, selectively demonstrated spontaneous production of IL-4, but not IFN-γ. These observations strongly support the concept that, in human allergic diseases, immunological mechanisms exist to target memory Th2 cells to specific organs.

Studies on allergen-stimulated T-cells, at least in the acute and early stage of atopic dermatitis, reveal that IL-4 and IL-5 are over-produced relative to IFN-γ production. The paucity of IFN-γ in early lesions is supported by the fact that keratinocytes in epidermis of early atopic dermatitis do not express HLA-DR, a molecule that is induced by high levels of IFN-γ, such as occurs in psoriasis. This differs from the Th1 cells demonstrating increased IFN-γ, but not IL-4 and IL-5 in conventional DTH. Furthermore, Th2 cells are just as effective in inducing skin inflammation as Th1 cells. These data suggest that two indistinguishable cutaneous DTH reactions exist: the first is mediated by IFN-γ-secreting Th1 cells found in conventional DTH reactions; the second is mediated by IL-4- and IL-5-secreting Th2 cells and involves allergen-induced, cell-mediated reactions. Th2 dominance over Th1 in atopic dermatitis may be because of selective apoptosis of Th1 T cells.

A major consequence of IL-4 production during acute flares and lesion reinitiation is the effect on B lymphocytes to undergo isotype switching to IgE production, as well as upregulation of IL-4R and CD 23 (another IgE receptor) on B cells. Moreover, the high expression of B7.2 (CD86) on B cells of atopic dermatitis patients is correlated well with serum IgE levels, suggesting that CD86 plays a novel role in IgE synthesis.

IL-5 is another type-II immune response cytokine produced by T cells and elevated in early atopic dermatitis lesions, and is likely a critical factor in eosinophil participation in atopic dermatitis lesions.

GM-CSF produced by atopic dermatitis keratinocytes appears to be acting in conjunction with IL-5 to promote tissue and blood eosinophilia in atopic dermatitis. It is also important for basophil development and differentiation.

EOSINOPHILS Extracellular deposition of eosinophil, but not neutrophil, granule proteins can be found in atopic dermatitis lesional skin. These eosinophil granule proteins are also increased in the peripheral blood of patients with atopic dermatitis and are correlated with disease activity. Eosinophils also elaborate the lymphocyte chemoattractant factor, IL-16 (elevated in acute atopic dermatitis), and CCL5 (RANTES), a chemoattractant for lymphocytes as well as eosinophils. In addition, CCL11 (eotaxin), a chemokine specifically chemotactic for eosinophils, can be produced by various cells including eosinophils, lymphocytes, macrophages, and fibroblasts. Interestingly, human eosinophils can also produce biologically active IL-12 after treatment with type-II cytokines. Thus, IL-12 may promote switching of Th0 to Th1 subset in chronic lesions resulting in IFN-γ production. These data suggest that eosinophils play a pathogenic role in acute and chronic atopic dermatitis.

MAST CELLS/BASOPHILS Both mast cells and basophils originate from bone marrow progenitors, and mast cells complete their maturation after migrating into tissues. The number of mast cells may be increased in chronic lichenified lesions of atopic dermatitis. However, their significance in atopic dermatitis remains unclear. Both cells express high affinity FcεR1 on cell membranes. IgE crosslinking with FcεR1 on the cells results in histamine release and type I immediate hypersensitivity, but this is not directly relevant to atopic dermatitis skin lesions. Increased basophil histamine release occurs in atopic dermatitis, and may be related to the persistent pruritus in patients. This increased leukocyte histamine release is correlated with elevated cAMP-PDE activity, and could indicate that chronic intermittent mast cell degranulation is a continuous process in lesional atopic dermatitis, although mediators from mast cells other than histamine are likely related to the itch, because potent antihistamines do not result in clearing of atopic dermatitis pruritus.

Both mast cells and basophils, when activated, produce important type-II cytokines, such as IL-4 and IL-13. Mast cells also produce tumor necrosis factor (TNF)-α. These cytokines promote activation of B cells for IgE production and leukocyte migration through upregulation of adhesion molecules on endothelial cells. Mast cells and basophils also express the ligand for CD40 (CD40L), which contributes to B-cell IgE production independently of T cells.

Thus, the mononuclear cell infiltrate in the acute atopic dermatitis skin lesion likely reflects a combination of both IgE-dependent mast cell/basophil degranulation and Th2-cell-mediated responses elicited during acute exposures to allergen and other antigens or superantigens.

KERATINOCYTES Keratinocytes actively contribute to the pathogenesis of atopic dermatitis mainly by producing a diverse array of cytokines and chemokines. Keratinocytes are an important epidermal source of cytokines including IL-1, IL-6, IL-8, GM-CSF, and TNF-α. In this regard, any injury including mechanical trauma (rubbing and scratching) to the keratinocyte results in the release of cytokines that can induce inflammation through a number of actions, including the release of IL-1 and TNF-α. They are critical cytokines in the induction of adhesion molecules, such as endothelial cell leukocyte adhesion molecule-1, intercellular adhesion molecule (ICAM)-1, and vascular cell adhesion molecule (VCAM)-1, which allow adhesion to endothelial cells and egress of lymphocytes, macrophages, and eosinophils into cutaneous sites of inflammation. At this stage, a variety of resident and infiltrating cells are then capable of secreting cytokines and mediators that sustain the inflammation. Atopic dermatitis therefore results from a combination of specific and nonspecific cellular mechanisms that serve to trigger and maintain skin inflammation.

GM-CSF, particularly in the chronic stage, is overexpressed in atopic dermatitis keratinocytes, and can be enhanced by IFN-γ and IL-1α. GM-CSF also promotes the survival, recruitment, and activation of dendritic cells, monocytes, T cells, and eosinophils, thus providing yet another mechanism for perpetuation of inflammation.

In addition to cytokines, keratinocytes are a major source of chemokines in skin, particularly in atopic dermatitis. CCL5, a ligand for CCR3 that is expressed in Th2 T cells, is a major chemokine produced by keratinocytes of lesional atopic dermatitis skin. CCL17 (thymus and activation-regulated chemokine), a ligand for CCR4, is elevated in atopic dermatitis skin; CCL17 plays an important role in recruiting CD4+ Th2, CLA+ memory lymphocytes.

Other chemokines elevated in atopic dermatitis, such as CXCL9 (Mig), CXCL10 (IP-10), and CXCL11 (I-TAC) are ligands for CXCR3, a chemokine receptor expressed on Th1 cells; Th1 cell IFN-γ and TNF-α can further induce keratinocytes to produce these chemokines, thus establishing another self-perpetuating mechanism of inflammation. Similarly, CCL5 (RANTES), a ligand for CCR5 on Th1 cells and on eosinophils, is also elevated in atopic dermatitis skin, and its production can be enhanced in keratinocytes with cytokines such as TNF-α. Once Th1 cells are recruited, they can induce apoptosis of keratinocytes mediated by IFN-γ, possibly accounting for spongiosis in atopic dermatitis lesions.

ENDOTHELIAL CELLS The recruitment of inflammatory cells, as mentioned, into lesional skin of atopic dermatitis requires traverse of blood cells through dermal venules likely following a chemokine gradient, guided by adhesion molecules. Activation of dermal venular endothelial cells is an essential step in this process. The adhesion molecules of endothelial cells, such as ICAM-1, VCAM-1, and E-selectin, can be upregulated by CD40L on activated T cells, and are critical for memory T-cell infiltration. Cytokines, such as TNF-α and IL-1α, from various cell sources in atopic dermatitis skin, induce similar upregulations. Additionally, the type-II cytokines IL-4 and IL-13 contribute to upregulated VCAM-1 expression, which may promote monocyte infiltration via VLAα4. An overview of the above immunological features of atopic dermatitis is shown in Table 97-5.

Taken together, the immunopathogenesis of atopic dermatitis is a complicated molecular-based network, involving the interaction of diverse cells with cascades of cytokines and chemokines that promote the continuation of inflammation. The main interactions of the above cells associated with acute and chronic stages of atopic dermatitis (*see* Fig. 97-1).

"EXTRINSIC" VS "INTRINSIC"

Elevation of IgE is one hallmark feature of atopic dermatitis, especially in those patients who also have respiratory allergy. Elevated serum-IgE is also an important feature even in the patients without respiratory allergy. However, there is a group of atopic dermatitis patients in which serum IgE levels are within normal limits. Therefore, some authors have attempted to subtype

Table 97-5
Immunologic Features of Atopic Dermatitis

Phenotypically distinct and hyperstimulatory Langerhans and dendritic cells in atopic dermatitis epidermis and dermis
High expression and aggregation of the high-affinity IgE receptor FcεR1 on epidermal LC
Autoreactive T cells respond to lesional LCs
Increased IgE production (skin and blood)
Eosinophilia
Immediate skin-test reactivity to multiple allergens
Increased basophil spontaneous histamine release
Increased expression of CD23 on mononuclear cells
Expansion of lL-4-, IL-5-, and IL-13-secreting Th2-like cells
Chronic macrophage activation with increased secretion of GM-CSF, PGE2, and IL-10
Decreased numbers of IFN-γ-secreting Th1-like cells
Decreased CD8 suppressor/cytotoxic number and function
Partial attenuation of Th1 immune responses
Dysregulation of apoptosis in Th1 and Th2 cells
Increased soluble E-selectin, VCAM-1, and ICAM-1 levels in peripheral blood
Chemokine induction and release in the skin
Endothelial cell activation

atopic dermatitis in terms of the elevation of serum IgE. One group of atopic dermatitis patients has high levels of serum IgE, with polyvalent IgE sensitization against inhalant and/or food allergens in skin test, and this group is termed extrinsic atopic dermatitis (EAD). The other group has no specific IgE sensitization on skin testing or radioallergosorbent test and total serum IgE is not elevated; these patients are termed intrinsic atopic dermatitis (IAD).

Some clinical differences between IAD and EAD have been described. IAD tends to have later onset with mild female predominance. Eosinophilia is only moderate. The expression of IL-4 levels of T cells and CD23+ B cells in peripheral blood, IL-5 and IL-13 levels derived from lesional skin and FcεRI expression on epidermal dendritic cells, are all lower compared with EAD. The expression of FcεRI, FcεRII, and IL4 Rα by monocytes is upregulated in EAD but not in IAD, although high expression of CD40 is found on monocytes both in EAD and IAD. IL-5 levels are significantly elevated in serum in EAD relative to IAD and normal. By contrast, IL-13 is significantly elevated in IAD relative to EAD, although both IL-13 levels are significantly higher than normal. This differs from the findings in lesional skin, in which IL-5 and IL-13 levels are all similarly elevated. However, consensus on whether IAD and EAD are distinct clinical entities has not been achieved. A study on atopy patch tests with house dust mites (*Dermatophagoides pteronyssinus* and *D. farinae*) in adults with low IgE (IAD) and high IgE (EAD) contradicted this concept by showing that the atopy patch test was positive in 47% of EAD, in 67% of IAD, and in 12% of nonatopic healthy subjects. The positivity of atopic dermatitis compared with normal was highly significant, but, IAD patients had similar or even higher positivity than EAD patients.

Enhanced PTK activity for phosphorylation of phospholipase Cγ1 was found in FcεRIhigh LC from atopic dermatitis patients. However, the fact that FcεRIhigh IDECs displayed similar amounts of PTK to that of FcεRIlow LC from normal skin argues against the concept that PTK is a marker of IAD and EAD subgroups. Definitive segregation of subsets of atopic dermatitis will likely

desmosomal plaque proteins (desmoplakins, periplakins, and envoplakins), a hemidesmosomal component (BP230), and an unidentified 170-kDa protein. The whole IgG fraction as well as affinity purified anti-dsg3 antibodies from PNP patients are pathogenic when tested by passive transfer experiments in the mouse model. The animals develop the skin phenotype of PV and show suprabasilar acantholysis in histopathology. Moreover, immunoadsorption of the PNP sera with recombinant Dsg3 eliminates the sera's pathogenicity in the mouse model. These findings demonstrate the pathogenic role of anti-Dsg3 antibodies in PNP sera. However, it is not clear what causes the different clinical phenotypes of PNP and PV. It has been speculated that both humoral and cellular mediated immune responses play a role in the pathogenesis of PNP.

Because the development of a humoral response requires T-cell activity, the identification of T-cell epitopes is important to understanding how autoimmune disease develops and progresses. Although several investigative groups have reported that peptides derived from Dsg3 induce the proliferation of T cells isolated from PV patients, no immunodominant T-cell epitope has been identified. The ectodomain of Dsg1 is also capable of stimulating T-cell clones from FS patients. Furthermore, a peptide derived from the EC5 domain of Dsg1 causes T-cell proliferation isolated from a subset of PV patients who possess both anti-Dsg3 and anti-Dsg1 antibodies. The autoreactive T cells in PV as well as in FS all have Th2-like cytokine profiles and Th2-dependent IgG4 is the predominant IgG subclass found in PV and PF/FS. Taken together, this suggests that autoreactive Th2 responses play an important role in the pathogenesis of PV and PF/FS.

MANAGEMENT/TREATMENT Despite the tremendous advances in the understanding of the molecular pathogenesis of PV and PF, the mainstay of treatment remains corticosteroids and other immunosuppressive agents. Before immunosuppressive therapy, the 5-yr mortality of PV approached 100%. The prognosis in PF was slightly better, with a 40–60% mortality rate. Despite the effective steroid and immunosuppressive therapy, the 5-yr mortality remains between 5 and 15%. The majority of cases of PV and PF require initial systemic steroids in doses that vary from 0.5 to 1 mg/kg/d of prednisone. In the small number of patients within this group who enter into clinical and serological remission, the steroids may be gradually reduced. To prevent relapses, steroid tapering is conducted over several months. Once the patient reaches a prednisone dose of 30 mg/d, tapering is continued by alternate day dosing. Some patients require additional immunosuppressive agents. Cytotoxic agents including azathioprine (1–2 mg/kg/d), cyclophosphamide (1–2 mg/kg/d), methotrexate (5–15 mg/wk), and mycophenolate mofetil (1–3 g/d) have been used in conjunction with prednisone to effectively control the disease.

Parenteral gold has been successfully used in the therapy of PV, but because of the incidence of side effects over long-term therapy including dermatitis, nephrotoxicity, and blood dyscrasias, its use has been limited. Other drugs occasionally reported to be effective in pemphigus include cyclosporine, etretinate, and dapsone.

In patients with refractory disease, plasmapheresis can be used as an adjunct therapy to acutely decrease the titers of circulating antibody; however, a rebound rise in autoantibody titers will occur if the patient is not concurrently treated with systemic immunosuppressive agents. Several reports have described the beneficial effects of intravenous Ig as an effective therapy for treatment resistant PV and PF. The mechanism by which intravenous Ig induces clinical and serological disease remission has yet to be defined. Rituximab, a chimeric anti-CD20 monoclonal antibody

approved for use in CD20+ B-cell non-Hodgkins lymphoma, has shown promise for treatment refractory PV.

Patients on immunosuppressive therapy must be monitored for toxicity with a variety of laboratory tests including CBC, liver enzymes, creatinine, and urinalysis. Patients should be closely monitored for infection throughout the course of treatment. Patients on prednisone should be monitored for the development or worsening of conditions such as diabetes, hypertension, and osteoporosis that are exacerbated by systemic corticosteroids. Indirect IF studies of the patient's serum should be performed every 6–8 wk to monitor serological disease remission or relapse.

FUTURE DIRECTIONS There has been remarkable progress in characterizing the autoantibodies and target autoantigens in PV, PF, and PNP; however, the events that result in the production of these autoantibodies have not been defined. In essence, the etiology of pemphigus remains elusive. In this regard, because of the high incidence of disease and likely environmental factors that contribute to disease development, endemic PF offers a unique opportunity to identify the inciting agent and to begin to determine how cutaneous autoimmunity develops. Additional issues that need to be addressed include determining the (1) mechanism by which self-tolerance is broken, (2) T-cell epitope(s) implicated in promoting autoantibody production, and (3) the precise mechanism underlying acantholysis. The identification of B-cell and T-cell epitopes on Dsg3 and Dsg1 should pave the way for more specific therapies, including the induction of immunological tolerance. The availability of the active mouse model will be valuable for testing therapies including biological immunomodulatory agents.

BULLOUS PEMPHIGOID, CICATRICIAL PEMPHIGOID AND HERPES GESTATIONES

In 1953, Lever described the disease entity known as bullous pemphigoid (BP) as a subepidermal bullous dermatoses seen in the elderly. Subsequently IF techniques were used to demonstrate that BP patients have circulating and tissue-bound autoantibodies directed against antigens of the basement membrane zone (BMZ). The term "pemphigoid" applies to several different disorders that share the clinical appearance of vesicles and bullae, the histological finding of subepidermal blistering, and *in situ* deposition of autoantibodies at the BMZ (Table 98-1). Extensive skin involvement in the elderly population occasionally leads to significant morbidity. In addition, therapy with systemic corticosteroids and immunosuppressive agents may be associated with significant adverse effects.

CLINICAL FEATURES The precise incidence of pemphigoid is not known, but it is estimated to be twice that of PV. The incidence in Great Britain was estimated at 1/100,000/yr in 1985 and 7.63/million in France in 1995. There are three closely related pemphigoid diseases, namely BP, cicatricial (mucosal) pemphigoid (CP), and herpes gestationis (HG).

Bullous Pemphigoid BP appears to be a phenomenon of the aging immune system, with a peak incidence late in life. There is no known HLA class II gene that confers susceptibility for the disease; however, in the related disorder HG, approx 60–85% of patients are HLA-DR3 positive. Strikingly, approx 45% of women affected with HG are heterozygote HLA-DR3/DR4.

Often generalized BP has a predilection for the lower abdomen, inner thighs, groin, and axillae. The blisters are pruritic and appear on either normal skin or an erythematous, urticarial base (Fig. 98-6A). When blisters rupture, denuded areas may become crusted and occasionally invaded by pathogenic bacteria.

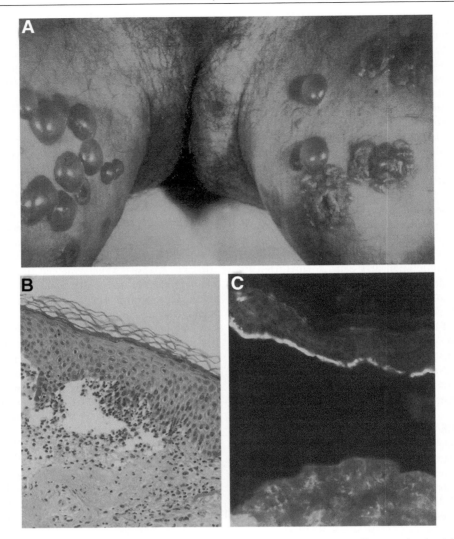

Figure 98-6 Clinical, histological, and immunological features of bullous pemphigoid. **(A)** Tense blisters and urticarial plaques develop on skin. **(B)** Histologically, biopsies of bullous pemphigoid show subepidermal bulla with an inflammatory infiltrate, including eosinophils, neutrophils, and lymphocytes. **(C)** Direct IF of skin section exhibits linear IgG deposition at the BMZ.

The course and prognosis of BP varies. Most treated patients go into a clinical remission within several months without need for further treatment.

Cicatricial Pemphigoid   CP is a relatively rare condition characterized by chronic blistering and scarring of mucosal surfaces covered by stratified squamous epithelium. Involved organs include the ocular conjunctiva, nasal pharynx, oral pharynx, larynx, upper esophagus, and anogenital mucosa. The marked tendency for scarring in this disorder leads to high morbidity secondary to loss of vision, esophageal strictures, and fibrotic scarring of other mucous membranes.

Herpes Gestationis   HG, also known as pemphigoid gestationis, is a relatively rare disease seen during pregnancy. The disorder often begins in the second or third trimester of pregnancy. It tends to recur in subsequent pregnancies and may be elicited by a challenge with oral contraceptives. Lesions tend to involve the abdomen and then spread peripherally. The lesion morphology is similar to that of BP.

LABORATORY DIAGNOSIS

Histopathology   The histopathology of BP, CP, and HG are similar; examination of an early intact blister reveals a subepidermal blister with a mixed inflammatory infiltrate rich in eosinophils. The blister cavity contains serum, fibrin, and inflammatory cells (Fig. 98-6B).

Direct IF   The ideal substrate for this test is a biopsy of normal-appearing skin adjacent to a lesion. A properly performed test from such a specimen is positive in essentially 100% of BP patients revealing a continuous linear deposition of C3 and IgG along the epidermal BMZ (Fig. 98-6C). Direct IF in HG and CP is similar to that of BP.

Indirect IF   The most commonly used substrate for this test is monkey esophagus, although other stratified squamous epithelia such as normal human skin may be used. Most patients with BP have circulating IgG autoantibodies against the BMZ. These antibodies bind to the basement membrane macromolecules of stratified squamous epithelia. By the use of 1 M NaCl-split human skin as substrate, BP autoantibodies have been shown to bind to the epidermal side of the artificial split, a test useful in distinguishing BP from epidermolysis bullosa acquisita, an autoimmune subepidermal blistering disease in which the autoantibodies bind to the dermal side of the cleavage plane of salt split skin. By standard methods, indirect IF for antibody deposition is usually negative in HG; however, anti-BMZ antibodies can be detected by complement-fixation amplification (HG factor assay) on intact or NaCl-split skin or by Western blotting. Of patients with CP, approx 25% have circulating anti-BMZ antibodies as detected by standard indirect IF. The site of autoantibody binding on NaCl-split human skin may be epidermal, dermal, or both.

Immunoelectromicroscopy On direct immunoelectromicroscopy (IEM), in vivo bound immune deposits (C3 and IgG) are seen in the lamina lucida of the BMZ as well as in the basal-cell hemidesmosomes. Similarly, circulating BP antibodies are directed against both the basal-cell hemidesmosomes as well as the lamina lucida on indirect IEM. The findings in HG are similar; however, in CP the autoantibodies localize to the hemidesmosomes, lamina lucida, and/or lamina densa.

AUTOANTIGENS AND AUTOANTIBODIES

Bullous Pemphigoid BP autoantibodies recognize two antigens, the hemidesmosome proteins BP180 and BP230. Both BP180 and BP230 have been cloned and characterized at the molecular level. The hemidesmosome is an organelle that mediates a stable interaction between the keratin intermediate filament proteins of the basilar pole of the keratinocyte and transmembrane adhesion molecules that anchor the basal cell to the underlying lamina densa of the basement membrane.

BP230 (also referred to as BPAg1) is an intracellular protein that localizes to the hemidesmosomal plaque and has significant homology with plectin and desmoplakins I and II. BP230 contains a central α-helical coiled–coil rod domain flanked by two globular domains. BPAg1 has been mapped to chromosome 6 (6p12-p11) in humans and to the proximal region of chromosome 1 in mice. BP230-specific autoantibodies recognize multiple epitopes on this molecule and belong to IgG and IgE immunoglobulin classes.

In contrast, BP180 (also referred to as BPAG2 and type XVII collagen) is a transmembrane protein with a type-II orientation (Fig. 98-7). Its amino-terminal region localizes to the intracellular hemidesmosomal plaque, whereas its carboxyl-terminal portion projects into the extracellular milieu of the BMZ. The extracellular region consists of 15 collagen domains separated from one another by noncollagen sequences. Mutations in the BP180 gene result in the nonlethal, but generalized blistering disease congenital epidermolysis bullosa, demonstrating the BP180's role in normal epithelial development. The BPAg2 has been mapped to chromosome 10 (10q24.3) in humans and to the distal end of chromosome 19 in mice. BP180-specific autoantibodies predominantly target epitopes located within the NC16A region of the molecule and are IgE, IgG1, and IgG4. Serum levels of anti-BP180 IgG and IgE are directly correlated with disease severity. Additionally, most BP patients have autoreactive T cells that recognize epitopes located in the extracellular region of BP180 and mainly in the NC16A domain. These T lymphocytes express CD4 memory T-cell surface markers and exhibit a Th1/Th2 mixed cytokine profile. These observations suggest that BP is a T- and B-cell-dependent and antibody-mediated skin autoimmune disease.

Herpes Gestationis HG autoantibodies react mainly with BP180 and, less frequently, with BP230. IgG autoantibodies in most HG sera recognize epitopes in the NC16A domain, which are different from those recognized by BP autoantibodies. Anti-NC16A autoantibodies belong to IgG1 and IgG3 subclasses. BP180-specific T cells react with NC16A and express a CD4+ Th1 memory phenotype.

Cicatricial Pemphigoid CP autoantibodies target multiple antigens, including BP180, laminin 5, laminin 6, β_4-integrin, and

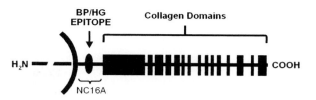

Figure 98-7 A schematic diagram of the structural organization of the human BP180 protein. The arch designates the transmembrane domain. The oval designates the NC16A antigenic site recognized by autoantibodies of bullous pemphigoid and herpes gestationis. The COOH-terminal extracellular region is made up of 15 interrupted collagen-like domains (black rectangles).

type-VII collagen. Isotypes of these autoantibodies are IgA and IgG. Among these autoantigens, BP180 is the most common. The majority of CP sera with BP180-specific CP autoantibodies react with epitopes in the C-terminal, NC16A, or central portion of the BP180 ectodomain. By indirect IEM, these anti-BP180 CP antibodies localize to the lamina lucida-lamina densa interface.

Laminin 5 (also referred to as epiligrin, kalinin, nicein, or BM600) is a heterotrimeric extracellular protein linking BP180 and α6β4 integrin with extracellular matrix components of the basement membrane. Anti-laminin 5 CP autoantibodies bind to the dermal side of NaCl-split human skin and localize to the lower region of the lamina lucida by IEM. Some CP patients have circulating autoantibodies reactive with the β_4-subunit of $\alpha_6\beta_4$-integrin or type-VII collagen.

IMMUNOPATHOLOGICAL MECHANISMS OF BLISTER FORMATION

BP and Herpes Gestationis Blister formation in BP and HG was thought to be an IgG autoantibody-mediated process; however, previous attempts to demonstrate the pathogenicity of patient autoantibodies had been unsuccessful. Antihuman BP180 NC16A autoantibodies fail to crossreact with the murine form of this autoantigen and thus cannot be assayed for pathogenicity in a conventional passive transfer mouse model. As an alternative, rabbit polyclonal antibodies were made against a segment of the murine BP180 protein homologous to human BP180 NC16A (mBP180 NC14A); purified rabbit anti-mBP180 IgG was then passively transferred to neonatal BALB/c mice. The injected animals developed a blistering disease that closely mimicked human BP, including in vivo deposition of rabbit IgG and mouse C3 at the BMZ and dermo-epidermal junction (DEJ) separation with an inflammatory cell infiltrate (Fig. 98-8). Further characterization of this IgG passive transfer model has revealed that subepidermal blistering is initiated by anti-BP180 antibodies and depends on complement activation, mast cell degranulation, and neutrophil infiltration.

Neutrophil infiltration is a prerequisite for experimental BP and the disease severity is directly correlated to the number of infiltrating neutrophils. Mice depleted of neutrophils are resistant to experimental BP. Blocking neutrophil infiltration abolishes subepidermal blistering. On activation through molecular interaction between Fc of pathogenic anti-mBP180 IgG and Fc receptors on the cell surface of neutrophils, infiltrating neutrophils release several proteolytic enzymes including neutrophil elastase (NE) and gelatinase B (GB). Mice lacking NE or GB are resistant to experimental BP. Although both GB and NE are capable of degrading the recombinant BP180 protein in vitro, only NE produces DEJ separation when incubated with skin sections. In vivo, NE compensates for the lack of GB, whereas GB cannot compensate for NE deficiency in the development of BP. In addition, the degradation of BP180

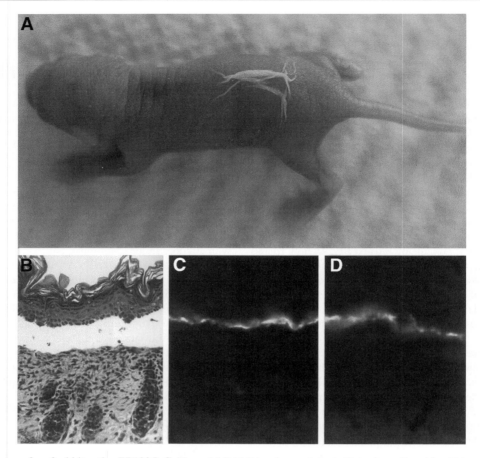

Figure 98-8   Passive transfer of rabbit anti-mBP180 IgG. Neonatal BALB/c mice are injected intradermally with rabbit anti-murine BP180 IgG. After 24 h, gentle friction elicits persistent epidermal wrinkling, producing the "epidermal detachment" sign (**A**). Histological examination of lesional skin reveals dermal–epidermal junction separation with an inflammatory infiltrate (**B**). Direct IF analysis shows deposition of anti-BP180 IgG (**C**) and murine C3 (**D**) at the BMZ.

in vivo depends on NE activity. Further dissection of this prote-olytic event in experimental BP reveals a functional relationship between GB and NE; GB proteolytically inactivates α1-proteinase inhibitor, the physiological inhibitor of NE. Unchecked NE then cleaves extracellular matrix proteins including BP180 antigen, resulting in DEJ separation. In total, these studies provide compelling evidence that anti-BP180 autoantibodies are pathogenic and suggest an immunopathological mechanism of subepidermal blistering in BP.

The pathogenic role of anti-BP180 antibodies has been confirmed by other in vitro and in vivo studies. BP180NC16A-specific autoantibodies purified from human BP sera induce dermal-epidermal separation in cryosections of human skin in the presence of neutrophils. This study confirms earlier findings in which BP autoantibodies induced DEJ separation in human skin sections only in the presence of both leukocytes (mostly neutrophils) and complement. Like the rabbit anti-mBP180 IgG passive transfer model, rabbit antibodies directed against the extracellular domain of hamster BP180 (NC16A region) trigger BP-like subepidermal blisters in neonatal hamsters. In addition, although human BP blister fluid has high levels of both NE and GB, BP180 degradation by blister fluid depends on NE activity.

It is not clear what role, if any, antibodies specific for the BPAg1 play in the development of lesions. Passive transfer of human antibodies against the BPAg1 does not produce inflammation in murine skin. Rabbits that are immunized to the antigen and have circulating anti-BPAg1 antibodies do not develop cutaneous lesions, although

these animals do exhibit an unusual inflammatory reaction to UV radiation. In this circumstance, erythematous doses of UV light produce marked epidermal inflammation and keratinocyte necrosis suggesting that antibodies against BPAg1 may result in secondary inflammatory events in vivo.

Cicatricial Pemphigoid   Although anti-BP180NC16A antibodies have been shown to be pathogenic in BP, the pathogenicity of CP autoantibodies directed against the central portion and C-terminal portion of the BP180 ectodomain has not been demonstrated. In contrast, anti-laminin 5 CP antibodies have been demonstrated to be pathogenic by IgG passive transfer:

1. Rabbit anti-laminin 5 induced a subepidermal blistering disease in neonatal mice.
2. Human anti-laminin 5 autoantibodies induce subepidermal blisters in an experimental human skin graft model.
3. Mice receiving rabbit anti-laminin 5 Fab fragments developed CP.

These studies demonstrated that neither complement activation nor crosslinking of laminin 5 in epidermal basement membranes was required for induction of subepidermal blister formation in this animal model of a human autoimmune bullous disease. When incubated with normal human conjunctiva tissue sections, β_4-integrin specific autoantibodies from ocular CP sera induce BMZ separation suggesting that circulating anti-β_4-integrin autoantibodies are pathogenic in ocular CP.

MANAGEMENT Pemphigoid, a disorder with prominent inflammatory features, results from an abnormal immune response. In the absence of effective therapy, elderly patients with extensive erosions may develop complications including fluid loss, electrolyte imbalance, bacterial colonization with potential sepsis, and scarring. Therapy for pemphigoid is directed at suppressing the inflammation and/or the immune response.

Patients with generalized BP require systemic therapy; the most commonly used agents are the corticosteroids. Immunosuppressive therapy with azathioprine, cyclophosphamide, mycophenolate mofetil, and methotrexate has been used as steroid-sparing agents. Similar precautions as described in the treatment of PV and PF should be followed. Dapsone is effective in controlling the diseases in some BP patients. Potential side effects of dapsone include hemolysis, hepatitis, and peripheral neuropathies; monitoring for the development of these effects includes laboratory and physical examination at initial and subsequent visits. High potency topical steroids (e.g., clobetasol) under occlusion and systemic intravenous Ig are two additional therapies effective in BP management, particularly in patients in whom comorbid conditions may restrict the use of systemic immunosuppressive therapy. Animal model studies show that intravenous Ig is effective in treating BP, PF, and PV. The mode of intravenous Ig action in these autoantibody-mediated bullous diseases is to accelerate clearance of pathogenic antibody by saturating the IgG protective receptor FcRn. The failure of tumor necrosis factor-α knockout mice to develop blisters by passive transfer of BP180 antibodies suggests that anti- tumor necrosis factor-α biologics may have a future therapeutic role in BP. The treatment of CP and HG follows the same principles as that of BP.

FUTURE DIRECTIONS Extensive information has been derived about the molecular structure and biological functions of autoantigens in BP, HG, and CP. Animal models have confirmed the pathogenic role of some of these autoantibodies in the induction of skin lesions. Future research should be directed toward further dissection of the mechanisms of antibody-mediated tissue injury and the immune response that results in the production of pathogenic autoantibodies. The goal of such studies is to develop treatments of greater specificity and potency that have a more tolerable risk-benefit profile.

ACKNOWLEDGMENTS

This work was supported in part by grants R01 AR40410, R01 AI40768, R01 AR32599, R37 AR32081, and T32 AR07577 from the National Institutes of Health.

SELECTED REFERENCES

Ahmed AR, Yunis EY, Khatri K, et al. Major histocompatibility complex haplotypes studies in Ashkenazi Jewish patients with pemphigus vulgaris. Proc Natl Acad Sci USA 1990;87:7658–7662.

Amagai M, Klaus-Kovtun V, Stanley JR. Autoantibodies against a novel epithelial cadherin in pemphigus vulgaris, a disease of cell adhesion. Cell 1991;67:869–877.

Anhalt GJ, Kim SC, Stanley JR, et al. Paraneoplastic pemphigus: an autoimmune mucocutaneous disease associated with neoplasia. N Engl J Med 1990;323:1729–1735.

Anhalt GJ, Labib R, Voorhees JJ, et al. Induction of pemphigus in neonatal mice by passive transfer of IgG from patients with the disease. N Engl J Med 1982;306:1189–1196.

Berkowitz P, Hu P, Liu Z, et al. Desmosome signaling: inhibition of p38MAPK prevents pemphigus vulgaris IgG induced cytoskeleton reorganization. J Biol Chem 2005;280:23778–23784.

Budinger L, Borradori L, Yee C, et al. Identification and characterization of autoreactive CD4+ T-cell responses to the extracellular domain of bullous pemphigoid antigen 2 in patients with bullous pemphigoid and normals. J Clin Invest 1998;102:2082–2089.

Chan RY, Bhol K, Tesavibul N, et al. The role of antibody to human beta4 integrin in conjunctival basement membrane separation: possible in vitro model for ocular cicatricial pemphigoid. Invest Ophthalmol Vis Sci 1999; 40:2283–2290.

Diaz LA, Ratrie H 3rd, Saunders WS, et al. Isolation of a human epidermal cNA corresponding to the 180-kD autoantigen recognized by bullous pemphigoid and herpes gestationis sera. Immunolocalization of this protein to the hemidesmosome. J Clin Invest 1990;86: 1088–1094.

Diaz LA, Sampaio SAP, Rivitti EA, et al. Endemic pemphigus foliaceous (fogo selvagem): II. Current and historical epidemiological studies. J Invest Dermatol 1989;92:4–12.

Domloge-Hultsch N, Gammon WR, Briggaman RA, Gil SG, Carter WG, Yancey KB. Epiligrin, the major human keratinocyte integrin ligand, is a target in both an acquired autoimmune and an inherited subepidermal blistering skin disease. J Clin Invest 1992;90:1628–1633.

Giudice GJ, Emery DJ, Zelickson BD, Anhalt GJ, Liu Z, Diaz LA. Bullous pemphigoid and herpes gestationis autoantibodies recognize a common non-collagenous site on the BP180 ectodomain. J Immunol 1993;151: 5742–5750.

Jordon RE, Kawana S, Fritz KA. Immunopathologic mechanisms in pemphigus and bullous pemphigoid. J Invest Dermatol 1985;85: 72s–78s.

Katz SI, Hertz KC, Yaoita H. Herpes gestationis: immunopathology and characterization of the HG factor. J Clin Invest 1976;57: 1434–1441.

Lazarova Z, Yee C, Darling T, Briggaman RA, Yancey KB. Passive transfer of anti-laminin 5 antibodies induces subepidermal blisters in neonatal mice. J Clin Invest 1996;98:1509–1518.

Lever WF. Pemphigus. Medicine 1953;32:1–123.

Lever WF. Pemphigus vulgaris. In: Lever WF, ed. Pemphigus and Pemphigoid. Springfield, IL: Charles C. Thomas, 1965:15–72.

Li N, Aoki V, Hans-Filho G, Rivittin EA, Diaz LA. The role of intramolecular epitope spreading in the pathogenesis of endemic pemphigus foliaceus (Fogo Selvagem) J Exp Med 2003;197:1501–1510.

Lin MS, Mascaro JM Jr, Liu Z, Espana A, Diaz LA. The desmosome and hemidesmosome in cutaneous autoimmunity. Clin Exp Immunol 1997; 107:9–15.

Liu Z, Diaz LA, Troy JT, et al. A passive transfer model for the organ-specific autoimmune disease, bullous pemphigoid, using antibodies generated against the hemidesmosomal antigen, BP180. J Clin Invest 1993;92:2480–2486.

Liu Z, Zhou X, Shapiro SD, et al. The serpin alpha1-proteinase inhibitor is a critical substrate for gelatinase B/MMP-9 in vivo. Cell 2000;102: 647–655.

Roscoe JT, Diaz LA, Sampaio SAP, et al. Brazilian pemphigus foliaceus autoantibodies are pathogenic to BALB/c mice by passive transfer. J Invest Dermatol 1985;85:538–541.

Stanley JR, Tanaka T, Mueller S, Klaus-Kovtun V, Roop D. Isolation of complementary DNA for bullous pemphigoid antigen by use of patients' autoantibodies. J Clin Invest 1988;82:1864–1870.

Verraes S, Hornebeck W, Polette M, Borradori L, Bernard P. Respective contribution of neutrophil elastase and matrix metalloproteinase 9 in the degradation of BP180 (type XVII collagen) in human bullous pemphigoid. J Invest Dermatol 2001;117:1091–1096.

99 Systemic Lupus Erythematosus

AMR H. SAWALHA, LUIS A. DIAZ, AND JOHN B. HARLEY

SUMMARY

Lupus is a serious, potentially life-threatening disease. Its natural history is to culminate in a crescendo of autoimmunity and organ involvement. Difficulty arriving at the diagnosis may delay institution of therapy, which although helpful brings new problems. The fundamental understanding of this disease has made major strides. There is no consensus on the likely etiological agent(s), though evidence implicates Epstein-Barr virus, and the genetic approach to understanding etiology is in its infancy. Nevertheless, efficacious treatments are anticipated in the plethora of new biologics likely to have therapeutic effects in lupus, essentially a disease of immune dysregulation.

Key Words: Clinical manifestations; EBV; genetics; lupus; serology; skin.

INTRODUCTION

Systemic lupus erythematosus (SLE) is multisystem autoimmune disease characterized by the production of autoantibodies against a host of nuclear antigens. *Lupus*, the Latin word for wolf, has been used for at least seven centuries to describe the malar rash that some think resembles an animal bite. The disease was recognized initially as a skin disease. Hebra and Kaposi were the first to report systemic involvement of the disease. Their work published in 1874 described the association of lupus with anemia, lung involvement, mental status changes, and death. In three papers published between 1895 and 1903, Sir William Osler described the systematic involvement of lupus, the first detailed description recognizing the multiple systems affected by the disease.

Lupus affects multiple organ systems including the skin, joints, mucous and serosal membranes, kidneys, blood, lungs, and nervous system. The disease is more common in females and in African Americans. Despite advances, the pathogenesis of SLE is still incompletely understood. This chapter discusses the epidemiology, clinical features, pathogenesis, etiology, and management of SLE.

EPIDEMIOLOGY

SLE is distributed worldwide and affects all ethnicities. Disease incidence in the United States ranges between 2 and 7.6/100,000/yr. The prevalence has been estimated between 12 and 50.8 lupus cases/100,000. As many as 85–90% of the lupus

From: *Principles of Molecular Medicine, Second Edition*
Edited by: M. S. Runge and C. Patterson © Humana Press Inc., Totowa, NJ

patients are females. The female predominance disappears in age groups younger than 14 yr and older than 64 yr, consistent with an important role for estrogens in this phenomenon, an idea that is also supported by data from animal models of lupus.

In the United States, SLE is more common and more severe in African Americans than in European Americans. Relative to European Americans, the African American lupus patients tend to have more discoid lupus (DLE), lupus nephritis, myositis, and pericarditis. However, African American lupus patients have less photosensitivity, malar rash, mouth ulcers, anticardiolipin, and lupus anticoagulant compared with European Americans. Interestingly, lupus appears to be much less common in Africa than it is in American blacks.

DIAGNOSIS AND CLASSIFICATION

There is no single test that establishes the diagnosis of SLE. Instead, the diagnosis rests on the presence of a complicated set of clinical and laboratory findings. Consequently, reliable diagnosis is usually the purview of an experienced clinician. Because lupus is so heterogeneous, patients may present with a range of different clinical findings. The American College of Rheumatology (ACR) classification criteria are used to standardize the various clinical features for research studies. According to these criteria, the patient is classified as having lupus if he or she meets at least four of the eleven criteria (Table 99-1). It should be remembered however, that the ACR criteria are classification and not diagnostic criteria. There are patients who well satisfy the criteria, but who do not have lupus and others who do not satisfy the ACR criteria, but clearly have lupus. As a guide to the scope and range of the usual manifestations of this disease, they are useful and have found their way into ordinary rheumatic disease clinical practice.

Several laboratory tests are useful in evaluating a patient suspected of having lupus. The most sensitive test for lupus is the presence of antinuclear antibodies (ANA), which is positive in approx 98% of lupus patients. ANA are present, however, in a variety of other autoimmune and infectious conditions, as well as in normal, especially older individuals. ANA are usually detected by indirect immunofluorescence (IF) assay using HEp-2 cell lines as substrate. The results are reported in titers and patterns. There are no ANA patterns that are diagnostic of lupus. Examples of immunofluorescent patterns found in lupus include speckled, homogeneous, rim or peripheral, nucleolar, and nucleolar with cytoplasmic IF (Fig. 99-1). Antidouble-stranded DNA (dsDNA) antibodies are also detected by indirect IF using Crithidia luciliae as substrate.

leukopenia (<4000/mcl), lymphopenia (<1500/mcl), or thrombocytopenia (<100,000/mcl). Anemia of chronic disease is probably the most common hematological manifestation in lupus. Idiopathic thrombocytopenic purpura can be especially deadly in lupus. About 10% of lupus patients who die do so with a process resembling idiopathic thrombocytopenia, and without effective intervention the process can be fulminant and rapidly evolving into a medical emergency. Idiopathic thrombocytopenic purpura and hemolytic anemia are formes frustes of lupus. Patients may present with idiopathic thrombocytopenia purpura or with hemolytic anemia without other signs or symptoms suggesting lupus and then develop other features of lupus in the subsequent months or years.

Thrombocytopenia is the most reliable predictor of death in lupus, having been found in virtually all of the reported studies of survival. The increased relative risk (RR) for death is as high as 40-fold in lupus patients with thrombocytopenia. There is no insight explaining why thrombocytopenia is associated with a poor prognosis.

OTHER FEATURES Abdominal pain may be explained by mesenteric vasculitis, pancreatitis, and lupus peritonitis. Budd-Chiari syndrome and splenic infarcts are associated with anticardiolipin antibodies. Patients with lupus can also present with lymphadenopathy, hepatomegaly or splenomegaly. Ocular findings can include keratoconjunctivits sicca, episcleritis, and retinal vasculitis.

Other features that can be seen in SLE are related to complications of treatment. These include gastrointestinal toxicity induced by the NSAIDs, various toxic effects resulting from prolonged use of systemic steroids including steroid-induced osteoporosis and avascular bone necrosis, and increased susceptibility to infections secondary to the various immunosuppressive medications used.

ETIOLOGY AND PATHOGENESIS

The etiology of SLE is poorly understood. Several genetic and environmental factors are thought to influence its development.

THE GENETICS OF LUPUS The evidence that lupus is a genetic disorder is convincing. First, familial aggregation is present in lupus families. Second, particular genetics associations are already known. Third, genetic linkage studies have consistently implicated a number of additional genes as fundamental to the pathogenesis of lupus. Fourth, many of the animal models of lupus have a genetic basis, consistent with genetic variation being important in lupus.

About 10% of lupus patients report a second family member with lupus and 20–40% of identical twins are concordant for lupus. Evidence for a genetic etiology for lupus is supported by familial clustering of the disease with the ratio of risk to a sibling being 10–20 times higher than the population risk of lupus.

The DR2 and DR3 alleles at human leukocyte antigen (HLA)-DR are clearly associated with lupus in Europeans. As is true for all human histocompatibility associations, the pathophysiology and mechanistic details that explain this association are not known.

Lupus is also associated with polymorphisms of at least *FcγRIIA* and *FcγRIIIA*, and perhaps other Fc receptor genes. In both cases the allele that binds IgG subtypes with lower affinity is associated with increased risk of lupus. These alleles are thought to have decreased capacity to clear immune complexes made up of the specific low affinity IgG subtypes. These genes are neighbors on the human genome at chromosome 1q22-24, in a region also known to have genetic linkage with lupus. These two Fc receptors are separated by only 20 kb of genomic DNA and are in linkage disequilibrium.

Alleles of *PDCD-1*, a T-cell transcription factor, have been implicated as responsible for the linkage at 2q37, first found in the Nordic pedigrees lupus multiplex directory.

Several other genes are thought to increase susceptibility to the development of lupus without producing consistently convincing evidence of genetic association. These include polymorphisms involving the *IL-10*, *FAS* and *FASL*, the mannose binding lectin genes, *Bcl-2*, *CTLA4*, the T cell receptors, prolactin, tumor necrosis factor, and its receptor.

Genome wide linkage studies for SLE have revealed some potentially important genetic polymorphisms that increase the susceptibility to lupus. At least five linkages have been established and confirmed including those at 1q23, 2q37, 4p16, 6p21, and 16q13, along with many others that have not produced such convincing results. Of these linkages convincing associations that may explain them are published with alleles at *FcγRIIIA* (1q23), *PDCD-1* (2q37), and *HLA-DR* (6q21). Many other genetic effects (>15) have been established and await confirmation. Completion of the human genome project and improved methods of analysis are anticipated to provide much more rapid progress toward a more complete genetic understanding than has been previously possible.

LUPUS AND THE COMPLEMENT SYSTEM The complement system is a key constituent of the immune response and plays a central role in protecting against infections. In lupus, the classic complement pathway is thought to have an essential role in the pathophysiology of the disease. Deposition of immune complexes in various tissues is followed by activation of the classic complement pathway that will induce inflammation, tissue injury, and damage characteristic of SLE. As a result, patients with active disease tend to have low complement components C3 and C4. Complement consumption is also measured by hemolysis of immunoglobulin-coated erythrocytes with the CH50 test. The use of complement assays to assess disease activity in patients with lupus has been controversial, but is a useful measure in some patients. In others complement assays are not very helpful for disease management.

Lupus is one of the diseases with depressed complement in the circulation. Others include some glomerulonephritides, cryoglobulinemia, and subacute bacterial endocarditis all diseases confused with lupus in other ways.

Interestingly, however, the relationship between lupus and the complement system is paradoxical. Deficiency in any of the components of the early classic complement pathway is associated with lupus. Patients with a complete deficiency of complement component C1q have greater than 90% probability of developing lupus. In addition, patients who have antibodies to C1q have a higher frequency of glomerulonephritis.

In complete complement component C4 deficiency, approx 75% of patients develop lupus. C4 is produced by two separate, but closely related and neighboring genes, *C4A* and *C4B*, located in the HLA region on 6p21, thereby confusing the complicated histocompatibility associations with lupus. Complete deficiency occurs when both genes on both chromosomes fail to produce the C4 proteins. Indeed, even partial deficiencies of C4 have been associated with lupus.

Complement component C2 is the most common of the lupus-associated deficiencies at about 1 in 10,000 persons. In C2 deficiency, skin manifestations are the predominant feature of a lupus-like picture. Anti-Ro autoantibodies may be more common in this form of complement deficiency. The penetrance for lupus in C2 deficiency is low because most C2 deficient individuals are asymptomatic.

A lupus-like illness characterized by skin rashes, pyogenic infections, and a membranoproliferative glomerulonephritis, develops in 23% of complement component C3 deficient patients, but is rare.

Abnormalities in the complement receptor 2 (CR2), are also thought to have a role in the development of lupus as supported by various lupus mouse models. However, only meager evidence supports polymorphisms of complement receptor 2 being susceptibility factors in man.

The theoretical background explaining the association between complement deficiencies and lupus rests on the role of complement in clearing immune complexes from both the circulation and tissues. In addition, failure to process apoptotic cells by the complement may encourage autoimmunity. The paradox of complement being consumed in most patients and yet its deficiency being a risk factor for disease is presumably explained by immune complex activation in the former situation and failure to process immune complexes through the complement and complement receptor mediated pathways in the latter.

ENVIRONMENTAL FACTORS ASSOCIATED WITH LUPUS

Several environmental factors have been associated with the development of SLE, including infectious and noninfectious agents.

Noninfectious Agents Hormones, especially estrogens, are thought to be important in the development of lupus. This idea is supported by the predominance of lupus in females and is supported by animal experiments that show worsening of lupus symptoms with estrogens and improvement with androgens. In addition, worsening of lupus during pregnancy suggests a role of estrogens in lupus.

Exposure to UV light is important in causing or worsening lupus, especially the cutaneous manifestations of lupus. It has been suggested that exposure to UV light accelerates apoptosis of the keratinocytes, which increases the binding of anti-Ro to induce inflammation and tissue injury. Photosensitive lupus patients should be advised to avoid sun exposure by wearing long sleeves and protective hats.

Other factors associated with lupus include smoking (RR approx 2–3), herpes zoster before lupus onset (RR approx 4.7), use of allergy medication (RR approx 4.7), night shift work (RR approx 5.7), asthma (RR approx 2.1), and hives (RR approx 1.8), though some of these have not been confirmed. Hair dyes and straighteners have been suspected, but are not established as risk factors for lupus.

Infectious Agents Several viral infections have been studied in the setting of SLE, including parvovirus, mumps, measles, the common human herpes viruses, and others. Results consistently and reproducibly suggesting association have not been obtained, and perhaps except for Epstein-Barr virus there is no strong evidence of viral involvement in the etiology of lupus. The data supporting Epstein-Barr virus in lupus are suggestive of a fundamental relationship with lupus, and these, along with the properties of the virus, make Epstein-Barr virus the strongest candidate for an important etiological factor.

The modern solid phase assay methods for viral infection are significant advances over the immunofluorescent and precipitin methods used previously. Indeed, association of Epstein-Barr virus has been shown in four different collections of lupus

patients. In children and teenagers the RR is approx 50 with virtually all lupus patients showing serological responses consistent with having been infected. Because Epstein-Barr virus infects more than 90% of adults, there must be much more to the relationship than just the infection. Immunochemistry data are consistent with a structural antigenic relationship between Epstein-Barr nuclear antigen-1 (EBNA-1) of Epstein-Barr virus and the Sm B/B′ component of the spliceosome. EBNA-1 is expressed in the latent phase of the viral infection, tethers the viral DNA episome to human chromatin and preserves the viral DNA so that the infection continues in the daughter cells after replication. EBNA-1 initiates the latent viral DNA transcription and determines whether the latent or lytic program is followed. EBNA-1 is highly antigenic in most normal subjects, but is present in virtually all lupus patients tested. These results and other evidence are construed to support the hypothesis that lupus autoimmunity arises out of the EBNA-1 humoral immune response. According to this hypothesis, the association of lupus with Epstein-Barr virus infection is observed only because Epstein-Barr virus infection is required in order to develop an anti-EBNA-1 response.

Other properties of Epstein-Barr virus make this virus an attractive candidate etiological agent. Epstein-Barr virus infects B cells, and lupus is a disease of humoral immune dysfunction. Epstein-Barr virus induces autoantibodies and lupus appears to be mediated by autoantibodies. Epstein-Barr virus infection prevents normal B-cell apoptosis and prevention of normal apoptosis in B cells induces lupus in animal models. One mechanism involves an Epstein-Barr virus viral homologue of *bcl-2*, which has been shown to induce lupus-like autoimmunity. Epstein-Barr virus also has a Th-2 cytokine, viral IL-10, which is similar to human IL-10 and is expected to enhance humoral immune responses. A surprisingly large proportion of the normal human T cell repertoire (approx 7%) is directed against Epstein-Barr virus and once infected with the virus a person remains infected for life constantly emerging from the latent infection at a level sufficiently low to avoid immune destruction of infected cells. These features are also expected of an etiological agent for lupus. Only a few of the immune avoidance mechanisms of Epstein-Barr virus are probably known. Because this virus has been evolving with humans and predecessors for tens of millions of years, a number of effective immune avoidance mechanisms are likely to be discovered. The inhibition of EBNA-1 antigen presentation via a repeat sequence of Gly-Ala amino acids in the middle of the EBNA-1 sequence is one of these; it prevents the development of cytotoxic T cell responses directed against EBNA-1.

DNA METHYLATION AND LUPUS DNA methylation refers to the addition of a methyl group to position 5 of the cytosine residues in the CG pairs. Promoters of the active genes are typically hypomethylated, whereas methylation of promoter sequences renders the genes transcriptionally inactive.

A series of reports demonstrate a role for abnormal T-cell DNA methylation in the pathogenesis of lupus. Indeed, in both drug-induced and idiopathic lupus decreased T-cell DNA methylation results in the overexpression of methylation sensitive T-cell genes that induce T-cell autoreactivity. T cells treated with the methylation inhibitor 5-azacytidine demonstrate overexpression of the methylation sensitive genes *ITGAL* (CD11a), *TNFSF7* (CD70) and PRF1 (perforin) similar to T cells from active lupus patients. Furthermore, these cells become autoreactive, responding to self-class II MHC without the presence of the appropriate antigen in the antigen-binding cleft of the class II molecule. The autoreactive cells also kill autologous or syngeneic antigen-presenting cells. Procainamide and hydralazine, two known lupus-inducing drugs, also inhibit T-cell DNA methylation and induce T-cell autoreactivity similar to 5-azacytidine-treated T cells. Subsequently, it was shown that procainamide directly inhibits the DNA methylating enzyme DNA methyltransferase 1 (Dnmt 1), whereas hydralazine inhibits signaling through the extracellular signal-regulated kinase (ERK) pathway, which regulates Dnmt 1 expression. Interestingly, T cells from patients with active lupus have reduced ERK signaling and a decreased Dnmt 1 activity, thus, resembling hydralazine-treated cells. Furthermore, inhibiting the ERK signaling pathway in T cells in vitro results in changes similar to those caused by 5-azacytidine, with the overexpression of the methylation-sensitive genes and T-cell autoreactivity in vitro. Moreover, T cells treated with either 5-azacytidine, procainamide or ERK pathway inhibitors, induce autoimmunity and a lupus like-disease when injected into syngeneic mice. These results suggest that changes in T-cell DNA methylation, when occurring in a genetically predisposed host, may be fundamental to lupus pathogenesis.

MANAGEMENT

The introduction of steroids in the 1950s had an enormous impact on survival in lupus patients. Steroid therapy appears to derail the crescendo of immune abnormalities and end organ injury that would otherwise be the disease's natural history in many patients. The introduction of various other therapeutic modalities has made further incremental progress such that survival is more than 90% 10 yr after diagnosis. The goal of management is to control the tissue injury and immune activation. Once the disease is controlled, the goal is to prevent relapses although minimizing risk from the side effects and toxicities of the medications. Several medications are used, including the nonsteroidal antiinflammatory medications, hydroxychloroquine, cyclophosphamide, azathioprine, methotrexate, and mycophenolate mofetil.

PREVENTION AND GENERAL MEASURES Education is an integral part in the management of SLE. Patients should be aware of various environmental factors that can trigger a relapse in their disease. Because many lupus patients are photosensitive, they should protect themselves from the sun or UV light exposure and should wear protective clothing and sunscreens. In addition, various photosensitizing drugs are better avoided, including thiazides, sulfonamides, tetracyclines, and amiodarone.

Pregnancy in lupus can be problematic. If the disease is in remission at conception or if the medical regimen that controls the disorder can be continued through the entire pregnancy, the chances are good that the pregnancy can be carried to term. If the underlying disease process is active at conception and is not or cannot be controlled, serious problems are more likely. Sometimes, physicians discontinue all of the lupus medications when patients become pregnant, which can have the unfortunate consequence of inducing disease activity that threatens the life of the mother and fetus.

Placentas are small in pregnancies; infarcts are often found. This problem is more frequent in patients with the antiphospholipid antibody, but occurs in other lupus patients, as well. The small placentas probably explain the difficulties that many mothers face in the third trimester with higher rates of toxemia and premature deliveries. Of course, other difficulties, such as renal insufficiency generate increased risk of complication from pregnancy, independent of the activity of the lupus that may have caused it.

Anti-Ro is associated with neonatal lupus, which consists of neonatal lupus dermatitis, congenital heart block, hepatitis, or thrombocytopenia. The rash spontaneously resolves without scarring. Heart block is permanent. In about equal shares, patients have hydrops fetalis, require pacemakers, or are asymptomatic. The spectrum of possible outcomes is extreme in this situation. Some experience has been interpreted to suggest that dexamethasone can delay or prevent complete heart block on the earliest evidence of a conduction abnormality (e.g., first or second degree heart block).

Poor social support is associated with poor prognosis in lupus patients. The factors responsible for this or for the more severe disease in lower socioeconomic groups are not known. Psychosocial and family support are important in the successful management of lupus.

MEDICAL TREATMENT NSAIDs are generally used in mild lupus symptoms. They are particularly helpful for musculoskeletal manifestations including arthralgia and arthritis, as well as fever and mild serositis. Iboprofen should be avoided because of its association with aseptic meningitis in lupus patients. To the extent possible, NSAIDs should be avoided in patients with lupus nephritis as they may further worsen renal function.

The natural history of SLE has changed significantly since the introduction of steroids in the early 1950s. However, the use of steroids is complicated by major toxic effects that limit use for prolonged periods. In general, high dose systemic steroids (60 mg/d) might be needed in a lupus exacerbation, but such high doses should not be continued more than 6–8 wk. However, high dose intravenous steroids can be lifesaving, as in the case of lupus central nervous system involvement or severe lupus pneumonitis. Side effects of systemic steroids are legion, but specifically include weight gain, hirsutism, diabetes, cataract, cardiovascular complications, and osteoporosis. Topical steroids are used to treat the various skin rashes associated with lupus, but can result in skin atrophy and telangectasias. For this reason, potent steroids are not usually used on the face, with the exception of DLE rash, which if left untreated can produce disfiguring scars.

Hydroxychloroquine is widely used in mild lupus, and it particularly improves the joint and skin manifestations. There is convincing evidence that hydroxychloroquine prevents lupus exacerbations in patients with relatively mild disease. Hydroxychloroquine can be associated with several side effects including gastrointestinal disturbance and skin rash. Though uncommon, the most feared complication is retinal toxicity and, therefore, most practitioners recommend periodic ophthalmological exam. Hydroxychloroquine may also be helpful in treating the dryness symptoms of secondary Sjögren's syndrome in lupus patients.

Several other medications used in the treatment of lupus include immunosuppressive therapies such as cyclophosphamide, azathioprin, and mycophenolate mofetil. Several promising biological agents are being actively evaluated for the treatment of lupus: rituximab, an anti-CD20 monoclonal antibody, anti-C5 complement monoclonal antibody and anti-IL-10 monoclonal antibody. Stem cell transplantation has been used with some success in treating severe lupus patients. Also, autologous stem cell transplantation is performed with high doses of immunosuppressive, cytotoxic agents.

ACKNOWLEDGMENTS

We appreciate support of the NIH (JBH: AR42460, AR12253, AI24717, AI31584, AR049084, RR020143, and AR048940, LAD: AR32599, AR32081, T32-AR07369; AHS: RR015577) and US Department of Veterans Affairs (CC103) for our work.

SELECTED REFERENCES

Cooper GS, Dooley MA, Treadwell EL, St Clair EW, Parks CG, Gilkeson GS. Hormonal, environmental, and infectious risk factors for developing systemic lupus erythematosus. Arthritis Rheum 1998;41(10):1714–1724.

Golan TD, Elkon KB, Gharavi AE, Krueger JG. Enhanced membrane binding of autoantigens to cultured keratinocytes of systemic lupus erythematosus patients after ultraviolet B/ultraviolet A irradiation J Clin Invest 1992;90:1067–1076.

Harley JB, Reichlin M, Arnett FC, Alexander EL, Bias WB, Provost TT. Gene interaction at HLA-DQ enhances autoantibody production in primary Sjögren's syndrome. Science 1986;232:1145–1147.

James JA, Harley JB, Scofield RH. Role of viruses in systemic lupus erythematous and Sjögren's syndrome. Curr Opin Rheum 2001;13:370–376.

James JA, Gross T, Scofield RH, Harley JB. Immunoglobulin epitope spreading and autoimmune disease after peptide immunization: Sm B/B(derived PPPGMRPP and PPPGIRGP induced spliceosome autoimmunity. J Exp Med 1995;181:453–461.

James JA, Kaufman KM, Farris AD, Taylor-Albert E, Lehman TJA, Harley JB. An increased prevalence of Epstein-Barr virus infection in young patients suggests a possible etiology for systemic lupus erythematosus. J Clin Invest 1997;100:3019–3026.

Kawashima T, Zappi EG, Lieu TS, Sontheimer RD. Impact of ultraviolet radiation on the cellular expression of Ro/SS-A-autoantigenic polypeptides. Dermatology 1994;189:6–10.

Kelly JA, Moser KL, Harley JB. The genetics of systemic lupus erythematosus: putting the pieces together. Genes Immun 2002;3(Suppl 1): S71–S85.

Molina H. Update on complement in the pathogenesis of systemic lupus erythematosus. Curr Opin Rheum 2002;14:492–497.

Reichlin M. Autoantibodies to the RoRNP particles. Clin Exp Immunol 1995;99(1):7–9.

Richardson B. DNA methylation and autoimmune disease. Clin Immunol 2003;109:72–79.

Sawalha AH, Richardson BC. DNA methylation in the pathogenesis of systemic lupus erythematosus. Current Pharmacogenomics 2005;3: 73–78.

Smoller BR, Horn TD. Lupus erythematosus. In: Smoller BR, Horn TD, eds. Dermatopathology in Systemic Disease, 1st ed. New York: Oxford, 2001, pp. 3–16.

Sontheimer RD, Provost TT. Lupus erythematosus. In: Sontheimer RD, Provost TT, eds. Cutaneous Manifestations of Rheumatic Diseases, 1st ed. Baltimore: Williams and Wilkins, 1996, pp. 1–71.

Srivastava M, Rencic A, Diglio G, et al. Drug-induced, Ro/SSA-positive cutaneous lupus erythematosus. Arch Dermatol 2003;139:45–49.

Wallace D. Management of lupus erythematosus: recent insights. Curr Opin Rheum 2002;14:212–219.

Yung RL, Quddus J, Chrisp CE, Johnson KJ, Richardson BC. Mechanism of drug-induced lupus. I. Cloned Th2 cells modified with DNA methylation inhibitors in vitro cause autoimmunity in vivo. J immunol 1995;154:3025–3035.

100 Systemic Sclerosis

CHRIS T. DERK AND SERGIO A. JIMENEZ

SUMMARY

Systemic sclerosis is an autoimmune disease of unknown origin characterized by excessive deposition of collagen and other connective tissue macromolecules in skin and multiple internal organs, severe alterations in the microvasculature, and humoral and cellular immunological abnormalities. Although the most apparent and almost universal clinical features of systemic sclerosis are related to the progressive thickening and fibrosis of the skin, some degree of involvement of multiple internal organs is uniformly present even when not clinically apparent. This chapter will examine the clinical aspects and pathogenesis of the disease and review some promising therapies that have been and are being developed that might modify the natural course of this serious and often lethal disorder.

Key Words: Raynaud's phenomenon; systemic sclerosis; skin; scleroderma; TGF-β.

INTRODUCTION

Systemic sclerosis (SSc) is an autoimmune disease of unknown origin characterized by excessive deposition of collagen and other connective tissue macromolecules in skin and multiple internal organs, severe alterations in the microvasculature, and humoral and cellular immunological abnormalities. SSc is the most common and important among a group of chronic diseases of unknown cause characterized by induration and thickening of the skin (scleroderma, derived from *skleros* [hard] and *derma* [skin]) (Table 100-1). SSc is a complex and clinically heterogeneous disease with clinical forms ranging from limited skin involvement (limited cutaneous SSc; lcSSc) to forms with diffuse skin sclerosis and severe internal organ disease (diffuse cutaneous SSc; dcSSc), and occasionally a fulminant course (fulminant SSc).

Although the most apparent and almost universal clinical features of SSc are related to the progressive thickening and fibrosis of the skin, some degree of involvement of multiple internal organs is uniformly present even when not clinically apparent. Morbidity and mortality in SSc are substantial, and are related to the extent of the fibrotic and microvascular alterations, as well as to the severity and extent of visceral organ involvement.

Even though the pathogenesis of SSc remains elusive, an increasing number of investigations has helped to understand better some of the pieces of this complex puzzle. It was not until 1972 that a landmark study by LeRoy demonstrated an increased production of collagen in fibroblast monolayer cultures obtained from skin biopsies from patients with SSc. A wealth of knowledge has been gained since then regarding the clinical aspects and pathogenesis of the disease and some promising therapies have been and are being developed that might modify the natural course of this serious and often lethal disorder.

EPIDEMIOLOGY

Although Hippocrates was among one of many physicians of ancient times who described patients with "hard" and "stretched" skin, it is remarkable that clear descriptions of a disease with such obvious and apparent clinical manifestations was not more widely recognized or more precisely described until the 18th century. Indeed, it appears that the first concise report of scleroderma as the disease known today was by Carlo Curzio in 1752 who described a 17-yr-old woman admitted to a hospital in Naples. However, the term scleroderma was not used until Giovambattista Fantonetti, a prominent physician in Milan, employed it in 1836 to describe a 30-yr-old peasant woman who developed dark, tense, leathery skin, sparing only her face and breasts, which resolved in 3 mo. Although many different terms have been used through the years for this disorder, scleroderma has been the preferred term until 1945 when Robert Goetz coined the term *SSc* to reflect the systemic nature of this disorder.

SSc is the third most common connective tissue disease (following rheumatoid arthritis and systemic lupus erythematosus). It occurs more commonly in females (4–8/1 female to male preponderance), affects all racial groups and can present at any age, although the peak of disease onset occurs in the fourth and fifth decades. Familial SSc is rare and there is no conclusive evidence of genetic transmission of the disease.

The prevalence of SSc in the United States is generally accepted to be as high as 242–286 cases/million of population although it varies by ethnic background and geographic region. Of note is the high prevalence of SSc in the population of Choctaw American Indians of Oklahoma in whom the prevalence is as high as 469 cases/million. Disease expression also appears to be different among different ethnic groups; for example, Caucasians more frequently display limited skin involvement with less severe systemic manifestations, whereas, African Americans manifest more frequently diffuse skin involvement and more severe pulmonary manifestations.

EARLY SIGNS AND SYMPTOMS

In its early stages SSc might mimic other connective tissue diseases. Raynaud's phenomenon, the initial symptom in the majority

From: *Principles of Molecular Medicine, Second Edition*
Edited by: M. S. Runge and C. Patterson © Humana Press, Inc., Totowa, NJ

Table 100-1
Classification of Scleroderma

Systemic scleroderma or SSc
Diffuse cutaneous SSc
Limited cutaneous SSc
Overlap syndromes: polymyositis, systemic lupus erythematosus,
    rheumatoid arthritis

Localized scleroderma
Morphea: localized or generalized
Linear scleroderma
Scleroderma "En coup de sabre"

Scleroderma-like syndromes
Eosinophilic fascitis
Graft-vs-host disease
Nephrogenic fibrosing dermopathy/nephrogenic systemic fibrosis

Chemically-induced scleroderma
Eosinophilia-myalgia syndrome
Toxic oil syndrome
Vinyl chloride
Organic solvents
Silica
Bleomycin
Pentazocine

Pseudoscleroderma
Scleredema, scleromyxedema, cutaneous, amyloidosis, and others

Table 100-2
Clinical Features of SSc

Cutaneous
Skin induration and sclerosis
Loss of skin appendages
Pigmentary changes
Telangiectasias
Calcinosis

Musculoskeletal
Polyarthralgia and arthritis
Digital flexion contractures
Tendon friction rubs
Myopathy/myositis
Acro-osteolysis

Gastrointestinal involvement
Esophageal reflux, stricture, dysplasia and cancer
Dysphagia and odynophagia
Delayed gastric emptying
Bacterial overgrowth and malabsorption
Alternating diarrhea and constipation
Gastric antral vascular ectasia (watermelon stomach)

Pulmonary
Alveolitis
Interstitial fibrosis
Pulmonary hypertension

Cardiac
Pericarditis
Myocardial fibrosis and heart failure
Conduction defects
Cor pulmonale

Renal
Renal crisis
Proteinuria
Chronic interstitial fibrosis

Others
Entrapment neuropathies (including carpal tunnel syndrome
    and trigeminal neuralgia)
Erectile dysfunction
Hypothyroidism (thyroid fibrosis)
Bladder fibrosis
Sicca syndrome

of patients, is characterized by cold- or emotion-induced episodic constriction of the digital arterioles, manifested by pallor, cyanosis and redness of the fingers or toes, accompanied by numbness, tingling, or pain. Raynaud's phenomenon might precede the onset of other SSc features by months or years; however, it ultimately develops in virtually all SSc patients. Although Raynaud's phenomenon is common among premenopausal women, only a minority of them develops a connective tissue disease, most commonly SSc. Puffy hands and forearms are often noted in early SSc. Arthralgia and sometimes a palpable tendon friction rub in wrists, ankles and other sites might be present at this stage of disease evolution. Diffuse hyperpigmentation and/or hypopigmentation of the skin accompanied by pruritus is a common early manifestation of SSc.

CLINICAL FEATURES

As mentioned, SSc displays both cutaneous and systemic visceral involvement. The most common clinical manifestations of SSc are shown in Table 100-2.

CUTANEOUS MANIFESTATIONS The most apparent and almost universal clinical manifestation of SSc is the progressive thickening and induration of the skin. Skin sclerosis is present in 95% of patients with SSc. In the remaining patients typical visceral involvement occurs in the absence of obvious skin sclerosis (scleroderma sine scleroderma). Thickened and hidebound skin generally first appears distally and progresses proximally. The skin is taut, shiny, and tightly adherent to the underlying subcutaneous tissues. The hands and face show the most pronounced changes, especially in the early stages of the disease. Early manifestations include pruritus and edema of the affected skin, which over time evolves into severely indurated skin that is firmly bound to the subcutaneous tissue. Skin involvement of the fingers (sclerodactyly) is accompanied by widening of the cuticles, and in the late stages, loss of soft tissue

at the fingertips. The face assumes an expressionless appearance with loss of wrinkles. The nose becomes beaked, and the lips are thin and tightly pursed with radial furrowing around them. The maximal oral aperture is diminished (microstomia). Fibrotic tissue encroachment of the local hair follicles and sweat glands causes hair loss and diminished perspiration. As the disease progresses the sclerotic changes might affect the entire body.

Diffuse hyperpigmentation, similar to that seen in Addison's disease, can precede the onset of detectable skin thickening. In some patients, hyperpigmented hair follicles are surrounded by depigmented areas of skin, resulting in the characteristic "salt-and-pepper" pattern. Telangiectasias, representing dilated capillary loops, can be found on the hands, face, lips, and tongue. Mucosal telangiectasias are common and have been implicated as a source of nasal and gastrointestinal bleeding. Painful recurrent ulcerations develop at the fingertips and other areas in which the skin is tightly stretched and can become infected. Cutaneous calcifications because of deposition of calcium hydroxyapatite are found at the fingertips, along the extensor surface of the forearms, and other periarticular and subcutaneous areas.

SKELETAL INVOLVEMENT Symmetric polyarthralgia involving the fingers, wrists, and ankles, occurs commonly in early SSc, but true arthritis and synovitis are rare. Contracture of the fingers resulting from fibrosis of the tendons as well as skin tightening can develop rapidly and result in loss of hand function. Carpal tunnel syndrome is occasionally seen in early SSc and might resolve spontaneously. Coarse leathery crepitus (tendon friction rub) can be palpated and often heard on active and passive motion of the wrists and ankles. Tendon friction rubs are virtually specific for diffuse SSc and might antedate progressive skin involvement. Roentgenograms might show characteristic resorption, and in advanced cases, complete dissolution of the distal end of the phalanx (acro-osteolysis). Many patients with diffuse SSc have an indolent myopathy, characterized by minimal elevation in serum muscle enzymes owing to focal muscle fibrosis and fiber atrophy. A minority of patients develop full-blown myositis with marked elevation in serum creatine phosphokinase and aldolase levels and typical inflammatory myopathy electromyographic changes.

VISCERAL INVOLVEMENT

Gastrointestinal Tract The gastrointestinal tract is the most frequent visceral organ involved in SSc. Esophageal abnormalities are found in up to 90% of patients. Incompetence of the lower esophageal sphincter and decreased or absent peristalsis in the lower two-thirds of the esophagus are characteristic of SSc. These abnormalities lead to symptoms of gastroesophageal reflux with intermittent retrosternal burning pain and regurgitation. The loss of coordinated and effective peristalsis affects the smooth muscle of the lower two-thirds of the esophagus and manifests as dysphagia and odynophagia. Chronic reflux and esophageal stasis might result in the development of esophagitis, Barrett's esophagus, and lower esophageal strictures. Reflux of gastric contents might result in hoarseness, cough, and aspiration pneumonitis. SSc is among the most common diseases associated with gastric antral vascular ectasia (watermelon stomach) and in some cases severe gastrointestinal hemorrhage might be caused by bleeding from these lesions. Barium esophagogram studies demonstrate incompetent lower esophageal sphincter, dilatation, and aperistalsis of the body of the esophagus, gastro-esophageal reflux and occasionally, lower esophageal strictures. Esophageal manometric studies are more sensitive and are particularly helpful in excluding other causes of dysphagia, such as polymyositis. Disordered motility might result in gastric distension, bacterial overgrowth in the small bowel with subsequent diarrhea and malabsorption, and pseudoobstruction. In long-standing colonic disease, wide-mouth sacculations (pseudodiverticula) are found.

Respiratory System Lung involvement is the leading cause of morbidity and mortality in SSc. Pulmonary fibrosis has an insidious onset and often a progressive course with increasing exertional dyspnea and limited exercise tolerance. Physical examination usually discloses fine inspiratory crackles at the lung bases. Pulmonary hypertension and cor pulmonale might develop in some patients even in the absence of pulmonary parenchymal involvement, particularly in those with limited SSc. Advanced pulmonary involvement can be detected as increased interstitial markings on a chest roentgenogram, but this is insensitive for detection of early lesions. High resolution CT of the chest is highly sensitivity for the diagnosis of SSc lung fibrosis and allows

the early detection of alveolitis. Pulmonary function studies, especially the single breath diffusing capacity, are more sensitive and, therefore, are useful in establishing the presence of pulmonary involvement at an earlier stage. An isolated reduction of diffusing capacity in a patient with SSc suggests pulmonary hypertension.

Renal Involvement Renal involvement, considered to be the most deadly complication of SSc, develops in 15–20% of patients and usually occurs with an abrupt onset (scleroderma renal crisis). Patients with diffuse and rapidly progressive skin involvement are at the highest risk of developing scleroderma renal crisis. Malignant hypertension with headache and retinopathy, acute cardiac failure, myocardial infarction, stroke, and oliguria with rapidly progressive renal insufficiency characterize scleroderma renal crisis. Progression to renal failure and death occurs rapidly unless the diagnosis of renal crisis is established and aggressive treatment instituted promptly. Less dramatic renal dysfunction occurs with greater frequency in SSc and manifests as a reduction in renal functional reserve and intermittent mild proteinuria.

Cardiac Involvement Laboratory or pathological evidence of heart involvement is noted in 70–80% of SSc patients but clinically significant primary cardiac dysfunction is less common. Tachyarrhythmias and cardiac conduction disturbances detected by ambulatory Holter monitoring are frequent and associated with increased mortality. Pericardial effusion is found by echocardiography in many patients, but symptomatic pericarditis is rare. Cor pulmonale with right ventricular failure occurs in patients with pulmonary hypertension.

Other Visceral Involvement Peripheral neuropathy, particularly trigeminal neuralgia and carpal tunnel syndrome can occur, but the central nervous system is spared. Erectile dysfunction develops in many male patients, and can precede other SSc manifestations. The sicca syndrome is frequently found. Hypothyroidism is detected in one-third of patients, but is generally mild. Primary liver disease is unusual, but the concomitant occurrence of primary biliary cirrhosis has been documented in some cases.

LABORATORY FINDINGS

The diagnosis of SSc is generally made on clinical grounds. Laboratory data help define the type and extent of visceral involvement. The erythrocyte sedimentation rate and the serum levels of C reactive protein are usually normal. The antinuclear antibody test is positive in more than 90% of patients, and most characteristically shows a speckled or nucleolar immunofluorescence pattern in diffuse SSc and a centromere pattern in limited SSc. Antibodies to native DNA and Sm are typically absent. Antibodies to the kinetochore (anticentromere antibodies) are found in more than 80% of patients with limited SSc, occasionally in patients with diffuse SSc, and only rarely in patients with other connective tissue disorders. Of patients with diffuse SSc, approx 30–40% have serum antibodies reactive with the enzyme DNA topoisomerase I (termed Scl-70). Anti-Scl-70 antibodies are rare in patients with limited SSc and are not present in patients with other connective tissue diseases. Anti-Scl-70 and anticentromere marker antibodies are mutually exclusive, coexisting in only a few patients. The titers of these antibodies are not associated with the clinical course of the disease. Their presence; however, is helpful in classification of SSc patients into the limited or diffuse cutaneous subsets of SSc. The presence of these antibodies in an individual with isolated Raynaud's phenomenon identifies a patient at high risk for the subsequent development of SSc.

CLINICAL SUBSETS OF SSc

SSc is a clinically heterogeneous disease, with a spectrum of severity ranging from minimal sclerodactyly or limited skin sclerosis (limited SSc) to extensive and rapidly progressive diffuse skin involvement with severe derangement of critical organs (diffuse SSc). The latter clinical subset is associated with much higher and earlier mortality. Several clinical and laboratory features allow the distinction of these two subsets of SSc (Table 100-3).

COURSE AND PROGNOSIS

Unlike other connective tissue diseases, the course of SSc is not one of flares and remissions, but is often characterized by relentless progression. The highest mortality is seen in the first 2–5 yr of the disease. The prognosis of SSc is related to the extent of visceral involvement. Limited SSc has low overall mortality, whereas diffuse SSc has 50–60% mortality at 5 yr.

A grave prognosis is closely correlated with the presence of renal, pulmonary, and cardiac involvement. Early diagnosis, detection of the extent and degree of organ involvement, and treatment of specific organ involvement offer the best hope for reducing morbidity and mortality.

HISTOPATHOLOGICAL ABNORMALITIES

The pathological changes in SSc encompass a spectrum reflecting variable stages of development and progression of three major processes occurring in the affected tissues:

1. Connective tissue alterations with increased deposition of collagen and other connective tissue components in the extracellular matrix (ECM).
2. Inflammation, occurring predominantly in the early stages of disease and characterized by infiltration with mononuclear cells, mostly of the macrophage and T-cell lineages.
3. Microvascular disease, characterized by intimal proliferation, concentric subendothelial deposition of collagen and mucinous material, and narrowing and thrombosis of the vessel lumen.

Progression of the vascular and fibrotic changes and decrease in the inflammatory component lead to end-stage fibrosis and atrophy of the affected organs.

Histopathological findings in the skin include marked thickening of the dermis with massive accumulation of dense collagen causing epidermal atrophy, flattening of the rete pegs, and replacement of sebaceous and sweat glands, as well as hair follicles. A prominent inflammatory infiltrate mostly consisting of CD4+ lymphocytes is often present at the dermal–adipose tissue interphase, especially in early lesions. The small vessels of the lower dermis show fibrous thickening but evidence of vasculitis is absent. In the lungs, fibrosis of the alveolocapillary membrane and the parenchymal interstitium accompanied by severe mononuclear cell infiltration and fibroblast proliferation occurs frequently, resulting in marked disruption of their architecture. Prominent vascular abnormalities with intimal proliferation and medial hypertrophy causing severe narrowing or complete obliteration of small vessels occur frequently. The renal lesions display severe narrowing and obliteration of the medium-sized arcuate arterioles from concentric medial hypertrophy, subintimal accumulation of loose connective tissue, and reduplication of the internal elastic lamina. The glomeruli frequently appear ischemic but there is no evidence of

Table 100-3
Clinical and Laboratory Test Differences Between Diffuse and Limited Cutaneous SSc

	Diffuse cutaneous SSc	Limited cutaneous SSc
Mortality	>60% at 7 yr	<15% at 7 yr
Raynaud phenomenon	<1 yr	>1 yr (decades)
Skin sclerosis	Truncal, acral	Acral
Lung involvement	Early: interstitial	Late: pulmonary hypertension
Renal involvement	Renal crisis	Rare
Cardiac involvement	Cardiac fibrosis	Rare
Autoantibodies (%)	90	90
Pattern (fluorescence)	Speckled/nucleolar	Centromere
Scl-70 (%)	30–40	0
Antitopoisomerase (%)	60	0
Anticentromere (%)	10	80–90
Antikinetochore (%)	5	95

glomerulitis. Severe interstitial, perivascular, and periglomerular fibrosis might be present in cases of long duration. The renal lesion of scleroderma renal crisis might be histologically indistinguishable from that of malignant hypertension, with intimal proliferation of the interlobular and arcuate arteries and fibrinoid necrosis of the media. All other affected organs show various degrees of fibrosis and mononuclear inflammatory cell infiltration.

MOLECULAR PATHOGENESIS

The pathogenesis of SSc is extremely complex; numerous studies have examined several aspects of its intricate picture. Although the exact mechanisms involved are not well understood, three outstanding features are responsible for the clinical and pathological manifestations of the disease: excessive deposition of collagen and other connective tissue macromolecules in skin and internal organs, vascular lesions of small arteries and arterioles, and alterations of humoral and cellular immunity. It is not clear which of these factors is of primary importance or how they interrelate to cause the progressive fibrotic process in SSc. However, a crucial component in the pathogenesis of SSc is the persistent and unregulated activation of genes encoding various collagens and other ECM proteins. This is the most important difference between normal fibroblasts that promote normal wound healing and SSc fibroblasts that demonstrate an uncontrolled collagen production and tissue deposition resulting in pathological organ fibrosis.

POSSIBLE CAUSATIVE AGENTS   It has been postulated that infectious agents might be the initial causative agents of autoimmune responses that result in autoimmune disorders including SSc. Autoantibodies in SSc have been considered to result from an antigen driven response either from an unspecified tissue injury or from "molecular mimicry." The concept of "molecular mimicry" suggests that the production of autoantibodies against self antigens is directed against these antigens because they contain epitopes that share structural similarities to viral or bacterial proteins. In the immunopathogenesis of SSc, herpesviruses, retroviruses, and human cytomegalovirus (HCMV) infections, among others, have been suggested as causative agents. Evidence supporting the role of retroviruses includes the demonstration of sequence homologies between the p30^{gag} protein of retroviruses that cause leukemia in rodents and felines and the DNA topoisomerase I antigen, which is the target of SSc-specific anti-Scl-70 antibodies, the demonstration that expression of certain retroviral proteins in normal human dermal fibroblasts causes increased expression of several ECM protein genes, and the detection of antibodies to specific retroviral proteins in the sera of SSc patients. The possible involvement of HCMV is supported by the observations of a higher prevalence of IgG anti-HCMV antibodies capable of binding the HCMV late protein UL94 and inducing apoptosis in human endothelial cells in patients with SSc, the increased prevalence of IgA HCMV in patients positive for Scl-70 autoantibodies, and the severe fibroproliferative vascular changes observed in HCMV infections. However, despite intensive study, there is no definitive evidence to conclude that SSc has a viral etiology.

Environmental agents have also been implicated in the development of SSc. Silica and metal dust exposure had been shown in case studies to be related to SSc, but studies have failed to confirm an association. However, exposure to organic solvent might be an important environmental factor triggering SSc. Indeed, some individuals exposed to vinyl chloride develop skin thickening, Raynaud's phenomenon, and digital ulcers. Other environmental factors implicated in the pathogenesis of SSc or SSc-like syndromes include certain pesticides, hair dyes, and exposure to fuel-derived fumes.

GENETIC FACTORS The contribution of genetic factors in the development and expression of SSc is strongly supported by the observation of familial clustering of the disease, the high frequency of other autoimmune disorders and autoantibodies in SSc family members, differences in prevalence and clinical manifestations among different ethnic groups, and the increased prevalence of certain human leukocyte antigens and major histocompatibility complex (MHC) alleles among different ethnic groups and among patients with different clinical types of disease or different pattern of autoantibodies. Although the concordance of SSc among identical twins is only 5.9%, suggesting that the heritability component is rather low; this frequency is still approx 300 times higher than that expected by chance alone. Furthermore, only a small group of twins has been studied (34 pairs) rendering it difficult to draw definitive conclusions.

The differences of MHC and human leukocyte antigen allele expression are evident when comparing the different haplotypes that have been identified to be linked to SSc expression among different ethnic groups. In the Choctaw American Indians, the human leukocyte antigen haplotypes related with disease expression are DRB1*1602, DQA1*0501, DQB1*0301, whereas in Caucasian populations from the United States and from Europe they are DRB1*1101, DRB1*1104, DQA1*0501, DQB1*0301, DRB1*0301, DQA1*0501, and DQB1*0201. Disease expression also appears to be different among different ethnic groups. African-Americans are more likely to harbor antitopoisomerase 1 antibodies and to present more severe visceral manifestations including a higher frequency of pulmonary fibrosis. In contrast, anticentromere antibodies are more common in Caucasians who also display higher frequency of limited disease with less severe systemic manifestations.

ROLE OF CELLULAR MICROCHIMERISM One hypothesis in the causality of SSc suggests that during pregnancy allogenic fetal or maternal cells cross the placenta in a bidirectional traffic and persist in the circulation and tissues of the mother or child, respectively, and that these engrafted foreign cells might become activated by a second event and might mount a graft-vs-host

reaction that manifests as SSc. There are remarkable clinical, histopathological, and serological similarities between graft-vs-host disease and SSc, including esophageal, lung, and skin involvement, lymphocytic infiltration and fibrosis of affected organs and production of autoantibodies. Strong support to this hypothesis was provided by the demonstration of Y-chromosome sequences in DNA extracted from peripheral blood cells and in affected skin samples from women with SSc who had a previous male pregnancy. Microchimeric cells of maternal origin have also been identified in the circulation of offspring. These findings might explain, according to this hypothesis, the occurrence of SSc in nulliparous women and men.

Although some studies found that the frequency of Y-chromosome sequences in the skin of SSc women who had male offspring was similar to that of normal controls, quantification of microchimeric fetal cells showed significantly higher numbers in SSc patients indicating that it is the quantity and not only the mere presence of fetal cells that might contribute to the pathogenesis of SSc.

HUMORAL IMMUNE SYSTEM ALTERATIONS The presence of specific autoantibodies is one of the most common manifestations of SSc and more than 90% of SSc patients have antinuclear antibodies in their serum. Numerous autoantibodies have been described in SSc patients. Some of these are highly specific for SSc, whereas others are associated with different clinical manifestations of the disease (Table 100-4). Anti-Scl-70 antibodies were initially described to recognize a 70-kDa nuclear protein. Subsequently, it was shown that these antibodies react with a 110-kDa protein identified as DNA topoisomerase 1. These antibodies are almost exclusively present in sera from patients with the diffuse form of SSc. About 30–40% of patients with diffuse SSc harbor these autoantibodies with a higher prevalence seen in African-American patients. Anticentromere antibodies recognize several protein components of the trilaminar kinetochore. The most common anticentromere antibodies recognize three different antigens: a 17-kDa (CENP-A), an 80-kDa (CENP-B), and a 140-kDa (CENP-C) centromere protein. These antibodies are usually present in patients with the limited form of SSc and are seen in 80–90% of these patients. In contrast to anti-Scl-70 antibodies, anticentromere antibodies are only found in approx 10% of patients with diffuse SSc. These two autoantibodies are mutually exclusive, coexisting in the same patient only in rare instances. Several other autoantibody systems with various levels of specificity for SSc and organ involvement have been described in SSc patients.

ABNORMALITIES IN THE CELLULAR IMMUNE SYSTEM The presence of mononuclear cell infiltrates in affected skin and visceral organs from SSc patients has long been recognized. Early in the presentation of SSc, biopsies from affected skin show prominent macrophage and T-cell lymphocytic infiltrates. The cells in these early infiltrates are CD14+ and express Class II MHC, suggesting that they are activated. Prior activation of peripheral blood T cells in patients with SSc is also evident by the increased expression of high affinity interleukin (IL)-2R on the T-cell membranes and the observation that sera from SSc patients contains a threefold higher level of serum IL-2. In more advanced stages of SSc, the majority of tissue-bound T-cell lymphocytes is CD4+ (helper T-cells) expressing the activation marker class II MHC antigen DR. Although true in most cases, a few studies have shown an increased prevalence of CD8+ cells in lymphocytic infiltrates from the skin and lungs. Most of the tissue infiltrating cells express α/β receptors

Table 100-4
Principal Autoantibodies in SSc

Autoantibody	Target antigen	Clinical association	ANA pattern
Anti-Scl-70	DNA topoisomerase I	Diffuse SSc	Speckled
Anticentromere	Kinetochore proteins CENP A (17 kDa) CENP B (80 kDa) CENP C (140 kDa)	Limited SSc	Centromere
Anti-RNA polymerase I	Complex of 210-14-kDa proteins	Progressive SSc, organ involvement	Speckled Nucleolar
Antifibrillin (U3 RNP)	Nucleolar protein of 34 kDa component of U3-RNP	Diffuse SSc	Nucleolar
Anti-PM-Scl	Complex of 110-20 kDa nucleolar and nuclear proteins	Polymyositis/SSc overlap	Nucleolar
Anti-nRNP	Nuclear ribonucleoprotein	Mixed connective tissue disease	Speckled
Anti-7-2-RNP	Nucleolar protein of 40 kDa complexed with 7-2 and 8-2 RNAs	Limited SSc	Nucleolar
Anti-NOR-90	Protein of 90 kDa localized to the nucleolar organizer region	Lung involvement	Nucleolar
Antimitochondrial	M2 complex of 70 kDa and 47 kDa proteins	Limited SSc associated with PBC	None
Anti-Ku	Nucleolar heterodimer of 70 kDa and 80 kDa polypeptide chains	Polymyositis/SSc overlap	Nucleolar
Anti-Th/To	RNAse MRP and RNAse P ribo-nucleoprotein complexes	Pulmonary hypertension	Nucleolar

rather than γ/δ receptors although γ/δ receptor bearing T cells appear to be predominant in bronchial alveolar lavage fluids of patients with SSc interstitial lung disease. Further expansion of T cells within the affected tissues appears to be oligoclonal as shown in studies of T-cell receptor transcripts in SSc skin. The expanded T-cell populations in affected SSc tissues are thought to release cytokines that initiate and/or perpetuate the fibrotic process as well as the endothelial and vascular alterations. Indeed, clones of T cells established from infiltrating lymphocytes isolated from affected SSc skin produce cytokines capable of modulating fibroblast proliferation and collagen production, as well as various endothelial cell functions.

Cytokines   Numerous cytokines have been shown in in vitro studies to exert potent effects on various fibroblast functions and on the production and/or degradation of collagens. However, it is likely that the ultimate effects of these cytokines on fibroblast proliferative and biosynthetic activities depend on their concentration in the pericellular environment and on the relative proportions among a mixture of a large number of cytokines that often have opposing effects. The cytokines with most potent effects on connective tissue metabolism are ILs-1, -4, -8, and -10, the interferons (IFNs), particularly IFNγ, and tumor necrosis factor α and β (lymphotoxin).

IL-1 has been shown in some studies to stimulate the synthesis of type I collagen, whereas in others, to inhibit it. IL-1 inhibits collagen production by lung and dermal fibroblasts, whereas it causes an increased production of collagen by kidney fibroblasts and synovial cells. The mechanisms involved in IL-1 modulation of type I collagen synthesis appear to be different among different cell types and are not clearly understood. The role of IL-1 in SSc pathogenesis has not been established.

IL-4 is considered to be one of the most important profibrotic cytokines. It stimulates fibroblast proliferation, chemotaxis, and ECM production. Furthermore, IL-4 has potent effects on adhesion molecule expression, a property of great relevance to the vascular alterations of SSc. IL-4 levels are increased in peripheral blood of SSc patients. Most of this increase appears to be related to an increase in an alternatively spliced form of the molecule, IL-4δ2. Functionally, IL-4δ2 acts as an IL-4 antagonist in the stimulation of human T and B cells whereas, on the contrary, it acts as an agonist in its effects on fibroblasts. The activation of T cells and the upregulation of IL-4 and IL-4δ2 in SSc provide further support for the crucial role that inflammatory cells play in the pathogenesis of the disease.

IFNγ is secreted by activated T cells and is the most potent collagen synthesis inhibitory cytokine known. It causes a remarkable inhibition of fibroblast proliferation and collagen production, decreasing mRNA levels of the interstitial collagens in normal as well as SSc fibroblasts, both in vivo and in vitro. IFN-γ also abrogates the stimulatory effects of transforming growth factor (TGF)-β on fibroblast collagen production. These effects appear to be mediated by transcriptional mechanisms. Although it was suggested that IFN-γ production by SSc lymphocytes was decreased, a direct role of this cytokine on the pathogenesis of SSc has not been demonstrated.

TNFα, a major cytokine product of macrophages is also released by activated T cells. TNFα has similar effects to those of IFN-γ on fibroblast proliferation and collagen production causing a dose-dependent inhibitory effect on types I and III collagen production at the transcriptional level, as well as an inhibitory effect on TGF-β stimulation of fibroblasts. The role of TNFα in the pathogenesis of tissue fibrosis in SSc remains controversial. Although in vitro studies have shown a potent antifibrotic effect, in vivo studies have suggested that it is required for the production of pulmonary fibrosis in animal models. Given the availability of potent and specific antiTNFα biological agents, it is crucial to determine the precise role of this cytokine in the pathogenesis of SSc.

Growth Factors Since the discovery of the potent profibrotic and immunomodulatory activities of TGF-β, this growth factor has been considered one of the most likely molecules involved in the pathogenesis of SSc and other fibroproliferative diseases, and a plethora of publications have described studies focused on this subject. Three functionally and structurally similar isoforms of TGF-β exist in humans and they play important roles in embryonic development, immune responses, and regulation of tissue repair following injury. Activated monocytes from SSc patients secrete increased amounts of TGF-β and the upregulation of this cytokine/growth factor appears to play a crucial role in the development of fibrosis in patients with SSc. One of the most important effects of TGF-β is the stimulation of ECM synthesis as evidenced by a remarkable increase in the production of numerous molecules including collagens types I, III, V, and VI, as well as of other matrix proteins such as fibronectin and matrix glycoproteins. TGF-β also decreases the synthesis of collagen-degrading metalloproteinases and stimulates the production of protease inhibitors such as the tissue inhibitor of metalloproteinases-1. Small amounts of TGF-β appear to sensitize fibroblasts to its own effects and maintain them in a persistently activated state involving an autocrine mechanism that causes further production of TGF-β. It also appears that SSc fibroblasts express increased numbers of TGF-β receptors on their surface, which might account for the increased TGF-β-induced signaling and the resulting increased collagen production in these cells. Bioactive TGF-β binds to cell surface TGF-β II receptors (TβRII) in target cells to form a receptor complex. This receptor complex becomes activated and, in turn, it transphosphorylates the TGF-βI receptor (TβRI) causing its activation. Signaling from the phosphorylated TGF-βI receptor to the nucleus then occurs through the Smad family of proteins. Smad2 and Smad3 bind to the activated TGF-β receptor complex and they also become phosphorylated. Phosphorylation allows these proteins to form a complex with Smad4, which is a cytoplasmic protein involved in the translocation of the complex into the nucleus. Smad7 is an inhibitory Smad that can bind to the TGF-β receptor complex and prevent Smad2 or Smad3 phosphorylation. Once in the nucleus, Smad2/Smad4 or Smad3/Smad4 complexes bind directly to specific DNA binding sites in the promoter regions of target genes and activate their expression. The Smad3 complex binds to DNA sites in the promoter region of responsive genes with the help of intranuclear proteins that act as transcriptional partners. In contrast, Smad2 complexes do not appear to be able to directly bind to DNA promoter sites but instead exert their effect through other unidentified transcription factors or coactivator proteins. A diagrammatic representation of the TGF-β/SMAD pathway is shown in Fig. 100-1. More recent studies have provided additional details regarding the complex pathways of TGF-β modulation of expression of extracellular matrix genes and numerous other participating proteins such as SARA, smurfs, coactivators and corepressors, and others have been identified. Furthermore, it has become apparent that important TGF-β effects might be mediated by protein cascades independent of those of the classic SMAD pathway. These nonSMAD pathways involve members of the Rho family of proteins, numerous other intermediary steps such as protein prenylation, and kinase cascades involving novel proteins such as protein kinase Cδ, PKN, Rho kinase, and so on.

Connective tissue growth factor (CTGF) is another growth factor that appears also to play a crucial role in tissue fibrosis. In addition to a potent profibrotic effect, CTGF participates in angiogenesis, axial development of the musculoskeletal system, structural organization of connective tissue, and embryo implantation. TGF-β stimulates CTGF synthesis in fibroblasts, vascular smooth muscle cells, and endothelial cells. The CTGF produced by these cells in response to TGF-β stimulation in turn stimulates the synthesis of such ECM components as type I collagen and fibronectin in dermal and lung fibroblasts and very likely in endothelial cells.

Platelet-derived growth factor (PDGF) is a key inducer of monocyte chemoattractant protein 1 in SSc pathogenesis. In addition to its chemotactic properties, evidence suggests that monocyte chemoattractant protein 1 might participate in the fibrotic process by inducing the secretion of ECM components. The demonstrated overexpression of PDGF in SSc lesions and the selective upregulation of PDGF α receptors by TGF-β in SSc fibroblasts, indicate that PDGF ligand/receptor pathways are activated in these fibroblasts. Also, PDGF induces the profibrotic cytokine IL-6 in cultured SSc fibroblasts and is known to be a chemoattractant and potent mitogen for skin fibroblasts.

Finally, insulin-like growth factor-I is partially responsible for fibroblast proliferation in SSc patients with interstitial lung disease, thus playing a pathogenic role in the development of fibrotic lung changes in these patients. Insulin-like growth factor-I binding protein-5, which is the most conserved of the six identified IGFBPs, exhibits particularly high levels in affected skin fibroblasts from SSc patients as compared with unaffected and healthy control skin fibroblasts. Insulin-like growth factor-I binding protein-5 binds to collagen, fibronectin, and glycosaminoglycans such as heparan sulfate. Its binding to these ECM components decreases its affinity for insulin-like growth factor-I, resulting in increased biological activity of insulin-like growth factor-I, including its promotion of wound healing and increased tissue deposition.

DYSREGULATION OF CONNECTIVE TISSUE METABOLISM The most prominent clinical manifestations of SSc are caused by the exaggerated accumulation of collagen in the affected organs. The excessive collagen deposition in SSc is because of overproduction of this protein by fibroblasts. Regardless of the etiological event, the resulting alterations in the biosynthetic phenotype of collagen producing cells are crucial in the pathogenesis of SSc. Despite advances in the understanding of the regulation of collagen gene expression under normal conditions or under the effects of various cytokines and growth factors, the intimate mechanisms responsible for the pathological increase in the expression of collagen genes in SSc remain obscure. The exaggerated production of collagens by SSc fibroblasts largely results from increased transcription rates of their corresponding genes, although in certain conditions alterations in the stability of their mature transcripts might also contribute. Collagen is the most abundant protein in the body, and 28 different types have been described. Each has a highly specialized function in addition to providing the extracellular framework and tensile strength for such structures as tendons, skin, bone, blood vessels, and joint cartilage. Type I collagen is the most abundant collagen of the ECM of skin, and it represents 90% of the body's total collagen. In SSc it is mainly the upregulation of this collagen that produces the characteristic clinical findings. Although in the initial stages of fibrosis there is an increase in the proportion of type III collagen, eventually type I collagen becomes quantitatively the most abundant collagenous species and is, therefore,

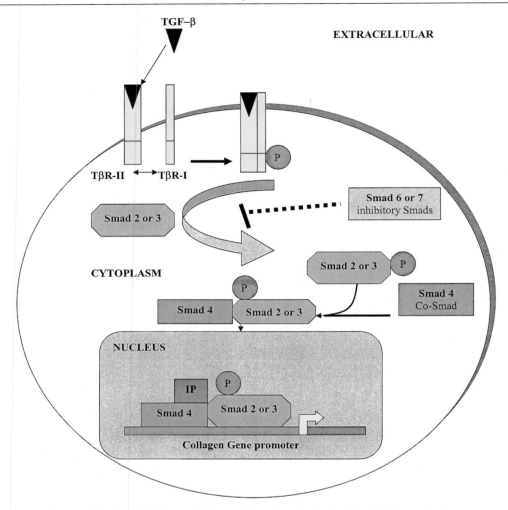

SSc = systemic sclerosis; TGFβ = transforming growth factor beta; P = phosphorylation; TβRII = transforming growth factor beta receptor 2; TβRI = transforming growth factor beta receptor 1; IP = intranuclear proteins

Figure 100-1   Diagrammatic representation of the TGF-β/Smad cascade of collagen gene activation.

largely responsible for the functional failure of the affected organs. Normal fibroblasts are capable of regulating collagen production according to the dynamic requirements of the ECM during development, differentiation, and repair. The regulatory mechanisms involved are complex: transcriptional regulation, modulation of mRNA stability and translation rates, and variation in the fraction of the newly synthesized collagen that is degraded before being secreted out of the cell.

Numerous studies have examined the normal mechanisms that regulate the initiation and rates of transcription of various collagen genes and their alterations in pathological states. As for most eukaryotic genes, the regulation of transcription rates of collagen genes involves precise interactions between specific nucleotide sequences present in the promoters and, often, in their first introns, with various transcription factors capable of recognizing and binding specifically to these sequences. The entire complement of regulatory elements in collagen genes and of transcription factors interacting with these elements is unknown.

One of the most extensively studied transcription factors is Sp1, a ubiquitously expressed zinc-finger protein that recognizes a GGGCGG sequence (GC box) widely distributed in the promoters of various Sp1-responsive cellular and viral genes. Several studies on the basal regulation of COL1A1 expression support the crucial importance of Sp1 in collagen gene expression regulation. Similar studies examining the role of Sp1 in the pathogenesis of SSc have shown that Sp1 appears to play a pivotal function in the activated expression of COL1A1. Increased Sp1 binding activity has been demonstrated in SSc fibroblast nuclear extracts in comparison to nuclear extracts from normal cells and increased Sp1 phosphorylation associated with increased expression of type I collagen genes has been found in these cells. Binding of Sp1 to its recognition sites has also been implicated in the regulation of expression of type I collagen genes under the influence of TGF-β. Indeed, a synergistic cooperative interaction between Sp1 and the TGF-β intracellular transduction pathways mediated by Smad3/Smad4 proteins in the stimulatory effects of the growth factor on COL1A2 transcriptional activity has been shown. Furthermore, specific inhibition of Sp1 and binding to its cognate elements within COL1A1 and COL1A2 employing DNA intercalators such as mithramycin, mitoxanthrone, and the doxyrubicin derivative, WP631, caused potent and selective inhibition of collagen gene expression in normal and SSc fibroblasts.

Sp1 binding and its transcriptional effects appear to be modulated by interactions with other nuclear proteins and coactivators involving protein–protein contacts between DNA-bound Sp1 and TATA-associated factors (TAFs) such as TAF110. Therefore, cell-specific differences in the activity of Sp1 might be because of the presence of different coactivators in different cells, or because of differential posttranslational modifications of Sp1.

Another transcription factor that appears to play an important role in collagen gene regulation is the CCAAT-binding factor (CBF). It has been demonstrated that CBF interacts with TAF110. Thus, both CBF and Sp1 transcription factors are involved in a protein–protein interaction in the initiation complex of the collagen core promoter as shown in studies demonstrating that nuclear extracts from normal and SSc dermal fibroblasts contained COL1A1 protein complexes corresponding to Sp1 and CBF. These results strongly indicate that CBF and Sp1 play a crucial role in the regulation of COL1A1 transcriptional activity under normal conditions and in SSc.

In contrast with the stimulatory effects of Sp1 and CBF, another transcription factor, c-Krox, represses COL1A1 transcription through its binding to a specific region of the proximal human COL1A1 promoter.

Transcription factors might also bind to enhancer elements in the first intron of collagen genes to bring about transcriptional regulation. It is likely that interactions between transcription factors and these intronic elements might cause profound effects on the regulation of COL1A1 transcriptional activity in SSc. Indeed, intronic sequences cause a potent stimulation of the transcriptional activity of the COL1A1 promoter and these effects are even more noticeable in SSc fibroblasts.

ENDOTHELIAL CELL ABNORMALITIES Vascular dysfunction is one of the earliest clinical manifestations of SSc. Small blood vessels in affected tissues from SSc patients show perivascular cellular infiltration with activated T cells similar to that present in affected skin and internal organs. It has been postulated that cytokines or growth factors, such as TGF-β, secreted by these activated lymphocytes cause activation and injury of small vessel endothelial cells inducing their expression of MHC classes I and II antigens and adhesion ligand ICAM-1, and secretion of increased amounts of von Willebrand factor. As described, TGF-β causes an upregulation of CTGF that in turn induces an increased production of ECM components as well as an upregulation of PDGF. PDGF is a potent endothelial cell mitogen that causes increased endothelial cell proliferation. Also, in SSc a downregulation of vascular endothelial growth factor results in decreased and impaired neovascularization. Chemo-attraction of fibroblasts into the vessel wall and transdifferentiation of resident vessel wall fibroblasts into myofibroblasts occurs as a result of the effects of the locally secreted cytokines and growth factors, leading to increased collagen synthesis and deposition. Endothelial injury causes the subendothelium to be exposed to circulating platelets that eventually adhere to it and initiate fibrin deposition and intravascular thrombus formation. SSc vascular fibroproliferative lesions and intravascular platelet thrombosis inevitably result in a state of local hypoxia in affected tissues. Studies have demonstrated that local hypoxia can further cause tissue fibrosis by activation of collagen and TGF-β genes.

Vasodilation also appears to be impaired in SSc patients. Vasodilation is usually controlled by both endothelial and nonendothelial (neurological) mechanisms. Endothelial cells regulate vascular tone by secreting vasoactive substances such as nitric oxide and calcitonin-related peptide that are vasodilatory, as well as endothelin-I that is a potent vasoconstrictor. It appears that in SSc a relative deficiency of vasodilator molecules and a relative increase of vasoconstrictor ones in turn causes further vascular hypoxia and endothelial injury resulting in the production and release of additional cytokines from the activated inflammatory cells, thus maintaining the vicious cycle of endothelial injury and fibrosis. Indeed, several studies have demonstrated increased production of endothelin-I in affected SSc microvasculature as well as in parenchyma of affected tissues. The effects of vascular dysfunction in patients with SSc are most dramatic when they involve the pulmonary and renal arterioles, causing endothelial injury with subsequent intravascular thrombus formation as well as fibrous tissue deposition in the myointimal region of the vessels. The constellation of these multiple vascular alterations leads to renal crisis and pulmonary hypertension, respectively, which are the most prevalent causes of morbidity and mortality in patients with SSc. The novel therapeutic agents for pulmonary hypertension such as endothelin inhibitors have been generated from the understanding of its pathogenesis.

DIFFERENTIAL DIAGNOSIS

The diagnosis of SSc is based on the physical examination and presence of specific and characteristic clinical findings. Localized scleroderma (morphea and linear scleroderma) can generally be diagnosed by clinical examination. Other diseases characterized by skin thickening confined to the hands that need to be considered as part of the differential diagnosis include cutaneous amyloidosis, diabetic cheiropathy, vibration-related acrosclerosis, and reflex sympathetic dystrophy. Generalized skin thickening might also be seen in eosinophilia-fasciitis, the eosinophilic-myalgia syndrome, scleromyxedema, scleredema adultorum of Buschke, cutaneous amyloidosis, porphyria cutanea tarda, nephrogenic fibrosing dermopathy/nephrogenic systemic fibrosis, and human graft-vs-host disease. Although laboratory data is helpful in confirming the diagnosis, a full thickness skin biopsy including subcutaneous tissue and fascia is often necessary to exclude these diseases.

MANAGEMENT

Although numerous agents have been employed for the treatment of SSc no studies have conclusively proven the benefit of any one agent. Although some clinicians follow a minimalist approach and do not prescribe potentially effective disease modifying therapies, others have used such agents especially in patients with rapidly progressive diffuse disease. D-Penicillamine has been widely used to treat SSc owing to its potent inhibition of collagen crosslinking that causes an increase in the degradation of newly synthesized, noncrosslinked collagen molecules. Although several uncontrolled studies have shown improvement in the extent and severity of skin thickening and improvement in the overall survival rates, one prospective study comparing low vs a high dose of D-penicillamine failed to show a difference among the two therapies. Therefore, a placebo-controlled study is required to answer this question. Other immunosuppressive agents such as methotrexate have been used but have been shown to be ineffective in controlled trials. IFN-γ, one of the most potent inhibitors of collagen production by fibroblasts known, decreases skin thickening although its administration is complicated by an exacerbation of vascular events. Other immunosuppressive agents studied as disease modifying agents for this disorder have been chlorambucil, azathioprine, 5-fluorouracil, relaxin, photophoresis, and cyclosporine, all of which are ineffective. Other agents that modify collagen biosynthetic pathways have been studied with questionable results, including colchicine, N-acetylcysteine, potassium aminobenzoate and minocycline. Aggressive therapy with immunoablation and autologous stem cell transplantation has also been employed but the procedure carries a high risk of severe side effects and high mortality.

Major strides in SSc management have been in the treatment of the various symptoms of SSc. Raynaud's phenomenon can often be improved by the use of sustained release calcium-channel blockers, α-adrenergic blockers, or both. Platelet inhibitors such as low-dose aspirin and/or dipyrimadole might also be added to the regime. In severe cases, stellate ganglion blockade or digital sympathectomy might provide significant symptom relief. In critical situations in which an acute ischemic event is threatening the viability of a digit, intravenous alprostadil has been used with varying success.

For the esophageal manifestations of SSc, the introduction of H_2 blockers and proton-pump inhibitors has dramatically decreased symptoms of gastroesophageal reflux and chronic esophagitis and stricture. Regarding diminished gastic emptying and decreased intestinal peristalsis, a setback occurred with the withdrawal of cisapride from the market although metoclopramide is used with some beneficial results. Bacterial overgowth caused by decreased peristalsis in the small intestine often results in weight loss, chronic diarrhea, and even malabsorption. Two weeks of alternating cyclic courses of broad spectrum antibiotics such as metronidazole, tetracycline, and amoxicillin might help decrease these symptoms. Persistent abdominal distention with nausea and vomiting suggests an intestinal pseudoobstruction in these patients and surgical exploration should be avoided.

Pulmonary fibrosis is common in SSc patients with the diffuse form of the disease and early signs of lung involvement should be suspected in patients with dyspnea and a decreasing forced vital capacity or diffusing capacity for carbon dioxide on pulmonary function testing. Early evaluation by high-resolution CT and/or bronchoalveolar lavage might identify patients with alveolitis who are amenable to therapy with oral or intravenous pulse cyclophosphamide. Corticosteroids and other immunosuppressive drugs have proven remarkably ineffective in improving or preventing progression of interstitial fibrosis in SSc although numerous recent studies suggest that the oral or intravenous pulse administration of cyclophosphamide can stabilize or improve the pulmonary involvement in SSc. Pulmonary hypertension might occur as a complication of long-standing pulmonary fibrosis and in patients with limited SSc. Early evaluation by two-dimensional echocardiography and confirmation by right heart catherization is required to clearly define the severity of pulmonary hypertension. Calcium channel blockers do not affect the survival of these patients. In contrast, administration of prostacyclin analogs results in a reduction of mortality in this group of patients, although the need for a continued intravenous infusion is limiting. A longer acting prostacyclin analog, treprostenil, is more advantageous because it might be given by a subcutaneous pump-infusion. A remarkable improvement in the treatment of pulmonary hypertension, currently the most fatal complication of SSc, has been obtained following the introduction of an orally effective endothelin-1 receptor antagonist, bosentan. This drug has been shown to cause significant functional improvement and a remarkable prolongation in the survival of these patients.

The greatest success in the management of scleroderma has been in the treatment of scleroderma renal crisis. Before the advent of angiotensin converting enzyme inhibitors, the 1-yr survival of these patients was 16%. Today with the widespread use of angiotensin converting enzyme inhibitors in patients with early signs of scleroderma renal crisis, treated promptly and aggressively with these drugs, the survival rate has improved to 76%.

The study of SSc has evolved from the concept that the disease was purely because of collagen overproduction by affected fibroblasts to where it is possible to postulate distinct processes occurring in the initiating phases of this disease. The knowledge acquired in this search has already and undoubtedly will continue to uncover novel therapeutic targets that might result in the development of long awaited and effective therapeutic options.

SELECTED REFERENCES

Arnett FC, Cho M, Chatterjee S, et al. Familial occurrence frequencies and relative risks for systemic sclerosis (scleroderma) in three United States cohorts. Arthritis Rheum 2001;44(6):1359–1362.

Artlett CM, Smith JB, Jimenez SA. Identification of fetal DNA and cells in skin lesions from women with systemic sclerosis. N Engl J Med 1998;338:1186–1191.

Cheema GS, Quismorio FP Jr. Interstitial lung disease in systemic sclerosis. Curr Opin Pulm Med 2001;7:283–290.

Cepeda EJ, Reveille JD. Autoantibodies in systemic sclerosis and fibrosing syndromes: clinical indications and relevance. Curr Opin Rheumatol 2004;16:723–732.

Clark DA, Coker R. Transforming growth factor-beta (TGF-β). Int J Biochem Cell Biol 1998;30:293–298.

Coghlan JG, Mukerjee D. The heart and pulmonary vasculature in scleroderma: clinical features and pathobiology. Curr Opin Rheumatol 2001;13:495–499.

Derk CT, Jimenez SA. Systemic sclerosis: current views of its pathogenesis. Autoimmun Rev 2003;2:181–191.

Derynck R, Zhang YE. Smad-dependent and smad-independent pathways in TGFβ family signalling. Nature 2003;425:577–584.

Dong C, Zhu S, Wang T, et al. Deficient Smad 7 expression: a putative molecular defect in scleroderma. Proc Natl Acad Sci USA 2002; 99:3908–3913.

Ferri C, Valentini G, Cozzi F, et al. Systemic sclerosis: demographic, clinical and serologic features and survival in 1,012 Italian patients. Medicine 2002;81:139–153.

Ghosh AK. Factors involved in the regulation of type I collagen gene expression: implication in fibrosis. Exp Biol Med (Maywood) 2002; 227(5):301–314.

Ihn H, Yamane K, Kubo M, et al. Blockade of endogenous transforming growth factor β signaling prevents up-regulated collagen synthesis in scleroderma fibroblasts: association with increased expression of transforming growth factor β receptors. Arthritis Rheum 2001;44:474–480.

Jimenez SA, Derk CT. Following the molecular pathways toward an understanding of the pathogenesis of systemic sclerosis. Ann Intern Med 2004;140:37–50.

Johnson RW, Tew MB, Arnett FC. The genetics of systemic sclerosis. Curr Rheumatol Rep 2002;4:99–107.

Lally EV, Jimenez SA, Kaplan SR. Progressive systemic sclerosis: mode of presentation, rapidly progressive disease course, and mortality based on an analysis of 91 patients. Semin Arthritis Rheum 1988;18:1–13.

LeRoy EC. Connective tissue synthesis by scleroderma skin fibroblasts in cell culture. J Exp Med 1972;135:1351, 1352.

LeRoy EC, Black C, Fleischmajer R, et al. Scleroderma (systemic sclerosis): classification, subsets and pathogenesis. J Rheumatol 1988;15:202–205.

MacGregor AJ, Canavan R, Knight C, et al. Pulmonary hypertension in systemic sclerosis: risk factors for progression and consequences for survival. Rheumatology 2001;40:453–459.

Moustakas A, Heldin C-H. Non-Smad TGF-β signals. J Cell Sci 2005; 118:3573–3584.

Nietert PJ, Silver RM. Systemic sclerosis: environmental and occupational risk factors. Curr Opin Rheumatol 2000;12:520–526.

Rose S, Young MA, Reynolds JC. Gastointestinal manifestations of scleroderma. Gastroenterol Clin North Am 1998;27:563–594.

Rosenbloom J, Saitta B, Gaidarova S, et al. Inhibition of type I collagen gene expression in normal and systemic sclerosis fibroblasts by a specific inhibitor of geranylgeranyl transferase I. Arthritis Rheum 2000; 43:1624–1632.

Rubin LI, Badesch DB, Barst RJ, et al. Bosentan therapy for pulmonary arterial hypertension. N Engl J Med 2002;346:896–903.

Shi-Wen X, Denton CP, Dashwood MR, et al. Fibroblast matrix gene expression and connective tissue remodeling: role of endothelin-1. J Invest Dermatol 2001;116:417–425.

Steen VD. Scleroderma renal crisis. Rheum Dis Clin North Am 1996; 22:861–878.

Steen VD, Medsger TA Jr. Severe organ involvement in systemic sclerosis with diffuse scleroderma. Arthritis Rheum 2000;43: 2437–2444.

Ten Dijke P, Hill CS. New insights into TGF-β-Smad signalling. Trends Biochem Sci 2004;29:265–273.

Varga J. Scleroderma and smads: dysfunctional smad family dynamics culminating in fibrosis. Arthritis Rheum 2002;46:1703–1713.

Whitman M, Raftery L. TGFβ signaling at the summit. Development 2005;132:4205–4210.

NONIMMUNE

101 Diseases With Signaling and Transcriptional Abnormalities

DAVID S. RUBENSTEIN, AMY STEIN, AND LOWELL A. GOLDSMITH

SUMMARY

Tuberous sclerosis, neurofibromatosis 1 and 2, hereditary hemorrhagic telangiectasia, anhidrotic ectodermal dysplasia, and icontinentia pigmenti are pathological processes that affect signal transduction and transcriptional regulation. Elucidation of the molecular defects underlying these disorders has led to a better understanding of the mechanisms by which the skin and other organ systems develop and regulate cell growth and differentiation.

Key Words: Activin receptor-like kinase-1; connexin-30; endoglin; ectodysplasin; hamartin; merlin; NEMO; neurofibromin-1; tuberin.

INTRODUCTION

To coordinate their function within multicellular organisms, individual cells communicate with one another. Signal transduction is the process by which they transmit information. It can occur within both solid organ and bone marrow derived tissues. Because cells are enclosed by a lipid bilayer, the cell membrane, specific mechanisms have evolved to enable cells to transmit signals across this membrane, whether the flow of information is from the outside in or the inside out. The variety of mechanisms by which cells transduce information across the cell membrane includes classic single pass or multipass transmembrane protein receptors, ion channels, and cell-adhesion proteins. Activation of these transmembrane signaling events typically initiates activation of second messenger systems or post-translational modification of cellular proteins that activate intracellular cascades to alter gene transcription or the structural biology and behavior of cellular machinery. This chapter reviews several skin diseases in which alterations in signaling systems result in skin disease.

TUBEROUS SCLEROSIS

CLINICAL PRESENTATION   Tuberous sclerosis (TS) is an autosomal-dominant inherited disorder that involves the skin and internal organs. Typical cutaneous manifestations include angiofibromas (adenoma sebaceum), Shagreen patches (connective tissue nevi), periungual fibromas (Koenen tumors), ash leaf macules, and confetti style hypopigmented macules. TS-associated CNS tumors and hamartomas include cortical tubers, astrocytomas, and subependymal nodules. Clinical manifestations of CNS involvement include seizure disorder and mental retardation. Lymphangioleiomyomatosis of the lungs, almost always seen in women with TS, may result in repeat episodes of spontaneous pneumothorax. Renal angiomyolipomas and cardiac rhabdomyomas can also occur. The incidence of TS is estimated at 1 in 6000 live births. Approximately two-thirds of patients represent new mutations.

MOLECULAR BASIS AND DEFECTS   Mutations in either the TSC1 or TSC2 tumor suppressor genes have been identified as the cause of TS. TSC1, which maps to chromosome 9q34, encodes the protein hamartin, whereas TSC2 maps to chromosome 16p13.3 and encodes the protein tuberin. The structure of these two proteins reflects their interaction with a variety of cellular signaling and structural proteins. Structure function analysis of the 130-kDa hamartin protein has demonstrated an N-terminal Rho GTPase-activating region that overlaps a tuberin binding site; regions in the hamartin C-terminus bind the ezrin-radixin-moezin (ERM) family of actin binding proteins. This ERM site overlaps a neurofilament-L binding site. Tuberin is a 198 kDa protein whose N-terminus binds hamartin. Tuberin also contains several coiled-coil domains, a leucine zipper, Akt/PKB-dependent phosphorylation sites, phosphorylation-dependent 14-3-3-binding sites, and potential transcriptional activation domains at the C-terminus. Hamartin and tuberin form a complex that inhibits cell growth by negatively regulating the function of S6 kinase 1 and the eukaryotic initiation factor 4E-binding protein 1. Additionally, through interactions with ERM family proteins, hamartin signaling regulates the formation of focal adhesions. In vivo work in the fruit fly *Drosophila melanogaster* has demonstrated a role for TSC genes in cell-cycle regulation and cell-size control.

DIAGNOSIS: CLINICAL AND LABORATORY   The cutaneous manifestations of TS, particularly the hypopigmented macules, may be present at birth or develop as the child ages. The presence of hypopigmented macules and seizure disorder in an infant should alert the physician to the potential for TS. Because approximately two-thirds of new patients represent spontaneous mutations, a family history may not necessarily be elicited. Diagnostic criteria for TS include both major and minor features with a definite diagnosis requiring confirmation of either two major features or one major and two minor features. Major features include facial angiofibromas, periungual fibromas, three or more hypomelanotic macules,

From: *Principles of Molecular Medicine, Second Edition*
Edited by: M. S. Runge and C. Patterson © Humana Press, Inc., Totowa, NJ

991

Shagreen patch, retinal nodular hamartomas, cortical tubers, subependymal nodules, subependymal giant cell astrocytoma, cardiac rhabdomyoma, lymphangiomyomatosis, and renal angiomyolipomas. Minor features include pitting of the dental enamel, hamartomatous rectal polyps, bone cysts, cerebral white matter radial migration lines, gingival fibromas, nonrenal hamartomas, retinal achromia, confetti-like hypopigmentation, and renal cysts. In addition to full skin and ocular exams, the diagnostic workup should include an ECG, renal ultrasound, cranial CT or MRI, and neurodevelopmental testing.

MANAGEMENT/TREATMENT The management of TS involves diagnosing and treating the complications that arise from internal organ involvement. Involvement of multiple organ systems dictates a multispecialty approach including neurologists, cardiologists, nephrologists, and dermatologists. Infants suspected of having TS should be evaluated by CT or MRI to look for neurological changes such as subependymal calcifications and cortical tubers. Renal ultrasounds and echocardiograms aid in identifying renal angiomyolipomas and cardiac rhabdomyomas, respectively. Seizure disorders may be amenable to medical management. Surgical intervention may be considered for intractable seizures. Treatment strategies for managing the renal involvement include observation of small asymptomatic renal angiomyolipomas and selective arterial embolization or partial nephrectomy for hemorrhage or spontaneous rupture of larger tumors. The development of acute dyspnea should alert the clinician to the possibility of spontaneous pneumothorax with a chylous pleural effusion.

NEUROFIBROMATOSIS 1

CLINICAL PRESENTATION Also known as von Recklinghausen Disease, neurofibromatosis 1 (NF1) is an autosomal-dominant disorder of complete pentrance and variable expressivity characterized by neurocutaneous tumors and pigmentary alterations. Patients may have only a few clinical findings at birth or during childhood, but develop more characteristic lesions with age. One of the earliest findings that may be present at birth is light tan pigmented macules called café au lait macules. Axillary and inguinal freckling typically appears during late childhood or early adulthood. The pigmentary changes are thought to be a consequence of increased numbers of melanocytes and abnormal melanogenesis with the presence of giant pigment granules in lesional skin. Neurofibromas, benign tumors derived from the nerve sheath, may be numerous and have the appearance of pigmented skin tags, pedunculated masses, or subcutaneous nodules. Plexiform neurofibromas, which may mimic the appearance of a "bag of worms" beneath the skin, can undergo malignant degeneration to a neurofibrosarcoma (malignant peripheral nerve sheath tumor). Sudden growth and/or pain in a plexiform neurofibroma should alert the clinician to malignant degeneration. NF1 patients with NF1 microdeletions have a higher risk of developing neurofibrosarcoma.

Lisch nodules, small yellow-brown pigmented iris hamartomas, are an additional clinical feature present in more than 90% of affected individuals 6 yr of age and older. Optic gliomas may result in progressive vision loss. Although true mental retardation is uncommon, occurring in 4–8% of individuals, as many as 50% of NF1 patients experience variations in cognitive function that may manifest as a mild learning diasability. NF1 is associated with an increased risk of developing certain malignancies, including neurofibrosarcoma, malignant glioma, pheochromocytoma, carcinoid, rhabdomyosarcoma, and juvenile chronic myeloid leukemia.

Hypertension and hypoglycemia appear to be more common in this disorder. The incidence of NF1 is estimated at 1 in 3000; approximately half of new NF1 cases may represent new mutations.

MOLECULAR BASIS AND DEFECTS NF1 results from mutations in the gene encoding neurofibromin-1 localized to chromosome 17q11.2. Neurofibromin-1 is a large multidomain cytoplasmic protein that regulates the ERK MAP kinase signaling cascade (Fig. 101-1), adenyl cyclase, and the cytoskeleton. The central region of neurofibromin-1 contains sequence similarity to the GTPase-activating protein family (GAP); neurofibromin GAP activity promotes formation of inactive ras-GDP. In this capacity, neurofibromin-1 functions as a tumor suppressor and downregulates mitogenic signaling mediated by the ras/ERK signaling cascade. Ras is inactive when bound to GDP. Signaling through transmembrane receptors activates ras through guanine nucleotide exchange factors in which GTP is exchanged for bound GDP on ras. Active ras-GTP then leads to activation of downstream components including Raf, MEK, and ERK through a series of sequential phosphorylation events, that results in activation of CBP/CREB mediated transcription and altered gene expression. Mutations resulting in NF1 are distributed throughout the coding sequence and lead to decreased ras inhibition. The resulting increase in ras signaling activates cellular proliferation and tumor formation in NF1.

DIAGNOSIS: CLINICAL AND LABORATORY The clinical diagnosis of NF1 requires two or more of the following features:

1. Six or more café au lait macules (each >5 mm in prepubescent children, but >1.5 cm in diameter in postpubescent individuals).
2. Two or more neurofibromas or at least one plexiform neurofibroma.
3. Axillary or inguinal freckling.
4. Optic gliomas.
5. Lisch nodules.
6. Osseus lesion (sphenoid dysplasia or long bone cortical thinning).
7. A first degree relative with NF1.

Commercial testing for NF1 concentrates on the neurofibromin truncations resulting from many NF1 mutations; however, a negative result by this approach does not exclude the diagnosis.

MANAGEMENT/TREATMENT Management of NF1 is focused on early detection and intervention for complications arising from the disorder. Screening for learning disabilities may be warranted in children who experience difficulties in school. Routine ophthalmolgic examination may identify early visual changes owing to optic gliomas. Painful or rapidly growing tumors require biopsy to exclude neurofibrosarcoma. Pedunculated neurofibromas are readily removed by simple surgical excision and may be warranted for tumors in areas prone to frictional trauma such as waistbands or for improved cosmesis.

NEUROFIBROMATOSIS 2

CLINICAL PRESENTATION Neurofibromatosis 2 (NF2) is an autosomal-dominant disorder of high penetrance (>95%) that manifests clinically as deafness owing to tumors of the eighth cranial nerve as well as CNS meningiomas and schwannomas, usually of the brain and spinal cord dorsal roots, respectively. The acoustic neuromas, which are more correctly termed vestibular schwannomas, are usually bilateral. Patients experience tinnitus and diminished hearing with the growth of these tumors.

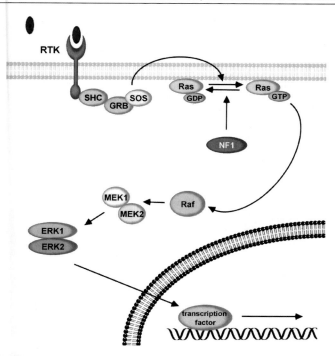

Figure 101-1 Mitogen activated protein kinase signaling and NF1. In this pathway, Ras is inactive when bound to GDP. Signaling through transmembrane receptor tyrosine kinases activates Ras through guanine nucleotide exchange factors in which GTP is exchanged for bound GDP on Ras. Active Ras-GTP then leads to activation of downstream components including Raf, MEK1/2, and ERK1/2 through a series of sequential phosphorylation events that results in activation of CBP/CREB mediated transcription and altered gene expression. NF1 contains GTPase activity, promotes formation of inactive Ras-GDP, and downregulates mitogenic signaling mediated by the Ras/ERK signaling cascade.

Some patients experience a distal symmetric sensorimotor neuropathy that may clinically manifest as muscle weakness or wasting. NF2 patients are predisposed to cataract formation. Skin findings in NF2 are much less numerous than in NF1, but include café au lait macules, and cutaneous and subcutaneous schwannomas. Neurofibromas are much less common in NF2. There does not appear to be a significantly increased risk of malignant tumor formation.

The incidence of NF2 is estimated to be 1 in 40,000. The rate of spontaneous mutation is high and up to 75% of patients with no family history may represent new mutations.

MOLECULAR BASIS AND DEFECTS NF2 is owing to mutations in the merlin (neurofibromin-2) gene that maps to chromosome 22q12.2. More severe forms of the disease arise from truncating mutations. Mutations resulting in single amino acid substitutions are associated with mild phenotypes. Merlin can be categorized as a tumor suppressor because of the resultant tumor formation with inactivation of merlin function. Merlin is structurally similar to the ERM family of proteins that mediates interactions between cell membrane glycoproteins and the actin cytoskeleton. Merlin has dual structural and signaling roles and may function as an adaptor protein that mediates signals allowing the cell to co-ordinate changes in adhesive state and differentiation. The precise mechanism of signaling is being studied and may involve signaling via PI3-kinase. Hepatocyte growth factor (HGF) stimulates schwann cell proliferation. By binding to the HGF-regulated tyrosine kinase substrate, merlin may function to downregulate signaling through the HGF-receptor (HGF-R).

DIAGNOSIS: CLINICAL AND LABORATORY The clinical diagnosis of NF2 can be made by the demonstration of bilateral cranial nerve masses by either MRI or CT, the presence of a unilateral cranial nerve mass and a first degree relative with NF2, or a first degree relative with NF2 and two or more of the following clinical features: neurofibroma, meningioma, glioma, schwannoma, and juvenile posterior subcapsular lenticular opacities.

Evaluation should include audiometry and ophthalmalogic evaluation with slit lamp examination and gadolinium, enhanced MRI of the brain and spine or CT. Nerve conduction studies and electromyography are useful in screening for neuropathy. Early diagnosis in some familial variants may be possible with linkage analysis or direct sequencing.

MANAGEMENT/TREATMENT Stereotactic radiosurgery and microsurgical resection have been used to treat acoustic neuromas.

HEREDITARY HEMORRHAGIC TELANGIECTASIA

CLINICAL PRESENTATION Hereditary hemorrhagic telangiectasia (HHT), an autosomal-dominant inherited disorder of high penetrance, also known as Osler-Weber-Rendu, is characterized by mucocutaneous telangiectases whose clinical manifestations include epistaxis and gastrointestinal hemorrhage. Punctate to several millimeters red, telangiectatic macules, or vascular papules are commonly found on the tongue, lips, conjunctiva, ears, and fingers. The vascular lesions typically appear during childhood and increase in size as the child grows to adulthood; approx 90% of patients have experienced an episode of epistaxis by 16 yr of age with a median age of onset at 12 yr. Arteriovenous malformations (AVMs) can be found in other tissues including the CNS, lungs, and liver. Migraine headaches occur with increased frequency; approx 50% of patients report a history of migraine with aura. Additionally, HHT has been associated with an increased incidence of spontaneous abortion. Pulmonary AVMs may result in heart failure; emboli originating from pulmonary AVMs can cause CNS infarcts and be a source for CNS abscess formation. Severe gastrointestinal hemorrhage requiring transfusions is not uncommon. Iron deficiency anemia may result from chronic hemorrhage.

The incidence of HHT is estimated to be 1 in 10,000.

MOLECULAR BASIS AND DEFECTS HHT results from aberrations in the transforming growth factor (TGF)-β signaling pathway (Fig. 101-2) resulting from mutations in either of two genes encoding (1) endoglin (ENG or HHT1) localized to chromosome 9q34.1 or (2) activin receptor-like kinase-1 (ACVRLK1, *ALK1*, HHT2) localized to chromosome 12q11-q14. Endoglin, expressed primarily on vascular endothelial cells, is a homodimeric membrane glycoprotein of 90 kDa subunits that binds to TGF-β1, TGF-β3, activin-A, BMP2, and BMP7. Endoglin antagonizes the inhibitory signaling of TGF-β1. *ALK1* encodes a protein that regulates blood vessel growth and repair. ALK1 is a type I serine-threonine kinase belonging to the TGF-β superfamily that is expressed primarily on vascular endothelial cells. ALK1 initiates signaling in response to both TGF-β1 and TGF-β3 and has been shown in vitro to bind activin-A. ALK1 signaling is mediated by phosphorylation of SMAD1 and SMAD5.

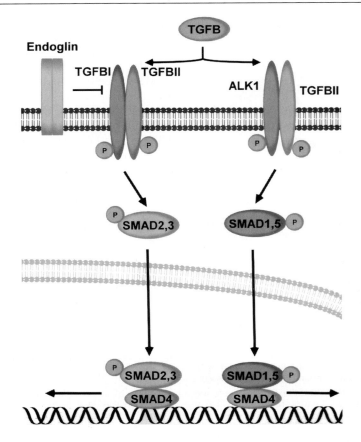

Figure 101-2 The TGF-β signaling pathway and HHT. The TGF-β superfamily (TGF-β) is comprised of a variety of related cytokines including TGF-β isoforms, activins, bone morphogenetic proteins, growth and differentiation factors, nodal and dorsalin. Members of this ligand super-family activate signaling pathways by binding to heterodimeric cell surface receptors. In this model of HHT, vascular endothelial differentiation is regulated by two alternative signaling pathways. Extracellular TGF-β binds to TGF-β receptor I/II heterodimers (TGF-βI/TGF-βII) and activates transcriptional events, mediated by SMAD2,3/SMAD4 heterodimers, that regulate the resolution phase of angiogenesis. Alternatively, TGF-β binding to ALK1/TGF-β receptor II heterodimers results in activation of angiogenesis via SMAD1,5/SMAD4 heterodimeric regulation of transcription. Endoglin negatively regulates TGF-βI/II signaling. HHT results from mutations in either ALK1 or endoglin that increase SMAD2,3/SMAD4 mediated transcription relative to SMAD1,5/SMAD4.

Patients with defects in endoglin may have earlier onset and more severe disease than those with mutations in ALK1. For example, pulmonary AVMs appear to be much more common in patients with endoglin mutations.

DIAGNOSIS: CLINICAL AND LABORATORY Criteria for the diagnosis of HHT include a positive family history, frequent epistaxis, the presence of mucocutaneous telangiectases, and the presence of visceral AVMs. HHT Foundation International, Inc., consensus clinical diagnostic criteria require at least three features for a definitive diagnosis of HHT. With only two criteria, the diagnosis is not definitive, but should be suspected and patients monitored closely for the development of additional features and/or clinical complications. HHT is considered unlikely with less than two features, although special consideration for additional screening should be considered if one of the criteria is a positive family history. Work-up should include imaging studies to assess for the presence of AVMs in the CNS, lungs, and liver. Endoscopy may reveal gastrointestinal telangiectases. The diagnosis of HHT should alert the physician to monitor the patient for potential complications arising from involvement of internal organs. In young children of affected individuals, the presence of capillary nail-fold telangiectases should increase the index of suspicion for HHT as these nail-fold changes may precede the development of telangectases in other areas.

Genetic testing via sequencing of the entire suspected coding region as well as prenatal diagnosis is available. Select laboratories that offer this testing can be found by searching Online Mendelian Inheritance in Man.

MANAGEMENT/TREATMENT Management attempts to minimize and treat the complications arising from the vascular malformations and hemorrhage. Larger AVMs are sometimes amenable to surgical intervention. Iron deficiency should be treated with supplementation.

ANHIDROTIC ECTODERMAL DYSPLASIA

CLINICAL PRESENTATION Also called hypohidrotic ectodermal dysplasia or Christ-Siemens-Touraine Syndrome, anhidrotic ectodermal dysplasia is characterized by a markedly reduced ability to sweat. X-linked recessive is the most common inheritance pattern; however, autosomal-dominant and autosomal-recessive forms have been reported. Male infants may present at birth with a colloidon membrane or scaling that may be misinterpreted as a manifestation of ichthyosis. An additional

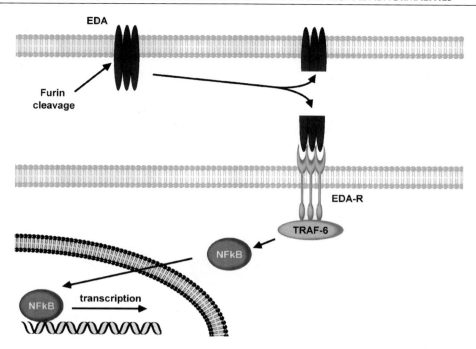

Figure 101-3 EDA signaling and anhidrotic ectodermal dysplasia. EDA is a transmembrane protein that forms homotrimers. Cleavage of EDA trimers by furin proteinases releases soluble trimeric EDA ligand that binds to the extracellular region of the trimeric EDAR, a member of the TNF-receptor protein family. When bound to EDA, the cytoplasmic tail of EDAR associates with TNF-receptor-associated factor-6 to initiate a signaling cascade that regulates NFκB-mediated transcription of target genes essential for the development of epithelial adnexal structures. Mutations in EDA result in the failure to activate this signaling pathway during the development of epithelial adnexal structures and cause anhidrotic ectodermal dysplasia.

feature is fine sparse blonde hair. Sweat pores are absent on physical exam and palmar creases are lost on the finger tips. Nail changes occur in 50% and include brittleness and ridging, but they are usually grossly normal. Recalcitrant atopic dermatitis is common. Because of the decreased ability to sweat, patients manifest elevated temperatures in warm environments. Infants may initially present because of repeated hospitalizations for high fevers with no identifiable infectious etiology. Other features include sebaceous hyperplasia as affected individual's age, hypodontia characterized by a few peg-shaped teeth or oligodontia, and focal patches of eczematous dermatitis. Frontal bossing, maxillary hypoplasia, saddle nose, and periorbital wrinkles characterize the typical facies. Affected males manifest the full clinical pattern, whereas the disorder is partially penetrant in female heterozygotes. Female carriers may be normal or manifest some features, predominately patchy focal hypotrichosis, in a distribution consistent with Barr body inactivation (lyonization). Female carriers may also demonstrate focal hypohidrosis and abnormal dentition. The incidence is estimated to be 1 in 100,000 live male births. All races are affected.

MOLECULAR BASIS AND DEFECTS Anhidrotic ectodermal dysplasia represents an inherited disorder in which transmembrane signaling is disrupted because of the failure to make a functional ligand capable of activating a receptor signaling pathway (Fig. 101-3) that is critical for development of epithelial adnexal structures. Anhidrotic ectodermal dysplasia has been mapped to the ectodysplasin-A (EDA) gene on chromosome Xq12-13.1. ED functions in the development of epithelial adnexal structures and its absence results in decreased numbers of hair follicles and sebaceous glands and reduced or absent

eccrine sweat glands. ED is the ligand for the ED-A receptor (EDAR), a member of the tumor necrosis factor (TNF) receptor protein family. EDA is a transmembrane protein that forms homotrimers. Cleavage of EDA trimers by furin proteinases releases soluble trimeric EDA ligand that binds to the extracellular region of the trimeric EDAR. Occupancy of the extracellular ligand binding site of EDAR by EDA results in the binding of TNF receptor-associated factor-6 to the cytoplasmic portion of the EDAR. Subsequent transcriptional regulation is thought to be mediated by nuclear factor (NF)κβ.

The Lyon hypothesis explains why a heterozygous female can display a range of clinical abnormalities, including none. In females, there is early, random inactivation of one X-chromosome; therefore, the adult female is a mosaic of two populations of cells, those in which the maternal X is the active chromosome and those in which the paternal X is the active one. For instance, there may be an individual in which inactivation occurs in cell lines with the mutated X-chromosome; in this case, there are no abnormalities detected. However, in many X-linked diseases such as anhidrotic ectodermal dysplasia, some carrier females display clinical abnormalities; this implies that inactivation occurs in the mutant X-chromosome in some cell lines but in the normal chromosome in others.

DIAGNOSIS: CLINICAL AND LABORATORY The diagnosis can be established by the typical clinical features described. Prenatal diagnosis has been performed by skin biopsy and by fetoscopy and shows a complete absence of pilosebaceous units. Fetal analysis has been performed by chorionic villus biopsy.

MANAGEMENT/TREATMENT Because of their reduced ability to sweat, affected individuals are susceptible to hot

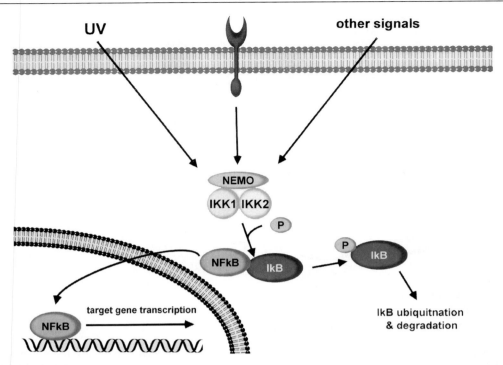

Figure 101-4   NFκB/IκB signaling. NFκB is a transcription factor that regulates a large number of genes implicated in apoptosis, cell growth, differentiation, and inflammation. NFκB is activated by many stimuli including UV light, growth factor receptors, and a variety of other signals (cytokines, lymphokines, drugs, and stress). NFκB activity prevents apoptosis induced by TNF-α. Various stimuli, including UV exposure and engagement of the TNF-α receptor, initiate a signaling cascade in which a multiprotein complex made up of NEMO, IKK1 and IKK2 phosphorylates IκB. Phosphorylated IκB releases NFκB, which subsequently translocates to the nucleus to regulate transcription of a variety of target genes that protect the cell against apoptosis. Loss of NEMO function results in the inability to transduce this antiapoptotic signal and renders mutant cells much more susceptible to apoptosis. The vesicular inflammatory phase of icontinentia pigmenti represents increased apoptosis of keratinocytes harboring NEMO mutations.

environments that may raise their core body temperature. Avoidance of such environments or modification by use of air conditioning is helpful. Referral for dental restoration is suggested in individuals with hypodontia.

RELATED DISORDERS   Two other ectodermal dysplasia variants deserve mention. *Hidrotic ectodermal dysplasia* is an autosomal-dominant disorder resulting from mutations in the gene encoding connexin-30, a protein constituent of gap junctions. Patients with this disorder have normal sweating and teeth, but have sparse hair that may progress to total alopecia of the scalp and body as adults. In infancy and early childhood, the nails may be white, but become thick and dystrophic with time. Persistent paronychial infections are common and the palms and soles develop hyperkeratosis.

Hypohidrotic ectodermal dysplasia with immune deficency (HED-ID) is an X-linked recessive disorder that manifests clinically as an immune deficiency and developmental disorder of teeth, hair, and eccrine sweat glands. Affected male patients have low Ig levels and suffer from recurrent infections. Intravenous Ig and prophylactic antibiotics may be of benefit in treating the immune deficiency; however, the life expectancy is markedly shortened. Similar to anhidrotic ectodermal dysplasia, HED-ID results from defective ED signaling; however, the defect is in a downstream mediator of the EDA/EDAR signaling pathway. HED-ID is caused by mutations in the gene encoding NEMO (IKKγ) localized to chromosome Xq28. NEMO is a component of the multiprotein complex that phosphorylates IκB and results in

release and translocation to the nucleus of the NFκβ transcription factor (Fig. 101-4). Interestingly, mutations in the gene encoding NEMO are also responsible for incontinentia pigmenti (IP, *see* next section). Mutation mapping has suggested that HED-ID may be caused by mutations affecting the C-terminus of the expressed NEMO protein, whereas the mutations resulting in IP have more marked effects on the structure and function of the NEMO protein resulting in male prenatal lethality.

INCONTINENTIA PIGMENTI

CLINICAL PRESENTATION   IP is an X-linked dominant disorder also called Bloch-Sulzberger Syndrome characterized by the evolution of cutaneous lesions through four distinct stages. The first stage, consisting of erythema and vesicles, is present at birth or shortly thereafter and is followed by a second stage of verrucous papules and hyperkeratoses, a third stage of hyperpigmentation in adolescents and adults, and a fourth stage in which atrophy or scarring may be appreciated. The swirling patterns of involved skin in affected females represent the pattern of X-chromosome inactivation in postzygotic somatic cells, a process referred to as lyonization; normal skin represents cells in which the X-chromosome carrying the mutation is inactivated. The disease causes prenatal lethality in affected males. Additional clinical findings include nail dystrophy, abnormal teeth, and coloboma.

IP usually causes prenatal lethality in affected male fetuses; therefore, the disorder is seen in females. The few cases of affected males are owing to Klinefelter's syndrome in which a second X-chromosome is present. The prevalence of IP is not known.

MOLECULAR BASIS AND DEFECTS Familial IP results from mutations in the NEMO gene (IKKγ) localized to chromosome Xq28. NEMO functions in NFκβ-IκB mediated signaling (Fig. 101-4). NFκβ activity prevents apoptosis induced by TNF-α. Various stimuli, including UV exposure and engagement of the TNF-α receptor, initiate a signaling cascade in which a multiprotein complex made up of NEMO, IKK1, and IKK2 phosphorylates IκB. Phosphorylated IκB releases NFκβ, which subsequently translocates to the nucleus to regulate transcription of a variety of target genes that protect the cell against apoptosis. Loss of NEMO function results in the inability to transduce this anti-apoptotic signal and renders mutant cells much more susceptible to apoptosis. The vesicular inflammatory phase of IP represents increased apoptosis of keratinocytes harboring NEMO mutations. New mutations may result from partial deletions of the NEMO gene secondary to genomic rearrangements during paternal meiosis.

DIAGNOSIS: CLINICAL AND LABORATORY The diagnosis is made by the typical staged progression of vesiculobullous lesions, followed by verrucous, whorled hyperpigmented and atrophic, hypopigmented phases, although patients without all stages are common. Deletion of exons 4–10 in the NEMO gene

reportedly account for 80% of all mutations and serve as the basis for genetic screening and prenatal diagnosis.

MANAGEMENT/TREATMENT The initial vesiculobullous skin lesions, often misdiagnosed as herpesvirus infection, are self limiting and managed with local wound care. Patients with IP are at increased risk for seizure disorder and visual disturbances and should be monitored and treated accordingly.

SELECTED REFERENCES

Berlin AL, Paller AS, Chan LS. Incontinentia pigmenti: a review and update on the molecular basis of pathophysiology. J Am Acad Dermatol 2002;47:169–187.

Gutman DH. The neurofibromatosis: when less is more. Hum Mol Genet 2003;10:747–755.

Krymskaya VP. Tumor suppressors hamartin and tuberin: intracellular signaling. Cell Signal 2003;15:729–739.

Online Mendelian Inheritance in Man. McKusick-Nathans Institute for Genetic Medicine, Johns Hopkins University (Baltimore, MD), National Center for Biotechnology Information, National Library of Medicine (Bethesda, MD). http://www.ncbi.nlm.nih.gov/omim/. May 31, 2004.

Weeber EJ, Sweatt JD. Molecular neurobiology of human cognition. Neuron 2002;33:845–848.

Wisniewski SA, Kobielak A, Trzeciak WH, Kobielak K. Recent advances in understanding of the molecular basis of anhidrotic ectodermal dysplasia: Discovery of a ligand, EDA and its two receptors. J Appl Genet 2002;43:97–107.

102 Genetic Skin Diseases With Neoplasia

DAVID S. RUBENSTEIN

SUMMARY

The relationship between the molecular defects and cutaneous neoplasia in several genetic syndromes illustrates the key role played by a variety of proteins in cell growth, proliferation, and the repair of acquired genetic damage.

Key Words: ATM; *Adenomatous polyposis coli*; β-catenin; CYLD1; Gli1; helicase; kinase; nuclease; nucleotide excision repair; patched; smoothened; sonic hedgehog; tumor suppressor; XP complementation group.

INTRODUCTION

Multicellular organisms tightly regulate cell growth, proliferation, and migration. Without such regulation, rogue cells can disrupt the well-coordinated biology that enables these organisms to function. Such is the pathological phenomenon of neoplastic transformation that results in cancer. Genetic diseases in which the affected genes are involved in such regulatory processes lead to cancer. This chapter focuses on several genetic skin diseases as examples of this process. Tumor suppressors encode gene products in which inactivating mutations result in cancer. In contrast, cellular oncogenes encode gene products in which activating mutations result in cancer. Several examples of genetic lesions targeting tumor suppressors and cellular oncogenes highlight how disruption of these regulatory processes results in malignant transformation.

BASAL CELL NEVUS SYNDROME

CLINICAL PRESENTATION Basal cell nevus syndrome (BCNS), also known as Gorlin's syndrome, is an autosomal-dominant inherited disorder that presents with various developmental defects including frontal bossing, palmar and plantar pits, ondontogenic cysts, and bifid ribs. Additionally, there is an increased risk of developing some neoplasias, including medulloblastoma, meningioma, and rhabdomyosarcoma. Patients develop numerous basal cell carcinomas (BCC) of the skin at an early age.

Approximately one-third of patients may represent new sporadic mutations. In general, BCNS is a rare disorder. Despite the genetic predisposition to developing numerous BCCs, environmental factors, particularly exposure to ultraviolet (UV) radiation/natural sunlight and X-irradiation, are associated with increased numbers of tumors.

From: *Principles of Molecular Medicine, Second Edition*
Edited by: M. S. Runge and C. Patterson © Humana Press, Inc., Totowa, NJ

MOLECULAR BASIS AND DEFECTS The *PTCH1* gene (chromosome 9q22.3) is the mammalian homolog of the *Drosophila melanogaster ptc* gene that functions in hedgehog signaling during epithelial development and differentiation (Fig. 102-1). *PTCH1* encodes a multipass transmembrane protein that is the cell membrane receptor for the extracellular protein morphogen encoded by the sonic hedgehog gene. In the membrane, patched laterally associates with another transmembrane protein called smoothened. In this state, patched inhibits smoothened from activating downstream elements of the hedgehog-signaling pathway. When hedgehog binds to patched, the three-dimensional structure of patched is altered such that its affinity for smoothened is decreased, resulting in the dissociation of patched and smoothened. When not associated with patched, smoothened is then activated to initiate an intracellular signaling cascade that culminates in target gene regulation by Gli family member transcription factors.

PTCH1 mutations in BCNS result in a protein that can no longer bind to and prevent smoothened from activating this signaling cascade. One consequence of the inability to regulate this pathway is malignant transformation of the population of cells within the epidermis that give rise to BCCs. Because humans are diploid, patients with BCNS typically have one normal copy of the *PTCH1* gene in addition to the mutated gene. In BCNS, BCCs develop in cells in which this second copy of *PTCH1* is mutated, as often results from UV induced mutagenesis from natural sunlight exposure.

DIAGNOSIS: CLINICAL AND LABORATORY The diagnosis of BCNS is straightforward in patients presenting with the characteristic developmental abnormalities and a positive family history of the syndrome; however, new cases may represent sporadic mutations, so it is not always possible to elicit a positive family history. Nevertheless, in addition to the patient, it is worthwhile examining first-degree relatives for the presence of numerous BCCs, palmar and plantar pits, and frontal bossing. Histological examination of skin biopsies of suspected BCCs reveals the typical characteristics of BCC as seen in sporadic nonsyndromic BCCs, namely, a well circumscribed tumor of basaloid cells with peripheral palisading and often a retraction artifact during fixation that results in the appearance on H&E stains of a cleft between the tumor and the adjacent dermal stroma. X-rays can reveal skeletal abnormalities such as jaw cysts, rib defects, and calcification of the falx cerebri.

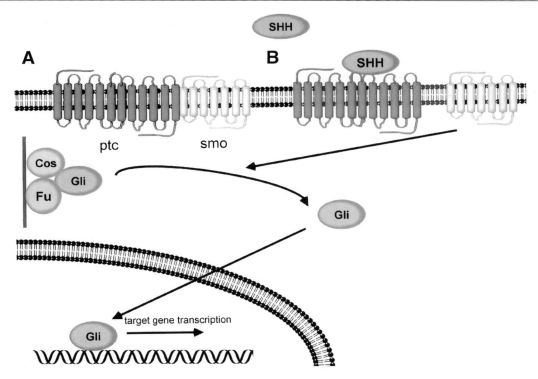

Figure 102-1   The hedgehog-patched signaling pathway and basal cell nevus syndrome. (**A**) Patched (ptc) is a multipass transmembrane receptor that laterally associates with and inactivates smoothened (smo). Gli, a transcription factor, is held inactive in a microtubule associated complex with Costal (Cos) and Fused (Fu). (**B**) When ptc is bound to its extracellular ligand Sonic Hegehog (SHH), smo is released and becomes activated to transduce a signal that results in release of Gli from the Cos/Fu complex. Gli translocates to the nucleus to regulate transcription of target genes. Ptc mutations in basal cell nevus syndrome and sporadic basal cell carcinomas prevent ptc from inhibiting smo with the result that this signaling pathway is constitutively active in mutant cells.

MANAGEMENT   Management focuses on early diagnosis of the syndrome and photoprotective measures to minimize the risk of acquiring secondary UV-induced inactivating mutations in *PTCH1*. Avoidance of radiotherapy is advised; patients receiving X-ray therapy for medulloblastoma have developed numerous BCCs within the radiation field. Frequent full body skin examinations should be performed for the early diagnosis of BCCs. Traditional treatment methods for BCC include electrodessication and curettage, excisional surgery, and Mohs surgery. Because patients often present with numerous BCCs, on the order of hundreds, excision of all tumors by electrodessication and curettage or surgery may be impractical. Other modalities more amenable to treating numerous tumors include destruction by freezing with liquid nitrogen (cryotherapy) or topical application of the base pair analog 5-flourouracil. The use of the topical immunomodulatory agent imiquimod has garnered favor for the treatment of BCCs. Imiquimod stimulates the local production of interferon α; the activation and targeting of natural killer cells to the tumor may be one mechanism by which imiquimod works against BCCs. Topical vitamin A derivatives are being studied to determine their effectiveness for treating BCCs. Inhibitors of hedgehog signaling may also prove useful in the treatment of BCCs arising from BCNS as well as in the treatment of nonsyndromic sporadic UV-induced BCCs occurring within the general population. One such agent is a derivative of the plant alkaloid cyclopamine. As with the other disorders described in this chapter, patients and their families should be referred for genetic counseling. In some cases, fetal diagnosis has been performed with genetic techniques.

XERODERMA PIGMENTOSA AND RELATED GROUPS

CLINICAL PRESENTATION   Xeroderma pigmentosa (XP) is a group of related autosomal-recessive genetic disorders that share an increased photosensitivity and a 1000-fold increased incidence in developing cutaneous malignancies as a result of genetic defects in the enzymes responsible for repairing damage to DNA. Signs of photodamage and aging, including numerous freckles, hypopigmentation and hyperpigmentation, xerosis, atrophy, and telangiectasia, appear within the first year of life. Patients characteristically develop premalignant actinic keratoses and numerous malignant cutaneous neoplasms such as BCCs and squamous cell carcinomas of the skin within the first decade of life; this contrasts sharply with the general US population in whom the median age of onset for nonmelanoma skin cancers is 60. Clustering of these neoplasms is noted on sun-exposed surfaces, particularly the face, head, and neck. Melanomas are reported in approx 5% of XP patients. Ocular findings occur in as many as 40% and include conjunctivitis, keratitis, ectropion, and corneal opacities that can lead to loss of vision. Ocular and oral cavity tumors, particularly squamous cell carcinomas of the anterior portion of the tongue, are also typical. Internal malignancies affecting both solid organs and the lymphoreticular system occur with increased frequency. Mild to severe neurological disease secondary to progressive axonal loss occurs in approximately one-third of patients, typically in XP complementation group A, and less so in C, D, and G. Neurological manifestations include hyporeflexia, mental retardation, seizure disorder, and hearing loss. Patients with XP have a shortened life span with an estimated survival rate of 70% at age 40. Death is typically owing to invasive, metastatic neoplastic disease. The incidence of XP worldwide is estimated to be 4 per million, although the incidence in certain populations such as the Middle East may approach 25 per million. Within the United States, XPC is the most common XP complementation group.

MOLECULAR BASIS AND DEFECTS   Seven complementation groups including genes encoding protein components of the DNA excision repair machinery have been described. Nucleotide exchange repair defective XP cells cannot repair pyrimidine/cyclobutane dimers. XP variant has the clinical features of XP, but has normal DNA excision repair, and results from defects in the gene encoding the DNA polymerase pol-η.

XPA and the *XPC* complex (along with the non-XP related *DDB* complex and *RPA*) encode nucleotide excision repair factors that are responsible for binding to and recognizing damaged DNA. *XPB* (3′ to 5′ DNA helicase) and *XPD* (5′ to 3′ DNA helicase) encode DNA helicases that are required to unwind the DNA prior to endonuclease cleavage of the damaged DNA. *XPG* and *XPF* (*ERCC1*) encode the nucleases. XPG is responsible for catalyzing the 3′ cleavage, whereas XPF (along with the ERCC1-subunit) catalyze the 5′ cleavage.

XPG may also serve as a cofactor for the hNTH1 glycosylase by facilitating the localization of the hNTH1 glycosylase onto damaged DNA containing oxidized pyrimidines in base excision repair. This additional non-nucleotide exchange repair function is likely responsible for the unique clinical phenotype of XPG patients who have features of traditional XP, developmental defects, as well as features of Cockayne Syndrome.

DIAGNOSIS: CLINICAL AND LABORATORY   The diagnosis of XP should be considered when there is a history of severe photosensitivity with minimal exposure to natural sunlight or in those patients who have early onset photodamage as described. Cultured cells from XP patients demonstrate increased sensitivity to UV radiation. PCR based diagnostic tests are available for some XP complementation groups.

MANAGEMENT   Minimizing the effects of UV radiation by photoprotection is critically important in the management of XP. Patients should undergo routine screening for early diagnosis and treatment of cutaneous malignancies. Chemoprophylaxis with systemic retinoids or cyclo-oxygenase-2 (COX-2) inhibitors should be considered. A strategy aimed at repairing UV-induced pyrimidine dimers using topical recombinant liposome encapsulated T4 endonuclease V is being investigated.

RELATED SYNDROMES   Several other rare genetic disorders have been described in which mutations in helicases predispose the affected individuals to UV induced damage and neoplasia, including *Bloom syndrome, Werner's syndrome,* and *Rothmund-Thomson Syndrome.* Each of these disorders is from a genetic defect in one of the RecQ DNA helicases. The RecQ DNA helicases have been characterized in model systems. DNA helicases improve DNA replication accuracy during DNA elongation. Mutations that inactivate these proteins result in defective DNA repair and increased chromosome rearrangements. The resulting inability to repair UV induced mutations leads to the increased numbers of skin cancers observed in patients with these disorders.

Bloom syndrome, an autosomal-recessive disorder, is due to mutations in the gene encoding the BLM DNA helicase, and is characterized by photosensitivity and premature photoaging of the skin including facial erythema and telangiectasia. An additional feature includes a partial immunodeficiency manifested by increased frequency of respiratory and gastrointestinal infections. Systemic malignancies are common and include lymphoreticular malignancies, adenocarcinoma, and squamous cell carcinoma of the oropharyngeal and esophageal mucosa.

Werner's syndrome, an autosomal-recessive disease resulting from mutations in the gene encoding the WRN DNA helicase, causes premature aging of the skin and internal organ systems. In the skin, extreme early photoaging is characterized by premature graying and balding, atrophy, telangectasia, skin ulcers, and dyspigmentation. Affected individuals have an increased incidence of melanoma. Systemic involvement includes advanced atherosclerotic changes during childhood.

Rothmund-Thomson, an autosomal-recessive disorder caused by mutations in the *RecQL4* DNA helicase gene, is characterized by photosensitivity. Clinical features include poikiloderma (the triad of skin atrophy, pigmentary change, and telangiectasia) and limb defects.

ATAXIA TELANGIECTASIA

CLINICAL PRESENTATION   Ataxia telangiectasia (AT), an autosomal-recessive disorder, results from inactivating mutations in the tumor suppressor gene that encodes the *ATM* gene. Patients develop progressive cerebellar dysfunction, ocular telangiectases usually by 3–5 yr of age, immune defects, gonadal dysfunction/infertility, and malignancies, typically B-cell lymphomas and T-cell leukemias. Immune defects include thymic hypoplasia, decreased serum Ig levels (IgG2 and IgA), and decreased cellular immunity. Frequent sinopulmonary infections is one of the more common manifestations of the immunodeficiency seen in AT. AT patients have elevated blood levels of alpha-fetoprotein.

The incidence of AT in the United States is estimated to be as high as 1 in 100,000 live births. Heterozygote AT carriers have an increased predisposition to developing a variety of cancers.

MOLECULAR BASIS AND DEFECTS   Mutations in the *ATM* gene found on chromosome 11q23.3 are responsible for this disorder. *ATM* encodes a 3056 amino acid protein of 350 kDa that is constitutively expressed and localized to the cell nucleus. ATM is a protein kinase belonging to the phosphatidylinositol-3 kinase protein family. The *ATM* gene is large and numerous mutations have been described in this disorder, the majority of which result in premature termination and inactivation of the kinase activity of the ATM protein. ATM phosphorylates p53 at Ser15 and promotes p53 activation and stabilization during DNA responses induced as a result of exposure to ionizing radiation. ATM is one of the protein constituents of the BRCA1-associated genome surveillance complex that functions in sensing aberrant DNA structures and in regulating post replication DNA repair. The BRCA1-associated genome surveillance complex is made up of tumor suppressors, DNA damage sensors and signaling proteins.

ATM activation is one of the earliest cellular events in the response pathway to ionizing radiation (Fig. 102-2). Ionizing radiation results in double stranded breaks and changes in chromatin structure that are thought to activate ATM. Irradiation of cells in culture results in ATM autophosphorylation at serine[1981] and subsequent dimerization. Cell cycle arrest is because of a series of phosphorylation events initiated by ATM. ATM phosphorylation of p53 causes activation of p21 and cell cycle arrest. Additionally, ATM binds to and phosphorylates BLM, the helicase that is defective in

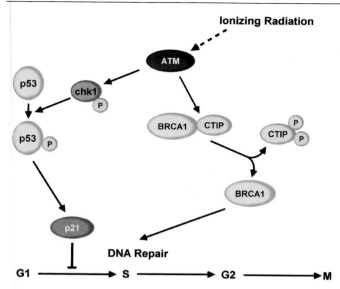

Figure 102-2 The ATM tumor suppressor. ATM, constitutively expressed and localized to the nucleus, is a protein kinase. ATM activation is one of the earliest cellular events in the response pathway to ionizing radiation. ATM phosphorylation of p53 causes activation of p21 and cell cycle arrest. Additionally, ATM phosphorylates CTIP resulting in release of BRCA1 and subsequent activation of DNA repair processes. Loss of ATM function disrupts this cell cycle arrest and DNA repair mechanism resulting in the accumulation of additional oncogenic mutations.

Bloom's syndrome. *ATM* knockout mice recapitulate many of the features of the human disorder demonstrating that loss of ATM function in AT leads to the observed phenotype. Loss of ATM results in increased sensitivity to ionizing radiation, and oxidation of macromolecules has been suggested to be one mechanism by which target organs are damaged in AT. In a mouse *ATM* knockout model of AT, cerebellar Purkinje cells were particularly susceptible to oxidative damage, which may suggest a mechanism for the ataxic phenotype observed in this disorder. Blockade of oxidative damage may provide an approach for treating this disease.

DIAGNOSIS: CLINICAL AND LABORATORY The diagnosis is suggested by early onset ataxia and oculocutaneous telangiectases. As described, elevated serum α-fetoprotein levels can aid in the diagnosis. Direct screening for specific mutations is of limited value; the *ATM* gene is large, approx 66 exons spanning 150 kb of DNA. Mutations that result in dysfunctional protein in a host of AT patients have been mapped throughout the *ATM* locus.

MANAGEMENT Because of the immune deficiency, AT patients should be closely monitored for infections and treated appropriately. AT patients are at increased for the development of lymphoreticular malignancies. The marked sensitivity to X-ray makes avoidance of this treatment modality essential in the management of neoplastic disease. Survival to adulthood is uncommon.

GARDNER'S SYNDROME

CLINICAL PRESENTATION This autosomal-dominant inherited disorder is a variant of the colon cancer associated syndrome familial adenomatous polyposis (FAP). It is completely penetrant and of variable expressivity. In addition to the numerous intestinal polyps that undergo malignant degeneration that characterize FAP, additional features of Gardner's syndrome include multiple epidermal inclusion cysts and intestinal and fibrous tumors. Congenital hypertrophy of the retinal pigment epithelium, jaw cysts, osteomas, and desmoid tumors, often at sites of surgical intervention, are other features of Gardner's syndrome. Patients develop malignant colonic tumors as young adults. Other associated malignant tumors include fibrosarcoma, meningioma, and leiomyosarcoma. The prevalence of FAP is estimated to be approx 1 in 13,500, although regional variation in prevalence rates has been observed. As many as 30% of cases may represent new mutations.

MOLECULAR BASIS AND DEFECTS Gardner's results from mutations in the gene encoding the APC protein. The gene localizes to chromosome 5q21. Various mutations have been described. Those within the central portion of the encoded polypeptide result in more severe phenotypes than those occurring in either the amino- or carboxy-termini. APC is a component of the Wnt signaling pathway (Fig. 102-3) and forms part of the multicellular protein complex that targets cytoplasmic β-catenin for ubiquitination and subsequent proteoosome mediated degradation. In the absence of functional APC, cytoplasmic and nuclear β-catenin accumulate, driving formation of a bipartite transcription factor between β-catenin and TCF/LEF family member proteins. Subsequent activation of target genes containing TCF/LEF response elements, such as c-*myc*, drives the proliferative changes that characterize the malignant phenotype observed in FAP/Gardner's. In addition, APC associates with microtubules. Mutant APC in FAP has decreased affinity for kinetochore associated microtubules and likely is responsible for the chromosome instability and aberrant chromosome segregation observed in APC mutant cells. Less severe FAP phenotypes result from mutations in the 5′ region of the gene encoding the N terminus of the protein, whereas more severe phenotypes result from inactivating mutations that affect the β-catenin binding function localized to the central region of the encoded APC protein. Other than the retinal pigmented lesions, no significant associations have been observed between the extraintestinal manifestations of FAP and specific *APC* mutations. Environmental factors and/or modifying genes may influence the presence of extraintestinal disease.

DIAGNOSIS: CLINICAL AND LABORATORY Diagnosis is based on the intestinal and extraintestinal clinical manifestations as described. The diagnosis is relatively straightforward in known kindreds; however, about 30% of FAP patients may represent new mutations. Gardner's syndrome should be considered in patients presenting with numerous epidermal inclusion cysts. A history of altered bowel habits and/or rectal bleeding should be queried and followed by screening colonoscopy. Palpation of nodules along the jaw should initiate a search for jaw osteomas using dental panoramic tomography; Gardner's syndrome is suggested by the finding of three or more jaw osteomas. Funduscopic examination for congenital hypertrophy of the retinal pigment epithelium is helpful in the diagnosis of suspected Gardner's syndrome, particularly in infants and young children because this finding may precede the development of intestinal polyps and epidermal cysts. Patients suspected of harboring mutations in the *APC* gene can be tested by screening for mutations in *APC* from peripheral blood lymphocytes. Direct sequencing for *APC* mutations in known kindreds facilitates prenatal diagnosis.

MANAGEMENT Because of the essentially 100% risk of developing colorectal carcinoma, annual screening colonoscopies are recommended in affected individuals from the age of 12 onward. The risk of developing gastric and duodenal tumors

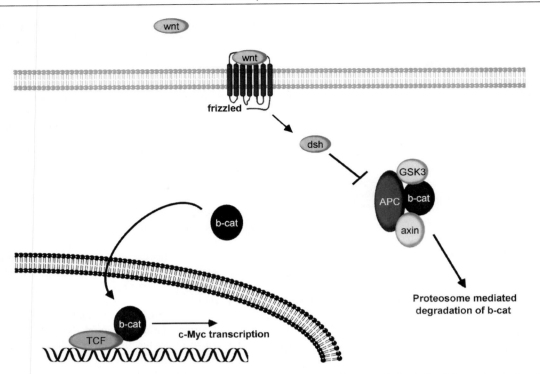

Figure 102-3 Wnt signaling and Gardner's Syndrome. β-catenin (b-cat) is constitutively synthesized, but fails to accumulate in the cytoplasm or nucleus because it is targeted for proteosome mediated degradation by a complex of proteins including APC, the serine threonine kinase GSK3, and axin. Wnts, a family of secreted polypeptides, bind to the cell membrane frizzled receptor to initiate a signal mediated by disheveled (dsh) that inhibits the APC/GSK3/axin mediated targeting and degradation of β-catenin. Cytoplasmic and nuclear β-catenin accumulate, driving formation of a bipartite transcription factor with TCF/LEF family proteins and transcription of a variety of target genes including c-*myc*. In Gardner's Syndrome, APC mutations result in constitutive activation of the downstream elements of the Wnt signaling pathway.

requires upper gastrointestinal endoscopic screening as well. Prophylactic colectomy has been advocated, but such patients still require surveillance for rectal and upper GI tumors. The use of nonsteroidal antiinflammatory drugs and in particular COX-2 inhibitors has been advocated for chemoprophylaxis. In vitro work has suggested that inhibition of COX-2 inhibits metastatic potential and promotes apoptosis of malignant cells.

FAMILIAL CYLINDROMATOSIS

CLINICAL PRESENTATION Familial cylindromatosis is an autosomal-dominant condition characterized by the appearance of multiple flesh colored papules, nodules, and tumors predominantly on the scalp and face. The tumors originate in skin structures such as hair follicles, eccrine, and apocrine glands. Cylindromas tend to affect the scalp, whereas trichoepitheliomas are found on the face. Confluent involvement of the scalp, which mimics the appearance of a turban, gives rise to the alternative designation of turban tumor syndrome. Although the cylindromas are benign neoplasms, malignant degeneration has been observed and the syndrome has been associated with other malignant neoplasms including BCCs.

Familial cylindromatosis is a rare disorder whose incidence has not been defined.

MOLECULAR BASIS AND DEFECTS Familial cylindromatosis is linked to a gene on chromosome 16q12-q13. The loss of the tumor suppressor CYLD1 is responsible for causing this disorder. Loss of heterozygosity in the *CYLD1* gene has been implicated in the development of nonsyndromic sporadic cylindromas. Mutations in the *CYLD1* gene result in either truncated nonfunctional protein or the absence of the encoded protein. *CYLD1* encodes a deubiquitinating

enzyme that negatively regulates nuclear factor (NF)-κβ. NF-κβ has been well characterized as a critical component in signaling cascades that regulate cellular inflammatory responses. Engagement of transmembrane tumor necrosis factor receptor by tumor necrosis factor α causes tumor necrosis factor receptor trimerization. This results in TRAF recruitment; activation of the IκB kinase complex, phosphorylation and subsequent polyubiquitination and degradation of IκB. Degradation of IκB releases NF-κβ to translocate to the nucleus in which it activates transcription of target genes. CYLD1 catalyzes the removal of the polypeptide ubiquitin from lysine 63 of TRAF2, which prevents IκB phosphorylation, and dissociation of the NF-κβ–IκB complex. Activation of this pathway inhibits apoptosis. The growth of benign tumors in familial cylindromatosis is thought to be due to the inhibition of apoptosis resulting from loss of CYLD1.

DIAGNOSIS CLINICAL AND LABORATORY The diagnosis is straightforward in patients presenting with the characteristic clinical pattern of multiple scalp papules, nodules, and tumors. Biopsy of the scalp lesions reveals the typical histology of a cylindroma, namely irregular islands of basaloid cells within the dermis and subcutaneous tissues mimicking the pattern of a jigsaw puzzle. The facial lesions demonstrate numerous well-circumscribed dermal aggregates of basaloid cells with horn cysts and a fibrous stroma that characterizes trichoepitheliomas.

MANAGEMENT Surgical excision of the scalp tumors may improve cosmesis. The ability of aspirin or prostaglandin A1 to reverse the antiapototic effects of *CYLD1* mutations has suggested that these agents may be useful in the treatment of familial cylindromatosis.

SELECTED REFERENCES

Barth AIM, Nelson WJ. What can humans learn from flies about *Adenomatous polyposis coli*? BioEssays 2002;24:771–774.

Bienz M. The subcellular destinations of APC proteins. Nat Rev Mol Cell Biol 2002;3:328–338.

Brummelkamp TR, Nijman SM, Dirac AM, Bernards R. Loss of the cylindromatosis tumour suppressor inhibits apoptosis by activating NF-kappaB. Nature 2003;424:797–801.

Johnson RL, Rothman AL, Xie J, et al. Human homolog of patched, a candidate gene for the basal cell nevus syndrome. Science 1996;272:1668–1671.

Mullor JL, Sanchez P, Ruiz I, Altaba A. Pathways and consequences: Hedgehog signaling in human disease. Trends Cell Biol 2002;12:562–569.

Online Mendelian Inheritance in Man. McKusick-Nathans Institute for Genetic Medicine, Johns Hopkins University (Baltimore, MD), National Center for Biotechnology Information, National Library of Medicine (Bethesda, MD). http://www.ncbi.nlm.nih.gov/omim/. May 31, 2004.

Shiloh Y. ATM and related protein kinases: Safeguarding genome integrity. Nat Rev Cancer 2003;3:155–168.

Van Steeg H, Kraemer KH. Xeroderma pigmentosum and the role of UV-induced DNA damage in skin cancer. Mol Med Today 1999;5:86–94.

103 Melanoma and Nevi

NANCY E. THOMAS

SUMMARY

Melanoma, which is increasing in incidence, is the most lethal skin cancer. Risk factors for melanoma include genotypic and phenotypic characteristics combined with environmental exposures. Germline mutations in *CDKN2A* and *CDK4* are thought to confer high susceptibility for melanoma. Polymorphisms in the melanocortin receptor-1 gene, which is central to melanin synthesis, confer low susceptibility for melanoma. In addition to germline alterations, somatic mutations in either *BRAF* or *NRAS* mutations have been found in a high percentage of melanomas. Nevi, which are one of the strongest risk factors for melanoma, also have *BRAF* mutations. Prevention, early diagnosis, and treatment remain important areas for future advancements.

Key Words: Braf; dysplastic nevus; early diagnosis; epidemiology; melanoma; mutation; nevus; pathology; p53; ras; somatic; staging.

INTRODUCTION

Melanoma is rapidly increasing in incidence and remains a potentially fatal disease with poor medical treatment options and controversial methods of prevention. Melanoma likely results from a series of mutations in critical genes (Table 103-1), with tumors emerging as a result of selection. Nevi (moles are synonymous), in particular dysplastic nevi, are thought to represent precursors for some melanomas. The risks for development of nevi and melanoma include both genetic and environmental factors.

CLINICAL FEATURES

The four clinical subtypes of melanoma have variable radial growth phases (Fig. 103-1). During radial growth phase, the melanoma is either *in situ* or has only single or small clusters of melanoma cells without mitoses in the papillary dermis. Superficial spreading melanoma is the most common subtype representing 60–70% of melanomas. Its location can be any anatomic site, and the radial growth phase is months to years. Nodular melanoma is less common, comprising approx 10% of melanomas. It also can be located at any anatomic site, but the radial growth phase is brief or unrecognized. Lentigo maligna melanoma consists of approx 10–15% of melanomas. It usually occurs on sun-exposed sites such as the head or neck and has a long radial growth phase (lentigo maligna) that extends, at times, to 15–20 yr.

From: *Principles of Molecular Medicine, Second Edition*
Edited by: M. S. Runge and C. Patterson © Humana Press, Inc., Totowa, NJ

Clinically, it can mimic a solar lentigo. Acral lentiginous melanoma is the least common, representing approx 5% of melanomas, and occurs with relatively increased frequency in African American and Asian populations. It characteristically occurs on the palms, soles, or underneath the nail plate. For all subtypes of melanoma, the prognosis is closely related to the depth of the lesion at the time of initial excision.

Cutaneous melanoma, owing to loss of growth controls, generally presents as a changing, irregular pigmented papule or plaque. The *ABCDE* clinical criteria for diagnosis include asymmetry, irregular borders, color variegation, diameter greater than 6 mm, and evolution of the lesion. Melanomas are usually asymptomatic, with bleeding and ulceration typically only occurring as late changes. Of note, amelanotic melanoma, comprising 2–8% of melanomas, lacks visible pigment and can be any of the previously mentioned subtypes. Because most of the visual clues are absent in amelanotic melanoma, it is frequently misdiagnosed.

Benign acquired melanocytic nevi tend to be symmetric with smooth well-defined borders and homogeneous pigmentation. Acquired nevi develop after birth with a peak incidence between ages 22 and 25, with few developing after age 40. As nevi age, they are thought to evolve from junctional to compound to intradermal nevi, and then ultimately involute. Individuals older than 90 yr have few, if any, nevi.

Clinically, dysplastic nevi are moles with some of the *ABCD* characteristics of melanomas, but which generally are not as atypical clinically as melanomas. Histologically, dysplastic nevi are compound nevi with histological, cytological, and/or architectural atypia that is not as severe as that found in melanoma. However, poor correlation exists between the clinical and the histological criteria for dysplastic nevi; therefore, dysplastic nevi are not considered to be a distinct clinicopathological entity. However, the increased risk of melanoma based on clinical criteria for dysplastic nevi is consistent in diverse populations.

Congenital melanocytic nevi (CMN) are benign melanocytic neoplasms apparent at or shortly after birth. Congenital nevi are often larger than acquired nevi and can be classified into small (1.5 cm), intermediate (1.5–20 cm), or large (>20 cm). The color can range from tan to dark brown with various hues found within the same lesion. The surface can be papillated or smooth, and terminal hairs can be present.

The Spitz nevus, a benign melanocytic lesion, is most commonly a pink, red, or tan dome-shaped firm nodule; however a Spitz nevus can be macular, polypoid, or verrucous. Spitz nevi

Table 103-1
Genes Found to be Altered in Primary Melanomas

Tumor suppressor genes	Oncogenes
CDKN2A (p16 and ARF)	CDK4
p53	RAS
PTEN/MMAC1	BRAF

often initially grow rapidly and then stabilize. The differential diagnosis histopathologically and clinically between Spitz nevi and melanoma can, at times, be extremely challenging. Despite well-established histopathological criteria for distinguishing Spitz nevi from melanoma, there are some atypical cases with overlap in features in which the diagnosis between a Spitz nevus and melanoma cannot unequivocally be made. Historically, Spitz nevi were called juvenile melanoma, adding to the confusion.

EPIDEMIOLOGY

Melanoma more than tripled in incidence among Caucasians between 1980 and 2003, bringing the estimated number of new invasive melanomas to 54,200 and *in situ* melanomas to 37,700, with 7600 deaths for the year 2003 in the United States. Melanoma is the fifth and seventh most common cancer in men and women, respectively. The lifetime risk of melanoma is 1.75% (1 in 57) in males and 1.23% (1 in 81) in females.

Melanoma risk is associated with genetic and environmental factors that are likely interrelated. Inherited risk factors include the fair phenotypic traits of red/blond hair, fair skin, easy burning/inability to tan, and light eye color. Red hair, fair skin, and freckling are associated with variants of the melanocortin receptor 1 (MC1R) gene, a low penetrance melanoma susceptibility gene. One-third of melanomas in Queensland, Australia may be attributable to *MC1R* variants. In addition, *MC1R* may increase melanoma risk in individuals with medium to dark complexions.

CDKN2A and *CDK4* are high penetrance melanoma susceptibility loci associated with proteins regulating the cell cycle. In melanoma-prone families, mutations in the *CDKN2A* gene, which codes for *p16* and the alternate reading frame protein (*ARF*) have been identified. *ARF* and *p16* are involved in the *p53* pathway and cell cycle control, respectively. *CDKN2A* mutations have been found in approx 5% of families with two or more affected first-degree relatives and 20–40% of families with three or more affected first-degree relatives. In a Queensland population-based melanoma study, 10.3% of high-risk families had a *CDKN2A* germline mutation, but mutations were rare (0.2%) among total cases. Germline mutations in *CDK4* have been identified in a few melanoma-prone families. In addition, melanoma risk is increased in xeroderma pigmentosum, heritable retinoblastoma, Li-Fraumeni syndrome (germline *p53* mutation), and Werner syndrome (Table 103-2).

Worldwide, the rate of melanoma tends to be higher in populations living closer to the equator and those living at higher altitude. Sun exposure is an important acquired risk factor for melanoma, with intermittent, recreational type exposure increasing the risk of superficial spreading melanoma and total sun exposure likely increasing the risk of lentigo maligna melanoma. In addition, the number of sunburns, especially severe childhood sunburn, is associated with increased risk of melanoma. PUVA, a treatment for psoriasis involving administration of ultraviolet (UV) A in combination with psoralen, increases the risk of melanoma above a certain number of treatments. Immunosuppression is also an acquired risk factor for melanoma.

Risk factors that could either be genetic or environmental include a personal history of melanoma and/or nonmelanoma skin cancer, a family history of melanoma, number of sunburns, and the number and type nevi. Familial melanoma, as defined by two or more first-degree relatives having melanoma, consists of 0.6–12.5% of melanoma depending on the geographic area, generally with higher percentages occurring in areas of higher melanoma incidence. An individual with a first-degree relative newly diagnosed with melanoma is considered to have a twofold increased risk of melanoma. However, family members who develop melanoma tend to have earlier age of onset, thinner melanomas, and be more likely to develop multiple primaries than sporadic cases. When family history is defined as three or more living relatives with a history of melanoma, familial melanoma consists of approx 1% of melanomas. Number of nevi is the most significant factor in predicting risk of melanoma in high-risk families.

Essentially, every study assessing nevi in association with melanoma risk has found number of nevi to be one of the strongest risk factors for melanoma. Although common nevi increase the risk of melanoma roughly two- to fourfold, dysplastic nevi (*see* clinical features) are associated with a greatly increased risk factor for melanoma in prospective clinical and cohort studies. Dysplastic nevi are relatively common, with an estimated prevalence of 7–18% in Caucasian controls from different populations. Although frequent in melanoma prone families, dysplastic nevi do not cosegregate with *CDKN2A* or *CDK4* mutations. The significance of an isolated dysplastic nevus is controversial; however, there is consensus that the lifetime risk of developing malignant melanoma is increased when many atypical moles occur in a person with a family history of melanoma.

Nevi may arise from a genetic-environmental interaction. Case–control studies show evidence of a role for sun exposure in the development of both common and atypical nevi. In Australia, children with increased numbers of nevi had more sun exposure and were more likely to have been sunburned than those with fewer nevi. Other studies also link sun exposure with number of nevi in children, adolescents, and adults using surveys. In addition, sun protection in children and adolescents decreases the number of nevi that develop. However, in highly sun protected children, different patterns of the distribution of nevi in males and females suggest that hormones may play a role. In addition, twin studies provide evidence of a genetic component in the development of common nevi. One twin study showed that the region containing the *CDKN2A* gene may also contain a locus affecting number of nevi.

Estimates of the incidence of congenital nevi vary from 1 to 2.5% of newborn infants. The risk of melanoma is highest in large congenital nevi and decreases as the size decreases. The risk is felt to be proportional to the number of melanocytes. Between 5 and 20% of patients with large congenital nevi will develop a melanoma within the nevus during their lifetime. The malignant potential of small and medium congenital nevi is more controversial.

Spitz nevi can occur at any age but are more frequent before age 30. The true incidence in the population is unknown, but it has been estimated that they constitute 1–10% of melanocytic nevi in children.

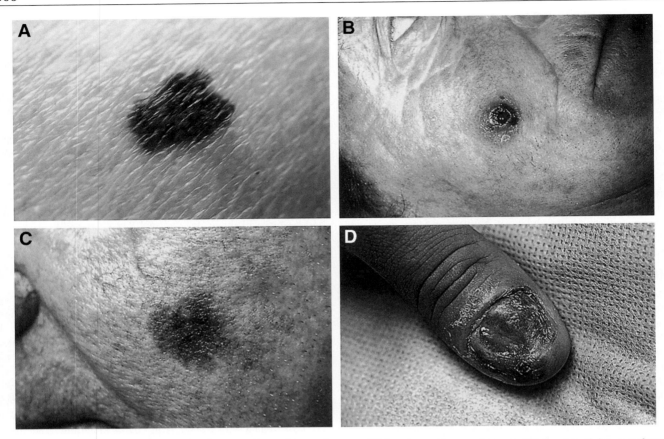

Figure 103-1 (**A**) Superficial spreading melanoma. (**B**) Nodular melanoma. (**C**) Lentigo maligna melanoma. (**D**) Acral lentiginous melanoma.

Table 103-2
Syndromes With Increased Melanoma Risk

Syndrome	Gene defect	Functional deficiency
Familial retinoblastoma	*Rb*	Cell cycle control at G1
Li-Fraumeni syndrome	*p53*	DNA integrity and genomic stability
Xeroderma pigmentosum	*XP*	DNA excision repair
Werner syndrome	*WRN*	DNA helicase with roles in multiple DNA metabolic processes

MOLECULAR BASIS AND DEFECTS

MELANOMA

Germline Mutations *CDKN2A*, located at 9p21, is a major susceptibility gene for melanoma. It is transmitted as an autosomal-dominant trait in most affected families. It codes for two overlapping gene products, p16INK4A and p14ARF, that are differentially spliced and read on alternating reading frames such that they do not share the same amino acid sequence. Different first exons are utilized by the *INK4A* and *ARF* transcript, although both *INK4A* and *ARF* use the same second and third exons. Mutations in exon 1A affect only *INK4A*, whereas mutations in exon 2 can affect either of the two gene products. Some melanoma families also have a mutation in the 5'UTR of *CDKN2A*, which results in an aberrant initiation codon.

The p16INK4A gene product is a cell cycle inhibitor that binds to CDK4 and functions as a tumor suppressor. p16 has four ankyrin repeats that bind to CDK4, and the tumorigenic mutations map to sites of contact between p16 and CDK4. CDK4, with its regulatory subunit Cyclin D1, is required for the kinase activity. CDK4 is the key kinase that phosphorylates the tumor suppressor retinoblastoma protein (Rb), thereby freeing the transcription factor E2F. Rb is a tumor suppressor that is defective in hereditary retinoblastoma and central to arresting the cell cycle at G1. The Rb protein can interact with several members of E2F family to repress the transcription from E2F regulated promoters. E2F responsive genes include *Cyclin E, Cyclin A* and other gene encoding proteins and enzymes required for DNA replication.

p14ARF, also a tumor suppressor, works by a different mechanism. Human double minute 2 (HDM2- MDM2 in mice) binds to p53, targeting it for degradation. The ARF protein binds to HDM2, abrogating the degradation of p53. Mitogenic signals upregulate ARF, promoting p53-dependent apoptosis or arrest in cells with unscheduled proliferation. Mutations that affect ARF without affecting p16 are much less common than those affecting p16 alone or affecting both p16 and ARF.

CDKN2A mutations include more than 14 different mutations or small deletions. Mutations in the *p16* gene open reading frame are highly penetrant, with melanoma eventually occurring in 55–100% of individuals with these mutations. Residence in a country with a high incidence of melanoma increases the penetrance, possible evidence for a role for UV.

An excess of pancreatic cancer has been found in some families with *CDKN2A* mutations. In families in which the mutation affects the ARF protein and not p16, there may be an association with neural tumors including astrocytomas.

CDK4, located at 12q14, has been reported to be mutated in three melanoma-prone families. The mutations occur in the p16 binding region of CDK4, rendering CDK4 resistant to p16 inhibition. Because there are few affected families, there is not much data; however, the penetrance, number of primary melanomas, risk of melanoma, and age at diagnosis for *CDK4* have been estimated to be similar to that for *CDKN2A* alterations.

Genetic Polymorphisms MC1R is a seven-pass transmembrane G protein-coupled receptor that controls the switch from pheomelanin (red/yellow pigments) to eumelanin (brown/black pigments) in mice. Stimulation of the *MC1R* receptor leads to activation of adenylate cyclase, resulting in an increase in cAMP production. This activation favors eumelanogenesis, which is important for the tanning response. Certain MC1R variants apparently are not as effective at switching from pheomelanin to eumelanin production.

Although there are more than 30 *MCR1* variants, most of the effect is because of a subset of variants. In humans, red hair, a recessive trait, and fair skin are significantly associated with three *MC1R* gene alterations (R151C, R160W, D294H). In addition, heterozygous *MC1R* variant carriers are at a two- to threefold increased risk of freckling, when controlling for skin type and hair color.

The three *MC1R* variants noted each confers a two- to threefold increased melanoma risk, with the effects from more than one affected allele being additive. In light skin individuals, when controlling for skin and hair type, the association between melanoma and *MC1R* variants disappears; however, in individuals with medium or olive/dark skin types, which normally are considered protective, carrying these particular *MC1R* variants may increase melanoma risk in comparison with individuals with similar skin types. It is possible that eumelanin is better at blocking UV than pheomelanin; that pheomelanin, its precursors or photoproducts are directly harmful by producing free radicals in response to UV; or that MC1R is involved in the modulation of growth and differentiation.

The estimated melanoma risk for *MC1R* variant carriers is 14% by age 50. *MC1R* increases p16 penetrance. *CDKN2A* mutation with consensus *MC1R* has 50% penetrance, whereas *CDKN2A* mutation with variant *MC1R* has 84% penetrance.

Somatic Mutations *BRAF* and *RAS* somatic mutations have been found in approx 60% and 10–30% of melanomas, respectively. *NRAS* mutations are much more common than *K* or *HRAS* mutations. Activating *BRAF* mutants can transform certain cell lines and activate kinase activity. *BRAF* V600E and *NRAS* mutations do not occur simultaneously in melanomas but, instead, have a reciprocal relationship. *BRAF* and *RAS* mutations have also been found in nevi.

RAS gene products, including HRAS, KRAS, and NRAS, are membrane-bound GTPases found mutated in several types of tumors. Based on mouse models, oncogenic *RAS* is important for both the genesis and maintenance of murine melanoma. In cultured human melanocytes, expression of *RAS* oncogenes can cause induction of complete melanoma phenotype and genotype.

The RAF family proteins, including RAF1, ARAF, and BRAF, are cytoplasmic serine/threonine kinases that phosphorylate

mitogen-activated protein/extracellular signal-regulated kinases (MEKs) in the *RAF-MEK-extracellular signal-regulated kinase* (ERK)-MAP membrane-to-nucleus signaling module. RAF is recruited to the membrane by GTP-loaded RAS and then phosphorylated, resulting in the activation of the RAS-RAF-MEK-ERK-MAP pathway.

The RAS-RAF-MEK-ERK-MAP module transmits extracellular signals from the membrane to ERKs, which then translocate into the nucleus in which they phosphorylate and regulate transcription factors affecting cell cycle entry, differentiation, migration, adhesion, and gene regulation induced by growth factors. In addition, RAS is a known positive upstream regulator of phosphatidylinositol (3,4,5) triphosphate kinase (*PI3K*), which activates the survival kinase, serine/threonine kinase (Akt).

PTEN/MMAC1 (PTEN—phosphatase tensin and MMAC1—mutated in multiple advanced cancers), found at 10q23.3, is a tumor suppressor gene located on chromosome 10q23. It has homology with tyrosine protein phosphatases and tensin, the cytoskeletal protein that interacts with actin filaments at focal adhesions. PTEN, a dual lipid and protein phosphatase, is a tumor suppressor gene that reverses the growth signals induced by tyrosine kinases. PTEN is also involved in apoptosis and inhibition of cell spreading, migration and focal adhesion formation.

Germline mutations occur in Cowden disease, an autosomal-dominant syndrome in which there is an increase risk for breast and thyroid cancer, and in Bannayan-Zonana kindred, who have intestinal polyposis, vascular malformation, and hamartomatous growths such as subcutaneous and visceral lipomas.

PTEN mutations are found in approx 30–50% of melanoma cell lines. About 5–20% of uncultured metastatic melanomas have *PTEN* alterations; but only one in over 30 primary melanomas tested has an intragenic *PTEN* alteration. Allelic losses of the *PTEN* gene were found in 3/8 (38%) primary melanomas analyzed in one study.

PTEN protein expression, as detected by immunohistochemistry, was absent in 15% (5/34) and low in 50% (17/34) of melanoma samples in one study. However, metastatic melanomas were found with no PTEN expression that had no mutation or deletion of PTEN. Also metastatic melanomas were found that had weak *PTEN* staining. Of these, some had hemizygous allelic loss of *PTEN*, and others had no identifiable alterations. Based on these results, an epigenetic biallelic functional inactivation may occur in *PTEN*. In addition, lack of PTEN nuclear expression is associated with mitotic index, anatomic site, and presence of p53 expression.

A relative reciprocity of *NRAS* and *PTEN* mutations has been found in cutaneous melanoma cell lines, in which 51% had an alteration in either *PTEN* or *RAS*. Of these, 30% had an alteration in *PTEN*, 21% had a mutation in *NRAS*, and only one cell line had alterations in both *PTEN* and RAS alterations.

p53, known as the "guardian of the genome," helps maintain DNA integrity and genomic stability through cell cycle arrest. p53 senses genetic injury and arrests the cell at multiple cell cycle check-points, allowing cells time to repair damaged DNA. If genetic injury is too severe or cellular proliferation cannot be blocked, p53 can cause programmed cell death (apoptosis).

Approximately 20–25% of metastatic melanomas have *p53* mutations. The frequency of *p53* mutations in primary melanomas is not as well elucidated, but is reported to range from 1 to 2% to as high as approx 25%. In a study of nodular melanomas, 5 of 21 primary tumors (24%) were mutated. In addition, in a study of archived primary melanoma tissue, 28.5% of 35 mucosal tumors and 17.6% of 34 head or neck tumors had *p53* mutations. Some of the mucosal and cutaneous melanomas had more than one *p53* mutation, some of which were on the same allele. One mucosal melanoma was found with mutations on different alleles. Mutations at dipyrimidine sites, considered UV fingerprints, were found in both mucosal and cutaneous melanomas.

Nearly all melanoma cell lines have mutations, deletions, or methylations of the *CDKN2A* gene. In primary melanomas, somatic mutations in *CDKN2A* are found in approx 10–30%. In addition, homozygous deletions of *CDKN2A* have been found in 10% primary melanomas. Also, approx 10% of primary melanomas and cell lines have hypermethylation of a 5′ CpG island of p16, causing silencing. Mutations and deletions in *CDKN2A* have also been found in metastases. A 540 C > T polymorphism in the 3′UTR of the *CDKN2A* gene, which may affect expression of both *p16* and *p14ARF* transcripts, was significantly higher in sporadic primary melanomas than in normal controls.

In melanoma cell lines, homozygous deletions of *CDKN2B*, which encodes *p15^INK4b* have been found. In addition, rare *CDK4* mutations have been found in melanoma cell lines and sporadic melanoma tumors.

Other Genes A new melanoma susceptibility locus was found at 1p22, with linkage being strongest for families with an early age at diagnosis. Genes that may be affected in this region are those that code for the cell division *CDC7* (cycle 7–related kinase) and *TGFBR3* (transforming growth factor b receptor 3).

In addition, it has been suggested that in individuals with red, reddish-brown, or blond hair, *GST* (glutathione *S*-transferase) M1 null, *GSTT1* null, and *GST* null may be associated with an increased risk of melanoma.

Occasionally breast cancer families with *BRCA2* mutations have ocular melanomas that segregate with *BRCA2* mutations. In addition, a few sporadic ocular melanoma cases have *BRCA2* mutations.

Acral melanomas tend to show frequent gene amplifications occurring early in their progression. Using comparative genomic hybridization (CGH), amplifications have been found at *HRAS*, *cyclin D1*, *CDK4*, and the catalytic subunit of telomerase, *hTERT*. *Cyclin D1*, a subunit of *CDK4* and *6*, is required for making the holoenzyme needed for kinase activity and can act as an oncogene when amplified. A smaller proportion of superficial spreading melanomas have amplifications that tend to occur later in their progression. Also the *c-MET* is on 7q33, a region that is amplified in some human melanomas.

In 7% of melanomas, mutations of *FAS* (Apo-1/CD95), a cell-surface receptor in a cell death signaling pathway, have been found. These mutations are in the death domain, a region of the protein that is highly conserved and necessary for apoptotic signaling. In addition, other melanoma cases have shown *FAS* allelic loss. Silencing of the *FAS* promoter in melanoma can also occur by hypermethylation or through cooperating transcription factors.

In addition, some melanoma cells have completely lost expression of *TRAIL* receptors, which can be from the loss chromosome 8p22–21 or an epigenetic silencing mechanism. Upregulation of β-catenin mutations, through faulty mRNA splicing, or adenomatous polyposis coli tumor suppressor protein inactivation, can also occur in melanomas and may play a role in progression.

MELANOCYTIC NEVI Although it is suggestive, based on their frequent histological association and epidemiological data, that some melanomas arise from nevi, it is unproven. In addition it is unknown whether nevi are clonal. X-linked genes have been

examined looking at X-inactivation, but conflicting results have been presented in different studies. There is also controversy regarding the importance of *p53* and *CDKN2A* alterations in dysplastic nevi, with different authors getting conflicting results. *BRAF* has been found in 86% of 7 congenital nevi, 88% of 42 intradermal nevi, 70% of 23 compound nevi, and 80% of 5 dysplastic nevi. *NRAS* mutations were found in 10/18 (56%) of congenital nevi in codon 61. One *NRAS* mutation in a dysplastic nevus has been reported. In a study of nevi histologically associated with melanoma, six out of seven associated nevi carried the same *NRAS* sequence (mutated or wild type) as the primary melanoma implying a clonal relationship.

CMN are generally larger than nevi acquired later in life. It has been theorized that this is from a longer period of proliferation because of telomeres being longer earlier in life. A mutation could result in a clonal proliferation of nevic cells; however, proliferation would stop because of the telomere checkpoint. Using CGH, proliferations arising in CMN have been analyzed and compared. In 86% of CMN with benign atypical nodular proliferations, numerical chromosome aberrations were found, which were not found in CMNs without these proliferations. These aberrations are different than those found in melanoma, which tends to have structural aberrations and different patterns of numerical aberrations. About 20% of Spitz nevi show multiple copies of an isochromosome 11p. Of the Spitz nevi with 11p copy increases, 70% have mutations in *HRAS,* codons 12, 13, or 61, which maps to 11p. In addition, one Spitz nevus without increase copy number of 11p also had a mutation in *HRAS*. No melanomas with histological features of Spitz nevi have been shown to have this alteration.

DIAGNOSIS: CLINICAL AND LABORATORY

The clinical *ABCDE* criteria, as noted, are used in the diagnosis of melanoma. Dermoscopy, a method combining surface magnification and either polarization or oil to eliminate reflection and refraction, improves diagnostic accuracy further. However, the gold standard for diagnosis remains pathological examination of biopsy specimens. Whenever feasible, the biopsy should be an excision or punch biopsy with complete removal of the lesion with narrow margins. An incisional biopsy that removes a portion of the lesion can be done when complete excision of the lesion for biopsy purposes would be difficult because of size or location. If the initial biopsy specimen is not adequate for diagnosis or staging, it should be repeated. The pathology should be read by a physician experienced in the histological diagnosis of melanoma.

MANAGEMENT

MELANOMA Genetic testing for melanoma susceptibility genes is not recommended.

The rationale is that most *CDKN2A* carriers, based on risk factors assessed by phenotype, family and personal history, are already known to be at increased risk of melanoma. These individuals should be counseled regarding sun avoidance and protection, self-examination, signs of melanoma, and encouraged to have yearly skin examinations. In addition, although the risk of disease based on *CDKN2A* has been studied, mutations are extremely rare (Table 103-3), confidence limits on estimates of risk are large, and penetrance varies with location in the world. Also, the risk of other cancers besides melanoma in *CDKN2A* mutation carriers is not well defined. Knowledge of mutation would not be expected to change clinical care, but instead might provide mutation negative

Table 103-3
Estimate of Percent Positive *CDKN2A* Mutations
That Would be Found With Testing

Group	% *CDKN2A* mutations
Sporadic melanoma	0.2[a]
≥2 Affected first-degree relatives	<5
≥3 Affected first-degree relatives	20–40
Multiple primary melanomas	9–15
Patients with melanoma age <40	2[b]

[a]J Natl Cancer Inst;1999;91:446–452.
[b]Arch Derm 2000;136:1118–1122.
Adapted from J Clin Oncol 1999;17:3245–3251.

individuals with a false sense of security. Mutation negative individuals in *CDKN2A* melanoma families are at increased risk of melanoma, possibly because of shared environmental risks and less penetrant genes.

Once a diagnosis of melanoma has been confirmed by biopsy, the disease should be staged. The updated AJCC staging system takes into account the Breslow depth (the depth from the epidermal granular layer to the deepest point of tumor invasion), Clark level if the depth is ≤1 mm, ulceration, whether in transit or satellite metastases are present, whether lymph node involvement involving micro- or macrometastases are present and whether distant metastases have occurred. At many centers, patients with a new diagnosis of invasive melanoma are offered lymphatic mapping and sentinel node procedure to determine if the melanoma has spread to the lymph nodes. If a sentinel lymph node biopsy is performed, it should be done before the wide excision.

The mainstay of treatment for melanoma remains surgical, with wide margins being taken around the melanoma or around the biopsy site, with the size of the margins determined by the depth of the melanoma. Additional surgical procedures may be indicated such as lymph node dissection if lymph node micro- or macrometastases are present. Surgical removal of isolated distant metastases may also be warranted.

High risk patients such as those with intermediate-thickness melanomas (1.0–4.0 mm) that are ulcerated, with deep primary melanomas (>4.0 mm), stage III disease, or who have had resection of distant metastases (stage IV) may be offered chemotherapy, treatment with biological agents or the option of a clinical trial. Once melanoma is found outside the regional nodal basis, prognosis is poor, with only 5% of patients being long-term survivors.

NEVI Management of nevi, especially dysplastic nevi, is controversial. Although dysplastic nevi may represent a precursor state for melanoma, it is likely rare that any one dysplastic nevus progresses to melanoma. Further work is needed in identifying how melanoma might arise from nevi and which nevi warrant removal.

Regarding giant CMN, in which there is a known increase in melanoma risk, the pros and cons of prophylactic excision must take into account melanoma risk, cosmetic outcome, and surgical complexity. Whether small congenital nevi should be prophylactically removed is controversial.

In addition, management of Spitz nevi is also controversial because of the diagnostic difficulty in discriminating them from melanoma. Atypical Spitz nevi warrant complete excision; at times, sentinel lymph node biopsy should be considered.

SELECTED REFERENCES

Aitken J, Welch J, Duffy D, et al. CDKN2A variants in a population-based sample of Queensland families with melanoma. J Natl Cancer Inst 1999;91:446–452.

Akslen LA, Monstad SE, Larsen B, et al. Frequent mutations of the p53 gene in cutaneous melanoma of the nodular type. Int J Cancer 1998; 79:91–95.

Balch CM, Buzaid AC, Soong SJ, et al. Final version of the American Joint Committee on Cancer staging system for cutaneous melanoma. J Clin Oncol 2001;19:3635–3648.

Barrett JH, Gaut R, Wachsmuth R, et al. Linkage and association analysis of nevus density and the region containing the melanoma gene CDKN2A in UK twins. Br J Cancer 2003;88:1920–1924.

Bastian BC. Understanding the progression of melanocytic neoplasia using genomic analysis: from fields to cancer. Oncogene 2003;22: 3081–3086.

Bastian BC, Xiong J, Frieden IJ, et al. Genetic changes in neoplasms arising in congenital melanocytic nevi: differences between nodular proliferations and melanomas. Am J Pathol 2002;161: 1163–1169.

Birck A, Ahrenkiel V, Zeuthen J, et al. Mutation and allelic loss of the PTEN/MMAC1 gene in primary and metastatic melanoma biopsies. J Invest Dermatol 2000;114:277–280.

Box NF, Duffy DL, Chen W, et al. MC1R genotype modifies risk of melanoma in families segregating CDKN2A mutations. Am J Hum Genet 2001;69:765–773.

Cachia AR, Indsto JO, McLaren KM, et al. CDKN2A mutation and deletion status in thin and thick primary melanoma. Clin Cancer Res 2000;6: 3511–3515.

Casso EM, Grin-Jorgensen CM, Grant-Kels JM. Spitz nevi. J Am Acad Dermatol 1992;27:901–913.

Davies H, Bignell GR, Cox C, et al. Mutations of the BRAF gene in human cancer. Nature 2002;417:949–954.

Demunter A, Stas M, Degreef H, et al. Analysis of N- and K-ras mutations in the distinctive tumor progression phases of melanoma. J Invest Dermatol 2001;117:1483–1489.

Elwood JM, Jopson J. Melanoma and sun exposure: an overview of published studies. Int J Cancer 1997;73:198–203.

Gillanders E, Juo SH, Holland EA, et al. Localization of a novel melanoma susceptibility locus to 1p22. Am J Hum Genet 2003;73: 301–313.

Hayward NK. Genetics of melanoma predisposition. Oncogene 2003;22: 3053–3062.

Ivanov VN, Bhoumik A, Ronai Z. Death receptors and melanoma resistance to apoptosis. Oncogene 2003;22:3152–3161.

Jemal A, Murray T, Samuels A, et al. Cancer statistics, 2003. CA Cancer J Clin 2003;53:5–26.

Kefford R, Bishop JN, Tucker M, et al. Genetic testing for melanoma. Lancet Oncol 2002;3:653, 654.

Kefford RF, Mann GJ. Is there a role for genetic testing in patients with melanoma? Curr Opin Oncol 2003;15:157–161.

Kefford RF, Bishop JA, Bergman W, Tucker MA. Counseling and DNA testing for individuals perceived to be genetically predisposed to melanoma: a consensus statement of the Melanoma Genetics Consortium. J Clin Oncol 1999;17:3245–3251.

Maitra A, Gazdar AF, Moore TO, Moore AY. Loss of heterozygosity analysis of cutaneous melanoma and benign melanocytic nevi: laser capture microdissection demonstrates clonal genetic changes in acquired nevocellular nevi. Hum Pathol 2002;33:191–197.

Palmer JS, Duffy DL, Box NF, et al. Melanocortin-1 receptor polymorphisms and risk of melanoma: is the association explained solely by pigmentation phenotype? Am J Hum Genet 2000;66:176–186.

Papp T, Pemsel H, Rollwitz I, et al. Mutational analysis of N-ras, p53, CDKN2A (p16(INK4a)), p14(ARF), CDK4, and MC1R genes in human dysplastic melanocytic naevi. J Med Genet 2003;40:E14.

Papp T, Pemsel H, Zimmermann R, et al. Mutational analysis of the N-ras, p53, p16INK4a, CDK4, and MC1R genes in human congenital melanocytic naevi. J Med Genet 1999;36:610–614.

Pollock PM, Harper UL, Hansen KS, et al. High frequency of BRAF mutations in nevi. Nat Genet 2003;33:19, 20.

Polsky D, Cordon-Cardo C. Oncogenes in melanoma. Oncogene 2003;22: 3087–3091.

Ragnarsson-Olding BK, Karsberg S, Platz A, Ringborg UK. Mutations in the TP53 gene in human malignant melanomas derived from sun-exposed skin and unexposed mucosal membranes. Melanoma Res 2002;12:453–463.

Rao UN, Jones MW, Finkelstein SD. Genotypic analysis of primary and metastatic cutaneous melanoma. Cancer Genet Cytogenet 2003;140: 37–44.

Sharpless E, Chin L. The INK4a/ARF locus and melanoma. Oncogene 2003;22:3092–3098.

Sober AJ, Chuang TY, Duvic M, et al. Guidelines of care for primary cutaneous melanoma. J Am Acad Dermatol 2001; 45:579–586.

Soufir N, Avril MF, Chompret A, et al. Prevalence of p16 and CDK4 germline mutations in 48 melanoma-prone families in France. The French Familial Melanoma Study Group. Hum Mol Genet 1998; 7:209–216.

Tsao H. Update on familial cancer syndromes and the skin. J Am Acad Dermatol 2000;42:939–969.

Tsao H, Zhang X, Kwitkiwski K, et al. Low prevalence of germline CDKN2A and CDK4 mutations in patients with early-onset melanoma. Arch Dermatol 2000;136:1118–1122.

Tucker MA, Fraser MC, Goldstein AM, et al. A natural history of melanomas and dysplastic nevi: An atlas of lesions in melanoma-prone families. Cancer 2002;94:3192–3209.

Wu H, Goel V, Haluska FG. PTEN signaling pathways in melanoma. Oncogene 2003;22:3113–3122.

Zhang H, Li Z, Viklund EK, Stromblad S. P21-activated kinase 4 interacts with integrin alpha v beta 5 and regulates alpha v beta 5-mediated cell migration. J Cell Biol 2002;158:1287–1297.

Zhang H, Schneider J, Rosdahl I. Expression of p16, p27, p53, p73 and Nup88 proteins in matched primary and metastatic melanoma cells. Int J Oncol 2002;21:43–48.

Zhou X-P, Gimm O, Hampel H, et al. Epigenetic PTEN Silencing in malignant melanomas without PTEN mutation. Am J Pathol 2000; 157:1123–1128.

104 Disorders of Hypopigmentation

JULIE V. SCHAFFER AND JEAN L. BOLOGNIA

SUMMARY

This chapter reviews the clinical features and genetic bases of classic genodermatoses such as oculocutaneous albinism, piebaldism, and Waardenburg syndrome, with an emphasis on the understanding of their molecular pathophysiology. Other disorders of hypopigmentation with known genetic defects, such as Griscelli syndrome, are also briefly discussed, as is pigmentary mosaicism. The chapter is divided into three sections: oculocutaneous albinism, other inherited disorders characterized by diffuse pigmentary dilution, and inherited disorders characterized by circumscribed or linear hypopigmentation.

Key Words: Albinism-deafness syndrome; Chédiak-Higashi syndrome (CHS); Cross syndrome; Griscelli syndrome (GS); Hermansky-Pudlak syndrome (HPS); oculocutaneous albinism (OCA); piebaldism; Waardenburg syndrome (WS).

INTRODUCTION

The study of patients and animal models of inherited disorders of hypopigmentation has led to important advances in melanocyte biology and cell biology as a whole, from signaling pathways in embryonic development to mechanisms of intracellular organelle biogenesis and trafficking to the regulation of melanogenesis. The elucidation of the genetic bases of these conditions has provided insight into the pathogenesis of the individual disorders as well as important lessons in molecular medicine.

This chapter reviews the clinical features and genetic bases of classic genodermatoses such as oculocutaneous albinism (OCA), piebaldism and Waardenburg syndrome (WS), with an emphasis on the understanding of their molecular pathophysiology. Other disorders of hypopigmentation with known genetic defects, such as Griscelli syndrome (GS), are also briefly discussed, as is pigmentary mosaicism. The chapter is divided into three sections: OCA, other inherited disorders characterized by diffuse pigmentary dilution, and inherited disorders characterized by circumscribed or linear hypopigmentation. (Tuberous sclerosis is covered in Chapter 101).

OCULOCUTANEOUS ALBINISM

OCA represents a group of autosomal-recessive disorders characterized by diffuse pigmentary dilution of the skin, hair, and eyes. Although affected individuals have a normal number of

From: *Principles of Molecular Medicine, Second Edition*
Edited by: M. S. Runge and C. Patterson © Humana Press, Inc., Totowa, NJ

melanocytes, the ability of these cells to produce melanin is either absent or reduced. Historically, OCA was divided into two major forms: tyrosinase negative and tyrosinase positive. Tyrosinase, the key enzyme in the melanin biosynthetic pathway (Fig. 104-1), catalyzes the initial rate-limiting conversion of tyrosine to dihydroxyphenylalanine (DOPA). In addition to this essential role as a tyrosine hydroxylase, human tyrosinase has DOPA oxidase, 5,6-dihydroxyindole oxidase, and perhaps 5,6-dihydroxyindole-2-carboxylic acid (DHICA) oxidase activities that regulate several other steps in the pathway. Patients with OCA were classically categorized based on clinical appearance, with tyrosinase-negative individuals having a more severe phenotype, as well as by the presence (tyrosinase positive) or absence (tyrosinase negative) of melanin production when anagen hair bulbs were incubated with tyrosine.

With the advent of molecular biology, determination of the genetic bases of the various forms of OCA has enabled more precise classification. As predicted, mutations in the tyrosinase (*TYR*) gene were found to be responsible for tyrosinase-negative OCA and a subset of tyrosinase-positive OCA (designated as OCA1A and OCA1B, respectively). Furthermore, mutations in several other genes cause tyrosinase-positive OCA, including *P* (OCA2), *tyrosinase-related protein 1* (*TYRP1*; OCA3), and *membrane-associated transporter protein* (*MATP*; OCA4). In addition, the molecular bases of disorders of intracytoplasmic organelle biogenesis and trafficking, which result in an OCA phenotype (because of defective melanosomes) as well as other manifestations such as a bleeding diathesis (because of defective platelet dense granules), have been elucidated. Mutations in the *LYST* gene were found to cause Chédiak-Higashi syndrome (CHS), and mutations in eight different genes have been reported in patients with Hermansky-Pudlak syndrome (HPS).

CLINICAL FEATURES

Ocular Manifestations The presence of ocular stigmata is necessary for the diagnosis of OCA, and the severity generally correlates with the overall degree of reduction in melanin pigment. Because of a decreased amount of melanin in the retinal pigment epithelium (RPE) and in particular the fovea (Fig. 104-2A), patients with OCA have foveal hypoplasia and impaired visual acuity that ranges from 20/40 to legal blindness. Photophobia also occurs from the discomfort associated with excess light scatter in a hypopigmented fundus. In addition, patients exhibit nystagmus, strabismus, and a lack of stereoscopic vision, which are thought to be related to misrouting of optic fibers at the chiasm during development.

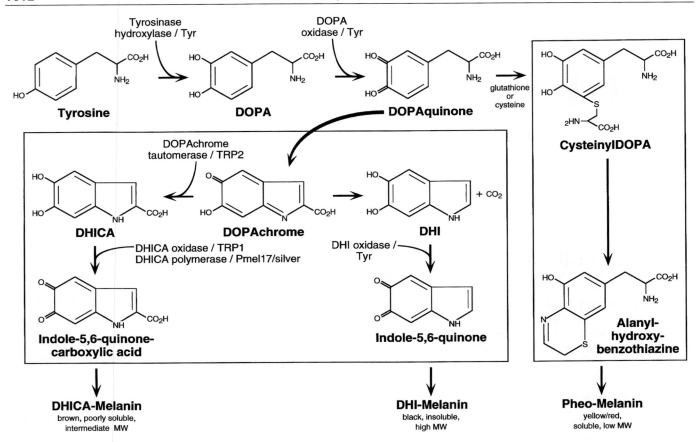

Figure 104-1 The melanin biosynthetic pathway, which includes the sites of dysfunction in OCA1 (tyrosinase) and OCA3 (TRP1). The two major forms of melanin in the skin and hair are brown-black eumelanin and yellow-red pheomelanin. Tyr, tyrosinase; DOPA, dihydroxyphenylalanine; DHI, 5,6-dihydroxyindole; DHICA, 5,6-dihydroxyindole-2-carboxylic acid; TRP, tyrosinase-related protein; MW, molecular weight. (Courtesy of Dr. Vincent Hearing.)

OCA1 In this autosomal-recessive disorder caused by mutations in both copies of the *TYR* gene, the clinical features reflect the amount of pigment that is produced in the skin, hair, and eyes. There are two subtypes of OCA1, depending on whether tyrosinase activity is reduced (OCA1B) or absent (OCA1A).

Individuals with OCA1A have pink skin, white hair, and gray-blue eyes at birth and throughout life (Fig. 104-2B). These are the patients who were previously referred to as having tyrosinase-negative OCA and, even with increasing age, they fail to produce any pheo- or eumelanin (*see* Fig. 104-1). Of all the patients with OCA, this group is the most susceptible to the development of cutaneous neoplasms, primarily squamous cell carcinomas, which can metastasize and lead to premature death, especially in those who reside in the tropics. Patients with OCA1A also have significant ocular manifestations including poor visual acuity (20/200–20/400+), and many are legally blind.

As expected, some mutations in *TYR* lead to a decrease rather than a complete lack of tyrosinase activity. Neonates with OCA1B are similar in appearance to those with OCA1A, i.e., they have pink-white skin and their hair is usually snow-white in color. However, as patients with OCA1B age they acquire more pigmentation (primarily via the production of pheomelanin, which requires less tyrosinase activity than the production of eumelanin); depending on their ethnic background, their hair can develop a yellow to reddish color, pigmented nevi can appear, and a tan can even develop in sun-exposed skin. This phenomenon, initially described

in an Amish family, accounts for the term "yellow mutant" that was previously used in reference to patients with OCA1B. As with OCA2 (*see* below), some patients may not have a striking albino phenotype, but do exhibit characteristic ocular abnormalities. However, the ocular findings are less severe than in OCA1A.

In a variant of OCA1B referred to as the temperature-sensitive phenotype, patients have lightly colored hair in warm areas of the body such as the axilla, but darkly pigmented hair in cooler parts of the body such as the leg. First described in 1991, this phenotype is analogous to that of the Himalayan mouse or the Siamese cat in which darkly pigmented hairs on the ears, paws, and nose reflect a tyrosinase enzyme that has minimal activity at 37°C, but some activity at 35°C. Most patients with OCA1 are compound heterozygotes (different maternal and paternal alleles) and, as some patients have one "yellow mutant" allele and one temperature-sensitive allele, the boundary between these variants has become blurred. The degree of pigmentary dilution in OCA1B depends on the severity of the mutations (i.e., their impact on tyrosinase activity) as well as the ethnic background of the patient. The clinical spectrum also includes phenotypes previously referred to as minimal pigment OCA and platinum OCA.

OCA2 Two observations strengthened the hypothesis that there was at least one gene other than *TYR* involved in the pathogenesis of OCA: (1) the localization of *TYR* to human chromosome 11q; and (2) the pigmentary dilution seen in some patients with Angelman and Prader-Willi syndromes, both of which are associated with deletions

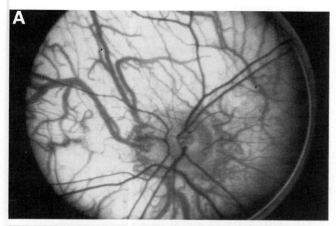

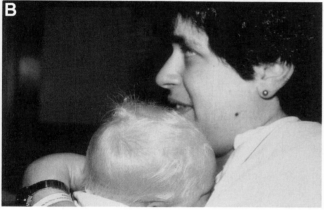

Figure 104-2 **(A)** Hypopigmented fundus in a patient with OCA1A. The vasculature is prominent because of the lack of pigment production in the retinal pigment epithelium. **(B)** A newborn with OCA1A who has white hair and pink skin. The pigmentary dilution is obvious when compared to her mother. (Courtesy of the Yale Residents' Slide Collection.)

of chromosome 15q11-q13. OCA2 is an autosomal-recessive disorder in which patients have mutations in both copies of the *P* gene located on chromosome 15q.

The phenotype of OCA2 is generally less severe than that of OCA1A, although an occasional patient has profound pigmentary dilution. As with OCA1B, the skin, hair, and eyes become darker as the patient ages; however, in contrast to OCA1B, the hair is usually not white at birth. The eventual level of pigmentation depends on the ethnic background of the patient, and some individuals, especially adults, may remain undiagnosed unless compared with first-degree relatives. A rather striking clinical finding seen in approx 1/2 of patients with OCA2 is the development of multiple large (5 mm–2 cm), stellate solar lentigines. The spectrum of pigmentation associated with OCA2 in Africa includes *brown albinism*, which manifests with light brown skin and hair together with ocular findings.

OCA3 Mutations in the *TYRP1* gene on chromosome 9p result in OCA3, also called *rufous* or *red albinism*. This condition, which has been described primarily in individuals of African or New Guinean heritage, typically results in brick- to mahogany-red or bronze skin, reddish-ginger hair, and red–brown to brown irides together with mild ocular abnormalities. Of note, one African-American infant with diffuse pigmentary dilution (compared to his fraternal twin) characterized by light brown skin and hair was

found to have mutations in both copies of the *TYRP1* gene and no detectable TYRP1. Marked hypopigmentation of the skin and hair was also reported in two siblings with 9p- syndrome, a disorder characterized by craniosynostosis, midfacial hypoplasia, abdominal wall defects, and mental retardation. An explanation for the associated hypopigmentation was not obvious, given that only one copy of *TYRP1* was deleted in these children.

OCA4 In OCA4, the degree of diffuse pigmentary dilution of the skin, hair, and eyes varies depending on the underlying mutations in the *MATP* gene. Hair color ranges from white to yellow-brown, and patients may or may not develop increased pigmentation of the skin and hair over time.

Hermansky-Pudlak Syndrome In HPS, an autosomal-recessive disorder, diffuse pigmentary dilution of the skin, hair, and eyes as well as ocular findings resulting from defective melanosomes are accompanied by a bleeding diathesis secondary to an absence of platelet dense granules. In addition, an accumulation of ceroid lipofuscin because of defective lysosomes can result in pulmonary fibrosis and granulomatous colitis.

Chédiak-Higashi Syndrome Patients with CHS have mild diffuse pigmentary dilution (often with areas of hyperpigmentation in sun-exposed sites), silvery-blonde hair that is characterized by small, regularly spaced clumps of melanin microscopically, ocular findings, and recurrent pyogenic infections because of abnormal function of neutrophils, cytotoxic T cells, and natural killer cells. Abnormally large melanosomes and lysosomal granules are seen in the perinuclear area of melanocytes and granulocytes, respectively. Additional manifestations include a bleeding diathesis, progressive neurological deterioration, and an "accelerated phase" characterized by pancytopenia and lymphohistiocytic infiltration of the liver, spleen, lymph nodes, and other organs. The latter, which results from uncontrolled T cell and macrophage activation and may be associated with Epstein-Barr viral infection, typically leads to death by the age of 10 yr unless bone marrow transplantation is performed. However, approx 10% of patients with CHS follow a less severe clinical course and survive to adulthood, but eventually develop debilitating neurologic dysfunction.

EPIDEMIOLOGY It has been estimated that OCA1 and OCA2 account for 40% and 50% of OCA worldwide, respectively. In Caucasian Americans, both OCA1 and OCA2 have an incidence of approx 1/36,000. However, OCA2 is more common among African-Americans, with an incidence approaching 1/10,000, and in certain African tribes its frequency is as high as 1/1000. In addition, the frequency of OCA2 in the Native American Navajo population was reported to be at least 1/2000. OCA3 (rufous/red albinism) has an estimated incidence of 1:8500 in southern Africa, but thus far it has not been described in Caucasians or Asians. OCA4 accounts for approx 25 and 5% of albinism in Japan and Germany, respectively.

Although rare in most populations, the frequency of HPS is approx 1/1800 in the Arecibo region of northwest Puerto Rico; this disorder also has an increased incidence in individuals from certain areas of Holland. CHS is a rare disorder, and approx 300 cases have been reported.

MOLECULAR BASIS AND GENETIC DEFECTS

OCA1 Patients with OCA1 have mutations in both copies of the *TYR* gene located on chromosome 11q14–q21. There are five exons in *TYR*, and the entire gene spans more than 65 kb of genomic DNA. Translation of tyrosinase mRNA results in a 529-amino acid polypeptide, which contains two copper-binding sites, a transmembrane domain at the carboxy-terminal end, and an 18-amino

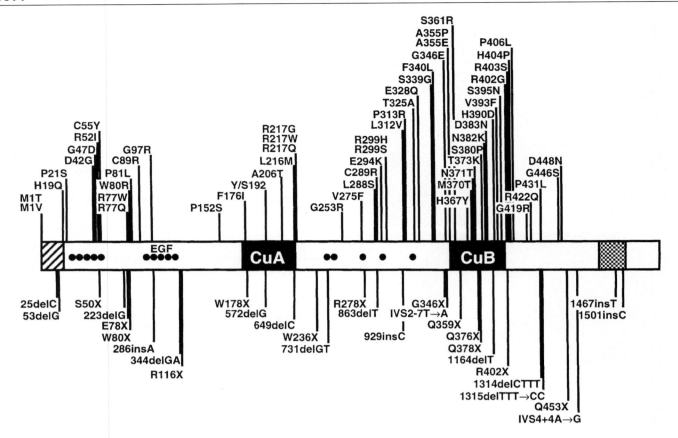

Figure 104-3 Locations of mutations in the tyrosinase gene that are associated with OCA1. CuA and CuB represent the copper-binding sites; *striped area*, signal peptide; *checkered area*, transmembrane region; *black dots*, locations of cysteine residues. *EGF*, epidermal growth factor-like region. *Top*, missense mutations; *bottom*, nonsense, frameshift, and splice-site mutations. (Reproduced from Oetting WS, King RA. Molecular basis of albinism: mutations and polymorphisms of pigmentation genes associated with albinism. Hum Mutat 1999;13:99–115. Copyright 1999 John Wiley and Sons. Reprinted with permission of Wiley-Liss, Inc., a subsidiary of John Wiley and Sons.)

acid leader peptide that is eventually cleaved. At least 115 different *TYR* mutations have been reported in patients with OCA1, and the associated phenotype depends on whether the mutations lead to a lack of enzyme activity (OCA1A) or a decreased level of enzyme activity (OCA1B). As noted, the majority of patients with OCA1 are compound heterozygotes and there is no predominant mutant allele in the general population.

Several types of *TYR* mutations have been described, including missense, nonsense, and splice-site mutations (Fig. 104-3). Some patients have also had frameshift mutations, but deletions are rare. In addition, two nonsynonymous polymorphisms (Ser192Tyr and Arg402Gln) are fairly common in Caucasian populations, with the latter resulting in temperature-sensitive enzyme activity. When the locations of *TYR* mutations are mapped, there is an obvious clustering near the amino-terminal end as well as within and flanking the two copper-binding domains (*see* Fig. 104-3). Tyrosinase is a copper-dependent enzyme, which makes the copper-binding sites logical locations for mutations in OCA1A and explains the diffuse pigmentary dilution seen in Menkes kinky-hair syndrome (which is caused by mutations in a copper-transporting ATPase) and rare cases of copper deficiency.

Although it was previously assumed that OCA1 resulted from catalytic malfunction of mutant tyrosinases, it is clear that the pathogenesis is more closely associated with tyrosinase processing in the endoplasmic reticulum (ER). During its synthesis by

ribosomes, tyrosinase is translocated into the lumen of the rough ER, where molecular chaperones (e.g., calnexin) bind the nascent glycoprotein and regulate its folding. In patients with OCA1A and OCA1B, quality-control mechanisms "trap" misfolded mutant tyrosinase within the ER compartment, and it is subsequently degraded by proteasomes rather than being sorted to melanosomes.

A specific chaperone-assisted interaction between the two copper-binding domains of tyrosinase is essential for the acquisition of an ER-exit-competent conformation and enzymatic activity. *TYR* mutations that prevent this interaction, and thus the subsequent conformational change, result in ER retention and degradation of tyrosinase, whereas missense mutations in a histidine residue critical to copper binding do not interfere with export of tyrosinase to melanosomes. This explains the apparent paradox of severe OCA phenotypes resulting from mutations predicted to have minimal effects on tyrosinase structure and function, and mild OCA phenotypes associated with mutations at key sites of catalytic activity. Lastly, in vitro studies show that temperature-sensitive tyrosinase mutants fail to exit the ER at 37°C, but are properly folded and sorted to melanosomes at 31°C or with coexpression of wild-type tyrosinase.

Murine tyrosinase has been mapped to the *albino* or *c* locus on mouse chromosome 7. Pigment production has been observed in albino mice following the introduction of a minigene that contained mouse tyrosinase cDNA plus the genomic 5′ noncoding flanking region.

OCA2   OCA2 is caused by mutations in both copies of the *P* gene, which spans 250–600 kb in chromosomal segment 15q11–q12 and contains 25 exons. The *P* gene is the human orthologue of the murine *pink-eyed dilution (p)* gene, and its 838-amino acid protein product has 12 membrane-spanning domains (Fig. 104-4A).

The P protein has an important role in eumelanogenesis, although its exact function is not known. Because its amino acid sequence is homologous to that of transmembrane transporters of small molecules and high concentrations of tyrosine can increase pigment production in *P*-null melanocytes, it was initially predicted that the P protein might serve to transport tyrosine across the melanosomal membrane. However, kinetic studies showed no difference between the melanosomes of wild-type and *P*-null melanocytes in the rate of tyrosine uptake. A second hypothesis is that the P protein regulates the pH of melanosomes and/or other organelles, potentially mediating neutralization of pH to optimize the activity and/or folding of tyrosinase. The restoration of pigment production in *P*-null cells by vacuolar H⁺-ATPase inhibitors (e.g., bafilomycin A1) that are known to alkalinize (i.e., neutralize) organelles supports this theory. The majority of the P protein in melanocytes is actually located in the ER rather than in melanosomes, and abnormal processing and trafficking of tyrosinase occurs when the P protein is absent. In addition, it was observed that the P protein facilitates vacuolar accumulation of glutathione, a major redox buffer that is required for the folding of cysteine-rich proteins such as tyrosinase. The P protein may thus regulate the processing of tyrosinase via control of glutathione.

As with OCA1, most patients with OCA2 are compound heterozygotes. The types of mutations described include missense and splice-site mutations, in-frame deletions, and frameshifts. An intragenic deletion of the *P* gene involving exon 7 is a commonly observed mutant allele in Africans with OCA2. Many of the *P* missense mutations occur at residues that are conserved among homologous transmembrane transporter proteins, whereas some mutations that result in a milder phenotype occur at less well-conserved residues. In contrast to *TYR*, the *P* gene has >40 non-pathogenic DNA sequence polymorphisms. When Caucasians with tyrosinase-positive OCA are evaluated, an equal number have *TYR* gene mutations as have *P* gene mutations. In contrast, *P* gene mutations are found in the vast majority of Africans and African-Americans with tyrosinase-positive OCA.

Patients with Angelman or Prader-Willi syndrome plus OCA2 have a deletion in the maternal or paternal copy of chromosome 15, respectively, in addition to a mutation in the second copy of the *P* gene. Uniparental disomy is a less common cause of this constellation of findings. Conversely, generalized cutaneous hyperpigmentation has been reported in a patient with a *P* gene duplication.

OCA3   OCA3 (rufous/red albinism) is caused by mutations in both copies of the *TYRP1* gene on chromosome 9p23, a member of the *TYR* family that spans approx 25 kb and contains 9 exons. Although the murine *Tyrp1* gene maps to the *brown* locus, in humans brown albinism results from mutations in the *P* gene (*see* OCA2). TYRP1, a transmembrane protein with approx 40% amino acid sequence homology with tyrosinase, represents the most abundant melanosomal protein. Also known as gp75, it is detected by MEL-5 immunohistochemical staining. In mice and humans, the major function of TYRP1 is to promote eumelanogenesis by

stabilizing tyrosinase, whereas in mice Tyrp1 also acts as a DHICA oxidase (*see* Fig. 104-1).

Only two mutations in the *TYRP1* gene have been reported (1104delA and S166X), both of which produce a truncated protein. Interestingly, these mutations result in the ER retention and early degradation of both mutant TYRP1 and wild-type tyrosinase, suggesting that tyrosinase and TYRP1 form a complex early during their processing in the ER.

OCA4   OCA4 is caused by mutations in both copies of the *MATP* (solute carrier family 45 member 2, *SLC45A2*) gene, which spans a region of approx 40 kb on chromosome 5p and contains 7 exons. Initially identified by its expression in melanoma cell lines and called *a*ntigen *i*n *m*elanoma-1 (*AIM1*), the *MATP* gene represents the human orthologue of the murine *underwhite* (*uw*) gene. A conserved mutation in the *Matp* gene causes the cream coat color in horses and diffuse pigmentary dilution in the mouse as well as the OCA4 phenotype in humans, and *Matp* mutations also result in generalized hypopigmentation in medaka fish. In addition, polymorphisms in the *MATP* gene are associated with physiologic variation in human pigmentation.

The MATP, like the P protein, is predicted to have 12 transmembrane domains (Fig. 104-4B), and it demonstrates homology to plant sucrose transporters. The expression of *MATP* during embryological development is similar to that of *TYRP1* and *TYRP2*, and there is evidence that its transcription is regulated by *m*icrophthlamia-associated *t*ranscription *f*actor (MITF), the "master gene" for melanocyte survival and melanogenesis. In melanocytes from mice with a homozygous mutation at the *uw* locus, tyrosinase processing and trafficking is disrupted and the enzyme is abnormally secreted from the cells within vesicles rather than being sorted to early melanosomes. Similar abnormalities have been observed in the setting of *p* gene mutations.

Several missense and frameshift mutations have been identified in patients with OCA4. A founder effect for the D157N mutation may account for the relatively high prevalence of OCA4 in East Asia.

Hermansky-Pudlak Syndrome   HPS is an autosomal-recessive disorder that results from defective trafficking of organelle-specific proteins to melanosomes, lysosomes, and platelet dense granules. Mutations in eight different genes cause HPS in humans (Table 104-1). As at least 16 loci exist for HPS-like phenotypes in mice, additional genes are likely to be discovered in patients with this disorder.

Mutations in the *HPS1* and *HPS4* genes (corresponding to the murine *pale ear* and *light ear* genes, respectively) are the most common causes of HPS, and both result in a relatively severe phenotype with a significant risk of developing pulmonary fibrosis and granulomatous colitis. HPS patients from northwest Puerto Rico are homozygous for a 16-bp duplication in exon 15 of *HPS1*, which represents a founder mutation in this population. The *HPS1* and *HPS4* genes encode novel nonmembrane proteins that are components of *b*iogenesis of *l*ysosome-related *o*rganelles *c*omplex (BLOC)-3 and BLOC-4 (the latter representing a discrete module within the former). These complexes are involved in the trafficking of proteins to newly synthesized organelles.

The heterotetrameric adaptor protein-3 (AP-3) facilitates protein sorting to organelles via a different mechanism, in particular by binding to a di-leucine motif in the cytoplasmic domain of tyrosinase. Mutations in the *AP3B1* gene (*HPS2*; murine *pearl*), which encodes the β3A subunit of adaptor protein-3, have been reported in three HPS patients.

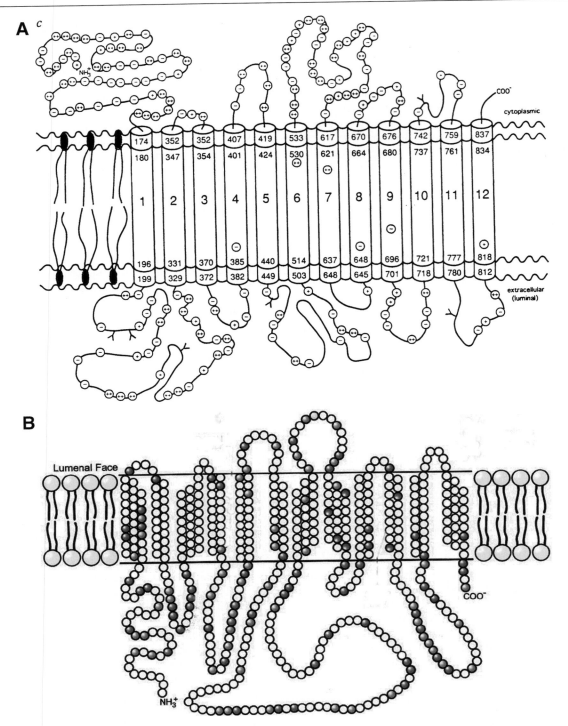

Figure 104-4   Proposed models for the arrangements of the P protein and membrane-associated transporter protein within the lipid bilayer. **(A)** The P protein, which is defective in OCA2, has 12 transmembrane domains. (Adapted from Rinchik EM, Bultman SJ, Horsthemke B, et al. A gene for the mouse pink-eyed dilution locus and for human type II oculocutaneous albinism. Nature 1993;361:72–76. Copyright Nature Publishing Group.) **(B)** The membrane-associated transporter protein, which is defective in OCA4, also has 12 transmembrane domains. (Adapted from with permission from the University of Chicago, Newton JM, Cohen-Barak O, Hagiwara N, et al. Mutations in the humanorthologue of the mouse underwhite gene (uw) underlie a new form of oculocutaneous albinism, OCA4. Am J Hum Genet 2001; 69:981–988.)

Mutations in the *HPS3* gene (murine *cocoa*) cause a relatively mild form of HPS. Initially described in a genetic isolate from central Puerto Rico, *HPS3* mutations have also been reported in Ashkenazi Jews and other non-Puerto Rican patients. The HPS3 protein is a member of the BLOC-2 complex and associates with clathrin, the main component of protein coats that assist in the budding of vesicles from the trans-Golgi network.

Table 104-1

Mouse Coat Color Genes That Have Been Cloned, Their Human Orthologues, and Associated Diseases

Murine locus	Human locus	Human chromosome	Protein	Function	Associated human disease or phenotype
Proteins with a role in melanogenesis					
Albino (c)	TYR	11q14-q21	Tyrosinase	Key melanogenic enzyme	OCA1A, OCA1B
Pink-eyed dilution (p)	P	15q11-q12	P protein	Tyrosinase processing via control of organelle pH and/or glutathione accumulation	OCA2
Brown (b)	TYRP1	9p23	Tyrosinase-related protein 1	Tyrosinase stabilization; DHICA oxidase (in mice)	OCA3 (rufous/red)
Underwhite (uw)	MATP (SLC45A2)	5p	Membrane-associated transporter protein	Tyrosinase processing and trafficking	OCA4; physiologic variation in pigmentary phenotype
Extension (e)	MC1R	16q24.3	Melanocortin-1 receptor	Stimulates eumelanogenesis	Red-hair-color phenotype, fair skin/hair, freckling; increased risk of melanoma and nonmelanoma skin cancers
Pomc1	POMC	2p23.3	POMC cleavage products include MSH and ACTH	Stimulates eumelanogenesis	Red hair, obesity, and adrenocortical insufficiency
Gray lethal (gl)	GGT	22q11	γ-glutamyl transpeptidase	Role in glutathione metabolism	Glutathionuria
	GL	6q21	Gray lethal	Role in pheomelanogenesis	Severe recessive osteopetrosis
Mottled (mo)	ATP7A	Xq12-q13	Copper-transporting P-type ATPase 7A	Copper transport	Menkes kinky hair syndrome; occipital horn syndrome
Toxic milk (tx)	ATP7B	13q14.3-q21.1	Copper-transporting P-type ATPase 7B	Copper transport	Wilson disease
Proteins with a role in organelle biogenesis (e.g., melanosomes, platelet dense granules)					
Pale ear (ep)	HPS1	10q23.1-q23.2	HPS1 (component of BLOC-3, -4)	Trafficking of organelle-specific proteins to melanosomes, lysosomes, and cytoplasmic granules (including platelet dense granules)	Hermansky-Pudlak syndrome
Pearl (pe)	AP3B1	Chr. 5	β3A subunit of adaptor protein-3		
Cocoa (coa)	HPS3	3q24	HPS3 (component of BLOC-2)		
Light ear (le)	HPS4	22q11.2-q12.2	HPS4 (component of BLOC-3, -4)		
Ruby-eye 2 (ru2)	HPS5	11p15-p13	Ru2 (component of BLOC-2)		
Ruby-eye (ru)	HPS6	10q24.32	Ru (component of BLOC-2)		
Sandy (sdy)	DTNBP1	6p22.3	Dysbindin (component of BLOC-1)		
Reduced pigmentation (rp)	BLOC1S3	19q13	BLOC1S3 (component of BLOC-1)		
Proteins with a role in organelle trafficking (affecting melanosomes, platelet dense granules and/or lysosomes, e.g., of leukocytes and natural killer cells)					
Beige (bg)	LYST	1q43	(cytosolic protein that interacts with SNARE proteins)	Regulates vesicle fission/fusion	Chédiak-Higashi syndrome
Oa1	OA1	Xp22.3	(G protein-coupled receptor)	May regulate vesicle fission/fusion in melanosome development	Ocular albinism 1
Proteins with a role in organelle transport (e.g., attachment of organelles to the actin cytoskeleton)					
Ashen (ash)	RAB27A	15q21	Rab27A	Ras-like GTPase; present in mature melanosomes	Griscelli syndrome 2
Dilute (d)	MYO5A	15q21	Myosin Va	Molecular motor that moves along the actin cytoskeleton	Griscelli syndrome 1
Leaden (ln)	MLPH	2q37	Melanophilin	Links Rab27A to myosin Va	Griscelli syndrome 3
Shaker-1 (sh1)	MYO7A	11q13.5	Myosin VIIa	Molecular motor that moves along the actin cytoskeleton; functions in the retinal pigment epithelium	Usher syndrome, type IB

Proteins with a role in melanocyte development (e.g., survival, proliferation, migration and differentiation)

Dominant white spotting (W)	KIT	4q12	KIT receptor	Tyrosine kinase receptor	Piebaldism; adult mastocytosis; gastrointestinal stromal tumors
Splotch (Sp)	PAX3	2q35	Paired-box gene 3	Transcription factor	WS1, WS3; alveolar rhabdomyosarcomas
Microphthalmia (mi)	MITF	3p14-p12	Microphthalmia-associated transcription factor	Transcription factor	WS2
Slugh	SLUG (SNAI2)	8q11	Snail homolog 2	Transcription factor	WS2
Piebald spotting (s)	EDNRB	13q22	Endothelin B receptor	G protein-coupled receptor on melanoblast/ganglion cell precursors	WS4
Lethal spotting (ls)	EDN3	20q13.2-q13.3	Endothelin-3	Ligand of endothelin B receptor	WS4
Dominant megacolon (dom)	SOX10	22q13	SRY box-containing gene 10	Transcription factor	WS4
	ECE1	1p36.1	Endothelin-converting enzyme 1	Proteolytic processing of endothelin-1, -3	Hirschsprung disease
Bcl2	BCL2	18q21.33	Bcl2	Inhibits apoptosis	B cell chronic lymphocytic leukemia or lymphoma
Other					
	DKC1	Xq28	Dyskerin	Telomere maintenance; associates with the telomerase RNA component	Dyskeratosis congenita, X-linked recessive
	TERC	3q21-q28	Telomerase RNA component	Telomere maintenance	Dyskeratosis congenita, autosomal-dominant
	IKBKG	Xq28	Inhibitor of κB kinase, γ subunit (NEMO)	Required for NF-κB activation	Incontinentia pigmenti; hypohidrotic ectodermal dysplasia with immune deficiency

OCA, oculocutaneous albinism; BLOC, *biogenesis of lysosomal related organelles complex*; NEMO, *Nuclear factor-κB essential modulator*.

Positional candidate and transgenic rescue approaches were used to identify the genes mutated in the ruby-eye-2 and ruby-eye mouse models of HPS (*ru2* and *ru*), and the human orthologues, *HPS5* and *HPS6*, were shown to be mutated in patients with a mild form of HPS. The Ru and Ru2 proteins directly interact in the BLOC-2 complex. In addition, mutations in the *DTNBP1* gene (murine *sandy*), which encodes the dysbindin protein, and the *BLOC1S3* gene (murine *reduced pigment*) have been reported in patients with HPS (HPS7 and HPS8, respectively). Dysbindin and BLOC1S3 represent the first components of the BLOC-1 complex shown to be defective in human HPS, whereas mutations in several other components of BLOC-1 underlie HPS-like phenotypes in mice.

Chédiak-Higashi Syndrome   CHS is caused by mutations in both copies of the *LYST* (*l*ysosomal *t*rafficking regulator, *LYST*) gene on chromosome 1q43, the human orthologue of the murine *beige* gene. Frameshift and nonsense mutations that result in a truncated protein lead to a severe phenotype in which there is progression to a fatal accelerated phase during childhood, whereas missense mutations are associated with a milder phenotype and survival to adulthood.

The exact function of CHS1, a 3801-amino acid cytosolic protein that is expressed by most cell types, is not known. The amino-terminus contains a series of α-helical ARM/HEAT repeats thought to mediate membrane associations and vesicle transport, and the carboxy terminus contains a *b*eige *a*nd *C*hédiak-*H*igashi syndrome (BEACH) domain conserved within a family of proteins that regulates vesicle morphology. The CHS1 protein interacts with SNARE proteins, which play an important role in the fusion of intracellular organelles. In addition, an association between ceramide-induced protein kinase C down-regulation and organelle dysfunction in CHS has been proposed. Cells from patients with CHS have abnormally large, centrally located lysosomes and melanosomes, whereas over-expression of *CHS1* in fibroblasts results in unusually small, peripherally located lysosomes. CHS thus appears to be a disorder of vesicle trafficking, resulting from aberrant fission/fusion in a step downstream from the vesicle formation that is defective in HPS. In addition, generalized impairment of plasma membrane repair may contribute to the pathogenesis of CHS.

Diagnosis   The diagnosis of OCA1A can be made on the basis of clinical findings in a child or adult and then confirmed by molecular analysis of the *TYR* gene. However, the latter is not necessary unless it provides information required for future prenatal screening or genetic counseling of family members. In patients in whom there is some pigment production, albeit reduced, clinical clues (e.g., color of hair at birth) can help to distinguish OCA1B from OCA2, but molecular analysis of the *TYR* and *P* genes is the most exact method for confirming the clinical diagnosis. Of note, approx 17% of individuals with OCA1 have only one identifiable *TYR* mutation, rather than the expected two.

If there is a clinical suspicion of OCA, but the patient has a rather subtle form of the disease (i.e., one that is associated with a significant level of pigment production), it is important to evaluate the first-degree relatives and to have an ophthalmologist perform a complete eye examination. In addition, a thorough medical history should be taken in patients with OCA, with special attention to recurrent infections or a bleeding tendency suggestive of CHS or HPS. Simple screening laboratory tests for these syndromes include examination of a peripheral blood smear for giant lysosomal granules within leukocytes and performance of a bleeding time. If the latter is prolonged, an absence of platelet dense granules on wet-mount electron microscopy can establish the diagnosis of HPS.

Other causes of diffuse pigmentary dilution of the skin, hair, and occasionally eyes should be considered and then excluded by lack of associated findings; these include Angelman, Prader-Willi and Apert (craniosynostosis, syndactyly, and acneiform eruptions) syndromes, phenylketonuria, histidinemia, homocystinuria, and infantile sialic acid storage disease. Pigmentary dilution limited to the skin and hair is seen in GS, *e*ctrodactyly, *e*ctodermal dysplasia, and *c*lefting (EEC) syndrome and Menkes kinky hair syndrome; copper or selenium deficiency, and kwashiorkor.

Another entity that overlaps clinically with OCA is ocular albinism (OA), a disorder that is usually inherited in an X-linked recessive fashion. The gene responsible for the most common form of X-linked OA (OA1; Nettleship-Falls) encodes a transmembrane protein thought to represent an intracellular G protein-coupled receptor that transduces a lumenal-to-cytosolic signal. The OA1 protein plays a role in melanosomal development, possibly regulating the budding of vesicles from the endolysosomal compartment or their fusion with melanosomes (functions that are especially critical in RPE cells). Microscopic examination of both RPE cells and melanocytes in patients with OA1 reveals macromelanosomes with a multivesicular appearance (reminiscent of the giant organelles seen in CHS). Interestingly, as occurs with abnormal tyrosinase in OCA1, mutations in *OA1* result in retention of the aberrant OA1 protein within the ER. Classically, individuals with OA were considered to have the eye, but not the cutaneous, findings of albinism. However, some patients with OA1 have hypomelanotic macules or a mild generalized pigmentary dilution when compared with unaffected siblings. It is important to note that mutations in the *TYR* and *P* genes have been described in the smaller group of patients with autosomal-recessive OA.

Prenatal screening for OCA1A and OCA1B has been performed successfully via molecular analysis of the *TYR* gene in amniotic cells after predetermination of the responsible mutations. Although not reported in the literature, such an analysis could potentially be utilized for other forms of OCA in which the genetic defect is known. Previously, scalp biopsies were performed between weeks 17 and 20 of gestation, and the diagnosis of OCA1A was based on the presence or absence of melanized melanosomes. Prenatal diagnosis of CHS by examining cultured amniotic fluid cells or chorionic villus cells for the presence of abnormally large acid phosphatase-positive lysosomes has also been reported.

Management   The earlier in life the diagnosis of OCA is established, the sooner interventions that have an impact on development can be instituted. It is critical to assess visual acuity in each child and to provide corrective eyewear as well as access to products such as large-print materials that are specially designed for a visually impaired person. In addition, it is important to identify ocular abnormalities such as strabismus that can be corrected medically or surgically.

Because of the markedly increased risk for the development of ultraviolet radiation-induced cutaneous carcinomas, a sun-protection program needs to be instituted early in life. Most individuals receive the majority of their cumulative lifetime sun exposure by the age of 18 yr, which underscores the need for early intervention. Effective measures include avoidance of midday sun, application of sunscreens, and the use of hats and clothing made of tightly woven material. The closer a patient lives to the equator, the more important this aspect of clinical care becomes. For example, in a study of albinos from Tanzania, patients commonly developed advanced (>4 cm) cutaneous squamous cell carcinomas by their late 20s, and <10% survived beyond the age of 30 yr.

In patients with HPS, 1-desamino-8D-arginine (DDAVP) has been reported as a treatment for the associated bleeding diathesis, and the results of a clinical trial suggested that the antifibrotic agent pirfinidone may help to prevent pulmonary fibrosis. Allogeneic bone marrow transplantation has been used successfully in patients with CHS as well as GS (see GS).

Genetic counseling should be made available to all OCA families. Prenatal diagnosis of OCA1 can be performed as outlined above. Because there is no treatment that reverses the major forms of this genetic disorder, both patients and their parents can receive valuable information and support by joining the National Organization for Albinism and Hypopigmentation (http://www. albinism.org/).

OTHER INHERITED DISORDERS CHARACTERIZED BY DIFFUSE PIGMENTARY DILUTION

GRISCELLI SYNDROME   GS is a rare autosomal-recessive disorder of organelle transport characterized by mild pigmentary dilution and silvery-colored hair with irregularly distributed clumps of melanin on microscopic examination, but not the ocular findings that are required for classification as OCA. Melanocytes in patients with GS are characteristically "stuffed" with melanosomes because of a failure of transfer to keratinocytes. Mutations in the *MYO5A* (murine *dilute*; encodes myosin Va), *RAB27A* (murine *ashen*), and *MLPH* (murine *leaden*; encodes melanophilin) genes cause GS1, GS2, and GS3, respectively. Primary neurological abnormalities occur in patients with GS1, whereas recurrent infections and an "accelerated phase" of pancytopenia and lymphohistiocytic infiltrates of multiple organs ("hemophagocytic syndrome"; see CHS) develop in those with GS2. Neither of these manifestations has been observed in individuals with GS3. It has been proposed that Elejalde syndrome (neuroectodermal melanolysosomal disorder) and GS1 represent the same entity.

Myosin Va, a dimeric molecular motor that moves along the actin meshwork beneath the plasma membrane, normally captures melanosomes when they reach the cell periphery. This occurs by linkage of Rab27A, a Ras-like GTPase present in mature melanosomes, to myosin Va via melanophilin. In GS, failure to securely attach melanosomes to the actin cytoskeleton causes them to "slip back" and accumulate in the center of the melanocyte. Mutations in *RAB27A*, but not *MYO5A* or *MLPH,* lead to defective secretion of lytic granules by cytotoxic T cells; this suggests that Rab27a function is mediated by different effectors in melanocytes and T cells.

Cross Syndrome   Cross syndrome is a rare autosomal-recessive disorder of diffuse pigmentary dilution, with or without ocular findings such as nystagmus, in association with mental and growth retardation, spasticity, and athetosis. Patients may have silvery-blonde hair or an admixture of lightly and darkly pigmented strands of scalp, eyebrow and eyelash hairs. The molecular basis of Cross syndrome has not yet been determined.

ALBINISM-DEAFNESS SYNDROME (ZIPRKOWSKI-MARGOLIS SYNDROME)   Albinism-deafness syndrome is a rare X-linked recessive disorder in which patients have diffuse pigmentary dilution of the hair and skin, with exception of the buttocks and genitalia. Over time, multiple hyperpigmented macules appear, resulting in a leopard-like appearance. Patients may also have congenital sensorineural deafness and heterochromia irides. The gene for this syndrome has been mapped to Xq26.3– q27.1.

INHERITED DISORDERS CHARACTERIZED BY CIRCUMSCRIBED OR LINEAR HYPOPIGMENTATION

PIEBALDISM

Clinical Features   In contrast to OCA and its variants, piebaldism is an autosomal-dominant disorder characterized by discrete, circumscribed areas of leukoderma that are devoid of melanocytes. The lesions are present at birth and generally remain stable, with an increase in size in proportion to the growth of the child; an occasional patient has expansion or limited contraction of the areas of leukoderma over time. Piebaldism has a distinctive distribution pattern, involving the ventral trunk and mid portions of the extremities but sparing the dorsal midline, hands, and feet. The depigmented patches of piebaldism characteristically contain islands of normally pigmented or hyperpigmented skin. These café-au-lait-like macules sometimes line up at the border of the lesions, and may also be seen in uninvolved skin; the latter should not be misinterpreted as a sign of neurofibromatosis.

The frontal white forelock represents a classic finding in piebaldism that is present in 80–90% of patients. The underlying scalp is amelanotic, and there is often an associated V-shaped area of leukoderma on the mid forehead. Patients may also have poliosis of the medial eyebrows and eyelashes, and premature graying of scalp hair can occur. Associated systemic abnormalities are uncommon, and include Hirschsprung disease, mental retardation, cerebellar ataxia, and sensorineural deafness; although some cases of the latter may represent a forme fruste of WS or Woolf syndrome (piebaldism and deafness described in two native American brothers), at least one patient has been documented to have a *KIT* mutation.

The incidence of piebaldism in Caucasians is estimated to be approx 1/20,000–1/40,000, with an equal frequency in men and women. It can occur in all races.

Molecular Basis and Genetic Defects   Piebaldism is caused by mutations in the *KIT* gene on chromosome 4q12, which encodes a transmembrane tyrosine kinase receptor that is expressed by melanoblasts, melanocytes, and other cell types such as mast cells. The extracellular ligand for the KIT receptor is steel factor (stem cell factor, mast cell growth factor), and its binding induces receptor activation via dimerization and autophosphorylation. During embryogenesis, the survival and migration of melanoblasts derived from the neural crest depend on interactions between the KIT receptor and steel factor.

As piebaldism is an autosomal-dominant disorder, a mutation in only one of the two copies of the *KIT* gene is required to give rise to the disease. A frameshift mutation that results in half of the KIT receptors being severely truncated and nonfunctional typically produces a mild phenotype, whereas a missense mutation that results in a single amino acid substitution can lead to a severe phenotype. Because dimerization is involved in receptor activation, a population of dysfunctional mutant receptors that "bind up" normal receptors, referred to as the dominant negative effect, is worse than a complete loss of mutant receptor function that leaves half of the normal level of receptor activity, referred to as haploinsufficiency.

In addition, heterozygous deletions of the *SLUG* (*SNAI2*) gene (also mutated in WS2) have been identified in patients with classic features of piebaldism who lacked a *KIT* mutation. Of note, mutations in either the *Kit* gene or the *steel* gene can lead to dominant white spotting in mice, but no mutations in the latter locus have

Table 104-2
Waardenburg Syndrome and its Variants: Inheritance, Associated Genes, and Clinical Features

Type	Inheritance	Gene (locus)	Classic WS features	Other features
WS1	AD	PAX3 (2q35)	Dystopia canthorum (>95%) Increased frequency of white forelock, skin lesions of piebaldism, and synophrys	Spinal dysraphism, e.g., myelomeningocele (*rare*) Facial clefts (*rare*)
WS2	AD AR	MITF (3p14.1–p12.3) SLUG (8q11)	*Absence* of dystopia canthorum Increased frequency of deafness and heterochromia irides	
WS3 (Klein-WS)	AD[a]	PAX3 (2q35)	As in WS1	Musculoskeletal anomalies of the upper extremities, e.g., hypoplasia, fusion of carpal bones, flexion contractures, syndactyly
WS4 (Shah-WS)	AR AR AD	EDN3 (20q13.2) EDNRB (13q22) SOX10 (22q13)	As in WS2	Hirschsprung disease (aganglionic megacolon) Central and autonomic nervous system dysfunction, neonatal hypotonia, arthrogryposis (*SOX10* mutations; *rare*)
Other variants				
Tietz syndrome	AD	MITF (3p14.1-p12.3)	Deafness	*Diffuse* pigmentary dilution of the skin, hair, and eyes Sparse eyebrows
Albinism, *b*lack lock, *c*ell migration disorder of the neurocytes of the gut, and *d*eafness (ABCD) syndrome	AR	EDNRB (13q22)	Deafness	*Diffuse* pigmentary dilution of the skin, hair and eyes Black lock in the temporo-occipital region Hirschsprung disease and total absence of nerve fibers in the small intestine Macrosomia
Yemenite deaf-blind hypopigmentation syndrome	AD	SOX10 (22q13)	Deafness White forelock and skin lesions of piebaldism	Nystagmus *No* Hirschsprung disease

AD, autosomal-dominant; AR autosomal-recessive; WS, Waardenburg syndrome.
[a]At least one patient has been found to be homozygous for a *PAX3* mutation.

been described in humans with piebaldism. However, somatic *activating* mutations in the *KIT* gene are often found in adult human patients with mastocytosis/mast cell leukemia and gastrointestinal stromal tumors.

Diagnosis The diagnosis of piebaldism is usually straightforward. As the major entity in the differential diagnosis is WS, patients should be evaluated for evidence of heterochromia irides, facial dysmorphism, and deafness.

Management The application of sunscreens and use of protective clothing should be encouraged. Successful treatment with autologous transplantation techniques (e.g., skin grafts or suspensions containing melanocytes) has been reported.

WAARDENBURG SYNDROME

Clinical Features The classic sextad of clinical features, as described by Waardenburg in 1951, is

1. Dystopia canthorum (increased distance between the inner canthi with relatively normal interpupillary distance; less of the medial portion of the sclera is visible and there is lateral displacement of the inferior lacrimal punctum).
2. A broad nasal root and hypoplastic alae nasi.
3. Synophrys.

4. Heterochromia irides (partial or total, or isohypochromia).
5. Congenital sensorineural deafness.
6. Cutaneous lesions of piebaldism.

WS has been divided into four subtypes that differ in their clinical manifestations and genetic bases. In addition to the findings noted in Table 104-2, premature graying of scalp hair, palmoplantar keratoderma and congenital heart defects have been reported.

The incidence of WS is estimated to be approx 1/50,000, and is equal in men and women. WS has been described in individuals of various ethnic backgrounds.

Molecular Basis and Genetic Defects Mutations in at least six different genes have been shown to cause WS (*see* Table 104-2). These genes encode regulatory proteins with important functions in embryonic development, including critical roles in the survival, proliferation, migration, and/or differentiation of neural crest-derived melanocyte precursors destined for the inner ear (in which melanocytes are critical to the ability to hear), iris and skin. Furthermore, melanocytes and enteric ganglion cells share a dipotent precursor in the developing neural crest, and interactions between endothelin-3 (EDN3) and endothelin B receptors (EDNRB) are found on these melanoblast/ganglion cell precursors. It is therefore not surprising that mutations in both alleles of the *EDN3* gene or the *EDNRB* gene can produce a combination of WS and Hirschsprung disease (congenital megacolon because of lack of myenteric ganglion cells; WS4).

In addition to such receptor-ligand interactions, several transcription factors (i.e., proteins with the ability to bind to DNA and influence the activity of other genes) have functions essential to melanocyte development. MITF, the earliest known marker of commitment to the melanocyte lineage, has been implicated as the "master gene" for melanocyte survival as well as a key regulator of the promoters of the genes encoding tyrosinase and other melanogenic proteins. Heterozygous mutations in the *MITF* gene can result in WS2. MITF is also thought to transactivate the *SLUG* gene, which encodes another transcription factor expressed by neural crest-derived cells; homozygous loss-of-function *SLUG* mutations represent a second cause of WS2. Other transcription factors expressed by melanocyte precursors include paired box gene-3 (PAX3) and SRY box-containing gene 10 (SOX10), which have a synergistic role in regulating the expression of *MITF*. Mutations in the *PAX3* gene can result in WS1 or WS3, and the expression of *PAX3* in other neural crest derivatives such as craniofacial cells (e.g., those of the frontonasal prominence) and in the limb buds accounts for the facial dysmorphism and musculoskeletal abnormalities seen in these WS subtypes. Lastly, SOX10 plays a role in the development of melanoblast/ganglion cell precursors via activation of *RET* (the major gene implicated in Hirschsprung disease) as well as *MITF*, and it is also expressed in glial cells of the central nervous system (CNS). As a consequence, heterozygous *SOX10* mutations can produce a WS4 phenotype that is associated with neurological abnormalities.

Diagnosis   Although the diagnosis is clear in patients with the complete syndrome, it can be more difficult to establish in forme fruste cases. An evaluation of hearing is important, and calculating the W index (a composite of the inner pupillary, inner canthal, and outer canthal distances) can help determine whether dystopia canthorum is present. Examination of family members can also be useful, as they may have other features of WS.

Management   Early detection of associated deafness allows intervention via hearing aids and specialized education. Patients with Hirschsprung disease require surgical resection of the involved intestinal segment. Treatment options for associated leukoderma are as described for piebaldism.

PIGMENTARY MOSAICISM (HYPOMELANOSIS OF ITO)
A variety of names have been used for hypopigmented patches resulting from cutaneous mosaicism. Hypomelanosis of Ito, qualified as *with* or *without* systemic abnormalities, was previously the preferred term for patients with linear streaks and whorls of hypopigmentation. This pigmentary disorder overlaps considerably with systematized nevus depigmentosus, with presence at birth and stability over time as the only distinguishing features of the latter. However, this represents an artificial categorization, for both conditions are manifestations of mosaicism. Furthermore, as the genetic defects that cause hypomelanosis of Ito are extremely heterogeneous and, as a consequence, it is no longer thought to be a discrete neurocutaneous syndrome, the use of a more descriptive term such as pigmentary mosaicism with nevoid hypopigmentation has been advocated.

Clinical Features   Nevoid hypopigmentation resulting from cutaneous mosaicism is often noted at birth, but may not become apparent until infancy or childhood. Classically, hypopigmented streaks and swirls follow Blaschko's lines as narrow bands. Hypopigmented patches with a block-like or phylloid configuration can also be seen. The latter pattern, which has a particular association with mosaic trisomy 13, is characterized by an arrangement of hypomelanotic lesions reminiscent of a floral ornament; it consists of leaf-like ovals and large pear-shaped or oblong elements. The hypopigmented lesions of cutaneous mosaicism can be widespread or limited in extent, with a unilateral or bilateral distribution. When the scalp is involved, circumscribed areas or whorls of lighter-colored hairs may be seen.

Associated systemic findings include central nervous system disorders (e.g., mental retardation and seizures), ocular, craniofacial, and musculoskeletal abnormalities. Of children who presented to a pediatric dermatologist at a tertiary care center with a diagnosis of hypomelanosis of Ito, approx 1/3 had systemic abnormalities, which usually became clinically apparent by early childhood. However, as localized areas of nevoid hypopigmentation in otherwise normal individuals, especially those with lightly pigmented skin, are often overlooked, the occurrence of systemic features in the general population is likely to be even lower.

Molecular Basis and Genetic Defects   Mosaicism implies the presence of at least two clones of genetically different cells, which can arise via mechanisms including post-zygotic mutations, gametic half-chromatid mutations, somatic nondysjunction, and lyonization (functional mosaicism because of random inactivation during embryogenesis of one of the two X chromosomes in females). In the case of nevoid hypopigmentation, the clones have different pigment potentials. Because many genes have a role in the production, storage, and distribution of melanin, these processes can be disturbed by a variety of chromosomal rearrangements and gene mutations, and the cytogenetic abnormalities that have been detected in patients with nevoid hypopigmentation are highly heterogeneous. Of note, chromosomal mosaicism involving 15q11–q12, the location of the *P* gene, has been reported in at least two patients. In one study, 60% of patients with a diagnosis of hypomelanosis of Ito had evidence of mosaicism when karyotype analyses of both circulating lymphocytes and dermal fibroblasts were performed. Most of these patients were mosaic for aneuploidy or unbalanced translocations. In cases of nevoid hypopigmentation in which no mosaicism is demonstrated by cytogenetic examination, it is likely that either minor chromosomal abnormalities or mosaicism at the level of genes rather than chromosomes is present.

Hypopigmentation distributed along the lines of Blaschko, which reflect the streams of growth of embryonic tissues, typically occurs if two cell clones with different pigment potentials are established early in embryonic development. Differences between the rates of proliferation and the migration potential of the two cell clones, or a different time of origin of the mosaicism, may produce other configurations such as the checkerboard pattern or the phylloid pattern. As noted, the phylloid configuration of hypopigmentation has a particular association with mosaic trisomy 13.

Diagnosis   In some cases with widespread involvement, determination of whether the patient has hypopigmented or hyperpigmented streaks can be difficult. As both are manifestations of cutaneous mosaicism, the distinction is not critical. Hypopigmentation along Blaschko's lines can also be seen in female carriers of Menkes kinky hair syndrome as a reflection of lyonization. It is important to exclude the fourth stage of incontinentia pigmenti (IP) by the lack of a history of vesicles, verrucous lesions, or hyperpigmentation following the lines of Blaschko. In

Physiology

Pathology

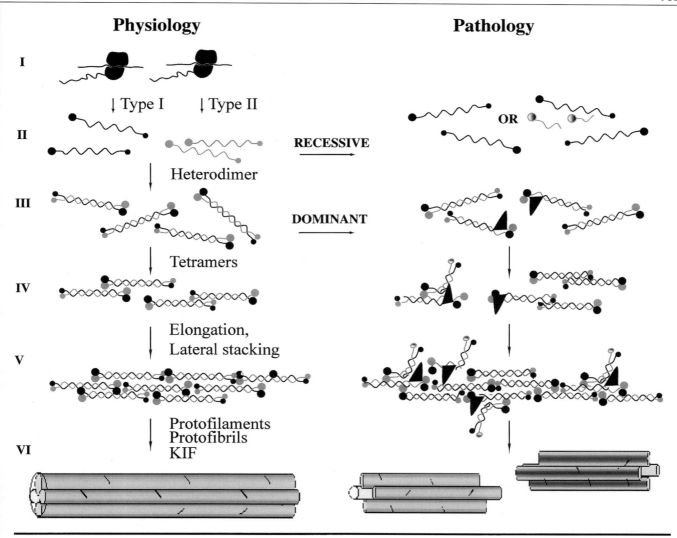

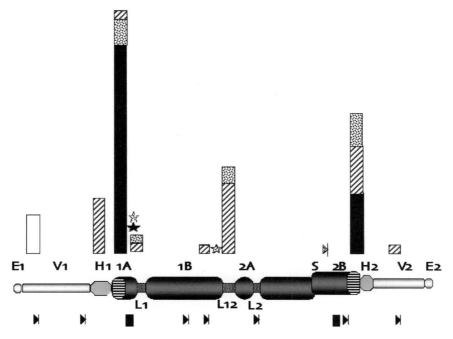

Figure 105-3 *(Continued)*

disorder owing to fragility of basal cells of the epidermis. Three major subtypes have been recognized and share a common disease pathology with an abnormal KIF network, cytolysis of basal cells leading to intraepidermal blister formation and skin fragility, whereas the differentiation of keratinocytes in the upper layers of the epidermis remains largely undisturbed. The structural abnormalities confined to the basal compartment of the epidermis and mucous membranes result from faulty K5/K14 heterodimers because of mutations in their corresponding genes, *KRT5* and *KRT14*. Mutations in either gene can produce a comparable phenotype reflecting the genetic heterogeneity of EBS. *KRT5* and *KRT14* mutations are usually inherited in an autosomal-dominant manner and lead to substitution of conserved amino acid residues, having a deleterious, dominant-negative effect on the assembly of KIF and causing weakening of the cytoskeleton and cell fragility.

More than 80 distinct pathogenic mutations have been identified in EBS. The majority (up to 80%) are sporadic new mutations, which are not present in one of the parents of an affected person. Mutations are clustered at seven defined regions (*see* Fig. 105-3, bottom), and their relative position seems to dictate the severity of disease. Most mutations (approx 60%) occur at two "hot spots" corresponding to the beginning and end of the central rod domain, known as helix initiation peptide and helix termination peptide. Functional in vivo and in vitro studies have demonstrated that the helix boundaries are zones of overlap between keratin heterodimers during filament assembly and that mutant keratin molecules perturb proper keratin alignment, and thereby oligomerization, filament assembly, and integrity (*see* Fig. 105-3, top). Consequently, these "hot spot" mutations are consistently associated with a severe phenotype. Other mutation sites, such as the homologous domain in the head of type-II keratins or nonhelical linker and stutter motifs, are associated with a milder phenotype. The former region has been implicated in filament assembly and contains major phosphorylation sites whereas the latter regions provide crucial flexibility to the otherwise rigid α-helical rod. In addition, a few rare autosomal-recessive mutations leading to the "knockout" of a keratin in the basal epidermis have also been described in EBS.

EBS DOWLING-MEARA EBS Dowling-Meara (EBS-DM) is a common and the most severe subtype manifesting at birth with erythema, widespread blistering, erosions, and areas of denuded skin (*see* Fig. 105-2). Although spontaneous development of grouped blisters at any body site slowly improves with age, a progressive palmoplantar keratoderma becomes the chief complaint in adulthood. Other features of EBS-DM include involvement of mucous membranes, secondary skin infections and sepsis, nail dystrophy, milia, and healing with hypo- and hyperpigmentation of the skin. Typically, pathogenic defects are heterozygous missense mutations clustering at the highly conserved boundaries of the α-helical rod of K5 or K14. An arginine codon of the helix initiation peptide in K14 (R125) is most commonly mutated (>30% of patients), probably because it contains a hypermutable CpG dinucleotide. As a result, the arginine codon (CGC) is replaced either by one for cysteine (TGC) or histidine (CAC). Although most keratin gene mutations in EBS are dominant, recessive *KRT14* mutations have been identified in seven families, including predominantly nonsense and splice site mutations leading to premature termination of protein translation and ablation of the affected keratin. Although the "knockout" of *KRT14* usually results in severe EBS-DM, mutations in three families were noted to have a milder phenotype with minimal extracutaneous involvement.

KÖBNER SUBTYPE OF EBS The Köbner subtype of the simplex forms of EB is characterized by milder, generalized blistering of the skin without apparent clustering, often in response to minor trauma and induced by increased ambient temperature. Hands, feet, and extremities are most consistently affected, probably because of the greater mechanical trauma at these body sites. *KRT5* or *KRT14* mutations appear more widely distributed across the keratin polypeptides and may lie within and outside the highly conserved helix boundaries as well as in nonhelical linker segments.

EBS WEBER-COCKAYNE The simplex form of EB—Weber-Cockayne is the most common, relatively mild, localized subtype of EBS, in which serous blisters are confined to the hands, feet, and areas of friction or trauma. In contrast to the other EBS subtypes, blisters are usually not present at birth but develop later in life in response to mechanical trauma to the skin. The disorder worsens with sweating and at increased ambient temperature. Ultrastructural abnormalities of the cytoskeleton are far less severe than those seen in EBS-DM, and even essentially normal KIF ultrastructure has been reported. In this relatively mild form

Figure 105-3 (*see Opposite Page*) Physiology and pathophysiology of KIFs (top panel). Synthesis of type-I and type-II keratin polypeptides and their assembly into KIFs are depicted on the left side of the figure. The keratin mRNAs are translated on the ribosomes of epithelial cells, which synthesize these keratins (I). In the cytoplasm, a type-I and a type-II keratin polypeptide align in parallel and register (II) and oligomerize to obligate heterodimers (III). Pairs of heterodimers align in an antiparallel, mostly overlapping fashion to tetramers (IV), which subsequently polymerize to elongated chains packed into KIFs (V). The presence of a mutation in a keratin gene can lead to different pathological processes depicted on the right side of the figure. For example, mutations that introduce a PTC or affect mRNA splicing result in the synthesis of truncated polypeptides. Subsequent nonsense-mediated mRNA decay or enhanced degradation of the truncated polypeptide results in absence of the mutant protein and lack of formation of corresponding heterodimers and KIF, usually associated with severe disease (the simplex form of EBS-DM) (I). Alternatively, the truncated or altered keratin polypeptides can prevent the heterodimer formation and KIFs assembly (II). In autosomal-dominant keratin disorders, most mutations result in nonconservative amino acid replacements at sites of high sequence conservation (helix boundaries) (III). The mutant keratin polypeptides interfere in a dominant negative manner with head-to-tail interactions and proper alignment of heterodimers (IV) as well as elongation and lateral packing during KIF assembly (V), thus producing a severe phenotype. Mutations with a less severe phenotype reside outside the helix boundaries and may have a more subtle effect on KIF assembly or affect keratin phosphorylation or interaction with other proteins. Schematic diagram of a keratin protein depicting the structural domains and common mutation sites in EBS (bottom panel). The nonhelical head domain consists of E1, V1, and H1 (only in type-II keratins). The α-helical rod domain is composed of four segments, 1A, 1B, 2A, and 2B (with stutter-S), which are interrupted by nonhelical linker domains L1, L12, and L2. H2 (only in type-II keratins), V2, and E2 form the nonhelical tail domain. The highly conserved helix initiation and termination motifs (the regions containing the mutational hot spots) are striped. Common sites of dominant mutations and their EBS phenotypes are depicted above the diagram; the location of recessive mutations is shown below. The relative height of the bars reflects the relative frequency of mutations. White symbols: EBS with MP; Dashed symbols: EBS Weber-Cockayne; Black symbols: EBS-DM; Dotted symbols: Köbner subtype of EBS. The nature of mutations is indicated by the symbols: bars represent missense mutations, triangles represent nonsense and frameshift mutations leading to PTC, and stars represent splice site mutations.

of EBS, pathogenic mutations lie in most cases outside of the helix boundaries, elsewhere in the rod domain of K5 or K14, including the nonhelical L12 linker motif or in the amino-terminal homologous domain of K5. Dominant point mutations usually result in amino acid substitutions, but a small in-frame deletion in *KRT14* has also been described.

EBS WITH MOTTLED PIGMENTATION The simplex form of EB with mottled pigmentation (EBS-MP) is a rare form of EBS with generalized or acral blistering and small hyper- and hypopigmented spots that form a reticulate pattern. This variant is also associated with thickened, dystrophic nails and punctate palmoplantar keratoderma. The MP seems unrelated to skin blistering and corresponds with an increased number of melanosomes within basal keratinocytes, dermal macrophages and Schwann cells, as observed by electron microscopy. EBS-MP is caused by a heterozygous missense mutation in exon 1 of *KRT5* that results in substitution of proline 25 with leucine in the nonhelical head domain of K5. This mutation was consistently detected in each of seven unrelated families with EBS-MP tested to date. Preliminary investigations of this mutation revealed that the keratin 5 head domain might directly bind to a cytoplasmic dynein cargo complex transporting melanosomes, thus unraveling the basis for abnormal pigment distribution in this rare disorder.

JUNCTIONAL FORMS OF EB

JEB display a remarkable degree of genetic heterogeneity, with seven different genes implicated in its pathogenesis thus far. In JEB, tissue cleavage occurs within the dermal–epidermal basement membrane at the level of the lamina lucida or the overlying HDs, and ultrastructural abnormalities are evident in the HD–AF complexes.

THE HEMIDESMOSOME-ANCHORING FILAMENT COMPLEX The HDs extend from the intracellular compartment of the basal keratinocytes to the lamina lucida in the upper portion of the dermal–epidermal basement membrane. Within the lamina lucida, the HDs attach to AFs, thread-like structures that tend to concentrate below the HDs. Early biochemical studies identified five major components of the HDs, consisting of polypeptides with molecular masses of 500, 230, 200, 180, and 120 kDa; these were originally designated as HD1–HD5, respectively. HD2 and HD4 have since been shown to be identical to BPAG1 and BPAG2/COL17A1, respectively. HD3 and HD5 correspond to the β_4 and α_6-integrins, respectively, and HD1 corresponds to plectin. Plectin is localized to the cytoplasmic side of the HDs, in a distribution slightly above, yet almost indistinguishable from BPAG1, at the level of the cytoplasmic periphery of the HD inner plaque. The intracellular hemidesmosomal plaque is comprised of BPAG1, a noncollagenous protein of the plakin family, which serves as an autoantigen in an acquired autoimmune disease, bullous pemphigoid. BPAG2, a transmembrane collagen also known as COL17A1, together with $\alpha_6\beta_4$-integrin, extends from the intracellular compartment into the extracellular space, thus stabilizing the association of basal keratinocytes to the underlying basement membrane. Consequently, mutations resulting in abnormalities in any one of the protein components of the HD–AF network can give rise to the different forms of JEB.

MOLECULAR HETEROGENEITY OF JUNCTIONAL EB JEB display a considerable range of phenotypic heterogeneity, and on the basis of clinical severity, the disease has been traditionally divided into the classic, Herlitz (lethal) type, and a variety of non-Herlitz (nonlethal) forms. Within the nonlethal forms, several subtypes have been described based on the associated extracutaneous manifestations and the extent and severity of the blistering tendency. Three of these subtypes traditionally classified as non-Herlitz JEB have since been considered as the HD variants of EB (*see* below). The clinical heterogeneity of JEB reflects the repertoire of underlying genetic lesions demonstrated in as many as seven different genes. Mutations in different forms of JEB (including the hemidesmosomal variants) have been identified in the known genes encoding the macromolecular components of the HD–AF complex, with the exception of BPAG1. Careful examination of the mutation database in these genes reveals genotype–phenotype correlations that reflect the expression of the mutated genes, the types and combinations of the mutations, and the consequences at the mRNA and protein levels.

HERLITZ JEB: PREMATURE TERMINATION CODON MUTATIONS IN THE LAMININ-5 GENES Historically, electron microscopic studies on the skin of JEB patients first revealed ultrastructural abnormalities in the HD–AF complexes, and specifically, the HDs were found to be rudimentary and poorly formed. In the most severe, clinically devastating Herlitz type of JEB, immunofluorescence staining for laminin-5 epitopes suggested the complete absence of this protein. Subsequent to the cloning of genes encoding the three constitutive polypeptides of laminin 5, mutation detection strategies have revealed genetic mutations in each of the three genes, *LAMA3*, *LAMB3*, and *LAMC2*, encoding the α_3, β_3, and γ_2 chains, respectively. Most of these mutations are located in the LAMB3 gene, owing to the presence of two mutational hotspots (R635X and R42X) leading to recurrent mutations. It is noteworthy that in the Herlitz form of JEB, all mutations disclosed result in premature termination codons (PTC) in one of the laminin-5 chains, leading to markedly reduced levels of the corresponding mRNA transcript via nonsense-mediated mRNA decay, and the virtual absence of the corresponding protein.

NON-HERLITZ JEB: COMPOUND HETEROZYGOUS MUTATIONS IN THE LAMININ-5 GENES Laminin-5 gene mutations have been also discovered in the some of the nonlethal forms of JEB, however, the type and combinations of mutations specify a milder clinical phenotype. In some cases, only one of the mutations is a PTC in one of the laminin-5 genes. However, the other genetic lesion may consist of a missense mutation or an in-frame exon-skipping mutation, each of which would encode for some laminin-5 protein, albeit with impaired function. These observations suggest that polypeptides with an intact carboxy-terminal end are able to assemble into trimer molecules, which serve a partial function in the AFs. This interpretation is consistent with the observation that immunofluorescence microscopy performed with an antilaminin-5 antibody, such as GB3, is positive, although frequently attenuated, in the skin of nonlethal JEB patients.

LAMA3 mutations have been disclosed in laryngo-onychocutaneous syndrome or Shabbir syndrome, a recessively inherited disorder with some features of skin fragility. The disorder is typified by skin erosions, nail dystrophy and exuberant granulation tissue in specific epithelia, particularly the conjunctiva and larynx. Linkage mapping localized the gene to chromosome 18q11.2 in a region including the laminin-α_3 gene (*LAMA3*). Further analysis revealed that the *LAMA3* gene encodes three distinct proteins generated by alternative promoter utilization and internal splicing, which are designated laminin-α_{3a}, -α_{3b1}, and -α_{3b2}. The identical causative mutation in 15 LOC families is a frameshift mutation that is specific only to the laminin-α_{3a}-isoform. Thus, in LOC, only one LAMA3 isoform is affected, whereas in Herlitz JEB, the mutations reside in a commonly utilized region among the three isoforms, leading to complete absence of all LAMA3 chains. These studies provide insight into the specific role of the N-terminal domain of laminin-α_{3a} in the granulation tissue response noted in Herlitz-JEB.

HEMIDESMOSOMAL VARIANTS OF JEB Whereas the molecular basis of many of the classic forms of Herlitz and non-Herlitz JEB are well defined on the basis of laminin-5 mutations, there is a group of patients in whom blisters form in and around the HD, and have therefore been called the "hemidesmosomal variants." Ultrastructural classification initially identified at least three groups of patients with EB whose blisters form at the level of the HD, and whose clinical phenotype is unlike any of the "classic" forms of EB. These three subtypes include GABEB, EB-PA, and EB-MD. Mutations have been identified in four HD-associated structural genes in patients with these rare forms of EB.

MUTATIONS IN BPAG2 IN GABEB Underscoring the genetic heterogeneity of the JEB is the demonstration of specific mutations in genes encoding structural components of the HDs. Specifically, mutations have been identified in the *COL17A1* gene in a subset of patients originally classified as a nonlethal JEB variant, known as GABEB. Clinically, these patients demonstrate a moderate blistering tendency associated with a characteristic constellation of extracutaneous involvement, including dystrophy of the fingernails, focal scarring alopecia of the scalp, loss of eyelashes, dental anomalies, and patchy macular hyperpigmentation. The mutation in the original GABEB family, described in a geographically limited area in Austria, is a PTC transmitted through many branches of the large inbred family. Subsequently, many different types of mutations in *COL17A1* have been observed in GABEB, including missense, nonsense, splice-site and insertions/ deletions, resulting in PTCs. Although there is slight variation in phenotypic severity, GABEB is uniformly nonlethal, and there does not appear to be a strict genotype–phenotype correlation with respect to *COL17A1* mutations, as compared with the laminin-5 genes. A dominantly inherited glycine substitution mutation in *COL17A1* was identified in a GABEB family, in which the proband had inherited a PTC on the second allele. Interestingly, all heterozygous carriers of the glycine substitution alone had markedly abnormal dentition and enamel pitting. Clearly, the glycine substitution mutation in COL17A1 also affects the basement membrane of the developing tooth, a previously undisclosed function for this transmembrane collagen.

IDENTIFICATION OF $\alpha_6\beta_4$-INTEGRIN MUTATIONS IN EB-PA EB-PA another rare subtype of EB, characterized by blistering of the skin and congenital PA, EB-PA, was previously classified as a nonlethal form of JEB, although the phenotypes can range from moderate to early postnatal demise. Mutations in the genes encoding the two polypeptides of the $\alpha_6\beta_4$-integrin receptor (*ITGA6* and *ITGB4*) have been identified in EB-PA. A survey of the reported mutations indicates that PTCs are associated predominantly with the lethal EB-PA variants, whereas missense mutations are more prevalent in nonlethal forms. However, the consequences of the missense mutations are position dependent, and substitutions of highly conserved amino acids within the individual integrin receptors may have lethal consequences. The phenotypic manifestation of PA from mutations in the *ITGB4* and *ITGA6* genes suggest a tissue-specific role for this integrin both in the skin and the gastrointestinal tract.

PLECTIN MUTATIONS IN EB-MD To determine which of the candidate proteins of the HD (BPAG1 or plectin) is responsible for making the connection between the HD and the keratinocyte

intermediate-filament network, a knockout mouse was created targeting *BPAG1*. Whereas the HDs in these mice were largely normal, they lacked the inner plate and demonstrated a complete severance of the connection between the HD with the intermediate-filament network. The zone of mechanical fragility of the basal keratinocytes was restricted to the region of the HD, distinct from the ultrastructural findings in classic EB simplex, yet strikingly similar to the cleavage plane reported in "pseudojunctional" (now called HD variants) EB. Unexpectedly, the *BPAG1* knockout mice also developed late-onset muscular dystonia and neurodegeneration, and were found to be allelic to a naturally occurring mouse, dystonia musculorum. This constellation of phenotypic features together with the ultrastructural findings was highly reminiscent of the pathogenesis of EB-MD. On the basis of the striking similarities in the clinical phenotype of EB-MD and the *BPAG1* knockout mouse, it appeared likely that one of the two components of the hemidesmosomal inner plaque, BPAG1 or HD-1, would be involved in the pathogenesis of this disorder. Subsequently, BPAG1 was excluded as the cause of EB-MD, and it remains the only known hemidesmosomal component without an associated human genetic disease.

HD-1 was first described as an approx 500-kDa component of the HD, and was subsequently shown to be identical with plectin, an exceptionally large intermediate filament interacting protein, that was cloned independently. Plectin is a plakin family member with similarities to both desmoplakin and BPAG1, is highly conserved between rat and human, and has a wide tissue distribution, including the central nervous system and muscle. Plectin has a remarkable number of versatile binding affinities for other proteins, including vimentin, glial fibrillary acidic protein, the neurofilament protein triplet, keratin 5 and 14, and lamin B, suggesting that it can tether one filamentous network to another. Although plectin is expressed in nearly all cell types, its precise cytoplasmic localization is cell-type specific, and it can appear diffuse throughout the cell as a cytomatrix component, or in a restricted distribution as a focal adhesion protein.

Initial examination of biochemical and synthetic properties of cultured keratinocytes from patients with EB-MD using antibodies against plectin showed that this protein was completely absent in the cells of several patients with EB-MD. Typical presentation of EB-MD is neonatal blistering and late-onset muscular dystrophy with nail and tooth abnormalities. Severe mucocutaneous involvement, including laryngeal webs and urethral strictures, has also been reported. Although EB-MD is rare, most of the mutations reported result in PTCs on both alleles of plectin, either by nonsense, insertion/deletion or splicing mutations, and the phenotype in these patients is remarkably consistent manifesting with neonatal blistering and progressive muscle weakness from the first or second decade of life and thereafter. In some patients, small inframe deletions or insertions have been disclosed with significantly milder phenotype and the onset of the muscle weakness on the third or fourth decade of life. Thus, continued identification of plectin mutations in patients with EB-MD will provide further insights into the phenotype–genotype correlations in this disorder as well as the relationship between the skin, the musculoskeletal and the nervous systems.

EB OGNA VARIANT: CAUSED BY A PLECTIN MISSENSE MUTATION Although several mutations in the plectin gene have been identified in recessively inherited EB-MD, a different type of mutation in plectin leads to a rare, dominant form of EB, known as the Ogna variant. The EB Ogna phenotype is owing to a specific missense mutation (R2110W) within the rod domain of plectin. EB Ogna is not restricted to single Norwegian kindred as previously believed, because a German family with this phenotype was found to carry the identical mutation. Clinically, the EB Ogna patients demonstrate hemorrhagic blistering of the skin, but unlike patients with EB-MD, there is no muscle phenotype, and muscle biopsies from several EB Ogna patients revealed normal staining patterns with antibodies against plectin. Clearly, the genotype–phenotype relationships among plectin mutations in the different forms of EB are unusually complex and still emerging.

CONCLUSION JEB, including the HD variants, reflect mutations in at least seven different genes, and the specific clinical constellations result from the combination of different types of mutations within the mutated genes (*see* Table 105-1). Whereas the mechanistic consequences of these mutations have been explored at the mRNA and protein levels in many studies, the functional role of these components in HD assembly is also becoming increasingly clear through biochemical studies of protein–protein interactions. For example, an interaction between BPAG2 and α_6-integrin has been described, the disruption of HD assembly by a tailless β_4-integrin subunit was reported, and roles for the integrin receptors in mediating signal transduction continue to emerge. Whereas these components clearly represent functionally interdependent structural macromolecules in the dermal–epidermal adhesion zone, studies suggest a functionally dynamic and interactive role of some of these proteins in cell–matrix communication. Finally, it is noteworthy that despite an extensive survey of the seven genes involved in JEB, several families have proven negative for mutations, suggesting additional undisclosed candidate genes and uncharacterized protein components for this increasingly heterogeneous group of disorders.

DEB: COL7A1 MUTATIONS RESULT IN A SPECTRUM OF CLINICAL SEVERITY

DEB, which can be inherited in either an autosomal-dominant or autosomal-recessive pattern, demonstrate extensive variability in the clinical spectrum of severity. The less severe forms, such as dominantly inherited dystrophic EB (DDEB) or the mitis type of recessively inherited dystrophic forms of EB (M-RDEB), are characterized by a significant blistering tendency, but they lack the extensive mutilating scarring that is the hallmark of the severe, generalized, Hallopeau-Siemens type of recessive dystrophic EB (HS-RDEB). In addition to cutaneous manifestations, the dystrophic forms, particularly HS-RDEB, are associated with scarring of the esophagus and corneal erosions. Furthermore, the patients with HS-RDEB develop unusually aggressive, rapidly metastasizing squamous cell carcinomas primarily in the hands and feet. Thus, the combination of cutaneous and extracutaneous manifestations is associated with considerable morbidity and mortality in the most severely affected patients with DEB.

MOLECULAR GENETICS OF DYSTROPHIC EB Several lines of evidence initially suggested that type-VII collagen is the candidate gene/protein system harboring mutations in DEB. First, the ultrastructural diagnostic hallmark of DEB is an abnormality in anchoring fibrils, attachment structures that are made up of predominantly, if not exclusively, of type-VII collagen. In different variants of DEB, the anchoring fibrils can be shown by transmission electron microscopy to be morphologically abnormal, reduced in number, or even completely absent. Second, these ultrastructural observations are reflected by changes in the immunofluorescence pattern when antitype-VII antibodies are used for staining of the skin. In normal individuals, type-VII collagen epitopes are readily

evident in a linear pattern at the dermal–epidermal junction, whereas the immunostaining is entirely negative in generalized HS-RDEB patients. In DDEB, the immunostaining reveals a near-normal pattern and intensity, whereas in M-RDEB, the staining can be attenuated, although clearly positive. These ultrastructural and immunofluorescent findings suggested that type-VII collagen was a candidate gene for mutations in the DEB. This suggestion was subsequently strengthened by demonstration of genetic linkage between the *COL7A1* locus on chromosome 3p21 and both dominantly and recessively inherited forms of DEB.

Subsequent cloning of the human type-VII collagen cDNA sequences allowed determination of the normal structure of type-VII collagen polypeptides. Elucidation of the intron–exon organization of the entire human type-VII collagen gene has revealed that the gene is highly complex, consisting of a total of 118 exons. However, *COL7A1* is relatively compact, and the exons are contained within approx 32 kb of human genomic DNA. The elucidation of the intron–exon organization of COL7A1 has provided necessary information to undertake mutation analysis of this gene in families with DEB. In fact, specific mutations have now been disclosed in >300 kindreds with different forms of DEB.

The wealth of information on specific mutations has allowed establishment of genotype–phenotype relationships in different forms of DEB. In normal skin, type-VII collagen molecules form antiparallel dimers that associate through their overlapping carboxy-terminal ends (Fig. 105-4). This association is stabilized by interchain disulfide bonds, and such stable type-VII collagen dimer molecules laterally aggregate to form anchoring fibrils. Thus, following the synthesis of type-VII collagen, several critical steps are required for proper assembly of anchoring fibrils. Consequently, mutations affecting the synthesis of type-VII collagen at the transcriptional or translational level, or those interfering with its supramolecular assembly to anchoring fibrils can result in DEB phenotype (*see* Fig. 105-4).

GENOTYPE/PHENOTYPE CORRELATIONS IN DEB

Severe, Mutilating HS-RDEB: PTC Mutations In COL7a1 In most HS-RDEB patients, the consistent genetic lesion is a PTC in both alleles of the affected individual. The major effect of a PTC mutation is reduction in mRNA abundance as a result of nonsense-mediated mRNA decay. This phenomenon is coupled to the splicing process itself, because the levels of unspliced, heteronuclear RNA are equivalent for both the mutant and wild-type alleles, and the decay is evident only on comparison of processed mRNA. The PTCs result in perturbations in synthesis of type-VII collagen mRNAs at the transcriptional level, which are then unable to provide templates for translation of functional polypeptides. Even if the mutant allele containing a PTC is expressed at reduced levels, the translated protein is truncated at its carboxy terminus and is unable to assemble into anchoring fibrils. These interpretations are consistent with the ultrastructural demonstration of complete absence of the anchoring fibrils in HS-RDEB, and negative immunofluorescence for type-VII collagen, thus explaining the extreme fragility of the skin, so characteristic of this phenotype (*see* Fig. 105-4).

Mitis RDEB: Missense and In-Frame Deletion Mutations In the mitis forms of RDEB, at least one, and in some cases both, alleles encode for a full length type-VII collagen polypeptide. However, this allele usually contains a missense mutation that can change the conformation of the protein such that the anchoring fibril assembly is perturbed. In some cases, one allele contains a missense mutation or in-frame deletion, whereas the second allele

Physiology　　　　　　　　　　　　　　　　**Pathology**

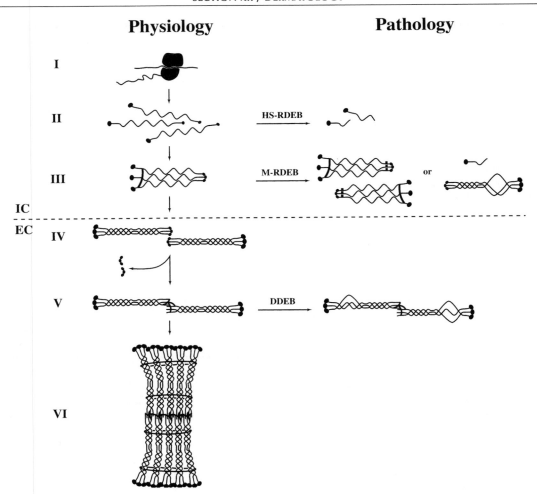

Figure 105-4　The physiology and pathology of type-VII collagen. Synthesis of pro-α_1(VII)-collagen polypeptides and their assembly into anchoring fibrils is depicted on the left side of the figure. The mRNA, approx 9 kb in size, is translated on the ribosomes of cells, such as basal keratinocytes, synthesizing type-VII collagen (I). Within the extracellular space (EC), two of these triple-helical type-VII collagen molecules align into an antiparallel tail-to-tail orientation with overlapping carboxy termini (IV). The molecules are processed by proteolytic removal of the NC-2 domains (•), and the association of the dimer is stabilized by disulfide bonding (V). Subsequently, a large number of the dimer molecules laterally assemble into anchoring fibrils that contain at both ends intact amino-terminal NC-1 domains with adhesive properties (VI). In the presence of genetic lesions in COL7A1, type-VII collagen pathology can manifest as different variants of DEB. For example, PTC mutations result in synthesis of truncated polypeptides unable to form anchoring fibrils, causing severe Hallopeau-Siemens type of recessive dystrophic EB (HS-RDEB). In a milder autosomal-recessive form, known as the mitis variant (M-RDEB), missense mutations of either the homozygous or compound heterozygous state, or in combination with a PTC *in trans* prevent the assembly of type-VII collagen dimers. In cases of dominant dystrophic EB (DDEB), glycine substitution mutations affecting the collagenous domain of type-VII collagen interfere with packing of the anchoring fibrils (Modified with permission of the McGraw-Hill companies, from Uitto J, Pulkkinen L. Epidermolysis bullosa: The Disease of the cutaneous basement membrane zone. In: Scriver CR, Beaudet A, Valle D, et al., eds. The Metabolic and Molecular Bases of Inherited Disease, 8th ed. New York: McGraw Hill, 2001; pp. 5655–5674.)

contains a PTC. The net result of the latter combination of mutations is a reduction in mutant RNA from the PTC allele at the transcriptional level, together with a mutation on the second allele, which is transcribed and presumably translated at normal rate, yet is likely to affect nucleation and assembly of anchoring fibrils (*see* Fig. 105-4). As a result of these more subtle mutations, combined with a PTC on the other allele, mutant full length type-VII collagen molecules may be able to assemble into anchoring fibrils, which are, however, unlikely to be stabilized by disulfide bonding (*see* Fig. 105-4). Thus, these attachment structures, although present, are weakened, resulting in moderately severe fragility of the skin, as observed in M-RDEB.

Dominant Dystrophic EB: Glycine Substitution Mutations In One Allele　In dominantly inherited forms of EB, the recurrent theme of mutations is missense substitutions of glycine residues that

occur within the collagenous domain of the type-VII collagen molecule, a region characterized by the repeating Gly-X–Y amino acid sequence. These mutated molecules are able to associate with polypeptides synthesized from the normal allele and interfere with their assembly through a mechanism known as dominant-negative interference (*see* Fig. 105-4). The glycine substitutions, therefore, destabilize the collagen triple helix, interfere with the secretion of the molecules, and render them susceptible to intracellular degradation, thus exerting their effect at the posttranslational level. Because type-VII collagen is a homotrimer consisting of three identical α_1(VII)-polypeptides, only one out of eight triple-helical molecules (12.5%) is entirely normal, assuming equal expression of the mutant and wild-type alleles. As a result, some normal type-VII collagen homotrimers can be assembled, consistent with ultrastructural demonstration of thin anchoring fibrils, positive immunofluorescence for type-VII collagen, and the relatively mild clinical phenotype in DDEB. In addition to the classic forms of DDEB, glycine substitution mutations have been demonstrated in two clinical variants known as pretibial DEB and the Bart syndrome, proving that these subtypes are allelic to DDEB with mutations in COL7A1.

Collectively, the type and combination of mutations are able to predict, in general terms, the clinical severity and natural history of DEB. Because clinical severity represents a continuum in the spectrum of manifestations, the precise nature of the genetic lesions, their positions along the type-VII collagen gene, and the dynamic interplay of the two mutant alleles on the individual's genetic background, coupled with environmental influences, will determine the precise phenotype of the patient in DEB.

REVISIONS IN GENETIC COUNSELING IN DYSTROPHIC EB
As indicated, DEB can be inherited in an autosomal-dominant or autosomal-recessive fashion. The diagnosis of classic HS-RDEB in a patient with severe, mutilating scarring, with clinically unaffected parents, is usually made without difficulty. Similarly, inheritance of a blistering tendency and a relatively mild scarring phenotype, with multiple affected family members in several generations, allows unequivocal diagnosis of dominantly inherited DEB.

The difficulties arise during the diagnosis and ascertainment of the inheritance pattern in patients with a relatively mild phenotype and clinically normal parents. By ultrastructural analyses, these patients often demonstrate the presence, but a reduced number, of anchoring fibrils, and immunofluorescence shows positive staining for type-VII collagen. Consequently, these cases are often diagnosed as dominant DEB, and were presumed to be caused by a new dominant mutation or reflecting parental germline mosaicism. This diagnosis has implications in terms of genetic counseling of the affected individuals. If their disease is truly a new dominant mutation, the risk of their offspring being affected is one in two (50%). In contrast, in cases of a recessively inherited M-RDEB, which can be clinically indistinguishable from de novo DDEB, the risk of their offspring being affected is low, approximately the same as in the general population, with the exception of consanguineous matings.

Unexpectedly, determination of the genotype and mutation analysis of several patients with relatively mild disease and ultrastructurally detectable anchoring fibrils with positive immunofluorescence staining for type-VII collagen has demonstrated that many of them are compound heterozygotes or have homozygous missense mutations inherited in a recessive manner and therefore the diagnosis is M-RDEB. For example, the first demonstration of type-VII collagen mutations in M-RDEB revealed the presence of a homozygous missense mutation, a methionine-to-lysine substitution (M2798K) at the carboxy terminal end of the molecule. Similarly, in other cases, a missense mutation in one allele, including a glycine substitution in the collagenous domain, together with a PTC mutation on the other allele, can result in M-RDEB. Finally, in a survey of a cohort of more than 400 families, in which distinct COL7A1 mutations were identified, only a limited number of cases appeared to be de novo dominant mutations, at least one of them being derived from the maternal germline.

Based on these considerations, for genetic counseling purposes, it is appropriate to consider each "new" case as a recessively inherited condition, unless proven to be dominant by mutation analysis. Reclassification of DEB on the basis of the underlying mutations clearly affects the likelihood of the affected individual having an affected offspring.

APPLICATIONS OF MUTATION ANALYSIS IN PRENATAL DIAGNOSIS

Precise understanding of the underlying mutations in different forms of DEB has several translational implications in terms of genetic counseling, DNA-based prenatal diagnosis, and gene therapy. Most immediately relevant to patient care is the development of DNA-based prenatal diagnosis, which can be performed as early as the 10th gestational week through chorionic villus sampling, or through amniocentesis from the 15th wk and beyond. In the severe DEB, such analyses can be performed either by direct mutation analyses or by genetic-linkage approaches, taking advantage of the fact that no evidence for locus heterogeneity has been observed in DEB. In contrast, in the case of JEB or EBS, in which significant locus heterogeneity exists, prenatal testing must be based on identification of specific mutations. These approaches have already been applied with outstanding success to DNA-based prenatal diagnosis in more than 200 families at risk for recurrence of the severe forms of EB, mostly HS-RDEB and hemidesmosomal junctional EB. Efforts are in progress to establish noninvasive prenatal testing by detection of mutations in fetal DNA present in the maternal circulation during the early stages of gestation. The genetic information also provides the basis for development of preimplantation genetic diagnosis through blastomere analysis, a technological advance that would obviate the necessity of termination of the pregnancy in case of an affected fetus, if elected.

GENE THERAPY APPROACHES

Precise understanding of the underlying mutations and subsequent demonstration of the functional consequences of such mutations at the mRNA and protein levels are obligatory prerequisites for the development of gene therapy approaches for this group of devastating skin diseases. It is conceivable that several forms of EB are realistic targets for genetic therapies of different forms of EB. Significant progress has been made to transduce keratinocytes cultured from patients with different forms of EB with transgene constructs using either viral vectors or nonviral approaches. However, because of the concern for mutagenesis resulting from integration of the viral vectors into the genome, exploration of alternative technologies has begun, including direct introduction of genetic material into the skin cells by biolistic particle bombardment ("gene gun"), use of ribozyme-mediated repair of mutant mRNAs by trans-splicing, and application of single-stranded oligonucleotides for targeted gene correction. Thus, establishing the genetic basis of different forms of EB has provided the necessary foundation for development of rationally designed gene therapy approaches to counteract these devastating skin diseases in the future.

ACKNOWLEDGMENTS

Carol Kelly assisted in preparation of this manuscript. The original work by the authors was supported by the National Institutes of Health grant P01AR38923 and by The Dystrophic Epidermolysis Bullosa Research Association.

SELECTED REFERENCES

Ashton GH, Sorelli P, Mellerio JE, Keane FM, Eady RA, McGrath JA. Alpha 6 beta 4 integrin abnormalities in junctional epidermolysis bullosa with pyloric atresia. Br J Dermatol 2001;144:408–414.

Baldeschi C, Gache Y, Rattenhall A, et al. Genetic correction of canine dystrophic epidermolysis bullosa mediated by retroviral vectors. Hum Mol Genet 2003;12:1897–1905.

Coulombe PA, Omary MB. 'Hard' and 'soft' principles defining the structure, function and regulation of keratin intermediate filaments. Curr Opin Cell Biol 2002;14:110–122.

Fine JD, Eady RA, Bauer EA, et al. Revised classification system for inherited epidermolysis bullosa: report of the Second International Consensus Meeting on diagnosis and classification of epidermolysis bullosa. J Am Acad Dermatol 2000;42:1051–1066.

Guo L, Degenstein L, Dowling J, et al. Gene targeting of BPAG1: abnormalities in mechanical strength and cell migration in stratified epithelia and neurologic degeneration. Cell 1995;81:233–243.

Irvine AD, McLean WH. Human keratin diseases: the increasing spectrum of disease and subtlety of the phenotype–genotype correlation. Br J Dermatol 1999;140:815–828.

Koss-Harnes D, Hoyheim B, Anton-Lamprecht I, et al. A site-specific plectin mutation causes dominant epidermolysis bullosa simplex Ogna: two identical *de novo* mutations. J Invest Dermatol 2002;118:87–93.

Lane EB. Keratin diseases. Curr Opin Genet Dev 1994;4:412–418.

Lin MTS, Pulkkinen L, Uitto J. Cutaneous gene therapy: principles and prospects. Clin Dermatol 2000;18:177–188.

McLean WH, Irvine AD, Hamill KJ, et al. An unusual N-terminal deletion of the laminin α3a isoform leads to the chronic granulation tissue disorder laryngo-onycho-cutaneous syndrome. Hum Mol Genet 2003; 12:2395–2409.

Nakano A, Pulkkinen L, Murrell D, et al. Epidermolysis bullosa with congenital pyloric atresia: Novel mutations in the beta 4 integrin gene (ITGB4) and genotype/phenotype correlations. Pediatr Res 2001;49: 618–626.

Ortiz-Urda S, Lin Q, Yant SR, Keene D, Kay MA, Khavari PA. Sustainable correction of junctional epidermolysis bullosa via transposon-mediated nonviral gene transfer. Gene Ther 2003;1099–1104.

Pfendner E, Nakano A, Pulkkinen L, Christiano AM, Uitto J. Prenatal diagnosis for epidermolysis bullosa: a study of 144 consecutive pregnancies at risk. Prenat Diagn 2003,23:447–456.

Pfendner EG, Sadowski SG, Uitto J. Epidermolysis bullosa simplex: recurrent and *de novo* mutations in the KRT5 and KRT14 genes, phenotype/genotype correlations, and implications for genetic counseling and prenatal diagnosis. J Invest Dermatol 2005;125:239–243.

Pulkkinen L, Ringpfeil F, Uitto J. Progress in heritable skin diseases: molecular bases and clinical implications. J Am Acad Dermatol 2002; 47:91–104.

Pulkkinen L, Uitto J. Hemidesmosomal variants of epidermolysis bullosa. Mutations in the α6β4 integrin and the 180-kD bullous pemphigoid antigen/type XVII collagen genes. Exp Dermatol 1998;7: 46–64.

Pulkkinen L, Uitto J. Mutation analysis and molecular genetics of epidermolysis bullosa. Matrix Biol 1999;18:29–42.

Steinert PM, Marekov LN, Fraser RD, Parry DA. Structure, function, and dynamics of keratin intermediate filaments. J Invest Dermatol 1993; 100:729–734.

Uitto J, Christiano AM. Molecular genetics of the cutaneous basement membrane zone. Perspectives on epidermolysis bullosa and other blistering skin diseases. J Clin Invest 1992;90:687–692.

Uitto J, Pulkkinen L. Epidermolysis bullosa: the disease of the cutaneous basement membrane zone. In: Scriver CR, Beaudet A, Valle D, et al., eds. The Metabolic and Molecular Bases of Inherited Disease, 8th ed. New York: McGraw Hill, 2001; pp. 5655–5674.

Uitto J, Pulkkinen L. Molecular genetics of heritable blistering disorders. Arch Dermatol 2001;137:1458–1461.

Uitto J, Pfendner E, Jackson LC. Probing the fetal genome: progress towards non-invasive prenatal diagnosis. Trends Mol Med 2003;9: 339–343.

Uitto J, Pulkkinen L, McLean WHI. Epidermolysis bullosa: a spectrum of clinical phenotypes explained by molecular heterogeneity. Mol Med Today 1997;3:457–465.

Uitto J, Pulkkinen L, Ringpfeil F. Progress in molecular genetics of heritable skin diseases: the paradigms of EB and PXE. J Invest Dermatol Symp Proc 2002;7:6–16.

Uitto J, Pulkkinen L, Smith FJD, McLean WHI. Plectin and human genetic disorders of the skin and muscle. The paradigm of epidermolysis bullosa with muscular dystrophy. Exp Dermatol 1996;5: 237–246.

Varki R, Sadowski S, Pfendner E, Uitto J. Epidermolysis bullosa. I. Molecular genetics of the junctional and hemidesmosomal variants. J Med Genet (in press), 2006.

107 Genetic Epidermal Diseases

AMY STEIN AND LOWELL A. GOLDSMITH

SUMMARY

Profound changes in the epidermis occur associated with abnormal epidermal structural proteins and lipids. Abnormal suprabasal keratins cause blistering and scaling: epidermolytic hyperkeratosis. Other abnormal keratins are associated with marked deformed nails and prenatal teeth: pachyonychia congenita. Deficient transglutaminase an enzyme that cross-links epidermal proteins is associated with generalized scaling: lamellar ichthyosis. Males with deficient steroid sulfatase have associated brown epidermal scales. Defective fatty acid alcohol metabolism in addition to scaling has associated mental retardation and spastic diplegia: Sjogren-Larsson syndrome. Mutations in different calcium pumps are associated with scaling and sun sensitivity (Darier disease) or blistering especially in intertriginous areas (Hailey-Hailey disease). Connexins, when mutated, are associated with scaling of the skin and sometimes associated deafness.

Key Words: Cell envelope; connexins; Darier-White disease; epidermolytic hyperkeratosis; erythrokeratodermia variablis; Hailey-Hailey disease; harlequin ichthyosis; hidrotic ectodermal dysplasia; ichthyosis vulgaris; keratins; lamellar ichthyosis; Netherton's syndrome; pachyonychia congenita; Palmoplantar keratoderma; Sjogren-Larsson syndrome; trichothiodystrophy; X-linked ichthyosis.

INTRODUCTION

A large number of genetic defects, mediated through alterations of different biological molecules, affect the structure and function of the epidermis. Many of these diseases fit into classic clinical categories, which have been called ichthyosis, keratosis palmaris and palmaris for hundreds of years, or ectodermal dysplasias for many decades. The clinical classifications are still useful because they define the "forest" in which biochemistry and genetics identify the "trees."

Ichthyosis, derived from the Greek *ichthys,* fish, is not one disease but a heterogeneous group of skin disorders characterized by abnormal or altered epidermal differentiation (or cornification) resulting in generalized or localized scaly skin. Ichthyosis can present at birth or less frequently later in life. The disease can be limited to the skin or simultaneously involve internal organs, and phenotypically patients are similar despite different genotypes. These disorders have been classified clinically and histologically;

the genetics and underlying pathophysiology allow better understanding and integration of genotype–phenotype relationships and development of novel therapies including targeting the mutated gene or resultant abnormal proteins.

PALMOPLANTAR KERATODERMA Palmoplantar keratoderma (PPK) is a heterogenous group of disorders characterized by hyperkeratosis or thickening of the palms and soles. The genetic mutations underlying many of these disorders have been elucidated. These genes encode structural proteins (including keratins and cornified cell envelope proteins), gap junction components, enzymes and desmosomal proteins.

CLINICAL PRESENTATION Age of onset, location and quality of scale, involvement of other areas of the body, family history, and histological features of the abnormal skin differentiate many of the different disorders of cornification and can focus the genetic testing. Specific diagnosis aids prognosis, treatment, and assessment of family members' risks of developing disease. Because of the frequent clinical heterogeneity and other variable factors that influence disease expression, precise diagnosis in some patients may be difficult.

PRENATAL DIAGNOSIS Molecular analysis of chorionic villus sampling or amniocentesis fluid can be done early in pregnancy when the given gene defect is known and the specific mutation is already identified in the family. Fetoscopy and fetal skin biopsy is rarely needed.

Prenatal diagnosis by mutational analysis has been successfully performed in epidermolytic hyperkeratosis (EHK), lamellar ichthyosis (LI) (transglutaminase 1 [*TGM1*]), Sjögren-Larsson syndrome *(fatty aldehyde dehydrogenase [FALDH])*, ichthyosis bullosa of Siemens (*K2e*), PIBI(D)S *(ERCC2/XPD, ERCC3/XPB)*, autosomal-recessive rhizomelic chondrodysplasia punctata (CDPX2) *(PEX7)*, X-linked CDPX2 (arylsulfatase gene cluster at Xp22) and Netherton's syndrome *(SPINK5)*. Sjögren-Larsson syndrome can be detected by measuring the FALDH enzyme activity in cultured amniocytes. The carrier status can be assessed for relatives with autosomal-recessive (AR) disorders with an identified mutation.

TREATMENT Therapies for the disorders of keratinization are symptomatic with the main goal of hydration, lubrication and desquamation (often incorrectly called keratolysis). Patients can thin some areas of hyperkeratosis with hydration followed by mild abrasives (sponges, buff puffs, or pumice stones). Humidifiers should be used in cold, dry environments. Patients need to avoid hot environments and moisten their skin to cool it to decrease heat stress associated with decreased sweating. Caution is advised with

From: *Principles of Molecular Medicine, Second Edition*
Edited by: M. S. Runge and C. Patterson © Humana Press, Inc., Totowa, NJ

widespread topical applications (i.e., salicylic acid) to prevent systemic toxicity owing to increased absorption secondary to the markedly abnormal barrier function. Nutrition is paramount as increased epidermal proliferation causes increased nutritional requirements. Percutaneous water loss can lead to increased caloric and protein requirements in childhood. A high degree of suspicion and subsequent treatment of secondary fungal infections is important; sometimes, the only sign is pruritus or a localized area of hair loss. Oral retinoids, usually necessary for years, can be particularly helpful in LI, bullous congenital ichthysiform erythroderma and erythrokeratoderma variablis (EKV), but the risks (including fetal abnormalities in pregnant women) vs the benefits need careful evaluation.

DISEASES WITH ABNORMAL STRUCTURAL PROTEINS

Disorders of two classes of structural proteins, the intracellular keratins—a large number of proteins within the intermediate filament suprafamily of proteins—and proteins composing the cell envelope, produce a variety of phenotypes that result in ichthyosis or keratoderma.

KERATINS

EHK/Bullous Congenital Ichthyosiform Erythroderma EHK is a rare disorder, occurring in 1/200,000– 300,000 births, with equal gender predilection. It is autosomal-dominant (AD) with up to 50% spontaneous mutations. There are reports of patients with EHK born to parents with linear epidermal nevi (hamartomas of the epidermis) along the lines of Blaschko, showing EHK on pathology and abnormal *K10* or *K1* expression. These epidermal nevi may represent somatic mosaicism for the gene for bullous congenital ichthysiform erythroderma.

At birth, EHK presents with generalized erythematous blisters, erythroderma, erosions, peeling, and some hyperkeratotic areas. These patients have an increased risk of cutaneous infections and sepsis. Over time, blister formation decreases but ichthyosis increases and becomes warty. These grayish brown verrucous scales often mainly involve the flexures and intertriginous areas. The hyperkeratotic areas have a corrugated pattern. Erythroderma lessens but remains throughout life. Patients often have a pungent odor resulting from colonization by *Staphylococcus* and fungi. EHK has striking clinical heterogeneity.

Although teeth, nails, and hair are usually normal, secondary alopecia may occur because of infection/hyperkeratosis, and heat intolerance is common. Palmoplantar hyperkeratosis is present in up to 60% of patients.

Mutations in K1 and K10, proteins that confer structural stability to keratin intermediate filaments in suprabasal keratinocytes, lead to keratinocyte fragility (particularly of the upper epidermis). There is increased epidermal proliferation. Many of the mutations are within residues of the highly conserved helical rod portions of the molecule responsible for intermolecular associations of the keratins.

Prenatal diagnosis is possible by direct DNA analysis of chorionic villus sampling or amniocentesis. Hyperkeratosis with lysis and tonofilament clumping in the granular layer is characteristic but not pathognomonic.

For newborns, monitoring of water/electrolyte balance and infection prevention is the primary approach.

Oral retinoids can be effective in decreasing the hyperkeratosis and rate of infection but caution is advised owing to the increased possibility of blistering. A mixture of 60% propylene glycol and water under plastic occlusion for 4–12 h several times weekly can be helpful. LacHydrin, 10% urea cream, 10% lactic acid in eucerin, glycolic acid lotions, topical Retin-A cream are also used. Soaks and gentle debridement of scale can aid patient comfort. Intermittent antibiotics (topical and oral) may be needed as bacterial infections are common and can lead to increased blistering.

Vorner's Syndrome (Diffuse Epidermolytic PPK) Vorner's Syndrome, also called diffuse epidermolytic PPK, has an AD inheritance. Disease presents at birth or during the first few months of life with well-demarcated, symmetric, yellowish thickening of the palms and soles with erythematous bases, and margins. Elbows and knees can be mildly involved. The skin is often described as having a "dirty" snake skin appearance. Occasional blistering on the hands and feet occurs. There are no associated internal manifestations.

Mutations in K9, a keratin specific to palmoplantar epidermis, have been identified. In addition, a K1 mutation has been reported in families with milder disease.

Biopsy of a weight bearing region on the thenar or hypothenar eminence reveals hyperkeratosis, acanthosis, papillomatosis, and epidermolysis in the spinous and granular cell layer.

Oral retinoids can be useful but can also lead to erosions. Topical therapies are often adequate.

Diffuse Nonepidermolytic PPK (Unna-Thost Disease) Diffuse nonepidermolytic PPK, also called Unna-Thost disease, is the most common inherited PPK. Its inheritance is AD with high penetrance and expressivity.

Patients present at birth or in infancy with well-demarcated, symmetric, often "waxy" appearing yellow thickening of the entire palms and soles with a sharp cut off at the wrist. Often there is a scleroderma-like constriction and tapering because of the skin thickening distal to the proximal interphalangeal joint. The dorsal hand is often affected. The fingernails have been likened to "parrot beaking" and display widening of the onychocorneal band. Marked hyperhidrosis is typical and secondary dermatophyte infection is frequent (reported in approximately one-third of patients). Hair and teeth are normal.

Mutations have been identified in an area on chromosome 12 containing a type-II keratin gene cluster. In addition, a mutation was detected in one family in the V1 region of K1, an area speculated to be involved in keratin–loricrin interaction.

Oral retinoids have favorable responses in some patients. Long-term systemic antifungals (i.e., itraconazole 100 mg daily) are useful when secondary dermatophyte infections occur. Topical salicylates are helpful.

Ichthyosis Bullosa of Siemens In ichthyosis bullosa of Siemens, inheritance is AD with variable expression between families. Similar to EHK, patients are usually normal at birth and in infancy, blistering occurs after minor trauma, usually localized to hands, feet and extensor arms, and legs. Blisters are usually small. Over time, patients develop dark brown hyperkeratosis primarily over the knees, elbows, dorsal wrists and hands, ankles and feet. About 50% have periumbilical hyperkeratosis. Many patients display characteristic erosion termed moulting/mausering (superficial shedding of the skin) given the higher level of epidermal involvement. There is no erythroderma.

Mutations in keratin 2e (type-II keratin cluster on12q11-13) expressed in the more superficial epidermis cause disruption of normal filament assembly. Emollients and keratolytics are used. The disorder is responsive to systemic retinoids.

Jadasshon-Lewandowsky Syndrome (Pachyonychia Congenita Type I) Pachyonychia congenita (PC) type-I inheritance is AD with more than 100 case reports described. The disorder mostly involves plantar surfaces. Plantar calluses over pressure points form as late as 7 yr of age. Manual workers develop palmar calluses. Nail changes are present from birth to the first few months of life and are characterized by an upward "angulation" of the distal ends of all nails owing to wedge-shaped subungual hyperkeratosis. Paronychial infections occur in up to 70% of patients. Blistering may occur on the plantar surfaces. There are associated patchy or streaky thickened white areas of nonmalignant leukokeratosis of the mucous membranes. Follicular keratoses on the elbows, knees, and extensor extremities are seen.

Mutations occur in K6 and K16, keratins that normally are located in the palmoplantar epidermis, nail plate, hair follicle, sweat gland, oral mucosa, and larynx. K6 and K16 levels are increased in hyperproliferative epidermal cells such as occur in psoriasis.

Jackson-Sertoli Syndrome, and Jackson-Lawler PC (PC Type II)   PC type II has AD inheritance. There are focal areas of often minor plantar keratoderma. Nail changes similar to PC type 1 are present at birth to the first few months of life. Multiple steatocystomas and epidermal cysts are seen. There is variable appearance of natal teeth but no oral lesions are seen. Some patients have been described with wooly or frizzy scalp hair and full eyebrows growing straight out.

Mutations occur in K6b and K17, keratins that are normally located in the outer root sheath of the hair follicle, nails, and basal layer of the palmoplantar epidermis. For mild cases, emollients and keratolytics are helpful. Retinoids have been used to improve the keratoderma and flatten the nails with some success.

CELL-ENVELOPE COMPONENTS

Lamellar Ichthyosis   LI occurs in 1/300,000–500,000 births with an equal gender predilection. Almost all cases display an AR inheritance, although rare reports of AD transmission exist. At birth, patients' skin is erythrodermic and scaling; they often display ectropion and eclabium secondary to skin tautness. Affected infants often present with a *collodion membrane*, a translucent encasement. This membrane is taut and can interfere with respiration. It desquamates over the first 10–14 d of life, commonly leaving fissures and increasing the potential for dehydration, electrolyte imbalance, infection, and thermoregulation problems. They have large, dark, plate-like firmly adherent scales greatest over their lower extremities but also present in the flexures. Over time, the erythroderma fades in varying degrees but the scaling remains.

Patients may have mild or moderate PPK. There is no associated blistering, and lips and mucous membranes are usually spared. Teeth and nails are normal. Hair may appear thin, sparse, or absent (especially at the periphery) because of thick scale encasement. Patients are prone to secondary infections, especially fungal in origin. There is often associated heat intolerance because of thicker scales impairing the ability to sweat. Involvement is severe throughout life.

Mutations in *TGM1* have been identified in some families. This enzyme is important in the cornified cell envelope structure; mutations result in failure to properly crosslink cellular proteins, including involucrin, loricrin, and small proline-rich proteins. Transglutaminase also crosslink extracellular lipids, ceramides to cornified envelope proteins, particularly involucrin. There is increased epidermal proliferation. DNA analysis by sequencing confirms biopsy diagnosis in 70% of cases.

Lactic acid, urea, glycolic acid, calcipitriol, and tazarotene have been used topically. Systemic retinoids are used in severe cases. Typical collodion baby management should be implemented and includes monitoring of water/electrolyte loss and temperature.

Newborns should be kept in a humidified incubator. Lubrication (wet compresses followed by bland emollients, i.e., Eucerin) of the membrane is important to help with desquamation. The patient should receive careful eye exams and may need artificial tears during the day and lubricants at night to avoid exposure keratitis. Overheating should be avoided.

Gottron's Syndrome (Symmetrical Progressive Erythrokeratodermia)   Gottron's syndrome has AD inheritance with incomplete penetrance and variable expressivity. Up to 50% of cases are sporadic. This disorder is characterized by large, well-demarcated, fixed, symmetric, erythematous, hyperkeratotic plaques on the extremities, buttocks, and often on the face. Half of patients have palm/sole involvement. The trunk is usually spared. It appears shortly after birth, progresses slowly and then stabilizes in early childhood. Disease activity may decrease after puberty. There is a lack of variable, migratory erythema that is seen in EKV (discussed later). An insertional mutation has been identified in one family of loricrin (a cell envelope component). Standard keratolytics (lactic acid, glycolic acid, urea) are minimally effective. Psoralen ultraviolet A and oral retinoids may be useful.

Nonbullous Congenital Icthyosiform Erythroderma   This disorder is considered to be a milder, erythrodermic variant of lamellar icthyosis. It occurs in 1/180,000–300,000 births. Incidence is equal in males and females. AR inheritance is displayed. Disease is apparent at birth with a common collodion membrane presentation. After shedding, the skin usually remains red, with generalized, fine, white scale. Generalized involvement of the face, palms, soles, and flexures occurs, but the mucous membranes are usually spared. There is minimal to no ectropion, eclabium, or alopecia.

Heat intolerance, owing to hypohidrosis from sweat duct obstruction by the hyperkeratosis, varies. Secondary dermatophyte infections of the skin and nails are common. The disorder is usually persistent but may improve after puberty.

A subset of patients with mutations in TGM1 has been identified. Two siblings with a defect in loricrin, a cornified cell envelope protein have been examined. Increased epidermal proliferation is a feature. Owing to increased epidermal proliferation, patients should be monitored for anemia and treated with iron if deficient. Simple emollients are useful. It is important to maintain a humid environment and monitor fluid and electrolytes.

DISEASES OWING TO DEFECTIVE CONNEXINS

Connexins are a family of proteins that aggregate and form intercellular gap junctions, important channels spanning the cell membrane between adjacent cells enabling cell–cell signaling. A gap junction is made up of two adjoining connexins on adjacent cells. This intercellular communication is vital for maintaining tissue homeostasis, growth development and control, as well as regulated cell response to stimuli.

Connexins 26, 30, 31 are found in stratified epithelia of the cochlea and epidermis; abnormalities can result in sensorineural deafness and/or skin disease. Connexin mutations have been identified in patients with EKV, deafness, and peripheral neuropathy, as well as Vohwinkel's syndrome and hidrotic ectodermal dysplasia (discussed later). Because connexin 26 is the predominant connexin in cochlear cells, these mutations are the leading cause of nonsyndromic AR hereditary hearing loss.

ERYTHROKERATODERMIA VARIABLIS, MENDES DE COSTA TYPE ERYTHROKERATODERMIA   EKV is rare; approx 150 cases have been reported. It has AD inheritance with variable expression and equal gender predilection. EKV usually presents at or shortly after birth and progresses until puberty. Two skin changes, usually involving the face, extensor extremities, trunk, buttocks, axilla, and groin, predominate: (1) migratory, sharply demarcated erythematous patches of varying shapes and sizes (few to many cm) that last for minutes to months and may be triggered by trauma and change in temperature, and (2) hyperkeratotic, sharply demarcated and often polycyclic, usually fixed plaques with a yellow–brown–gray scale.

Keratoderma of palms and soles and hyperhidrosis may occur. Hair, nail, and mucous membranes are normal.

Mutations have been found in *GJB3* (the gene encoding connexin 31) and *GJB4* (the gene encoding connexin 30.3), resulting in abnormal intercellular communication. Pathological changes include retention hyperkeratosis with normal epidermal proliferation. Isotretinoin and acitretin have resulted in complete clearing of the hyperkeratotic plaques and partial clearing of the erythematous patches. However, patients often relapse when off treatment.

KERATITIS-ICHTHYOSIS-DEAFNESS (KID) SYNDROME CONGENITAL ICHTHYOSIFORM SYNDROME WITH DEAFNESS AND KERATITIS

Inheritance of keratitis-ichthyosis-deafness (KID) syndrome is most consistent with sporadic AD, but cases of AR inheritance have been suggested. It has equal gender predilection. Presenting at birth, patients have keratitis (with progressive corneal opacification), icthyosis, and deafness (most with severe neurosensory loss). Well-demarcated, orange to erythematous, keratotic, spiny plaques appear on the face and extremities more than the trunk. There is variable mild generalized hyperkeratosis.

Prominent follicular hyperkeratosis can cause scarring alopecia of the body, scalp, eyelashes, and eyebrows. Nails and teeth may be abnormal. Patients have increased risk of bacterial, viral, and fungal infections. PPK develops with a reticulated appearance resembling grained leather. Some patients experience hypohidrosis owing to occlusion. Dominant mutations have been discovered in *GJB2* (the gene encoding connexin 26) leading to disruption of intercellular signaling.

Unlike patients with other disorders of keratinization, these patients rarely benefit and may even worsen (i.e., corneal neovascularization) with systemic retinoids. Topical antibiotic therapy is often necessary and helpful. Patients should be referred to an ophthalmologist and otolaryngologist for frequent eye and audiological assessment and treatment of deficits (i.e., hearing aids, cochlear implants).

VOHWINKEL'S SYNDROME (KERATODERMA HEREDITARIA MUTILANS)

Vohwinkel's syndrome, a rare disorder with AD inheritance, may be more frequent in females and whites.

Diffuse, honeycombed palmoplantar hyperkeratosis develops in early infancy. Patients often develop flexion contractures and constricting bands of the digits, especially the fifth digit, resulting in spontaneous autoamputation (pseudoainhum). The dorsal hands, fingers, and toes develop characteristic "starfish" keratoses; the extensor surfaces of the knees and elbows display linear keratoses. There is often associated mild to moderate, nonprogressive high-frequency sensorineural hearing loss. There are descriptions of nail changes, alopecia, onychogryphosis, spastic diplegia, and myopathy in some cases.

Mutations in connexin 26 are characteristic in the classic form of Vohwinkel's syndrome. Mutations in loricrin have been found in a patient with Camisa disease, a form of Vohwinkel's with normal hearing and diffuse, generalized ichthyosis associated with mutilating keratoderma.

Characteristic hyperkeratosis and "round" retained nuclei with hypergranulosis is seen on pathology. Oral retinoids are helpful for the keratoderma and pseudoainhum. Patients should have audiological testing.

PPK WITH DEAFNESS   PPK presents in mid childhood and patients may also have involvement of the elbows and knees. Progressive sensorineural hearing loss presents at birth or infancy and may result in complete deafness.

There is an AD form that also has an associated connexin 26 mutation. Mutations in a mitochondrial gene encoding a mitochondrial serine tRNA (whose role is to add serine to protein chains during mitochondrial protein synthesis) have been identified.

Variable success has been reported with oral retinoids. Topical therapies used include saline compresses followed by gentle debridement and 60% propylene glycol in water under plastic occlusion overnight weekly. Hidrotic ectodermal dysplasia, owing to connexin mutations, is discussed later.

DEFECTS OF LIPID METABOLISM

X-LINKED ICHTHYOSIS (STEROID SULFATASE DEFICIENCY)   X-linked ichthyosis occurs in 1/2000–9500 male births. It has an X-linked recessive inheritance, and thus is transmitted only to males by heterozygous normally appearing females. Patients have large, yellow-brown, firmly adherent scales on all body surfaces involved except the face, palms, and soles. The antecubital and popliteal fossae are relatively spared. The disorder is often regarded as the "dirty-neck disease" because of the clinical appearance of scale and the invariable lateral neck involvement. Skin peeling may occur within the first few days of life and is most apparent on extensor surfaces, although flexural areas are also involved. After this desquamation, disease is often not again apparent until 3–6 mo of age. Most female carriers exhibit minimal to no cutaneous changes. There is a seasonal variation but no improvement with age.

There is no associated keratosis pilaris or increased risk of atopy. Asymptomatic, diffuse corneal opacities in the posterior capsule or Descemet's membrane are seen on slit-lamp examination in 25–50% of males and some female carriers. Approximately one-third of patients are born after a pregnancy characterized by failure of spontaneous initiation or progression of labor; this results in postterm delivery and is because of the absence of placental sterol sulfatase. Cryptorchidism occurs in up to half of patients and there is an increased risk of testicular cancer independent of cryptorchidism.

In more than 80% of patients, there is a gene deletion at the STS locus on the short arm of the X-chromosome. Steroid sulfatase is one of a group of aryl sulfatases and its deficiency leads to an inability to hydrolyze cholesterol sulfate, causing an accumulation of cholesterol sulfate with a concomitant decrease in cholesterol and abnormal cornification; in addition, maternal urinary and serum estrogens are decreased. The disorder is characterized as a retention hyperkeratosis with normal epidermal proliferation.

Pedigree and clinical characteristics are usually sufficient to make a diagnosis. The disease is usually not severe enough to require prenatal diagnosis. Cholesterol sulfate levels are increased in serum, epidermis and scale. A diagnostic clue is increased motility of β-lipoproteins (low-density lipoproteins) on electropheresis. However, confirmation of the diagnosis requires an increased cholesterol sulfate level of serum, erythrocyte membranes and keratin. Decreased enzyme activity can be demonstrated in fibroblasts, keratinocytes, leukocytes, and prenatally in amniocytes.

Topical keratolytics (urea and lactic acid creams) or 60% propylene glycol under plastic occlusion overnight weekly are often helpful (earlier in treatment course, may require 5–7 nights/wk to remove excess scale). Testicular self-exam should be performed and patients should be referred to urologists when necessary.

KALLMAN'S SYNDROME   Kallman's syndrome is characterized by anosmia (secondary to absence of olfactory lobe formation) and hypogonadotropic hypogonadism. Several patients have been found to demonstrate a contiguous gene syndrome that involves a number of nearby gene loci, including that of steroid sulfatase. As a result, these patients have X-linked recessive ichthyosis.

CHONDRODYSPLASIA PUNCTATA   CDPX2 is a group of diverse diseases sharing common skin changes and congenital stippled epiphyses and skeletal alterations that affect growth. AR, X-linked dominant and X-linked recessive forms exist.

CONRADI-HUNERMANN-HAPPLE SYNDROME (LINKED DOMINANT CDPX2)   Conradi-Hunermann-Happle syndrome is the most common form of CDPX2 seen by dermatologists. It presents in a mosaic pattern in females. Cutaneous changes are seen in almost all patients. At birth, patients exhibit icthyosiform erythroderma or a collodion membrane, which is replaced with linear hyperkeratosis or fine scale, follicular atrophoderma, pigmentary changes and variable hair problems usually along Blaschko's lines. Affected individuals may have asymmetric, mild lower extremity shortening. Stippled calcifications may no longer be present after puberty. Congenital, asymmetric cataracts occur in approximately two-thirds of patients.

CDPX2 may show anticipation, with increasing disease severity in successive generations. Mutations have been identified in a gene encoding emopamil-binding protein.

The disorder usually requires no treatment owing to resolution of the icthyosis over the first year. If any treatment is necessary, emollients are appropriate. Ophthalmology and orthopedics referrals are warranted.

RHIZOMELIC CDPX2 (PEROXISOMAL BIOGENESIS DISORDER COMPLEMENTATION GROUP 11)   Rhizomelic CDPX2 is an AR, rare multisystem disorder characterized by rhizomelia (symmetric and severe dwarfism), stippled calcifications in cartilage because of premature calcification, joint contractures, congenital cataracts, severe mental retardation, and ichthyosis (in 25%, appearing as a fine "feather-like" scaling).

Mutations have been found in *PEX7*, a gene encoding Peroxin 7, a receptor that enables enzymes to function in the peroxisome. This leads to decreased levels of RBC plasmalogens and buildup of phytanic acid over time. Phytanic acid increases are characteristic of Refsum's disease.

REFSUM'S DISEASE (HEREDOPATHIA ATACTICA POLYNEURITIFORMIS, PHYTANIC ACID STORAGE DISEASE)   Refsum's disease is a rare disorder with approx 100 cases reported, mostly in Scandinavians and people from Northern Europe. It has equal gender predilection and AR inheritance. Patients usually present in the first two to three decades with peripheral neuropathy, cerebellar ataxia, increased CSF protein, cranial nerve abnormalities (sensorineural deafness, tinnitus, and anosmia), retinitis pigmentosa with salt and pepper pigmentation, night blindness, miosis, ECG abnormalities, cardiomyopathy, renal tubular abnormalities, epiphyseal dysplasia, and other skeletal abnormalities. Variable ichthyosis, most similar to ichthyosis vulgaris, develops in adulthood after the eye and nervous system changes occur.

Mutations in *PAHX* (a gene encoding phytanoyl-CoA hydroxylase) and *PEX7* gene have been found, leading to deficiency in

phytanoyl-CoA hydroxylase, a peroxisomal protein that catalyzes the oxidation of phytanic acid. As a result, there is an accumulation of phytanic acid in serum and tissues and replacement of the normal fatty acids in epidermal lipids and other body tissues. Phytanic acid is a fatty acid found in different dietary products including dairy sources, ruminant fats, and green vegetables. Increased epidermal turnover occurs as well. There are increased levels of plasma phytanic acid and lipid vacuoles in the basal and suprabasal layers of the epidermis.

Treatment consists of dietary restriction of foods containing phytanic acid and its precursors (green vegetables and animal fat) to less than 5 mg/d. Plasmapheresis and lipapheresis rapidly decreases phytanic acid levels. Therapy can arrest progression of skin and cardiac changes as well as neuropathy, but retinitis pigmentosa and hearing loss continues. Patients should be referred to a nutritionist, neurologist, cardiologist, ophthalmologist, and dermatologist.

X-LINKED RECESSIVE CDPX2   Skin changes are multiple: erythroderma, possible remnants of collodion membrane, whorled or linear atrophic or icthyosiform hyperkeratosis and follicular atrophoderma. Hair is often sparse, coarse, wiry, and lusterless; some patients develop scarring alopecia. Skeletal abnormalities observed include short stature and vertebral coronal clefting. Cataracts and deafness also occur.

A deletion has been detected in a gene encoding steroid sulfatase on Xp22. In addition, mutations in *ARSE* have been identified in five patients.

SJÖGREN-LARSSON SYNDROME   Sjögren-Larsson syndrome is rare, with approx 200 cases reported. Inheritance is AR. At birth, patients display fine to generalized scaling. Erythema, if present, fades and is no longer present by 1 yr of age. Generalized ichthyosis with characteristic velvety orange or brown lichenification of the lateral and posterior neck, lower abdomen, and flexures is often present. The central face, scalp hair, and nails are usually spared. Patients often complain of intense pruritus, although sweating is normal. Spastic diplegia or tetraplegia with a scissor gait and mild to severe mental retardation (+/–grand mal seizures and altered speech) develop during the first 2–3 yr of life. Many patients are wheelchair bound by adolescence. Glistening white dots can be seen in the macula of the retina in 50–80% of patients after age 1 and are characteristic eye findings.

The defect leads to an accumulation of long chain fatty alcohols because of a deficiency in a *FALDH* gene, which codes for a microsomal enzyme that catalyzes the oxidation of medium and long-chain aliphatic aldehydes generated from the metabolism of fatty alcohol, phytanic acid, ether, glycerolipids, and leukotriene B4.

On electron microscopy (EM), epidermal cells display prominent golgi apparatus and increased density of mitochondria. In addition, there are abnormal lamellar inclusions in the cytoplasm of corneocytes. Dietary restriction of long chain fatty acids may help. Emollients and keratolytics can be useful. Patients should be referred to a nutritionist, neurologist and opthalmologist.

CHILD SYNDROME (CONGENITAL HEMIDYSPLASIA WITH ICHTHYOSIFORM ERYTHRODERMA AND LIMB DEFECTS)   CHILD syndrome is apparent at birth. Inflammatory hyperkeratotic plaques with sharp midline demarcation and minimal contralateral involvement in a linear or segmental pattern are seen. The limb defects are ipsilateral to the ichthyosis and range from digital hypoplasia to complete absence of an extremity. There is variable internal involvement of the musculoskeletal, cardiovascular, central nervous system, renal, and genitourinary systems.

Mutations in two peroxisomal genes involved in cholesterol biosynthesis have been described. These genes encode emopamil binding protein (EBP) (3β-hydroxysteroid-δ-8-δ-7-isomerase) and NSDHL (NAD(P)H steroid dehydrogenase-like protein encoding a 3β-hydroxysteroid dehydrogenase).

Lyonization may occur producing a clinical pattern involving Blaschko's lines.

Treatment consists of referral to a dermatologist for topical treatment (although disease is difficult to control with the usual agents) and to an orthopedist and organ-specific specialist depending on internal organ involvement. CT/MRI should be performed on the side ipsilateral to the icthyosis.

CHANARIN-DORFMAN SYNDROME (NEUTRAL LIPID STORAGE DISEASE) Chanarin-Dorfman syndrome is rare; approx 30 cases, mainly from the Mediterranean, have been reported. Patients appear most similar to those with nonbullous congenital ichthyosiform erythroderma. They display generalized, fine white-gray scaling with varying degrees of erythema. At birth, affected individuals often present as a collodion baby with ectropion and eclabium. Variable, progressive extracutaneous disease develops later and includes cataracts, neurosensory deafness, psychomotor retardation, myopathy with elevated muscle enzymes, and abnormalities of the nervous system.

A mutation has been identified in *CGI-58* gene in nine families. CGI-58 is a member of a large group of proteins, mostly enzymes with unknown functions, but defects result in an alteration in the rates of synthesis and degradation of the major cellular phospholipids. Triglycerides accumulate in the cytoplasm of leukocytes, muscle, liver, fibroblasts, and other tissues in affected individuals. However, serum lipid levels are normal.

Peripheral blood smear demonstrates lipid vacuoles within granulocytes, eosinophils, monocytes, dermal cells, keratinocytes, and acrosyringia in patients and sometimes in carriers. On EM, electron lucent nonmembrane bound lipid droplets may be identified. Dietary intervention and keratolytics are the mainstays of treatment.

DISORDERS OF CALCIUM METABOLISM

DARIER-WHITE DISEASE (KERATOSIS FOLLICULARIS)
Darier-White disease (DWD) has an AD inheritance with a high penetrance. The prevalence ranges from 1 in 50,000–100,000 individuals.

DWD is characterized by abnormal keratinization of the epidermis, nails, and mucous membranes. It usually begins in the first or second decades, often around puberty. There are multiple yellowish tan-brown greasy and pruritic papules on the nasolabial folds, forehead, scalp, chest, back, ears, and groin; these may coalesce into large, warty, malodorous plaques. The hair is intrinsically normal but there may be an abnormality resulting from the thick scale and crust. Punctate keratoses (raised or depressed) occur on the palms and soles. Nails are thin and may display a characteristic V-shaped scalloping and subungual thickening, longitudinal ridges, and red and white longitudinal bands. White, centrally depressed papules resembling cobblestones can be seen on the buccal mucosa, cheeks, hard and soft palate, and gums (larynx, esophagus, and rectum in rare cases). Patients display discrete hyperkeratotic papules on the dorsal hands and feet.

Disease activity frequently worsens with heat and humidity, ultraviolet B light, mechanical trauma, and lithium. Frequent bacterial and generalized herpes simplex infections can occur, but no immune abnormalities have been consistently reported. Recurrent parotid gland swelling often occurs from squamous metaplasia of the lining leading to obstruction. Affective disorders and diminished intelligence have been reported. There is a variant of DWD described with hemorrhagic macules and vesicles often in an acral distribution.

Multiple mutations (missense, alternative splicing, deletions, insertions, frameshift, and premature codon mutations) of the Ca^{2+}-ATPase isoforms (*SERCA2* and *SERCA2b*) have been identified. In contrast to the usual situation with enzyme defects in which the heterozygote is usually clinically normal, DWD exhibits haploinsufficiency whereby a deficiency of one copy of a gene leads to a genetic disease. This implies that the ATPases involved are not present in great quantities such that an insult (i.e., ultraviolet B or heat/humidity) on 50% the normal amount of enzyme results in phenotypic abnormalities.

Patients should wear sunscreens and avoid mechanical triggers. Topical (tazarotene, adapalene) and systemic (acitretin, isotretinoin) retinoids have been useful. Antibiotics are necessary for infections that cause disease exacerbations. Dermabrasion, lasers and surgical excision, and grafting have been utilized for hypertrophic lesions.

HAILEY-HAILEY DISEASE (BENIGN FAMILIAL PEMPHIGUS) Hailey-Hailey disease is of AD inheritance with variable penetrance. There is an equal gender distribution. Onset of disease is typically in the third to fourth decades. Patients develop flaccid blisters on an erythematous background; on presentation, these most often appear as fissured plaques in the axillae, groin, inframammary region, neck, and antecubital and popliteal fossae. Activity is often precipitated by friction, heat, and infection. The nails may have longitudinal white streaks.

Patients complain of severe pain, itching, and odor owing to the lesions. There are no extracutaneous manifestations and the disease generally becomes less problematic with time. A mutation has been described in *ATP2C1*, a gene that encodes an adenosine triphosphate-calcium pump in the golgi apparatus. It results in abnormal adhesion and acantholysis.

Topical (tetracyclines, fusidic acid, imidazoles) and oral (tetracyclines) antimicrobials are useful in some patients. Topical steroids can occasionally provide relief. Methotrexate and systemic retinoids have been used in recalcitrant disease.

One patient had brown papules characteristic of Darier's disease on the central chest and flanks as well as linear erosions and maceration in the axillae, groin and suprapubic region typically observed in Hailey-Hailey disease, which may imply that the signaling is not exclusive. This patient's particular mutation has not been characterized, but there may be a motif on the affected proteins that determines the final destination in the endoplasmic reticulum (as in Darier's) or the golgi (as in Hailey-Hailey); perhaps there is an enzyme in both locations such that the patient has both disorders.

OTHER MECHANISMS

NETHERTON'S SYNDROME (ICHTHYOSIS LINEARIS CIRCUMFLEXA)
A rare disorder of AR inheritance, Netherton's syndrome is mainly described in case reports. Its incidence is estimated at 1/100,000 births.

Ichthyosis linearis circumflexa is characterized by the coexistence of ichthyosis, structural hair shaft abnormalities and atopy. It may present as a collodion baby or with generalized erythroderma at or around birth. Ichthyosis linearis circumflexa develops and is characterized by migratory, polycyclic and serpiginous plaques of erythema with a double-edged scale at the periphery; this usually does not occur until age two.

Affected individuals often have lichenification over popliteal and antecubital fossae and often complain of pruritus. There is often thick seborrheic dermatitis-like scaling on the scalp, eyebrows, and face. The hair is thin, slow growing, lusterless and fragile; the classic finding is trichorrhexis invaginata ("ball and socket" where the distal hair segment intussuscepts into the proximal part) or bamboo hairs from abnormal cornification of the internal root sheath. Trichorrhexis nodosa and pili torti can also be seen on examination of the hair shafts.

Atopy, manifested by atopic dermatitis, urticaria, and angioedema (especially to nuts and fish) and/or asthma, is a key component. Hypernatremia and dehydration can occur, secondary to transepidermal water loss in the neonatal period. Eosinophilia and increased IgE levels are often seen. There is mild to severe intellectual impairment. Patients are often of short stature and display failure to thrive in approximately one-third of cases. Recurrent skin and lung bacterial and candidal infections are often a problem. There have been early reports of patients with generalized aminoaciduria.

Mutations have been identified in *SPINK5*, a gene encoding lympho-epithelial-kazal-type related inhibitor, a serine protease inhibitor that may be involved in dampening the inflammatory response.

In the neonatal period, fluid and electrolyte support and monitoring for infections is of utmost importance to prevent dehydration. Treatment has included emollients for mild disease. There is an increased risk for systemic toxic effects with tacrolimus ointment and generalized topical steroids. Referral to an allergist for RAST testing may be appropriate.

TRICHOTHIODYSTROPHY (TAY'S SYNDROME AND IBIDS) Etymology of trichothiodystrophy reveals that tricho refers to hair, thio to sulfur, dys means faulty and trophy means nourishment. A rare syndrome of AR inheritance, less than 100 cases have been reported. Males and females are affected equally.

IBIDS refers to ichthyosis, brittle hair, intellectual impairment, decreased fertility, and short stature. At birth, patients may have a collodion membrane, but redness fades and a generalized ichthyosis develops varying from fine, translucent scaling to large, dark yellow–brown hyperkeratosis. The flexures may be spared. Patients may have irregular nails and PPK. Hypogonadism is manifested as cryptorchidism in males and impaired sexual maturation in females. There is an increased risk of infections. Scalp hair, eyelashes, and eyebrows are short, sparse, and brittle. Examination of hair shafts under light microscopy reveals trichoschisis (transverse fractures), pili torti, or trichorrhexis nodosa (transverse, frayed fractures). Under polarized light, the hair shaft has a tiger tail appearance with alternating light and dark bands. There is an abnormally low (<50% of normal) sulfur content in the hair. Some patients have been reported to have eczema, severe nail abnormalities, palmoplantar hyperkeratosis, and flexion contractures.

A spectrum of related syndromes is described with variable involvement of different systems. For instance, Tay's syndrome and photosensitivity is known is PIBI(D)S syndrome. These patients have mild, noncongenital ichthyosis. They usually lack hypogonadism and do not have an increased risk of skin cancer.

Mutations in the basal transcription factor TFIIH have been identified. It plays a role in the nucleotide excision repair of ultraviolet-induced damage (identical to xeroderma pigmentosa [XP] Group D but without cancers). Mutations have been found in *XP group D helicase gene (ERCC2/XPD)* and *XP Group B helicase gene (ERCC3/XPB)*. Amino acid analysis and micro-

scopic evaluation of hair, DNA studies and phototesting can aid in the diagnosis.

Emollients and photoprotection are treatment approaches. Patients should be referred to dermatologists and other specialists based on symptoms and organ involvement.

PROTEOLYTIC ENZYME DEFECTS

PAPILLON-LEFEVRE SYNDROME (PPK WITH PERIODONTITIS) Papillon-Lefevre syndrome is of AR inheritance. There is an estimated prevalence of 1 in 4,000,000 and an equal gender distribution. In the first few months of life, patients develop symmetric involvement of palms and soles with punctiform accentuation especially along the palmoplantar creases. The dorsal hands, posterior heels including the Achilles tendon, elbows, and knees are involved occasionally. Severe periodontitis of primary and secondary dentition begins at 2–3 yr of age and is accompanied by generalized whitish discoloration of the oral mucosa, which resolves after all teeth are shed. An increased frequency of skin and systemic infection is reported.

There are reports of transverse grooves in nails, onychogryphosis, follicular hyperkeratosis, and hyperhidrosis. Calcification of the falx cerebri and choroid plexus is common and increases with age.

A mutation in the gene encoding a lysosomal protease cathepsin C has been identified. Cathepsins are thought to mediate enzymes integral in the formation and degradation of the cornified cell envelope.

Retinoids have been helpful for the PPK and periodontitis. Elective extraction of the affected teeth may prevent increased alveolar bone resorption. Antibiotics may be needed for recurrent infections.

DISEASES OWING TO SECRETED PROTEINS

MAL DE MELEDA (KERATODERMA PALMOPLANTARIS TRANSGRADIENS, ACROERYTHROKERATODERMA) Mal de Meleda is marked by AR inheritance. Most cases originate in the island of Meleda in the Adriatic Sea or southern Italy. At birth or early infancy, redness of the palms and soles develops and progresses to a diffuse, symmetric thickening that spreads to the dorsal hands and feet in a "glove and stocking" distribution. Knuckles, knees, and elbows can be affected. Constricting bands (pseudoainhum) around the digits leading to autoamputation have been described in a few patients.

Nail changes include koilonychia, subungual hyperkeratosis, longitudinal grooving, and onychogryphosis. Angular cheilitis and perioral erythema have occurred in some patients. Hyperhidrosis with bromhidrosis is a complaint occasionally. EEG abnormalities have been reported.

Mutations in the gene encoding SLURP1 (secreted mammalian Ly-6/uPAR-related protein 1) have been identified. SLURP1 is a secreted protein thought to be involved in cell adhesion and signaling.

Retinoids are helpful for the keratoderma and pseudoainhum but not the erythema. If there is no relief, surgery may be necessary to relieve the constriction.

RECENT FINDINGS

ICHTHYOSIS VULGARIS Ichthyosis vulgaris is the most common inherited disorder of cornification. It has AD inheritance with variable expression and equal gender distribution. Incidence is as high as 1 in 250 (to 1/2000).

Ichthyosis vulgaris often becomes clinically apparent within the first year (usually 3–12 mo) as mild to moderate scaling primarily involving extensor surfaces with sparing of flexures and the neck. Scale may be centrally attached but turned up at edges. Facial involvement is common, but legs are often the most severely involved. This disorder improves with age and in warmer, humid environments.

Keratosis pilaris is common. Hyperlinear palms/soles may be seen, but there is no underlying erythroderma. Up to 50% of patients have atopy (hayfever, asthma, eczema, or urticaria).

Molecular origin of ichthyosis vulgaris is unknown. There is decreased to no filaggrin and its precursor, profilaggrin. Filaggrin is an epidermal protein localized to keratohyaline granules important in the aggregation of keratin intermediate filaments. Recent finding implicate loss-of-function mutations in filaggrin. Homozygous mutations and compound heterozygotes were identified and 4% of Europeans had mutant alleles.

Biopsy reveals mild hyperkeratosis and an absent granular layer. On EM, there are small, poorly formed keratohyaline granules. Simple emollients (especially Vaseline after epidermal hydration) or those with alpha hydroxy acids or urea are helpful. The associated eczema requires treatment as well as the ichthyosis.

HARLEQUIN ICHTHYOSIS Harlequin ichthyosis occurs in less than 1 in 300,000 individuals. It has equal gender predilection and is most likely a heterogeneous mode of inheritance; AR and X-linked recessive reports exist, but most cases are sporadic.

Harlequin ichthyosis presents as massive, shiny, thick plates of red fissuring and cracking scale with sausage-like encasement of hands and feet, ectropion, and eclabium. Ears are deformed or absent; the nasal tip is flattened with eversion of nares. Mortality is high within the first few days to weeks and is usually from respiratory and feeding problems owing to severe constriction from the encasement. Eyebrows and eyelashes are usually absent. Patients are frequently premature. Those that survive the neonatal period usually display the phenotype of severe congenital ichthysiform erythroderma. A skin biopsy at 20–22 wk demonstrates premature keratinization. EM demonstrates an absence of lamellar bodies. Mutations in *ABCA12* cause the disease.

Etretinate (approx 1 mg/kg/d) and isotretinoin treatment within the first few days of life has been associated with desquamation of the membrane and subsequent survival in reported patients. Patients require close monitoring of fluid and electrolytes, temperature regulation, and signs/symptoms of infection.

ECTODERMAL DYSPLASIA

Ectodermal dysplasia is used to describe a diverse group of disorders characterized by aberrant development of the epidermal appendages or oral mucosa (hair, sebaceous glands, teeth, nails, or mucosal glands). Recalcitrant atopic dermatitis is common. Hypohidrotic ectodermal dysplasia, anhidrotic ectodermal dysplasia, Christ-Siemens-Touraine syndrome is discussed in Chapter 101.

CLOUSTON SYNDROME (HIDROTIC ECTODERMAL DYSPLASIA) Clouston syndrome is characterized by AD inheritance with variable penetrance. There is an equal gender distribution.

Hidrotic ectodermal dysplasia is marked by defects of the hair and nails and PPK. The scalp hair is patchy, wiry, brittle, and pale. Over time, this may result in complete alopecia of the scalp, body, and face. In infancy and early childhood, the nails may be white. Eventually, they may thicken and become dystrophic or absent.

Nail plates are thick, short, slow growing, and onycholytic. Persistent paronychial infections are common.

Progressive palmoplantar thickening is frequent. Of note, sweating and teeth are normal.

Conjunctivitis and blepharitis, possibly secondary to lack of protection from eyelashes, occur. Patients have normal facial features.

Mutations in *GJB6* or *connexin 30* gene have been reported. Patients occasionally undergo nail matrix ablation for palliation. Wigs are often beneficial for cosmetic purposes.

AEC SYNDROME (ANKYLOBLEPHARON FILIFORME, ADENATUM-ECTODERMAL DEFECTS, CLEFT LIP AND/OR PALATE SYNDROME/HAY WELLS SYNDROME)

Ankyloblepharon Filiforme Adenatum-Ectodermal Defects, Cleft Lip and/or Palate Syndrome is associated with AD inheritance with complete penetrance and variable expression. At birth the condition resembles epidermolysis bullosa or congenital ichthyosis with erythematous, fissured, peeling skin, and superficial erosions. This sheds in 1–2 wk, leaving dry, thin skin. The scalp is almost always involved, often with chronic, erosive crusting dermatitis with granulation tissue. Recurrent bacterial infections are common. There may be patchy alopecia with remaining wiry, coarse, pale scalp hairs. Body hair is minimal to nonexistent. There is complete or partial fusion of the eyelids (ankyloblepharon filiforme adnatum) in approx 70% of infants. The strands may separate spontaneously or require surgical correction. Lacrimal obstruction or atresia occurs in approx 66% of patients.

A constellation of nail findings range from normal nails to thickened and hyperconvex to absent to deformed. Sweating is usually unimpaired but patients may describe subjective heat intolerance.

Cleft lip and/or palate affects 80% of patients. There may be malformed auricles and mild syndactyly of the second and third toes. Patients may have a decreased quantity or abnormally shaped and spaced teeth. Recurrent otitis media and secondary hearing loss are problematic. There are reports of associated hypospadias.

Mutations in the tumor suppressor gene *p63* (also known as *p51* or *KET*) have been discovered in affected patients. Light emollients are useful until the membrane sheds. Surgery may be necessary for ankyloblepharon, followed by proper ocular hygiene.

Continued meticulous scalp care with early treatment of infection is of utmost importance. Affected individuals benefit most from a multidisciplinary approach, involving a dermatologist, surgeon, nutritionist, speech therapist, orthodontist, and otolaryngologist.

SELECTED REFERENCES

Atlas of Genetics and Cytogenetics in Oncology and Haematology http://www.infobiogen.fr/services/chromcancer/. Accessed Jan. 12, 2006.

Fitzpatrick TB, Eisen AZ, Wolff K, eds. Fitzpatrick's Dermatology in General Medicine, 6th ed. New York: Mc-Graw Hill, Inc., 2003.

Foundation for Ichthyosis and Related Skin Types (First). http://www.scalyskin.org/. Accessed Jan. 12, 2006.

Gene Tests. National Institutes of Health, Health Resources and Services Administration, US Department of Energy (Seattle, WA). http://www.geneclinics.org/. Accessed Jan. 12, 2006.

GeneDx: DNA Diagnostic Services. http://www.genedx.com/. Accessed Jan. 12, 2006.

Kelsell DP, Norgett EE, Unsworth H, et al. Mutations in ABCA12 underlie the severe congenital skin disease harlequin ichthyosis. Am J Hum Genet 2005;76:794–803.

Kimyai-Asadi A, Kotcher L, Jih M. The molecular basis of hereditary palmoplantar keratodermas. J Am Acad Dermatol 2002;47:327–343.

Mutation Data Base. http://www.mutdb.org. Accessed Jan. 12, 2006.

109 Metabolic Genetic Disorders With Prominent Skin Findings

CHRISTOPHER B. MIZELLE AND LOWELL A. GOLDSMITH

SUMMARY

Specific skin lesions associated with internal disorders result from metabolic defects. Excesses in specific aromatic amino acids owing to autosomal-recessive diseases cause distinctive skin lesions. Excess phenylalanine is associated with decreased hair and skin pigment, tyrosine excess with skin blisters and hyperkeratosis of the palms and soles, and homogentisic acid excess with deposition of colored polymers in the skin and cartilage. Excessive iron stimulates melanin synthesis in hemochromatosis. Storage of complete carbohydrates is responsible for vascular lesions in Fabry disease and fucosidosis. Genetic defects of porphyrin synthesis causes increased sensitivity to visible light leading to blisters. A defect in a urea cycle enzyme causes fragile hair in argininosuccinic aciduria.

Key Words: Alkaptonuria; argininosuccinic aciduria; erythropoietic protoporphyria; Fabry disease: fucosidosis; hemochromatosis; phenylketonuria; porphyria cutanea tarda; porphyrias; tyrosinemia II.

INTRODUCTION

Genetic disorders of general metabolism may have prominent skin manifestations; several of these diseases are discussed in this chapter. Three disorders are caused by enzymatic defects in aromatic amino acid metabolism: phenylketonuria (PKU), tyrosinemia II, and alkaptonuria. Two are storage diseases caused by disorders of lysosomal carbohydrate degrading enzymes: Fabry disease and fucosidosis. One is a defect in the urea cycle with distinctive hair findings. Iron storage in hemochromatosis leads to a prominent skin phenotype. Finally, enzymatic defects in the complex process of porphyrin synthesis lead to diseases with prominent photosensitivity.

PHENYLKETONURIA

PKU is an autosomal-recessive disease resulting from a deficiency of hepatic phenylalanine hydroxylase or its required cofactors and the resulting plasma and tissue levels of phenylalanine. Mental retardation, seizures, hypopigmentation, and eczematous dermatitis may result.

CLINICAL FEATURES PKU occurs in 1:10,000 births and is usually detected with neonatal screening. The characteristic cutaneous manifestations are blond hair, blue eyes, and fair skin that is often eczematous. These findings may be subtle and apparent only with comparison to other family members. The more serious problems occurring with untreated disease involve the central and peripheral nervous system with mental retardation, athetosis, restlessness, increased tendon reflexes and muscle tone, hyperkinesis, tremors, and seizures. Sclerodermatous skin changes are rare but striking and commonly present as indurated plaques on the thighs during the first year of life. They resolve with a phenylalanine-restricted diet.

GENETICS A single 100-kb gene on chromosome 12 codes for a 452 amino acid peptide. Pterin tetrahydrabiopterin is an essential component of the reaction and defects in its metabolism can increase phenylalanine levels. Mutations include null alleles without enzymatic activity, kinetic alleles with altered substrate or cofactor activity, and unstable alleles with increased turnover.

TREATMENT A low-phenylalanine diet prevents the neurological complications including the mental retardation.

TYROSINEMIA II

Tyrosinemia type II, Richner-Hanhart Syndrome, is resulting from an autosomal-recessive deficiency of hepatic tyrosine aminotransferase. The eyes, epidermis, and central nervous system are typically affected. This rare disorder has less than 100 reported patients with about half of Italian descent. The syndrome is found worldwide, with equal distribution among men and women.

CLINICAL FEATURES Skin manifestations are limited to acral surfaces with erosions or hyperkeratotic lesions of the palms and soles. Painful, nonpruritic, and often hyperhidrotic lesions typically begin during the first year of life. The pain can limit mobility and lead patients to continue crawling to avoid direct pressure.

Ophthalmological findings usually precede the skin involvement by weeks to months and early findings are tearing, redness, pain and photophobia. Corneal clouding and central or paracentral opacities are later signs. Mental retardation as well as normal mental development has been reported.

LABORATORY AND PATHOLOGICAL FINDINGS The hallmark finding is elevated blood and urine tyrosine levels. Deficient hepatic tyrosine aminotransferase leads to all of the metabolic effects including high levels of tyrosine and its metabolites. Routine histopathology of the skin or conjunctiva is typically nondiagnostic.

From: *Principles of Molecular Medicine, Second Edition*
Edited by: M. S. Runge and C. Patterson © Humana Press, Inc., Totowa, NJ

DIFFERENTIAL DIAGNOSIS Neonatal tyrosinemia is a common transient condition with decreased levels of p-hydroxy-phenylpyruvic acid oxidase apoenzyme and a relative ascorbic acid deficiency contributing to the tyrosinemia, tyrosinuria, and increased tyrosine metabolite excretion. Treatment includes low protein diet and ascorbic acid supplementation. Hereditary tyrosinemia (tyrosinemia type I, tyrosinosis) is an autosomal-recessively inherited defect in fumaryl-acetoacetate hydrolase deficiency with severe liver and renal disease. Early in life, affected patients develop fever, edema, vomiting, a boiled-cabbage odor, hematuria, diarrhea, jaundice, hepatosplenomegaly, and Fanconi's syndrome. These patients are also at increased risk for development of hepatocellular carcinoma.

GENETICS The 454 amino acid tyrosine aminotransferase protein is cytoplasmic and is coded by a 10.9-kb gene at 16q22.1-22.3. R57Y is the common mutant allele in Italy but there are multiple mutations in the gene. There are no definitive genotype–phenotype relationships.

TREATMENT AND PROGNOSIS All patients presenting with atypical bullous and hyperkeratotic disease of the acral surfaces needs to be evaluated for possible tyrosinemia II as it is easily treatable. Dietary restriction of tyrosine and phenylalanine leads to rapid reversal of the skin and ocular findings with normalization of tyrosine levels. Early treatment prevents the associated mental retardation.

ALKAPTONURIA

Alkaptonuria is a rare (1:250,000) autosomal-recessive metabolic disorder resulting from a deficiency of homogentisic acid oxidase (HGO), the sole enzyme catabolizing homogentisic acid (HGA). Excessive HGA is excreted in the urine and accumulates in connective tissues. The disease is distributed worldwide with a higher incidence in certain areas such as Slovakia and Santa Domingo. Men and women are affected equally.

PATHOGENESIS HGO is an enzyme in the catabolic pathway of phenylalanine and tyrosine. Its cofactors include oxygen, ferrous iron, and sulfhydryl groups. HGO is inhibited by the quinones producing pseudo-ochronosis. HGA is colorless until oxidized when it obtains a black pigment. Patients with alkalinized urine are more likely to develop dark urine. A decrease in urinary pH prevents the oxidation of HGA after tubular secretion. The deposition in connective tissues is not well understood. HGA inhibits lysyl hydroxylase in chick embryos and weakens collagen. In addition, HGA may form crosslinks with collagen further decreasing its strength.

CLINICAL FEATURES Dark urine is dependent on oxidation that occurs after tubular secretion. Oxidation usually requires a urinary pH >7.0 or the absence of reducing substances such as ascorbic acid. A presumptive diagnosis is made under from a positive family history and discoloration of diapers with the use of alkaline soap. Before glucose oxidase urinary analysis, testing for urinary glucose with Benedict's solution produced an orange precipitate that turned black. Although the diagnosis can be made during childhood, it is typically made in the third or fourth decades with the presentation of connective tissue changes.

Clinically visible hyperpigmentation occurs in several organs including the skin, eyes, and various cartilaginous structures. Dark brown or black cerumen may be the presenting symptom. Some patients develop axillary hyperpigmentation especially in a glandular orifice pattern. The ear can be affected in several ways ranging from cartilage and tympanic membrane discoloration

to calcification. Patients may complain of tinnitus or hearing loss. Cartilage in the larynx and trachea may be involved, but remains asymptomatic. Ocular findings include grayish-black scleral pigmentation, as well as corneal, conjunctival, and tarsal findings.

Disabling arthritis of multiple joints presents with recurring bouts of inflammation typically in the third to fourth decades. X-rays show early calcification of the intervertebral disk with narrowing of the intervertebral spaces. There may be eventual disk collapse with gradual decrease in height. Pseudogout may coexist with ochronosis.

The prostate and kidneys are frequently affected with pigmentation.

LABORATORY AND PATHOLOGICAL FINDINGS Alkaptonuric patients show no abnormalities on routine lab testing except for excretion of HGA. Sodium hydroxide added to a patient's urine leads to darkening of the urine and provides a presumptive diagnosis.

Skin biopsy can show yellow to light brown pigmented granules in dermal macrophages. Routine stains for melanin are positive and the pigment is resistant to 10% hydrogen peroxide.

GENETICS A 60-kb gene on 3q21-23 codes for HGA oxidase. Multiple mutations have been reported and in a large series, 81% of patients were compound heterozygotes.

The gene is at 3q21-q23.66 and has multiple mutations.

DIFFERENTIAL DIAGNOSIS The other main causes of dark urine are melaninuria, porphyria, myoglobinuria, bilirubinaria, and hematuria that should not be confused with alkaptonuria. Pseudo-ochronosis has been reported in blacks using hydroquinones for depigmentation and in patients treating their skin with carbolic acid.

TREATMENT AND PROGNOSIS Symptomatic relief with rest and analgesics is required for the arthritis, although many patients eventually need prosthetic joint replacement. Life-span is not typically affected despite the unremitting and progressive disease course. Nitisinone, a reversible inhibitor of 4-hydoxy-phenylpyruvate (the enzyme proximal to HGA oxidase in the catabolic pathway), decreases HGA levels and is being evaluated clinically. Oral ascorbic acid is not an effective treatment.

FABRY DISEASE: β-GALACTOSIDASE A DEFICIENCY

Fabry disease is an X-linked recessive inborn error of glycosphingolipid metabolism resulting from abnormal β-galactosidase A, a lysosomal enzyme. Incidence is 1:40,000–60,000 in males. The enzymatic defect leads to deposition of neutral glycosphingolipids in lysosomes of most visceral tissues, especially the vascular endothelium.

CLINICAL FEATURES Males are almost solely affected with minimal manifestations in carrier females. Disease onset begins in childhood with periodic acroparesthesias, appearance of angiokeratomas, hypohidrosis, and characteristic corneal and lenticular opacities. With aging, the continued glycosphingolipid deposition leads to severe renal, cardiac and cerebrovascular involvement.

Severe and debilitating pain characterized as episodic crises or persistent burning pain begins early in the disease initially involving the palms and soles. The constant pain may be slightly less debilitating but is a nagging, persistent tingling or burning sensation in the hands and feet. Pain crises may be triggered by exercise, fatigue, emotional stress, or rapid changes in temperature or humidity. With advancing age, the periodic crises decrease in frequency.

Angiokeratomas progressively increase with age in size and number and are dark red to blue-black clusters of individual, punctate lesions. They tend to be symmetric and can be nonblanching macules or slightly raised papules. Common locations are the hips, lower abdomen and back, thighs, buttocks, penis, scrotum, oral mucosa, and conjunctiva. Anhidrosis or hypohidrosis from neuropathy are common.

The progressive infiltration of glycosphingolipid in the vascular system produces a variety of cardiac, cerebral, and renal manifestations including angina, myocardial ischemia and infarction, mitral valve prolapse, congestive heart failure, hypertension, mitral insufficiency, and cardiomegaly. Hypertension from renal vascular compromise may accentuate or accelerate these finding. Cerebrovascular disease resulting from multifocal small vessel disease leads to thromboses, basilar artery ischemia and aneurysm, seizures, hemiplegia, hemianesthesia, aphasia, labyrinthine disorders, or frank cerebral hemorrhage. Psychiatric disorders may also occur. Renal disease presents as proteinuria with gradual deterioration of renal function resulting in azotemia. In childhood, polarization microsocopy reveals birefringent lipid globules with characteristic Maltese cross structures both free in the urine and within desquamated urinary sediment cells. Death is commonly from vascular disease involving the kidneys, heart or brain.

Ocular involvement is most common in the cornea, lens, conjunctiva, and retina. A characteristic corneal opacity visualized with slit-lamp microscopy is evident in males and heterozygous females. This corneal dystrophy of Fabry disease is characteristic, but indistinguishable from the drug-induced phenocopy of chloroquine and amiodarone. Lenticular changes include a granular anterior/subcapsular deposit or a posterior cortex deposit. Visual impairment is uncommon despite the involvement of the cornea, retina, and conjunctiva. However, acute visual loss as a result of total central retinal artery occlusion is reported.

Pulmonary effects include chronic bronchitis, wheezing, or dyspnea. Lymphedema and priapism can result secondary to obstruction of lymphatics from glycosphingolipid deposition.

Cardiac Variants This phenotypic variant presents in affected males usually after age 40, later than the classic disease. Patients have retained β-galactosidase A activity. They have 1–5% of residual α-galactosidase activity, and usually have cardiac effects but not cutaneous manifestations.

Carrier Females The clinical course and prognosis of carriers differs greatly from the affected males. Females do not experience the ill effects of the disease as early as their male counterparts. Some patients eventually experience some renal and cardiac effects. About 30% of the females develop angiokeratomas and acroparesthesias, whereas most have the classic corneal dystrophy. Clinical findings depend on random X-inactivation and most obligate carrier females have no clinical manifestations.

GENETIC COUNSELING Both females and males can transmit the enzymatic defect as a typical X-linked recessive gene. Fabry disease has been detected prenatally with amniocentesis and chorionic villus sampling.

GENETICS β-Galactosidase A is coded by a single copy, seven exon gene at Xq21. There are no characteristic mutations and the disease is owing to multiple missense or nonsense mutations, splice defects or gene rearrangements.

DIFFERENTIAL DIAGNOSIS The use of a skin biopsy, ophthalmological examination, and demonstration of the birefringent inclusions in urinary sediment can help solidify a presumptive diagnosis. Deficient or absent β-galactosidase A on biochemical analysis is needed to confirm the diagnosis. Prenatal diagnosis can be performed by chorionic villus sampling at 9–10 wk of pregnancy.

TREATMENT Pain is the single most debilitating symptom; carbamazepine, diphenylhydantoin and gabapentin have been shown to decrease pain severity. Renal transplantation is likely to be required as renal insufficiency is the most frequent late complication. β-Galactosidase A replacement with recombinant enzyme has been approved, is effective and is under long-term study. Skin biopsy is useful for following the response to gene therapy.

FUCOIDOSIS AND OTHER GLYCOPROTEIN DISORDERS

Fucoidosis is a rare autosomally recessive lysosomal storage disease similar to Fabry disease and because of deficiency of β-L-fucosidase with accumulation of certain fucose-containing complex compounds in various tissues. It is divided into two forms: type-I (without angiokeratomas) and -II (with angiokeratomas).

CLINICAL FEATURES Accumulation of the fucose-containing compounds leads to many clinical findings. Major findings are mental retardation, seizures, and progressive neurological deterioration including anhidrosis. Visceromegaly, course facial features, angiokeratomas, delayed psychomotor development, cardiac problems, and an unusual variant of spondylometaphyseal dysplasia are often found.

Type I is the most severe, typically becomes apparent within the first 6 mo of life, and progresses with death usually before the age of 10. These infants have severe mental and growth retardation with continued deterioration of the brain and spinal cord. They may also have multiple gastrointestinal complications.

Type II also presents in the first year of life but is less progressive; patients live to their twenties. The clinical findings are the same as type I, but with the addition of angiokeratomas.

Angiokeratomas are described in β-mannosidosis (onset 1–6 yr) and juvenile sialidosis (onset 2–20 yr).

ARGININOSUCCINIC ACIDURIA

Argininosuccinic aciduria is an autosomal-recessive disorder characterized by cutaneous and systemic findings because of argininosuccinate lyase deficiency. This enzyme is essential in the urea cycle and its deficiency leads to citrullinemia and elevated blood ammonia levels. Hepatomegaly, mental retardation, lethargy, and ataxia are the main systemic findings, whereas brittle hair characterized as trichorrhexis nodosa is the major dermatological finding.

Argininosuccinic aciduria typically presents with failure to thrive and ammonia intoxication in neonates or during the second year of life with seizures, psychomotor retardation, and ataxia. The characteristic hair findings with trichorrhexis nodosa usually have a later onset.

HEMOCHROMATOSIS

Hereditary hemochromatosis (HH) is an autosomal-recessive inherited disease of iron deposition in multiple tissues throughout the body. Whites are most commonly affected. It is a relatively common inheritable disorder with approx 10% of the general population having an abnormal allele for the hemochromatosis gene. Major complications are from visceral deposition of iron, but cutaneous involvement is also seen. The classic tetrad includes cirrhosis, diabetes mellitus, skin hyperpigmentation, and cardiac failure.

Less common consequences include hepatocellular carcinoma, impotence, and arthritis.

HH is a genetically heterogeneous disorder with three different described subsets. Hemochromatosis type 1 is the most common and its gene, *HFE1,* is telomeric to the HLA-A locus on 6p. Two mutations in *HFE* have been described and both are missense mutations with resulting single amino acid substitutions. Juvenile hemochromatosis or type 2 has been mapped to1q21, whereas hemochromatosis type 3, an adult form, is located on 7q22. The clinical appearance of these variants can be similar except for their clinical onset. The underlying pathophysiology of all three is iron overload. Neonatal hemochromatosis is the most severe with rapid progression to death soon after birth.

CLINICAL FEATURES   The classic tetrad of cirrhosis, diabetes mellitus, bronze hyperpigmentation of the skin, and cardiac failure may be the presenting findings, but earlier complaints should be investigated. Patients with solated asthenia, asthenia with arthralgia, or hypertransaminasemia should be screened for hemochromatosis. Other findings include amenorrhea, loss of libido, impotence, and symptoms of hypothyroidism.

General symptoms include chronic fatigue, weakness, lethargy, and apathy. Hepatomegaly is seen in more than 95% of affected patients and may be associated with other complaints of chronic liver disease. Until testing for the *HFE* gene was developed, liver biopsy and histological evaluation of tissue iron accumulation were required for diagnosis.

Cutaneous hyperpigmentation is seen in more than 90% of patients with idiopathic hemochromatosis. Skin discoloration is one of the earliest signs and is resulting from accumulation of hemosiderin-laden macrophages. The color has been described as slate gray, but is classically a brownish bronze. The color tends to be darker and more pronounced in sun exposed areas. Non-sun exposed areas that may be involved include the flexural folds, scars, and nipple areolae. Ichthyosiform alterations (in up to half of patients), skin atrophy, koilonychia, and hair loss may also be present.

Differential diagnosis of the cutaneous pigmentation is extensive and including drug-induced hyperpigmentation, actinic reticuloid, porphyria cutanea tarda (PCT) and other forms of liver disease such as alcoholic liver disease, nonalcoholic steatohepatitis and chronic viral hepatitis.

LABORATORY FINDINGS   Screening tests include serum iron, ferritin, and transferrin. Genetic tests for C282Y and H63D mutations are available. Testing for these mutations is carried out as confirmation of diagnosis or screening in asymptomatic patients. Liver biopsy is no longer obligatory to establish the diagnosis, but may be needed in cases of cirrhosis.

Skin biopsy may confirm the diagnosis of HH if iron deposition is found in any area except the lower extremities where stasis could produce a false positive.

Serum iron is usually more than 150 mcg/dL with a transferring saturation of more than 45%. Ferritin is more than 500 ng/mL.

GENETICS   A mutation (845 G to A) causes an amino acid change, C282Y, which is the most common mutation. Of the US white population, 61.5% are homozygous for the normal allele, 23.5% are heterozygous for the H63D allele and 10.3% are heterozygous for the C282Y allele. Other rarer alleles are also present. Occasionally heterozygotes have clinical hemochromatosis.

TREATMENT AND PROGNOSIS   Once the diagnosis is confirmed, treatment is fairly direct. Phlebotomy is the sole recommended treatment and is effective if able to be used. Genetic

counseling is also recommended as well as screening for *HFE* mutations in first-degree relatives. Prognosis depends on the extent of organ involvement. Increased awareness and initiation of early treatment has led to higher survival rates than those treated inadequately.

PORPHYRIAS

The porphyrias are a group of acquired and inherited diseases involving the porphyrin-heme biosynthetic pathway. Eight enzymes contribute to the pathway and their deficiency or defectiveness produces an accumulation of specific porphyrin intermediate(s) and clinical disease (Table 109-1). Diagnosis of any of the porphyrias includes measurement of urinary, fecal, and plasma porphyrins. Table 109-1 lists the known porphyrias and their respective enzymes; those with skin involvement are shown in bold type. Except for PCT and erthropoietic protoporphyria (EPP), most of these diseases are rare. This section reviews PCT and EPP.

PORPHYRIA CUTANEA TARDA   PCT (type 1, symptomatic porphyria, acquired hepatic porphyria, and chemical porphyria) is the most common of all the porphyrias and occurs as an inherited or acquired form. It is found worldwide with most studies demonstrating a male predominance. Urogen decarboxylase is deficient or nonfunctional. Three categories of PCT have been described. The most common is the sporadic form or PCT type-I, which has a deficiency of hepatic urogen decarboxylase restricted to the liver or resulting from hepatotoxic substances. Type II has autosomal-dominant inheritance and demonstrates urogen decarboxylase deficiency in all tissues. The third subset includes patients having a positive family history of disease as in type II, but with normal concentrations of a probably dysfunctional enzyme. PCT features are found in patients with variegate poryphyria.

Most of the PCT in the United States are of the type-I pattern and are often alcohol related. Other compounds and conditions that can produce PCT are estrogens (including treatment of men who have prostate cancer), hexachlorobenzene, iron, tetra-chlorodibenzo-*p*-dioxin, and hemodialysis. Clinical findings are similar for all forms of PCT.

PCT patients have vesicles and blisters resulting from repeated trauma and sun exposure. The chronic damage with subepidemal blistering leads to scarring and milia formation. These two latter findings, useful to the attentive clinician, are seen even when the disease is quiescent. Unlike other porphyrias, PCT patients are unaware of the role of sunlight because they are not as photosensitive. Other clinical findings include hypertrichosis, hyperpigmentation, hypopigmentation, and sclerodermoid changes. Some or all of these may exist in any patient. Some studies have shown a direct correlation between elevated urinary uroporphyrins and sclerodermoid changes. The hypertrichosis is mainly facial and improves slowly with treatment of PCT. When these findings are seen in the clinic, a Wood's light can be used to fluorescence the patient's urine. The elevated urinary uroporphyrin demonstrates pink to orange fluorescence if the concentration is more than 1 mg/L.

Coexisting diseases can produce PCT or have been associated with it. Underlying infections need to be excluded in patients with PCT. Both HIV and hepatitis C has been reported in patients with PCT. PCT has been reported before the known infection and vice versa. Therefore, any patient with newly diagnosed PCT should be screened for possible hepatitis C and HIV. Diabetes mellitus and hemochromatosis are two systemic diseases that need consideration.

Table 109-1
Human Porphyrias and Related Enzyme Defects

Tissue	Porphyria	Inheritance	Enzyme
Erythyropoietic	**Congenital Erythropoietic Porphyria**	Autosomal-recessive	Uroporphyrinogen III (Urogen III) cosynthase
	Erythropoietic Protoporphyria (EPP)	Autosomal-dominant	Ferrochelatase
Hepatic	Acute Intermittent Porphyria	Autosomal-dominant	Porphobilinogen deaminase
	Variegate Poryphyria	Autosomal-dominant	Protoporphyrinogen (Protogen) oxidase
	Hereditary coproporphyria	Autosomal-dominant	Coproporphyrinogen (Coprogen) oxidase
	Porphyria Cutanea Tarda (PCT)	Autosomal-dominant, variable	Uroporphyrinogen (Urogen) decarboxylase
	ALA-dehydratase Poryphyria	Autosomal-recessive	ALA-dehydratase
Hepatoerythropoietic	**Hepatoerythropoietic porphyria**	Autosomal-recessive	Uroporphyrinogen (Urogen) decarboxylase

Diseases with skin manifestation are in bold type.

The frequency of the most common mutant hemochromatosis allele (C282Y) is increased in both Types-I and -II PCT.

Laboratory Findings The laboratory findings of PCT include elevated total body iron stores as seen in increased serum iron, ferritin, and transferrin. About 25% of patients have abnormal serum glucose and glucose tolerance tests. PCT patients excrete increased amounts of porphyrins in the urine. The three main features of abnormal excretion are:

1. Increased urinary excretion of uroporphyrin and other acetate-substituted porphyrins.
2. A distinctive pattern of isomer series I and III porphyrins (I > III).
3. Increased excretion of fecal isocoproporphyrin. A complete work-up includes analysis of liver transaminases, liver function tests, CBC, and serology for viral infections. Histopathology is also helpful demonstrating a pauciimmune subepidermal blister. Other characteristic findings include festooning, and thickened papillary vessel walls with a periodic acid–Schiff stain. Direct immunofluorescence shows deposition of C3 and IgG in a granular pattern at the dermal-epidermal junction and around vessel walls.
4. Plasma testing for most porphyrins simplifies diagnosis.

Treatment The treatment of PCT is often effective with the use of phlebotomy. The goal of phlebotomy is to induce an iron deficiency as iron can impede hepatic urogen decarboxylase. Iron also has other functions such as enhancing δ-aminolevulinic acid (ALA) synthases and irreversible binding to uroporphyrin, thus increasing levels of uroporphyrin. Antimalarials are used in patients where phlebotomy is not an option. Although it is thought that the antimalarials have photoprotective properties, their effect in the porphyrias is thought to derive from binding with porphyrins leading to rapid sequestration and excretion by the liver.

ERTHROPOIETIC PROTOPORPHYRIA The second most common porphyria is EPP (erythrohepatic porphyia, protoporphyria), which was first clearly defined in 1961 by Magnus et al. Ferrochelatase is the enzyme defect for this porphyria and is deficient in erythrocytes, mitogen-stimulated lymphocytes, and skin fibroblasts. Family studies have shown genetic heterogeneity with both autosomal-dominant and recessive patterns. EPP has been reported worldwide without any racial predilection.

EPP, unlike PCT, begins early in life with characteristic cutaneous photosensitivity and elevated protoporphyrin in erythrocytes, feces, and plasma. Owing to its insolubility, protoporphyrin is rarely found in urine. Acute attacks of EPP are characterized by marked photosensitivity including burning, stinging and pruritus. The affected areas are obviously photoexposed, but the nose, cheeks, and dorsal hands are particularly involved. The symptoms are usually seasonal, most frequent in spring and summer. The skin lesions include erythema, edema, urticarial lesions, and purpura. Resolution of these acute lesions usually leaves atrophic, waxy or pitted scars. The lips may have a pursed appearance and the dorsal hands may have dramatic scarring with a waxy appearance. Vesicular or bullous lesions are typically seen in temperate climates, but have been reported in the tropics. Patients seem to have a hardening effect as symptoms decrease with age. There is no erythrodontia, hypertrichosis, milia, sclerodermoid changes, or hyperpigmentation as in other porphyrias. Approximately 11% of patients develop a hemolytic anemia. Gall stones and hepatic failure have also has been reported, but seem to be relatively rare.

Laboratory Findings The diagnosis of EPP is made by measuring elevated levels of protoporphyrin in feces, erythrocytes and plasma. There may be elevated fecal and erythrocyte coproporphyrin. A blood smear may show red fluorescent erythrocytes. Histopathlogy may reveal endothelial cell damage, mast cell degranulation, and a polymorphonuclear cell infiltrate in the dermis. There is also marked thickening of the vessels in the papillary dermis as well as perivascular deposits mimicking lipoid proteinosis. The differential diagnosis includes polymorphous light eruption, hydroa vacciniforme, idiopathic solar urticaria, and the other porphyrias.

Treatment Treatment of EPP consists of β-carotene, topical sunscreens, antimalarial drugs, cholestyramine, and vitamins E and C. β-Carotene doses of 60–180 mg/d have been the most effective. The mechanism is thought to be β-carotene's ability to bind free oxygen radicals produced by the photo-excited porphyrins. Future therapies may include enzymatic replacement with ferrochelatase.

SELECTED REFERENCES

Bickers DR, Frank J. The porphyrias. In: Freedberg IM, Eisen AZ, Wolff K, Austen KF, Goldsmith LA, Katz SI, eds. Fitzpatrick's

Dermatology in General Medicine, 6th ed. New York: McGraw-Hill, 2003; pp. 1766–1803.

Britton RS, Fleming RE, Parkkila S, Waheed A, SlyWS, Bacon Br. Pathogenesis of hereditary hemochromatosis: genetics and beyond. Semin Gastrointest Dis 2002;13:68–79.

de Haas V, Carbasius Weber EC, de Klerk JB. The success of dietary protein restriction in alkaptonuria patients is age-dependent. J Inherit Metab Dis 1998;21:791–798.

Desnick RJ, Banikazemi M. Fabry disease: α-galactosidase a deficiency (angiokeratoma corporis diffusum universale). In: Freedberg IM, Eisen AZ, Wolff K, Austen KF, Goldsmith LA, Katz SI, eds. Fitzpatrick's Dermatology in General Medicine. 6th ed. New York: McGraw-Hill, 2003; pp. 1474–1486.

Goldsmith LA. Cutaneous changes in errors of amino acid metabolism: tyrosinemia II, phenylketonuria, argininosuccinic aciduria, and alkaptonuria. In: Freedberg IM, Eisen AZ, Wolff K, Austen KF, Goldsmith LA, Katz SI, eds. Fitzpatrick's Dermatology in General Medicine, 6th ed. New York: McGraw-Hill, 2003:1418–1428.

Goldsmith LA, Thorpe J, Roe Cr. Hepatic enzymes of tyrosine metabolism in tyrosinemia II. J Invest Dermatol 1979;73:530–532.

Imperatore G, Pinsky LE, Motulsky A, Reyes M, Bradley LA, Burke W. Hereditary hemochromatosis: perspectives of public health, medical genetics, and primary care. Genet Med 2003;5:1–8.

Mohrenschlager M, Ring J, Abeck D. Options in the treatment of Fabry Disease. Pediatr Dermatol 2003;20:373, 374.

Phornphutkul C, Introne WJ, Perry MB, et al. Natural history of alkaptonuria. N Engl J Med 2002;347(26):2111–2121.

Pietrangelo A. Hereditary Hemochromatosis—A New Look at an Old Disease.N Engl J Med 2004;350:2383–2397.

Scriver CR, Kaufman S, Eisensmith RC, Woo SLC. The hyperphenylalaninemias. In: Scriver CR, Beaudet AL, Sly WS, et al, eds. The Metabolic and Molecular Basis of Inherited Disease, 8th ed. New York: McGraw-Hill, 2001; pp. 1667–1724.

Thurberg BL, Byers HR, Granter SR, Phelps RG, Gordon RE, O'Callaghan M. Monitoring the 3-yr efficacy of Enzyme Replacement Therapy in Fabry disease by repeated skin biopsies. J Investig Dermatol 2004:122:900–908.

110 Heritable Conditions Affecting Tissues of the Oral Cavity

J. TIM WRIGHT

SUMMARY

The oral cavity is made up of complex and diverse tissues that provide a variety of highly specialized functions ranging from nuerosensory (e.g., taste) to nutritional/digestive functions (e.g., salivary digestion and mastication). Not surprisingly there is a substantial portion of the human genome used in making these unique diverse structures and allowing them to function appropriately. Consequently there are hundreds of conditions affecting the soft and hard tissues of the oral cavity. Some of these conditions affect primarily or only the oral cavity, although others are associated with significant somatic manifestations. This chapter reviews some of these conditions providing the reader a framework for understanding hereditary pathologies of the oral cavity.

Key Words: Amelogenesis; cementum; dentin; dentinogenesis; ectodermal dysplasia; enamel; epidermolysis bullosa; gingival; hair; hypodontia; oral epithelium; teeth.

INTRODUCTION

The oral cavity is a complex system characterized by unique sensory and functional activities that involve highly specialized soft and hard tissues. The mucosal lining of the oral cavity is diverse in its structure depending on its location and function. For example, the tissue directly adjacent to the teeth and on the palate is highly keratinized to protect it from the mechanical and thermal trauma involved in mastication and eating. In contrast, mucosa lining the inner surfaces of the cheeks and the dental vestibules (trough between cheeks and teeth) has little or no surface keratin, has a flexible underlying dermis and is thus mobile allowing the tissues to move for functioning during swallowing, clearing food, and speech. The tongue is a highly muscular appendage that has a unique neurosensory system providing the mechanism for taste.

Complementing the sophisticated soft tissues of the oral cavity is the dental complex. Normally, humans have 20 primary teeth that are lost in childhood and 32 permanent teeth. Teeth are made up of highly specialized mineralized tissues (e.g., enamel, dentin, and cementum) that are supported by pulpal tissue internally and held in the jaws by the periodontal ligament. Each of

From: *Principles of Molecular Medicine, Second Edition*
Edited by: M. S. Runge and C. Patterson © Humana Press, Inc., Totowa, NJ

these tissues is critical to normal function of the dentition and can be affected by hereditary conditions that produce unique structural and compositional defects. Clinical genetic studies coupled with knowledge derived from the Human Genome Project have tremendously advanced the understanding of the molecular basis and associated phenotypes for many hereditary conditions affecting the oral cavity. This chapter presents several of the more common hereditary conditions affecting the hard and soft tissues and provides tables listing other conditions and their associated genes.

HERITABLE CONDITIONS INVOLVING ORAL SOFT TISSUES

Multitudes of diverse hereditary conditions (Table 110-1) affect the soft tissues of the oral cavity and present unique and potentially devastating manifestations. For example, palmar-plantar hyperkeratosis (Papillon Lefevre syndrome), caused by mutations in the cathepsin C gene, is characterized by hyperkeratosis of the palms and soles of the feet and frequently knees and elbows. Interestingly this mutation is associated with severe and rapid periodontal destruction that leads to rapid loss of all the primary teeth and eventually the permanent teeth. The gingiva around the teeth becomes highly inflamed beginning shortly after tooth eruption, the periodontal attachment is destroyed and the teeth loosen and exfoliate with little or no root resorption. Other conditions such as epidermolysis bullosa (EB) can cause severe destruction of the oral soft tissues because of recurrent blistering whereas other disorders are associated with pigmentation changes of the mucosa that can be associated with increased risk for malignancy (e.g., Peutz–Jeghers syndrome, dyskeratosis congenita).

EPIDERMOLYSIS BULLOSA EB is a clinically diverse group of disorders having blister formation as their common feature and is discussed in detail in Chapter 105.

Depending on the specific protein involved and the associated abnormality, the clinical presentation variably affects soft as well as hard tissues in the oral cavity. All of the defective proteins responsible for skin fragility in EB are expressed in the oral soft tissues, although, because of the oral epithelium's unique structural and compositional characteristics, the oral mucosa may or may not display fragility similar to the skin. As with the skin, the

Table 110-1
Simple and Complex Hereditary Conditions Associated With Periodontal Disease, Mucosal Ulceration
and Pigmentation, and Head and Neck Cancer

Condition	Inheritance	Protein/function	Gene
Periodontitis			
Papillon-Lefèvre syndrome	AR	Cathepsin C, lysozomal protease	CTSC
Haim Munk syndrome	AR	Cathepsin C, lysozomal protease	CTSC
Ehlers-Danlos IV	AD	Type-III Collagen	COL3A1
Leukocyte adhesion deficiency I	AD	Integrin-B2, neutrophil dysfunction	ITGB2
Mucosal blistering and ulceration			
Dystrophic epidermolysis bullosa	AD/R	Type VII collagen, anchoring fibrils	COL7A1
Junctional epidermolysis bullosa	AR	Laminin 5, anchors cells in basement membrane area by interaction with integrin B4	LAMA3, LAMB3, LAMC2, ITGB4
Mucosal pigmentation			
Peutz-Jeghers syndrome	AD	Serine threonine protein kinase	STK11
Dyskeratosis congenita	X-linked AD	Dyskerin, cell cycle function	DKC1
		Telomerase RNA component	TERC
Head and neck cancer			
Squamous cell carcinoma	Complex	Tumor necrosis factor family member	TNFRSF10B
Cowden disease	AD	Phosphatase and tensin homolog	PTEN
Basal cell nevus syndrome	AD	Patched-transmembrane transcription repressor	PTCH
Bloom syndrome	AR	RecQ protein-like 3-DNA dependent ATPase	RECQL3
Beckwith-Wiedemann syndrome	AD	Cyclin-dependent kinase inhibitor 1C, negative regulator of cell proliferation	CDKN1C

AR, autosomal-recessive; AD, autosomal-dominant.

frequency, magnitude, and depth of lesion formation and tissue separation ultimately determines the progression of the oral soft tissue manifestations in the different EB types and whether lesion healing is associated with scarring.

In the milder forms (e.g., most simplex subtypes) of inherited EB, there is only occasional blistering of the oral mucosa with small discrete vesicles that heal rapidly without scarring. Generalized recessive dystrophic EB has the most severe involvement of the oral mucosa characterized by microstomia, complete obliteration of the vestibule, and ankyloglossia (Fig. 110-1). With increasing age, structures such as the palatal rugae and lingual papilla typically become unrecognizable because of the presence of continuous blister formation and scarring. In contrast, localized or less severe cases of generalized recessive dystrophic EB do not show the same severity of oral scarring observed in the severe, generalized forms. For example, although the recessive dystrophic EB inversa subtype has marked oral involvement, there tends to be less scarring, with only mild to moderate microstomia, ankyloglossia, and vestibular obliteration. Although different mutations in the type-VII collagen gene have been related to the variable expression observed in EB, the relationship between genotype and phenotype has not been fully characterized.

Individuals with recessive dystrophic and junctional EB are at increased risk for the development of squamous cell carcinomas. Squamous cell carcinomas do occur in the oral cavity of these individuals necessitating diligent oral cancer examinations beginning in early to mid adolescence. Recessive dystrophic and junctional EB are often associated with severe dental problems including the development of rampant dental caries requiring aggressive preventative and restorative approaches. Affected individuals should be counseled regarding optimal caries prevention (e.g., fluoride consumption and dietary considerations regarding frequency and amount of carbohydrate ingestion) beginning by 1 yr of age.

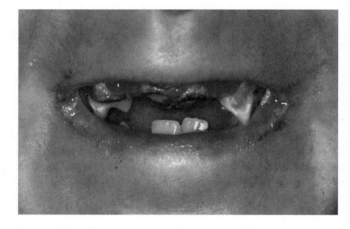

Figure 110-1   The oral cavity of this young child with generalized recessive dystrophic epidermolysis bullosa (EB) displays the marked microstomia, severe dental crowding and rampant caries frequently associated with this form of EB.

HERITABLE CONDITIONS AFFECTING THE HUMAN DENTITION

Development of the human dentition involves a highly orchestrated series of events under strict genetic control. The developmental timing, location, morphology, structure, and composition of teeth are all primarily determined by cascades of molecular events that are regulated by hundreds of genes. Early embryonic requisites for tooth development include the differentiation of the oral ectoderm and the migration of neural crest cells into the craniofacial region in which tooth buds will ultimately form. By approx 6 wk of age (*in utero*) the oral ectoderm begins to proliferate at the future sites of primary teeth. As the oral ectoderm proliferates, it invaginates

Abbreviations

XIII. NEUROLOGY

AChR	acetylcholine receptor
AD	Alzheimer's disease
ADNFLE	autosomal-dominant nocturnal frontal lobe epilepsy
AICD	amyloid intracellular domain
ALS	amyotrophic lateral sclerosis
APLP1	amyloid precursor-like protein 1
APOE	apolipoprotein E
APP	amyloid precursor protein
AR	androgen receptor
AR-JP	autosomal-recessive juvenile parkinsonism
AS	Andersen's syndrome
$A\beta$	amyloid-β-peptide
BACE 1	β-secretase
βAPP	β-amyloid precursor protein
BFNC	benign familial neonatal convulsions
BFPP	bilateral frontoparietal polymicrogyria
BPNH	bilateral periventricular nodular heterotopia
BSE	bovine spongiform encephalopathy
CAE	childhood absence epilepsy
CBP	CREB-binding protein
CHN	congenital hypomyelinating neuropathy
CJD	Creutzfeldt-Jakob disease
CMD	congenital muscular dystrophy
CMS	congenital myasthenic syndrome
CMT	Charcot-Marie-Tooth disease
CMT1	Charcot-Marie-Tooth disease type 1
CMT1A	Charcot-Marie-Tooth disease type 1A
CMT1A-REP	CMT1A repeat sequence
CMT1B	Charcot-Marie-Tooth disease type 1B
CMT2	Charcot-Marie-Tooth disease type 2
CNS	central nervous system
CNTF	ciliary neurotrophic factor
CoQ10	coenzyme Q10
COX 2	cyclooxygenase-2
CRB	CREB-binding protein
CSF	cerebrospinal fluid
CSPGs	chondroitin sulfate proteoglycans
CUG-BP	CUG-binding protein
DCX	doublecortin
DM	myotonic dystrophy
DMH	dorsomedial nucleus of the hypothalamus
DMPK	myotonin protein kinase
DR	dorsal raphe
DRPLA	dentatorubropallidoluysian atrophy
DSN	Dejerine-Sottas neuropathy
EA	episodic ataxia
EA1	episodic ataxia, Type 1
EA2	episodic ataxia, Type 2
EDMD	Emery-Dreifuss muscular dystrophy
EPP	end plate potential
ERM	ezrin-radixin-moesin
ETC	electron transport chain
FAD	familial Alzheimer's disease
FALS	familial amyotrophic lateral sclerosis
FBD	familial British dementia
fCJD	familial Creutzfeldt-Jakob disease
FDCs	follicular dendritic cells
FEN1b	Familial Encephalopathy with Neuroserpin inclusion Bodies
FERM	Four.1-ezrin-radixin-moesin
FFI	fatal familial insomnia
FHM	familial hemiplegic migraine
FISH	fluorescent *in situ* hybridization
FKRP	fukutin-related protein
FLNA	filamin A
FMRP	FMR1 gene product
FRAXA	fragile X, type A
FRAXE	fragile X, type E
FRDA	Friedreich ataxia
FS	febrile seizures
FTD	Frontotemporal dementias
GABA	γ-aminobutyric acid
GABA$_A$	γ aminobutyric acid receptor type A
GAPs	GTPase-activating proteins
GDNF	glial cell-derived neurotrophic factor
GEFS+	generalized epilepsy with febrile seizures plus
GLRA1	α1 subunit of the glycine receptor
GPe	external segment of the globus pallidus
GPI	glycosyl phosphotidylinositol
GPi	internal segment of the globus pallidus
GSS	Gerstmann-Sträussler-Scheinker
HD	Huntington's disease
HDAC	histone deacetylase
HLA	human leukocyte antigen
HMSN	hereditary motor and sensory neuropathies
HNPP	hereditary neuropathy with liability to pressure palsies
HRS	Haw River syndrome
HSP	hereditary familial spastic paraplegia
HyperPP	hyperkalemic periodic paralysis
HypoPP	hypokalemic periodic paralysis
ICEGTC	intractable childhood epilepsy with generalized tonic-clonic seizures

IDE	insulin-degrading enzyme		REM	rapid eye movement
IGE	idiopathic generalized epilepsy		RFLP	restriction fragment length polymorphic
IL	interleukin		RLS	restless legs syndrome
IR	insulin receptor		ROS	reactive oxygen species
JME	juvenile myoclonic epilepsy		SALS	sporadic amyotrophic lateral sclerosis
LBs	Lewy bodies		SBH	subcortical band heterotopia
LBV	Lewy body variant		SBMA	spinobulbar muscular atrophy
LC	locus coeruleus		SCA	spinocerebellar ataxias
LCH	lissencephaly with cerebellar hypoplasia		SCA1	SCA type 1
LNs	Lewy neurites		SCA17	SCA type 17
LRP	lipoprotein-related		SCA2	SCA type 2
LVH	left-ventricular hypertrophy		SCA6	SCA type 6
MAG	myelin-associated glycoprotein		SCA7	SCA type 7
MBM	meat and bone meal		SCI	spinal cord injury
MC	myotonia congenita		sCJD	sporadic Creutzfeldt-Jakob disease
MCDs	malformations of cortical development		SCN	suprachiasmatic nucleus
MJD	Machado-Joseph disease		Sinc	scrapie incubation
MPNST	malignant peripheral nerve sheath tumor		SMA	spinal muscular atrophy
MPP$^+$	1-methyl-4-phenylpyridium		SMEI	severe myoclonic epilepsy of infancy
MPTP	1-methyl-4-phenyl-1,2,3,6-tetrahydropyridine		SMN	survival motor neuron protein
MSLT	Multiple Sleep Latency Test		SN	substantia nigra
NAIP	anti-apoptotic protein		SNpc	substantia nigra pars compacta
NCVs	nerve conduction velocities		SNpr	substantia nigra pars reticulata
NF	neurofibromatosis		SOD1	superoxide dismutase
NF-H	heavy neurofilament subunit		SOD2	Mn-dependent superoxide dismutase
NF-L	light neurofilament subunit		SOD3	Cu/Zn-dependent superoxide dismutase
NGF	nerve growth factor		SPZ	subparaventricular zone
NgR	Nogo-66 receptor		STN	subthalamic nucleus
NREM	non-rapid eye movement		TBP	TATA-binding protein
OEC	olfactory ensheathing cell		TGFα	transforming growth factor α
OMgp	oligodendrocyte myelin glycoprotein		TMN	tuberomammillary nucleus
PAB2	poly A binding protein 2		TNFα	tumor necrosis factor-α
PAEL-R	parkin-associated endothelin-like receptor		Tr	Trembler
PAM	potassium aggravated myotonia		TSEs	transmissible spongiform encephalopathies
PD	Parkinson's disease		UCH	ubiquitin C-terminal hydrolase
PK2	prokineticin 2		vCJD	variant Creutzfeldt-Jakob disease
PLMS	periodic limb movements of sleep		VEGF	vascular endothelial factor
PLS	primary lateral sclerosis		VLPO	ventrolateral preoptic area
PMC	paramyotonia congenita		Vm	membrane potential
PNS	peripheral nervous system		VS	vestibular schwannomas
PPT/LDT	pedunculopontine and laterodorsal tegmental nuclei		WHO	World Health Organization
			WT	wild-type
PrD	prion-forming domain		XLAG	X-linked lissencephaly with abnormal genitalia
PS1	presenilin 1			
PS2	Presenilin 2		X-SBMA	X-linked spinal bulbar muscular atrophy
RAGs	regeneration-associated genes		ZNF9	zinc finger protein 9
RBD	rapid eye movement sleep behavior disorder			

111 The Genetic Basis of Human Cerebral Cortical Malformations

BERNARD S. CHANG AND CHRISTOPHER A. WALSH

SUMMARY

Malformations of cortical development occur when the normal process of brain development is disrupted. With the widespread use of high-resolution neuroimaging, brain malformations are increasingly being recognized as a relatively common cause of refractory epilepsy, mental retardation, and other neurological disorders. The molecular and genetic bases of many cortical malformations have been elucidated in recent years, both expanding our understanding of the underlying biological processes in brain development and informing our approach to these disorders in clinical practice. This chapter highlights some of these malformations, including disorders of microcephaly, gray matter heterotopia, lissencephaly syndromes, and polymicrogyria.

Key Words: Cobblestone complex syndromes; heterotopia; lissencephaly; malformation of cortical development; microcephaly; neuronal migration disorder; polymicrogyria.

INTRODUCTION

The development of the cerebral cortex is an intricate process that culminates in the formation and organization of the most complex network in the human body, that of the neurons that reside in the ribbon of gray matter at the surface of the brain. Understanding of this developmental process has taken on new clinical importance, as disorders caused by disruptions in this process, termed malformations of cortical development (MCDs), are substantially more prevalent than previously recognized. In fact, MCDs are now a common diagnosis in cases of refractory epilepsy and mental retardation that were previously unexplained. The elucidation of MCDs on a molecular and genetic level has thus expanded understanding of the underlying biological processes at work, and influenced the approach to these disorders in common neurological practice. This chapter highlights some of the MCDs whose genetic foundations have been elucidated.

DEVELOPMENT OF THE CEREBRAL CORTEX

Initially, neuronal precursors proliferate in regions deep in the brain; most excitatory pyramidal neurons originate in a region lining the lateral ventricle (the ventricular zone), whereas inhibitory interneurons appear to originate from precursors in the ganglionic eminences of the embryonic brain. Neuronal precursors then migrate outward toward the brain surface to form the neurons of the developing cortex. The molecular mechanisms underlying this migration are still being elucidated, but the process extends over a long period spanning much of the first half of human gestation. Finally, the cerebral cortex, once populated with neurons, undergoes organizational changes during which gyration, lamination, and the formation of proper synaptic connections occur.

CLASSIFICATION OF MCDS

Although the steps described earlier temporally overlap to a significant extent, and some disorders may result from abnormalities in more than one successive step, MCDs are often classified according to the developmental stage that is disrupted in their pathogenesis. Disorders of neuronal proliferation include both those with increased proliferation (such as megalencephaly, characterized by a larger cerebral cortex than normal) and those with decreased proliferation (such as microcephaly vera or small cortex). Disorders of neuronal migration lead to some of the most striking abnormalities of cerebral cortical architecture, because failure of some neurons to migrate properly to the brain surface can result in regions of misplaced neurons called gray matter heterotopia. Finally, disorders of cortical organization include those in which gyration and lamination are disrupted, such as polymicrogyria, as well as disorders of neuronal specification and/or maturation, such as focal cortical dysplasia.

DISORDERS OF PROLIFERATION

Primary Microcephaly (Microcephaly Vera) Microcephaly refers to the presence of a small head circumference, generally more than two or three standard deviations below the mean, and implies an underlying disorder of abnormally small brain size. Many forms of microcephaly have associated cortical abnormalities or dysmorphic features, but primary microcephaly (microcephaly vera) refers to those in which the gyral pattern and other aspects of brain anatomy are relatively preserved and other syndromic features are absent. Most patients have mild-to-moderate mental retardation as the predominant clinical finding. Radiologically, brain volumes are reduced but other anatomical abnormalities are absent.

Primary microcephaly is etiologically diverse and many cases likely arise from environmental insults during gestation. Most familial cases of primary microcephaly, however, appear to be inherited in an autosomal-recessive fashion. Five separate loci (MCPH1–MCPH5) have been mapped by homozygosity in consanguineous pedigrees (Table 111-1). No obvious clinical or

From: *Principles of Molecular Medicine, Second Edition*
Edited by: M. S. Runge and C. Patterson © Humana Press, Inc., Totowa, NJ

Table 111-1

Selected Genetic Disorders of Human Cerebral Cortical Development

Name	Clinical features	Radiological features	Inheritance pattern	Chromosome locus	Gene	Molecular pathogenesis
Primary microcephaly	Small head circumference; mild-to-moderate mental retardation	Small brain volumes with anatomy otherwise preserved	Autosomal-recessive	MCPH1 (8p23), MCPH2 (19q13), MCPH3 (9q34), MCPH4 (15q14), MCPH5 (1q31)	Microcephalin (at MCPH1), ASPM (at MCPH5)	Disorder of neuronal progenitor proliferation or survival (because of cell cycle, mitotic, or apoptotic mechanisms)
Cohen syndrome	Microcephaly, facial dysmorphism, joint laxity, retinal dystrophy	Small brain volumes, ?relatively enlarged corpus callosum	Autosomal-recessive	8q22	COH1	?
Bilateral periventricular nodular heterotopia	Seizures; normal cognitive function	Heterotopic gray matter nodules lining the ventricles	X-linked dominant (most common), autosomal-recessive	Xq28	Filamin A	Disorder of neuronal migration (?because of actin cytoskeletal mechanisms)
Subcortical band heterotopia	Mental retardation, cerebral palsy, seizures	Heterotopic gray matter bands between cortex and ventricles	X-linked dominant	Xq22	DCX/XLIS	Disorder of neuronal migration (because of microtubule-associated mechanisms)
Classic lissencephaly	Mental retardation, cerebral palsy, seizures	Smooth brain surface with increased cortical thickness	X-linked, autosomal-recessive	Xq22, 17p13	DCX/XLIS, LIS1	Disorder of neuronal migration (because of microtubule-associated mechanisms) or progenitor proliferation and survival (for LIS1)
Lissencephaly with cerebellar hypoplasia	Cognitive and motor delay, ataxia, seizures	Lissencephaly with dysplastic hippocampi and severe cerebellar hypoplasia	Autosomal-recessive	7q22	RELN	Disorder of neuronal migration (because of detachment from radial glial cells and/or microtubule-associated mechanisms)
X-linked lissencephaly with abnormal genitalia	Mental retardation, epilepsy, ambiguous genitalia	Lissencephaly with absence of corpus callosum	X-linked recessive	Xp22	ARX	Disorder of neuronal migration
Cobblestone complex syndromes (Walker-Warburg syndrome, muscle-eye-brain disease, Fukuyama congenital muscular dystrophy)	Developmental delay, congenital muscular dystrophy, eye abnormalities (in some)	Cobblestone appearance to cortex, often brainstem abnormalities and cerebellar microcysts	Autosomal-recessive	WWS: 9q34; MEB: 1p33-34; FCMD: 9q31	WWS: POMT1; MEB: POMGnT1; FCMD: fukutin	Disorder of neuronal overmigration resulting from dysfunctional glial limiting membrane (?because of impaired glycosylation of α-dystroglycan)
Bilateral perisylvian polymicrogyria	Oromotor dysfunction (predominant), developmental delay, seizures	Polymicrogyria around Sylvian fissures	Autosomal-dominant (most common), X-linked	?, Xq28	?	?
Bilateral frontoparietal polymicrogyria	Developmental delay, dysconjugate gaze, seizures, cerebellar signs	Polymicrogyria of frontoparietal predominance, ventriculomegaly, small brainstem and cerebellum	Autosomal-recessive	16q12.2-21	GPR56	?

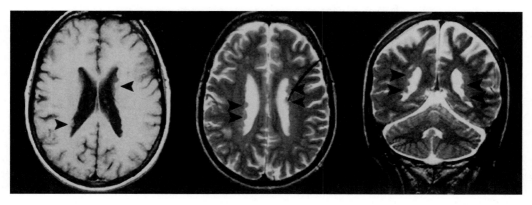

Figure 111-1 MRI appearance of bilateral periventricular nodular heterotopia. From left to right, the T1-weighted axial; T2-weighted axial; and T2-weighted coronal images demonstrate the heterotopic gray matter nodules that line the ventricular wall and protrude into the ventricular lumen (arrowheads). The black streak in the middle image is a mark made by the radiologist on the image to indicate one of the nodules.

radiological signs differentiate among cases linked to these different loci.

Understanding of the molecular pathogenesis of primary microcephaly has been advanced by the identification of the responsible genes at two of the MCPH loci. A novel gene at the MCPH1 locus encodes a protein, microcephalin, which contains a BRCA C-terminal domain. Such domains are present both in proteins controlling the cell cycle and in those involved in DNA repair. Because microcephalin is highly expressed in the ventricular zone of fetal mouse brain (in which neuronal progenitors proliferate), it is reasonable to speculate that disturbances of the progenitors' cell cycle or ability to repair lethal DNA mutations may lead to impaired proliferation or increased cell death and thus, ultimately, decreased brain size.

The second cloned gene, called *ASPM* and located at the MCPH5 locus, is the human orthologue of a *Drosophila* gene that is essential for normal mitotic spindle formation in neuronal progenitors. Because ASPM is highly expressed in the ventricular zone and ganglionic eminences of fetal mouse brain, impaired cell division in neuronal progenitors because of a mitotic spindle abnormality may also be a molecular mechanism leading to the phenotype of decreased cerebral cortical size. A hint at the importance of ASPM in cortical development comes from a comparison of the predicted protein structures of its homologues across multiple species. Progressing from the *C. elegans* homologue to asp in *Drosophila* to Aspm in mice and finally human ASPM, the salient difference is a marked increase in the number of repeated calmodulin-binding "IQ" domains, whereas the remainder of the protein is generally conserved. Although the function of these "IQ" domains is not known, these findings suggest that they play a key role in determining brain size.

Cohen Syndrome Many syndromic disorders feature small head size as an important clinical characteristic. One of these, Cohen syndrome, is an autosomal-recessive disorder over-represented in Finland that is characterized by cognitive and motor retardation, microcephaly, unusual facial features, joint laxity, retinochoroidal dystrophy, and intermittent neutropenia. Mutations in a novel gene called *COH1*, located on chromosome 8q22, have been found in patients with the classic Cohen syndrome phenotype. Analysis of the predicted protein sequence suggests that COH1 may have a role in intracellular protein transport and sorting. Further investigation into the genetic etiologies of other syndromic microcephaly disorders

may reveal common molecular features that help to explain how cerebral cortical size is determined.

DISORDERS OF MIGRATION

Bilateral Periventricular Nodular Heterotopia Bilateral periventricular nodular heterotopia (BPNH) is characterized by the presence of heterotopic, or misplaced, nodules of gray matter that line the lateral ventricles deep in the brain, typically in a bilaterally symmetric fashion (Fig. 111-1). Patients most commonly have normal intellectual and neurological function except for seizures, which typically begin during the adolescent years. Pathologically, these nodules contain mature neurons with normal morphology but varying orientations and no laminar organization, whereas the cerebral cortex appears to maintain its normal six-layered architecture.

Early reports of families with BPNH described the presence of multiple affected females, a higher-than-expected rate of spontaneous abortions, and a shortage of male offspring, suggesting an X-linked dominant inheritance pattern. Subsequently, the responsible gene for BPNH was identified as *filamin A* (*FLNA*), located on chromosome Xq28. FLNA is an intracellular actin-crosslinking protein that is essential for cell locomotion. The leading pathogenetic explanation for BPNH is that heterozygous females (who express the mutant *FLNA* allele in half of their neurons because of X-inactivation) exhibit these periventricular nodules because some of their neurons fail to migrate away from the ventricular surface, whereas the remaining neurons migrate properly and form the normally layered cerebral cortex. Males hemizygous for the mutation (who carry the mutant *FLNA* allele on their only X chromosome and must express the mutant protein in all of their neurons) usually demonstrate prenatal lethality.

There is both genetic and phenotypic heterogeneity to this disorder, however. An autosomal-recessive form of periventricular heterotopia has been described, for example. In addition, it appears that prenatal lethality is mostly associated with null *FLNA* mutations, whereas males with less severe *FLNA* mutations (such as those that lead to distal truncation of the protein) may survive and demonstrate a typical X-linked BPNH phenotype similar to that seen in females. The phenotypic spectrum of FLNA abnormalities has been expanded further by the identification of *FLNA* mutations in patients with a number of congenital malformations affecting non-nervous system organs, including the craniofacial structures, skeleton, viscera, and genitourinary tract.

Subcortical Band Heterotopia Subcortical band heterotopia (SBH) or "double cortex" syndrome is a cortical malformation in which heterotopic bands of gray matter are present
bilaterally, traversing the white matter between the cerebral cortex
and the lateral ventricle in an orientation generally parallel to the
ventricle. Most patients with SBH are females who have mental
retardation, cerebral palsy, and epilepsy to varying degrees.

The responsible gene for this disorder was identified on chromosome Xq22 and labeled *doublecortin (DCX)* or *XLIS,* as males
with mutations in this gene have a separate phenotype called
X-linked lissencephaly, discussed later. In an analogous fashion to
the suspected pathogenesis of BPNH, females may express the
mutant *DCX/XLIS* allele in half of their neurons, which presumably fail to migrate fully to the cortical surface and form the subcortical heterotopic band of gray matter, whereas hemizygous
males express the mutant allele in all neurons and demonstrate a
more severe phenotype with a generalized disorder of migration
affecting all cerebral cortical neurons.

The role of the DCX protein in neuronal migration has become
increasingly clear. DCX is associated with microtubules and
appears to serve a stabilizing function; its structure features novel
microtubule-binding domains that occur in tandem. It physically
interacts with LIS1, another microtubule-associated protein associated with a lissencephaly phenotype when mutated (*see* Classical
Lissencephaly). LIS1 interacts with a complex of proteins that play
a role in regulating microtubule dynamics. Therefore, the likely
molecular mechanism of SBH pathogenesis is an alteration in
microtubule function that impairs neuronal migration.

Non-Mendelian factors, such as reduced penetrance and
somatic mosaicism, are commonly present in those with
DCX/XLIS mutations and thus affect the clinical expression of
these mutations. These findings have a significant impact on the
questions of whether asymptomatic parents of children with SBH
should be radiologically and genetically tested and how SBH
patients and their parents should be counseled about recurrence
risks in future offspring.

Classical Lissencephaly Classical lissencephaly is characterized by a smooth brain surface with an absence of gyri and sulci and
by an abnormal cortical lamination, usually featuring four rather
than six layers. The clinical presentation of lissencephaly involves
mental retardation, cerebral palsy to varying degrees, and epilepsy
including a number of different seizure types. Radiologically, the
cortical thickness is increased and the gyral/sulcal pattern is simplified, with a smooth appearance to the cortical surface.

Two separate genetic etiologies lead to classical lissencephaly
in its isolated form: hemizygous mutations in *DCX/XLIS,* described
earlier, and heterozygous (dominantly inherited) mutations in *LIS1,*
on chromosome 17p13. Although some radiological features help
differentiate between *DCX/XLIS* and *LIS1* cases, in particular an
anterior vs posterior predominance to the malformed cortex, the
phenotypes are broadly similar. It was the study of Miller-Dieker
syndrome, characterized by the combination of severe classical
lissencephaly and associated facial dysmorphism, that led to the
initial identification of the autosomal 17p locus for lissencephaly;
it now appears that Miller-Dieker syndrome is caused by chromosome 17p deletions that encompass both *LIS1* and other neighboring
genes.

As described earlier, the LIS1 protein (also known as
PAFAH1b1 or the platelet-activating factor acetylhydrolase β-1
subunit) appears to interact both with DCX and with other mem-

bers of a microtubule-associated complex, including NudE and
NudEL. However, its other functions may be relevant to earlier
steps in cortical development, particularly neuronal proliferation
and survival. Therefore, although classical lissencephaly is usually
thought of as primarily a migration disorder, it may be that two
sequential molecular mechanisms play a role in this malformation's pathogenesis.

Lissencephaly With Cerebellar Hypoplasia Lissencephaly
with cerebellar hypoplasia (LCH) is characterized by lissencephaly
that is more severe frontally than posteriorly and is accompanied
by severe hypoplasia of the cerebellum (often to the extent that
only a portion of the vermis is present), dysplastic-appearing hippocampi, and a small pons. Clinical features in two original families who demonstrated LCH with autosomal-recessive inheritance
consisted of severe cognitive and motor delay and seizures.

The identification of the gene responsible for LCH as *RELN*
(located on chromosome 7q22) represented the culmination of a
long series of investigations beginning with the reeler mouse, a
spontaneously occurring mutant so called because of a staggering
gait and originally described more than 50 yr ago. The reeler
mouse exhibits an unusual cerebral cortical architecture, consisting
of an "upside-down" cortex in which the normal six layers are
essentially inverted. Cerebellar and hippocampal abnormalities
are also present. Mutations in a mouse gene termed *Reln* were
identified in reeler, and the discovery of the human orthologue followed. Because of the similarities between the reeler mouse and
human LCH phenotypes, the human *RELN* locus was tested for
linkage to this disorder and *RELN* gene mutations subsequently
found in affected LCH patients.

The function of the reelin protein has been the subject of interest and investigation. Reelin binds the very low-density lipoprotein receptor, apolipoprotein E receptor 2, and extracellular matrix
proteins such as integrins and protocadherins. In vitro experiments
have demonstrated that reelin appears to cause migrating neurons
to detach from the radial glial cells that serve as their guideposts,
possibly through its interaction with integrins, which mediate
cell–cell adhesion. In addition, reelin also participates in a signaling
pathway through the transmembrane receptors listed earlier that
may eventually affect proteins known to be associated with microtubule organization. Thus, the molecular pathogenesis of LCH
may involve disrupted neuronal migration through more than one
mechanism, including both cell locomotion and adhesion to radial
glial guideposts.

X-Linked Lissencephaly With Abnormal Genitalia X-linked
lissencephaly with abnormal genitalia (XLAG) is characterized by
a distinctive form of lissencephaly that is worse posteriorly than
anteriorly and features only a moderately increased cortical thickness. In addition, the clinical syndrome includes absence of the
corpus callosum, hypothalamic dysfunction, severe epilepsy, and
ambiguous male genitalia. Multiple loss-of-function mutations in
ARX, the human orthologue of the Aristaless-related homeobox
gene in *Drosophila,* have now been identified in patients with X-
linked lissencephaly with abnormal genitalia. The predicted
ARX protein contains two conserved domains, a DNA-binding
homeodomain and a C-peptide (aristaless) domain whose function is not known, and is likely to play a role in transcriptional
regulation.

Mutations in the *ARX* gene are one of the most striking examples of allelic heterogeneity in the field of developmental brain
disorders. The range of phenotypes now linked to *ARX* mutations

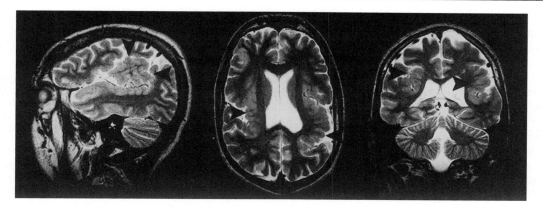

Figure 111-2   MRI appearance of bilateral perisylvian polymicrogyria. From left to right, T2, weighted sagittal, axial, and coronal images demonstrate the excessive number of small gyri (and irregular appearance of the gray–white junction) in the regions around the Sylvian fissure bilaterally (arrowheads).

encompasses such diverse disorders as infantile spasms, Partington syndrome (mental retardation with hand and wrist dystonia), nonsyndromic mental retardation, and autism. In one case, bilateral cerebral and cerebellar cysts, presumably developmental in origin, were seen.

Many of the documented *ARX* mutations lead to predicted polyalanine tract expansions, raising the possibility that toxic protein aggregation, similar to that seen in polyglutamine neurodegenerative disorders, might play a role in their pathogenesis.

Cobblestone Complex Syndromes   Cobblestone complex (formerly "cobblestone lissencephaly" or type II lissencephaly) is a term applied to a group of brain malformations that are distinctly different from classical lissencephaly histologically. In cobblestone syndromes, the brain surface actually has an irregular appearance in some places, because of the presence of heterotopic tissue. This tissue consists of glioneuronal elements that appear to have overmigrated out of the brain through discontinuities in the glial limiting membrane at the brain surface. Cobblestone complex is typically seen in association with congenital muscular dystrophy (CMD) and is a defining part of the phenotype of such disorders as Walker-Warburg syndrome, muscle-eye-brain disease, and Fukuyama CMD. Clinically, these disorders range widely in severity: Walker-Warburg patients typically die in infancy, for example, whereas Fukuyama patients can survive into young adulthood. On radiological images, cobblestone complex is often associated with brainstem abnormalities and cerebellar microcysts.

Understanding of these syndromes' molecular pathogenesis has begun to coalesce with the identification of genes responsible for all three prototypic disorders. Fukuyama CMD is caused by mutations in the *fukutin* gene; the founder mutation present in Japanese patients is a retrotransposal insertion that leads to decreased protein expression. Muscle-eye-brain disease is associated with loss-of-function mutations in a gene called *POMGnT1*. Some patients with Walker-Warburg syndrome have mutations in the *POMT1* gene, although this disorder is genetically heterogeneous and other Walker-Warburg genes remain unidentified.

These three genes all appear to encode glycosyltransferases, enzymes that chemically modify other proteins by adding sugar groups. In these cobblestone disorders, one target, if not the major one, of these glycosyltransferases appears to be α-dystroglycan, a protein that forms part of the laminin-associated complex linking the cytoskeleton to the extracellular matrix. Because laminin abnormalities occur in CMD, the natural implication is that defi-cient glycosylation of α -dystroglycan is the molecular mechanism underlying the muscle disorder in these conditions.

Whether faulty α-dystroglycan modification is also responsible for the apparent overmigration of neurons in the brain is being investigated. The finding that mutations in a gene encoding a fukutin-related protein lead to CMD without any brain malformation suggests that the specific molecular defect underlying the migrational disorder may be elucidated by detailed functional studies of the glycosyltransferases encoded by these genes.

DISORDERS OF CEREBRAL CORTICAL ORGANIZATION

Bilateral Polymicrogyria Syndromes   Polymicrogyria is a cortical malformation characterized by an excessive number of abnormally small gyri. Histologically, affected cortex is usually disorganized and lacks a normal six-layered architecture. Radiologically, polymicrogyria may be distinguished from other malformations such as pachygyria by the irregular "scalloped" appearance of the gray–white junction and an increase in the apparent cortical thickness. Although polymicrogyria can arise from environmental insults, several syndromes of region-specific symmetric polymicrogyria have been described, some or all of which are genetic.

Bilateral perisylvian polymicrogyria, for example, is a disorder in which the cortex surrounding the Sylvian fissure is polymicrogyric; often, the Sylvian fissure is abnormally oriented as well (Fig. 111-2). Clinically, patients have a highly distinctive presentation dominated by oromotor dysfunction, ranging in severity from a mild speech impediment to life-threatening feeding difficulties in infancy. Many patients also have mental retardation and seizures. The disorder appears to be genetically heterogeneous, with the most common inheritance pattern being autosomal-dominant. X-linked inheritance has also been seen in some families, and a locus on Xq28 has been reported.

Another region-specific symmetric syndrome, bilateral frontoparietal polymicrogyria, is an autosomal-recessive disorder characterized clinically by developmental delay, seizures, dysconjugate gaze, and cerebellar signs. Radiologically, the polymicrogyria is generalized but exhibits a decreasing anterior-posterior gradient, such that the frontoparietal regions are most severely affected. In addition, white matter signal changes, ventriculomegaly, and hypoplasia of the brainstem and cerebellum are also seen. Bilateral frontoparietal polymicrogyria is caused by mutations in *GPR56*, a gene on chromosome 16g that encodes an orphan G-protein-coupled receptor.

The regional specificity of the malformation in both these syndromes raises the possibility that the genes responsible for their pathogenesis may have an anatomic gradient of expression, or may interact with or be regulated by other factors that may have such a gradient. Alternatively, it may be that particular regions of the cerebral cortex have specific developmental features that make them more susceptible to certain malformative processes.

CONCLUSION

The elucidation of the genetic and molecular basis for many developmental malformations of the brain has been one of the most exciting and important advances in molecular neurology. Major strides in the use of two key investigative tools, magnetic resonance technology and molecular biology, have led to better understanding of how the cerebral cortex normally develops and an appreciation for the myriad consequences that can result when this process is disrupted. With the growing importance of MCDs in the diagnosis and treatment of epilepsy, mental retardation, and other neurological disorders, knowledge gained in this field has immediate relevance to clinical care. Future work on cortical development may allow us to provide more refined treatments and prognoses for those afflicted by these disorders.

ACKNOWLEDGMENTS

B.S.C. was supported by the Clinical Investigator Training Program of Beth Israel Deaconess Medical Center, Harvard-MIT Division of Health Sciences and Technology, and Pfizer, Inc. C.A.W. was supported by grants from the National Institute of Neurological Disorders and Stroke (R37 NS35129), the McKnight Foundation, and the March of Dimes, and is an Investigator of the Howard Hughes Medical Institute.

SELECTED REFERENCES

Aigner L, Uyanik G, Couillard-Despres S, et al. Somatic mosaicism and variable penetrance in doublecortin-associated migration disorders. Neurology 2003;60:329–332.

Anton ES, Kreidberg JA, Rakic P. Distinct functions of a3 and av integrin receptors in neuronal migration and laminar organization of the cerebral cortex. Neuron 1999;22:277–289.

Barkovich AJ. Imaging of the cobblestone lissencephalies. AJNR Am J Neuroradiol 1996;17:615–618.

Barkovich AJ, Kuzniecky RI. Neuroimaging of focal malformations of cortical development. J Clin Neurophysiol 1996;13:481–494.

Barkovich AJ, Kuziecky RI. Gray matter heterotopia. Neurology 2000;55:1603–1608.

Barkovich AJ, Kuzniecky RI, Jackson GD, Guerrini R, Dobyns WB. Classification system for malformations of cortical development: Update 2001. Neurology 2001;57:2168–2178.

Beltrán-Valero de Bernabé D, Currier S, Steinbrecher A, et al. Mutations in the O-Mannosyltransferase gene POMT1 give rise to the severe neuronal migration disorder Walker-Warburg syndrome. Am J Hum Genet 2002;71:1033–1043.

Bienvenu T, Poirier K, Friocourt G, et al. ARX, a novel Prd-class-homeobox gene highly expressed in the telencephalon, is mutated in X-linked mental retardation. Hum Mol Genet 2002;11:981–991.

Bond J, Roberts E, Mochida GH, et al. ASPM is a major determinant of cerebral cortical size. Nat Genet 2002;32:316–320.

Brockington M, Blake DJ, Prandini P, et al. Mutations in the fukutin-related protein gene (FKRP) cause a form of congenital muscular dystrophy with secondary laminin a2 deficiency and abnormal glycosylation of a-dystroglycan. Am J Hum Genet 2001;69:1198–1209.

Cardoso C, Leventer RJ, Ward HL, et al. Refinement of a 400-kb critical region allows genotypic differentiation between isolated lissencephaly,

Miller-Dieker syndrome, and other phenotypes secondary to deletions of 17p13.3. Am J Hum Genet 2003;72:918–930.

Caspi M, Atlas R, Kantor A, Sapir T, Reiner O. Interaction between LIS1 and doublecortin, two lissencephaly gene products. Hum Mol Genet 2000;9:2205–2213.

Chang BS, Piao X, Bodell A, et al. Bilateral frontoparietal polymicrogyria: Clinical and radiological features in 10 families with linkage to chromosome 16. Ann Neurol 2003;53:596–606.

Corbin JG, Nery S, Fishell G. Telencephalic cells take a tangent: nonradial migration in the mammalian forebrain. Nat Neurosci 2001;4:1177–1182.

Couillard-Despres S, Winkler J, Uyanik G, Aigner L. Molecular mechanisms of neuronal migration disorders, quo vadis? Curr Mol Med 2001;1:677–688.

Crino PB, Miyata H, Vinters H. Neurodevelopmental disorders as a cause of seizures: neuropathologic, genetic, and mechanistic considerations. Brain Pathol 2002;12:212–233.

D'Arcangelo G, Miao GG, Chen SC, et al. A protein related to extracellular matrix proteins deleted in the mouse mutant reeler. Nature 1995;374:719–723.

des Portes V, Pinard JM, Billuart P, et al. A novel CNS gene required for neuronal migration and involved in X-linked subcortical laminar heterotopia and lissencephaly syndrome. Cell 1998;92:51–61.

DeSilva U, D'arcangelo G, Braden UV, et al. The human reelin gene: isolation, sequencing, and mapping on chromosome 7. Genome Res 1997;7:157–164.

Dobyns WB, Berry-Kravis E, Havernick NJ, Holden KR, Viskochil D. X-linked lissencephaly with absent corpus callosum and ambiguous genitalia. Am J Med Genet 1999;86:331–337.

Dobyns WB, Truwit CL, Ross ME, et al. Differences in the gyral pattern distinguish chromosome 17-linked and X-linked lissencephaly. Neurology 1999;53:270–277.

Eksioglu YZ, Scheffer IE, Cardenas P, et al. Periventricular heterotopia: an X-linked dominant epilepsy locus causing aberrant cerebral cortical development. Neuron 1996;16:77–87.

Fox JW, Lamperti ED, Eksioglu YZ, et al. Mutations in filamin 1 prevent migration of cerebral cortical neurons in human periventricular heterotopia. Neuron 1999;21:1315–1325.

Gambello MJ, Darling DL, Yingling J, Tanaka T, Gleeson JG, Wynshaw-Boris A. Multiple dose-dependent effects of Lis1 on cerebral cortical development. J Neurosci 2003;23:1719–1729.

Gleeson JG. Classical lissencephaly and double cortex (subcortical band heterotopia): LIS1 and doublecortin. Curr Opin Neurol. 2000;13:121–125.

Gleeson JG, Walsh CA. Neuronal migration disorders: from genetic diseases to developmental mechanisms. Trends Neurosci 2000;23:352–359.

Gleeson JG, Allen KA, Fox JW, et al. Doublecortin, a brain-specific gene mutated in human X-linked lissencephaly and double cortex syndrome, encodes a putative signaling protein. Cell 1998;92:63–72.

Guerreiro MM, Andermann E, Guerrini R, et al. Familial perisylvian polymicrogyria: a new familial syndrome of cortical maldevelopment. Ann Neurol 2000;48:39–48.

Guerrini R, Barkovich AJ, Sztriha L, Dobyns WB. Bilateral frontal polymicrogyria: a newly recognized brain malformation syndrome. Neurology 2000;54:909–913.

Guerrini R, Dubeau F, Dulac O, et al. Bilateral parasagittal parietooccipital polymicrogyria and epilepsy. Ann Neurol 1997;41:65–73.

Harding B, Copp AJ. Malformations. In: Graham DI, Lantos PL, eds. Greenfield's Neuropathology, 6th ed., London: Arnold, 1997; pp. 397–533.

Hong SE, Shugart YY, Huang DT, et al. Autosomal recessive lissencephaly with cerebellar hypoplasia is associated with human RELN mutations. Nat Genet 2000;26:93–96.

Huyton T, Bates PA, Zhang X, Sternberg MJ, Freemont PS. The BRCA1 C-terminal domain: structure and function. Mutat Res 2000;460:319–332.

Jackson AP, Eastwood H, Bell SM, et al. Identification of microcephalin, a protein implicated in determining the size of the human brain. Am J Hum Genet 2002;71:136–142.

Jackson AP, McHale DP, Campbell DA, et al. Primary autosomal recessive microcephaly (MCPH1) maps to chromosome 8p22-pter. Am J Hum Genet 1998;63:541–546.

Jamieson CR, Fryns JP, Jacobs J, et al. Primary autosomal recessive microcephaly: MCPH5 maps to 1q25-q32. Am J Hum Genet 2000; 67:1575–1577.

Jamieson CR, Govaerts C, Abramowicz MJ. Primary autosomal recessive microcephaly: homozygosity mapping of MCPH4 to chromosome 15. Am J Hum Genet 1999;65:1465–1469.

Kim MH, Cierpicki T, Derewenda U, et al. The DCX-domain tandems of doublecortin and doublecortin-like kinase. Nat Struct Biol 2003; 10:324–333.

Kitamura K, Yanazawa M, Sugiyama N, et al. Mutation of ARX causes abnormal development of forebrain and testes in mice and X-linked lissencephaly with abnormal genitalia in humans. Nat Genet 2002;32:359–369.

Kivitie-Kallio S, Norio R. Cohen syndrome: essential features, natural history, and heterogeneity. Am J Med Genet 2001;102:125–135.

Kobayashi K, Nakahori Y, Miyake M, et al. An ancient retrotransposal insertion causes Fukuyama-type congenital muscular dystrophy. Nature 1998;394:388–392.

Kolehmainen J, Black GCM, Saarinen A, et al. Cohen syndrome is caused by mutations in a novel gene, COH1, encoding a transmembrane protein with a presumed role in vesicle-mediated sorting and intracellular protein transport. Am J Hum Genet 2003;72:1359–1369.

Leventer RJ, Cardoso C, Ledbetter DH, Dobyns WB. LIS1: from cortical malformation to essential protein of cellular dynamics. Trends Neurosci 2001;24:489–492.

Marin O, Rubenstein JLR. A long, remarkable journey: tangential migration in the telencephalon. Nat Rev Neurosci 2001;2:780–790.

Mercuri E, Sewry C, Brown SC, Muntoni F. Congenital muscular dystrophies. Semin Pediatr Neurol 2002;9:120–131.

Michele DE, Barresi R, Kanagawa M, et al. Post-translational disruption of dystroglycan-ligand interactions in congenital muscular dystrophies. Nature 2002;418:417–422.

Mochida GH, Walsh CA. Molecular genetics of human microcephaly. Curr Opin Neurol 2001;14:151–156.

Moore SA, Saito F, Chen J, et al. Deletion of brain dystroglycan recapitulates aspects of congenital muscular dystrophy. Nature 2002;418:422–425.

Moynihan L, Jackson AP, Roberts E, et al. A third novel locus for primary autosomal recessive microcephaly maps to chromosome 9q34. Am J Hum Genet 2000;66:724–727.

Nadarajah B, Parnavelas JG. Modes of neuronal migration in the developing cerebral cortex. Nat Rev Neurosci 2002;3:423–432.

Olson EC, Walsh CA. Smooth, rough and upside-down neocortical development. Curr Opin Genet Dev 2002;12:320–327.

Pattison L, Crow YJ, Deeble VJ, et al. A fifth locus for primary autosomal recessive microcephaly maps to chromosome 1q31. Am J Hum Genet 2000;67:1578–1580.

Piao X, Basel-Vanagaite L, Straussberg R, et al. An autosomal recessive form of bilateral frontoparietal polymicrogyria maps to chromosome 16q12.2-21. Am J Hum Genet 2002;70:1028–1033.

Piao X, Hill RS, Bodell A, et al. G protein-coupled receptor-dependent development of human frontal cortex. Science 2004;303:2033–2036.

Pilz D, Stoodley N, Golden JA. Neuronal migration, cerebral cortical development, and cerebral cortical anomalies. J Neuropathol Exp Neurol 2002;61:1–11.

Raybaud CGN, Canto-Moreira N, Poncet M. High-definition magnetic resonance imaging identification of cortical dysplasias: micropolygyria versus lissencephaly. In: Guerrini R, Canapicchi R, Zifkin BG, et al., eds. Dysplasias of Cerebral Cortex and Epilepsy. Philadelphia: Lippincott-Raven, 1996, pp. 57–64.

Reiner O, Carrozzo R, Shen Y, et al. Isolation of a Miller-Dieker lissencephaly gene containing G protein ß-subunit-like repeats. Nature 1993;364: 717–721.

Rice DS, Curran T. Role of the reelin signaling pathway in central nervous system development. Annu Rev Neurosci 2001;24:1005–1039.

Roberts E, Hampshire DJ, Pattison L, et al. Autosomal recessive primary microcephaly: an analysis of locus heterogeneity and phenotypic variation. J Med Genet 2002;39:718–721.

Roberts E, Jackson AP, Carradice AC, et al. The second locus for autosomal recessive primary microcephaly (MCPH2) maps to chromosome 19q13.1-13.2. Eur J Hum Genet 1999;7:815–820.

Robertson SP, Twigg SR, Sutherland-Smith AJ, et al. Localized mutations in the gene encoding the cytoskeletal protein filamin A cause diverse malformations in humans. Nat Genet 2003;33:487–491.

Sheen VL, Dixon PH, Fox JW, et al. Mutations in the X-linked filamin 1 gene cause periventricular nodular heterotopia in males as well as in females. Hum Mol Genet 2001;10:1775–1783.

Sheen VL, Topcu M, Berkovic S, et al. Autosomal recessive form of periventricular heterotopia. Neurology 2003;60:1108–1112.

Stossel TP, Condeelis J, Cooley L, et al. Filamins as integrators of cell mechanics and signalling. Nat Rev Mol Cell Biol 2001;2:138–145.

Stromme P, Bakke SJ, Dahl A, Gecz J. Brain cysts associated with mutation in the Aristaless related homeobox gene, ARX. J Neurol Neurosurg Psychiatry 2003;74:536–538.

Stromme P, Mangelsdorf ME, Scheffer IE, Gecz J. Infantile spasms, dystonia, and other X-linked phenotypes caused by mutations in Aristaless related homeobox gene, ARX. Brain Dev 2002;24:266–268.

Stromme P, Mangelsdorf ME, Shaw MA, et al. Mutations in the human ortholog of Aristaless cause X-linked mental retardation and epilepsy. Nat Genet 2002;30:441–445.

Turner G, Partington M, Kerr B, Mangelsdorf M, Gecz J. Variable expression of mental retardation, autism, seizures, and dystonic hand movements in two families with an identical ARX gene mutation. Am J Med Genet 2002;112:405–411.

Villard L, Nguyen K, Cardoso C, et al. A locus for bilateral perisylvian polymicrogyria maps to Xq28. Am J Hum Genet 2002;70:1003–1008.

Yoshida A, Kobayashi K, Manya H, et al. Muscular dystrophy and neuronal migration disorder caused by mutations in a glycosyltransferase, POMGnT1. Dev Cell 2001;1:717–724.

Zoghbi HY, Orr HT. Glutamine repeats and neurodegeneration. Annu Rev Neurosci 2000;23:217–247.

112 Muscular Dystrophies
Molecular Diagnosis

ERIC P. HOFFMAN AND ERYNN S. GORDON

SUMMARY

Muscular dystrophies are generally genetic changes resulting in degeneration (and regeneration) of muscle. Mutations of 29 different genes can cause specific types of muscular dystrophy. The most common form of muscular dystrophy is Duchenne muscular dystrophy, caused by mutations in the dystrophin gene on the X-chromosome, resulting in an absence of the protein dystrophin. Mutations in the same gene cause the less common and less severe Becker muscular dystrophy, characterized by a partial deficiency of the dystrophin protein.

Key Words: Becker; Duchenne; Emery-Dreifuss muscular dystrophy; facioscapulohumeral; merosin; muscular dystrophy; myotonic dystrophy.

INTRODUCTION

Muscular dystrophies are generally genetic changes resulting in degeneration (and regeneration) of muscle. Mutations of 29 different genes can cause specific types of muscular dystrophy. The most common form of muscular dystrophy is Duchenne muscular dystrophy, caused by mutations in the dystrophin gene on the X-chromosome, resulting in an absence of the protein dystrophin. Mutations in the same gene cause the less common and less severe Becker muscular dystrophy, characterized by a partial deficiency of the dystrophin protein. Although mutations in dystrophin are commonly associated with muscular dystrophy in males, approx 10% of females with muscular dystrophy have a mutation in dystrophin resulting in symptoms because of skewed X-inactivation. The pathophysiology of dystrophin abnormalities involves instability of the plasma membrane of myofibers with chronic muscle deterioration leading to weakness. Two other relatively common types of muscular dystrophy include myotonic dystrophy and facioscapulohumeral dystrophy. Presentations of myotonic dystrophy vary greatly, ranging from neonatal lethality, to childhood mental retardation, adult distal weakness with myotonia, or early onset cataracts. Caused by an increase in size of a trinucleotide repeat (CTG) in the 3′ untranslated region of a protein kinase, it is dominantly inherited, with considerable variation in phenotype within families. The size of the expansion generally correlates with disease severity. The mechanism by which the expansion mutation causes the observed multisystemic and variable clinical features appears to be consequential to altered mRNA metabolism within cells. Facioscapulohumeral dystrophy is dominantly inherited and involves a deletion of a subtelomeric region of 4q, with a complex molecular pathophysiology.

Mutations of 26 additional genes for less common forms of muscular dystrophy have been identified. Many of these involve components of the myofiber plasma membrane and extracellular basal lamina (dysferlin [involved in vesicle traffic]; four different sarcoglycan genes [interact with dystrophin]; caveolin 3 [vesicle traffic]; fukutin, and fukutin-related protein [glycosidases]; collagen VI [three subunit genes]; and integrin α7).

One of the major structural components of the myofiber basal lamina, α2 laminin, causes approx 40% of neonatal onset disease, congenital muscular dystrophy. In addition to profound weakness at birth, these patients show marked abnormalities of white matter by MRI studies, yet are intellectually normal. Abnormalities in two nuclear membrane components cause either X-linked recessive (emerin protein) or autosomal-dominant (lamin A/C) Emery-Dreifuss muscular dystrophy (EDMD) with contractures and cardiac conduction defect. Another nuclear protein, poly(A)-binding protein (PAB) 2 shows a late-onset oculopharyngeal dystrophy. Mutations of calpain III, a muscle-specific membrane-bound protease, might be a relatively common cause of dystrophy in patients with normal dystrophin. Of the 29 genes causing muscular dystrophies, 15 fall under the umbrella of limb-girdle muscular dystrophy. Most patients carrying the descriptive diagnosis of limb-girdle muscular dystrophy have a recessively inherited disease, although rare families with late-onset dominant inheritance have been described.

Of the 29 genes for which mutations cause subtypes of muscular dystrophy, 13 result from abnormalities of the plasma membrane and adjacent basal lamina. Myofibers likely have a stringent requirement for a durable and resilient plasma membrane based on two features of its normal physiology and function. First, each contraction of the myofibrils leads to a rapid and dramatic redistribution of the cytoplasm, resulting in changes of the shape of the myofiber. These shape changes would be expected to impart considerable stresses on the plasma membrane. Second, the force generated by the myofibrils must be transduced to the extracellular matrix so that the muscle group can contract and generate force as a single coordinated unit. Thus, this force transduction must be transmitted through the plasma membrane, which must be strongly

From: *Principles of Molecular Medicine, Second Edition*
Edited by: M. S. Runge and C. Patterson © Humana Press, Inc., Totowa, NJ

reinforced to withstand these sheer forces. The study of human disease has been critical in both identifying components of the myofiber membrane cytoskeleton and in determining the relative functions of many of the components. Six distinct human inherited muscular dystrophies have been identified which are caused by deficiencies of the membrane cytoskeleton: one intracellular component (dystrophin; Duchenne muscular dystrophy), four trans-membrane components (α-, β-, γ-, and δ-sarcoglycans) and one extracellular component (α2 laminin). The muscular dystrophies caused by deficiency of dystrophin or any of the four sarcoglycans are similar histologically and clinically. This observation suggests that the progressive muscle diseases caused by these proteins might all share a similar pathogenesis, namely, chronic membrane instability leading to progressive dysfunction of the muscle, and that all of the sarcoglycans and dystrophin are required for membrane stability. The deficiency of the extracellular component, α2 laminin, results in a more complicated and severe phenotype (congenital muscular dystrophy), with apparent involvement of the immune system in tissue pathology, and also abnormalities of myofiber regeneration. Other neonatal onset congenital muscular dystrophies result from defects in glycosylation of proteins, and thus their appropriate interaction between the myofiber plasma membrane and extracellular basal lamina.

PLASMA MEMBRANE PROTEIN DEFECTS IN CHILDHOOD AND ADULT ONSET DYSTROPHIES

Duchenne muscular dystrophy is one of the most common inherited disorders of humans and is the most frequent muscle disease (1/3500 live born males). Its high frequency in all world populations is a result of the high mutation rate of the gene, which in turn is largely a consequence of the enormous size of the gene (2.5×10^6 bp). Affected children are predominantly male, because of the X-linked recessive inheritance pattern, and appear normal until about 4–5 yr of age, when muscle weakness becomes obvious. Thereafter, weakness and muscle wasting progress relentlessly, leading to wheelchair confinement by age 14 yr, and death in the mid 20s.

The biochemical deficiency causing the disorder remained obscure until 1987, when the Duchenne muscular dystrophy gene was identified by positional cloning techniques. The gene, 10 times larger than the next largest gene, encodes a 427-kDa protein dubbed "dystrophin"; dystrophin deficiency is recognized to define Duchenne muscular dystrophy at the biochemical level. Mutations of the gene are deletions (55%), duplications (5%), and point mutations (40%). Partial dystrophin deficiency, often the result of in-frame deletion mutations compatible with production of dystrophin that lacks segments of amino acids, is diagnostic of the milder and more variable Becker muscular dystrophy. Presentations of Becker dystrophy include proximal weakness, myoglobinuria, myalgias, hyper- CKemia, and cardiac failure, and some patients might remain asymptomatic at advanced ages.

Female homozygotes do not exist because of the relative rarity of the disorder; females generally act as heterozygous gene carriers. However, approx 10% of females with unknown forms of muscular dystrohy express their symptoms as a consequence of heterozygosity for a dystrophinopathy. Most of these females show preferential inactivation of the X-chromosome containing the normal dystrophin gene (skewed X inactivation). Presentations of isolated female carriers vary as much as Becker muscular dystrophy in males, although the progression is often mitigated in the female patients. Overall, approx 20% of adult female carriers of Duchenne and Becker muscular dystrophy show some symptoms,

including muscle weakness of varying severity, cardiomyopathy and left ventricle dilation.

Molecular diagnosis, genetic counseling, and prenatal diagnosis are well established in the dystrophinopathies. Dystrophin protein analysis of muscle biopsy, mutation analysis, and gene linkage analysis are all routinely used. The gene's large size complicates the use of linkage analysis in genetic counseling and prenatal diagnosis due to the 10% recombination within the gene, which results in some uncertainty in all linkage analysis. The high mutation rate leads to many "new mutations," which might affect a single egg or sperm or several eggs leading to the issue of gonadal mosaicism, in which a parent might have multiple affected children (because of multiple affected eggs) yet not be a carrier herself. Owing to the high production rate of sperm, gonadal mosaicism is not an issue for men but must be considered for all at risk carriers. The identification of dystrophin as a major component of the membrane cytoskeleton of muscle fibers permitted use of the dystrophin protein as a probe to isolate and characterize other components. Research has identified three complexes of proteins that interact with dystrophin near the plasma membrane and appear to provide one type of connection between the intracellular contractile myofibrils and the extracellular matrix (Fig. 112-1). Rare childhood-onset muscular dystrophies with autosomal-recessive inheritance patterns have been shown to be caused by mutations of four of the sarcoglycan proteins (Table 112-1). No disorders have been associated with the primary defects in any of the syntrophins or dystroglycan components, although dystroglycan is a target of specific glycosylation modifications, and deficiencies in these enzymes cause severe congenital muscular dystrophy (see Basal Lamina and Glycosylation Defects in Neonatal Onset Congenital Muscular Dystrophy).

The clinical and histopathological consequences of primary disorders of dystrophin and the sarcoglycans are similar, and it can be safely assumed that they share a common molecular pathogenesis. Models suggest that deficiencies of these proteins lead to membrane instability, which initiates acute (hyperCKemia, myofiber necrosis) and chronic responses (progressive fibrosis, failure of myofiber regeneration, and muscle wasting/weakness). The immune system might play a role in both the acute and chronic responses, and immune suppressants such as prednisone show some effect in slowing disease progression. Efforts at gene therapy are underway, although the refractory nature of mature myofibers to viral delivery systems and the unique nature and large amount of the target muscle tissue are hurdles facing this approach.

Three additional plasma membrane proteins cause muscular dystrophy: dysferlin, integrin α7, and caveolin 3. Dysferlin and caveolin 3 directly interact with each other, and caveolin 3 also binds to dystroglycan. Indeed, caveolin 3 and dystrophin appear to compete for the same binding site on dystroglycan, and might represent alternative microdomains providing support to the plasma membrane. Caveolins form lipid rafts and "caveolae" (invaginations of the plasma membrane), and are likely involved in regulating aspects of cell signaling. Integrins interact directly with laminins in the basal lamina, and provide a membrane cytoskeleton that appears complementary to that of the dystrophin membrane cytoskeleton. Consistent with the partial redundancy of the integrin- and dystrophin-based cytoskeletons, overexpression of integrin α7 rescues the pathology of dystrophin deficiency in mice.

BASAL LAMINA AND GLYCOSYLATION DEFECTS IN NEONATAL ONSET CONGENITAL MUSCULAR DYSTROPHY

In 1994, a subset of congenital muscular dystrophy patients were identified who showed complete lack of immunostaining for the

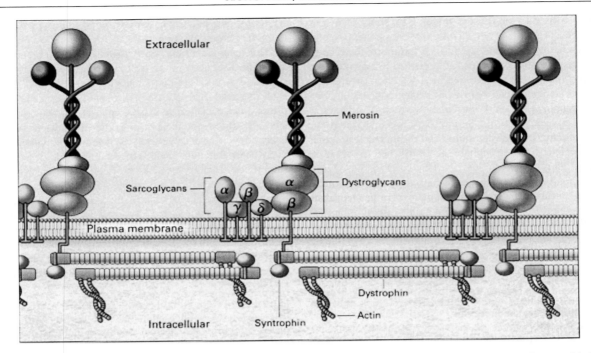

Figure 112-1 Schematic of proteins involved in muscular dystrophies. Shown is a segment of a myofiber plasma membrane, with the intracellular dystrophin-based membrane cytoskeleton, transmembrane sarcoglycans and dystroglycans, and extracellular basal lamina with laminin 2. Male Duchenne/Becker muscular dystrophy and isolated female dystrophinopathy patients are the result of abnormalities of the dystrophin protein, a common X-linked recessive disease. Rare autosomal-recessive childhood-onset dystrophies are caused by mutations in any one of the sarcoglycan proteins (α-sarcoglycan [adhalin], β-sarcoglycan, γ-sarcoglycan, and δ-sarcoglycan). Many cases of neonatal onset severe congenital muscular dystrophy are caused by deficiency of α2 laminin (merosin), which is the large subunit of laminin in the myofiber basal lamina. (From ref. Duggan DJ, Gorospe JR, Fanin M, Hoffman EP, Angelini C. Mutations in the sarcoglycan genes in patients with myopathy. N Engl J Med 1997;336:618–624. Copyright © 1997 Massachusetts Medical Society. All rights reserved.)

α7-laminin chain in their muscle biopsy. The α2-laminin gene has been mapped to chromosome 6q22-23, and mutations have been identified in affected patients. Merosin-deficient patients are relatively uniform in clinical presentation and progression: patients are floppy at birth, unable to raise limbs against gravity. Serum creatine kinase levels are elevated to 2000–10,000 IU/L (normal <200 IU/L). The muscle biopsy shows a dystrophic process, with degeneration of myofibers, and a marked increase in endomysial and perimysial connective tissue with fatty infiltration. One study found that 3 of 10 merosin-deficient patients were initially given the diagnosis of infantile polymyositis because of the presence of significant populations of inflammatory cells. This study documented focal inflammatory reaction in a young patient's muscle, with concentrations of B- and T cells resembling primary follicles, generally seen in spleen. These results suggested that earlier reports of the diagnosis of infantile polymyositis, with a presumed autoimmune etiology, could represent a possible histological finding in inherited α2-laminin deficiency. Both CD4+ and CD8+ cells are seen in large numbers, both distributed throughout the biopsy and in focal aggregates.

α2 laminin is one of the three components of the heterotrimeric muscle laminin molecule (*see* Fig. 112-1). The α2-subunit is present in muscle, the central nervous system (CNS), and Schwann cells, and replaces the more ubiquitous α$_1$ chain during the development of muscle tissue. The other two components, laminin β$_1$ and γ$_1$, are not tissue specific. Laminin is a major constituent of basal lamina of most cells, in which it complexes with collagen IV and other proteins to anchor cells in their tissue environment. α$_2$ laminin is involved in neurite outgrowth in the peripheral and CNS. Patients with α$_2$ laminin deficiency show dramatic white-matter changes

by MRI, although there is no overt CNS dysfunction or intellectual impairment. There is a mouse model for merosin deficiency, dy/dy, and the mutation in the milder of two alleles have been identified. These mice show a phenotype similar to the human disease.

Three different muscle glycosylase have been found to cause congenital muscular dystrophy. Each appears to disrupt specific types of glycosylation, particularly of dystroglycan, leading to abnormal binding of dystroglycan to the extracellular basal lamina. The first identified was the "fukutin" protein; named after the disease subtype, Fukuyama congenital muscular dystrophy, that it causes. This congenital muscular dystrophy is seen almost exclusively in Japan and shows high serum creatine kinase levels at birth and atrophic brain. A protein identified based on structural homology to fukutin, fukutin-related protein, was also found to cause both congenital and adult onset forms of muscular dystrophy. Finally, mutations of yet another glycosidase, *O*-mannoside *N*-acetylglucosaminyltransferase, cause a syndromic type of muscular dystrophy dubbed "Muscle Eye Brain Disease."

NUCLEAR MEMBRANE DEFECTS: EDMD AND OCULOPHARYNGEAL DYSTROPHY

A rare X-linked-recessive disorder, EDMD, is clinically distinct from the dystrophinopathies resulting from the early presence of contractures and cardiac conduction defects requiring placement of a pacemaker. Linkage studies had mapped the gene to Xq28, and the responsible gene was found to encode a novel protein, emerin, which is a component of the nuclear envelope. A second nuclear membrane component, lamin A/C, was found to harbor missense mutations in autosomal-dominant families showing a phenotype indistinguishable

Table 113-2
Epilepsies Established as Channelopathies of the CNS

Gene	Channel	Syndrome
CHRNA4	α_4-subunit, nicotinic acetylcholine receptor	ADNFLE
CHRNB2	β_2-subunit, nicotinic acetylcholine receptor	ADNFLE
GABRA1	α_1-subunit, GABA$_A$ receptor	Autosomal-dominant JME
GABRG2	γ_2-subunit, GABA$_A$ receptor	GEFS+/FS/CAE
SCN1A	α-subunit, Na$_V$1.1 sodium channel	GEFS+/intractable childhood epilepsy with generalized tonic–clonic seizures/severe myoclonic epilepsy of infancy
SCN2A	α-subunit, Na$_V$1.2 sodium channel	GEFS+/benign familial neonatal convulsions
SCN1B	β_1-subunit, sodium channel	GEFS+
KCNQ2	KCNQ2 potassium channel	Benign familial neonatal convulsions
KCNQ3	KCNQ3 potassium channel	Benign familial neonatal convulsions
CLCN2	ClC-2 voltage-gated chloride channel	CAE/juvenile absence epilepsy/JME/epilepsy with grand mal seizures on awakening

A (GABA$_A$) (Table 113-2). The identification of the molecular defect for all of the CNS channelopathies was achieved by linkage analysis followed by positional cloning and mutational analysis of candidate genes.

EPILEPSY Idiopathic generalized epilepsy (IGE), defined as epilepsy of unknown cause and the absence of associated neurological features, is presumed to have a genetic basis. In the last decade, ten ion-channel genes have been implicated in monogenic IGE syndromes (see Table 113-2). The mutations have been identified in fast ligand-gated (ionotropic) channels (nicotinic AChR, GABA$_A$), and voltage-gated ion channels (sodium channel, M-type potassium channel, chloride channel).

Sodium Channel Epilepsies Neuronal voltage-gated sodium channels are heterotrimeric complexes of the main pore-forming α-subunit, an accessory β_1 (or possibly β_3) and covalently linked β_2-subunits. Sodium channels are closed in resting cells and generate the action potential by opening rapidly as threshold is approached and thereby conducting inward sodium current that strongly depolarizes the cell. Sodium channels inactivate once depolarized, which allows the more slowly activating potassium channels to repolarize the cell and also produces the refractory period wherein sodium channels must recover from inactivation to enable the generation of subsequent action potentials.

Three sodium channel genes (SCN1A, SCN2A, and SCN1B) have been associated with idiopathic epilepsy syndromes. The pore-forming α-subunit genes (SCN1A and SCN2A) and accessory β_1-subunit gene (SCN1B) are expressed throughout the brain, with the SCN1A channels localized to neuronal cell bodies and SCN2A being axonal. Mutations in all three of these sodium channel genes are established causes of GEFS+. GEFS+ is a common epilepsy syndrome of childhood, which encompasses a wide range of seizure types and phenotypic variability within families. The most common presentation is febrile seizures (FS) "plus," where the + indicates that generalized tonic–clonic seizures may also occur without fever or after the age of 6 yr, in distinction from classic FS. The inheritance pattern in GEFS+ is autosomal-dominant, but segregation analysis and phenotypic variability suggests interactions with additional modifying genes in most pedigrees. Based on a few index GEFS+ families with monogenic autosomal-dominant inheritance, missense mutations were identified in SCN1A, SCN2A, and SCN1B. In subsequent studies, these sodium channel subunits were screened as candidate disease genes in additional GEFS+ pedigrees and other familial epilepsies with

FS (severe myoclonic epilepsy of infancy, SMEI, and intractable childhood epilepsy with generalized tonic–clonic seizures, ICEGTC). Defects in SCN1A are the most common known genetic cause of familial epilepsy, with over 150 reported mutations. Nearly 80% of families with SEMI or ICEGTC have known mutations in SCN1A and most are catastrophic, with nonsense mutations, frameshift and premature stops.

Expression studies of mutant sodium channels suggest a common gain-of-function defect underlies GEFS+. Inactivation is impaired, as demonstrated by small persistent sodium currents during maintained depolarization (SCN1A mutants), a slower rate of inactivation (SCN2A mutants), or a shift in the voltage dependence of inactivation toward more positive potentials (SCN2A mutant). All of these inactivation defects are predicted to aberrantly depolarize the cell and thereby enhance excitability. In theory, antiepileptic drugs that work by preferentially blocking depolarized sodium channels, such as phenytoin, carbamazepine, or valproate, are predicted to be especially efficacious in preventing seizures produced by this pathomechanism. Improvement with valproate has been reported, but controlled pharmacogenetic studies are not available.

Most mutations of SCN1A associated with the more severe SMEI phenotype are predicted to result in nonfunctional channels, because of nonsense mutations or frameshift mutations with premature stop codons. This observation led to the hypothesis that SCN1A haploinsufficieny resulting from a nonfunctional allele predisposes to SMEI whereas gain-of-function defects resulting from missense mutations cause GEFS+. The pathomechanism may not be so straightforward, because many missense mutations in SCN1A have subsequently been found in SMEI families. A targeted disruption of SCN1A in mice has not been done, so it remains to be tested whether haploinsufficiency in +/– SCN1A knockout mice will produce epilepsy.

Potassium Channel Epilepsies Two potassium channel genes, KCNQ2 and KCNQ3, have been implicated in familial epilepsy. The KCNQ channels are members of the six-transmembrane voltage-dependent family of potassium channels. KCNQ2 and KCNQ3 subunits are highly homologous and co-assemble to form a heterotetrameric potassium channel, which recapitulates the properties of the so-called M-current first identified in sympathetic neurons. The M-current is a subthreshold potassium current that exerts a strong inhibitory influence on neuronal excitability and in turn is inhibited by G-protein coupled receptors, such as the muscarinic AChR, from which the name M-current is derived.

The initial cloning and characterization of KCNQ2 and KCNQ3 was a direct result of linkage analysis and positional cloning to identify disease genes in benign familial neonatal convulsions (BFNC). BFNC is a rare syndrome of autosomal-dominant inherited multifocal or tonic–clonic seizures that begin within the first few days to months of life. The prognosis is good, with seizures spontaneously disappearing after weeks to months. BFNC was one of the first idiopathic epilepsies to be linked to a candidate region (20q13.3, reported in 1989), and a second minor locus was discovered 4 yr later at 8q24. Characterization of cDNAs from these regions led to the discovery of two new postassium channel genes that were most similar to the cardiac potassium channel responsible for the long-QT syndrome, and thereby became the second and third members of this subfamily, KCNQ2 and KCNQ3. Over a dozen mutations in KCNQ2 and a handful in KCNQ3 have been isolated in BFNC families. Missense mutations are concentrated in the pore-loop between the fifth and sixth transmembrane segments and as frameshift or truncation defects that occur in the long cytoplasmic carboxyl tail, which is thought to be important in directing subunit assembly. Expression studies have shown homomeric mutant channels are nonfunctional. Coexpression of mutant and wild-type channels, to mimic the heterozygous state in patients, results in about 50% reduction in current density consistent with haploinsufficiency rather than a dominant negative effect. The relatively mild effect of haploinsufficiency, as compared with some deleterious alteration in gating, may explain the benign course of BFNC. A reduction in the M-current is expected to increase neuronal excitability, but the mechanism whereby convulsions are limited to the first months of life is unknown. One proposal is that the immature brain has an increased susceptibility to seizures. Alternatively, another potassium channel may be expressed later in life that replaces or compensates for the reduced M-current.

Genetic heterogeneity beyond the KCNQ family has been established for BFNC. Missense mutations in the SCN2A sodium channel have been identified in two families with a BFNC-like syndrome, albeit with somewhat later onset of 4–8 mo.

Chloride Channel Epilepsies   Several of the more common forms of IGE were recently mapped to 3q26. A voltage-gated chloride channel at this locus, CLCN2, was screened as a candidate disease gene in 46 IGE families. Mutations were identified in three families: one with an insertion leading to frameshift and premature stop, one with an 11-base deletion, and a third with a missense mutation. The IGE seizure phenotypes were varied within each family and included childhood absence epilepsy (CAE), juvenile absence epilepsy, juvenile myoclonic epilepsy (JME), and epilepsy with grand mal seizures on awakening. Expression studies showed the deletion and insertion mutations were nonfunctional and had a dominant negative effect when coexpressed with wild-type channels. In neurons responsive to GABA, the ClC-2 channel is thought to be an important efflux pathway for chloride ions. A rise in intracellular chloride because of reduced ClC-2 activity would depolarize the reversal potential for $GABA_A$ channels, and may thereby produce seizures by converting the response at $GABA_A$ synapses from inhibitory to excitatory.

$GABA_A$ Receptor Epilepsies   GABA is the major inhibitory neurotransmitter in the CNS. The fast ligand-gated $GABA_A$ receptors are pentameric complexes consisting of subunits from up to seven families (α, β, γ, δ, ϵ, π, θ), although most receptors are thought to be $\alpha\beta\gamma$- or $\alpha\beta\delta$-isoforms. Epilepsy-associated mutations in $GABA_A$ receptors were found first in GABRG2, which codes for the γ_2-subunit. Missense mutations were identified in families with GEFS+ and CAE. Expression studies in $\alpha_1\beta_2\gamma_2$-channels showed loss-of-function changes, either faster deactivation or reduced expression level. More severe mutations in GABRG2 that produced nonfunctional channels because of frameshift/truncation mutations or splice defects were found in families with GEFS+ and SMEI, or with CAE and FS. Mutation of a second $GABA_A$ receptor gene, GABRA1 encoding the α_1-subunit, was identified in a family with autosomal-dominant JME. The missense mutation caused a loss-of-function defect with reduced current amplitude and a 150-fold reduction in sensitivity to GABA. A reduction of inhibitory synaptic activity for mutant $GABA_A$ receptors is expected to predispose to hyperexcitability and epilepsy, but the mechanisms by which distinct seizure phenotypes arise from mutations in the same gene (allelic heterogeneity) remain to be determined.

Acetylcholine Receptor Epilepsies   Neuronal nicotinic AChRs are heteropentameric complexes of α- and β-subunits. Numerous isoforms of α- and β-subunit genes have been identified with the predominantly expressed isoforms in brain being α_4 and β_2. Missense mutations in either the α_4 (CHRNA4) or β_2 (CHNRB2) subunits have been identified in families with autosomal-dominant nocturnal frontal lobe epilepsy (ADNFLE). The mutations are clustered in the second transmembrane segment, which lines the ion-conducting pore of the channel. Seizures occur most often during sleep onset, often in clusters of spells, with an onset in the first or second decade of life. Electroencephalographic studies show a frontal localization of the seizure focus. Expression studies have revealed mixed effects of the mutations on channel function. A loss-of-function is implicated by reduced single-channel conductance, drastically reduced permeability to Ca^{2+}, and augmented desensitization. Conversely, other mutants increased the sensitivity to agonists and impaired desensitization. The pathogenic basis of seizures in ADNFLE remains to be elucidated. The cholinergic system has been implicated in sleep, which may be a factor in the nocturnal occurrence of seizures. The mechanism whereby the seizure focus is localized to the frontal lobe is unclear, because α_4- and β_2-subunits are expressed diffusively throughout the CNS.

EPISODIC ATAXIA TYPE 1   EA is a rare autosomal-dominant neurological disorder, which presents with recurrent attacks of generalized ataxia that may affect the limbs, trunk, speech, and eye movements. Attacks last for minutes to hours and are triggered by emotional or physical stress. The carbonic anhydrase inhibitor, acetazolamide, is effective at reducing attack frequency and severity. Two forms of EA were distinguished clinically and mapped genetically to different loci. The distinguishing feature of EA Type 1 (EA1) is a coincident interictal rippling of muscles because of spontaneous discharges of the distal motor neuron (neuromyotonia). EA1 maps to chromosome 12p, and screening of a candidate potassium channel gene, KCNA1 encoding the voltage-dependent potassium channel KV1.1, has revealed over ten missense mutations and one premature stop in the cytoplasmic carboxyl terminus. Expression studies have shown mixed effects. Loss-of-function was demonstrated by dominant negative suppression of potassium current density, haploinsufficiency, or accelerated kinetics of deactivation on hyperpolarization. Conversely, other mutations

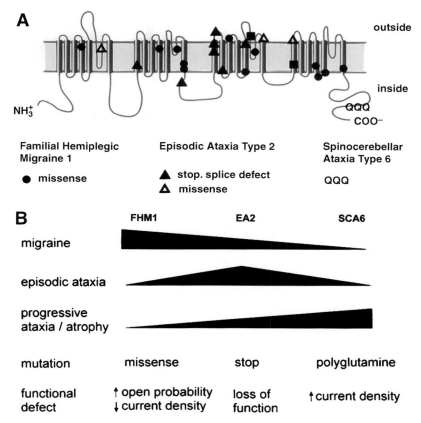

Figure 113-2   Allelic disorders from mutations of CACNA1A encoding the α_1-subunit of the P/Q-type Ca channel. **(A)** Location and type of mutations are shown on the schematic representation of the membrane folding pattern for the P/Q-type α_1-subunit. Filled circles show missense mutations in FHM1. Triangles show position of truncations because of stop/splice errors (filled) or missense mutations found in EA2. Site of the polyglutamine expansion associated with SCA6 is indicated by the symbol QQQ. **(B)** Spectrum of molecular defects, clinical features and disease severity for FHM1, EA2 and SCA6.

slowed the rate of inactivation or accelerated the rate of recovery, both of which imply a gain-of-function defect. Neuronal firing patterns are very sensitive to small changes in potassium currents at subthreshold voltages, and so it is likely that either gain- or loss-of-function defects could be deleterious to neuronal activity. Partial epilepsy has been observed in several EA1 families with known mutations in KCNA1, suggesting that alterations in the Kv1.1 potassium channel may also increase the susceptibility to partial seizures.

FHM, EA2, AND SCA6: ALLELIC DISORDERS OF THE P/Q CA CHANNEL   Migraine is a common neurological disorder, characterized by recurrent disabling headache that is typically unilateral with involvement of retroorbital or fronto-temporal regions and associated with vomiting, photophobia and general malaise. Family and population-based studies have suggested a genetic component to migraine, most likely as a polygenic multifactorial mechanism. FHM is a rare autosomal-dominant form of migraine that presents as migraine with aura plus ictal hemiparesis. The trait maps to chromosome 19p13 in about 50% of families, and patients with this so-called FHM1 often develop late-onset cerebellar atrophy. A second locus is at chromosome 1q23, where loss-of-function mutations in the α_2-subunit of the Na^+/K^+ pump produce FMH2. Another autosomal-dominant neurological disorder, EA2, also maps to chromosome 19p13. Like EA1, the predominant feature of EA2 is recurrent attacks of ataxia and dysarthria that are

alleviated by the carbonic anhydrase inhibitor acetazolamide. The episodes of ataxia in EA-2 tend to be longer (hours), and there is associated interictal nystagmus, cerebellar atrophy, and increased propensity for migraine.

A candidate disease gene encoding the pore-forming α_1-subunit a P/Q-type Ca channel, CACNA1A, was identified by exon trapping at19p13. This initial report identified four missense mutations in CACNA1A associated with FMH1 and two mutations disrupting the reading frame in families with EA2 (deletion and splice error). Subsequently, a total of 14 missense mutations have been identified in FHM1 families, with the threonine to methionine substitution in the pore region at position or T666M being the most common. The majority of EA2 mutations are predicted to result in a nonfunctional subunit resulting from frame shift–truncation mutations or splice site errors. In a few families with EA-2, missense mutations in CACNA1A have been detected.

A third class of genetic lesion, expansion of a CAG repeat, has been identified in the CACNA1A gene in SCA6. Autosomal-dominant cerebellar ataxia has been recognized clinically for more than a century, and subclasses were first distinguished clinically on the basis of age of onset, severity, or associated degeneration of specific neuronal populations. Subsequently more than 14 different SCAs have been delineated genetically. SCA6 has a late onset in the third or fourth decade with mildly progressive ataxia of limbs and eye movements, and cerebellar atrophy without other regions of tissue loss by MRI. The CAG polymorphism is in a variably spliced region of the carboxyl cytoplasmic tail of the P/Q-type Ca channel. The normal allele has 4–18 repeats, whereas repeats of 21–33 in number cause SCA6.

The genotype-phenotype correlations observed in these allelic disorders has led to the proposal that increasing severity of the molecular lesion in CACNA1A (missense, nonsense/truncation, and CAG expansion) results in a spectrum of increasingly severe clinical phenotype: FHM1, EA-2, SCA6, respectively, as depicted in Fig. 113-2. CACNA1A is expressed diffusely in the nervous system, and P/Q-type Ca channels are located both presynaptically at the vesicle release site and on neuronal soma and dendrites. Targeted disruption of the CACNA1A homolog in mice causes severe ataxia and dystonia with cerebellar atrophy. Numerous alterations in channel function have been reported in expression studies of α1A-mutants. A common defect for the missense mutations that cause FHM1 is a shift in the voltage dependence of opening, such that mutant channels open more readily for mild depolarization from the resting potential. Other effects are more variable and include decreased density of functional channels, reduced flow of Ca^{2+} through the open channel, and altered kinetics of inactivation. In principle, such varied effects could produce either loss- or gain-of-function changes (i.e., too much or too little Ca^{2+} entry). These alterations in Ca^{2+} signaling and therefore of transmitter release are proposed to underlie the cortical spreading depression responsible for local transient neuronal dysfunction that manifest as the aura of migraine. The majority of EA2 mutations result in truncations because of frame shifts and premature stop codons or splicing defects that are not expected to code for functional subunits. A few missense mutations have been reported in EA2 families, and expression testing of one (F1491S) has shown a complete loss of P/Q-type Ca channel activity. The CAG repeat expansion in SCA6 codes for a polyglutamine track in the cytoplasmic carboxyl tail of the α1A-subunit. The consensus on the effect of this expansion is a gain-of-function change either through increased functional protein levels, a hyperpolarized shift of activation or slower inactivation. The CACNA1A splice variant that includes the polyglutamine track is expressed at high levels in the cerebellum, especially in Purkinje cells, and may explain the selective vulnerability resulting from Ca^{2+} overload.

HYPEREKPLEXIA Hereditary startle disease, or hyperekplexia, is a rare familial disorder with autosomal-dominant or autosomal-recessive inheritance. The core features are an enhanced startle response to environmental stimuli (especially auditory or tactile) often followed by sustained stiffness, nocturnal myoclonus, and neonatal hypertonia. Mutations in the α1-subunit of the glycine receptor (GLRA1) have been identified in both familial and sporadic hyperkplexia. Glycine receptors are heteropentamers consisting of three α1- and two β-subunits, and are the major effectors of fast inhibitory neurotransmission in the spinal cord and brainstem. Dominant and recessive missense and nonsense mutations of the α1-subunit have been reported. Expression studies of mutant channels have shown loss-of-function defects with reduced glycine affinity and a lower conductance of the chloride channel. Interestingly, a transgenic mouse model of a dominant GLRA1 mutation (R271Q) produced a decrease in GABA-ergic inhibitory transmission in the ventral horn of the spinal cord, and diminished glycine receptor transmission. Compound heterozygous mutations in the β1-subunit (missense and splice mutations of GLRB) have been reported in one boy with transient hyperekplexia. Augmentation of GABA-ergic inhibition with clonazpepam alleviates many of the symptoms in hyperekplexia.

SELECTED REFERENCES

Ashcroft FM. Ion Channels and Disease. San Diego: Academic Press, 2000.

Cannon SC. An expanding view for the molecular basis of familial periodic paralysis. Neuromuscul Disord 2002;12(6):533–543.

Engel AG, Ohno K, Sine SM. Neurological diseases: sleuthing molecular targets for neurological diseases at the neuromuscular junction. Nat Rev Neurosci 2003;4(5):339–352.

Hille B. Ion Channels of Excitable Membranes. Sunderland, MA; Sinauer, 2001.

Lehmann-Horn F, Jurkat-Rott K. Voltage-gated ion channels and hereditary disease. Physiol Rev 1999;79(4):1317–1372.

Mulley JC, Scheffer IE, Petrou S, Berkovic SF. Channelopathies as a genetic cause of epilepsy. Curr Opin Neurol 2003;16(2): 171–176.

Pietrobon D, Striessnig J. Neurological diseases: neurobiology of migraine. Nat Rev Neurosci 2003;4(5):386–398.

114 Charcot-Marie-Tooth Disease and Related Peripheral Neuropathies

JAMES R. LUPSKI

SUMMARY

Molecular genetic analysis of the demyelinating neuropathies Charcot-Marie-Tooth disease and hereditary neuropathy with liability to pressure palsies has uncovered a novel mutational mechanism whereby a reciprocal recombination involving a misaligned flanking repeat sequence results in both the Charcot-Marie-Tooth disease type-1A duplication and hereditary neuropathy with liability to pressure palsies deletion. These studies have illuminated the role that gene dosage may play in causing a disease phenotype, which has important implications for therapeutic strategies, and which may underlie the basis of the extreme clinical variability. The identification of these rearrangement mutations (duplication and deletion) has resulted in the availability of molecular procedures for establishing or excluding a secure diagnosis, enabling presymptomatic and prenatal diagnosis, and providing prognostic information.

Key Words: Charcot-Marie-Tooth disease; congenital hypomyelinating neuropathy; Dejerine-Sottas neuropathy; hereditary neuropathy with liability to pressure palsies; Roussy-Lévy syndrome.

INTRODUCTION

Charcot-Marie-Tooth disease (CMT) is the most common inherited peripheral neuropathy, affecting at least 1 in 2500 individuals. CMT represents a heterogeneous collection of disorders of the peripheral nerve. It can be inherited as an autosomal-dominant, autosomal-recessive, or X-linked trait, and isolated or sporadic cases also occur. The autosomal-dominant segregation pattern is the most frequently observed, and molecular studies identified a novel mutational mechanism for this form—the Charcot-Marie-Tooth disease type 1A (CMT1A) duplication. It is intriguing that for one of the most common dominant disorders affecting humans, no mutant gene is involved in the majority of cases. Instead, the disease phenotype results from having three copies of a normal nonmutated gene or a gene dosage affect secondary to an inherited or *de novo* DNA duplication. Furthermore, an intrinsic structural property of the human genome, a low-copy CMT1A repeat sequence (CMT1A-REP) flanking the duplicated region, acts as a substrate for homologous recombination and an unequal crossover

From: *Principles of Molecular Medicine, Second Edition*
Edited by: M. S. Runge and C. Patterson © Humana Press, Inc., Totowa, NJ

event. This recombination among misaligned flanking CMT1A-REP repeats appears to have a sex predilection and to occur preferentially during male gametogenesis. The identification of the CMT1A duplication has potent implications for clinical diagnosis, clinical management with respect to prognosis, counseling regarding recurrence risk, and the rational design of therapy geared at normalizing the levels of gene expression.

Hereditary neuropathy with liability to pressure palsies (HNPP) (OMIM 162500) is a less frequently diagnosed autosomal-dominant peripheral neuropathy, which usually presents with a milder clinical phenotype than CMT. The patient inherits a tendency to nerve injury after mild trauma; it is likely that many affected individuals remain undiagnosed because they are clinically asymptomatic or only minimally aware of functional disabilities. Carpal tunnel syndrome and other entrapment neuropathies are frequent manifestations of HNPP, making it sometimes difficult to distinguish from an acquired neuropathy. In the majority of cases, HNPP results from DNA deletion of the same genetic region duplicated in CMT1A. Molecular detection of the HNPP deletion secures a diagnosis suspected clinically and can be useful for distinguishing HNPP from acquired neuropathies.

The Dejerine-Sottas neuropathy (DSN) (OMIM 145900) is a rare and severe neuropathy. Though it was initially thought to be an autosomal-recessive trait, molecular studies have identified mutations in only one copy of the two homologues of the same genes that when mutated can lead to a CMT phenotype. These heterozygous mutations presumably represent dominant alleles. However, the DSN phenotype in some cases may result from recessive mutations in select genes (e.g., *PRX* and *GDAP1*). Congenital hypomyelinating neuropathy (CHN) (OMIM 605253) represents the most severe form of hereditary motor and sensory neuropathy (HMSN). The clinical features are present at birth with marked hypotonia, areflexia, and distal muscle weakness. Thus, instead of being completely distinct entities, CHN, DSN, and CMT may more accurately represent a spectrum of related clinical findings owing to allelic heterogeneity underlying the disorders; many CHN and DSN cases may result from new mutant dominant alleles. Roussy-Lévy syndrome (OMIM 180800) combines the CMT1 phenotype with marked tremor and sensory ataxia. It may not be a distinct clinical entity, but rather may represent the spectrum of the CMT1 phenotype.

Molecular analyses have identified some thirty genes wherein mutations, or altered dosage of the normal gene in the case of *PMP22*, lead to inherited neuropathies. These genes provide critical reagents to study the biology of peripheral nerves. Each gene product is important for proper structure or function of the Schwann cell, neuron or communication between the two. Molecular genetic studies of CMT and related neuropathies have given new insights into the biology of the human peripheral nervous system and have important implications for patient care.

CLINICAL FEATURES AND PATHOGENESIS

CMT polyneuropathy syndrome, or the HMSNs, are genetically and clinically heterogeneous disorders of the peripheral nerves characterized by an insidious onset and slowly progressive weakness of the distal muscles and mild sensory impairment. Symptoms typically appear in the first or second decade but may appear later. Children with CMT often walk on their toes, and adults consult a physician because of abnormalities of gait from a dropped foot resulting from dorsiflexor weakness, foot deformities such as pes cavus, or loss of balance. Cramps are a frequent complaint, are worse after long walks, and are sometimes exacerbated by cold weather. The most frequent complaint concerning hand function that may occur later in the disease is difficulty with fine finger movements. Deep tendon reflexes disappear early at the ankle and later at the patella and the upper limb.

Electrophysiological and neuropathological studies distinguish two major forms. CMT1 (OMIM 118200), also called HMSNI, is a demyelinating neuropathy with moderately to severely decreased motor nerve conduction velocities (NCVs, usually <38 m/s). The conduction deficit is uniform from nerve to nerve and from nerve segment to nerve segment, suggesting a cell-autonomous defect involving the Schwann cell. CMT1 is characterized by hypertrophic nerves, which may be visualized in some patients under the skin (greater auricular nerve) or palpated (ulnar and peroneal nerves). Peripheral nerve pathology shows segmental demyelination and remyelination and frequent "onion bulb" formation, which consists of circumferentially directed Schwann cells and their processes. CMT has been characterized further with genetic linkage studies, which demonstrate the involvement of over 30 loci. The first three type-1 loci identified include CMT1A at 17p11.2–p12, Charcot-Marie-Tooth disease type 1B (CMT1B) on 1q21.2–q23, and CMTX at Xq13.1.

Charcot-Marie-Tooth disease type 2 (CMT2) (OMIM 118210), also called HMSN type II, is characterized by normal or slightly reduced motor NCVs with decreased amplitudes and neuropathology that shows axonal loss with few if any onion bulbs. DSN (or motor and sensory neuropathy type III) is a demyelinating neuropathy with clinical electrophysiological and histopathological features similar to, but of more severe and earlier onset than CMT1. CHN is at the most severe end of the clinical spectrum with NCVs less than 10 m/s. However, the clinical distinction between CHN and DSN is often difficult. The diagnosis is confirmed by nerve biopsy showing hypomyelination with only a few thin myelin lamellae left without active myelin degradation products and early onion bulb formations. These classifications appear to reflect primary pathological involvement of the myelin (CMT1, DSN, and CHN) or the axon (CMT2) of the peripheral nerve. The clinical distinction of CMT1 vs CMT2 is important both for diagnosis and directing molecular testing. Nevertheless, it has become clear from molecular studies that for some "CMT disease genes" different

mutations in the same gene can result in either a type-1 or type-2 CMT phenotype.

HNPP may manifest clinically as periodic episodes of numbness, muscular weakness, atrophy, and in some cases palsies that follow relatively minor compression or trauma to the peripheral nerves. HNPP may present as multifocal neuropathy. Electrophysiological studies sometimes show mildly slowed NCV in clinically affected individuals as well as in asymptomatic "carriers." Conduction blocks can also be observed. Peripheral nerve pathology shows segmental demyelination and remyelination with tomacula or "sausage-like" focal thickenings of the myelin sheath. Ultrastructural studies reveal frequent occurrence of uncompacted myelin, particularly in the inner lamellae, because of separation of the major dense line with widened islands of cytoplasm in the Schwann cell.

MOLECULAR MECHANISMS

DNA DUPLICATION ASSOCIATED WITH CMT1A   The CMT1A duplication (OMIM 118220) was identified initially in multiple US and European CMT1 families, wherein it was found to cosegregate with the disease in familial cases and as a new mutation in many isolated or sporadic cases. The segregation of marker genotypes from within the duplicated segment in the new mutation individual suggested a mechanism of unequal crossover or nonsister chromatid exchange for the duplication. Demonstration of the CMT1A duplication in affected individuals was carried out by the following methods: detection of three alleles at a highly polymorphic dinucleotide repeat locus, dosage differences at restriction fragment length polymorphic (RFLP) alleles, detection of a duplication-specific junction fragment of 500 kb with pulsed field gel electrophoresis to separate large-molecular-weight fragments of SacII digested genomic DNA from the affected individual, and microscopically by two-color fluorescent *in situ* hybridization (FISH) of interphase nuclei. Failure to recognize the molecular duplication can lead to misinterpretation of marker genotypes for affected individuals, identification of false recombinants, and incorrect localization of the disease locus. The CMT1A duplication, confirmed subsequently by many laboratories in patients from varied ethnic background, occurs in approx 70% of unrelated CMT1 cases, and was found in 76–90% sporadic CMT1 cases. The junction fragment appeared to be identical in multiple CMT1A duplication patients of varied ethnicity, suggesting a precise recombination event to generate the duplication. Taken together, these observations suggested that the CMT1A duplication was a frequent cause of CMT that appears to have occurred *de novo* multiple and independent times in different genetic backgrounds.

Patients with the CMT1A duplication exhibit typical neuropathology of CMT1. Electrophysiological studies in families segregating the CMT1A duplication demonstrated a clear bimodal distribution of abnormally decreased motor NCV in individuals with the CMT1A duplication, although normal NCVs appeared in those shown not to have inherited the CMT1A duplication. However, a remarkable range of motor NCV was observed in CMT1A duplication patients that were not related to age or clinical severity. Longitudinal electrophysiological studies performed 22 yr apart in one family segregating the CMT1A duplication demonstrated little change in NCV and only mild increased motor impairment. Thus, the CMT1A duplication is a good biological marker for the disease with clinical utility for diagnosis and prognosis.

A

Reactions of Wild-type Cu/Zn SOD1

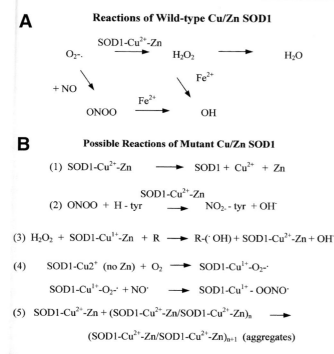

B

Possible Reactions of Mutant Cu/Zn SOD1

(1) $SOD1-Cu^{2+}-Zn \longrightarrow SOD1 + Cu^{2+} + Zn$

(2) $ONOO + H - tyr \xrightarrow{SOD1-Cu^{2+}-Zn} NO_2 - tyr + OH^-$

(3) $H_2O_2 + SOD1-Cu^{1+}-Zn + R \longrightarrow R-(^{\cdot}OH) + SOD1-Cu^{2+}-Zn + OH^-$

(4) $SOD1-Cu2^+ (no\ Zn) + O_2 \longrightarrow SOD1-Cu^{1+}-O_2^{-\cdot}$

$SOD1-Cu^{1+}-O_2^{-\cdot} + NO^{\cdot} \longrightarrow SOD1-Cu^{1+} - OONO^{\cdot}$

(5) $SOD1-Cu^{2+}-Zn + (SOD1-Cu^{2+}-Zn/SOD1-Cu^{2+}-Zn)_n \longrightarrow$

$(SOD1-Cu^{2+}-Zn/SOD1-Cu^{2+}-Zn)_{n+1}$ (aggregates)

Figure 115-1 (**A**) Selected reactions of cytosolic copper, zinc super-oxide dismutase (SOD1). SOD1 catalyzes the conversion (dismutation) of O_2^- to H_2O_2. H_2O_2 is converted to water by catalase and glutathione peroxidase. O_2^- can combine noncatalytically with NO to form ONOO–. ONOO– and H_2O_2 can interact with reduced metals such as Fe^{2+} or Cu^{1+} to hydroxyl radicals. (**B**) Putative reactions of mutant Cu/Zn SOD1. (1) Familial amyotrophic lateral sclerosis (FALS)-associated mutations may lessen the affinity of SOD1 for copper and zinc. (2) Nitronium anions may be formed more rapidly by the reaction of ONOO– with mutant SOD1 in the presence of FALS mutations; this may accelerate transfer of nitrate groups to tyrosines. (3) FALS-associated mutations may favor the reduction of Cu^{2+}, enhancing the ability of SOD1 to reduce substrates like H_2O_2 and thereby act as a peroxidase. (4) In the absence of zinc, oxygen can reduce Cu^{2+} in SOD1 to produce O_2^- within the active channel; this can potentially interact with nitric oxide to form ONOO–. (5) Mutant SOD1 may be unstable and aggregate, both with itself and with wild-type SOD1.

Reports documenting that SOD1 activity is decreased in tissues of patients with SOD1-associated FALS initially raised the possibility that motor neuron death is a direct consequence of this loss of SOD1 function. For example, as reviewed later, studies of motor neurons in vitro show that diminished superoxide activity initiates programmed cell death of neurons. However, several arguments strongly favor the view that the mutant SOD1 protein has acquired properties that are lethal for the motor neuron. Strong support for this view is the observation that SOD1 knock-out mice do not develop motor neuron cell death in the first few months of life. Oppositely, overexpression of FALS-related mutant SOD1 protein (with FALS mutations) causes a lethal, paralytic disorder in mice beginning at 3–5 mo of age, and in rats.

These considerations indicate that the mutant SOD1 molecule is cytotoxic. Although the basis for this novel activity is not yet well established, several possible adverse functions for the mutant molecule have been proposed (Fig. 115-1B). One possibility is that metal binding properties of some mutants (e.g., G85R and G93A) are abnormal, and that either copper or zinc acts as a toxin for motor neurons. It also has been reported that deficiency of zinc

from SOD1 enhances its potential toxicity, both in the wild type (WT) and mutant form. Indeed, in neurons in cell culture, zinc-deficient apoprotein is as toxic as the zinc-deficient mutant protein; when fully zinc-loaded, neither form of the protein is toxic in this system. Another hypothesis is that nitration of critical tyrosine residues is a key event. High-pressure liquid chromatography and immunochemical studies indicate that levels of nitrotyrosine are augmented in human and mouse ALS brains. A fourth hypothesis is that the mutant SOD1 protein has an enhanced ability to act as a peroxidase with H_2O_2 as a substrate. This hypothesis is consistent with reports that levels of production of hydroxyl radicals are increased in ALS mice.

Distinct from the foregoing proposals is the alternative suggestion that the critical effect of mutations in this abundant SOD1 protein (up to 0.5% of intracellular proteins) is to cause misfolding, leading to the accumulation of unstable, mutant protein, perhaps as insoluble toxic aggregates. The stability of many of the mutant SOD1 proteins are reduced when expressed in mammalian cells. More recent studies document that the most, if not all, of the mutant SOD1 proteins are unstable either at baseline or with minimal physiological stresses. Such aggregates might be directly injurious; they might also act by impairing normal endogenous mechanisms for protein reutilization. It is proposed that through one or more of these adverse biochemical reactions, the mutant SOD1 protein is directly or indirectly toxic to the cell. Whether oxidative pathology is critical for the cytotoxic effects of mutant SOD1 is unclear. An elegant study documented that elimination in the ALS mice of a protein responsible for loading copper into the active site of SOD1 does not ameliorate the disease; this has been interpreted as excluding a role for copper-mediated oxidative pathology; however, this view has been challenged on the grounds that there may be residual copper associated with the SOD1 molecule either in the normal active site or at an atypical but potentially toxic site.

Several possible targets exist for this toxicity. One intensively studied target is the astroglial glutamate transporter, EAAT2 or GLT1. This protein is strongly implicated as a factor in ALS pathogenesis both because glutamate toxicity has generally been incriminated in the disease and because studies have documented a decrease in both astroglial glutamate transport activity and levels of EAAT2 protein. It has been suggested that the latter might be a consequence of altered splicing of the RNA transcript for EAAT2. Studies show that EAAT2 is susceptible to inactivation by mutant SOD1, particularly in the face of oxidative challenge by H_2O_2 or iron. Another molecular target of mutant SOD1 protein is the voltage-sensitive Na^+ channel, which shows diminished Na^+ current and a depolarizing shift of the voltage dependence of activation in the presence of mutant SOD1. A third important target is the Na^+/K^+ pump; one report documents a marked reduction in subunits of this pump in spinal cords of mice expressing high levels of mutant $SOD1^{G93A}$.

At the level of subcellular organelles, another important target of mutant SOD1 protein are mitochondria. High levels of the protein, as expressed in different lines of transgenic ALS mice, trigger striking morphological changes in mitochondria selectively in motor neurons. It is clear that high levels of both WT and mutant SOD1 are evident in mitochondria. Moreover, mutant SOD1 is apparently more toxic when localized to mitochondria than in other organelles. The mutant SOD1 protein within mitochondria disrupts electron transport and ATP generation at the time of disease onset but not in presymptomatic stages. The process by which SOD1 enters the mitochondrion is not clear, although this may be enhanced by demetallation; entry of mutant SOD1 into mitochondria is blocked by binding to heat shock proteins, a process that may divert these proteins from critical antiapoptotic functions.

In addition to specific molecules and subcellular organelles, some subcellular processes are deficient in the presence of aberrant SOD1. Important among these is axonal transport, which may decline many weeks before motor neuron degeneration becomes evident. In turn, this diminishes peripheral transport of critical proteins such as tubulin and neurofilaments.

It became apparent from several lines of study that whatever the specific target or mechanism of its action, mutant SOD1 protein can markedly induce activity of cell death genes in neurons. This is particularly remarkable because WT SOD1 is antiapoptotic. The proapoptotic properties of mutant SOD1 were first explored in a variety of cell types in vitro, including yeast cells and diverse types of neuronal cells. In one model, the proapoptotic mutant SOD1 protein aggregates within the cytosol of motor neurons. Oxidative stress can activate the cell death gene caspase-1 (IL-1β converting enzyme) and thereby lead to increased formation and secretion of IL-1β; this change is also seen in the spinal cords of ALS mice. Subsequently, it was shown that both caspase-1 and -3 are activated sequentially in the spinal cords of the SOD1^{G93A} mice. The activation of caspase 3 appears to invoke a pathway of programmed cell death that implicates mitochondria, with increased expression of BAX, release of cytochrome-c and activation of caspase 9.

The prediction from these observations that inhibition of caspases might slow the motor neuron disease has been tested in some experiments. Inactivation of caspase 1 slightly prolongs survival in ALS mice bearing the glycine 93 to alanine mutation. Similarly, overexpression of the antiapoptotic protein (NAIP) bcl-2 slows the onset of the disease in these mice. Moreover, infusion of tetrapeptide pan-caspase inhibitors into the spinal fluid of ALS mice prolongs survival by approx 25%. Analogously, treatment with minocycline is also beneficial. These findings are of general interest in understanding cell death in neurodegenerative disorders, as activation of caspase-1 and elevation of IL-1β levels have also been detected in the brains of patients with Huntington's disease.

Non-neuronal cells are abnormal in ALS. There is, for example, intense microglial proliferation and some astrogliosis, in both human and murine ALS. In fact, astroglial proliferation is one of the earliest microscopic changes in murine ALS. Numerous studies have found evidence for activation of inflammatory cascades in spinal cord in transgenic and human ALS. For example, the observation that COX2 is elevated in ALS mice led to studies confirming its elevation in humans with sporadic ALS. One view is that elevated spinal cord COX 2 activity generates elevated levels of prostaglandin that, in turn, enhance glutamate release. In this context, it was of considerable importance that inhibition of COX 2 retarded motor neuron cell death in a Petri dish model of motor neuron degeneration. A subsequent studied showed that COX 2 inhibition prolongs survival in ALS mice. This striking finding has, in turn, led to a multicenter trial of celecoxib in human ALS.

A central issue in understanding the pathogenesis of mutant SOD1-mediated neuronal death is the degree to which it reflects cascades of events evolving selectively within the motor neuron (a cell autonomous death process). The activation of inflammatory cells and molecular cascades suggests that abnormal biological properties of activated non-neuronal cells that surround the motor neuron might contribute to the death of neuronal cells. Three centers published a joint report that demonstrated, using chimeric mice with varying contributions of WT and mutant SOD1-bearing cells, that surprisingly small fractions of WT cells in the spinal cord (e.g., 15–20%) can rescue the motor neuron death phenotype. Particularly striking is that the rescue is not attributable simply to survival of WT motor neurons. Rather, the presence of the WT cells allows the motor neurons bearing mutant SOD1 to avoid cell death. In a chimeric mouse with equal numbers of WT SOD1 and G93A-mutant SOD1 cells, there was no weakness at more than 1 yr of age, whereas the all-mutant G93A-mutant SOD1 transgenic mouse died at 135 d. Moreover, in that chimeric mouse, equal numbers of WT SOD1 and G93A-SOD1 spinal motor neurons were evident at more than 1 yr of age. Also remarkable in these studies was that the presence of mutant-SOD1-positive cells was injurious to WT motor neurons, as assessed by the presence of ubiquitin-positive inclusions.

TREATMENT OF ALS Regrettably, there is no therapy that substantially augments survival in ALS. Riluzole, which is thought to act primarily but not exclusively through inhibition of glutamate, has repeatedly been documented to prolong survival in ALS by approx 10–15%. The availability of mouse and now cell-based models for cytotoxicity by mutant SOD1 protein should accelerate the search for effective therapies. An extensive series of compounds and manipulations have proven statistically if not biologically significant in extending the life span of the ALS mice. A partial list includes the following categories of compounds: antioxidants (vitamin E, buckminsterfullerine, lyophilized red wine, and gingseng root); copper chelating agents (d-penicillamine, trientine, and ascorbate); antiglutamate compounds (riluzole, gabapentin), and agents that augment cellular energy production (coenzyme Q10, creatine). Beneficial genetic approaches to ameliorating the disease in mice have consisted of overexpression of the major astroglial glutamate transporter, EAAT2, and forced expression of two compounds that inhibit apoptosis, bcl-2 and a dominant negative inhibitor of caspase-1. As noted, infusion of tetrapeptide inhibitors of caspases also slowed the course of the disease in the mice. Particularly exciting has been the observation that activity of the enzyme COX2 is elevated in spinal cords of ALS patients and in ALS mice. This has a direct implication for therapy, as potent cyclo-oxygenase inhibitors are already in widespread use in such disorders as arthritis. The observation that the cyclooxygenase inhibition can slow the course of motor neuron disease in ALS mice has led to a multicenter human trial of this drug in ALS.

Several genetic manipulations that alter levels of expression of subunits of neurofilaments in the motor nerve axons have also had significant impact on the survival of the transgenic ALS mice. For example, expression of high levels of the heavy neurofilament subunit (NF-H) increases the lifespan of the G37R mice by approx 65%. Analogously, blocking expression of any axonal neurofilament subunits by knocking out the light neurofilament subunits (NF-L) also prolongs survival. This apparent paradox may be resolved by the observation that in both of these mouse strains neurofilament aggregates accumulate within the soma of the motor neuron. The prediction of this finding is that genetic manipulations that stoichiometrically reduce NF-L, medium neurofilament subunits, and NF-H should reduce axon NF burden (and axonal caliber) without causing NF accumulations in the cell body. If the NF aggregates protect the G37R mice, these mice should have the typical, shorter survival of the unmanipulated

G37R mice. However, if the critical factor is the diminution in axonal NF burden, these mice should have enhanced survival. When this painstaking experiment was completed, it favored the former view. The resulting mice had no accumulation of NF protein in the motor neuron cell body, and they showed no prolongation in survival. Why the aggregated NF protein in the cell body might partially rescue the ALS phenotype is not clear, although studies in progress suggest the accumulated proteins may act as a sink or buffer for one or more adverse substances.

At least two other strategies for treating the ALS mice have been attempted. Gene therapy has been attempted with cautiously encouraging results. Two groups have shown a modest benefit from administration of, glial cell-derived neurotrophic factor, GDNF. When myoblasts transduced with GDNF ex vivo are implanted in the ALS mice, a modest but statistically significant benefit resulted. Intramuscular, segmental administration of GDNF via adenoviral vectors also produced a modest survival benefit in the ALS mice. Dramatic prolongation of survival of the G93A ALS transgenic mice has been afforded by retrograde delivery of insulin-like growth factor-1 via an adeno-associated virus vector.

The other, dramatically different therapy used in the ALS mice was systemic administration of human umbilical cord blood cells. It was reported that intravenous infusion of 30–70 million cord blood cells into ALS mice that have been exposed to near lethal irradiation extends the life of some of the recipients by as much as 50%. A positive but less pronounced benefit was reported in a second study of human umbilical cord blood therapy in the G93A ALS mice.

NON-SOD1, DOMINANTLY INHERITED ALS—THE ROLE OF MOTOR PROTEINS

Because most cases of dominantly inherited, adult-onset ALS are not associated with mutations in the SOD1 gene, there is an intense effort to identify the underlying ALS-associated gene defects. In a family with a slowly progressive form of ALS, characterized by vocal cord involvement and prominent bulbar features, a mutation has been identified in the gene encoding the motor protein dynactin. The causative missense mutations are predicted to alter binding microtubules and thereby adversely affect axonal transport. This signal observation was noteworthy for three reasons. First, it is the first evidence for direct involvement of motor abnormalities of motor transport in ALS. Second, that motor proteins are pivotal in the viability of motor neurons is further underscored by the observations that three forms of kinesin are mutated in three forms of motor neuropathy, KIF1Bβ in Charcot-Marie Tooth type 2A, KIF21A in congenital fibrosis of the extraocular muscles because of absence of the superior division of the third nerve, and KIF5A in a form of hereditary spastic paraparesis. Third, almost simultaneously with the report of the dynactin mutation in human motor neuron disease, it was reported that a mouse model of motor neuron disease ("legs at odd angles") is caused by mutations in the gene that expresses dynein, a dynactin binding protein.

DOMINANTLY INHERITED, JUVENILE-ONSET ALS

A single large family with a slowly evolving disorder of both upper and lower motor neurons has been mapped to a single a large pedigree with this disease to chromosome 9. The linked locus has been successfully narrowed and studies show that the causative mutation is in the gene encoding the gene for sentaxin, a DNA helicase.

RECESSIVELY INHERITED, JUVENILE-ONSET ALS

In recessively inherited juvenile ALS, there is very slowly progressive degeneration of both upper and lower motor neurons and a survival of several decades. This "juvenile ALS" appears to be recessively inherited. Most affected individuals have limb atrophy, reflecting both disuse and some degree of denervation. In two small families, the disease is predominantly because of degeneration of the corticospinal and corticobulbar tracts; these features have suggested this disorder should be designated juvenile primary lateral sclerosis (PLS). In some families, this disorder is mapped to chromosome 2q33; in others the disorder maps to chromosome 15q. The 2q33 locus has been fully cloned; several candidate genes within it have been identified. The gene defect in these families has been attributed to mutations in gene encoding a protein with domains that show homology to guanine nucleotide exchange factors. This gene is therefore thought to regulate activity of one or more GTPases.

DISORDERS OF THE LOWER MOTOR NEURON

SPINAL MUSCULAR ATROPHY

The spinal muscular atrophies (SMAs) are characterized by progressive death of lower motor neurons in the brainstem and spinal cord. SMA is inherited as an autosomal recessive trait. Type I SMA (Werdnig-Hoffmann disease) begins very early (and may be evident *in utero* as diminished fetal movement in the weeks before birth). Werdnig-Hoffmann infants are weak, floppy, and suck and cry feebly. They never develop enough strength to sit up and they rarely survive beyond 2 yr. SMA I is relatively common, affecting up to 1/20,000 babies. The carrier frequency for SMA I is 1/80. Type II SMA begins clinically before 18 mo of age but is associated with long-term survival. Unlike SMA I patients, those with SMA II can sit but they cannot stand or walk. Patients with SMA III, which begins after 18 mo, are able to walk. In late-onset SMA (Kugelberg-Welander disease), weakness may be more evident proximally than distally; often the legs are more severely involved than the arms. The hallmark of SMA microscopically is lower motor neurons cell death.

Genetically, all forms of SMA are linked to chromosome 5. The critical gene appears to be a novel protein of 294 amino acids designated the "survival motor neuron" protein or SMN. The locus encoding SMN and NAIP is complex; it is duplicated such that there are at least two copies SMN (telomeric or centromeric). These copies differ only in that one exon (exon 7) is spliced out of the centromeric copy. SMN has been localized both to the nucleus and cytoplasm in cells in vitro. Its function is not entirely clear although several elegant studies have documented that it complexes with several ribonuclear proteins in spliceosomes and may be important in the shuttling of RNA between the nucleus and cytoplasm. The fundamental defect in SMA may involve aberrant splicing and trafficking of mRNA species. The telomeric copy of SMN is deleted in 98% of SMA patients. In the remaining approx 2%, it has undergone gene conversion such that it has the sequence of the centromeric copy of the protein. The severity of SMA is probably modified by several factors including the overall level of expressed SMN, the number of intact copies of SMN_t, and the presence or absence of neighboring genes that are commonly deleted with SMN. These include a NAIP and a second protein even more closely associated with SMN designated 4F5. Mouse models of SMA have been developed. Two entail dual genetic manipulations: knocking out the single native SMN gene in mice (a change that, by itself, is lethal because mice have only one copy of SMN), and expressing a transgenic copy of the human centromeric SMN gene. The third involves a motor neuron specific deletion of exon 7 from the endogenous SMN gene. The phenotype of the resulting animals rather closely resembles SMA.

ADULT-ONSET TAY SACH'S DISEASE Infrequently, patients with G_{M2} gangliosidosis develop a slowly progressive motor neuropathy characterized by lifelong motor clumsiness and later development of frank proximal muscle weakness. These individuals may also manifest some upper motor neuron signs, cerebellar features and behavioral features such as an altered attention span or even psychotic episodes. Bulbar features such as dysphagia and some dysarthria may become apparent. The critical defect in Tay-Sach's disease is an accumulation of G_{M2} ganglioside that develops because of deficiency of activity of the proteins that metabolize G_{M2} ganglioside, N-acetyl-hexosaminidase A and B. These dimeric enzymes consist of an α and a β subunit (hexosaminidase A), or two β subunits (hexosaminidase B). Each dimer is complexed with a third protein, G_{M2}activator, which modulates the activity of both enzymes.

X-LINKED SPINAL BULBAR MUSCULAR ATROPHY This is a slowly progressive, familial motor neuropathy that affects only males. In addition to motor weakness, there may be subtle gynecomastia and testicular atrophy, as well as low-grade sensory findings. The molecular defect in X-linked spinal bulbar muscular atrophy (X-SBMA) is an expansion of a CAG repeat in exon 1 of the androgen receptor gene. This produces an expanded polyglutamine tract within the receptor. In general, the longer is the tract of repeated CAGs, the more severe the illness. The mechanism of neurotoxicity of the CAGs is not known, although data suggest that the expanded polyglutamine tract may aggregate to form nuclear inclusions in these CAG-expansion diseases. In neurons in cell culture, expanded polyglutamine tracts induce apoptosis through activation of a specific cell death gene, caspase 8. Data suggest that in X-SBMA and other CAG repeat diseases, accumulation of CREB-binding protein (CRB) in the intranuclear aggregates may be a pivotal element in the pathogenesis of the disease; forced expression of CREB-binding protein can correct the neurotoxicity of the expanded androgen receptor glutamine repeat domain. The availability of transgenic mice with expanded androgen receptor polyglutamine tract should facilitate studies of pathogenesis and therapy of X-SBMA.

DISORDERS OF THE UPPER MOTOR NEURON

PRIMARY LATERAL SCLEROSIS PLS is a disorder that selectively targets the upper motor neuron. It usually occurs as a sporadic disease. Its main clinical feature is slowly progressive weakness without atrophy but with marked limb spasticity. Laboratory studies (electromyography and muscle biopsies) do not detect denervation of muscles. Although long-term survival is reported in PLS, the disease may run its course aggressively with 3–4 yr survival from onset to death. Autopsy shows loss of pyramidal cells in the motor cortex with corresponding degeneration of the corticospinal and corticobulbar projections. Early PLS raises the diagnostic possibility of multiple sclerosis or other demyelinating diseases, although these diagnoses are usually clarified over time.

HEREDITARY FAMILIAL SPASTIC PARAPLEGIA Hereditary familial spastic paraplegia (HSP) is an autosomal dominant trait with a clinical picture marked by spastic weakness beginning in the distal legs. The crucial neuropathological abnormality is corticospinal tract degeneration that is more pronounced caudally. In "complicated" HSP progressive spasticity is accompanied by findings not confined to the corticospinal tract. These include amyotrophy, mental retardation, optic atrophy, and sensory neuropathy; the corresponding pathology is not confined to the corticospinal tracts. In the more common, "uncomplicated" form, HSP is purely a corticospinal disease. Fortunately, genetic studies are illuminating some of these clinical distinctions. At least 10 HSP genes are identified (*see* Table 115-3). An early onset pedigree with spastic gait, relatively little weakness, and a very slow disease course is mapped to chromosome 14q and encodes the protein spastin, whose mutation is implicated in approx 40% of HSP. A large family with uncomplicated HSP has also been linked to chromosome 15q. This family has a more variable age of onset and a more aggressive course than the 14q family. Both early and late-onset families map to a third HSP locus on chromosome 2p. The defective gene at this locus has been identified and termed "spastin;" this protein may play a role in the metabolism of nucleoproteins. Table 115-3 enumerates the other known HSP genes. As described, one involves a gene that encodes a kinesin, further implicating motor protein dysfunction in motor degeneration. Also of interest is the involvement of a possible heat shock protein HSPD1 in another form of HSP. There is extensive genetic heterogeneity in dominantly inherited, uncomplicated HSP. Moreover, other HSP loci remain to be identified.

There are early onset forms of recessively inherited HSP. One locus, on chromosome 16, encodes a novel gene, "paraplegin," whose gene product is thought to function within mitochondria and to have homology to a yeast ATPase. A locus for uncomplicated, recessive HSP has been reported on chromosome 8q. X-linked recessive forms are also reported. One is caused by mutations in the gene encoding proteolipid protein. It is intriguing that other mutations within this gene cause the more fulminant Pelizaeus-Merzbacher disease. Another type of complicated, infantile-onset HSP is caused by mutations in the gene encoding the adhesion molecule L1CAM. Finally, there are rare cases of adult-onset, X-linked HSP-like disorders that are allelic forms of adrenoleukodystrophy.

OTHER INHERITED MOTOR NEURON DISEASES

Other inherited motor neuron diseases are recognized. Some affect only the motor system; others are complex, multisystem degenerations. Fazio-Londe disease (progressive juvenile bulbar palsy) is a bulbar motor neuronopathy that begins before the third year. The arthrogryposes are a complex set of disorders with contractures at birth from motor neuron cell loss. These may be either sporadic or inherited as autosomal recessive, autosomal dominant, or X-linked traits. In the scapuloperoneal muscular atrophies there is neuropathic weakness in the shoulders muscles and the peroneal groups. This disease also shows considerable diversity with dominantly inherited midlife onset and early onset and possible X-linked forms.

ALS RISK FACTORS: A BRIDGE BETWEEN INHERITED AND SPORADIC ALS

Although most cases of ALS are not familial, it remains plausible that many individuals with sporadic ALS may have heightened susceptibility to factors such as environmental insults and the consequences of aging that challenge and ultimately disrupt motor neuron function and viability. Many such putative ALS risk factors have been considered. The status of polymorphisms in ApoE has been investigated because the ApoE4 allele confers a distinct risk for early onset in Alzheimer's disease. Studies do not clearly implicate ApoE as an ALS risk factor. However, in one large series, the rate of progression in sporadic ALS was more rapid in a cohort with higher levels of total serum apolipoprotein E. Ciliary neurotrophic factor (CNTF) is a potent trophic substance for motor neurons in vitro; inactivation of the CNTF gene in mice

FRDA is most commonly caused by expansion of an unstable GAA repeat in the first intron of the *FRDA* (*X25*) gene. Normal alleles have 7–34 repeats whereas disease alleles are typically more than 100 repeats. Rare patients are compound heterozygotes for a repeat expansion and sequence alteration. The gene product frataxin is a widely expressed mitochondrial protein and is usually drastically reduced in FRDA because the expansion interferes with its transcription. A strong correlation exists between GAA repeat size and disease severity: the longer the repeat the lower the levels of frataxin and the more severe the disease. Studies of a yeast frataxin homolog (Yfh1) focused attention on the role of frataxin in iron homeostasis. That mice lacking frataxin develop a deficiency in respiratory chain complex activities and have intramitochondrial iron accumulation further refined the site and mechanism of pathogenesis within the cell. The iron accumulation in mitochondria of animal models and human FRDA hearts was associated with increased sensitivity to oxidative stress. These findings inspired therapeutic strategies aimed at boosting antioxidant activity in the cell by providing antioxidants such as coenzyme Q10 (CoQ10) and its short-chain analog idebenone. Treatment of FRDA patients with CoQ10 and vitamin E for 6 mo improved muscle mitochondrial ATP production, but a functional significance of this change was not demonstrated. Three studies used idebenone at 5 mg/kg/d for several months to 1 yr. Two of these were open label and one was a placebo-controlled, double blind study. All three studies demonstrated significant reduction in interventricular septum thickness and/or left-ventricular mass index. The clinical significance of the reduction in LVH was not demonstrated and there was no evidence of an effect on the ataxia. Although a change in the clinical and neurological course was not demonstrated, the preliminary findings of reduced LVH after idebenone therapy are encouraging and call for additional clinical studies designed to assess cardiac and neurological outcome measures in FRDA.

SPINOCEREBELLAR ATAXIA TYPE 8 AND TYPE 12 Two SCAs are caused by expansion of trinucleotide repeats that are outside the coding region of the respective gene. SCA8 is caused by expansion of an untranslated CTG repeat in the 3′ end of a processed noncoding mRNA. The 5′ end of the SCA8 gene overlaps, in the opposite direction, the 5′ end of Kelch-like 1 that encodes an actin-binding protein. Normal alleles have 20–50 repeats and disease-causing alleles contain 100–250 repeats. Intriguingly, very large alleles (250–800 repeats) do not cause a phenotype. Exactly why large expansions are not deleterious is not known, but one hypothesis is that such expansion may interfere with RNA processing or stability thus a toxic expanded RNA will not be generated or is rapidly degraded. SCA12 is a rare SCA caused by expansion of an untranslated CAG repeat in the 5′ untranslated region of the brain-specific regulatory subunit of the protein phosphatase PP2A (PPP2R2B). The normal range of CAG repeat is 7–28 whereas expanded alleles have 66–78 repeats. The pathogenic mechanism in SCA12 is not yet understood and it is not known if the repeat expansion affects the function of PPP2-R2B or that of another gene.

DISEASES CAUSED BY CODING TRINUCLEOTIDE REPEATS: THE POLYGLUTAMINE DISORDERS

The polyglutamine neurodegenerative disorders include SBMA, HD, DRPLA, and various SCAs. All these diseases result from an expansion of an unstable CAG repeat that encodes a glutamine tract in the respective protein. This group of diseases shares many clinical and pathophysiological features in spite of the diverse group of genes involved. First, all these diseases are inherited in an autosomal-dominant manner except SBMA, which is X-linked but dominant at the cellular level. Second, all these disorders are late onset with most patients developing symptoms in the third or fourth decade. There is an inverse correlation between repeat size and age of onset for each of these disorders. The intergenerational repeat instability, particularly expansions of paternally transmitted repeats, leads to anticipation in successive generations and to the juvenile onset of disease. Third, a gain of function mechanism is responsible for the neurodegenerative phenotype given that loss of function or haploinsufficiency of several of these genes leads to a phenotype that is distinct from that caused by CAG repeat expansion. Last, all these disorders appear to share at least one common pathogenic mechanism at the cellular level: the expanded polyglutamine tract is thought to alter the conformation, folding, and/or degradation pattern of the native protein thus leading to its accumulation. These accumulated proteins have various toxic effects depending on their normal function, interacting partners, and subcellular localization patterns.

It is curious that in each of these disorders there is a group of particularly vulnerable neurons in spite of the overlapping and wide expression patterns of the various gene products. As the CAG repeat size expands beyond 80–100 repeats to cause childhood or infantile disease the selective neuronal vulnerability disappears and the overlap in clinical and neuropathological findings becomes apparent. These findings highlight a commonality to some of the pathogenic mechanisms and raise the possibility that most neurons become equally vulnerable if sufficient levels of the misfolded mutant proteins accumulate in them. The following section provides an overview of each disorder, followed by a discussion of pathogenic mechanisms and translational research efforts.

SPINOBULBAR MUSCULAR ATROPHY (KENNEDY DISEASE) SBMA is an X-linked disorder characterized by proximal muscle weakness, bulbar dysfunction, and partial loss of secondary sexual characteristics. The clinical findings of lower motor neuron disease, gynecomastia, and impotence led to the hypothesis that SBMA may result from dysfunction of the androgen receptor (AR) given that this receptor is expressed in spinal and cranial motor neurons. The SBMA locus has been mapped to the long arm of the X chromosome and subsequently determined the mutation in SBMA to be an expansion of the CAG repeat within the first exon of the *AR* gene. Normal alleles contain 9–36 repeats, and expanded alleles contain 38–66 repeats.

The AR is a member of the steroid hormone receptor family and typically on binding of their ligand (androgen in the case of AR) in the cytoplasm, the complex is translocated to the nucleus in which it regulates transcription of hormone responsive genes. The expansion may cause partial loss of receptor function given some signs of androgen insensitivity in males but the predominant effect is a toxic gain of function because total lack of AR causes testicular feminization and not motor neuron degeneration. Several transgenic mouse models using portions or full-length AR with variable lengths of the CAG tract have been generated. One study demonstrated that when full-length AR with 97 CAG repeats is expressed at sufficiently high levels in mice, the SBMA phenotype is reproduced in a sex-limited pattern. Male mice developed motor neuron disease that resolved on castration; female mice were spared unless they were treated with testosterone. This study demonstrated the importance of androgen and the translocation of the hormone/receptor complex to the nucleus for pathogenesis.

Based on these findings interventional trials that reduce the male hormones are being investigated to see if they will curb the toxicity of the mutant AR in SBMA patients.

HUNTINGTON DISEASE   HD is characterized by chorea, memory deficits, affective disturbance, and changes in personality. Dystonia, rigidity, and other involuntary motor impairments may occur. Patients with juvenile-onset suffer from rigidity, epilepsy, severe dementia, and rapid disease progression. Neuropathologically, HD is characterized by severe atrophy of the neostriatum (worse in the caudate), volume loss in the globus pallidus, and some cortical atrophy. The medium-sized spiny striatal neurons appear to be the most vulnerable neurons in HD. Purkinje cells are vulnerable in juvenile-onset cases. HD is caused by expansion of a CAG repeat in the first exon of the *HD* gene. Normal alleles have 6–34 repeats whereas disease causing alleles range from 36 to 121. The *HD* gene encodes for huntingtin, a protein that is essential for normal neuronal development and viability of the organism as demonstrated from studies of various knock-out mouse models. Gain of function animal models that express full length or truncated portions of HD with varying length repeats reproduce features of HD. Abnormal nuclear and neuropil aggregation of huntingtin has been documented in both postmortem human tissues and tissues from various mouse models. A HD-like 2 disorder has been reported in patients that have features of HD but no evidence of CAG repeat expansion at the HD locus. HD-like 2 is caused by expansion of a trinucleotide repeat in an alternatively spliced exon of the gene encoding junctophilin-3. The repeat is predicted to be either translated or in a 3' untranslated region depending on which splice acceptor site is used during RNA processing. Thus the mechanism mediating the pathogenesis of HD-like 2 is not yet understood.

Various clinical trials in transgenic mouse models and human patients include treatment protocols using CoQ10, creatine, minocycline, remacemide, and riluzole. Although several of these therapies showed benefit in the mouse models, the data in humans have not demonstrated significant effects for CoQ10 or remacemide. Studies with riluzole, creatine, and minocycline continue.

DENTATORUBROPALLIDOLUYSIAN ATROPHY   DRPLA is a rare autosomal-dominant neurodegenerative disorder, characterized by progressive ataxia, myoclonus, epilepsy, chorea, athetosis, and dementia. The mutation causing DRPLA was identified using the candidate gene approach and determined to involve an expansion of a CAG repeat within a novel gene that maps to human chromosome 12p. DRPLA patients have an expanded allele in the 49–88 repeat range in addition to the normal allele, which typically contains 6–35 repeats. The size of the expanded allele typically increases when paternally transmitted, with larger alleles causing juvenile-onset cases. The DRPLA mutation was found in an African American family with Haw River syndrome (HRS). HRS differs from DRPLA in the absence of myoclonic epilepsy and presence of demyelination of the subcortical white matter.

The DRPLA gene product, atrophin-1, is a widely expressed protein that localizes to both the cytoplasm and nucleus. Studies of its *Drosophila* homolog suggest that atrophin-1 may function as a transcriptional repressor. Patients with DRPLA suffer from neuronal loss in the dentate nucleus, globus pallidus, thalamus, and subthalamic nucleic. Severe demyelination and axonal degeneration is documented in the superior cerebellar peduncle and subcortical white matter. Basal ganglia calcifications are also noted.

Transgenic mice expressing full-length atrophin-1 develop ataxia, tremors, seizures, and premature death. Abnormal accumulation of atrophin-1 is noted in the nuclei of several neuronal populations similar to what is observed in postmortem human tissue.

SPINOCEREBELLAR ATAXIA TYPE 1   The main clinical features in SCA type 1 (SCA1) include gait ataxia, dysarthria, and dysmetria. As the disease progresses, brainstem involvement results in facial weakness, tongue atrophy, severe dysarthria, and dysphagia. Hyperreflexia may be detected early in the course of the disease, but in later stages the patients develop muscular atrophy, hypotonia, and hyporeflexia. Other, less consistent findings observed in some patients include optic nerve atrophy, ophthalmoparesis, and loss of proprioception and vibration sense. The disease typically manifests in the third to fourth decade, progresses over 10–15 yr, and results in death from brainstem dysfunction. Earlier age of onset and increase in the severity of the phenotype is observed in later generations of SCA1 kindreds.

Imaging studies in SCA1 patients reveal atrophy of the brachia pontis and anterior lobe of the cerebellum and enlargement of the fourth ventricle. Typical neuropathological findings in SCA1 include cerebellar atrophy with loss of Purkinje's cells and dentate nucleus neurons, presence of "torpedoes," which are swollen axons of degenerating Purkinje's cells, and severe neuronal degeneration in the inferior olive and to a lesser degree in cranial nerve nuclei III, IV, IX, X, and XII. Demyelination in the restiform body, brachium conjunctivum, spinocerebellar tracts, and posterior columns is frequently noted.

SCA1 results from expansion of a highly polymorphic CAG repeat that encodes a polyglutamine tract in the protein ataxin-1. Normal alleles contain 6–44 repeats that typically have 1–4 CAT interruptions when beyond 20 repeats. Disease alleles have a pure tract of uninterrupted CAG trinucleotides ranging from 39 to 82 repeats. Ataxin-1 is a protein of unknown cellular function. Loss of function in mice causes impaired motor learning but no ataxia. Transgenic and knock-in mouse models reproduce clinical and pathological features of SCA1. Mutant ataxin-1 localizes to a single ubiquitin-positive nuclear inclusion in neurons of SCA1 patients and mice. Studies of SCA1 transgenic mice and flies provided insight about the importance of protein folding and degradation in SCA1 pathogenesis as discussed later.

SPINOCEREBELLAR ATAXIA TYPE 2   SCA type 2 (SCA2) is characterized by ataxia, dysarthria, tremor, nystagmus, and slow saccades. Hyporeflexia occurs in later stages of the disease and some patients suffer cognitive impairment. Infantile SCA2 has been documented and is characterized by neonatal hypotonia, developmental delay, bulbar dysfunction, and retinitis pigmentosa. Neuropathologically SCA2 is characterized by loss of cerebellar Purkinje cells and brainstem neurons. Atrophy of fronto-temporal lobes and loss of nigral neurons have also been reported. The SCA2 CAG repeat is not very polymorphic with the majority of alleles containing 22 or 23 repeats; normal range is 14–31 repeats interrupted by two CAA triplets. Disease alleles contain a pure CAG tract that ranges from 33 to 200 repeats. A patient with 33 repeats has onset at 86 yr of age whereas the one with 200 repeats has neonatal onset. The SCA2 gene product, ataxin-2, is a novel protein of unknown function. Genetic studies in *Drosophila* provided insight about the function of the fruit fly homolog of ataxin-2 (Datx2). Flies lacking Datx2 manifest sterility, abnormal bristle morphology, cellular degeneration and lethality. These phenotypes appear to result from defects in actin filament formation raising the possibility that Datx2 is a regulator of actin filament formation. Like other mutant polyglutamine proteins, ataxin-2 accumulates in SCA2 brains and in Purkinje cells of mice that overexpress a mutant allele. Interestingly, mutant ataxin-2 predominantly accumulates in the cytoplasm in contrast to most other polyglutamine disorders in which the mutant proteins accumulate in the nucleus. This is most likely because of ataxin-2's normal cytoplasmic subcellular localization.

MACHADO-JOSEPH DISEASE/SPINOCEREBELLAR ATAXIA TYPE 3 Machado-Joseph disease (MJD) is characterized by progressive ataxia, external ophthalmoplegia, bulging eyes, facial and lingual fasciculations, muscle atrophy, dystonia, and spasticity. Dementia and extrapyramidal findings occur in approx 20% of patients. Neuropathological findings include severe neuronal loss in the striatum and substantia nigra, with moderate abnormalities in the dentate nucleus and red nucleus. The mutational mechanism in MJD involves the expansion of a CAG repeat that lies within a novel gene on chromosome 14q32.1. Normal alleles contain 12–40 repeats, whereas expanded alleles contain 55–84 repeats. SCA3, clinically distinct from MJD and resembling SCA1, is also caused by CAG expansions within the *MJD* gene.

Ataxin-3 is a predominantly cytoplasmic protein, although when mutated it accumulates in nuclei of neurons. Transgenic mice and flies harboring truncated ataxin-3 with expanded polyglutamine tracts revealed the toxicity of such expanded tracts and highlighted the importance of protein misfolding in the pathogenesis of polyglutamine-induced degeneration.

SPINOCEREBELLAR ATAXIA TYPE 6 Patients with SCA type 6 (SCA6) present with mild, slowly progressive ataxia and dysarthria; as the disease worsens, patients suffer from pronounced incoordination, tremor, and dysphagia. Some patients exhibit horizontal gaze-evoked and vertical nystagmus and some develop mild neuropathy.

Neuropathological findings in SCA6 include marked cerebellar atrophy with severe loss of cerebellar Purkinje cells and moderate loss of cerebellar granule cells, dentate nucleus neurons, and neurons of the inferior olive.

SCA6 is caused by a CAG repeat expansion in the α_{1A}-voltage dependent calcium channel (*CACNA1A*). Voltage-sensitive calcium channels are multimeric complexes made of the pore-forming α_{1A}-subunit and several regulatory subunits. These channels mediate calcium entry into neurons and are abundant in cerebellar Purkinje cells and granule neurons. Consistent with this, the mutant α_{1A} calcium channels aggregate in the cytoplasm of SCA6 Purkinje cells. These accumulations occur in the peripheral perikaryal cytoplasm and in the proximal dendrites but not in the nucleus.

The CAG repeat in *CACNA1A* is exceptionally small, with fewer than 18 repeats on normal alleles. Disease-causing alleles are also small and contain 20–33 CAG repeats. These small expansions, however, are sufficient to increase α-1A protein expression at the cellular surface and thus Ca^{2+} current. Missense, splice, and protein-truncating mutations in *CACNA1A* have been reported in episodic ataxia type 2 (EA2) and familial hemiplegic migraine. Furthermore, the tottering and tottering-leaner mice bear nonexpansion mutations in the mouse homolog. That some patients with SCA6 experience episodic ataxia in the early stages of their disease raises the possibility that SCA6 and EA2 may represent different points along a phenotypic continuum of the same disease.

SPINOCEREBELLAR ATAXIA TYPE 7 Of the patients with SCA type 7 (SCA7), approximately half present with cerebellar ataxia and visual deficits; the majority of the remaining half present with cerebellar ataxia but may develop visual dysfunction after decades of disease. SCA7 patients lose visual acuity because of a progressive pigmentary macular degeneration. Patients initially lose central vision but have intact peripheral and night vision. Secondary optic atrophy and bilateral blindness occur in the disease's later stages. Additional features of SCA7 include increased reflexes and spasticity, slow saccades, ophthalmoplegia, and hearing deficits. Behavioral disturbances such as auditory hallucinations, progressive psychosis, depression, and delusions have been reported. Infantile SCA7 is severe and characterized by severe hypotonia, patent ductus arteriosus, congestive heart failure, and the visual and neuronal deficits. These infants typically die in the first year of life.

Neuronal loss occurs primarily in the cerebellum, inferior olive, and some cranial nerve nuclei. Degeneration of cones and rods as well as hypomyelination of the optic tract and gliosis of the lateral geniculate body and visual cortex are also characteristics of SCA7. Electron microscopy studies of skeletal muscles of SCA7 patients reveal mitochondrial abnormalities, such as subsarcolemmal accumulations of rounded mitochondria and frequent autophagic vacuoles.

The polyglutamine tract is near the amino terminus of the *SCA7* gene product, ataxin-7. Normal alleles contain pure CAG tracts ranging from 4 to 35 repeats whereas expanded alleles contain 37–460 repeats. The SCA7 mutation is highly unstable and manifests the most extreme intergenerational CAG repeat instability, with an expansion of 263 repeats in one paternal transmission.

Ataxin-7 is of very low abundance in the cell, probably because of its rapid degradation. Ataxin-7, is a component of a protein complex that has a histone acetyl transferase activiy, and thus must play a role in transcriptional regulation. The *SCA7* RNA shows ubiquitous expression, with high levels in the heart, placenta, skeletal muscle, pancreas, and brain. Within the central nervous system, the *SCA7* transcript is most abundant in the cerebellum. In SCA7 patients, ataxin-7 nuclear aggregates were observed in the brainstem, especially pons and inferior olive and, in one juvenile-onset patient, in the cerebral cortex. Studies in several transgenic models of SCA7 and a knock-in model of the disease demonstrate that mutant ataxin-7 alters transcription of at least photoreceptor-specific genes, suggesting that transcriptional dysregulation is an important component of pathogenesis.

SPINOCEREBELLAR ATAXIA TYPE 17 SCA type 17 (SCA17) manifests with ataxia, dementia or features of Parkinsonism, such as truncal dystonia, dysmetria, bradykinesia, accelerated gait, and retropulsion. Epilepsy is typically a late feature but rarely occurs early in the course.

Imaging studies of SCA17 patients reveal diffuse cortical and cerebellar atrophy. Neuropathological examination reveals loss of small neurons in the thalamus, frontal and temporal cortical regions, caudate nucleus, and putamen. The cerebellum shows moderate Purkinje cell loss and increased gliosis.

SCA17 is caused by a CAG repeat expansion in the gene encoding the TATA-binding protein (TBP), a general transcription initiation factor. Normal repeat tracts contain 29–42 CAGs whereas disease alleles range from 47 to 55 repeats. TBP is the DNA-binding subunit of RNA polymerase II transcription factor D, a multi-subunit complex critical for the transcription of most genes.

PATHOGENESIS OF POLYGLUTAMINE DISORDERS

The presence of abnormal protein aggregates in neurons is common in polyglutamine disorders. This feature is shared with other neurodegenerative disorders such as Alzheimer's disease, Parkinson's disease, frontotemporal dementia, amyotrophic lateral sclerosis and prion encephalopathies. Studies in cell culture, animal models, and human tissues led to the discovery that the nuclear protein aggregates stain positively for ubiquitin, molecular chaperones, and components of the proteasome. These findings led to the hypothesis that the expanded polyglutamine tracts alter the conformation of the host protein causing it to misfold and resist degradation. Data from an SCA7 knock-in mouse model that carries an expanded CAG tract within the endogenous SCA7 locus revealed gradual accumulation of mutant ataxin-7. Because wild-type ataxin-7 is normally rapidly degraded, the gradual increase in the levels of the mutant protein is consistent with the hypothesis that the expanded protein resists degradation.

Other evidence in support of the importance of the ubiquitin-proteasome pathway in pathogenesis comes from cellular and genetic studies. Decreasing the amounts of ubiquitin and/or some of the enzymes typically involved in ligating ubiquitin to protein substrates (so that they can be targeted for proteasomal degradation) enhanced the neurodegenerative phenotypes in *Drosophila* and mouse SCA1 models. To boost the cells' ability to deal with mutant polyglutamine proteins, several investigators overexpressed chaperones in cells and in model organisms of the polyglutamine proteinopathies. Molecular chaperones are proteins that typically promote proper folding of newly synthesized or misfolded proteins or usher them to be degraded by the proteasome if they cannot be folded properly. Chaperone overexpression clearly suppressed the neurodegenerative phenotypes in flies expressing either an expanded polyglutamine tract, a portion of mutant ataxin-3, or full-length ataxin-1. Chaperone overexpression also improved the motor function in SCA1 mice. These data provide evidence in support of a common pathogenic mechanism in polyglutamine disorders and identify chaperones as a potential therapeutic target in this class of disorders. If the chaperone activity of neurons can be boosted pharmacologically, disease progression might be slowed.

Exactly how the expanded polyglutamine protein induces neuronal dysfunction and degeneration in each of the disorders is not understood but some implicated mechanisms are being investigated. Because many of the protein accumulations occur in the nucleus, several investigators focused on the role of transcription in pathogenesis. Transcriptional dysregulation has been confirmed in mouse models of SCA1, SCA7, and HD. Alterations in the nuclear distribution and activity of the transcriptional activator CREB-binding protein (CBP) in mouse and cellular models and in human tissues made it an excellent candidate for mediating some of the pathogenic effects. CBP is known to enhance transcription through enhancing histone acetylation and thus rendering chromatin more open and accessible to the transcriptional machinery. Alterations found in CBP activity in some polyglutamine disorders raised the question of whether decreasing histone deacetylation would have beneficial effects. This proved to be the case in *Drosophila* and in mouse models bearing exon 1 of huntingtin with an expanded repeat tract and in cells expressing mutant AR and HD proteins. The histone deacetylase inhibitors suberolylamide hydroxamic acid and sodium butyrate suppressed neuronal degeneration and improved the viability in these model systems. Thus histone deacetylase inhibitors constitute another potential therapeutic target for this class of diseases.

Studies of ataxin-1, its modifications and interactions revealed another potential pathway for intervention. Ataxin-1 is phosphorylated by Akt protein kinase, allowing ataxin-1 to interact with the protein 14-3-3, which in turn hinders its degradation. Genetic studies

in mice and flies revealed that interfering with this phosphorylation by mutating the amino acid that is normally phosphorylated by Akt or by decreasing Akt levels suppresses neuronal degeneration in SCA1 mice and flies, respectively. These findings point to inhibitors of Akt (and its upstream activator phosphotidyl inositol 3-kinase) as potential therapeutic targets for evaluation in SCA1 mice.

SUMMARY AND CLINICAL IMPLICATIONS

The finding that expansion of trinucleotide repeats is the mutational mechanism in the described neurological disorders greatly facilitates the diagnosis of these diseases and provides options for genetic counseling. In the case of dominantly inherited ataxias, the identification of these mutations allows a rational classification of this highly heterogeneous group of diseases in addition to facilitating diagnosis. Molecular testing for trinucleotide repeat expansions should be considered as the leading diagnostic test in trying to evaluate patients with dominantly inherited ataxia, progressive degenerative disorders characterized by chorea, dementia with or without seizures, X-linked patterns of lower motor neuron disease, congenital muscle disorders and suspected DM, and mental retardation. Testing for the HD, DRPLA, and SCA mutations in asymptomatic individuals who are at risk should be restricted to adults who have undergone extensive psychological and genetic counseling, given the devastating nature of these diseases. In children these tests should be limited to those already symptomatic. In the case of FRAXA, the molecular analysis of the CGG repeat is superior to the cytogenetic approach traditionally used for identifying the fragile site, owing to its sensitivity and accuracy. However, chromosomal analysis in patients with mental retardation is still extremely valuable given the relative high likelihood of identifying other cytogenetic abnormalities. The finding that male patients with premutation alleles at FMR1 develop a late onset progressive ataxia and tremors should entice clinicians to obtain careful family history about mental retardation and ovarian failure in the descendents of these males. Importantly, a DNA test in these patients might prove beneficial for diagnosing this new emerging clinical entity and for counseling their descendents about risk of future expansions. The progress in pathogenesis studies has been hastened by the power of genetic models and cell and molecular biology techniques. These studies are revealing pathways that are potential therapeutic targets. Ongoing interventional trials in FRDA and potentially in several of these diseases are encouraging.

The availability of excellent mouse models for several polyglutamine disorders and the identification of several potential therapeutic targets will allow rigorous design of preclinical trials to evaluate safety and efficacy. In the case of SBMA, preclinical data suggest that manipulating androgen levels in affected males is a therapeutic strategy. The finding that neurons can recover if the production of the mutant protein is halted in conditional mouse models of HD and SCH provide hope that some treatments might reverse aspects of the disease in symptomatic individuals. The delayed onset of these diseases provides a window of opportunity to intervene before clinical symptoms become apparent. The challenge, however, is identifying outcome measures and biological markers that can be used to gage the effect of interventional trials because of the variable onset in this group of diseases and because their course typically spans decades.

SELECTED REFERENCES

Brown V, Jin P, Ceman S, et al. Microarray identification of FMRP-associated brain mRNAs and altered mRNA translational profiles in fragile X syndrome. Cell 2001;107:477–487.

Buyse G, Mertens L, Di Salvo G, et al. Idebenone treatment in Friedreich's ataxia: neurological, cardiac, and biochemical monitoring. Neurology 2003;60:1679–1681.

Chantrel-Groussard K, Geromel V, Puccio H, et al. Disabled early recruitment of antioxidant defenses in Friedreich's ataxia. Hum Mol Genet 2001;10:2061–2067.

Chen HK, Fernandez-Funez P, Acevedo SF, et al. Interaction of Akt-phosphorylated ataxin-1 with 14-3-3 mediates neurodegeneration in spinocerebellar ataxia type 1. Cell 2003;113:457–468.

Cleary JD, Nichol K, Wang YH, Pearson CE. Evidence of cis-acting factors in replication-mediated trinucleotide repeat instability in primate cells. Nat Genet 2002;31:37–46.

Cummings CJ, Sun Y, Opal P, et al. Over-expression of inducible HSP70 chaperone suppresses neuropathology and improves motor function in SCA1 mice. Hum Mol Genet 2001;10:1511–1518.

Darnell JC, Jensen KB, Jin P, Brown V, Warren ST, Darnell RB. Fragile X mental retardation protein targets G quartet mRNAs important for neuronal function. Cell 2001;107:489–499.

Dedeoglu A, Kubilus JK, Yang L, et al. Creatine therapy provides neuroprotection after onset of clinical symptoms in Huntington's disease transgenic mice. J Neurochem 2003;85:1359–1367.

Emamian ES, Kaytor MD, Duvick LA, et al. Serine 776 of ataxin-1 is critical for polyglutamine-induced disease in SCA1 transgenic mice. Neuron 2003;38:375–387.

Fernandez-Funez P, Nino-Rosales ML, de Gouyon B, et al. Identification of genes that modify ataxin-1-induced neurodegeneration. Nature 2000;408:101–106.

Gatchel JR, Zoghbi HY. Diseases of unstable repeat expansion: mechanisms and common principles. Nat Rev Genet 2005;6:743–755.

Greco CM, Hagerman RJ, Tassone F, et al. Neuronal intranuclear inclusions in a new cerebellar tremor/ataxia syndrome among fragile X carriers. Brain 2002;125:1760–1771.

Hagerman RJ, Leehey M, Heinrichs W, et al. Intention tremor, parkinsonism, and generalized brain atrophy in male carriers of fragile X. Neurology 2001;57:127–130.

Helmlinger D, Hardy S, Abou-Sleymane G, et al. Glutamine-Expanded Ataxin-7 Alters TFTC/STAGA Recruitment and Chromatin Structure Leading to Photoreceptor Dysfunction. PLoS Biol 2006;4:e67.

Hockly E, Richon VM, Woodman B, et al. Suberoylanilide hydroxamic acid, a histone deacetylase inhibitor, ameliorates motor deficits in a mouse model of Huntington's disease. Proc Natl Acad Sci USA 2003;100:2041–2046.

Holmes SE, O'Hearn EE, McInnis MG, et al. Expansion of a novel CAG trinucleotide repeat in the 5' region of PPP2R2B is associated with SCA12. Nat Genet 1999;23:391–392.

Huber KM, Gallagher SM, Warren ST, Bear MF. Altered synaptic plasticity in a mouse model of fragile X mental retardation. Proc Natl Acad Sci USA 2002;99:7746–7750.

Hughes RE, Olson JM. Therapeutic opportunities in polyglutamine disease. Nat Med 2001;7:419–423.

Huynh DP, Del Bigio MR, Ho DH, Pulst SM. Expression of ataxin-2 in brains from normal individuals and patients with Alzheimer's disease and spinocerebellar ataxia 2. Ann Neurol 1999;45:232–241.

Huynh DP, Figueroa K, Hoang N, Pulst SM. Nuclear localization or inclusion body formation of ataxin-2 are not necessary for SCA2 pathogenesis in mouse or human. Nat Genet 2000;26:44–50.

Jin P, Warren ST. New insights into fragile X syndrome: from molecules to neurobehaviors. Trends Biochem Sci 2003;28:152–158.

Klesert TR, Cho DH, Clark JI, et al. Mice deficient in Six5 develop cataracts: Implications for myotonic dystrophy. Nat Genet 2000;25:105–109.

Koob MD, Moseley ML, Schut LJ, et al. An untranslated CTG expansion causes a novel form of spinocerebellar ataxia (SCA8). Nat Genet 1999;21:379–384.

Kopito RR. Aggresomes, inclusion bodies and protein aggregation. Trends Cell Biol 2000;10:524–530.

La Spada AR, Fu YH, Sopher BL, et al. Polyglutamine-expanded ataxin-7 antagonizes CRX function and induces cone-rod dystrophy in a mouse model of SCA7. Neuron 2001;31:913–927.

Liquori CL, Ricker K, Moseley ML, et al. Myotonic dystrophy type 2 caused by a CCTG expansion in intron 1 of ZNF9. Science 2001; 293:864–867.

Luthi-Carter R, Strand AD, Hanson SA, et al. Polyglutamine and transcription: gene expression changes shared by DRPLA and Huntington's disease mouse models reveal context-independent effects. Hum Mol Genet 2002;11:1927–1937.

Lynch DR, Farmer JM, Balcer LJ, Wilson RB. Friedreich ataxia: effects of genetic understanding on clinical evaluation and therapy. Arch Neurol 2002;59:743–747.

Mankodi A, Logigian E, Callahan L, et al. Myotonic dystrophy in transgenic mice expressing an expanded CUG repeat. Science 2000;289:1769–1773.

Mankodi A, Urbinati CR, Yuan QP, et al. Muscleblind localizes to nuclear foci of aberrant RNA in myotonic dystrophy types 1 and 2. Hum Mol Genet 2001;10:2165–2170.

Mariotti C, Solari A, Torta D, Marano L, Fiorentini C, Di Donato S. Idebenone treatment in Friedreich patients: one-year-long randomized placebo-controlled trial. Neurology 2003;60:1676–1679.

McMahon SJ, Pray-Grant MG, Schieltz D, Yates JR 3rd, Grant PA. Polyglutamine-expanded spinocerebellar ataxia-7 protein disrupts normal SAGA and SLIK histone acetyltransferase activity. Proc Natl Acad Sci USA 2005;102:8478–8482.

Nakamura K, Jeong SY, Uchihara T, et al. SCA17, a novel autosomal dominant cerebellar ataxia caused by an expanded polyglutamine in TATA-binding protein. Hum Mol Genet 2001;10:1441–1448.

Nemes JP, Benzow KA, Moseley ML, Ranum LP, Koob MD. The SCA8 transcript is an antisense RNA to a brain-specific transcript encoding a novel actin-binding protein (KLHL1). Hum Mol Genet 2000;9:1543–1551.

Nucifora FC Jr, Sasaki M, Peters MF, et al. Interference by huntingtin and atrophin-1 with cbp-mediated transcription leading to cellular toxicity. Science 2001;291:2423–2428.

Orr HT. Beyond the Qs in the polyglutamine diseases. Genes Dev 2001;15:925–932.

Palhan VB, Chen S, Peng GH, et al. Polyglutamine-expanded ataxin-7 inhibits STAGA histone acetyltransferase activity to produce retinal degeneration. Proc Natl Acad Sci USA 2005;102:8472–8477.

Philips AV, Timchenko LT, Cooper TA. Disruption of splicing regulated by a CUG-binding protein in myotonic dystrophy. Science 1998;280:737–741.

Puccio H, Koenig M. Friedreich ataxia: a paradigm for mitochondrial diseases. Curr Opin Genet Dev 2002;12:272–277.

Puccio H, Simon D, Cossee M, et al. Mouse models for Friedreich ataxia exhibit cardiomyopathy, sensory nerve defect and Fe-S enzyme deficiency followed by intramitochondrial iron deposits. Nat Genet 2001;27:181–186.

Reddy S, Smith DB, Rich MM, et al. Mice lacking the myotonic dystrophy protein kinase develop a late onset. Nat Genet 1996;13:325–335.

Richards RI. Dynamic mutations: a decade of unstable expanded repeats in human genetic disease. Hum Mol Genet 2001;10:2187–2194.

Sarkar PS, Appukuttan B, Han J, et al. Heterozygous loss of Six5 in mice is sufficient to cause ocular cataracts. Nat Genet 2000;25:110–114.

Satterfield TF, Jackson SM, Pallanck LJ. A Drosophila homolog of the polyglutamine disease gene SCA2 is a dosage-sensitive regulator of actin filament formation. Genetics 2002;162:1687–1702.

Savkur RS, Philips AV, Cooper TA. Aberrant regulation of insulin receptor alternative splicing is associated with insulin resistance in myotonic dystrophy. Nat Genet 2001;29:40–47.

Shan DE, Soong BW, Sun CM, Lee SJ, Liao KK, Liu RS. Spinocerebellar ataxia type 2 presenting as familial levodopa-responsive parkinsonism. Ann Neurol 2001;50:812–815.

Steffan JS, Thompson LM. Targeting aggregation in the development of therapeutics for the treatment of Huntington's disease and other polyglutamine repeat diseases. Expert Opin Ther Targets 2003;7:201–213.

Steffan JS, Bodai L, Pallos J, et al. Histone deacetylase inhibitors arrest polyglutamine-dependent neurodegeneration in Drosophila. Nature 2001;413:739–743.

Sullivan AK, Crawford DC, Scott EH, Leslie ML, Sherman SL. Paternally transmitted FMR1 alleles are less stable than maternally transmitted alleles in the common and intermediate size range. Am J Hum Genet 2002;70:1532–1544.

Taylor JP, Fischbeck KH. Altered acetylation in polyglutamine disease: an opportunity for therapeutic intervention? Trends Mol Med 2002;8:195–197.

The Dutch-Belgian fragile X consortium. Fmr1 knockout mice: a model to study fragile X mental retardation. Cell 1994;78:23–33.

Warren ST, Sherman SL. The fragile X syndrome. In: Scriver CR, ed. The Metabolic and Molecular Bases of Inherited Deisease, Vol. 1. New York: McGraw-Hill Companies, 2001; pp. 1257–1290.

Warrick JM, Chan HY, Gray-Board GL, Chai Y, Paulson HL, Bonini NM. Suppression of polyglutamine-mediated neurodegeneration in Drosophila by the molecular chaperone HSP70. Nat Genet 1999;23:425–428.

Watase K, Weeber EJ, Xu B, et al. A long CAG tract in the mouse Sca1 locus replicates human SCA1 and reveals the impact of mutant protein solubility on selective neuronal vulnerability. Neuron 2002;34:905–919.

Willemsen R, Hoogeveen-Westerveld M, Reis S, et al. The FMR1 CGG repeat mouse displays ubiquitin-positive intranuclear neuronal inclusions; implications for the cerebellar tremor/ataxia syndrome. Hum Mol Genet 2003;12:949–959.

Yamamoto A, Lucas JJ, Hen R. Reversal of neuropathology and motor dysfunction in a conditional model of Huntington's disease. Cell 2000; 101:57–66.

Yoo SY, Pennesi ME, Weeber EJ, et al. SCA7 knockin mice model human SCA7 and reveal gradual accumulation of mutant ataxin-7 in neurons and abnormalities in short-term plasticity. Neuron 2003;37:383–401.

Young AB. Huntingtin in health and disease. J Clin Invest 2003;111: 299–302.

Zhang S, Xu L, Lee J, Xu T. Drosophila atrophin homolog functions as a transcriptional corepressor in multiple developmental processes. Cell 2002;108:45–56.

Zoghbi HY, Botas J. Mouse and fly models of neurodegeneration. Trends Genet 2002;18:463–471.

Zu T, Duvick LA, Kaytor MD, et al. Recovery from polyglutamine-induced neurodegeneration in conditional SCA1 transgenic mice. J Neurosci 2004;24:8853–8861.

117 Parkinson's Disease

Deepak M. Sampathu and Virginia M.-Y. Lee

SUMMARY

Parkinson's disease (PD), which is the most common neurodegenerative movement disorder, is clinically characterized by resting tremor, rigidity, bradykinesia, and postural instability. The pathological hallmarks of PD include loss of dopaminergic neurons in the substantia nigra pars compacta as well as the presence of abnormal protein deposits known as Lewy bodies in some of the surviving nigral neurons. The loss of dopaminergic neurons in the substantia nigra pars compacta results in striatal dopamine deficiency, which accounts for the motor impairments of patients with PD. Although the precise etiology remains unclear, several environmental and genetic factors have been implicated in the molecular pathogenesis of PD. This chapter will systematically discuss each of these factors and their putative pathogenic mechanisms.

Key Words: Basal ganglia; dopamine; L-DOPA; Lewy body; neurodegeneration; oxidative stress; parkin; Parkinson's disease; substantia nigra; α-synuclein.

INTRODUCTION

Descriptions of what may have been Parkinson's disease (PD) are found in traditional Indian medical (*Ayurvedic*) texts written long ago (approx 4500 BCE–1000 BCE). The Sanskrit term *kampavata* described a clinical syndrome consisting of tremor and akinesia, which remarkably was treated with a formulation made using beans from the plant *Mucuna pruriens*, now known to contain L-DOPA. Although such descriptions and others point to the existence of PD before the industrial revolution, the first formal description of the disorder came in 1817, when the English physician James Parkinson wrote a short pamphlet entitled "An Essay on the Shaking Palsy," in which he described resting tremor, flexed posture, festinating gait, and "lessened muscular power" in six patients, some of whom he had only casually observed on the streets of London. Beginning in 1861, a series of landmark publications by the French physician Jean-Martin Charcot expanded on Parkinson's description and clarified the cardinal features, emphasizing that "slowness in execution of movement" (or bradykinesia), rather than weakness, contributed to the disorder. Charcot suggested the term "Parkinson's disease" to replace the earlier designation of "shaking palsy," perhaps to reflect that marked weakness is not a feature and patients do not always have tremor.

From: *Principles of Molecular Medicine, Second Edition*
Edited by: M. S. Runge and C. Patterson © Humana Press, Inc., Totowa, NJ

In spite of Charcot's detailed clinical descriptions of PD, he never fully comprehended its neuroanatomic basis. In 1893, Blocq and Marinesco suggested that a lesion of the substantia nigra (SN) might be responsible, based on a case of hemiplegic parkinsonism in which a tuberculoma had destroyed the region. Subsequent pathological investigation confirmed this idea, as a 1919 study by Tretiakoff found degeneration of the SN a constant feature of PD. Tretiakoff also reported that surviving nigral neurons could contain eosinophilic intraneuronal inclusions (Lewy bodies [LBs]), which had been previously described in the dorsal motor nucleus of the vagus and substantia innominata of PD patients by Friedrich Lewy in 1912.

CLINICAL AND PATHOLOGICAL FEATURES

PD is the most common neurodegenerative movement disorder and a significant burden to society, afflicting at least 1% of individuals greater than 65 yr. The major triad of classic signs of PD is resting tremor, rigidity, and bradykinesia, but additional cardinal features include flexed posture, loss of postural reflexes, and the freezing phenomenon. The clinical diagnosis of parkinsonism requires at least two of these features, with at least one being bradykinesia or resting tremor. As the disease progresses, PD patients may suffer from behavioral and cognitive disturbances, including dementia, which is increasingly recognized in the elderly. Idiopathic PD can be best differentiated clinically from secondary causes of parkinsonism by the combination of the presence of resting tremor, asymmetry of signs and symptoms, and a good response to L-DOPA. Although clinical diagnosis of PD is fairly accurate (approx 75% in some reports), misdiagnosis, even by well-trained neurologists, is still a significant problem because of the existence of many secondary causes of parkinsonism, and neuropathological confirmation is required for definitive diagnosis.

The pathological hallmarks of PD include dopaminergic neuronal loss in the substantia nigra pars compacta (SNpc) and the presence of fibrillar proteinaceous inclusions known as LBs in the cytoplasm some of the surviving nigral neurons (Fig. 117-1A). LBs, which are easily detected by α-synuclein immunostaining and to a lesser extent by ubiquitin immunoreactivity, can also be found in other brainstem nuclei, cortical regions, and autonomic ganglia. In addition to LBs in affected areas, proteinaceous deposits termed Lewy neurites (LNs) are found in neuronal processes (Fig. 117-1B). The loss of dopaminergic neurons in the SNpc results in a profound deficiency in striatal dopamine, which underlies the classic motor signs and symptoms of PD, particularly

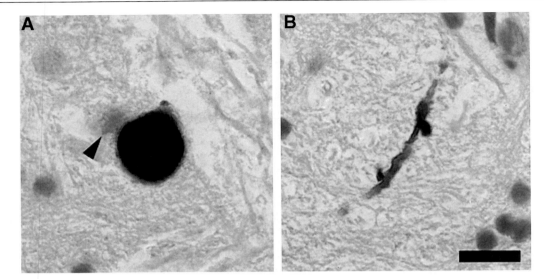

Figure 117-1   Lewy bodies and Lewy neurites are pathological hallmarks of Parkinson's disease. α-Synuclein is the main component of the intra-neuronal inclusions termed Lewy bodies (LBs) and Lewy neurites (LNs). **(A)** A LB and **(B)** a LN in the substantia nigra pars compacta of a patient with Parkinson's disease stained with an antibody specific for α-synuclein. The sections were counterstained with hematoxylin, and the arrowhead in **(A)** indicates the nucleus of the neuron containing a LB. Scale bar = 20 μm.

bradykinesia and rigidity. Involvement of other neuronal systems may be responsible for cognitive, behavioral, and autonomic symptoms, although definitive clinicopathological correlations have not yet been made.

NEUROPHYSIOLOGICAL BASIS OF MOTOR IMPAIRMENT

To understand how loss of nigral dopaminergic neurons and striatal dopamine deficiency result in the motor impairments of PD, a discussion of the basal ganglia and its connections to other brain regions follows (Fig. 117-2). The term "basal ganglia" refers to a set of subcortical nuclei (including the striatum, globus pallidus, and subthalamic nucleus [STN]) that are functionally important in coordinating motor functions via connections with other regions of the brain, including the SN, thalamus, and cerebral cortex. The main region of the basal ganglia receiving input from motor cortex is the striatum. The striatum influences both the output nucleus of the basal ganglia (the internal segment of the globus pallidus [GPi]) and the substantia nigra pars reticulata (SNpr) via direct and indirect connections. The GPi and SNpr, in turn, make connections with the motor nuclei of the thalamus, which contains efferents projecting to the motor cortex, completing the so-called "motor loop."

Dopaminergic neurotransmission from the SNpc influences the so-called "direct" and "indirect" pathways that emanate from the striatum. The direct pathway consists of inhibitory connections from the striatum directly to the GPi and SNpr. The indirect pathway, however, consists of two sequential inhibitory connections, one from the striatum to the external segment of the globus pallidus (GPe) and the second from the GPe to the STN, followed by excitatory connections from the STN to the GPi and SNpr. Therefore, the net effect of connections within the indirect pathway is excitation of the GPi and SNpr.

Dopamine has opposite effects on the direct and indirect pathways because of the different types of dopamine receptors expressed in subpopulations of neurons in the striatum. D1 type receptors are expressed in striatal neurons signaling through the direct pathway, and D2 type receptors are expressed in striatal neurons that initiate the indirect pathway. Normally, neurons expressing D1 type receptors are activated by dopamine, leading to activation of the direct pathway, whereas neurons with D2 type receptors are inhibited by dopamine, leading to inhibition of the indirect pathway. Thus, dopaminergic transmission has a normal inhibitory effect on activity of the GPi and SNpr, leading to normal motor control (Fig. 117-2A).

The dopamine-deficiency state in PD, however, is associated with abnormally elevated activity of the GPi and SNpr, which underlies the motor impairments of PD. The decreased signaling through striatal D1 and D2 receptors in PD leads to a decrease in the inhibitory activity of the direct pathway and increased excitation via the indirect pathway. The characteristic loss of SNpc neurons in PD, therefore, ultimately leads to overactivity of the GPi and SNpr, resulting in excessive inhibition of thalamic nuclei and dysfunctional motor control (Fig. 117-2B).

Although the earlier discussion of the cortico-basal ganglia-thalamo-cortical motor loop is simplified and does not account for all connections between basal ganglia nuclei, it serves as a basic framework for understanding PD treatments. Because dopamine deficiency appears to be instrumental in the motor phenotype of PD, the main therapeutic strategy is dopamine replacement. L-DOPA, a dopamine precursor used routinely in PD treatment for several decades, remains the most efficacious treatment available. Its main drawback is that with increasing duration of treatment, patients develop motor complications, including dyskinesias and fluctuations in L-DOPA response. Within 5 yr of treatment, up to 80% of patients develop dyskinesias, abnormal purposeless movements and abnormal sustained muscle contractions. Because of this potential for debilitating motor complications, dopamine agonists are often used as alternative or ancillary treatment to L-DOPA. Although dopamine agonist therapy may result in a lower incidence of complications, it is also less effective in treating PD's motor symptoms.

The understanding of the neuroanatomic basis of the motor symptoms of PD serves as the basis for therapeutic neurosurgical

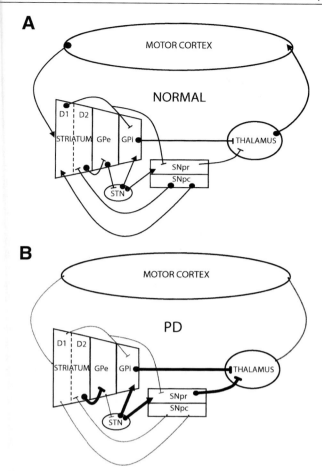

Figure 117-2   Simplified schematic of the "motor loop" under normal conditions and in Parkinson's disease. The excitatory and inhibitory connections between the components of the cortico-basal ganglia-thalamo-cortical motor loop are depicted (see text for details). **(A)** Under normal conditions, neurotransmission within the motor loop results in appropriate motor control. **(B)** In Parkinson's disease, loss of SNpc neurons causes dopamine deficiency in the striatum, leading to increased inhibitory transmission to the motor nuclei of the thalamus from the GPi and SNpr. The dysfunction of these pathways is a major contributor to the loss of motor control in Parkinson's disease. Thicker lines represent increased transmission within pathways whereas thinner lines indicated decreased transmission. Note that this schematic omits other existing connections within depicted brain regions for the sake of simplicity. D1, type-D1 dopamine receptors; D2, type-D2 dopamine receptors; GPe, external segment of globus pallidus; GPi, internal segment of globus pallidus; SNpc, substantia nigra pars compacta; SNpr, substantia nigra pars reticulata; STN, subthalamic nucleus.

options. Targets of surgical procedures include the GPi or the STN. Although such treatment is far from risk-free, ablation of the GPi or STN normalizes the abnormal neuronal firing patterns associated with dopamine deficiency and thus ameliorates the motor symptoms of PD. Bilateral ablative therapies are particularly associated with a significant risk of long-term complications, so an increasingly used alternative is deep brain stimulation. It involves long-term electrical stimulation of the GPi or STN through implanted deep-brain electrodes, which allows for adjustment and reversibility of the exogenous manipulation.

Although dopamine replacement and surgical options are effective treatment, they are purely symptomatic and do not slow disease progression. Ideal treatments would be protective and/or restorative rather than simply targeting symptoms. Allo-transplantation of fetal dopaminergic neurons seems to be a promising restorative possibility but remains investigational.

PATHOGENESIS

The relative importance of environmental vs genetic factors in the pathogenesis of PD is debatable. Inconclusive results from early twin studies and the discovery of toxins capable of causing parkinsonism have favored environmental causes. Nevertheless, twin studies utilizing functional imaging to detect presymptomatic dopaminergic deficits in siblings, as well as the linkage of several genes and loci to rare familial forms of PD, have suggested that the genetic contribution to PD is significant. Although idiopathic PD most likely has a multifactorial etiology in which undefined environmental insults and genetic predisposition interact to cause disease, knowledge about the roles of individual pathogenic factors may lead to the identification of targets amenable to therapy and useful insights into the disease process.

ENVIROMENTAL FACTORS AND OXIDATIVE STRESS

MPTP and Parkinsonism   In 1979, a group of young adults in California developed severe parkinsonism after intravenous use of contaminated synthetic heroin. The agent responsible for the parkinsonism was identified as 1-methyl-4-phenyl-1,2,3,6-tetrahydropyridine (MPTP), a byproduct in the synthesis of a meperidine analog. This finding lent credibility to the idea that an environmental toxin could be involved in the pathogenesis of parkinsonism. MPTP is a lipophilic molecule that readily crosses the blood-brain barrier and is enzymatically converted to 1-methyl-4-phenylpyridium (MPP^+) by monoamine oxidase type B in glia. MPP^+ is selectively taken into dopaminergic neurons via its high affinity for the dopamine transporter and exerts its toxicity through binding and inhibition of NADH ubiquinone reductase (complex I) of the mitochondrial electron transport chain. Because electron transport chain function is necessary for oxidative phosphorylation, it has been suggested that reduction in complex I activity may lead to suboptimal ATP production and subsequent negative effects on cellular functions because of energy failure. In addition, it is thought that complex I inhibition by MPP^+ exerts toxic effects on neurons via the production of reactive oxygen species that can interfere with normal cellular functions by damaging proteins, nucleic acids, and lipids. The effects of MPTP have been confirmed in animal models, including mice, cats, and primates. Nonhuman primate models develop the cardinal parkinsonian signs (tremor, bradykinesia, rigidity, and postural instability) associated with SNpc degeneration following administration of MPTP. Although the MPTP models of parkinsonism have been useful in the development and testing of symptomatic therapies for PD, they have several drawbacks, and MPTP toxicity may not truly represent idiopathic PD. Most importantly, MPTP parkinsonism occurs shortly following an acute exposure to the toxin, whereas in PD neuronal death is progressive and occurs over many years. Further, MPTP exposure results in selective degeneration of dopaminergic neurons whereas both dopaminergic and nondopaminergic neuronal death is responsible for the variety of symptoms idiopathic PD patients suffer. The absence of fibrillar inclusions resembling LBs in MPTP parkinsonism also suggests that MPTP models provide an incomplete representation of idiopathic PD, or alternatively, that idiopathic PD is the result of a distinct pathogenetic process.

Pesticides   Epidemiological studies suggest that exposure to pesticides may be a risk factor for PD development. The herbicide

1,1'-dimethyl-4,4'-bipyridinium (paraquat), when injected systemically into mice, causes dose-dependent death of dopaminergic nigral neurons associated with decreased locomotor activity. Because of its structural similarity to MPP⁺, paraquat may induce oxidative stress via effects on mitochondrial electron transport. Additionally, the pesticide manganese ethylenebisdithiocarbamate (or maneb) potentiates the toxic effects of paraquat on the nigrostriatal dopaminergic pathway in mice. This suggests the possibility that mixtures of environmental toxins may be pertinent to PD etiology.

The idea that pesticides increase PD risk is further supported by the finding that the compound rotenone, often used as an insecticide in vegetable gardens or to kill fish in lakes and water reservoirs, can cause a PD-like syndrome in a rat model. In this paradigm, chronic low-dose exposure to rotenone results in complex I inhibition throughout the rat brain, but nigrostriatal dopaminergic neurons selectively degenerate. Fibrillar inclusions closely resembling LBs form in nigral cell bodies, and behaviorally, hypokinesia, flexed posture, rigidity, and tremor are variably present in exposed rats. Thus, the rotenone model demonstrates that systemic complex I inhibition can recapitulate key PD features. This rat model, however, is limited because greater than 50% of rotenone-exposed rats develop the pathological and clinical PD-like features.

Oxidative Stress in Idiopathic PD   Subsequent to the discovery of MPTP's mode of action, it was found that idiopathic PD patients exhibit reduced mitochondrial complex I activity in the brain and peripheral tissues. This has led to the hypothesis that mitochondrial dysfunction and the resultant oxidative stress may play a role in the selective degeneration of vulnerable neurons in PD. Oxidative injury occurs when the antioxidant capacity of neurons is overwhelmed by the production of destructive reactive oxygen species. Complex I inhibition leads to the production of superoxide radicals, which can react with nitric oxide to form peroxynitrite. Peroxynitrite, which readily modifies native tyrosine residues in proteins to form 3-nitrotyrosine, may be a critical oxidant, as 3-nitrotyrosine is increased in PD brains and a subset of α-synuclein (the main component of LBs and LNs, *see* Implicated Genes) in PD inclusions is nitrated. Dopaminergic neurons may be particularly vulnerable to oxidative stress because the degradation of dopamine by monoamine oxidase produces hydrogen peroxide (H_2O_2), which can be converted to hydroxyl radicals that can damage cellular constituents.

IMPLICATED GENES   Although most PD research focused on possible environmental factors involved in the pathogenesis of PD, the discovery of mutations in several different genes (α-*synuclein, parkin, ubiquitin C-terminal hydrolase* [UCH]-*L1, DJ-1*, and *NR4A2/NURR1, PINK1, LRRK2*, and *synphilin-1*), and additional loci with unidentified genes, involved in familial forms of PD has shifted much attention to the role of genetic factors. Although familial forms of PD are rare compared with idiopathic PD, research has focused on these genes with the hope that understanding rare forms of PD will yield insights into the pathogenesis of idiopathic PD.

α-Synuclein   α-synuclein is a 140 amino acid residue neuronal cytoplasmic protein predominantly localized to presynaptic terminals in the CNS and loosely associated with synaptic vesicles. Its normal function remains unclear, although studies in songbirds suggest it may play a role in synaptic plasticity, and results from knockout mice indicate that it may be involved in activity-dependent negative regulation of dopamine neurotransmission. Two seminal findings clearly linked α-synuclein

to PD: the discovery that point mutations in the α-synuclein gene are causative of familial forms of PD, and the demonstration that α-synuclein is the major component of LBs and LNs in familial forms of PD and in idiopathic PD.

Three missense mutations in the α-*synuclein* gene, as well as triplication of the locus containing the α-*synuclein* gene, have been identified in familial forms of PD. One of the missense mutations, resulting in the substitution of threonine for alanine at amino acid position 53 (A53T), causes autosomal-dominantly inherited PD in several families of Greek and Italian origin that are thought to have a common founder. Several clinical features may distinguish patients with the A53T mutation from those with idiopathic PD, including slightly earlier onset (mean age of onset is 46 yr), more rapid disease progression, lower prevalence of tremor, and noncardinal features such as dementia and myoclonus earlier in the disease course. A second mutation in α-synuclein (A30P) has been found in one German family, in which the autosomal-dominantly inherited PD clinically resembles idiopathic PD. Although no neuropathological reports on patients with the A30P mutation have been reported, postmortem examination of A53T brains revealed SNpc degeneration and an abundance of LBs and LNs.

More recently, a third mutation in α-synuclein (E46K) was found in a Spanish family with autosomal-dominant inheritance of PD. Interestingly, this family exhibits the clinical features of dementia and visual hallucinations in addition to parkinsonism, and neuropathologically, LBs were present in neurons of the SN as well as the cortex. Finally, the finding in an Iowa kindred that triplication of the α-synuclein gene locus can cause autosomal-dominant PD implicates gene dosage effects in the pathogenesis of PD. Neuropathological analysis of patients from this kindred has revealed extensive LB pathology.

Immunohistochemical studies show that antibodies to α-synuclein intensely stain LBs and LNs in PD as well as in other neurodegenerative disorders, such as dementia with LBs, suggesting that aggregation of α-*synuclein* may be a key event in the process of neurodegeneration. Furthermore, it is known that α-synuclein is the major building block of LBs, as immunoelectron microscopic studies have indicated that LB filaments specifically react with α-synuclein antibodies, and α-synuclein filaments assembled in vitro from recombinant protein closely resemble those in pathological inclusions. The A53T mutation accelerates fibril formation in the test tube, suggesting that accelerated polymerization of α-synuclein may be responsible for disease in patients harboring this mutation. Many other factors and events have been reported to influence the fibrillogenesis of α-synuclein in vitro, and these could be involved in the formation of α-synuclein inclusions in sporadic PD. Post-translational modification of α-synuclein (such as C-terminal truncation and phosphorylation), incubation with metals (such as aluminum, copper, and iron), and oxidative challenge (hydrogen peroxide) may accelerate fibril formation. A30P α-synuclein has been reported to bind poorly to vesicles compared with the wild-type protein, although it is not clear how this is related to disease because the autosomal-dominant mode of inheritance suggests a gain of toxic function for α-synuclein. One possibility is that impaired binding of A30P α-synuclein to vesicles hinders axonal transport of the protein, leading to accumulation of and aggregation of α-synuclein in cell bodies and processes.

Several α-synuclein animal models have been reported. Expression of wildtype and mutant α-synuclein using promoters in mice has yielded differing results. Use of the platelet-derived growth factor promoter to overexpress wild-type α-synuclein results in a mild motor phenotype associated with dopaminergic nerve terminal loss in the striatum and inclusion formation in the SN, cortex, and hippocampus. Although these inclusions contain α-synuclein and ubiquitin, they are unlike the LBs of PD because they are granular rather than fibrillar, and some inclusions are nuclear. Expression of wildtype or mutant forms of α-synuclein by the Thy1 promoter also results in a mild motor phenotype with nonfilamentous accumulation of α-synuclein in various brain regions. Surprisingly, no differences between mice expressing wildtype and mutant forms occur. Mice expressing A53T α-synuclein under control of the mouse PrP promoter, however, develop filamentous α-synuclein inclusions, primarily in brainstem and spinal cord, which correlate with the expression of a severe, complex motor phenotype leading to paralysis and death. Although these mice have provided a model that exhibits α-synuclein inclusion formation and associated neuronal dysfunction, the SN of these mice is unaffected. Therefore, transgenic mice models have failed to provide a compelling model that recapitulates the major neurodegenerative features of PD. Results from transgenic *Drosophila*, however, may be more promising. Pan-neuronal overexpression of wildtype or mutant α-synuclein resulted in age-dependent degeneration of a subset of dopaminergic neurons, formation of filamentous α-synuclein inclusions, and locomotor dysfunction. Thus, this model exhibits key features of PD and may serve as a powerful tool in the discovery of genetic factors or pharmacological agents that influence the pathogenic process.

Parkin   A number of missense, nonsense, and exon deletion mutations in the *parkin* gene can cause autosomal-recessive juvenile parkinsonism (AR-JP). Although rare in comparison to idiopathic PD, it is thought that *parkin* mutations are responsible for approx 50% of autosomal-recessively inherited parkinsonism in families in which at least one patient exhibited onset before 45 yr of age. In addition to early age of onset, AR-JP sometimes may be distinguished clinically from idiopathic PD by its slow progression and presence of features such as benefit from sleep and foot dystonia. Although AR-JP patients show good initial response to L-DOPA, they are more prone to the development of dyskinesias as a side effect of therapy. A limited number of cases in which *parkin* mutations are responsible for disease have been examined postmortem. A constant finding is loss of dopaminergic neurons in the SN, and LBs have not been found in most cases. LBs were, however, described in one patient with compound heterozygous mutations in parkin. The lack of LBs may reflect the loss of functional parkin activity in the brains of AR-JP patients. The finding that one case did show LBs, however, suggests that LBs may form early on in disease, but may not be found at autopsy because of the passage of many decades between onset and death in *parkin* cases, although this is speculative. Alternatively, the pathogenic process in *parkin* cases may be distinct from idiopathic PD. If this is the case, the compound heterozygous patient with LBs may have been affected by more than one disease process.

Parkin is a 465 amino acid residue protein that contains a ubiquitin-like domain at its N-terminal end and two RING (Really Interesting New Gene) motifs in its C-terminal half. The presence of these motifs initially suggested involvement in the process of ubiquitination, in which enzymes known as E3 ligases participate in the covalent conjugation of one or more molecules of a small protein called ubiquitin to selective lysine residues in intracellular proteins. Such tagging with ubiquitin can serve as a signal for

proteasomal degradation as well as for other functions in the cell. Parkin has the ability to function as an E3 ligase, and several possible substrates have been identified, including parkin-associated endothelin-like receptor (PAEL-R), cdc-rel1, synphilin, cyclin E, a putative glycosylated form of α-synuclein, and tubulin. Thus, parkin may be a multifunctional E3 ligase involved in the clearance of many different proteins. A possible explanation for the development of AR-JP is that parkin function may be critical in the clearance of abnormal proteins that are toxic to dopaminergic neurons. For example, in cell culture, parkin suppresses the endoplasmic reticulum-stress related toxicity associated with overexpression of PAEL-R, presumably through polyubiquitination and proteasomal degradation of this misfolded protein. Furthermore, overexpression of parkin in *Drosophila* engineered to pan-neuronally express PAEL-R mitigates the dopaminergic degeneration caused by PAEL-R. It is unknown whether PAEL-R or other putative parkin substrates are significant in the pathogenesis of idiopathic PD.

Drosophila flies in which the fly *parkin* ortholog was knocked out exhibit reduced life span and locomotor dysfunction associated with apoptotic muscle degeneration. Mitochondrial abnormalities were noted in degenerating muscle, suggesting that parkin may be involved in clearance of a protein that is important for the integrity of mitochondrial function, or alternatively that parkin itself is critical to mitochondrial function. Although the role of parkin and putative substrates in the pathogenesis of idiopathic PD remains unclear, it is possible that a normal role for parkin in the clearance of toxic proteins is compromised in PD.

UCH-L1   UCH-L1 is one member of a family of deubiquitinating enzymes that is capable of cleaving ubiquitin C-terminal adducts to serve critical functions in the cell. UCH-L1 is abundant in brain (approx 1–2% of neuronal protein), and its activity is thought to be important in regenerating free ubiquitin for utilization in subsequent rounds of ubiquitin-mediated degradation via proteasomes. An amino acid residue substitution in UCH-L1 (I93M) has been identified in two siblings from a German family exhibiting presumed autosomal-dominantly inherited PD with incomplete penetrance. The clinical phenotype resembled idiopathic PD and ages of onset in the siblings were 49 and 51 yr. Neuroradiological and neuropathological data are not available, and the I93M substitution has not been reported in other PD patients. The S18Y polymorphism in UCH-L1, however, is a protective factor against PD in some populations, lending further support to the idea that UCH-L1 might be involved in PD pathogenesis. In vitro, the I93M substitution reduces the catalytic hydrolase activity of UCH-L1 toward an artificial substrate by approx 50%. It is unclear how this may result in a dominant phenotype in patients heterozygous for the I93M, unless the presence of only approx 75% UCH-L1 activity is lower than the threshold for maintenance of normal functions in aging neurons. Perhaps a slight reduction in deubiquitinating activity can lead to inefficient protein clearance by the ubiquitin-proteasomal pathway and accumulation of abnormal protein species, which are toxic.

DJ-1   Mutations in the *DJ-1* gene were found in patients with autosomal-recessive parkinsonism. One kindred from a genetically isolated Dutch population had a large deletion removing five of seven exons in the *DJ-1* gene, whereas an L166P missense mutation was found in an Italian family. Clinically, DJ-1 parkinsonism is characterized by early age of onset, slow progression, and lasting response to L-DOPA treatment. Focal dystonia and behavioral

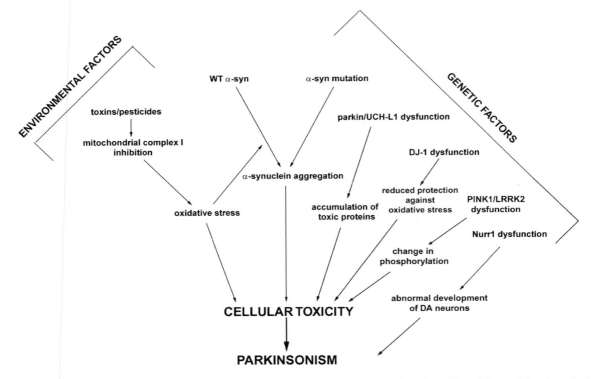

Figure 117-3   Environmental and genetic factors can contribute to the development of parkinsonism. The etiology of Parkinson's disease (PD) is thought to be multifactorial, with contributions from environmental and genetic factors. This model depicts many of the known factors that have been implicated in PD and their possible contribution(s) to PD pathogenesis. α-syn, α-synuclein; DA, dopaminergic.

disturbances have occurred in both families. Neuropathological data on patients with DJ-1 mutations have not been reported.

Although the normal function of DJ-1 is unclear, it was first identified as an oncogene, and subsequent studies suggested that it may be part of an RNA-binding protein complex. DJ-1 interacts with a protein called PIAS (protein inhibitor of activated STAT [signal transducer and activator of transcription protein]), which belongs to a family of ligases that covalently attach SUMO-1 (small ubiquitin-like modifier) to protein substrates, and DJ-1 itself may be sumoylated. Sumoylation (covalent attachment of SUMO to lysine residues in proteins) occurs in a number of transcription factors, suggesting that DJ-1 may have a role in transcriptional regulation. Some evidence suggests that DJ-1 may be involved in cellular responses to oxidative stress, and therefore dysfunction of DJ-1 could potentially make neurons more vulnerable to oxidative and nitrative damage. A role for any of these potential normal functions of DJ-1 remains to be explored further, as does a possible role for dysfunction of DJ-1 in the pathogenesis of PD.

NR4A2/NURR1   Another gene to be linked to familial PD is *NR4A2*, also known as *NURR1*. Previous evidence had suggested that *NR4A2* could be a genetic risk factor for PD, as *NURR1* deficient mice failed to develop dopaminergic neurons in the SN and midbrain dopaminergic neurons are more susceptible to MPTP-mediated toxicity in heterozygous mice (*NURR1* +/–). Nurr1 acts as a transcription factor thought to be important in the differentiation and maintenance of dopaminergic neurons.

Genetic screening of European individuals with familial PD has revealed two heterozygous mutations in exon 1 of *NR4A2*, upstream of the translational initiator codon of the gene. The 10 patients identified with either of these two mutations have a clinical

phenotype that is similar to idiopathic PD and without atypical features, and neuropathology has not been reported in any cases. Based on studies with lymphocytes from these affected individuals, these heterozygous mutations result in a significant decrease in the levels of *NR4A2* mRNA, although the mechanism of this reduction is unclear. Further work is necessary to determine if a downregulation of *NR4A2* expression occurs in idiopathic PD and how neuronal dysfunction/degeneration may occur as a downstream consequence.

PINK1 and LRRK2   Recently, mutations in two genes whose gene products putatively function as kinases have been found in inherited forms of PD, implicating dysregulation of phosphorylation as a possible mechanism in the pathogenesis of PD. Mutations in the PTEN-induced putative kinase 1 *(PINK1)* gene are associated with an early onset autosomal-recessive form of PD characterized by typical parkinsonism but with slow progression. The encoded PINK1 protein is predicted to be a Ser/Thr protein kinase targeted to mitochondria. The autosomal-recessive inheritance suggests that loss of function of the PINK1 protein may play a role in the pathogenesis. Neuropathological data on patients with *PINK1* mutations has not yet been reported.

Furthermore, it has been discovered that mutations in the leucine-rich repeat kinase 2 *(LRRK2)* gene cause an autosomal-dominant form of PD in several families. Neuropathological analysis of patients with *LRRK2* mutations has revealed variable pathology. Although the brains of patients with *LRRK2* mutations all exhibit neuronal degeneration in the SN, some brains exhibit an absence of LB pathology, with other brains having varying degrees of LBs, LNs, and aggregates containing the microtubule-associated protein tau. As many as 5% of PD patients with a family history and >1% of sporadic idiopathic PD patients harbor a mutation in the *LRRK2* gene, with the G2019S being the most common. Further research on the normal and abnormal forms of these presumed kinases will likely yield useful insights into molecular events which could go awry in PD.

Synphilin-1 One mutation (R621C) in the *synphilin-1* gene has been identified in two apparently independent German patients with sporadic PD. These patients had no family history of PD or other movement disorders. Whereas the significance of this finding is still unclear, synphilin-1 protein had been previously implicated in PD as it was identified as an α-synuclein interacting protein, and synphilin-1 appears to be present in a small percentage of LBs. Furthermore, studies have revealed that cotransfection of synphilin-1 and α-synuclein in cell culture results in intracellular protein deposits containing both proteins. Whereas this is an intriguing finding, how closely these aggregates resemble the LBs characteristic of PD is debatable.

CONCLUSION

Idiopathic PD likely represents a complex disease in which many factors interact in pathogenic pathways to cause disease. Clues from known environmental and genetic factors suggest roles for oxidative stress, protein aggregation, and impaired protein clearance in the pathogenesis of parkinsonism (*see* Fig. 117-3). Such events need not be mutually exclusive and may all contribute to the development of sporadic PD. As more knowledge is gained about the identity and effects of individual environmental and genetic factors, further investigation will be necessary to determine how these entities may interact to produce the neuronal dysfunction and death that underlies the phenotype of PD. Researchers have begun to pursue studies in which transgenic animals are exposed to environmental toxins. As understanding of the molecular events underlying the pathogenesis of PD improves, the development of therapeutic interventions that can potentially prevent disease initiation and/or progression will become more of a reality.

SELECTED REFERENCES

Betarbet R, Sherer TB, MacKenzie G, Garcia-Osuna M, Panov AV, Greenamyre JT. Chronic systemic pesticide exposure reproduces features of Parkinson's disease. Nat Neurosci 2000;3:1301–1306.

Betarbet R, Sherer TB, Greenamyre JT. Animal models of Parkinson's disease. Bioessays 2002;24:308–318.

Bonifati V, Rizzu P, van Baren MJ, et al. Mutations in the DJ-1 gene associated with autosomal recessive early-onset parkinsonism. Science 2003;299:256–259.

Chung KK, Dawson VL, Dawson TM. The role of the ubiquitin-proteasomal pathway in Parkinson's disease and other neurodegenerative disorders. Trends Neurosci 2001;24:S7–S14.

Cookson MR. Pathways to parkinsonism. Neuron 2003;37:7–10.

Dawson TM, Dawson VL. Rare genetic mutations shed light on the pathogenesis of Parkinson disease. J Clin Invest 2003;111:145–151.

Dawson TM, Mandir AS, Lee MK. Animal models of PD: pieces of the same puzzle? Neuron 2002;35:219–222.

Dekker MC, Bonifati V, van Duijn CM. Parkinson's disease: piecing together a genetic jigsaw. Brain 2003;126:1722–1733.

Duvoisin RC. A brief history of parkinsonism. Neurol Clin 1992;10: 301–316.

Fukuda T. Neurotoxicity of MPTP. Neuropathology 2001;21:323–332.

Giasson BI, Lee VM-Y. Parkin and the molecular pathways of Parkinson's disease. Neuron 2001;31:885–888.

Goedert M. α-Synuclein and neurodegenerative diseases. Nat Rev Neurosci 2001;2:492–501.

Gwinn-Hardy K. Genetics of parkinsonism. Mov Disord 2002;17:645–656.

Ischiropoulos H, Beckman JS. Oxidative stress and nitration in neurodegeneration: cause, effect, or association? J Clin Invest 2003;111: 163–169.

Kitada T, Asakawa S, Hattori N, et al. Mutations in the parkin gene cause autosomal recessive juvenile parkinsonism. Nature 1998;392: 605–608.

Kruger R, Kuhn W, Muller T, et al. Ala30Pro mutation in the gene encoding a-synuclein in Parkinson's disease. Nat Genet 1998;18:106–108.

Lang AE, Lozano AM. Parkinson's disease—first of two parts. N Engl J Med 1998;339:1044–1053.

Lang AE, Lozano AM. Parkinson's disease—second of two parts. N Engl J Med 1998;339:1130–1143.

Langston JW, Ballard P, Tetrud JW, Irwin I. Chronic parkinsonism in humans due to a product of meperidine-analog synthesis. Science 1983;219:979, 980.

Le W, Xu P, Jankovic J, et al. Mutations in NR4A2 associated with familial Parkinson disease. Nat Genet 2003;33:85.

Leroy E, Boyer R, Auburger G, et al. The ubiquitin pathway in Parkinson's disease. Nature 1998;395:451, 452.

Moore DJ, West AB, Dawson VL, Dawson TM. Molecular pathophysiology of Parkinson's disease. Annu Rev Neurosci 2005;28:57–87.

Polymeropoulos MH, Lavedan C, Leroy E, et al. Mutation in the a-synuclein gene identified in families with Parkinson's disease. Science 1997; 276:2045–2047.

Siderowf A, Stern M. Update on Parkinson disease. Ann Intern Med 2003; 138:651–658.

Takahashi H, Wakabayashi K. The cellular pathology of Parkinson's disease. Neuropathology 2001;21:315–322.

118 Genetics and Neurobiology of Alzheimer's Disease and Frontotemporal Dementias

PETER H. ST. GEORGE-HYSLOP

SUMMARY

Alzheimer's Disease (AD), Lewy body variant of AD, and the frontotemporal dementias are the three most common causes of adult onset dementia. This chapter will examine the genetic basis of AD and Lewy body variant, familial British dementia and familial encephalopathy with neuronal dementia with neuroserpin deposits, tau mutations in FTDP-17, and the practical implications of genetic testing.

Key Words: Alzheimer's disease; frontotemporal dementias; Lewy body variant of Alzheimer disease.

INTRODUCTION

Alzheimer's Disease (AD), Lewy body variant (LBV) of AD, (which is now referred to as Dementia with Lewy Bodies [DLB]) and the frontotemporal dementias (FTD) are the three commonest causes of adult onset dementia. These diseases present in mid to late adult life with progressive defects in memory and higher cognitive functions such as the performance of complex, learned motor tasks (apraxias), reasoning, and so on. The clinical features of AD and DLB (deficits in recent and immediate memory deficits, praxis, reasoning and judgment, and so on) stem from involvement of the temporal lobe, hippocampus, and the parietal association cortices, with lesser involvement of frontal lobes until late in the disease. DLB overlaps with AD, sharing most of the clinical and neuropathological features of AD, but differentiated by prominent visual hallucinations, sensitivity to phenothiazine tranquilizers, and the presence of Lewy bodies (α-synuclein containing intraneuronal inclusions) in neocortical neurons. In contrast, in FTD, the clinical syndrome is overshadowed by behavioral disturbances (disinhibition, aggressivity, and so on) and speech disturbances (aphasia), which arise from involvement of the frontal neocortex. The FTD symptom complex frequently also includes additional features such as muscle rigidity, tremor, bradykinesia (Parkinsonism), and muscle weakness (amyotrophy).

All three diseases have a characteristic set of neuropathological changes including prominent loss of neurons in selected cerebral

From: *Principles of Molecular Medicine, Second Edition*
Edited by: M. S. Runge and C. Patterson © Humana Press, Inc., Totowa, NJ

cortical regions (e.g., hippocampus and temporoparietal neocortices in AD and DLB; frontal neocortices in FTD) (Figs. 118-1 and 118-2). In AD and DLB, the second prominent neuropathological feature is complex, extracellular, fibrillar deposits in the cortex, termed senile or amyloid plaques. These plaques contain a number of proteins including apolipoprotein E (APOE) and 1-antichymotrypsin, but the principal protein is amyloid-β (Aβ)-peptide, which is derived from proteolytic cleavage of a longer precursor β-amyloid precursor protein (APP). Finally, AD, DLB and FTD are characterized by neurofibrillary tangles, intraneuronal inclusions made up of phosphorylated forms of tau, a microtubule associated protein. These intraneuronal phosphorylated tau aggregates are also called neurofibrillary tangles. The overlap between AD and DLB is considerable in their major clinical and neuropathological features, and in their genetic bases (i.e., both show associations with the APOE ε4 variant—*see* Apolipoprotein E). As a result, the genetics of AD and DLB are discussed together.

GENETIC BASIS OF AD AND DLB

A number of genetic epidemiology studies have been undertaken on probands with AD and their families. Cumulatively, these studies strongly argue that the familial aggregation of AD is not simply because of the high frequency of AD in the general population. They reveal that the overall lifetime risk for AD in first-degree relatives of AD probands is approx 38% by age 85 yr. They also demonstrate that most cases of familially aggregated AD probably reflect a complex mode of transmission such as one or more common independent, but incompletely penetrant, single-autosomal gene defects; a multigenic trait; or a mode of transmission in which both genetic and environmental factors interact. Nevertheless, a small proportion of AD cases (approx 10%) appear to be transmitted as pure autosomal-dominant Mendelian traits with age-dependent but high penetrance. Molecular genetic studies on pedigrees with the latter type of familial AD (FAD) has led to the discovery of four different genetic loci associated with inherited susceptibility to AD. It is suspected that at least two, and possibly several additional AD susceptibility loci remain to be identified because the four known FAD loci account for only approx 50% of FAD cases.

THE AMYLOID PRECURSOR PROTEIN The first gene to be identified in association with inherited susceptibility to AD was

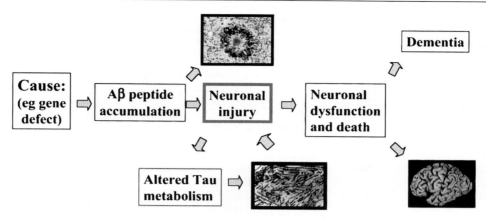

Figure 118-6   Schematic for the putative "amyloid cascade" in which accumulation of neurotoxic Aβ initiates a series of downstream events, some of which are also neurotoxic themselves (e.g., misprocessing and accumulation of tau).

Table 118-2
Mutations in the Presenilin Genes

Codon	Location	Mutation	Phenotype
PRESENILIN I			
79	N-term loop	Ala→Val	FAD, onset 64 yr
82	TM1	Val→Leu	FAD, onset 55 yr
96	TM1	Val→Phe	FAD, onset 53 yr
113–114 (ins)	TM1/TM2 loop	Leu-Thr(ins)-Ile	FAD, onset 35 yr
115	TM1/TM2 loop	Tyr→His	FAD, onset 37 yr
115	TM1/TM2 loop	Tyr→Cys	FAD, onset 42 yr
116	TM1/TM2 loop	Thr→Asn	onset 37 yr
117	TM1/TM2 loop	Pro→Leu	FAD, onset 28 yr
120	TM1/TM2 loop	Glu→Asp	FAD, onset 48 yr
120	TM1/TM2 loop	Glu→Lys	FAD, onset 37 yr
123	TM1/TM2 loop	Glu→Lys	
135	TM2	Asn→Asp	FAD, onset 36 yr
139	TM2	Met→Thr	FAD, onset 49 yr
139	TM2	Met→Val	FAD, onset 40 yr
139	TM2	Met→Ile	FAD,
139	TM2	Met→Lys	FAD, onset 37 yr
143	TM2	Ile→Thr	FAD, onset 35 yr
143	TM2	Ile→Phe	FAD, onset 55 yr
146	TM2	Met→Leu	FAD, onset 45 yr
146	TM2	Met→Val	FAD, onset 38 yr
146	TM2	Met→Ile	FAD, onset 40 yr
147	TM2	Thr→Ile	FAD, onset 42 yr
163	TM3 interface	His→Arg	FAD, onset 50 yr
163	TM3 interface	His→Tyr	FAD, onset 47 yr
165	TM3	Trp→Cys	FAD, onset 42 yr
169	TM3	Ser→Leu	
169	TM3	Ser→Pro	onset 35 yr
171	TM3	Leu→Pro	FAD, onset 40 yr
173	TM3	leu→Trp	FAD, onset 27 yr
177	TM3	Phe→Ser	
178	TM3	Ser→Pro	
206	TM4	Gly→Ser	
209	TM4	Gly→Val	FAD
209	TM4	Gly→Arg	onset 49 yr
213	TM4 interface	Ile→Thr	FAD
213	TM4 interface	Ile→Leu	
219	TM4 interface	Leu→Pro	
222	TM5	Gln→Ala	
231	TM5	Ala→Thr	FAD, onset 52 yr

(Continued)

Table 118-2 *(Continued)*

Codon	Location	Mutation	Phenotype
233	TM5	Met→Thr	FAD, onset 35 yr
235	TM5	Leu→Pro	FAD, onset 32 yr
246	TM6	Ala→Glu	FAD, onset 55 yr
250	TM6	Leu→Ser	onset 53 yr
260	TM6	Ala→Val	FAD, onset 40 yr
261	TM6	Val→Phe	
262	TM6	Leu→Phe	onset 50 yr
263	TM6/TM7 loop	Cys→Arg	FAD, onset 47 yr
264	TM6/TM7 loop	Pro→Leu	FAD, onset 45 yr
267	TM6/TM7 loop	Pro→Ser	FAD, onset 35 yr
269	TM6/TM7 loop	Arg→Gly	
269	TM6/TM7 loop	Arg→His	onset 47 yr
278	TM6/TM7 loop	Arg→Thr	onset 37 yr
280	TM6/TM7 loop	Glu→Ala	FAD, onset 47 yr
280	TM6/TM7 loop	Glu→Gly	FAD, onset 42 yr
282	TM6/TM7 loop	Leu→Arg	onset 43 yr
285	TM6/TM7 loop	Ala→Val	FAD, onset 50 yr
286	TM6/TM7 loop	Leu→Val	FAD, onset 50 yr
291–319	TM6/TM7 loop	short loop	FAD,
318	TM6/TM7 loop	Glu→Gly	onset 35–64 yr, polymorphism?
378	TM6/TM7 loop	Gly→Glu	onset 35 yr
384	TM6/TM7 loop	Gly→Ala	FAD, onset 35 yr
390	TM6/TM7 loop	Ser→Ile	FAD, onset 39 yr
392	TM6/TM7 loop	Leu→Val	FAD, onset 25–40 yr
410	TM7	Cys→Tyr	FAD, onset 48 yr
418	TM7	Leu→Phe	
424	TM7	Leu→Arg	onset 33 yr
426	TM7	Ala→Pro	
431	C-term loop	Ala→Glu	
434	C-term loop	Ala→Cys	
436	C-term loop	Pro→Ser	
436	C-term loop	Pro→Gln	
439	C-term loop	Ile→Val	
PRESENILIN II			
62	N-term loop	Arg→His	Sporadic AD, onset 62 yr
141	TM2	Asn→Ile	FAD, onset 50–65 yr
239	TM5	Met→Val	FAD, onset variable 45–84 yr

giving rise to the substitution of a single amino acid. A few in-frame splicing, deletion or insertion defects have also been identified. However, nonsense mutations resulting in truncated proteins, which would cause loss-of-function mutations, have yet to be found in AD-affected subjects.

All of the PS1 mutations associated with AD increase γ-secretase cleavage of β-APP and preferentially increase the production of toxic long-tailed Aβ-peptides ending at residue 42. However, some investigators think that like the β-APP mutations, PS1 and presenilin 2 (PS2) mutations may also cause neurodegeneration by modulating cellular sensitivity to apoptosis induced by a variety of factors, including Aβ-peptide.

PRESENILIN 2 During the cloning of the PS1 gene on chromosome 14, an homologous sequence, PS2, was identified on chromosome 1. PS2 encodes a polypeptide whose open reading frame contains 448 amino acids, with substantial sequence similarity to PS1 (overall identity approx 60%), and a similar structural organization. Despite this similarity, PS1 and PS2 are likely to have distinct but overlapping functions. For instance, PS2 does not functionally repair either the APP or Notch processing defects in PS1⁻/⁻ animals, yet PS2 mutations, like PS1 mutations, increase the secretion of long-tailed Aβ-peptides.

Mutational analyses have uncovered a small number of missense mutations (approx 9) in the PS2 gene in families segregating early-onset forms of AD (http://molgen-www.uia.ac.be/ADMutations). The phenotype associated with PS2 mutations is much more variable. Thus, the majority of heterozygous carriers of missense mutations in the β-APP and PS1 genes develop the illness between ages 35 and 55 yr for PS1 mutations, and between 45 and 65 yr for β-APP mutations. In contrast, the range of age-of-onset in heterozygous carriers of PS2 mutations is between 40 and 85 yr, and there is at least one instance of apparent nonpenetrance in an asymptomatic octogenarian transmitting the disease to affected offspring. Furthermore, in contrast to APP mutations, the effect of APOEε4 on the age-at-onset in PS2 mutations is either absent or less profound. Modifier loci other than APOE probably account for much of this variation.

OTHER GENES FOR AD Large surveys of patients with familial AD indicate that the APP, APOE, PS1, and PS2 genes account for about half of the genetic risk factors for AD. It is therefore likely that there are several additional AD susceptibility genes. Some of these loci will be associated with additional rare, but highly penetrant defects similar to those seen with mutations in PS1 and APP. Other genes may result in incompletely penetrant autosomal-dominant traits like those associated with PS2. However, it is likely that a significant proportion of the remaining genes will have low-effect sizes similar to APOE, and in which the ultimate phenotype is likely to be influenced by the presence or absence of other genetic and environmental risk factors.

Multiple strategies have been deployed to map these additional AD susceptibility genes. Genetic linkage studies and family based association analyses have been employed on datasets with pedigrees multiply affected with AD, and have led to the suggestion that additional susceptibility loci may exist in the pericentromeric region of chromosome 12 and the long arm and pericentromeric region of chromosome 10. However, the genes in these regions that cause susceptibility to AD have not been identified.

A second strategy to identify AD genes has been to use cohorts of sporadic AD cases and age/sex-matched controls in a case-control association design. This has led to a long list of potential candidate genes, most of which have not been robustly replicated. A partial list of candidate genes provisionally identified as putative AD susceptibility loci includes α1-chymotrypsin, very low density lipoprotein receptor, low-density lipoprotein receptor related protein, butyrylcholinesterase, bleomycin hydroxylase; IL4, and so on. However, in contrast to APOE ε4, most of these candidate genes have not received widespread confirmation when tested in independent but comparable datasets. A number of obvious candidate genes involved in APP processing, including BACE (β-secretase involved in Aβ generation), neprilysin and insulin degrading enzyme (involved in Aβ-degradation) have been screened, but have not been widely found to have genetic variants associated with increased risk for AD.

FAMILIAL BRITISH DEMENTIA AND FAMILIAL ENCEPHALOPATHY WITH NEURONAL DEMENTIA WITH NEUROSERPIN DEPOSITS

Two very rare forms of inherited dementia—familial British dementia and familial encephalopathy with neuroserpin inclusions (FEN1b)—have been described that support the emerging concept that many inherited dementias are disorders of protein processing in which there is intracellular or extracellular accumulation of toxic misfolded/misprocessed proteins—a theme common to all the diseases discussed here.

Familial British dementia is characterized by spasticity, ataxia, and progressive dementia accompanied by widespread demyelination and distinctive perivascular fibrous deposits. A T→A transversion mutation in the stop codon of the BRI gene on chr 13 causes the addition of several amino acids at the C-terminus of the BRI protein. Although the normal function of the BRI protein is unknown, the presence of the extra C-terminal amino acids causes the protein to be misprocessed by a furin-mediated cleavage. This results in the accumulation of a 34 amino acid C-terminal derivative (the ABRI peptide) that assembles into toxic amyloid deposits through mechanisms yet to be elucidated.

Missense mutations in Neuroserpin, a neuron specific serine protease inhibitor (serpin), have been described in two pedigrees with a familial dementia. In these families with FEN1B, the mutant neuroserpin forms typical serpin loop-sheet polymers that assemble into fibrous aggregates, which appear as 5–50 μm PAS-positive eosinophilic inclusions, called "Collins bodies," in the deep layers of the cerebral cortex, subcortical nuclei, and substantia nigra.

FRONTOTEMPORAL LOBE DEMENTIA   FTD is a pleomorphic neurodegenerative illness that typically begins before age 65. In a minority of cases, the disease is inherited as an autosomal-dominant trait. FTD often begins with personality and behavioral changes including disinhibition manifest by alcoholism, hyperreligiosity, hypersexuality, hyperphagia (elements of the Kluver-Bucy syndrome) and stealing. As the disease progresses, further abnormalities in judgment, language, and praxia develop. In addition to these cognitive changes, some patients also developed Parkinsonism and amyotrophy, and presentations with primary progressive aphasia, dystonia, and/or oculomotor disturbances are not infrequent. Neuropathologically, the illness is typified by frontotemporal atrophy with severe neuronal loss, spongiform change in the superficial layers of the neocortex of the temporal lobe and frontal cortex, neuronal loss, and gliosis in the substantia nigra and amygdala, and anterior horn cell loss in the spinal cord. In some cases, notably those arising from mutations in the tau gene (*see* Tau Mutations in FTDP-17) the other prominent neuropathological feature is the presence of tau fibrils in neurons and/or glia.

Genetic linkage studies in the subset of FTD cases showing autosomal-dominant inheritance revealed that 10–40% of these familial FTD cases showed genetic linkage to DNA markers on chromosome 17 near the tau gene (*see* Tau Mutations in FTDP-17). It was also apparent that a significant proportion of autosomal-dominant FTD pedigrees did not show linkage to this region. Genetic linkage studies in these cases subsequently led to the discovery of an additional, but uncloned genetic locus associated with autosomal-dominant FTD with amyotrophic lateral sclerosis on chromosome 9q. Other loci are expected to exist.

TAU MUTATIONS IN FTDP-17

Sequencing of the tau gene led to the discovery of several different mutations in some families with FTDP-17. Tau is an abundant phosphoprotein predominantly expressed in both central and peripheral nervous systems. In brain it is found predominantly in axons of neurons, with lower levels in some glial cells. The major physiological function of Tau is to bind to and stabilize microtubules, and it may play a role in microtubule-dependent axoplasmic transport. Microtubule binding is mediated by three or four "microtubule-binding domain" repeats (depending on alternative splicing of the tau mRNA); these isoforms are therefore known as 3-repeat or 4-repeat isoforms.

Tau phosphorylation is developmentally regulated. Phosphorylation is thought to be regulated by one or more of several kinases including mitogen-activated protein kinase, glycogen synthase kinase-3, neuronal cdc2-like kinase and stress-activated protein kinases. The phosphorylation state of tau is balanced by the dephosphorylating activity of protein phosphatase 2A. Hyperphosphorylation is an invariant feature of the filamentous tau deposits that characterize a number of neurodegenerative diseases including AD and FTD.

Tau mutations causing FTDP-17 have generally been missense and deletion mutations in the coding region or intronic mutations located close to the 5′-splice site of the intron following exon 10. The tau missense mutations have generally been located in the microtubule-binding repeat region or close to it. Most of these missense mutations reduce the ability of tau to interact with microtubules, as reflected by a marked reduction in the ability of mutated tau proteins to promote microtubule assembly. Intronic

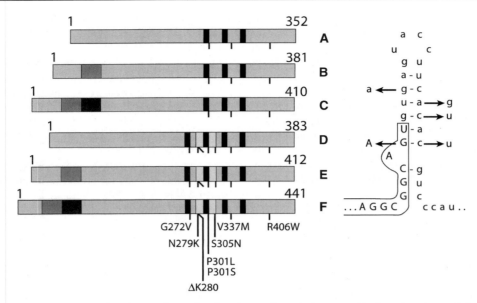

Figure 118-7   Diagram of the various splice forms of tau showing three microtubule repeat binding domains and four microtubule binding domains. The site of some of the mutations causing FTDP-17 is depicted.

mutations are located at positions +3, +13, +14, and +16, relative to the first nucleotide of the splice-donor site of the intron following exon 10. These intronic mutations disrupt an RNA stem-loop structure at the exon 10/5′-intron boundary and lead to increased production of transcripts encoding exon 10, which is reflected by a net overproduction of tau isoforms containing four rather than three microtubule binding repeats.

Validation of the hypothesis that overexpression of wild-type tau with four microtubule binding repeats or overexpression of mutant tau can cause intracellular accumulation of fibrillar deposits of tau and neurodegeneration has been obtained from the analysis of transgenic mice. Overexpression of either wild-type four repeat tau, or of P301L mutant tau transgenes results in neurodegeneration with NFT and spheroids particularly in the amygdala, brainstem, and cerebellar nuclei, and spinal cord. These neuropathological changes were associated with hindlimb weakness, amyo-trophy, and dystonic posturing.

The mechanism by which tau mutations or overexpression of specific isoforms of tau, cause neurodegeneration is unclear. There is some evidence that they alter the binding of tau to microtubules, causing increased amounts of free tau, which then inhibits kinesin-dependent intracellular transport of organelles, neurofilaments and cargo vesicles (including those carrying APP).

Cross breeding transgenic mice overexpressing mutant human tau transgenes with transgenic mice expressing mutant APP transgenes, and giving intracerebral injections of Aβ42 into these tau mice has resulted in a modest exacerbation of the tau pathology. This supports the idea that defects in APP processing in AD may initiate a cascade of other events (Fig. 118-7), which add to the neurotoxic cascade (i.e., tau misprocessing) and lead to neurodegeneration. If correct, this brings together the final common pathways for several neurodegenerative diseases.

PRACTICAL IMPLICATIONS: GENETIC TESTING

The discovery that mutations in specific genes are associated with inheritable susceptibility to AD and FTD, together with increasing public awareness of genetics as a cause of illness, and of familial aggregation of these diseases in particular, has led to the frequent need for physicians to consider the merits of genetic counselling and genetic testing. In the absence of clearly effective preventative or curative treatments without significant side effects, the main reason for genetic counselling and testing is currently to provide information only. However, although such information can be empowering, it also has the potential to be misused to the patient's disadvantage.

There is relatively little practical experience with genetic counselling of members of families multiply affected with AD or FTD. Consequently, most of the paradigms for genetic counselling of members of AD families are based on similar paradigms used in the counselling of subjects with Huntington's disease. The Huntington's disease model is useful for counselling of members of families with early-onset FAD or FTD because the age-of-onset is often similar (30–65 yr of age) and has a similar pattern of transmission (highly penetrant, age-dependent penetrance, autosomal-dominant segregation). Thus, it is possible to screen at-risk family members for the presence of mutations detected in affected individuals, and to counsel these family members based on the concept that β-APP, PS1 and tau mutations are highly penetrant (approx 95%) with typical age-of-symptom-onset between 35 and 65 yr. PS2 mutations on the other hand have a lower penetrance and a more variable age-of-onset (45–85 yr). Using the Huntington's disease paradigm, members of a small number of families with PS1 and β-APP mutations have been counselled without significant problems. Screening for PS1 mutations is cost effective when done on symptomatic cases with a positive family history of AD and onset before the age of 60 yr.

Although use of the Huntington's disease paradigm will probably work well for PS1, PS2, and β-APP mutations, mutations in these genes are a comparatively rare cause of FAD, cumulatively accounting for approx 50% of early-onset FAD (which itself accounts for approx 5% of all AD). A much more common clinical experience is the presence of two or three affected family members with late-onset AD in a small nuclear pedigree. Frequently, in these "multiplex" late-onset AD pedigrees, the disease does not inherit as a classic autosomal-dominant trait. As a result, in any given family, it is frequently unclear whether the multiplex pedigree structure reflects an incompletely penetrant autosomal-dominant trait, or a more complex mode of transmission involving either the additive effects of several genes or the interaction of genes and environment. Empirical counselling of pedigrees of this type is difficult and must largely be based on epidemiological studies. Although the use of molecular genetic studies would clearly facilitate counselling in such pedigrees, the only locus that has shown robust association with late-onset AD is the APOE gene. Retrospective studies, in autopsy and clinical series, have suggested that the cumulative lifetime risk for AD in subjects homozygous for APOE ε4 may be as high as 90% by age 90 yr. However, even from these retrospective studies, it is apparent that there is a huge variation in the age-of-onset of AD even in subjects who are homozygous for APOE ε4 (50–90 yr). To confound matters further, a small number of limited prospective studies suggest that the APOE genotype is a relatively poor predictor of the onset of AD even in high-risk groups such as those with age-associated memory loss. Consequently, a number of research groups have recommended that the APOE genotype not be used for presymptomatic testing. The question of whether the APOE genotype may be of assistance in establishing the diagnosis of AD in demented patients undergoing diagnostic workup is under discussion. Most experts agree that although the APOE genotype studies might form a part of the diagnostic armamentarium, they are unlikely by themselves to be the only test that should be done even in individuals with classic clinical features of AD.

It is likely that additional AD and FTD susceptibility genes will be identified. However, until most or all of these genes are identified, and their relative frequencies as a cause of dementia in specific populations can be defined, genetic testing of at-risk family members can only be reasonably performed if there is a testable, clinically affected member available. If an affected pedigree member is available, their DNA can be screened for mutations in the known susceptibility genes. If mutations are found, this information can be used for testing at-risk family members. Where no mutations in the affected subject's DNA are found, it can be reasonably assumed that the disease is caused by mutations or polymorphisms in other genes yet to be identified, and mutation screening studies in at-risk family members would not be indicated. However, in the absence of a living affected member who can be tested, the screening for mutations in the DNA of at-risk family members is likely to be unproductive because the failure to discover disease-related polymorphisms or mutations in the known AD or FTD genes can give no reassurance that the at-risk family member is not a carrier of a mutation in another susceptibility gene.

SELECTED REFERENCES

Alberts MJ, Graffagnino C. ApoE genotype and survival from intracerebral hemorrhage. Lancet 1995;346:575.

Arispe N, Pollard HB, Rojas E. Giant multilevel cation channels formed by Alzheimer disease amyloid B protein in a bilayer membrane. Proc Natl Acad Sci USA 1993;90:10,573–10,577.

Bales KR, Verina T, Dodel RC, et al. Lack of apolipoprotein E dramatically reduces amyloid beta-peptide deposition. Nat Genet 1997;17:254–256.

Bertram L, Blacker D, Mullin K, et al. Evidence for genetic linkage of Alzheimer's disease to chromosome 10q. Science 2000;290:2302–2303.

Bird TD. Familial Alzheimer's disease in American descendents of the Volga Germans: probable genetic founder effect. Ann Neurol 1988; 23:25.

Bird TD, Levy-Lehad E, Poorkaj J, et al. Wide range in age of onset for chromosome 1 related familial AD. Ann Neurol 1997;40:932–936.

Bird TD, Sumi SM, Nemens EJ, et al. Phenotypic heterogeneity in familial Alzheimer's disease: a study of 24 kindreds. Ann Neurol 1989;25: 12–25.

Boulianne G, Livne-Bar I, Humphreys JM, Rogaev E, St George-Hyslop P. Cloning and mapping of a close homologue of human presenilins in D. Melanogaster. Neuroreport 1997;8:1025–1029.

Cao X, Sudhof TC. A transcriptionally active complex of APP with Fe65 and histone acetyltransferase Tip60. Science 2001;293:115–120.

Checler F. The multiple paradoxes of presenilins. J Neurochem 2001;76: 1621–1627.

Copley TT, Wiggins W, Dufrasne S, et al. Are we all of one mind? Canadian Collaborative study for predictive testing for Huntington disease. Am J Med Genet 1995;58:59–69.

Corder EH, Saunders AM, Risch NJ, et al. Apolipoprotein E type 2 allele decreases the risk of late-onset Alzheimer disease. Nat Genet 1994;7: 180–184.

Corder EH, Saunders AM, Srittmatter WJ, et al. Gene dosage of apolipoprotein E type 4 allele and the risk for Alzheimer's disease in late-onset families. Science 1993;261:921–923.

Cupers P, Orlans I, Craessaerts K, Annaert W, De Strooper B. The amyloid precursor protein (APP)-cytoplasmic fragment generated by gamma-secretase is rapidly degraded but distributes partially in a nuclear fraction of neurones in culture. J Neurochem 2001;78:1168–1178.

Davis RL, Shrimpton AE, Holohan PD, et al. Familial demnetia caused by polymerization of mutant neuroserpin. Nature 1999;401:376–379.

De Strooper B, Annert W, Cupers P, et al. A presenilin dependent gamma-secretase-like protease mediates release of Notch intracellular domain. Nature 1999;398:518–522.

De Strooper B, Beullens M, Contreras B, et al. Posttranslational modification, subcellular localization and membrane orientation of the Alzheimer's disease associated Presenilins. J Biol Chem 1997;272: 3590–3598.

Ertekin-Taner N, Graff-Radford N, Younkin LH, et al. Linkage of plasma Abeta42 to a quantitative locus on chromosome 10 in late-onset Alzheimer's disease pedigrees. Science 2000;290:2303–2304.

Fassbender K, Simons M, Bergmann C, et al. Simvastatin strongly reduces levels of Alzheimer's disease beta—amyloid peptides Abeta 42 and Abeta 40 in vitro and in vivo. Proc Natl Acad Sci USA 2001;98: 5856–5861.

Gotz J, Chen F, van Dorpe J, Nitsch RM. Formation of neurofibrillary tangles in P301l tau transgenic mice induced by Abeta 42 fibrils. Science 2001;293:1491–1495.

Gu Y, Chen F, Sanjo N, et al. APH-1 interacts with mature and immature forms of presenilins and nicastrin and may play a role in maturation of presenilin-nicastrin complexes. J Biol Chem 2003;278:7374–7380.

Hendrie HC, Hall KS, Hui S. Apolipoprotein E genotypes and Alzheimer's disease in a community study of elderly African Americans. Ann Neurol 1995;37:118–121.

Herreman A, Hartmann D, Annaert W, et al. Presenilin 2 deficiency causes a mild pulmonary phenotype and no changes in amyloid precursor protein processing but enhances the embryonic lethal phenotype of presenilin 1 deficiency. Proc Natl Acad Sci USA 1999;96:11,872–11,877.

Jarrett JT, Lansbury PT. Seeding one-dimensional crystallization of amyloid: A pathogenic mechanism in Alzheimer's disease and scrapie? Cell 1993;73:1055–1058.

Jick H, Zornberg GL, Jick SS, Seshadri S, Drachman DA. Statins and the risk of dementia. Lancet 2000;356:1627–1631.

Kamal A, Almenar-Queralt A, LeBlanc JF, Roberts EA, Goldstein LS. Kinesin-mediated axonal transport of a membrane compartment containing beta-secretase and presenilin-1 requires APP. Nature 2001;414: 643–648.

Kang J, Lemaire HG, Unterbeck A, et al. The precursor of Alzheimer disease amyloid A4 protein resembles a cell surface receptor. Nature 1987; 325:733–736.

Katzman R, Kawas C. The epidemiology of dementia and Alzheimer disease. In: Terry RD, Katzman R, Bick KL, eds. Alzheimer Disease. New York: Raven Press, 1994; pp. 105–122.

Kim SH, Wang R, Gordon DJ, et al. Furin mediates enhanced production of fibrillogenic ABri peptides in familial British dementia. Nat Neurosci 1999;2:984–988.

Kounnas MZ, Moir RD, Rebeck GW, et al. LDL receptor related protein, a multifunctional ApoE receptor binds secreted bAPP and mediates its degradation. Cell 1995;82:331–340.

Kwok JB, Tadder K, Fisher C, et al. Two novel PS1 mutations in early-onset Alzheimer disease: evidence for association of PS1 mutations with a novel phenotype. Neuroreport 1997;8:1537–1542.

Lautenschlager NT, Cupples LA, Rao VS, et al. Risk of dementia among relatives of Alzheimer disease patients in the MIRAGE study: what is in store for the oldest old? Neurology 1996;46:641–650.

Levitan D, Greenwald I. Facilitation of lin-12-mediated signalling by sel-12, a Caenorhabditis elegans S182 Alzheimer's disease gene. Nature 1995;377:351–354.

Lewis J, Dickson DW, Lin WL, et al. Enhanced neurofibrillary degeneration in transgenic mice expressing mutant tau and APP. Science 2001; 293: 1487–1491.

Lewis J, McGowan E, Rockwood J, et al. Neurofibrillary tangles, amyotrophy and progressive motor disturbance in mice expressing mutant (P301L) tau protein. Nat Genet 2000;25:402–405.

Lorenzo A, Yanker BA. B-amyloid neurotoxicity requires fibril formation and is inhibited by Congo red. Proc Natl Acad Sci USA 1994;91: 12,243–12,247.

Lu DC, Rabizadeh S, Chandra S, et al. A second cytotoxic proteolytic peptide derived from amyloid beta-protein precursor. Nat Med 2000; 6:397–404.

Lynch T, Sano M, Marder K, et al. Clinical characteristics of a family with chromosome 17-linked disinhibition–dementia–parkinson–amyotrophy complex. Neurology 1994;44:1878–1884.

Maestre G, Ottman R, Stern Y, Mayeux R. Apolipoprotein E and Alzheimer disease: ethnic variation in genotype risks. Ann Neurol 1995;37: 254–259.

Mandelkow E, Mandelkow EM. Kinesin motors and disease. Trends Cell Biol 2002;12:585–591.

Mattson MP, Cheng B, Davis D, Bryant K, Lieberburg I, Rydel R. Beta-amyloid peptides destabilize calcium homeostasis and render human cortical neurons vulnerable to excitotoxicity. J Neurosci 1992;12: 376–389.

Mattson MP, Goodman Y. Different amyloidogenic peptides share a similar mechanism of neurotoxicity involving reactive oxygen species and calcium. Brain Res Brain Res Rev 1995;676:219–224.

Mayeux R, Ottman R. Synergistic effects of traumatic head injury and ApoE e4 in patients with Alzheimer's disease. Neurology 1995;45: 555–557.

Mayeux R, Saunders M, Shea S, et al. Utility of the apolipoprotein E genotype in the diagnosis of Alzheimer's disease. N Engl J Med 1998;338:506–511.

McKeith IG, Burn DJ, Ballard CG, et al. Dementia with Lewy bodies. Semin Clin Neuropsychiatry 2003;8:46–57.

Myers A, Holmans P, Marshall H, et al. Susceptibility locus for Alzheimer's disease on chromosome 10. Science 2000;290:2304–2305.

Newman MF, Croughwell ND. Predictors of cognitive decline after cardiac operation. Ann Thorac Surg 1995;59:1326–1330.

Olichney JM, Hansen LA, Galasko D, et al. The ApoE e4 allele is associated with increased neuritic plaques and cerebral amyloid angiopathy in AD and in Lewy body variant. Neurology 1996;47:190–196.

Perez-Tur J, Froelich S, Prihar G, et al. A mutation in Alzheimer's disease destroying a splice acceptor site in the presenilin 1 gene. Neuroreport 1996;7:297–301.

Pericak-Vance MA, Bass MP, Yamaoka LH, et al. Complete genomic screen in late-onset familial Alzheimer disease. Evidence for a new locus on chromosome 12. JAMA 1997;278:1282–1283.

Pericak-Vance MA, Bedout JL, Gaskell PC, Roses AD. Linkage studies in familial Alzheimer disease—evidence for chromosome 19 linkage. Am J Hum Genet 1991;48:1034–1050.

Pike CJ, Burdick D, Walencewicz AJ, Glabe CG, Cotman CW. Neurodegeneration induced by beta-amyloid peptides in vitro: the role of peptide assembly state. J Neurosci 1993;13:1676–1678.

Poorkaj P, Bird TD, Wijsman E, et al. Tau is a candidate gene for chromosome 17 frontotemporal dementia. Ann Neurol 1998;43:815–825.

Qiu WQ, Walsh DM, Ye Z, et al. Insulin-degrading enzyme regulates extracellular levels of amyloid beta-protein by degradation. J Biol Chem 1998;273:32,730–32,738.

Rebeck GW, Perls T, West H, Sodhi P, Lipsitz LA, Hyman BT. Reduced apolipoprotein e4 allele in the oldest old Alzheimer's patients and cognitively normal individuals. Neurology 1994;175:46–48.

Relkin N, Breitner J, Farrer L, et al. Apolipoprotein E genotyping in AD. Lancet 1996;347:1091–1095.

Rogaev EI, Sherrington R, Rogaeva EA, et al. Familial Alzheimer's disease in kindreds with missense mutations in a novel gene on chromosome 1 related to the Alzheimer's disease type 3 gene. Nature 1995;376:775–778.

Rogaeva E, Premkumar S, Song Y, et al. Evidence for an Alzheimer disease susceptibility locus on chr 12, and for further locus heterogeneity. JAMA 1998;280:614–618.

Rogaeva EA, Fafel KC, Song YQ, et al. Screening for PS1 mutations in a referral-based series of AD cases: 21 novel mutations. Neurology 2001; 57:621–625.

Roses AD, Saunders AM. Head injury, amyloid B and Alzheimer's disease. Nat Med 1995;1:603–604.

Runz H, Rietdorf J, Tomic I, et al. Inhibition of intracellular cholesterol transport alters presenilin localization and amyloid precursor protein processing in neuronal cells. J Neurosci 2002;22:1679–1689.

Sastre M, Steiner H, Fuchs K, et al. Presenilin-dependent gamma-secretase processing of beta-amyloid precursor protein at a site corresponding to the S3 cleavage of Notch. EMBO Rep 2001;2:835–841.

Sato S, Kamino K, Miki T, et al. Splicing mutation of presenilin 1 gene for early onset familial Alzheimer's disease. Hum Mutat 1998;1: 91–94.

Saunders A, Strittmatter WJ, Schmechel S, et al. Association of apolipoprotein E allele e4 with the late-onset familial and sporadic Alzheimer disease. Neurology 1993;43:1467–1472.

Scheuner D, Eckman L, Jensen M, et al. Secreted amyloid-b protein similar to that in the senile plaques of Alzheimer disease is increased in vivo by presenilin 1 and 2 and APP mutations linked to FAD. Nat Med 1996;2:864–870.

Schmechel DE, Saunders AM, Strittmatter WJ, et al. Increased vascular and plaque beta-A4 amyloid deposits in sporadic Alzheimer's disease patients with apolipoprotein e4. Proc Natl Acad Sci USA 1993;90: 9649–9653.

Selkoe DJ. Normal and abnormal biology of B-amyloid precursor protein. Ann Rev Neurosci 1994;17:489–517.

Sherrington R, Froelich S, Sorbi S, et al. Alzheimer's disease associated with mutations in presenilin-2 are rare and variably penetrant. Hum Mol Genet 1996;5:985–988.

Sherrington R, Rogaev E, Liang Y, et al. Cloning of a gene bearing missense mutations in early onset familial Alzheimer's disease. Nature 1995; 375:754–760.

Sima AA, Defendini R, Keohane C, et al. The neuropathology of chromosome 17 linked dementia. Ann Neurol 1996;39:734–743.

Spittaels K, Van den Haute C, Van Dorpe J, et al. Prominent axonopathy in the brain and spinal cord of transgenic mice overexpressing four-repeat human tau protein. Am J Pathol 1999;155:2153–2165.

St. George-Hyslop PH, Tsuda T, Crapper McLachlan DR, Karlinsky H, Pollen D, Lippa C. Alzheimer's disease and possible gene interaction. Science 1994;263:536–537.

Strittmatter WJ, Saunders AM, Schmechel D, et al. Apolipoprotein E: High affinity binding to B/A4 amyloid and increased frequency of type 4 allele in familial Alzheimer's disease. Proc Natl Acad Sci USA 1993; 90:1977–1981.

Strittmatter WJ, Weisgraber KH, Huang DY, Schemechel D, Saunders AM, Roses AD. Binding of human lipoprotein E to synthetic amyloid beta peptide: Isoform-specific effects and implications for late onset AD. Proc Natl Acad Sci USA 1993;90:8098–8102.

Thinakaran G, Borchelt DR, Lee MK, et al. Endoproteolysis of presenilin 1 and accumulation of processed derivatives in vivo. Neuron 1996;17: 181–190.

Tierney M, Szalai JP, Snow WG, et al. A prospective study of the clinical utility of ApoE genotypes in the prediction of outcome in patients with memory impairment. Neurology 1996;46:149–154.

Van Duijn CM, de Knijff P, Crutts M, et al. Apolipoprotein E4 allele in a population based study of early onset Alzheimer disease. Nat Genet 1994;7:74–78.

Vassar R, Bennett BD, Babu-Kahn S, et al. Beta-secretase cleavage of Alzheimer's amyloid precursor protein by the transmembrane aspartic protease BACE. Science 1999;286:735–741.

Vidal R, Frangione B, Rostagno A, et al. A stop-codon mutation in the BRI gene associated with familial British dementia. Nature 1999;399: 776–781.

Wolfe MS, Presenilin and gamma-secretase: structure meets function. J Neurochem 2001;76:1615–1620.

Wolfe MS, Xia W, Ostaszewski BL, Diehl TS, Kimberly WT, Selkoe DS. Two transmembrane aspartates in presenilin 1 required for presenilin endoproteolysis and gamma-secretase activity. Nature 1999;398: 513–517.

Wong PC, Zheng H, Chen H, et al. Functions of the presenilins: generation and characterization of presenilin-1 null mice. Society for Neuroscience 1996;22:728.

Wolozin B, Kellman W, Ruosseau P, Celesia GG, Siegel G. Decreased prevalence of Alzheimer disease associated with 3-hydroxy-3-methyglutaryl coenzyme A reductase inhibitors. Arch Neurol 2000;57:143–943.

Yankner BA, Duffy LK, Kirschner DA. Neurotrophic and neurotoxic effects of amyloid B protein: reversal by tachykinin neuropeptides. Science 1990;250:279–282.

Yasojima K, Akiyama H, McGeer EG, McGeer PL. Reduced neprilysin in high plaque areas of Alzheimer brain: a possible relationship to deficient degradation of beta-amyloid peptide. Neurosci Lett 2001; 297:97–100.

Ye Y, Lukinova N, Fortini ME. Neurogenic phenotypes and altered Notch processing in Drosophila presenilin mutants. Nature 1999;398: 525–529.

Yu G, Nishimura M, Arawaka S, et al. A novel protein (nicastrin) modulates presenilin-mediated Notch/Glp1 and betaAPP processing. Nature 2000;407:48–54.

Zheng H, Jiang M, Trumbauer ME, et al. Mice deficient for the amyloid precursor protein gene. Ann NY Acad Sci 1996;777:421–426.

119 Prion Diseases

Adriano Aguzzi

SUMMARY

Considerable experimental and theoretical evidence supports the proposition that the prion (i.e., the transmissible entity of transmissible spongiform encephalopathies) is made up of a self-propagating isoform of PrP, and that informational nucleic acids are not required for transmissibility. Many questions still need to be elucidated, such as the mechanism and the requirements for the conversion reaction, the portals of entry of prions into the body, the transport of prions from periphery to CNS, and the mechanism of pathogenesis. Clinically, early diagnosis of prion disease and treatments aiming to arrest or cure prion disease in humans are important goals.

Key Words: Bovine prion disease; central nervous system; Creutzfeldt-Jakob disease; fatal familial insomnia; Gerstmann-Sträussler-Scheinker; transmissible spongiform encephalopathies.

INTRODUCTION

Prion diseases, or transmissible spongiform encephalopathies (TSEs), are CNS degenerative disorders of sporadic, familial, or acquired nature. They include Creutzfeldt-Jakob disease (CJD), Gerstmann-Sträussler-Scheinker (GSS) syndrome, Kuru, and fatal familial insomnia (FFI) in humans, and a number of encephalopathies of animals. The latter comprise scrapie of sheep, bovine spongiform encephalopathy (BSE) or "mad cow disease," chronic wasting diseases of deer and elk, and similar diseases of exotic ungulates. A large body of circumstantial evidence has accumulated indicating that BSE prions can provoke a variant form of CJD in humans. This chapter describes the nature of the infectious agent along with its molecular and biochemical properties, and gives a synopsis on clinical, histopathological, and genetic features of TSEs.

The TSEs, or prion diseases (Table 119-1), represent a group of diseases with unique clinical and histological features, the transmission of which can be genetic or infectious. According to most available evidence, the agent causing TSEs, termed prion, is devoid of informational nucleic acids and consists of an "infectious" protein capable of converting a normal host protein called PrP^C, PrP-sen, or simply PrP, into a likeness of itself (called PrP^{Sc} or PrP-res).

From: *Principles of Molecular Medicine, Second Edition*
Edited by: M. S. Runge and C. Patterson © Humana Press, Inc., Totowa, NJ

The only organ system in which histopathological damage with its clinical effects is visible as a consequence of prion infection is the nervous system. This applies to all human TSEs and to all known prion encephalopathies of animals. However, it is apparent that prions can colonize organs other than the central and peripheral nervous system, and can be demonstrated in extracerebral compartments. A large body of incidental evidence has accumulated indicating that BSE prions can provoke new variant Creutzfeldt-Jakob disease (vCJD), although no ultimate proof has been presented—perhaps resulting from limitations of the analytical assays used for determining the characteristics of prions. Although most cases of human prion diseases are sporadic, about 10% run within family trees with a dominant pattern of transmission, and linked to one of a number of mutations in the gene encoding PrP. It is believed that these mutations allow spontaneous conversion of PrP^C into PrP^{Sc} with a frequency sufficient to cause disease within the lifetime of an individual.

HUMAN PRION DISEASES

Because the first description of CJD by Jakob and Creutzfeldt, five human diseases have been identified as TSEs (*see* Table 119-1). A striking hallmark applying to all TSEs is that the brain is heavily affected in sharp contrast to the extraneural tissues, which remain unharmed. To ultimately diagnose human prion diseases, a histopathological assessment of the CNS is essential. The communal lesions are neuronal loss, spongiosis, and astrogliosis, accompanied by an accumulation of microglia and, occasionally, the presence of amyloid plaques and various kinds of small deposits immunolabeled with anti-PrP antibodies (Fig. 119-1). These deposits are variable in their number and topography, hence representing one in a number of phenotypic variations typical of the various forms of human prion disease. The classifications of these disorders are being revised to incorporate genetic and biochemical data in addition to clinical and histopathological parameters.

CJD occurs sporadically with an incidence of approx 1–1.5 cases/million/yr, although higher incidence was reported in countries carrying out intensive surveillance programs. CJD may be transmitted through injection of infected tissues, and has a genetic basis in roughly 10% of all cases. Clinically, patients suffering from CJD show a wide spectrum of diversely associated symptoms. Besides the typical rapidly progressive form including dementia, myoclonia, cerebellar ataxia, visual disturbances, and periodic EEG

Table 119-1
Classification of Prion Diseases

Disease	Host	Mechanism of pathogenesis
Iatrogenic Creutzfeldt-Jakob disease	Humans	Infection from prion-contaminated pituitary hormones, dura mater grafts, and so on.
vCJD	Humans	Infection from BSE prions (hypothesized)
Familial CJD	Humans	Germ-line mutations in *PRNP* gene
sCJD	Humans	Unknown. Possibly somatic mutations resulting in spontaneous conversion of PrP^C into PrP^{Sc}?
Kuru	Fore people	Infection through ritualistic cannibalism
GSS disease	Humans	Germ-line mutations in *PRNP* gene
FFI	Humans	Germ-line mutations in *PRNP* gene
Fatal sporadic insomnia	Humans	Unknown
Scrapie	Sheep	Infection in genetically susceptible sheep
BSE	Cattle	Infection with prion-contaminated meat-and-bone meal
Transmissible mink encephalopathy	Mink	Infection with prions from sheep or cattle
Chronic wasting disease	Mule deer, white-tail deer, elk	Unknown
Feline spongiform encephalopathy	Cats	Infection with prion-contaminated bovine tissues or MBM
Exotic ungulate encephalopathy	Greater kudu, nyala, oryx	Infection with prion-contaminated MBM

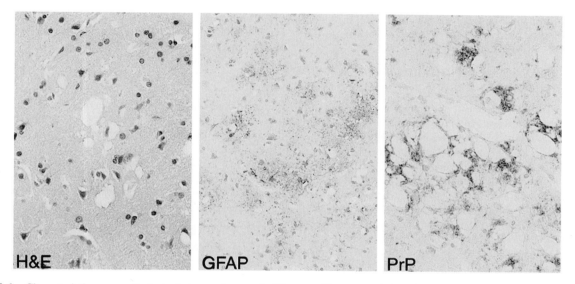

Figure 119-1 Characteristic neuropathologic features of transmissible spongiform encephalopathies. Grey matter of the brain of a Creutzfeldt-Jakob disease patient stained with hematoxylin-eosin (H&E) displaying the characteristic spongiform morphology (left). The normal texture is disturbed by the presence of coarse vacuoles. Antibodies against glial fibrillary acidic protein (GFAP; brown color, middle) allow for visualization of activated, proliferated reactive, swollen astrocytes. The immunohistochemical stain with anti-PrP antibodies evidences perivacuolar prion protein deposits (brown color, right). (Please *see* color insert.)

changes, other forms of the disease exist and may give rise to diagnostic difficulties. Albeit not completely diagnostic, periodic sharp wave complexes detected by EEG and 14-3-3 protein detection in spinal fluid are sometimes helpful for diagnosis, when clinical symptoms are present. There is no validated diagnostic procedure that would allow for confirmation of sporadic Creutzfeldt-Jakob disease (sCJD) in a patient short of brain biopsy, although it was reported that prions can be detected in the nasal mucosa of sCJD patients. Interestingly, there are no general symptoms such as fever or leukocytosis reminiscent of a humoral immune response.

The most recently recognized form of CJD in humans, vCJD, was first described in 1996 and has been linked to BSE. vCJD represents a distinct clinico-pathological entity characterized at onset by psychiatric abnormalities, sensory symptoms, and ataxia, eventually leading to dementia with other features usually observed in sCJD. What distinguishes vCJD from sporadic cases is that the

age of patients is abnormally low (vCJD: 19–39 yr; sCJD: 55–70 yr) and duration of the illness is rather long (vCJD: 7.5–22 mo; sCJD: 2.5–6.5 mo). Moreover, the vCJD displays a distinct pathology within the brain characterized by abundant "florid plaques," decorated by a daisy-like pattern of vacuolation. Most cases of vCJD have been observed in the United Kingdom.

Other genetic diseases in humans are GSS syndrome and FFI. GSS is transmitted by autosomal-dominant inheritance. It is characterized by missense mutations of the gene encoding PrP (Fig. 119-2), associated with specific neuropathological lesions, and by multicentric amyloid plaques that can be visualized by antibodies directed against the prion protein. This restrictive definition justifies retaining the name of GSS syndrome and excludes observations of hereditary prion diseases without multicentric amyloid plaques, as well as sporadic forms with multicentric plaques. It has been possible to transmit GSS to chimpanzees

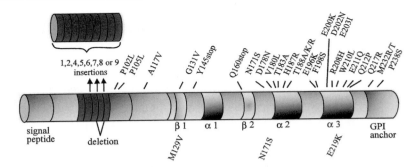

Figure 119-2 Schematic drawing of the coding region of the human PRNP gene. Mutations that segregate with inherited prion diseases are shown in the figure, as well as nonpathogenic polymorphisms and silent mutations. The N- and C-terminal domains are signal peptides that are cleaved off during maturation of PrP^C. Octa repeat regions are represented by dark gray boxes, and pathogenic octa repeat insertions of 16, 32, 40, 48, 56, 64, and 72 amino acids are shown in the figure. Deletion of one octa repeat stretch does not appear to segregate with a neurodegenerative disorder. The light gray box indicates a conserved region and β-sheet domains. There is an apparent clustering of pathogenic mutations associated with a Creutzfeldt-Jakob disease phenotype around the α-helical domains (H1, H2, H3, dark gray), whereas amino acid exchanges associated with a Gerstmann-Sträussler-Scheinker phenotype are located further upstream around the conserved region.

and to mice. An additional member of the group of TSEs, FFI, was also transmitted experimentally in at least three instances to mice. Kuru is a form of spongiform encephalopathies transmitted by ritual cannibalism, which affected the Fore population in the Northern provinces of New Guinea.

THE MOLECULAR BASIS OF BRAIN DAMAGE IN PRION DISEASES

Protease-resistant prion protein (PrP^Sc) deposits in the brain in most prion diseases. However, in some inherited cases PrP^Sc is hardly detectable, whereas ^CTMPrP, a transmembrane form of the prion protein, is abundant and may represent the prime pathogenetic moiety. This applies to a subset of people with GSS syndrome carrying a distinct mutation in the PrP gene, namely a substitution of alanine to valine at position 117 (*see* Fig. 119-2). Interestingly, this mutation, which leads to the irreversible neurodegeneration characteristic for prion diseases, is neither producing conventional PrP^Sc nor transmittable to laboratory rodents. It has been claimed that the effectiveness of accumulated PrP^Sc in causing neurodegenerative disease depends on the predilection of host-encoded PrP to be made in the ^CTMPrP form. In addition, the time course of PrP^Sc accumulation seems to modulate the events involved in generating ^CTMPrP suggesting a common mechanism in the pathogenesis of both genetic and acquired prion diseases—thus, possibly presenting not an exception but an explanation to the rule. This might explain why in many instances of human and experimental TSE extremely little PrP^Sc can be detected, even in terminal disease.

Cytosolic translocation of PrP^C has also been suggested to be involved in spongiform damage. A significant proportion of misfolded, secreted proteins can undergo retrotranslocation from the lumen of the endoplasmic reticulum to the cytosol, and targeting of a PrP^C variant to the neuronal cytosol was reported to be extremely neurotoxic in transgenic mice. It is conceivable that pathogenic missense mutations lead to enhanced production of misfolded prion protein and induce a late-onset metabolic disease by this mechanism. However, the exact biochemical pathways by which cytosolic PrP^C may arise are unclear and controversially debated.

THE BASIS OF PRION NEUROTROPISM

Although the prime target of damage seems to be neuronal, profound neuronal loss is not always seen in TSEs. Instead, activation of astrocytes, a brain-specific cell type, occurs early and in

an extremely consistent fashion (*see* Fig. 119-1). It can be easily reproduced in vitro, and leads to significant physiological effects such as impairment of the blood–brain barrier. Additionally, astrocytes belong to the few cell types identified that are capable of supporting prion replication.

Growing evidence incriminates another cell type in brain damage, not only in TSEs but in diseases ranging from Alzheimer's to multiple sclerosis and even stroke: microglial cells, the brain's immunocompetent macrophages. In vitro experiments suggest that activation of microglia may be pivotal in effecting neuronal damage in TSEs, and that this phenomenon is dependent on expression of PrP^C; however, both claims have been subsequently challenged. The detailed pathways of neuronal cell death, therefore, still escape understanding. Future strategies to investigate the function of microglial cells in prion diseases may necessitate conditional lineage ablation strategies in trangenic mice.

HORIZONTAL TRANSMISSION OF PRIONS AMONG HUMANS

Prion diseases of humans are undeniably transmissible. But transmission is accomplished only under certain conditions, thus fulfilling the characteristics of transmissibility delineated by Semmelweiss for puerperal fever, prions are infectious but not contagious. Direct transmissions of brain-derived material from a patient suffering from CJD to other persons have proven to result in transmission of disease. A particularly tragic case occurred in the early seventies in Zurich, when electrodes used for cortical recordings from Creutzfeldt-Jakob patients were sterilized using formaldehyde vapors and alcohol, and used in additional patients. Disease was transmitted to two very young recipients. Moreover, several thousand patients, predominantly in Japan, may have been exposed to the CJD agent via preparations of prion-contaminated dura mater, although less than 2% of those exposed have developed disease so far. Also cornea transplantation likely resulted in transmission in the United States decades ago.

The largest problem with iatrogenic transmission of CJD has occurred as result of peripheral administration of pituitary hormones of cadaveric origin. Preparations of growth hormone and of gonadotropins contaminated with human prions have caused the death of more than 80 persons, of which most were children. Nonetheless, iatrogenic transmission is a rare event. This can be explained in two nonexclusive ways, either by the long incubation time of prion diseases, especially in the earlier described case of extracerebrally administered growth hormones, assuming that further cases may arise within the future, or that some concomitant cofactors and endogenous modifiers, in addition to the virulence of prions, may affect the probability that infection takes place, thus either protecting or sensitizing individuals exposed to CJD prions.

The observations that latency after intracerebral contamination (such as cornea and dura mater transplants) is much shorter than latency after peripheral infection (as in the case of extracerebral application of pituitary hormones) is in agreement with experimental data from animal models, and suggest that a rather prolonged period of extracerebral events possibly including replication of the agent and invasion of specific extraneuronal systems may be a precondition to prion neuroinvasion.

NEUROINVASION–HOW PRIONS PAVE THEIR WAY TO THE CNS

Although prions are most effective when directly administered to the brain of their hosts, this situation occurs mainly in experimental lab work, and does not reflect the reality of the common routes of prion infections. Acquired forms of prion diseases are largely transmitted through oral uptake of the agent or peripheral administration—such as intramuscular injection of growth hormone and, to a lesser extent, pituitary gonadotropins—raising the question as to how prions find their way to the CNS.

Neuroectodermal tissue of $Prnp^{+/+}$ mice postnatally grafted into the brain of $Prnp^{o/o}$ mice develops into differentiated $Prnp^{+/+}$ nervous tissue. Intracerebral inoculation of such engrafted mice leads to typical scrapie pathology within the graft but not in the surrounding $Prnp^{o/o}$ tissue, whereas intraperitoneal infection does not, suggesting that prion transport from periphery to CNS requires interposed PrP-bearing tissue. Because no pathologies can be identified in organs other than the CNS it is of great importance to identify "reservoirs" within the periphery in which prions multiply (silently) during the incubation phase of the disease.

One such reservoir of PrP^{Sc} or infectivity is doubtlessly the immune system; studies point to the importance of prion replication in lymphoid organs. The nature of the cells supporting prion replication within the lymphoreticular system, however, is still uncertain. Inoculation of various genetically modified immunodeficient mice lacking different components of the immune system with scrapie prions revealed that the lack of B-cells renders mice unsusceptible to experimental scrapie. Whereas defects affecting only T lymphocytes had no apparent effect, all mutations affecting differentiation and responses of B-lymphocytes prevented development of clinical scrapie. Because absence of B-cells and of antibodies correlates with severe defects in follicular dendritic cells (FDCs), the lack of any of these three components may prevent clinical scrapie. FDCs have been incriminated, because PrP^{Sc} accumulates in FDCs of wild-type and nude mice (which suffer from a selective T-cell defect). Depletion of FDCs can block the replication of prions in the spleen.

Repopulation of immunodeficient mice with fetal liver cells from either PrP-expressing or PrP-deficient mice and from T-cell deficient mice, but not from B-cell deficient mice, is equally efficient in restoring neuroinvasion after intraperitoneal inoculation of scrapie prions. This suggests that cells whose maturation depends on B cells or their products (such as FDCs) may enhance neuroinvasion. Alternatively, B cells may transport prions to the nervous system by a PrP-independent mechanism, because PrP expression in B cells is not required for prion neuroinvasion. Interestingly,

components of the complement system appear to play an important modulatory role in susceptibility to prion infection.

However, immune cells are unlikely to transport the agent all the way from the lymphoreticular system to the CNS, because prion replication occurs first in the CNS segments to which the sites of peripheral inoculation project. This implies that the agent may spread through other compartments, such as the peripheral nervous system (Fig. 119-3). There is experimental evidence implicating both the sympathetic and the parasympathetic nervous systems.

APPROACHES TO THE THERAPY OF PRION DISEASES

Despite that no patient and no experimental animal were ever rescued from manifest prion disease, developments appear to suggest that immunological and pharmacological interventions may bear some potential for pre-exposure and postexposure prophylaxis. Although no realistic prospect for curing the clinically overt stages of prion diseases exists, an increasing arsenal of palliative and even life-prolonging interventions is being tested in experimental and clinical settings.

Preincubation with anti-PrP antisera reduces the prion titer of infectious hamster brain homogenates and anti-PrP antibodies inhibit formation of PrP^{Sc} in a cell-free system. Also, antibodies and F(ab) fragments raised against certain domains of PrP can suppress prion replication in cultured cells. However, it is difficult to induce humoral immune responses against PrP^{C} and PrP^{Sc} because of tolerance to PrP^{C}, which is expressed almost ubiquitously. Ablation of the $Prnp$ gene, which encodes PrP^{C}, renders mice highly susceptible to immunization with prions. However, $Prnp^{o/o}$ mice are unsuitable for testing vaccination regimens because they do not support prion pathogenesis.

Introduction of the epitope-interacting region, the heavy chain of a high-affinity anti-PrP monoclonal antibody, into the germ line of mice induced spontaneous anti-PrP^{C} immunity. Most intriguingly, expression of the 6H4μ heavy chain blocked peripheral prion pathogenesis on intraperitoneal inoculation of the prion agent. This delivers proof-of-principle that a protective humoral response against prions can be mounted by the mammalian immune system, and suggests that B cells are not intrinsically tolerant to PrP^{C}. These data were confirmed by passive transfer of immunoglobulins.

If the antiprion effect of anti-PrP^{C} antibodies is generally true, lack of immunity to prions may be resulting from T-helper tolerance. The latter problem is not trivial, but may perhaps be overcome by presenting PrP^{C} to the immune system along with highly active adjuvants. These findings, therefore, encourage a reassessment of the possible value of active and passive immunization, and perhaps of reprogramming B-cell repertoires by μ chain transfer, in prophylaxis or in therapy of prion diseases.

The possibility of producing protective immunity against prions has, in the meantime, captured the imagination of a considerable number of scientists, and additional reports are appearing of original ways to break tolerance and induce an immune response in animals that express the normal prion protein, including passive immunization and mixing of the immunogenic moiety with bacterial chaperons.

It was claimed that chronic administration of CpG-containing oligodeoxynucleotides, which stimulate the innate immunity receptor TLR9, can accomplish postexposure prophylaxis against prion diseases. Details of this surprising phenomenon show that

Possible actors of neuroinvasion

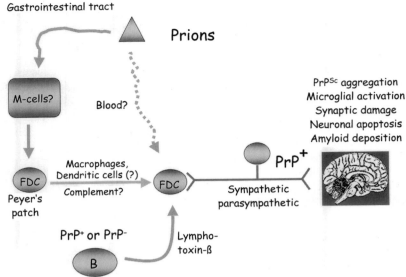

Figure 119-3   Possible models for prion neuroinvasion. In the upper panel, B lymphocytes, which may be genotypically PrP-positive or PrP-negative, physically carry prions to their sites of replication in spleen. These may be represented, in part or entirely, by FDCs. Neuroinvasion proper then occurs preferentially along fibers of the peripheral nervous system, which may support transfer of prions to the CNS depending on their own expression of PrP^C. The lower panel illustrates a second possibility, i.e., that B cells are not directly involved in neuroinvasion. In this instance, the crucial role of B-cells in neuroinvasive scrapie relies on their function in inducing maturation of FDCs.

this treatment abolishes germinal center networks and ablates FDCs, which are the major reservoir of prion infectivity in the periphery. CpG oligodeoxynucleotide protect against prions by virtue of their toxic side effects, and therefore are hardly suitable for clinical applications in this context.

MOLECULAR BIOLOGY OF PRIONS

PrP^C has been identified in all mammals and birds examined, and it is anchored to the external surface of cells by a glycolipid moiety. Its function is unknown. Attempts to identify a post-translational chemical modification that distinguishes PrP^{Sc} from PrP^C have been unsuccessful. PrP^C contains approx 45% α-helix and is virtually devoid of β-sheet. Conversion to PrP^{Sc} creates a protein that contains approx 30% α-helix and 45% β-sheet. The mechanism by which PrP^C is converted into PrP^{Sc} remains unknown but PrP^C seems to bind to PrP^{Sc} and to form an intermediate complex during the formation of nascent PrP^{Sc}. Transgenic mouse studies have demonstrated that PrP^{Sc} in the inoculum interacts preferentially with homotypic PrP^C during the propagation of prions.

Prnp is transcribed in brain and many other cells of the body in both prion-infected and noninfected animals. Removal of *Prnp* from the mouse genome leads to complete immunity from prions. The emergence of a vCJD in young people in the UK has raised the possibility that BSE has spread to humans by dietary exposure. Experimental evidence claiming that the agent causing BSE is indistinguishable from the vCJD agent has supported this view.

THE CONVERSION OF PRP^C INTO PRP^{SC}

Accumulation of an abnormal isoform (PrP^{Sc}) of the host encoded PrP^C in the CNS is a hallmark of prion diseases. Because no chemical differences were found between PrP^C and PrP^{Sc}, the two species are believed to differ in their conformation. The fine 3D structure of PrP^C has been resolved at the atomic level using both nuclear magnetic resonance spectroscopy and X-ray diffraction crystallography. Instead, only low-resolution structural data exist for PrP^{Sc}, which have been extended to electron crystallography. The β-sheet content of PrP^{Sc} was found to be high, whereas PrP^C contains only a very short β-sheet stretch. Conversion of PrP^C into PrP^{Sc} in prion-infected cells is known to be a late post-translational process, occurring after PrP^C has reached its normal extracellular location.

To explain the mechanism by which a misfolded form of PrP might induce the refolding of "native," normal PrP molecules into the abnormal conformation, two distinct models have been postulated: the template assistance or "refolding" model, and the nucleation-polymerization or "seeding" model (Fig. 119-4). In the first model, the conformational change is kinetically controlled; a high activation energy barrier prevents spontaneous conversion at detectable rates. Interaction with exogenously introduced PrP^{Sc} causes PrP^C to undergo an induced conformational change to yield PrP^{Sc}. This reaction may involve extensive unfolding and refolding of the protein to explain the postulated high energy barrier and could be dependent on an enzyme or chaperone, provisionally designated as protein X. In the second model, PrP^C and PrP^{Sc} are in equilibrium strongly favoring PrP^C. PrP^{Sc} is only stabilized when it adds onto a crystal-like aggregate of PrP^{Sc} acting as a seed in a nucleation-dependent polymerization process. Cell-free conversion studies suggest that PrP^{Sc} aggregates are able to convert PrP^C into a protease-resistant PrP isoform.

THE PRION PROTEIN

The cellular prion protein PrP^C contains two N-linked complex-type oligosaccharides at positions 181 and 197. Accordingly, Western blot analysis of PrP reveals three major bands, reflecting PrP that has two, one, or no glycosylation signals occupied. On translocation of PrP into the endoplasmic reticulum, an NH$_2$-terminal secretory

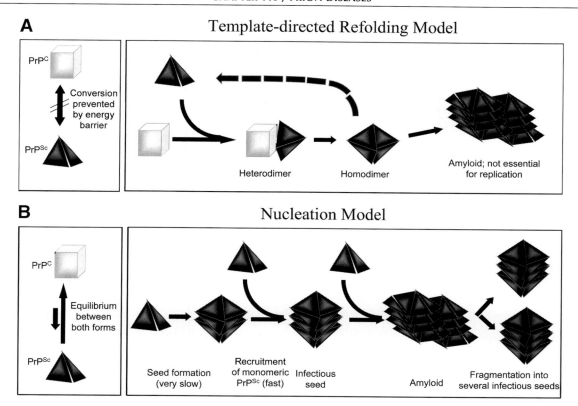

Figure 119-4 Models for the conformational conversion of PrP^C into PrP^{Sc}. **(A)** The "refolding" or template assistance model postulates an interaction between exogenously introduced PrP^{Sc} and endogenous PrP^C, which is induced to transform itself into further PrP^{Sc}. A high energy barrier may prevent spontaneous conversion of PrP^C into PrP^{Sc}. **(B)** The "seeding" or nucleation-polymerization model proposes that PrP^C and PrP^{Sc} are in a reversible thermodynamic equilibrium. Only if several monomeric PrP^{Sc} molecules are mounted into a highly ordered seed, further monomeric PrP^{Sc} can be recruited and eventually aggregates to amyloid. Within such a crystal-like seed, PrP^{Sc} becomes stabilized. Fragmentation of PrP^{Sc} aggregates increases the number of nuclei, which can recruit further PrP^{Sc} and thus results in apparent replication of the agent.

signal peptide of 22 amino acids is cleaved from PrP, and twenty-three COOH-terminal residues are processed during addition of the GPI-anchor to the amino acid residue serine at position 231. Mature mouse PrP contains 209 amino acids.

PrP^{Sc}, which accumulates in TSE-affected organisms is a modified form of PrP^C. PrP^C and PrP^{Sc} have an identical amino acid sequence and share the same posttranslational modifications as assessed by available methodology, but differ in their secondary and (presumably) tertiary structure. The physiological isoform PrP^C is protease-sensitive (consequently sometimes designated as PrP^{sen}), whereas the pathological isoform PrP^{Sc} is partially protease-resistant (thus also called PrP^{res}). The protease-resistant core of PrP^{Sc}, designated PrP$^{27-30}$ according to its molecular weight on SDS-PAGE, provides a specific and reliable molecular marker for the presence of the infectious agent (Fig. 119-5).

Because of its location at the outer surface of cells, anchored by phosphatidyl inositol glycolipid, PrP is a candidate for signaling, cell adhesion, or perhaps even for some transport functions. PrP is expressed on many cell types, including neurons, glial cells, and lymphocytes and appears to be developmentally regulated during mouse embryogenesis. All prion proteins investigated contain 4-5 "octa repeats," repetitive sequences of eight amino acids. Amplification of the number of octa repeats has been found in hereditary prion diseases such as Familial CJD and GSS syndrome. Several studies have established that mammalian and chicken prion protein octa repeats bind up to four copper atoms. It has been suggested from studies with peptides based on the octa

repeat region of PrP that the four highly conserved histidines in the repeat region coordinate four copper atoms suggest that binding of copper may be essential for the function of PrP^C. PrP refolded with copper has been purported to have an antioxidant activity similar to superoxide dismutase, but these claims were not independently reproduced and there is no evidence that PrP^C acts as a superoxide dismutase in vivo.

Although PrP is predominantly found in brain tissue, high levels are also present in heart, skeletal muscle and kidney whereas it is barely detectable in the liver. Several candidate proteins that bind PrP^C have been reported. Among them are a member of the amyloid precursor protein, the amyloid precursor-like protein 1 (APLP1), the antiapoptotic protein bcl-2, and the 37 kDa human laminin receptor precursor. The observation that PrP binds to APLP1 is intriguing in light of potential analogies of TSEs to Alzheimer's disease. Evidence that any of these interactions are of physiological relevance is, however, still amiss.

PRNP—THE GENE ENCODING PRP

The gene encoding the cellular isoform of the prion protein is located on chromosome 20 in humans and on chromosome 2 in mice, and is termed *Prnp* in mouse and *PRNP* in humans. In all known mammalian and avian *Prnp* genes, PrP^C is encoded by a single open reading frame. The *Prnp* genes of mouse, sheep, and cattle contain 3 exons, although those of hamsters and humans span over 2 exons. PrP expression seems to be controlled by the SP1 transcription factor that binds to G+C rich nonamer-regions

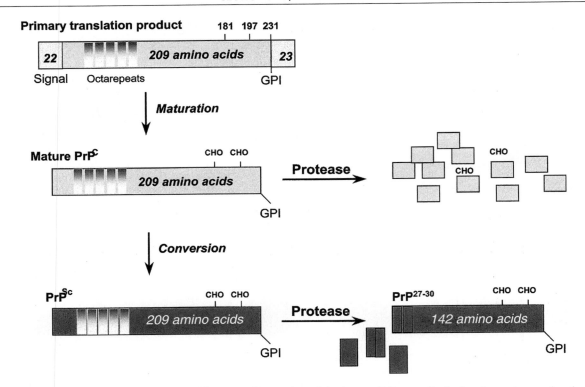

Figure 119-5   Post-translational processing of PrP^C. The coding region of the human PrP gene displaying the amino- and carboxy-terminal signal sequences; the five internally shaded boxes indicate the "octa repeats," sequences of eight amino acids. On reaching its destination on the cell surface, an amino-terminal secretory signal peptide of 22 amino acids is cleaved from the 254 amino acid PrP^C precursor protein. Twenty-three carboxy-terminal residues are also processed during addition of the GPI-anchor to a serine residue at position 231. On completion of these modifications, mature PrP^C contains 209 amino acids. PrP^{Sc} is a modified form of PrP^C. PrP^C and PrP^{Sc} have an identical amino acid sequence and share the same post-translational modifications, but differ in their secondary and (presumably) tertiary structure. The physiologic isoform PrP^C is protease-sensitive, whereas the pathological isoform PrP^{Sc} is partially protease-resistant displaying a protease-resistant core of PrP^{Sc}, designated PrP 27-30.

upstream of exon 1. Within the genome, *Prnp* is present as a single copy gene. A partial homologue gene termed *Prnd*, and encoding the *Dpl* protein ("downstream of the *Prnp* locus"), was identified approx 16 kb 3′ from the *Prnp* locus. No evidence incriminates *Dpl* in the pathogenesis of transmissible prion diseases, and the physiological function of *Dpl* seems to be related to male reproduction.

Prnp mRNA is constitutively expressed in the adult organism and developmentally regulated during mouse embryogenesis. Mutations in the host-encoded PrP gene are genetically linked to human prion diseases. In addition, polymorphisms in the PrP gene control many features of prion diseases including incubation time, species barrier, and specificity of recovered prion strain. Mice that lack PrP^C (denominated *Prnp*$^{o/o}$ or *Prnp*$^{-/-}$) are resistant to infection with prions.

Interestingly, *Prnp*$^{o/o}$ mice of an amino proximally truncated transgene encoding PrP devoid of the octa repeats and the conserved 106-126 region suffer from ataxia and degeneration of the cerebellar granule cells shortly after birth. Similar (but not identical) phenotypes are observed in mice overexpressing Dpl, which experience degeneration of cerebellar Purkinje cells. Introduction of a single intact PrP allele largely rescues this phenotype. These findings may be explained by postulating that PrP interacts with a ligand to obtain an essential signal. In the absence of PrP, a notional PrP-like molecule with lower binding affinity may arguably supply the missing PrP function. According to this hypothesis, in PrP knockout mice by interacting with the ligand the truncated PrP could displace the PrP-like molecule without eliciting a survival

signal. In case PrP has the highest affinity for the ligand, it would replace its truncated equivalent and restore function.

An alternative explanation posits that Dpl or amino-terminally truncated PrP^C can exist as transmembrane proteins and form oligomers. Lack of the amino terminus may create a toxic channel that would be patent for ions and lead to osmotic or excitotoxic damage. Single molecules of PrP^C containing its amino-terminal tail may block such channels in a transdominant fashion, and thereby abrogate neurotoxicity.

THE SPECIES BARRIER

Transmission of prions from one species to another is usually accompanied by a prolongation of the incubation period in the first passage and incomplete penetrance ("attack rate") of the disease. This phenomenon is called the "species barrier." Subsequent passage in the same species occurs with high frequency and shortened incubation times. In the case of prion transmission from hamster to mice, this species barrier was overcome by introducing hamster *Prnp* transgenes into recipient wild-type mice. Crucially, the properties of the prions produced were compatible with the prion species used for inoculation; infection with hamster prions led to production of hamster prions, whereas infection with mouse prions gave rise to mouse prions. With respect to the protein-only hypothesis these findings can be interpreted as follows: hamster PrP^C but not murine PrP^C (the latter differing from the former by 10 amino acids) is an appropriate substrate for conversion to hamster PrP^{Sc} by hamster prions and vice versa. Intriguingly, susceptibility of mice to prions

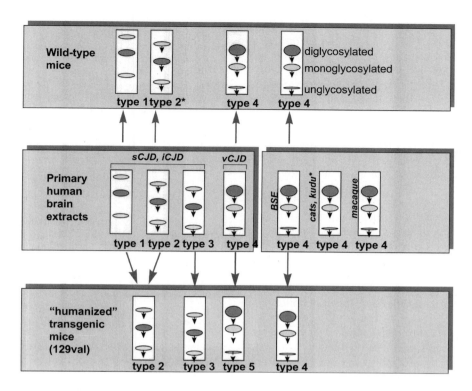

Figure 119-6 Patterns of PrP glycosylation. Representation of the three glycosylated PrP^{Sc} moieties (non-, mono-, and diglycosylated PrP^{Sc}) in immunoblots of brain extracts after digestion with proteinase K. Different inocula result in specific mobilities of the three PrP bands as well as different predominance of certain bands (middle panel). These characteristic patterns can be retained, or changed to other predictable patterns after passage in wild-type (upper panel) or humanized mice (PrP-deficient mice bearing a human PrP transgene, lower panel). Based on the fragment size and the relative abundance of individual bands, three distinct patterns (PrP^{Sc} types 1–3) were defined for sporadic and iatrogenic Creutzfeldt-Jakob disease cases. In contrast, all cases of variant Creutzfeldt-Jakob disease displayed a novel pattern, designated as type-4 pattern.

from other species is increased when the corresponding PrP trans-gene is introduced into a PrP knockout mouse, suggesting that the resident murine gene inhibits the propagation of the alien prions.

UNDERSTANDING PRION STRAINS

In 1961, distinct isolates or strains of prions were first described in scrapie-diseased goats, in which two dissimilar clinical manifestations ("scratching" and "drowsy," respectively) were identified. These strains differ in their incubation times in various inbred mouse lines and by their lesion pattern in the brain. Strikingly, distinct strains of prions can be propagated in an inbred mouse strain that is homozygous with respect to *Prnp*, a perplexing finding regarding the protein-only hypothesis, meaning that an identical polypeptide chain is able to mediate different strain phenotypes. Both the "refolding" and the "seeding" model propose that each strain is associated with a distinct conformation of PrP^{Sc} and that each of these can convert PrP^{C} of its host into a likeness of itself. Indeed, PrP^{Sc} species associated with two hamster-adapted scrapie strains, hyper and drowsy, proved to display characteristic clinical and histopathological properties as well as distinct biochemical patterns with respect to proteinase K digestion, which may be explainable by the presence of different conformations of PrP^{Sc}. Analogous findings have been made with other prion strains propagated in mice. In addition, PrP^{Sc} of certain strains differ in the ratio of diglycosylated to the monoglycosylated form. Based on the fragment size and the relative abundance of individual bands, three distinct patterns

(PrP^{Sc} types 1–3) were defined for sporadic and iatrogenic CJD cases. In contrast, all cases of vCJD displayed a novel pattern, designated type-4 by Collinge, and type III by Parchi and Gambetti (Fig. 119-6). Interestingly, brain extracts from BSE-infected cattle and BSE-inoculated macaques exhibited a type-4 pattern. Even more intriguingly, transmission of BSE or vCJD to mice produced mouse PrP^{Sc} with a type-4 pattern indistinguishable from the original inoculum–findings that impressively support the hypothesis that vCJD is the human counterpart to BSE. An additional tool, which may eventually serve to characterize prion strains, utilizes the differential affinity of certain antibodies for properly folded and denatured isoforms of PrP, thereby differentiating as many as eight different conformers. This provides further circumstantial evidence for the assumption that strain specificity is encrypted within the physical structure of PrP.

Studies of scrapie in inbred mice led to identification of a single autosomal gene, termed *Sinc* (*scrapie incubation*), controlling incubation time of mice infected with mouse prion strains. Soon after, a link between *Sinc* and a polymorphism in the mouse *Prnp* gene was discovered. Elegant knock-in experiments, in which *Prnp* alleles of inbred mice were swapped, have provided strong support for the contention that *Sinc* is identical to *Prnp*.

YEAST PRIONS

For more than 20 yr the genetic analysis of two unrelated mutants of the fission yeast *Saccharomyces cerevisiae* caused a substantial dilemma to yeast researchers. The two mutants in question, the [*PSI*⁺] mutant (modifying the efficiency of nonsense suppression) and the [*URE3*] mutant (causing an alteration in nitrogen metabolism) failed to behave according to Mendel's laws. The unusual genetic properties of both mutants were explained by a prion-like behavior of two previously identified yeast proteins: [*PSI*⁺] is associated with Sup35p (also known as eRF3), an essential component of the translation termination machinery, whereas [*URE3*] is associated with Ure2p, a protein that negatively regulates nitrogen metabolism. Further yeast proteins with a prion-like behavior have been discovered; among them is Rnq1p fulfilling all diagnostic criteria of yeast prions, although obviously not associated with a specific phenotype.

Strikingly, the prion-forming domain (PrD) of Sup35p is both modular and transferable. An artificial prion was generated by fusing a recombinant version of a mammalian receptor to the Sup35p-PrD. The fusion protein altered the biochemical properties of yeast cells in ways that could be inherited by progeny cells. The modular and transferable properties of yeast PrD provide strong support for the "yeast protein only" hypothesis, and may have considerable evolutionary and biotechnological implications, if broadly applicable.

In a further set of experiments, both yeast and a neural tumor cell line cytoplasmically expressing mouse PrP acquired the characteristics of PrP^Sc, detergent insolubility and resistance to protease digestion. Cytosolic PrP was shown to be selfsustaining (however, only within one single cell, and not from one individual to another, which is what would be expected from real prions) and highly neurotoxic when expressed in transgenic mice.

Overall, yeast is providing a powerful and experimentally testable paradigm for prions, although caution must be taken in directly extrapolating from findings with yeast prions to the mammalian system.

SELECTED REFERENCES

Aguzzi A, Brandner S, Marino S, Steinbach JP. Transgenic and knockout mice in the study of neurodegenerative diseases. J Mol Med 1996;74:111–126.

Aguzzi A, Glatzel M, Montrasio F, Prinz M, Heppner FL. Interventional strategies against prion diseases. Nat Rev Neurosci 2001;2:745–749.

Aguzzi A, Heikenwalder M. Prion diseases: cannibals and garbage piles. Nature 2003;423:127–129.

Aguzzi A, Heppner FL. Pathogenesis of prion diseases: a progress report. Cell Death Differ 2000;7:889–902.

Aguzzi A, Montrasio F, Kaeser PS. Prions: health scare and biological challenge. Nat Rev Mol Cell Biol 2001;2:118–126.

Aguzzi A, Weissmann C. Sleepless in Bologna: transmission of fatal familial insomnia. Trends Microbiol 1996;4:129–131.

Basler K, Oesch B, Scott M, et al. Scrapie and cellular PrP isoforms are encoded by the same chromosomal gene. Cell 1986;46:417–428.

Beekes M, McBride PA, Baldauf E. Cerebral targeting indicates vagal spread of infection in hamsters fed with scrapie. J Gen Virol 1998;79 Part 3:601–607.

Behrens A, Aguzzi A. Small is not beautiful: antagonizing functions for the prion protein PrP(C) and its homologue Dpl. Trends Neurosci 2002;25:150–154.

Behrens A, Brandner S, Genoud N, Aguzzi A. Normal neurogenesis and scrapie pathogenesis in neural grafts lacking the prion protein homologue Doppel. EMBO Rep 2001;2:347–352.

Behrens A, Genoud N, Naumann H, et al. Absence of the prion protein homologue Doppel causes male sterility. EMBO J 2002;21:3652–3658.

Belay ED. Transmissible spongiform encephalopathies in humans. Annu Rev Microbiol 1999;53:283–314.

Bessen RA, Marsh RF. Biochemical and physical properties of the prion protein from two strains of the transmissible mink encephalopathy agent. J Virol 1992;66:2096–2101.

Bessen RA, Marsh RF. Distinct PrP properties suggest the molecular basis of strain variation in transmissible mink encephalopathy. J Virol 1994;68:7859–7868.

Bessen RA, Raymond GJ, Caughey B. *In situ* formation of protease-resistant prion protein in transmissible spongiform encephalopathy-infected brain slices. J Biol Chem 1997;272:15,227–15,231.

Brandner S, Isenmann S, Raeber A, et al. Normal host prion protein necessary for scrapie-induced neurotoxicity. Nature 1996;379:339–343.

Brandner S, Raeber A, Sailer A, et al. Normal host prion protein (PrPC) is required for scrapie spread within the central nervous system. Proc Natl Acad Sci USA 1996;93:13,148–13,151.

Brown DR, Schmidt B, Kretzschmar HA. A neurotoxic prion protein fragment enhances proliferation of microglia but not astrocytes in culture. Glia 1996;18:59–67.

Bruce ME, Will RG, Ironside JW, et al. Transmissions to mice indicate that 'new variant' CJD is caused by the BSE agent. Nature 1997;389:498–501.

Budka H, Aguzzi A, Brown P, et al. Neuropathological diagnostic criteria for Creutzfeldt-Jakob disease (CJD) and other human spongiform encephalopathies (prion diseases). Brain Pathol 1995;5:459–466.

Büeler HR, Aguzzi A, Sailer A, et al. Mice devoid of PrP are resistant to scrapie. Cell 1993;73:1339–1347.

Büeler HR, Fischer M, Lang Y, et al. Normal development and behaviour of mice lacking the neuronal cell-surface PrP protein. Nature 1992; 356:577–582.

Chesebro B, Race R, Wehrly K, et al. Identification of scrapie prion protein-specific mRNA in scrapie-infected and uninfected brain. Nature 1985;315:331–333.

Collinge J, Sidle KC, Meads J, Ironside J, Hill AF. Molecular analysis of prion strain variation and the aetiology of 'new variant' CJD. Nature 1996;383:685–690.

Creutzfeldt HG. Über eine eigenartige herdförmige Erkrankung des Zentralnervensystems. Z Neurol U Psychiatr 1920;57:1–19.

Cuille J, Chelle PL. Experimental transmission of trembling to the goat. C R Seances Acad Sci 1939;208:1058–1160.

Drisaldi B, Stewart RS, Adles C, et al. Mutant PrP is delayed in its exit from the endoplasmic reticulum, but neither wild-type nor mutant PrP undergoes retrotranslocation prior to proteasomal degradation. J Biol Chem 2003;278:21,732–21,743.

Gabizon R, McKinley MP, Groth D, Prusiner SB. Immunoaffinity purification and neutralization of scrapie prion infectivity. Proc Natl Acad Sci USA 1988;85:6617–6621.

Gajdusek DC, Gibbs CJ, Alpers M. Experimental transmission of a Kuru-like syndrome to chimpanzees. Nature 1966;209:794–796.

Gibbs CJ Jr, Gajdusek DC, Asher DM, et al. Creutzfeldt-Jakob disease (spongiform encephalopathy): transmission to the chimpanzee. Science 1968;161:388–389.

Glatzel M, Heppner FL, Albers KM, Aguzzi A. Sympathetic innervation of lymphoreticular organs is rate limiting for prion neuroinvasion. Neuron 2001;31:25–34.

Glatzel M, Pekarik V, Luhrs T, Dittami J, Aguzzi A. Analysis of the prion protein in primates reveals a new polymorphism in codon 226 (Y226F). Biol Chem 2002;383:1021–1025.

Griffith JS. Self-replication and scrapie. Nature 1967;215:1043–1044.

Hadlow WJ. Scrapie and kuru. Lancet 1959;2:289–290.

Hegde RS, Mastrianni JA, Scott MR, et al. A transmembrane form of the prion protein in neurodegenerative disease. Science 1998;279:827–834.

Heppner FL, Christ AD, Klein MA, et al. Transepithelial prion transport by M cells. Nat Med 2001;7:976–977.

Heppner FL, Musahl C, Arrighi I, et al. Prevention of scrapie pathogenesis by transgenic expression of anti-prion protein antibodies. Science 2001;294:178–182.

Hill AF, Desbruslais M, Joiner S, et al. The same prion strain causes vCJD and BSE. Nature 1997;389:448–450 (letter) (see comments).

Horiuchi M, Caughey B. Specific binding of normal prion protein to the scrapie form via a localized domain initiates its conversion to the protease-resistant state. EMBO J 1999;18:3193–3203. (In Process Citation)

Hsiao K, Baker HF, Crow TJ, et al. Linkage of a prion protein missense variant to Gerstmann-Straussler syndrome. Nature 1989;338:342–345.

Hsich G, Kinney K, Gibbs CJ, Lee KH, Harrington MG. The 14-3-3 Brain protein in cerebrospinal fluid as a marker for transmissible spongiform encephalopathies. N Engl J Med 1996;335:924–930.

Jakob A. Über eigenartige Erkrankungen des Zentralnervensystems mit bemerkenswertem anatomischem Befunde. (Spastische Pseudosklerose-Encephalomyelopathie mit disseminierten Degenerationsherden). Dtsch Z Nervenheilk 1921;70:132–146.

Jarrett JT, Lansbury PT Jr. Seeding "one-dimensional crystallization" of amyloid: a pathogenic mechanism in Alzheimer's disease and scrapie? Cell 1993;73:1055–1058.

Kahana E, Alter M, Braham J, Sofer D. Creutzfeldt-jakob disease: focus among Libyan Jews in Israel. Science 1974;183:90, 91.

Klein MA, Frigg R, Flechsig E, et al. A crucial role for B cells in neuroinvasive scrapie. Nature 1997;390:687–690.

Klein MA, Frigg R, Raeber AJ, et al. PrP expression in B lymphocytes is not required for prion neuroinvasion. Nat Med 1998;4:1429–1433.

Klein MA, Kaeser PS, Schwarz P, et al. Complement facilitates early prion pathogenesis. Nat Med 2001;7:488–492.

Knaus KJ, Morillas M, Swietnicki W, Malone M, Surewicz WK, Yee VC. Crystal structure of the human prion protein reveals a mechanism for oligomerization. Nat Struct Biol 2001;8:770–774.

Koller MF, Grau T, Christen P. Induction of antibodies against murine full-length prion protein in wild-type mice. J Neuroimmunol 2002;132:113–116.

Korth C, Stierli B, Streit P, et al. Prion (PrPSc)-specific epitope defined by a monoclonal antibody. Nature 1997;390:74–77.

Kretzschmar HA, Prusiner SB, Stowring LE, DeArmond SJ. Scrapie prion proteins are synthesized in neurons. Am J Pathol 1986;122:1–5.

Kreutzberg GW. Microglia: a sensor for pathological events in the CNS. Trends Neurosci 1996;19:312–318.

Kunz B, Sandmeier E, Christen P. Neurotoxicity of prion peptide 106-126 not confirmed. FEBS Lett 1999;458:65–68 (see comments).

Lacroute F. Non-Mendelian mutation allowing ureidosuccinic acid uptake in yeast. J Bacteriol 1971;106:519–522.

Li L, Lindquist S. Creating a protein-based element of inheritance. Science 2000;287:661–664 (see comments).

Ma J, Lindquist S. Conversion of PrP to a self-perpetuating PrPSc-like conformation in the cytosol. Science 2002;298:1785–1788.

Ma J, Lindquist S. De novo generation of a PrPSc-like conformation in living cells. Nat Cell Biol 1999;1:358–361.

Ma J, Lindquist S. Wild-type PrP and a mutant associated with prion disease are subject to retrograde transport and proteasome degradation. Proc Natl Acad Sci USA 2001;98:14,955–14,960.

Ma J, Wollmann R, Lindquist S. Neurotoxicity and neurodegeneration when PrP accumulates in the cytosol. Science 2002;298:1781–1785.

Mabbott NA, Bruce ME, Botto M, Walport MJ, Pepys MB. Temporary depletion of complement component C3 or genetic deficiency of C1q significantly delays onset of scrapie. Nat Med 2001;7:485–487.

Meier P, Genoud N, Prinz M, et al. Soluble dimeric prion protein binds PrP(Sc) in vivo and antagonizes prion disease. Cell 2003;113:49–60.

Montrasio F, Frigg R, Glatzel M, et al. Impaired prion replication in spleens of mice lacking functional follicular dendritic cells. Science 2000;288:1257–1259.

Moore RC, Hope J, McBride PA, et al. Mice with gene targetted prion protein alterations show that Prnp, Sinc and Prni are congruent. Nat Genet 1998;18:118–125.

Moore RC, Lee IY, Silverman GL, et al. Ataxia in prion protein (PrP)-deficient mice is associated with upregulation of the novel PrP-like protein doppel. J Mol Biol 1999;292:797–817.

Oesch B, Westaway D, Walchli M, et al. A cellular gene encodes scrapie PrP 27-30 protein. Cell 1985;40:735–746.

Pan KM, Baldwin M, Nguyen J, et al. Conversion of alpha-helices into beta-sheets features in the formation of the scrapie prion proteins. Proc Natl Acad Sci USA 1993;90:10,962–10,966.

Parchi P, Castellani R, Capellari S, et al. Molecular basis of phenotypic variability in sporadic Creutzfeldt-Jakob disease. Ann Neurol 1996;39:767–778.

Parchi P, Giese A, Capellari S, et al. Classification of sporadic Creutzfeldt-Jakob disease based on molecular and phenotypic analysis of 300 subjects. Ann Neurol 1999;46:224–233.

Pattison IH. The relative susceptibility of sheep, goats and mice to two types of the goat scrapie agent. Res Vet Sci 1966;7:207–212.

Pattison IH, Jones KM. Modification of a strain of mouse-adapted scrapie by passage through rats. Res Vet Sci 1968;9:408–410.

Peoc'h K, Guerin C, Brandel J, Launay J, Laplanche J. First report of polymorphisms in the prion-like protein gene (PRND): implications for human prion diseases. Neurosci Lett 2000;286: 144–148.

Peretz D, Williamson RA, Kaneko K, et al. Antibodies inhibit prion propagation and clear cell cultures of prion infectivity. Nature 2001;412: 739–743.

Prusiner SB. Creutzfeldt-Jakob disease and scrapie prions. Alzheimer Dis Assoc Disord 1989;3:52–78.

Prusiner SB. Novel proteinaceous infectious particles cause scrapie. Science 1982;216:136–144.

Prusiner SB, Scott M, Foster D, et al. Transgenetic studies implicate interactions between homologous PrP isoforms in scrapie prion replication. Cell 1990;63:673–686.

Raeber AJ, Race RE, Brandner S, et al. Astrocyte-specific expression of hamster prion protein (PrP) renders PrP knockout mice susceptible to hamster scrapie. EMBO J 1997;16:6057–6065.

Riek R, Hornemann S, Wider G, Billeter M, Glockshuber R, Wuthrich K. NMR structure of the mouse prion protein domain PrP(121-321). Nature 1996;382:180–182.

Rossi D, Cozzio A, Flechsig E, Klein MA, Aguzzi A, Weissmann C. Onset of ataxia and Purkinje cell loss in PrP null mice inversely correlated with Dpl level in brain. EMBO J 2001;20:1–9.

Safar J, Wille H, Itri V, et al. Eight prion strains have PrP(Sc) molecules with different conformations. Nat Med 1998;4:1157–1165 (see comments).

Sailer A, Büeler H, Fischer M, Aguzzi A, Weissmann C. No propagation of prions in mice devoid of PrP. Cell 1994;77:967–968.

Sakaguchi S, Katamine S, Nishida N, et al. Loss of cerebellar purkinje cells in aged mice homozygous for a disrupted Prp gene. Nature 1996;380:528–531.

Scott M, Groth D, Foster D, et al. Propagation of prions with artificial properties in transgenic mice expressing chimeric PrP genes. Cell 1993;73:979–988.

Sethi S, Lipford G, Wagner H, Kretzschmar H. Postexposure prophylaxis against prion disease with a stimulator of innate immunity. Lancet 2002;360:229–230.

Shmerling D, Hegyi I, Fischer M, et al. Expression of amino-terminally truncated PrP in the mouse leading to ataxia and specific cerebellar lesions. Cell 1998;93:203–214.

Sondheimer N, Lindquist S. Rnq1: an epigenetic modifier of protein function in yeast. Mol Cell 2000;5:163–172.

Stahl N, Baldwin MA, Teplow DB, et al. Structural studies of the scrapie prion protein using mass spectrometry and amino acid sequencing. Biochemistry 1993;32:1991–2002.

Stahl N, Borchelt DR, Hsiao K, Prusiner SB. Scrapie prion protein contains a phosphatidylinositol glycolipid. Cell 1987;51:229–240.

Telling GC, Scott M, Mastrianni J, et al. Prion propagation in mice expressing human and chimeric PrP transgenes implicates the interaction of cellular PrP with another protein. Cell 1995;83: 79–90.

Weissmann C. Spongiform encephalopathies. The prion's progress. Nature 1991;349:569–571.

Weissmann C, Aguzzi A. Bovine spongiform encephalopathy and early onset variant Creutzfeldt- Jakob disease. Curr Opin Neurobiol 1997; 7:695–700.

Weissmann C, Aguzzi A. Perspectives: neurobiology. PrP's double causes trouble. Science 1999;286:914–915.

Wells GA, Scott AC, Johnson CT, et al. A novel progressive spongiform encephalopathy in cattle. Vet Rec 1987;121:419–420.

Westaway D, Carlson GA. Mammalian prion proteins: enigma, variation and vaccination. Trends Biochem Sci 2002;27:301–307.

White AR, Enever P, Tayebi M, et al. Monoclonal antibodies inhibit prion replication and delay the development of prion disease. Nature 2003;422:80–83.

Wickner RB. [URE3] as an altered URE2 protein: evidence for a prion analog in Saccharomyces cerevisiae Science 1994;264:566–569.

Will R, Zeidler M. Diagnosing Creutzfeldt-Jakob Disease—case identification depends on neurological and neuropathological assessment. BMJ 1996;313:833–834.

Will RG, Ironside JW, Zeidler M, et al. A new variant of Creutzfeldt-Jakob disease in the UK. Lancet 1996;347:921–925.

Will RG, Zeidler M, Stewart GE, et al. Diagnosis of new variant Creutzfeldt-Jakob disease. Ann Neurol 2000;47:575–582.

Wille H, Michelitsch MD, Guenebaut V, et al. Structural studies of the scrapie prion protein by electron crystallography. Proc Natl Acad Sci USA 2002;99:3563–3568.

Zanusso G, Ferrari S, Cardone F, et al. Detection of pathologic prion protein in the olfactory epithelium in sporadic Creutzfeldt-Jakob disease. N Engl J Med 2003;348:711–719.

120 Narcolepsy and Other Neurological Sleep Disorders

Thomas E. Scammell

SUMMARY

Sleep disorders are among the most common clinical ailments, and molecular research is beginning to shed light on the neurobiology of sleep and the mechanisms underlying specific disorders of sleep. This chapter focuses on sleep disorders with a neurological basis, particularly those in which recent discoveries have realed the underlying molecular biology.

Key Words: Arousal; circadian rhythms; hypocretin; insomnia; narcolepsy; orexin; REM behavior disorder; sleep; sleep disorders; suprachiasmatic nucleus; wakefulness.

NEUROBIOLOGICAL CONTROL OF SLEEP AND WAKEFULNESS

Sleep consists of two major states: rapid eye movement (REM) sleep and nonrapid eye movement (NREM) sleep. REM sleep is characterized by cortical activation with vivid dreams, brief saccadic eye movements, and intense paralysis of most voluntary muscles. In NREM sleep, cortical activity and mentation are minimal, and autonomic activity is low.

To understand the basis of many sleep disorders, it is helpful to review some of the pathways involved in the control of behavioral state. Normal wakefulness requires the coordinated activity of several ascending arousal systems located in the rostral brainstem and posterior hypothalamus (Fig. 120-1). Cholinergic innervation of the thalamus from the pedunculopontine tegmental and laterodorsal tegmental nuclei (PPT/LDT) facilitates thalamocortical signaling and activates the cortex during wakefulness. During NREM sleep, these cholinergic neurons are much less active, thus decreasing thalamic and cortical activity. A separate population of cholinergic neurons in the basal forebrain helps to generate full attention and cortical functioning, but it is unclear whether these cells are required for the production of wakefulness itself.

Monoaminergic neurons also are essential for the production of wakefulness. The noradrenergic neurons of the locus ceruleus (LC), serotonergic neurons of the dorsal raphe (DR) nuclei, and histaminergic neurons of the tuberomammillary nucleus (TMN) diffusely innervate and activate much of the forebrain, firing most rapidly during wakefulness, slower in NREM sleep, and then becoming silent in REM sleep. The role of dopaminergic neurons

From: *Principles of Molecular Medicine, Second Edition*
Edited by: M. S. Runge and C. Patterson © Humana Press, Inc., Totowa, NJ

is less clear, but one cell group in the ventral periaqueductal gray is active during wakefulness and may be a critical site for dopaminergic effects on wakefulness.

These cholinergic and monoaminergic regions interact to produce REM sleep. A distinct population of REM-on cholinergic neurons in the PPT/LDT activates the thalamus during REM sleep, producing cortical activation and atonia through descending spinal projections. The LC, DR, and TMN inhibit the REM sleep-producing neurons during wakefulness and NREM sleep, but during REM sleep, these monoaminergic nuclei become inactive, thus disinhibiting the REM-generating neurons.

NREM sleep is produced by neurons in the preoptic area and brainstem. The dorsal vagal complex, raphe nuclei, and ventral midbrain contain some NREM-generating cells, but the ventrolateral preoptic area (VLPO) is the best characterized sleep-producing region. VLPO neurons are active during NREM and REM sleep and are necessary for sleep because lesions of the VLPO produce marked insomnia. These γ-aminobutyric acid-containing neurons help maintain sleep by inhibiting neurons in the TMN, LC, and DR. In turn, VLPO neurons are inhibited by monoamines during wakefulness, thus creating a reciprocally inhibitory circuit in which wake- and sleep-promoting regions inhibit one another.

Two major factors influence the timing of sleep and wakefulness. Homeostatic sleep drive increases with prolonged wakefulness, and rising levels of sleep-promoting factors such as adenosine and prostaglandin D2 provide part of this drive. When cats are kept awake for several hours, the concentration of the neuromodulator adenosine rises in the basal forebrain. This adenosine disinhibits the sleep-producing neurons of the VLPO, thus, promoting sleep. Caffeine probably promotes wakefulness by blocking this adenosine signaling. The timing of sleep and wakefulness is also strongly influenced by circadian rhythms.

CIRCADIAN RHYTHMS

Nearly all living organisms organize their physiology and behavior around the daily cycle of light and darkness. However, these circadian rhythms are not simply driven by the ambient light cycle; they are endogenously generated rhythms that persist in constant darkness. In mammals, circadian rhythms are controlled by the suprachiasmatic nucleus (SCN), a small cluster of neurons just above the optic chiasm in the anterior hypothalamus. The SCN acts as a master clock, keeping time with an accuracy of a few

Wakefulness

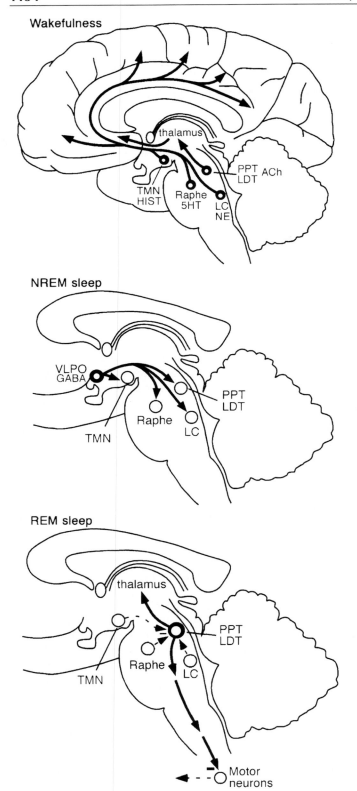

Figure 120-1 Pathways for the production of wakefulness, NREM sleep, and REM sleep. During wakefulness, the forebrain is widely activated by projections from aminergic nuclei including the noradrenergic LC, serotonergic (5HT) raphe nuclei, and histaminergic (HIST) tuberomammillary nucleus. Cholinergic (ACh) fibers from the PPT/LDT innervate the thalamus to promote thalamocortical signaling. During NREM sleep, γ-aminobutyric acid (GABA)-containing neurons of the VLPO inhibit these aminergic and cholinergic regions to promote

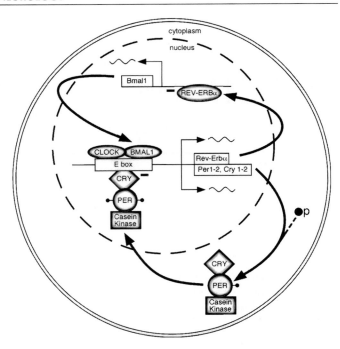

Figure 120-2 Molecular mechanism of circadian rhythmicity in SCN neurons. CLOCK and BMAL1 act on an E box enhancer to increase the expression of *per* and *cry* mRNAs. In the cytoplasm, PER forms a complex with CRY and is phosphorylated by casein kinase. This complex moves back into the nucleus and inhibits expression of the *per* and *cry* genes, thus forming a negative feedback loop. REV-ERBα inhibits the expression of *Bmal1*, but the PER/CRY complex also decreases expression of *Rev-Erbα*, thus, allowing production of BMAL1. These positive and negative feedback loops most likely generate daily rhythms in SCN neurons.

minutes each day, and adjusting bodily rhythms to seasonal variations in day length. Most likely, each SCN neuron is a competent circadian pacemaker, and the coordinated activity of all SCN neurons results in highly accurate 24-h rhythms. The importance of this nucleus is apparent in people and animals with lesions of the SCN who may sleep and wake at any time of day.

MOLECULAR BIOLOGY OF CIRCADIAN RHYTHMS

Molecular biological studies have identified the fundamental mechanisms that generate daily rhythms in SCN neurons. The core mechanism involves daily cycles of gene expression that are driven by autoregulatory feedback loops in which clock gene products regulate the expression of their own mRNA (Fig. 120-2).

Two transcription factors, CLOCK and BMAL1, provide the basic drive to these rhythms. CLOCK/BMAL1 heterodimers constitutively bind to E box enhancers to increase the production of *period* (*Per1*, *Per2*, and *Per3*) and *cryptochrome* (*Cry1* and *Cry2*) transcripts. The PER and CRY proteins form a complex that inhibits expression of the *per* and *cry* genes by interfering with the enhancing effects of CLOCK and BMAL1. Thus, rising levels of PER eventually shut down the expression of *per* and *cry*, and PER and CRY protein levels fall. Phosphorylation of the PER/CRY

sleep. In REM sleep, a specific set of cholinergic neurons in the PPT/LDT activates the thalamus and also inhibits motor neurons through a series of descending projections. These REM-active PPT/LDT neurons are inhibited by aminergic brain regions during wakefulness. Nuclei with thick outlines are active during each state.

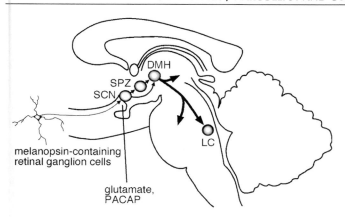

Figure 120-3 Pathways that govern circadian rhythms. The SCN is the master regulator of circadian rhythms. The phase of SCN activity is adjusted to the ambient light–dark cycle by luminance information from melanopsin-containing retinal ganglion cells. The SCN sends timing signals to the SPZ and DMH. The DMH then relays these signals to the LC and other state-regulatory brain regions. PACAP, pituitary adenylate cyclase activating peptide.

complex by casein kinase (CKIɛ and CKIδ) hastens the degradation of PER, thereby slowing the rate of this negative feedback loop.

A positive feedback loop occurs when CLOCK and BMAL1 increase the transcription of a nuclear receptor, REV-ERBα. REV-ERBα inhibits the transcription of *Bmal1*. However, the PER/CRY complex inhibits expression of *Rev-Erbα*, thus disinhibiting BMAL1 production. This positive (double negative) feedback loop allows *Bmal1* mRNA levels to peak 12 h out of phase with those of the *per* and *cry* genes.

The functional importance of these genes has been demonstrated in several lines of knockout mice. In the absence of environmental time cues, mice lacking both *per1* and *per2* or both *cry* genes cannot generate circadian rhythms. Similar behavior is seen in mice lacking the genes for *Bmal1* or *clock*. In hamsters, a mutation in the gene for *casein kinase Iɛ* results in very short rhythms, probably because poorly phosphorylated PER and CRY degrade more slowly, accumulate rapidly, and, thus, inhibit their own expression more quickly.

MELANOPSIN AND THE RETINOHYPOTHALAMIC TRACT The SCN receives photic information directly from the retina, and these signals help synchronize SCN neuronal activity with the ambient light–dark cycle (Fig. 120-3). Unlike the more familiar pathways that mediate visual perception, the retinohypothalamic tract carries luminance information from the retina to the SCN and other diencephalic and midbrain regions. These fibers release glutamate and pituitary adenylate cyclase-activating peptide onto SCN neurons which markedly increases the expression of PER, shifting the phase of the molecular clock.

Surprisingly, this photoentrainment does not require rods and cones, but studies have identified a novel photopigment known as melanopsin that helps generate this luminance signal. In contrast to the classic photopigments found in rods and cones, melanopsin is produced in a small subset of retinal ganglion cells with large dendritic fields. These ganglion cells project directly to the SCN, and in isolated retinal preparations, the firing rate of these neurons increases in response to light, even when synaptic transmission has been blocked. Thus, these inherently photoreceptive ganglion cells are well positioned to transmit luminance information to the SCN. The functional importance of this system has been

demonstrated in mice lacking melanopsin. In response to a 15-min pulse of light, these mice have much smaller shifts in their circadian rhythms than normal mice. Because some shifts still occur, rods, cones, and the melanopsin system probably work together to entrain circadian rhythms.

PATHWAYS THROUGH WHICH THE SCN MAY CONTROL BEHAVIORAL STATE The SCN drives circadian rhythms through synaptic and humoral processes. The SCN heavily innervates several hypothalamic regions, especially an area just dorsal to the SCN known as the subparaventricular zone (SPZ). Lesions of the SPZ block circadian rhythms of sleep/wake behavior and body temperature. The SPZ projects to the dorsomedial nucleus of the hypothalamus (DMH), and DMH lesions also block sleep/wake rhythms. The DMH then relays these timing signals to wake-promoting regions such the orexin neurons and LC, which help promote wakefulness and suppress REM sleep during the day.

Humoral factors secreted from the SCN also influence the timing of sleep. SCN-lesioned animals lack circadian rhythms, but rhythms can be restored with SCN transplants. This restoration of rhythmicity does not require synaptic connections because the daily rhythm of locomotor activity can be partially restored with SCN transplants encased in a polymer that blocks the outgrowth of neurites but allows passage of small molecules. These secreted timing factors include transforming growth factor (TGF)-α and prokineticin 2 (PK2). In nocturnal rodents, TGF-α and PK2 expression is high during the day, and infusion of these peptides suppresses locomotor activity. TGF-α and PK2 receptors are expressed in targets of the SCN, including the SPZ and DMH. Chronic infusions of TGF-α block the circadian variation in sleep/wake behavior in a pattern similar to that seen with lesions of the SPZ. Thus, release of TGF-α and PK2 from the SCN may act on nearby hypothalamic regions to inhibit the circadian rhythms of locomotor activity and wakefulness.

CLINICAL DISORDERS OF CIRCADIAN RHYTHMS The importance of circadian rhythms in humans is apparent to everyone who has worked a night shift or crossed several time zones. The pressure to sleep is often intense around one's usual bedtime, but even after remaining awake all night it can be difficult to fall asleep in the late morning. Because of this circadian promotion of wakefulness during the day, many shift workers have difficulty obtaining adequate amounts of sleep.

Abnormal timing of sleep is a common presentation of circadian rhythm disorders. Delayed Sleep Phase Syndrome is widespread in teens and young adults and helps explain the propensity of many young people to stay up late and then sleep late in the morning. Although this is sometimes a behavioral choice, for many it results from a delay in their endogenous rhythms that substantially interferes with morning activities. Exposure to bright light in the morning often helps entrain these individuals to a normal schedule.

For years, people believed that rising early in the morning was a matter of will power, but genetic studies have shown that genes involved in the timing of circadian rhythms play a critical role. Advanced Sleep Phase Syndrome (OMIM 604348) is uncommon, but can occur in families in an autosomal-dominant fashion. Affected individuals fall asleep around 7:30 PM and awaken around 4:30 AM and their rhythms of body temperature and melatonin are also advanced about 3–4 h. One affected family carries a mutation (S662G) in the *per2* gene that interferes with phosphorylation by casein kinase Iɛ. Deficient phosphorylation of this site probably hastens the accumulation of PER2, thus, phase advancing its rhythm and producing very early bedtimes.

Polymorphisms in the *clock* gene also affect the timing of circadian rhythms. People with a C to T substitution at position 3111 in the 3′ UTR of the *clock* gene are more likely to be early risers. Unlike mice in which mutations in the coding region of *clock* produce large shifts in the timing of rhythms, this polymorphism only shifts preferred awakening times 10–44 min earlier. However, it clearly demonstrates the importance of CLOCK in the circadian regulation of human sleep.

NARCOLEPSY

CLINICAL FEATURES Narcolepsy (OMIM 161400) is characterized by chronic sleepiness and a marked disorganization of sleep/wake behavior. It commonly begins with mild to severe daytime sleepiness and unintentional naps in the teens and early twenties, though symptoms can begin in young childhood or after the age of 40. In contrast to sleep apnea and other disorders with poor quality sleep, the sleepiness of narcoleptics is often improved temporarily by a brief nap.

Narcoleptics usually have abnormal manifestations of REM sleep that intrude into wakefulness, including hypnagogic hallucinations, sleep paralysis, and cataplexy. Hypnagogic hallucinations are dream-like, often frightening hallucinations that typically occur with drowsiness or the onset of sleep. Sleep paralysis is profound weakness that occurs at the onset of sleep or on awakening. This is probably a persistence of REM sleep atonia into wakefulness, and during these episodes the individual feels awake but is unable to move. Cataplexy is sudden muscle weakness brought on by strong emotions, particularly joking, laughter, or anger. Most likely, this also is an intrusion of REM sleep atonia into wakefulness, but in contrast to sleep paralysis, cataplexy occurs almost exclusively in narcolepsy. Sixty percent of narcoleptics develop cataplexy, usually around the onset of sleepiness or within 3–5 yr.

The history alone is often very suggestive of narcolepsy, but a complete evaluation includes an overnight polysomnogram to exclude other causes of sleepiness followed by a multiple sleep latency test. During the daytime nap opportunities of the multiple sleep latency test, narcoleptics usually fall asleep in less than 5 min and have sleep-onset REM periods in two or more naps. Such daytime episodes of REM sleep are rare in normal individuals as REM sleep is under tight circadian control.

EPIDEMIOLOGY AND GENETICS Narcolepsy occurs in about 1 in 2000 individuals. Most cases occur sporadically, but genetic causes are likely to play an important role because first degree relatives have a 40-fold increased risk of developing narcolepsy. Nevertheless, these genetic factors are only a partial influence as even among monozygotic twins in which one has narcolepsy, the second twin is affected only about 25% of the time.

The most robust of these genetic factors are specific human leukocyte antigens (HLAs). Early studies using low resolution serological techniques found that narcolepsy is associated with two HLA class II antigens, DR2 and DQ1. This association varies with ethnicity; DR2 is found in 100% of Japanese, 90–95% of Caucasian, and 60% of African American narcoleptics with cataplexy. High resolution mapping of these regions demonstrated the existence of numerous alleles, and the 0602 allele of DQB1 (a DQ1 subtype), has been strongly linked with narcolepsy. DQB1*0602 is found in 88–98% of narcoleptics with unambiguous cataplexy, whereas it is found in only 12% of Caucasian

American and 38% of African-American controls. Further susceptibility may be conferred by another allele, DQA1*0102, with an increase in risk when both DQA1*0102 and DQB1*0602 are present. A two- to fourfold increase in susceptibility is also seen in subjects homozygous for DQB1*0602. These associations do not prove an involvement of these alleles in the development of narcolepsy because the actual susceptibility could be because of nearby genes. However, extensive sequencing of this region has failed to reveal any new genes or narcolepsy linkages, suggesting that DQB1*0602 and DQA1*0102 directly influence the development of narcolepsy. Testing for DQB1*0602 can be helpful, particularly in individuals with questionable cataplexy, but this allele is hardly predictive of narcolepsy as over 99% of DQB1*0602 positive individuals do not have narcolepsy.

The genes for tumor necrosis factor (TNF)-α and the TNF receptor 2 also have been implicated in narcolepsy. TNF-α promotes sleep in laboratory animals, and *TNF-α* polymorphisms increase the risk of other HLA-linked diseases such as multiple sclerosis or systemic lupus erythematosis. The *TNF-α* gene sits within the HLA class III region on chromosome 6, and polymorphisms in the promoter regions of the *TNF-α* gene are associated with narcolepsy in Japan. A polymorphism in the *TNF receptor 2* gene on chromosome 1 also occurs more frequently among Japanese narcoleptics with cataplexy. This susceptibility appears especially strong among narcoleptics who have specific polymorphisms in both the *TNF-α* gene and the *TNF receptor 2* gene. Plasma TNF-α levels are normal in narcolepsy, but these polymorphisms may still affect TNF-α signaling, thus contributing to an autoimmune process or directly influencing the activity of sleep/wake regulatory pathways in the brain.

Familial narcoleptics are often DQB1*0602 negative and have an earlier onset of symptoms. The genes underlying these familial cases are generally unknown, but eight Japanese families with narcolepsy showed linkage to a site on chromosome 4p13-q21 that may act in concert with the HLA-influenced predisposition. Another family showed linkage to a site on chromosome 6 near the HLA region.

NEUROBIOLOGY OF OREXIN/HYPOCRETIN AND NARCOLEPSY Substantial evidence indicates that the neuropeptide orexin (also known as hypocretin) plays a critical role in the neurobiology of narcolepsy. One group named this peptide orexin for its presumed role in appetite, whereas another group named it hypocretin as a hypothalamic peptide with a resemblance to secretin. This peptide exists in two forms, orexin-A and orexin-B, which are derived from the same precursor and are colocalized in the same neurons. Orexin-containing neurons are found only in the lateral and posterior hypothalamus, but they project widely throughout the central nervous system (CNS), innervating the monoaminergic and cholinergic regions that promote wakefulness (Fig. 120-4).

The orexins are potent regulators of sleep/wake behavior. Injection of orexin into the CNS of rats increases wakefulness and markedly suppresses REM sleep. Orexin is released during wakefulness and acts through the type-1 and type-2 orexin receptors to directly excite neurons of the LC, DR, TMN, and PPT/LDT. Increased activity of aminergic arousal regions may directly promote wakefulness and inhibit the REM-producing cells of the LDT, thus stabilizing and sustaining wakefulness. Conversely, an absence of orexin signaling would weaken or otherwise alter the activity of the aminergic arousal regions, producing a destabilization of this circuit and abrupt fluctuations in behavioral state.

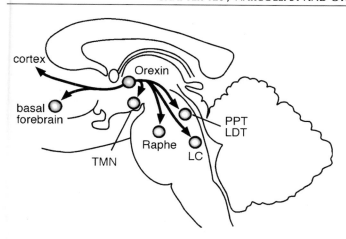

Figure 120-4 Orexin/hypocretin neurons in the lateral hypothalamus heavily innervate and excite many state-regulatory brain regions including the aminergic arousal regions, cholinergic PPT/LDT neurons, and basal forebrain. Orexin also may have direct effects on the cortex. LC, locus coeruleus; TMN, tuberomammillary nucleus.

IMPAIRED OREXIN SIGNALING CAUSES NARCOLEPSY

After an extensive linkage analysis, mutations in the *orexin type-2 receptor* gene of dogs with autosomal-recessive narcolepsy were found. The more common mutation in these dogs probably produces a nonfunctional receptor because of skipping of exon 4. Simultaneously, other researchers found that orexin knockout mice have a phenotype strongly resembling human narcolepsy, with brief periods of wakefulness, rapid transitions into REM sleep, and behavior resembling cataplexy.

These studies demonstrated that congenitally impaired orexin signaling can produce symptoms of narcolepsy, but human narcolepsy is usually an acquired disease. To create a mouse model similar to human narcolepsy, mice were produced in which the orexin promoter drives the expression of ataxin-3, a truncated Machado–Joseph disease gene product that induces apoptosis in neurons. These orexin/ataxin-3 mice have a normal number of orexin neurons at birth, but as they reach adulthood, the orexin neurons degenerate. This acquired loss of orexin neurons roughly parallels the typical timing of human narcolepsy, and just as in humans, these mice cannot remain awake for long periods, rapidly enter REM sleep, and have behavioral arrests resembling cataplexy.

The importance of orexin in human narcolepsy has been established by several findings. About 90% of narcoleptics with cataplexy have no detectable orexin-A in their cerebrospinal fluid. Most likely, this is because of a loss of the orexin-producing neurons as 90% or more of the orexin neurons are absent from the brains of narcoleptics with cataplexy. This neuronal loss appears highly specific as other neurons in the same region are present in normal numbers.

Although this decrease in orexin is most likely because of a loss of the orexin-producing neurons, other causes are possible. One individual has been identified with a mutation in the *prepro-orexin* gene that probably produces inappropriate trafficking of the peptide. This exceptional patient has severe cataplexy and sleepiness that first became evident at the age of 6 mo. The adult onset of symptoms in the majority of narcoleptics makes orexin gene mutations an unlikely contributor in most cases, though a slow, degenerative process is possible. Alternatively, impaired transcription of the *prepro-orexin* gene could produce a loss of orexin without

a loss of the orexin neurons. In support of this, a small number of narcoleptics may have a polymorphism in the 5′ untranslated region of the *prepro-orexin* gene, but this finding has not been confirmed by other studies. Many other polymorphisms have been identified in the *prepro-orexin* gene or in the genes coding for the orexin receptors, but none of these is linked with sporadic or familial narcolepsy. Thus, although some genetic factors such as HLA alleles clearly influence the occurrence of narcolepsy, mutations in the genes coding for orexin or its receptors are unlikely to be major contributors.

Narcolepsy is thought to result from an autoimmune or neurodegenerative process, but little evidence supports this idea. Markers of inflammation, analysis of spinal fluid, and neuroimaging are generally normal. Microglia and TNF-α mRNA are not increased in the brains of narcoleptics examined decades after the onset of symptoms, suggesting that there is no ongoing inflammation. The number of astrocytes may be moderately increased in the orexin neuron region, though one study found no gliosis. If supported by additional studies, this gliosis would be consistent with a neurodegenerative or inflammatory process.

These discoveries have markedly improved the understanding of narcolepsy with cataplexy, but the neurobiology of narcolepsy without cataplexy is still unknown. Narcoleptics without cataplexy are much less likely to carry DQB1*0602, and almost all have normal orexin levels. Possibly, these individuals simply have less extensive loss of the orexin neurons, with enough orexin production to stave off cataplexy, but the loss is still great enough to produce sleepiness and sleep-onset REM periods during their daytime naps. Alternatively, orexin may somehow be less effective in these individuals. Clearly, more research is needed to explain the varied causes of narcolepsy.

OTHER SLEEP DISORDERS RESULTING FROM CNS DYSFUNCTION

Landmark discoveries in the last few years have markedly improved our understanding of the molecular biology of narcolepsy and some disorders of circadian rhythmicity. This last section highlights other CNS sleep disorders for which new discoveries are beginning to reveal the underlying pathogenesis.

RESTLESS LEGS SYNDROME AND PERIODIC LIMB MOVEMENTS OF SLEEP

Restless legs syndrome (RLS) is characterized by nocturnal leg dysesthesias that are exacerbated by rest and relieved by movement or stretching. These uncomfortable sensations affect 10–20% of the population and can make it difficult to initiate or maintain sleep. Most patients with RLS also have periodic limb movements of sleep (PLMS) which are repetitive leg movements during NREM sleep. When they occur frequently, PLMS can disrupt sleep, producing mild to moderate daytime sleepiness.

Familial RLS usually begins before age 45 and is highly penetrant, often demonstrating an autosomal-dominant pattern. In some families, the disease may be recessive with linkage to chromosome 12q. Most cases of nonfamilial RLS results from iron deficiency, a peripheral neuropathy, or renal failure.

RLS and PLMS may be caused by brain iron deficiency and dysfunction of central dopaminergic pathways. Patients with RLS have low cerebrospinal fluid concentrations of iron, and iron levels are also low within the substantia nigra and possibly other brain regions. As iron is a necessary cofactor for tyrosine hydroxylase, this central iron deficiency may impair dopaminergic signaling. Dopamine agonists often improve RLS and PLMS, and dysfunction of descending dopaminergic pathways that regulate spinal cord excitability may produce the dysesthesias and limb movements.

REM BEHAVIOR DISORDER Potent descending pathways normally inhibit motor activity during REM sleep, but in REM sleep behavior disorder (RBD), individuals vigorously act out their dreams, often resulting in injury. Although RBD is occasionally familial, it usually occurs in elderly men with synucleinopathies such as Parkinson's disease, multiple system atrophy, and dementia with Lewy bodies, as well as in narcolepsy, spinocerebellar ataxia type 3, and other diseases. RBD patients are often HLA DQw1 positive, but they do not have a high incidence of DR2. Neuropathological studies have yet to identify a consistent anatomic substrate, but identical behavior occurs in cats with lesions of the dorsal pons that interrupt descending inhibitory projections from the PPT/LDT to the medulla and spinal cord.

FATAL FAMILIAL INSOMNIA Most insomnia is caused by psychiatric or psychological disorders, but fatal familial insomnia (FFI; OMIM 600072) is characterized by progressive, severe insomnia in association with autonomic hyperactivity, dementia, and death within a few years. These rare patients often present with a striking loss of sleep, particularly deep NREM sleep, and in the later stages of the disease, they spend much of their time in a state of persistent drowsiness and dream-like hallucinations.

Like familial Creutzfeld–Jacob disease, FFI is produced by a D178N mutation of the *prion protein* gene that results in a protease-resistant prion protein. However, all FFI patients also have a 129M polymorphism that predisposes them to early severe insomnia, particularly with 129M homozygosity.

Pathologically, most cases have severe atrophy and gliosis of the anterior ventral and mediodorsal thalamic nuclei and olivary nuclei, with less substantial involvement of cortical and subcortical regions. Because the thalamus is essential in the generation of cortical slow waves, degeneration of this region may contribute to the intense insomnia of FFI. However, the insomnia also may be caused by injury to hypothalamic and brainstem regions.

NOCTURNAL FRONTAL LOBE EPILEPSY Nocturnal frontal lobe epilepsy begins around age 10 and is manifested by complex partial seizures that occur most commonly in light NREM sleep. The clinical spectrum ranges from paroxysmal dystonia to behavior resembling nightmares or sleepwalking.

Autosomal-dominant nocturnal frontal lobe epilepsy (ADNFLE) is caused by mutations in the genes coding for the α- or β-subunits of the nicotinic acetylcholine receptor. In type 1 ADNFLE (OMIM 600513), the α4-subunit contains single nucleotide mutations (S248F, S252L) or a 3 base insertion that results in the addition of a leucine (L-776ins3). Type 2 ADNFLE (OMIM 603204) is linked to a site on chromosome 15 near the α3-, α5-, and β4-subunit genes. In type 3 ADNFLE (OMIM 605375), the β2 gene on chromosome 1 contains single base substitutions (V287L, V287M).

All of these mutations affect the transmembrane ionic pore region of the nicotinic receptor, but how these mutations produce seizures during sleep is unknown. α- and β-subunits assemble to form pentameric nicotinic channels, and the most common form in the brain is α4/β2. Most of these mutations increase receptor sensitivity to acetylcholine. Mice with gain-of-function mutations in the α4-subunit similar to the S248F mutation are more sensitive to the seizure-inducing effects of nicotine. Possibly, abnormal thalamo-cortical signaling during stage 2 NREM sleep triggers these seizures, but the precise electrophysiology is unknown.

FUTURE DIRECTIONS

Advances in the molecular biology of sleep disorders have shed light on the basic mechanisms of narcolepsy and other diseases, but many questions remain unanswered. Does an autoimmune or neurodegenerative process lead to orexin deficiency in narcolepsy? What is the cause of narcolepsy without cataplexy? What is the neurobiology of RLS and PLMS? Progress on these and other questions will improve understanding of these diseases and ultimately provide more effective therapies.

SELECTED REFERENCES

Aston-Jones G, Chen S, Zhu Y, Oshinsky M. A neural circuit for circadian regulation of arousal. Nat Neurosci 2001;4:732–738.

Chemelli RM, Willie JT, Sinton CM, et al. Narcolepsy in orexin knockout mice: molecular genetics of sleep regulation. Cell 1999;98:437–451.

Cheng M, Bullock C, Li C, et al. Prokineticin 2 transmits the behavioural circadian rhythm of the suprachiasmatic nucleus. Nature 2002;417: 405–410.

Chou T, Scammell T, Gooley J, Gaus S, Saper C, Lu J. Critical role of the dorsomedial hypothalamic nucleus in a wide range of behavioral circadian rhythms. J Neurosci 2003;23:10,691–10,702.

Crocker A, Espana RA, Papadopoulou M, et al. Concomitant loss of dynorphin, NARP, and orexin in narcolepsy. Neurology, 2005;65: 1184–1185.

Czeisler C, Duffy J, Shanahan T, et al. Stability, precision, and near-24-hour period of the human circadian pacemaker. Science 1999;284: 2177–2181.

Dauvilliers Y, Montplaisir J, Molinari N, et al. Age at onset of narcolepsy in two large populations of patients in France and Quebec. Neurology 2001;57:2029–2033.

de Lecea L, Kilduff TS, Peyron C, et al. The hypocretins: hypothalamus-specific peptides with neuroexcitatory activity. Proc Natl Acad Sci USA 1998;95:322–327.

Desautels A, Turecki G, Montplaisir J, Sequeira A, Verner A, Rouleau G. Identification of a major susceptibility locus for restless legs syndrome on chromosome 12q. Am J Hum Genet 2001;69:1266–1270.

Earley C, Connor J, Beard J, Malecki E, Epstein D, Allen R. Abnormalities in CSF concentrations of ferritin and transferrin in restless legs syndrome. Neurology 2000;54:1698–1700.

Erlich SS, Itabashi HH. Narcolepsy: a neuropathologic study. Sleep 1986; 9:126–132.

Gallopin T, Fort P, Eggermann E, et al. Identification of sleep-promoting neurons in vitro. Nature 2000;404:992–995.

Garcia J, Rosen G, Mahowald M. Circadian rhythms and circadian rhythm disorders in children and adolescents. Semin Pediatr Neurol 2001;8: 229–240.

Gencik M, Dahmen N, Wieczorek S, et al. A prepro-orexin gene polymorphism is associated with narcolepsy. Neurology 2001;56: 115–117.

Gooley JJ, Lu J, Chou TC, Scammell TE, Saper CB. Melanopsin in cells of origin of the retinohypothalamic tract. Nat Neurosci 2001;4:1165.

Hara J, Beuckmann CT, Nambu T, et al. Genetic ablation of orexin neurons in mice results in narcolepsy, hypophagia, and obesity. Neuron 2001;30:345–354.

Hinze-Selch D, Wetter TC, Zhang Y, et al. In vivo and in vitro immune variables in patients with narcolepsy and HLA-DR2 matched controls. Neurology 1998;50:1149–1152.

Hohjoh H, Nakayama T, Ohashi J, et al. Significant association of a single nucleotide polymorphism in the tumor necrosis factor-alpha (TNF-alpha) gene promoter with human narcolepsy. Tissue Antigens 1999; 54:138–145.

Hohjoh H, Terada N, Kawashima M, Honda Y, Tokunaga K. Significant association of the tumor necrosis factor receptor 2 (TNFR2) gene with human narcolepsy. Tissue Antigens 2000;56:446–448.

Hohjoh H, Terada N, Nakayama T, et al. Case-control study with narcoleptic patients and healthy controls who, like the patients, possess both HLA-DRB1*1501 and -DQB1*0602. Tissue Antigens 2001;57: 230–235.

Hungs M, Lin L, Okun M, Mignot E. Polymorphisms in the vicinity of the hypocretin/orexin are not associated with human narcolepsy. Neurology 2001;57:1893–1895.

Itier V, Bertrand D. Mutations of the neuronal nicotinic acetylcholine receptors and their association with ADNFLE. Neurophysiol Clin 2002;32:99–107.

Jones B. Basic mechanisms of sleep-wake states. In: Kryger M, Roth T, Dement W, eds. Principles and Practice of Sleep Medicine. Philadelphia: WB Saunders, 2000: pp.134–154.

Jones C, Campbell S, Zone S, et al. Familial advanced sleep-phase syndrome: A short-period circadian rhythm variant in humans. Nat Med 1999;5: 1062–1065.

Katzenberg D, Young T, Finn L, et al. A CLOCK polymorphism associated with human diurnal preference. Sleep 1998;21:569–576.

Kramer A, Yang FC, Snodgrass P, et al. Regulation of daily locomotor activity and sleep by hypothalamic EGF receptor signaling. Science 2001;294:2511–2515.

Lai YY, Shalita T, Hajnik T, et al. Neurotoxic N-methyl-D-aspartate lesion of the ventral midbrain and mesopontine junction alters sleep-wake organization. Neuroscience 1999;90:469–483.

Lin L, Faraco J, Li R, et al. The sleep disorder canine narcolepsy is caused by a mutation in the hypocretin (orexin) receptor 2 gene. Cell 1999;98: 365–376.

Lu J, Zhang Y, Chou T, et al. Contrasting effects of ibotenate lesions of the paraventricular nucleus and subparaventricular zone on sleep-wake cycle and temperature regulation. J Neurosci 2001;21: 4568–4576.

Lugaresi E, Medori R, Montagna P, et al. Fatal familial insomnia and dysautonomia with selective degeneration of thalamic nuclei. N Engl J Med 1986;315:997–1003.

Mignot E. Genetic and familial aspects of narcolepsy. Neurology 1998;50: S16–S22.

Mignot E, Lammers G, Ripley B, et al. The role of cerebrospinal fluid hypocretin measurement in the diagnosis of narcolepsy and other hypersomnias. Arch Neurol 2002;59:1553–1562.

Mignot E, Lin X, Hesla PE, Dement WC, Guilleminault C, Grumet FC. A novel HLA DR17, DQ1 (DQA1-0102/DQB1-0602 positive) haplotype predisposing to narcolepsy in Caucasians. Sleep 1993;16: 764, 765.

Mignot E, Lin L, Rogers W, et al. Complex HLA-DR and -DQ interactions confer risk of narcolepsy-cataplexy in three ethnic groups. Am J Hum Genet 2001;68:686–699.

Miyagawa T, Hohjoh H, Honda Y, Juji T, Tokunaga K. Identification of a telomeric boundary of the HLA region with potential for predisposition to human narcolepsy. Immunogenetics 2000;52:12–18.

Nakayama J, Miura M, Honda M, Miki T, Honda Y, Arinami T. Linkage of human narcolepsy with HLA association to chromosome 4p13- q21. Genomics 2000;65:84–86.

Nishino S, Ripley B, Overeem S, Lammers GJ, Mignot E. Hypocretin (orexin) deficiency in human narcolepsy. Lancet 2000;355:39, 40.

Okun ML, Lin L, Pelin Z, Hong S, Mignot E. Clinical aspects of narcolepsy-cataplexy across ethnic groups. Sleep 2002;25:27–35.

Olafsdottir BR, Rye DB, Scammell TE, Matheson JK, Stefansson K, Gulcher JR. Polymorphisms in hypocretin/orexin pathway genes and narcolepsy. Neurology 2001;57:1896–1899.

Panda S, Sato T, Castrucci A, et al. Melanopsin (Opn4) requirement for normal light-induced circadian phase shifting. Science 2002; 298: 2213–2216.

Pelin Z, Guilleminault C, Risch N, Grumet FC, Mignot E. HLA-DQB1 *0602 homozygosity increases relative risk for narcolepsy but not disease severity in two ethnic groups. US Modafinil in Narcolepsy Multicenter Study Group. Tissue Antigens 1998;51:96–100.

Peyron C, Faraco J, Rogers W, et al. A mutation in a case of early onset narcolepsy and a generalized absence of hypocretin peptides in human narcoleptic brains. Nat Med 2000;6:991–997.

Peyron C, Tighe DK, van den Pol AN, et al. Neurons containing hypocretin (orexin) project to multiple neuronal systems. J Neurosci 1998;18: 9996–10,015.

Porkka-Heiskanen T, Strecker RE, Thakkar M, Bjorkum AA, Greene RW, McCarley RW. Adenosine: a mediator of the sleep-inducing effects of prolonged wakefulness. Science 1997;276:1265–1268.

Reppert S, Weaver D. Coordination of circadian timing in mammals. Nature 2002;418:935–941.

Sakurai T, Amemiya A, Ishii M, et al. Orexins and orexin receptors: a family of hypothalamic neuropeptides and G protein-coupled receptors that regulate feeding behaviour. cell 1998;92:573–585.

Saper CB, Chou TC, Scammell TE. The sleep switch: hypothalamic control of sleep and wakefulness. Trends Neurosci 2001;24:726–731.

Schenck C, Mahowald M. REM sleep behavior disorder: clinical, developmental, and neuroscience perspective and neuroscience perspectives 16 years after its formal identification in SLEEP. Sleep 2002;25: 126–138.

Schmidauer C, Sojer M, Seppi K, et al. Transcranial ultrasound shows nigral hypoechogenicity in restless legs syndrome. Ann Neurol 2005;58:630–634.

Sherin JE, Shiromani PJ, McCarley RW, Saper CB. Activation of ventrolateral preoptic neurons during sleep. Science 1996;271:216–219.

Silver R, LeSaute RJ, Tresco P, Lehman M. A diffusible coupling signal from the transplanted suprachiasmatic nucleus controlling circadian locomotor rhythms. Nature 1996;382:810–813.

Steriade M, McCarley RW. Brainstem Control of Wakefulness and Sleep. New York: Plenum, 1990.

Steriade M, McCormick DA, Sejnowski TJ. Thalamocortical oscillations in the sleeping and aroused brain. Science 1993;262:679–685.

Thannickal T, Moore RY, Nienhuis R, et al. Reduced number of hypocretin neurons in human narcolepsy. Neuron 2000;27:469–474.

Toh K, Jones C, He Y, et al. An hPer2 phosphorylation site mutation in familial advanced sleep phase syndrome. Science 2001;291:1040–1043.

Willie JT, Chemelli RM, Sinton CM, Yanagisawa M. To eat or to sleep? orexin in the regulation of feeding and wakefulness. Annu Rev Neurosci 2001;24:429–458.

Winkelmann J, Muller-Myhsok B, Wittchen H, et al. Complex segregation analysis of restless legs syndrome provides evidence for an autosomal dominant mode of inheritance in early age at onset families. Ann Neurol 2002;52:297–302.

121 Neurofibromatosis 1 and 2

GREGORY J. ESPER AND DAVID H. GUTMANN

SUMMARY

Neurofibromatosis (NF) 1 and 2 are genetically and phenotypically distinct genetic disorders characterized by the development of benign and malignant tumors. Advances in molecular genetics have resulted in the identification of the *NF1* and *NF2* genes and their encoded proteins, neurofibromin, and merlin/schwannomin. Identification of these causative genes has led to an improved understanding of the molecular pathogenesis of NF1 and NF2, and has recently resulted in the development of targeted biologically based therapies for tumors in NF1. In this chapter, the epidemiology, clinical features, molecular pathogenesis, animal models, and therapeutic strategies for NF1 and NF2 will be discussed.

Key Words: Café-au-lait macule; juvenile cataract; meningioma; merlin; NF1; NF2; neurofibroma; neurofibromin; optic glioma; RAS; schwannoma; schwannomin.

INTRODUCTION

Neurofibromatosis (NF) 1 and 2 are genetically and phenotypically distinct diseases both characterized by the development of benign and malignant tumors. Advances in molecular genetics have resulted in the identification of the *NF1* and *NF2* genes and their encoded proteins, neurofibromin and merlin/schwannomin, respectively. Neurofibromin suppresses cell growth by downregulating RAS-GTPase mitogenic signaling, whereas merlin functions to negatively regulate cell growth and motility. Identification of these causative genes has led to an improved understanding of the molecular pathogenesis of NF1 and NF2, and has initiated the development of targeted therapies. This chapter discusses the epidemiology, clinical features, molecular pathogenesis, animal models, and therapeutic strategies for NF1 and NF2.

NEUROFIBROMATOSIS 1

EPIDEMIOLOGY   NF1 is known also as peripheral neurofibromatosis or von Recklinghausen's disease, to recognize Frederick von Recklinghausen who first described the cellular component of the neurofibroma in 1882. NF1 is inherited in an autosomal-dominant fashion. Although complete penetrance is the rule, wide phenotypic variation occurs, such that some patients are only mildly affected, whereas others may be severely affected. The prevalence of NF1 has been estimated between 1/2190 and

From: *Principles of Molecular Medicine, Second Edition*
Edited by: M. S. Runge and C. Patterson © Humana Press, Inc., Totowa, NJ

1/7800. NF1 affects both genders and all races and ethnic groups equally. Despite its autosomal-dominant inheritance pattern, approx 50% of individuals with NF1 have no positive family history and likely represent new mutations.

The clinical manifestations of NF1 are mostly frequently recognized in early childhood, and are evident in nearly all affected patients by age 20. Although the majority of individuals with NF1 are relatively healthy, they exhibit increased morbidity and mortality compared to people without NF1, and they typically have life expectancies 10–15 yr less than unaffected individuals in the general population.

CLINICAL FEATURES   The diagnosis of NF1 is based on the identification of two or more features from a defined list of NF1-associated clinical criteria (Table 121-1). Café-au-lait spots, skinfold freckling in the axillary, inguinal, and neck regions, and Lisch nodules or iris hamartomas are common pigmentary abnormalities. Cognitive dysfunction is also frequent, with more than 50% of affected individuals manifesting some form of specific learning disability. Skeletal dysplasia of the long bones or sphenoid ridge is distinctive in NF1, but much less common.

Tumors are among the most frequently observed manifestation of NF1. Benign peripheral nerve tumors, called neurofibromas, are seen in nearly all adults with NF1. Neurofibromas are Schwann cell tumors that grow from an associated nerve and contain other cell types, including fibroblasts and mast cells. In one-third of individuals with NF1, more diffuse neurofibromas (plexiform neurofibroma) that involve multiple nerve fascicles may be encountered. In contrast to discrete neurofibromas, plexiform neurofibroma tumors harbor a 5–10% lifetime risk for transformation into a malignant peripheral nerve sheath tumor (MPNST). MPNSTs occur in approx 8–13% of patients with NF1, and they are associated with a high mortality rate because they are poorly responsive to chemotherapy and radiation.

In addition to Schwann cell tumors, children with NF1 are at risk for the development of astrocytomas. Of children with NF1, 15–20% develop astrocytomas involving the optic pathway and hypothalamus. Continued growth of these tumors may result in visual loss, hydrocephalus, and hypothalamic dysfunction. Optic pathway gliomas are most frequently World Health Organization grade I pilocytic tumors. Typically, NF1-associated optic pathway tumors do not progress after 10 yr of age. Treatment is reserved for symptomatic tumors and most frequently involves carboplatin/vincristine chemotherapy.

Other cancers seen in individuals with NF1 include myeloid leukemias, myelodysplastic syndromes, and pheochromocytoma.

Table 121-1
Diagnostic Features for NF1

Two or more of the following features must be present for an individual to be diagnosed with NF1:

- Six of more café-au-lait spots with diameters more than 0.5 cm before puberty or 1.5 cm after puberty
- Two or more neurofibromas or a single plexiform neurofibroma
- Freckling in the axillary and inguinal regions (Crowe's sign)
- Optic pathway tumor
- Lisch nodules (hamartomas of the iris)
- A distinctive bony lesion: dysplasia of the sphenoid bone or dysplasia/thinning of long bone cortex
- A first-degree relative diagnosed with NF1

Data from Gutmann et al., 1997.

There are significant psychosocial issues affecting individuals with NF1 that relate to physical appearance. The presence of numerous pigmentary lesions and neurofibromas can result in a significant cosmetic burden, which can be detrimental to a patient's self image.

MOLECULAR PATHOGENESIS The *NF1* locus spans 350 kb of genomic DNA on chromosome 17q11.2 and encodes a large gene, with more than 60 exons. The *NF1* protein, neurofibromin, is expressed in Schwann cells, neurons, astrocytes, myeloid cells, adrenal medulla, and oligodendrocytes. Inspection of the coding sequence of neurofibromin revealed striking sequence similarities between a small portion of neurofibromin and the catalytic region of a family of proteins termed GTPase-activating proteins (GAPs).

Subsequent studies have shown that neurofibromin functions as a GAP for the proto-oncogene RAS. When in its active form, RAS is bound to GTP and stimulates cell growth. The neurofibromin GAP-related domain functions to accelerate the conversion of active GTP-bound RAS to its inactive GDP-bound form. When neurofibromin is not expressed in NF1-associated tumor cells, dysregulated cell growth results from increased RAS activity (Fig. 121-1). In this regard, increased RAS activity has been associated with neurofibromin loss in tumors from NF1 patients, including leukemias, MPNSTs, and gliomas.

As is true for other tumor predisposition syndromes, individuals with NF1 start life with one mutated, nonfunctional *NF1* gene in every cell in their bodies. This is insufficient for tumor formation. Tumorigenesis requires a second inactivating mutation in the one remaining functional *NF1* gene to result in total loss of *NF1* gene expression. The combination of the germline *NF1* mutation and the subsequent acquired somatic *NF1* loss is termed the "two hit" hypothesis and explains why individuals with these inherited tumor predisposition syndromes are at high risk for tumor development.

Malignant tumors associated with NF1 involve additional genetic changes. In the case of the MPNST, a number of additional genetic changes are observed in addition to *NF1* inactivation, including inactivation of the p53 and p16 tumor suppressor genes as well as overexpression of the epidermal growth factor receptor.

ANIMAL MODELS OF NF1 The understanding of the molecular pathogenesis of NF1-associated tumors has derived from elegant studies in mice. Mice in which one copy of the *NF1* gene was mutated (*Nf1*+/– mice) are viable, but they succumb to malignant tumors (leukemia, lymphoma, and pheochromocytoma) at 15–18 mo of life. Although these mice do not develop the tumors typically associated with the human disorder, *Nf1*+/– mice exhibit specific learning disabilities, reminiscent of those found in children with NF1.

To develop mouse models of NF1-associated tumors, three approaches have been taken. First, mice have been generated in which some of their cells lack neurofibromin expression. These mice develop leukemias and plexiform neurofibromas. Second, *Nf1*+/– mice have been bred with *p53*+/– mice to generate *Nf1*+/–;*p53*/– mice. These mice develop high-grade MPNSTs that appear histologically similar to human MPNSTs. Lastly, to circumvent the embryonic lethality of *Nf1*–/– mice, mice have been generated that lack neurofibromin expression in specific tissues. These conditional *Nf1* knockout mice include those that lack neurofibromin in neurons, astrocytes, or Schwann cells. Neuron-specific *Nf1* inactivation results in abnormal neuronal function and extensive brain astrogliosis and cortical abnormalities. Astrocyte-specific *Nf1* conditional knockout mice have more astrocytes in their brains, but do not develop astrocytomas. Schwann cell-specific *Nf1* inactivation is also not sufficient for neurofibroma formation.

Recently *Nf1*+/– mice have generated in which either astrocytes or Schwann cells lack neurofibromin expression. These *Nf1* genetically engineered mice develop optic glioma and plexiform neurofibroma, respectively.

POTENTIAL THERAPIES Therapies focus on surgery and limited chemotherapies. As the understanding of the molecular pathogenesis of NF1 improves and robust preclinical animal models become available, the ability to offer more targeted, tailored therapies for NF1 may be possible. One explored treatment entails pharmacologic inactivation of RAS. RAS activation requires further post-translational modification by farnesylation of its CAAX sequence. Inhibition of this process using farnesyl transferase inhibitors results in inactivation of RAS, and theoretically, inhibition of cell hyperproliferation. This approach is in clinical trial for NF1.

NEUROFIBROMATOSIS 2

EPIDEMIOLOGY Also known as central or bilateral neurofibromatosis, the incidence of NF2 is between 1/33,000 and 1/87,000, based on two population studies from the United Kingdom and Finland. In the United States, there are about 100 new cases per year, though the prevalence is about 0.5 million people. In this respect, NF2 is 10-fold less common than NF1. Patients generally manifest clinical signs or symptoms by age 60, but most frequently present in their 20s. As is true for NF1, NF2 is transmitted in an autosomal-dominant fashion, and penetrance is almost complete.

CLINICAL FEATURES The most common clinical features of NF2 are bilateral vestibular schwannomas (VS). Schwannomas may also affect other cranial or peripheral nerves, but the vestibular nerve is the most frequently affected nerve. Bilateral VS or a family history of NF2 combined with any two of the other associated features, including meningioma, glioma, schwannoma, or cataracts, are criteria used to establish the diagnosis of NF2 (Table 121-2). Patients with unilateral VS and one of the aforementioned tumors, or patients with multiple meningiomas should also be evaluated for NF2. Manifestations begin by the third decade of life and are usually related to the site of origin of the tumor. For instance, vestibular tumors cause vertigo, tinnitus, and hearing loss. The "Wishart" and "Gardner" variants differ in severity, the former occurring in younger patients and behaving more aggressively because of multiple tumors, whereas the latter tends to occur later in life with a less severe clinical course. Mononeuropathy affecting the facial nerve is also a presenting feature, and can occur before VS are present.

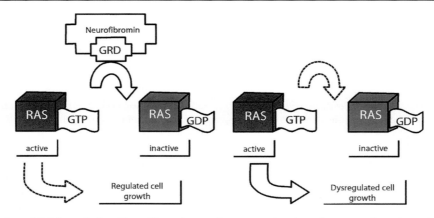

Figure 121-1   Neurofibromin and RAS regulation. Neurofibromin contains a central region of sequence homology shared with a family of proteins (GTPase activating proteins or GAPs) that accelerate the conversion of active RAS (bound to GTP to the inactive RAS-GDP molecule (left panel). Tight control of RAS activity results in regulated cell growth. In contrast, loss of neurofibromin results in increased RAS-GTP activity, facilitating cell growth and proliferation (right panel). GRD, neurofibromin GAP-related domain.

Table 121-2
Diagnostic Criteria for NF2

Confirmed (definite) NF2
    Bilateral VS
Or
    Family history of NF2 (first degree family relative) plus:
        Unilateral VS at less than 30-yr-old, or
        Any two of the following: meningioma, glioma, schwannoma,
            juvenile posterior subcapsular lenticular opacities/juvenile
            cortical cataracts
Individuals to be evaluated for NF2 (presumptive or probable)
    Unilateral VS at less than 30-yr-old, plus at least one of any of the
        following: meningioma, glioma, schwannoma, juvenile posterior
        subcapsular lenticular opacities/juvenile cortical cataracts
    Multiple meningiomas (two or more) plus unilateral VS at less
        than 30-yr-old, or
    Any one of the following: glioma, schwannoma, juvenile posterior
        subcapsular lenticular opacities/juvenile cortical cataracts

Data from Gutmann et al., 1997.

There are few cutaneous pigmentary features compared with NF1. Three different types of skin tumors are present: an intracutaneous, raised, pigmented, plaque-like lesion, a subcutaneous nodular tumor manifesting on peripheral nerves, and intracutaneous tumors, thought to be schwannomas, similar to those in NF1. There are also prominent eye features, including optic nerve meningiomas, retinal hamartomas, and posterior lenticular opacities (juvenile cataracts).

MOLECULAR PATHOGENESIS   The *NF2* locus spans 120 kb of DNA on chromosome 22q12.2. The *NF2* gene contains 17 exons that encode a 595 amino acid protein, termed merlin or schwannomin. Merlin is expressed in Schwann cells, neurons, lens fibers, blood vessels, and leptomeningeal cells. Analysis of the predicted protein sequence of merlin revealed striking sequence similarity to a family of proteins that link cell surface glycoproteins to the actin cytoskeleton. Merlin has homology to the ezrin, radixin, and moesin (ERM) subfamily of protein 4.1 molecules that contain three structural domains including the N-terminal

(or FERM) domain, a predicted α helix, and a unique carboxyl terminal domain (Fig. 121-2A). Merlin is different from the ERM proteins, however, in that it does not contain the conventional C-terminal actin-binding domain present in ERM proteins, and it binds weakly to the actin cytoskeleton.

Consistent with merlin's proposed function as an ERM tumor suppressor, overexpression of merlin results in reduced cell growth and motility. Loss of merlin in schwannoma cells is associated with dramatic alterations in the actin cytoskeleton and merlin-deficient mouse tumor cells have a highly motile and metastatic phenotype.

Although the exact mechanism underlying merlin growth regulation is unknown, merlin associates with a number of important proteins that may impact on its ability to function as a negative growth regulator (Fig. 121-2B). In this regard, merlin binds CD44, sodium–hydrogen exchange regulatory factor, hepatocyte growth factor-regulated tyrosine kinase substrate, β-integrin, paxillin, syntenin, and schwannomin interacting protein 1. Further studies will be required to define the mechanism of merlin growth suppression.

ANIMAL MODELS OF NF2   The understanding of the molecular pathogenesis of NF2-associated tumors has derived from mouse modeling studies in which the *Nf2* gene has been inactivated in Schwann and leptomeningeal cells. *Nf2*+/– mice do not develop tumors associated with the human condition. To circumvent the early embryonic lethality of *Nf2*–/– mice, conditional *Nf2* knockout mice (*Nf2*^{flox2}) have been generated. *Nf2*^{flox2}; *P0*-Cre mice manifest Schwann cell hyperplasia, schwannomas, cataracts, and cerebral calcifications. Additional mice have been generated in which homozygous *Nf2* inactivation occurs in the leptomeninges by adenoviral-Cre delivery. These mice developed meningioma subtypes histologically similar to human meningioma subtypes.

POTENTIAL THERAPIES   Management of NF2 is based on excision of tumors that result in hearing loss or other neurologic dysfunction. A combined medical and surgical approach by neurology, medical and radiation oncology, neurosurgery, otolaryngology, and other specialties is employed, and results are often better in centers with significant experience managing individuals with NF2. As the understanding of the function of merlin and its associated protein interactors improves, more promising therapies may be developed.

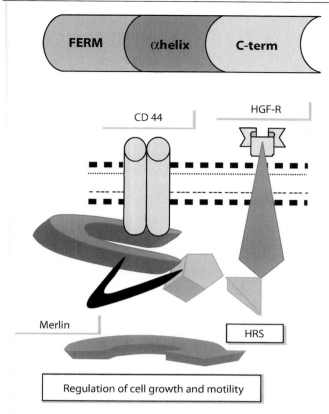

Figure 121-2 Merlin contains three predicted protein domains. **(A)** The FERM (four.1-ezrin-radixin-moesin) domain and the α-helical region are conserved among all ERM proteins, whereas the carboxyl terminus (C-term) is a unique region. **(B)** Merlin may regulate cell proliferation and motility by integrating mitogenic (cell growth) and motogenic (cell motility) signals emanating at the hyaluronic acid receptor (CD44) and hepatocyte growth factor receptor (c-met). Merlin has been shown to bind the cytoplasmic tail of CD44 and associates with one of the molecules (hepatocyte growth factor-regulated tyrosine kinase substrate) recruited by c-met activation.

CONCLUSIONS

Since the identification of the *NF1* and *NF2* genes, tremendous amounts have been learned of the normal function of neurofibromin and merlin relative to the pathogenesis of NF1- and NF2-associated features. Further research on the precise mechanisms underlying merlin and neurofibromin growth regulation will likely yield significant insights into targets for tailored drug design. The availability of robust mouse models for most of the NF-associated tumor features offers the exciting possibility of evaluating potential therapies in preclinical small animal models before testing in humans.

SELECTED REFERENCES

Antinheimo J, Sankila R, Carpen O, Pukkala E, Sainio M, Jaaskelainen J. Population based analysis of sporadic and NF2-associated meningiomas and schwannomas. J Neurol 2000;54:71–76.

Bajenaru ML, Hernandez MR, Perry A, et al. Optic nerve glioma in mice requires astrocyte Nf1 gene inactivation and Nf1 brain heterozygosity. Cancer Res 2003;63:8573–8577.

Bajenaru ML, Zhu Y, Hedrick NM, Donahoe J, Parada LF, Gutmann DH. Astrocyte-specific inactivation of the neurofibromatosis 1 gene (NF1) is insufficient for astrocytoma formation. Mol Cell Biol 2002;22: 5100–5113.

Birnbaum RA, O'Marcaigh A, Wardak Z, et al. Nf1 and Gmcsf interact in myeloid leukemogenesis. Mol Cell 2000;5:189–195.

Bollag G, Clapp DW, Shih S, et al. Loss of NF1 results in activation of the Ras signaling pathway and leads to aberrant growth in haematopoietic cells. Nat Genet 1996;12:144–148.

Bollag G, McCormick F. Regulators and effectors of ras proteins. Ann Rev Cell Dev Biol 1991;7:601–632.

Cawthon RM, Weiss R, Xu GF, et al. A major segment of the neurofibromatosis type 1 gene: cDNA sequence, genomic structure, and point mutations. Cell 1990;62:193–201.

Cichowski K, Shih TS, Schmitt E, et al. Mouse models of tumor development in neurofibromatosis type 1. Science 1999;286:2172–2176.

Claudio JO, Veneziale RW, Menko AS, Rouleau GA. Expression of schwannomin in lens and Schwann cells. Neuroreport 1997;8: 2025–2030.

Costa RM, Federov NB, Kogan JH, et al. Mechanism for the learning deficits in a mouse model of neurofibromatosis type 1. Nature 2002; 415:526–530.

Daston MM, Scrable H, Nordlund M, Sturbaum AK, Nissen LM, Ratner N. The protein product of the neurofibromatosis type 1 gene is expressed at highest abundance in neurons, Schwann cells, and oligodendrocytes. Neuron 1992;8:415–428.

Deballa K, Szudek J, Friedman JM. Use of the NIH criteria for diagnosis of NF1 in children. Pediatrics 2000;105:608–614.

DeClue JE, Papageorge AG, Fletcher JA, et al. Abnormal regulation of mammalian p21(ras) contributes to malignant tumor growth in von Recklinghausen (type 1) neurofibromatosis. Cell 1992;69:265–273.

Evans DG, Baser ME, McGaughran J, Sharif S, Howard E, Moran A. Malignant peripheral nerve sheath tumours in neurofibromatosis 1. J Med Genet 2002;39:311–314.

Evans DGR, Huson SM, Donnai D, et al. A clinical study of type 2 neurofibromatosis. QJM 1992;84:603–618.

Evans DGR, Newton V, Neary W, et al. Use of MRI and audiological tests in presymptomatic diagnosis of type 2 neurofibromatosis (NF2). J Med Genet 2000;37:944–946.

Feldkamp MM, Lau N, Provias JP, Gutmann DH, Guha A. Acute presentation of a neurogenic sarcoma in a patient with neurofibromatosis type 1: a pathological and molecular explanation. J Neurosurg 1996; 84:867–873.

Fernandez-Valle C, Tang Y, Ricard J, et al. Paxillin binds schwannomin and regulates its density-dependent localization and effect on cell morphology. Nat Genet 2002;31:354–362.

Ferner RE, Gutmann DH. International consensus statement on malignant peripheral nerve sheath tumors in neurofibromatosis. Cancer Res 2002;62:1573–1577.

Friedman JM. Epidemiology of neurofibromatosis type 1. Am J Med Genet 1999;89:1–6.

Giovannini M, Robanus-Maandag E, Niwa-Kawakita M, et al. Schwann cell hyperplasia and tumors in transgenic mice expressing a naturally occurring mutant NF2 protein. Genes Dev 1999;13:978–986.

Giovannini M, Robanus-Maandag E, van der Valk M, et al. Conditional biallelic Nf2 mutation in the mouse promotes manifestations of human neurofibromatosis type 2. Genes Dev 2000;14:1617–1630.

Goutebroze L, Brault E, Muchardt C, Camonis J, Thomas G. Cloning and characterization of SCHIP-1, a novel protein interacting specifically with spliced isoforms and naturally occurring mutant NF2 proteins. Mol Cell Biol 2000;20:1699–1712.

Gutmann DH, Aylsworth A, Carey JC, et al. The diagnostic evaluation and multidisciplinary management of neurofibromatosis 1 and neurofibromatosis 2. JAMA 1997:278:51–57.

Gutmann DH, Giovannini M. Mouse models of neurofibromatosis 1 and 2. Neoplasia 2002;4:279–290.

Gutmann DH, Haipek CA, Burke SP, Sun C-X, Scoles DR, Pulst SM. The neurofibromatosis 2 tumor suppressor protein interacts with hepatocyte growth factor regulated tyrosine kinase substrate. Hum Mol Genet 2000;9:1567–1574.

Gutmann DH, Wood DL, Collins FS. Identification of the neurofibromatosis type 1 gene product. Proc Natl Acad Sci USA 1991;88: 9658–9662.

Huson SM, Harper PS, Compston DAS. Von Recklinghausen neurofibromatosis: a clinical and population study in southeast Wales. Brain 1988;111:1355–1381.

Jacks T, Shih TS, Schmitt EM, Bronson RT, Bernards A, Weinberg RA. Tumour predisposition in mice heterozygous for a targeted mutation in Nf1. Nat Genet 1994;7:353–361.

Jannatipour M, Dion P, Khan S, et al. Schwannomin isoform-1 interacts with syntenin via PDZ domains. J Biol Chem. 2001;276:33,093–33,100.

Jhanwar SC, Chen Q, Li FP, Brennan MF, Woodruff JM. Cytogenetic analysis of soft tissue sarcomas. Recurrent chromosome abnormalities in malignant peripheral nerve sheath tumors (MPNST). Cancer Genet Cytogenet 1994;78:138–144.

Kalamarides M, Niwa-Kawakita M, Leblois H, et al. Nf2 gene inactivation in arachnoidal cells is rate limiting for meningioma development in the mouse. Genes Dev 2002;16:1060–1065.

Kourea HP, Cordon-Cardo C, Dudas M, Leung D, Woodruff JM. Expression of p27^{kip} and other cell cycle regulators in malignant peripheral nerve sheath tumors and neurofibromas: The emerging role of p27^{kip} in malignant transformation of neurofibromas. Am J Pathol 1999;155:1885–1891.

Kourea HP, Orlow I, Scheithauer BW, Cordon-Cardo C, Woodruff JM. Deletions of the *INK4A* gene occur in malignant peripheral nerve sheath tumors but not in neurofibromas. Am J Pathol 1999;155: 1855–1860.

Lau N, Feldkamp MM, Roncari L, et al. Loss of neurofibromin is associated with activation of ras/MAPK and PIS-K/akt signaling in a neurofibromatosis 1 astrocytoma. J Neuropathol Exp Neurol 2000;59:759–767.

Listernick R, Louis DN, Packer RJ, Gutmann DH. Optic pathway gliomas in children with neurofibromatosis 1: consensus statement from the NF1 Optic Pathway Glioma Task Force. Ann Neurol 1997;41:143–149.

Marchuk DA, Saulino AM, Tavakkol R, et al. cDNA cloning of the type 1 neurofibromatosis type 1 gene: complete sequence of the NF 1 gene product. Genomics 1991;11:931–940.

Matsui I, Tanimura M, Kobayashi N, Sawada T, Nagahara N, Akatsuka J. Neurofibromatosis type 1 and childhood cancer. Cancer1993;72: 2746–2754.

Mawrin C, Kirches E, Boltze C, Dietzmann K, Roessner A, Schneider-Stock R. Immunohistochemical and molecular analysis of p53, RB, and PTEN in malignant peripheral nerve sheath tumors. Virchows Arch 2002;440:610–615.

McClatchey AI, Saotome I, Mercer K, et al. Mice heterozygous for a mutation at the NF2 tumor suppressor locus develop a range of highly metastatic tumors. Genes Dev 1998;12:1121–1133.

Miles DK, Freedman MH, Stephens K, et al. Patterns of hematopoietic lineage involvement in children with neurofibromatosis type 1 and malignant myeloid disorders. Blood 1996;88:4314–4320.

Morrison H, Sherman LS, Legg J, et al. The NF2 tumor suppressor gene product, merlin, mediates contact inhibition of growth through interactions with CD44. Genes Dev 2001;15:968–980.

Murthy A, Gonzalez-Agosti C, Cordero E, et al. NHE-RF, a regulatory cofactor for Na$^+$–H$^+$ exchange, is a common interactor for merlin and ERM (MERM) proteins. J Biol Chem 1998;273:1273–1276.

Nielsen GP, Stemmer-Rachamimov AO, Ino Y, Møller MB, Rosenberg A, Louis DN. Malignant Transformation of Neurofibromas in Neurofibromatosis 1 is associated with CDKN2A/p16 inactivation. Am J Pathol 1999;155:1879–1884.

North KN, Riccardi V, Samango-Sprouse C, et al. Cognitive function and academic performance in neurofibromatosis 1: consensus statement from the NF1 cognitive disorders task force. Neurology 1997;48: 1121–1127.

Obremski VJ, Hall AM, Fernandez-Valle C. Merlin, the neurofibromatosis type 2 gene product, and beta1 integrin associate in isolated and differentiating Schwann cells. J Neurobiol 1998;37:487–501.

Ozonoff S. Cognitive impairment in neurofibromatosis type 1. Am J Med Genet 1999;89:45–52.

Packer RJ, Gutmann DH, Rubenstein A, et al. Plexiform neurofibromas in NF1: toward biologic-based therapy. Neurology 2002;58: 1461–1470.

Pelton PD, Sherman LS, Rizvi TA, et al. Ruffling membrane, stress fiber, cell spreading, and proliferation abnormalities in human schwannoma cells. Oncogene 1998;17:2195–2209.

Perry A, Kunz SN, Fuller CE, et al. Differential NF1, p16, and EGFR patterns by interphase cytogenetics (FISH) in malignant peripheral nerve sheath tumor (MPNST) and morphologically similar spindle cell neoplasms. J Neuropathol Exp Neurol 2002;61:702–709.

Rouleau GA, Merel P, Lutchman M, et al. Alteration in a new gene encoding a putative membrane-organizing protein causes neuro-fibromatosis type 2. Nature 1993;363:515–521.

Scharovsky OG, Rozados VR, Gervasoni SI, Matar P. Inhibition of ras oncogene: a novel approach to antineoplastic therapy. J Biomed Sci 2000;7:292–298.

Scoles DR, Huynh DP, Chen MS, Burke SP, Gutmann DH, Pulst SM. The neurofibromatosis 2 tumor suppressor protein interacts with hepatocyte growth factor-regulated tyrosine kinase substrate. Hum Mol Genet 2000;9:1567–1574.

Silva AJ, Elgersma Y, Friedman E, Stern J, Kogan J. A mouse model for learning and memory defects associated with neurofibromatosis type I. Pathol Biol (Paris) 1998;46:697, 698.

Sørenson SA, Mulvihill JJ, Nielsen A. Long-term follow-up of von Recklinghausen neurofibromatosis: Survival and malignant neoplasms. N Engl J Med 1986b;314:1010–1015.

Stemmer-Rachamimov AO, Gonzalez-Agosti C, Xu L, et al. Expression of NF2-encoded merlin and related ERM family proteins in the human central nervous system. J Neuropathol Exp Neurol 1997;56: 735–742.

Strauss BL, Gutmann DH, Dehner LP, et al. Molecular analysis of malignant triton tumors. Hum Pathol 1999;30:984–988.

Trofatter JA, MacCollin MM, Rutter JL, et al. A novel moesin-, ezrin-, radixin-like gene is a candidate for the neurofibromatosis 2 tumor suppressor. Cell 1993;72:791–800.

Tsukita S, Oishi K, Sato N, Sagara J, Kawai A, Tsukita S. ERM family members as molecular linkers between the cell surface glycoprotein CD44 and actin-based cytoskeletons. J Cell Biol 1994;126:391–401.

Viskochil D, Buchberg AM, Xu G, et al. Deletions and a translocation interrupt a cloned gene at the neurofibromatosis type 1 locus. Cell 1990;62:187–192.

Vogel KS, Klesse LJ, Velasco-Miguel S, Meyers K, Rushing EJ, Parada LF. Mouse tumor model for neurofibromatosis type 1. Science 1999; 286:2176–2179.

Xu GF, O'Connell P, Viskochil D, et al. The neurofibromatosis type 1 gene encodes a protein related to GAP. Cell 1990;62:599–608.

Xu HM, Gutmann DH. Merlin differentially associates with the microtubule and actin cytoskeleton. J Neurosci 1998;51:403–415.

Zhu Y, Ghosh P, Charnay P, Burns DK, Parada LF. Neurofibromas in NF1: Schwann cell origin and role of tumor environment. Science 2002; 296:920–922.

Zhu Y, Romero MI, Ghosh P, et al. Ablation of NF1 function in neurons induces abnormal development of cerebral cortex and reactive gliosis in the brain. Genes Dev 2001;15:859–876.

Zöller M, Rembeck B, Akesson HO, Angervall L. Life expectancy, mortality and prognostic factors in neurofibromatosis type 1: a twelve-year follow-up of an epidemiological study in Göteborg, Sweden. Acta Derm Venereol (Stockh) 1995;75:136–140.

122 Axonal Regeneration and Recovery From Chronic Central Nervous System Injury

STEPHEN M. STRITTMATTER

SUMMARY

Damage to the adult brain or spinal cord commonly produces persistent dysfunction without recovery. To replace lost neurons, stem cells, trophic factors, and transplantation of neural-competent cells might be relevant. Treatment of dysfunction based on the disconnection of surviving neurons requires the axonal regeneration from remaining neurons and a degree of plasticity in neuronal connectivity. Those neurological conditions in which axonal regeneration and plasticity are most relevant are reviewed here. Recent scientific advances are likely to lead to the development of a novel group of therapeutics targeting axonal regeneration for the recovery of function in chronic neurological dysfunction.

Key Words: Axon; cerebrovascular accident; head trauma; multiple sclerosis; neural repair; Nogo; physical therapy; regeneration; spinal cord injury; stroke.

INTRODUCTION

Damage to the brain or spinal cord of adults commonly produces persistent dysfunction with limited recovery regardless of whether the insult is traumatic, ischemic, immunological, genetic, degenerative, toxic, metabolic, or nutritional in origin. One method to classify the basis of persistent deficits is cellular; either neuronal cell bodies are lost, or neurons survive but are functionally disconnected because of axonal or myelin loss. Therapeutic replacement or compensation for lost neurons poses a different problem than restoring functional connectivity between remaining neuronal populations. To replace lost neurons, stem cells, trophic factors, and transplantation of neural-competent cells might be relevant. Conversely, treatment of dysfunction based on the disconnection of surviving neurons requires the promotion of axonal regeneration from remaining neurons and a degree of plasticity in neuronal connectivity. This chapter reviews the neurological conditions in which axonal regeneration and plasticity are most relevant. Advances likely to lead to the development of a novel group of therapeutics targeting axonal regeneration for the recovery of function in chronic neurological dysfunction are summarized.

From: *Principles of Molecular Medicine, Second Edition*
Edited by: M. S. Runge and C. Patterson © Humana Press, Inc., Totowa, NJ

AXONAL DISCONNECTION AFTER CHRONIC CENTRAL NERVOUS SYSTEM INJURY

SPINAL CORD INJURY Axonal disconnection is most obviously the proximate cause of persistent disability after spinal cord injury (SCI). In the United States, approx 10,000 new cases occur each year, with a total prevalence of 250,000 individuals suffering disability from SCI. The two primary causes are motor vehicle accidents and gunshot wounds. Sporting accidents are the third most common cause. Most patients are young adults at onset and males are more commonly affected than females.

Spinal cord trauma selectively damages nervous system tissue at one to several spinal levels, but not throughout the cord. Although only a small segmental group of neurons are lost, functional deficits can be complete at all levels below the injury owing to the inability of descending motor and autonomic systems to connect with remaining caudal circuitry. Similarly, ascending sensory neurons caudal to the injury site might survive but cannot communicate with the supratentorial structures owing to axonal disruption. Functional axonal disconnection can result from both physical separation of distal axonal segments and from demyelination with conduction failure in remaining axons near the site of the trauma. It is clear that re-establishment of functional axonal connections between neuronal populations rostral and caudal to a SCI site is the most direct means of restoring function.

HEAD TRAUMA Head trauma with persistent deficits in motor or cognitive or emotional dysfunction is at least five times more common than spinal cord trauma. Pathophysiological mechanisms include skull fracture, epidural hemorrhage, subdural hemorrhage, and hydrocephalus. In addition, diffuse axonal injury secondary to acceleration/deceleration shearing of long axons in the forebrain is also recognized as a significant cause of long-term global cognitive dysfunction. In this case, multiple tracts in the subcortical white matter are disconnected and global functions dependent on interconnectivity are impaired.

STROKE Ischemic damage in the central nervous system (CNS) has multiple effects. A primary aspect of many "large vessel" hemispheral strokes is the loss of neuronal populations in discrete areas of the brain. Plasticity of remaining axonal connections is likely to play a critical role in the degree of functional recovery, but the primary insult in these cases is not the axon. In contrast, most "small vessel" lacunar strokes occur in the white matter and, therefore, these events disrupt axonal connectivity to a greater extent than neuronal survival.

CHRONIC PROGRESSIVE MULTIPLE SCLEROSIS
Recurrent immunological attack on CNS myelin is the principal pathophysiological process in relapsing remitting multiple sclerosis (MS). In chronic progressive MS, the accumulation of functional deficits is best correlated with axonal damage as sites of immunological myelin damage. Axonal retraction balls provide histological evidence for axonal interruption.

NATURAL HISTORY OF RECOVERY AFTER CHRONIC CNS INJURIES

MINIMAL IMPROVEMENT   After traumatic SCI, the natural history of recovery follows a relatively predictable path. The level and distribution of injury in the cord determines the balance and distribution of motor deficits, sensory deficits, autonomic disturbance, and pain associated with the injury. On the American Spinal Injury Association clinical rating scale of functional performance from A (no function) to E (normal function), most patients improve by one point from their level at 3 d after injury to their level at 6 or 12 mo after injury. This modest improvement occurs over 1–6 mo but little further improvement, or decline, occurs after 6–12 mo. Few patients improve by two points, and essentially no patients improve by three or more points in large clinical studies.

The basis of the recovery that does occur spontaneously after SCI is not clear. It is unlikely to relate to axonal regeneration. More likely, plastic changes in the function and anatomy of uninjured circuitry are likely to account for enhanced clinical performance. For example, there are caudal intrinsic circuits in the spinal cord that can generate locomotor patterns. In tetrapedal vertebrates, the operation of these circuits in the absence of descending inputs can produce a degree of locomotion. This central pattern generator in the spinal cord of bipedal humans is less effective in the absence of descending input. However, modestly improved function might result from its enhanced function through anatomical plasticity in the months following an injury.

Clinical deficits after head trauma are much more variable than after SCI. However, the time-course for significant improvement matches the primary 1–6 mo window observed after SCI. Cognitive and emotional disturbances after head trauma are likely to improve to a greater extent than are motor deficits. This might reflect greater degrees of plasticity in these circuits.

Recovery from stroke is also variable but typically follows a time-course similar to the 1–6 mo course described earlier. It is not unusual for focal motor paralysis after lacunar strokes to completely resolve after several months, leaving only trace spasticity. Larger hemispheral strokes produce more persistent deficits, sometimes with minimal recovery of function. To the extent that recovery occurs, function appears to be redistributed to parallel pathways and/or to new alternate pathways. For example, partial recovery from the contralateral hemiplegia associated with a hemispheral stroke can involve activation of regions in the opposite, undamaged hemisphere. This shift of cerebral activity has been documented in functional MRI studies and if a second hemispheral stroke occurs contralateral to the first stroke, then recovered function is frequently lost. This redistribution is determined in large part by the age of the individual. Whereas robust in infants, plasticity is severely curtailed in adults. It is likely that both anatomic

changes and altered electrical patterns in persistent connections account for these shifts in activation patterns during specific tasks.

Deficits in chronic progressive MS are by definition permanent. Continued disease activity and the accumulation of new lesions might be one explanation for the absence of recovery. In addition, the presence of widespread lesions is likely to limit compensation by parallel pathways.

PHYSICAL TRAINING   Medical treatment to enhance recovery from chronic neurological injuries is severely limited. Physical and occupational therapy is the primary mode of treatment for the chronic deficits associated with the conditions described. Active physical therapy regimens do enhance the increase in functional status at 6 or 12 mo after one of these insults. The cellular or molecular mechanism by which this improvement occurs is not clear. The optimal form of training is also less than clear. Specific body weight-supported treadmill training has achieved much attention for SCI patients. Clinical trials to verify these benefits and optimize training regimens are underway.

PHARMACOLOGY   No pharmaceutical agents are known to enhance the modest degree of functional recovery that occurs spontaneously and through optimal physical therapy. Some studies have suggested that amphetamines might enhance the benefits of physical therapy, but more definitive data are required to confirm or refute this effect. No pharmacological agents are in use to directly promote axonal regeneration or plasticity in the adult CNS after injury.

MOLECULAR DETERMINANTS OF AXON REGENERATION

EVIDENCE FOR EXTRINSIC DETERMINANTS   *A priori*, one might imagine that adult CNS neurons have lost the capacity for axonal growth. However, adult mammalian CNS axons can grow extensively if their environment is altered. Transplantation of sciatic nerve segments into various regions of the CNS is followed by dramatic axonal growth into the peripheral tissue. Although cell-autonomous factors might limit the rate of maximal axonal regeneration in the CNS, extrinsic factors play a critical role in preventing axonal regeneration after SCI, head trauma, stroke and chronic progressive MS (Fig. 122-1).

GROWTH PROMOTING FACTORS IN THE PERIPHERY
Extrinsic controls on adult CNS axon regeneration might include the presence of inhibitory factors limiting growth and the absence of factors that promote growth. Neurotrophic axon-growth promoting factors that are not expressed at adequate levels in the CNS to promote robust regeneration are potentially numerous. For specific neuronal populations, nerve growth factor (NGF), brain-derived neurotrophic factor, neurotrophic-3 play some role in regulating short-range sprouting in the adult CNS. However, data suggest that the neurotrophic factors alone cannot support long-distance axonal growth in the adult CNS. Glial-derived neurotrophic factor family ligands and gp130 cytokines have also been implicated in regulating the axonal growth potential of certain adult neurons. Although these factors clearly regulate the potential for growth, they appear inadequate to explain the great disparity between rapid peripheral nerve regenerative extension and absent CNS axonal regeneration.

INHIBITORS IN CNS: ASTROCYTES AND OLIGODENDROCYTES   The presence of axon growth inhibitors in the adult CNS appears to play a more prominent role in limiting axonal regeneration after injury. Growth inhibitors can be separated as CNS myelin-derived or astrocyte glial-scar derived. The astrocytic

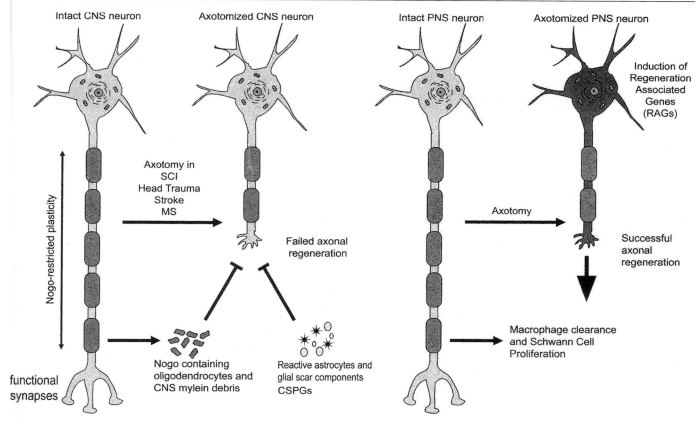

Figure 122-1   Molecular determinants of axonal regeneration and recovery from axotomy. Axonal regeneration after CNS injury is limited by CNS myelin and astrocytic scars. Regeneration-associated genes activated during peripheral nerve regeneration fail to be induced after central axotomy.

glial reaction is localized at the site of injury whereas myelin inhibition might be widespread and play a role in regulating CNS plasticity in the absence of injury. Although CNS oligodendrocyte-derived myelin is inhibitory of axonal growth in vitro, peripheral nervous system (PNS) Schwann-cell-derived myelin is much less of an impediment for axonal growth.

OVERCOMING CNS INHIBITION OF AXONAL GROWTH: GLIAL SCAR

CHONDROITIN SULFATE PROTEOGLYCANS   Astrocytic scar tissue in sections or in tissue culture limits axon growth. Several products of the astrocyte are implicated in mediating this inhibition. Most prominent are a class of proteoglycans containing chondroitin sulfate (Fig. 122-2). Astrocytes also secrete the inhibitory extracellular matrix (ECM) protein tenascin. The chondroitin sulfate proteoglycans (CSPGs) exist in secreted, ECM-bound and cell surface forms and include Neurocan, Phosphocan, neuroglian 2, Aggrecan, and others. Immobilized CSPGs can inhibit axonal growth in tissue culture and, in vivo, those CNS axons that do not regenerate are frequently observed to be halted at a zone of increased CSPG. There is evidence that the glycosaminoglycan side chains of these molecules are the primary determinant of their inhibitory activity. However, the exact determinants of activity regarding side chain length, diffusibility, and structure are not well defined.

SIGNALING MECHANISMS   Although an axonal cell surface receptor for CSPGs has not been described, there is evidence that they limit axonal growth by activating an intracellular signaling

protein, Rho (*see* Fig. 122-2). Rho is a GTP-binding protein that is active in the GTP-bound state and plays a prominent role in regulating filamentous actin cytoskeleton dynamics. CSPG exposure activates Rho in neurons. Activated Rho signals to the cytoskeleton through a Rho-associated kinase, ROCK. In this regard, axonal growth inhibition by astrocytic CSPG and oligodendrocyte myelin-derived inhibitors converge on one pathway (*see* Fig. 122-2). Inhibition of either Rho or ROCK stimulates axon growth in vitro and overcomes axon inhibition by CSPGs.

TREATMENT OPTIONS   Two methods have been developed in preclinical studies to perturb astrocytic CSPG inhibition of axon regeneration. The first involves digesting the CSPGs with a bacterial enzyme, chondroitinase. The second method is to inhibit Rho or ROCK activity. Both methods reportedly alleviate some CNS inhibition and promote anatomical axonal regeneration of some fibers and behavioral recovery in rodent SCI studies. Regeneration is by no means complete in these studies, but the regeneration of a small portion of axons has pronounced effects on locomotor recovery. To the extent that different methods can be compared, the results are similar to those observed with various myelin perturbations described in the next section.

OVERCOMING CNS INHIBITION OF AXONAL GROWTH: CNS MYELIN

NOGO   In defining the molecules underlying the inhibition of adult CNS axonal regeneration by CNS myelin, protein fractionation and molecular cloning identified Nogo (*see* Fig. 122-2).

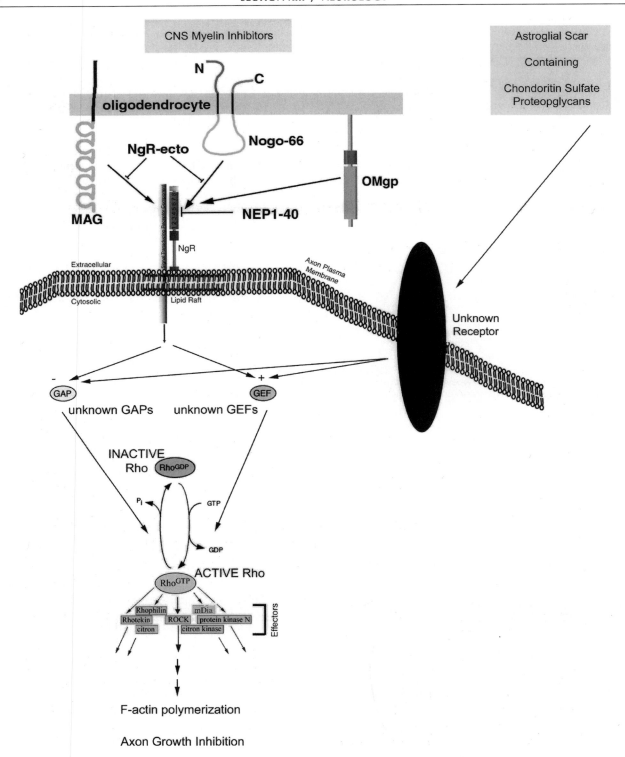

Figure 122-2   Molecular pathways limiting axonal regeneration and points of intervention. The myelin proteins, Nogo, MAG, and oligodendrocyte myelin glycoprotein bind to an axonal Nogo-66 receptor to limit axonal regeneration in the CNS through Rho/ROCK activation. CSPGs produced at high concentrations in glial scars also inhibit CNS regeneration by activating the Rho pathway. MAG, myelin-associated glycoprotein; GAP, GTPase-activating protein; GEF, guanine nucleotide exchange factor; NEP1-40; NgR, Nogo-66 receptor; OMgp, oligodendrocyte myelin glycoprotein.

Nogo is a member of the reticulon family of genes, which appear to play a role in endoplasmic reticulum function in neurons and endocrine cells. All reticulons have two hydrophobic domains and no signal sequence, suggesting that the amino and carboxyl termini might be located in the cytoplasm. Nogo (or reticulon 4) exists in three isoforms derived from alternate splicing and promotor usage.

Only Nogo-A ·of the reticulon family has been detected in the oligodendrocyte in which a fraction of the protein reaches the cell surface rather than being confined to the endoplasmic reticulum. Peripheral Schwann cells do not express Nogo, providing a molecular basis for the selectivity of axonal regeneration.

Recombinant purified Nogo protein has two inhibitory domains, termed Amino-Nogo and Nogo-66. The Nogo-66 domain specifically inhibits axonal growth, whereas the Amino-Nogo domain acts to inhibit cell spreading from multiple cell types as well as axonal outgrowth. Nogo-66 action is mediated by the Nogo-66 receptor (NgR) described later. The mechanism of Amino-Nogo action is not known. CNS myelin lacking Nogo is much less inhibitory for axonal growth in culture, suggesting that Nogo accounts for much of the inhibitory activity of CNS myelin. Significant degrees of axonal regeneration and functional locomotor recovery after SCI have been observed in some mouse strains lacking the Nogo-A/B isoforms.

MYELIN-ASSOCIATED GLYCOPROTEIN Alternative protein fractionation methods applied to CNS myelin led to the recognition that a second protein, myelin-associated glycoprotein (MAG), is also inhibitory for axonal growth. MAG, an immunoglobulin superfamily protein with a single transmembrane domain, is found on the surface of myelinating cells and localized in perinodal regions. The relative importance of MAG vs Nogo is not entirely clear. Because MAG is expressed in both the peripheral and central myelin fractions its expression does not correlate with regenerative potential, suggesting that it might be less relevant than Nogo-A. However, the MAG expression in Schwann cells might be compensated by a more rapid clearance of MAG in the periphery than in the CNS during Wallerian degeneration. The fact that mice lacking MAG do not show evidence for CNS axonal regeneration after SCI demonstrates that MAG is not necessary to prevent CNS axonal regeneration.

OLIGODENDROCYTE-MYELIN GLYCOPROTEIN By focusing selectively on the glycosyl phosphotidylinositol (GPI)-linked proteins of CNS myelin, investigators identified a third axonal growth inhibitory protein, termed oligodendrocyte myelin glycoprotein (OMgp). OMgp is a leucine-rich repeat cell surface protein, attached to the plasma membrane through a GPI lipid anchor. This inhibitor is selectively expressed in the CNS, and is found in both neurons and oligodendrocytes. No genetic studies of OMgp's role in axonal regeneration in vivo have been reported.

RECEPTOR MECHANISMS NgR was identified as a necessary mediator of Nogo-66 neuronal binding and axonal inhibition (see Fig. 122-2). NgR is expressed only in mature neurons and localizes to axons. The protein is made up of eight leucine-rich repeats of defined structure and the polypeptide is anchored to the plasma membrane through a GPI lipid moiety. After NgR was identified as a mediator of Nogo-66 action, it became clear that the protein also mediates the action of MAG and OMgp through high affinity binding. Thus, one receptor is the focus of action for three CNS myelin-derived axonal growth inhibitors. In the human genome there are two NgR-related genes, but neither protein encoded by these genes interacts with myelin inhibitors.

SIGNALING MECHANISMS Because the NgR is GPI-anchored to the outside of the plasma membrane, it is not immediately obvious by what means signals are transduced to the cell interior in order to limit axonal growth. The most possible mechanism for signal transduction is a second receptor subunit that functions in transduction but not ligand recognition. For some neurons, the p75-NTR low affinity NGF receptor might play this

role, but the role of p75-NTR in axonal regeneration has not been examined in vivo. Although the mechanisms by which myelin inhibitory signals reach from the NgR to the cytoplasm is not completely clear, NgR signals activate the GTP binding protein Rho and its downstream kinase ROCK inside of the neuron. This provides a point of convergence between inhibitory signaling by myelin and scar-derived CSPGs (see Fig. 122-2).

TREATMENTS TARGETING MYELIN-BASED INHIBITION Because the molecular basis of CNS myelin inhibition of adult axonal regeneration is defined molecularly, several opportunities for intervention have been developed. One method is to mask the inhibitors with antibodies. Either antiNogo antibodies or immunization with myelin to generate auto-antibodies has been effective in producing a degree of axonal regeneration and functional recovery after experimental SCI. Given the possibility that immunoreactivity to myelin might produce MS or experimental allergic encephalitis-like side effects, the determinants of beneficial and deleterious myelin immunoreactivity will have to be explored carefully. A variant of the antimyelin antibody method that has produced axonal regeneration in rodent models is the CNS delivery of autologous macrophages or dendritic cells primed with myelin in vitro in order to clear myelin and promote regeneration.

The NgR is a prime target for intervention to promote axonal regeneration because it is an extracellular neuronal protein and a focal point for the action of three inhibitory ligands in myelin. A peptide antagonist of the NgR has been identified that blocks Nogo action in vitro. In vivo, this peptide promotes the regeneration of descending corticospinal tract fibers and raphe spinal fibers after experimental rodent SCI. The axonal regeneration is accompanied by significant functional improvement in locomotion. The therapeutic time window is broad for this compound, with high effectiveness when treatment is begun at 1 wk postinjury. Furthermore, this compound is effective when administered systemically, accessing the spinal cord through an interrupted blood–brain barrier during the weeks after SCI. NgR antagonists that block the action of MAG and OMgp as well as Nogo at the NgR might have even greater effectiveness. Soluble fragments of the NgR itself can serve as decoy receptors blocking all three myelin inhibitors, and are likely to be more efficacious in vivo than the Nogo-selective NgR peptide antagonist.

The myelin inhibition system might also be blocked at the level of intracellular signaling through the Rho-ROCK pathway. Small molecule ROCK antagonists have been identified, and are in development for therapeutic use in humans. The advantage of this method for promoting axonal regeneration and functional recovery is that CSPG inhibition might be blocked as well as myelin inhibition. The disadvantage is that Rho and ROCK are expressed in many cell types and unwanted side effects might occur. ROCK inhibitors have produced a degree of axonal regeneration and functional improvement in rodent SCI studies.

OVERCOMING CNS INHIBITION OF AXONAL GROWTH: TRANSPLANTATION

SCHWANN CELLS The sciatic nerve transplantation studies make clear that the peripheral nerve environment is conducive to CNS axonal regeneration, suggesting that transplantation of isolated Schwann cells into sites of CNS axotomy might alter the environment and allow long-distance growth of axons to improve recovery. This altered environment might include the masking of inhibitors, the substitution of a noninhibitory environment and the secretion of growth-promoting factors. It is clear that transplanted Schwann cells

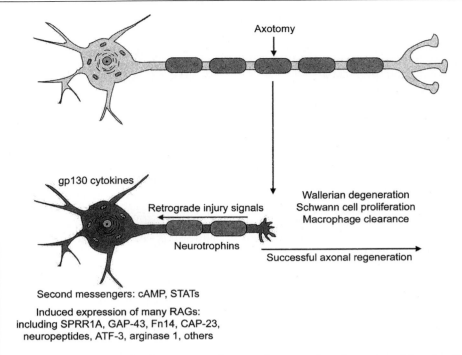

Figure 122-3   Regeneration-associated genes and pathways promoting axonal regeneration of recovery of function. In the PNS, regeneration-associated gene products such as GAP-43, CAP-23, galanin, SPRR1A, and Fn14 are induced by axotomy and support rapid axonal regeneration. Cytokine, neurotrophin, and cAMP signaling play roles in supporting rapid axonal outgrowth.

can promote a degree of axonal regeneration and can myelinate injured axons in rodent SCI models. To a somewhat lesser extent, regenerating axons leave a site of transplantation to enter the uninjured CNS to provide functional connections. Although any transplantation methodology raises issues related to rejection, there is a possibility that autologous transplantation from expanded cultures of peripheral Schwann cells from the sural nerve might avoid this issue.

OLFACTORY ENSHEATHING CELLS   The olfactory system is unique in the adult mammalian CNS in that axons continue to possess regenerative capacity in the adult. Rather than Schwann cells or oligodendrocytes, primary olfactory neurons are surrounded by a specialized olfactory ensheathing cell (OEC). When transplanted into adult rodent SCI sites, the OEC survives and migrates into surrounding uninjured tissue. Several laboratories have documented dramatic axonal regeneration and remyelination of injured axons after OEC transplantation in rodent SCI. Even after chronic complete spinal transection injuries, OEC transplantation is reported to improve substantially the degree of functional recovery in rodent locomotion. Human trials of OEC transplantation are being conducted in China.

BIOPOLYMERS   Bioengineering has the potential to provide synthetic materials with axonal growth promoting surfaces and with diffusible growth-promoting factors that might bridge a CNS axotomy site. Numerous versions of such materials are being developed. Although many such polymers might promote growth, a major unresolved obstacle is that axons growing into a graft must leave the graft and reenter inhibitory CNS tissue if they are to perform any useful function.

PROMOTING THE GROWTH POTENTIAL OF CNS NEURONS

REGENERATION-ASSOCIATED GENES   Apart from the preferential expression of inhibitory myelin and scar inhibitors in

the CNS, the differential growth of CNS and PNS neurons is explained in part by cell-autonomous factors. After PNS injury, but not after CNS injury, changes in gene expression within injured neurons support robust axonal regeneration, irrespective of extracellular factors (Fig. 122-3). One demonstration of this principle comes from "preconditioning" peripheral nerve lesions. If a sciatic nerve axotomy precedes a SCI by a few days, then the central process of the sensory neuron that was previously injured in the periphery exhibits a marked degree of axonal regeneration at the SCI site. It is clear that the peripheral injury induces changes in second messengers and gene expression in the dorsal root ganglion neurons that allow CNS growth.

A number of genes exhibit altered expression after peripheral nerve injury. Among the regeneration-associated gene products (RAGs) that alter the growth state of the sensory neuron are GAP-43, CAP-23, SPRR1A, Fn14, *galanin*, *arginase* I, and HSP-27. It is unclear if the enhanced expression of one or more of these genes is sufficient for CNS axonal regeneration in vivo. There are data that combined transgenic expression of GAP-43 and CAP-23 can drive a limited degree of CNS axonal growth under certain circumstances in the CNS. It might be that multiple genes must be expressed coordinately to fully mimic the rapid growth of peripheral neurons.

SIGNALING MECHANISMS   Several signaling cascades have been demonstrated to participate in the enhanced growth state of the "preconditioned" growth state and to contribute to enhanced axonal growth. cAMP is present at high levels in developing neurons and decreases postnatally, only to be increased selectively after peripheral axonal injury. Pharmacological elevation of cAMP increases the growth of axons in culture on permissive and nonpermissive substrates. Furthermore, in vivo elevation of cAMP levels in sensory neurons allows a degree of sprouting and growth at SCI sites. These changes might be mediated at least in part through the induction of arginase I expression and increased polyamine levels.

Cytokines of the gp130 class, including LIF and IL-6, are increased in the stump of an injured peripheral nerve and in vitro application promotes axonal growth in vitro through Stat-dependent signaling. In vivo studies with knockout mice support the notion that these cytokines play a critical role in rapid peripheral axonal regeneration and contribute to the "preconditioning" effects. Because these cytokines have prominent roles in immunological responses and axonal regeneration, it is not obvious how they might alter recovery if administered locally in the brain or spinal cord.

TREATMENT OPTIONS The potential for mimicry of peripheral gene expression and second messenger changes as a therapeutic modality is large, but untested in most cases. Methods for increasing the function of individual RAGs are not well developed so in vivo data about their ability to increase CNS regeneration are few. Methods to promote cAMP and thereby enhance the growth state of neurons have received the most attention. At least for ascending sensory fibers, acute cAMP elevation appears to produce some local sprouting of injured fibers. Rolipram is a cAMP phosphodiesterase type 4 inhibitor developed originally as an antidepressant that might be most useful in testing the efficacy of this mode of therapy.

CONCLUSION

Axonal disconnection plays a major role in the persistent disability following a number of CNS injuries of traumatic, ischemic, and immunological nature. For many years, the possibility of promoting recovery from these injuries by axonal regeneration has been considered to be nil. This pessimism has been relieved by the scientific developments described. It is reasonable to suggest that rational molecular therapies will someday be employed to improve recovery. The molecular understanding of the limits on the axon regeneration process has advanced rapidly. Moreover, it has led to several methods for promoting adult CNS axonal regeneration in preclinical studies. Enhancement of axonal regeneration can be considered a novel therapeutic target for recovery from SCI, head trauma, stroke and chronic progressive MS. Treatment modalities might be developed to reduce the effectiveness of myelin inhibitors such as Nogo, MAG and OMgp acting at the NgR and of the glial scar containing CSPG inhibitors. Alternatively, enhancement of the intrinsic growth state of neurons by increasing the expression or function of RAGs might be effective. Cell transplantations might have the capacity to alter the CNS environment and support maximal axonal regeneration. Because these different potential treatments attack semi-independent mechanisms, they might have synergistic effects on improving recovery from chronic CNS axonal disconnection.

ACKNOWLEDGMENT

This work was supported by grants to S.M.S. from the National Institutes of Health (NIH), the McKnight Foundation for Neuroscience. S.M.S. is an Investigator of the Patrick and Catherine Weldon Donaghue Medical Research Foundation.

SELECTED REFERENCES

Barton WA, Liu BP, Tzvetkova D, et al. Structure and axon outgrowth inhibitor binding of the Nogo-66 receptor and related proteins. EMBO J 2003;22(13):3291–3302.

Bartsch U, Bandtlow CE, Schnell L, et al. Lack of evidence that myelin-associated glycoprotein is a major inhibitor of axonal regeneration in the CNS. Neuron 1995;15(6):1375–1381.

Bomze HM, Bulsara KR, Iskandar BJ, Caroni P, Skene JH. Spinal axon regeneration evoked by replacing two growth cone proteins in adult neurons. Nat Neurosci 2001;4(1):38–43.

Bonilla IE, Tanabe K, Strittmatter SM. Small proline-rich repeat protein 1A is expressed by axotomized neurons and promotes axonal outgrowth. J Neurosci 2002;22(4):1303–1315.

Bradbury EJ, Moon LD, Popat RJ, et al. Chondroitinase ABC promotes functional recovery after spinal cord injury. Nature 2002;416(6881): 636–640.

Cafferty WB, Gardiner NJ, Gavazzi I, et al. Leukemia inhibitory factor determines the growth status of injured adult sensory neurons. J Neurosci 2001;21(18):7161–7170.

Cai D, Deng K, Mellado W, Lee J, Ratan RR, Filbin MT. Arginase I and polyamines act downstream from cyclic AMP in overcoming inhibition of axonal growth MAG and myelin in vitro. Neuron 2002;35(4): 711–719.

Chen MS, Huber AB, van der Haar ME, et al. Nogo-A is a myelin-associated neurite outgrowth inhibitor and an antigen for monoclonal antibody IN-1. Nature 2000;403(6768):434–439.

Dergham P, Ellezam B, Essagian C, Avedissian H, Lubell WD, McKerracher L. Rho signaling pathway targeted to promote spinal cord repair. J Neurosci 2002;22(15):6570–6577.

Dou CL, Levine JM. Inhibition of neurite growth by the NG2 chondroitin sulfate proteoglycan. J Neurosci 1994;14(12):7616–7628.

Fournier AE, GrandPre T, Strittmatter SM. Identification of a receptor mediating Nogo-66 inhibition of axonal regeneration. Nature 2001;409(6818):341–346.

Fournier AE, Takizawa BT, Strittmatter SM. Rho kinase inhibition enhances axonal regeneration in the injured CNS. J Neurosci 2003;23(4): 1416–1423.

GrandPre T, Li S, Strittmatter SM. Nogo-66 receptor antagonist peptide promotes axonal regeneration. Nature 2002;417(6888):547–551.

GrandPre T, Nakamura F, Vartanian T, Strittmatter SM. Identification of the Nogo inhibitor of axon regeneration as a Reticulon protein. Nature 2000;403(6768):439–444.

He XL, Bazan JF, G M, et al. Structure of the Nogo receptor ectodomain: a recognition module implicated in myelin inhibition. Neuron 2003; 38:177–185.

Kim JE, Li S, GrandPre T, Qiu D, Strittmatter SM. Axon regeneration in young adult mice lacking Nogo-A/B. Neuron 2003;38(2):187–199.

Li S, Strittmatter SM. Delayed systemic Nogo-66 receptor antagonist promotes recovery from spinal cord injury. J Neurosci 2003;23(10): 4219–4227.

Liu BP, Fournier A, GrandPre T, Strittmatter SM. Myelin-associated glycoprotein as a functional ligand for the Nogo-66 receptor. Science 2002;297(5584):1190–1193.

Liu RY, Snider WD. Different signaling pathways mediate regenerative Vs developmental sensory axon growth. J Neurosci 2001;21(17):RC164.

McKerracher L, David S, Jackson DL, Kottis V, Dunn RJ, Braun PE. Identification of myelin-associated glycoprotein as a major myelin-derived inhibitor of neurite growth. Neuron 1994;13(4):805–811.

Merkler D, Metz GA, Raineteau O, Dietz V, Schwab ME, Fouad K. Locomotor recovery in spinal cord-injured rats treated with an antibody neutralizing the myelin-associated neurite growth inhibitor Nogo-A. J Neurosci 2001;21(10):3665–3673.

Monnier PP, Sierra A, Schwab JM, Henke-Fahle S, Mueller BK. The Rho/ROCK pathway mediates neurite growth-inhibitory activity associated with the chondroitin sulfate proteoglycans of the CNS glial scar. Mol Cell Neurosci 2003;22(3):319–330.

Mukhopadhyay G, Doherty P, Walsh FS, Crocker PR, Filbin MT. A novel role for myelin-associated glycoprotein as an inhibitor of axonal regeneration. Neuron 1994;13(3):757–767.

Neumann S, Bradke F, Tessier-Lavigne M, Basbaum AI. Regeneration of sensory axons within the injured spinal cord induced by intraganglionic cAMP elevation. Neuron 2002;34(6):885–893.

Neumann S, Woolf CJ. Regeneration of dorsal column fibers into and beyond the lesion site following adult spinal cord injury. Neuron 1999;23(1):83–91.

Niederost B, Oertle T, Fritsche J, McKinney RA, Bandtlow CE. Nogo-A and myelin-associated glycoprotein mediate neurite growth inhibition by antagonistic regulation of RhoA and Rac1. J Neurosci 2002;22(23):10,368–10,376.

Prinjha R, Moore SE, Vinson M, et al. Inhibitor of neurite outgrowth in humans. Nature 2000;403(6768):383–384.

Qiu J, Cai D, Dai H, et al. Spinal axon regeneration induced by elevation of cyclic AMP. Neuron 2002;34(6):895–903.

Richardson PM, McGuinness UM, Aguayo AJ. Axons from CNS neurons regenerate into PNS grafts. Nature 1980;284(5753):264, 265.

Schnell L, Schwab ME. Axonal regeneration in the rat spinal cord produced by an antibody against myelin-associated neurite growth inhibitors. Nature 1990;343(6255):269–272.

Simonen M, Pedersen V, Weinmann O, et al. Systemic deletion of the myelin-associated outgrowth inhibitor Nogo-A improves regenerative and plastic responses after spinal cord injury. Neuron 2003;38:201–211.

Tanabe K, Bonilla I, Winkles JA, Strittmatter SM. Fibroblast growth factor-inducible-14 is induced in axotomized neurons and promotes neurite outgrowth. J Neurosci 2003;23(29):9675–9686.

Wang KC, Kim JA, Sivasankaran R, Segal R, He Z. P75 interacts with the Nogo receptor as a co-receptor for Nogo, MAG and OMgp. Nature 2002;420(6911):74–78.

Wang KC, Koprivica V, Kim JA, et al. Oligodendrocyte-myelin glycoprotein is a Nogo receptor ligand that inhibits neurite outgrowth. Nature 2002;417(6892):941–944.

Wiessner C, Bareyre FM, Allegrini PR, et al. Anti-Nogo-A antibody infusion 24 h after experimental stroke improved behavioral outcome and corticospinal plasticity in normotensive and spontaneously hypertensive rats. J Cereb Blood Flow Metab 2003;23(2):154–165.

Zheng B, Ho C, Li S, Keirstead H, Steward O, Tessier-Lavigne M. Lack of enhanced spinal regeneration in Nogo-deficient mice. Neuron 2003;38:213–224.

PSYCHIATRY | XIV

SECTION EDITORS:
KERRY J. RESSLER AND CHARLES B. NEMEROFF

Abbreviations

XIV. PSYCHIATRY

5HT$_{1A}$	serotonin receptor
5HT1b	serotonergic autoreceptor
5HTT	serotonin transporter
ACC	anterior cingulate cortex
ACTH	adrenocorticotropic hormone
AMPA	α-amino-3-hydroxy-5-methyl-4-isoxazole propionate
ASD	acute stress disorder
AVP	arginine vasopressin
BDNF	brain-derived neurotrophic factor
BDZ	benzodiazepine
BNST	bed nucleus of the stria terminalis
BPD	borderline personality disorder
CC	corpus callosum
CCK	cholecystokinin
CCK-4	cholecystokinin tetrapeptide
Cdk5	cyclin-dependent kinase 5
CENTG2	centaurin γ-2
CNS	central nervous system
CPZ	chlorpromazine
CREB	cAMP response element-binding protein
CRF	corticotropin-releasing factor
CRH	corticotropin-releasing hormone
CRHR1	corticotropin-releasing hormone receptor 1
CSF	cerebrospinal fluid
DA	dopamine
DARPP-32	dopamine and cAMP-regulated phosphoprotein 32
DAT	DA transporter
DRD3	dopamine receptor D3
DSM-IV	*Diagnostic and Statistical Manual of Mental Disorders*
EAA	excitatory amino acid
EEG	electroencephalographic
FDG	fluorodeoxyglucose
FMRP	Fragile X mental retardation protein
GABA	γ-aminobutyric acid
GAL	galanin
GAP	GTPase-activating protein
GR	glucocorticoid receptor

GRKs	G protein receptor kinases
HPA	hypothalamic–pituitary–adrenal
HVA	homovanillic acid
LC-NE	*locus ceruleus*-based noradrenergic
LTP	long-term potentiation
MAO-A	monoamine oxidase A
MAOIs	monamine oxidase inhibitors
MAP1B	microtubule associated protein 1B
MeCP2	methyl-CpG-binding protein 2
MHC1-R	melanin-concentrating hormone receptor
MR	mineralocorticoid receptor
NAc	nucleus accumbens
NE	norepinephrine
NK-1	neurokinin 1
NMDA	*N*-methyl-D-aspartate
NPY	neuropeptide Y
OCD	obsessive-compulsive disorder
OTR	oxytocin receptor
PCP	phencyclidine
PDD-NOS	pervasive developmental disorders not otherwise specified
PDE	Phosphodiesterase
PFC	prefrontal cortex
PKA	protein kinase A
PP-1	protein phosphatase 1
PTSD	posttraumatic stress disorder
PVN	paraventricular nucleus
rCBF	regional cerebral blood flow
RGS	regulators of G protein signaling
SERT	serotonin transporter
SMC	sensorimotor control
SNPs	single-nucleotide polymorphisms
SNRIs	selective norepinephrine reuptake inhibitors
SRR	sibling relative risk
SSRI	selective serotonin reuptake inhibitor
SSRIs	selective serotonin reuptake inhibitors
V1aR	vasopressin receptor
V1b	AVP receptorWnt w/e
VTA	ventral tegmental area of the midbrain

123 Molecular Mechanisms Regulating Behavior

Focus on Genetic and Environmental Influences

KERRY J. RESSLER AND CHARLES B. NEMEROFF

SUMMARY

This chapter outlines how the preclinical fields of molecular biology and neuroscience are converging to allow for meaningful answers relevant to the molecular foundations of psychiatry. Advances over the next decades will undoubtedly provide novel and powerful tools that advance the treatment, if not cure, of devastating psychiatric disorders that not that long ago were thought to be untreatable. This introduction will examine how molecules act at different organizational levels within the brain to influence behavior. Specifically, this chapter examines how both genetic and environmental influences can alter the molecular milieu of individual neurons, discrete neural circuits, and neuromodulation throughout the brain.

Key Words: Anxiety; behavior; corticotrophin releasing factor; environment; Fragile X; gene; oxytocin; psychiatry; serotonin; synaptic plasticity; vasopressin.

INTRODUCTION

Perhaps the most complicated problem in biology is how molecules, interacting through the laws of physics, create complex behavior in animals. The molecular mechanisms that create thought, emotion, self-awareness, and consciousness in humans seem impossibly complex, and yet progress is being made. This chapter outlines how the preclinical fields of molecular biology and neuroscience are converging to begin to allow dissection of these questions in ways that provide meaningful answers relevant to the molecular foundations of psychiatry. Such advances over the next decades will undoubtedly provide novel and powerful tools that advance the treatment, if not cure, of devastating psychiatric disorders previously thought to be untreatable.

The following chapters outline first how to approach complex genetic mechanisms in psychiatry followed by discussion of the current state of knowledge regarding the molecular and genetic bases of depression, anxiety, schizophrenia, autism, post-traumatic stress disorder, and addictive disorders. This chapter examines

how molecules act at different organizational levels within the brain to influence behavior and how both genetic and environmental influences can alter the molecular milieu of individual neurons, discrete neural circuits, and neuromodulation throughout the brain.

The external environment, through various mechanisms combined under the term "stress," is known to affect the risk of psychiatric disease. However, the relative roles of environment and genetics have been heatedly debated. The pendulum of thought in psychiatry has swung from an entirely environmentally based process with the more extreme views of psychoanalysis, to a sometimes extreme biological determinism view of genetics in the latter half of the 20th century. The fields of psychology, behavioral neuroscience, molecular neuroscience, and genetics are now sufficiently advanced that a rapproachment may be possible, in which whether nature vs nurture determines behavior is no longer the question. Instead, acceptance that both clearly do create an exciting series of questions in examining, through their molecular mechanisms, "How do genes and environment work together to create behavior?"

THE COMPLEXITY OF BRAIN AND BEHAVIOR

The biological rules that govern brain function are uniquely complicated compared with other organ systems because of the biological complexity of the brain (it expresses more of the total genetic information encoded in DNA than any other organ in the body) and because the brain is continuously being molded by the environment. In fact, the most critical function of the brain may be to alter itself, i.e., to learn, through interaction with the external environment.

Furthermore, brain function cannot be inferred directly from neuronal function. This is in contrast with most other organ systems within medicine in which molecular medicine = cellular medicine = medicine. This is because in most organs, the function of the organ straightforwardly represents the function of its component cells. For example, a molecular understanding of hepatocytes or cardiac myocytes readily leads to direct predictions regarding the physiology and pathophysiology of the liver and heart, respectively. In contrast, although th̲e̲ b̲r̲a̲i̲n̲ i̲n̲c̲l̲udes neurons and glia, and the function of neurons and g̲l̲i̲a̲ i̲s̲ u̲n̲d̲e̲r̲standable, that understanding alone does not directly re̲l̲a̲t̲e̲ t̲o̲ b̲r̲a̲i̲n̲ function.

From: *Principles of Molecular Medicine, Second Edition*
Edited by: M. S. Runge and C. Patterson © Humana Press, Inc., Totowa, NJ

1175

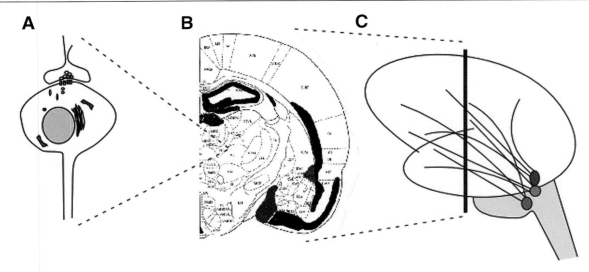

Figure 123-1 Levels of brain organization. This schematic diagram illustrates different levels of neuronal and brain organization that must be appreciated to understand the molecular mechanisms by which genes and environment influence behavior. (**A**) Cellular biology of individual neurons as well as the molecular mechanisms mediating formation and maintenance of the synapse (specialized cellular connections that permit rapid transfer of information between neurons). (**B**) Discrete neural systems perform separate functions and express different sets of genes as illustrated by this coronal section of a rodent brain in which a subset of different brain regions are highlighted. (**C**) Modulation of the different neural systems within the brain occurs at a whole brain level in part owing to neuromodulatory neurotransmitters that are released from mid-brain nuclei such as the raphe nucleus that releases serotonin, the ventral tegmental area that releases dopamine, and the locus ceruleus that releases norepinephrine.

This dissociation between neuronal cellular function and behavior occurs for several reasons. As mentioned, the complexity of gene expression in the brain is as complex as the remainder of the body. This results from genetic heterogeneity among hundreds of different types of neurons and supporting glial cells. Furthermore, groups of different neurons are molecularly, anatomically, and functionally clustered such that it may be sometimes more useful to consider each nucleus in the brain as a separate functional "organ system." For example, the striatal system appears to mediate motor learning and coordination, the amygdala system mediates fear and other emotions, and the hippocampal system mediates multiple aspects of memory formation. Even with this perspective, the complexity of these discrete brain nuclei is still more than the molecules and genes that compose them because of the nearly infinite combination of neuronal connections that occur between the 100 billion neurons and their 100 trillion synapses in the human brain.

Therefore, an effort to understand molecular mechanisms of behavior actually requires an effort to understand multiple levels of functional organization:

1. How molecules mediate individual neuronal function and connectivity.
2. How molecules influence processing of information within discrete nuclei.
3. How molecules modulate interaction between neurons and brain regions in the formation of behavior.

An understanding of the physiology and pathophysiology of behavior thus requires an integration of molecular and systems level neurobiology.

MOLECULAR MECHANISMS OF BEHAVIOR OCCUR AT MULTIPLE LEVELS OF BRAIN ORGANIZATION To understand the genetic and environmental mechanisms by which molecules affect behavior, the primary levels of organization that are differentially influenced must be clarified (Fig. 123-1). This section outlines how molecules influence cellular connectivity, regional brain specialization, and neuromodulation of multiple brain circuits. Table 123-1 summarizes the examples described below of how both genes and environmental influences are able to act through different molecular mechanisms to result in similar physiological and pathophysiological outcomes at each level of organization. These examples illustrate the multiple complex, yet eventually understandable, mechanisms by which genes and environment may interact to regulate behavior.

INFLUENCES ON NEURON FUNCTION AND CONNECTIVITY: THE ROLE OF SYNAPTIC PLASTICITY

The principle cellular function of the neuron is to receive chemical and electrical neural signals and to pass similar signals to other neurons. As with all cell types, a large variety of ion channels and pumps, neurotransmitter receptors, growth factor receptors, transcription factors, and other molecules are required for normal cellular functions. In addition to these proteins, the neuron also requires specialized machinery for the development, maintenance, and ongoing plasticity of its synapses, the specialized cellular regions in which signals are transmitted from one neuron to the next (Fig. 123-1A).

The ability to form, maintain, and eliminate synapses has tremendous importance for animal behavior. These cellular functions provide the underpinnings of learning and memory and, thus, the basis for animals to react to situations based on previous experience. Evidence suggests that cellular synaptic plasticity can be modulated by both genetic and environmental influences. One method to examine synaptic plasticity in the brain involves the visualization of synaptic spines, the dendritic specializations for synaptic inputs (Fig. 123-2A). Evidence suggests that with learning and following periods of enhanced synaptic plasticity, the number, size, and shape of synaptic spines are altered on neurons that are undergoing neural plasticity. The following two examples illustrate genetic and environmental mechanisms by which synaptic spine regulation is altered contributing to altered synaptic plasticity.

Table 123-1
Genetic Bases for Behavior

Level of organization	Gene function (example)	Behavioral function	Genetic influence	Environmental influence	Associated disorder
Intracellular/synaptic plasticity	FMR-1/FMRP is involved in dendritic translation and synaptic plasticity	Learning and memory	CGG expansion diminishes FMRP production and leads to immature spines	Enrichment enhances FMRP production and synaptic spine density	FMR1 mutation leads to Fragile X inherited mental retardation
Regional brain function	OTR/V1aR regional patterns of expression influence level of parental care and pair bonding	Social memory and behavior	Promoter polymorphisms lead to different expression patterns	Maternal Care influences levels of expression in different brain regions	Alterations in levels of oxytocin or OTR are implicated in autism and affective disorders
Central modulation of neuronal activity	5HT transporter removes synaptic 5HT 5HT1b is a 5HT autoreceptor	Behavioral state	5HTT "l" vs "s" Polymorphism. Short allele diminishes 5HTT expression	Acute stress increases 5HT1b receptor expression	Increased risk for anxiety and depression have been shown with short promoter allele of 5HTT

FRAGILE X, A GENETIC MECHANISM OF IMPAIRED PLASTICITY Fragile X syndrome is the most common form of inherited mental retardation, occurring in 1:4000 males and 1:8000 females. It is characterized by a cluster of signs in addition to mental retardation, including stereotyped facial features, macroorchidism, and abnormalities in attention and short-term memory. The disorder is now known to result from an unstable trinucleotide repeat within the gene that leads to variable lengths of repeats in different individuals. The presence of 5–50 repeats of the nucleotide sequence "CGG" leads to normal Fragile X mental retardation protein (FMRP) function. Longer series of repeats, in some individuals as many as 200 repeats, lead to a "premutation" that is still without phenotype. But in the next generation, a dramatic expansion of the repeat region occurs that is up to several thousands of nucleotides, leading to the full phenotype of Fragile X mental retardation. This occurs owing to the lack of functional FMRP.

FMRP is known to encode a mRNA binding protein that serves as a chaperone to carry mRNA from the nucleus to the cytoplasm. This function is important for many mRNAs, but particularly for dynamically regulated mRNAs such as the mRNA for microtubule associated protein 1B (MAP1B). MAP1B is one of many proteins implicated in the normal synaptic plasticity mechanisms required for normal synaptic spine function. Absence of FMRP is thought to lead to inappropriate or dysregulated MAP1B expression at the dendritic synapse, which may contribute to dysregulated synaptic plasticity, and abnormalities in dendritic spines that occur in Fragile X syndrome (Fig. 123-2B,C). The inability to form normal mature synaptic spines likely leads to dysfunctional neuronal communication in the brain and may underlie the short-term memory, attentional, and cognitive deficits seen in Fragile X syndrome.

EARLY ENRICHMENT: AN ENVIRONMENTAL MECHANISM OF ENHANCED PLASTICITY Results from several experiments suggest that following a learning event, there may be enhanced neural plasticity to alter the structure and synaptic contacts of neurons involved in this plasticity. In fact, animals that have an enriched and complex environment during development have a higher synaptic spine density in certain cortical areas than animals that were raised in standard housing containing minimal sensory stimulation. Animal data consistently shows that early

enrichment leads to more plastic brains and more dendritic spine density (Fig. 123-2D).

What leads to this increased density of synaptic spines? Early environmental enrichment likely enhances the availability of a neurotrophic growth factor in the brain, brain-derived neurotrophic factor (BDNF), which has been implicated in enhancing the learning process and synaptic spine density in certain brain areas. Furthermore, clinical depression has been associated with lowered BDNF levels in certain regions of the brain, and data suggest that the complex phenotype of depression results partly from lowered synaptic plasticity during the depressed phase. Certain animal models of depression also are characterized by decreased BDNF concentrations, and early environmental enrichment appears to partially prevent depression-like phenotypes in those animals.

INFLUENCES ON REGION-SPECIFIC BRAIN FUNCTION: THE ROLE OF NEUROPEPTIDE SPECIALIZATION

Regional circuits contribute to specific brain functions resulting in distinct behaviors. Some genes, such as the homeobox family and other similar transcription factors, act during development to determine regional brain specialization. Differential gene expression in the adult contributes to the specialized connectivity and function of different brain regions. Despite this developmental determination of regional function, the levels and patterns of expression of certain genes can still be influenced by environmental experience. The following examples of genetic and environmental control of regional gene expression involve the vasopressin receptor (V1aR) and oxytocin receptor (OTR) genes. These neuropeptide receptors have significant influence on sexual and social behavior, and are implicated in the stress response and the biology of depression.

GENETIC CONTROL OF REGIONAL NEUROPEPTIDE RECEPTOR EXPRESSION DETERMINES SEXUAL BEHAVIOR Exclusive mating for life between a male and female of the same species is called pair bonding. This occurs in some monogamous species, whereas other species are entirely polygamous. How does this difference arise? One particularly powerful model of pair bonding is the vole, a rodent species slightly larger than a mouse. Remarkably, behavioral scientists observing animal behavior in the

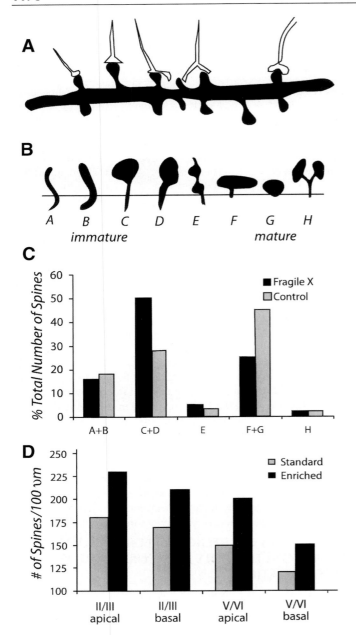

Figure 123-2 Development of synaptic spines as a marker of synaptic plasticity. **(A)** Schematic illustration of the many synaptic contacts (on the order of 1000 per neuron) that occur between presynaptic axon terminals connecting onto synaptic spines of a region of a pyramidal neuron dendrite within the brain. **(B)** Synaptic spines have different morphologies at different times following their induction as illustrated by spines A–H. **(C)** Graph illustrating the relative immaturity of synaptic spines in Fragile-X syndrome as compared to control human brains (B,C adapted from Greenough et al. 2001 with permission.). **(D)** Total number of synaptic spines in different layers of cortex (II, III, V, VI) of rats that were housed in standard conditions vs those housed in enriched environments. (Adapted from Johansson and Belichenko, 2002 with permission.) This illustrates the enhancement of synaptic connectivity that occurs with environmentally enriched stimuli.

wild noted that one species (the prairie vole) pair bonded, whereas a very similar species (montane vole) was highly polygamous. Gene expression was examined in the brains of these animals looking for correlations between pair bonding and gene expression. Although

the animals were almost identical in their genomes and in their brain expression pattern, they exhibited one critical difference. In males, it is known that the neuropeptide vasopressin is critical for sexual behavior and is released with mating, whereas in females, the neuropeptide oxytocin has a similar role. In the brains of the monogamous species, the V1aR in males and the OTR in females was found to be highly expressed in a region of the brain called the ventral striatum or nucleus accumbens, an area known to be involved in appetitive learning and reward (Fig. 123-3A). In contrast, the polygamous species had similarities in patterns of vasopressin and OTR expression in many areas of the brain, except for the ventral striatum, in which there was very little or no receptor expression.

Further experiments suggest that this differential expression pattern may lead to a conditioned learning event following mating. Thus the monogamous animals may associate their partner as a highly rewarding neural signal whereas the polygamous animals do not undergo that conditioning event. This difference in expression pattern is in part because of variation in the promoter regions of these receptors. These results imply that genetic control of regional expression of neuropeptide receptors can exert profound effects on the behavioral state of the organism.

Oxytocin is likely involved in many social behaviors in addition to pair bonding. Autism is a highly genetic disorder that involves profound disruption of social learning. Autism has recently been suggested, at least in some cases, to involve disruption within the oxytocin system.

ENVIRONMENTAL CONTROL OF NEUROPEPTIDE RECEPTOR EXPRESSION BY VARIATION IN MATERNAL CARE

Despite the previously mentioned data that neuropeptide receptor expression, specifically the OTR, is highly genetically controlled, there is now considerable evidence that environmental signals also exert control over expression of this receptor during development. In addition to its role in pair bonding, OTR levels may be involved in differential sensitivity to experimental measures of anxiety as well as other social behaviors. Numerous environmental effects have been identified that influence social behavior and anxiety measures. One of the most interesting and clinically relevant models is of variations in maternal care. Within the same species of lab rats, there are individual variations in levels of maternal nurturing as measured by licking, grooming, and nursing behaviors. Adult offspring of mothers that were observed to have high levels of nurturing maternal care (e.g., high levels of licking/grooming and arched-back nursing), are consistently found to appear less anxious in numerous behavioral models, even though there are no obvious differences in health, weight, or other general physical measures.

Their data suggest that such variation in maternal care lead to early developmental changes in gene expression within the brain. In fact OTR levels in females and V1aR levels in males are increased within the central nucleus of the amygdala in offspring of more nurturing mothers (Fig. 123-3B). It is important to note that these variations in maternal care can be entirely different based on early environmental exposure, independent of genotype. Cross-fostering studies show that animals raised by highly nurturing foster mothers are more social, less anxious, and express more OTR or V1aR than do those raised by less nurturing foster or natural mothers. These findings suggest that variations in maternal care may influence the expression of oxytocin and vasopressin in a gender-specific manner. Although the genetic mechanisms have not yet been elucidated, it is likely that such dynamic regulation of these neuropeptide receptors involves both genetically determined promoter polymorphisms and

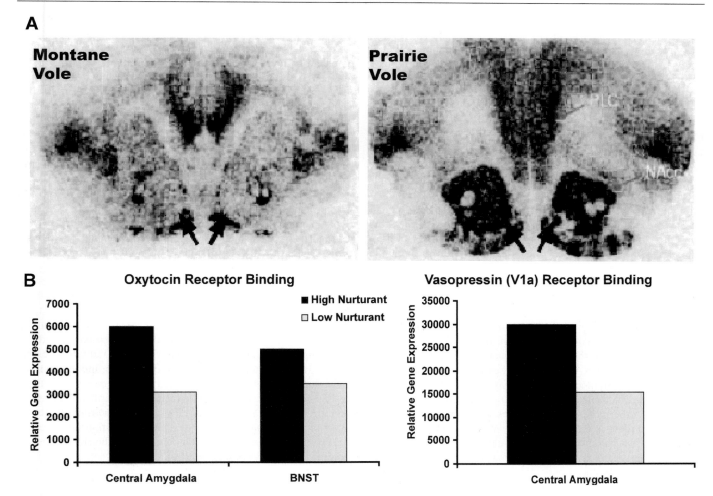

Figure 123-3 Oxytocin and vasopressin receptor expression in specific brain regions. (**A**) Figure showing expression of the oxytocin receptor, as demonstrated with receptor binding autoradiography, in the polygamous montane vole or the monogamous prairie vole. This genetic control increased receptor expression in the nucleus accumbens, a brain region important in reward, is thought to contribute to the monogamous sexual behavior of the prairie vole. (Adapted from Insel and Young, 2001.) (**B**) Total level of oxytocin receptor in female rats (left graph) or vasopressin receptor in male rats (right graph) is partially a function of rearing environment. The animals raised by mothers that were highly nurturant (as indicated by increased licking, grooming, and arched-back nursing behavior), had offspring with higher levels of oxytocin and vasopressin receptor gene expression in the central amygdala and nucleus of the stria terminalis (BNST), two regions implicated in emotional and social learning and behavior. (Adapted from Francis et al. 2002.)

environmentally determined molecular factors that provide modulatory control over the expression of these receptors.

INFLUENCES ON NEUROMODULATORY CIRCUITS: THE ROLE OF CENTRALLY ACTING NEUROTRANSMITTERS

This chapter has focused on the roles of individual neuron function and connectivity and the importance of regional gene expression in contributing to behaviorally important functions. The broadest mechanism by which genes and molecules can influence behavior is through action at the level of the entire brain. In fact the majority of psychiatric medications are active at this level—on the neuromodulatory neurotransmitters, specifically monoamines such as serotonin, norepinephrine, and to a somewhat lesser extent, dopamine. These three neurotransmitter systems are similarly organized anatomically, with their primary releasing neurons located in the midbrain, and their axonal projections reaching throughout the entire brain. The regulated firing of these modulatory systems has

tremendous impact on "states" of brain function such as level of arousal, attention, sleep/wake, vigilance, or relaxation. Central neuromodulation of multiple brain circuits occurs to coordinate activity of different brain regions and circuits. Genes determine aspects of this modulation, yet the *tone* of these systems is regulated through environmental experience.

Although there are many different neuropeptide and neurotransmitter modulatory systems within the brain, the following examples illustrate how the serotonin transporter and a specific serotonin receptor are regulated. Serotonin is produced by the raphe nuclei within the midbrain and is released by raphe neuronal projections throughout the brain. Serotonin neurotransmission is clearly dysregulated in depression and anxiety-related disorders. In general, cerebrospinal fluid measurements have revealed decreased concentrations of serotonin, or its major metabolite, 5-hydroxy-indoleacetic acid. There is also evidence of brain alterations from postmortem studies and functional brain imaging studies in serotonin receptor binding in depression. In general, antidepressants enhance serotonergic transmission by a variety of mechanisms throughout the brain. Although serotonin clearly has many functions, one of its roles is the proper modulation of limbic circuits, including the hippocampus and amygdala, during the experience of emotional stimuli. Alterations in the serotonin system, both in the raphe neurons and in target postsynaptic neurons can have profound effects on emotional behavior.

GENETIC CONTROL OF SEROTONIN TRANSPORTER EXPRESSION INFLUENCES ANXIETY The primary mechanism of action of the selective serotonin reuptake inhibitor antidepressants is binding and inhibiting the serotonin transporter (5HTT). The 5HTT protein is located primarily on presynaptic nerve terminals, and plays a critical role in removing serotonin from the synapse and thus in terminating the neurotransmitter signal. Selective serotonin reuptake inhibitors, through inhibiting this transporter, initially enhance serotonin release throughout the brain. After several weeks of treatment with this class of medication, the serotonergic system shows altered firing patterns. It is thought that this long-term adaptation is integral for the antidepressant effect.

Studies examining polymorphisms of the 5HTT gene have revealed interesting aspects of its regulation and potential effects of this regulation on mood and anxiety disorders. The long (l) variant of a promoter polymorphism within the 5HTT gene is more than twice as active as the short (s) variant. This is because of differences in 5HTT mRNA synthesis and expression resulting from the promoter polymorphism. Increased anxiety traits and increased traits of "neuroticism" are associated with the less active "s" allele. Furthermore in some studies, the response to antidepressant treatment is different in patients with homozygous "s" alleles such that patients with the "s" allele are more resistant to antidepressant treatment. Another approach to examining antidepressant function has been to deplete the availability of the amino acid tryptophan, a precursor to serotonin, during the treatment response period on antidepressants. Patients with the "s" allele of 5HTT are more likely to experience a rapid return of depressed symptoms during tryptophan depletion than are patients with the more active "l" allele. Through such mechanisms of altered promoter regulation of 5HTT, genetic control over the central serotonergic modulatory system can significantly influence risk for depression and anxiety, as well as response to treatment.

ENVIRONMENTAL REGULATION OF SEROTONIN RECEPTORS IN ANIMAL MODELS OF STRESS Through genetic knockout models and by examination of levels of receptor expression, the serotonergic autoreceptor (5HT1b) has also been implicated in response to stress and antidepressant action. The 5HT1b receptor is located on presynaptic axon terminals of raphe neurons and is involved in regulating serotonin release onto target neurons. Decreased 5HT1b binding intensity has been demonstrated in cortex, hippocampus, and septum after acute stress in rats. These changes were seen in conjunction with decreased 5HT1b mRNA expression in the dorsal raphe nucleus.

5HT1b expression was measured within the dorsal raphe nucleus in two different rodent models of differential stress sensitivity, congenital learned helplessness and maternal separation. The congenital learned helplessness model involves the development of two lines of rats through differential breeding that are either highly susceptible or resistant to developing learned helplessness. Learned helplessness is a model in which rats receive repeated inescapable shocks resulting in behavior that appears less active and socially withdrawn and is accompanied by neurochemical indicators of

depression. It is an often-utilized model of depression that exhibits antidepressant responsiveness.

Maternal separation is another widely-used model in which rat pups are removed from their mother for 3 h daily from postnatal d 2–14. As adults, these animals are then compared on a number of behavioral measures with controls that were removed from their mother for only 15 min daily over the same time period. This maternal separation paradigm leads to reproducible behavioral effects mimicking depression and anxiety in the adult. Interestingly, the animals removed for only 15 min daily appear to have more resistance to depressive symptoms following stress than do control (animal facility reared) animals. This suggests that such environmental models may model risk for depression following stress, but may also provide a model of resilience.

A number of molecular studies have been performed with the learned helplessness and maternal separation models of depression. These studies have clearly demonstrated that chronic inescapable stress leading to learned helplessness as well as early alterations in maternal care can both have profound effects on the molecular milieu within the brain. In particular, the levels of 5HT1b-receptor expression have been examined in both of these models of depression. There are differences in levels of 5HT1b-receptor expression in acutely stressed animals vs unstressed animals, suggesting that there are rapid changes in serotonin receptor levels in the aftermath of environmentally induced stress. Receptor levels were also examined in both models of stress-resilience, the line of rats that is resistant to learned helplessness and the rat pups that experienced 15 min of maternal separation. Both models of stress resilience showed elevations in levels of 5HT1b-receptor gene expression compared to the stress-sensitive controls. These results suggest that there are differences in 5HT1b levels in animals that are sensitive vs those that are resilient to stressful situations.

The two different approaches also provide for interesting interaction between genetic differences (as seen in the congenital learned helplessness lines) or environmental insult (maternal separation) and environmental stress experienced in adulthood. It is remarkable that the genetic model exhibiting lowered activity of 5HTT and the environmental model with less 5HT1b may both result in similar neural phenotypes—decreased feedback control of serotonin levels at the synapse.

ENVIRONMENTAL REGULATION OF CORTICOTROPIN-RELEASING FACTOR IN ANIMAL MODELS OF STRESS Another neuromodulatory neurotransmitter that clearly shows environmental regulation is the corticotropin-releasing factor (CRF) neuropeptide. There is abundant evidence that CRF and related peptides are the primary CNS mediators of stress. Stress generally is defined as extraordinary demand on the organism or alterations in psychological homeostatic processes. Initially its importance was thought to be primarily endocrine via activation of adrenocorticotropic hormone from the pituitary, with subsequent release of cortisol and other glucocorticoids from the adrenal gland. However, its role in the brain independent of the hypothalamus–pituitary–adrenal axis has been firmly established. Consistent with its role as a neurotransmitter mediating complex repertoires, CNS administration of CRF mimics many of the behaviors and autonomic responses seen with physiological stress.

There are multiple experimental paradigms implicating the central CRF system as the prime mediator of the acute and prolonged stress response. Rodents administered CRF directly into the CNS

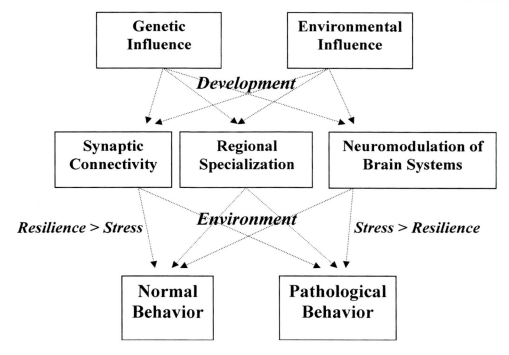

Figure 123-4 Interaction of genetic and environmental influences on behavior. Schematic diagram illustrating the interaction through development of genetic and environmental influences on different levels of brain organization. Interplay between developmental genetic programs and environmental insults leads to differential effects on synaptic connectivity, regional neural systems, and brain-wide neuromodulation. Normal behavior results when the genetic and environmental influences lead to resilience outweighing stress effects on brain and behavior. Alternatively, when either too much stress or too little resilience interact pathological behavior arises in the form of psychiatric syndromes.

show decreased reproductive behaviors, altered sleep, increased grooming, increased signs of despair, increased neophobia, and altered appetite, all of which mimic the behavioral stress response. Furthermore, rodents raised with early life-stress hypersecrete CRF from the hypothalamus and amygdala, both during the stress and later as adults. The maternal separation paradigm previously described leads to offspring with enhanced levels of apparent anxiety and depressive symptoms. Such animals have enhanced levels of CRF mRNA expression as well as enhanced release of CRF. Early untoward life events associated with development of depression and anxiety in adulthood give rise to long-lasting changes in CRF neurons, thus, increasing individual vulnerability for affective and anxiety disorders.

INFLUENCE OF GENETICS, DEVELOPMENT, AND ENVIRONMENT TO CREATE INDIVIDUAL BEHAVIOR

Considerable effort has been expended to develop a valid animal model of depression. Virtually all of the extant models have focused on either developmental (maternal separation) or environmental (learned helplessness) chronic unpredictable stress to generate a depressed phenotype. Additional animal models have been created through the use of mice with transgenic DNA insertion or homologous recombination (knockouts). One of the most impressive models is the serotonin receptor ($5HT_{1A}$) knockout. Mice lacking this receptor exhibit anxiety and fear behavior in several behavioral paradigms. Elegant molecular biology techniques have been used to "rescue" the phenotype of these knockout animals. In a $5HT_{1A}$ mutant mouse background strain, a tissue specific promoter is used to replace the $5HT_{1A}$ gene within neurons of the hippocampus,

amygdala, and forebrain, but specifically not the raphe nuclei in which serotonin is produced. This limited expression is sufficient to normalize the behavioral phenotype of $5HT_{1A}$ knockout mice. This suggests that it is the $5HT_{1A}$ gene in postsynaptic neurons within these target areas that contributes to the development of anxiety-like behavior, and not its role in auto-feedback on the raphe neurons themselves. Finally, use of a conditional gene that can be replaced for a limited period of time has shown that the replacement is only necessary during development. If the $5HT_{1A}$ gene is replaced only during the first month of life, but is absent again in adulthood, the animal shows normal levels of anxiety-like behavior as an adult. However, if it is replaced only in adulthood and not earlier during development, the behavioral phenotype is not restored. These data reveal how a specific interaction between a gene and development can lead to establishing normal and abnormal adult anxiety-like behavior in the context of stressful environments.

PSYCHOPATHOLOGY RESULTS FROM INTERACTION OF GENETIC RISK FACTORS WITH ENVIRONMENTAL INSULTS

Neither genetics nor environmental influences alone lead to behavior. Rather, both normal and abnormal states of behavior result from an intricate interaction in which environmental influences are limited by genetic programs to produce a functioning brain and its resultant behavior. Figure 123-4 illustrates schematically how these different influences combine to produce behavior, both normal and pathological.

The relative contributions of genetics, development, and stress contributing to illness are becoming understood in terms of brain biology. Temperamental influences clearly place "reactive" infants and behaviorally inhibited children at higher later risk for anxiety and affective disorders. Substantial data is accumulating supporting the preeminent role of early adverse experience in increasing vulnerability for mood and anxiety disorders. The complex interaction of environment with the 5HTT gene, specifically this "l" vs "s" promoter polymorphism discussed above, affects the risk of depression. This polymorphism moderated the influence of stressful life events on depression. Individuals with one or two copies of the short allele of the 5HTT exhibited more depressive symptoms than did those homozygous for the long allele. However, this difference in depression symptomatology was only seen in individuals who reported early stressful life events. Furthermore, there was a clear interaction between number of stressful life events and depressive symptoms in the "s" allele carriers, but not in the "l" allele homozygotes.

Through molecular mechanisms that affect the way neurons communicate with each other, the way region-specific genes are regulated, and the way in which brain-wide neuromodulation occur, genetic constraints interact with environmental influences to produce behavior, both normal and abnormal. Abnormalities in behavior lead to the symptom clusters that occur in psychiatric disease. For example, in clinical depression, patients are generally hypersensitive to stress and fear states. They are more likely to experience anxiety, defeat, and anger as well as having decreased attention and concentration. They are unable to experience pleasure and have very low self esteem. They also show neurovegetative signs of altered appetite, libido, and energy. The paragraph below outlines how these symptom clusters can arise from the impaired neural pathways that result during depression.

Genetic predispositions and environmental influences affect the neural circuits that mediate stress responsiveness and modulation of emotion. The alterations in midbrain neuromodulatory systems likely contribute to these increased vulnerabilities. With sufficient stress, these systems are dysregulated, leading to increased stress and fear responsiveness. Hypersensitive limbic pathways lead to experiences of defeat, anxiety, anger, negative mood, and aggression. Abnormal cortical regulation through altered plasticity mechanisms and abnormal neuromodulation likely underlies impaired concentration and memory, worry, and inability to control negative thoughts. Hypothalamic abnormalities likely contribute to altered appetite, libido, energy, and autonomic symptoms. Brainstem and thalamic abnormalities likely contribute to altered sleep and arousal states.

Treatment of depression and anxiety with antidepressants leads to alterations in these and related abnormal circuits, not necessarily resulting in normalization of the circuitry, but with amelioration in the symptoms. It is likely that there are many different pathways for the brain to become dysregulated leading to a syndrome of depression, and that different combinations of genetic and environmental influences can interact. Treatment may now appear similar for all types of depressive syndromes, but new data suggest that subtypes of depression indeed respond differentially to different treatments, for example, psychotherapy vs pharmacotherapy.

CHALLENGES FOR THE FUTURE

A primary goal of psychiatry is to continue to uncover the molecular mechanisms underlying mental health diseases. As these mechanisms are further elucidated, they will provide further understanding of the role of both environment and genetics in the molecular underpinnings of psychiatry. More importantly with such an understanding, more will be possible in prevention of environmental insults as well as in the availability of novel molecular targets for drug development.

Further understanding of genetic contributions to psychiatric illness will also provide powerful tools for evaluating an individual's genetic risk. Understanding risk may help physicians counsel patients to help them reduce subsequent environmental insults. Further understanding of genetic and environmental molecular mechanisms may help guide pharmacotherapy and psychotherapy in determining optimal individualized treatment.

Finally for the more severe psychiatric illnesses such as schizophrenia and bipolar disorder, knowing significant risk might be helpful for prevention through both pharmacological and psychotherapeutic means. Additionally, such awareness of risk would assist in initial diagnosis, helping to significantly curb illness onset and severity when symptoms first appear.

A much greater understanding of brain function may allow for the eventual combined understanding of genetic and environmental influences on molecules, cells, circuits, and systems within the brain. Through such advances in understanding, more powerful models of psychiatric disease are possible, with the effect of eventually developing psychopharmacological agents that target only the specific molecular "lesions" affected in the individual patient. As the brain is an organ for learning, there may be new approaches using combined pharmacotherapy with psychotherapy, in which the pharmacological approach is aimed specifically at enhancing the learning and utilization of the psychotherapy tools. Through such approaches, ways may be found to use the molecules of pharmacology to target the molecular deficits and new "environmental" experiences that allow the brain to correct itself in individual-specific ways.

ACKNOWLEDGMENT

The authors are in part supported by grants from NIMH, NARSAD, and the Rockefeller Brother's fund Culpeper scholarship.

SELECTED REFERENCES

Avissar S, Schreiber G. Toward molecular diagnostics of mood disorders in psychiatry. Trends Mol Med 2002;8(6):294–300.

Blakely RD. Physiological genomics of antidepressant targets: keeping the periphery in mind. J Neurosci 2001;21(21):8319–8323.

Bucan M, Abel T. The mouse: genetics meets behaviour. Nat Rev Genet 2002;3:114–123.

Caldji C, Tannenbaum B, Sharma S, Francis D, Plotsky PM, Meaney MJ. Maternal care during infancy regulates the development of neural systems mediating the expression of fearfulness in the rat. Proc Natl Sci USA 1998;95:5335–5340.

Caspi A, Sugden K, Moffitt TE, et al. Influence of life stress on depression: moderation by a polymorphism in the 5-HTT gene. Science 2003;301(5631):386–389.

Chakravarti A, Little P. Nature, nurture and human disease. Nature 2003;421:412–414.

Francis DD, Diorio J, Plotsky PM, Meaney MJ. Environmental enrichment reverses the effects of maternal separation on stress reactivity. J Neurosci 2002;22(18):7840–7843.

Francis DD, Young LJ, Meaney MJ, Insel TR. Naturally occurring differences in maternal care are associated with the expression of oxytocin and vasopressin (V1a) receptors: gender differences. J Neuroendocrinol 2002; 14:349–353.

Gingrich JA, Hen R. Dissecting the role of the serotonin system in neuropsychiatric disorder using knockout mice. Psychopharmacology (Berl) 2001;155:1–10.

Greenough WT, Klintsova AY, Irwin SA, Galvez R, Bates KE, Weiler IJ. Synaptic regulation of protein synthesis and the fragile X protein. Proc Natl Acad Sci USA 2001;98(13)7101–7106.

Gross C, Zhuang X, Stark K, et al. Serotonin1A receptor acts during development to establish normal anxiety-like behaviour in the adult. Nature 2002;416:396–400.

Hariri AR, Mattay VS, Tessitore A, et al. Serotonin transporter genetic variation and the response of the human amygdala. Science 2002; 297(5580):400–403.

Heim C, Nemeroff CB. Neurobiology of early life stress: clinical studies. Semin Clin Neuropsychiatry 2002;7:147–159.

Heim C, Nemeroff CB. The role of childhood trauma in the neurobiology of mood and anxiety disorders: preclinical and clinical studies. Biol Psychiatry 2001;49:1023–1039.

Insel TR, Young LJ. The neurobiology of attachment. Nat Rev Neurosci 2001;2:129–136.

Johansson BB, Belichenko PV. Neuronal plasticity and dendritic spines: effect of environmental enrichment on intact and postischemic rat brain. J Cereb Blood Flow Metab 2002;22:89–96.

Kagan J, Snidman N. Early childhood predictors of adult anxiety disorders. Biol Psychiatry 1999;46:1536–1541.

Kandel E, Schwartz J, Jessell T. Principles of Neural Science. New York: McGraw-Hill, 2000.

King JA, Campbell D, Edwards E. Differential development of the stress response in conditional learned helplessness. Int J Dev Neurosci 1993;11:435–442.

Lesch KP, Bengel D, Heils A, et al. Association of anxiety-related traits with a polymorphism in the serotonin transporter gene regulatory region. Science 1996;274(5292):1527–1531.

Lombroso PJ. Genetics of childhood disorders: XLVIII. Learning and memory, part 1: Fragile X syndrome update. J Am Acad Child Adolesc Psychiatry 2003;42(3):372–375.

MacGregor AJ, Sneider H, Schork MH, Spector TD. Twins: novel uses to study complex traits and genetic diseases. Trends Genet 2000;16(3): 131–134.

Manji HK, Drevets WC, Charney DS. The cellular neurobiology of depression. Nat Med 2001;7(5) 541–547.

Mann JJ, Huang YY, Underwood MD, et al. A serotonin transporter gene promoter polymorphism (5-HTTLPR) and prefrontal cortical binding in major depression and suicide. Arch Gen Psychiatry. 2000;57(8): 729–738.

Meaney MJ. Maternal care, gene expression, and the transmission of individual differences in stress reactivity across generations. Annu Rev Neurosci 2001;24:1161–1192.

Nemeroff CB, Owens MJ. Treatment of mood disorders. Nat Neurosci 2002;5(Suppl):1068–1070.

Neumaier JH, Edwards E, Plotsky PM. 5-HT1b mRNA Regulation in two animal models of altered stress reactivity. Biol Psychiatry 2002;51: 902–908.

Ressler KJ, Nemeroff CB. Role of serotonergic and noradrenergic systems in the pathophysiology of depression and anxiety disorders. Depress Anxiety 2000;12:2–19.

Rutter M. The interplay of nature, nurture, and developmental influences. Arch Gen Psychiatry 2002;59:996–1000.

Sanchez MM, Ladd CO, Plotsky PM. Early adverse experience as a developmental risk for later psychopathology: evidence from rodent and primate models. Dev Psychopathol 2001;13:419–449.

Seong E, Seasholtz AF, Burmeister M. Mouse models for psychiatric disorders. Trends Genet 2002;18(12):643–650.

Tamminga CA, Nemeroff CB, Blakely RD, et al. Developing novel treatments for mood disorders: Accelerating discovery. Biological Psych 2002;52(6)589–609.

Volkmar FR, Greenough WT. Rearing complexity affects branching of dendrites in the visual cortex of the rat. Science 1972;176:1445–1447.

124 The Complex Genetics of Psychiatric Disorders

MING T. TSUANG, STEPHEN J. GLATT, AND STEPHEN V. FARAONE

SUMMARY

Unlike many single-gene neurological disorders such as Huntington's disease, neurofibromatosis, and Rett syndrome, most psychiatric illnesses are etiologically complex. It is this complexity that stands as the major obstacle hindering risk-gene identification in psychiatry, and all of the diagnostic, therapeutic, and preventive advances that such discoveries might engender. Linkage and association analyses will probably be able to resolve some of the genetic complexity of many psychiatric conditions; but it is also likely that emerging disciplines, such as systems biology and functional genomics, will inform traditional genomic methods to hasten the compilation of a full catalog of susceptibility genes for psychiatric illness.

Key Words: Heterogeneity; oligogenic; polygenic; pooling; psychiatric disorders; splitting.

INTRODUCTION

The methods of genetic epidemiology, particularly twin and adoption studies, have unequivocally demonstrated that most if not all psychiatric disorders have some genetic basis. However, the relative contribution of genetic and nongenetic factors to the development of each of these illnesses varies widely. For conditions such as autism, bipolar disorder, and schizophrenia, genes are responsible for the majority of total illness susceptibility, whereas the genetic contribution to risk for other conditions such as social phobia and several personality disorders is low (Table 124-1). For the more genetically driven psychiatric illnesses, it was anticipated that the unraveling of the human genome would facilitate the determination of their genetic underpinnings, but this idea is largely unrealized. Few specific genetic risk factors for even the most heritable and most commonly studied psychiatric conditions (e.g., autism, bipolar disorder, and schizophrenia) have been identified; even fewer have been validated in independent samples, and none have been evaluated prospectively.

Although much more genetic and genomic analysis of psychiatric illnesses remains to be done, it is apparent at this relatively early stage of inquiry that traditional gene-finding strategies will not easily yield the goal of psychiatric genetic inquiry—a specific genetic etiology for a given illness. If the emergent harnessing of the human genome is expected to produce dividends for the diagnosis, treatment, and ultimately prevention of psychiatric disorders, understanding of these illnesses must grow, along with the scope of genetic epidemiological methods used. Unlike many single-gene neurological disorders such as Huntington's disease, neurofibromatosis, and Rett syndrome, most psychiatric illnesses are etiologically complex. It is this complexity that stands as the major obstacle hindering risk-gene identification in psychiatry, and all of the diagnostic, therapeutic, and preventive advances that such discoveries might engender.

THE GENETIC COMPLEXITY OF PSYCHIATRIC DISORDERS

The main factors contributing to the complexity of psychiatric disorders can be broadly divided into those that relate to the small size and great quantity of risk factors for these conditions, and those that produce various types of heterogeneity. Of note, both classes of complicating factors are problematic because of their effects on inferential power. For example, regarding the first complicating factor, genetic epidemiological methods and molecular genetic techniques consistently demonstrate that psychiatric illnesses are not caused by single genes that always precipitate illness in all individuals possessing the gene. Rather, these procedures typically yield evidence for multiple (sometimes many) susceptibility genes, each of which may have a relatively restricted effect on the total risk for a given disease. Regarding the second factor, the complexity introduced by heterogeneity can come from the nonuniformity of the phenotype, whereby the same genes can produce numerous distinct clinical pictures, or from the nonuniformity of the etiological factors, which can produce different paths to the same disease.

Psychiatric geneticists now appreciate that even the most advanced molecular and statistical genetic techniques will not have optimal power unless each of these complicating factors—multiple risk genes with small effects, and heterogeneity—are adequately addressed in research studies even before the first piece of data is collected. Common strategies for overcoming these obstacles to risk-gene discovery are discussed later, along with the negative consequences that may be realized if these steps are not taken.

From: *Principles of Molecular Medicine, Second Edition*
Edited by: M. S. Runge and C. Patterson © Humana Press, Inc., Totowa, NJ

Table 124-1
Heritability and Status of Association Testing of Various Psychiatric Disorders

Psychiatric disorder	Heritability (%)	Allelic association studies (n)
Autism	93	56
Tourette's disorder	90	27
Schizoaffective disorder	85	34
Bipolar disorder	84	287
Schizophrenia	84	487
Narcissistic personality disorder	79	–
Obsessive-compulsive personality disorder	78	–
Cannabis abuse	76	–
Attention-deficit/hyperactivity disorder	75	114
Conduct disorder	74	10
Anorexia nervosa	71	29
Stuttering	70	5
Antisocial personality disorder	69	35
Borderline personality disorder	69	4
Obsessive-compulsive disorder	68	43
Histrionic personality disorder	67	–
Stimulant abuse	66	1
Hallucinogen abuse	65	–
Gender identity disorder	62	–
Oppositional defiant disorder	61	2
Nicotine dependence	60	15
Sleepwalking	60	–
Sedative abuse	59	–
Alzheimer's disease	58	894
Dependent personality disorder	57	–
Bulimia nervosa	55	7
Dyslexia	53	3
Post-(assaultive)traumatic stress disorder	53	4
Dissociative identity disorder	48	–
Pathological gambling	46	5
Panic disorder	43	38
Suicide	43	73
Nightmare disorder	41	–
Agoraphobia	38	6
Opiate (heroin) abuse	38	30
Postpartum psychosis	38	2
Major depression	37	139
Narcolepsy	37	32
Alcohol abuse	36	256
Cocaine abuse	32	10
Generalized anxiety disorder	32	7
Insomnia	32	–
Schizoid personality disorder	29	–
Seasonal affective disorder	29	3
Simple phobia	29	7
Avoidant personality disorder	28	–
Paranoid personality disorder	28	–
Schizotypal personality disorder	28	–
Social phobia	25	6
Enuresis	24	1

THE COMPLEX, MULTIFACTORIAL POLYGENIC ETIOLO-GIES OF PSYCHIATRIC DISORDERS The greatest contributions of the molecular genetic revolution to medicine have been in the identification of individual genes that are solely responsible for the development of hundreds of devastating diseases, including cystic fibrosis, phenylketonuria, thalassemias, myotonic dystrophy, fragile-X syndrome, and some forms of breast cancer, in addition to the neurological disorders introduced previously. The practical impact of these discoveries is realized on a daily basis in the forms of increased diagnostic certainty for these diseases, targeted treatments at the molecular level, prenatal diagnoses, and personal and familial risk assessments. These are also the ambitious goals of those who study psychiatric conditions, but these objectives can only be reached after the elusive genes underlying these conditions are finally isolated, and this task has proven far more difficult than initially anticipated.

Before modern molecular genetic techniques made genome-wide DNA analysis possible, the mathematical analysis of illness transmission through pedigrees was used to test hypotheses about the number and mode of inheritance of genes underlying these disorders. These mathematical techniques, collectively known as segregation analysis, generally did not support single-gene inheritance models of autism, Tourette's disorder, bipolar disorder, schizophrenia, schizoaffective disorder, attention-deficit/hyperactivity disorder, or alcohol abuse, among other psychiatric illnesses. Instead, the etiologies of these disorders were more often found to be consistent with oligogenic (caused by a few genes) or polygenic (caused by many genes) inheritance patterns; however, the precise number of risk genes estimated to be responsible for each disorder typically varied across studies. Today, most cases of psychiatric illness are presumed to have multifactorial polygenic etiologies, in which numerous genetic and environmental risk factors interact; however, a small fraction of families exhibit evidence for rare single-gene forms of some psychiatric illnesses, including bipolar disorder, major depression, obsessive–compulsive disorder, dyslexia, and panic disorder.

Because the previously mentioned psychiatric disorders were known from twin studies to have such a strong genetic component (Table 124-1), the technological advances in molecular genetics made during the 1970s and 1980s ushered in a period of great optimism in the possibility of finally localizing and identifying their causative genes. Initially, the chromosomal loci of the genes for autism, bipolar disorder, and schizophrenia were sought by methods of linkage analysis, which correlate phenotypic and genetic similarity among family members to allow the identification of broad chromosomal regions that may be involved in the disease. Evidence suggesting genetic linkage to these and other disorders soon followed, generating a great deal of excitement that the genes underlying these disorders were finally within reach. However, as attempts were made to replicate these findings, a disturbing pattern emerged: very few of the initially implicated chromosomal regions showed evidence of linkage with these diseases in other samples, although loci previously determined to be unlinked showed evidence for linkage. This problem of nonreplication increased as more reports emerged, suggesting the possibility that these studies were actually underpowered to produce similar patterns of results if these disorders were, in fact, polygenic. For example, simulated data has been used to show that typically designed linkage studies have adequate power to detect any one out of a number of linked loci, but low power to detect a particular target locus (as might be the goal of a replication study).

The shortcomings of linkage analysis have been demonstrated through the use of simulated data; between 185 and 4260 families (depending on the frequency of the disease allele) would be needed to detect a locus containing a gene with a relative risk of 4 by linkage analysis; yet the vast majority of linkage studies of psychiatric disorders have sampled far fewer than 200 families each. Hence at best, such studies may be detecting those chromosomal loci harboring the genes with the greatest effects on risk but, presumably, the numerous genes that confer less than a fourfold increase in disease risk would go undetected. In fact, to detect linkage at a chromosomal locus harboring a gene that confers a relative risk of 1.5 for a given disease (i.e., the gene increases risk by 50%), the number of families needed for analysis becomes unreasonably large; the number is so excessive (between approx 18,000 and 4.6 million families, depending on the disease-allele frequency) that such a quantity of eligible pedigrees would likely never be attainable for even the most common psychiatric conditions. Thus, it would not be expected that the loci of genes that carry a relative risk of 1.5 would ever be implicated in individual linkage studies of even several hundred families.

For this reason, allelic association analysis, which directly tests for linkage disequilibrium between a genetic marker and a disease gene, has been advanced by some as a more powerful gene-finding strategy for complex disorders with presumed polygenic etiologies. For example, a gene carrying a relative risk of 1.5 for a given disorder would be detectable by allelic association testing in as few as 949 or as many as 19,320 parent–child trios (depending on the proportion of heterozygous parents in the sample). Even in the worst-case scenario, this sample size compares favorably with the more than 4.6 million families that would be needed to detect this locus by linkage analysis, especially when considering the relative ease of ascertaining trios with one affected offspring for association analysis vs ascertaining families with affected sibling-pairs for linkage analysis.

Psychiatric geneticists have tried to leverage the greater power and efficiency of allelic association analysis to find genes for many psychiatric illnesses, including each of those disorders that had previously been examined for genome-wide linkage and many other disorders that had not yet been the subject of linkage analysis. The results of more than 2600 allelic association studies of psychiatric disorders have been published (Table 124-1), and many significant associations have been noted. However, as with linkage analyses, allelic association analyses also suffer from a bewildering propensity for nonreplication. This phenomenon is especially frequent for complex diseases, including psychiatric disorders. In some instances, nonreplication of a documented association becomes so frequent that the initial finding of association becomes rightly seen as a type-I inferential error. Other apparent nonreplications are simply resulting from random sampling errors around a small but real effect. Thus, although one study may detect an association that is slightly larger (and more significant) than the true association, another study will detect a smaller (and nonsignificant) effect. The true nature and magnitude of such associations may be eventually clarified after several replication studies have been conducted; but for some associations, even numerous replication efforts fail to clarify the issue. This variability illustrates the need for strategies that maximize the power to detect genes with very small effects on risk, even within the relatively powerful association analysis paradigm.

Thus, some of the great etiological complexity of psychiatric disorders is a function of the large number and small magnitude of their underlying genetic risk factors. The shortcomings of linkage and association analyses for identifying the risk genes for these disorders (or even their general chromosomal location) are most visible as a chronic failure to replicate even the strongest evidence for the involvement of particular genes or loci. This, however, does not necessarily indicate that these methods are somehow faulty and will never be used to successfully locate the risk genes for psychiatric disorders. On the contrary, these methods may ultimately prove to be the best possible means of accomplishing this goal. However, there clearly is room to improve on these methods, and to implement them in more powerful ways in order to hasten the discovery of the risk genes for this group of complex disorders.

THE HETEROGENEITY OF PSYCHIATRIC DISORDERS   In addition to the fact that most psychiatric disorders have multifactorial polygenic etiologies with multiple underlying risk genes of small effect, the heterogeneity of these disorders contributes to the difficulties experienced in isolating their risk genes. Two main types of heterogeneity can be delineated: clinical heterogeneity and causal heterogeneity. Clinical heterogeneity exists in which more than one condition can be brought about by the same cause, although causal heterogeneity exists in which two or more causes can independently lead to the same condition. Through different means, both forms of heterogeneity serve to obscure the effects of risk genes, delaying and sometimes even preventing their identification.

Clinical heterogeneity is a problem for psychiatric genetics because it complicates the proper identification and ascertainment of individuals who may be carrying the same risk genes. For example, in a given family through which several risk genes for schizophrenia are segregating, the individual family members may present with a wide range of illness, from full schizophrenia through none at all. Between these extremes, other family members may display varying degrees of illness, receiving diagnoses of conditions that appear to be more or less related to schizophrenia. For example, some individuals may be diagnosed with schizoaffective disorder, whereas others receive a diagnosis of schizotypal personality disorder, and still others do not qualify for any commonly accepted diagnosis but still show subtle signs of disruption in particular domains of social and neuropsychological functioning. These intermediate conditions, or schizophrenia-spectrum conditions, are more common among the biological relatives of schizophrenic patients than among the relatives of control subjects or in the general population, suggesting that they share some genetic basis with schizophrenia. It is also common for schizophrenia and other psychiatric conditions to show some degree of discordance between monozygotic twins, who share 100% of the same genes. Findings such as these evoke a critical question: Why do related individuals who share the same genetic risk factors (to a greater or lesser degree, depending on the nature of their relationship) have different psychiatric outcomes?

To answer this question, the multifactorial polygenic nature of psychiatric disorders must be considered; that is, even the most heritable of these conditions have some environmental underpinnings. Thus, in families in which risk genes for a highly genetically based disorder are shared, the resulting differences in the degree of psychiatric impairment among individual family members are governed by environmental factors, in which the most severely affected members may be those who, in addition to possessing the risk genes, also were subjected to unfavorable environmental circumstances. The combination of enough detrimental genetic and environmental risk factors may ultimately cause an individual's total susceptibility to surpass some threshold level, beyond which the full disorder (in this case, schizophrenia) would be expressed. Conversely, psychiatrically well members of families with a high genetic propensity toward illness may not have experienced any such environmental circumstances or, indeed, may have been exposed to protective environmental factors. Those family members expressing varying degrees of schizophrenia-spectrum deficit may have varying combinations of these risk factors, some individuals with more genetic risk and others with more environmental risk. Such a "multifactorial threshold" model fits familial patterns of illness for many complex psychiatric disorders, including schizophrenia.

Thus, the possession of specific risk genes for a complex illness (or a specific environmental factor, for that matter) does not place an individual at absolute risk for that disorder; this is the essence of complex diseases. Possessing such risk factors may place an individual along a continuum of risk for that illness, which may or may not correspond to the actual presentation of some or all of the features of the illness. This information is reassuring to those individuals from affected families, as they can recognize that their genetic susceptibility to disease is not absolute and can be modified by environmental variables. However, such phenomena make the identification of risk genes much more difficult than would be the case if every individual with the same genes exhibited the same phenotype. Thus, in linkage and association studies, the incomplete penetrance of risk genes (i.e., their less-than-absolute causation of disease) will lead some subjects who possess those risk genes to be labeled as well. Consequently, the possession of those particular risk genes in well individuals will cause the evidence for the involvement of those genes in the disease to appear weaker.

The other dimension of heterogeneity—causal heterogeneity—is probably common in psychiatric disorders. If these disorders are caused by the interaction of many genetic and environmental factors, it is likely that no single factor is either necessary or sufficient to produce disease. If each genetic and environmental risk factor independently increases risk by a small amount, it may be the total liability that is achieved (rather than the identity of its constituent factors) that determines illness. For example, if there were 10 risk factors that predisposed to schizophrenia-spectrum illness (five genes and five environmental experiences), but only four of these (in any combination) were needed to reach the threshold for full schizophrenia, there would be 210 different routes to schizophrenia. Some of these etiological paths would overlap almost entirely, some only partially, and others not at all. In addition, some of these paths to schizophrenia would be entirely genetically determined, whereas others would be produced by a combination of genes and environmental factors. Other cases (called phenocopies) might be caused solely by environmental factors. Phenocopies are particularly problematic for genetic studies because they will be counted as affected individuals but will show no evidence implicating the risk genes that underlie the true genetic or partially genetic forms of the disease, with a net effect of reducing the strength of genetic linkage or association detected in the group of affected individuals.

Alzheimer's disease is a prototypical example of a psychiatric illness with heterogeneous causation. For example, mutations in any one of three different genes (amyloid-β precursor protein, presenilin-1, or presenilin-2) will almost invariably cause Alzheimer's disease, independent of the presence of other risk genes or deleterious environmental circumstances. To add to this complexity, the familial, early-onset forms of the disorder caused by mutations in any of these genes only account for a small fraction of the total cases of Alzheimer's disease. In fact, the majority of cases are probably attributable to an unknown combination of genetic and environmental factors, although several specific risk genes are becoming recognized, including α-2-macroglobulin, angiotensin I converting enzyme 1, and apolipoprotein E.

The presence of multiple genetic paths to psychiatric illness will have clear detrimental effects on the power of positional cloning studies. For example, the genetic signals obtained in an unfocussed search for genetic risk factors, as typically conducted by linkage analysis, might go unnoted unless specific allowances for heterogeneity are built into the underlying statistical models of inheritance. Furthermore, the genetic signals obtained from a focused examination of a candidate gene, as in an allelic association study, could be reduced or potentially eliminated if, for example, the cause of the illness in the sampled population is a gene or genes other than the candidate gene being investigated.

UNRAVELLING THE COMPLEX GENETICS OF PSYCHIATRIC DISORDERS

It is clear that the multifactorial polygenic etiologies and heterogeneity of psychiatric disorders obscure the discovery of their underlying genetic bases. The multifactorial polygenic nature of these diseases dictates that the "signals" obtained in linkage and association studies will be numerous and of very low intensity, although the heterogeneity of these disorders increases the "noise" against which these already-faint signals must be detected. Some of the most effective ways of combating these complexities are through the maximization of power, both by increasing sample size and by studying homogeneous groups of affected individuals. To identify the numerous genes with small effects on the risk of psychiatric illness, various data-pooling strategies (collectively referred to as "pooling") are particularly effective. However, to overcome the obstacles introduced by heterogeneity, delineating and studying smaller, more homogeneous subgroups of affected individuals (called "splitting") may have the greatest beneficial effects on power. When used in tandem, the practices of pooling and splitting yield maximal power in genetic studies.

POOLING STRATEGIES FOR RESOLVING THE MULTIFACTORIAL POLYGENIC NATURE OF PSYCHIATRIC ILLNESSES As previously illustrated, statistical simulations indicate that the power of typically designed linkage and association studies is woefully inadequate for detecting genes with very small effects on disease risk (e.g., relative risk = 1.5). Unfortunately, the genes underlying most psychiatric disorders are likely to have relative risks on approximately this order of magnitude. Thus, one of the greatest challenges to the successful implementation of these methods is their low power, limited by the typically low sample size of individual studies. Large collaborative studies and meta-analyses of existing datasets offer opportunities to overcome this obstacle.

Indeed, the psychiatric linkage analysis literature has already been clarified by meta-analyses of linkage studies for schizophrenia, bipolar disorder, and autism, which have revealed strong evidence for multiple linked loci for each disorder. For example, individual linkage analyses of schizophrenia have found at least suggestive (if not significant) evidence for linkage with the disease in no less than 16 distinct chromosomal regions (Fig 124-1). However, two different meta-analytic pooling techniques have produced evidence for only three strongly linked loci, one of which (centromeric region of chromosome 2p) was in a location not strongly implicated in any of the individual linkage analyses. The meta-analyses of bipolar disorder and autism linkage analysis

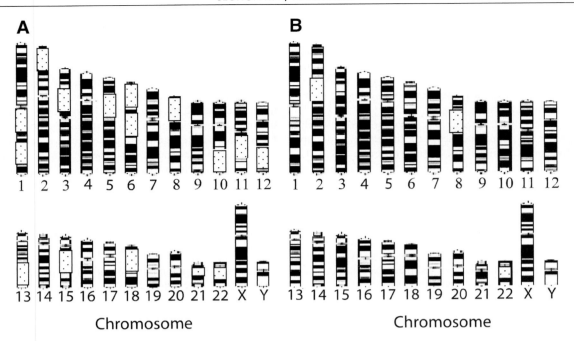

Figure 124-1   Chromosomal loci showing at least suggestive evidence for linkage (⬚) with schizophrenia in at least one individual linkage study (**A**) and in both meta-analyses of linkage studies (**B**).

datasets have been equally enlightening, and suggest clear targets for further analysis by both linkage and association methods.

Although these meta-analyses provide useful directions for future positional cloning efforts, they are unlikely to have detected all the genes involved in these disorders. Linkage methods and the resulting meta-analyses of their data may detect loci that harbor genes with the largest effects on disease susceptibility, but other disease loci with smaller yet meaningful effects on risk will elude detection. For example, recalling that between 185 and 4260 families would be needed to detect a locus containing a gene with a relative risk of 4.0 by linkage analysis, it is reasonable to presume that these meta-analyses (which have pooled data from 700 or fewer families) did not detect all susceptibility loci for these diseases. Again, the number of families needed to detect a chromosomal locus harboring a gene with a relative risk of 1.5 (between 18,000 and 4.6 million families) is not even approached in these meta-analyses.

The tangible impact of this "power failure" can be seen in a concrete example from the psychiatric genetic literature. For example, not a single linkage analysis for schizophrenia, nor either of the meta-analyses of these linkage studies, identified chromosome 3q as a strong candidate locus for the disease; yet, the gene that codes for dopamine receptor D3 (DRD3, chromosome 3q13.3) carries a relative risk for schizophrenia of 1.3 or less, an effect which has been repeatedly demonstrated by allelic association, and confirmed in separate meta-analyses of these association studies. This finding is a direct result of the greater power of association studies relative to linkage studies and, consequently, the greater power of meta-analyses of association studies as well. Again, recalling that a gene conferring a relative risk of 1.5 can be detected in as few 949 trios by allelic association (as opposed to 18,000 or more families for linkage analysis), many associations with psychiatric disorders have already been tested often enough to yield pooled samples with enough power to detect these small but important associations; the

meta-analyses of the association between DRD3 and schizophrenia, each with pooled sample sizes of greater than 2600 patients and 2500 control subjects, again provides a compelling example. Thus, it appears that one of the simplest ways to overcome the fact that most psychiatric disorders have numerous risk genes with small effects is to maximize inferential power by increasing sample size. However, such maximization of power, either through collaborative studies or meta-analysis, is not the only option for improving risk-gene detection methods when individual genetic effects are small. In fact, the ability to identify risk genes with small effects can be enhanced as a byproduct of implementing procedures that also overcome the difficulties introduced by clinical and causal heterogeneity.

SPLITTING STRATEGIES FOR OVERCOMING THE HETEROGENEITY OF PSYCHIATRIC DISORDERS   Clinical and causal heterogeneity are detrimental to gene-finding efforts for complex diseases to the degree that they obscure detection of the effects of individual risk genes by increasing the "noise" surrounding them. In the case of clinical heterogeneity, the improper or incomplete specification of the affected phenotype may cause misclassification of subjects, allowing some overlap of risk genes to be detected in affected and unaffected individuals in which no such overlap truly occurs. Similarly, the apparent effects of genes are reduced in the presence of causal heterogeneity: because several nonoverlapping or partially overlapping genetic etiologies may exist in a population, a given genetic risk factor may not be present in a large proportion (perhaps even the majority) of individuals with a disorder.

In overcoming these difficulties, simply increasing sample sizes by pooling may not be enough. Instead, splitting techniques (e.g., cluster analysis, recursive partitioning, and classification and regression trees) may yield greater gains in power through the delineation of smaller (rather than larger) groups of subjects. The objective of this splitting strategy is to delineate homogeneous subgroups of a disorder that are clinically distinct from each other, under the assumption that clinical homogeneity within groups reflects (at least to some degree) underlying etiological or causal homogeneity. Within such causally homogeneous subgroups, the genetic risk should be more uniform and, thus, the effects of risk genes will be more pronounced and easily detected. In essence, this strategy is designed to maximize the observable genetic signal within a given subgroup although minimizing the noise that might typically arise from jointly examining groups of individuals whose seemingly identical conditions are caused by partially or entirely distinct etiologies.

In practice, splitting techniques are most effective when used in conjunction with (not in opposition to) pooling techniques. The maximization of sample size through pooling affords greater power and reliability to the splitting methods that will be subsequently employed. In addition, pooling before splitting will ensure that delineated subgroups have large enough sample sizes to be powerful samples on their own. The pooling-then-splitting method can be applied in single studies, given that they have large enough samples; however, power will be greatest when data can be directly pooled from multiple samples. These methods can also be applied to published studies through the use of meta-analytic methods, whereby studies can be divided into subgroups based on some design feature, or heterogeneity among the pooled studies can be explained by regressing the size of the genetic effect obtained in each study against key characteristics of those studies, such as sample ethnicity or age-at-onset in the patient group.

THE FUTURE OF GENE-FINDING EFFORTS FOR PSYCHIATRIC DISORDERS

It is likely that even if the pooling and splitting strategies advocated above are implemented, other methods will be needed to comprehensively delineate the genetic contributions to psychiatric disorders. Methods in use in other fields of medical research, such as immunology, cell biology, and physiology, may be used to meaningfully contribute to the search; however, it is also likely that new and developing methods will lead to gene discovery. A brief review of some of these promising techniques clearly shows that emerging methods of genomic and postgenomic analysis emphasize high throughput and comprehensiveness, allowing research to remain hypothesis-driven whereas simultaneously employing broader, more inclusive standards in identifying potential "candidate" genes for study.

MINING THE TRANSCRIPTOME, THE PROTEOME, AND BEYOND As twin and adoption studies clearly show, most psychiatric illnesses have a genetic component, i.e., at least some of the susceptibility to these illnesses is passed vertically through generations by the inheritance of particular DNA sequence variations. For this reason, the search for risk genes for these disorders naturally began with the study of DNA sequence variation in multiply affected pedigrees by linkage analysis and in nuclear families and individuals by association analysis. However, the analysis of DNA sequence variations does not tap all of the complexity of the human genome, and cannot account for heritable variations in gene expression that may also play a critical role in disease development. These so-called epigenetic phenomena may be better understood by analyzing the RNA transcripts and proteins specified by genes.

DNA sequence variations dictate which RNA transcripts and, ultimately, which proteins can be produced by cells. However, other factors govern these processes as well, and the rate and location of

transcript and protein production may also be influenced by extragenomic factors. Transcripts and proteins can be viewed as more proximal than genes to the disease state, which has made them logical targets for study in postgenomic analyses. Microarray technologies, in which the expression levels of thousands of genes can be simultaneously examined, are now being used to assess altered patterns of gene regulation in various psychiatric illnesses, including autism, major depression, schizophrenia, and bipolar disorder.

Microarray analyses are valuable because the expression of many genes can be examined simultaneously. Unfortunately, because of alternate splicing of transcripts and post-translational modifications in proteins, the number of transcripts and proteins available for study is far greater than the number of genes in the genome. Thus, these procedures, although potentially powerful, further illustrate the potential genomic and extragenomic complexity that may be encountered in the comprehensive analysis of psychiatric disorders at the molecular level.

MULTI-INFORMANT ANALYSIS No existing or forthcoming genetic analysis method is likely to solve all of the problems encountered while hunting the genes for mental illnesses. More likely, as when studying other difficult problems in science, a combination of approaches will prove the most useful in understanding psychiatric phenomena in all of their complexity. Researchers are becoming increasingly aware that individual methods employed at a single level of analysis cannot hope to capture the essence of these disorders, which most likely involves changes at many levels of numerous biological systems. Also, adopting an interdisciplinary perspective allows optimal utilization of valuable research resources; the richness of samples collected for genetic studies (from clinical data, to pedigree structures, to biological samples) is too great to be analyzed by a single method.

The field of psychiatric genetics is gravitating toward systems biological and integrative behavioral genomic approaches wherein multiple sources of information are used to build a preponderance of evidence implicating particular risk genes. Historically, the results of linkage analyses (i.e., linked chromosomal loci) have been used to inform the approach of association studies (i.e., targeted gene analysis within the linked region). This approach is now expanding to incorporate the findings from many other sources, including gene expression data and animal models of psychiatric illness. For example, in a typical microarray analysis of several thousand genes, many may appear to be differentially expressed in brain tissue from patients and control subjects. Although ideally each of these genes would then be investigated further for association with the disorder, practical constraints may hinder the implementation of this plan. Instead, the genomic location of each differentially expressed gene can be examined within the context of previous findings from linkage analyses of the disorder under investigation. Thus, those genes coding to a chromosomal region previously found linked to the illness can be given the highest priority for association analysis. If significance is observed in association analysis, the functional consequences of the responsible polymorphism can be investigated in transgenic or knockout animal models of the disease.

The advantages of employing such an integrative approach are clear. First, the inclusion of high-throughput methods in the chain of research will allow the identification of novel, previously unsuspected candidate genes for further analysis. Indeed, one of the major drawbacks of traditional allelic association testing is the paucity of objective criteria (aside from being in a linked chromosomal region) for selecting candidate genes for study. In addition, relying solely on the results of linkage analysis to inform association testing is far from optimal because, as illustrated, linkage analysis is not very sensitive for detecting genes with very small effects on risk and, furthermore, association can sometimes occur in the absence of linkage. Second, the analysis of functional consequences of gene variation or epigenetic modification on transcription, translation, and behavior in animal models will provide some insights into the molecular mechanisms of these diseases. Finally, and perhaps most critically, a multidisciplinary and integrative approach will allow for the assessment and establishment of concurrent validity for genes putatively identified as risk factors by one method, thus, ensuring greater accuracy and reliability in classifying susceptibility genes for psychiatric disorders.

CONCLUSIONS

Psychiatric disorders are undeniably complex diseases. The etiology of all but a few of these conditions remain unknown, despite profound advances in the methods of psychiatric genetic epidemiology and statistical and molecular genetics. The tools of modern molecular genetic inquiry are useful in establishing the genetic bases of disorders caused exclusively by individual disease-genes; however, these tools may be suboptimal (at least as they are currently employed) for unraveling the multiple complex interactions of genetic and environmental risk factors that determine the liability toward most psychiatric illnesses. Yet, these methods should not be disregarded; rather, they should be utilized in a manner that maximizes their power. Two general methods to enhance the power of positional cloning methods such as linkage and allelic association analyses include pooling methods, in which raw data or individual studies are combined in collaborative studies or meta-analyses, and splitting methods, in which the genetic signal-to-noise ratio is maximized by delineating homogeneous subgroups of affected individuals that may have shared paths to disease. When these strategies are implemented jointly, linkage and association studies of complex psychiatric conditions will be maximally—if not optimally—powered to identify risk genes. However, until these disorders are more thoroughly investigated with positional cloning methods, it will remain unknown if maximal power equals adequate power for accomplishing these objectives. Linkage and association analyses will probably be able to resolve some of the genetic complexity of many psychiatric conditions; but it is also likely that emerging disciplines, such as systems biology and functional genomics, will inform traditional genomic methods to hasten the compilation of a full catalog of susceptibility genes for psychiatric illness.

ACKNOWLEDGMENTS

Preparation of this chapter was supported in part by the National Institute of Mental Health Grants 1R01MH41879091, 5 U01 MH4631820, 1R37MH4351801, and R25 MH60485 to Dr. Ming T. Tsuang and the Veterans Administration's Medical Research, Health Services Research and Development and Cooperative Studies Programs, and by a NARSAD Distinguished Investigators Award to Dr. Tsuang.

SELECTED REFERENCES

Bunney WE, Bunney BG, Vawter MP, et al. Microarray technology: a review of new strategies to discover candidate vulnerability genes in psychiatric disorders. Am J Psychiatry 2003;160:657–666.

Dubertret C, Gorwood P, Ades J, Feingold J, Schwartz JC, Sokoloff P. Meta-analysis of DRD3 gene and schizophrenia: Ethnic heterogeneity and significant association in Caucasians. Am J Med Genet (Neuropsychiat Genet) 1998;81:318–322.

Faraone SV, Tsuang MT. Familial links between schizophrenia and other disorders: application of the multifactorial polygenic model. Psychiatry 1988;51:37–47.

Faraone SV, Tsuang D, Tsuang MT. Genetics of mental disorders: A guide for students, clinicians, and researchers. New York: Guilford, 1999.

Hanash S. Disease proteomics. Nature 2003;422:226–232.

Kendler KS. Twin studies of psychiatric illness: an update. Arch Gen Psychiatry 2001;58:1005–1014.

Kendler KS, Karkowski-Shuman L, O'Neill A, Straub RE, MacLean CJ, Walsh D. Resemblance of psychotic symptoms and syndromes in affected sibling pairs from the Irish study of high-density schizophrenia families: evidence for possible etiologic heterogeneity. Am J Psychiatry 1997;154:191–198.

Niculescu AB, Segal DS, Kuczenski R, Barrett T, Hauger RLK, Jr. Identifying a series of candidate genes for mania and psychosis: a convergent functional genomics approach. Physiol Genomics 2000;4:83–91.

Rao DC, Province MA, eds. Genetic Dissection of Complex Traits. San Diego, CA: Academic Press, 2000.

Reich T, Rice J, Cloninger CR, Wette R, James JW. The use of multiple thresholds and segregation analysis in analyzing the phenotypic heterogeneity of multifactorial traits. Ann Hum Genet 1979;42:371–389.

Risch N, Merikangas K. The future of genetic studies of complex human diseases. Science 1996;273:1516, 1517.

Suarez BK, Hampe CL, Van Eerdewegh P. Problems of replicating linkage claims in psychiatry. In: Gershon ES, Cloninger CR, Barrett JE, eds. Genetic Approaches in Mental Disorders. Washington, DC: American Psychiatric Press, 1994; pp. 23–46.

Van Duijn CM, Van Broeckhoven C, Hardy JA, et al. Evidence for allelic heterogeneity in familial early-onset Alzheimer's disease. Br J Psychiatry 1991;158:471–474.

125 Treating Depression

Antidepressant-Activated Signaling Pathways as a Source for Novel Drug Targets

MARCELO PÁEZ-PEREDA AND FLORIAN HOLSBOER

SUMMARY

Different hypotheses explain the etiology of depression. Each focuses on different biological processes that contribute to explain the clinical manifestation of depression and connect the regulation of mood to other biological processes such as the stress response and feeding behavior. Most likely, these different signaling pathways converge at a certain point to specifically control mood. This convergence point may control neurotransmission, in particular, long-term potentiation in the hippocampus. This opens the possibility that by dissecting pathways activated by antidepressants it would be possible to find new targets for novel drugs with a direct and specific mechanism of action, likely producing novel antidepressants with a higher potency, a faster action and fewer side effects.

Key Words: Antidepressant; calcium signaling; corticosteroid receptor; depression; monoamine.

INTRODUCTION

Current antidepressant treatments are efficacious. However, they work in only 70–80% of patients and often take often more than 5–8 wk to elicit patient response. Moreover, current treatment modalities are burdened by adverse effects and often produce only a partial remission, a risk factor for early relapse. To overcome these constraints, new molecular targets for antidepressant compounds are needed. Possible strategies to find these targets can be grouped into hypothesis-based and unbiased approaches. One possible strategy is to take advantage of the dissection of the signal transduction pathways that mediate the effects of the current antidepressants beyond the membrane receptor level. Alternative strategies are based on unbiased approaches that use gene expression profiling with DNA microarrays and proteomics or genome-wide genetic linkage.

There are examples that suggest that both approaches, hypothesis-based and unbiased, can be successful to find candidate targets. The pathway dissection of the monoamine-directed antidepressants led to the identification of the cAMP pathway as a key transduction mechanism. This led to the proposal that the use of phosphodiesterase (PDE) inhibitors would increase the effectiveness of monoamine therapies, which proved to be true. In another example, derived from the corticosteroid receptor hypothesis of depression, the use of glucocorticoid receptor (GR) antagonists may exert antidepressant effects. A pitfall of hypothesis-based approaches is that they suffer from the intrinsic limitations of the hypothesis on which they are based. It is not always straightforward to conclude that the function of a candidate target gene is involved in the control of mood or whether it is involved in related mechanisms that could produce side effects. Therefore, better drugs could be designed if the molecular pathways of the successful antidepressants are better known and new targets are identified. The use of unbiased approaches offers the possibility of overcoming these limitations. They also offer the theoretical possibility of finding targets that avoid side effects produced by known antidepressants. Unbiased approaches could be based on the identification of specific gene expression patterns using DNA microarrays or proteomics. As a proof of concept, an unbiased approach using gene expression profiling by microarrays identified components of the Wnt pathway as responsive to antidepressant treatment. Independent evidence proved that the mood stabilizer lithium chloride regulates the Wnt pathway. Yet another unbiased approach is the genome-wide scanning for DNA markers that could be associated with depression. There is evidence that risk factors for depression have genetic components. The use of genetic linkage studies may, therefore, identify these genes, providing more insight into the mechanisms that control mood, which could be used as novel targets to develop antidepressants. After the candidate gene identification process, further experimental proof of the specific involvement of these genes in the control of mood is required. Particularly in the case of unbiased approaches, the large amount of candidate targets poses the problem of prioritizing and selecting the best candidates for further studies.

This chapter explores different approaches to define the signal transduction pathways involved in antidepressant action and proposes criteria to prioritize candidate targets for antidepressant compounds.

From: *Principles of Molecular Medicine, Second Edition*
Edited by: M. S. Runge and C. Patterson © Humana Press, Inc., Totowa, NJ

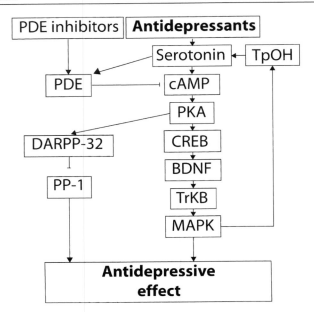

Figure 125-1   Schematic diagram of the signaling pathway mediated by monoamines activated by antidepressant treatment. BDNF, brain-derived neurotrophic factor; DARPP-32, dopamine and cAMP-regulated phosphoprotein 32; MAPK, mitogen-activated protein kinase; PP-1, protein phosphatase 1; PDE, phosphodiesterase; CREB, cAMP-response element-binding protein; PKA, protein kinase A.

THE MONOAMINE HYPOTHESIS

The first tricyclic antidepressants and monoamine oxidase inhibitors were discovered by serendipity. Both classes empirically showed improvement of symptoms in depressive patients. Later, the discovery of these compounds' biochemical mechanism of action led to the monoamine hypothesis of depression. Both types of antidepressants increase the levels of monoamines either by inhibiting their uptake by monoamine transporters (tricyclic antidepressants) or by inhibiting their inactivation (monoamine oxidase inhibitors). The development of selective serotonin or norepinephrine reuptake inhibitors has produced improved antidepressants, at least regarding their side-effect profiles. All of these compounds produce an increase in the extracellular levels of serotonin, norepinephrine, or dopamine. These monoamines, in turn, bind to their specific receptors at the plasma membrane and modulate the adenylate cyclase. Therefore, long-term antidepressant treatment results in the activation of the cAMP signal transduction pathway, mainly in the hippocampus and the forebrain (Fig. 125-1). This pathway further leads to the activation of protein kinase A (PKA) and the activation of the transcription factor cAMP-response element-binding protein (CREB). The involvement of this signal transduction pathway in chronic antidepressant action and its relevance for drug discovery is further emphasized by the fact that PDE inhibitors that increase cAMP levels, such as rolipram, increase the efficacy of antidepressants in clinical trials. CREB overexpression in the hippocampus driven by a viral vector produces antidepressant effects. However, the null mutation of CREB also produces antidepressant-like effects. Therefore, CREB activity in different brain areas might have opposite impacts on mood. One of the target genes of CREB is brain-derived neurotrophic factor (BDNF) (see Fig. 125-1). Antidepressant treatment results in the upregulation of BDNF, which is mediated by CREB. The administration of antidepressants together with the

PDE inhibitor rolipram produces a strong increase in BDNF expression, supporting the involvement of the cAMP pathway in the effects of antidepressants on BDNF expression (see Fig. 125-1). BDNF itself has antidepressant actions when injected in high doses in the rat midbrain, suggesting that BDNF may mediate the antidepressant effects on mood. A proposed mechanism for BDNF antidepressant action involves its effects on neural plasticity and survival (see Fig. 125-1). BDNF also enhances long-term potentiation (LTP) and other forms of synaptic plasticity. The extrapolation of these results supports the view that BDNF could promote cell survival and neurogenesis in the hippocampus. Therefore, BDNF could hypothetically contribute to prevent or repair the neuronal damage induced by stress. However, definitive evidence that BDNF expression in the hippocampus is involved in antidepressant mechanisms is still missing. An alternative explanation for the antidepressant-like effects produced by BDNF in the hippocampus is that BDNF could increase the expression of tryptophan hydroxylase, which would increase serotonin levels and produce an indirect antidepressant effect (see Fig. 125-1).

BDNF knockout mice show an obese phenotype, suggesting that the induction of BDNF expression by antidepressants might be involved in the coordination between anxiety and appetite instead of the direct control of mood. Other proteins phosphorylated by PKA, independently from CREB and BDNF, could mediate the effects of antidepressants on mood. One of the PKA substrates activated in response to antidepressants is the dopamine and cAMP-regulated phosphoprotein 32 (DARPP-32) (see Fig. 125-1). Fluoxetine, serotonin, and serotonin receptor agonists cause phosphorylation of DARPP-32. At least some of the effects of DARPP-32 are mediated by protein phosphatase 1 (PP-1), which, in turn, regulates c-fos. This pathway is also reduced in DARPP-32-deficient mice but definite proof of this pathway's involvement in antidepressant effects is still needed.

THE CORTICOSTEROID RECEPTOR HYPOTHESIS

One of the main components of the stress response is the activation of the hypothalamic–pituitary–adrenal (HPA)-axis. Corticotropin-releasing hormone (CRH) is produced in the hypothalamus, and it stimulates the release of adrenocorticotropic hormone (ACTH) in the pituitary gland, which, in turn stimulates the production of glucocorticoids (Fig. 125-2). CRH production in response to stress is controlled by the hippocampus and the amygdala. An excessive activation of the HPA-axis is one of the main neuroendocrine alterations in patients with depression. CRH administration in different areas of the brain in rodents induces many of the symptoms observed in depressive patients. The ACTH increase in response to CRH injection and the suppression of cortisol in response to dexamethasone are absent in patients with depression. These responses follow the disease's clinical course and the improvement of these parameters precedes a successful response to antidepressant treatment. Therefore, CRH overproduction is thought to play a causative role in the development of depression. According to the Munich vulnerability study, the alterations in the HPA-axis also happen in healthy relatives of depressive patients. This strongly indicates that risk factors for depression have genetic components. The corticosteroid receptor hypothesis provides a mechanistic basis to explain the involvement of CRH in depression (see Fig. 125-2). Mineralocorticoid receptors (MRs) are localized in the hippocampus and control the inhibitory tone on hypothalamic CRH production by binding to endogenous glucocorticoids. CRH, in turn, also controls the levels

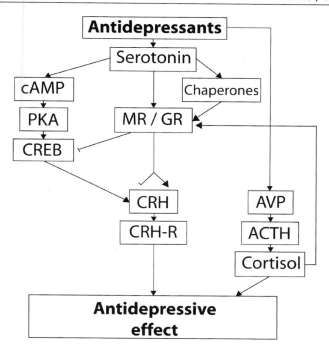

Figure 125-2 Diagram of the interactions between the corticosteroid receptors, the HPA-axis and the signaling pathways activated by antidepressants. ACTH, adrenocorticotropic hormone; CREB, cAMP-response element-binding protein; PKA, protein kinase A; MR/GR, mineralocorticoid receptor/glucocorticoid receptor; CRH, corticotrophin-releasing hormone; CRH-R, corticotrophin-releasing hormone receptor; AVP, arginine vasopressin; HPA, hypothalamic–pituitary–adrenal.

of corticosteroid receptors. Therefore, CRH overproduction in depressive patients could result from a dysfunction of MR inhibitory mechanism or from a dysfunction of corticosteroid receptors caused by CRH overproduction. In any case, the interaction between corticosteroid receptors and CRH plays a central part in the pathogenesis of depression. Further supporting evidence is the fact that long-term antidepressant treatment increases the mineralocorticoid and GR levels in the hippocampus and normalizes the levels of CRH production (*see* Fig. 125-2). Two possibilities that are not mutually exclusive may explain the antidepressant-induced reduction of CRH. Chemically enhanced activation of biogenic amine receptors (adrenergic and serotoninergic) through reuptake transporter inhibition results in desensitization followed by reduced PKA-mediated CREB phosphorylation and thus to decreased CRH gene activation via phospho-CREB action on the cAMP response element present in the CRH promoter. Concomitantly, antidepressants are able to increase GR function resulting in suppression of CRH gene expression. The administration of the MR antagonist, spironolactone, before antidepressant treatment with amitriptyline blocks the therapeutic response, indicating that MR function mediates antidepressant effects. A meta-analysis of antiglucocorticoid treatment of patients with major depression concluded that antidepressant effects happen in around 70% of the cases.

However, another study indicates that mifepristone, an antagonist of the GR, reduces symptoms in patients with psychotic depression. Therefore, the effects of glucocorticoids on depression seem to be dual. However, the effect of mifepristone might be limited to psychotic depression, in which many symptoms are

explained by the high levels of cortisol, which is believed to activate dopaminergic neurotransmission.

CRH receptor1 (CRHR1) knockout mice show a clear low-anxiety phenotype. Based on this experimental and clinical evidence, the CRHR1 receptor has been proposed as a target for antidepressants (*see* Fig. 125-2). CRHR1 knockout mice are viable and show no pathological symptoms that could indicate that CRHR1 antagonists would produce significant side effects. In fact, CRHR1 antagonists have antidepressant effects on many experimental models of depression. An early open clinical trial with a potent CRHR1 antagonist, NBI 30775, suggested antidepressant efficacy whereas no side effects were observed. Therefore, different compounds with CRHR1 antagonist activity have been developed by the pharmaceutical industry.

Another component of the HPA-axis also regulated by the MR is arginine vasopressin, which regulates ACTH production and potentiates CRH effects (*see* Fig. 125-2). The arginine vasopressin receptor (V1b) is expressed in brain areas involved in mood and anxiety. An orally active nonpeptide inhibitor of V1b, SSR149415, produces anxiolytic and antidepressive-like effects in a rat model. Therefore, V1b is another component of the HPA-axis with a promising potential as an antidepressant target.

THE CALCIUM SIGNALING HYPOTHESIS

One of the cellular mechanisms thought to be involved in the etiology as well as the therapeutic treatment of depression is LTP. This phenomenon consists in the long term, activity-dependent enhancement of the synaptic response. The mechanism requires the entry into the cell of calcium current. There are many ways in which calcium can enter cells; the one most commonly associated with LTP is the glutamate *N*-methyl-D-aspartate (NMDA) receptor. However, other calcium channels could also play a part in LTP. Inside the postsynaptic terminal, calcium binds to calmodulin and activates α-Ca^{2+}/calmodulin-dependent protein kinase (CaM kinase) II, the most abundant neuronal kinase (Fig. 125-3). CaM kinase phosphorylates itself to maintain an activated state and also phosphorylates other substrates such as α-amino-3-hydroxy-5-methyl-4-isoxazolepropionate receptors, providing a molecular basis for the increased conductance at the synaptic terminals during LTP. Many studies link LTP and calcium signaling to stress, anxiety, and depression as well as concerning antidepressant effects. Stress induced by inescapable electric shocks reduces LTP in the rat hippocampus. Within the hippocampus, the dentate gyrus seems to play a particularly important role in the vulnerability to stress. An increased synaptic efficacy in the dentate gyrus is associated with successful coping with stressful experiences. The calcium signaling hypothesis proposes that antidepressant treatment works by restoring a normal mechanism of coping with stressful events at the hippocampal level (*see* Fig. 125-3). This mechanism requires calcium signaling and LTP that in turn modulate the effects of monoamine neurotransmission in the hippocampus. In support of this hypothesis, monoaminergic afferent pathways modulate the induction and decay of LTP in the dentate gyrus. Fluoxetine treatment and electroconvulsive shock, which produce antidepressant-like effects, modulate LTP in the dentate gyrus.

One mechanism through which antidepressants could modulate LTP is the regulation of calcium entry through NMDA receptors. In fact, several antidepressants downregulate NMDA-subunit expression, including the glycine-binding sites. Interestingly, these effects happen mainly in the cerebral cortex but not in the

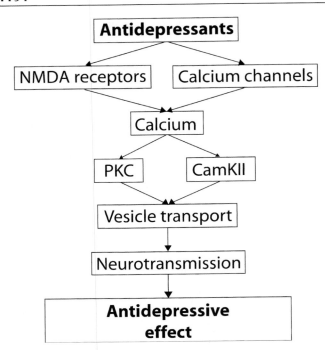

Figure 125-3 Schematic diagram of the role of calcium signaling activated by antidepressants in the regulation of neurotransmission and mood. PKC, protein kinase C; NMDA, *N*-methyl-D-aspartate; CAMK II, Ca^{2+}/calmodulin-responsive kinase II.

hippocampus. Only imipramine inhibits ε2 expression in the hippocampus but this inhibition does not happen in the dentate gyrus. Therefore, other antidepressant-regulated targets should regulate calcium currents in the dentate gyrus. The identification of tissue-specific and drug-responsive targets in the calcium signaling remains a challenge that could lead to novel antidepressant compounds.

UNIFYING THEMES IN ANTIDEPRESSANT SIGNAL TRANSDUCTION

The major components in the monoamine mechanism, the corticosteroid and calcium signaling pathways, show a high degree of crosstalk. As mentioned, an important interaction between the corticosteroid and monoamine pathways derives from different antidepressants' ability to induce an early increase in the mineralocorticoid binding capacity that is necessary for CRH downregulation by antidepressants and precedes the antidepressant effect. Initial clinical data further emphasize the importance of MR upregulation for the antidepressant effects because spironolactone, an MR antagonist, impairs the therapeutic effects of amitryptiline on patients with major depression. One mechanism by which antidepressants modulate the activity of corticosteroid receptors is through the regulation of chaperones, which bind corticosteroid receptor and control their activity and trafficking. Antidepressants can also modulate the expression of CRH through the cAMP pathway that leads to CREB activation. A functional site for CREB has been described in the CRH promoter. Therefore, a desensitization of this mechanism could play a role in antidepressant effects. More extensive and complex are the effects of glucocorticoids at different levels of the monoamine and BDNF cascade. The antidepressant venlafaxine may counteract an altered crosstalk between both pathways by inhibiting CREB phosphorylation and,

therefore, could produce an antidepressant effect. All these data together indicate that antidepressants modulate the negative feedback of the HPA-axis at different levels resulting in a normalization of this axis that correlates with therapeutic effects.

PATHWAYS THAT BLOCK ANTIDEPRESSANT ACTION The most direct way to define the pathways that are specific for the regulation of mood without affecting other biological processes is to analyze the effects of the blockade of these pathways and observe the impact on the antidepressant effects. Transgenic mice with a 90% reduction in CREB activity are viable and do not show an overt phenotype. Surprisingly, these mice show a therapeutic response after antidepressant treatment although they do not show an increase in BDNF. Therefore, in these mice, the therapeutic effect of antidepressants seems to be independent from BDNF upregulation by CREB. BDNF deficient mice develop hyperphagia and aggressiveness related to alterations in serotonergic neurons. However, depressive-like symptoms and antidepressant effects at the behavioral level have not been examined.

Therefore, if the phosphorylation of CREB by PKA and subsequent BDNF upregulation do not play a role in antidepressant action, other PKA substrates might mediate the therapeutic effects of antidepressants. One such PKA substrate is DARPP-32, which is phosphorylated by PKA in response to dopamine and cAMP or in response to antidepressant treatments. Importantly, the knockout of DARPP-32 shows a significant reduction in the therapeutic action of antidepressants. Therefore, DARPP-32 mediates at least in part the antidepressant effects of monoamines. However, DARPP-32 might not be a good drug target because it acts as a potent PP-1 inhibitor through protein–protein interactions that are not easily pharmacologically manipulated. Moreover, the inhibition of PP-1 results in the alteration of many important biological functions as demonstrated by the lethality of the PP-1-deficient mouse.

However, transgenic mice with altered expression of factors related to the corticosteroid hypothesis provide evidence in favor of the involvement of this pathway in antidepressant action. CRHR1-deficient mice show reduced anxiety-related behavior. Consistent with these observations, CRH overexpressing mice show increased anxiety-related behavior. Loss of GR function in the nervous system impairs the HPA-axis regulation, resulting in increased glucocorticoid levels that lead to an impaired behavioral response to stress and display reduced anxiety. The specific overexpression of GR in the brain leads to an increase in anxiety-like behavior. Moreover, clinical evidence indicates that a normalization of the HPA-axis precedes the successful response to antidepressant therapy.

OTHER MECHANISMS OF ANTIDEPRESSANT ACTION Substance P (neurokinin 1) and its receptor (NK1) are involved in the etiology of depression and NK1 antagonists have shown antidepressant-like effects. Substance P and NK1 are expressed at high levels in the brain, including brain areas thought to be involved in depression such as the amygdala. Anxiety-like behavior is produced by the administration of NK1 receptor agonists, which is indirect evidence that NK1 is involved in depression. Moreover, some reports show antidepressive-like effects of NK1 antagonists although there is still controversy in the field. An initial clinical study with the NK1 antagonist MK-869 showed antidepressive effects similar to that of paroxetine. However, the antidepressant effects of NK1 antagonists have not been confirmed in other clinical settings.

Different components of the Wnt signal transduction pathway are connected to mechanisms that control mood. *Wnt* genes encode secreted proteins that bind to membrane receptors of the Frizzled family. The stimulation of this pathway leads to the activation of the lymphocyte enhancer factor (LEF)/T-cell factor-β-catenin system. A mediator of this pathway is the glycogen synthase kinase 3b. This enzyme is a target for the mood stabilizer lithium chloride. However, there is controversial evidence about the involvement of this pathway in psychiatric disorders.

Melanin-concentrating hormone and its receptor are involved in the control of food intake. MCH1-R is expressed in brain areas that control not only feeding behavior but also mood and stress, including the hippocampus and amygdala. Recently, a melanin-concentrating hormone antagonist has been developed and tested in mice showing a decrease in body weight as well as anxiolytic and antidepressant effects. Therefore, the melanin-concentrating hormone and its receptor defines a novel pathway having antidepressive effects and it constitutes a further mechanism that coordinates feeding behavior and mood.

CONCLUSIONS

After target identification, the relatively large number of candidate genes requires a selection and prioritization process. Criteria to select candidates for further validation should include drug responsiveness as the highest priority. Therefore, the prioritized targets should belong to categories of genes known to be modulated by small compounds such as G protein-coupled receptors or protein kinases. To ensure a reduced number of side effects after long-term treatment, a target gene should have an expression pattern specific for the brain structures involved in depression. One further criterion to validate candidate targets is their regulation by stress, anxiety and antidepressant treatment. If the activity of a target gene is important for the control of mood, this activity should correlate with different alterations of mood as they happen in models of stress and anxiety. Genes found by unbiased approaches should be validated using accepted models of depressive-like behavior. These models are based on the previously discussed hypotheses, such as CRH overexpressing mice, which have high anxiety. Therefore, a combination between unbiased and hypothesis-driven research is needed to accomplish the complete process of functional target validation. The gold standard for a candidate target to be validated for the treatment of depression would be the observation of the specific impact that its modulation has on mood. To prove this point, it is necessary to produce transgenic mice with an altered expression of the candidate target and examine the effects of this alteration in depressive-like behavior.

Some of the target identification and validation approaches have intrinsic advantages. For example, genetic linkage results in targets related to depression in the human population. Targets found by other means need to be validated in humans. This procedure can be achieved using single nucleotide polymorphism analysis and association studies to complement neuroanatomic and behavioral data from animal models.

Different hypotheses explain the etiology of depression. Each focuses on different biological processes that contribute to explain the clinical manifestation of depression and connect the regulation of mood to other biological processes such as the stress response and feeding behavior. Most likely, these different signaling pathways converge at a certain point to specifically control mood. This convergence point may control neurotransmission, in particular,

LTP in the hippocampus. This opens the possibility that by dissecting pathways activated by antidepressants it would be possible to find new targets for novel drugs with a direct and specific mechanism of action, likely producing novel antidepressants with a higher potency, a faster action and fewer side effects.

SELECTED REFERENCES

Arborelius L, Owens MJ, Plotsky PM, Nemeroff CB. The role of corticotropin-releasing factor in depression and anxiety disorders. J Endocrinol 1999;160:1–12.

Beasley C, Cotter D, Everall I. An investigation of the Wnt-signalling pathway in the prefrontal cortex in schizophrenia, bipolar disorder and major depressive disorder. Schizophr Res 2002;58:63–67.

Belanoff JK, Flores BH, Kalezhan M, Sund B, Schatzberg AF. Rapid reversal of psychotic depression using mifepristone. J Clin Psychopharmacol 2001;21:516–521.

Borowsky B, Durkin MM, Ogozalek K, et al. Antidepressant, anxiolytic and anorectic effects of a melanin-concentrating hormone-1 receptor antagonist. Nat Med 2002;8:825–830.

Brown JD, Moon RT. Wnt signaling: why is everything so negative? Curr Opin Cell Biol 1998;10:182–187.

Chen AC, Shirayama Y, Shin KH, Neve RL, Duman RS. Expression of the cAMP response element binding protein (CREB) in hippocampus produces an antidepressant effect. Biol Psychiatry 2001;49:753–762.

Conti AC, Cryan JF, Dalvi A, Lucki I, Blendy JA. cAMP response element-binding protein is essential for the upregulation of brain-derived neurotrophic factor transcription, but not the behavioral or endocrine responses to antidepressant drugs. J Neurosci 2002;22:3262–3268.

Gould TD, Manji HK. The Wnt signaling pathway in bipolar disorder. Neuroscientist 2002;8:497–511.

Greengard P, Allen PB, Nairn AC. Beyond the dopamine receptor: the DARPP-32/protein phosphatase-1 cascade. Neuron 1999;23:435–447.

Heuser I, Yassouridis A, Holsboer F. The combined dexamethasone/CRH test: a refined laboratory test for psychiatric disorders. J Psychiatr Res 1994;28:341–356.

Holsboer F. The corticosteroid receptor hypothesis of depression. Neuropsychopharmacology 2000;23:477–501.

Holsboer F. The rationale for corticotropin-releasing hormone receptor (CRH-R) antagonists to treat depression and anxiety. J Psychiatr Res 1999;33:181–214.

Holsboer F, Barden N. Antidepressants and hypothalamic-pituitary-adrenocortical regulation. Endocr Rev 1996;17:187–205.

Klein PS, Melton DA. A molecular mechanism for the effect of lithium on development. Proc Natl Acad Sci USA 1996;93:8455–8459.

Kramer MS, Cutler N, Feighner J, et al. Distinct mechanism for antidepressant activity by blockade of central substance P receptors. Science 1998;281:1640–1645.

Landgrebe J, Welzl G, Metz T, et al. Molecular characterisation of antidepressant effects in the mouse brain using gene expression profiling. J Psychiatr Res 2002;36:119–129.

Lauer CJ, Schreiber W, Modell S, Holsboer F, Krieg JC. The Munich vulnerability study on affective disorders: overview of the cross-sectional observations at index investigation. J Psychiatr Res 1998;32:393–401.

Lyons WE, Mamounas LA, Ricaurte GA, et al. Brain-derived neurotrophic factor-deficient mice develop aggressiveness and hyperphagia in conjunction with brain serotonergic abnormalities. Proc Natl Acad Sci USA 1999;96:15,239–15,244.

Müller M, Holsboer F, Keck ME. Genetic modification of corticosteroid receptor signalling: novel insights into pathophysiology and treatment strategies of human affective disorders. Neuropeptides 2002;36:117–131.

Nestler EJ, Barrot M, DiLeone RJ, Eisch AJ, Gold SJ, Monteggia LM. Neurobiology of depression. Neuron 2002;34:13–25.

Nestler EJ, Gould E, Manji H, et al. Preclinical models: status of basic research in depression. Biol Psychiatry 2002;52:503–528.

Nibuya M, Nestler EJ, Duman RS. Chronic antidepressant administration increases the expression of cAMP response element binding protein (CREB) in rat hippocampus. J Neurosci 1996;16:2365–2372.

Patterson SL, Abel T, Deuel TA, Martin KC, Rose JC, Kandel ER. Recombinant BDNF rescues deficits in basal synaptic transmission and hippocampal LTP in BDNF knockout mice. Neuron 1996; 16:1137–1145.

Qu D, Ludwig DS, Gammeltoft S, et al. A role for melanin-concentrating hormone in the central regulation of feeding behaviour. Nature 1996; 380:243–247.

Reul JM, Gesing A, Droste S, et al. The brain mineralocorticoid receptor: Greedy for ligand, mysterious in function. Eur J Pharmacol 2000; 405:235–249.

Reul JM, Holsboer F. Corticotropin-releasing factor receptors 1 and 2 in anxiety and depression. Curr Opin Pharmacol 2002;2:23–33.

Reul JM, Labeur MS, Grigoriadis DE, De Souza EB, Holsboer F. Hypothalamic-pituitary-adrenocortical axis changes in the rat after long-term treatment with the reversible monoamine oxidase-A inhibitor moclobemide. Neuroendocrinology 1994;60: 509–519.

Rossby SP, Manier DH, Liang S, Nalepa I, Sulser F. Pharmacological actions of the antidepressant venlafaxine beyond aminergic receptors. Int J Neuropsychopharmacol 1999;2:1–8.

Rupniak NM, Carlson EJ, Webb JK, et al. Comparison of the phenotype of NK1R–/– mice with pharmacological blockade of the substance P (NK1) receptor in assays for antidepressant and anxiolytic drugs. Behav Pharmacol 2001;12:497–508.

Spengler D, Rupprecht R, Van LP, Holsboer F. Identification and characterization of a 3′,5′-cyclic adenosine monophosphate-responsive element in the human corticotropin-releasing hormone gene promoter. Mol Endocrinol 1992;6:1931–1941.

Stambolic V, Ruel L, Woodgett JR. Lithium inhibits glycogen synthase kinase-3 activity and mimics wingless signalling in intact cells. Curr Biol 1996;6:1664–1668.

Stout SC, Owens MJ, Nemeroff CB. Neurokinin(1) receptor antagonists as potential antidepressants. Annu Rev Pharmacol Toxicol 2001; 41:877–906.

Svenningsson P, Tzavara ET, Witkin JM, Fienberg AA, Nomikos GG, Greengard P. Involvement of striatal and extrastriatal DARPP-32 in biochemical and behavioral effects of fluoxetine (Prozac). Proc Natl Acad Sci USA 2002;99:3182–3187.

Teixeira RM, Santos AR, Ribeiro SJ, Calixto JB, Rae GA, De Lima TC. Effects of central administration of tachykinin receptor agonists and antagonists on plus-maze behavior in mice. Eur J Pharmacol 1996; 311:7–14.

Timpl P, Spanagel R, Sillaber I, et al. Impaired stress response and reduced anxiety in mice lacking a functional corticotropin-releasing hormone receptor 1. Nat Genet 1998;19:162–166.

Tronche F, Kellendonk C, Kretz O, et al. Disruption of the glucocorticoid receptor gene in the nervous system results in reduced anxiety. Nat Genet 1999;23:99–103.

van Gaalen MM, Stenzel-Poore MP, Holsboer F, Steckler T. Effects of transgenic overproduction of CRH on anxiety-like behaviour. Eur J Neurosci 2002;15:2007–2015.

Wolkowitz OM, Reus VI. Treatment of depression with antiglucocorticoid drugs. Psychosom Med 1999;61:698–711.

Yamada M, Higuchi T. Functional genomics and depression research. Beyond the monoamine hypothesis. Eur Neuropsychopharmacol 2002;12:235–244.

Zeller E, Stief HJ, Pflug B, Sastre-y-Hernandez M. Results of a phase II study of the antidepressant effect of rolipram. Pharmacopsychiatry 1984;17:188–190.

Zobel AW, Yassouridis A, Frieboes RM, Holsboer F. Prediction of medium-term outcome by cortisol response to the combined dexamethasone-CRH test in patients with remitted depression. Am J Psychiatry 1999;156:949–951.

126 Anxiety Disorders

Gregory M. Sullivan and Jack M. Gorman

SUMMARY

The anxiety disorders involve dysfunctional brain processes that offer prime targets for molecular therapeutics borne from neuroscience research. First, a brief historical overview of existing therapeutic agents for anxiety disorders is provided, and phenomenological descriptions of the major anxiety disorders are summarized. Next, brain circuitry relevant to the anxiety disorders is described, emphasizing the findings of neuroscience research on stress and conditioned fear. Molecular targets in the brain's neuropeptide and amino acid transmitter systems are then detailed, and plausible future targets are discussed. This chapter is intended to impart some of the exciting translational research advances and drug development in the anxiety disorders.

Key Words: PTSD; panic disorder; social anxiety disorder; generalized anxiety disorder; obsessive-compulsive disorder; amygdala; hippocampus; prefrontal cortex; neurokinins; corticotropin-releasing factor; GABA; glutamate.

INTRODUCTION

Sigmund Freud believed that the basis of mental illness would eventually be shown to lie in aberrant brain function. Yet the tools were not available in his time to understand or treat behavioral pathology through a physiological approach. A century later the understanding of brain function has grown immensely, and there is a boom of pharmacological research and drug development aimed at targeting the disabling symptoms of psychiatric disorders.

It is well established that anxiety disorders occur at high prevalence and impose significant health burdens. Medication management of the symptoms is often necessary, and, although there are several medication classes with proven efficacy, available treatments have significant drawbacks and do not work for all patients. Therefore, there is an ongoing need for improved anti-anxiety agents. It is desirable to target the dysfunctional neurobiological systems responsible for the disorders in the most specific manner, and, ideally, anxiolytics should have high therapeutic efficacy for a large percentage of patients with a given anxiety disorder although being safe and tolerable. This chapter presents a brief history of anxiolytic medications, reviews developments in the neurobiological understanding of anxiety disorders, and indicates what anxiolytic drug developments to expect in this age of molecular medicine.

From: *Principles of Molecular Medicine, Second Edition*
Edited by: M. S. Runge and C. Patterson © Humana Press, Inc., Totowa, NJ

HISTORICAL OVERVIEW OF ANXIETY DISORDER THERAPEUTICS

In the second half of the last century the "psychopharmacological revolution" in psychiatry began with a series of serendipitous discoveries of the medications with therapeutic efficacy for particular psychiatric disorders. These early discoveries provided the forerunners of virtually all-available medications for anxiety and affective illnesses. Through such discoveries it became evident that symptoms of particular "psychological" disorders, including anxiety disorders, could be reversed by administration of a medicinal agent. This implied that the neurobiological substrates affected by these medications were likely involved in the disorders treated. For example, in the 1950s iproniazid, then in use as an antituberculosis agent, was noted to have mood elevating properties by investigators in the United States. This led to the eventual understanding that drugs like it acted as antidepressants by inhibition of monoamine oxidase, an enzyme responsible for degradation of several monoamine neurotransmitters. In 1957, the antidepressant properties of the tricyclic compound imipramine, an agent that inhibits neuronal reuptake of the monoamines serotonin and norepinephrine, were reported by a Swiss clinical researcher. A few years later in the United States, imipramine was reported as a treatment for the anxiety condition that was to become known as panic disorder, and French clinicians had begun using monamine oxidase inhibitors (MAOIs) for this condition. Establishment of the tranquilizing properties of meprobamate in the 1950s was shortly followed by the introduction of another class of anxiolytic agents, the benzodiazepines (BDZs); and soon BDZ agents such as chlordiazepoxide and diazepam were widely available therapeutic options for anxious behaviors. This era firmly established that the anxiety disorders had a basis in abnormal brain function.

Unfortunately, these treatments were not without liabilities. The side effect profiles of the tricyclic antidepressants and MAOIs were often undesirable. Moreover, the tricyclics could produce deadly cardiotoxicity in overdose of less than 10 times a typical daily dose, a particularly critical issue when treating patients at risk for suicide attempt. The MAOIs could lead to a deadly hypertensive crisis by ingestion of common foods containing high amounts of the vasoactive amine tyramine, which would otherwise be metabolized by MAO in the gut. The addicting qualities of BDZs such as the infamous "mother's little helper," diazepam, also soon became apparent. The subsequent decades saw introduction of "me too" drugs, i.e., the development of agents based on the molecular structures and pharmacodynamics of the agents already identified. Even the more recent introductions of the selective serotonin reuptake inhibitors (SSRIs), selective norepinephrine reuptake inhibitors, and newer agents with both properties can be considered simply as improved versions of the tricyclic antidepressants.

Diverse scientific disciplines are presently converging on common understanding of behavioral pathology in the anxiety disorders in terms of brain dysfunction. These disorders are particularly well positioned among psychiatric conditions to benefit from this second stage of the psychopharmacological revolution. In particular, there are validated animal models for anxious, fearful, and avoidant behaviors, making drug design and development more like that found in other areas of medicine in which basic models often drive development of therapeutics. Neuroscience research has been providing a rapidly improving understanding of the neural circuits, cellular events, and molecular mediators of cognitive functions, emotional expressions, and behavioral adaptations to stressors. At the same time, biological studies of particular anxiety disorders have identified involved neurochemical, endocrine, and autonomic systems. Advances in neuroimaging techniques are beginning to allow in vivo quantitative assessment of regional structural, functional, and neurochemical abnormalities in the brains of patients with a wide array of psychiatric conditions including the anxiety disorders. Therefore, with these developments, a rational scientific approach to the anxiety disorders is made possible by immensely improved understanding of brain pathophysiology in the anxiety disorders and many novel approaches are on the horizon.

CLINICAL PRESENTATIONS OF THE ANXIETY DISORDERS

Post-traumatic stress disorder (PTSD) is characterized by a symptom constellation that develops following an emotionally traumatic event that involves threat of injury, bodily harm, or death to oneself or others. The emotional response to the event should by definition involve intense fear or helplessness. Importantly, three main categories of symptoms should result: re-experiencing of the trauma in the form of images, nightmares, or flashbacks; persistent avoidance of trauma-related thoughts, activities, situations, or people, including detachment from others or psychological numbing; and symptoms of hyperarousal such as exaggerated startle, insomnia, irritability, or hypervigilance.

Panic disorder has as its core clinical feature the occurrence of panic attacks, bursts of rapidly developing fear or discomfort occurring in a crescendo pattern and accompanied by distressing cognitive and somatic symptoms. Often these include dyspnea, heart pounding or racing, sweats, trembling, dizziness, gastrointestinal disturbance, and feelings of unreality or urge to flee. Essential for a diagnosis of panic disorder is interpanic attack worry about the occurrence of future attacks or the medical implications of the attacks, or there is phobic avoidance of situations in which another attack is believed likely to occur. Avoidance of situations that have become associated with attacks, such as crowds, elevators, bridges, is common.

Social anxiety disorder is characterized by excessive fear of social or performance situations. The fear centers around behaving in social situations in a way that will be humiliating or embarrassing, and the situations are avoided or else endured with intense distress or anxiety.

Generalized anxiety disorder is characterized by excessive anxiety or worry about a number of events or situations that occur more days than not for at least 6 mo. The patient has difficulty controlling the worry and there are several associated symptoms such as becoming easily fatigued, irritability, poor concentration, muscle tension, and sleep disturbance.

Obsessive-compulsive disorder (OCD) is characterized by the presence of intrusive thoughts or impulses. The obsessions, although usually recognized by the patient as excessive and products of their own mind, are usually accompanied by anxiety. This in turn often prompts ritualized behaviors that are performed in an effort to neutralize the obsessions or the associated anxiety. The obsessions and compulsions cause marked distress and consume significant amounts of time. Obsessions typically fall into several broad categories, including checking, ordering, or counting; preoccupation with contamination; aggressive or horrific impulses (such as hurting one's own child); or sexual imagery. In all of these anxiety disorders the impairment should be of a substantial level such that the disorder directly results in significant interference with work and/or social functioning.

BRAIN CIRCUITRY AND ANXIETY

An understanding of the neural correlates of anxiety is facilitated by an understanding of the stress response systems. An inherent assumption in this approach to anxiety disorders is that they involve dysfunction in phylogenetically conserved systems for response to adversity, whether real or imagined. Stress comes in many forms including physiological stressors, such as hemorrhage or ingestion of a toxin, and psychological stressors, such as sensory stimuli that the brain has learned are predictive of imminent danger. Over 50 yr ago, Hans Selye made the seminal observation that rather diverse stressors appear to activate a common stress response system with resulting hypertrophy of the adrenal glands and involution of immune structures such as the thymus gland. Although there are elements of differential physiological response that depend on the nature of the stressor, central commonalities are more the rule. For example, the hypothalamic–pituitary–adrenal (HPA) axis and the *locus ceruleus*-based noradrenergic system are the two main arms of a common stress system response to diverse stressors. Efferent neurons from the locus ceruleus activate the autonomic nervous system through both the sympathetic-adrenomedullary branch and the parasympathetic branch. HPA activation results in systemic glucocorticoids release whereas *locus ceruleus*-based noradrenergic system activation results in systemic release of epinephrine. The multiorgan pathology observed by Selye is explained by excessive activity of the HPA axis, leading to adrenal hyperplasia, and the inhibitory effects of an activated stress system on aspects of immune function, resulting in immune organ involution. Exposure to stress, particularly of an uncontrollable type, also results in increased release of the neurotransmitter norepinephrine in stress-responsive brain regions that include prefrontal cortex (PFC), hypothalamus, amygdala, hippocampus, and locus ceruleus. Many aspects of anxiety disorders' pathophysiology appear related to overactivity of components of the stress response system.

Neuroscience study of the emotional circuits underlying fear and anxiety has largely focused on Pavlovian fear conditioning and fear-potentiated startle, in part because the brain processes underlying these behavioral phenomena are readily studied in rodent models at anatomical, cellular, and molecular levels. These types of fear learning involve a coordinated network of brain structures, and the temporal lobe structure known as the amygdala plays a central role. Sensory information is relayed to the amygdala via two main

127 Trauma Spectrum Disorders

Christine Heim, J. Douglas Bremner, and Charles B. Nemeroff

SUMMARY

Exposure to trauma and pathological responses are influenced by genotype. Despite the inherent difficulties of studying the genetics of trauma-related disorders, the field has exhibited remarkable advances. Identification of polymorphisms in critical genes that influence neurotransmitter systems involved in the stress response is rapidly progressing and will elucidate the nature of gene-by-environment interactions that determine whether an individual develops a disorder in response to trauma. This chapter provides an overview of the status of genetic research on trauma spectrum disorders and discusses clinical implications.

Key Words: Amygdala; comorbidity; depression; endophenotype; gene-environment interaction; hippocampus; hypothalamic-pituitary-adrenal axis; neurobiology; polymorphisms; post-traumatic stress disorder; startle; trauma.

INTRODUCTION

The deleterious effects of stress have become increasingly evident. Surprisingly high rates of traumatic stress occur in our daily lives. Childhood abuse, car accidents, terrorism, combat, rape, assault, and a variety of severe traumas can all be associated with lasting effects on the individual. The American Psychiatric Association defines a traumatic event as an experience that is threatening to the self or someone close to you, accompanied by intense fear, horror, or helplessness. The definition of a traumatic event is outlined in the Diagnostic and Statistical Manual of Mental Disorders (DSM-IV). Exposure to a traumatic event, defined in this way, is required for the diagnosis of post-traumatic stress disorder (PTSD), making PTSD a psychiatric disorder that by definition is related to, and occurs as a consequence of, a stressful or traumatic event. In addition to PTSD, patients with other disorders exhibit high rates of trauma, including depression, substance and alcohol abuse, anxiety disorders, borderline personality disorder (BPD), and somatic disorders. The diagnosis of these latter disorders does not necessarily require exposure to a traumatic event. However, epidemiological studies have provided strong evidence that stressful life experiences and trauma represent major risk factors for the development of these disorders.

There is a great deal of comorbidity among these disorders, so that a traumatized individual is most likely to fulfill diagnostic criteria for several disorders, for example, PTSD and depression, or PTSD and alcoholism, and so on. The development of the DSM from its inception after World War II has led to a progressive "splitting" of psychiatric disorders into finer and finer categories, from the initial broad psychoanalytical categorization of "neurosis" vs "psychosis." The swing of the pendulum toward this pattern of progressive splitting may have gone too far. Psychiatric disorders may be better represented to the "neurosis-psychosis" dichotomy than the fine-tuned current psychiatric nosology. The neurosis concept would encompass depression, anxiety disorders (including panic disorder, generalized anxiety disorder, and PTSD), personality disorders (including BPD), the somatic disorders, and to a certain extent alcohol and substance abuse disorders, suggesting that there are not separate distinct disorders, but spectra of disorders that have been improperly categorized as distinct disorders by the current diagnostic schema. One such spectrum would be to a variable extent associated with trauma. Taken together, these considerations support the existence of a central "core" disorder that underlies several disorders. Evidence from studies employing neurobiological assessment methods suggests that this underlying core disorder might consist of specific neurobiological alterations that, in the genetically vulnerable individual, are induced by stress or trauma resulting in physiological and behavioral patterns that represent the clinical phenotypes of trauma spectrum disorders. These two views are not mutually exclusive.

Not all individuals who experience a traumatic event subsequently develop psychopathology. Why some individuals develop a psychiatric disorder after trauma whereas others do not remains obscure. Moreover, it is not well understood why some develop PTSD, although others develop depression or another disorder. In most cases, the manifestation of one or more trauma spectrum disorders in response to trauma is influenced by a complex interplay of preexisting vulnerabilities, including genetic predispositions, personality styles, and experiences, as well as psychological and situational factors at the time of the trauma and in the trauma's aftermath. Because the majority of trauma survivors do not develop a disorder, it is crucial to identify vulnerability and resilience factors, including genetic factors. Studies on the genetics of trauma spectrum disorders have been hampered by many factors, such as genetic heterogeneity (e.g., a similar phenotype develops from different genotypes) and incomplete penetrance of the phenotype (e.g., a person with genetic risk for PTSD, who is not exposed to trauma, will not develop PTSD). Despite these difficulties, evidence is accumulating that exposure to trauma and pathological responses to trauma are influenced by genetic composition. There are also advances in identifying molecular genetic

From: *Principles of Molecular Medicine, Second Edition*
Edited by: M. S. Runge and C. Patterson © Humana Press, Inc., Totowa, NJ

variations that confer risk to develop disorders in response to trauma. Elucidation of the genetics of neurobiological traits that determine to what extent and in which way the brain will respond to a stressor or a frightening situation is progressing. Finally, researchers are beginning to disentangle the continuous interplay between genetic make-up and environmental influences across the life span in shaping phenotypic expressions with vulnerability to stress and disease. This chapter provides an overview of the status of genetic research on trauma spectrum disorders with a focus on PTSD, including the genetics of comorbidity among related disorders. Other disorders frequently related to trauma, such as depression and alcoholism, are covered elsewhere in this section.

POST-TRAUMATIC STRESS DISORDER

According to the DSM-IV, PTSD is characterized by a set of symptoms that develop and persist in relation to the experience of one or more severely stressful or traumatic events. To be diagnosed with PTSD, a person must have experienced a traumatic event. Criterion A in the DSM-IV specifies that a stressful experience is classified as a "traumatic" event if the person experienced an event that involved actual or threatened death or serious injury, or a threat to the physical integrity of the person or others, and if the person responded with fear, helplessness, or horror to the event. Criteria B, C, and D of the DSM-IV define three symptom clusters comprising three types of symptoms that occur in response to the traumatic event in PTSD. These symptom clusters include re-experiencing the event, avoidance of reminders of the event, and hyperarousal. Re-experiencing, also called intrusion, involves recurrent or unwanted memories of the event, such as images, thoughts or perceptions, nightmares or flashbacks related to the event, or intense psychological distress or physiological reactions to reminders of the event. Symptoms of avoidance involve efforts to avoid reminders of the event, such as people, places, thoughts or feelings that are associated with the event. Symptoms of hyperarousal include disturbed sleep, impaired concentration, hypervigilance, and exaggerated startle responses. A diagnosis of PTSD requires at least one symptom from the re-experiencing category, three symptoms from the avoidant category, and two symptoms from the hyperarousal category. The symptoms must last a month or longer and must be associated with significant disturbance or distress in work, family, or social functioning. Chronic PTSD is diagnosed if these symptoms persist for 3 mo or longer. Delayed onset PTSD refers to symptoms developing at least 6 mo after the event. If a person develops similar symptoms within a month after the traumatic event, acute stress disorder (ASD) may be diagnosed. ASD requires three to five dissociative symptoms, one or more of each of the re-experiencing, avoidance, and hyperarousal symptoms, as well as functional impairment. ASD is associated with increased risk to later develop PTSD, though PTSD does not necessarily follow ASD.

PREVALENCE AND RISKS Epidemiological studies in the United States, including the National Comorbidity Study, report that up to 90% of Americans experience a traumatic event in their lifetime. Events reported include life-threatening accidents, natural disasters, combat, rape, physical attacks, child abuse, witnessing the death or injury of another person, and traumatic loss of a loved one. With a lifetime prevalence of about 10% in women and 5% in men, PTSD is among the most common psychiatric disorders. The likelihood to develop PTSD in response to a trauma varies considerably depending on the specific type of event experienced. For example, about half of all rape victims develop PTSD compared

with 14% of individuals who suddenly lose a loved one, 7.5% of accident victims, and 2% of individuals who learn about a trauma.

Based on the lifetime prevalence rates, female gender appears to be a risk factor for PTSD. This risk might reflect increased vulnerability of women to the effects of trauma or gender differences in the prevalence of types of events that are more frequently associated with PTSD, or the interaction of both. For example, women more often experience molestation than men and are also more likely to develop PTSD related to molestation. Rape is 10 times more common in women compared with men, but men are more likely than women to develop PTSD in response to being raped. Women, in contrast, are more likely than men to develop PTSD after physical assault, though physical assault is less common in women. Because of the high frequency of these specific traumas experienced by women, or to which women more frequently respond with PTSD, overall lifetime prevalence of PTSD is higher in women than in men.

Because not all women or men who experience traumatic events continue to develop PTSD, additional factors appear to moderate a person's risk to develop PTSD. Factors that increase the risk to develop PTSD include severity and duration of the trauma, proximity to the event, degree of danger, repetition of a trauma, infliction by other people (social trauma, such as rape or molestation), and negative reactions from family and friends. Perceived vulnerability and lack of control are important factors that might increase the risk for later PTSD. In general, events that involve an interpersonal component (e.g., rape, assault, or terrorist attacks) more likely induce PTSD than traumas that are not inflicted by persons (e.g., natural disaster). In addition to these factors that describe characteristics of the traumatic event, characteristics of the person exposed to the trauma also play a role. For example, previous or comorbid psychiatric illness, certain personality disorders, low intelligence, poor coping abilities and other factors increase the likelihood to develop PTSD. As discussed next, a family history of psychiatric illness (especially anxiety disorders and depression) and previous stressful experiences (particularly early in life) further increase individual risk to develop PTSD in response to given events, suggesting that genetic and environmental factors may influence susceptibility to PTSD.

NEUROBIOLOGY Because the development of PTSD by definition is related to extreme stress experiences, changes in neurobiological systems that participate in the mediation of stress responses have been extensively studied in patients with PTSD. One of the key mediators of stress in the central nervous system (CNS) is corticotropin-releasing factor (CRF). CRF neurons and receptors are heterogeneously distributed throughout the brain and are found in brain regions integral to cognitive and emotional processing, as well as autonomic and neuroendocrine regulation. Microinjections of CRF into the CNS of laboratory animals produces integrated endocrine, autonomic and behavioral responses that parallel signs of stress, depression and anxiety, including loss of appetite, sleep disruption, decreased sexual behavior, despair, increased motor activity, neophobia, facilitated fear conditioning, and enhanced startle reactivity. Treatment with CRF receptor antagonists or CRF receptor knockouts exhibit attenuated stress responses. A circuit connecting the amygdala and the hypothalamus with the locus ceruleus, in which CRF and norepinephrine (NE) are the major neurotransmitters, participates in the regulation of vigilance, anxiety and fear, and the integration of endocrine and autonomic responses. Given the pre-eminent role of CRF in mediating stress and anxiety, it is understandable that the hypothesis that PTSD patients exhibit CRF hypersecretion has been promulgated. Indeed, patients with combat-related PTSD exhibit marked and sustained elevations of CRF concentrations in cerebrospinal fluid (CSF), obtained by a single lumbar puncture or by using an indwelling subarachnoid catheter for collection of CSF over 6 h. PTSD patients also exhibit elevated CSF NE concentrations. Elevated CRF and NE availability plausibly explains many core symptoms of PTSD, such as sleep disruption, increased autonomic arousal, imprinted emotional memories, and enhanced startle reactivity.

CRF neurons in the hypothalamic paraventricular nucleus (PVN) form the CNS component of the hypothalamic-pituitary-adrenal (HPA) axis, the major stress system in mammals. When exposed to stress, CRF is secreted from nerve terminals in the median eminence into the hypothalamus–hypophyseal portal circulation and activates CRF receptors on corticotrophs stimulating the production and release of adrenocorticotropic hormone from the anterior pituitary. Adrenocorticotropic hormone in turn stimulates release of glucocorticoids (cortisol in humans) from the adrenal cortex. Glucocorticoids exert marked effects on metabolism, immune function and the CNS. Cortisol secretion is essential for successful adaptation of the organism to stress. Although there is evidence for hyperactivity of CNS CRF systems in PTSD, paradoxically, basal cortisol secretion appears to be reduced in PTSD patients compared with healthy volunteers, though this finding has not been consistently replicated. However, even normal cortisol output reported in some studies for PTSD patients is inappropriately low in the face of elevated CRF secretion. Low basal cortisol secretion may reflect increased negative feedback sensitivity of the HPA axis, though mild adrenal insufficiency might also play a role. Low cortisol secretion in PTSD might represent a counter-regulatory adaptation to central hyperactivity. Cortisol is also known to inhibit the NE-CRF feedforward loop in the brain. Therefore, perhaps reduced cortisol availability (as a consequence of genetic disposition or prior experience) before a given trauma and/or too rapid shutdown of the peripheral cortisol response might represent risk factors leading toward disinhibition and perpetuation of CNS responses to stress, which might ultimately evolve into PTSD symptoms. Indeed, increased endocrine responses to laboratory stress and imagery of the trauma have been documented in PTSD patients.

Several brain pathways modulate HPA axis activity. The hippocampus and the prefrontal cortex inhibit the HPA axis, whereas the amygdala and monoaminergic input from the brainstem stimulate PVN CRF neurons. Sustained excessive glucocorticoid exposure is known to produce adverse effects on hippocampal neurons, including reduction in dendritic branching, loss of dendritic spines, and impairment of neurogenesis. Glucocorticoids also adversely affect the prefrontal cortex. Although basal plasma cortisol concentrations are low in PTSD, relatively small hippocampal volumes are seen in patients with PTSD. Functional neuroimaging studies provide evidence for altered activity of the hippocampus, which is likely related to cognitive deficits in PTSD. These structural changes could be secondary to increased cortisol secretion at the time of the trauma or in response to repeated stresses, or they could reflect a pre-existing vulnerability marker for the development of PTSD. Other studies document decreased activity in frontal cortical regions and increased amygdala responses to traumatic or emotional stimuli in PTSD patients.

OTHER TRAUMA SPECTRUM DISORDERS

Experiences of extreme stress or trauma are also associated with several disorders other than PTSD, including depression, other anxiety disorders, alcoholism, substance abuse, personality disorders, and somatoform disorders. Trauma exposure not an essential diagnostic requirement in these disorders, and these disorders often occur in individuals who did not experience a major trauma. However, stress and trauma dramatically increase an individual's risk to develop these disorders, particularly when experienced early in life. Episodes of these disorders are often precipitated by stressful life events in adulthood. A complex interplay between stresses across the life span, coupled with genetic vulnerabilities and other risk factors, is thought to underlie these disorders' manifestation.

Trauma spectrum disorders, including PTSD and the previously mentioned disorders, often occur together in one individual. For example, the National Comorbidity Study reports that lifetime comorbidity rates of PTSD patients are 49% for major depression, 40% for alcohol abuse, 31% for drug abuse, 28% for social phobia, 16% for generalized anxiety disorder, and 10% for panic disorder. About half of individuals with a lifetime history of PTSD have three or more comorbid additional Axis I disorders. In trauma survivors, PTSD often precedes the onset of mood and alcohol abuse disorders. In Axis II disorders show a high comorbidity rate between BPD and PTSD, prompting suggestions that BPD might represent a chronic form of PTSD. However, because almost half of patients with BPD do not have a lifetime history of PTSD, it appears that BPD is more closely related to trauma experience itself rather than PTSD, though many patients with BPD do not have any trauma history. Many patients with PTSD and other trauma spectrum disorders also have multiple somatic symptoms, including chronic pain symptoms, which also appear to be associated with traumatic experiences. These findings lend substantial support to the concept of trauma spectrum disorders. Certain personality traits, such as neuroticism, are risk factors for many of these disorders. Substantial support for the existence of a spectrum of trauma-related disorders, which likely share the same common pathophysiology, has emerged.

Are there neurobiological similarities among the various trauma spectrum disorders and PTSD? All trauma spectrum disorders have been associated with HPA axis alterations, though the nature of the alterations varies in the different disorders. Thus, severe major depression, for example, melancholia, has been associated with increased cortisol output and HPA feedback resistance, opposing the findings in PTSD. Despite these discrepancies, depression and PTSD share many CNS alterations, including increased CRF and NE activity, smaller than normal hippocampus volumes, and functional alterations in limbic and prefrontal cortical areas. Other trauma spectrum disorders, such as BPD and chronic pain syndromes, have been associated with low cortisol levels and increased HPA feedback sensitivity, similar to the findings in PTSD. Basal cortisol output may be decreased in nonpsychotic depression, particularly if the depression is associated with trauma and PTSD. These examples demonstrate considerable overlap in the neurobiological alterations of several trauma-related disorders. These overlapping pathophysiologies might reflect effects of trauma and/or neurobiological correlates of symptoms, which overlap among these disorders. Alternatively these commonalities might reflect underlying stress vulnerability, which might confer risk to develop an array of symptoms and syndromes on trauma exposure. Inherent stress vulnerability is likely the result of a complex interplay of genetic factors, experiences and other factors.

PROBLEMS IN STUDYING THE GENETICS OF TRAUMA SPECTRUM DISORDERS

Because trauma spectrum disorders are complex behavioral disorders, many factors complicate studies on underlying genetic vulnerability. One major problem is that an epigenetic factor in the form of a severely stressful event is required to "uncover" the susceptibility to trauma spectrum disorders and, for PTSD, to develop or be diagnosed with the disorder. Following is an overview on these problems using PTSD as the prototype. Genetic vulnerability for PTSD, like those for other major psychiatric disorders (schizophrenia, depression, and bipolar disorder) is likely not determined by a single gene inherited in a Mendelian pattern. High rates of comorbidity between PTSD and other (trauma spectrum) disorders, variability of symptoms within the PTSD category, and multiple psychopathologies in family members of patients with PTSD are consistent with a complex mode of inheritance. Thus, several genes likely "collaborate" in defining the vulnerability and the phenotype, and different genes may contribute to the same phenotype. The latter phenomenon is referred to as "genetic heterogeneity."

The development and diagnosis of PTSD, in contrast to other trauma spectrum disorders, depends on a trauma exposure. Because not all individuals in the population experience a trauma capable of inducing PTSD, not all individuals can or will be diagnosed with PTSD, even if they carry high genetic risk. Thus, even if an individual is at high genetic risk for PTSD, the disorder might actually never develop because the traumatic triggering event never occurs. This is referred to as "incomplete penetrance," which considerably complicates research on the genetics of PTSD.

The phenotype definition of PTSD according to DSM-IV is also problematic for genetic research. For example, the dichotomous categorization of whether an individual has PTSD or does not have PTSD is highly arbitrary and leads to a loss of information. This is also true for categorical distinctions between PTSD and other trauma-spectrum disorders. DSM-IV criteria are not designed to minimize false-positives, and are unrelated to specific pathophysiological mechanisms. There is as yet no marker of genetic risk for PTSD to detect vulnerable patients who never experienced a trauma.

Especially pertinent for trauma spectrum disorders are observations that genes for psychiatric disorders may be pleiotropic; the same gene contributes to the manifestation of several different disorders. The facts that PTSD patients have extremely high rates of comorbid psychiatric disorders and that certain psychiatric disorders are over represented among the relatives of patients with PTSD, are consistent with the presence of a pleiotropic gene. Such a pleiotropic gene may underlie genetic vulnerability for a "core" disorder common to the spectrum of disorders that are manifested after exposure to stress and trauma. Additional genes might modify this phenotype, leading to specific clinical expressions categorized as separate disorders in DSM-IV.

Considerable evidence exists that the risk to develop PTSD or other trauma spectrum disorders increases with the severity of trauma. This suggests that the genetic risk for PTSD is particularly important at the lower end of the trauma severity continuum, whereas toward the higher end of the severity continuum, individuals without any genetic risk might develop the disorder. Thus, it is possible that some persons develop PTSD or another trauma spectrum disorder following very severe traumas without any significant genetic contribution. Moreover, resilience and the possible existence of resilience genes may contribute to invulnerability to PTSD development. It is also likely that the impact of an environmental event on a specific disease is moderated by age at the time of the event, type of the event or pre-existing disorders.

Genetic research on trauma spectrum disorders, including PTSD, is complicated by the circumstance that some types of exposure, such as child abuse or going to war, are heavily influenced by genetic dispositions or certain personality traits that are in turn genetically influenced.

GENETICS OF TRAUMA SPECTRUM DISORDERS

FAMILY STUDIES Family studies have been used to elucidate the potential genetic contributions to PTSD and other trauma spectrum disorders. The first family studies on PTSD-like symptoms were performed after World Wars I and II. Remarkably, these studies found that immediate relatives of soldiers, who suffered from PTSD-like symptoms, more often had psychiatric problems, such as "insanity," nervousness, alcohol abuse, and neurasthenia. Familial aggregation of PTSD and the prevalence of other psychiatric disorders in family members of PTSD patients have been examined. For example, the offspring of a parent with PTSD has a fivefold increased risk of PTSD development. The risk of developing PTSD is two- to threefold higher if a family member suffers from depression, an anxiety disorder other than PTSD, or a personality disorder. A family history of alcohol or substance abuse, surprisingly, was not found to be associated with an increased risk for PTSD, though an increased prevalence rate of these disorders was found in siblings of patients with chronic PTSD.

Similar patterns of familial aggregation are also found among trauma spectrum disorders other than PTSD. For example, familial aggregation and transmission of BPD has been reported, but so has only a familial relationship for individuals who had BPD and comorbid depression. It is assumed that, when all family studies are combined, the morbid risk of BPD in first-degree relatives is 11.5%. There is also a suggestion that BPD has a familial relationship to alcoholism and substance abuse. Interestingly, relatives of BPD patients show increased rates of impulsive or affective personality traits, suggesting that familial relationship might be stronger for dimensions such as impulsiveness/aggression and affective instability than for the diagnostic entities. In sum, it appears that a cluster of disorders and traits run in families. This cluster resembles the spectrum of trauma-related disorders, and also seems to include traits that are risk factors for them.

These and other findings from family studies suggest a genetic susceptibility for PTSD and other trauma spectrum disorders. However, family studies are difficult to interpret because it is uncertain whether the aggregation observed is resulting from genetic factors, other biological factors, or shared experience. The association of familial psychopathology and PTSD may be mediated by increased risk of traumatic exposure and by pre-existing psychopathology. More valid approaches to detect genetic contributions to trauma spectrum disorders involve studies in twin populations.

TWIN STUDIES Several twin studies provide considerable evidence of a hereditary predisposition for PTSD. The first substantial data on PTSD in twins were results from the Vietnam Era Twin Registry project, which included more than 4000 male–male pairs of Vietnam Era veteran twins. When adjusting for variance in the heritability of trauma exposure, it was estimated that genetic factors accounted for approx 30% of the variance in liability for most of the PTSD symptoms in all symptom clusters (intrusion: 13–30%; avoidance: 30–34%; hyperarousal: 28–32%). Interestingly, shared family environment, such as parental style among others, did not contribute to susceptibility to PTSD. The remaining variance was resulting from nonshared, unique environmental experiences. Because this study recruited solely male twins and focused exclusively on the trauma of combat exposure, the findings cannot be generalized to women and other types of trauma. Twins in another study of 406 male and female twin pairs from the general population in Canada did not experience combat trauma, but an array of civilian traumas, including robbery, assaults, violent family death, accidents, fire, and natural disasters. This study confirmed a moderate heritable component for the development of PTSD symptoms and, again, the remaining variance was accounted for by unique environmental experiences.

As for trauma spectrum disorders other than PTSD, twin studies show that 40–50% of the risk to develop depression is genetic, even higher for bipolar disorder. Other anxiety disorders have somewhat less of a genetic component, but it is substantial. Alcohol and substance abuse disorders are moderately heritable (for genetics of these disorders, *see* Chapter 129). There is also evidence for a genetic component in the development of BPD. In a Norwegian twin study of 221 twin pairs, about 60% of the BPD liability was genetic and about 10% was resulting from common environmental experiences. If replicated, this would suggest that BPD is a highly heritable disorder. Interestingly, using the twin approach, several studies determined to what extent genetic contributions overlap between PTSD and other disorders that often co-occur in trauma survivors, such as alcoholism, drug dependence, or other anxiety disorders. For example, one study made up of a small number of subjects found that PTSD was only present in cotwins of twins with anxiety disorders, and was twice as prevalent in monozygotic twins compared with dizygotic twins. In another study using the Vietnam Era Twin Registry, the liability for PTSD was partially resulting from a 15.3% genetic contribution common to alcoholism and drug dependence and a 20% genetic contribution specific to PTSD. The genetic risk for alcoholism or drug dependence were the same genetic contributions common to PTSD and drug dependence, or PTSD and alcoholism, respectively, as well as specific risk for each disorder. Shared environment contributed to risk for drug abuse. Similar associations were found for genetic overlap between PTSD, generalized anxiety disorder and panic disorder. Another study evaluating twin pairs discordant for combat exposure found that monozygotic combat-unexposed cotwins of subjects with PTSD had significantly more symptoms of mood disorders than monozygotic cotwins of combat controls, suggesting that genetic vulnerability contributes to the association between PTSD and depression or dysthymia. These studies suggest that there is overlap in genetic predisposition to develop a spectrum of disorders and that each of these disorders also has some specific genetic liability. These findings are not discordant with the concept of trauma spectrum disorders.

MOLECULAR GENETIC STUDIES Although there is evidence from family and twin studies for an inherited vulnerability to develop trauma spectrum disorders in response to severe stress exposure, little is known about the molecular bases of this vulnerability. Although there are no linkage studies in PTSD, most of the small number of association studies in PTSD focused on variations of genes that are involved in dopamine (DA) neurotransmission. The rationale for studying genetic variations in DA systems is based on previous findings that PTSD patients, and stressed animals, show increased DA neuronal reactivity and that stress-induced alterations of brain DA reactivity are at least in part genetically determined. Comparison of 37 drug-dependent Vietnam

veterans with PTSD with 19 drug-dependent veterans without PTSD showed that the A1 allele of the DA-2 receptor was more common in those with PTSD. These results suggested that a variant in the DA receptor gene might confer an increased risk for PTSD, whereas the absence of the variant might confer resistance. However, another study failed to replicate these findings. These conflicting results are likely resulting from small sample sizes and the presence of substance dependence in the first study, which might also be associated with the A1 allele. In the second study, trauma exposure was not controlled for in the non-PTSD group. This might have resulted in the inclusion of subjects in the control group with inherited vulnerability to PTSD, which was not expressed because of lack of trauma exposure. Based on these findings, a gene coding for the DA transporter (DAT) was investigated that is located on the nerve terminals of DA neurons, except prefrontal cortical DA neurons. The DAT is responsible for the presynaptic reuptake of DA released into the synaptic cleft, thereby controlling the availability of DA in the synapse to activate postsynaptic DA receptors. A common mutation in the DAT gene was more frequent in trauma survivors who developed chronic PTSD compared with trauma survivors who did not. These findings suggest that a genetically determined variation in DA neurotransmission may participate in shaping pathological responses to trauma, and, in general, vulnerability to the effects of stress. Future studies should also evaluate genetic polymorphisms in critical components of other neural systems that are implicated in stress responses, such as the CRF systems (CRF, CRF receptor subtypes, CRF binding protein), and their role in conferring risk for PTSD. They should also attempt to elucidate a potential molecular basis of the common comorbidity among the spectrum of trauma-related disorders. Interestingly, one study showed that a polymorphism of the γ-amino butyric acid$_A$ receptor β 3-subunit gene is associated with comorbid somatic symptoms and depression among PTSD patients.

GENETICS OF THE BIOLOGICAL FOUNDATIONS OF TRAUMA SPECTRUM DISORDERS

It has become increasingly clear that the classification of psychiatric disorders on the basis of symptomatic phenotypes is not ideal for genetic research trying to dissect vulnerabilities for these disorders. This is particularly true for PTSD and other trauma spectrum disorders mainly because of the wide range of the symptomatic phenotypes and the incomplete penetrance of the phenotype depending on the occurrence of a triggering event, which might in turn be genetically influenced. Therefore, it might be more fruitful for genetic research to focus on internal changes or biological markers that are associated with a given disorder. Such internal biological states are also referred to as "endophenotypes." Although these biological traits might be correlates or consequences of the disease, there may also be preexisting biological vulnerabilities that confer risk to develop a disorder, if trauma occurs. Such underlying biological vulnerabilities might be genetic in nature, be shaped by the person's environment, or both. With advances in detecting biological underpinnings of PTSD and other trauma spectrum disorders, there are exciting possibilities to explore the genetics of the neurobiological mechanisms involved in pathological stress responses, such as deficits in hippocampal structure, fear responses, and sensitization of CRF systems.

HIPPOCAMPUS SIZE LINKED TO PATHOLOGICAL VULNERABILITY TO TRAUMA Preclinical studies show that stress can damage the brain, particularly the hippocampus. The hippocampus is a brain structure important for declarative memory, contextual aspects of fear conditioning and control of the HPA axis. Overexposure of the hippocampus to high concentrations of glucocorticoids during states of ongoing stress is thought to lead to atrophy and neuronal loss in the hippocampus, which in turn contributes to the symptoms of stress-related disorders. In fact, structural MRI shows the hippocampus to be smaller in patients with PTSD compared with controls. Similar findings exist in patients with major depression. The size of the hippocampus in PTSD has been a "chicken-or-egg" question. Whether this region shrinks as a result of the trauma exposure (and presumed HPA axis activation) or because of the presence of PTSD itself, or whether it might already be smaller before a person undergoes a traumatic event has been debated. The latter suggests that a small hippocampus is a risk factor for PTSD. Researchers have been able to address this question using a twin study design of 40 pairs of identical twins, including Vietnam veterans who were exposed to combat trauma and their cotwins who did not go to Vietnam, by measuring the size of the hippocampus in all the twins. As expected, among Vietnam veterans, the hippocampus was smaller in those with PTSD compared with those who did not develop the disorder. However, this brain region was also smaller in the cotwins of the men with PTSD, suggesting that a smaller hippocampus is a preexisting, potentially genetic, vulnerability factor that predisposes to PTSD and other trauma spectrum disorders, after exposure to stress or trauma.

A GENE BIASES THE AMYGDALA TO OVER-REACT TO FRIGHTENING FACES

Functional brain imaging has provided compelling evidence of a strong genetic component to the extent to which the amygdala reacts to emotional stimuli. The amygdala is a limbic brain structure integral to fear responses. Its response to pictures of frightening faces depends on which form of a gene involved in serotonergic neurotransmission is present. Subjects who had one or two copies of the short variant of the human serotonin transporter (SERT) gene, associated with reduced serotonergic transmission, showed greater activation of the amygdala to fearful faces compared with those who had two copies of the long variant of the gene. In previous studies, variations of this gene have been associated with increased trait-like anxiety and heightened stress reactivity. Thus, this gene might be associated with a phenotype with particular vulnerability to pathological responses to stress, which might promote the development of emotional disorders, if trauma occurs.

"JUMPINESS" AS AN INHERITED VULNERABILITY MARKER FOR PTSD

Exaggerated startle reactivity is one of the diagnostic criteria for PTSD. PTSD patients exhibit greater than normal physiological reactions, such as eye-blink, heart pounding and sweating, when exposed to loud or sudden tones, or to unexpected touch. The startle response is a reflex common to all mammals. Interestingly, the amplitude of the startle reflex can be modulated by the induction of emotional states. In the context of fear, the startle reflex is enhanced. In contrast, twin studies revealed high rates of concordance in startle reactivity among healthy identical twins in general. Based on the previously mentioned and similar to discussions regarding the origin of a small hippocampus in PTSD, it has been debated whether an exaggerated startle reactivity might be a consequence of trauma exposure or a correlate of having PTSD, or whether it might be a pre-existing vulnerability factor that increases the risk of a person to develop PTSD on trauma exposure. A study in identical twin pairs discordant for Vietnam combat exposure helped address this question.

Combat-exposed Vietnam veterans with PTSD showed exaggerated responses to loud and sudden tones. However, their nonexposed cotwins showed responses similar to combat veterans without PTSD and their nonexposed cotwins. These results strongly suggest that increased startle reactivity is secondary to PTSD rather than a preexisting vulnerability trait.

HIGHER THAN NORMAL STRESS HORMONE RESPONSES IN FAMILIES

Stress activates the HPA axis, which is mainly controlled by hypothalamic CRF. Increased activation of CRF and sensitization of the HPA axis have been measured in patients with in PTSD and other stress-related disorders. The behavioral effects of CRF at extrahypothalamic sites, together with the manifold effects of cortisol on the brain, are thought to underlie many of the symptoms of trauma spectrum disorders, including anxiety and depression. Although severe and ongoing stress can markedly alter the activity of CRF neurons and the dynamics of the HPA axis, less is known about the extent to which CRF and HPA axis function are shaped by genetics. Heightened reactivity of CRF systems and the HPA axis to a given stressor or trauma might confer increased risk to develop pathological conditions related to stress. A study of first-degree relatives of depressed patients who never suffered from a psychiatric disorder themselves, showed increased cortisol responses to a pharmacological challenge test (the dexamethasone-CRF test) that is highly sensitive to detect HPA axis hyperactivity. Increased reactivity in this test was found to be constant overtime, possibly reflecting an inherited trait, though experiences shared within families might contribute to these results. These findings are complemented by reports from studies in healthy twin pairs that revealed moderate heritability of HPA reactivity to laboratory stress. Inherited neuroendocrine stress reactivity might be based on polymorphisms of genes that participate in the regulation of neuroendocrine stress responses, such as glucocorticoid receptor and CRF receptor genes. Whether inherited neuroendocrine sensitization contributes to the risk for the development of PTSD and other trauma spectrum disorders after trauma exposure is unknown.

INTERACTION OF GENOTYPE AND EXPERIENCES ACROSS THE LIFE SPAN

INFLUENCE OF LIFE EXPERIENCES

Trauma spectrum disorders, in particular PTSD, by definition occur in the context of a traumatic experience. Because not everyone exposed to such an experience develops PTSD or a related disorder, the manifestation of these illnesses depends on the interaction of the traumatic experience with dispositions of the person and other situational factors that a person is exposed to surrounding the traumatic experience. Thus, the manifestation of trauma spectrum disorders probably reflects a complex gene by environment interaction. The severity and nature of the index trauma itself plays a major role in determining whether the victim develops PTSD or another disorder. However, experiences other than the index trauma also shape the risk to develop a trauma spectrum disorder. The effects of early developmental experiences on later vulnerability to subsequent stresses and its relationship to the development of psychiatric disorders have been studied. Compelling evidence from epidemiological, twin, and case–control studies suggests that adverse experiences during childhood have pronounced and long-term effects on later stress vulnerability, and represent major risk factors for the development of mood and anxiety disorders in adulthood. There is a complex relationship between early-life stress and PTSD. A traumatic event experienced early in life surely is a form of early stress, but not all forms of early-life stress are necessarily traumatic events. For example, chronic demands of a young child to manage a family household would not meet the DSM-IV A criterion, but may exert pronounced influences on the child's subsequent vulnerability to stress and PTSD. Thus, the relationship between early-life stress and PTSD can be direct or indirect. In the direct relationship, the early stress experience itself represents the index trauma to which PTSD symptoms are related. Indirect relationships between early-life stress and PTSD occur in at least two ways. Early-life stress increases the risk of later trauma that may, in turn, elicit PTSD and early-life stress also increases the risk for the development of PTSD in response to traumas occurring in adulthood, such as combat. Such sensitization of responses to trauma has been observed after child abuse experiences, but also after more subtle instances of early stress, such as negative parenting style or neglect. In addition, acute or chronic life stresses in adulthood that are not traumatic also exacerbate or aggravate PTSD. Similar relationships exist for other disorders that are often precipitated by stressful events, such as depression.

The pronounced effects of early-life stress on vulnerability to stress and psychopathology are surely mediated by the substantial plasticity of the developing brain as a function of experience. During such critical periods, certain brain regions are particularly sensitive to adverse experiences, which may then lead to major, perhaps irreversible, alterations. Findings from laboratory animal studies have provided direct evidence that stress or trauma during development permanently shapes the structure and function of brain regions involved in the mediation of stress and emotion, leading to altered emotional processing and heightened responsiveness to stress. Adult rats separated from their mothers for brief periods of time in the first 2 wk of life exhibit up to threefold increases in HPA axis responses to mild stressors and develop marked behavioral changes including increased anxiety-like behavior, anhedonia, alcohol preference, sleep disruption, and cognitive impairment. Many of these changes resemble cardinal symptoms of trauma spectrum disorders. Evidence exists that similar changes occur in humans after early-life traumatic events. Thus, women abused as children exhibit greater HPA axis and autonomic responses to a standardized psychosocial laboratory stress, the Trier Social Stress Test, compared with controls, and the increase is more pronounced in those abused women with current depression. Taken together, these and other findings from developmental neurosciences strongly suggest that endophenotypes, which underlie manifestations of psychiatric disorders, do not necessarily reflect genetic variations influencing the blueprint of the brain, but that the structure and function of the brain is profoundly shaped by experiences throughout development, which is then expressed into behaviors.

INTERACTION OF GENES AND ENVIRONMENT   Not all individuals exposed to trauma develop a trauma spectrum disorder. Similarly, not every child who experiences adverse life events, such as abuse, neglect or loss, will be sensitized to stress and or develop certain stress- or trauma-related disorders, even on further stress challenge. In addition to protective environmental and psychological factors, genetic vulnerability and resiliency factors must be considered. For instance, the risk to develop PTSD in response to combat exposure is moderated by the presence or absence of polymorphisms in genes involved in DA neurotransmission. Such genetic moderation might also occur related to the effects of early-life stress on later stress vulnerability/resistance

and risk/resilience for stress-related disorders. One study provided particular insight. A prospective-longitudinal study of a representative birth cohort sought to determine why stressful experiences lead to depression in some individuals but not in others by evaluating the presence or absence of the functional polymorphism in the promoter region of the SERT. This polymorphism moderates the influence of stressful life events on depression. Individuals with one or two copies of the short allele of the SERT promoter exhibited more depressive symptoms, diagnosable depression, and suicidality in relation to stressful life events, including child maltreatment, than individuals homozygous for the long allele. As noted, individuals with the same genetic variation also exhibited traits of anxiety, heightened stress reactivity, and increased amygdala responses to frightening faces. Thus, the gene-by-environment interaction in this epidemiological study likely reflects genetic moderation of the brain's functional response to stress, including child maltreatment, which translates into psychiatric symptoms. Similarly, the same investigators studied a large sample of male children from birth to adulthood to determine why some maltreated children grow up to develop antisocial behavior, whereas others do not. In that study, a functional polymorphism in the gene coding for the neurotransmitter-metabolizing enzyme monoamine oxidase A (MAO-A) moderated the effects of maltreatment. Maltreated children with a genotype conferring high levels of MAO-A expression were less likely to develop antisocial disorder.

IS EXPOSURE TO TRAUMA GENETICALLY DETERMINED?
Two twin studies provided evidence that exposure to trauma is moderately heritable. For example, it was shown in the Vietnam era Twin Registry project that genetic factors accounted for 36% of the variance in volunteering for service and 47% of the variance in combat exposure. In the Canadian PTSD twin study, similar heritability rates were found for exposure to assaultive traumas, but not nonassaultive traumas. There is also evidence that, in addition to trauma, exposure to any type of stressful life events is influenced by genetic factors. Findings from several twin populations suggest that exposure to childhood maltreatment, abuse or parental loss is, in part, genetic. For example, data obtained from the Virginia Twin Registry reflects that 20–30% of the variance in the exposure to a disturbed family environment, sexual abuse, or parental loss is explained by genetic loading for depression. These relationships might be explained by the genotype of the parents or the child. Parents of twins with depression would have high liability to major depression, which would likely predispose directly to family discord and divorce. Also, childhood temperament, influenced by genetic factors, could contribute to familial discord, abuse, and loss. It indeed appears that persons with high genetic risk for depression self-select into stressful environments, which in turn increases the risk for depression. A major challenge for future studies will be the task of separating genetic heritability factors for stress or trauma exposure from heritability factors for developing symptoms in response to these insults, and to elucidate the underlying neurobiological mechanisms.

CLINICAL IMPLICATIONS

Trauma spectrum disorders are complex disorders related to the experience of severe stress. The concatenation of findings strongly supports a developmental model that combines genetic and environmental factors across the life span to explain individual risk and resilience of developing adult psychopathology in response to a trauma. Despite the inherent difficulties of studying the genetics of trauma-related disorders, the field has exhibited remarkable advances. Particularly exciting are those of the genetic and environmental contributions to functional brain mechanisms that underlie the symptoms of trauma spectrum disorders. With the identification of polymorphisms in critical genes that influence the availability of certain neurotransmitters involved in the stress response, a rapid increase in knowledge on the nature of gene-by-environment interactions that determine whether an individual will develop a disorder in response to trauma has occurred. Rapid advances in the discovery of the precise genetic contributions to environmental or trauma-related disorders are anticipated. Discovery of the genetic bases of trauma spectrum disorders will aid in accurate diagnosis of persons at risk, even before trauma exposure. Such strategies will allow for effective prevention and, if trauma occurs, for direct treatment of pathological responses based on an accurate understanding of the biological pathways implicated in the "core trauma disorder" and the cognate trauma spectrum disorders. Some of the polymorphisms that confer risk to develop disorders in response to trauma may even be amenable to gene therapy.

ACKNOWLEDGMENTS AND DISCLOSURES

The authors are supported in part by the Emory Conte Center for the Neuroscience of Mental Disorders NIH MH-58922 (CBN), NIH R01 MH-56120 and VA Merit Award (JDB) and a NARSAD Young Investigator Award (CH).
Financial Interest Disclosures of Dr. Nemeroff:

Grants/Research	Abbott Laboratories; AFSP; AstraZeneca; Bristol-Myers-Squibb; Eli Lilly; Forest Laboratories; GlaxoSmithKline; Janssen Pharmaceutica; Merck; NARSAD; NIMH; Pfizer Pharmaceuticals; Stanley Foundation/NAMI; Wyeth-Ayerst
Consultant	Abbott Laboratories; Acadia Pharmaceuticals; AstraZeneca; Bristol-Myers-Squibb; Corcept; Cypress Biosciences; Cyberonics; Eli Lilly; Forest Laboratories; GlaxoSmithKline; Janssen Pharmaceutica; Merck; Neurocrine Biosciences; Novartis; Organon; Otsuka; Sanofi; Scirex; Somerset; Wyeth-Ayerst
Speakers Bureau	Abbott Laboratories; AstraZeneca; Bristol-Myers-Squibb; Eli Lilly; Forest Laboratories; GlaxoSmithKline; Janssen Pharmaceutica; Organon; Otsuka; Pfizer Pharmaceuticals; Wyeth-Ayerst
Stockholder	Corcept; Neurocrine Biosciences
Patents	Method and devices for transdermal delivery of lithium (US 6,375,990 B1) Method to estimate serotonin and norepinephrine transporter occupancy after drug treatment using patient or animal serum (provisional filing April, 2001).

SELECTED REFERENCES

Arborelius L, Owens MJ, Plotsky PM, Nemeroff CB. The role of corticotropin-releasing factor in depression and anxiety disorders. J Endocrinol 1999;60:1–12.
Bremner JD. Neuroimaging studies in post-traumatic stress disorder. Curr Psychiatry Rep 2002;4:254–263.
Bremner JD, Saigh PA. Posttraumatic Stress Disorder: a Comprehensive Text. Needham Heights, MA: Allyn and Bacon, 1999.
Breslau N, Kessler RC, Chilcoat HD, Schultz LR, Davis GC, Andreski P. Trauma and posttraumatic stress disorder in the community: the 1996 Detroit Area Survey of Trauma. Arch Gen Psychiatry 1998;55:626–632.
Caspi A, McClay J, Moffitt TE, et al. Role of genotype in the cycle of violence in maltreated children. Science 2002;297:851–854.
Caspi A, Sugden K, Moffitt TE, et al. Influence of life stress on depression: moderation by a polymorphism in the 5-HTT gene. Science 2003;301:386–389.
Gilbertson MW, Shenton ME, Ciszewski A, et al. Smaller hippocampal volume predicts pathologic vulnerability to psychological trauma. Nat Neurosci 2002;5:1242–1247.
Gottesman II, Gould TD. The endophenotype concept in psychiatry: etymology and strategic intentions. Am J Psychiatry 2003;160:636–645.
Hariri AR, Mattay VS, Tessitore A, et al. Serotonin transporter genetic variation and the response of the human amygdala. Science 2002;297:400–403.
Heim C, Ehlert U, Hellhammer DH. The potential role of hypocortisolism in the pathophysiology of stress-related bodily disorders. Psychoneuroendocrinology 2000;25:1–35.
Heim C, Newport DJ, Heit S, et al. Pituitary-adrenal and autonomic responses to stress in women after sexual and physical abuse in childhood. JAMA 2000;284:592–597.
Holsboer F. The corticosteroid receptor hypothesis of depression. Neuropsychopharmacology 2000;23:477–501.
Kascow JW, Baker D, Geracioti TD Jr. Corticotropin-releasing hormone in depression and post-traumatic stress disorder. Peptides 2001;22:845–851.
Kendler KS, Gardner CO, Prescott CA. Toward a comprehensive developmental model for major depression in women. Am J Psychiatry 2002;159:1133–1145.
Kessler RC, Sonnega A, Bromet E, Hughes M, Nelson CB. Posttraumatic stress disorder in the National Comorbidity Survey. Arch Gen Psychiatry 1995;52:1048–1060.
Orr SP, Metzger LJ, Lasko NB, et al. for the Harvard/Veterans Affairs Post-traumatic Stress Disorder Twin Study Investigators. Physiologic responses to sudden, loud tones in monozygotic twins discordant for combat exposure: association with posttraumatic stress disorder. Arch Gen Psychiatry 2003;60:283–288.
Radant A, Tsuang D, Peskind ER, McFall M, Raskind W. Biological markers and diagnostic accuracy in the genetics of posttraumatic stress disorder. Psychiatry Res 2001;102:203–215.
Sanchez MM, Ladd CO, Plotsky PM. Early adverse experience as a developmental risk factor for later psychopathology: evidence from rodent and primate models. Dev Psychopathol 13:419–449.
Seedat S, Niehaus DJ, Stein DJ. The role of genes and family in trauma exposure and posttraumatic stress disorder. Mol Psychiatry 2001;6:360–362.
Segman RH, Cooper-Kazaz R, Macciardi F, et al. Association between the dopamine transporter gene and posttraumatic stress disorder. Mol Psychiatry 2002;7:903–907.
Stein MB, Jang KL, Taylor S, Vernon PA, Livesley WJ. Genetic and environmental influences on trauma exposure and posttraumatic stress disorder symptoms: a twin study. Am J Psychiatry 2002;159:1675–1681.
True WR, Rice J, Eisen SA, et al. A twin study of genetic and environmental contributions to liability for posttraumatic stress symptoms. Arch Gen Psychiatry 1993;50:257–264.
Yehuda R. Current status of cortisol findings in post-traumatic stress disorder. Psychiatr Clin North Am 2002;25:341–368.
Yehuda R. Post-traumatic stress disorder. N Engl J Med 2002;346:108–114.
Zanarini MC, Frankenburg FR, Dubo ED, et al. Axis I comorbidity of borderline personality disorder. Am J Psychiatry 1998;155:1733–1739.

slow eye movements used to track a small moving object. The smooth pursuit eye movement abnormality has been documented in schizophrenia, is stable, and cannot be explained by disease related factors or overt psychotic symptoms. Nonpsychotic family members of schizophrenic probands also show poor pursuit globally, by pursuit gain, or by other measures. Often family members with abnormalities in smooth pursuit eye movements also have spectrum personality symptoms, although not all studies find such an association. Those studies in individuals with schizophrenia spectrum personality, with and without a known family history of schizophrenia, have noted smooth pursuit deficits only in subjects with a positive family history of schizophrenia. Smooth pursuit eye movement abnormality has been linked to chromosome 6p21 in relatives of patients with schizophrenia. Some investigators have argued that there is a deficit in motion processing in schizophrenia, thus explaining the smooth pursuit eye movement abnormality. But, because saccadic eye movements to a moving target are normal in schizophrenia, others have argued that the underlying deficit must be subsequent to the motion processing, either during the integration of motion signal into a smooth pursuit response, or the holding of the motion signal "online" for the smooth pursuit maintenance. The latter hypothesis implicates lesion(s) in posterior parietal and/or frontal cortical ocular motor regions associated with the smooth pursuit abnormality in schizophrenia, and is supported by functional imaging studies in schizophrenia spectrum.

In addition to changes in smooth pursuit, additional, subtle abnormalities in saccadic measures exist in schizophrenic patients, including failure on performing an antisaccade task in which the subject needs to look in the opposite direction of a target jump. Patients with schizophrenia made significantly more errors (i.e., made saccades to the target rather than away from the target) than the comparison groups. Nonpsychotic relatives, like schizophrenia probands themselves, also show an inability to inhibit an inappropriate saccade toward the target. This "antisaccade" deficit is modestly correlated with the smooth pursuit abnormality in the relatives of schizophrenic patients. These saccadic changes implicate dysfunction of the frontal cortex, especially the frontal eye fields in schizophrenia.

Neurophysiological studies identify abnormalities in information processing that can be elicited in the absence of a conscious behavioral response. Signal averaging of electroencephalographic (EEG) changes that are time-locked to sensory or cognitive events have been used. Such event-related potentials have several time bound segments (e.g., P50 or P300) that facilitate the examination of distinct aspects of information processing. P300 evoked potential response is a reliable positive change in an electrical potential occurring about 300 ms after a task-relevant or unexpected stimulus. P300 shows increased latency and decreased amplitude in persons with schizophrenia. Although specific EEG measures might vary with changes in symptoms, the P300 amplitude is consistently small in schizophrenia even during relative remission of psychotic symptoms. In addition, other components of evoked potential are abnormal in schizophrenia. Mismatched negativity response, an evoked EEG response occurring earlier than P300 has smaller amplitude in schizophrenia, suggesting an abnormal electrical response to stimulus novelty.

It is unclear what, if any, role these information processing deficits play in the development of clinical symptoms within the schizophrenia phenotype. However, neurophysiological paradigms that measure sensory gating provide a theoretical framework for understanding the development of the core symptoms of schizophrenia. Measures of sensory gating are obtained by examining a process called prepulse inhibition. In this paradigm, a person's ability to inhibit a startle response to a strong sensory stimulus in the presence of a preceding weak "prepulse" stimulus is evaluated. In contrast to a normal comparison group, persons with schizophrenia show poor prepulse inhibition. Schizophrenia might be associated with a reduced ability to gate sensory information, leading to a condition of sensory overload; positive symptoms could develop because of misinterpretation of unfiltered sensory information. Negative symptoms might occur due to the withdrawal from the sensory overload.

Sensory gating is also evaluated by using positive change in the evoked potentials 50 ms (P50) after each of the two auditory stimuli presented about 500 ms apart. Normal subjects show a diminished evoked potential response to the second compared with the first stimulus. In contrast, in persons with schizophrenia, the P50 evoked potential response is of similar amplitude as the response to the preceding stimulus. The ratio of amplitude of P50 response of the second (test) stimulus to the amplitude of the first (conditioning) stimulus is generally used as a measure of gating. A segregation analysis in the families of patients with schizophrenia suggested that P50 gating deficit is the result of autosomal-dominant effect of a single gene. Subsequent linkage analysis showed evidence for linkage of the gating deficit in families of schizophrenic patients with markers of location in the chromosome 15q14 region. This region has been shown to be the locus of α-7 nicotinic cholinergic receptor subunit gene, although no molecular abnormality has been found in this region of linkage.

FUNCTIONAL BRAIN ACTIVITY: rCMRglu AND rCBF

Initial studies with the early low-resolution PET cameras reported several different cortical and subcortical findings in schizophrenia. Studies reported relative hypometabolism in frontal cortex, a finding consistent with earlier SPECT blood flow studies. Early Xenon-133 rCBF studies identified and then extended the observation of frontal cortex blood flow abnormalities especially associated with impaired task performance. Schizophrenic subjects failed to activate frontal cortex areas when performing a task known to involve frontal cortex activity (e.g., Wisconsin card sort). Subsequent PET/fluorodeoxyglucose (FDG) studies in schizophrenia inconsistently detected frontal cortex hypometabolism, with some studies continuing to find it, others reporting no change in the measure, and still others finding frontal hypermetabolism. These inconsistencies can be partially explained by two plausible confounding conditions: an antipsychotic drug effect and a skewed schizophrenia target population. Antipsychotic drugs reduce cerebral metabolism in (among several sites) frontal cortex, thus possibly producing confound in the early studies that compared drug-treated schizophrenic persons with normal (untreated) controls. Also, because frontal cortical hypometabolism is associated with deficit (negative) type schizophrenia, a population skew might alter results. The composition of a patient group with drug-treated, deficit-type schizophrenics (often available for study) could skew results to identify frontal hypometabolism. Other results at first associated with the disease (e.g., elevated caudate/putamen metabolism), are now known to be a neuroleptic effect.

Studies using PET/FDG were conducted in drug-free, young, floridly psychotic schizophrenic individuals. The initial study detected metabolic differences in schizophrenia in limbic structures (anterior cingulate and hippocampal cortices) showing reduced regional metabolism in both structures. No other differences were apparent between the schizophrenic individuals and normal volunteers. However, within the schizophrenic group in this study, primary negative symptom patients showed additional changes of reduced metabolism in frontal and parietal cortex compared with the nonnegative symptom group. Both of these findings (limbic changes overall in schizophrenia, and frontal/parietal cortex reductions in negative symptoms) are consistent with other literature in their regional localization.

Blood flow studies in normal and schizophrenic persons performing hierarchical tasks within a single task modality and using contemporary scanning and analytic techniques, have begun to suggest human cerebral activation strategies associated with task performance. Because schizophrenia individuals characteristically perform many tasks more poorly than normal individuals, imaging experiments conducted without some attention to matching performance usually include a performance confound. The use of a variable error-rate task with all subjects fixed to the same performance level has been an innovation in this area, allowing comparisons across groups without a prominent performance confound. An rCBF comparison between schizophrenic patients and matched normal controls has been generated while both groups are performing a practiced auditory recognition task at a similar performance level (e.g., with task difficulty set to an 80% error level). The task involves discriminating between two auditory tones; the decibel difference in tone frequency can be varied to fix performance at 80% accuracy. There are also sensorimotor control (SMC) and rest conditions. Image analysis used in the Statistical Parametric Mapping software localized areas of activation associated with sensorimotor performance and decision during the control condition (SMC minus rest) and during the decision (decision minus SMC) condition, respectively. In the auditory recognition decision task, normal individuals activated the anterior cingulate, right insula, and right middle frontal cortex. The schizophrenic subjects had considerably more activation in extent and magnitude of response in the SMC task, showing activation not only in the superior temporal auditory cortex (left > right) but also in the left premotor cortex, left parietal cortex, right insula, and the cingulate cortex. In the decision task, especially in the ACC, schizophrenic participants showed no significant increase in activation except for a mild flow increase in right frontal cortex. Overall, in comparing the "decision minus rest" subtraction between groups, the schizophrenic patients show activation of more or less the same areas as normals. However, significantly more of this activation (which accompanied only the decision task in normals) was recruited for the relatively easy SMC task in the schizophrenic subjects. Moreover when the difficulty of the task increased and volunteers needed to increase performance, patients failed to provide additional blood flow to the ACC as did normals. Because the patients were performing this task at a similar accuracy level as controls, they must have been using other, presumably less efficient (possibly less consistent) brain regions for the task. One explanation of these data is that schizophrenic persons need "full effort" to perform the easiest of tasks. Another explanation could be that the schizophrenia volunteers all used different brain regions without consistency. One could expect a good deal of mental inefficiency

with this abnormality, no matter what its explanation. These data are concretely consistent with the psychological and symptomatic abnormalities of the illness.

Other laboratories have applied this method to the localization and type of functional defects in schizophrenia. The correlation between well-delineated symptom clusters in schizophrenia (negative symptoms, hallucinations/delusions, and disorganization) and rCBF has been studied. In vivo functional manifestations associated with schizophrenia are diverse. Negative symptoms were negatively associated with rCBF in left frontal cortex and left parietal areas. Hallucinations/delusions were positively associated with flow in the left parahippocampal gyrus and the left ventral striatum. Disorganization was associated with flow in anterior cingulate and mediodorsal thalamus. This analysis shows that different brain areas are likely to be differently involved in symptom manifestations in schizophrenia, perhaps either as a cause or effect of the disorder. A subsequent PET/H$_2$^{15}O study of hallucinating schizophrenic persons noted several CNS regions associated with the presence of hallucinations: the left and right thalamus, right putamen, left and right parahippocampal area, and right anterior cingulate. Cortical activations were present, but their localizations were variable between the subjects and not significant in group analysis. Another study showed that apomorphine (an antipsychotic in schizophrenia, despite being a dopamine agonist) improves (i.e., "normalizes") the anterior cingulate blood flow of schizophrenic persons during verbal fluency task performance.

Additional studies have localized changes to limbic cortex as well in schizophrenia both at rest and with cognitive challenge. Reduced hippocampal activation has been reported in schizophrenic subjects during a memory retrieval task of previously learned words. These findings (earlier) complement postmortem and structural imaging studies of abnormalities in medial temporal lobe structures of schizophrenics. A complex motor task was studied in schizophrenia during an acute illness exacerbation and 4–6 wk later after symptoms had improved. While the subjects were acutely ill, they showed signs of prefrontal hypometabolism. When the schizophrenic volunteers' symptoms improved, the prefrontal regions were normal. However, when the schizophrenic volunteers were less symptomatic, rCBF in the anterior cingulate and bilateral parietal regions was still decreased. These limbic regions' abnormalities might be the result of a dysfunctional network of regions and not a series of separate lesions.

Abnormal functional connectivity between brain regions might also explain abnormal rCBF patterns in schizophrenia. In studies of verbal fluency and semantic processing a network analysis revealed a functional disconnection between the anterior cingulate and prefrontal regions of schizophrenic subjects. Frontal lobe functional connectivity was abnormal in the schizophrenic subjects even though they had significantly activated the regions and their behavior on the tasks was not impaired. The normal circuits putatively mediating an auditory task specifically failed in connectivity between hippocampus and ACC and in influencing the prefrontal cortex. These findings are consistent with the view that the abnormalities seen in the frontal lobes of schizophrenics might be a circuitry problem of integration across regions and not a specific regional abnormality.

Several fMRI studies have explored whether rCBF changes produced by simple motor tasks are normal in schizophrenic volunteers. No rCBF differences were found between first episode, never medicated schizophrenic volunteers and normal volunteers while were performing a sequential finger–thumb apposition task. In the same study, a decrease in the blood oxygen level dependent response in the sensorimotor cortices of schizophrenic volunteers treated with traditional (first generation) antipsychotic drugs was found. Other studies found no differences, increased rCBF in the sensorimotor cortices of the schizophrenics, or decreases in those regions. Because the schizophrenic volunteers were medicated with both traditional and atypical neuroleptics, these results suggest that previous exposure to antipsychotics can have an interactive effect with task performance and brain activation patterns.

In more cognitively demanding tasks, such as working memory tasks, fMRI results remain inconsistent. The Sternberg Item Recognition working memory paradigm was used, requiring subjects to remember either two or five digits. Unlike many PET studies of working memory, an increase was found instead of a decrease in prefrontal rCBF in the schizophrenic volunteers compared with normal controls. Use of the N-back task and the Word and Tone serial position task revealed decreases of rCBF in inferior frontal regions of the schizophrenia group. The task performance of the schizophrenia volunteers was significantly worse on the N-back and word serial position task, but was matched on the tone task. Although rCBF increases in prefrontal regions with greater working memory demands, if working memory capacity is exceeded, the activation decreases. The discrepant findings in schizophrenia might be explained by an overload of working memory in the schizophrenia group.

CLINICAL PHARMACOLOGY

Clinical therapeutics of psychotic illness began in the second half of the 20th century with the discovery of chlorpromazine's (CPZ) antipsychotic properties. All treatment advances have been based on empiric observation, not theoretical prediction. CPZ was first tested in people with schizophrenia because of its known sedative properties as a preanesthetic agent. Its selective antipsychotic activity was noticed by informed clinical observation and was subsequently demonstrated empirically. This observation became the springboard for hypotheses of altered dopaminergic transmission in schizophrenia, once the mechanism of CPZ action was identified as dopamine receptor blockade. It has generated decades of research in therapeutics, but also was pivotal in promoting pharmacological approaches to the exploration of schizophrenia pathophysiology and to its biological formulations. Drug development in schizophrenia has focused almost entirely on dopamine receptor blockade, and has been highly productive, though empiric. Many potent, clinically effective selective dopamine receptor antagonists were developed and marketed after CPZ's discovery, and are available for clinical use. The drugs are similar in their primary actions but distinctive in side effect profile. Not until the controlled study of clozapine in the late 1980s in the United States was it clearly demonstrated that this neuroleptic had a unique superior antipsychotic action in the illness. This demonstration implied that potential therapeutic gains can be expected from new pharmacological approaches. Clozapine has a unique and superior antipsychotic action in neuroleptic nonresponding schizophrenic individuals and in partially responding schizophrenics compared with CPZ. Also, clozapine produces only a very low level of motor side effects (despite its other serious side effects), thus increasing patient comfort, social adjustment, and medication compliance. Based on these clarified clinical actions of clozapine, several new clozapine-like

compounds with fewer side effects, called "atypical" or second generation antipsychotics, have been developed and are available. All have reduced motor side effects, but with the exception of clozapine, do not show an advantage in treating psychosis better than first generation drugs. The pharmacological characteristics important in determining the clinical actions of the second generation antipsychotic drugs include (1) a restricted action on dopamine neurons as reflected in a limited expression of depolarization inactivation in A10 but not A9 dopamine cell body areas, (2) multiple monoamine (especially serotonin) receptor blockade, and (3) a lower dopamine receptor affinity. These second generation drugs, including risperidone, olanzapine, quetiapine, ziprasidone, and aripiprazole, have a primary antipsychotic action at least equivalent to first generation drugs, but have considerably lower motor side effects (parkinsonism, and akathisia) and possibly improved effects on cognition. Where available, use has switched completely from first to second generation drugs with considerable increases in patient satisfaction. Other improvements in medication compliance and clear improvements in psychosocial function remain to be demonstrated. Only dopamine receptor antagonists and a partial dopamine agonist of the dopamine$_2$-family show broad and potent antipsychotic efficacy in schizophrenia.

To understand the cerebral mechanisms of antipsychotic drug action, PET with FDG was used to study the localization of haloperidol action in the schizophrenic brain. Reports of the increase in glucose metabolism in the caudate and putamen with typical neuroleptics, were confirmed. It also found an increase in metabolism in the anterior thalamus and a decrease in metabolism in the frontal cortex (middle and inferior gyri) and anterior cingulate areas. Based on the known anatomic connections between basal ganglia structures and neocortex, these data can be interpreted as showing a primary drug action of haloperidol in the basal ganglia (caudate and putamen) with secondary and tertiary effects being propagated to these other related brain areas over the cortical-subcortical parallel-distributed neuronal circuits. This interpretation of haloperidol action is consistent with the idea that the drug acts primarily in the caudate-putamen with that action distributed to other related brain areas through the well-described parallel segmented cortical–subcortical motor circuit. This theory of anti-dopaminergic antipsychotic drug mechanisms needs expansion and further testing. Other mechanisms also known to diminish dopamine-mediated neurotransmission have been shown to be antipsychotic, although they do not seem as potent or as consistently effective as the dopamine$_2$-family receptor antagonists. An effect was initially demonstrated with tetrabenazine, a dopamine synthesis inhibitor; co-treatment with this drug decreased the dose of thioridazine required for full schizophrenia treatment, tested in a case-controlled study. Also reserpine, which depletes dopamine stores from nerve terminals, shows antipsychotic activity in schizophrenia and other psychoses. This action of reserpine, known before the discovery of neuroleptics, was used to treat acute psychosis, but with considerable side effect burden. The evaluation of full and partial dopamine agonists has been tested theoretically in schizophrenia. Dopamine agonists reduce dopamine synthesis and release by their action at the dopamine autoreceptor. The antipsychotic actions of drugs like apomorphine and (-)-3-hydroxyphenyl-N-propyl piperidine in schizophrenia might be based on an autoreceptor mechanism, namely a stimulation of dopamine autoreceptors to diminish dopamine release and thereby diminish dopamine mediated neurotransmission. These strategies for therapeutics have now been translated into clinical practice with the development of aripiprazole, a partial dopamine agonist.

There is no clear evidence from multicenter trials that glutamatergic drugs are therapeutic in schizophrenia, but there are reasons to be interested in this system's pharmacology in the illness. First, the excitatory amino acid (EAA) system with glutamate is ubiquitous in the brain; nearly every CNS cell bears EAA-sensitive receptors, indicating the extent of this system's influence. It is a complex system with at least two major transmitters (glutamate and aspartate) and probably several minor ones; it has at least four families of receptors, three ionotropic (NMDA-sensitive, AMPA, and kainate) and several metabotropic families with each receptor having a unique distribution, pharmacology, and probably distinctive functions. EAAs are the chief excitatory neurotransmitters in brain. They mediate fast information transmission functions and are also thought to be involved in other kinds of brain activity, such as developmental pruning, learning and memory, and neuronal plasticity. A therapeutic action of d-cycloserine (an NMDA-sensitive glutamatergic coagonist at the glycine receptor) and high doses of glycine (precursor) as a cotreatment for negative schizophrenic symptoms with first generation antipsychotics has been reported. Certainly the EAAs must mediate some aspects of psychosis due to their ubiquitous involvement in the CNS. Whether they might be involved in schizophrenia in a more primary way is speculation.

A connection between a part of the glutamate system, the NMDA-sensitive glutamate receptor system, and schizophrenia can be suspected because of the actions of PCP and its congener ketamine on human cognition. PCP produces a complex array of behaviors in humans including a psychotomimetic state. It can induce a psychotic state in normal persons (without delirium) characterized by many signs and symptoms often found in schizophrenia. Moreover, PCP and ketamine can both selectively exacerbate a patient's psychotic symptoms in schizophrenia, suggesting an action on (or near) the site of schizophrenia pathophysiology. Associated with the NMDA-sensitive glutamate receptor is a PCP recognition site located inside the NMDA-gated ion channel; the PCP site antagonizes ionic flow through the channel. This is a complex receptor site where NMDA, glycine, and polyamines positively gate ion flow into the cell and PCP, Zn^{2+}, and Mg^{2+} inhibit flow. It is presumed that PCP and ketamine both exert several important behavior actions through effects at this NMDA receptor.

Ketamine causes psychosis-like experiences in normal persons, exacerbates psychosis in schizophrenia, and functionally affects rCBF directly in those brain areas already identified as abnormal in schizophrenia, the ACC and hippocampus. Behaviorally, ketamine increases psychosis at subanesthetic doses in both neuroleptic-treated and neuroleptic-free schizophrenic patients to approximately the same degree. Ketamine stimulates positive symptoms in schizophrenia, and its action is not blocked by dopamine receptor antagonism. Ketamine stimulates a person's characteristic set of schizophrenic hallucinations, delusions, and/or thought disorder without totally inducing a new psychotomimetic state. This is unlike other psychotomimetics (e.g., amphetamine or muscimol), which stimulate psychotomimetic symptoms typical of the drug, not the illness. This ketamine action would be most parsimoniously explained by assuming that the drug stimulates a brain system that is already active in mediating the psychosis.

CONCLUSION

Schizophrenia is a serious mental illness. Persons with this illness are severely disadvantaged in life to the extent they cannot hold a job or maintain a family structure because of the breadth of mental symptoms influencing thought structure, thought content, affect, and cognition. Drug treatments reduce symptoms and blunt manifestations, but do not eliminate disease features. New therapeutics research needs to build on a known pathophysiology with well-supported molecular targets for drug discovery.

SELECTED REFERENCES

Altshuler LL, Conrad A, Kovelman JA, Scheibel A. Hippocampal pyramidal cell orientation in schizophrenia: a controlled neurohistologic study of the Yakovlev collection. Arch Gen Psychiatry 1987;44(12): 1094–1098.

Andreasen NC, Arndt S, Swayze VW II, et al. Abnormalities in schizophrenia visualized through magnetic resonance image averaging. Science 1994;266(5183):294–298.

Andreasen NC, Rezai K, Alliger RJ, et al. Hypofrontality in neuroleptic-naive patients and in patients with chronic schizophrenia. Arch Gen Psychiatry 1992;49:943–958.

Arolt V, Lencer R, Nolte A, Pinnow M, Schwinger E. Eye tracking dysfunction in families with multiple cases of schizophrenia. Eur Arch Psychiatry Clin Neurosci 1996;246(4):175–181.

Barta PE, Pearlson GD, Powers RE, Richards SS, Tune LE. Auditory hallucinations and smaller superior temporal gyral volume in schizophrenia. Am J Psychiatry 1990;147(11):1457–1462.

Benes FM, Vincent SL, Alsterberg G, Bird ED, SanGiovanni JP. Increased GABAA receptor binding in superficial layers of cingulate cortex in schizophrenics. J Neurosci 1992;12(3):924–929.

Bogerts B, Ashtari M, Degreef G, Alvir JM, Bilder RM, Lieberman JA. Reduced temporal limbic structure volumes on magnetic resonance images in first episode schizophrenia. Psychiatry Res 1990;35(1):1–13.

Braff DL. Information processing and attention dysfunctions in schizophrenia. Schizophr Bull 1993;19(2):233–259.

Braff DL, Heaton R, Kuck J, et al. The generalized pattern of neuropsychological deficits in outpatients with chronic schizophrenia with heterogeneous Wisconsin card sorting test results. Arch Gen Psychiatry 1991;48(10):891–898.

Breier A, Buchanan RW, Elkashef A, Munson RC, Kirkpatrick B, Gellad F. Brain morphology and schizophrenia: a magnetic resonance imaging study of limbic, prefrontal cortex, and caudate structures. Arch Gen Psychiatry 1992;49(12):921–926.

Buchsbaum MS, DeLisi LE, Holcomb HH, et al. Anteroposterior gradients in cerebral glucose use in schizophrenia and affective disorders. Arch Gen Psychiatry 1984;41:1159–1166.

Carpenter WT Jr, Buchanan RW. Schizophrenia. N Engl J Med 1994; 330:681–690.

Chen Y, Nakayama K, Levy DL, Matthysse S, Holzman PS. Psychophysical isolation of a motion-processing deficit in schizophrenics and their relatives and its association with impaired smooth pursuit. Proc Natl Acad Sci USA 1999;96(8):4724–4729.

Cleghorn JM, Kaplan RD, Nahmias C, Garnett ES, Szechtman H, Szechtman B. Inferior parietal region implicated in neurocognitive impairment in schizophrenia. Arch Gen Psychiatry 1989;46(8):758–760.

Condray R, Steinhauer SR, van Kammen DP, Kasparek A. Working memory capacity predicts language comprehension in schizophrenic patients. Schizophr Res 1996;20(1–2):1–13.

Crawford TJ, Sharma T, Puri BK, Murray RM, Berridge DM, Lewis SW. Saccadic eye movements in families multiply affected with schizophrenia: the Maudsley family study. Am J Psychiatry 1998;155(12): 1703–1710.

Deutsch SI, Mastropaolo J, Schwartz B, Rosse RB, Morihisa JM. A glutamatergic hypothesis of schizophrenia. Clin Neuropharmacol 1989;12:1–13.

Dolan RJ, Fletcher P, Frith CD, Friston KJ, Frackowiak RSJ, Grasby PM. Dopaminergic modulation of impaired cognitive activation in the anterior cingulate cortex in schizophrenia. Nature 1995;378: 180–182.

Faraone SV, Seidman LJ, Kremen WS, Pepple JR, Lyons MJ, Tsuang MT. Neuropsychological functioning among the nonpsychotic relatives of schizophrenic patients: a diagnostic efficiency analysis. J Abnorm Psychol 1995;104(2):286–304.

Freedman R, Coon H, Myles-Worsley M, et al. Linkage of a neurophysiological deficit in schizophrenia to a chromosome 15 locus. Proc Natl Acad Sci USA 1997;94(2):587–592.

Gold JM, Hermann BP, Randolph C, Wyler AR, Goldberg TE, Weinberger DR. Schizophrenia and temporal lobe epilepsy: a neuropsychological analysis. Arch Gen Psychiatry 1994;51(4):265–272.

Goldberg TE, Ragland JD, Torrey EF, Gold JM, Bigelow LB, Weinberger DR. Neuropsychological assessment of monozygotic twins discordant for schizophrenia. Arch Gen Psychiatry 1990;47(11):1066–1072.

Green MF, Nuechterlein KH, Breitmeyer B. Backward masking performance in unaffected siblings of schizophrenic patients: evidence for a vulnerability indicator. Arch Gen Psychiatry 1997;54(5):465–472.

Gur RE, Resnick SM, Alavi A, et al. Regional brain function in schizophrenia. Arch Gen Psychiatry 1987;44:119–125.

Harding CM, Brooks GW, Ashikaga T, Strauss JS, Breier A. The Vermont longitudinal study of persons with severe mental illness, II: long-term outcome of subjects who retrospectively met DSM-III criteria for schizophrenia. Am J Psychiatry 1987;144(6):727–735.

Harrison PJ, McLaughlin D, Kerwin RW. Decreased hippocampal expression of a glutamate receptor gene in schizophrenia. Lancet 1991; 337(8739):450–452.

Heckers S, Goff D, Schacter DL, et al. Functional imaging of memory retrieval in deficit Vs nondeficit schizophrenia. Arch Gen Psychiatry 1999;56(12):1117–1123.

Heckers S, Rauch SL, Goff D, Savage CR, Schacter DLFAJ, Alpert NM. Impaired recruitment of the hippocampus during conscious recollection in schizophrenia. Nature 1998;1(4):318–323.

Holcomb HH, Cascella NG, Thaker GK, Medoff DR, Dannals RF, Tamminga CA. Functional sites of neuroleptic drug action in the human brain: PET/FDG studies with and without haloperidol. Am J Psychiatry 1996;153(1):41–49.

Issa F, Gerhardt GA, Bartko JJ, et al. A multidimensional approach to analysis of cerebrospinal fluid biogenic amines in cchizophrenia: I comparisons with healthy control subjects and neuroleptic-treated/unmedicated pairs analyses. Psychiatry Res 1994;52(3): 237–249.

Javitt DC, Zylberman I, Zukin SR, Heresco-Levy U, Lindenmayer JP. Amelioration of negative symptoms in schizophrenia by glycine. Am J Psychiatry 1994;151(8):1234–1236.

Johnstone EC, Crow TJ, Frith CD, Husband J, Kreel L. Cerebral ventricular size and cognitive impairment in chronic schizophrenia. Lancet 1976;2(7992):924–926.

Kane J, Honigfeld G, Singer J, Meltzer H. Clozapine for the treatment-resistant schizophrenic: a double-blind comparison with chlorpromazine. Arch Gen Psychiatry 1988;45:789–796.

Kendler KS, Diehl SR. The genetics of schizophrenia: a current, genetic-epidemiologic perspective. Schizophr Bull 1993;19(2):261–285.

Kety SS. The significance of genetic factors in the etiology of schizophrenia: results from the national study of adoptees in Denmark. J Psychiatr Res 1987;21(4):423–429.

Kornhuber J, Mack-Burkhardt F, Riederer P, et al. [3H] MK-801 binding items in postmortem brain regions of schizophrenic patients. J Neural Transm 1989;77:231–236.

Lahti AC, Holcomb HH, Medoff DR, Weiler MA, Tamminga CA, Carpenter WT Jr. Abnormal patterns of regional cerebral blood flow in schizophrenia with primary negative symptoms during an effortful auditory recognition task. Am J Psychiatry 2001;158(11):1797–1808.

Liddle PF, Friston KJ, Frith CD, Hirsch SR, Jones T, Frackowiak RS. Patterns of cerebral blood flow in schizophrenia. Br J Psychiatry 1992;160:179–186.

Lidow MS, Goldman-Rakic PS. A common action of clozapine, haloperidol, and remoxipride on D1- and D2-dopaminergic receptors in the primate cerebral cortex. Proc Natl Acad Sci USA 1994;91(10): 4353–4356.

Mackay AV, Iversen LL, Rossor M, et al. Increased brain dopamine and dopamine receptors in schizophrenia. Arch Gen Psychiatry 1982;39(9): 991–997.

McCarley RW, Shenton ME, O'Donnell BF, et al. Auditory P300 abnormalities and left posterior superior temporal gyrus volume reduction in schizophrenia. Arch Gen Psychiatry 1993;50(3):190–197.

Memo M, Kleinman JE, Hanbauer I. Coupling of dopamine D1 recognition sites with adenylate cyclase in nuclei accumbens and caudatus of schizophrenics. Science 1983;221(4617):1304–1307.

Nishikawa T, Takashima M, Toru M. Increased [3H] kainic acid binding in the prefrontal cortex in schizophrenia. Neurosci Lett 1983;40(3): 245–250.

Owen F, Cross AJ, Crow TJ, Longden A, Poulter M, Riley GJ. Increased dopamine-receptor sensitivity in schizophrenia. Lancet 1978;2(8083): 223–226.

Pogue-Geile MF, Garrett AH, Brunke JJ, Hall JK. Neuropsychological impairments are increased in siblings of schizophrenic patients. Schizophr Res 1991;4:390.

Reynolds GP. Increased concentrations and lateral asymmetry of amygdala dopamine in schizophrenia. Nature 1983;305(5934):527–529.

Rosenthal R, Bigelow LB. Quantitative brain measurements in chronic schizophrenia. Br J Psychiatry 1972;121(562):259–264.

Ross DE, Thaker GK, Holcomb HH, Cascella NG, Medoff DR, Tamminga CA. Abnormal smooth pursuit eye movements in schizophrenic patients are associated with cerebral glucose metabolism in oculomotor regions. Psychiatry Res 1995;58(1):53–67.

Schwarcz R, Rassoulpour A, Wu HQ, Medoff D, Tamminga CA, Roberts RC. Increased cortical kynurenate content in schizophrenia. Biol Psychiatry 2001;50(7):521–530.

Seeman P, Guan HC, Van Tol HH. Dopamine D4 receptors elevated in schizophrenia. Nature 1993;365(6445):441–445.

Shenton ME, Dickey CC, Frumin M, McCarley RW. A review of MRI findings in schizophrenia. Schizophr Res 2001;49(1–2):1–52.

Shirakawa O, Tamminga CA. Basal ganglia GABAA and dopamine D1 binding site correlates of haloperidol-induced oral dyskinesias in rat. Exp Neurol 1994;127(1):62–69.

Silbersweig DA, Stern E, Frith C, et al. A functional neuroanatomy of hallucinations in schizophrenia. Nature 1995;378(6553):176–179.

Stevens AA, Goldman-Rakic PS, Gore JC, Fulbright RK, Wexler BE. Cortical dysfunction in schizophrenia during auditory word and tone working memory demonstrated by functional magnetic resonance imaging. Arch Gen Psychiatry 1998;55(12):1097–1103.

Suddath RL, Christison GW, Torrey EF, Casanova MF, Weinberger DR. Anatomical abnormalities in the brains of monozygotic twins discordant for schizophrenia. N Engl J Med 1990;322(12):789–794.

Tamminga CA. Schizophrenia and glutamatergic transmission. Crit Rev Neurobiol 1998;12(1,2):21–36.

Tamminga CA, Thaker GK, Buchanan R, et al. Limbic system abnormalities identified in schizophrenia using positron emission tomography with fluorodeoxyglucose and neocortical alterations with deficit syndrome. Arch Gen Psychiatry 1992;49(7):522–530.

Thaker GK, Ross DE, Cassady SL, et al. Smooth pursuit eye movements to extraretinal motion signals: deficits in relatives of patients with schizophrenia. Arch Gen Psychiatry 1998;55(9):830–836.

Toru M, Watamabe S, Shibuya H, et al. Neurotransmitters, receptors and neuropeptides in post-mortem brains of chronic schizophrenic patients. Acta Psychiatr Scand 1988;78:121–137.

Tsuang MT, Woolson RF, Fleming JA. Long-term outcome of major psychoses. I. schizophrenia and affective disorders compared with psychiatrically symptom-free surgical conditions. Arch Gen Psychiatry 1979;36(12):1295–1301.

Ulas J, Cotman CW. Excitatory amino acid receptors in schizophrenia. Schizophr Bull 1993;19(1):105–117.

Volk DW, Austin MC, Pierri JN, Sampson AR, Lewis DA. Decreased glutamic acid decarboxylase67 messenger RNA expression in a subset of prefrontal cortical gamma-aminobutyric acid neurons in subjects with schizophrenia. Arch Gen Psychiatry 2000;57:237–245.

Weinberger DR, Berman KF, Suddath R, Torrey EF. Evidence of dysfunction of a prefrontal-limbic network in schizophrenia: a magnetic resonance imaging and regional cerebral blood flow study of discordant monozygotic twins. Am J Psychiatry 1992;149(7):890–897.

129 Disorders of Substance Abuse and Dependence

Eric J. Nestler and Jennifer Chao

SUMMARY

Drug addiction continues to exact enormous human and financial costs on society, at a time when available treatments remain inadequately effective for most people. Given that advances in treating other medical disorders have resulted directly from research of the molecular and cellular pathophysiology of the disease process, an improved understanding of the basic neurobiology of addiction should likewise translate into more efficacious treatments. This chapter reviews our knowledge of circuits in the brain that mediate addiction and the changes in these circuits, induced by drugs of abuse at the molecular level, which represent the pathophysiology of addiction.

Key Words: Brain reward regions; cAMP; cocaine; CREB (cAMP response element binding protein); dopamine; drug addiction; drugs of abuse; ΔFosB; gene expression; nucleus accumbens; opiates; transcription factors; ventral tegmental area.

INTRODUCTION

According to the *Diagnostic and Statistical Manual of Mental Disorders*, drug addiction is referred to as *"substance dependence,"* the essential characteristic of which is a compulsive pattern of drug-seeking and drug-taking behavior that continues despite adverse consequences of drug use. Addiction, however, is by far the preferable term, because dependence—a pharmacological term—describes just one of many types of adaptations to drug exposure that includes addiction. *Dependence* refers to drug-induced adaptations that compensate for drug exposure and lead to an array of *withdrawal* symptoms when drug use ceases. Withdrawal symptoms vary based on the substance, but usually involve a significant negative affective state (dysphoria), and in some cases profound somatic abnormalities. *Tolerance* refers to drug-induced adaptations that lead to diminishing effects of a constant drug dose. *Sensitization*, or reverse tolerance, is caused by drug-induced adaptations that enhance drug responsiveness with repeated drug exposure. Many drugs cause both tolerance and sensitization, with some drug effects decreasing over time whereas others increase.

The complex syndrome of addiction is believed to be caused by a compilation of these types of pharmacological adaptations to

From: *Principles of Molecular Medicine, Second Edition*
Edited by: M. S. Runge and C. Patterson © Humana Press, Inc., Totowa, NJ

repeated drug exposure that occur in many brain regions important for the regulation of reward, motivation, and affective state. This chapter reviews the advances that have been made over the past several decades to understand the initial mechanisms by which drugs of abuse influence reward centers in the brain, and provides a progress report of efforts to identify the precise adaptations to repeated drug exposure that are responsible for addiction.

ACUTE MECHANISMS OF DRUG ACTION

The acute protein targets for most drugs of abuse are known as is considerable detail about how those actions perturb synaptic transmission after initial exposure to the drugs (Table 129-1). For example, opiates are agonists at opioid receptors, and cocaine binds to and inhibits the nerve terminal transporters for dopamine or other monoamine neurotransmitters. Thus, drugs of abuse comprise chemically divergent molecules with different initial activities. Yet, each of these drugs can produce addiction, which shares key features. Each drug, despite many distinct actions in the brain, converges in producing some common actions.

Prominent among these common actions is activation of the mesolimbic dopamine system (Fig. 129-1), which involves increased dopaminergic transmission from the ventral tegmental area (VTA) of the midbrain to the nucleus accumbens (NAc) (also called ventral striatum) and other regions of the limbic forebrain (e.g., prefrontal cortex). Several drugs of abuse also converge by mimicking (opiates) or activating (alcohol, nicotine) endogenous opioid pathways that innervate the VTA and NAc. Other drugs appear to act directly in the NAc via other mechanisms (e.g., cannabinoids, phencyclidine). These several actions appear to produce some similar net effects (generally inhibition) on medium spiny neurons of the NAc, in part because opioid, cannabinoid, and certain dopamine receptors, all of which are Gi-coupled (*see* Table 129-1), are expressed by some of the same NAc neurons. There is compelling evidence that these various mechanisms play a central role in mediating the acute rewarding properties shared by all drugs of abuse. The mesolimbic dopamine system and its forebrain targets are very old from an evolutionary point of view and are part of the brain's motivational system that regulates responses to natural rewards such as food, drink, sex, and social interaction. It is thought that drugs of abuse affect this pathway with a power and persistence probably not seen in response to natural rewards and, consequently, induce chronic adaptations that underlie addiction.

Table 129-1
Acute Actions of Some Drugs of Abuse

Drug	Action	Receptor signaling mechanism
Opiates	Agonist at μ, δ, and κ opioid receptors[a]	Gi
Cocaine	Indirect agonist at dopamine receptors by inhibiting dopamine transporters[b]	Gi and Gs[c]
Amphetamine	Indirect agonist at dopamine receptors by stimulating dopamine release[b]	Gi and Gs[c]
Ethanol	Facilitates $GABA_A$ receptor function and inhibits NMDA glutamate receptor function[d]	Ligand-gated channels
Nicotine	Agonist at nicotinic acetylcholine receptors	Ligand-gated channels
Cannabinoids	Agonist at CB_1 and CB_2 cannabinoid receptors[e]	Gi
Phencyclidine	Antagonist at NMDA glutamate receptors	Ligand-gated channels
Hallucinogens	Partial agonist at $5HT_{2A}$ serotonin receptors	Gq
Inhalants	Unknown	

[a]Activity at μ (and possibly) δ receptors mediates the reinforcing actions of opiates; κ receptors mediate aversive actions.

[b]Cocaine and amphetamine exert analogous actions on serotonergic and noradrenergic systems, which may also contribute to the reinforcing effects of these drugs.

[c]Gi couples D_2-like dopamine receptors, and Gs couples D_1-like dopamine receptors, both of which are important for dopamine's reinforcing effects.

[d]Ethanol affects several other ligand-gated channels, and at higher concentrations voltage-gated channels, as well. In addition, ethanol is reported to influence many other neurotransmitter systems, including serotonergic, opioidergic, and dopaminergic systems. It is not known whether these effects are direct or achieved indirectly via actions on various ligand-gated channels.

[e]Activity at CB_1 receptors mediates the reinforcing actions of cannabinoids; CB_2 receptors are expressed in the periphery only. Proposed endogenous ligands for the CB_1 receptor include the arachidonic acid metabolites, anandamide, and 2-arachidonylglycerol.

GABA, γ-aminobutyric acid; NMDA, N-methyl-D-aspartate.

Although the field has focused primarily on the VTA–NAc pathway as a key mediator of acute drug reward and addiction, several other brain regions are also important, and recent work has begun to examine these regions for chronic adaptations to repeated drug exposure (*see* Fig. 129-1). The amygdala is particularly important for conditioned aspects of drug exposure, for example, establishing associations between environmental cues and both the rewarding actions of acute drug exposure and the aversive symptoms of drug withdrawal. The hippocampus, a traditional memory circuit, is no doubt critical for memories of the context of drug exposure and withdrawal. The hypothalamus is important for mediating vast effects of drugs on the body's physiological state. Probably the most important, but least understood, are frontal regions of cerebral cortex, such as medial prefrontal cortex, anterior cingulate cortex, and orbitofrontal cortex, which provide executive control over drug use, which is severely impaired in many addicts. Of course, these various brain regions, and many more, do not function separately.

Rather, they are parts of a complex and highly integrated circuit that is profoundly altered by drug exposure.

CHRONIC ADAPTATIONS TO DRUG EXPOSURE

Drugs of abuse change literally hundreds of proteins in the various reward-related brain regions previously mentioned. Rather than providing a comprehensive review of such drug-induced changes, this chapter focuses on well-characterized changes that contribute to particular features of the behavioral syndrome of addiction.

UPREGULATION OF THE cAMP PATHWAY One of the best-established adaptations to chronic drug exposure is upregulation of the cAMP pathway after chronic opiate administration, illustrated in Fig. 129-2. Acutely, opiates inhibit the functional activity of the cAMP pathway by inhibiting adenylyl cyclase, the enzyme that catalyzes the synthesis of cAMP. With continued opiate exposure, inhibition of the cAMP pathway gradually recovers, which can be viewed as a sign of tolerance. This recovery can also be viewed as a sign of dependence, because on removal of the opiate (e.g., by administration of an opioid receptor antagonist such as naloxone) activity of the cAMP pathway increases far above control levels (which can be viewed as a sign of withdrawal).

Upregulation of the cAMP pathway in response to chronic opiate administration was demonstrated in cultured neuroblastoma × glioma cells in culture, and later shown to occur in several brain regions in vivo. The molecular mechanisms by which this upregulation occurs are now partly understood (*see* Fig. 129-2). With chronic opiate administration there is a gradual induction of adenylyl cyclase and of cAMP-dependent protein kinase (protein kinase A), which mediates most of the effects of cAMP on neuronal function. Some of these effects occur at the level of gene expression (*see* Adaptations In Gene Expression). Induction of these enzymes opposes acute opiate inhibition of adenylyl cyclase and explains the recovery in the functional activity of the cAMP pathway with repeated opiate administration (tolerance and dependence). On removal of the opiate, the upregulated cAMP pathway is no longer inhibited and becomes fully activated functionally (withdrawal).

Opiate-induced upregulation of the cAMP pathway occurs in many regions of the brain, in which it is implicated in several features of addiction, depending on the role of that brain region (Table 129-2). Moreover, in at least one region, the NAc, several drugs of abuse in addition to opiates (e.g., cocaine and alcohol) cause a similar upregulation of the cAMP pathway. Thus, this molecular adaptation can be viewed as a common adaptation to drug exposure and perhaps a common mechanism of addiction. One of the consequences of cAMP pathway upregulation is the sustained activation of the transcription factor cAMP response element-binding protein (CREB). Evidence for a role of the cAMP pathway and CREB in the NAc in particular aspects of addiction is discussed later.

ADAPTATIONS IN RECEPTOR SENSITIVITY Several pharmacological adaptations thought to contribute to addiction (e.g., tolerance and sensitization) involve changes in the sensitivity of neurotransmitter receptor function. Hence, effort has been directed toward understanding the molecular basis of such changes.

The best-characterized mechanism concerns trafficking of the opioid receptor. When an opiate binds to an opioid receptor, it initiates a negative feedback pathway. The opiate-bound receptor becomes a good substrate for G protein receptor kinases (GRKs), a class of protein kinase that phosphorylates ligand-bound G protein-coupled receptors. This triggers the binding of the receptor to another protein, called arrestin, which then triggers internalization

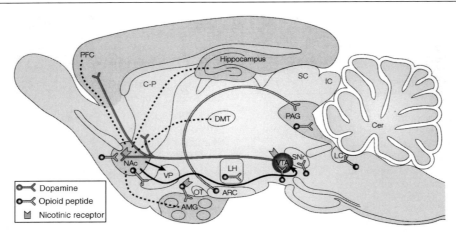

Figure 129-1   Key neural circuits of addiction. *Dotted lines* indicate limbic afferents to the NAc. *Arrows* represent efferents from the NAc thought to be involved in drug reward. *Dopamine pathways* indicate projections of the mesolimbic dopamine system thought to be a critical substrate for drug reward. This system originates in the VTA and projects to the NAc and other limbic structures, including olfactory tubercle (OT), ventral domains of the caudate-putamen (C-P), amygdala (AMG), and prefrontal cortex (PFC). *Opioid peptide pathways* indicate opioid peptide-containing neurons, which are involved in opiate, ethanol, and possibly nicotine reward. These opioid peptide systems include the local enkephalinergic circuits (short segments) and the hypothalamic midbrain beta-endorphin circuit (long segment). *Shaded areas* indicate the hypothesized distribution of GABA$_A$ receptor complexes, which may contribute to ethanol reward. *Nicotinic receptors* indicate nicotinic acetylcholine receptors hypothesized to be located on dopaminergic and opioid peptidergic systems. ARC, arcuate nucleus; Cer, cerebellum; DMT, dorsomedial thalamus; GABA, γ-aminobutyric acid; PFC prefrontal cortex; IC, inferior colliculus; LC, locus ceruleus; LH, lateral hypothalamus; PAG, periaqueductal gray; SC, superior colliculus; SNr, substantia nigra pars reticulata; VP, ventral pallidum. (Reproduced with permission from Nestler EJ. Molecular basis of long-term plasticity underlying addiction. Nat Rev Neurosci 2001;2:119–128. Copyright Nature Publishing Group.) (Please *see* color insert.)

of the receptor and receptor desensitization, contributing to receptor tolerance. Such receptor internalization is dependent on G protein βγ-subunits and appears to be a dynamin-mediated process. Indeed, mice lacking certain arrestins or GRKs show reduced opiate tolerance. Interestingly, dopamine receptors are regulated by analogous mechanisms. Accordingly, mice lacking arrestins or GRKs also showed abnormal behavioral adaptations to cocaine and other stimulants.

Drug-induced adaptations in G proteins or proteins that regulate G proteins—for example, regulators of G protein signaling (RGS) proteins—represent additional mechanisms of altered receptor sensitivity. Drug-induced changes in particular G protein subunits occur in specific brain regions and in some cases relate to drug tolerance or sensitization. RGS proteins serve as GTPase activating proteins; they activate the GTPase activity intrinsic to G protein α-subunits, which normally terminates the G protein signal. Over 25 forms of RGS proteins are known and most show highly restricted patterns of expression in brain. Chronic exposure to opiates, cocaine, or other drugs of abuse alters levels of particular RGS subtypes in brain regions important for addiction, such as the NAc. Moreover, such changes have been directly implicated in mechanisms of drug tolerance or sensitization depending on the brain region involved.

ADAPTATIONS IN NEUROTRANSMITTER SYSTEMS

Implicit in this discussion is the idea that chronic drug exposure alters the activity of particular neurotransmitter systems in the brain and that such alterations contribute to addiction. Changes in receptor sensitivity, presented in the previous section, are just one possible mechanism of adaptations in neurotransmitter systems. Although numerous neurotransmitter systems undergo such drug-induced adaptations, this chapter focuses on three neurotransmitters.

Dopamine   A widely held view is that repeated exposure to a drug of abuse produces some of its behavioral effects, for example,

drug craving and locomotor sensitization, by facilitating drug-induced dopamine release in the NAc. However, literature on this subject is inconsistent and confusing, given that these drugs both increase and decrease synaptic levels of dopamine depending on the drug treatment regimen employed and the time of withdrawal studied. Further work, therefore, is needed to understand precisely how altered regulation of dopamine release in the NAc or other brain regions contributes to the behavioral abnormalities of addiction. Further investigation is also needed to identify the molecular targets of drugs of abuse that mediate the altered synaptic levels of dopamine observed. Possibilities include drug regulation of the dopamine transporter and dopamine synthetic enzymes, such as tyrosine hydroxylase.

Glutamate   Drug-induced adaptations in glutamate systems have gained significant attention because of their prominent interactions with VTA and NAc function: projections from amygdala, frontal cortical regions, and hippocampus, which regulate the mesolimbic dopamine system, are largely glutamatergic. Accordingly, glutamate receptor antagonists can block the development of locomotor sensitization to stimulants and opiates, as well as some electrophysiological perturbations in mesolimbic dopamine function that accompany repeated stimulant exposure. Moreover, repeated stimulant exposure increases and decreases, respectively, the electrophysiological responsiveness of VTA dopamine neurons and NAc neurons to glutamate. Supersensitivity of VTA dopamine neurons to glutamate could be mediated via upregulation of specific glutamate receptor subunits in this region, specifically glutamate receptor 1, which has been seen after chronic cocaine, opiates, or ethanol administration. Altered levels of glutamate receptor subunits in the NAc are more variable, with both decreases in early withdrawal and increases in late withdrawal reported.

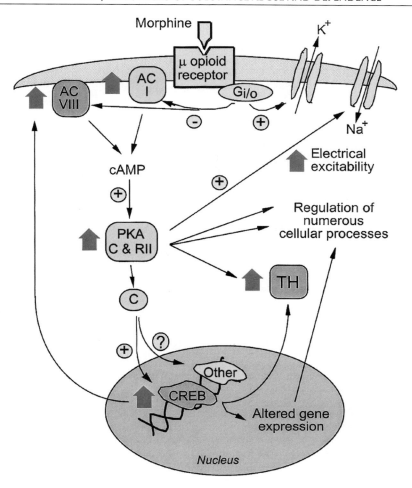

Figure 129-2 Scheme illustrating upregulation of the cAMP pathway in the locus ceruleus (LC), one target for opiates in the brain. Opiates acutely inhibit LC neurons by increasing the conductance of an inwardly rectifying K^+ channel via coupling with subtypes of Gi/o, and by decreasing a Na^+-dependent inward current via coupling with Gi/o and the consequent inhibition of adenylyl cyclase. Reduced levels of cAMP decrease PKA activity and the phosphorylation of the responsible channel or pump. Inhibition of the cAMP pathway also decreases phosphorylation of numerous other proteins and thereby affects many additional processes in the neuron. For example, it reduces the phosphorylation state of CREB, which may initiate some of the longer-term changes in locus ceruleus function. Upward bold arrows summarize effects of chronic morphine in the locus ceruleus. Chronic morphine increases levels of types I (ACI) and VIII (ACVIII) adenylyl cyclase, PKA catalytic (C) and regulatory type II (RII) subunits, and several phosphoproteins, including CREB and tyrosine hydroxylase (TH), the rate-limiting enzyme in norepinephrine biosynthesis. These changes contribute to the altered phenotype of the drug-addicted state. For example, the intrinsic excitability of LC neurons is increased via enhanced activity of the cAMP pathway and Na^+-dependent inward current, which contributes to the tolerance, dependence, and withdrawal exhibited by these neurons. Upregulation of ACVIII and TH is mediated via CREB, whereas upregulation of ACI and of the PKA subunits appears to occur via a CREB-independent mechanism not yet identified. (Reproduced with permission from Nestler EJ, Aghajanian GK. Molecular and cellular basis of addiction. Science 1997;278:58–63.)

Interest in drug-induced adaptations in glutamatergic systems has been sparked in part by the increasing evidence that such changes in glutamate transmission resemble changes in other brain regions that have been implicated in cellular mechanisms of learning and memory. For example, long-term potentiation in the CA1 region of hippocampus involves NMDA glutamate receptor-mediated changes in sensitivity of α-amino-3-hydroxy-5-methyl-4-isoxazole propionate (AMPA) glutamate receptors. This may occur via activation of Ca^{2+}-activated protein kinases, the phosphorylation of AMPA receptors, and the subsequent activation of the receptors as well as their delivery to the plasma membrane from intracellular stores. Research has demonstrated long-term potentiation and related forms of synaptic plasticity at glutamatergic synapses in the VTA and NAc and their regulation by drugs of abuse. An attractive hypothesis is that aspects of addiction are driven by memory-like processes within the reward regions of brain. This principle is discussed later.

Corticotropin-Releasing Factor Corticotropin-releasing factor (CRF) is best known as the hypothalamic peptide that regulates adrenocorticotropin hormone from the pituitary, part of the classic stress response. However, hypothalamic neurons that express CRF also influence many brain regions, and CRF is a prominent transmitter elsewhere in brain, for example, the amygdala. In both locations, CRF would be expected to influence the effects of drugs of abuse on the brain. Indeed, drug-induced alterations in CRF systems in the hypothalamus and the amygdala have been implicated in mediating the ability of stress to induce relapse to drug use. CRF systems also contribute to the negative emotional systems of drug withdrawal, a role documented for several drugs of abuse.

Table 129-2
Upregulation of the cAMP Pathway and Opiate Addiction

Site of upregulation	Functional consequence
Locus ceruleus[a]	Physical dependence and withdrawal
Ventral tegmental area[b]	Dysphoria during early withdrawal periods
Periaqueductal gray[b]	Dysphoria during early withdrawal periods, and physical dependence and withdrawal
Nucleus accumbens	Dysphoria during early withdrawal periods
Amygdala	?Conditioned aspects of addiction
Dorsal horn of spinal cord	Tolerance to opiate-induced analgesia
Myenteric plexus of gut	Tolerance to opiate-induced reductions in intestinal motility and increases in motility during withdrawal

[a]The cAMP pathway is upregulated within the principal noradrenergic neurons located in this region.

[b]Indirect evidence suggests that the cAMP pathway is upregulated within GABAergic neurons that innervate the dopaminergic (ventral tegmental area) and serotonergic (periaqueductal gray) neurons located in these regions. During withdrawal, the upregulated cAMP pathway would become fully functional and could contribute to a state of dysphoria by increasing the activity of the GABAergic neurons, which would then inhibit the dopaminergic and serotonergic neurons.

GABA, γ-aminobutyric acid.

ADAPTATIONS IN GENE EXPRESSION   The precise molecular mechanisms by which chronic drug exposure alters levels of specific proteins in the VTA–NAc pathway are still unknown, but gene expression may be involved. Such studies have focused on the role of two families of transcription factors: CREB family proteins, and Fos and Jun family proteins, in particular ΔFosB. CREB proteins regulate transcription by binding as dimers to specific DNA sequences termed cAMP response element sites, whereas Fos and Jun proteins form heterodimeric complexes that bind to DNA sequences named activator protein-1 sites. Most genes likely contain numerous response elements for these and many other transcription factors, suggesting that complex interactions among multiple mechanisms control the expression of a given gene.

CREB   As mentioned, chronic exposure to opiates, cocaine, or alcohol upregulates the cAMP pathway in the NAc and, as expected, this is associated with sustained activation of CREB in this region. Perspective into the functional role of the upregulated cAMP pathway and CREB in addiction has come from a series of studies examining the behavioral manifestations of a localized increase in CREB activity in the NAc. First, bilateral intra-NAc infusions of a PKA activator decreased cocaine reward in rats, whereas infusion of PKA inhibitors increased cocaine reward. Studies overexpressing CREB in the rat NAc via viral-mediated gene transfer have provided more direct evidence of the effects of CREB activity on reward. Increased CREB expression decreases the rewarding effects of cocaine, opiates, and sucrose, a natural reward, whereas expression of a dominant-negative mutant form of CREB resulted in opposite effects. Similarly, inducible transgenic mice overexpressing CREB in the NAc and dorsal striatum exhibit decreased drug reward, and mice lacking CREB show the opposite responses. Together, these data indicate that upregulation of the cAMP pathway and CREB in the NAc as a result of chronic drug administration decreases the rewarding effects of drugs of abuse and can be viewed as a mechanism of tolerance.

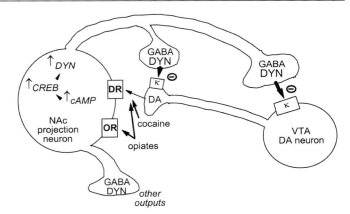

Figure 129-3   Regulation of CREB by drugs of abuse. The figure shows a VTA (ventral tegmental area of the midbrain) dopamine (DA) neuron innervating a class of NAc GABAergic projection neuron that expressed dynorphin (dyn). Dynorphin serves a negative feedback mechanism in this circuit; dynorphin, released from terminals of the NAc neurons, acts on κ opioid receptors located on nerve terminals and cell bodies of the DA neurons to inhibit their functioning. Chronic exposure to cocaine or opiates upregulates the activity of this negative feedback loop via upregulation of the cAMP pathway, activation of CREB, and induction of dynorphin. (Reproduced with permission from Nestler EJ. Molecular basis of long-term plasticity underlying addiction. Nat Rev Neurosci 2001;2:119–128. Copyright Nature Publishing Group.) CREB, cAMP response element-binding protein; DR, dopamine receptor; GABA, γ-aminobutyric acid; OR, opioid receptor.

Efforts are underway to identify target genes for CREB in the NAc. One apparent target is dynorphin, an opioid peptide expressed in a subset of medium spiny neurons in the NAc, which is induced in this region after chronic drug exposure (Fig. 129-3). Dynorphin release from the NAc is implicated in mediating dysphoria during withdrawal through a negative feedback loop to VTA dopamine neurons. Dynorphin binds to κ opioid receptors on VTA dopamine neuron cell bodies and terminals to inhibit their activity and decrease DA release in the NAc. The cocaine aversion caused by CREB overexpression in the NAc can be attenuated with a κ opioid antagonist.

ΔFosB   Acute exposure to drugs of abuse rapidly (1–4 h) induces all Fos family members in the NAc and dorsal striatum (Fig. 129-4). Even with continued drug exposure, levels of these proteins decline rapidly toward basal levels within 8–12 h. Biochemically modified isoforms of ΔFosB (a truncated splice variant of the FosB gene) exhibit a different expression pattern. Acutely, ΔFosB expression is only modestly induced, but it persists long after the other Fos family members have returned to basal levels. This persistence is mediated by the high level of stability of the ΔFosB isoforms. As a result, ΔFosB levels gradually accumulate after repeated drug exposure and can persist for weeks after withdrawal, dynamics that allow it to play a longer-term role in drug regulation of gene expression. Also, ΔFosB expression is induced in response to chronic exposure to several drugs of abuse, including cocaine, amphetamine, opiates, nicotine, ethanol, and phencyclidine. Such induction is most prominent in the NAc and dorsal striatum, but is seen to a lesser extent in other brain regions known to be important in addiction, including the amygdala and prefrontal cortex. Further, ΔFosB accumulates in the NAc after excessive running behavior, suggesting that such induction may occur in response to many types of compulsive behaviors.

Based on its unique properties, the functional significance of ΔFosB in drug-related behaviors has been studied extensively.

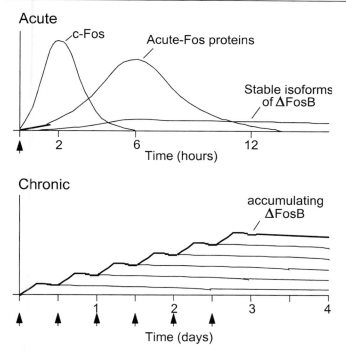

Figure 129-4   Scheme for the gradual accumulation of ΔFosB vs the rapid and transient induction of acute Fos family proteins in brain. **(A)** Several waves of Fos-like proteins are induced in neurons by acute stimuli. c-Fos is induced rapidly and degraded within several hours of the acute stimulus, whereas other "Acute Fos proteins" (i.e., FosB, ΔFosB, and Fos-related antigen [Fra]-1 and -2) are induced somewhat later and persist somewhat longer than c-Fos. Stable isoforms of ΔFosB are also induced at low levels following a single acute stimulus but persist in brain for long periods. In a complex with Jun-like proteins, these waves of Fos proteins form activator protein-1 binding complexes with shifting composition over time. **(B)** With repeated (e.g., twice daily) stimulation, each acute stimulus induces low levels of stable ΔFosB isoforms. This is indicated by the lower set of overlapping lines, which indicate ΔFosB induced by each acute stimulus. The result is a gradual increase in the total levels of ΔFosB with repeated stimuli during a course of long-term treatment, indicated by the increasing stepped line in the graph. The increasing levels of ΔFosB with repeated stimulation would result in the gradual induction of significant levels of a long-lasting AP-1 complex, which is hypothesized to underlie persisting forms of neural plasticity in the brain. (Reproduced with permission from Nestler EJ. Molecular basis of long-term plasticity underlying addiction. Nat Rev Neurosci 2001;2: 119–128. Copyright Nature Publishing Group.)

Transgenic mice were generated that confer inducible expression of ΔFosB primarily in the NAc and dorsal striatum. On ΔFosB expression, the mice show increased sensitivity to the locomotor activating and rewarding properties of cocaine and morphine. The mice also self-administer cocaine at lower doses and work harder for cocaine self-administration. These findings indicate that ΔFosB may play a role in sensitizing animals to the rewarding effects of cocaine and opiates as well as in increasing relapse when the drug is withheld. In addition, ΔFosB expression increases running activity, demonstrating a similar effect on natural rewards. Finally, mice that inducibly express a dominant negative antagonist of ΔFosB in the NAc and dorsal striatum show a decrease in cocaine reward, as expected. Thus, ΔFosB accumulation could amount to a "molecular switch," whose uniquely stable expression bridges the gap between acute responses to drug exposure and long-term adaptations in the neural and behavioral plasticity of addiction.

A major goal of research is to identify ΔFosB target genes. Using the candidate gene approach, two target genes have been identified. ΔFosB mediates the ability of cocaine to upregulate the AMPA glutamate receptor subunit glutamate receptor 2 in the NAc and could thereby mediate some of the drug-induced changes in glutamatergic transmission discussed earlier. Another potential target gene of ΔFosB is dynorphin. In contrast to CREB's induction of dynorphin, ΔFosB decreases expression of the neuropeptide, which could further contribute to the enhancement of reward sensitivity seen with ΔFosB induction.

Another approach to identifying potential ΔFosB target genes has been through the use of DNA microarrays. Inducible overexpression of ΔFosB regulates the expression of several genes in the NAc and other regions. The transcriptional regulation of these genes by ΔFosB requires additional confirmation, and their significance to drug-related plasticity has yet to be elucidated. However, one putative ΔFosB target gene identified by DNA microarray analysis is cyclin-dependent kinase 5 (Cdk5), which was subsequently found to be induced in the NAc and dorsal striatum by chronic cocaine. A possible function of Cdk5 in addiction plasticity is discussed later in this chapter; however, it is significant that its identification and subsequent characterization was enabled through the use of DNA microarrays.

CONSOLIDATION OF DRUG-INDUCED ADAPTATIONS

Although induction of ΔFosB is the most long-lived molecular adaptation known to occur in response to a drug of abuse, it does undergo proteolysis at a finite rate and therefore cannot underlie the near-permanent changes in behavior that are seen in many addicted individuals. This dilemma is analogous to challenges faced in the learning and memory field: although there are many elegant molecular and cellular models of memory, no long-lived molecular adaptations have yet been identified that could account for highly stable behavioral memory. By analogy with the learning and memory field, an evolving view in the addiction field is that some form of consolidation is needed, in the context of chronic drug exposure, to cause particularly long-lived adaptations in the brain.

One possibility, which remains highly speculative, is that such consolidation is mediated by structural changes in neurons. Indeed, drugs of abuse produce morphological changes in particular neuronal cell types after long-term administration. Repeated opiate exposure decreases the size and caliber of dendrites and soma of midbrain dopamine neurons that innervate the NAc. The functional consequences of these changes are unknown, but they could reflect a downregulation of dopaminergic activity and contribute to the dysphoria of drug withdrawal states. In contrast, repeated stimulant exposure increases the number of dendritic spines and dendritic branch points both of medium spiny neurons in the NAc and of pyramidal neurons in the medial prefrontal cortex (both of which receive dopaminergic inputs) (Fig. 129-5). These latter changes persist for at least 1 mo after the last drug exposure. It has been proposed that such structural changes could represent the neural substrates for the near-permanent sensitization in drug responsiveness seen in some models of addiction.

Of course, these various observations raise the critical question of the underlying molecular and cellular mechanisms that mediate such alterations in neural structure. Studies of the VTA–NAc pathway suggest that neurotrophic factors could be involved. Infusion of brain-derived neurotrophic factor into the VTA promotes the

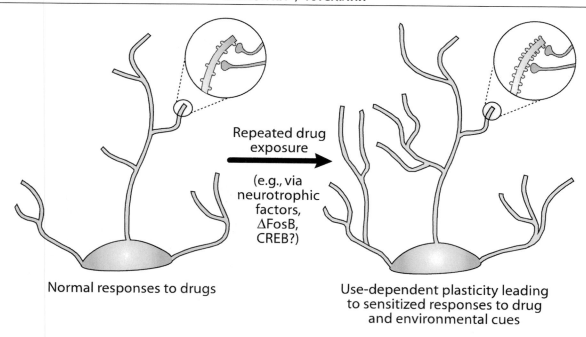

Figure 129-5 Regulation of dendritic structure by drugs of abuse. Expansion of a neuron's dendritic tree after chronic exposure to a drug of abuse, as has been observed in the NAc and prefrontal cortex for cocaine and related psychostimulants. The areas of magnification show an increase in dendritic spines, which is postulated to occur in conjunction with activated nerve terminals. Such alterations in dendritic structure, which are similar to those observed in some learning models (e.g., long-term potentiation), could mediate long-lived sensitized responses to drugs of abuse or environmental cues. (Reproduced with permission from Nestler EJ. Molecular basis of long-term plasticity underlying addiction. Nat Rev Neurosci 2001;2:119–128. Copyright Nature Publishing Group.) CREB, cAMP response element-binding protein.

behavioral actions of drugs of abuse, whereas infusion of glial cell line-derived neurotrophic factor exerts the opposite effect. Moreover, chronic administration of opiates or cocaine causes alterations in the intracellular signaling cascades for both of these neurotrophic factors, as well as changes in other neurotrophic factor systems. The results suggest a scheme whereby drug exposure perturbs neurotrophic factor signaling, which then disrupts the homeostatic role normally subserved by these factors in maintaining neuronal function. Given the ability of neurotrophic factors to mediate permanent changes in the brain during development, it is possible that analogous mechanisms contribute to stable changes in the adult brain that are related to addiction.

Although the molecular mechanisms underlying cocaine-induced changes in dendritic structure in the NAc and prefrontal cortex are not known, research has suggested one possible scheme. Chronic cocaine administration, via ΔFosB, increases levels of Cdk5 within the NAc and related striatal regions, and infusion of an inhibitor of Cdk5 into the NAc prevents the ability of cocaine to increase dendritic spine density in this brain region. The implication of these findings is that some of the structural changes caused by repeated cocaine administration may be mediated via induction of ΔFosB and may persist long after the ΔFosB signal itself dissipates (*see* Fig. 129-5).

FUTURE CONSIDERATIONS

Schemes discussed in this chapter are under evaluation to explain, at the molecular and cellular level, the highly stable behavioral abnormalities that define an addicted state. As knowledge of the neurobiological basis of addiction becomes more complete, it can be exploited to develop more effective treatments and ultimately preventive measures for addictive disorders.

Answers to another key question in the study of addiction will be critical for the understanding of addiction and for the development of new strategies for clinical management: Why do some individuals transition from casual drug use to compulsive use (addiction) so readily, yet others are highly resistant? Epidemiological studies show that addiction is highly heritable, with 40–60% of the risk for addiction to opiates, cocaine, nicotine, and alcohol being genetic. However, the individual genetic variations that comprise this risk have not been identified. Discovery of the genes involved will make it possible to better grasp the nongenetic factors that are also important. Such discoveries may allow individuals at risk for addiction to be targeted for prevention, and treatments for addiction to be targeted to certain individuals based on the underlying pathophysiology of their disorder.

ACKNOWLEDGMENT

Preparation of this review was supported by grants from the National Institute on Drug Abuse.

SELECTED REFERENCES

Barrot M, Olivier JD, Perrotti LI, et al. CREB activity in the nucleus accumbens shell controls gating of behavioral responses to emotional stimuli. Proc Natl Acad Sci USA 2002;99:11,435–11,440.

Berke JD, Hyman SE. Addiction, dopamine, and the molecular mechanisms of memory. Neuron 2000;25:515–532.

Bibb JA, Chen J, Taylor JR, et al. Effects of chronic exposure to cocaine are regulated by the neuronal protein Cdk5. Nature 2001;410:376–380.

Bohn LM, Gainetdinov RR, Lin FT, Lefkowitz RJ, Caron MG. Mu-opioid receptor desensitization by beta-arrestin-2 determines morphine tolerance but not dependence. Nature 2000;408:720–723.

Carlezon WA Jr, Nestler EJ. Elevated levels of GluR1 in the midbrain: a trigger for sensitization to drugs of abuse? Trends Neurosci 2002; 25: 610–615.

Table 130-1
Chromosomal Regions Implicated by Multiple Genome Scans

Chromosomal region	Markers	Position (cM)	Research group	Highest lod score
7q	D7S530–D7S684	134.5–147.2	IMGSAC et al. (2001)[a]	3.63
	D7S486	124	Philippe et al. (1999)[b]	0.83
	D7S1804	136.9	Risch et al. (1999)[c]	0.93
	D7S1813	103.6	CLSA et al. (1999)[d]	2.20
	D7S502	78.7	Buxbaum et al. (2001)[e]	1.30
	D7S684	147	Buxbaum et al. (2001)[e]	1.53
	D7S495	144.7	Ashley-Koch et al. (1999)[f]	1.47–1.66
	D7S2527	129	Ashley-Koch et al. (1999)[f]	1.77
	D7S2640		Ashley-Koch et al. (1999)[f]	2.01
2q	D2S364–D2S335	186.2-	Buxbaum et al. (2001)[e]	Hlod 1.96–2.99 NPL 2.39–3.32
	D2S2188	180.8	IMGSAC et al. (2001)[a]	3.74–4.8
	D2S382–D2S364	169.4–186.2	Philippe et al. (1999)[b]	0.64
	D2S116	198.7	Shao et al. (2002)[f]	1.12
16p	D16S3102	24.5	IMGSAC et al. (2001)[a]	2.93
	D16S407–D16S3114	18.1–23.3	IMGSAC et al. (2001)[a]	1.51
	D16S2619	28.3	Liu et al. (2001)[g]	1.93
	D16S3075–D16S3036	23.3–39.0	Philippe et al. (1999)[b]	0.74
19p	D19S221–D19S49	36.2–50.8	IMGSAC et al. 2001[a]	0.99
	D19S226	42.3	Philippe et al. (1999)[b]	1.37
	D19S216–D19S226	20.0–42.3	Buxbaum et al., 2001[e]	1.13
	D19S714		Liu et al. (2001)[g]	2.53
15q	D15S975	13.06	CLSA et al., 1999[d]	0.51
	D15S217	14.5	Shao et al. (2002)[f]	1.37

[a]International Molecular Genetic Study of Autism Consortium.
[b]Paris Autism Research International Sib-pair Study.
[c]This research group is led by Neil Risch of Stanford University.
[d]Collaborative Linkage Study of Autism.
[e]This research group is led by Joe Buxbaum at the Seaver Autism Research Center, Mount Sinai School of Medicine.
[f]This research group is led by Margaret Pericak-Vance, director of the Center for Human Genetics at Duke University.
[g]Autism Genetic Resource Exchange Consortium (AGRE).

individuals with the Broader Autism Phenotype are being implemented to address these difficulties.

Subgrouping involves categorizing families within a study sample based on endophenotypes that are suspected of having independent genetic etiologies. The most common endophenotypes used thus far in autism relate to language. Families in affected sib-pair linkage samples have been separated into two groups based on whether both children have severe phrase speech delay or not, with the hope that both subgroups will be more homogeneous than the combined group. Use of this specific endophenotype has dramatically influenced linkage data in at least three separate studies, with the language impaired subgroups demonstrating significantly stronger evidence for linkage than the combined samples from which they were drawn. Recently, "rigidity" in probands has been examined with similar benefit.

Similarly, the broader autism phenotype has been used to gain more information from pedigrees. For example, classifying parents in affected sib-pair families as *affected* or *unaffected* based on whether they had difficulties with specific aspects of language as children rather than as *unknown* significantly increased the linkage signals in a language impaired subgroup of families in two previously implicated regions of interest. Further, this approach elicited additional information from an existing sample without the expenditure of effort required to ascertain and enroll new families.

Molecular Approaches Improved statistical and phenotypic approaches will almost certainly enhance the ability to identify

autism disease genes. They are unlikely, however, to completely overcome the challenges named earlier; chromosomal regions of interest will continue to contain many candidate genes, all of equal merit, and genes of weak effect will thwart detection by current methods. However, additional molecular methods are being developed that will enhance the ability to overcome such challenges. These include enhanced detection of chromosomal abnormalities, case–control association studies using single-nucleotide polymorphisms (SNPs), and development of more appropriate animal models of autism.

Chromosomal abnormalities provide valuable clues to the location of potential susceptibility genes. With traditional karyotyping techniques, it is difficult to detect abnormalities that are smaller than 2 Mb, are in regions that are gene rich or have indistinct banding patterns, or are in telomeric and subtelomeric regions, which are prone to small deletions. Recently, panels of fluorescence-*in situ* hybridization probes specific for telomeres have been developed. Studies using them to screen populations of individuals with previously unexplained mental retardation have found that 5–20% have subtelomeric abnormalities that were not detected by high-resolution karyotyping. Small pilot studies have demonstrated this technology's efficacy in autism, and large-scale investigations are underway.

A case–control association study, which compares genotypes of probands and normal controls drawn from the same demographic population, is easier and less expensive to gather than affected sib-pair families. Such studies of closely spaced SNPs may enable more accurate refinement of initial linkage findings. Although unsuitable for linkage studies, case–control samples are useful for combing through regions of interest within linked intervals. SNPs are more common and more stable than the microsatellite polymorphisms typically genotyped in linkage studies, and therefore, enable more accurate and defined localization of disease gene variants.

Animal models of genetic abnormalities, which have assisted identification and characterization of numerous disease genes, have seldom been utilized in psychiatric disorders because of difficulties in defining the mouse phenotypes relevant for psychiatric disorders. However, assays for traits relevant to autism such as social activity, rigidity, and anxiety are being developed in mice. Technology is available that can limit the timing and location of altered genetic activity in mice, which is particularly important for neurodevelopmental disorders. Technologies have already generated data suggesting specific genes, such as those in the Wnt/disheveled/β-catenin and oxytocin/vasopressin biomolecular pathways, as candidate disease genes for autism.

NEUROPATHOLOGY OF AUTISM

Neuropathological studies in autism have been limited by the availability of only a small number of brains from individuals with this disorder. The brains studied have been from individuals of diverse ages, who are predominately mentally retarded. The two most comprehensive studies involve only 11 subjects. Despite this, a number of findings have emerged that suggest subtle, regional disruptions in the size and complexity of individual neurons, the number of neurons, and the organization of neurons. Although the cerebellum has consistently shown changes in autism, findings in other brain regions appear more variable. The number and density of cerebellar Purkinje cells was consistently reduced compared with controls. In other regions of the cerebellum, children were noted to have unusually large neurons, whereas adults had neurons with smaller cell bodies. Because there is a 1:1 correspondence between neurons in the inferior olive and the Purkinje cells, the normal numbers of inferior olive cells and absence of gliosis have been cited as evidence that brain abnormalities in autism occur very early in development. However, it is also possible that the inferior olive neurons survive because each inferior olive neuron connects to multiple Purkinje cells. In the hippocampus, amygdale, and entorhinal cortex, subjects had unusually small neurons. In the hippocampus, these neurons appeared to have less complex dendritic trees than neurons from control subjects. One research group found these neurons were densely packed although another study found no changes in unit density. There have also been isolated case reports of brainstem abnormalities.

Isolated areas of cortical dysgenesis with abnormal gyral patterns, disrupted laminar boundaries and abnormally oriented pyramidal cells have been noted in frontal, temporal, and cingulate regions. Advances in analysis methods show significant differences in cortical minicolums. These minicolumns appear to be the fundamental organizational unit of the cortex and consist of a neuron-rich core that also contains cortical efferents and cortico-cortical fibers, bounded by vertical, inhibitory fiber bundles from γ-aminobutyric acid (GABA)-ergic interneurons and surrounded by a cell-poor area that is rich in dendritic arborizations and unmyelinated axons. Minicolumn size is evolutionarily highly conserved. It has been hypothesized that minicolumns are critical in ensuring appropriate thalamocortical connectivity. Individuals with autism have more minicolumns per unit area and the core areas are larger with fewer cells, although the cell-poor areas are

significantly smaller than in matched controls. It is not yet known whether the total number of thalamic afferents is similar to controls. However, if it is, these changes in minicolumn organization would lead to innervation of a larger number of cortical units by the same thalamic afferent and reduce the specificity of inputs.

CHANGES IN PROTEINS AND NEUROTRANSMITTERS IN AUTISM Studies of specific proteins and neurotransmitters in autism have been limited by difficulties in assessing brain levels of molecules in vivo and/or by the scarcity of postmortem tissue. However, there have been a number of PET, serum, and postmortem studies examining various molecules thought to be important in neurodevelopment or neurotransmission. These studies have revealed modest differences, typically in the range of a 40–50% change in the level of several molecules. These molecules include reelin (which is important in cortical layering), B-cell leukemia/lymphoma 2 (an apoptosis regulator), and Neural Cell Adhesion Molecule (NCAM-180d form, which is involved in neurite outgrowth and synaptic plasticity).

Several systems show modest differences from control samples in the expression of neurotransmitter related molecules, although the significance of these findings is unclear. There appear to be changes in GABA-ergic transmission in the hippocampus with decreases in glutamic acid decarboxylase, which converts glutamate to GABA, and reduced binding to GABA(A) and benzodiazepine receptors reported. Changes in the cholinergic system have been reported in the frontal and parietal cortices. Specifically decreases in receptor binding of approx 30% for muscarinic M1 receptors and of approx 70% for nicotinic receptors have been reported. In cerebellar tissue, increased activity of the glutamate system has been reported with increased expression of the excitatory amino acid transporter 1 gene and the α-amino-3-hydroxy-5-methyl-4-isoxazole propionate 1 glutamate receptor. In contrast, no changes in the binding of serotonergic, cholinergic, and glutaminergic ligands in the hippocampi of autistic individuals were observed.

Changes have also been reported in the serotonergic system of individuals with autism. The observation that approx 33% of individuals with autism have hyperserotonemia is longstanding. However, PET scans studying serotonin synthesis in the brain revealed an abnormal spatial distribution of serotonin synthesis in a pathway connecting the dentate nucleus of the cerebellum, the thalamus, and frontal cortex with decreased levels of synthesis in the cortex and thalamus and increased levels in the contralateral cerebellum. A difference has been found in the developmental pattern of serotonin synthesis between individuals with autism and controls with typical development. Normally, serotonin synthesis is 200% the adult levels until 5 yr of age, and gradually falls to adult levels over the next several years. However, in individuals with autism levels are very low until approx 9 yr of age and then increase to about 150% of the normal adult levels. The typical developmental pattern of serotonin synthesis is very similar to the developmental patterns of synapse formation and elimination with many synapses during early childhood that are gradually eliminated during the second decade of life.

STRUCTURAL BRAIN IMAGING IN AUTISM

Structural imaging of the brain is ideally suited for the study of a phenotypically complex, etiologically heterogeneous, neurodevelopmental disorder such as autism, where the changes in neuroanatomy over time can be characterized in large numbers of affected individuals from the earliest ages of diagnosis. However, as a result of a lack of standardized diagnostic criteria and assessment protocols, small sample sizes, inclusion of heterogeneous populations (e.g., autistic subjects with associated medical conditions), failure to account for a number of confounding factors (e.g., gender, IQ, overall brain size) and the technological limitations of the available MRI hardware and image processing software, early MRI studies of autism failed to generate consistent findings. More recent studies have documented an increase in brain size in autistic individuals along with abnormal size of other structures (e.g., basal ganglia, corpus callosum [CC]) that may provide important insights into the brain phenotypes and underlying neural development.

BRAIN SIZE IN AUTISM   About 20% of autistic individuals have macrocephaly. Increased brain size was reported in two independent samples of autistic individuals contrasted with independent comparison groups that were sensitive to gender, cognitive level, age, and socioeconomic status. Increased lateral ventricular size was proportionate to the overall increases in brain size.

TIMING OF BRAIN SIZE ENLARGEMENT   Chart reviews suggest that individuals with autism often have enlarged head circumference at birth, but do not develop frank macrocephaly until the first few years of life. Because the rate of brain growth may be increased during the early postnatal period, several groups have attempted to examine age effects. Brain volume on MRI was studied in a cross-sectional sample of 60 males with autism and 52 "normal" controls, all of whom were divided into two age groups: 2–4 and 5–16 yr of age. Analysis of the 2–4-yr-old group revealed significant brain volume enlargement in individuals with autism compared to controls, with significant increases in both gray and white matter volume; whereas in the older group, brain volumes in the autistic group were either smaller or no different than controls. Analysis of a subset of these subjects (12, 2–4-yr-old autistic individuals vs 8, 2–4-yr-old controls) showed an increased gray matter volume in the frontal and temporal lobes only and an increased white matter volume in frontal and parietal lobes. Brain volume enlargement on MRI has also been independently demonstrated in 3–4 yr olds with autism. Finally, enlargement of the total temporal and parietal lobe volumes, but not frontal lobe volumes, has been demonstrated in a sample of adolescents and adults with autism.

Overall these studies provide converging evidence for brain volume enlargement in autism. However, the timing and nature of this enlargement are unclear. Longitudinal studies will be necessary to clarify the timing of this phenomenon. Elucidation of the timing and pattern of enlargement across tissues and structures may provide insight into underlying mechanisms that may be responsible for the abnormality as well as clues for candidate genes involved in determining particular patterns of brain development.

CEREBELLUM   Although postmortem studies have consistently shown abnormal loss of Purkinje cells in the cerebellum, and a highly visible study reported decreased size of the neocerebellar vermis on MRI in autism, numerous independent attempts at replication have not provided support for the observation of neocerebellar hypoplasia in autism. However, two studies have found evidence for an increase in overall cerebellar volume that appears to be proportionate to the overall increase in total brain volume in autistic individuals.

MEDIAL TEMPORAL LOBE STRUCTURES   The medial temporal lobe has been implicated in autism because of its role in social behavior and cognition in human and animal lesion studies, and the finding of postmortem abnormalities. Increased amygdala volumes were found in 44, 3–4-yr-old children with autistic spectrum disorders compared to developmentally delayed, nonautistic controls. Further the increased amygdala volumes largely resulted from a subset of 31 children with autism and were not present in a more mildly affected group of 14 children with PDD-NOS. Results of other studies have varied, showing increases, decreases, and no differences in amygdala volume. No consistent volume abnormalities have been reported in MRI studies of the hippocampus in autistic individuals. Finally, consistent with PET and postmortem studies, the anterior cingulate was noted to show a decreased volume in autistic individuals on MRI in one study. Given the diversity of results, small sample sizes and lack of longitudinal examination across a range of ages, no firm conclusions can be drawn about the size of medial temporal lobe structures on MRI in autism.

BASAL GANGLIA   Structural studies of the basal ganglia in autism are particularly interesting because volumetric changes in these structures have been consistently described in obsessive-compulsive disorder and Tourette's syndrome, disorders that overlap phenomenologically with the ritualistic, repetitive behaviors seen in autism. Increased caudate volume and stereotyped behaviors have also been correlated in Fragile-X syndrome. Enlargement of the caudate, but not the globus pallidus or putamen, was detected in two independent samples of autistic individuals. In addition, there were significant correlations between caudate size and stereotyped-repetitive behaviors ($r = 0.5$), but not social or communication deficits. These data suggest the possibility that two different frontal—striatal mechanisms, one involved with motor stereotypies (positively correlated with caudate volume) and the other involved in compulsive and ritualistic behavior (negatively correlated with caudate volume), might be operating in autism.

CORPUS CALLOSUM   The CC is the major axonal pathway linking the two hemispheres. Abnormalities in the CC are hypothesized to index disruption in cortical connectivity. Further, the axons crossing in the CC are known to be topographically related to their origins in the cerebral cortex, providing the potential to narrow the cortical regions implicated through an examination of the size of subsections of the corpus callosum. A reduction in CC size in autism is well established. These findings are of increased interest because CC enlargement would be expected given the evidence for increased brain volume. The discrepant findings of enlarged brain volume and reduced CC size may provide an index of overall disconnectivity in autism, or provide clues to particular cortical layers that may be implicated in the increased brain size, as only selected layers (e.g., cortical layer III) contribute axons that cross at the CC. However, consistency is lacking regarding which subsections are implicated.

NEUROPSYCHOLOGICAL CHARACTERISTICS ASSOCIATED WITH AUTISM

Individuals with autism appear to have problems both attending to socially salient stimuli and making inferences about the mental states of others in specific social situations. In contrast to normal controls that focus on the eyes and mouth of people when looking at faces, individuals with autism focus on peripheral parts of the face such as the ears and chin and avoid the eyes (Fig. 130-1). This tendency is maintained when people with autism evaluate social interactions between people, in contrast to controls who focus on the eye gaze between people. Investigators have also found differences in the extent to which individuals with autism are aware that others

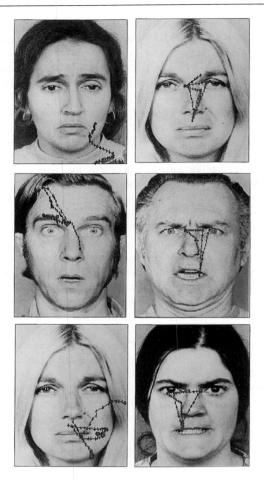

Figure 130-1 The visual scan paths utilized to inspect still pictures of faces by three individuals with autism are shown on the left. These scan paths avoid the eyes and nose in stark contrast to the scan paths of three typically developing controls (on the right). (Reproduced with permission from Pelphrey KA, Sasson NJ, Reznick JS, Paul G, Goldman BN, Piven J, Visual scanning of faces in adults with autism. J Autism Dev Disord 2002:32[4]:249–261.)

may have perceptions and beliefs that differ from their own because the others have access to different information or experiences. This awareness, known as a theory of mind, is critical to empathy and truly reciprocal interactions. However, this ability is clearly influenced by one's developmental level. Social cognition appears to involve a widely distributed neural network in which the amygdala, temporal cortex, and orbitofrontal regions play central roles.

Central coherence refers to the ability to process information within a contextual context. People with autism appear to show a processing bias in favor of featural information at the expense of configural information. They often excel at the Wechsler Block Design subtest and the embedded figures test, easily breaking the whole figures into parts. However, this detail-focused processing style leads to poor performance on other tasks in which processing in context is necessary. Prefrontal cortex appears important in the processing of contextual information in control subjects, whereas the right hemisphere, particularly the somatosensory cortex, has been implicated in problems of central coherence.

Executive function is specifically conceptualized as involving several overlapping, but potentially dissociable mental operations, such as cognitive flexibility, planning, inhibition of prepotent responses, and working memory. Executive functioning deficits are

observed in multiple neuropsychiatric and neurodevelopmental conditions, and do not appear directly related to IQ. Individuals with autism have been shown to have particular difficulty with cognitive flexibility as assessed by the ability to readily shift from one set of rules to another in multiple studies. In addition, autistic individuals also appear to perform poorly on tasks that simultaneously tax both planning and inhibitory control. Difficulties with cognitive flexibility, response inhibition, and working memory have been independently correlated with ritualistic and repetitive behaviors in autism. Difficulties in executive function have also been related to difficulties in social behavior in autism. Impairments of executive function in neurodevelopmental disorders appear to arise from abnormalities in the pathways connecting frontal cortex and subcortical structures (e.g., fronto-striatal system).

FUNCTIONAL NEUROIMAGING IN AUTISM

Functional neuroimaging findings in autism have been focused on studies of simple motor actions, the embedded figures task, language processing, and social cognition. The potential of functional neuroimaging studies to illuminate the neural basis of specific domains of behavior in autism is well illustrated by studies of social cognition. For example, neuroimaging studies of typically developing individuals have consistently identified a region on the lateral aspect of the fusiform gyrus that responds selectively to faces in contrast to nearby regions, including the inferior temporal gyrus, that are active during visual processing of nonface objects. In typically developing controls, activation of the fusiform gyrus is also modulated by the intentionality of socially relevant stimuli. The fusiform gyrus may be a critical component in the neural network involved in emotion recognition and social cognition. Specifically, the fusiform gyrus and the superior temporal cortices provide information about facial structure and movement to other brain structures especially the amygdala, which appears to connect the perceptual representation of a socially relevant stimulus to an emotional and social significance.

Individuals with autism have striking impairments in the processing of social and emotional information from faces. Three independent studies, all using slightly different face processing paradigms, have found that adult male participants with autism showed less activity in the fusiform gyrus and more activity in the inferior temporal gyrus than controls when looking at faces. The specific location of the evoked activity outside the fusiform gyrus was highly variable between different autistic subjects. These studies also demonstrated reduced amygdala activity during implicit processing of emotion from faces. Eye tracking studies also demonstrate that individuals with autism tend to inspect faces in an idiosyncratic, somewhat disorganized way in contrast to control subjects, who focus on the eyes and mouth. Collectively, these studies suggest a neural basis for the face processing deficits observed in individuals with autism. Based on these studies, postmortem studies in autism, and an animal model of early amygdala ablation, investigators have proposed that an early disruption in the amygdala and its connections to temporal cortices impairs the development of normal specificity in the fusiform gyrus.

Similarly, functional neuroimaging studies in individuals with typical development have found that frontal–temporal cortical regions and subcortical regions (including the left amygdala, hippocampus, and striatum; and the insula and superior temporal cortices bilaterally) are activated to a greater extent during theory of mind tasks than control tasks. However, when individuals with autism performed the same tasks, they failed to activate the amygdala and had reduced activation of frontal cortex. In a similar PET study, individuals with autism had marked difficulty when asked to identify the intentions of animated, nonhuman figures, and had hypoactivation of medial prefrontal cortex, the superior temporal cortices, and the temporal pole near the amygdala.

One study of motor activation in autism found reduced activation overall in individuals with autism relative to controls. In addition, there was less deactivation of prefrontal cortex and greater individual variability of regional activation among subjects with autism. The existing embedded figures study also suggests that individuals with autism may utilize different brain regions for detail-oriented processing than controls. In the autism group, reduced activation was observed overall, particularly in the right dorsolateral prefrontal cortex and parietal cortices. However, there was greater relative activation of the right ventral occipital region among subjects with autism. The limited studies of language processing also show atypical activation patterns. The atypical findings included reversed or reduced hemispheric specialization, anomalous activation of cingulate cortex during a tone perception task, and reduced activation of the frontal-thalamic-cerebellar pathway in which abnormal serotonin synthesis has been demonstrated. Studies of language processing in autism are likely to be greatly enhanced by research aimed at dissecting the neural bases of pragmatic and semantic language skills in normal individuals.

CONCLUSIONS

The search for the molecular basis of autism is challenging. The high heritability of the disorder led to great optimism that traditional linkage methods would rapidly identify disease genes for this phenotypically complex disorder and provide a means for understanding its underlying pathophysiology in the same way that the identification of the MeCP3 gene provided the impetus for major advances in the understanding of Rett Syndrome. Similarly, structural neuroimaging studies and neurochemical investigations of serotonin initially met with considerable optimism. In each of these cases, unexpected deficiencies of the methods coupled with heterogeneity in autism limited progress. Researchers have responded by developing more sensitive methods and by more precisely defining subject and control groups with particular attention to narrowly defined phenotypes, age, cognitive ability, and gender. There has been particular emphasis on taking a developmental perspective, especially regarding imaging and studies of brain chemistry and function.

Exciting research is aimed at elucidating both the neural systems involved in specific aspects of the behavioral phenotype and basic neurodevelopmental processes likely to underlie the disturbances in these neural systems. Functional imaging studies of several different cognitive processes have found activation patterns in individuals with autism that differ from those robustly observed in typically developing individuals. Highly specialized areas such as the temporal fusiform gyrus during facial perception and the amygdala in theory of mind tasks appear to be less active in autistic individuals than typically developing individuals. Functional imaging studies have also shown great individual variability in the activation patterns of autistic individuals, which raises the possibility that individuals with autism may have difficulties developing appropriate functional specialization of cortical regions. Synapse refinement through pruning is thought to play a crucial role in the functional specialization of the cortex. There are intriguing, but indirect, leads that synapse refinement may be impaired in autism. First, increased cortical size could result from persistence of inappropriately large dendritic

arbors during specific developmental periods. The changes described in the density and organization of cortical minicolumns in autism is also consistent with a reduction in cortical specialization. Finally, because serotonin plays a crucial role in cortical patterning, the developmental disturbances in serotonin synthesis reported in autism might lead to problems with synaptic pruning and cortical specialization. Similar problems might be caused by other abnormalities in neurotransmitter systems or neurodevelopmental molecules reported in autism. Aberrant synapse elimination might initially lead to more cells that receive less specific inputs and fail to establish appropriate and efficient connections with other components of key neural circuits (like the amygdala-temporal-frontal circuits involved in social cognition). Ultimately, cells with inadequate appropriate stimulation might atrophy or even die. Ongoing integration of the findings from genetic studies, structural, and functional neuroimaging and neurodevelopmental studies in relevant animal models and brain samples has great potential to provide insights into brain-behavior relationships and neural mechanisms in this complex neurodevelopmental disorder.

ACKNOWLEDGMENTS

The authors of this chapter have received support from the UNC STAART Center U54 MH066418. In addition, Dr Sikich is supported by K23 MH01802 and the Foundation of Hope, Dr Wassink is supported by 5K08 MH062123 and 5R01NS043550-02, Dr Pelphrey is supported by T32 HD40127, and Dr Piven is supported by K02 MH01562, R01 MH 616696, R01 MH55284, R01 MH64580, and 5 P30 HD03110.

SELECTED REFERENCES

Adolphs R. Cognitive neuroscience of human social behavior. Nat Rev Neurosci 2003;1:165–178.

Amir R, Van den Veyver I, Wan M, Tran C, Francke U, Zoghbi H. Rett syndrome is caused by mutations in X-linked MECP2, encoding methy-CpG-binding protein 2. Nat Genet 1999;23:185–188.

Armstrong D, Dunn JK, Antalffy B, Trivedi R. Selective dendritic alterations in the cortex of Rett syndrome. J Neuropathol Exp Neurol 1995;54:195–201.

Ashley-Koch A, Wolpert CM, Menold MM, et al. Genetic studies of autistic disorder and chromosome 7. Genomics 1999;61:227–236.

Bailey A, Luthert P, Dean A, et al. A clinicopathological study of autism. Brain 1998;121:889–905.

Bauman M, Kemper T. Histoanatomic observations of the brain in early infantile autism. Neurology 1985;35:866–874.

Buxbaum J, Silverman J, Smith C, et al. Evidence for a susceptibility gene for autism on chromosome 2 and for genetic heterogeneity. Am J Hum Genet 2001;68:1514–1520.

CLSA (Collaborative Linkage Study of Autism); Barrett S, Beck J, et al. An autosomal genomic screen for autism. Am J Med Genet (Neuropsychiat Genet) 1999;88:609–615.

Cody H, Pelphrey K, Piven J. Structural and functional magnetic resonance imaging of autism. Int J Dev Neurosci 2002;20:421–438.

Comery T, Harris J, Willems P, et al. Abnormal dendritic spines in fragile X knockout mice: maturation and pruning deficits. Proc Natl Acad Sci USA 1997;94:5401–5404.

Folstein SE, Rosen-Sheidley B. Genetics of autism: complex aetiology for a heterogeneous disorder. Nat Rev Genet 2001;2(12):943–955.

Fombonne E, Du Mazaubrun C, Cans C, Grandjean H. Autism and associated medical disorders in a French epidemiological survey. J Am Acad Child Adolesc Psychiatry 1997;36:1561–1569.

Huang J, Vieland V. Comparison of 'model-free' and 'model-based' linkage statistics in the presence of locus heterogeneity: single data set and multiple data set applications. Hum Heredity 2001;51:217–225.

Huttenlocher P, de Courten C, Garey L, Van Der Loos H. Synaptogenesis in human visual cortex—evidence for synapse elimination during normal development. Neurosci Lett 1982;33:247–252.

IMGSAC (International Molecular Genetic Study of Autism Consortium). A genomewide screen for autism: strong evidence for linkage to chromosomes 2q, 7q, and 16p. Am J Hum Genet 2001;69:570–581.

Irwin S, Patel B, Idupulapati M, et al. Abnormal dendritic spine characteristics in the temporal and visual cortices of patients with fragile-X syndrome: a quantitative examination. Am J Med Genet 2001;98:161–167.

Irwin S, Swain R, Christmon C, Chakravarti A, Weiler I, Greenough W. Evidence for altered Fragile-X mental retardation protein expression in response to behavioral stimulation. Neurobiol Learn Mem 2000;74:87–93.

Johnston M, Jeon O-H, Pevsner J, Blue M, Naidu S. Neurobiology of Rett syndrome: a genetic disorder of synapse development. Brain Dev 2001;23:S206–S213.

Kemper T, Bauman M. Neuropathology of infantile autism. Mol Psychiatry 2002;7(Suppl 2):S12–S13.

Liu J, Nyholt D, Magnussen P, et al. A genomewide screen for autism susceptibility loci. Am J Hum Genet 2001;69:327–340.

Nowaczyk M, Waye J. The Smith-Lemli-Opitz syndrome: a novel metabolic way of understanding developmental biology, embryogenesis, and dysmorphology. Clin Genet 2001;59:375–386.

Pelphrey KA, Sasson NJ, Reznick JS, Paul G, Goldman BN, Piven J. Visual scanning of faces in adults with autism. J Autism Dev Disord 2002;32(4):249–261.

Philippe A, Martinez M, Guilloud-Batallle M, et al. Genome-wide scan for autism susceptibility genes: Paris Autism Research International Sibpair Study. Hum Mol Genet 1999;8:805–812.

Pickles A, Bolton P, Macdonald H, et al. Latent-class analysis of recurrence risks for complex phenotypes with selection and measurement error: a twin and family history study of autism. Am J Hum Genet 1995;57:717–726.

Risch N, Spiker D, Lotspeich L, et al. A genomic screen of autism: Evidence for a multilocus etiology. Am J Hum Genet 1999;65:493–507.

Ritvo E, Freeman B, Scheibel A, et al. Lower Purkinje cell counts in the cerebella of four autistic subjects: initial findings of the UCLA-NSAC Autopsy Research Report. Am J Psychiatry 1986;143(7):862–866.

Shao Y, Cuccaro M, Hauser E, et al. Fine mapping of autistic disorder to chromosome 15q11-q13 by use of phenotypic subtypes. Am J Hum Genet. 2003;72(3):539–548.

Shao Y, Raiford K, Wolpert C, et al. Phenotypic homogeneity provides increased support for linkage on chromosome 2 in autistic disorder. Am J Hum Genet 2002;70:1058–1061.

Shao Y, Wolpert C, Raiford K, et al. Genomic screen and follow-up analysis for autistic disorder. Am J Med Genet (Neuropsychiat Genet) 2002;114:99–105.

Siegal M, Varley R. Neural systems involved in "theory of mind." Nat Rev Neurosci 2002;3(6):463–471.

Sutcliffe J, Nurmi E, Lombroso P. Genetics of childhood disorders: XLVII. Autism, part 6: duplication and inherited susceptibility of chromosome 15q11-q13 genes in autism. J Am Acad Child Adolesc Psychiatry 2003;42:253–256.

Wing L, Potter D. The epidemiology of autistic spectrum disorders: is the prevalence rising? Ment Retard Dev Disabil Res Rev 2002;8(3):151–161.

Index

About the Editors

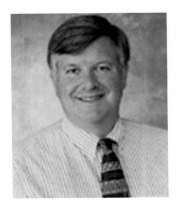

Marschall S. Runge, MD, PhD, was born in Austin, TX and graduated from Vanderbilt University with a BA in general biology and a PhD in molecular biology. He received his medical degree from the Johns Hopkins School of Medicine and trained in internal medicine at Johns Hopkins Hospital. He was a cardiology fellow and junior faculty member at the Massachusetts General Hospital. Dr. Runge's next position was at Emory University where he directed the Cardiology Fellowship Training Program. He then moved to the University of Texas Medical Branch in Galveston where he was Chief of Cardiology and Director of the Sealy Center for Molecular Cardiology. He joined the University of North Carolina (UNC) in 2000 as chairman of the Department of Medicine and in 2004 was also appointed president of UNC Physicians and Clinics. Dr. Runge is board certified in internal medicine and cardiovascular diseases and has spoken and published widely on topics in clinical cardiology and vascular medicine. He maintains an active clinical practice in cardiovascular disease and medicine, in addition to his teaching and administrative activities in the Department of Medicine.

Dr. Runge's basic research interests centers around atherosclerosis, thrombosis and vascular biology. He has published extensively and received both National Institutes of Health (NIH) and industry funding for his work in this area. He is a member of numerous grant review committees including those of the NIH and the American Heart Association.

Dr. Runge is also co-editor of *Netter's Internal Medicine, Netter's Cardiology,* and *Principles of Molecular Cardiology.* He has published nearly 175 articles in peer-reviewed journals, actively reviews articles for top publications, and serves on the Editorial Board for *Circulation, Circulation Research, Current Cardiology Reviews,* and *Arteriosclerosis, Thrombosis and Vascular Biology.* He is an active member of many prestigious academic medical societies and has given numerous lectures in the United States and abroad.

Cam Patterson was born in Mobile, AL and attended UMS Preparatory School, where he was a member of the state championship soccer team, class president, and valedictorian. He was a Harold Sterling Vanderbilt Scholar and studied psychology and English at Vanderbilt University, graduating Summa Cum Laude. He participated in the Honors Research Program at Vanderbilt and conducted research in behavioral pharmacology during that time. Dr. Patterson subsequently attended Emory University School of Medicine, graduating with induction in the Alpha Omega Alpha Honor Society, and completed his residency in internal medicine at Emory University Hospitals. He became the youngest ever chief resident at Grady Memorial Hospital at Emory University in 1992, supervising more than 200 house officers in four hospitals. He completed 3 years of research fellowship under the guidance of Edgar Haber at the Harvard School of Public Health, developing an independent research program in vascular biology and angiogenesis that was supported by an NIH fellowship.

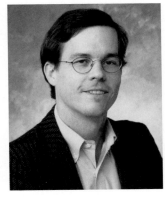

In 1996, he accepted his first faculty position at the University of Texas Medical Branch, and in 2000 Dr. Patterson was recruited to the UNC at Chapel Hill to become the founding director of the Carolina Cardiovascular Biology Center. In 2005, he also became the chief of the Division of Cardiology at UNC. Dr. Patterson is the Ernest and Hazel Craige Distinguished Professor of Cardiovascular Medicine, and he has been recognized at UNC with the Ruth and Phillip Hettleman Prize for Artistic and Scholarly Achievement. He is an established investigator of the American Heart Association and a Burroughs Wellcome Fund Clinical Scientist in Translational Research.

Dr. Patterson is a member of several editorial boards, including *Circulation* and *Circulation Research,* and is an elected member of the American Society of Clinical Investigation and the Association of University Cardiologists. Dr. Patterson maintains active research programs in the areas of angiogenesis and vascular development, cardiac hypertrophy, protein quality control, and translational genomics and metabolomics. He is also the director of the Cardiac Genetics Clinic. He is married to Kristine Blair Patterson, MD, who is a member of the Division of Infectious Diseases at UNC and the medical director of the Wake County Health Department. They have three children, Celia Blair, Anna Alyse, and Graham Gehring.